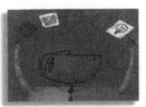
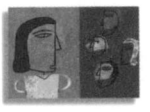
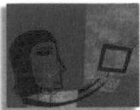
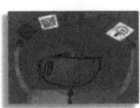
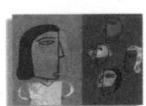

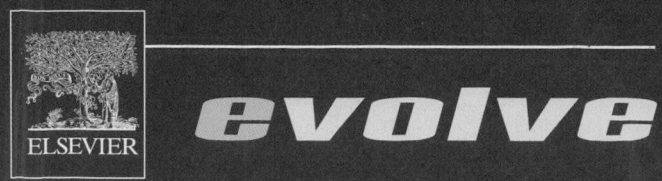

ELSEVIER

evolve

To access your Student Resources, visit the Web address below:

http://evolve.elsevier.com/Kinn

- **Content Updates**

  The latest content updates from the authors of the textbook to keep you current with recent developments in medical assisting, updated procedures, and more!

- **Online Quizzes**

  Quizzes for each chapter are set up for instant feedback, any time you want a little practice.

- **Chapter Resources**

  Additional materials, including chapter summaries & suggested readings, to enhance each chapter.

- **External and Career Tips**

  Get advice on surviving an externship and starting a career as an MA! The authors provide interview tips, possible scenarios you'll encounter on the job, and additional advice on how to succeed on the job.

KINN'S
THE Medical Assistant

AN APPLIED LEARNING APPROACH

NINTH EDITION

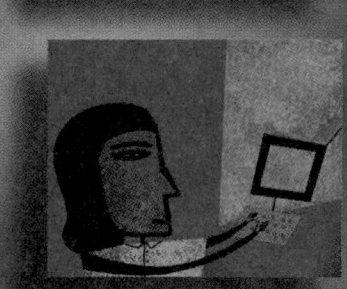

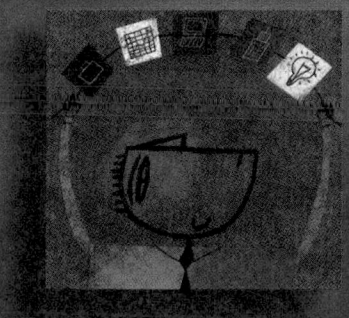

KINN'S
THE Medical Assistant

AN APPLIED LEARNING APPROACH

NINTH EDITION

Alexandra Patricia Young, BBA, RMA, CMA

Director of Admissions
Parker College of Chiropractic
Dallas, Texas;
Former Program Director, Health Information Specialist Division
Former Lead Medical Assisting Instructor
Ultrasound Diagnostic School
Dallas, Texas

Deborah B. Kennedy, EdD, RN, CMA

Associate Professor and Director
Medical Assisting Program
Butler County Community College
Butler, Pennsylvania

with over 1200 illustrations

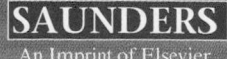
SAUNDERS
An Imprint of Elsevier

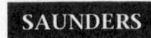

An Imprint of Elsevier

11830 Westline Industrial Drive
St. Louis, Missouri 63146

Kinn's The Medical Assistant: An Applied Learning Approach   ISBN 0-7216-9012-2
Copyright © 2003, Elsevier. All rights reserved.

CPT only © Current Procedural Terminology, 2002, Professional
Edition, American Medical Association. All rights reserved.

NOTICE

Medical assisting is an ever-changing field. Standard safety precautions must be followed, but as
new research and clinical experience broaden our knowledge, changes in treatment and drug
therapy may become necessary or appropriate. Readers are advised to check the most current
product information provided by the manufacturer of each drug to be administered to verify the
recommended dose, the method and duration of administration, and contraindications. It is the
responsibility of the licensed medical assistant, relying on experience and knowledge of the patient,
to determine dosages and the best treatment for each individual patient. Neither the publisher nor
the author assumes any liability for any injury and/or damage to persons or property arising from
this publication.

Previous editions copyrighted 1999, 1993, 1988, 1981, 1974, 1967, 1960, 1956 by W.B. Saunders
Company.

International Standard Book Number 0-7216-9012-2

Executive Editor: Adrianne Cochran
Associate Developmental Editor: Beth LoGiudice
Publishing Services Manager: Pat Joiner
Project Manager: David Stein
Senior Designer: Mark A. Oberkrom
Designer: Bill Donnelly

Printed in the United States of America
Last digit is the print number: 9 8 7 6 5 4 3

Dedication

It is with great honor that the publisher and authors dedicate the ninth edition of this textbook, and its Administrative and Clinical spin-off publications, to Mary E. Kinn, CPS, CMA-A. Mary's contribution to quality medical assisting education spans nearly half a century, starting in 1954 with a telephone crusade to bring medical office "girls," as they were then called, together to create a local medical assistant's association in Southern California. Her contribution continued right through the publication of this edition, with Mary's oversight and review of the text and supplement manuscripts.

A devoted wife and mother, Mary gave generously of her time to furthering the professionalism of her chosen career. She provided leadership and vision to every organization in which she became involved, first as president of a local medical office worker's organization in Southern California, to the second president of the California Medical Assistant's Association, to helping establish a national association, the American Association of Medical Assistants and serving as its president from 1958 to 1959, and finally in 1959 to helping establish a certifying program for members, and serving as its first chairman.

During her time as chairman of the Certifying Board of AAMA, from 1959 to 1967, Mary also became active in the California Association of Medical Assisting Instructors (CAMAI) because of her keen interest in the training and competency of medical assisting instructors. Her work within that organization led her to be hand-selected by the publisher of Frederick and Towner's *The Office Assistant in Medical Practice* in 1967 to replace Carol Towner, who was an executive assistant at the American Medical Association, and who was retiring from the project. Mary's classroom experience, combined with her work on the state and national level to further the interests of the medical assisting profession, made her an ideal choice to co-author this textbook for W.B. Saunders, and she applied her classroom experience into infusing the text with the sound educational principles of competency-based learning, together with a real-world approach to the presentation of material.

In over six editions and 32 years, Mary Kinn's contribution to both the textbook and her profession would have a profound impact on the training of several generations of medical office personnel. Today, there are nearly 350,000 medical assistants, many of whom have Mary Kinn to thank for paving the way for them to enjoy a career with unlimited possibilities due to the professional recognition of the certification credential, as well as the breadth of skills that have all become part of the medical assisting curriculum. Medical assisting is a viable career for the thousands of women and men who have entered it, and it provides a solid springboard from which to launch a career in medical office management, insurance billing and coding, phlebotomy, medical laboratory technician, and even nursing.

It is therefore both fitting and right that the ninth edition of Mary Kinn's textbook, as well as its Administrative and Clinical spin-off publications, bear her name from this edition forward. Few have earned that honor, but then few have provided so much to so many for so long as has Mary Kinn. The new author team of Alexandra Patricia Young and Deborah B. Kennedy, the publisher, particularly Mary's editors Adrianne Cochran, Andrew Allen, and Helaine Tobin, and the thousands of instructors and students whose lives Mary has affected over the years thank her for all her years of dedication to quality medical assisting education. Enjoy your well-deserved retirement, Mary, but know you will be greatly missed.

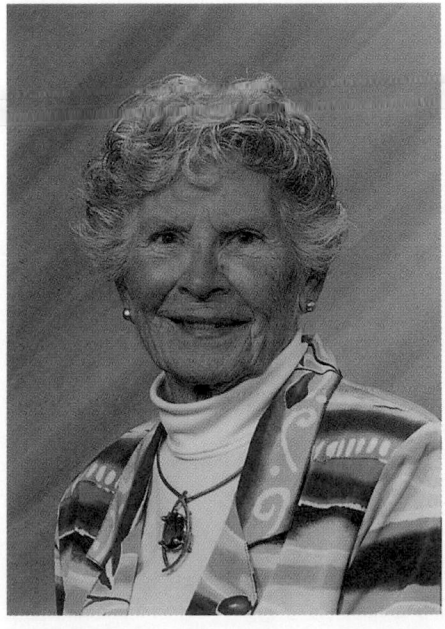

Foreword

Medical assisting as a profession has changed dramatically in the 36 years since I became involved as co-author with Portia Frederick of the third edition of *The Office Assistant in Medical Practice* in 1967. That was a time of tremendous change, both for our nation, and for the field of medical assisting. John Dusseau, our editor at WB Saunders, was the chief medical editor and a most remarkable individual. It was John who encouraged me to become involved in this project, and who nurtured me as a fledgling author through that first edition. At that time, WB Saunders had no Health-Related Professions publishing department as it does today, and the Nursing department wanted nothing to do with medical assistants. John lobbied the medical editorial staff at the publishing house to continue supporting this book in its third edition because he knew as Portia and I did that properly trained medical assistants can "make or break" a medical office.

My first professional career started as a legal assistant. I had no interest in the medical field, and no inclination to even explore it as a potential profession. But in 1950, after my children reached school age, and with legal support positions limited, I took a job as an office manager, working for a young surgeon in Southern California who had just opened his first solo medical practice. Office management, I figured, was something I could do, a piece of cake. My first professional shock was discovering that if you worked in a medical practice back then, but were not the nurse, you were simply referred to as "the girl." My second shock was discovering there were no textbooks or reference manuals to guide me, and no educational opportunities in this area. It was all on-the-job training; we "girls" learned as we gained experience, and we learned from one another.

It was out of that dearth of training materials that in 1954, with the encouragement of the local medical society, a few of us "girls" who had become acquainted by telephone, got together and developed a countywide medical assistant's association. Our initial membership of 200 medical assistants met with opposition from some physicians, who were afraid we were trying to *unionize*. As the group's first president, it was my job to change that attitude, which eventually happened over the course of several subsequent and rocky years. Concurrently, there was action taking place on the state level in California, and I became the second president of the California Medical Assistant's Association.

It was through these activities that I became acquainted with Portia Frederick, the daughter of a physician who had developed a course for medical assistant training in a nearby community college. Portia had been requested by an official of the American Medical Association to co-author a textbook with Carol Towner, an executive assistant in the AMA's Department of Public Relations. The result of their efforts was the first edition of *The Office Assistant in Medical and Dental Practice,* published in 1956 by WB Saunders, which was the forerunner of today's *Kinn's The Medical Assistant: An Applied Learning Approach, Ninth Edition.* Simplistic and chatty, that first edition had a few poorly drawn illustrations and no color. The entire book, including the index, contained 351 pages, but it covered the necessary information and was the best and only book to address the training needs of medical office supportive personnel. The Foreword, written by George F. Lull, MD, then the secretary and general manager of the AMA, stated "*The modern day physician runs a constant race against the clock. As his practice grows, the demands of his patients for medical services increase. In order to make the best use of his time, he continually seeks ways to run his practice more efficiently. At least 75% of all practicing physicians in this country have found that one logical answer is to employ a girl in the office to whom many routine duties can be delegated...it is becoming quite apparent that the ideal assistant should be trained to handle efficiently both medical assisting and medical secretarial duties in the office.*"

At about the time of the second edition of this text, which was retitled *The Office Assistant in Medical Practice,* I had become involved with others in establishing a national association, the American Association of Medical Assistants, and served as its president in 1958-1959. At the 1959 AAMA meeting in Philadelphia, at the end of my term, a resolution was adopted to establish a certifying program for our members, and I was appointed its first chairman. I served as founding chairman of the Certifying Board from 1959 through 1967, and became deeply interested in the training and competency of medical assistants.

About that time, a new organization for instructors was coming to life, named California Association of Medical Assisting Instructors (CAMAI), and Portia Frederick invited me to attend the early informal meetings. The contacts I met at that meeting increased my interest in medical assistant training, and I was thrilled to be asked to co-author the next edition of the text, to replace Carol Towner who had answered the call to motherhood. I began my teaching career in 1970 using the third edition that John Dusseau had so clairvoyantly lobbied to preserve, and began to realize how the book could be enlarged and improved as a teaching tool and a reference. As an instructor, I was eligible to become a full-fledged member of CAMAI, and I jumped in with both feet. Because of my involvement in that organization, this third edition had more information about medical assisting associations, and of course the certified medical assistant credential. Management, medical ethics, and law were also expanded and given more attention, and a chapter on medical emergencies was added.

The fourth edition, published in 1974, was retitled *The Medical Office Assistant: Administrative and Clinical,* and the book was reorganized into its three sections of general, administrative, and clinical. Government-sponsored health insurance was dominating office practice, and we greatly expanded this section of the book to reflect the impact of Medicare and Medicaid. Nutrition and diet therapy and microbiology were added, the clinical section was divided into the various medical specialties, now a hallmark of the text. Still no color was added, but the book topped out at 742 pages and was a vast improvement over the previous edition in terms of its integration in the training program.

The fifth edition, in 1981, is still my favorite edition because the manuscript was updated and enlarged to better reflect the changing face of the profession. Different print font and margin width, as well as thinner paper, allowed for the inclusion of extended content without requiring more pages. Color was used for marginal paragraph headings, and many photographs appeared throughout the text. But the joy of achievement in that edition was overshadowed by the sudden and unexpected death of my friend, Portia Frederick, before the new edition had gone to press.

Major changes were taking place within the medical assisting profession at that time. The 1984 DACUM Analysis of the Medical Assisting Profession had been circulated. More and more physicians were using computers in their practice. The sixth edition of the text brought in Eleanor Derge to help completely update the content and format, which included a vocabulary list at the beginning of each chapter, learning objectives for both didactic and practical application, and step-by-step procedures covering all essential entry-level skills, including terminal performance objectives and current safety precautions for the prevention of AIDS transmission. This edition also saw the debut of the first *Student Review and Activities Manual* and an instructor's manual added to the package.

The seventh edition, authored by Kinn, Derge, and Dr. MaryAnne Woods, was published in 1993 and topped out over 900 pages. The book had a whole new look and a fresh approach. Personal communication, dictation, and transcription were added to the Administrative section. More color was used, and more emphasis was placed on personal communications and the medical

specialty chapters. The accompanying ancillaries were updated and improved to reflect the expanded text content.

When the eighth edition of Kinn and Woods published in 1999, I turned to my editor, Adrianne Cochran, and announced that I was done. It had been a long road from the time John Dusseau had flown to San Francisco in 1965 to meet with Portia Frederick and me, to "look me over" as a suitable candidate for co-authoring this text. In the ensuing years, the book had grown to 1144 pages, had collected a student workbook, instructor's manual, text software, and a dedicated website. I felt I'd made a real contribution to the text at the publication of the eighth edition, and had made a difference in the training of thousands of medical assistants over the 22 years in which I was involved. But I had things I still wanted to do in life, I'd retired from teaching, and I felt it was time to pass along the torch to others with a similar devotion to quality medical assisting education.

I feel that the publisher has found those individuals in Tricia Young and Debby Kennedy, and it was with a mix of nostalgia, sadness, and excitement that I relinquished my participation in the future of this text and turned it over to these two very capable and dedicated medical assisting instructors.

Alexandra Patricia Young, BBA, CMA, RMA, is the former program director of the Health Information Specialist program and the former lead instructor for the Medical Assisting program at Ultrasound Diagnostic School, a large vocational chain of schools with campuses all over the country. She was also the director of education for allied health for Bryan Institute. Tricia's natural writing gift, her love of the subject material, and her devotion to medical assisting training have infused the Administrative section of this textbook with a brilliance that reflects current practice and a sensitivity to topics that are crucial to quality medical assisting education. Tricia has done a wonderful job of updating the material and bringing together both her mastery of current information and her creative instincts. As this was the section for which I was responsible for so many years, I feel particularly good about the chapters I reviewed that Tricia authored.

Deborah B. Kennedy, EdD, RN, CMA, the new author of the clinical section, is the Director and Associate Professor of the Medical Assistant Program at Butler County Community College, in Butler, PA. Debby brings particularly excellent credentials to the half of the book that requires a keen knowledge of patient interaction, current medical diagnostic and therapeutic practice, and instructional expertise in order to convey particularly difficult subjects in a straightforward, retainable way. This is not an easy task given how complicated the clinical portion of the medical assisting curriculum has become today. Medical assistants are now the primary patient educators. They must reason, problem-solve, and react to patients during sometimes difficult and trying times in the patients' lives with a sensitivity and grace that is often difficult to convey in a textbook. From the chapters I reviewed of Debby's work, I was extremely pleased to see she has raised the level of the clinical chapters to a quality of training that is not just nice to have, but required in today's demanding medical office.

Although it was over 36 years ago, I well remember the anticipation of that first publication and seeing the cover on which my name would be listed as a co-author. Students were going to read what I wrote, and that both thrilled and intimidated me, but as Tricia and Debby have discovered, it's an experience of a lifetime to be involved in a project with such a worthy cause. Tricia and Debby have done an exemplary job at completely rewriting the entire textbook; reorganizing chapters; adding new chapters, photos, and illustrations; and integrating an innovative new "applied" approach; and have taken the training a step beyond with the new Study Skills and Career Development and Life Skills chapters that bookend the primary material.

Tammy B. Morton, MS, RN, CS, CMA, has also written the revision of the *Student Study Guide* and *Instructor's Curriculum Resource with CD-ROM*. Not only are her exercises creative examples of learning by doing, Tammy understands that not all students learn the same way, and she has integrated a unique identification classification so that no matter how a student learns there is something available in this *Study Guide* to help them master the material. She has also written some beautiful PowerPoint slides, and helpful instructor tools that will make planning interesting and motivating classroom presentations easier for instructors. Tammy's educational background, like that of Tricia and Debby, is evident throughout both of these supplements, and I'm pleased to see they are some of the best I've seen on the market.

In my lifetime it is also wonderful to witness two new exciting supplements that have been added to the package that reflect the technical revolution that is happening in America's learning institutions. The EVOLVE learning management system now gives instructors and students a new platform for communication with one another, one that simulates a means of communicating that will dominate the medical assistant's professional career, as email and the digital age are so prevalent in the medical office. And the online courses for both Administrative and Clinical Medical Assisting now provide students with a convenient, anytime/anywhere opportunity to become confident in mastering the key concepts and skills they need to know, in order to prove competence when they reach the practice lab. This new learning platform reaches out to the many medical assisting students who would otherwise not be able to find the time to attend class, and it brings learning to life as only the Internet and its three-dimensional format can.

My heartfelt congratulations are extended to both Tricia Young and Debby Kennedy on the publication of their first textbook, and to Tammy Morton on the publication of the supplements. I also congratulate their advocates behind the scenes at WB Saunders/Elsevier who believe, as John Dusseau believed over 42 years ago, that success in life starts with the power of knowledge, and that that power comes in creating the right combination of training materials that together can turn a novice student into a highly qualified professional medical assistant ready to meet the challenges of today's busy and complicated medical office practice.

Mary E. Kinn, CPS, CMA-A
San Clemente, California
February 2003

Preface to the Ninth Edition

Medical assisting as a profession has changed dramatically since *The Office Assistant in Medical and Dental Practice,* by Portia Frederick and Carol Towner, was first published in 1956. Each subsequent edition of this textbook has reflected the age in which it was published. Now, 47 years and nine editions later, *Kinn's The Medical Assistant: An Applied Learning Approach, Ninth Edition* continues to represent a long-standing commitment to quality medical assisting education with its engaging, straightforward writing style and demonstrated positive outcomes. Hundreds of instructors in classrooms all across the country have used this text to teach thousands of students over the years. Many of these students have gone on to teach students of their own with this very same trusted resource. To continue the use and growth of this text and its features, the ninth edition has undergone a massive revision in an effort to offer you the most comprehensive, up-to-date, and innovative approach to teaching this subject today. We appreciate the opportunity to explore the existing field of medical assisting with you!

DISTINCTIVE FEATURES OF OUR APPROACH

This textbook has endured throughout the years because it has been able to keep pace with an ever-changing profession while producing students who are well trained and qualified to enter medical practices across the country. This dependability is why the market continues to rely on this text edition after edition. Underlying this dependability is a foundation of pedagogical features that has stood the test of time and that has been expanded and improved upon yet again in this new edition. Such pedagogical features include the following:

- An easy-to-read, highly interactive writing style that engages students through practical applications of medical assistant competencies.
- An emphasis on skill development with procedural steps outlining each skill, supported by rationales that provide meaning to each step.
- An organizational approach that addresses each body system with its own chapter, with additional chapters dedicated to specialty medical assistant skills.
- Each clinical chapter begins with a review of that system's anatomy and physiology, then moves to the common disorders found in that system, with the chapter concluding with patient education and legal and ethical issues.
- A pedagogical framework based on the use of learning objectives, vocabulary terms, and supportive student supplements.
- A package of supportive materials to accommodate a wide variety of student learning types and instructor teaching styles.

NEW FEATURES IN THIS EDITION

The medical field is an ever-changing one, with constant advances in diagnostic procedures and treatment protocols. Accrediting agencies, including the Committee on Accreditation of Allied Health Programs (CAAHEP) and the Accrediting Bureau of Health Education Schools (ABHES), place demands on faculty and medical assistant programs to maintain accreditation standards. The influence of current risk management practices and the potential of electronic technology as a resource for student and patient education have both complicated and expanded the opportunities available to medical assistant professionals.

To build on the long-established strengths of the Kinn textbook, the ninth edition expands and supplements the techniques used so successfully in past editions. The combination of many talented individuals on the editorial and production staffs working with two new authors from varying backgrounds has resulted in a text that adheres to the Kinn tradition while meeting the needs of a new generation of medical assistant educators and students. The result is an innovative text that comprehensively meets the educational and accreditation needs of all types of medical assistant programs while effectively training tomorrow's medical assisting professionals.

The new edition of *Kinn's The Medical Assistant* incorporates a unique new approach that is reflected in the subtitle that has been added to the book for this edition: *An Applied Learning Approach.* It is believed that learning takes place only when students are engaged and when the learning requires something from them in response to information that is being imparted to them. We therefore attempt to provide meaningful thought in the form of realistic scenarios that put information in context and provide a way for students to directly apply concepts they're learning by challenging them to consider how they would behave in certain situations.

This "applied" theme is set up-front in the first chapter, which introduces students to the concepts of critical thinking and the impact of individual learning styles on student success. This in turn transitions into time management and problem-solving skills, as well as effective study skills and test-taking strategies. The text develops from there true to the original Kinn textbook, with its distinctive Administrative and Clinical sections, and is rounded out by the last chapter that helps students focus on preparing for and nurturing their career as a medical assistant.

This pedagogical theme and other new enhancements can be found throughout the book and its supplements in the following features:

- Each chapter opens with a scenario related to the chapter's focus that introduces students to a medical assistant and a situation, or situations, that the medical assistant must approach.

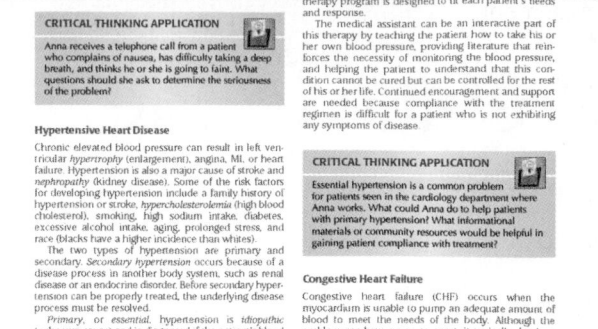

CHAPTER 29

Scenario

Felicia Grand, a newly hired certified medical assistant (CMA), is working for Dr. Anna Kosto. Dr. Kosto is part of a busy multiphysician primary care practice. One of Felicia's chief responsibilities is to assist Dr. Kosto with physical examinations. Her duties include preparing and maintaining the examination room and equipment as well as preparing the patient for specific physical examinations.

- Throughout the chapter, Critical Thinking Applications are designed to allow the student to use a concept that has just been learned in the context of the overall chapter scenario. These exercises help students look at the big picture and consider various angles, or approaches, to the challenges in which they will

eventually find themselves in the medical office. These exercises provide a wonderful opportunity for discussion and further reflection.

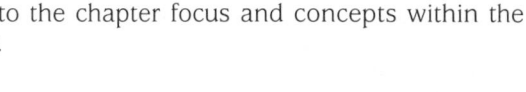

therapy program is designed to fit each patient's needs and response.

CRITICAL THINKING APPLICATION

Anna receives a telephone call from a patient who complains of nausea, has difficulty taking a deep breath, and thinks he or she is going to faint. What questions should she ask to determine the seriousness of the problem?

The medical assistant can be an interactive part of this therapy by teaching the patient how to take his or her own blood pressure, providing literature that reinforces the necessity of monitoring the blood pressure, and helping the patient to understand that this condition cannot be cured but can be controlled for the rest of his or her life. Continued encouragement and support are needed because compliance with the treatment regimen is difficult for a patient who is not exhibiting any symptoms of disease.

Hypertensive Heart Disease

Chronic elevated blood pressure can result in left ventricular *hypertrophy* (enlargement), angina, MI, or heart failure. Hypertension is also a major cause of stroke and *nephropathy* (kidney disease). Some of the risk factors for developing hypertension include a family history of hypertension or stroke, *hypercholesterolemia* (high blood cholesterol), smoking, high sodium intake, diabetes, excessive alcohol intake, aging, prolonged stress, and race (blacks have a higher incidence than whites).

The two types of hypertension are primary and secondary. *Secondary hypertension* occurs because of a disease process in another body system, such as renal disease or an endocrine disorder. Before secondary hypertension can be properly treated, the underlying disease process must be resolved.

Primary, or *essential*, hypertension is *idiopathic* (unknown cause) and is diagnosed if the patient's blood pressure is consistently above 140/90. The diastolic number is especially important because it reflects the level of peripheral resistance and the resultant workload of the left ventricle. The general rule in diagnosis is that the patient's blood pressure is elevated in two or more

CRITICAL THINKING APPLICATION

Essential hypertension is a common problem for patients seen in the cardiology department where Anna works. What could Anna do to help patients with primary hypertension? What informational materials or community resources would be helpful in gaining patient compliance with treatment?

Congestive Heart Failure

Congestive heart failure (CHF) occurs when the myocardium is unable to pump an adequate amount of blood to meet the needs of the body. Although the problem can have an acute onset, it typically develops over time because of weakness in the left ventricle from chronic hypertension or MI of the ventricular wall, valvular heart disease, or pulmonary complications. Typically, heart failure initially occurs on one side of the heart, followed by the other side. Left-sided heart failure

- Chapters end with a Summary of Scenario that identifies concepts for student focus, as well as a discussion, where relevant, of patient education as it relates to the chapter focus and concepts within the chapter.

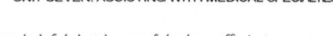

698   UNIT SEVEN: ASSISTING WITH MEDICAL SPECIALTIES

is always helpful, but be careful when offering encouragement about the course and outcome of their treatment. No treatment can restore youth. The improvement achieved may be slow and gradual. Keep encouragement on a positive level. Compliment the patient on small improvements, but let the physician describe the possible course and outcome of the prescribed treatment.

SUMMARY OF SCENARIO

Melissa enjoys her work with Dr. Lee but recognizes the need to keep up with new developments in the field of dermatology. She has learned the importance of giving patients accurate information while conducting telephone screening and always referring questions or concerns to Dr. Lee. [...] the patient education aspects of [...]gist, including the importance of [...]ntrolling sun exposure, and [...] the warning signs of cancer. [...] how to assist Dr. Lee with derma[...] ncluding allergy skin testing, [...]s, and assisting with biopsies, [...]asions, and laser resurfacing.

Patient Education

The medical assistant should take every opportunity to educate his or her patient on the infection process and ways of preventing disease transmission. The best time to instruct your patient in aseptic techniques that can be used at home is while you are performing the aseptic procedure. For example:

- While hand washing, explain to the patient that this routine is part of daily hygiene and is particularly important for patients who are very young or old or who seem to get sick frequently. Discuss with the patient that hands should be washed before and after meals; after sneezing, coughing, or nose blowing; after using the bathroom; before and after changing a dressing; and after changing an infant's diaper.
- Explain to the patient how using disposable tissues to cover the nose and mouth when coughing or sneezing decreases the possibility of transmitting illness between household members.
- Discuss proper ways for disposing of used tissues, especially when one member of the household is suspected of having a communicable disease.
- Instruct the patient regarding the differences between sterile and clean dressings and bandages. Show him or her step by step how to change a dressing properly and then how to dispose of the contaminated items.

There are many ways that a medical assistant can help the patient. Here are a few more suggestions to educate and inform the patient about asepsis and infection control:

- There is improved integration of concepts that transcend chapter topics, such as legal and ethical issues, communications, professionalism, and office management.

- The artwork throughout has been updated and modernized, providing a more attractive textbook for student use. Many new photographs throughout better support the revised content and are more relevant to the actual medical office. Many old photos were replaced with new photos that show more updated equipment, provide more disease examples, and better illustrate key procedural steps.

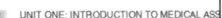

can be frustrating for patients when they must list their address and phone numbers on each of several forms. Review and revise the forms used in the office often so that they are user-friendly for the office and patient alike.

Patients may need reassurance that each staff member in the physician's office is committed to complete patient confidentiality. Always be open to answering questions regarding the patient medical record.

Legal and Ethical Issues

The authority to release information from the medical record lies solely with the patient unless required by law by subpoena. Ownership of the record is often a subject of controversy. The record belongs to the physician; the information belongs to the patient.

When a medical record is used as evidence in a court case, the person who entered information in the chart must be able to read it, no matter how much time has lapsed since the entry was created. When a chart is corrected, the proper method must be followed and the record should never be obliterated.

Be sure to understand the laws concerning records retention. Records should be kept through the period of the statute of limitations, and possibly longer in certain situations. Take care with the medical chart, as it is the lifeline of patient care in the medical facility.

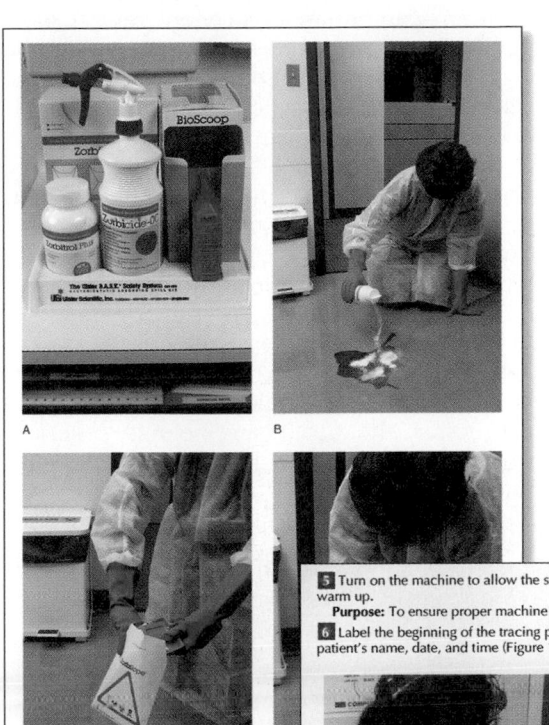

56   UNIT ONE: INTRODUCTION TO MEDICAL ASSISTING

Credibility

Credibility is the perceived **competence** or character of a person. It leads to the belief that the person can be trusted. Since trust is a vital component of the physician-patient relationship, the credibility of the physician and those who assist in the office should be strong. The information provided to patients must be accurate. Patients expect that the physician and medical assistant will instruct them in a manner that will enhance their health and provide positive results. One must take care in giving any advice to patients, because they view the medical assistant as an agent of the physician. Patients may not distinguish between the medical assistant's advice and the physician's orders. To avoid charges of practicing medicine without a license, a medical assistant must be sure to suggest only what the physician has authorized.

Confidentiality

The importance of confidentiality cannot be stressed enough in the medical environment. Patients are entitled to privacy where their health is concerned, and they should be confident that medical professionals use information only to care for them. One must never reveal any information about any patient to anyone without specific permission to do so. If in doubt, be conservative and verify that the person seeking information has the right to see it. Casual conversations in hallways, elevators, and break rooms between staff can be overheard by a family member or friend of the patient.

The rules regarding confidentiality extend beyond the medical office. While at home, medical assistants should not discuss details about patients with their families and friends. Those outside the medical profession do not understand how vital it is to keep information confidential. Never pass along damaging facts to others. Medical [...] make it a rule never to discuss a patient [...] must be shared for [...]

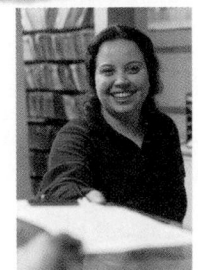

FIGURE 4–4   A good attitude goes a long way in patient and staff relationships.

and it can be hard to maintain a professional attitude in these cases. Some of the obstructions to professional behavior are discussed in this section.

Personal Problems and "Baggage"

Everyone has a life outside of the workplace, and sometimes we face challenges and difficult times that are hard to put aside. During working hours our thoughts should be on the job at hand, especially when we are dealing with patients. However, there may be situations in our lives that are so critical or important that we find ourselves [...] *personal baggage*, as it

5 Turn on the machine to allow the stylus to warm up.
Purpose: To ensure proper machine performance.

6 Label the beginning of the tracing paper with the patient's name, date, and time (Figure 1).

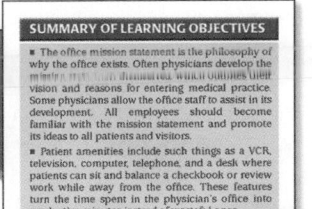

Figure 1

- Well-developed learning objectives emphasize the cognitive and performance objectives addressed in the chapter, and are summarized at the end of each chapter for student review of learning.

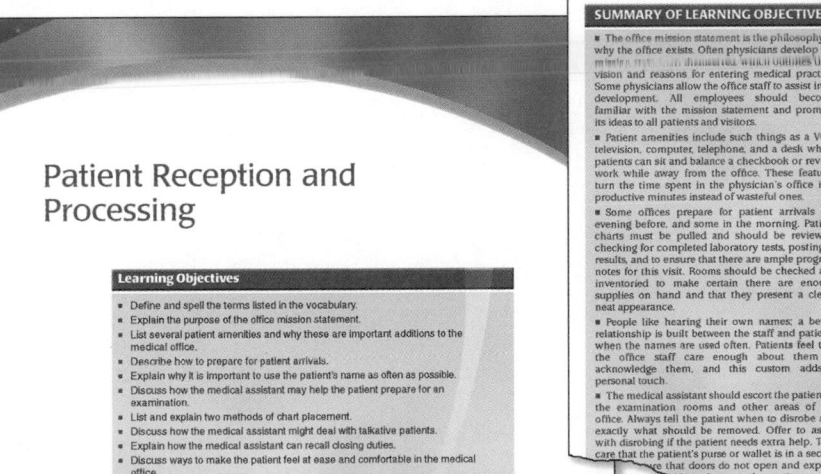

Patient Reception and Processing

Learning Objectives

- Define and spell the terms listed in the vocabulary.
- Explain the purpose of the office mission statement.
- List several patient amenities and why these are important additions to the medical office.
- Describe how to prepare for patient arrivals.
- Explain why it is important to use the patient's name as often as possible.
- Discuss how the medical assistant may help the patient prepare for an examination.
- List and explain two methods of chart placement.
- Discuss how the medical assistant might deal with talkative patients.
- Explain how the medical assistant can recall closing duties.
- Discuss ways to make the patient feel at ease and comfortable in the medical office.
- Correctly prepare charts for registered patients who are scheduled.
- Demonstrate the correct way to register a new patient.

SUMMARY OF LEARNING OBJECTIVES

■ The office mission statement is the philosophy of why the office exists. Often physicians develop the mission statement, a document which outlines their vision and reasons for entering medical practice. Some physicians allow the office staff to assist in its development. All employees should become familiar with the mission statement and promote its ideas to all patients and visitors.

■ Patient amenities include such things as a VCR, television, computer, telephone, and a desk where patients can sit and balance a checkbook or review work while away from the office. These features turn the time spent in the physician's office into productive minutes instead of wasteful ones.

■ Some offices prepare for patient arrivals the evening before, and some in the morning. Patient charts must be pulled and should be reviewed, checking for completed laboratory tests, posting of results, and to ensure that there are ample progress notes for this visit. Rooms should be checked and inventoried to make certain there are enough supplies on hand and that they present a clean, neat appearance.

■ People like hearing their own names; a better relationship is built between the staff and patients when the names are used often. Patients feel that the office staff care enough about them to acknowledge them, and this custom adds a personal touch.

■ The medical assistant should escort the patient to the examination rooms and other areas of the office. Always tell the patient when to disrobe and exactly what should be removed. Offer to assist with disrobing if the patient needs extra help. Take care that the patient's purse or wallet is in a secure [...] make that doors do not open and expose [...] Instruct the patient as to [...] leave or should wait after

- Chapter 5 now includes an expanded and much more comprehensive discussion of interpersonal skills and human relations. This chapter provides information about the communication process, listening and observation skills, defense mechanisms, dealing with conflict, and perception. There is an emphasis on communication during difficult times, as well as a discussion about health self-esteem, self-improvement, and comfort zones.

- Chapter 8 on computers has been revised and thoroughly updated to include timely information to reflect the more sophisticated computer systems found in today's busy medical practice. It provides easy-to-understand details about subjects such as the elements of microprocessors, an "inside-the-computer" section, file formats, internet connectivity, networking basics, computer security, and ergonomics. The medical records management and health information chapters also include an in-depth discussion of computer-based medical records.

- More than any previous edition, customer service is stressed throughout the chapters. As patients become more involved in their healthcare, medical assistants must realize that the healthcare field is a service industry and that patients should be treated more like customers. Chapter 21 is devoted to practice marketing and customer service, and several sections stress the need for concern for the patient's time and for working efficiently.

- New compliance regulations in medical billing and coding have lent a far greater emphasis on reimbursement than ever before. Both billing and coding have been expanded and three new coding chapters have been added: Basics of Diagnostic Coding (Chapter 15), Basics of Procedural Coding (Chapter 16), and The Health Insurance Claim Form (Chapter 17).

- The clinical section includes four new chapters: Patient Education (Chapter 26), Pharmacology Math (Chapter 31), Assisting in Endocrinology (Chapter 42), and Principles of Electrocardiography (Chapter 46). Other chapters, including those addressing medical laboratory procedures, Nutrition and Health Promotion (Chapter 27), and Assisting in Neurology and Mental Health (Chapter 41), introduce material not included in previous editions.

- New to this edition is the integration of administrative concepts into the discussions of the various diseases and conditions within each medical specialty, including application of telephone screening situations and related medical documentation. This innovative feature transcends the traditional separation of administrative and clinical and brings them together in the context of real-world application.

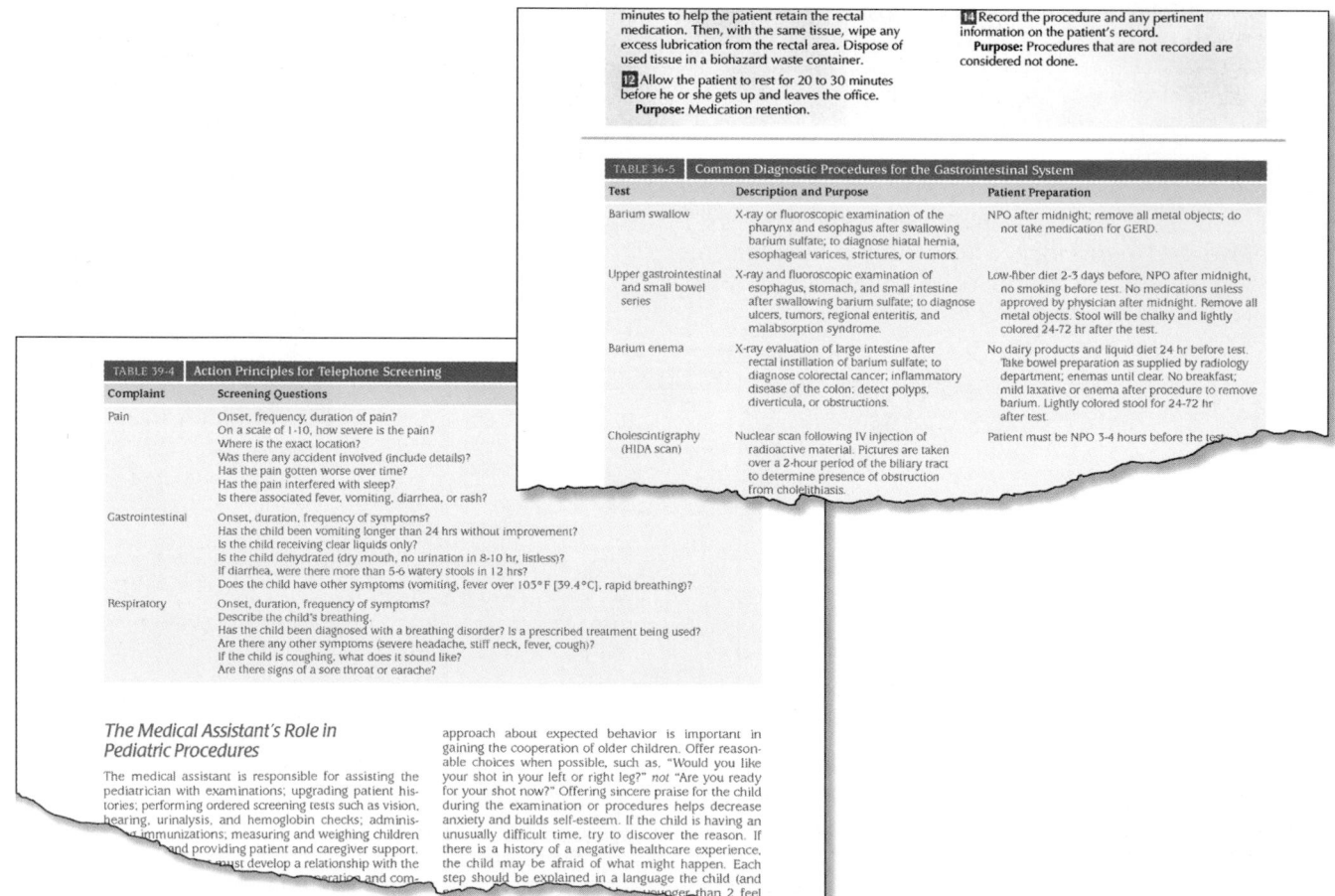

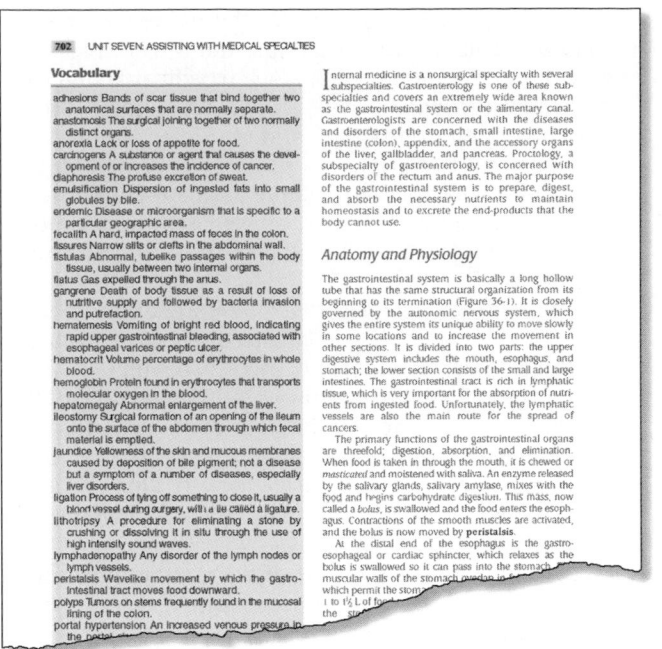

NEW INTERNET RESOURCE

Stay current with trends, developments, and news in the medical field, as well as access additional chapter supplemental features, advice on your externship, interviewing techniques, and more through EVOLVE, the website that is provided complimentary to this textbook. This exciting website is your gateway to the World Wide Web. It is an interactive learning environment that adds an incredibly powerful set of instructional resources to your classroom experience. EVOLVE works in coordination with *Kinn's The Medical Assistant: An Applied Learning Approach, Ninth Edition* by providing Internet-based course content and Internet web links to reinforce and expand your learning experience.

The EVOLVE Course Management System (CMS) is also available to instructors who adopt this textbook. In addition to the Evolve Learning Resources available to students, there is an entire suite of tools available to instructors that allow for communication between instructors and students, including discussion boards, e-mail, chat rooms, and more.

- Each clinical specialty chapter has been completely revised and has expanded its focus on medical terminology, anatomy and physiology, and pathophysiology. In addition to focusing on the diagnostic and therapeutic interventions that are most frequently used in each specialty, there is also a discussion of the equipment and pharmacology that students can expect to encounter when working in that specialty, including drug types and dosage calculations.

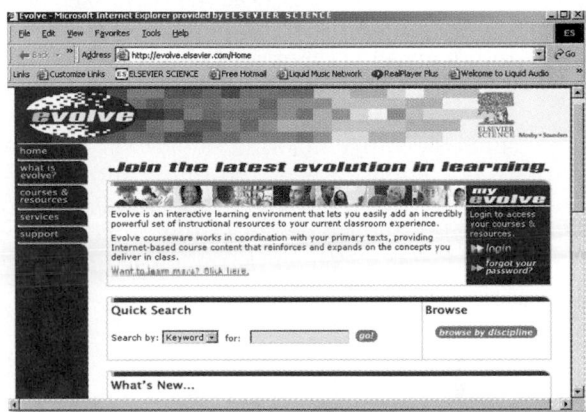

To access this comprehensive online resource, simply go to the EVOLVE Home Page at http://evolve.elsevier.com and enter your user name and password provided to you from your instructor. If your instructor has not set up a Course Management System, you can still access all the learning resources available free with this textbook by going to http://evolve.elsevier.com/Kinn/.

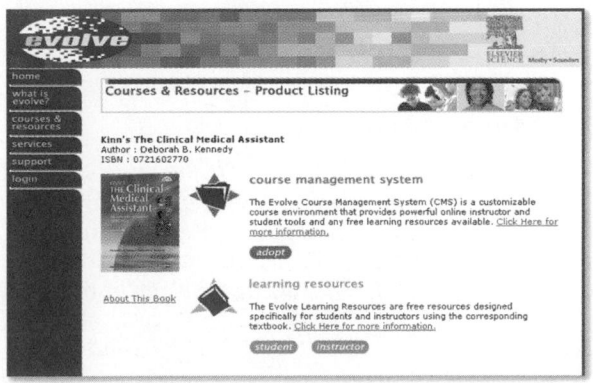

- Major Internet sites relating to each chapter are provided for students to expand their understanding of chapter concepts and stay current on medical news and industry developments through research on the World Wide Web.

EXTENSIVE SUPPLEMENTAL RESOURCES

The diversity of students, instructors, programs, institutions, and teaching environments using this textbook required that we develop an integrated, comprehensive, and flexible package of supplements to support *Kinn's The Medical Assistant: An Applied Learning Approach, Ninth Edition.* Each of these innovative supplements is designed to enhance the teaching and learning experience, with the outcome of producing students well equipped to pass any certification examination, and who will go on to experience successful professional careers in medical assisting. These supplements and their unique features include:

Student Software Program

The free CD-ROM that comes with your textbook includes three programs designed for you to apply the key content and skills you've learned throughout the textbook. *The Virtual Medical Office Challenge* provides four realistic scenarios, with you making the decisions and getting feedback on each decision you make, plus a skill-building section that lets you practice both administrative and clinical competencies. All forms used throughout are included for reference in a format suitable for printing. *The Body Spectrum,* an interactive Anatomy and Physiology coloring book, will help you strengthen your knowledge of the body and medical terminology. *Lytec Medical 2001,* a real medical office software program, lets you practice front office skills on the computer. A user's manual for the *Lytec* program is included in a format suitable for printing.

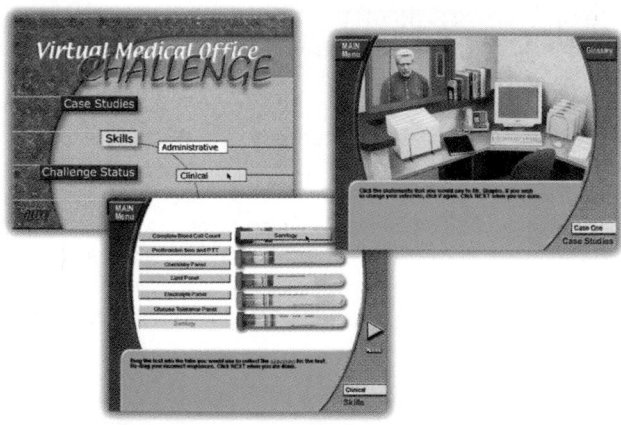

Student Study Guide
Tammy B. Morton, MS, RN, CS, CMA

This practical tool takes the "applied learning approach" to a whole new level, giving you the opportunity to apply the knowledge and skills you're learning in the textbook. Some of the outstanding features of this study guide include:

- Learning style icons that identify the targeted learning style of each exercise. Find out which learning style works best for you!
- Reinforcement of anatomy and physiology with extensive labeling exercises.
- Procedure checklists that serve as a valuable tool for checking your competency, as well as a tool for your instructor to gauge your skill level and proficiency for each skill in the textbook.
- A multitude of exercises to reinforce key content throughout the textbook, including vocabulary exercises that help you recall and apply medical terms.
- Coding applications, documentation scenarios, and telephone screening examples provide you with the opportunity to apply administrative concepts to clinical situations.
- Instrument identification, as well as a review of disease-specific skills, further reinforces clinical material.
- Chapter quizzes at the end of each chapter exercise set allow you to further test your knowledge.
- Study tips for all medical assisting students, as well as a section on study tips specifically designed for ESL (English-as-a-Second-Language) students, written by an ESL consultant.
- A glossary of English-Spanish terms, based on the text glossary, gives students an excellent resource for working with patients who speak English as a second language. This glossary is likewise extremely helpful for those medical assisting students who themselves speak English as a second language.

Instructor's Curriculum Resource
Tammy B. Morton, MS, RN, CS, CMA

This complete instructor teaching tool includes extensive curriculum materials in both print and electronic formats. Beginning and veteran instructors alike will be able to easily prepare their lectures, presentations, labs, and assessments with an extensive course syllabus, multiple course outlines, individual chapter lesson plans, chapter Internet addresses, and ready-made tests for each chapter. Answer keys for all text and Student Study Guide questions are also included. In addition, special tips for instructors with ESL (English-as-a-Second-Language) students have been provided, written by an ESL consultant. All of the printed materials from the Instructor's Curriculum Resource are also available in Word format on the free CD-ROM, making them fully customizable for use in any classroom.

Test Bank
Tammy B. Morton, MS, RN, CS, CMA

Our test bank provides an accurate and exhaustive source of test items for a wide variety of examination styles. It contains more than 1,900 questions, and is available in both printed, and electronic format so you can easily prepare your quizzes and exams, tailored to your classroom format.

PowerPoint Presentation Slides
Tammy B. Morton, MS, RN, CS, CMA

The instructor CD-ROM includes a PowerPoint viewer and a set of over 1,400 PowerPoint slides. The slides include a summary of key chapter material, and can easily be customized to support your lectures and enhance your classroom presentation. All slides have been formatted to reflect the text design, and include nearly 300 images from the text. These slides can also be easily formatted within the PowerPoint program for student note taking or as overhead transparencies.

KINN'S MEDICAL ASSISTING ONLINE

Today's educational environment has the potential to be more interactive than ever before. The more resources available to facilitate learning, and the more varied those resources are, the greater the chances are for material to be comprehended and retained.

Kinn's Medical Assisting Online has been developed with this creative approach to education in mind. Offering a multidimensional experience that is not possible in a traditional classroom setting, these unique and innovative new products are complete courses that simulate the externship experience by creating a virtual medical practice where students have an opportunity to learn by doing.

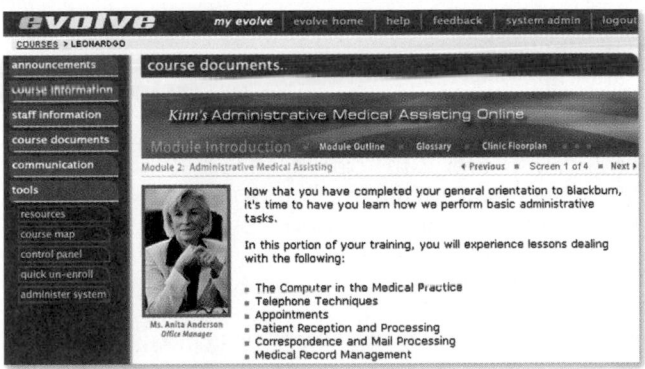

Designed to be used together with *Kinn's The Medical Assistant: An Applied Learning Approach, Ninth Edition,* this set of two courses is divided by administrative (available summer 2003) and clinical (available winter 2003) information. Lessons draw upon the text for reading assignments, then provide an opportunity for you to apply text content by entering the simulated environment of "Blackburn Primary Care Associates," complete with an office manager who acts as your supervisor/mentor through the courses, other office personnel, physicians, and realistic patient cases. This environment is an exciting way for you to discover what it is like to work in the field of medical assisting before you ever enter your externship.

A wide range of visual, auditory, and interactive elements create this exciting environment and work together to amplify key learning objectives from the textbook, giving you the opportunity to practice key skills first by being guided through a practice of each skill, then by trying to perform that skill in a realistic application exercise. This combination of guided practice and application of skills gives you the *confidence* to perform these skills with *competence* in the lab or on the job.

Providing a myriad of learning opportunities, *Kinn's Medical Assisting Online* accommodates diverse learning styles and circumstances through the use of a sophisticated learning management system that lets your instructor tailor the program's content either to support a traditional classroom learning experience or as a true distance education course. You log on through the Evolve portal to complete lessons, take quizzes and exams online, participate in threaded discussions, post assignments to your instructor, or chat with your instructor or fellow classmates, all from any location that has an Internet connection.

DEVELOPMENT OF THIS EDITION

To ensure continuous improvement and accuracy of the material presented throughout this textbook, an extensive review and development process was utilized for each of the past editions. Building on that history, the ninth edition developmental process included several phases of evaluation by a variety of medical assisting instructors. The first phase of the review process asked instructors who both used and did not use the text to suggest improvements to the organization of the text, to the text material, to the figures and tables throughout, and to the supplements. The second phase encompassed a more detailed review of each chapter as material was being prepared.

We are deeply grateful to the numerous people who have shared their comments and suggestions on this edition. Reviewing a book or supplement takes an incredible amount of energy and attention, and we are glad so many of our colleagues were able to take time out of their busy schedule to help ensure the validity and appropriateness of content in this edition. The reviewers provided us with additional viewpoints and opinions that combine to make this text an incredible learning tool.

We wish to thank the following editorial reviewing team:

Kim Anthony Aaronson, BS, DC
Adjunct Instructor
Anatomy and Physiology and Medical Terminology
Truman College;
Adjunct Instructor
Pacific College of Oriental Medicine
Chicago, Illinois

Jannie Adams, PhD, RN, BSN, MSHA
Director/Assistant Professor
Medical Assisting
Clayton College and State University
Morrow, Georgia

Laura Baumgardner, CPC, CPC-H, CCS-P, CCS
Instructor, Health Careers Division
Harrisburg Area Community College
Harrisburg, Pennsylvania

Deborah Bedford, CMA, AAS
Program Coordinator and Instructor
Medical Assisting Program
North Seattle Community College
Seattle, Washington

Crystal Dawn Bennett, CMA, AAS
Instructor, Medical Assisting
Hocking College
Nelsonville, Ohio

Kathy Bonewit-West, BS, MEd, CMAC
Professor, Medical Assistant Technology
Hocking College
Nelsonville, Ohio

Carol J. Buck, MS, CPC
Program Director (Ret.)
Medical Secretary Programs
Northwest Technical College
East Grand Forks, Minnesota

Wendy Campbell, ADN
Medical Assistant Program Director
Concorde Career Institute
Portland, Oregon

Diana L. Carroll, CMA, CPC
Assistant Professor
Salt Lake City Community College
Salt Lake City, Utah

Janet Haggerty Davis, BSN, MS, MBA, PhD, RN
Dean, School of Health Studies
Robert Morris College
Chicago, Illinois

Judy Ehninger, RN, BS, CMA
Coordinator and Assistant Professor
Medical Assisting Program
Lehigh Carbon Community College
Schnecksville, Pennsylvania

Eugenia M. Fulcher, RN, BSN, MEd, EdD
Program Director, Medical Assisting
Swainsboro Technical College
Swainsboro, Georgia

Marti Garrels, MSA, MT, CMA-C
Medical Assistant Program
Ivy Tech State College
South Bend, Indiana

Jesse Green, JD
General Counsel
Parker College of Chiropractic
Dallas, Texas

Helen Houser, RN, MSHA
Program Director
Medical Assisting Program
Phoenix College
Phoenix, Arizona

Carol Lee Jarrell, MLT, OPT
Instructor
Commonwealth Business College
Merrillville, Indiana

Peggy M. Krueger, MEd, RN, BSN, CMA
Program Coordinator
Medical Assisting Program
Linn-Benton Community College
Albany, Oregon

Karen D. Lockyer, BA, RHIT, CPC
Instructor
Montgomery College
Takoma Park, Maryland;
Administrative Assistant,
National Institutes of Health,
Bethesda, Maryland

Joseph E. McCann, BA, LVN, CMA
Medical Assisting Program Coordinator
San Antonio College
San Antonio, Texas

Catherine McCartney, MA, RN, CMA
Program Director/Instructor
Medical Assistant Program
Henry Ford Community College
Health Careers Division
Dearborn, Michigan

Shirley Jordan Oktay, BA, CMA, POLT(AAB)
Instructional Specialist III, Health Professions
Richland College
Dallas, Texas

Lauren Perlstein, RN, MSN
Coordinator of Medical Assistant Program
Norwalk Community Technical College
Norwalk, Connecticut

Janet Sesser, RMA(AMT), CMA, BSEd Admin
Director of Education for Allied Health
High-Tech Institute, Inc.
Phoenix, Arizona

Jane A. Shingler
Allied Health Department Chair
Allentown Business School
Allentown, Pennsylvania

Nina Thierer, CMA, BS, CPC-A
Associate Professor and Instructor
Medical Assisting Program
Ivy Tech State College—Fort Wayne
Fort Wayne, Indiana

Jana W. Tucker, CMA, LPRT
Medical Assistant Program Coordinator
Assistant Professor
Salt Lake City Community College
Salt Lake City, Utah

CONTRIBUTORS TO THIS EDITION

The preceding section demonstrates the amount of feedback and developmental input that went into shaping the ninth edition of this textbook. Because the medical assisting curriculum is so broad in scope, no individual can be an expert in all areas. We therefore extend a special acknowledgment to the following people who brought their expertise to bear by contributing one or more chapters to this edition:

Kim Anthony Aaronson, BS, DC
Adjunct Instructor
Anatomy and Physiology and Medical Terminology
Truman College;
Adjunct Instructor
Pacific College of Oriental Medicine
Chicago, Illinois

Janet Beik, MEd
Administrative Instructor
Medical Assistant Program
Southeastern Community College
West Burlington, Iowa

Brenda K. Burton
President
Medextend, Inc.
Cazenovia, New York

Ruth Ann Ehrlich, RT(R)
Senior Instructor, Radiology
Western States Chiropractic College
Portland, Oregon

Robin R. Patterson, BS, MT(ASCP), MS, EdD
Associate Professor
Department of Technology and Natural Science
Butler County Community College
Butler, Pennsylvania

Carol A. Turiello, RN, RDMS, CPC
Administrator
Cardiology Division
Department of Medicine
State University of New York
Upstate Medical University
Syracuse, New York

Carole Stemple Zeglin, BS, MT(AMT)
Adjunct Faculty
Westmoreland Community College
Youngwood, Pennsylvania

Author Acknowledgments

It takes a dedicated group of individuals to produce an outstanding textbook such as this. I am thankful for the Elsevier team for the tireless work that was put into *Kinn's The Medical Assistant: An Applied Learning Approach, Ninth Edition.* Adrianne Cochran, Executive Editor for Vocational Publishing, provided encouragement, ideas, and a healthy dose of confidence as we undertook the project and throughout its development. I will be forever grateful for her belief in my ability as a writer. Beth LoGiudice, Associate Developmental Editor, was a tremendous asset to the project as we progressed from chapter to chapter. Her enthusiasm, sense of humor, and support were unending and greatly appreciated. It seemed that she was never frazzled, no matter what the challenge was before us. David Stein, Project Manager, was courteous and helpful as our project manager through the production process. The photographer, Jack Foley of Jack Foley Photography, his team, and the Elsevier design team of Bill Donnelly and Mark Oberkrom all did a superb job in turning this book into a beautiful work of art. Finally, thanks also to Anne Rowe for introducing me to Adrianne Cochran and jump-starting my writing career. I could not have asked for a better team. Thanks to you all for your part in making this project become a reality.

Special thanks go to Debby Kennedy and Tammy Morton. I am privileged to know such talented individuals. You both did a wonderful job on this text and its supplements. Thanks also to Brenda Burton, Carol Turiello, and Janet Beik for writing the contributed chapters. They are truly fantastic.

I would like to thank my dad, Jim Crumley, attorney-at-law, for giving me a sense for law and ethics, and for allowing me to interrupt his black-and-white TV shows with my questions for the book. Without my mom, Patricia Crumley, I would have never made it through school and learned to spell and pronounce medical terms like "otorhinolaryngologist." Thanks to my sisters, Alisha and Karry, for their encouragement. I would also like to thank the physicians that I have worked with in the past, especially Dr. Brad Burns, Dr. Robert Wray, and my brother, Dr. Terry Watson, for their willingness to share and teach so that I might have a greater understanding of the healthcare industry. I would never have entered the medical field were it not for the foresight of Harry and Zylphia Dickerson, who founded the school where I obtained my medical assistant training. Without their dream of educating medical assistants, I would not have had the opportunities that have been placed before me over the years. It was with Carole Cannefax in mind that I pictured this book in use. She made my medical assistant courses intriguing, and without a great instructor, the textbook cannot take on life and reach the students.

Last, my family deserves so many thanks, because they allowed me to work on this text when they would rather have had me to themselves. My children—Jimmie, Jonathan, and Jessica—inspire me daily. Yes, Jonathan, the book is finished now. And to my precious husband, Jerry Homolka, thank you for your love and for encouraging me to do what I love the most in life—to write.

Alexandra Patricia Young, BBA, CMA, RMA
Dallas, Texas
February 2003

A huge task such as this major revision to the long-standing Kinn text can only be accomplished through the efforts of a dedicated and talented team of individuals. I have been very fortunate to work with such an outstanding team, led by the experienced and creative voice of Adrianne Cochran. Adrianne was always available with support and encouragement as well as an excellent comprehensive view of the project. She managed to keep us focused on the work at hand while providing a creative and unique approach to the text and its support materials. Her efforts were reinforced by Beth LoGiudice, who consistently provided research, editorial support, comfort, and encouragement during the more trying times in the project. The individuals who worked so diligently at the Boston photo shoot, especially Jack Foley, provided the exceptional figures seen throughout the text. The Elsevier team was completed by the proof king, David Stein. Although David and I have never met, we have shared endless correspondence over e-mail in the last year, and while I dreaded receiving another of those FedEx packages, it was comforting to know that David was working hard on completing the editorial phase of the text.

I have also had the privilege to work with an exceptional author team. Tricia Young, who is responsible for the administrative portion of the text, and Tammy Morton, who accomplished major revisions to the text support materials, have each made indispensable contributions to the overall project. They have helped make the ninth Kinn an excellent comprehensive textbook and I am very grateful for their dedication and expertise. A special thank you goes to the contributing authors, especially Dr. Robin Patterson, for providing their outstanding talents in the specialty chapters.

My primary focus throughout this project was my students. I have been fortunate to interact with a dedicated, sincere group of students who are willing to work hard to achieve their goals. Throughout the critical thinking applications I repeatedly considered how my students would best understand the material and benefit from the learning experience. Chapter 1 was developed specifically with my students in mind. More than anything else I hope this textbook helps students gain confidence in their ability to be successful learners. I have also been very fortunate to have the support of my home institution, Butler County Community College, which lives its mission of promoting teaching and learning in a community education environment.

And finally, my children—Sara, Erin, and Sean—have served as sounding boards and cheerleaders over the last 2 years, offering their love and appreciation of my efforts. I am very blessed to have them as an integral part of my life and I do promise an outstanding family vacation very soon. And to my soon-to-be husband, Timothy Shields Proctor, who has been with me throughout this project—at the initial authors' meeting in Annapolis, the photo shoot in Boston (even doing a cameo appearance in many of the photos as "Dr. Proctor"), and with me through those long nights and weekends of endless work—it is FINALLY done, honey. The question is....what to do now with all of this free time?

Deborah B. Kennedy, EdD, RN, CMA
Butler, Pennsylvania
February 2003

Contents

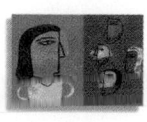

UNIT ONE
Introduction to Medical Assisting

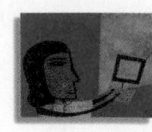

UNIT TWO
Administrative Medical Assisting

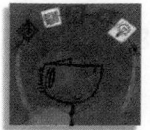

UNIT THREE
Financial Management

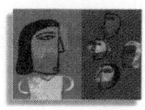

UNIT FOUR
Medical Practice and Health Information Management

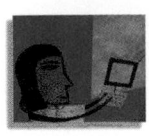

UNIT FIVE
Fundamentals of Clinical Medical Assisting

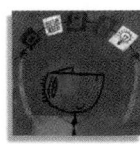

UNIT SIX
Assisting With Medications

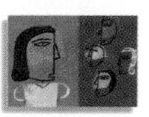

UNIT SEVEN
Assisting With Medical Specialties

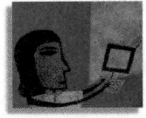

UNIT EIGHT
Diagnostic Procedures

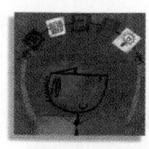

UNIT NINE
Assisting With Surgeries

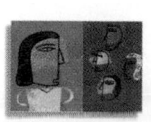

UNIT TEN
Career Development

List of Procedures

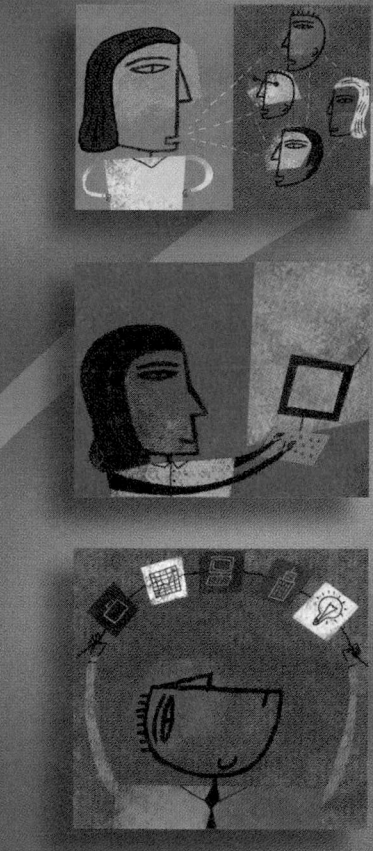

Introduction

CHAPTER 1

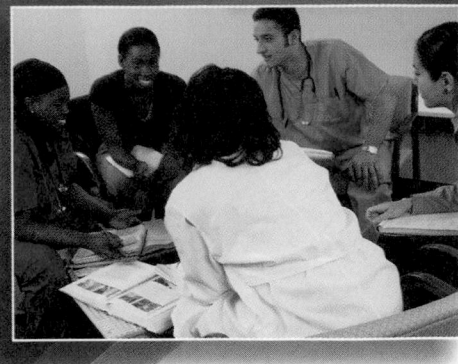

Scenario

Shawna Long is a newly admitted student in a medical assistant program at your school. Shawna is anxious about starting classes and very concerned that she may not be a successful student. She had trouble with some of her classes in high school and must continue to work part-time while taking medical assistant classes. Based on what you discover about the learning process in this chapter, see if you can help Shawna take steps toward success.

Becoming a
Successful Student

Vocabulary

critical thinking The constant practice of considering all aspects of a situation when deciding what to believe or what to do.

empathy Sensitivity to the individual needs and reactions of patients.

learning style The way that an individual perceives and processes information to learn new material.

perceiving How an individual looks at information and sees it as real.

processing How an individual internalizes new information and makes it his or her own.

professional behaviors Those actions that identify the medical assistant as a member of a healthcare profession including dependability, respectful patient care, initiative, positive attitude, and teamwork.

reflection The process of considering new information and internalizing it to create new ways of examining information.

You have taken the first step to becoming a successful student by choosing your profession and field of study. The medical assistant profession is both challenging and rewarding. Becoming a medical assistant opens the doors to a wide variety of opportunities in both administrative and clinical practice at ambulatory or institutional healthcare settings. Medical assistants are important members of the healthcare team, and as a healthcare professional you will be expected to practice certain **professional behaviors** (Figure 1-1). These professional behaviors, which are discussed in depth in Chapter 4, include dependability, respectful patient care, **empathy**, initiative, positive attitude, and teamwork. In order to become a successful medical assistant you must first become a successful student. This chapter helps you to discover the way that you learn best and provides multiple strategies to assist you in your journey toward success.

Who You Are As a Learner: How Do You Learn Best?

Think about what you do when you are faced with something new to learn. How do you go about understanding and learning the new material? Over time you have developed a method for **perceiving** and **processing** information. This pattern of behavior is called your **learning style.** There are many different ways of examining learning styles, but most professionals agree that the success of students depends more on whether they can "make sense" of the information rather than on whether or not they are "smart." Education that is based on attention to individual learning styles is sensitive to the different ways that students learn and approaches new material with a wide variety of methods so that all students have the opportunity to learn. Determining your individual learning style and understanding how it applies to your ability to learn new material are the first steps to becoming a successful student (Figure 1-2).

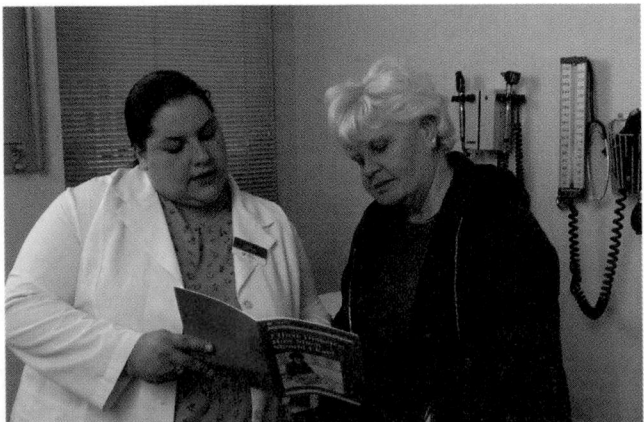

FIGURE 1-1   Professional interaction with patient.

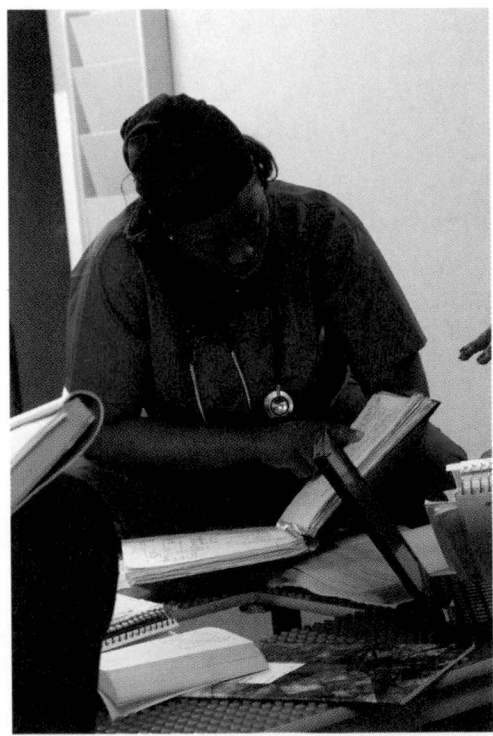

FIGURE 1-2   Student learning.

Learning Style Inventory

For you to learn new material, two things must happen. First you must perceive the information. This is the method you have developed over time that helps you examine the material and recognize it as real. Then you must process the information. Processing the information is how you internalize it and make it your own. By investigating various learning styles, you can figure out how to combine different methods of perceiving and processing information. In his book *Becoming a Master Student*, David Ellis discusses these different methods of information perception, processing, and learning.*

Information perception involves how you go about examining new material and making it real. There are two ways learners perceive new material. Some people are concrete perceivers who learn information through direct experience by doing, acting, sensing, or feeling. *Concrete* learners prefer to learn things that have a personal meaning or things that they feel are relevant. Other learners are *abstract* perceivers who take in information through analysis, observation, and **reflection.** Abstract learners like to think things through. They analyze the new material and build theories to help understand it. They prefer structured learning situations and use a step-by-step approach to problem solving.

Information processing is how you internalize the new information and make it your own. There are also two different methods for processing material. *Active* processors prefer to jump in and start doing things immediately. They make sense of the new material by immediately using it. They look for practical ways to apply the new material and typically do not mind taking risks to get the desired results. They learn best with practice and hands-on activities. *Reflective* processors, however, have to think about the information before they can internalize it. They prefer to observe and consider what is going on. The only way they can make sense of new material is to spend time thinking and learning a great deal about it before acting.

CRITICAL THINKING APPLICATION

- Consider the two ways to perceive new material. Are you a concrete perceiver who ties the information to a personal experience or do you prefer abstract perception in which you like to analyze or reflect on the meaning of the material? Choose which one you think most accurately describes your method of investigating new information.
- Then think about the way you process learning. Are you an active processor who is always looking for the practical application of what you learn or are you a reflective processor who has to think about new material before internalizing it?
- After completing this activity write down the combination of your perceiving/processing learning style and share it with your instructor.

*Ellis D: *Becoming a master student*, ed 10. Boston, 2002, Houghton Mifflin.

Using Your Learning Profile to be a Successful Student: Where Do I Go from Here?

No one falls completely into one or the other of these categories. However, by being aware of how we generally prefer to first perceive information and then process it, we can be more sensitive to our learning style and can approach new learning situations with a plan for learning the material in a way that best suits our learning preferences. Your preferred perceiving/processing learning profile will fall into one of the following stages in the Learning Style Inventory created by David Kolb of Case Western Reserve University.

Learners in *Stage 1* have a concrete/reflective style. These students want to know the purpose of the information and have a personal connection to the content. They like to consider a situation from many different points of view, observe others, and plan before taking action. Their strengths are in understanding people, brainstorming, and recognizing and creatively solving problems. If you fall into this stage, you enjoy small group activities and learn well in study groups.

Stage 2 learners have an abstract/reflective style. These students are eager to learn just for the sheer pleasure of learning rather than because the material relates to their personal lives. They like to learn lots of facts and arrange new material in a logical and clear manner. Stage 2 learners plan studying and like to create ways of thinking about the material but do not always make the connection with the practical application of the material. If you are a Stage 2 learner, you prefer organized, logical presentations of material and therefore enjoy lectures and generally dislike group work. You also need time to process and think about the new material before applying it.

Learners in *Stage 3* have an abstract/active style. Learners with this combination of learning style want to experiment and test the information that they are learning. If you are a Stage 3 learner, you want to know how techniques or ideas work and you also want to practice what you are learning. Your strengths are in problem solving and decision making, but you may lack focus and be hasty when making decisions. You learn best with hands-on practice by doing experiments, projects, and lab activities. You also enjoy working alone or in small groups (Figure 1-3).

Stage 4 is made up of concrete/active learners. These students are concerned about how they can use what they learn to make a difference in their lives. If you fall into this stage, you like to relate new material to other areas of your life. You have leadership capabilities, can create on your feet, and are usually vocal in a group, but you may have difficulty completing your work on time. Stage 4 learners enjoy teaching others and working in groups and learn best when they can apply the new information to real-world problems (Figure 1-4).

To get the most out of knowing your learning profile, you need to apply this knowledge to how you approach learning. There are pluses and minuses to each of the learning stages. When faced with a learning situation that does not match your learning preference, see how you can adapt your individual learning to make the best of the information. For example, if you are bored by lectures, look for an opportunity to apply the information being

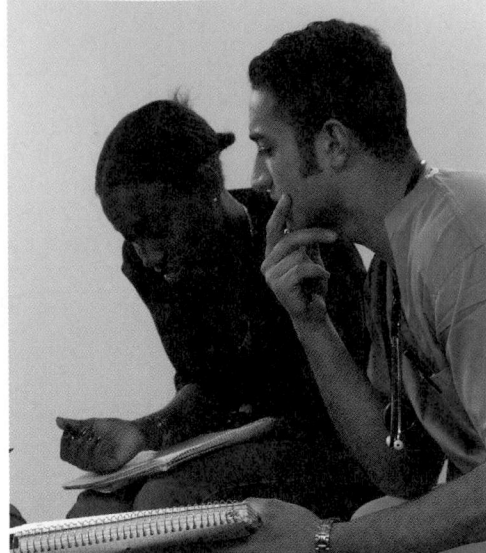

FIGURE 1-3   Learning in a small group.

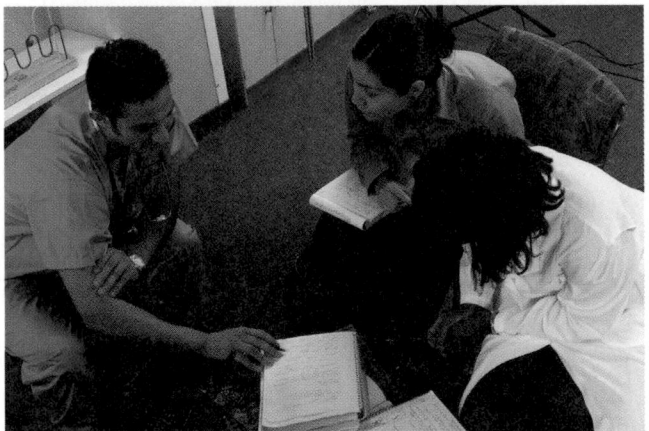

FIGURE 1-4   Teaching and working with others.

presented to a real problem you are facing in the classroom or at home. If you are an abstract perceiver, take time outside of class to think about new information so that you are ready to process it into your learning system. If you benefit from learning in a group, make the effort to organize review sessions and study groups. If you learn best by teaching others, offer to assist your peers with their learning. By taking the time now to investigate your preferred method of learning, you will perceive and process information more effectively throughout your school career.

CRITICAL THINKING APPLICATION

Take a few minutes to reflect on a time when you really enjoyed learning about something new. How was the material presented and what did you do to "make it your own"? What do you need to do to become a more effective learner?

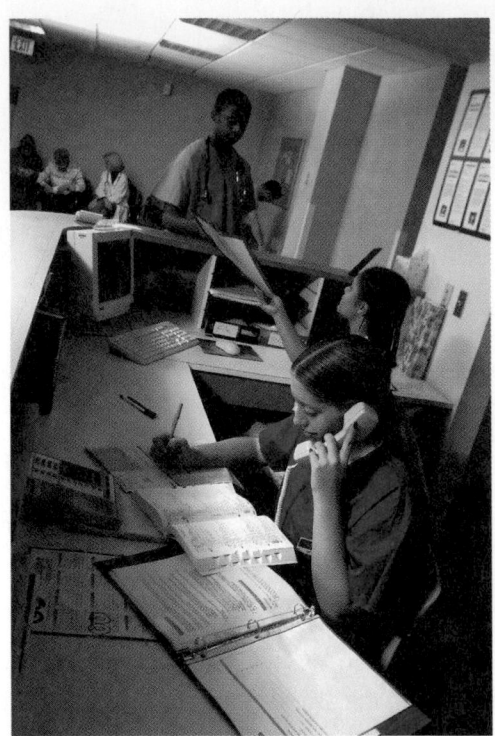

FIGURE 1-5   Time management in a busy medical practice.

Time Management: Putting Time on Your Side

One of the most complicated tasks for a professional medical assistant is to effectively manage time. No other workplace can compete with the distractions and demands of a busy healthcare setting. Do you think that you practice effective time management skills? Do you believe that you are in control of your time or do you think that other people or situations control it? How frequently do you say that you just do not have enough time to do what you are supposed to do, let alone those things you would like to do? Time management gives you the opportunity to spend time in the way you choose. Effective time management is also crucial to your success as a student and as a future healthcare professional (Figure 1-5).

How to Put Time on Your Side

The following time management skills are designed to help you effectively deal with the demands on your time. Highlight the ones that you think will be most useful in helping you deal with your situation.

1. *Determine your purpose.* What do you want to accomplish this semester, in this course, or in this unit of study? What do you want to achieve as a student? What is one thing you can do to help achieve your goals?
2. *Identify your main concern.* Besides school, what other demands do you have on your time? Based on the learning goals you have established, what do you need to do to accomplish your goals?

- Plan time: Schedule projects in advance with notes to yourself on deadlines.
- Use down time: Take your work with you everywhere you go. Do small bits at every opportunity.
- Guard time: Avoid distractions (e.g., television, music) that will interfere with your concentration. Notice how others abuse your time. Learn to say no to outside demands on your time.
- Discover time: Steal time from other activities in your schedule.
- Assign time: Ask for help when you need it from friends and family.

3. *Be organized.* What materials (e.g., books, research, supplies) do you need to have an effective study session? What preparation is needed to make the most of your time?
   - Record time: Use a day planner or calendar to write down due dates for assignments and tests.
   - Optimal time: Take advantage of the time of day when you study and learn the best.

4. *Stop procrastinating.* If you avoid working on your goals, you may not achieve them. Examine the following suggestions as ways to break the procrastination cycle.
   - Make the work meaningful: What is important about the work you are putting off and what are the benefits of getting it done?
   - Plan work deadlines: Break assignments into achievable sections that can be completed in the time slots available.
   - Ask for help: Let your support system know you have work to get done. Ask them for encouragement to stay on track.
   - Prioritize: If you keep avoiding a certain task, re-evaluate its priority. If it is really worth worrying about, get started now not later.
   - Reward yourself: Create a reward that is meaningful and something you will work for. If you want to spend time with your family or friends on the weekend, develop a plan and stick to it so you can share that special time as a reward.

5. *Remember you.* It is very easy to become overwhelmed with responsibilities both in school and at home. Part of successful time management includes setting aside time to do things you enjoy. You have chosen a profession that can be very demanding. Now is the time to remember that you have to take care of yourself as well as meet your professional and personal responsibilities. So remember to plan some time for yourself as well (Figure 1-6).

CRITICAL THINKING APPLICATION

How do you spend your time? Over 3 days this week write down the amount of time you spend on each activity. How much TV do you watch? How much time do you talk on the phone? How about driving time, visiting time, work time, time for family and friends, and so on? At the end of the 3-day period, add up the various categories of time. Do you

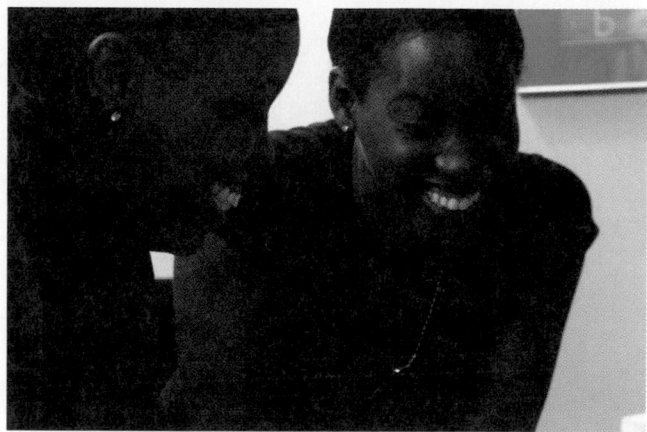

FIGURE 1-6   Making time for you.

recognize any time you might be wasting? Can you implement any of the suggested time management strategies to make more time available?

Problem Solving and Conflict Management

As a future member of the healthcare team, you will frequently face problems and conflict. Although we usually look at these situations as negative factors in our lives, problem solving and conflict management actually give us the opportunity to positively impact a potentially negative situation. Learning how to manage problems can be very useful for your practice as a medical assistant, as well as for your success as a student.

The first step in reaching an equitable solution to a problem or conflict situation is to identify the central issue. How many times have you known that you were upset about something but were not really sure why? You cannot solve a problem or a negative situation unless you are sure what is at the root of your feelings. You need to understand the problem and gather as much information about the situation as possible before you decide to act. One way of doing this is to ask yourself these questions:

- When does the situation occur and under what circumstances?
- Is there someone else involved?
- What interferes with making a decision or solving the conflict?

Once you understand the situation and how you feel about it, you need to decide if it is worth the effort to solve it. Prioritize your involvement. Sometimes there are situations and problems that you are unable to solve or ones that you decide are not important enough for you to act on.

After you have gathered the details about the problem or conflict, and you have decided to act, it is time to determine possible solutions. One way to do this is to ask for advice or brainstorm ideas with individuals you respect. Sometimes another person can give you special insight into the problem that you were unable to see on your own. After brainstorming for possible solutions, get feedback regarding the workability of the suggested solutions. Another way of approaching the problem is to list the pros and cons of possible solutions. Simply looking at a list of the positive and negative aspects of the solution may clarify how you should solve the problem. Before deciding on a solution, critically analyze the consequences of each proposed solution: Which one best meets your needs and has the potential of providing an outcome you can live with?

Finally you are ready to implement the chosen solution. However, your work is not over yet. You need to evaluate the outcome of your decision and see if it truly did meet your needs. If not, it may be time to review possible solutions and try another approach.

Conflict management requires some additional consideration. If you are in conflict with a peer, instructor, or co-worker, it is important to follow certain guidelines. You should attempt to solve the conflict in a private place at a prescheduled time. This ensures that the person will meet with you and that neither one has to worry about others overhearing the conversation. At the meeting clearly state your feelings about the conflict and how you would like it solved. Then try to come to an agreeable solution. The best way to deal with conflict situations is through open, honest, assertive communication. However, just as with problem solving, it is important to follow up on the decided course of action to see if it effectively dealt with the source of the conflict (Figure 1-7).

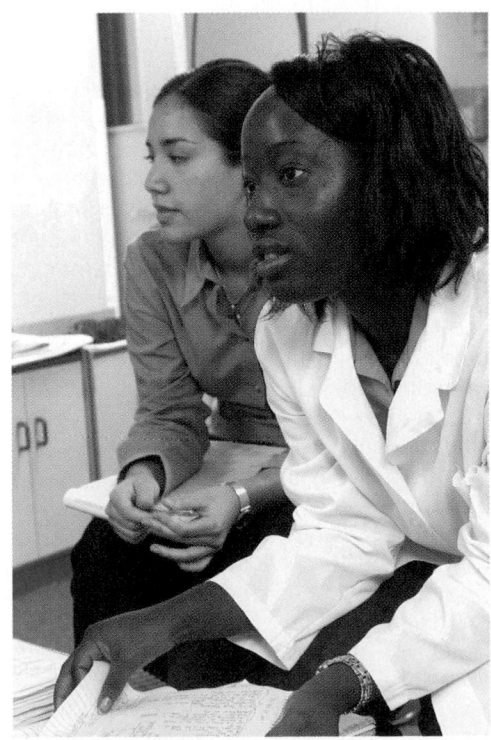

FIGURE 1-7 Dealing with conflict.

CRITICAL THINKING APPLICATION

Think about a serious problem you are currently facing. Utilize the brainstorming and/or pros-and-cons method for creating solutions to the problem. Implement your chosen solution and follow up on its effectiveness. Did the problem-solving process help you manage the situation more effectively?

Study Skills: Tricks to Becoming a Successful Student

So far in this chapter we have looked at the influence of individual learning styles and time management on learning success. Now we will investigate some ideas that are useful in learning new material. These study skills include memory techniques, active learning, brain tricks, reading methods, and note-taking strategies.

There are several techniques you can utilize to help you store and remember information. The first of these involves organizing information into recognizable groups so the brain can easily find it. You can organize information by getting the big picture first before trying to learn the details. One way to implement this strategy is to skim a reading assignment before actually reading and taking notes on the material, thus getting a general impression of what you need to learn before tackling the details. Depending on your learning style, it may also help to find a way of making the new information meaningful. Think about your educational goals and how the new material will help you achieve those goals. Another way of remembering material is to create an association with something you already know. By grouping new material with already stored material, your brain will remember it much easier.

A useful study skill for some learners is to be physically active while learning. Some students learn best if they walk or talk out loud while studying. Besides encouraging learning, moving and talking while studying relieve boredom and keep you awake. Another way to be actively involved in learning is to use pictures or diagrams to represent the material you are studying. Some people are visual learners, and creating pictures of the material is the easiest method for them to retain the information. Other students find that rewriting notes or making lists of information helps them retain the material. Writing also helps those students who need to "do" something in order to learn.

Studying will go much smoother if you work with your brain rather than against it. If you tend to get anxious and worried while studying, you may act as your own worst enemy. One way of dealing with a topic that you find anxiety producing is to overlearn it. If material is overlearned, you are much less likely to experience test anxiety. Another method for remembering material is to quickly review it after class. This mini-review will help the new information become part of your long-term memory system. Many students find creating songs, dances, or word associations an effective way to learn and remember new material. Putting details into a familiar song and moving to it can help trick the brain into remembering the information. This is especially helpful when trying to learn anatomy and physiology. Another excellent way of learning information is to actually teach it to someone else. Teaching requires you to have a good understanding of the material as well as the ability to describe it for others. It can be an effective reinforcer of complicated material (Figure 1-8).

A great deal of the learning process is expected to take place from assigned readings. There are methods that you can use to make reading assignments more meaningful. If you find a reading assignment challenging or difficult to understand, the first step is to take the time to read it again. Sometimes the first time through the material is not enough to gain understanding. As you read, highlight important words or thoughts and stop periodically to summarize the material. If you get bored while reading, use your body—walk or talk your way through the assignment. Take the time to look up words or terms you do not understand or ask your instructor or tutor for help. Outlining the material can help you create a brief overview of what you need to learn. And finally, the best way to determine if you learned anything from your reading is to try to explain it to someone else. If that is effective, you know you acquired the knowledge needed from the reading assignment.

Many students find effective note taking a challenge. The big question is, "How much of what the instructor says do I actually need to write down?" The first step in effective note taking is to come to class prepared. The more familiar you are with the material, the easier it will be to determine the important parts of the instructor's lecture. Pay attention to the instructor and look for clues about what he or she thinks is important. Ask questions about the material if you do not understand it rather than writing down information that makes no sense to you. Think critically about what you hear before you write it down so you can start to build relationships between what you want or need to know.

When it comes to actual note taking, there are some strategies that can make the process of recording notes an active learning tool. Organize the information as much as possible while you are writing in either an outline or paragraph format. Use only one side of the paper for easier reading and leave blank spaces where needed to fill in details later. Use key words to help you remember the material and create pictures or diagrams to help visualize it. If permitted, use tape recorders when appropriate and make sure you have either handouts or notes that cover material written on the board, in an overhead, or in a PowerPoint presentation. Another helpful tool is to develop your own system of abbreviations to help simplify the writing load.

The most effective way to use your notes is to review them shortly after class. This is the time to add details, clarify information, or make notes about asking the instructor for explanations during the next class. You could even exchange notes with students you trust to compare information (Figure 1-9). Some students find it beneficial to type or rewrite their notes. This can give you an opportunity to learn the material as you are transcribing it. As you are reviewing your notes you can also draw mind maps of the information or diagram outlines to help you better understand and remember the material.

Creating mind maps is a way of representing the main idea of the topic and supporting important details with a figure or picture. Healthcare textbooks are made up of complicated concepts with multiple main ideas, each with its own important details. Mind maps are a way of consolidating complex details and organizing them into a format that is easier to remember. The Spider map example in Figure 1-10 presents a method for including several main ideas with details in one study guide. The Fishbone map in Figure 1-11 can be used to learn complicated causes of disease. The Chain of Events map in

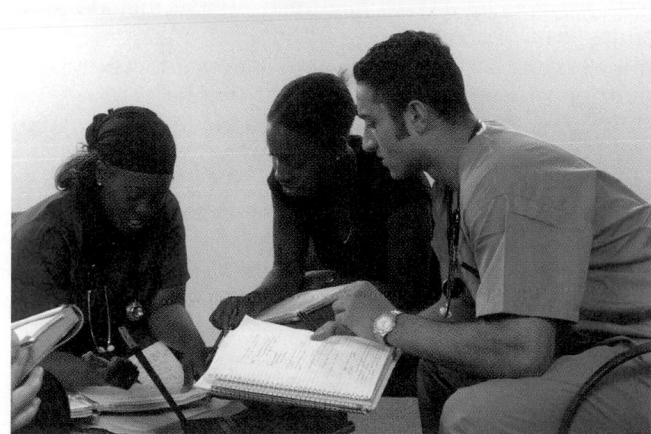

FIGURE 1-8   Effective study skills.

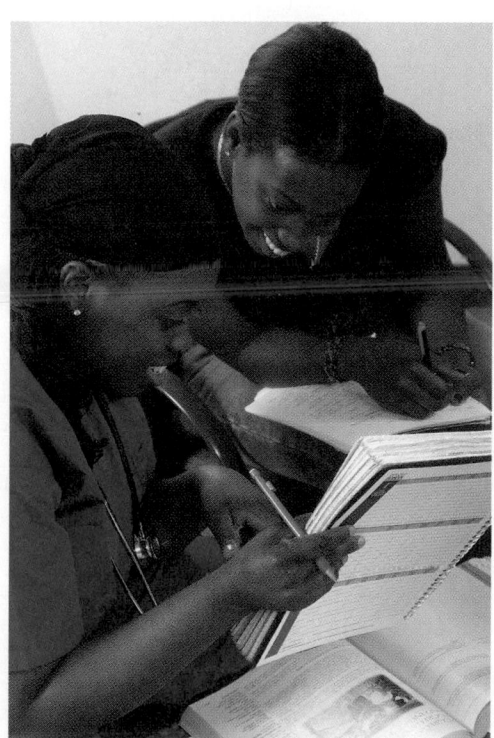

FIGURE 1-9   Sharing notes.

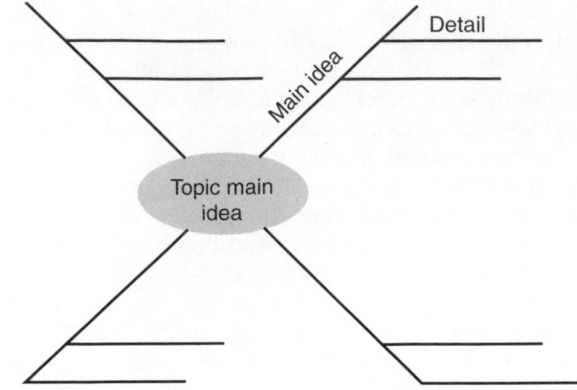

FIGURE 1-10 Spider map displays multiple main ideas with supporting details.

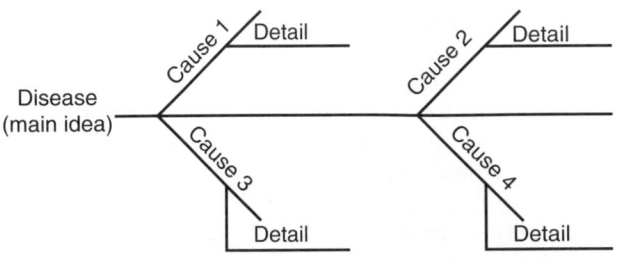

FIGURE 1-11 Fishbone map used to describe causes of disease.

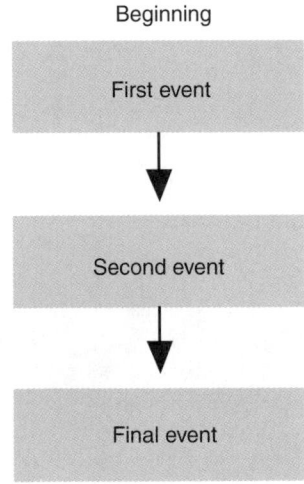

FIGURE 1-12 Chain of events map displays the cause and effect of events.

Figure 1-12 displays the cause and effect of events such as infection control or the history of medicine. The Cycle map in Figure 1-13 shows the connection between factors such as with the chain of infection. Creating your own mind maps is a way of making the information more meaningful and easier for you to understand.

Although there are many techniques you can use to help you study, perhaps the most important one is your attitude toward learning. Some students fall into the "I can't possibly learn this material" trap. That type of attitude only leads to self-defeat. The way to solve barriers is to first recognize that they exist. Once you know your weak spots, use the suggested study skills to improve in those areas. Do not be afraid to ask questions or to seek

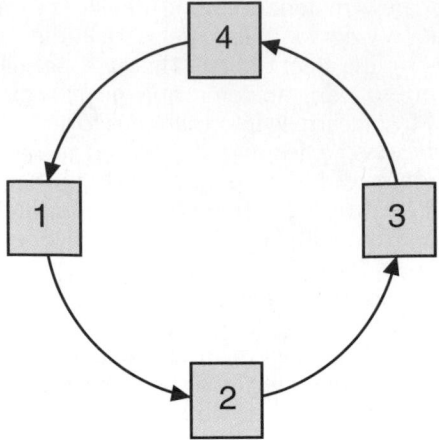

FIGURE 1-13 Cycle map shows how one action leads to another.

out help if you do not understand the material. Employ as many different strategies as necessary to become a successful student.

CRITICAL THINKING APPLICATION

Write down at least two barriers to your learning. Review the study skill suggestions above and choose four you want to try out. Use them over the next week to help you when learning new material. Reflect on whether the chosen study skills helped you learn the material better.

Test-Taking Strategies: Taking Charge of Your Success

What happens when you do not know the answer to the first question on a test? What if you do not know the next one? Are you able to go on without panicking? Many people find taking tests the most challenging part of being successful students. There are multiple approaches that you can employ to take charge of your success and improve your ability to take tests. These include such strategies as adequate preparation, controlling negative thoughts during test time, and understanding how to manage various types of questions.

The first step is to go into a test adequately prepared. Use the time management skills already outlined in this chapter to get prepared for the big day. Recognize and employ your preferred learning style to overlearn the material and increase your confidence. Use memory tools like flash cards, checklists, and mind maps to help visualize the material. Form a study group if you are the type of learner who benefits from studying in groups (Figure 1-14). Schedule and plan study time and reward yourself for your hard work. It is also important to go into the test rested and relaxed, so eat, exercise to relieve stress, and sleep before the test so that you are as alert as possible.

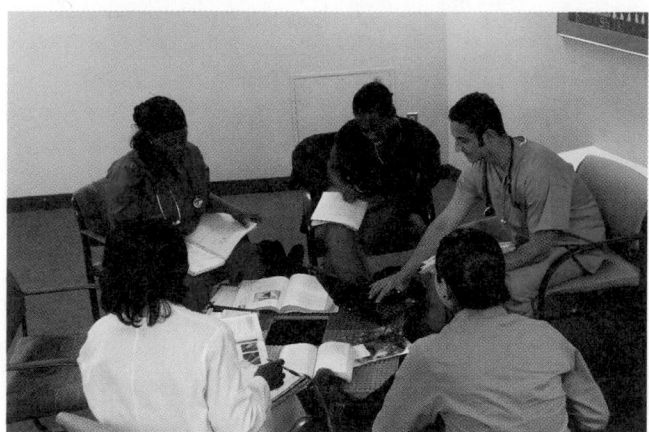

FIGURE 1-14   Study group.

Before you start the test make sure you read directions carefully and, if possible, begin with the easiest or shortest questions to build your confidence. Be aware of the amount of time allotted for the examination and pace yourself accordingly. As you go through the test, look for clues to answers in other questions. During test time remember to use positive self-talk at the first indication of panic. Repeatedly remind yourself that you are well prepared, relax, and think about the material before you get worried. You need to stop negative thoughts as soon as they arise, and instead visualize yourself being successful. Use slow deep breathing to relax and, if helpful, close your eyes for a minute and visualize a relaxing place before you go on with the test. You may find it helpful to wear a thick rubber band on your wrist and snap it as soon as you start to think negatively. This will provide a physical reaction to interfere with the power of your negative thoughts and serve as a reminder of what you should be concentrating on.

There are some strategies that you can employ when answering certain types of questions. With multiple choice questions, try to identify key words or clues in each question. Read the question carefully and answer it in your head before you review the provided answers. If you are not absolutely sure of the answer, make an educated guess or follow your instincts in choosing an answer. "True/false" questions give you a "50/50" chance of being correct. Remember that if any part of the question is not true, then the statement is false. Again, check the statements for key words that will help indicate the direction of the answer. Look for qualifying terms (e.g., "always," "never," "sometimes") that are key to understanding the meaning of the true/false statement.

CRITICAL THINKING APPLICATION

Think about a time you experienced test anxiety. Write down the details about the situation and how you felt. Choose four test-taking strategies that you think would be beneficial in handling similar situations in the future.

Becoming a Critical Thinker: Making Mental Connections

The ability to process information and arrive at reasonable conclusions is crucial to all healthcare workers. The process of **critical thinking** involves sorting out conflicting information, weighing the knowledge you possess about that information, ignoring or letting go of personal biases, and deciding on a reasonable belief or action. Critical thinking is actually an active search for the truth. Critical thinking could be described as thorough thinking because it requires learners to be open-minded to all possibilities. Successful students are thorough thinkers because they must determine the facts about the topic being learned and come to logical conclusions about the material. Critical thinkers are also inquisitive learners who are constantly in the process of analyzing and sorting out conflicting information to reach conclusions. A crucial step in critical thinking is evaluating the results of your learning. Reflection is key to critical thinking. "How did I learn what I learned" and "What does it mean in my life" are questions that must be consistently asked in order to continue to learn. Becoming a successful student and, ultimately, a successful member of the allied health team requires the possession of critical thinking skills. Both the material presented in this chapter and the critical thinking application exercises are designed to encourage you along this life-long learning path of critical thinking.

SUMMARY OF SCENARIO

One of the things Shawna can do to improve her learning is to determine her individual learning style. By understanding how she typically perceives and processes new information she can plan the best methods for learning the material. In addition to understanding who she is as a learner, Shawna needs to practice successful time management skills to keep up with school and work responsibilities. Effective problem solving and developing study skills that work for her are also key to her success as a student.

SUMMARY OF LEARNING OBJECTIVES

■ Medical assistants play a vital role in the healthcare team and are expected to display such professional behaviors as dependability, respectful patient care, empathy, initiative, positive attitude, and teamwork.

■ Critical thinkers can evaluate conflicting information and make a decision to act based on their knowledge and willingness to be open-minded to all possibilities.

■ Learning preferences are the ways that you like to learn and have proven successful in the past.

■ Learning styles are determined by your individual method of perceiving or examining new material and the way that you process it or make it your own. People are either concrete or abstract perceivers and either active or reflective processors.

■ Effective time management strategies such as setting goals, prioritizing, getting organized, and avoiding procrastination will make you a more successful student as well as an effective medical assistant.

■ Problem-solving and conflict-management techniques are key to your success. First, identify the central issue and how you feel about it; then consider possible solutions and their potential results, implement the chosen solution, and analyze the results.

■ Study skills such as memory techniques, active learning, brain tricks, effective reading methods, note-taking strategies, and mind maps all help students to be more successful.

■ Test-taking strategies include preparing adequately for the examination, controlling negative thoughts during the examination, and understanding how to deal with different types of questions.

■ Critical thinking can be described as thorough thinking because it considers all sides of the information without bias. Reflection is the process of thinking about or reviewing information before acting.

KEY INTERNET WEBSITES

LEARNING STYLES

- Coastline Community College. Online Study Skill Module.
- Fastrack Consulting. Online Learning Styles.
- Funderstanding. About Learning Theories.
  For active weblinks to each website visit
  http://evolve.elsevier.com/Kinn/

TIME MANAGEMENT

- Learning Skills Program
- Time Management Resources
  For active weblinks to each website visit
  http://evolve.elsevier.com/Kinn/

STUDY SKILLS

- Memory Improvement
- Strategies for Success
  For active weblinks to each website visit
  http://evolve.elsevier.com/Kinn/

TEST-TAKING STRATEGIES

- Academic Success-CAPS
- Study Guides and Test-taking Strategies
- Test Taking Strategies
  For active weblinks to each website visit
  http://evolve.elsevier.com/Kinn/

CHAPTER 2

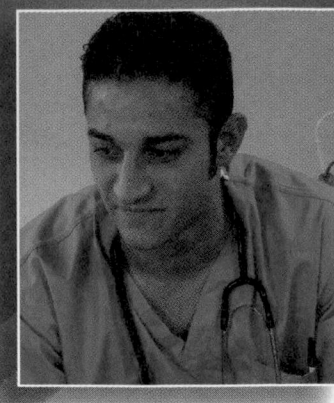

Scenario

Carlos Santos, CMA, is a medical assisting instructor with 10 years' experience in the clinical area. He has worked for a group of family practitioners and for an allergist during his career as a medical assistant. Mr. Santos believes that it is very important to give his students an overview of the healthcare industry early in their training. He feels that it is exciting to show them the history and progress of medicine and introduce them to the current types of facilities available for patient care on both a national and local level. This helps the student to understand where he or she fits in the whole picture as a medical assistant. Often Mr. Santos assigns the students a short report on one person who contributed to the growth of medicine. He finds that this is a good way to encourage the students to use the Internet right from the start of their training. It also offers the student a chance to grow more comfortable in speaking in front of a group. The knowledge that the students will learn about the different areas of patient care will be very useful once they graduate and begin working in a healthcare facility. They will frequently be required to provide patients with information about health and community resources. All of these skills will make Mr. Santos' students more versatile and valuable to their eventual employer.

The Healthcare Industry

Learning Objectives

- Define and spell the terms listed in the vocabulary.
- Identify the two ancient mythologies that contributed a major portion of our medical terminology.
- Distinguish between and describe the two medical symbols in general use today.
- Name and briefly explain the content of the oath that is often administered to new physicians.
- Explain the impact of Johns Hopkins on medical education in the United States.
- List at least five medical pioneers and their contributions to the medical profession.
- Explain the role of the world healthcare organizations.
- Discuss the various types of ambulatory care.
- Distinguish among the different types of doctors as presented in the chapter.
- Discuss the accomplishments of one of the medical leaders of the millennium.

National Curriculum Competencies

TRANSDISCIPLINARY COMPETENCIES

3e. Identify community resources

Vocabulary

accreditation The process through which an organization is recognized for adherence to a group of standards that meet or exceed expectations of the accrediting agency.

advent A coming into being or use.

allopathy A word coined by Samuel Christian Hahnemann to contrast homeopathic medicine with mainstream medicine; medicine supposedly characterized by an effort to counteract the symptoms of a disease by administration of treatments that produce an opposite effect from the symptoms.

ambulatory Able to walk about and not be bedridden.

amenities Something that contributes to comfort, enjoyment, or convenience.

cardiac arrhythmias Irregular heartbeat resulting from a malfunction of the electrical system of the heart.

case management The process of assessing and planning patient care, including referral and follow-up to ensure continuity of care and quality management.

chiropractic A medical discipline in which chiropractic physicians focus on the nervous system and painlessly, manually adjust the vertebral column to affect the nervous system, resulting in healthier patients.

cited Quoted by way of example, authority, or proof or mentioned formally in commendation or praise.

contamination A process by which something is made impure, unclean, or unfit for use by the introduction of unwholesome or undesirable elements.

credentialing The act of extending professional or medical privileges to an individual; the process of verifying and evaluating that person's credentials.

dissection Separation into pieces and exposure of parts for scientific examination.

encounter Any contact between a healthcare provider and a patient that results in treatment or evaluation of the patient's condition; not limited to in-person contact.

fermentation An enzymatically controlled transformation of an organic compound.

holistic Related to or concerned with all of the systems of the body, rather than breaking it down into parts.

indicators An important point or group of statistical values that, when evaluated, indicate the quality of care provided in a healthcare institution.

indicted Charged with a crime by the finding or presentment of a jury with due process of law.

indigent Totally lacking in something of need.

innate Existing in, belonging to, or determined by factors present in an individual since birth.

mysticism The experience of seeming to have direct communication with God or ultimate reality.

naturopathy An alternative to conventional medicine in which holistic methods are used, as well as herbs and natural supplements, with the belief that the body will heal itself. Naturopathic physicians can currently be licensed in 12 states.

osteopathy A medical discipline based primarily on the manual diagnosis and holistic treatment of impaired function resulting from loss of movement of all kinds of tissues.

pandemic Affecting the majority of the people in a country or a number of countries.

peer review organizations A group of medical reviewers contracted by the Centers for Medicare and Medicaid Services (CMS) (formerly HCFA) to ensure quality control and medical necessity of services provided by a facility.

philanthropist An individual who makes an active effort to promote human welfare.

putrefaction Decomposition of animal matter that results in a foul smell.

robotics Technology dealing with the design, construction, and operation of robots in automation.

staff privileges Allowance of a healthcare professional to practice within a specific facility.

standards Item or indicator used as a measure of quality or compliance with a statutory or accrediting body's policies and regulations.

subluxations Slight misalignments of the vertebrae or a partial dislocation.

telemedicine The use of telecommunications in the practice of medicine, in which great distances can exist between healthcare professionals, colleagues, patients, and students.

teleradiology The use of telecommunications devices to enhance and improve the results of radiological procedures.

treatises Systematic expositions or arguments in writing including a methodical discussion of the facts and principles involved and the conclusions reached.

triage The sorting of and allocation of treatment to patients according to a system of priorities designed to maximize the number of survivors and treat the sickest patients first.

In the first decade of the new millennium, the growth of the healthcare industry seems unstoppable. Thanks to modern technological advances, medicine speeds forward faster than ever in its quest to improve the health of humankind. **Telemedicine** is experiencing a significant growth spurt, and the images produced with **teleradiology** have vastly improved in their resolution. **Robotics** is assisting healthcare professionals in surgery and even delivers drugs to hospital floors using laser sensors. Education in medicine has grown exponentially: computers, the Internet, and video have enabled an instructor in New York to communicate with a student in Los Angeles. The key to this technology lies within the development and widespread use of elaborate information systems that have revolutionized the way that medicine is practiced today. The rate at which technology is advancing is clearly far ahead of the pace of 20 years ago, and we can barely imagine the benefits to healthcare of the future. This chapter looks back at the history of medicine, gazes at its present, and glances toward its future.

The History of Medicine

Medical Language and Mythology

Today's medicine uses words whose origins stem from the romance and fantasy of classical and ancient languages. In particular, the study of anatomy reaches back to the dawn of recorded history, and today's modern terms are almost unchanged from their original version. Some terms are inaccurate when translated literally, because the ancients did not fully understand body functions. For example, *artery*, which comes from the Greek word *arteria*, literally means "a windpipe." The Greeks believed that the arteries carried air, not blood. Greek and Roman mythology has contributed a major portion of our medical terminology, but we have also borrowed liberally from Arabic, Anglo-Saxon, and German sources. Several terms originate from the Bible.

The human head rests on the first cervical vertebra, which is called the *atlas*. Atlas was the famous Greek titan who was condemned by Zeus to bear the heavens on his shoulders. Achilles was held by the heel by his mother and dipped into the river Styx so that he would become invulnerable. However, his heel was not immersed, and he later died from a wound in that area. Thus a common expression used today to show a point of weakness is "Achilles heel." Aphrodite, the Greek goddess of love and beauty, is the source of the name for drugs used to enhance sexual arousal, called *aphrodisiacs*. The equivalent Roman goddess of love, Venus, is associated with lustful desires. A portion of the female anatomy, the mons veneris (mons pubis), as well as venereal diseases, was named after her. Venus carried quite a legacy into future centuries!

Aesculapius, the son of Apollo, was revered as the god of medicine. The early Greeks worshiped the healing powers of Aesculapius and built temples in his honor, where patients were treated by trained priests. His daughters were Hygeia, goddess of health, and Panacea, goddess of all healing and restorer of health. Our modern word "*hygiene*" has its origin in Hygeia, and the modern meaning for *panacea* is "a remedy for all ills and difficulties." A common medical icon is the staff of Aesculapius. It depicts a serpent encircling a staff and signifies the art of healing. The staff of Aesculapius has been adopted by the American Medical Association as the symbol of medicine. The mythological staff belonging to Apollo, the caduceus, which is a staff encircled by two serpents, is the medical insignia of the U.S. Army Medical Corps and is often misused as a symbol of the medical profession (Figure 2-1).

Medicine in Ancient Times

Although religious and mythological beliefs were the basis of care for the sick in ancient times, there is evidence of the use of drugs, surgery, and other treatments based on theories about the body from as early as 5000 BC. In the well-developed societies of the Egyptians, Babylonians, and Assyrians, certain men acted as physicians and used the little knowledge they had to try to treat illness and injury.

Moses presented rules of health to the Hebrews about 1205 BC. He was thus the first advocate of preventive medicine and is considered the first "public health officer." Moses knew that some animal diseases could be passed to humans and that **contamination** existed, so a religious law was developed forbidding humans to eat or drink from dirty dishes. The people of that era believed that doing so would defile their bodies, and they would lose their souls.

Hippocrates, known as the Father of Medicine, is the most famous of the ancient Greek physicians (Figure 2-2). He was born in 450 BC on the island of Cos in Greece. He is best remembered for the Hippocratic Oath, which his pupils repeated. This oath has been administered to physicians for more than 2000 years. Hippocrates is

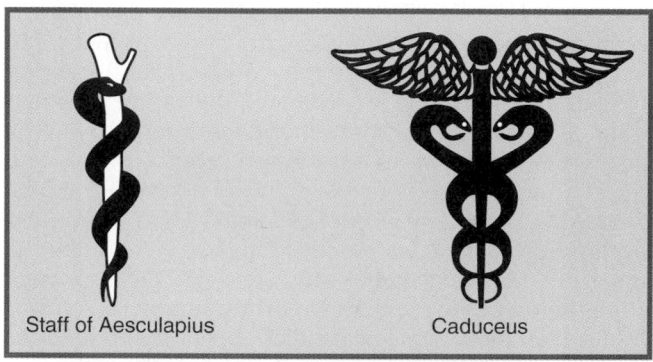

FIGURE 2-1   Staff of Aesculapius and the caduceus.

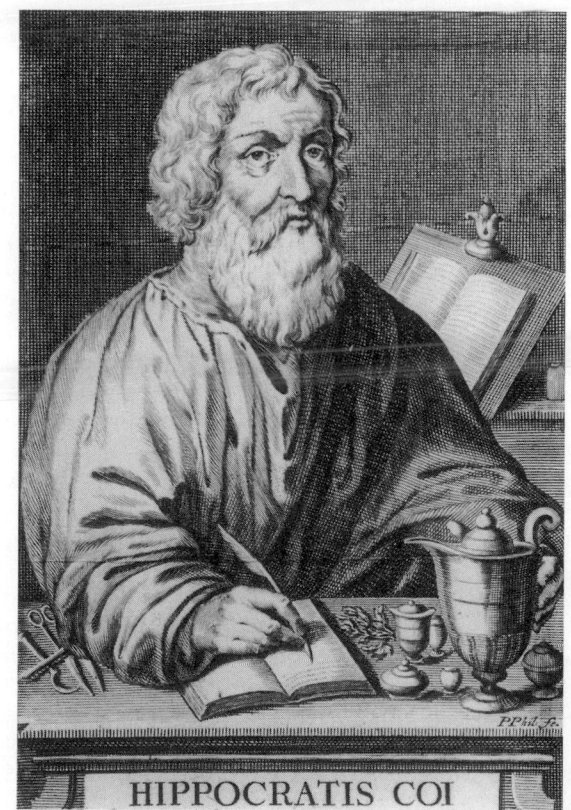

FIGURE 2-2   Hippocrates is known as the Father of Medicine. (Courtesy the National Library of Medicine.)

credited with taking medicine from **mysticism** and giving it a scientific basis. During this period of history, most believed that illness was caused by demon possession, and to cure the illness, the demon must be removed from the body. Hippocrates' clinical descriptions of diseases and his volumes on epidemics, fevers, epilepsy, fractures, and instruments were studied for centuries. He believed that the body had the capacity to heal itself and that the physician's role was to help nature. Very little was known about anatomy, physiology, and pathology, and there was no knowledge of chemistry. Despite these limitations, many of the classifications of diseases and descriptions of symptoms that Hippocrates developed are still being used today.

Galen was a Greek physician who migrated to Rome in 162 AD and became known as the Prince of Physicians. He is said to have written more than 500 **treatises** on medicine. He wrote an excellent summary on anatomy as it was known at the time, but his work was faulty and inaccurate, because it was largely based on the **dissection** of apes and swine. He is considered the Father of Experimental Physiology and the first experimental neurologist. He was the first to describe the cranial nerves and the sympathetic nervous system, and he performed the first experimental section of the spinal cord, producing hemiplegia. Galen also produced aphonia by cutting the recurrent laryngeal nerve, and he gave the first valid explanation of the mechanism of respiration. Galen was also a champion of medical ethics: he felt that physicians "must learn to despise money," and that if a physician was interested in profit, he was not serious in his devotion to the art of medicine. His thoughts parallel those of many modern leaders in the healthcare industry. Although much of what he believed about the body was incorrect, his teachings remained intact until human dissections began, when physicians were able to visualize exactly what was inside the human body.

Because both Hippocrates and Galen were highly respected, the authority of their observations went unquestioned, and this had a negative effect on the progress of science throughout the Dark Ages and well into the sixteenth century. Their theories and descriptions were considered immutable principles, so few physicians were innovative and curious enough to challenge them. Those who did experiment in medicine were scorned by their colleagues, and physicians continued to use methods that were at best ineffectual or innocuous and at worst harmful to the patient. However, the establishment of universities led to a study of theories of disease rather than observation of the sick.

Early Development of Medical Education

Medical knowledge developed slowly, and distribution of such knowledge was poor. Before the printing press was invented in the mid-fifteenth century, there was very little exchange of scientific knowledge and ideas, and scientists were not well informed about the investigations of others. The printing press allowed books to be distributed faster and over a widespread area. Another development important to science occurred in the seventeenth century, when European academies or societies were established, consisting of small groups of men who met to discuss subjects of mutual interest. The academies provided freedom of expression that, with the stimulus of exchanging ideas, contributed significantly to the development of scientific thought.

One of the earliest of the academies was the Royal Society of London, formed in 1662. A significant aspect of this organization was their publications, such as *Philosophical Transactions*. The development of communications during this era was important.

Society became more complex over the centuries, which prompted a greater need for regulation. The passage of the Medical Act of 1858 in Great Britain was considered one of the most important events in British medicine. It established a statutory body, the General Medical Council, which controlled admission to the medical register and had great power over medical education and examinations.

In the United States, medical education was greatly influenced by the Johns Hopkins University Medical School in Baltimore, Maryland. The school admitted only college graduates with a year's training in the natural sciences. Its clinical work was superior because the school partnered with Johns Hopkins Hospital, which had been created expressly for teaching and research by members of the medical faculty. The first four professors at Johns Hopkins were Sir William Osler (Professor of Medicine), William H. Welch (Chief of Pathology), Howard A. Kelley (Chief of Gynecology and Obstetrics), and William D. Halsted (Chief of Surgery). Together these four men transformed the organization and curriculum of clinical teaching and made Johns Hopkins the most famous medical school in the world. The earliest medical school **accreditation** resulted from a report published by Abraham Flexner. He received a grant from the Carnegie Foundation Commission to study the quality of medical colleges in the United States and Canada. His report, called the Flexner Report, resulted in the closure of many low-ranking schools and the upgrading of others. These events legitimized medical education and opened new doors for many individuals to the world of medicine.

CRITICAL THINKING APPLICATION

- Mr. Santos asks his class to identify which of the individuals involved in early medicine have had the most impact on modern healthcare. Which would you choose and why?
- The students point out that early research was often viewed in a negative manner. How does research affect us now and how is it viewed by the public?

Early Medical Pioneers

Andreas Vesalius (1514 to 1564) was a Belgian anatomist known as the Father of Modern Anatomy (Figure 2-3). At the age of 29 he published his great *De Corporis Humani Fabrica*, in which he described the structure of the human body. This work marked a turning point by

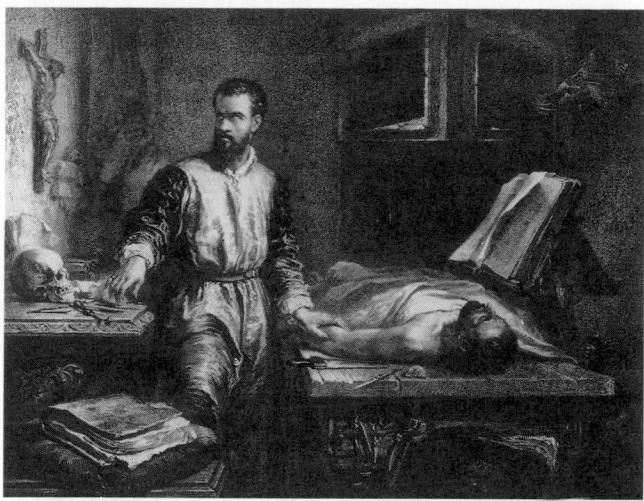

FIGURE 2-3   Andreas Vesalius is known as the Father of Modern Anatomy. (Courtesy National Library of Medicine.)

breaking with past traditional beliefs in Galen's theories. Vesalius introduced many new anatomical terms, but because of his radical approach, he was subjected to some persecution from his colleagues, teachers, and pupils. Despite his great contributions to the science of anatomy, his name is not used to identify any important anatomic structures.

Other important advances and discoveries took place throughout the world. Gabriele Fallopius (1523 to 1562), an Italian student of Vesalius, was also an accurate dissector. He described and named many parts of the human anatomy. He named the oviducts, or fallopian tubes, after himself, and also named the vagina and placenta. In 1628 William Harvey (1578 to1657) announced his discovery that the heart acts as a muscular pump, forcing and propelling the blood throughout the body. He revealed that the blood's motion is a continuous cycle, basing his conclusion on his experimental vivisection, ligation, and perfusion as well as brilliant reasoning. Harvey's writings were recognized in Germany before the English permitted their publication at home. Modern England now considers Harvey to be its medical Shakespeare.

There were few great advances in medicine for a century or more, but the unseen world of microorganisms was first revealed by Anton van Leeuwenhoek (1632 to 1723), a Dutch linen draper and haberdasher. Haberdashers made their living dealing in men's clothing and accessories, but Leeuwenhoek's hobby of grinding lenses eventually led to his discovery of the magnification process. He ground more than 400 lenses during his lifetime, some of which were no larger than a pinhead. In the grinding process, Leeuwenhoek learned how to use a simple biconvex lens to magnify the minute world of organisms and structures, which had never been seen before. Leeuwenhoek was the first to ever observe bacteria and protozoa through a lens, and his accurate interpretations of what he saw led to the sciences of bacteriology and protozoology.

Marcello Malpighi (1628 to 1694) was born near Bologna, Italy and attended the University of Bologna, where he earned a doctorate in both medicine and philosophy. He pioneered the use of the microscope in the study of plants and animals, after which microscopic anatomy became a prerequisite for advances in physiology, embryology, and practical medicine. In 1661 he described the pulmonary and capillary network connecting the smallest arteries with the smallest veins. This was one of the most important discoveries in the history of science, and it validated Harvey's work. Malpighi is commonly regarded as the first histologist.

Scientific Advances in the Eighteenth and Nineteenth Centuries

English scientist John Hunter (1728 to 1793) is known as the Founder of Scientific Surgery. An army surgeon, he became an expert on gunshot wounds and experimented with tissue transfer. His surgical procedures were soundly based on pathological evidence. He was the first to classify teeth in a scientific manner and introduced artificial feeding by means of a flexible tube passed into the stomach. He provided a classic description of the syphilitic chancre, which is sometimes called a *hunterian* chancre. During his studies of venereal diseases, he inoculated himself with what he thought was gonorrhea, but instead he acquired syphilis. His results in this study actually caused confusion in the medical community, because he mistakenly thought that gonorrhea was a symptom of syphilis. This confusion was not corrected until the beginning of the twentieth century. His collection of anatomic and animal specimens formed the basis for the museum of the Royal College of Surgeons. After Hunter's death he was buried in St. Martin. His remains were later moved, however, to Westminster Abbey as a gesture of honor, and a tablet was placed over his grave by the Royal College of Surgeons to "record their admiration of his genius as a gifted interpreter of the Divine Power and Wisdom at work in the laws of Organic Life and their grateful veneration for his services to mankind as the Founder of Scientific Surgery." Today in Australia, the John Hunter Hospital serves more than 570 inpatients and 980 outpatients per day.

Edward Jenner (1749 to 1823) was a student of John Hunter and a country physician from Dorsetshire, England. He is considered one of the immortals of preventive medicine for his development of the smallpox vaccine. While Jenner was serving as an apprentice, he assisted in treating a dairymaid. Smallpox was mentioned and she commented, "I cannot take that disease, for I have had cowpox." Smallpox at that time was a deadly **pandemic**. Jenner observed that those who had contracted cowpox never contracted smallpox. Later, as a practicing physician, Jenner continued investigating the relationship between cowpox and smallpox almost obsessively, and the medical society members grew bored with his obsession and threatened to expel him from their ranks. On May 14, 1796 Dr. Jenner took purulent matter from a pustule on the hand of Sarah Nelmes, a dairymaid, and inserted it through two small superficial incisions into the arm of James Phipps, a healthy 8-year-old boy. This was the first vaccination. On July 1 a virulent dose of smallpox matter was given to the boy in the same arm. Phipps' vaccination kept him safe from the dreaded disease, and Jenner's method of vaccination spread throughout the world. The results of his experiments were published in 1798. He called this method of protection *vaccination*, from the Latin word *vacca*, which means "cow," and at that time, cowpox was called *vaccinia*. Today smallpox has been eradicated throughout the world as a result of a planned program of world vaccination.

Austrian physician Leopold Auenbrugger (1722 to 1809) developed the use of percussion in diagnosis. He became physician-in-chief to the Hospital of the Holy Trinity at Vienna in 1751, and there he tested his discovery. Although scorned and ignored by his contemporaries, his techniques later made him famous and are still used today during physical examinations. René Laennec (1781 to 1826) was a French physician who developed the stethoscope in 1819. At first, he used only a cylinder of rolled paper in his hands, then a wooden device was used for its sound-conducting properties. With today's sophisticated stethoscopes physicians are able to hear sounds in the body, including a fetus inside the mother. Laennec's book, *Treatise on Mediate Auscultation and Diseases of the Chest*, was readily accepted and translated into many languages. It is said to be the most important treatise on diseases of the thoracic organs ever written.

Several men of the early 1800s are remembered for their fight against puerperal fever and their concern for women's health. Puerperal fever, an infectious disease that can be contracted during childbirth, was also called *puerperal sepsis* or *childbed fever*. The term *puerperal*, denoting a woman in childbed, originates from the Latin *puer*, "a child," and *pario*, "to bring forth." The word *puerperium* now designates the period from delivery to the time the uterus returns to normal size (about 42 days after childbirth).

The best known of these men was the Hungarian physician Ignaz Philipp Semmelweis (1818 to 1865); history has called him the Savior of Mothers. His fight against puerperal fever is a sad story of hardships. His theories were resisted by many professionals, including his instructors. Semmelweis noted that the fever often attacked women who were delivered by medical students coming straight from the autopsy or dissecting rooms. Semmelweis directed that in his wards, the students were to wash and disinfect their hands before going to examine the women and deliver the children. This process brought about a marked reduction of cases of puerperal fever on his ward, but he still faced unrelenting opposition. As his theories were proved correct, Semmelweis felt an incredible guilt that the doctors themselves had caused so many deaths. He died at the age of 47—ironically, from the very infection he had fought. He was infected with puerperal fever from a cut on his finger during an autopsy. His grave had hardly been closed when scientists began to understand the causes of this disease, largely as a result of the investigations of two great scientists, Louis Pasteur and Joseph Lister.

Pasteur (1822 to 1895) was a Frenchman who did brilliant work as a chemist, but it was his studies in bacteriology that made him one of the most famous men in medical history (Figure 2-4). He was bestowed the title of Father of Bacteriology and has also been honored as

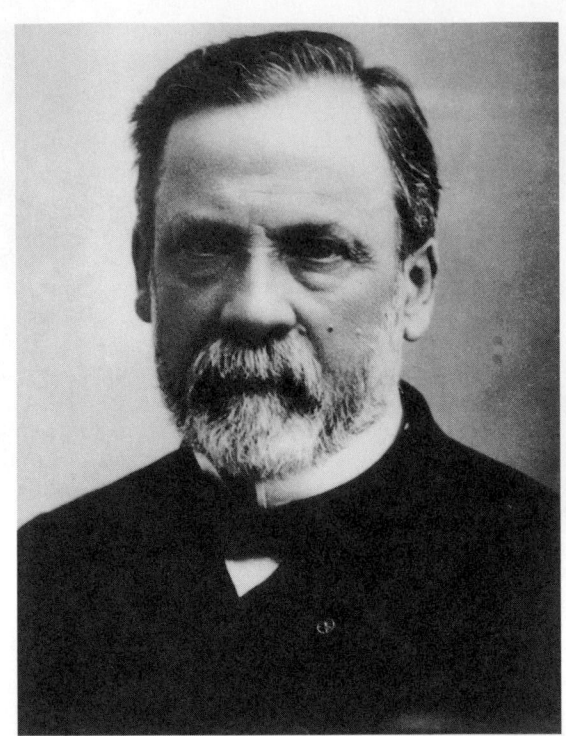

FIGURE 2-4 Louis Pasteur was a brilliant chemist who made numerous contributions to medicine. (Courtesy National Library of Medicine.)

the Father of Preventive Medicine. He gave unselfishly of his time outside his profession to help others solve problems. Pasteur's adventures included studying the difficulties in the **fermentation** of wine. He averted disaster in the most important industry of France at that time, winemaking, by a process he developed, now called *pasteurization*; this achievement alone would have made him an immortal among the French. Through a process of supplying enough heat to destroy microorganisms, wine was prevented from turning to vinegar. The French people called on Pasteur again to help the ailing silkworm industry. He devoted 5 years to the conquest of diseases that infected the silkworm. His efforts were impeded when he was stricken with hemiplegia, but after a long, difficult recovery, he was able to continue with a stiff hand and a limp.

Convinced that the infinite world of bacteria held the key to the secrets of contagious diseases, Pasteur left chemistry again to continue studying his theory. Many renowned scientists denied the germ theory of disease and devoted themselves to degrading Pasteur's theories and experiments. In the midst of this controversy, he became involved in the prevention of anthrax, which threatened the health of cattle and sheep. Pasteur was eventually honored for his work on many other diseases, such as rabies, chicken cholera, and swine erysipelas. He devoted the last 7 years of his life to the Pasteur Institute, which was founded as a clinic for rabies treatment, a research center for infectious disease, and a teaching center. The Pasteur Institute still exists today. He died in 1895, with his family at his bedside. It is said that his last words were, "There is still a great deal to do."

Joseph Lister (1827 to 1912) revolutionized surgery through the application of Pasteur's discoveries. He understood the similarity between infections in postsurgical wounds and the processes of **putrefaction**. Pasteur had proved that these processes were caused by microorganisms. Before this time surgeons had accepted that infections in surgical wounds were inevitable. Lister reasoned that microorganisms must be the cause of infection and should be kept out of wounds. His colleagues were indifferent to his theories, because most believed infections were God-given and natural. Lister disagreed, and he developed antiseptic methods by using carbolic acid for sterilization. By spraying the rooms with a fine mist of the acid, soaking the instruments in carbolic solutions, and washing his hands in a similar solution, he was able to prove his theories. He is honored as the Father of Sterile Surgery. Pasteur and Lister met after years of great mutual admiration. The meeting was filled with emotion, and it was written in *Pathfinders in Medicine* that "a new star should have appeared in the heavens to commemorate the event." Medicine truly owes a deep gratitude to these two pioneers for the knowledge they imparted to the art.

Robert Koch (1843 to 1910) is a familiar name to all bacteriologists, because of his famous Koch's Postulates. These are his theory of rules that must be followed before an organism can be accepted as the causative agent in a given disease. Koch was a German physician who earned great honors in bacteriology and public health. He introduced many of the tools used in the laboratory, such as the culture-plate method for isolation of bacteria. He discovered the cause of cholera and demonstrated its transmission by food and water. This discovery completely transformed health departments and proved the importance of bacteriology in everyday life. Koch's greatest disappointment was his failure to find a cure for tuberculosis, but in his attempt he isolated tuberculin, the substance produced by tubercle bacteria. Its use as a diagnostic aid was of immense value to medicine. In 1885 the University of Berlin created the Chair of Hygiene and Bacteriology in honor of Robert Koch. He became the Nobel Laureate in 1905.

One of Koch's students was a German physician named Paul Ehrlich (1854 to 1915). He pioneered the fields of bacteriology, immunology, and especially chemotherapy, which was a new science. He was only 20 when he wrote his first paper on typhoid, but his greatest gift to humanity was called his "magic bullet," or formula 606, which was designed to fight syphilis. With the organism identified by scientists Bordet and Wasserman, Ehrlich set out to find a chemical that would destroy the organism but not harm the host, specifically, the human body. The six hundred-sixth drug that Ehrlich tried finally brought about healing. He called it *salvarsan* because he believed that it offered mankind salvation from the disease. This endeavor also marked the beginning of the practice of injecting chemicals into the body to destroy a specific organism. In 1908 Ehrlich shared the Nobel Prize with Eli Metchnikoff, who is remembered for his theory of phagocytosis and immunology.

Crawford Williamson Long (1815 to 1878) was the first to employ ether as an anesthetic agent. Early in 1842 a group of students would have a social gathering after chemistry lectures and inhale ether, a chemical commonly found in chemistry labs, as a form of amusement. Ether, a similar intoxicant to nitrous oxide, functions as a soporific, or sleep-inducing agent. However, at one of these "ether frolics," as they were called, Dr. Long also observed that people under the influence of ether did not seem to feel pain. After considerable thought, he decided to use ether for a surgical operation. In March 1842 he removed a tumor from the neck of James M. Venable after placing him under the influence of ether. Dr. Horace Wells was a dentist who reported using nitrous oxide as an anesthetic in 1844. Another dentist, Dr. William T.G. Morton, reported using ether in 1846 when he extracted a tooth from a patient, and he also used the gas at Massachusetts General Hospital for a surgical procedure.

Surgeons are grateful to Wilhelm Konrad Roentgen (1845 to 1922), a professor of physics at the University of Wurzburg, Germany. Roentgen discovered the x-ray in 1895 while experimenting with electrical currents passed through sealed glass tubes. He was awarded the Nobel Prize in Physics in 1901. Although he called it an *x-ray*, history has honored him by calling it the *roentgen ray*. Marie and Pierre Curie discovered radium in 1898, and they were awarded the 1902 Nobel Prize in Physics for their work on radioactivity. Unfortunately, Pierre was killed 3 years later while crossing a street in a rainstorm. Marie was awarded his teaching position at the Sorbonne, a medical university in France, where no woman had taught in its 650-year history. In 1911 she was awarded the Nobel Prize for her discoveries of radium and polonium, the first person to receive the award twice. She died in 1934 from pernicious anemia, which was believed to have been caused by her overexposure to radiation and years of overwork.

Nineteenth Century Women in Medicine

Many other women made great contributions to medicine in the early nineteenth century. Florence Nightingale (1820 to 1910) is known as the founder of nursing and fondly called the Lady With the Lamp (Figure 2-5). She was of noble birth, and somewhat late in life she sought nurse's training in both England and Europe. By the dawn of the Crimean War in 1854, she had established a fine reputation for her work in hospital organization. She was invited by the British Secretary of War to visit the Crimea to help correct the terrible conditions that existed in caring for the wounded. She created the Women's Nursing Service in Scutari and Balaklava. The physicians treated her and the other 38 nurses poorly, until a crisis brought thousands of wounded and sick soldiers to the army hospitals. The bravery and competence of the nurses helped the doctors realize their value to the medical profession. In 1860 she founded the Nightingale School and Home for Nurses in London, which marked the beginning of professional nursing education.

Clara Barton (1821 to 1912), an American, began her nursing career early in life. When she was 11 years of age her brother fell from the roof of their barn, and

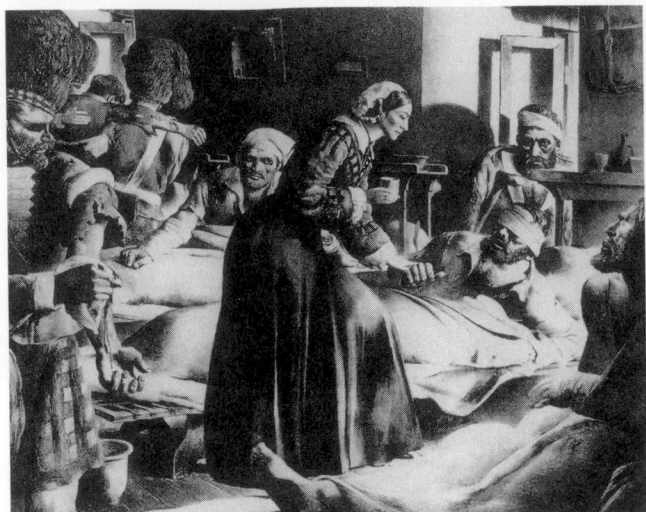

FIGURE 2-5   Considered the founder of nursing, Florence Nightingale is also known as the Lady With the Lamp. (Courtesy National Library of Medicine.)

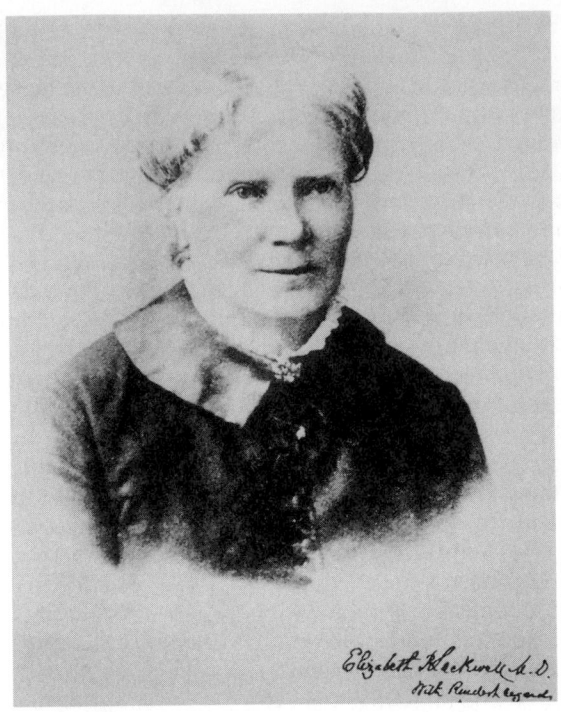

FIGURE 2-6   Elizabeth Blackwell was the first female to receive a degree as a medical doctor in the United States. (Courtesy National Library of Medicine.)

Clara nursed him back to health over a 2-year period. She later was a battlefield nurse and **philanthropist** whose work during the Civil War led her to recognize that very poor records were kept in Washington to aid in the search for missing men who were wounded or killed in combat. Her efforts to remedy this led to the formation of the Bureau of Records. Her organization and recruitment of supplies for the wounded led to her eventual involvement with the Red Cross in the Franco-Prussian War. In 1881 she organized a Red Cross Committee in Washington, forming the American Red Cross. She served as its first president from 1881 to 1904. Her retirement came at the age of 82, just after personally leading dangerous expeditions to help victims of fires, hurricanes, and floods.

Elizabeth Blackwell (1821 to 1910) was the first woman in the United States to receive the Doctor of Medicine degree from a medical school (Figure 2-6). Blackwell's family immigrated to New York from England in 1832. She began her medical education by reading medical books and later obtained private instruction. Medical schools in New York and Pennsylvania initially refused her applications for formal study, but finally in 1847 she was accepted at the Geneva Medical College in New York. Ten years later, as she was practicing medicine, she established the New York Infirmary for Indigent Women and Children, the first hospital staffed entirely by women. In 1869 Blackwell returned to her native England and became a professor of gynecology at the London School of Medicine for Women, of which she was a founder.

Lillian Wald (1867 to 1940), a social worker and nurse, made great contributions to medical care when she founded the Henry Street Settlement in New York City. Wald operated a visiting nurse service from this establishment. When one of her nurses was assigned to the city's public schools in 1902, the New York City Municipal Board of Health established the world's first public school nursing system.

Margaret Sanger (1883 to 1966) was born in Corning, New York and trained as a nurse at the White Plains Hospital. She became the American leader of the birth control movement. While working among the poor in New York City, she came to understand the public's need for information about contraception. She left nursing to devote herself to that objective. In 1873 the federal Comstock law declared it illegal to import or distribute any device, medicine, or information designed to prevent conception or induce abortion, or to mention in print the names of sexually transmitted diseases. Nurses and physicians were legally prohibited from providing this information to their patients. In 1914 Sanger was **indicted** for circulating the magazine *The Woman Rebel*, in which she attacked the legislative restrictions of the Comstock law. The case was dismissed 2 years later. In the same year she established the first American birth control clinic; this led to her arrest, conviction, and time in the county jail. She continued her work, and after World War II, she successfully advocated research into hormonal contraception, because of the newfound concern about population growth. This research ultimately led to development of the birth control pill. When the Planned Parenthood Federation of America was formed in 1941, she was named honorary chairperson.

CRITICAL THINKING APPLICATION

- Mr. Santos asks his students to tell him which of these early pioneers they would most like to have worked with. Which would you choose and why?

Twentieth Century Medicine

In recognition of the achievements of scientists of the past, Sir Isaac Newton said of our ability to discover and innovate, "We stood on the shoulders of giants." Great strides in medicine accompanied the twentieth century, and technology began to advance rapidly. Medical leaders continued their contributions, and knowledge, treatment, and research grew by leaps and bounds. Walter Reed was a U.S. Army pathologist and bacteriologist who proved that yellow fever was transmitted by the bite of a mosquito. Persons with diabetes should be grateful to Sir Frederick Grant Banting, a Canadian physician who isolated insulin for treatment, along with Charles Herbert Best, a Canadian physiologist. In 1928 Sir Alexander Fleming discovered penicillin accidentally while researching influenza and working with staphylococcal bacteria. He found a substance in mold that prevented growth of bacteria even when the substance was diluted 800 times. Children born with cyanosis resulting from a malformed heart benefit from the work of cardiologist Helen Taussig of Baltimore, who developed a lifesaving operation for "blue babies" while working with surgeon Alfred Blalock. This became known as the Blalock-Taussig procedure, first performed at Johns Hopkins University. Jonas Edward Salk and Albert Sabin almost eradicated poliomyelitis, once the killer and crippler of thousands in the United States. Salk's injectable vaccine was developed in 1952, and following wide-scale testing in 1954, it was distributed nationally, greatly reducing the incidence of the disease. Sabin's live-virus vaccine, in a form that could be swallowed, became available less than a decade later. Werner Forssmann, a German surgeon, originated a cardiac technique called *catheterization* that is used in the diagnosis and treatment of heart disease. Christiaan Barnard, a South African surgeon, performed the first human-heart transplant in 1967. Dr. Elisabeth Kübler-Ross, a Swiss-born psychiatrist, was shocked at the treatment of terminally ill patients at her hospital in New York. She wrote the best-selling book *On Death and Dying*, which helped professionals and laypersons alike to understand the stages of grief.

Leaders of the Millennium

Dr. David Ho. Dr. David Ho (Figure 2-7) is considered by many to be one of the most brilliant minds today helping to piece together the puzzle of the human immunodeficiency virus (HIV). Ho is the scientific director and chief executive officer (CEO) of the Aaron Diamond AIDS Research Center in New York City and is also a professor at Rockefeller University. He was born in Taiwan in 1952, and his family immigrated to the United States when he was 12 years of age. He eventually entered college to study physics—medicine was actually his second choice—but once he discovered molecular biology and the concept of gene splicing, he decided to become a researcher. He still does calculations in Chinese. Ho was named *Time* magazine's "Man of the Year" in 1996 for his work in the battle against HIV and acquired immunodeficiency syndrome (AIDS).

Dr. Eve Slater. Dr. Eve Slater serves as the Assistant Secretary for Health at the U.S. Department of Health

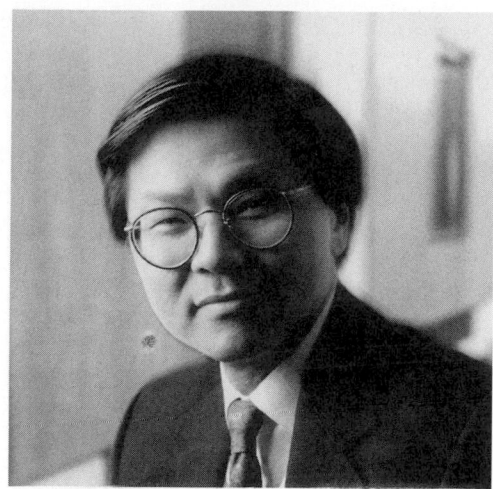

FIGURE 2-7   David Ho. (Courtesy David Ho, MD.)

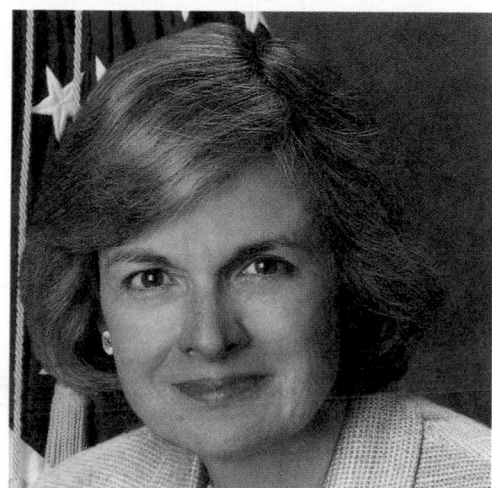

FIGURE 2-8   Eve Slater (Courtesy Eve Slater, MD.)

and Human Services (DHHS). She assumed this position in February 2002. Dr. Slater serves as Secretary Tommy G. Thompson's primary advisor on matters regarding issues concerning the nation's public health and oversees DHHS's U.S. Public Health Service (PHS). Before she joined DHHS, Dr. Slater served as a senior vice president of Merck Research Laboratories' external policy, and also as Vice President of Corporate Public Affairs. Dr. Slater was the first woman to hold this rank. During her time with Merck, she spearheaded the approval of major medicines used to treat the HIV infection, osteoporosis, cardiovascular disease, arthritis, chickenpox, and many others. In 1976, Dr. Slater became the first woman appointed chief resident in medicine at Massachusetts General Hospital. She served as an assistant professor at Harvard Medical School and directed laboratory research funded by the National Institutes of Health (NIH) and the American Heart Association.

Dr. C. Everett Koop. Dr. Koop (Figure 2-9) was graduated from Cornell University as a medical doctor in 1941 and spent most of his career as a pediatric surgeon. During his terms as the U.S. Surgeon General, he became a proponent of tobacco awareness, insisting that tobacco

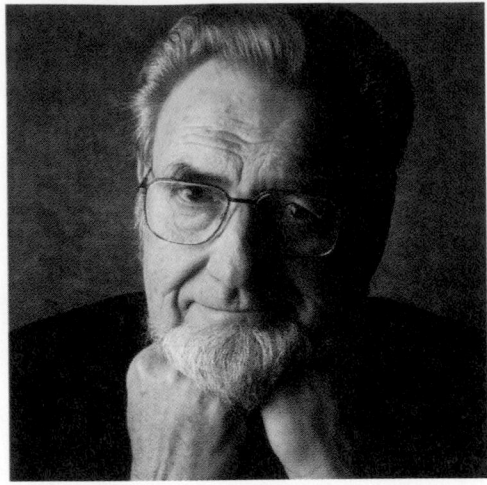

FIGURE 2-9   C. Everett Koop. (Courtesy C. Everett Koop, MD.)

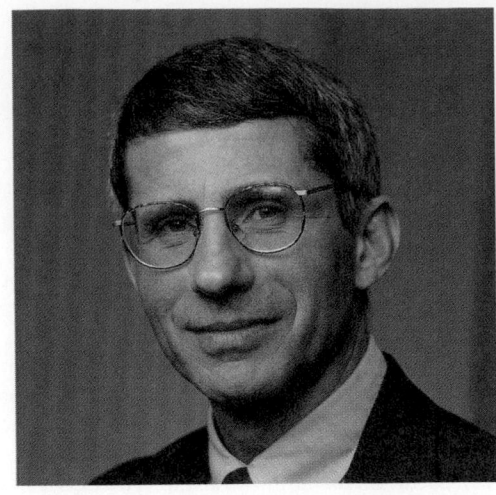

FIGURE 2-11   Anthony Fauci. (Courtesy Anthony Fauci, MD.)

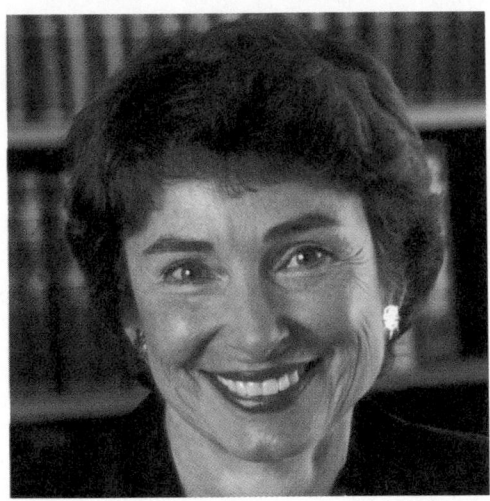

FIGURE 2-10   Marcia Angell. (Courtesy Marcia Angell, MD.)

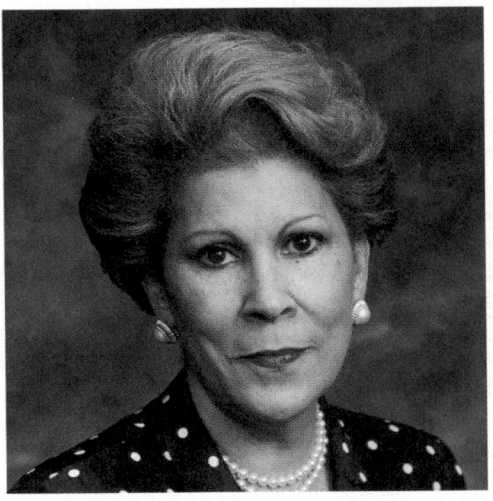

FIGURE 2-12   Antonia Novello. (Courtesy Antonia Novello, MD.)

advertisements must be less attractive to the youth of today. Dr. Koop is a professor at Dartmouth Medical School. He founded the Koop Institute, an organization whose mission is to "promote the health and well-being of all people." Dr. Koop has been honored with many awards, including 41 honorary doctorates.

Dr. Marcia Angell. Dr. Marcia Angell (Figure 2-10) is the former editor-in-chief of the *New England Journal of Medicine* (NEJM), one of the most prestigious medical publications in the United States. Her career with NEJM began in 1979, and her excellent articles spanned a variety of subjects, from the pharmaceutical companies' profit margins to the effects of socioeconomic status on Americans seeking healthcare services. Angell was named one of the 25 most influential Americans in 1997 by *Time* magazine. She has written and contributed to several books, including *Science on Trial: the Clash of Medical Evidence and the Law in the Breast Implant Case*. Angell is a board-certified pathologist and currently serves as senior lecturer in the Department of Social Medicine at Harvard Medical School.

Dr. Anthony S. Fauci. As the director of the National Institute of Allergy and Infectious Diseases at the NIH, Dr. Anthony Fauci leads research efforts on immune–medicated disorders. His scientific leadership has resulted in major advances in several diseases, such as polyarteritis nodosa and Wegener's granulomatosis. Many of his studies now relate to HIV and the body's response to the AIDS virus, and ways to improve HIV treatment and prevention, including HIV vaccine development. Out of more than one million scientists who published during the period between 1981 and 1994, Dr. Fauci was the fifth most cited. He received his MD from Cornell University Medical College, and his career with the NIH has spanned more than 30 years.

Dr. Antonia Novello. Dr. Antonia Novello (Figure 2-12) was the first woman, and the first Hispanic, to be honored with the post of Surgeon General. She served at the NIH and was the honorary chairperson of the National Youth Summit for Mothers Against Drunk Driving (MADD). Novello played a key role in writing the warning labels on cigarette packages. She supported and promoted the National Organ Transplant Act of 1984 and has contributed to the efforts of the United Nations Children's Fund (UNICEF). Novello was a clinical professor at Georgetown University Hospital and in 1994 was inducted into the National Women's Hall of Fame. She currently serves as New York State's health commissioner.

CRITICAL THINKING APPLICATION

- During class discussion, Mr. Santos points out that these Leaders of the Millennium had specific goals for their career and achieved worldwide recognition for their contributions. What other individuals not listed have made contributions to medicine in recent years?
- How can the individual medical assistant make a contribution to medicine?

The National View of Healthcare

World Health Organization

The World Health Organization (WHO), founded in 1948, is a specialized agency of the United Nations. The organization promotes cooperation between nations in their efforts to control and eliminate diseases worldwide. The purposes of WHO are to give worldwide guidance in the field of health; set global standards for health; cooperate with governments in strengthening national health programs; and develop and transfer appropriate health technology, information, and standards. One of the greatest accomplishments of this agency was the eradication of smallpox. Other diseases, such as polio and leprosy, are on the verge of eradication. WHO is committed to research and delivery of needed drugs and medical supplies to various areas of the world. In addition, WHO promotes the sharing of health information, and WHO officials meet with the leaders of the worldwide health industry to discuss various ethical and moral implications that face today's healthcare professionals.

Department of Health and Human Services

DHHS is the principal U.S. agency for providing essential human services and protecting the health of all Americans, especially those who are unable to help themselves. DHHS is made up of more than 300 programs that comprise medical and social science research, immunization services, financial assistance for low-income families, child support enforcement services, improvement of infant and maternal health, child and elder abuse prevention services, and various programs for elderly Americans. DHHS also oversees the Medicare and Medicaid programs. Medicare is the nation's largest health insurer, and DHHS processes more than 900 million claims every year. It is the largest grant-making agency in the federal government, providing approximately 60,000 grants annually. With a budget of more than $429 billion and more than 63,000 employees, DHHS works side by side with local and state governments in its effort to serve the healthcare needs of the public.

U.S. Army Medical Research Institute of Infectious Diseases

The primary focus of the U.S. Army Medical Research Institute of Infectious Diseases (USAMRIID) is protecting military service members, but the Institute conducts key research programs in national defense and infectious diseases that benefit everyone. USAMRIID, located at Ft. Detrick in Maryland, works extensively with the Centers for Disease Control and the World Health Organization (Figure 2-13). USAMRIID also controls an internationally known reference laboratory with state-of-the-art facilities. This laboratory is instrumental in identifying biological threats and the diseases those threats produce. USAMRIID is the only laboratory facility operated by the Department of Defense that is equipped to study Biosafety Level IV viruses and pathogens.

There are four Biosafety Levels commonly accepted among laboratory professionals. Biosafety Level I consists of well-known agents that have a minimal or low biohazard potential to laboratory personnel and to the environment as a whole. At this level, the laboratory is not necessarily separated from the regular areas of the facility. Examples of Level I pathogens include *Pneumococcus* and *Salmonella*. In the Biosafety Level II section of the laboratory, substances with a moderate biohazard potential are studied. At Levels I and II, laboratory personnel have specific training in handling pathogens, and specialized equipment is used to avoid splashes and splatters. Pathogens classified as Biosafety Level II are hepatitis, the Lyme disease virus, and influenza virus.

Personnel working in Biosafety Level III have very specific training in working with the potentially deadly pathogens found at this level. All procedures performed on Level III have a high biohazard risk and are done inside protective safety cabinets. Laboratory personnel are required to wear heavy personal protective equipment. Special regulations concerning exhaust air and ventilation are strictly followed, and there is limited access to the laboratory when work is in progress. HIV, anthrax, and typhus are some of the pathogens classified as Biosafety

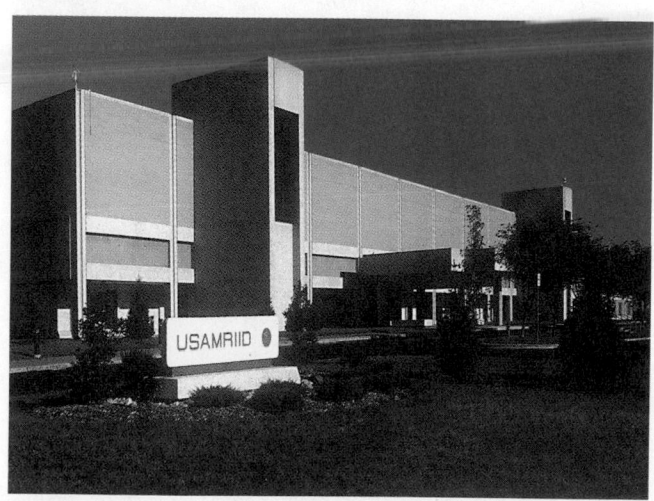

FIGURE 2-13   U.S. Army Medical Research Institute of Infectious Diseases in Fort Detrick, Maryland.

Level III. Biosafety Level IV contains the most deadly pathogens, which often produce incurable diseases. There is an extreme biohazard risk of transmission of these agents, including the risk of airborne transmission. Laboratory personnel are highly trained in the manipulation and handling of these dangerous pathogens. Laboratory access is strictly controlled in this section. Some of the pathogens studied at Biosafety Level IV include *Ebola*, *Lassa*, and the *Hantavirus*.

Centers for Disease Control and Prevention

The headquarters for the Centers for Disease Control and Prevention (CDC) are located in Atlanta, Georgia (Figure 2-14). The CDC is the principal U.S. federal agency concerned with the health and safety of people throughout the world. It is a clearinghouse for information and statistics associated with healthcare. There are 12 divisions within the CDC that focus on specific health-related issues, such as the National Center for HIV, STD, and TB Prevention; the Public Health Practice Program Office; the National Center on Birth Defects and Developmental Disabilities; and the National Center for Health Statistics. Branch offices are located throughout the United States and in several foreign countries. The CDC has approximately 8600 employees who are dedicated to public health. Extensive publications and information services provide healthcare professionals all over the world with the information needed to care for patients.

The agency conducts research into the origin and occurrence of diseases and develops methods for their control and prevention. Additionally, it develops immunization services and aids in the training of healthcare workers. In recent years the CDC has been intricately involved in the battle against HIV, the human immunodeficiency virus, which in its advanced form is called AIDS. The agency has developed guidelines emphasizing that universal blood and body fluid precautions be used in all situations where the risk of contamination by body fluids exists. These recommended precautions are the basis for the laws enforced by the Occupational Safety and Health Administration (OSHA) regarding bloodborne pathogens.

National Institutes of Health

The National Institutes of Health (NIH) began as a one-room laboratory in the marine hospital on New York's Staten Island in 1887. Its first major contribution to medicine was the isolation of the bacterium that causes cholera. Tuberculosis was the number one cause of death at that time. There were few drugs that could alleviate or cure diseases, and there were no vaccines, except for smallpox vaccine. There were no antibiotics, and even aspirin was not yet available. Doctors could diagnose some conditions but fell short on treatments. In 1891 the laboratory moved from Staten Island to Washington, DC. In 1930 this laboratory became the National Institutes of Health, an agency of the U.S. Department of Health and Human Services. The mission of the NIH is to uncover new knowledge that will lead to better health for everyone. As a part of the public health service, it seeks to improve the health of the American people, supports and conducts biomedical research into the causes and prevention of diseases, and uses a modern communications system to furnish biomedical information to the healthcare professions.

The NIH moved from Washington, DC to Bethesda, Maryland in 1938 and today occupies more than 60 buildings covering 30 acres. It consists of 27 different Institutes and Centers, and the National Library of Medicine. Thousands of research projects are under way in NIH laboratories and clinics at any given time. The NIH also provides support to other research projects conducted at universities, medical schools, and hospitals.

Health Industry Councils

Health industry councils are organizations that seek to organize and unify all of the entities providing healthcare in a certain region or community. These organizations keep statistical records about the medical trends in the area and are an important factor in drawing new businesses related to the medical field to the area that they represent. These councils are designed to function as a developmental group that promotes the industry in their area and works together for the good of all those involved in healthcare. The organizations represented within the council may fiercely compete in the area market, but they work together to promote the healthcare industry in the region in which they are located. The councils usually are made up of task forces and committees that study communications concepts, home health, managed care, membership and development, new business promotion, and design and construction. They also are an excellent source of medical information and trends in medicine locally, statewide, and nationally. These councils are valuable assets to any region that wishes to remain on the cutting edge of healthcare.

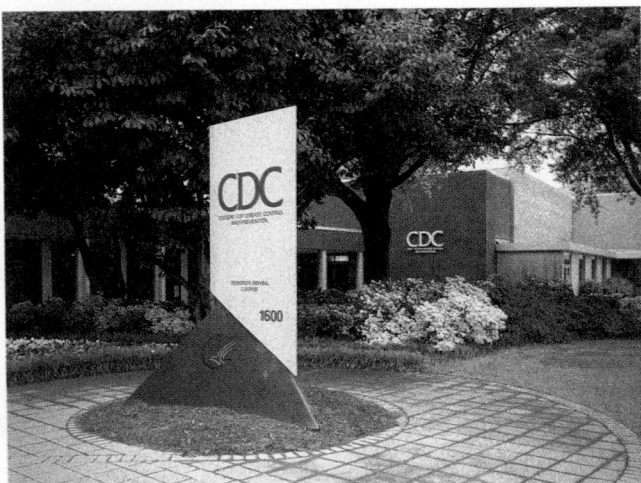

FIGURE 2-14 The headquarters of the Centers for Disease Control and Prevention (CDC) are located in Atlanta, Georgia. (Courtesy Centers for Disease Control and Prevention, Atlanta, GA.)

Types of Healthcare Facilities

Hospitals

There are several different types of hospitals. They are classified according to the type of care and services that they provide to patients. Acute care hospitals offer intensive care units and emergency or trauma departments and are equipped to handle the most severely ill or injured patients. Subacute hospitals offer patient care for those who do not require extensive services but still need hospital supervision and treatment. Specialty hospitals offer specific services, such as a psychiatric hospital. Teaching hospitals provide a learning environment and often have research departments as well. These hospitals are usually affiliated with medical schools, and interns or residents provide care supervised by licensed physician instructors. Community hospitals provide care in rural areas or in specific areas within a metropolis. Regional hospitals are usually acute care facilities and serve a large area that may not offer intensive care in its local communities.

Private hospitals are run by a corporation or other organization and are usually designed to produce a profit for the owners or stockholders. Nonprofit hospitals exist to serve the community in which they are located and are normally run by a board of directors. The term *nonprofit* is sometimes misleading, because there is a difference in "profit" and "making money." A nonprofit hospital or organization may make money in a campaign or fund-raiser, but all of the money is returned to the organization. Nonprofit hospitals and organizations must follow strict guidelines in the area of finance and must account to the government how much money is brought in and for what purposes it is used. Sometimes the term *county hospital* is used to designate the hospital to which **indigent** patients are taken. These are hospitals that will provide emergency care to those who cannot pay for medical expenses. Today, however, many people without insurance go to the emergency department for routine illnesses. This is one reason that emergency departments are busy and full. If patients have no other options, the emergency department physicians become the primary care providers, and this is a major cause of the long waiting times experienced in hospital emergency departments. Managed care has eased this problem somewhat by refusing to cover visits to the ER that are not true emergencies. **Triage** procedures are used to determine which patients have the most severe conditions and should be seen first.

Hospitals have various departments that are organized to provide efficient patient care. The admissions department gathers information and enters it into a computer for use by the rest of the hospital staff. Nursing service supervises all of the nursing care given to the patients and is involved in **case management**. The laboratory provides diagnostic testing on blood, body fluids, and tissues, while the radiology or nuclear medicine department offers diagnostic imaging and x-ray services. Respiratory services offers a broad spectrum of diagnostic tests and various treatments. Most hospitals also have a physical medicine and rehabilitation department, which offers both physical and occupational therapy. The dietary department employs professionals who carefully plan menus to meet the needs of each patient served. Most modern hospitals have a surgery department, and many offer day surgery services, which allow patients to have a procedure performed and go home the same day, if they recover as expected. The medical records department is responsible for the patient records related to every **encounter** that takes place in the facility. Social services works with patients to ensure continuity of care, patient education, and social intervention to assist the patient with emotional, economic, and social concerns.

The hospital administrators manage the hospital on a day-to-day basis, and human resources is usually a part of the administration department. Almost every hospital has a board of directors to assist the administrators in governing the hospital, and there is usually a medical staff committee, led by the hospital's chief of staff, who assist in the management of the facility and the **credentialing** process for the physicians that have **staff privileges** there. Credentialing involves determining whether a practitioner should be allowed to practice medicine in a facility, based on his or her education, license, past performance, and other qualifications.

The National Practitioner Data Bank also gathers information that helps healthcare facilities identify physicians who are incompetent. It provides information about physicians who have had licensure problems, made malpractice payments, had clinical privileges revoked or restricted, or had action taken against them by a professional society. This is an incredibly important process, because if an incompetent physician is allowed to have staff privileges at a hospital, patients could be harmed, and the facility could easily be held liable for the physician's actions and named as a codefendant in medical professional liability cases. Physicians' backgrounds should be carefully scrutinized by the credentialing committee and staff to avoid this threat of liability. Various types of **peer review organizations (PROs)** are also critical to good healthcare facility management.

Accreditation is considered the highest form of recognition for the quality of care that a facility or organization provides. Not only does it indicate to the public that the facility is concerned with offering quality care, it also provides professional liability insurance benefits and plays a role in regulatory agency relicensure and certification efforts. Hospitals and other healthcare facilities are often accredited by the Joint Commission on Accreditation of Healthcare Organizations (JCAHO), an organization that is concerned with the quality of care given in healthcare facilities. **Standards** or **indicators** have been developed that help to determine when patients are receiving quality care. There is much more to the term *quality* than whether the patient liked the food served or had to wait to have a procedure or test performed. Categories of compliance include such areas as the assessment and care of patients; use of medication; plant, technology, and safety management; orientation, education, and training of staff; medical staff qualifications; and patient rights. Ratings from 1 to 5 are given to the facility on their performance in specific areas. A "1" rating means that the facility is in full compliance with that standard, and the other ratings indicate different levels of non-compliance. DHHS also regulates healthcare facilities, as does the Occupational Safety and Health Administration (OSHA).

Ambulatory Care

There are many other types of healthcare facilities that operate in the industry today. **Ambulatory** care centers includes a wide range of facilities that offer healthcare services to patients who are able to walk around and are not bedridden. Physician's offices, group practices, and multispecialty group practices are a common type of ambulatory care facility. Group practices may be of a single specialty, such as pediatrics, or may be multispecialty. A multispecialty practice might consist of an internal medicine specialist, an oncologist, a family practitioner, and an endocrinologist. Usually the physicians within the practice refer to each other, where indicated. This is not only more convenient for the patients, but also more profitable for the physicians.

Occupational health centers are concerned with helping the patient return to work and productive activity. Often physical therapy is used in conjunction with rehabilitation services that assist the patient in regaining as much of their previous ability as possible. There are also freestanding rehabilitation centers that assist patients with a wide range of services. Pain management centers help patients deal with the pain associated with their condition. Sleep centers diagnose and treat people who have sleep problems. Difficulty in sleeping is a symptom, like pain, and the cause of the disturbance must be found so that proper treatment can be provided. Freestanding urgent or emergency care centers provide patients with an alternative to hospital emergency departments. They are less expensive, have a shorter waiting time, and are conveniently located in many areas. Most have flexible hours, often are open well into the evening hours, and walk-in appointments are usually accepted.

Surgery has become easier and more convenient because of the number of ambulatory surgical centers that exist today. Day surgery performed in hospitals has continued to provide patients with better alternatives than overnight hospital care after surgery. Many insurance companies now prefer day surgery, because it is more cost effective. Not many years ago, however, the only alternative to inpatient surgery was that hospital's day surgery department. Today there are an ever-increasing number of freestanding surgical centers. Patients can be treated with laser surgery, radial keratotomy, and cataract removal during the day and recover at home that same evening. Plastic surgeons are becoming very innovative in the physical structure of their offices and the types of surgery they offer on an outpatient basis. Many plastic surgeons offer breast augmentation and reduction and even abdominoplasty (tummy tuck) and liposuction in the office setting. It was not long ago that a tummy tuck surgical procedure meant several days in the hospital. This new trend is becoming more accepted partially as a result of the new "office-based surgery" accreditation offered by the Ambulatory Care Accreditation Program of the JCAHO.

Dialysis centers offer services to patients with severe kidney disorders, and many of the larger cities across the country offer cancer centers for patients who need treatment by oncologists. There are many other types of ambulatory care facilities, including centers that provide magnetic resonance imaging (MRI), student health clinics, dental clinics, endoscopy centers, community health centers, mobile health services, podiatric care centers, and women's health centers.

Geriatric and long-term patients have more options today for ambulatory care than ever before. In the past, nursing homes were the only alternative to keeping an elderly patient in their own home. These nursing homes provided care for residents that needed more than just assistance with day-to-day activities. Now there are many attractive options to traditional nursing homes, or skilled nursing facilities. One of the most popular is assisted living. Most assisted living facilities provide 24-hour supervision of their residents, all meals, and a broad range of services, from the very basic, such as transportation to physician office visits, to the extravagant, such as shopping trips taken by limousine. Most also provide exercise programs, social services, laundry and linen services, and housekeeping. The cost ranges from approximately $1000 to $3000 per month, depending on the location and the **amenities** desired by the resident. There are many new assisted-living facilities specifically designed for Alzheimer's or other memory-care patients.

Independent retirement communities offer residents the opportunity to come and go as they please. Many have a resortlike design, catering to the desire of retirees to enjoy their golden years. Usually the communities consist of apartments or duplex units, and some even offer small cottages. Activities are planned to enhance the social life of the residents, and some offer libraries with computer access, restaurant-style dining, beauty salons, and even gardens to grow food. Keeping safety in mind, the units usually have special emergency call bells and other protective devices.

Other Healthcare Facilities

Several other types of healthcare facilities deserve attention in the broad overview of the healthcare industry. Diagnostic laboratories offer testing services for patients referred by their physician. Since the enactment of the Clinical Laboratory Improvement Act (CLIA) in 1967 and its amendment in 1988, many physician offices stopped providing laboratory tests that were performed inside their offices. These types of labs are called physician office laboratories (POLs). The regulations set forth by both OSHA and CLIA rules made it more cost-effective to have the patient go to an outside laboratory to have tests done. It should be noted that OSHA is an organization and division of the U.S. Department of Labor. CLIA is a law, not an agency. However, both influence workplace safety and quality testing.

Home health agencies were tremendously successful in the late 1980s to the mid-1990s, but cuts in Medicare funding have caused them to suffer severe losses in recent years. This concept of care is very popular, but the influx of too many agencies and the subsequent drop in payments made to them have resulted in fewer home healthcare providers today. In addition, many hospitals began offering home healthcare, which added to the already heavy competition that smaller firms faced. Home healthcare offers its patients home care, therapy services, administration and assistance with medications, and other services so that the patient can remain at home yet still obtain the care that is needed.

Medical suppliers are retail operations that offer all types of medical devices and products. Diabetic patients can purchase glucose monitoring machines. Special hospital beds can be ordered for those who need them. All types of durable medical equipment (DME), such as bedpans, crutches, bathing assistance devices, wheelchairs, and walkers, are available, often without a physician's prescription. Most medical suppliers serve both the public and the profession.

Medical Practices

Three general types of business structure exist in medical practices today: the sole proprietorship, the partnership, and the corporation. Sole proprietorships dominated medical practice until the last quarter of the twentieth century. These practices are on the decline as a result of the **advent** of managed care and its favor of the multispecialty group practice.

The Sole Proprietorship

A sole proprietor is an individual who holds exclusive right and title to all aspects of the medical practice. The sole proprietor may employ other physicians to participate in the practice. The employed physician is entitled to employee benefits, but by contrast, the owner is not considered an employee, and is not so entitled. Additionally, the owner would be potentially liable for all of the acts of his or her professional employees and staff members. Although there are many advantages to practicing alone, including flexibility and independence, there are also heavy disadvantages. The drawbacks include having total responsibility for the practice 24 hours a day, 7 days a week. In an unincorporated solo practice, the business dies when the owner leaves it, unless it is sold to someone else. Many modern physicians do not see the sole proprietorship as an avenue for a decent income as a doctor, because so many of the managed care companies have selectively chosen to offer participation to group practices over the single-practice physician. Some doctors organize associate practices. In this case, physicians share office space, and often equipment and employees, but they operate their practices as sole proprietorships. Agreements such as these should always be in writing to avoid misunderstandings and legal concerns.

The Partnership

When two or more physicians elect to associate in the practice of medicine, they may enter into a partnership agreement. This agreement specifies all of the rights, obligations, and responsibilities of each partner. They have more potential for profit as a partnership than they would in practice as sole proprietors. Each of the physicians has more freedom, because the doctors rotate an "on-call" schedule so that there is some time away from the office and patients. However, one disadvantage of the partnership is the liability of each for the actions and conduct of all the others. In a partnership arrangement, the partners often pool employees, equipment, insurance, facilities, and even profits, and these resources are divided according to the specifications of the partnership agreement or contract.

A group practice is a body of at least three licensed physicians who engage in full-time practice in a formally organized and legally recognized entity. A group practice may take the form of a partnership, or it may be formed as a corporation. The group may share income and expenses, equipment, records, and personnel, and may combine patient care and business management. The group practice may be an association of the same specialty or be a multispecialty organization. Usually, a group practice will take the form of a partnership or a corporation.

The Corporation

A corporation may be defined as an artificial entity having a legal and business status that is independent of its shareholders or employees. Corporations are regulated by statutes of the state in which the incorporation takes place. In most cases, the physician shareholders are employees of the corporation. Even one physician in a solo practice can incorporate the practice. All employees of the corporation receive income and tax advantages. Corporations are usually able to offer better benefit packages, which may include pension and profit-sharing plans, medical expense reimbursement, life insurance, disability income insurance, and many other benefits. Some offer *cafeteria plans*, which the employees can customize to their specific needs, including benefits such as child care reimbursement and tuition reimbursement. Most benefits are tax deductible to both the employer and employee, and some plans offer pretax benefit packages as well. Professional employees of a corporation are liable only for their own acts, although it is always a good idea for any professional in the medical field to carry their own malpractice insurance. Another advantage of the corporate entity is the continuous life of the corporation. It does not dissolve with a change in shareholders.

Healthcare Professionals

See Tables 2-1 to 2-3.

The Title of "Doctor"

Doctors of Medicine. Medical doctors, or MDs, are considered to be **allopathic** physicians and are the most

TABLE 2-1	Types of Medical Specialties Recognized by the American Board of Medical Specialties	
Specialty	**Title of Practitioner**	**Description of Specialty**
Allergy and immunology	Allergist/immunologist	An allergist/immunologist is trained to evaluate disorders and diseases of the immune system. This includes such conditions as adverse reactions to drugs and foods, anaphylaxis, problems related to autoimmune diseases, asthma, and insect stings.
Anesthesiology	Anesthesiologist	An anesthesiologist provides pain relief and management during surgical procedures and for patients with long-standing conditions accompanied by pain, such as cancer patients. Anesthesiologists also provide critical care and resuscitation for patients during cardiac or respiratory emergencies.
Colorectal surgery	Colorectal surgeon	This type of surgeon diagnoses and treats conditions affecting the intestines, rectum, and anal area, as well as organs that can cause intestinal disease. They often treat cancers that appear in these areas, as well as disorders such as hemorrhoids and fissures.
Dermatology	Dermatologist	The dermatologist works with adult and pediatric patients in treating disorders and diseases of the skin, hair, nails, and related tissues. Dermatologists are specially trained to manage conditions such as skin cancers, cosmetic disorders of the skin, scars, allergies, and other disorders, both malignant and benign.
Emergency medicine	Emergency physician	An emergency physician is an expert in triage and treating a patient to prevent the patient's death or serious disability. This physician gives immediate care to stabilize the patient and then refers the patient to the appropriate professional for further care. These physicians are usually found in hospital emergency rooms or freestanding emergency centers.
Family practice	Family practitioner	The family practitioner offers care to the whole family, from newborns to elderly adults, and is familiar with a wide range of disorders and diseases. Preventive care is of primary concern. This is one of the more common specialties that physicians choose.
General surgery	Surgeon	Surgery is the correction of deformities, defects, diseases, or injured parts of the body by means of operative treatment. A surgeon must be familiar with the various specialties to effectively treat patients. General surgery includes all of the aspects of surgery other than those separated into a subgroup specialty.
Internal medicine	Internist	Internists are concerned with comprehensive care, often diagnosing and treating those with chronic, long-term conditions. They also offer treatment for common illnesses and preventive care. Internists must have a broad understanding of the body and its ailments to diagnose and provide treatment to the patient.
Medical genetics	Geneticist	A geneticist is a physician trained to diagnose and treat patients who have conditions related to genetically linked diseases and may provide special genetic counseling when indicated. Often associated with research projects, this physician may participate in screening programs for defects and abnormalities, sometimes prior to birth of an infant.
Neurological surgery	Neurological surgeon	The neurological surgeon offers nonoperative and operative care for patients with conditions of the central, autonomic, and peripheral nervous systems. This includes the supporting structures and vascular supplies of related organs.
Neurology	Neurologist	The neurologist diagnoses and treats disorders of the brain, spinal cord, nerves, and the blood vessels that support those organs. Generally, the neurologist manages infectious, metabolic, degenerative, and systemic involvement of the nervous system.
Nuclear medicine	Nuclear medicine specialist	This specialist uses radioactive substances for the diagnosis and treatment of disease. Radiation and imaging devices are used to detect diseases, often before the organ is seen as abnormal by other methods. The nuclear medicine specialist is aware of the effects of radiation on various structures, as well as the fundamentals of the principles of radiation and physics.
Obstetrics and gynecology	Obstetrician/ gynecologist (OB/Gyn)	Obstetricians provide care to women of child-bearing age and monitor the progress of the developing child. They deliver the baby, and care for the mother for approximately 6 weeks after birth. Gynecologists are concerned with the diagnosis and treatment of the female reproductive system.

TABLE 2-1	Types of Medical Specialties Recognized by the American Board of Medical Specialties—cont'd	
Specialty	**Title of Practitioner**	**Description of Specialty**
Ophthalmology	Ophthalmologist	Ophthalmologists diagnose, treat, and provide comprehensive care to the eye and its supporting structures. These physicians also offer vision services, including corrective lenses. Screening tests are promoted as a measure of preventive care.
Otolaryngology	Otolaryngologist	These physicians treat diseases and conditions that affect the ear, nose, throat, and structures related to the head and neck. Problems that affect the voice and hearing are also referred to this specialist.
Pathology	Pathologist	Pathologists study the causes of diseases that affect the body, and determine what may have caused the death of a patient. These physicians study tissues and cells, body fluids, and actual organs to assist in diagnosing the patient's ailments. Pathologists often perform autopsies.
Pediatrics	Pediatrician	Pediatricians promote preventive medicine and treat diseases that affect children and adolescents. They monitor the child's growth and development, and provide a wide range of health services to keep their patients healthy.
Physical medicine and rehabilitation	Physiatrist	This specialty assists patients who have physical disabilities. This may include those with musculoskeletal disorders, or who are suffering from pain as a result of injury or trauma. Their primary goal is to restore the patient to his or her state of health prior to the injury or trauma as nearly as possible through rehabilitation.
Plastic surgery	Plastic surgeon	The plastic surgeon works with patients who have had some type of injury or condition that has left them with a physical defect. The surgeon performs reconstructive procedures, using grafts, flaps, and tissue transfer and replanting. These surgeons also provide cosmetic enhancements and procedures that are elective in nature.
Preventive medicine	Preventive medicine specialist	Preventive medicine is concerned with preventing the occurrence of both mental and physical illness and disability. Analysis of present health services and planning for future medical needs are part of this specialty. Preventive medicine consists of several components, including biostatistics, environmental studies, occupational studies, and clinical preventive medicine activities.
Psychiatry	Psychiatrist	A psychiatrist is a physician whose specialty is the diagnosis and treatment of persons with mental, emotional, or behavioral disorders. The psychiatrist is qualified to conduct psychotherapy and to prescribe medications when necessary.
Radiology	Radiologist	Radiology is a specialty in which x-rays are used for diagnosis and treatment of disease. A diagnostic radiologist specializes in using x-rays, ultrasound, nuclear medicine, computed tomography, and magnetic resonance imaging for detection of abnormalities throughout the body.
Thoracic surgery	Thoracic surgeon	This surgical specialty is concerned with the operative treatment of the chest and chest wall, lungs, and respiratory passages. Specialists in this field are involved with heart surgery, including both valvular and coronary heart surgery.
Urology	Urologist	Urology is a medical specialty concerned with the treatment of diseases and disorders of the urinary tract. Urologists diagnose and manage problems with the genitourinary system and practice endoscopic and percutaneous procedures related to these structures.

widely recognized type of physician. They diagnose illness and disease and prescribe treatment for their patients. MDs are allowed to write prescriptions and perform surgeries. They offer advice on nutrition and preventative medicine. To become a medical doctor, 4 years of undergraduate training (premed) usually precede 4 years of medical school. Some extraordinary students are allowed entry after 3 years of undergraduate studies, but competition for entry to medical school is intense, so grades and other experience in healthcare is strongly considered. Premed students study biology, physics, organic and inorganic chemistry, mathematics, English, humanities, and social sciences. There are approximately 125 allopathic medical schools in the United States. After medical school the student faces 3 to 8 years of internship and residency programs. An intern is a medical student still in training at medical school, but treating patients under the supervision of licensed doctors. A residency is a graduate medical education program, often in a specialty, and is usually a paid "on-the-job training" hospital position. Often MDs specialize in a certain field, such as cardiology or pediatrics. These doctors usually invest 3 to 6 years of training in the specialty after medical school and can obtain board certification in one or more of 24 different specialty areas recognized by the American Board of Medical Specialties (see Table 2-1). An MD must have a state license to practice, and continuing education is required to maintain the license. Graduates of foreign medical schools can usually obtain a license in the United States after passing an examination and completing a residency program in this country.

Doctors of Osteopathy. Osteopathic physicians, or DOs, complete similar requirements as medical doctors to graduate and practice medicine. Osteopaths use medicine and surgery, as well as osteopathic manipulative therapy (OMT), in treating their patients. Andrew Taylor Still is considered the originator of osteopathic medicine, which he began in 1874. He believed in a more **holistic** approach to medicine, and although he was an MD, he founded the American School of Osteopathy in Kirksville, Missouri. The school was originally chartered to offer an MD degree but later focused more on the osteopathic approach. DOs stress preventive medicine and holistic patient care, as well as a special focus on the musculoskeletal system and OMT. Osteopathic medicine also promotes the **innate** ability of the body to heal itself, and many osteopaths tend to take a more conservative approach to using medications and surgical procedures than allopathic physicians. Premed students moving toward osteopathic medicine also study biology, physics, organic and inorganic chemistry, mathematics, English, humanities, and social sciences. They also usually attend 4 years of undergraduate studies and then begin 4 years of medical studies at a school for osteopathic medicine. Most DOs participate in a 12-month rotating internship in the various specialty areas before entering a residency program lasting from 2 to 6 years, and they are eligible for board certification through either the American Board of Medical Specialists or the American Osteopathic Association. Approximately one in 20 physicians in the United States is an osteopathic physician. DOs participate in continuing education programs to renew their licenses annually.

Doctors of Chiropractic. Chiropractors, or DCs, are typically thought of as "bone doctors," but actually focus on the nervous system to help patients live healthier lives. The nervous system is the master system of the body, controlling and coordinating all the other systems. Information from the environment, both internal and external, moves through the spinal cord to get to the brain, and in the same manner, information from the brain moves through the spinal cord to reach the body in a two-way flow of communication. The intention of the **chiropractic** adjustment is to remove any disruptions or distortions of this energy flow that may be caused by slight misalignments called **subluxations**. Chiropractors are trained to locate these subluxations and remove them, using touch as well as x-ray films, thereby restoring the normal flow of nerve energy so that the entire body functions in an optimal fashion. They believe that the same innate inner intelligence that grows the body from a single cell into a complex human being can also heal the body if it is free of disturbance to the nervous system. The philosophy is that health, not merely absence of symptoms, comes from within the body, not from the outside. Chiropractic

colleges require undergraduate studies in biology, organic and inorganic chemistry, physics, English, and the humanities, and then 3 years are spent studying chiropractic. Each state offers licensing, and some devote their practices to a specific specialty, but more often practice general chiropractic. Continuing education is required for relicensure.

CRITICAL THINKING APPLICATION

- Mr. Santos challenges his new medical assisting students to interview several types of doctors at some point during their studies. The class discusses the different philosophies of medicine among allopathic, osteopathic, and chiropractic physicians. Discuss with your class the similarities and differences of these three aspects of medicine.
- Most of Mr. Santos' students have visited one or more of these types of doctors. What experiences have you had with MDs, DOs, or chiropractors?

Dentists. There are two basic types of dentists in the United States: Doctors of Dental Medicine (DMD) and Doctors of Dental Surgery (DDS). Dentists treat and prevent problems dealing with the teeth, gums, and tissue surrounding them. They can perform oral surgery and write prescriptions for antibiotics and analgesics. Some specialist dentists perform straightening, called *orthodontics*, and some perform root canal therapy, called *endodontics*. Dental school usually lasts 4 years after completion of undergraduate studies, and state licensing is required.

Optometrists. The optometrist (OD) is trained and licensed to examine the eyes to test visual acuity and to treat vision defects by prescribing correctional lenses and other optical aids. A program of exercise may be planned for the patient's eyes. Optometrists study at accredited schools for optometry for 4 years after completing undergraduate studies in the sciences, mathematics, and English. They must be licensed in the state in which they practice. Optometrists should not be confused with ophthalmologists, who are licensed MDs.

Podiatrists. Podiatrists, or Doctors of Podiatric Medicine (DPM), are educated in caring for the feet, including surgical treatment. Normal persons spend an extraordinary amount of time on their feet, resulting in wear and tear and chronic pain. Podiatrists are trained to find pressure points and weight distribution problems. These doctors train for 4 years at accredited colleges after undergraduate studies in the sciences.

Other Doctorates. Other individuals may be called "doctor" based on the degree they have earned in their field. For instance, a person with a PhD has a doctoral degree in philosophy, may be addressed as "doctor," and might work as a professor at a university or in a field related to his or her discipline. A PsyD is a doctor of psychology, and an EdD is a doctor of educational psychology. Doctors who practice **naturopathy** use only natural means to help the body to heal. These medical professionals are licensed in several states.

TABLE 2-2	Healthcare Occupations Accredited by the Commission on Accreditation of Allied Health Education Programs (CAAHEP)	
Occupation	**Credential**	**Brief Job Description**
Anesthesiologist assistant	AA	Functions under the direction of a licensed and qualified anesthesiologist. Assists in developing and implementing the anesthesia care plan.
Athletic trainer	AT	Functions under supervision of attending and/or consulting physician. Provides a variety of services, including injury prevention, recognition, immediate care, treatment, and rehabilitation after physical trauma.
Cardiovascular technologist	CVT	Performs diagnostic examinations at the request or direction of a physician in one or more of three areas: (1) invasive cardiology, (2) noninvasive cardiology, and (3) noninvasive peripheral vascular study.
Cytotechnologist	CT	Works with pathologist. Prepares cellular samples for study under the microscope and assists in the diagnosis of disease by examining the samples.
Diagnostic medical sonographer	DMS	Provides patient services using medical ultrasound under the supervision of a physician. Assists in gathering sonographic data necessary to diagnose a variety of conditions and diseases.
Electrodiagnostic technologist	EEG-T	Works in collaboration with the electroencephalographer. Possesses the knowledge, attributes, and skills to obtain interpretable recordings of patients' nervous system function.
Emergency medical technician–paramedic	EMT-P	Works under the direction of a physician—often through radio communication—and is able to recognize, assess, and manage medical emergencies of acutely ill or injured patients in prehospital care settings.
Health information administrator	RHIA	Manages health information systems consistent with the medical, administrative, ethical, and legal requirements of the healthcare delivery system. Works with medical and hospital administrative staff involving medical records.
Health information technician	RHIT	Maintains components of health information systems in all types of facilities including hospitals and ambulatory healthcare centers. Processes, maintains, compiles, and reports patient data.
Kinesiotherapist	KT	Provides rehabilitation exercise and education under the prescription of a licensed physician in an appropriate setting. Kinesiotherapists are qualified to implement exercise programs designed to reverse or minimize debilitation and enhance the functional capacity of medically stable patients in a wellness, subacute, or extended care setting.
Medical assistant	CMA	Multiskilled practitioner who works primarily in ambulatory settings such as physicians' offices and clinics, performing both administrative and clinical procedures.
Medical illustrator	MI	Working with many different media, medical illustrators create visual material designed to facilitate the recording and dissemination of medical, biological, and related knowledge.
Ophthalmic medical technician/technologist	OMT	Renders supportive services to the ophthalmologist. Administers diagnostic tests, takes ocular measurements, tests ocular functions, and performs other tasks assigned by the ophthalmologist.
Orthotist/prosthetist	OP	Both the orthotist and the prosthetist work directly with the physician in the rehabilitation of the physically challenged. The orthotist designs and fits orthoses to provide care to patients who have disabling conditions of the limbs and spine. The prosthetist designs and fits devices for patients who have partial or total absence of limb.
Perfusionist	PERF	A perfusionist operates extracorporeal circulation equipment during any medical situation in which it is necessary to support or temporarily replace the patient's circulatory or respiratory function (e.g., cardiopulmonary bypass).
Physician assistant	PA	The physician assistant is academically and clinically prepared to practice medicine with the supervision of a licensed doctor of medicine or osteopathy. The functions of the physician assistant include performing diagnostic, therapeutic, preventive, and health maintenance services.
Respiratory therapist	RRT	The respiratory therapist working under the supervision of a physician evaluates all data to determine the appropriateness of the prescribed respiratory care and participates in the development of the respiratory care plan.
Respiratory therapy technician	CRTT	The respiratory therapy technician works under the supervision of the respiratory therapist and a physician in administering general respiratory care.
Specialist in blood bank technology	SBB	Specialists in blood bank technology perform both routine and specialized tests in blood bank immunohematology in technical areas of the modern blood bank and perform transfusion services.

Continued.

TABLE 2-2	Healthcare Occupations Accredited by the Commission on Accreditation of Allied Health Education Programs (CAAHEP)—cont'd	
Occupation	**Credential**	**Brief Job Description**
Surgical Assistant	CSA	Assists surgeons in the performance of surgical procedures. Surgical assistants scrub for operative procedures, and assist in the positioning of patients and in the draping and preparation of the operative site. During procedures the surgical assistant retracts and exposes the operative field and assists in securing the best possible exposure of the anatomical site. With experience, the surgical assistant learns to anticipate the moves and needs of the surgeon as the operative procedure progresses.
Surgical technologist	ST/CST	Works in the surgical suite with surgeons, anesthesiologists, registered nurses, and other surgical personnel.

From *Allied Health and Rehabilitation Professions Education Directory*, ed 24. American Medical Association, Chicago, IL, 1996-1997.

TABLE 2-3	Healthcare Occupations Accredited by Agencies Other Than CAAHEP Under the AMA Umbrella

Occupational therapist
Occupational therapy assistant
Dietetic technician
Dietitian/nutritionist
Dental assistant
Dental hygienist
Dental laboratory technician
Audiologist
Speech-language pathologist
Radiation therapist
Radiographer
Nuclear medicine technologist
Clinical laboratory technician/medical laboratory
   technician—associate degree
Clinical laboratory technician/medical laboratory
   technician—certificate
Clinical laboratory scientist/medical technologist
Histologic technician/technologist
Pathologist's assistant

From *Allied Health and Rehabilitation Professions Education Directory*, ed 24, Chicago, 1996-1997.

Licensed or Certified Professionals

There are numerous categories of licensed or certified professionals who assist the physician in diagnosing and treating the patient. Some of the professionals that the medical assistant will commonly encounter are listed in this section.

Physician Assistants. Physician assistants (PAs) provide direct patient care services under the supervision of licensed physicians. They are trained to diagnose and treat patients as directed by the physician, and in 46 states and the District of Columbia, they are allowed to write prescriptions. These professionals take patient histories, order and interpret tests, perform physical examinations, and even make diagnosis decisions. They can be found in physician offices, hospitals, military bases, and other healthcare facilities.

Nurse Practitioners. Nurse practitioners (NPs) provide basic patient care services, including diagnosis and prescribing for common illnesses. These professionals must have advanced academic training beyond the RN degree and also have vast clinical experience. Usually the focus of nurse practitioners is on preventive care and disease prevention, and an NP is allowed to practice independently or as a part of a team of healthcare professionals.

Nurse Anesthetists. Nurse anesthetists are registered nurses who administer anesthetics to patients during care by surgeons, physicians, dentists, or other qualified health professionals. They practice in many different settings, including offices, traditional hospitals, labor and delivery units, ophthalmology offices, plastic surgery offices, and many others. This practice is quite advanced, and they are compensated well for their skills. Nurse anesthetists can be found in metropolitan and rural communities alike.

Registered Nurses. The registered nurse (RN) has many career options available. Many nurses work in an administrative capacity within hospitals or other types of healthcare facilities as managers. They also provide direct patient care, where they are vital in assessing the patient and providing a care plan. Usually nurses find a specialty area that they enjoy and practice within that area, although they may also "float" to different departments within the hospital. Some function as home health nurses, visiting the patients and providing home care. Some work in nursing homes or in public health, and others serve in physicians' offices.

Licensed Practical/Vocational Nurses. Licensed practical/vocational nurses (LVNs/LPNs) offer bedside care, assisting with the actual day-to-day personal care required by inpatients. They assess patients, chart their progress, and administer medications and intravenous fluids where allowed by law. They often work in hospitals or skilled nursing facilities and are also found in physicians' offices. They sometimes supervise nursing assistants and may also provide patient education services.

Medical Technologists. Medical technologists (MTs) perform diagnostic testing on blood, body fluids, and other types of specimens to assist the physician in obtaining a diagnosis. These professionals work with bacteria and viruses and use their technical skills combined with their knowledge of disease to perform their duties. They can make quality control decisions and can act independently within their profession. Hospitals, teaching universities, research organizations, and laboratories employ most of the medical technologists. Usually they have a bachelor of science (BS) degree in addition to their certification or license.

Medical Laboratory Technicians. Medical laboratory technicians (MLTs) perform most of the same test procedures that the medical technologist performs; the difference between the two is that they do not work independently. They are usually supervised by an MT and have at least an associates degree and a certification or license. MLTs work in the same types of facilities as MTs.

Physical Therapists. Physical therapists (PTs) assist patients in regaining their mobility and improving their strength and range of motion, which may have been impaired by an accident or injury, or as a result of disease. After assessing the patient, the physical therapist devises a treatment plan in conjunction with the patient's physician. The goal of the physical therapist is to improve how the patient functions at work and at home.

Respiratory Therapists. Most respiratory therapists (RTs) work in the hospital environment. All types of patients receive respiratory care, including newborns and geriatric patients. RTs commonly use oxygen therapy to assist with breathing, and they also perform diagnostic tests that measure lung capacity.

Occupational Therapists. Occupational therapists (OTs) work with patients who have developed conditions that disable them developmentally, emotionally, mentally, or physically. They assist in helping the individual to compensate for loss of function. The goal of OTs is to bring their patients to a level of living healthy, productive lives.

Diagnostic Cardiac Sonographers. Diagnostic cardiac sonographers (DCSs) assist in the diagnosis and treatment of cardiac and vascular diseases and disorders. They perform noninvasive tests, including echocardiographs and electrocardiographs. Often ultrasonography is used by the cardiovascular technician to assist the physician in discovering the malfunction of the heart and its structures.

Diagnostic Medical Sonographers. Diagnostic medical sonographers (DMS) assist physicians in the diagnosis of various disorders by means of ultrasound waves, which produce images of the internal structures of the body. These professionals are often called *sonographers*. Ultrasonography is used to assist the physician in many ways, including the monitoring of fetal development.

Radiology Technicians. Radiology technicians (RTs) use various machines to help the physician diagnose and treat certain diseases. These machines may include x-ray equipment, ultrasonographic machines, and magnetic resonance (MR) scanners. RTs explain procedures to patients and know correct positioning techniques, so that the images recorded are accurate and helpful for the diagnosing physician.

Paramedics. Paramedics are specially trained to provide emergency care to patients in life-threatening situations. Paramedics are highly efficient and well versed in the functions of the body. They perform advanced skills and, with more experience, are able to supervise or direct the operations of an emergency care ambulance facility.

Emergency Medical Technicians. Emergency medical technicians (EMTs) progress through several levels of training, each providing more advanced skills. Their medical education encompasses managing respiratory, cardiac, and trauma cases, and often emergency childbirth. There are also specialties within the EMT field in certain states, such as EMT Cardiac, which includes training in **cardiac arrhythmias**, and EMT Shock Trauma, which includes starting intravenous fluids and administration of medication.

Registered Dietitians. Registered dietitians (RDs) have thorough training in nutrition and the different types of diets that patients are placed on to improve or maintain their condition. They use the advice of the physician and information about the patient to design healthy diets during hospital stays and even help to plan menus for home use. They also provide education for the patient about the diet and alternatives that will help in choosing attractive foods.

Closing Comments

The healthcare industry is certainly one of the most exciting career fields to enter in today's world. The constant change and development of new technology and theories make medicine an attractive option for career choices. The needs of medicine extend far beyond the boundaries of the United States, and collaborative efforts between countries promote a faster move forward with new discoveries and hope for those affected by disease. New headlines grace the papers and computer screens daily, and stories of human cloning, designer babies, genetic discoveries, and computer capabilities amaze us all. Medications are being developed that bring us to the brink of eliminating certain diseases. The mapping of the human genome may lead to incredible breakthroughs in the study of colon cancer, breast and ovarian cancer, cystic fibrosis, neurological degeneration, sickle cell anemia, and countless other conditions. There has never been a more thrilling time to become a part of the world of medicine and make a contribution as a healthcare professional.

Patient Education

The medical assistant must be able to help patients find community resources to improve their quality of life and provide needed services. The office should keep a current listing of all of the local resources as well as state and national resources. Service agencies such as the American Heart Association, American Red Cross, American Cancer Society, and others provide assistance and literature, often at no charge. Remember that not all of the patients seen in the office will be Internet savvy. Phone numbers and literature will be helpful, as well as Internet addresses.

Information about these agencies can be found in the phone book, library, newspaper, local Chambers of Commerce, and Internet sites. The medical assistant can provide information to patients with written leaflets and correspondence, as well as in-person discussions and over the phone. It is critical that the office conducts follow-up to be sure that the patient acted on the suggestions of the physician. When a referral to an outside agency is made, documentation of such should be made in the patient's chart.

Legal and Ethical Issues

The medical assistant should have a good understanding of the history of medicine so that there is an appreciation of those who paved the way and pushed to achieve today's level of medical care. These pioneers of medicine and patient care should be respected for their efforts to expand and improve healthcare, because many of them sacrificed their reputations and even their lives to prove the theories in which they believed. Their historical legacy, often taken for granted, represents enormous endeavors by these discoverers of new principles and treatments.

The ethical medical assistant will always strive above and beyond the call of duty to assist patients. Having information on hand to use in referring patients to various agencies is a way to ensure the patient's health and well-being outside the physician's office.

SUMMARY OF SCENARIO

Mr. Santos is an effective instructor, and one who is concerned about providing interesting material for his students. He wishes to instill a strong respect in the students for the people who played a role in early medical advances. His classroom discussions will help the students to think about what it was like to present new ideas to the public and often be ridiculed.

While teaching them about the history of medicine and the state of healthcare today, he also provides opportunities for the students to work together in discussion groups and present information to the class. He also encourages Internet research, a valuable skill that will help the medical assisting student in many areas of their training. In allowing the students to speak in front of the classroom while giving reports on the medical forefathers, Mr. Santos teaches them to be more at ease when speaking in public and when articulating instructions and details to patients and co-workers. All of these skills make a well-rounded medical assistant who will become a great asset to the facility in which he or she is employed.

SUMMARY OF LEARNING OBJECTIVES

- Greek and Roman mythology contributed the major portion of the medical terms we use today. Terms have also been borrowed from Anglo-Saxon, German, Arabic, and other sources, including the Bible.

- The American Medical Association adopted the staff of Aesculapius as the symbol of medicine. It is a staff encircled by a serpent. The caduceus is often mistakenly used to represent medicine, but is actually the medical insignia of the U.S. Army Medical Corps. This is a staff encircled by two serpents, bearing wings at the top.

- The Oath of Hippocrates is still administered to new medical graduates of many medical schools. It was written by Hippocrates, and contained ethical guidelines for the art of medicine. Clearly, medicine was to be considered a highly respected profession and honor was of the utmost importance. The Oath of Hippocrates can be found in more detail in Chapter 6 of this text.

- Johns Hopkins University Medical School has been recognized as a leader in healthcare education for over a century and was one of the first institutions to partner with a hospital for training purposes. It contained a research department as well, where faculty members investigated new methods and treatments for patients. Today Johns Hopkins is a $2.25 billion organization, containing three acute care hospitals and other entities of an integrated healthcare system.

- Numerous early pioneers made tremendous contributions to the medical field. Constant growth and research have pressed the medical profession forward, and with the assistance of technology, the growth speeds along today, faster than ever.

- World healthcare organizations provide information, medication, and personnel to attempt to eradicate disease and treat those diseases for which there is no cure. Many of these organizations operate with restricted funding and rely often on volunteer donations and volunteer workers to operate. WHO and the CDC often work together in an effort to effectively solve problems of epidemics and learn more about diseases. These organizations are a vital part of the medical industry today.

- Physicians' offices, group practices, and multispecialty group practices are a few types of ambulatory care. This division of medicine also includes occupational health centers, dialysis centers, rehabilitation clinics, and sleep centers. Patients who are ambulatory are able to move from place to place, usually on their own or with the assistance of a wheelchair or walker.

- There are three main provider portals of entry into the healthcare system today, which include medical doctors, osteopathic physicians, and chiropractic physicians. These different disciplines have some similar training, but osteopathic physicians usually use a holistic approach, and chiropractors concentrate many of their efforts on the alignment of the spine in an effort to promote a healing of the body.

KEY INTERNET WEBSITES

- American Cancer Society
- American Chiropractic Association
- American Heart Association
- American Medical Association
- American Osteopathic Association
- American Public Health Association

- American Red Cross
- Centers for Disease Control and Prevention
- Department of Health and Human Services
- Hospice Foundation of America
- National Council on Aging
- National Institutes of Health
- U.S. Army Medical Institute of Infectious Diseases
- United Way of America
- World Health Organization
  For active weblinks to each website visit
  http://evolve.elsevier.com/Kinn/

UNIT one

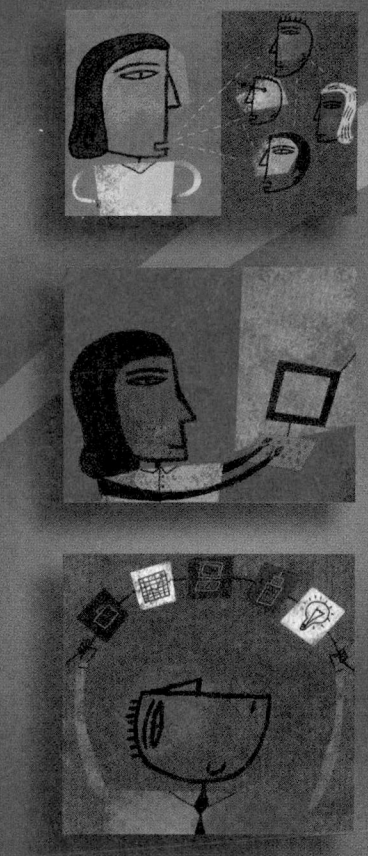

Introduction to Medical Assisting

CHAPTER 3

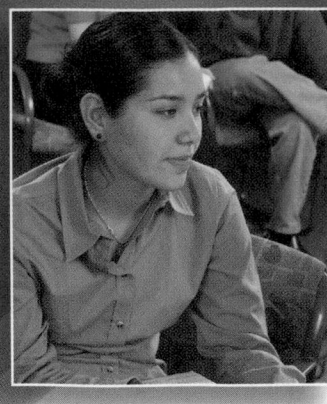

Scenario

Sandra Rameriz is a single mother who has decided on medical assisting as a career. She has always been interested in the medical field and wants a job that will allow her to spend evenings and weekends with her 3-year-old son, Roberto. The idea of working in a physician's office appeals to her, and she has applied to a school that is close to her apartment and day care provider. She plans to attend day classes and work part-time after school until it is time to pick up her son. Sandra is very excited about her new career and has set several goals for her training. First, she hopes to attain perfect attendance, and second, she would like to graduate with honors. She has budgeted her study time and plans to ask her instructors during the first 2 weeks of school for suggestions about how she can better prepare for classes and examinations. Sandra will find medical assisting to be a rewarding career and respected profession.

The Medical Assisting Profession

Learning Objectives

- Define and spell the terms listed in the vocabulary.
- Briefly discuss the history of medical assisting as a profession.
- Differentiate between administrative and clinical medical assisting duties.
- Discuss the versatility of a career in medical assisting.
- Explain the reasons that "bargain help" is often the most expensive.
- Identify several considerations when choosing a position as a medical assistant other than financial compensation.
- Discuss the aspects of the medical assistant's performance on a successful externship.
- List three unacceptable behaviors on the externship site.
- Explain why continuing education is so important to the medical assistant.
- Discuss the difference between a CMA and RMA.

Vocabulary

allied health fields Occupational disciplines in which professionals involved with the delivery of health-care or related services assist physicians with the diagnosis, treatment, and care of patients in many different specialty areas.

benefits Services or payments provided under a health plan, employee plan, or some other agreement, including programs such as health insurance, pensions, retirement planning, and many other options that may be offered to employees of a company or organization.

certification To attest as being true, as represented, or as meeting a standard; to have been tested, usually by a third party, and awarded a certificate based on proven knowledge.

continuing education units (CEUs) Credits for courses, classes, or seminars related to an individual's profession, designed to promote education and to keep the professional up-to-date on current procedures and trends in their field; often required for licensing.

cross-training Training in more than one area, so that a multitude of duties may be performed by one person, or so that substitutions of personnel may be made when necessary or in emergencies.

externship/internship A training program that is part of a course of study of an educational institution and is taken in the actual business setting in that field of study; these terms are often interchanged in reference to medical assisting.

intangibles Incapable of being perceived, especially by touch; incapable of being precisely identified or realized by the mind.

invasive Involving entry into the living body, as by incision or insertion of an instrument.

mandatory Containing or constituting a command.

perks Extra advantages or benefits from working in a specific job that may or may not be commonplace in that particular profession; a shortened form of *perquisites*.

phlebotomy The invasive procedure used to obtain a blood specimen for testing, experimentation, or diagnosis of disease.

profit sharing Offer of a part of the company's profits to employees or other designated individuals or groups.

stock option Offer of stocks for purchase to a certain group of individuals or certain groups, such as employees of a for-profit hospital.

versatile Embracing a variety of subjects, fields or skills; having a wide range of abilities.

According to the U.S. Department of Labor's *Occupational Outlook Handbook*, medical assisting is expected to be one of the ten fastest growing occupations through the year 2008. This exciting field is considered one of the most **versatile** of the healthcare professions. A career as a medical assistant is challenging and offers job satisfaction, opportunities for service, financial reward, and possibilities of advancement. Both men and women can be equally successful as medical assistants. Individuals considering the medical assisting discipline must be dedicated, committed, and have a strong desire to become *caregivers*. Caregivers are people who have the ability to put the needs of the patient first and have a sincere concern for those who are not at their best. A caregiver must feel an obligation to assist the patient in whatever way possible and have patience with those who, at times, are more difficult. This strong inner desire is one of the most important qualities of the successful, professional medical assistant. By developing this "caregiving" mentality, many personal rewards will follow, as will a long and beneficial career.

The History of Medical Assisting

The first medical assistant was probably a neighbor of a physician who was called on to help when an extra pair of hands was needed. As time passed and the practice of medicine became more organized and more complicated, some physicians hired registered nurses to help in their office practices. Gradually, record keeping, data reporting, and an increasing number of business details became important to physicians, and they realized a need for an assistant with both administrative and clinical training. Nurses were likely to have training only in clinical skills, so many physicians began training them or other individuals to assist with all of the office duties. Community and junior colleges began offering training programs that focused on both administrative and clinical skills in the late 1940s. Medical assistant organizations at the local and state level began developing around 1950, and soon after, certifying examinations were available. Today, medical assisting is one of the most respected **allied health fields** in the industry, and training is readily available through community colleges, junior colleges, and private educational institutions throughout the United States.

The Scope of Practice of a Medical Assistant

Versatile is an excellent descriptive term for today's medical assistant. The duties that medical assistants perform vary not only from office to office, but even within the same clinic. They perform routine duties within the offices of many types of health professionals, including physicians, chiropractors, podiatrists, and others. Individuals with medical assisting training can accomplish many jobs in the hospital environment, and some are employed by freestanding emergency centers or surgery centers. There are growing opportunities for medical assistants because of the constant change within the medical profession and the surge of **cross-training**, which means that one individual is trained to do a variety of duties. Medical assistants work under the direct supervision of a physician in the office and perform tasks delegated by the doctor or supervisor.

The American Association of Medical Assistants defines the scope of practice as the performance of delegated clinical and administrative duties within the supervising physician's scope of practice consistent with the medical assistant's education, training, and experience. The duties performed by the medical assistant do not constitute the practice of medicine.

There are two major categories of duties that medical assistants perform—administrative and clinical (Figure 3-1). On the administrative end of the spectrum, medical assistants greet patients who arrive in the office or clinic and obtain basic registration information from them. They may enter information into a computer and construct the patient's chart. They are trained to do office accounting, which may be done electronically or manually. The medical assistant is trained in filing procedures and in proper techniques for adding information to the patient's chart. A basic knowledge of procedure and diagnosis coding is important to today's medical assisting professional, and some medical assistants concentrate strictly on the billing and coding career option. The medical assistant is able to complete insurance claim forms and determine insurance coverage and limitations for the patient. Medical assistants answer telephones, schedule appointments, update medical records, and handle all types of correspondence. Often the medical assistant schedules outpatient procedures and hospital admissions, and may coordinate consultations with other physicians. Medical assistants who enjoy the administrative side of the profession often enter into office management positions.

The clinical duties that medical assistants perform are just as broad as the administrative duties. These professionals assist the physician with patient examinations and prepare the patient and the equipment needed before the examination. They assist with or perform basic testing procedures and are usually proficient in **phlebotomy**. Medical assistants are trained in first aid skills and cardiopulmonary resuscitation. They collect and prepare laboratory specimens and know how to adhere to OSHA and CLIA regulations. Often medical assistants working in the clinical area are responsible for inventorying and ordering supplies. If directed by a physician, they may administer various types of medications in most states. Medical assistants also perform electrocardiograms and prepare patients for x-ray evaluations. They assist in minor surgical procedures, prepare sterile trays, and perform autoclave sterilization procedures for instruments. Another clinical duty involves taking medical histories from patients, patient teaching, and obtaining and recording vital signs.

Medical assistants who enjoy the clinical side of the profession may also become office managers or may supervise other medical assistants. Duties and restrictions related to medical assisting vary from state to state, but in most of the United States, the medical assistant performs as an agent of the physician and is under the physician's supervision.

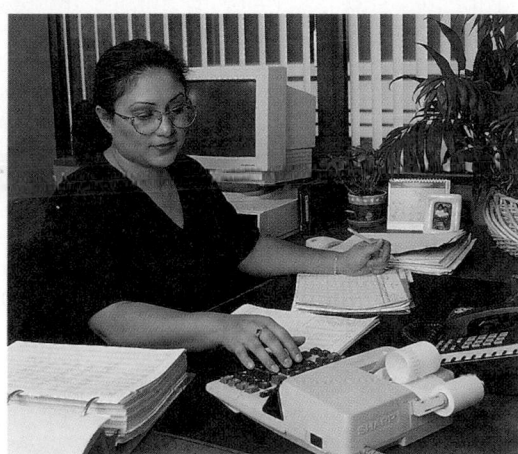
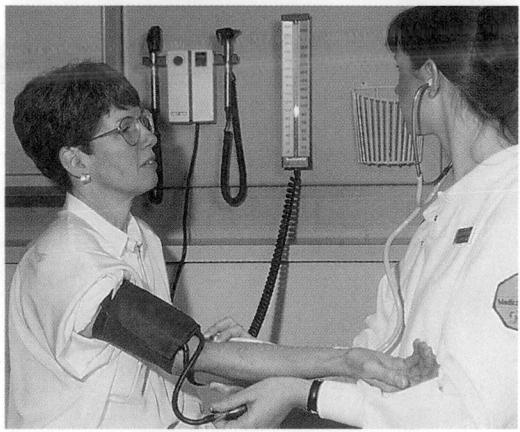

FIGURE 3-1   The responsibilities of a medical assistant include both administrative and clinical duties. (Bottom photo from Chester GA: *Modern medical assisting,* Philadelphia, 1998, WB Saunders.)

CRITICAL THINKING APPLICATION

- Sandra is not sure whether she will enjoy administrative or clinical assisting more. How can she begin to explore both avenues during her classroom training? During her externship/internship?
- How could Sandra explore the medical specialties and determine what areas might be of interest to her as a potential job site?

A Career in Medical Assisting

A trained medical assistant is equipped with a flexible, adaptable career (Figure 3-2). The skills acquired by the medical assistant are valuable, and employment is readily available anywhere in the world that medicine is practiced. Individuals working in the medical assisting field do not have a **mandatory** retirement age. Many medical assistants pursue their careers far beyond the usual retirement age, because physicians realize the value of the experienced, mature employee. This career attracts the nontraditional student who may be older than the average postsecondary student by a decade or more. Although many older students feel intimidated by the classroom, they normally have excellent experiences in school and become top in their class. Medical assisting is more than suitable for the student just exiting high school, who may plan on continuing his or her education and plans to use medical assisting as a viable income during further studies.

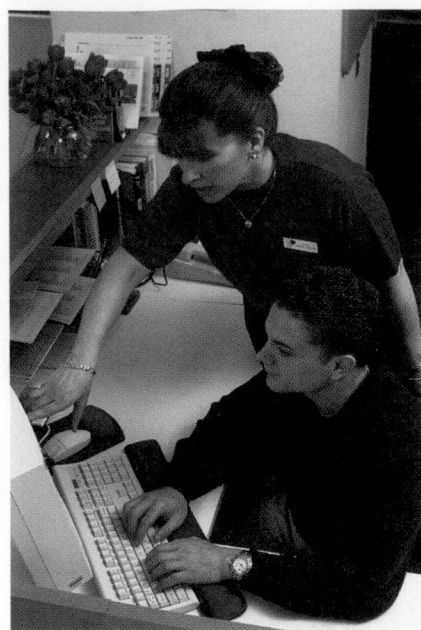

FIGURE 3-2 Medical assisting is a career with many benefits and perks, not to mention the internal rewards of assisting patients in need.

The practice of medicine has changed dramatically in the past several decades. Increasing costs have created a trend away from hospital-based treatment and moved toward the delivery of care in physicians' offices and in outpatient ambulatory clinics. Although physicians have employed medical assistants in their practices for many years, computerization and technologic advances have created more opportunities for formally trained medical assistants and their responsibilities have similarly increased. Clearly defined educational requirements have been determined by the nation's two certification organizations. These requirements have resulted in improvement of the quality and accessibility of medical assistant training, and have produced a healthy respect for medical assistants, who are considered a part of the allied health field.

Employment for medical assistants is abundant. There were 329,000 jobs held by medical assistants in the United States in 2000, and 60% of those were in physicians' offices, and 15% were in hospitals. Career opportunities abound in public health facilities, hospitals, laboratories, medical schools, research centers, voluntary health agencies, and medical firms of all kinds. Jobs may also be available with federal agencies such as the Department of Veterans Affairs, the U.S. Public Health Service, and armed forces clinics or hospitals.

Most medical assistants derive a high degree of satisfaction from their work. Job turnover among medical assistants is surprisingly low; some medical assistants begin working with a physician when the practice is opened and stay until the physician's retirement. Most physicians have learned that "bargain help" is often the most expensive, since untrained assistants often make errors that are costly to the practice. Formal training and certification is valuable not only to the medical assistant, but to the physician-employer.

Medical assistants are compensated in various ways, some hourly and some by salary. The earnings vary from place to place. Overall, medical assistants can expect a healthy return on their investment in training, experience, and skills. Most physicians realize that a good medical assistant is worth a higher-than-average wage, and a medical assistant with formal training often is compensated on a higher scale than one with no training. The *Occupational Outlook Handbook*, a Department of Labor publication, keeps statistics on the average salaries for many different career fields, including medical assisting. This information can be accessed at http://stats.bls.gov/ocohome.htm. More information on salaries may be obtained by monitoring the local help-wanted advertisements and by checking online job offer information on sites such as Yahoo! Careers. It is important to determine a realistic entering salary. Often graduates in many fields expect to make a much higher salary than is reasonable right after graduation.

The medical field often offers very good **benefits** to employees. Usually, the larger the organization, the better the benefits and **perks**. Most employers offer a health insurance plan or managed care plan to their employees. Often a moderate life insurance program is included, and dental insurance is always a valuable benefit. There are companies that have **profit sharing** plans and **stock options**. Some organizations give their employees access to credit unions, and many have discount options to local businesses, such as at a uniform shop. Remember that benefits and perks should be included when considering a certain job. Many medical assistants may choose to work for less money if the benefits and the opportunities for advancement are good. One should also consider driving time, holidays, paid parking, sick days, vacation days, and facilities when choosing a job. Do the co-workers seem to enjoy each other and get along? Is the physician friendly or more "stand-offish" and cold? All of these should be weighed carefully before making the final decision as to which position to accept. It is a truism that "money is a by-product of services rendered." Nowhere is this more accurate than in the medical field. When the patients are served well, the medical assistant becomes more and more valuable to the employer and is compensated accordingly.

CRITICAL THINKING APPLICATION

- Sandra knows that she needs certain benefits as a single mother. What might she need to look for in a potential job after her graduation?
- What are some ways that Sandra can compare positions and opportunities?
- What types of websites might help Sandra in learning about opportunities in her geographic location?

Education and Training

Ideally, a medical assistant should have both administrative and clinical skills, although he or she may have a personal preference for one or the other. The physician's staff must be able to handle all responsibilities of the office except those requiring the services of the physician or another licensed professional. Where there are several assistants, each should be able and willing to substitute in an emergency for any of the others and should be cross-trained on the basics of each other's duties. Teamwork is a very important part of any occupation, and even more so in the medical environment.

Certain knowledge and skills are expected of a trained medical assistant. The skills listed here are not all inclusive but suggest what may be expected on entry to employment as a professional medical assistant.

Classroom Training

Formal training is essential for today's medical assistant. Many community colleges, junior colleges, and private career institutions offer courses in medical assisting (Figure 3-3). After satisfactory completion of the program, the student receives a certificate or diploma. Students who attend community and junior colleges to study medical assisting may complete additional educational requirements to obtain an associate degree. Courses at the community college level usually take 1 to 2 years to complete, and offer enrollment two or three times per year. Private career institutions offer training that usually takes 7 to 10 months to complete, and offer enrollment as often as monthly.

Currently the trend is toward offering the medical assisting program in modules, so that the student receives some clinical training, some administrative training, and some theory in each module taken. Some classes are taught in traditional classrooms, and the clinical aspect is usually taught in a laboratory at the school. Much of the equipment that the medical assistant will use in practice is found in the laboratory, such as an autoclave, medical instruments and trays, and specimen collection equipment.

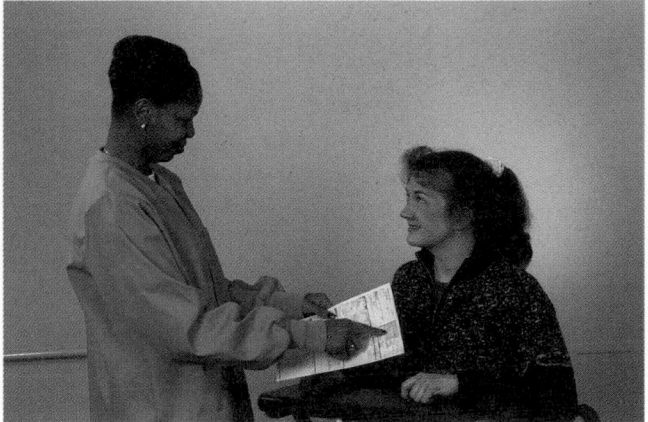

FIGURE 3-3   Get to know instructors and ask their advice on study habits and test preparation. Instructors are valuable references when the medical assistant begins the job search.

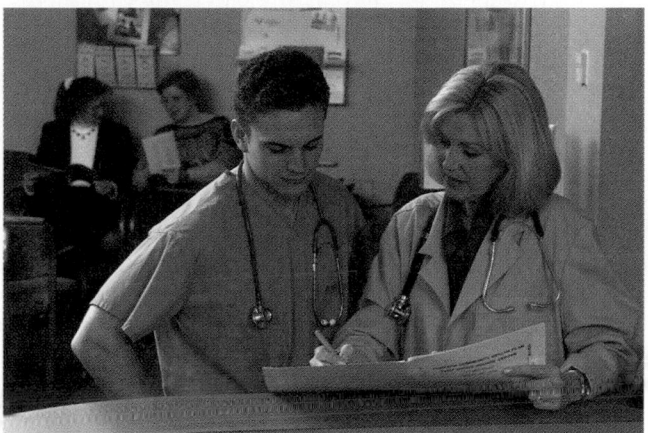

FIGURE 3-4   The externship/internship provides practical experience in the skills learned in the classroom. It is usually listed first on the resume once the medical assistant graduate prepares a resume, so it is vital to perform well and make a good impression.

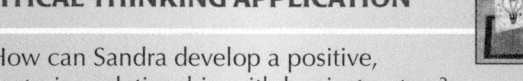

CRITICAL THINKING APPLICATION

- How can Sandra develop a positive, nurturing relationship with her instructors?
- What should she do if she has difficulty in the classroom or if her grades begin to fall?
- How can Sandra study effectively and prepare for examinations?

Externships/Internships

Most medical assisting training programs require an **externship** or **internship** before the student graduates. For the purposes of this text, the terms are interchangeable and have the same meaning. This is a type of on-the-job training that allows students to put the skills they have learned in the classroom setting to use with real patients and staff members. The physician, probably more than any other employer, expects employees to carry out their duties independently, with little or no direct supervision. Someone at the externship site will be designated as the

student's supervisor. The medical assisting student should consult frequently with the externship supervisor to determine what is expected of the student and what progress is being made (Figure 3-4).

The student must be open to constructive criticism and be a willing learner. Techniques may be learned on the externship that were not included in the classroom training, or optional methods may be taught for various procedures. The medical assistant should never argue with the staff at the clinical site that a method taught by the school is the only correct way. Often there are several methods available to obtain the same result. The medical assisting student should treat the externship experience as if it were a probationary period on an actual job. Remember, the externship is often the first medical reference that the student will be able to list on the resume.

There are several general rules to remember while on the externship site. First, the medical assistant will have to gain the trust of the employees there. This is done by willingly performing the duties assigned in a timely manner and performing those duties to the best of the student's ability. If there are any questions at any time, the student should ask the externship supervisor instead of assuming or performing the duties the wrong way.

It is often helpful to read the job description of the medical assistant so that the student will understand what is expected of him or her. The student medical assistant must show responsibility and dependability. There should never be a time that the student is not busy while at the externship site. If all assigned duties are completed, the extern should offer to assist others in their duties or ask for additional responsibilities. There is always a counter that can be cleaned or filing to be done. The student who does these duties without being told shows initiative and a strong work ethic.

There are a few other unwritten rules for externs to know. A medical assisting student must never attempt to form a romantic relationship with patients or co-workers on the externship site. Patient confidentiality must be respected at all times, and anything that the student discovers about a patient must not be revealed or discussed under any circumstances. The student must not use any of the drug samples at the office unless specifically given permission by the physician. The student should never go to the drug storage area alone without permission or unless directed by the supervisor or physician. Externs should be extremely careful if asked to handle petty cash in the office. No student wants to be accused of any impropriety while performing their externship hours. Students must never ask the physician to treat them or any members of their family or friends. If the physician offers this as a benefit, it is acceptable, but one must not assume the physician is available for and willing to give free treatment. An extern must not ask the physician to provide prescriptions; most physicians will not prescribe medications for people who are not their patients for liability reasons.

CRITICAL THINKING APPLICATION

- If Sandra has any difficulty on her externship, whom should she contact?
- What should Sandra do when she has completed her normal duties for the day at the externship, and it is not yet time to leave the clinic?
- How can Sandra glean more knowledge from her co-workers on the externship?

BENEFITS FROM AN EXTERNSHIP

- The school has a line of communication to the community and is better able to assess the needs and expectations of the public for which it is training prospective employees.
- The externship agency benefits from the new ideas and methods that the trainee may introduce. If the facility is looking for additional help, this is an ideal way to evaluate the performance of a trainee without involvement in the hiring process.
- The trainee benefits most of all by exposure to practical experience in a variety of settings. This experience in the real world removes a great deal of the anxiety that might otherwise be present in a first employment situation.

The externing student should bring many **intangibles** to the physician's office not found in any job description. Courtesy toward others and a capacity for teamwork, a positive attitude, enthusiasm, initiative, and dedication are important personal attributes for the professional medical assistant. After becoming comfortably acquainted with what is expected on the externship, the student should concentrate on developing his or her skills and learning as much as possible during this short period. An extern becomes a valuable team player by assisting others and being reliable. By performing at peak level, the student gains the respect and trust of those on the externship site, and these people can become an excellent reference to use in beginning the search for that first paid position. Remember, the professional services of a medical assistant are extremely personal. Therefore the manner in which these services are performed can affect the health and welfare of a patient in either a positive or a negative way. When medical assisting students do their best to be sure that all contact with patients is positive in nature, they win the praise of patients, supervisors, and co-workers alike.

Continuing Education

Education does not end with the completion of formal training. The amount of medical knowledge gained is said to double every 5 years. The practicing medical assistant must keep current with the rapid changes within the profession. Most physicians appreciate the medical assistant who asks questions about unfamiliar conditions and procedures and are willing teachers about the function of the body and treatments that benefit the patient. Much can be learned by reading or reviewing the medical literature that arrives in the daily mail or articles that appear in newspapers, magazines, and medically related newsletters.

Continuing education classes are available to enhance the knowledge of the professional medical assistant. **Continuing education units (CEUs)** may be required to maintain the medical assistant's certification. These credits can be obtained through many sources, including the American Association of Medical Assistants, the American Medical Technologists, and various other agencies and educational institutions. Professional seminars and workshops often offer CEUs. Notices of continuing education classes are sent in bulk to medical facilities and physicians' offices, so the staff should watch for courses that pertain to their particular job duties and take advantage of them as available.

Professional Appearance

A well-groomed medical assistant in appropriate attire has a positive psychological effect on patients. The essentials of a professional appearance are good health, good grooming, and suitable dress.

Good health requires getting adequate sleep, eating balanced meals, and exercising enough to keep fit. Medical assistants can set a good example by following a sensible and healthful lifestyle that includes regular checkups of their own physical condition, both medical and dental. A radiantly healthy office staff promotes the best possible public relations image for the physician.

Good grooming is little more than attention to the details of personal appearance. Personal cleanliness, which includes taking a daily bath or shower, using deodorant, and practicing good oral hygiene, is vital. The use of perfume or aftershave cologne should be avoided or limited, because patients and co-workers may be allergic to some scents. A female medical assistant's makeup should be conservative and moderately applied. Heavy or exaggerated makeup is out of place in the professional office; subtle eye and lip makeup is best for the physician's office. Clear or muted shades of nail polish are best, and long nails are not only inappropriate, but can be dangerous to the patient and the medical assistant. Nails must be kept clean and at a conservative length. Both male and female assistants should be sure that the hair is shiny clean, neatly styled, and off the collar.

The medical assistant usually wears a uniform or lab coat, which not only presents a professional appearance, but also identifies the assistant as a member of the health-care team (Figure 3-5). Fashionable styling makes it possible for the medical assistant's uniform to be both practical and attractive. Women may choose to wear pantsuits, which are available in white or a variety of colors; a two-piece dress uniform in white or a color; an attractively styled traditional white uniform; or a scrub set. Scrubs have become increasingly popular and much more attractive over the past decade. They are now often made of pretty fabrics in rich colors and patterns and are much better suited for the professional office than the old green or blue scrubs worn in the surgical suites of hospitals. Men may also wear the newer scrubs or may choose white

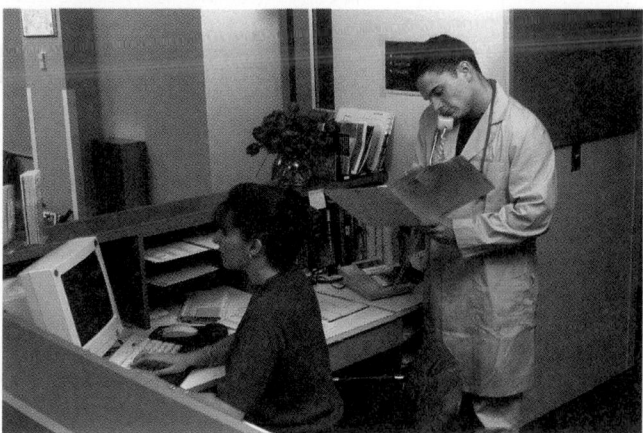

FIGURE 3-5   Medical assistants must have a professional appearance and demeanor in the medical office environment.

slacks with a white or colored shirt, jacket, or pullover top. If it is acceptable in the facility, a lab coat worn over street clothes may be worn, but it is important that the lab coat be buttoned when performing **invasive** procedures. Uniforms should be laundered daily, since medical assistants are exposed to ill patients throughout their workday. Shoes should be appropriate for a uniform and be spotless and comfortable. White shoes must be kept white by daily cleansing. Remember that if laced shoes are worn, the laces also need cleaning.

In some facilities, the physician prefers that the staff not wear uniforms. Some psychiatrists and some pediatricians, for example, believe that the clinical appearance of a uniform may affect patients adversely. However, today's uniforms reflect so many styles and patterns that the right one for the particular office should be readily available. Some of the fabrics depict cartoon characters or drawings that will appeal to children and still function as a durable uniform. A medical assistant who does not wear a uniform should follow the dictates of good taste and propriety in choosing a professional wardrobe.

The garments worn while on duty must be comfortable, allow easy movement, and still look fresh at the end of a busy day. Whatever uniform style the assistant chooses, it should be personally becoming and worn over appropriate undergarments. The lines, colors, and ornamentation of the undergarments should not be seen through the uniform; therefore it is best to wear a neutral color without a pattern. When wearing a uniform, jewelry should be limited to an engagement ring, wedding band, and professional pin. No more than two earrings per ear lobe should be worn, and the clothing or hairstyle should cover tattoos. A name badge worn on the right shoulder will help patients identify each staff person by name.

Be sure that there is a clear understanding of the dress code that is required in the office setting. Then adhere to that code as a demonstration of responsibility and the willingness to cooperate with office rules.

Professional Organizations

By joining a professional organization and taking part in the activities it affords, a medical assistant can grow personally and professionally, keeping abreast of current trends. Participation in a recognized professional organization shows that the employee takes the career seriously and wants to be an asset to the employer. There are national organizations, state chapters of these organizations, and local groups that meet to promote the profession of medical assisting. The organizations offer many benefits to members. Some offer health, disability, and malpractice insurance programs. Some offer VISA or MasterCard options and discount programs that are exclusive to their membership. All extend an opportunity for continuing education and learning beyond the classroom.

CRITICAL THINKING APPLICATION

- When should Sandra get involved with professional organizations for medical assistants?

American Association of Medical Assistants and Certified Medical Assistants

The AAMA was formally organized in 1956 as a federation of several state associations that had been functioning independently. Today the AAMA has 43 state societies and more than 350 local chapters. The organization, whose national headquarters are located in Chicago, Illinois, has been a driving force behind establishing a national certification program for medical assistants. It has also been instrumental in the accreditation of medical assisting training programs in community colleges and private career institutes and in setting the minimum standards for entry-level medical assistants. Meetings are held on a national, state, and local level, where medical assistants can participate in workshops, learn about all types of advancement in the field, hear prominent speakers, and network with other medical assistants from other parts of the country. AAMA publishes a bimonthly journal called *CMA Today*, which includes articles with tests that may be submitted for CEU credit.

Since 1963 the AAMA has administered the CMA examination. Those who pass the examination are awarded the certified medical assistant (CMA) credential (Figure 3-6). Examinations are given in January and June of each year at more than 280 centers throughout the United States. **Certification** is available to graduates of medical assisting programs accredited by the Commission on Accreditation of Allied Health Education Programs (CAAHEP) or by the Accrediting Bureau of Health Education Schools (ABHES). Recertification is required every 5 years and can be accomplished through CEUs or reexamination. More information is available at www.aama-ntl.org.

American Medical Technologists and Registered Medical Assistants

In the early 1970s the American Medical Technologists (AMT), a national certifying body for laboratory professionals, began offering a certifying examination for medical assistants. This led to the formation of the registered medical assistant (RMA) program within the AMT organization in 1976. AMT offers this national certification to medical assistants who meet established standards and pass the examination (Figure 3-7). There are several other certification examinations offered by AMT that may be of interest to medical assistants. The certified office laboratory technician (COLT) examination is available to those who have completed certain educational and work experience requirements. Most medical assistants who work in the clinical area and have at least 6 months' experience qualify to take the examination. Medical assistants may also qualify to take the phlebotomy technician certification examination (RPT) offered by AMT after meeting specific work-related requirements. AMT also provides

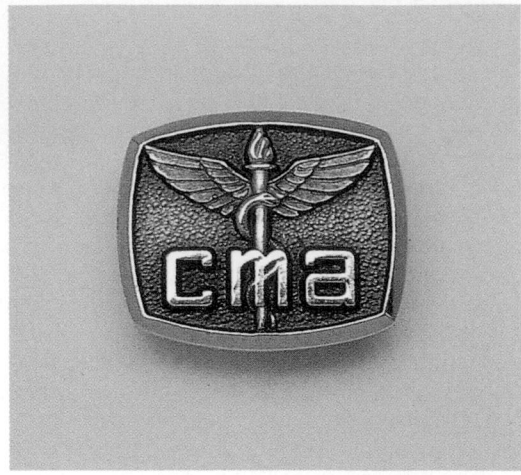

FIGURE 3-6   This pin is worn by the certified medical assistant. (Courtesy American Association of Medical Assistants, Chicago, Illinois.)

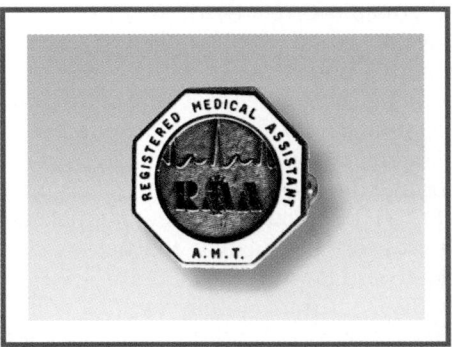

FIGURE 3-7   This pin is worn by the registered medical assistant. (Courtesy RMA/American Medical Technologists, Park Ridge, Illinois.)

societal benefits, including publications such as *AMT Events*, a quarterly magazine with useful information and articles relating to the professions served by the organization. AMT also offers national, state, and local meetings to enhance the knowledge and networking opportunities of its members. CEU credits are available to assist in increasing a medical assistant's level of competence.

The RMA examination can be scheduled nearly every day of the year other than Sundays and holidays at Prometric Testing Centers, with more than 300 locations throughout the United States. To find the nearest testing center, go to the Prometric website, which is www.2test.com. Applicants for the RMA examination must be graduates of a medical assisting course accredited by the Accrediting Bureau of Health Education Schools (ABHES) or by the Commission on Accreditation of Allied Health Education Programs (CAAHEP). The national headquarters for AMT are located in Park Ridge, Illinois, and more information about the RMA examination is available on their website, which is www.amt1.com.

National Healthcareer Association

Some schools also offer certification through the National Healthcareer Association. These include the Certified Medical Administrative Assistant (CMAA), the Certified Clinical Medical Assistant (CCMA), as well as the Certified Billing and Coding Specialist (CBCS) and Certified Medical Transcriptionist (CMT). The costs for these certification examinations range from $105 to $149.

The Difference Between CMAs and RMAs

Both of the certifying examinations are national credentials. The CMA credential is offered by the American Association of Medical Assistants, and the RMA credential is offered by the American Medical Technologists. Since medical assistants are not required to be licensed, both of these examinations are voluntary. A medical assistant may practice in the United States without either certification, but most employers today require at least one certification. Both organizations have committees that develop the examinations, and they are both based on the roles that medical assistants fulfill in the workplace. Graduates from CAAHEP- or ABHES-accredited schools are immediately eligible to take the CMA or RMA examination. Both organizations publish a list of the programs they have approved for accreditation.

The major difference between these two credentials and organizations is the cost. The CMA examination fee for the 2002 testing year is $80 for CAAHEP graduates, but ABHES graduates must be members of the AAMA to obtain the $80 fee. The membership fees vary from state to state and will be substantially less expensive if joined while one is still a student. Student membership costs range from $20 to approximately $32 but must be applied for before graduating. Nonmembers must pay $155 to take the CMA examination. Annual dues thereafter are between $67 and $92, depending on the state association joined. The RMA examination cost is $85, which includes the first year's dues. Annual dues thereafter are currently $48.

CRITICAL THINKING APPLICATION

- Why is it important for Sandra to obtain one of the medical assisting certifications after graduation?
- How might certification help her career as a medical assistant?
- When can the tests be taken in your area?

MEDICAL ASSISTANT'S CREED

I believe in the principles and purposes of the profession of medical assisting.
I endeavor to be more effective.
I aspire to render greater service.
I protect the confidence entrusted to me.
I am dedicated to the care and well-being of all patients.
I am loyal to my physician-employer.
I am true to the ethics of my profession.
I am strengthened by compassion, courage, and faith.

Closing Comments

This chapter has presented the advantages of becoming a trained medical assistant and some of the many career opportunities available. The necessary skills that must be developed and the general knowledge that must be acquired to function effectively have been presented. However, skills and knowledge alone do not ensure success.

Personality traits and professional appearance are also critical. Professional societies and continuing education are vital to the professional medical assistant. The individual who accepts this career must be willing to accept the responsibilities inherent in its standards. Whatever the career goals of the medical assistant, the ideas expressed in this chapter will be useful to all.

Patient Education

The medical assistant may find it necessary to educate the patient about the definition of what a medical assistant is and does. Often, patients assume that those assisting in the offices are nurses, but medical assistants should never represent themselves in this manner. When making introductions with the patient, one should state: "I am Sandra Rameriz, Dr. Patrick's medical assistant." These words accurately portray the duties performed and help the patient to know who is who in the physician's office.

Medical assisting has grown into one of the most respected professions in the allied health field. When asked about the field, one should share the role a medical assistant plays in the office and the training involved. Others may be interested in a career change or have a desire to enter the medical field. A medical assistant should always be a good ambassador for the profession.

Legal and Ethical Issues

In the course of a medical assistant's daily work, a vast amount of personal and intimate knowledge will surface about the patients who entrust their care to the physician and the practice. Such information must be held in strict confidence and never be discussed or relayed to others, including professional associates, unless the lack of knowledge will affect the patient's care in a negative way.

On an externship, a medical assisting student should expect to observe all the office protocols of regular attendance, being on time, and in appropriate attire. The extern should hold the rules and regulations of the office in high regard and not expect special treatment. One should never expect or ask for payment for serving as an extern, because this is usually a part of the school curriculum.

During the externship practice, medical assisting externs should restrict practice to areas in which they have been trained. If the state has a scope of practice for medical assistants, know the boundaries within which they are expected to perform and do not exceed them. Some medical assistants carry their own personal malpractice or medical liability insurance policies, and externing students may be covered under a blanket policy held by their school. Remember, if ever in doubt about what is acceptable during the externship, or even in actual practice as a medical assistant, ask the physician or supervisor.

SUMMARY OF SCENARIO

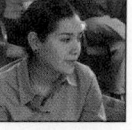

Sandra has chosen to embark on an exciting career and will find her work very rewarding. She knows that she will be proud of her efforts and looks forward to becoming a respected member of the healthcare team in a physician's office. She has set goals for her class work and attendance, and is determined to meet them.

There are many opportunities for the medical assistant in both administrative and clinical positions, and as Sandra progresses through her training, she will find areas that appeal to her more than others. All are vitally important so that she will be a versatile medical assistant, able to perform front and back office duties. More exposure to various duties will be provided during the externship, and these experiences will help her to determine where she might enjoy working once she graduates. It is important that Sandra glean as much experience and knowledge as possible while in school so that she will have more options after her training.

Sandra should develop a good relationship with her instructors and go to them when she has questions or concerns. These professionals are anxious to share their knowledge and experiences with students to best prepare them for the work environment. If there is ever a situation in which her grades drop or she is struggling, Sandra should seek the advice of the instructor to improve her performance. The externship is also critically important, because it is usually the first medical reference a new graduate will have. Any difficulties at the externship site should be brought to the attention of the externship supervisor or an instructor at her school.

There are many benefits to working in the medical field, and Sandra will need to carefully weigh what she needs for herself and her son before taking any position. She should look at all of her options and choose the best one after careful evaluation. This will result in her satisfaction with her job and new career.

SUMMARY OF LEARNING OBJECTIVES

- The first medical assistants were probably neighbors and friends of the physician. The field has grown into one of the most respected and versatile professions in allied health.

- Administrative duties are those that involve running the office, such as scheduling appointments and filing insurance. Administrative medical assistants usually spend most of their day in the front office of the facility. Clinical duties include more patient contact and assisting the physician in the back office. Often new graduates move toward one or the other divisions but should always be ready and willing to adapt to new duties or fill in other areas when necessary.

- Medical assistants are versatile enough to work in many different settings. Most often they are found in physician offices, but also work in hospitals, insurance companies, clinics, laboratories, and many other facilities. The combination of administrative and clinical training makes the medical assistant quite valuable to the employer.

- Medical assistants who have been formally trained certainly deserve a fair wage, comparable to the national average for a person in whatever position they hold. When a supervisor or employer attempts to find "bargain help" at a cheaper rate, often they do not hire the quality employee that is so necessary in the physician's office. Since medical assistants help care for the patient, they should be compensated well so that the retention of the office staff will be continuous and stable. This can only help the physician care for patients in a more effective manner and gives the patients a sense of familiarity and security as well.

- The medical assistant should consider many other factors than the salary when choosing a position. Location, perks, benefits, and the atmosphere of the office are all important. Many assistants are interested in growth within the organization and welcome those opportunities. Working for a friendly, caring physician and/or supervisor is invaluable. Sometimes, taking a lesser position in a well-known and reputable facility is temporarily worth a lower wage, because of future opportunities. Consider all aspects of a position before saying "Yes" to a job offer.

- The medical assisting externship offers the student an opportunity to put the skills learned in the classroom to good use. If completed successfully, this is an excellent reference for the resume. The student should perform at the optimal level and never hesitate to complete duties assigned. Offer to go above and beyond to secure the support of the externship site as the job search begins.

- An externing medical assistant should never attempt to form relationships with patients outside the office or view the chart for personal information. Do not ask the physician to treat family members or take medications without explicit permission from the physician or supervisor. Be very careful when handling cash and drugs in the office. The student should make every effort to never be late or tardy to the externship site, unless there is a severe emergency.

- Continuing education is important to medical assistants so that the latest trends and information are readily available and accessible. Take advantage of local seminars and continuing education classes. Often the employer will agree to pay for classes or seminars that the medical assistant takes if they relate to his or her employment at the facility. Some will provide tuition reimbursement for college expenses, often even if the college courses are not related to the position the employee holds at the facility.

■ The main difference between the CMA and RMA credentials is the agency that provides each certification. The CMA credential is awarded by the American Association of Medical Assistants, and the RMA is awarded by the American Medical Technologists. Both are nationally recognized certifications.

KEY INTERNET WEBSITES

- American Association of Medical Assistants
- American Medical Technologists
  For active weblinks to each website visit
  http://evolve.elsevier.com/Kinn/

CHAPTER 4

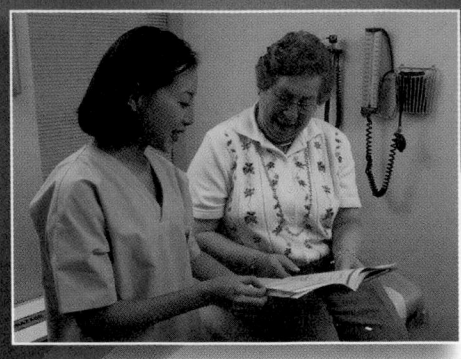

Scenario

Karen Yon has wanted to work in the medical field for most of her adult life. She volunteered in a local hospital during high school, and then after working for 3 years in the restaurant business, she enrolled in medical assistant classes. She studied very hard in school and graduated with honors. After her externship, she was asked to continue as a regular employee at a family practice in her area.

Karen strives to do all of her duties well in the physician's office. She wants to project a professional image to the patients and her co-workers. However, these are aspects of her job that are sometimes difficult to learn in the classroom setting. Since this is her first experience in the medical field, she wants to make a good impression on her employer and be a team player.

Professional Behavior in the Workplace

National Curriculum Competencies

TRANSDISCIPLINARY COMPETENCIES

2a. Identify and respond to issues of confidentiality
2b. Perform within legal and ethical boundaries
2d. Document appropriately

Vocabulary

characteristics Distinguishing traits, qualities, or properties.

commensurate Corresponding in size, amount, extent, or degree; equal in measure.

competence The quality or state of being competent; having adequate or requisite capabilities.

connotation An implication; something suggested by a word or thing.

credibility The quality or power of inspiring belief.

demeanor Behavior toward others; outward manner.

detrimental Obviously harmful or damaging.

discretion The quality of being discrete; having or showing good judgment or conduct, especially in speech.

disseminated To disburse; to spread around.

initiative To cause or facilitate the beginning of; to initiate something into happening.

insubordination Disobedience to authority.

morale The mental and emotional condition, enthusiasm, loyalty, or confidence of an individual or group with regard to the function or tasks at hand.

persona An individual's social facade or front that reflects the role in life the individual is playing; the personality that a person projects in public.

procrastination Intentionally putting off doing something that should be done.

professionalism The conduct or qualities characterized by or conforming to the technical or ethical standards of a profession; exhibiting a courteous, conscientious, and generally businesslike manner in the workplace.

reproach An expression of rebuke or disapproval; a cause or occasion of blame, discredit, or disgrace.

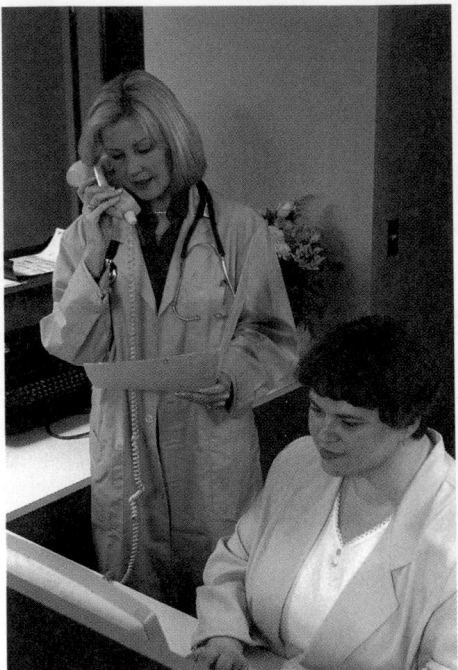

FIGURE 4-1 The professional medical assistant is an asset to the physician's office.

Characteristics of Professionalism

There are many **characteristics** that make up the professional posture required of medical assistants. It is critically important that a student medical assistant begin developing these characteristics while in school, because these qualities will not magically appear when the student begins working with actual patients. Although we might think that we would always behave appropriately during an externship or in a job setting, the habits developed in school will carry over into these experiences. If the behavior is unacceptable, it will be **detrimental** to the medical assistant's professional career. If the medical assistant wishes to advance and receive wage increases, promotions, and the trust of the employer, the following characteristics must be a part of his or her **persona**.

The word *professional* comes to mind when we think of physicians and those employed in their offices. What is professional behavior? We tend to hold medical personnel to a higher standard of **professionalism** than those in most other career fields. The medical assistant who works to improve his or her professional approach in the workplace will become quite valuable to the employer and will be promoted to positions of more responsibility more quickly within the healthcare industry.

The Meaning of Professionalism

Professionalism is defined as exhibiting a courteous, conscientious, and generally businesslike manner in the workplace. It is characterized by or conforms to the technical or ethical standards of a certain profession. Conducting oneself in a professional manner is essential for successful medical assistants. The attitude of those in the medical profession is generally more conservative than in other career fields. Patients expect professional behavior and will base much of their trust and confidence in those that exhibit this type of **demeanor** in the physician's office (Figure 4-1).

CRITICAL THINKING APPLICATION

- How can students practice professional behavior while still in the classroom experience?
- When students are practicing clinical skills, how can they demonstrate proficiency in professional behavior?

Loyalty

Loyalty is a faithfulness or allegiance to a cause, ideal, custom, institution, or product. Loyalty to an employer means that the employee is appreciative of the opportunity provided through the job and supports the company by giving the best effort possible. There are many

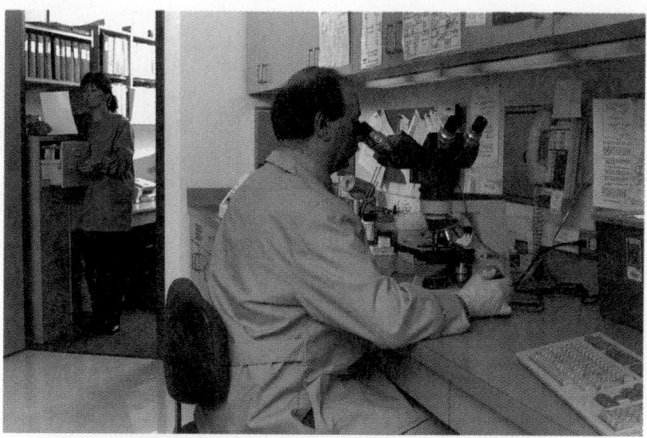

FIGURE 4-2 The physician will count on the dependability of the medical assistant to be at work on time and on each scheduled day. Absent or tardy employees cause scheduling difficulties and can greatly inconvenience the patients and remaining staff.

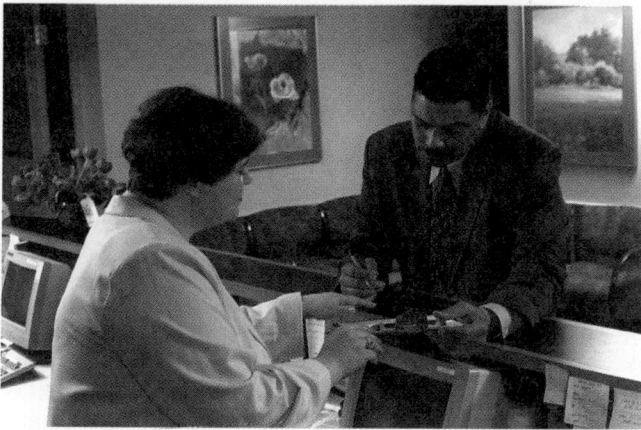

FIGURE 4-3 Taking a few moments to explain forms and bills to a patient is a courteous way to avoid misunderstandings and promote goodwill.

individuals today who are interested only in what the employer can provide them. However, this is an immature approach to take toward a job. When a person is employed by a company, there is an exchange of skills for different types of compensation. Each party benefits the other. Often we forget that experience alone is a great benefit from working. Loyalty to the employer is important, and the employee should feel a sense of loyalty from the company as well.

CRITICAL THINKING APPLICATION

- How can Karen demonstrate loyalty to her employer?
- What are some ways that her employer can reciprocate Karen's loyalty?

Dependability

One of the most valuable traits of a successful medical assistant is dependability. One should always be on time and make every attempt to be at work every day. When staff members arrive late, the entire day's schedule can be delayed (Figure 4-2). A medical assistant must follow through when the physician or supervisor gives an order. That person will count on the medical assistant to remember and complete all assigned duties. Supervisors should be confident that once given a task to do, the medical assistant will carry it out accurately and in a timely manner.

Courtesy

There is no excuse for not showing courtesy to the patients and co-workers in the physician's office. Kind words and compassion go far in building trust between the medical assistant and patients (Figure 4-3). It is essential that all visitors and staff members in the office be shown kindness and consideration. The fact that a medical assistant is having a bad day is no excuse for inflicting his or her

anger or irritation on patients. Always demonstrate a good attitude and offer patients and visitors a sincere smile.

Initiative

One of the more common complaints from supervisors is an employee's lack of **initiative**. Taking initiative means that the medical assistant looks for the opportunity to be of help, assisting others as the workload demands. Instead of waiting to be told to perform a task, look for jobs that need to be completed; never remain idle. There is always something that can be done in the medical office. There is never a lack of filing to be done. Inventories, supply ordering, or restocking can be performed when there is extra time in the medical facility. The medical assistant should also keep an eye on the reception area, since it may need to be tidied up several times during the day.

CRITICAL THINKING APPLICATION

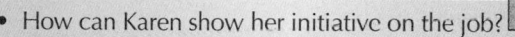

- How can Karen show her initiative on the job?
- What types of duties can she perform when she has finished her workload for the day and there is still time left before leaving the office?

Flexibility

A medical assistant must be able to adapt to a wide variety of situations. An emergency could occur in the office, and the staff must be flexible enough to adjust the schedule and care for all of the patients. Being flexible also means that there is a willingness among staff members to assist each other in the performance of their duties. No one in the physician's office should say, "That's not my job." The patients must come first, and every staff member must be willing to lend a hand where needed. Some medical assistants trade or rotate their duties. If there is a task that one assistant does not particularly enjoy doing, perhaps another assistant would be willing to trade tasks. This way, both are more satisfied with their jobs. Being able to adapt quickly and cheerfully will make the medical assistant a valuable asset to the office.

Credibility

Credibility is the perceived **competence** or character of a person. It leads to the belief that the person can be trusted. Since trust is a vital component of the physician-patient relationship, the credibility of the physician and those who assist in the office should be strong. The information provided to patients must be accurate. Patients expect that the physician and medical assistant will instruct them in a manner that will enhance their health and provide positive results. One must take care in giving any advice to patients, because they view the medical assistant as an agent of the physician. Patients may not distinguish between the medical assistant's advice and the physician's orders. To avoid charges of practicing medicine without a license, a medical assistant must be sure to suggest only what the physician has authorized.

Confidentiality

The importance of confidentiality cannot be stressed enough in the medical environment. Patients are entitled to privacy where their health is concerned, and they should be confident that medical professionals use information only to care for them. One must never reveal any information about any patient to anyone without specific permission to do so. If in doubt, be conservative and verify that the person seeking information has the right to see it. Casual conversations in hallways, elevators, and break rooms between staff can be overheard by a family member or friend of the patient.

The rules regarding confidentiality extend beyond the medical office. While at home, medical assistants should not discuss details about patients with their families and friends. Those outside the medical profession do not understand how vital it is to keep information confidential and may pass along damaging facts to others. Medical assistants must make it a rule never to discuss a patient with anyone unless information must be shared for patient care and treatment.

Attitude

Possibly the most important asset a medical assistant brings to the office is a good attitude. This trait alone can influence promotions, terminations, and the entire atmosphere of the office (Figure 4-4). We are able to control our attitude, with practice. It takes skill to react calmly to people who are very upset, rather than to respond in kind, especially if we are being harassed or accused. If you speak in an even tone and perhaps a little softer than normal, the listener will have to lower his or her voice to hear yours. Offer to help resolve the problem and attempt to move to a private room out of the hearing range of other patients to talk.

Obstructions to Professionalism

It is not always easy to be a professional. Sometimes patients, co-workers, and supervisors try our patience,

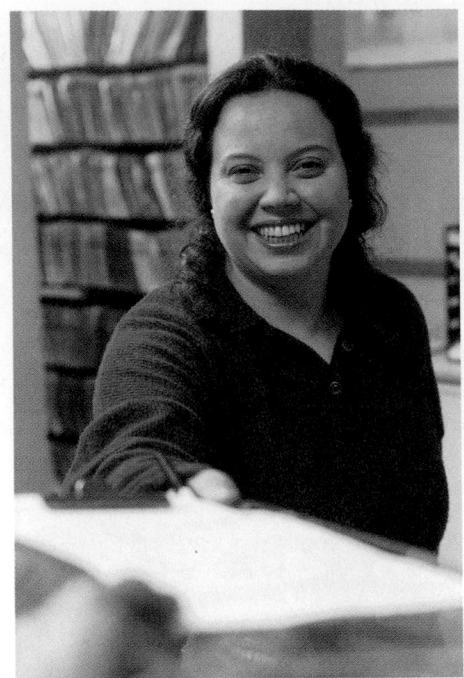

FIGURE 4-4 A good attitude goes a long way in patient and staff relationships.

and it can be hard to maintain a professional attitude in these cases. Some of the obstructions to professional behavior are discussed in this section.

Personal Problems and "Baggage"

Everyone has a life outside of the workplace, and sometimes we face challenges and difficult times that are hard to put aside. During working hours our thoughts should be on the job at hand, especially when we are dealing with patients. However, there may be situations in our lives that are so critical or important that we find ourselves thinking of them constantly. This personal *baggage*, as it is called, can interfere with our ability to properly perform job duties.

When there is a situation intruding on your thoughts at work, it is often best to take the time to talk with your supervisor. It is not necessary to share the intimate details, but a quick explanation that some difficulties are occurring outside of work will help the supervisor to understand any changes in your habit or attitude. However, there are some supervisors who are uncaring and are only concerned with satisfactory job performance. The medical assistant will have to use some **discretion** when discussing private affairs with the supervisor.

CRITICAL THINKING APPLICATION

- It is often hard to keep from thinking about a problem while you are working. How can Karen do this if she is concerned about a grandmother who is critically ill?

Rumors and the "Grapevine"

A rumor by definition is talk or widely **disseminated** opinion with no discernible source, or a statement that is not known to be true. The definition alone suggests that a rumor should be avoided. Most people enjoy working in an environment in which employees cooperate and get along with each other, but rumors can cause problems with employee **morale** and are often great exaggerations or manipulations of the truth. By promoting the grapevine, rumors are passed along and become more and more outrageous with each retelling. A medical assistant should refuse to participate in the office rumor-mill and attempt to be cordial and friendly to everyone at work (Figure 4-5). Supervisors regard those who spread or participate in rumors as unprofessional and untrustworthy.

Personal Phone Calls and Business

It is wise to avoid receiving unnecessary phone calls to the office from friends and family. The office phone should be considered a business line and must be used as such, except in emergencies. Visitors should not frequent the office, especially not in the area where the medical assistant is working. If someone must come to the office, always offer the reception area as a waiting room.

Checking personal email should also be avoided in the workplace. Any type of personal business, such as studying, looking up information on the Internet for personal use, or balancing a personal checkbook, should be done at home, not in the office setting. All of these distract the medical assistant from the job at hand; the focus should be on serving the patients in the office at all times.

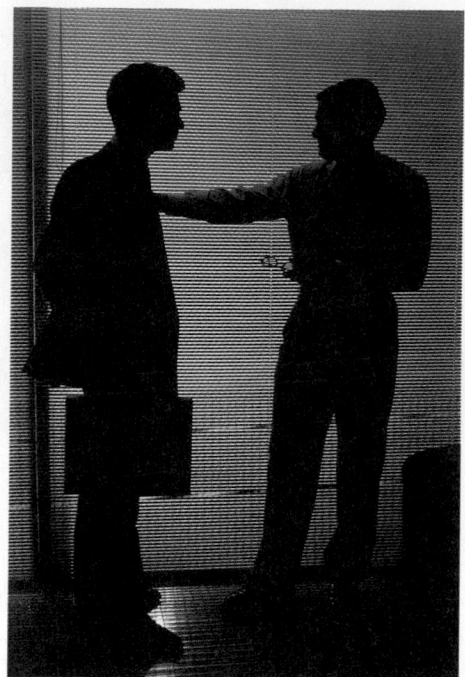

FIGURE 4-5   Gossip and rumors have no place in the medical profession. Avoid employees who participate in this type of activity.

productive workers, accept responsibility, be dependable, and always conduct themselves in a professional manner.

Procrastination

Procrastination is often a symptom of the fear of failure. Some people procrastinate because this gives them an excuse for failure. Others procrastinate because they are perfectionists and feel that only they can complete a project the right way. Procrastination is the surest way to see that goals remain unfulfilled. The best way to stop this habit is to DO something. Divide projects into small steps and complete one at a time. When a project is divided into small segments, it is much less overwhelming. The stronger the motivation, the easier it is to fight the urge to procrastinate.

CRITICAL THINKING APPLICATION

- Karen has a friend who works in a video store close to her office. Her friend has begun the habit of stopping in daily during her lunch hour to chat with Karen. How can Karen politely discourage her friend from doing this?
- Karen feels the need to check on her grandmother's condition as often as possible during the days she is ill. How might she accomplish this in a professional way?

Professional Attributes

Teamwork #1

If managers were asked what the most important attributes would be for medical professionals, teamwork would be high on the list (Figure 4-6). Staff members must work together for the good of the patients they care for. They must be willing to perform duties outside their formal job description if they are needed in other areas of the office. Many supervisors frown on employees who state, "That's not in my job description." Any order that is given by a supervisor becomes mandatory, and an individual who refuses to perform such a task can have his or her employment terminated for **insubordination**. A medical assistant should perform the duty and later discuss with

Office Politics

Most people associate office politics with some underhanded scheme or plans to move upward in the company in whatever way possible, whether the methods used are ethical or not. The tendency is to give the word *politics* a negative **connotation**. Politics can be defined as the art or science of influencing and guiding government or some other organization. The same can be applied to medical office politics. When an individual wishes to move upward in an organization, a certain strategy should be used. Many people develop a specific plan as to how they will advance, and in what time period they will accomplish this. Medical assistants who wish to advance should be

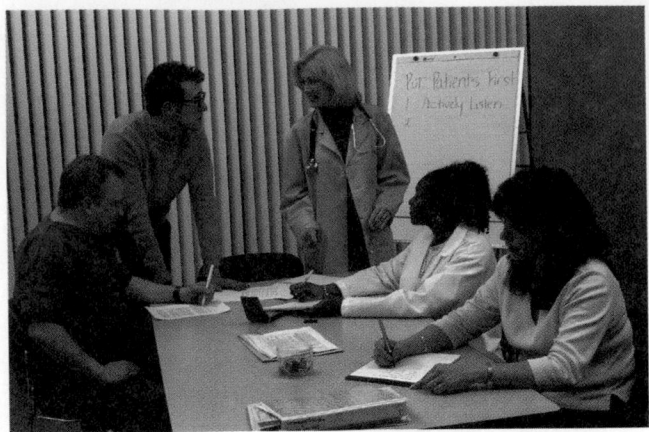

FIGURE 4-6   Teamwork is a vital part of the medical profession. All staff members must work together to care for the patient and perform required duties in the physician's office.

the supervisor any valid reasons that it should have been assigned to someone else.

Although we would all enjoy working in an office in which everyone gets along and likes every other employee, this does not always happen. Personal feelings must be set aside at work, and all employees must cooperate with others to get the job done efficiently. If a medical assistant has an issue with another employee, the first move would be to discuss it privately with the other person. Then, if the situation does not improve, perhaps a supervisor should be involved for further discussions.

Time Management

We have often heard the expression "work smart." This means that we are to use our time efficiently and concentrate on the duties that are most important first. To do this we must first prioritize our duties and arrange our schedule to ensure that these duties can be performed (see the next section). The first way to improve time management is to plan the tasks that need to be done that day. Taking 10 minutes to write down the day's tasks will help to ensure that they are done. Then it is important to stay on schedule throughout the day, unless emergencies disrupt the schedule. Even then, when office days are well planned, allowances can be made for emergencies, even if they happen often, and the majority of the tasks can still be completed. The key to managing time is prioritizing.

Prioritizing

Prioritizing is simply deciding which tasks are most important. Many people make a "to do" list for the day's activities, but the secret to success is prioritizing those activities into categories that give order to the tasks.

Most tasks can be prioritized into three general categories. There are activities that *must* be done that day, some that *should* be done that day, and those that *could* be done if there is time. Once you have a general list of tasks, review the list and further prioritize it, using a code such as *M* for must, *S* for should, and *C* for could (or this might be further simplified by using the letters

A, *B*, and *C*). Once the tasks are divided into these categories, they can be further classified within each section. For instance, if there are six A category duties, meaning they *must* be done today, these six can be numbered in the order they should be performed. The same process is completed with the B and C categories, and then as the tasks are completed, they are checked off for that day. Other categories can be added to customize the list. For example, an *H* category can be used for duties to perform at home, *P* could represent phone calls that need to be made, and *E* could represent errands to run. Customizing the categories will make the list more user-friendly.

Goal-Setting

Those who succeed in life are planners and goal-setters. The first step in becoming a proficient goal-setter is to take the time to really think about what is to be accomplished throughout one's lifetime. These goals must be written down and reviewed often. Goals should be set for all areas in a person's life, including personal growth, career, home life, family, spiritual needs, and any others that apply to the individual. The goals should not be unreasonable. They should be measurable and specific, with written steps detailing how they will be reached. Determination and persistence in reaching the goals will help to make them happen, along with a healthy dose of hard work. The goals should be reviewed often and progress evaluated; then goals can be reset as necessary.

Remember to celebrate the accomplishments and move past any goals that are missed, evaluating and restating the goals if necessary. Charles Kettering, an inventor who is most well-known for his invention of the automobile self-starter, once said, "The only time you can't afford to fail is the last time you try." Never quit trying to improve and experience personal growth.

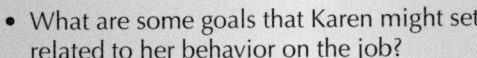

CRITICAL THINKING APPLICATION

- What are some goals that Karen might set related to her behavior on the job?
- List several goals for the new medical assistant to work toward during his or her first year in the field.

Knowing the Facility and its Employees

A much-circulated story tells of a college professor who used to end a critical test with the question, "What is the name of the woman who cleans our wing of the building?" This would perplex most students, but the question makes a good point. A professional medical assistant should attempt to get to know the people who work in the facility and should have a good idea of who handles which duties (Figure 4-7). When patients have specific problems with which they need help, they can be referred to the person

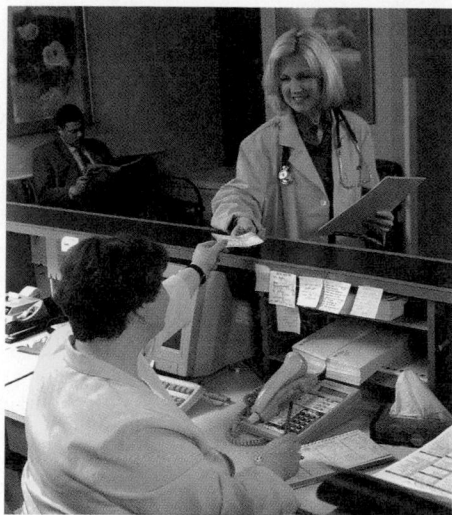

FIGURE 4-7   Knowing which employee to call when help is needed promotes goodwill among employees and often gets a task done more efficiently.

who knows the most about that particular issue. It is wise to express appreciation to others whenever possible. Say "thank you" often or "I appreciate your help" when working with others. This will make co-workers more likely to assist at other times when their help is needed.

Documentation

From the standpoint of professional behavior, documentation skills are vital to medical assistants. Charting accurately with legible, neat handwriting can make a difference in the perception of professionalism in the medical office. Be complete in any narrative regarding patients. Be sure to state facts, not opinions, and never use sarcastic remarks when charting. Phone messages must be documented carefully as well, and handled in a professional manner. Never use sarcasm when reporting messages to the physician or anyone else in the office. Use conservative speech and proper wording in all situations in the medical facility.

Note-Taking

Whenever office meetings or seminars are held, be prepared by having a pad and pencil ready for note-taking. A medical assistant should never be without paper and pen so that accurate information from the meeting can be jotted down for future reference. It is wise to keep a notebook or file on office meetings to refer to in case clarification of an order or a point is needed. Another good idea is to keep a small spiral notebook in a pocket with a pen, so that if an order is given in passing by the physician, the medical assistant will have a place to jot it down until he or she has access to the patient's chart. This avoids giving incorrect dosages of medication or forgetting to order a laboratory test, as well as many other errors that could be made by relying on memory.

Work Ethics

Work ethics can involve a whole range of activities, from individual acts to the philosophy of the entire facility. A person who has good work ethics is one who arrives on time, is rarely absent, and whose work output is **commensurate** with the pay received. Work ethics also involves other situations. If another employee is seen taking drugs from the supply cabinet or money from the cash box, the act should certainly be reported. However, if the guilty employee is also a close friend of the person who witnesses the act, an ethical dilemma is present. Ways to solve ethical problems will be discussed in Chapter 6. A medical assistant must always act in such a way that his or her actions are above **reproach**.

Communication

Communication skills are paramount in working with patients and other health professionals. A medical assistant should work hard to perfect his or her communication techniques. Often the success of a business is directly related to its ability to communicate effectively. Communication skills will be discussed in detail in Chapter 5.

Closing Comments

Patients expect and deserve professional behavior from those who work in medical facilities. Always show compassion, caring, and consideration for a person who comes to the office, whether a patient, visitor, or co-worker. By displaying these traits, the medical assistant will earn the respect of co-workers and become indispensable to the physician-employer.

Patient Education

When speaking to patients and providing them with information, remember that most do not have any medical background and do not understand many of the phrases used by the medical community. A medical assistant must be patient and explain in a courteous manner any aspect of the instructions or details that the patient does not understand. When educating the patient, the medical assistant should have a professional attitude of concern and helpfulness. Assure the patient that medical assistants and the rest of the staff in the facility are bound by rules of patient confidentiality if the patient seems concerned about revealing pertinent information.

Never transfer personal problems and baggage to the patient. A professional medical assistant does not share personal information with anyone at the medical facility. It is forbidden to pass along rumors of any type to patients or their families. The workday should be centered around patient care, so never allow personal business to impinge on time that should be spent assisting patients and the physician.

Legal and Ethical Issues

Behaving in a professional manner in the medical office will help to gain the patient's trust. Trust is one of the most important factors in avoiding cases of medical professional liability. Treating patients with care and not subjecting them to poor attitudes and unnecessary information will keep the patient-physician relationship a strong one, conducive to the health and recovery of the patient.

SUMMARY OF SCENARIO

Karen is happy to be employed in a family practice in which providing quality patient care is paramount. She is learning to be careful of what she says and to remain focused on the patient instead of any difficulties she may be having. She made an appointment to speak with her supervisor and explained the situation with her grandmother. The supervisor was very sympathetic and encouraged Karen to call and check on her grandmother whenever she felt she needed to, even offering the use of her phone and office. Karen was happy to find support in this area, and she has not taken advantage of the time she has been given to provide support to her own family.

Karen knows that it is her responsibility to be a team player and to assist the other staff members as much as possible. She maintains a good attitude, even when personal issues could distract her from her duties. Karen gets a strong sense of pride in being a part of the medical profession. She insists on a neat appearance and arriving on time for each scheduled workday. She always asks others if they need help when she has any extra time throughout the day. Karen looks forward to a long relationship with her employer. The rewards she feels as a member of the health team are second to none.

SUMMARY OF LEARNING OBJECTIVES

- Professionalism is the characteristic of being or conforming to the technical or ethical standards of a profession. It involves exhibiting courtesy, being conscientious, and conducting oneself in a business-like manner at the workplace. Professionalism is vitally important in the medical profession.

- Some of the characteristics of professionalism include loyalty, dependability, courtesy, initiative, flexibility, credibility, confidentiality, and a good attitude.

- Confidentiality is vitally important in the medical profession. Patients depend on medical personnel to keep their health information confidential and private. Breach of patient confidentiality is one reason that an employee could be immediately terminated from his or her position and can result in litigation between the patient and the physician-employer.

- Because most patients are not at their best when visiting the physician's office, the attitude of the staff plays an important role in patients' attitude while in the office. Medical assistants need patience when working with those who are ill. A smile or a reassuring pat on the back will go a long way and be encouraging.

- Office politics can be negative or positive. A person who uses others to be promoted through the company or takes credit for a team effort may be using office politics in a negative way; a person who strategically plans advancement by outstanding performance, dependability, and teamwork uses office politics in a positive manner. Knowing when to speak and when to listen will help the medical assistant to play the game of politics well in the medical facility.

- Teamwork makes any job easier to complete. By helping those who may be overwhelmed with duties, the medical assistant may find willing co-workers who will help when the situation is reversed in the future. If two assistants both have duties they dislike, they might trade the duties and both be satisfied.

- Insubordination can be used as grounds for immediate dismissal. Insubordination is being disobedient to any type of authority figure, usually the supervisor. When given a task to complete, the medical assistant should carry out the order unless it is unlawful or unethical. If the medical assistant feels that the duty should have been performed by someone else or there was some reason it should not have been performed, the supervisor should be consulted. Discuss the issue and attempt to reach an agreement about the appropriateness of performing the task in the future.

- Prioritizing tasks can help the medical assistant to accomplish more tasks. Prioritizing can be used for work, home, and extracurricular activities. Tasks can be identified as those that must, should, or could be done today. Then within each of these categories, the tasks can be numbered in the order they should be completed.

■ Goals should be written down and reviewed often to check progress. Taking small steps toward goals will help ensure that they are eventually reached.

Individuals should set goals in each area of their lives, breaking the tasks down into manageable parts. Goals should not be unreasonable or unattainable, but should provide the opportunity for small successes along the way to reaching the ultimate goal.

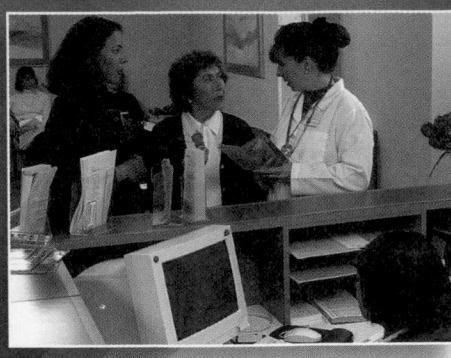

CHAPTER 5

Scenario

Many types of patients seek medical attention and care in the physician's office. Each will have different needs and different concerns, even when they have similar diagnoses. Communication and interpersonal skills are vitally important in meeting these needs and providing optimal care to the patient. However, the patient is not the only individual to consider. Family members are often instrumental in the health and well-being of the patient.

Lucille Cloyd is an 83-year-old patient who has been diagnosed with pancreatic cancer. Her daughter, Sarah Smithson, helps to care for her; she is very close to her mother emotionally. Sarah is also a patient of the same physician that cares for her mother. Although Sarah does not wish to see her mother in pain, she suffers with the knowledge that life will be very different without her. Mrs. Cloyd is widowed, and visits the physician once a month in addition to hospice services. She is a good-humored woman who feels she has led a fruitful life, yet she has moments of depression. She has been living with Sarah and her family for 2 months and enjoys interacting with her two grandchildren and the family's pets.

The medical assistant must consider not only Mrs. Cloyd, but also her extended family. Compassion and sensitivity will be necessary to care for this patient, as well as excellent listening skills. A good knowledge of human relations will help the medical assistant in making Mrs. Cloyd's medical care as pleasant as possible under the circumstances.

Interpersonal Skills and Human Behavior

Learning Objectives

- Define and spell the terms listed in the vocabulary.
- Explain why first impressions are critically important.
- Differentiate between verbal and nonverbal communication.
- Explain the different levels of spatial separation.
- Discuss the value of touch in the communication process.
- Describe the elements of the transactional communication model.
- Explain some of the barriers to effective communication.
- List and explain the levels of Maslow's hierarchy of needs.
- Discuss defense mechanisms and be able to recognize personal defense mechanisms you commonly use.
- Describe the value of listening.
- List several ways to deal with conflict.
- Explain the stages of grief.
- Discuss why physical and emotional needs affect our daily performance at work.

National Curriculum Competencies

TRANSDISCIPLINARY COMPETENCIES

1b. Recognize and respond to verbal communication
1c. Recognize and respond to nonverbal communication

Vocabulary

adage A saying, often in metaphorical form, that embodies a common observation.

aggression A forceful action or procedure intended to dominate; hostile, injurious, or destructive behavior, especially when caused by frustration.

ambiguous Capable of being understood in two or more possible senses or ways; unclear.

animate Full of life; to give spirit and support to expressions.

battery An offensive touching or use of force on a person without his or her consent.

caustic A remark or phrase marked by sarcasm.

channels Means of communication or expression; courses or directions of thought.

comfort zone A place in the mind where an individual feels safe and confident.

congruent Being in agreement, harmony, or correspondence; conforming to the circumstances or requirements of a situation.

decode To convert, as in a message, into intelligible form; to recognize and interpret.

defense mechanisms Psychological methods of dealing with stressful situations that are encountered in day-to-day living.

encode To convert from one system of communication to another; to convert a message into code.

encroachments That which advances beyond the usual or proper limits.

enunciate To utter articulate sounds; the act of being very distinct in speech.

external noise Sounds or factors outside the brain that interfere with the communication process.

externalization To attribute an event or occurrence to causes outside the self.

feedback The transmission of evaluative or corrective information to the original or controlling source about an action, event, or process.

grief An unfortunate outcome; a deep distress caused by bereavement.

internal noise Factors inside the brain that interfere with the communication process.

language barrier Any type of interference that inhibits the communication process that is related to languages spoken by the people attempting to communicate.

litigious Prone to engage in lawsuits.

malediction To speak evil of or curse.

media Term applied to agencies of mass communication, such as newspapers, magazines, and telecommunications.

paraphrasing To express an idea in different wording in an effort to enhance communication and clarify meaning.

perception Capacity for comprehension; an awareness of the elements of the environment.

physiological noise Physiological interferences with the communication process.

pitch Highness or lowness of a sound; the relative level, intensity, or extent of some quality or state.

proxemics The study of the nature, degree, and effect of the spatial separation individuals naturally maintain.

sarcasm A sharp and often satirical response or ironic utterance designed to cut or give pain.

stereotype Something conforming to a fixed or general pattern; a standardized mental picture that is held in common by many and represents an oversimplified opinion, prejudiced attitude, or uncritical judgment.

stressors Stimulus that causes stress.

subtle Difficult to understand or perceive; having or marked by keen insight and ability to penetrate deeply and thoroughly.

thanatology The description of the study of the phenomena of death and of psychological methods of coping with death.

vehemently Marked by forceful energy; intensely emotional.

volatile Easily aroused; tending to erupt in violence.

The interpersonal skills developed by the medical assistant help to set the tone of a medical office. Human relations can be defined as the study of the problems that arise from organizational and interpersonal contact. The two entities intersect each other, and a successful medical assistant will work to enhance these attributes on a continual basis. Patients who visit the healthcare facility may not be at their best, and the way in which the medical assistant reacts and interacts with them can make an incredible difference in their perception of the office, the physician, and the medical staff.

First Impressions

Our elders have stressed all of our lives that first impressions are lasting ones, and this old **adage** is still true! The opinions formed in the early moments of meeting someone remain in our thoughts long after the first words are spoken. The first impression is much more than just physical appearance or dress; it includes attitude and compassion, and the all-important smile (Figure 5-1)!

One of the primary objectives of the professional medical assistant is to care for and about the people that are being served. Patients are the reason for the existence of the facility, and they should be offered the best customer service available. They must be warmly welcomed, and it is important to call patients by their names. People enjoy hearing their name, and it gives the patient confidence that the medical staff knows whom they are caring for.

Although you may function comfortably in your facility, try to put yourself in the place of the new patient, who is entering unknown territory. As a staff member of the facility, you are in familiar surroundings and already have some information about the new patient. However, the patient knows nothing about you or the other staff members. One way to break that barrier is to have all staff members wear name badges, with letters large enough to be read at a distance of 3 feet. Include the staff position

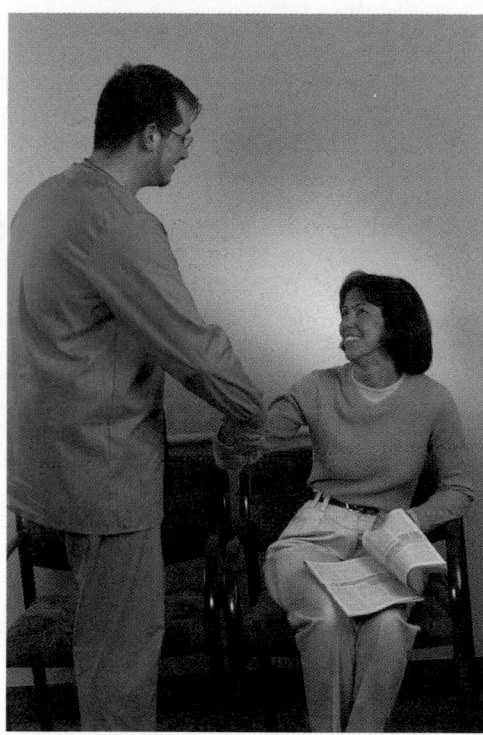

FIGURE 5-1   First impressions are critical in gaining the patient's trust.

if there are several divisions of responsibility; for instance, "medical assistant," "insurance biller," and "office manager." When the patient approaches, even though you are wearing a name badge, introduce yourself and smile. Let your smile show both facially and in your voice and eyes and genuinely welcome the patient to the office. This small effort will help to put the patient at ease in your environment.

Many physicians make brief notes in the chart about the personal lives of the patient. Then, when the patient arrives for the appointment, the physician can ask about his or her recent trip abroad or new grandchild. This tells the patient that the doctor and the office staff see him or her as more than just an illness or a chart number. It gives the impression that they truly care, and that impression should be an accurate one. Once an impression is formed in the patient's mind, it is very difficult to change, so make the first impressions of your office positive ones.

Communication Paths

Verbal Communication

Messages are conveyed by the use of language, which may be written, spoken, or communicated in another way. Verbal communication depends on words and sounds. The **pitch** of the voice is a part of verbal communication. The voice lifts at the end of a question. It drops at the end of a statement. Usually, when a speaker intends to continue a statement, the voice will hold the same pitch, the head will remain straight, and the eyes and hands will be unchanged. This is not an appropriate time to interrupt. If the message is interrupted, the train of thought may not be completed. Tone of voice and choice of words also affect messages.

The medical assistant should speak clearly and **enunciate** words properly. Speak loudly enough that the patients are able to hear clearly and pay particular attention to those who wear some type of hearing assistance device. It is wise to note this information on the patient's chart to jog the memory when a patient with a hearing problem visits the office. Never assume that just because a patient is elderly, he or she has a hearing problem. When talking with patients, be sure to use the volume of speech to an advantage. Always speak at a clearly audible level, but at times it will be necessary to increase or decrease the volume of speech. When a patient is upset, for instance, it often helps to lower the volume of speech, because the patient tends to get quieter to hear the person speaking.

Eye contact is critical. Look at the person being spoken to, and do not forget a genuine smile. Many people feel that a person who speaks and cannot look another in the eyes is being deceptive. It can also mean that the speaker is very shy and has little self-confidence. Use gestures where appropriate to liven speech and **animate** the conversation.

Medical assistants must become aware of how they express themselves and how they affect the feelings of others. The tone of voice is vitally important. There is no place for **sarcasm** or **caustic** remarks. For example, saying "I hope you can manage to be on time for your next appointment" to a patient is needless and rude. The medical assistant must be conservative when speaking and not be too familiar. The patient expects professionalism and has the right to demand this in the healthcare setting. Never make an inappropriate remark and follow with "I was just kidding." This has no place in a medical facility. Take special care not to hurt anyone's feelings with words and phrases. Be very careful about what is said, especially to patients.

Remember that patients are in the facility to be treated or cared for by the physician and staff. They are usually concerned about their illness and may have great apprehensions and fears about the future. It is completely out of place for the medical assistant to talk about his or her personal life and challenges with the patients. Allow the patient to speak, and listen instead of offering personal information. Often patients will casually mention things to the medical assistant that might influence their care. The saying that we are given "one mouth and two ears" stresses which should get more use!

Nonverbal Communication

Both verbal and nonverbal communications are important in the art of expression, and both are needed to succeed in the communication exchange. Nonverbal communications are messages conveyed without the use of words. They are transmitted by body language, gestures, and mannerisms that may or may not be in agreement with the words a person speaks. Body language is partly instinctive, partly taught, and partly imitative. It involves eye contact, facial expression, hand gestures, grooming, dress, space, tone of voice, posture, touch, and much more. We are often unaware of our own nonverbal signals and consciously recognize only a small number of the signals sent by others. Our ability to help others increases as we hone our own skills in interpreting nonverbal communication.

Appearance is an integral part of nonverbal communication. It influences the way others view us, and can present a conflicting message, or even a totally incorrect message. When we see someone who dresses or grooms in a way that is very different from our own style, we tend to assume that the personalities are opposite. This is not always true. Although we should not judge people by the way they dress, it is difficult not to form opinions based on what is seen. Visible piercings and tattoos are often looked on unfavorably in the medical profession, as are brightly painted long nails. Although these do not signify that the wearer is not professional, many patients, especially older patients, look on these trends unfavorably. For this reason alone, the medical assistant who is less conservative may be diminishing the chance for certain jobs and advancements. It is healthy to express oneself, yet in the medical profession, professional appearance is mandatory to avoid blocks in communications.

The successful medical assistant expresses self-esteem and confidence by stance, vocabulary, facial expression, and a caring attitude. The experience of speaking to someone who does not make eye contact helps one to realize the importance of greeting the patient with the eyes as well as the voice and body language. Facial expressions often convey our true feelings and are not masked by the words we use. Our eyes often tell the truth when our words are misleading or false. It is important to have an open body stance when dealing with patients. Crossed arms and legs hint that one is "closed" to the person being spoken to, and this may be construed as disinterest or disbelief. Nonverbal and verbal communications are dependent on one another (Figure 5-2). They must be in harmony to convey an accurate message, easily interpreted by the receiver. If the two are not **congruent**, the nonverbal is usually dominant and expresses the true message.

Our need for personal space is demonstrated by how patients in the reception area will choose a seat. **Proxemics** is defined as the study of the nature, degree,

and effect of the spatial separation individuals naturally maintain and how this separation relates to cultural and environmental factors. Seldom will a person sit in an adjoining seating space with a stranger, if there is another option. Although the need for space varies with the individual culture, some might even remain standing to satisfy the need for personal space. Public space is usually accepted as a distance of 12 to 25 feet, and social space is usually considered to be 4 to 12 feet. Personal space ranges from 1.5 to 4 feet, and intimate contact includes physical touching to about 1.5 feet. The medical assistant can often tell when he or she has invaded someone's personal space, because the person will tend to back up a step or two. If this happens, take a small step back and respect the boundaries that are being set. The more familiar and comfortable patients are with the medical assistant, the closer the space they will allow.

Touch is a powerful communicator. The soft acceptance of someone's hand in yours, to the good-natured pat on the back, to the harsh slap on the face, all relay different messages that need no words to accurately express. In the medical profession, as in any business, touch can be comforting or can promote a sexual harassment suit. Unfortunately, one must be extremely careful when using this effective communication tool. In today's **litigious** atmosphere, any nonconsensual touching may be considered **battery**, and touch should be used with great discretion and cautious care.

The medical assistant should not, however, be afraid to touch the patient appropriately, such as a pat on the back or a squeeze of the hand (Figure 5-3). Some patients are receptive to a brief sideways hug, whereas others would take this as an intrusion into their personal space. Certainly patients with serious illnesses appreciate touch as an expression of empathy. Never be afraid to touch sick patients, especially those with diseases such as AIDS, as long as proper precautions are followed where indicated. These individuals need to feel acceptance, and the attitude of the medical staff members they encounter will directly influence their adherence to keeping their appointments with the physician. If they do not feel accepted and cared for, they will not return to the physician's office. A gentle touch and a smile do wonders for showing that you care.

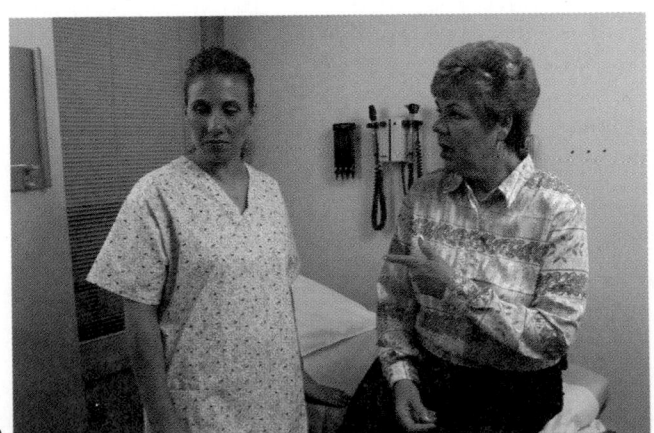
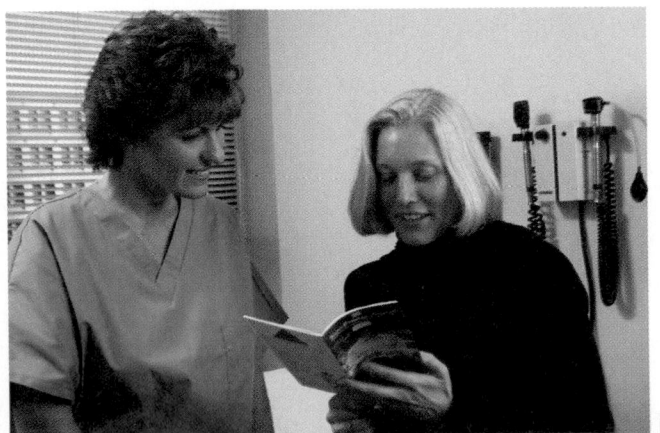

FIGURE 5-2   **A,** Pointing is often an accusatory gesture and causes discomfort. **B,** A bright smile helps to put the patient at ease and relax.

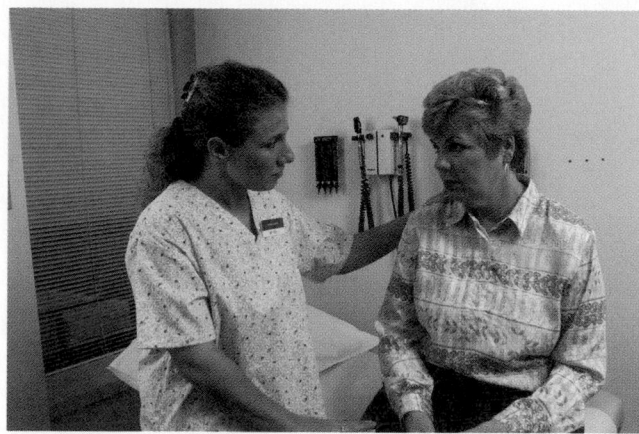

FIGURE 5-3 Touching the patient communicates care and compassion.

CRITICAL THINKING APPLICATION

- How might touch be an important communication tool with Mrs. Cloyd?
- How can Sarah be affected by using touch?
- Could laughter affect either of these women as they deal with death?

Posture can signal depression, excitement, anger, or even an appeal for help. When the physician sits at the front of the chair and leans forward, he or she is giving the message of caring and interest. Positioning is important as well. Sitting behind a desk promotes an air of authority. Standing or sitting across a room may convey a negative message of denying involvement or reluctance to talk. The medical assistant should practice good postural techniques as a part of projecting a positive image and for personal health reasons.

The Process of Communication

Anyone who works within the realm of public service should develop good communication skills. It is critically important to be able to interact with others and put them at ease, so that their comfort level increases and they develop trust. To communicate well, we must first have a general understanding of the process of communication. Once a message is sent, it cannot be retrieved and restated or expressed in a different way. Especially in the medical profession, communication must be clear and concise, and the message we intend to send must match what the receiver understands.

Although there are many different scientific models of communication, the one that best fits most types of communication is the *transactional communication model*. Before understanding how this model works, one must understand the elements we use to communicate.

Usually, when two people interact, both people act as a sender and as a receiver. The sender is the person who sends a message through a variety of different **channels**. Channels can be spoken words, written messages, and body language. The sender **encodes** the message, which simply means that he or she chooses a specific way of expression using words and other channels. The receiver **decodes** the message according to his or her understanding of what is being communicated. However, there are times that the receiver understands the message incorrectly. This is often because of noise, which is anything that interferes with the message being sent. It can be literal noise, such as a radio or a jackhammer on the street outside. This is called **external noise**. Or, it could be **internal noise**, which would include the receiver's own thoughts or prejudices and opinions. **Physiological noise** interferes with communication as well. This includes any biological factor that would preclude the communicator from sending or receiving accurate messages, such as not feeling well or being overly tired. **Feedback** can be verbal expressions or body language, such as a simple nod of understanding. The **perception** of the receiver is very important, and will be discussed later in this chapter.

The transactional communication model (Figure 5-4) depicts "communicators" instead of one sender and one receiver. If two people are communicating, both are sending and receiving messages and both are encoding and decoding what is being offered. Even when two people are speaking one at a time, messages are continually sent with words, body language, facial expressions, and gestures. Various channels of communication are used, and both communicators offer feedback, even if it is done subconsciously. Noise may or may not be present, but even the best communicators experience some type of noise, even if that is only thinking of what to say next.

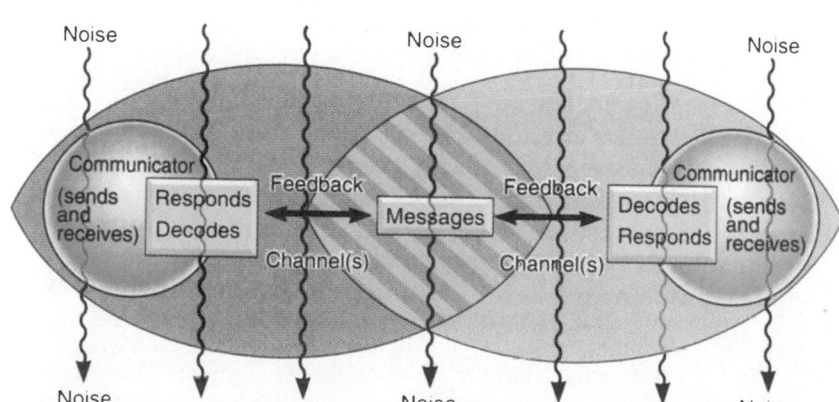

FIGURE 5-4 The transactional communication model. (From Adler RB, Towne N: *Looking out, looking in: interpersonal communication*, San Antonio, 1996, Harcourt Brace.)

Listening

Listening is just as important to good communication as the spoken word. People need to know that they are being heard. This is true in all interpersonal relationships, including husband/wife, parent/child, supervisor/employee, and doctor/patient interactions. When listening to someone who is attempting to communicate, the first rule is to look at the speaker and pay attention. Sometimes it is important not to respond immediately, but to remain silent and offer an understanding and reassuring nod.

There are times when it is hard to listen. We may not be able to listen effectively because we are distracted by our own thoughts. Perhaps the situations occurring in our own lives make the conversation we are hearing seem meaningless and unimportant. Or, there may be so many messages attacking at once that we are unable to focus on any specific one to hear what is being communicated. At other times, such as in anger, we are so rapidly preparing our response that we cannot hear what is being said. We may simply be too tired to listen or may have prejudged the speaker and decided that there is no need to listen. However, while working with patients, the medical assistant must be diligent in not only hearing the words being spoken, but also listening to them and what the patient is attempting to communicate.

Active listening is the skill whereby **paraphrasing** and clarifying what the speaker has said take place. Paraphrasing is listening to what the sender is communicating, analyzing the words, and then restating them to confirm that the receiver has understood the message as the sender intended it. This process clarifies the speaker's thoughts and helps to indicate that there is a common understanding of the message between both people. When communicating in this way, the receiver should reword what the sender has said and then ask a clarifying question. Consider the example below:

Patient: I have not been feeling well lately.
MA: You say you have not been feeling well. What exactly is the trouble?

This type of communicating may seem awkward at first, because most of us believe that listening involves lack of speech. Active listening means that the speaker's words are heard and there is a restatement that is used to verify that the message was understood correctly. This statement gives the speaker the opportunity to correct any misconceptions or misunderstandings. Consider the following example:

Patient: My back hurts.
MA: Where does it hurt?
Patient: In the middle.
MA: Can you point to exactly where it hurts?
Patient: Yes, right here (points).
MA: Is it a sharp or dull pain?
Patient: Very sharp.
MA: How often does it occur?
Patient: Several times a day.
MA: Can you tell me on an average day how many times it bothers you?
Patient: About six times.
MA: How long does it last?

Patient: About 10 or15 minutes.
MA: How long has this been a concern?
Patient: For about 2 weeks.
MA: So you have had a sharp pain in this part of your back, about six times a day lasting for up to 15 minutes for 2 weeks? Is that correct?
Patient: Yes.

It would have been easier for the patient to have said, "I have had a sharp pain in my back that lasts up to 15 minutes, and it happens about six times a day," but this example shows how the medical assistant can continue clarifying until the answer is specific enough. This is critical when obtaining information from the patient.

It is also helpful to ask "open" questions, as opposed to "closed" questions. An open question requires more than a "yes" or "no" answer. It forces the patient to provide more detail and expand on his or her thoughts. A closed question can be answered with "yes" or "no" and compel the medical assistant to spend more time obtaining the answers needed to accurately document the patient's needs.

CRITICAL THINKING APPLICATION

- How can the medical assistant be sure that Mrs. Cloyd understands how she is to take her medication?
- Often older patients do not appreciate instructions being given to their caregiver instead of directly to them. How can the medical assistant place the primary focus on communicating with Mrs. Cloyd, yet make sure that Sarah understands the instructions and care at the same time?

Often when a person or patient is talking with the medical assistant, he or she is looking for a specific type of response. Some patients want advice, some want sympathy, and others are looking for reassurance. Many patients will open up to the medical assistant faster and more completely than to the physician. Since it is important to build good rapport with patients, this can be a very positive aspect of the relationship the medical assistant has with the patient. However, the medical assistant should never agree to withhold information from the physician under any circumstances. If the patient asks that the assistant not reveal something to the physician, the medical assistant should politely explain that there is an ethical obligation to report any and all pertinent information to the physician, especially if it affects medical care. For example, if the patient asks the medical assistant not to tell the physician that the patient has been smoking against medical advice, the assistant could be jeopardizing the patient's care if the information is not reported.

This does not mean that specific details must always be aired. If the patient reveals that stress levels have been high because they have filed a sexual harassment suit against their boss, the medical assistant could report to the physician that the patient is having some legal problems, which have resulted in additional stress at work.

Never agree to lie to the physician! The patient must understand that if the physician questions any information given by the patient, it must be revealed so that the physician is assured that the care being provided is the right care. It is also critical to note that the physician may have worked with the patient for a long period and have a better understanding of the patient's needs than the medical assistant does. One patient may be able to handle a high degree of stress, and another may crumble at the first sign of stress. A good physician knows his or her patients and keeps accurate, complete records that will help with decision-making in these situations.

If ever in doubt about telling the physician something a patient has said, the best solution is to tell. Remember, medical professionals are legally bound to confidentiality, and the patient may need to be reminded of this. Encourage him or her to talk to the physician and communicate all of his or her concerns, no matter how insignificant they may seem. Never display a judgmental attitude or express negativity about the patient's activities, thoughts, or behavior. Offer to be with the patient, if he or she desires, as the patient discusses difficult issues with the physician, or to make arrangements for a special counseling session with the physician if this is indicated. Some patients are hesitant to initiate conversation with the physician because they feel they are taking too much time. The medical assistant can help to ensure that critical issues receive the doctor's attention.

Advising a Patient

The medical assistant must be extremely careful when giving advice to a patient in order to avoid legal accusations of practicing medicine without a license. Often a patient will ask for an opinion as to which course of action to take. Strict laws in most states prohibit anyone other than a licensed physician from giving medical advice. Even if the patient asks what the medical assistant would do if presented with the same options, the assistant cannot encourage the patient to choose one option over another. The assistant can offer a listening ear though, and help the patient process his or her own thoughts. This can be done in much the same way as using active listening techniques (Figure 5-5). When a patient expresses a concern, the medical assistant should restate the concern and then ask a clarifying question. For example:

> Patient: I don't know if I should take the chemotherapy treatments the doctor suggested.
> MA: You seem worried about the treatments. What are you concerned about specifically?

Patients must come to their own decisions about treatments and options that they have when faced with a medical decision. The medical assistant is often looked on not only as an authority figure, but also as an extension of the physician. Patients may mistakenly think that the medical assistant reflects the same opinion as the physician. Always attempt to get the patient to openly discuss all of his or her concerns and fears with the physician.

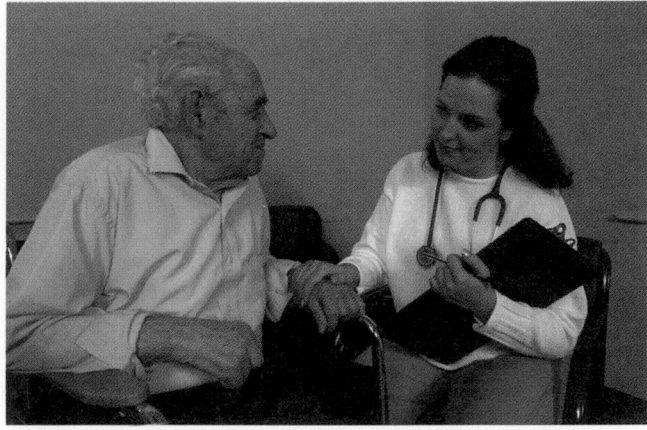

FIGURE 5-5   Careful listening and asking questions will help the patient express thoughts and feelings.

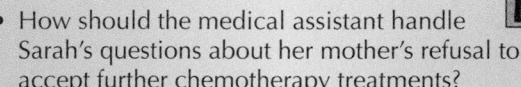

CRITICAL THINKING APPLICATION

- How should the medical assistant handle Sarah's questions about her mother's refusal to accept further chemotherapy treatments?
- How does this decision affect Sarah's ability to communicate with medical professionals? What barriers to communication might be present?

Observing Carefully

In the fast-paced world of medicine, there are times that nonverbal signals sent by patients are missed, which play a critical role in their care. Hesitancy while the patient is speaking may indicate that there is more to say. As mentioned previously, the inability to look a person directly in the eyes sometimes, but not always, indicates deception. The medical assistant must play close attention to what is seen as well as what is heard when communicating with the patient. Look in the eyes, and watch intently for signs of trouble.

When a patient cries, the medical assistant should always question what is causing the tears. Some patients may refuse to discuss the issue or insist that nothing is wrong, but tears are always a symptom of some emotion, whether it is anger, frustration, fear, pain, or some other concern. It is unwise to allow patients that are obviously emotionally upset to leave the office without reasonable assurance that they are going to be safe. The medical assistant might wish to suggest that a friend come to the office and escort the patient home. On rare occasions, it is better to be firm with the patient and insist on help getting home than later to find that the patient hurt herself or himself or someone else because of his or her **volatile** state. Careful observation of the patient as a whole is worth the time investment and may even save the patient's life.

Defense Mechanisms

Anxiety or stress causes the human body to react in many different ways. Some people handle **stressors** more easily than others. Most people use **defense mechanisms** during times in which they feel pressured or attacked in some way. These are often subconscious reactions designed for emotional protection; they help us to deal with whatever difficult event has triggered such a response. Often people may not even realize that they are using these mechanisms, and may even **vehemently** deny that they do so. There are many types of defense mechanisms, and the medical assistant should be familiar with them to better communicate with patients and others they come into contact with in the course of their duties.

Verbal Aggression

When a person verbally attacks another without addressing the original complaint, or disregards it, he or she is being verbally **aggressive** (Figure 5-6). Some individuals get very angry at any suggestion of wrongdoing; their response is to change the subject. They lash out, usually quite loudly, and attack back quickly in hopes of diminishing their role in any wrongdoing.

> "When are you going to clean the garage?"
> "Who are you to ask me that? You are late paying the rent again!"

Sarcasm

This word has its origin in the Greek *sarkasmos*, which means "to tear flesh" or "to bite the lips in rage." This is quite an accurate definition of the nature of sarcasm. It is a biting edge added to words that a person states with the intent to cause pain or anger. Sarcasm is hostile and cruel in most cases, and there are some individuals who use it constantly, thinking that it is quite witty. On the contrary, it often makes bitter enemies of its victims.

> "Of course it's a nice dress, if you like tents."

Rationalization

Rationalizing is attributing actions to rational and credible motives without analyzing underlying methods. When people rationalize their behavior, they are offering excuses for what has been done or said and trying to convince others that the behavior was completely justified.

> "He only hits me because he is stressed at work."

Compensation

A person who compensates makes up for one behavior by stressing another. Compensation is a psychological mechanism through which feelings of inferiority, frustration, or failure in one area are counterbalanced by achievement in another. Compensation is not always a negative response, but it is often used as an excuse for not accomplishing what should be accomplished.

> "I know I gained 5 pounds, Dr. George, but I exercised three times last week."

Regression

Regression is the reversion to an earlier mental or behavioral level. Some people regress to a childlike state or period or exhibit qualities inherent to an earlier time in life. This can include making excuses for not doing a certain thing, saying that it cannot be done, instead of the truth, which is that the person does not want to do it. Replacing the word "can't" with "won't" is a good gauge of using regression.

> "I'd like to get better grades, but I can't find time to study."

Repression

The process whereby unwanted desires or impulses are excluded from the consciousness and left to operate in the unconscious is called *repression*. Blocking a problem out of the mind, or changing the subject when it is mentioned, are both types of repression. The repressed urges or desires may seethe beneath the surface, absorbing energy, and force the continual repression of the desires, which takes more and more concentration to do successfully.

> "I should phone my brother since our fight, but I just can't deal with that now."

Apathy

Apathy is a lack of feeling, emotion, interest, or concern. It is an indifference to what is happening or a pretense of not caring about a situation. Usually, apathy is not a true reflection of the inner feeling. It is a defense mechanism that is similar to repression, but with a more flippant attitude.

> "I don't care what grade I made on the test, because I am not going to pass the class anyway."

Displacement

Displacement is defined as the redirection of an emotion or impulse from its original object, such as an idea or person, to another object. When challenged or attacked by one person or event, displacement is used to channel negative feelings to some other area, which gives a false

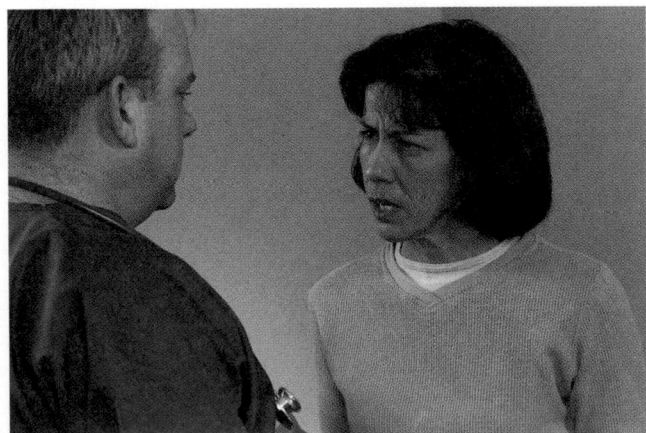

FIGURE 5-6 Remain calm even if a patient becomes verbally aggressive and attempt to calm him or her by listening and expressing empathy whenever possible.

sense of control over issues that may not be controllable. The venting of hostile feelings is directed somewhere other than where it should be directed, but usually this is a result of a lack of confidence in addressing the true issues at hand.

> "I have enough problems at work and don't need to come home to a nagging wife!"

Denial

Denial is a psychological defense mechanism in which confrontation with a personal problem or with reality is avoided by denying the existence of the problem or reality. This is where the common expression, "He's in denial" originates. For whatever reason, the individual is unable to cope with the stress of a situation and completely pushes it or any person or thing representing it away.

> "My husband can't have cancer. He is completely healthy."

Physical Avoidance

Some events are so painful for people that they completely avoid any representation of the event. This could be a person, a place, an object, or just about anything that serves as a reminder of the event that induces the negative feelings. If the problem is a person, that person may be avoided for the rest of their life. If it is a place, such as a home that a couple lived in before one of them died, the other person may physically move. In some cases, such as physical abuse, the avoidance may be necessary, but it can also be quite unhealthy and may need to be explored further through therapy.

> "I will never go to that restaurant again, because that is where my ex-husband proposed to me."

Projection

Projection as a defense mechanism is defined as the attribution of one's own ideas, feelings, or attitudes to other people or to objects. This especially includes the **externalization** of blame, guilt, or responsibility as a defense against anxiety. Some people project their feelings about a certain thing onto others, who may not be affected by the negative connotations the first person feels. Projection is a way to avoid dealing with the root issues of a problem.

> "Everyone else is always late, so why am I getting written up for it?"

Dealing with Conflict

Conflict is defined as the struggle resulting from incompatible or opposing needs, drives, wishes, or external or internal demands. We deal with conflict in our lives in some capacity almost daily. Knowing how to recognize the traits of conflict and what patterns people use to deal with conflict will be of great benefit to the medical assistant. This will enable the professional to be understanding and empathetic to patients, co-workers, supervisors, and others in the day-to-day work environment.

Conflict is not always negative; sometimes it is beneficial to relationships. It can be constructive and allow people to learn more about each other. This may promote a stronger understanding and deeper levels of intimacy. Unless both parties are aware that a problem exists between them, there is no conflict. The conflict begins when both realize there is a problem that needs resolution. People handle conflict in different ways. Some avoid it at all costs, and on the other end of the spectrum, some seem to thrive on it.

It is helpful to define some of the many types of conflict to understand the thought processes of others and how best to respond to them, as well as discerning how others respond. Of itself, assertion is not conflict; assertion is stating or declaring positively, often forcefully or aggressively. Being assertive or aggressive can be very productive. Assertive people often receive job promotions and reach the goals they set for their lives. Too much aggression can make a person seem pushy, so it should be controlled and used at the appropriate times. Remember, there is a difference between assertion and aggression, which will be discussed in the following paragraphs.

Nonassertion is the inability to express needs and thoughts or the refusal to express them. Some avoid conflict and some accommodate by putting others before their own desires. There are times that nonassertion is justifiable. Anyone who has been involved in a long-term relationship realizes that there will be occasions when the other person's needs must come first. Many have learned the truth of the old saying, "Choose your battles wisely."

CRITICAL THINKING APPLICATION

- Why might Mrs. Cloyd and Sarah experience conflict at this stage in their lives?
- How might each deal better with disagreements, especially regarding Mrs. Cloyd's decisions about her medical care?

Aggression is defined in several ways. It can be a hostile, injurious, or destructive behavior or outlook, especially when caused by frustration. It is also the practice of making attacks or **encroachments**, especially if the acts are unprovoked. In the realm of psychological studies, there are different types of aggression. Direct aggression occurs when a person directly attacks another, whether by criticism, **malediction**, ridiculing, or other methods. This behavior causes the victim to feel embarrassment, shame, anger, or a range of other emotions. *Passive aggression* is a familiar term, but most may not know its definition. A passive-aggressive person expresses himself or herself in an obscure, **ambiguous** way. People who experience passive aggression may have feelings or rage, inadequacy, or resentment that they cannot articulate in a direct manner. Unfortunately, this behavior usually will not provide the results that are needed or expected.

The Crazymakers: Passive-Aggressive Communications

In the book *Looking Out, Looking In: Interpersonal Communication* by Ronald B. Adler and Neil Towne, the concept of "Crazymakers" is discussed and credited to George Bach. Bach was a psychologist who developed the theory of creative aggression; he nicknamed this passive-aggressive behavior *crazymaking*. He said that there are two types of aggression—clean fighting and dirty fighting. Crazymaking was his name for dirty fighting, which is a detrimental behavior for all involved. The term *partner* is loosely used to indicate the opposite side or victim of the crazymaker.

Following are brief descriptions of the characteristic types of passive-aggressive persons described by Bach.*

The Avoider. Avoiders refuse to fight. When a conflict arises, they leave, fall asleep, pretend to be busy at work, or keep from facing the problem in some other way. This behavior makes it difficult for the partner to express feelings of anger and hurt, because the avoider will not fight back.

The Pseudoaccommodator. Pseudoaccommodators refuse to face up to a conflict either by giving in or pretending there is nothing wrong. This drives the partner crazy, who definitely feels there is a problem and causes feelings of guilt and resentment toward the accommodator for bringing up the situation in the first place.

The Guiltmaker. Instead of saying straight out that they don't want or approve of something, guiltmakers try to make their partners feel responsible for causing pain. A guiltmaker's favorite line is, "It's OK, don't worry about me..." followed by a long sigh.

The Subject Changer. Really an avoider, the subject changer escapes facing up to aggression by shifting the conversation whenever it approaches an area of conflict. Because of their tactics, subject changers and their partners never have the chance to explore their problems and do something about them.

The Distracter. Rather than come out and express their feelings about the object of their dissatisfaction, distracters attack other parts of their partner's life. Thus they never have to share what is really on their minds and can avoid dealing with painful parts of their relationships.

The Mind Reader. Instead of allowing their partners to express feelings honestly, mind readers go into character analysis, explaining what the other person really means or what is wrong with the other person. By behaving this way, mind readers refuse to handle their own feelings and leave no room for their partners to express themselves.

The Trapper. Trappers play an especially dirty trick by setting up a desired behavior for their partners and then when it's met, attacking the very thing they requested. An example of this technique is for the trapper to say, "Let's be totally honest with each other," and then attack the partner's words of honesty.

The Crisis Tickler. Crisis ticklers almost bring what is bothering them to the surface, but never quite come out and express it. Instead of admitting concern about the finances, they innocently ask, "Gee, how much did that cost?" dropping a rather obvious hint, but never really dealing with the crisis.

The Gunnysacker. Gunnysackers do not respond immediately when angry. Instead, they put their resentment into a gunnysack, which after a while begins to bulge with both large and small gripes. Then, when the sack is about to burst, the gunnysacker pours out all the pent-up aggressions on the overwhelmed and unsuspecting partner.

The Trivial Tyrannizer. Instead of honestly sharing their resentments, trivial tyrannizers do things they know will get their partner's goat—leaving dirty dishes in the sink, clipping fingernails in bed, belching out loud, turning up the television too loud, and so on.

The Beltliner. Everyone has a psychological "beltline," and below it are subjects too sensitive to be approached without damaging the relationship. Beltlines may have to do with physical characteristics, intelligence, past behavior, or deeply ingrained personality traits a person is trying to overcome. In an attempt to "get even" or hurt their partners, beltliners will use intimate knowledge to hit below the belt, where they know it will hurt.

The Joker. Because they are afraid to face conflicts squarely, jokers kid around when their partners want to be serious, thus blocking the expression of important feelings.

The Blamer. Blamers are more interested in finding fault than in solving a conflict. Needless to say, they usually do not blame themselves. Blaming behavior almost never solves a conflict and is an almost sure-fire way to make receivers defensive.

The Contract Tyrannizer. Contract tyrannizers will not allow their relationships to change from the way they once were. Whatever the agreements the partners had for roles and responsibilities at one time, they will remain unchanged.

The Kitchen Sink Fighter. Kitchen sink fighters are so named because in an argument they bring up things that are totally off the subject—as in everything including the kitchen sink. It may be the way the other person behaved last New Year's Eve, or bad breath, the unbalanced checkbook, any past imperfection is fair game.

The Withholder. Instead of expressing their anger honestly and directly, withholders punish their partners by keeping back something—courtesy, affection, good cooking, humor, sex. This is likely to build up even greater resentments in the relationship.

The Benedict Arnold. Benedict Arnolds get back at their partners by sabotage, by failing to defend them from attackers, and even by encouraging ridicule or disregard from outside the relationship.

Barriers to Communication

Physical Impairment

Patients may have physical troubles that impair their ability to communicate effectively. This could be a vision

---

*Modified from Adler RB, Towne N: *Looking out, looking in: interpersonal communication*, San Antonio, 1996, Harcourt Brace College.

or hearing problem, or one of many other conditions that makes communicating a bit more difficult than usual. The medical assistant should use more descriptive language when speaking with the patient who has a visual disturbance. This helps the patient to "see" what is being discussed in his or her thoughts. The person with diminished hearing may be very sensitive and in denial of the condition. Be certain that you have his or her attention and that you are face to face with the person while speaking. People who are hearing impaired are often very dependent on lip-reading for comprehension. Being elderly is not an impairment at all. Many older patients will be physically fit and mentally sharp and do not expect special treatment. Never increase the volume of your speech in an assumption that an older patient is hard of hearing.

CRITICAL THINKING APPLICATION

- What must be considered when communicating verbally with Mrs. Cloyd? With Sarah?
- How can the medical assistant show compassion to a terminally ill patient during her appointment when the office is extremely busy?

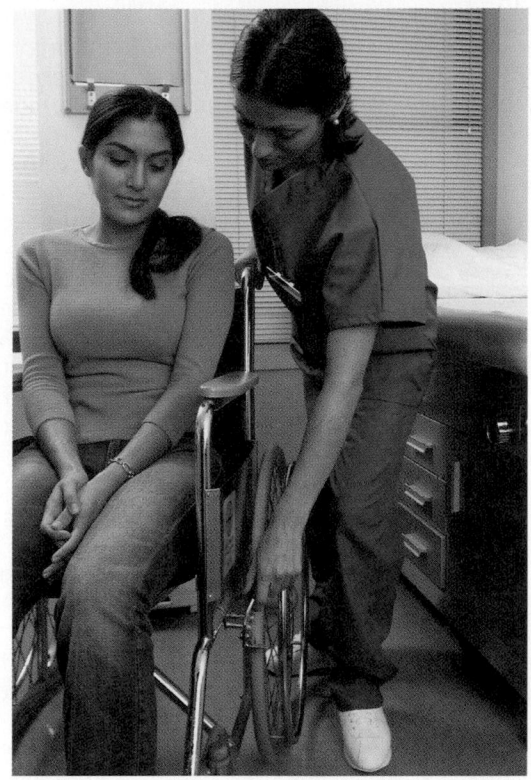

FIGURE 5-7   Bilingual staff members are valuable in ensuring accurate communications with patients who speak a different language.

Language

With non–English-speaking patients, the medical assistant may need to use gestures and more body language to convey messages. In such cases, be alert to the possibility of misunderstandings. Confirm that the message being sent is the message that the listener received by asking for feedback. Ask the listener to repeat the message, and if family members are present, be sure they have a good understanding of what is being communicated as well.

It is always helpful to have a bilingual staff member so that there is less chance of miscommunication with those who speak a different language (Figure 5-7). Many regions offer bilingual classes for medical professionals to assist them with basic communications with their patients. It would be well worth the time and financial investment to investigate such classes, because bilingual assistants are quite valuable to the physician and may be able to command a higher salary.

Prejudice

Personal and social bias, or prejudice, brings about discrimination. *Discrimination* is a word that is used to describe unfair treatment of a person because of race, gender, religious affiliation, handicap, or any other reason. Discrimination is unethical, morally and socially wrong, and in many situations, it is illegal. It also prevents us from communicating effectively.

Some discrimination is very **subtle**; it is not expressed openly or in a blatant manner. Subtle discrimination is based on a person's appearance, values, lifestyle, or some other personal factor. Examples include discrimination against those who are obese, divorced individuals, homo-sexuals, welfare recipients, or those with sexually transmitted diseases. Sometimes we are not aware that our words or actions reflect subtle discrimination against others.

Personal prejudices must be recognized before one can change them. Medical professionals are exposed to a wide variety of persons who need excellent medical care. The professional cannot allow personal prejudice to affect the care of any individual. Everyone has the right to be honored as a human being and treated respectfully. This enforces the Golden Rule, treating others as you would wish to be treated. Realize the worth of each individual person and allow that attitude to reflect in all of the actions taken with a patient.

Stereotyping

Stereotyping is defined as a standardized mental picture that is held in common by members of a group and that represents an oversimplified opinion, prejudiced attitude, or uncritical judgment. It is unfair to **stereotype** anyone or categorize him or her based on preconceived, often incorrect, assumptions. Although sometimes there is a degree of truth to the assumption based on stereotypical categories, people should not be judged before there has been an opportunity to get to know them as individuals. The medical assistant should push preconceived notions aside and look at the individual when forming and building a relationship. In the medical profession, stereotypical categories should not be considered when caring for patients and developing good rapport with them.

Perception

Perhaps one of the most important issues to consider when discussing barriers to communication is the concept of perception. *Perception* means the capacity for comprehension, or the discernment of what is being communicated, according to the message receiver's point of reference. When we discussed the transactional communication model earlier in the chapter, it was obvious that because of different types of noise and channels, there would be times that the message sent would be distorted; the receiver would not always get the message that the sender meant to send. The receiver's perceptions could completely alter the message, no matter how clearly it was sent. If the receiver believes that all attorneys are corrupt, he or she will probably be unable to get past this perception when speaking with a lawyer and therefore may not be able to trust.

Often our perceptions stem from some experience with a certain group of people from the past. This perception goes unresolved or has affected us so strongly that we group all people from that walk of life into a negative category. This is an unfair way to deal with people; everyone should be viewed as an individual, not as a part of a stereotypical group. Remember, perception is an individual's point of view, right or wrong. There is also the issue of interpretation and the determination of what is meant by a certain message. There must be an attempt to understand both points of view and be willing to discuss them calmly, even in the most heated of discussions. No one truly enjoys conflict, and we should have a healthy respect for others' opinions. The differences between individuals are part of what makes each of us unique.

Communication During Difficult Times

Communication is not an art that comes easily to everyone. It is often difficult to express feelings in an honest and open way. When a crisis occurs, it is much harder to communicate effectively and we sometimes say things that we do not mean. The medical assistant must develop communication skills that can be used in times of trouble. There must be an understanding of why a patient or co-worker is unable to communicate.

Patience is important, too, because people are not always at their best when they are concerned about their condition or that of a loved one. Always remain calm when dealing with a person who is experiencing a traumatic event or has any depressive condition. Remember that he or she may be reacting to many emotions—fear, anger, doubt, inadequacy, or many others. The key is to listen and determine the best way to help the patient out of any immediate danger, and help them establish some type of support system.

Anger

One of the most difficult times to communicate is when we are angry. Anger is a normal emotion that all of us feel at one time or another. Usually the expression of anger is a healthy thing. Some people bottle up their emotions and

do not express what they truly feel inside. If this is done repeatedly, at some point the anger will erupt, possibly over a tiny event. Others explode over every little situation, and people who do this need anger management skills and training.

Anger, like most emotions, can cause physiological changes. When a person feels anger, the blood pressure rises and the heart rate increases. Many things can trigger anger, from a simple traffic backup to a real or perceived betrayal, the diagnosis of a disease, or the death of a close relative. Road rage is one example of anger out of control and is a serious problem on our public highways today. Unexpressed anger can cause or contribute to all types of health problems, including depression and hypertension.

The medical assistant can help to calm an angry patient by speaking calmly and refusing to return the emotion. If the volume is gradually lowered with every sentence spoken, the angry person will have to lower the volume as well to hear what the assistant is saying. Suggest that the person breathe deeply and stop talking for a few minutes. Remember that the anger that is being expressed is usually not directed intentionally toward the medical assistant. Be a good listener and allow the person to speak as long as it is not abusive speech. Using logic with the angry individual may also help. Some will use words such as "never" and "always"; for example, "My wife never balances the checkbook!" or "You always make me wait for my appointment!" These statements are broad generalizations and usually untrue. Using a logical approach and maintaining a calm attitude will help the angry individual.

It is very important to address the root of the problem and be willing to admit if the office has made a mistake or contributed to a problem. Do not be afraid to say, "I'm sorry, we made an error." Arguing will never solve the situation and will only increase the intensity of the patient's feelings. Four words that will often disarm an angry person are "Let me help you." There will be times while working in the medical profession that a patient, co-worker, or even the physician will lash out, even though the medical assistant is not the source of their anger. Realize that this is a part of being human, and be as caring and kind as possible. If the anger becomes abusive, either refer the situation to a supervisor, or if that is not possible, tell the patient that you can no longer discuss the situation and offer to schedule an appointment so that the matter can be discussed at a later time. By then, the patient will probably have calmed down and will be able to discuss the situation rationally.

Shock

When an event or a circumstance arises that is especially painful, we may experience emotional shock. A person who has just been told that a family member has been killed in an automobile accident may go into what we call *shock*. There are many different types of shock, but in this chapter, the emotional aspect will be discussed. Often the person cannot think or move, and other coping reactions may take place. One person may scream in agony, whereas another may calmly sit down and begin to talk about a completely unrelated subject. The person who appears calm is probably more at risk, because in addition to shock, there may be a denial process. We never really know in advance how we will react to events that are traumatic. Also, our reactions may differ from time to time. So much depends on what else is happening in a person's life as to how they will be able to cope with a traumatic event.

The first rule is to never leave a person in emotional shock alone. If the healthcare professional cannot stay close by, arrangements should be made for someone to stay near, especially during the early stages, if at all possible. Since the thought processes the person is experiencing may not be under control, he or she could be a danger to himself or herself or others. People who are in shock have a strong need to get away from the situation they have found themselves in. They may try to literally run away, or may speed off in a car, which compounds the situation. The event does not have to be a life-threatening one, but the patient may perceive it as such. For instance, a teenager who becomes pregnant may not be able to focus on anything except her perception that her life is ruined. As with anger, listening is a good disarming tool for dealing with a person in emotional shock.

There are several symptoms of emotional shock that the medical assistant should watch for, including hyperactivity, disruptions in breathing patterns, a blank staring, sudden hysterics, and shaking. Humans have an innate sense of threat or danger, and this sense may initiate what psychologists call the "fight or flight" syndrome. When a person feels a threat of some kind, the hormone adrenaline is released in the body quickly, and this hormone promotes an increased heart rate and blood pressure. The oxygen level in the body increases, which prepares the muscles to help the body flee. Awareness is increased, as is energy and performance. The individual either runs, avoiding the danger, which is the "flight" aspect, or stays to "fight," facing the stressors or threat. With either choice, the body must have this increased energy level and awareness to deal with the situation. When the immediate period of shock abates, the individual may feel a debilitating, drained sensation as the hormonal levels return to normal.

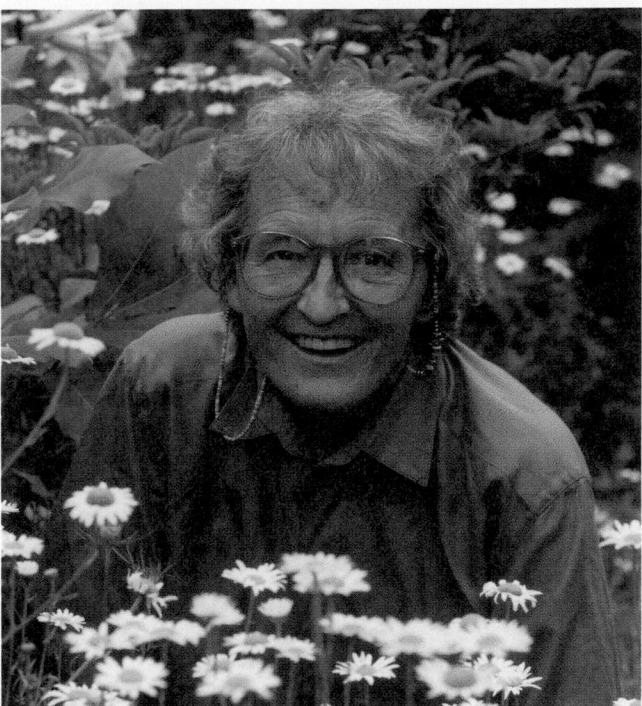

FIGURE 5-8   Dr. Elisabeth Kübler-Ross is the author of more than 20 books, many of which deal with the subject of death and dying, and is considered an international authority on the stages of grief. (Photograph copyright Ken Ross, 1985.)

CRITICAL THINKING APPLICATION

- Is it possible that Sarah might experience shock months after her mother's death?
- How can the medical assistant help Sarah to deal with these emotions?

Death and Dying

Years ago patients who were considered terminally ill were placed in hospital wards and left to their demise. The medical community did not focus on understanding the fears and concerns of the dying, and very few measures that preserved their dignity were offered to them. However, in 1969 a ground-breaking book, *On Death and Dying*, was published by Dr. Elisabeth Kübler-Ross, who studied **thanatology**. Kübler-Ross (Figure 5-8), a Swiss psychiatrist, realized that terminally ill patients were somewhat ignored, even by medical professionals, and she spent many hours interviewing these patients, discovering their fears and concerns. Kübler-Ross listened to them and realized that there were certain stages that patients passed through as they dealt with their impending death. She held seminars during which she interviewed dying patients as medical students listened. When the book was published, she was recognized internationally as an authority on the subject of death. She has written more than 20 books about the process of dying. Kübler-Ross's latest book is about the living. In *Life Lessons*, she shares many of the truths she has learned from the dying to encourage us to live.

Kübler-Ross states that there are five specific stages of the process of **grief**. These stages include denial, bargaining, anger, depression, and acceptance. She believes that all people go through each stage in the grieving process, but they may not go through the stages in the same order. A stage could take days to work through or several months. Although she relates these stages to dying patients, they are not exclusively limited to those who are dying. Anyone experiencing grief may progress through these five stages, and having a good understanding of them will help the medical assistant to better care for the patient.

Denial is the first stage, during which the patient or grieving person denies the issue that is causing the grief and thinks, "No, not me." The person is shocked and rejects the facts. The denial is a defense mechanism that helps the individual to deal with the news. The second stage is anger, when the dying patient begins to ask, "Why me?" The anger is often directed at others, and that may include the people in the family taking care of the patient, or may include healthcare workers who cannot present a cure. In the third stage, the patient begins to bargain in an attempt to postpone death or eliminate it altogether. This bargaining is usually with God, and the patient may pray to see a child marry or to witness some other upcoming event. The event is not the true hope of the patient, but life itself is. These patients say, "Yes, me, but…" in their attempt to postpone their death. The fourth stage is depression, and during this stage patients realize that they are going to die and may feel regret for the goals they did not accomplish or for not taking better care of themselves. These patients say, "Yes, it's me…." and they must be allowed this period of grieving. However, family and friends should watch the patient carefully for signs of deep depression. The final stage of grief is acceptance, during which the patient is able to say, "Yes, me, and I'm ready…." The reality of the impending death is accepted, and although the patient may continue to experience some depression, he or she is better equipped to deal with the arrangements that have to be made and may even demonstrate good humor during this time.

Patients who are dying must be treated with dignity and respect. This does not mean that they are unable to laugh and enjoy the life they are still living. Gentle touch and kind words will help patients to know the medical assistant cares for them. It is important to be careful with words and phrases around dying patients, but be natural in your conversations with them and do not be afraid to laugh. Never suggest to such patients that you "know how they feel." This phrase belittles their situation, and it is a fact that we will really never know how another person feels. Asking questions is a good method of communication when you are not sure what to say. Use questions such as, "How do you feel about that?" or "What does your family think about your plans to discontinue treatment?" Then listen to the patient and make eye contact with him or her as you listen. You may also ask, "How can I help you?" as opposed to "Is there anything I can do?" There will be a natural tendency for the patient to say "No" to the second question. However, if you ask specifically how to help, they may open up and allow you or the office staff to be of help. They may simply need suggestions about who could cut their grass or how to contact Meals on Wheels. Hospice services provide terminally ill patients and their families with care and support, often from the point of diagnosis to bereavement. Many have found hospice services invaluable in the process of coping with a loved one close to death. The medical office should have listings of community resources to assist in many types of situations.

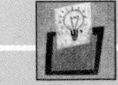

CRITICAL THINKING APPLICATION

- How can the medical assistant help Sarah to deal with her mother's impending death?
- What stage of grief might Mrs. Cloyd currently be experiencing? What stage might Sarah be experiencing?

CRITICAL THINKING APPLICATION

- Often people put off writing a will. Could this be procrastination or a fear of death?
- When is it important to have a will?

Multicultural Issues

Cultural differences influence the way we deal with those from various parts of the world. We often become isolated in our thinking and incorrectly assume that people all over the world think and do things the same way that we do. However, there are vast differences in cultures from country to country, and even from areas within the same country. In the United States we see a difference between Northerners and Southerners. The speech of people in New York is significantly different from that of people in south Texas, and there is still another change in dialect from Texas to the West Coast. We picture Texans with cowboy boots and hats, but that is not how most Texans dress. Some of us still associate Alaska with Eskimos and igloos. Perhaps this stems from the books we read in elementary school, but cultures today are much more widely mixed in the United States, and since many others immigrate to our country for various reasons and opportunities, it is wise to learn a bit more about the cultures and the variety of people that inhabit the world.

We sometimes stereotype people of other cultures and think that we understand what they are like and how they live. Often, some type of **media** has influenced our thinking. There is much to learn from other cultures, and sharing is a way to gain an understanding of the experiences in other places. This helps us to be more well-rounded individuals and to enjoy and appreciate our own cultural differences. Remember that those people who have come to the United States from other countries have to deal with their ideas of both their own homeland and this country as well. There may be significant misconceptions, so in the medical facility, patience will be necessary as explanations are provided. Take extra time and care with patients of other cultures without assuming they know or understand this culture. Also understand that culture is something that is passed from generation to generation, so many of the ideas people hold dear have been handed down for centuries.

Some people who enter a new country go through a period of what is called "culture shock," a state of being in unfamiliar surroundings and being away from the things that were present in everyday life in the homeland. Street signs are different; in some cases, people drive on the opposite side of the street. There is a quick realization that the person's "normal" way of doing things no longer works, and there must be some type of adaptation to survive. This adaptation may mean changing the habits and customs of a lifetime. This can be a very exciting prospect for some, but a very frightening prospect for others. Simple processes, such as enrolling in school, become difficult tasks. Patience is a critical tool to help others adjust to the American way of life.

WHAT OTHER CULTURES THINK OF AMERICANS

We are not the only ones with stereotypical ideas of other cultures—here is what some other cultures think of Americans!

- Outgoing and friendly
- Informal
- Loud, rude, and boastful
- Immature
- Hard-working
- Extravagant
- Wasteful
- Sure they have all the answers
- Disrespectful of authority
- Racially prejudiced
- Ignorant of other countries
- Wealthy
- Generous
- Promiscuous
- Always in a hurry
- Careless with money

From *www.studyabroad.com*.

EXAMPLES OF VARIOUS CULTURAL TRADITIONS

- A husband speaks for his wife. The wife does not speak to the physician.
- The palm of the hand, facing down, is used to beckon someone. The hand motion signaling one to come or follow, performed with the back of the hand toward the patient, is used only when calling an animal. An open hand is used to point, rather than one finger.
- A female's clothing is not removed without the presence of another female family member.
- Emotional crying and sobbing denote femininity.
- Going to the doctor is a sign of weakness.
- The female medical assistant never touches the male patient.
- Acquaintances are not permitted to stand within 3 feet of the patient; only immediate family members are permitted to stand within this space.
- The Chinese do not like to be touched by people they do not know.
- The Laotian's "yes" response may not mean "yes," because it is considered rude to say "no" to others or to cause conflict.
- A native of Cambodia, as well as a Laotian, will not look into the eyes of the person being addressed because long eye contact means disrespect and is impolite.
- Cambodians do not like to have their blood drawn because they believe it will weaken them.
- Afghans and Mexicans have a concept of time that is less precise than in the United States.
- Vietnamese consider the head to be a sacred part of the body and are offended by being touched on the head or shoulders. Only the elderly may touch the head of a child without giving offense.

Communicating With People of Other Cultures

People from other cultures want to be treated just as you would like to be treated if you were visiting another country; they wish to be respected and treated fairly. There is so much to learn about the background of others, and much to share about the culture we know, too. Cultural differences are responsible for many misunderstandings. We must make an attempt to understand people of other walks of life.

When speaking with those from a foreign country, there may be a **language barrier**. Even if the person knows some English, there will be words and phrases that do not make sense in the way that we use them in America. A period of time must pass when the words are heard frequently before they will take on meaning to a person who is unfamiliar with them. It is important to speak a little slower than usual to a person whose primary language is not English. This is not to insinuate they are less intelligent, but it does give them a chance to absorb the words and mentally translate them into their own language, then prepare a response. There is no need to increase the volume of speech—people from other cultures are not hard of hearing. They merely need a little more time to process the words that are said.

Medical assistants should have an awareness of the nonverbal messages being sent by the persons that are interacting. In our society, a simple up-and-down nod of the head means "yes" and a side-to-side shake means "no." However, in Bulgaria and among the Eskimos, these signals have the opposite meaning. It is important to be sensitive to and aware of the beliefs of the many cultures that will be represented in the patient population. If you work in a practice that predominantly serves a distinct ethnic group, discuss possible cultural differences with the physician and with influential people within the cultural group. Learning to understand cultural differences helps you to gain the confidence and respect of patients.

Emotional and Physical Needs

As human beings, there are certain emotional and physical needs that must be met for us to live balanced lives and a healthy existence. Many of us take these needs for granted until they become an absolute necessity, and then our focus becomes directed toward meeting the need. Few in the United States have faced hunger as those in some Third World countries have, and when hunger is our need, it suddenly becomes our prime concern. This section will provide some insight into the needs we have as humans and their role in the total health of the body, mind, and spirit.

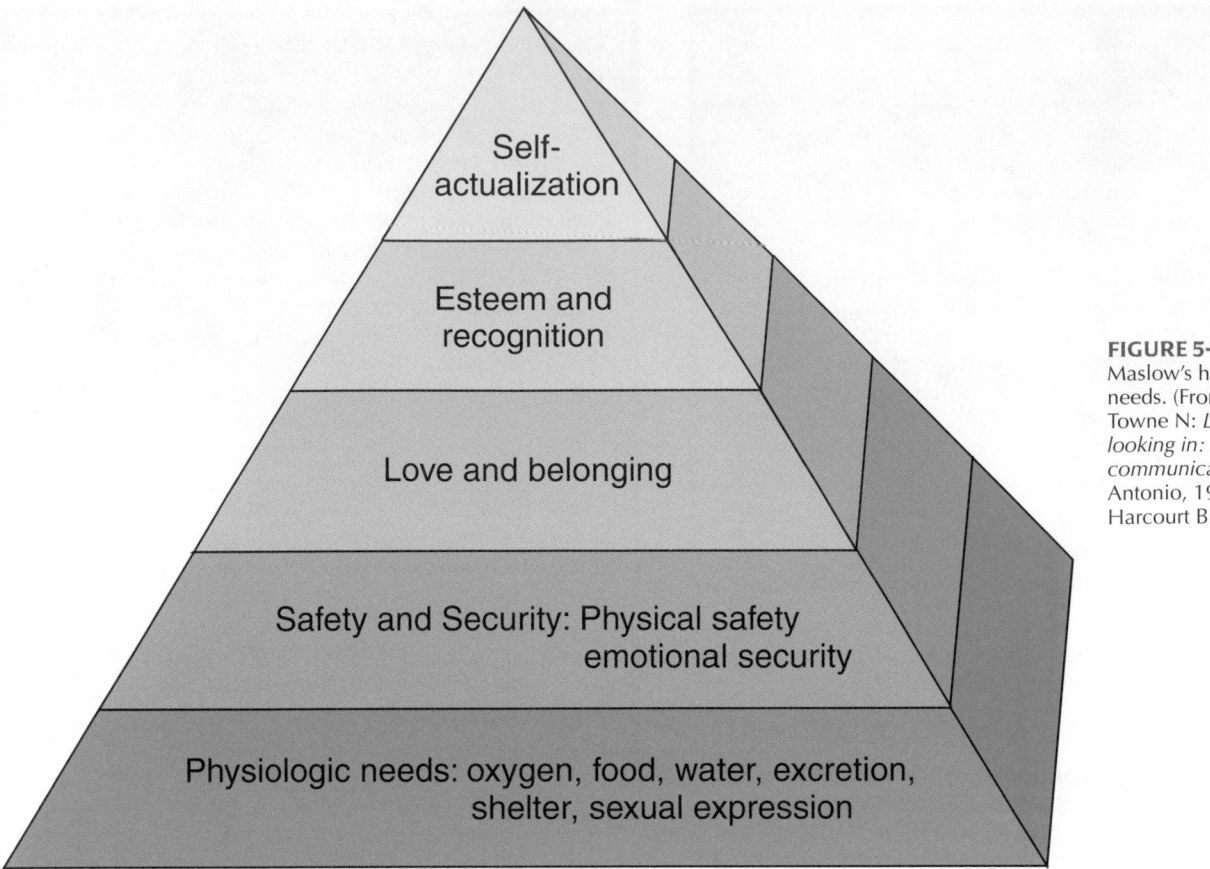

FIGURE 5-9
Maslow's hierarchy of needs. (From Adler RB, Towne N: *Looking out, looking in: interpersonal communication*, San Antonio, 1996, Harcourt Brace.)

Maslow's Hierarchy of Needs

Psychologist Abraham Maslow created what he called the *hierarchy of needs* (Figure 5-9). A hierarchy is defined as "things arranged in order, rank, or a graded series." Maslow believed that our human needs could be categorized into five levels and that the needs on each level had to be satisfied before moving to the next level. These levels are often depicted as a triangle, with the most basic needs at the bottom and the highest potential for growth as a human being at the top.

The needs we have as humans, at the most basic level, are those that involve our physical well-being. This includes food, rest, sleep, water, air, and sex. The second level includes issues related to our safety. We need to feel safe and secure in our homes and our environments, as well as the places where we work. The third level involves our social needs for love, a sense of belonging, and interaction with others. The fourth level relates to our self-esteem. We have an inner need to feel good about ourselves and to know that others view us in a positive manner. The last level is the self-actualization stage, in which we maximize our potential. In this level, we attempt to be at our best, and live our lives to the fullest extent possible.

Approval, Acceptance, and Achievement

There are three specific needs that we have, apart from Maslow's hierarchy of needs, that are critical to our happi-ness. These three needs include approval, acceptance, and achievement. Although most would agree that we do not need everyone's approval at all times, there are specific people whose approval we do seek. Children usually wish to please their parents, even when the child is an adult. We seek to please our supervisors, and even our own children. However, there is the danger of taking this need to please too far. There are books that address personal-ities called *pleasers*, who often place their own needs second to those they feel they must please.

We have a healthier self-esteem if we feel accepted by others. This is similar to the sense of belonging discussed earlier, but is a bit more extensive in nature. A feeling of acceptance includes the belief that our actions, words, dress, mannerisms, and other personality traits are accep-table to others we wish to impress.

Last, we have an inner need for achievement. Most humans want to do something great and contribute to their world in some way. A great thing to one person may be winning an Olympic race, but to another it may be reading to an elderly grandmother at a nursing home. We all enjoy praise for a job well done, or for losing weight, or for passing a difficult examination. It is beneficial to all when legitimate praise is shared freely and appreciated. This is especially true in our close relationships, but just as important in the workplace. It is much easier to work for a supervisor who praises for work well done than for one who never offers a pat on the back.

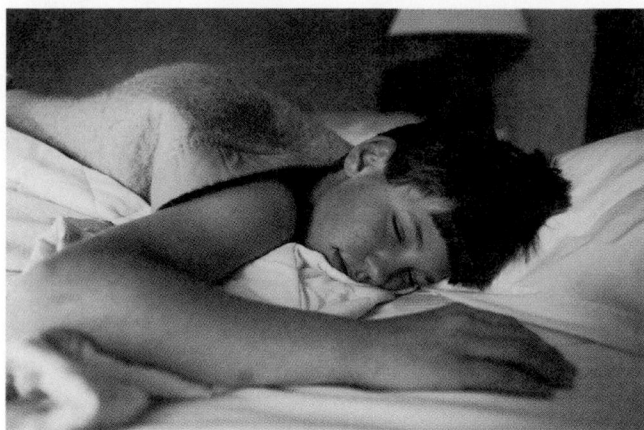

FIGURE 5-10   Sleep is a critically important physical need, the lack of which will eventually take a toll on the body, both physically and mentally.

A Good Night's Sleep

Many of us do not realize the value of our sleep time. Sleep is one of the most important physical needs that we have and is the one most often sacrificed during busy, stressful periods of life. This is called *sleep deprivation*. Human beings need about 8 hours of sleep each night, although many can function for a period of time with less sleep. Eventually this lack of sleep will take a physical and emotional toll on the body (Figure 5-10).

There are two main phases of sleep: nonrapid eye movement (NREM) and rapid eye movement (REM). During NREM sleep the eyes are fairly still and the body relaxes and slows down. There are four stages of NREM, which progress into a deeper sleep. After the body moves through the four stages of NREM, it enters REM sleep. During REM sleep the brain is highly active and the eyes move rapidly. Breathing is more irregular, and most people experience REM sleep in the last few hours of the sleep cycle. Dreaming occurs during REM sleep.

Many professionals who study and treat sleep disturbances agree that if an individual does not reach REM sleep, he or she will have provided physical rest for the body, but not mental rest. This rest is critical in stress management, and because it occurs at the end of most sleep cycles, or during its last hours, those who cut their sleep time short may not enter REM sleep often. Thus they do not get the mental rest that is needed to perform at optimal levels.

Healthy Nutrition

We have been taught since we were children that good nutrition is vital to healthy bodies. Our bodies are machines whose performance depends on good health. We care for the body with a balance of good nutrition, activity, and health care. A balanced diet is essential to ensure that the organs and systems within us function at optimal levels. When the body is not receiving the nutrients and vitamins that it needs, various parts may malfunction, and this can lead to conditions or diseases, or a worsening of the problems already present.

In today's diet-conscious society, some people attempt to lose weight by eating less food or cutting out meals altogether. This is a dangerous practice that prompts the body to hoard the fat stores it has built up, and there is no resulting weight loss. Losing weight quickly through fad diets and miracle supplements is usually a guarantee that the weight will eventually return.

One should always begin weight loss programs under the advice and care of a physician. Do not skip meals in an effort to lose weight and choose foods from the four basic food groups. Avoid unhealthy snacks and sodas, and drink at least 8 to 10 glasses of water every day. Exercise regularly and take walks to provide cardiovascular benefits to the body. By taking good care of your body, the chances are increased that it will function properly for a longer period of time, resulting in a longer, healthier lifetime to enjoy to the fullest.

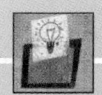

CRITICAL THINKING APPLICATION

- Could Sarah's sleep and nutrition habits affect her ability to care for her mother?
- How might these affect Sarah's personal stress levels and how can she ensure that she is caring for herself, when her thoughts are primarily on her mother?

Positive Relationships

As mentioned earlier in this chapter, all of us need to feel approval, acceptance, and achievement. This is a vital component within our relationships as well. When we are involved in a relationship that is not going well, it will naturally reflect in our attitude, our opinions, and our sense of self-esteem. This can greatly influence the performance we offer at work. Often, because of infatuation, we find ourselves in a situation that might not be a positive one. Once the relationship is in progress, it is sometimes hard to end it and find a connection with a supportive, caring individual.

Many individuals really have not determined what they need from a relationship. It is helpful to make a list of what you are looking for in a partner and commit not to compromise the critical points on the list. The sparks and fireworks that appear in the beginning of a relationship may lose their intensity as time goes on, and there must be a firm foundational base after the newness wears off. Choose carefully and wisely, and the chances of becoming involved in healthy relationships greatly increase. Additionally, more and more individuals are choosing to remain single and enjoying life to the fullest. Certainly this choice is better than being a part of a destructive partnership.

Harmful relationships are not always just between partners. Often we experience stress and strain with relatives, friends, and co-workers. There are times when contact with the person causing the discontent cannot be avoided, at least for a period of time. In these cases, we must learn coping techniques for dealing with the difficult relationship. Open, honest communication is of paramount importance.

Healthy Self-Esteem

Self-esteem is a confidence and satisfaction in oneself. To have good self-esteem, an individual must also be self-aware, and that takes some honesty. It means taking a look at your strengths and your weaknesses, and knowing what you have to offer as a person. To feel well and accomplish goals in life, you must develop positive attitudes and positive responses to the pressures in life (Figure 5-11). It can sometimes be difficult to keep a positive attitude when others around us are being negative. Some people believe that if they inflict their bad feelings on others, they will feel better about themselves. It is important to remember, though, that no one can make you feel a certain way; it is a choice that you make. Blaming others for our situation in life or our negative emotions is self-defeating.

There are two things in life that we are able to control—our attitude and our actions. Even when faced with a potentially volatile situation, our attitude and reactions are decisions that we make. These decisions should be made with careful thought, even if the reaction must be a swift one. Think before speaking. Pause a moment if needed, before reacting. Take a time out. Choose your battles wisely. All of these suggestions will help you to react in a more positive, constructive way when faced with a difficult situation.

Improving Yourself

No matter how great the training or how many opportunities are placed in front of a person, fear and doubt can sabotage efforts to improve the self-image, confidence, and future potential of an individual. Almost every failure or mistake experienced can be traced to fear or doubt; either we are afraid to take a specific action or we doubt our own abilities. Blaming the circumstances around us is no excuse for a poor performance. It is also important to remember that it is the small, daily decisions that make a huge impact on our lives, sometimes even more so than what we consider critical life decisions. For example, a student decides not to study for 30 minutes daily for an upcoming major examination, and then fails it. This small decision to do something other than study results in failing an examination that may force course repetition and delay the graduation date.

Self-esteem will improve if a person is able to adapt to situations well. To be human is to be a changing, growing, imperfect, but amazing living creation. Adapting means being flexible and open to the actions of others. Although we should have empathy for others, we cannot allow others to ruin our day or lower our confidence level. Inventor-philanthropist Charles Kettering once said, "The only time you can't afford to fail is the last time you try." Our failures often teach us much more than our successes. The important thing is to get up, evaluate why the failure occurred, and then move forward armed with the new knowledge gained from mistakes.

Procrastination is often a symptom of the fear of failure and the fear of success. Many people procrastinate because they feel it will give them an excuse for their failure. They say, "There is no way I could pass that test—I only had 2 days to study!" Others are perfectionists and put off doing a job or delegating because they feel no one can do it as well as they can. The best way to stop procrastinating is to do something! Divide projects into small steps and complete one at a time. This makes tasks much less overwhelming.

The self-improvement process is ongoing. Periodically stop and evaluate where you stand in relation to the goals you have set for your life. Set goals for all of the areas of life—short- and long-term—including career, relationships, and personal growth. Write the goals down and make them specific and measurable. Be sure that the goals are reasonable. Start with smaller, short-term goals and work toward long-term goals. Be persistent and never give up. Post a list of them on the refrigerator and note progress. Do not count on having a whole lifetime to pursue goals; instead, move toward them consistently and enthusiastically.

Comfort Zones

We all have comfort zones. When faced with new ideas or changes, many of us tend to be a bit unsure of ourselves. Think back to the first day at school, the first day on a new job, the first time going to a fancy restaurant, a first date—

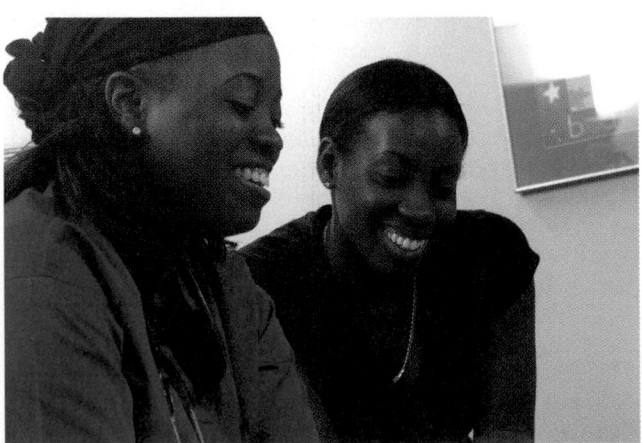

FIGURE 5-11 A healthy self-esteem will help the medical assistant keep a positive attitude and seek to improve performance. It will also encourage growth in the profession and personally.

these events often make us feel a bit uncomfortable. New experiences may be outside of our **comfort zone**. Psychologists often speak about a comfort zone, which is a place in the mind where we feel safe and comfortable, where we can perform comfortably and confidently. Most goals, however, require movement outside the comfort zone to reach them. Striving to reach a goal means trying new things, and this can be quite stressful. Since we do not want to become so stressed that we give up on our goals, we should take slow, small steps that are challenging and then move to the next step. Procrastination is a failure concept, but can be overcome through dedication and consistent planning.

Remember, too, that patients are usually outside of their comfort zones while visiting the physician's office. Do everything possible to make them feel at home and comfortable.

Closing Comments

Interpersonal skills are critically important to the successful medical assistant. Communication will be a part of all interactions throughout the day, and the better developed these skills are, the better the medical assistant will be able to serve the patients in the facility. Every attempt should be made to enhance the interpersonal and human relations skills that the medical assistant currently has, and strive to better these skills continually. This will ensure that effective communication will be a part of the relationship with patients as well as others with whom the medical assistant interacts.

Patient Education

The medical assistant has the opportunity to provide an educational service to every patient who enters the medical facility. Patients will often have questions about their care or treatment, and the medical assistant with good communication skills will be able to assist the patient in understanding.

Patients must have clear knowledge of the role they play in their own care. The medical assistant can communicate information to the patient in many ways other than verbally. Leaflets and brochures can help patients to understand their illness better and will educate them, but the medical assistant should always explain each piece of literature given to a patient. Never just hand them out and expect them to be read. Have patients clarify instructions given by repeating them if there is a question of their understanding.

Often patients will need to be educated about the community resources available to them. It is wise to keep an ongoing list of local community services and agencies that can assist patients. Remember that physical care is not the only aspect of patient care; they have emotional needs as well. Often the very things we take for granted, such as food and shelter, are struggles for patients, and this stress can worsen their physical condition. Ask questions and be aware of what the patient is communicating to the staff. This will help the medical assistant to best serve the patient.

Legal and Ethical Issues

Patients see the medical assistant as an extension of the physician, so it is important that all communication with the patient be professional and accurate. Never give a patient advice that is not approved by the physician to avoid accusations of practicing medicine without a license. Always discuss issues with the physician that affect the patient's care in any way. Never agree to withhold any information from the physician, because even a small piece of information could completely change his or her plan of treatment. When giving instructions to patients, it is always best to have them in writing and keep a copy for the patient's chart so that there is a written record of what was communicated to the patient. Use excellent documentation technique when adding information to the patient's chart. Remember that all of the patients in the facility deserve to be treated with respect and compassion. Help the physician to establish trust with the patient. An open, trusting relationship with the patient will help to avoid legal issues in the future.

SUMMARY OF SCENARIO

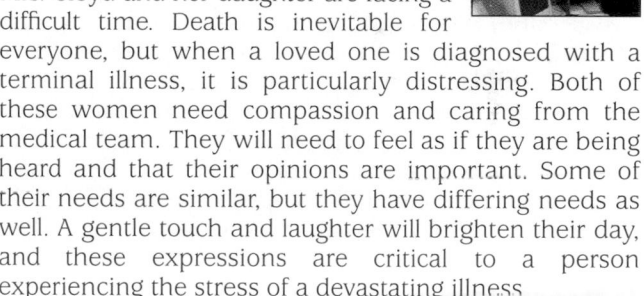

Mrs. Cloyd and her daughter are facing a difficult time. Death is inevitable for everyone, but when a loved one is diagnosed with a terminal illness, it is particularly distressing. Both of these women need compassion and caring from the medical team. They will need to feel as if they are being heard and that their opinions are important. Some of their needs are similar, but they have differing needs as well. A gentle touch and laughter will brighten their day, and these expressions are critical to a person experiencing the stress of a devastating illness.

The medical assistant must ensure that Mrs. Cloyd understands her medications and treatments. The office should assist her and her daughter in finding community resources for which she might be eligible. Be sure to instruct Mrs. Cloyd primarily, and make certain that Sarah also understands any directions her mother should follow. Sarah will need compassion as she deals with her mother's illness and impending death. Since she is also a patient of the clinic, she should be given care and attention and may have emotional needs or periods of great stress also. Even on the busiest of days, these two women deserve warmth from the staff and should be made as comfortable as possible as they seek medical care.

SUMMARY OF LEARNING OBJECTIVES

■ First impressions are critical in the medical profession. Dress, attitude, and appearance will all influence the credibility of the medical assistant. The medical assistant should always treat patients and visitors to the office as individuals who deserve the best in customer service.

■ Verbal communication depends on words and sound, while nonverbal communication is messages that are conveyed to another without the use of words. Body language, eye contact, facial expressions, and hand gestures are some of the many ways we use body language. Sometimes our body language conflicts with verbal communication and sends mixed signals to the receiver. Often we are unaware of nonverbal signals and notice only a small number of the signals that other people send.

■ Spatial separation can be defined as the space of comfort between individuals. Public space is usually considered to be 12 to 25 feet, whereas social space is about 4 to 12 feet. Personal space is the range of 1.5 to 4 feet, and intimate space would include touching up to about 1.5 feet.

■ Touch is important in the process of communication because it projects an air of care and compassion to the receiver. The medical assistant should never be afraid to touch patients, as long as precautions are taken with those who are contagious. Touching the patient shows empathy and often can be more eloquent than the spoken word.

■ The transactional communication model includes a sender and a receiver who both offer messages to each other using various channels. The sender encodes a message and then the receiver decodes it, to the best of his or her ability. Often some type of noise interferes as well, such as internal, external, and physiological noise. Perception is important when communicating because messages are sometimes easily misinterpreted.

■ Some of the barriers to communication include physical impairment, language differences, prejudice, stereotyping, and perception. Barriers may also be present during difficult times, such as a crisis, when angry or in shock, or when a patient or family member is experiencing an impending death or serious accident or illness.

■ Maslow's hierarchy of needs includes five levels, beginning with our most basic needs, such as food, rest, sleep, water, or anything that involves our physical well-being. The second level is related to safety issues, and the third, our social needs, such as love and interaction with others. The fourth level deals with our self-esteem, and the fifth is self-actualization, where our potential is maximized.

■ Defense mechanisms are psychological methods of dealing with stressful situations, and include sarcasm, denial, repression, compensation, and several others. Often these mechanisms are our only way of dealing with circumstances that are difficult to cope with.

■ Listening is one of the most important skills the medical assistant can possess. Listening involves not only silence, but active feedback as well. Open-ended questions help the medical assistant to restate what the patient is saying, to be sure that the patient is understood clearly.

■ Everyone experiences conflict in daily living, so it is necessary to develop skills in dealing with conflict in as positive a way as possible. Conflict is not always negative and can be quite beneficial to relationships. Knowing the different types of conflict, as well as how people attempt to process conflict, will help the medical assistant to recognize patterns and respond appropriately.

■ Elisabeth Kübler-Ross suggests that there are five stages to the process of grief, which include denial, bargaining, anger, depression, and acceptance. She believes that all stages are experienced while grieving, but not necessarily in the same order. The medical assistant can better care for the patient and the patient's loved ones when there is a good understanding of the grieving process.

■ Everyone needs physical and emotional rest to function throughout the day. A good night's sleep, consisting of at least 8 hours, regular exercise, and healthy nutrition will help to keep the medical assistant fit for duty.

KEY INTERNET WEBSITES

- Elisabeth Kübler-Ross
- Hospice Foundation of America
- Toastmasters International
  For active weblinks to each website visit
  http://evolve.elsevier.com/Kinn/

CHAPTER 6

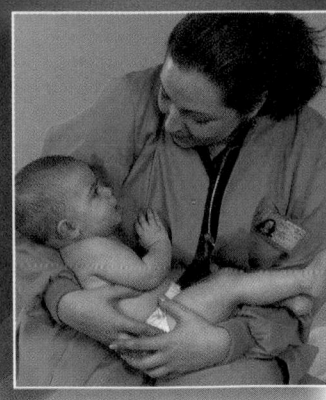

Scenario

Monica Johnson has been employed for 6 months as a medical assistant in a family practice. She works as the clinical medical assistant for Dr. Richard Wray. One of Dr. Wray's patients, Anna Walsh, recently adopted a baby after 8 years of trying to conceive a child. The baby, Delaney Gracelia, was born to a single mother, Susan, who participated in an open adoption in which she and the Walshes met and got to know each other during her pregnancy.

Dr. Wray performed some genetic testing on Delaney, and the adoptive parents were involved throughout the pregnancy, even meeting Delaney's birth mother for physician appointments from time to time. Monica observed both Susan and the Walshes and saw many benefits from the arrangement, noticing that everyone was primarily concerned with Delaney and her happiness and well-being. However, there were periods that were difficult as well for both sides. This prompted Monica to give some thought to her own feelings and ideas about many different ethical situations and issues and how she would react in the face of making ethical decisions.

Medicine and Ethics

Learning Objectives

- Define and spell the terms listed in the vocabulary.
- Explain rights and duties as related to ethics.
- List and define the four types of ethical problems.
- Discuss the process used for making an ethical decision.
- Detail the impact that the CEJA has on the ethical decisions made by healthcare professionals.
- Describe the way unique identifiers help HIV-positive patients to avoid some discrimination.
- Note some of the concerns regarding ethics that surround genetic information.
- Explain why confidentiality is an ethical issue.
- Discuss several of the CEJA opinions and how they might differ from the views of the class as a whole.

National Curriculum Competencies

TRANSDISCIPLINARY COMPETENCIES

2a. Identify and respond to issue of confidentiality
2b. Perform within legal and ethical boundaries

Vocabulary

allocating Apportioning for a specific purpose or to particular persons or things.

advocate One who pleads the cause of another; one who defends or maintains a cause or proposal.

annotation A note added by way of comment or explanation.

beneficence The act of doing or producing good, especially performing acts of charity or kindness.

clinical trials Research studies that test how well new medical treatments or other interventions work in the subjects, usually human beings.

disposition The tendency of something or someone to act in a certain manner under given circumstances.

duty Obligatory tasks, conduct, service, or functions that arise from one's position, as in life or in a group.

euthanasia The act or practice of killing or permitting the death of hopelessly sick or injured individuals in a relatively painless way for reasons of mercy.

fidelity Faithfulness to something to which one is bound by pledge or duty.

gametes Mature male or female germ cells usually possessing a haploid chromosome set and capable of initiating formation of a new diploid individual.

genome The genetic material of an organism.

idealism The practice of forming ideas or living under the influence of ideas.

infertile Not fertile or productive; not capable of reproducing.

introspection An inward, reflective examination of one's own thoughts and feelings.

nonmaleficence Refraining from the act of harming or committing evil.

opinion A formal expression of judgment or advice by an expert; the formal expression of the legal reasons and principles on which a legal decision is based.

philosopher A person who seeks wisdom or enlightenment; an expounder of a theory in a certain area of experience.

postmortem Done, collected, or occurring after death.

public domain The realm embracing property rights that belong to the community at large, are unprotected by copyright or patent, and are subject to use or appropriation by anyone.

ramifications Consequences produced by a cause or following from a set of conditions.

reparations The act of making amends, offering atonement, or giving satisfaction from a wrong or injury.

sociological Oriented or directed toward social needs and problems.

surrogate A substitute; to put in place of another.

unique identifiers Codes used instead of names to protect the confidentiality of the patient in a method of anonymous HIV testing.

veracity A devotion to or conformity with the truth.

*E*thics is defined as the thoughts, judgments, and actions on issues that have implications of moral right and wrong. The concept of ethics concerns itself with the philosophies underlying ideal relationships between human beings, as well as the promotion of the highest good for humanity as a whole. There are various beliefs about what is and is not ethical in everyday life and in the medical profession. The decisions that people make based on ethical beliefs can quite possibly alter the course of human existence.

A medical assistant must not only have a strong knowledge base about ethical issues that might be faced throughout the profession, but must also come to terms with some of the deeply rooted value systems that have been a part of his or her life since youth. The trials and tribulations we have experienced, as well as the joys, will all influence our thought patterns when we are faced with an opportunity to make a good ethical decision.

History of Ethics in Medicine

From earliest recorded history, humans have pondered ethics—the judgment of right and wrong. Ethics should not be confused with etiquette. *Etiquette* refers to courtesy, customs, and manners, whereas ethics explores the moral right or wrong of an issue. It is not surprising that for centuries the field of medicine has set for itself a rigid standard of ethical conduct toward patients and professional colleagues.

The earliest written code of ethical conduct for medical practice was conceived about 2250 BC by the Babylonians and was called the Code of Hammurabi. It elaborated on the conduct expected of a physician and even set the fees that a physician could charge. The Code was quite lengthy and detailed, which is the probable reason it did not survive the ages. About 400 BC Hippocrates, the Greek physician known as the Father of Medicine, developed a brief statement of principles that remains an inspiration to the physicians of today. The Oath of Hippocrates has been administered to many medical graduates (Figure 6-1). The most significant contribution to medical ethics after the time of Hippocrates was that of Thomas Percival. Percival was a physician, **philosopher**, and writer from Manchester, England. In 1803 he published his Code of Medical Ethics. Percival was very interested in **sociological** matters and took a great interest in the study of ethical concepts as related to the medical profession.

In 1846, as the American Medical Association (AMA) was being organized in New York City, medical education and medical ethics were already considered important aspects of the profession. At the first annual AMA meeting in 1847, a Code of Ethics was formulated and adopted. It specifically acknowledged Percival's code as its foundation, and this document became a part of the fundamental standards of the AMA and its component parts. Even today there are sections of the AMA Code of Ethics that stem from Percival's writings.

Who Decides What is Ethical?

When we weigh the question of who decides what is ethical, the answer is evident: you do. Every day medical professionals face the task of making ethical decisions.

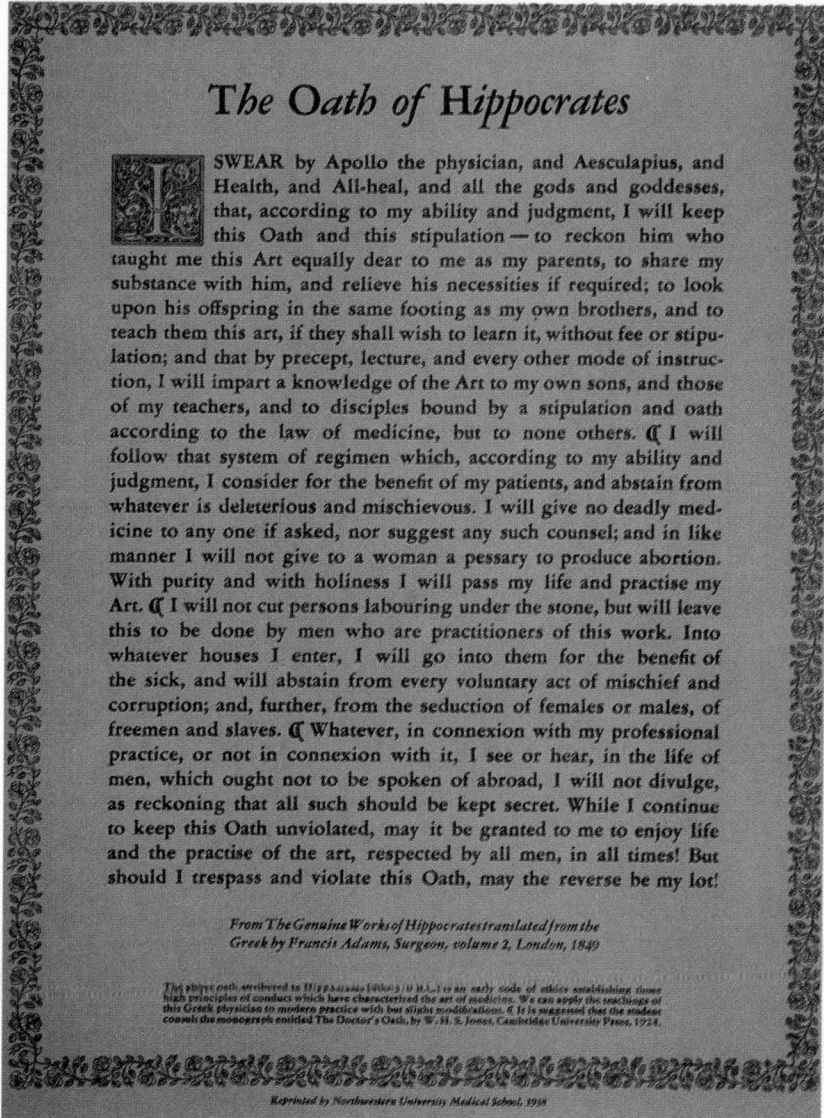

The Oath of Hippocrates

I SWEAR by Apollo the physician, and Aesculapius, and Health, and All-heal, and all the gods and goddesses, that, according to my ability and judgment, I will keep this Oath and this stipulation — to reckon him who taught me this Art equally dear to me as my parents, to share my substance with him, and relieve his necessities if required; to look upon his offspring in the same footing as my own brothers, and to teach them this art, if they shall wish to learn it, without fee or stipulation; and that by precept, lecture, and every other mode of instruction, I will impart a knowledge of the Art to my own sons, and those of my teachers, and to disciples bound by a stipulation and oath according to the law of medicine, but to none others. ❡ I will follow that system of regimen which, according to my ability and judgment, I consider for the benefit of my patients, and abstain from whatever is deleterious and mischievous. I will give no deadly medicine to any one if asked, nor suggest any such counsel; and in like manner I will not give to a woman a pessary to produce abortion. With purity and with holiness I will pass my life and practise my Art. ❡ I will not cut persons labouring under the stone, but will leave this to be done by men who are practitioners of this work. Into whatever houses I enter, I will go into them for the benefit of the sick, and will abstain from every voluntary act of mischief and corruption; and, further, from the seduction of females or males, of freemen and slaves. ❡ Whatever, in connexion with my professional practice, or not in connexion with it, I see or hear, in the life of men, which ought not to be spoken of abroad, I will not divulge, as reckoning that all such should be kept secret. While I continue to keep this Oath unviolated, may it be granted to me to enjoy life and the practise of the art, respected by all men, in all times! But should I trespass and violate this Oath, may the reverse be my lot!

From The Genuine Works of Hippocrates translated from the Greek by Francis Adams, Surgeon, volume 2, London, 1849

The above oath attributed to Hippocrates (460-370 B.C.) is an early code of ethics establishing those high principles of conduct which have characterized the art of medicine. We can apply the teachings of this Greek physician to modern practice with but slight modifications. It is suggested that the student consult the monograph entitled The Doctor's Oath, by W. H. S. Jones, Cambridge University Press, 1924.

Reprinted by Northwestern University Medical School, 1958

FIGURE 6-1   The Oath of Hippocrates. (Courtesy National Library of Medicine.)

Although many different groups of people meet to discuss the ethics of a procedure or decision from the local level to national and worldwide levels, fundamentally, each individual decides what is ethical and what is not for him or her and the individuals these decisions will affect. As with any important choice, one must consider the short- and long-term effects and consequences. Although it is a completely acceptable practice to depend on groups and committees to guide ethical decisions, the responsibility for making these decisions ultimately rests with the individual (Figure 6-2).

Organizations that study ethical dilemmas may decide that a concept such as abortion is an ethical medical practice. But if an individual does not find abortion to be an acceptable practice for religious or other reasons, abortion is not ethical for that individual. A great freedom that Americans often take for granted is that we can exercise free will in decisions related to individual conscience in this country, that we can choose from a variety of options—but we must exercise this responsibility carefully.

CRITICAL THINKING APPLICATION

- Monica knows that she has deep-rooted thoughts and ideas about many ethical matters. However, she has never really thought about where she formed her ideas. Where do we get most of our opinions on ethical or moral issues?
- What is the difference between an opinion's being "our own" and being someone else's?

The Role of the AMA and CEJA Regarding Ethics

The AMA serves physicians as a national organization providing various types of information and support. One of the most important facets of the AMA is its Council on Ethical and Judicial Affairs (CEJA). The CEJA consists of

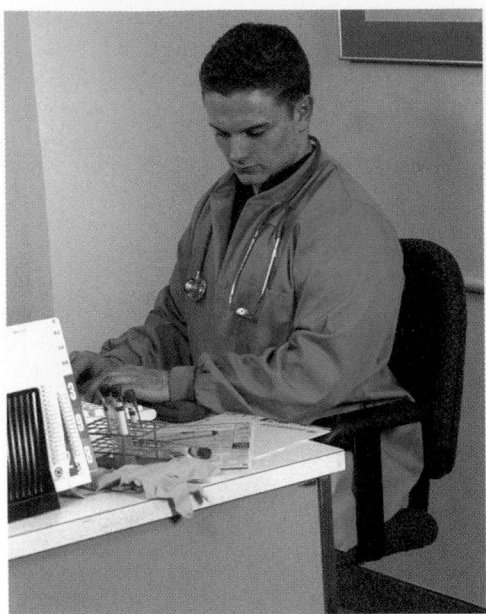

FIGURE 6-2 Medical assistants may find themselves making ethical decisions on a daily basis.

nine active members of the AMA, including one resident physician member and one medical student member, and is responsible for interpreting the Principles of Medical Ethics as adopted by the House of Delegates of the AMA. The AMA's Code of Ethics has four components:

- Principles of medical ethics
- The fundamental elements of the patient-physician relationship
- Current opinions of the CEJA with **annotations**
- Reports of the CEJA

The *Code of Medical Ethics: Current Opinions with Annotations* is a publication that contains the first three components, with discussion of more than 135 ethical issues encountered in medicine. A separate publication, *Reports of the Council on Ethical and Judicial Affairs*, discusses the rationale of the Council's **opinions** (Figure 6-3).

The AMA Principles of Medical Ethics has been revised several times to follow current trends in medicine, but there has never been a change in the moral intent or overall **idealism** of the statements. In 1957 the AMA Principles of Medical Ethics was condensed to a preamble and ten sections. In 1980 the principles were reduced to seven sections to clarify and update the language, eliminate ref-

---

FUNDAMENTAL ELEMENTS OF THE PATIENT-PHYSICIAN RELATIONSHIP

From ancient times, physicians have recognized that the health and well-being of patients depend on a collaborative effort between physician and patient. Patients share with physicians the responsibility for their own healthcare. The patient-physician relationship is of greatest benefit to patients when they bring medical problems to the attention of their physicians in a timely fashion, provide information about their medical condition to the best of their ability, and work with their physicians in a mutually respectful alliance. Physicians can best contribute to this alliance by serving as their patients' advocates and by fostering these rights:

1. The patient has the right to receive information from physicians and to discuss the benefits, risks, and costs of appropriate treatment alternatives. Patients should receive guidance from their physicians as to the optimal course of action. Patients are also entitled to obtain copies or summaries of their medical records, to have their questions answered, to be advised of potential conflicts of interest that their physicians might have, and to receive independent professional opinions.

2. The patient has the right to make decisions regarding the healthcare that is recommended by his or her physician. Accordingly, patients may accept or refuse any recommended medical treatment.

3. The patient has the right to courtesy, respect, dignity, responsiveness, and timely attention to his or her needs.

4. The patient has the right to confidentiality. The physician should not reveal confidential communications or information without the consent of the patient, unless provided for by law or by the need to protect the welfare of the individual or the public interest.

5. The patient has the right to continuity of healthcare. The physician has an obligation to cooperate in the coordination of medically indicated care with other healthcare providers treating the patient. The physician may not discontinue treatment of a patient as long as further treatment is medically indicated, without giving the patient reasonable assistance and sufficient opportunity to make alternative arrangements for care.

6. The patient has a basic right to have available adequate healthcare. Physicians, along with the rest of society, should continue to work toward this goal. Fulfillment of this right is dependent on society providing resources so that no patient is deprived of necessary care because of an inability to pay for the care. Physicians should continue their traditional assumption of a part of the responsibility for the medical care of those who cannot afford essential healthcare. Physicians should advocate for patients in dealing with third parties when appropriate.

FIGURE 6-3 Fundamental elements of the patient-physician relationship. (From *Report of the Council on Ethical and Judicial Affairs of the American Medical Association*. Originally adopted June 1990; last updated August 2001. http://www.ama-assn.org/ama/pub/category/5425.html Report #26 1990.)

erence to gender, and seek a proper and reasonable balance between professional standards and contemporary legal standards in our changing society. The most recently adopted changes, presented at the 2001 Annual Meeting of the AMA House of Delegates, reflect wording consistent with today's privacy issues and stress the importance of informed consent in DNA database information in genomic research. Several opinions were issued at the 2001 Interim meeting involving filming patients in healthcare settings, performing procedures on newly deceased persons for training purposes, and confidentiality of health information **postmortem**.

Making Ethical Decisions

Before discussing the opinions of AMA's Council on Ethical and Judicial Affairs, it is best to understand a few of the elements of ethics, the different types of ethical problems, and how a good ethical decision is made. Then, as some of the opinions are presented in this text, students can begin to evaluate their own positions regarding each issue. This section will enable the medical assistant to recognize the type of ethical problem that might present in the physician's office and provide a pattern to follow when making an ethical decision.

Elements of Ethics

Ruth Purtilo, in her book, *Ethical Dimensions in the Health Professions*, presents three general elements of ethics: duties, rights, and character traits. A **duty** is an obligation that a person has or perceives himself or herself to have. A daughter may feel the obligation to care for her elderly parents, or a husband who has hurt his spouse may feel an obligation to somehow make up for his act.

There are several types of duties that Purtilo mentions that relate to the medical profession. **Nonmaleficence** refers to refraining from harming the self or another person. **Beneficence** refers to bringing about good. **Fidelity** is the concept of promise-keeping, and **veracity** refers to the duty of telling the truth. Justice, in relation to medical ethics, deals with the fair distribution of benefits and burdens among individuals or groups in society having legitimate claims on those benefits. When a person has wronged another, he or she has a duty to make **reparations**, or right the wrong. Last, a person should feel grateful after being the beneficiary of someone else's goodness. This is also a type of duty.

Rights are defined as claims that a person or group makes on society, a group, or an individual. The Bill of Rights appended to the U.S. Constitution guarantees certain liberties that we enjoy as American citizens. However, some individuals think that they have rights that are really privileges. For instance, Americans do not have the "right" to healthcare services. There are some countries that provide medical care to all its citizens, but the United States is not one of those countries. A right applies to all people within a group, without prejudice. One of the most intense ethical arguments faced today is the right-to-life concept. If our Constitution states that we all have the right to life, liberty, and the pursuit of happiness, how can abortion be considered ethical? Or if an individual is trying to end his

or her suffering from a terminal illness, could the "pursuit of happiness" be interpreted to include seeking a physician's help in committing suicide? These are the types of ethical questions that arise in the healthcare field.

Character traits are defined in Purtilo's book as a **disposition** to act in a certain way. A person who feels honesty is an important character trait can usually be trusted to speak the truth. One who feels that it is acceptable to take small items from work for use at home may not be able to resist an opportunity to take something more valuable. Character traits will certainly not always provide an indication of how a person will react in all situations. No human being is perfect, and we are sometimes unpredictable. Stress can also interfere with our normal reactions, and there are other factors, such as depression or anger, that will influence how we act as well. The phrase that someone is acting "out of character" usually means that he or she is deviating from his or her normal behavior patterns.

With an understanding of these basic elements of ethics, we have a good foundation that will help us to look more objectively at ethical problems and then solve them to the best of our ability.

Types of Ethical Problems

Purtilo presents four basic types of ethical problems (Figure 6-4). They are:
- Ethical distress
- Ethical dilemmas
- Dilemmas of justice
- Locus of authority issues

Ethical distress is the type of problem faced when a certain course of action is indicated, but there is some type of hindrance or barrier preventing that action. A professional knows the right thing to do, but for whatever reason, cannot do it.

An ethical dilemma is a situation in which an individual is faced with two or more choices that are acceptable and correct, but doing one precludes doing another. A choice must be made, and there may be a loss of something of value if a second choice is eliminated. This could be viewed as the proverbial "being caught between a rock and a hard place," whereby a choice must be made that has more of an affect than what may be seen on the surface.

The third type of ethical problem is the dilemma of justice. This problem focuses on the fair distribution of benefits to those who are entitled to them. Choices must be made as to who receives these benefits and in what portion. A few examples of the dilemma of justice would include organ donations and distribution of scarce or pricey medications.

In locus of authority issues, there are two or more authority figures with their own ideas about how a situation should be handled, but only one of those authorities will prevail. If one physician feels a patient should have surgery and another does not, how does the patient decide (Figure 6-5)?

Recognizing the type of ethical problem is not always easy. Sometimes a medical professional is faced with an issue that is a mixture of one or more types of ethical problems. When possible, it is wise to take some time in weighing the right course of action to take before making

---

WHAT SHOULD BE DONE?

---

1. **Ethical Distress**
   I know which course of action I (the "agent") should take for the patient's benefit, but there is a structural barrier to my being able to do it.

   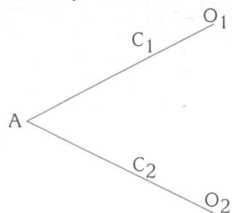

   A = Agent
   C = Course of Action
   O = Outcome

2. **Ethical Dilemma**
   There are two (or more) courses of action, each of which is right (or wrong). No matter which one I (the "agent") choose, something of value will be compromised.

3. **Distributive Justice**
   There are benefits to be distributed among several potential beneficiaries. Not everyone can receive a full measure of the benefit. On what basis should the distribution be made?

   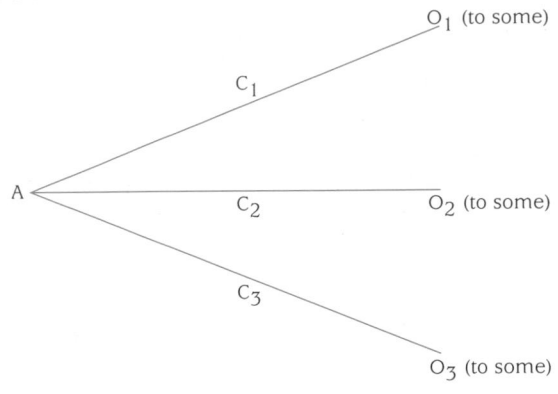

WHO SHOULD DO IT?

---

4. **Locus of Authority**
   There are 2 (or more) agents or "authorities" in this situation. Each believes he or she knows what outcome will benefit the patient the most, but only one authority will prevail.

   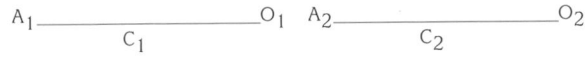

FIGURE 6-4 Summary of types of ethical problems. (From Purtilo R: *Ethical dimensions in the health professions*, ed 3, Philadelphia, 1999, WB Saunders.)

an important decision. Unfortunately, this is not always possible in the fast pace of the medical profession. Some decisions must be made in a split second, so it is wise to have a thorough grasp of ethical decision-making before the need arises.

The Ethical Decision-Making Process

Purtilo presents a five-step process for ethical decision-making in her book. The steps include:

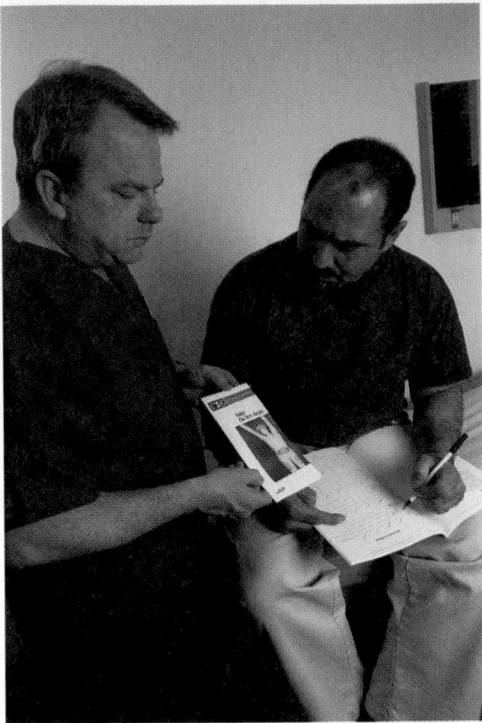

FIGURE 6-5 One of the duties of a medical assistant is to ensure that the patient understands the instructions given.

- Gathering relevant information
- Identifying the type of ethical problem
- Determining the ethics approach to use
- Exploring the practical alternatives
- Completing the action

While gathering information, a medical professional should ask questions, review charts, talk to the patient and other professionals, and search for other data so that the full view of the situation is available for scrutiny. Once the information is gathered, the medical professional must decide which ethical problem or problems are being presented. In determining the ethical approach to use, we must consider duties, rights, and character traits of all the individuals involved with this issue, paying close attention to the **ramifications** of all possible decisions. All of the alternatives must be considered and evaluated, and then an action should be taken.

CRITICAL THINKING APPLICATION

- What are the ramifications of an open adoption such as Delaney's? What problems might occur during the first year of her life?
- How might these problems be avoided?
- What are the positive aspects of the adoption?

Although it is best to have a space of time to give these areas some thought, this may not always be possible. It is a good practice for those entering the medical profession to take stock of what their core beliefs are. Scan the news-

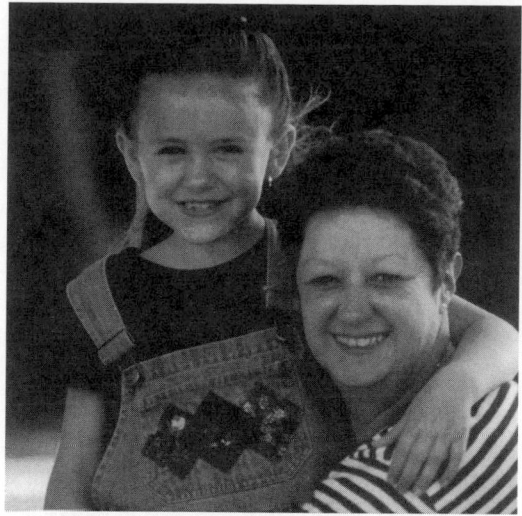

FIGURE 6-6   Norma McCorvey was "Jane Roe" in *Roe v. Wade*, the Supreme Court decision that legalized abortion. More than 20 years later, she became one of the pro-life movement's biggest advocates.

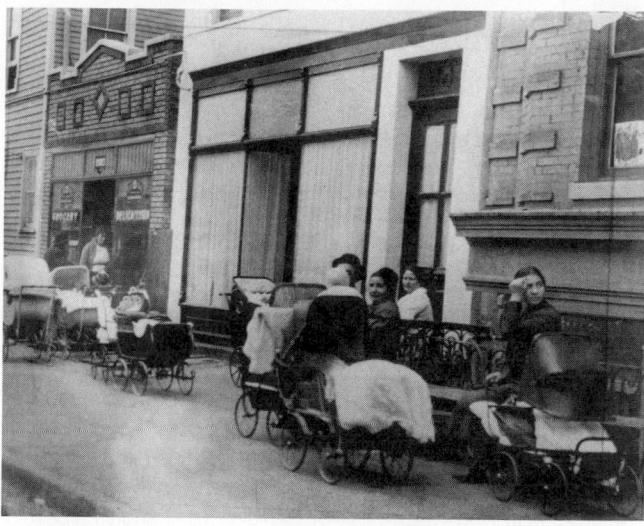

FIGURE 6-7   Margaret Sanger and her associates opened America's first birth control clinic on October 16, 1916, and women lined up on the street before the doors opened. The police closed the clinic on its tenth day, after providing advice and counseling to just 488 women. (Photo from Margaret Sanger Papers, Sophia Smith Collections, Smith College.)

papers and search professional journals for ethical situations, think about the facts, and then decide how you would react to each one. This is excellent preparation for the day that you will be faced with making a quick ethical decision.

Current Opinions of the CEJA and Medicine's Ethical Issues

Now, armed with a basic knowledge about the types of ethical problems and the process used to solve them, we will take a look at some of the Council opinions. Remember, physicians and other medical professionals are not bound to abide by the CEJA opinions. They have the freedom to make their own decisions, but many of the medical professionals in our country tend to agree with the decisions made by the committee.

Abortion

In 1973 the U.S. Supreme Court heard the case of *Roe v. Wade*. Since that ruling, abortion has been one of the most volatile issues with which the CEJA deals. According to the Principles of Medical Ethics, the AMA does not prohibit a physician from performing an abortion in accordance with good medical practice and under circumstances that do not violate the law (Figure 6-6). In recent years laws have been passed in some states requiring mandatory parental notification of a minor's intent to have an abortion. In some cases this means that the minor must have parental consent, and in others, parents must only be notified of their daughter's intent to have an abortion. Some states also require a 24-hour or more waiting period after the notification has been made.

The AMA strongly encourages physicians to persuade the minor toward seeking counseling with someone she trusts, such as a school counselor, teacher, or relative, if the minor's parent is not to be involved in the abortion

decision. However, the AMA agrees that the physician should not feel compelled to require minors to involve the parent in the decision. Medical professionals must be aware of the laws in their respective states that deal with the mandatory notification requirements and should contact the medical societies in their region to determine what constitutes proper notification.

In early 2002 the Bush administration proposed a change in the regulations of the Department of Health and Human Services (DHHS) that would give states the right to classify a fetus as an unborn child eligible for some government-paid health assistance, including prenatal care. This move enraged abortion supporters, who felt that the prenatal care definition could have been extended to pregnant women instead of the unborn child, which they felt sets the stage for anti-choice legislation. The change would alter the definition so that states would be able to provide coverage for children from *conception* to age 19, instead of the current wording, which defines a child as an individual under the age of 19. The issue of abortion continues to spark disagreement in the United States and abroad (Figure 6-7).

Case to Discuss: Should a woman who has been raped and become pregnant seek an abortion?

Abuse

The AMA requires that a physician be familiar with the signs of physical, psychological, and sexual abuse of spouses, children, mentally incompetent persons, and the elderly. Discovery of abuse creates a difficult situation for a medical professional. The patient may be the object of abuse but deny its existence because of fear of further attacks. The law requires that abuse be reported, and if the physician does not report abuse, ethical standards have also been breached. In addition, the abuse may continue. Any medical assistant who suspects abuse must report this information to the physician first, who must determine whether the incident is reportable by law and take action. If action is not taken, the medical assistant is responsible for making a report.

Case to Discuss: What harm can come to a patient's family if the medical professionals are incorrect about their assessment of abuse?

Allocation of Health Resources

Sometimes society must decide who will receive care when serving all who need care is not possible. Decisions must be made fairly and should be weighed carefully. The criteria to consider when **allocating** health resources include urgency of need, likelihood of benefit, duration of benefit, amount of resources required for successful treatment, and potential for change in quality of life. Nonmedical criteria should not be considered, such as ability to pay, social worth of the individual, age, obstacles to treatment, or the patient's contribution to the illness. The physician who is treating the patient must remain the **advocate** of the patient and should not be involved in making allocation decisions for that patient. Procedures for such allocations are determined in an objective manner by the institutions involved in the patient care.

Case to Discuss: If the CEO of American Airlines, the winner of last year's Academy Award for Best Actor, and a drug-abusing mother of three all were equally ill and needed a liver transplant, which should receive the organ, and on what would you base the decision?

Artificial Insemination

Any individual or couple considering artificial insemination must be thoroughly counseled and endure a lengthy group of screening procedures for infections, such as HIV, and genetic diseases and disorders that the donor and/or recipient may have. Informed consent must be provided, and there are further regulations based on the marital status of the people involved. If the recipient is married to the donor, the resultant child will have all of the rights of a child naturally conceived. If the donor is anonymous, the husband must sign consent if he is to become the legal father of the resultant child. If the donor and recipient are not married, the recipient is considered the sole parent, unless both parties agree to recognize a right to paternity.

There is much discussion on the use of extra embryos that are harvested for reproductive purposes. The control and use of these **gametes** should logically be left to the man and woman who produced them, but the AMA agrees that both must give their consent as to how they are used. In vitro fertilization is considered an ethical procedure, but there are new discussions as to stem cell research, which is done using human embryos. Many organizations feel that using human embryos for stem cell research destroys the most vulnerable of beings, and laws are designed to protect them. Others want to explore the possibility of developing cures from this research for diseases such as Alzheimer's disease, diabetes, Parkinson's disease, and heart disease.

Case to Discuss: If a man dies who fertilized eggs that were frozen for later use, but he made no provision for the use of those eggs before his death, should the wife be able to use those eggs after her marriage to a second man?

Surrogate Motherhood

Surrogate motherhood introduces many different ethical, legal, and social problems to the individuals involved. However, this could be the only opportunity for **infertile** couples to have a child. The risks of **surrogacy** must be heavily weighed against the possible problems that might arise. The AMA feels that the birth mother must be given a period of time during which she can reverse her decision to give up the child she has delivered and void the contract. However, in cases of gestational surrogacy, the legality and ethical implications are more complicated. In gestational surrogacy, the child is not genetically linked to the birth mother. Usually the couple engaging the surrogate mother would be the genetic parents of the resultant child. One must also consider what would happen if the child is born with a deformity or handicap. This is a contract that should never be entered into without strong forethought and counseling.

Case to Discuss: What is a fair length of time to give a surrogate mother to petition to void a surrogacy contract?

Human Cloning

The AMA agrees that physicians should not at this time participate in human cloning, or *somatic cell nuclear transfer*, because of the numerous legal and moral issues that must be explored. Most agree that our current ethical and moral standards would interpret that a "cloned human" be granted the same rights as "normal humans," much in the same way as an adopted child is accepted legally and socially as part of a family. The AMA does not feel there has been nearly enough research into the long-term effects of cloning and therefore does not advocate the practice today.

Case to Discuss: If a couple loses a child through death but it were possible to clone the child, what concerns would be present for the family?

Genetic Counseling

Genetic counseling is also an area in which the AMA recommends caution. Through genetic counseling, parents of tomorrow may be able to choose eye color, talents, and intellect levels for their children (Figure 6-8). There are already humans who were conceived as "designer babies" in the world today. In 1980 the Repository for Germinal Choice (more commonly known as the "Genius Sperm Bank") was founded. Although it was not established to create a perfect "master race," it did attempt to produce leaders and creators. As with cloning, the AMA recommends that much more research be done before instituting genetic counseling on a global scale.

Case to Discuss: What could happen if parents "designed" a baby, but it arrived flawed in some way or did not meet their expectations?

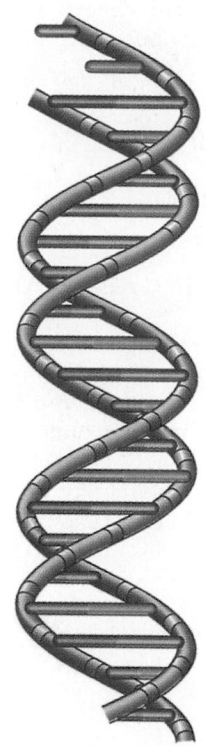

FIGURE 6-8   DNA, known as the "blueprint of the body," contains all the genes and chromosomes that make each human a unique creation, unlike any other human. (From Chester GA: *Modern medical assisting*, Philadelphia, 1998, WB Saunders.)

CRITICAL THINKING APPLICATION

- How might the genetic testing done in Delaney's case have caused an ethical dilemma?
- Discuss whether genetic testing can be counted on to predict disease.
- How many in your class would have genetic testing done on their own child before birth?

Physician-Assisted Suicide

The AMA believes that physician-assisted suicide interferes with the fundamental purpose of being a physician—being a healer. The CEJA advocates that physicians aggressively provide care and alternatives in treatment for those who are near the end of life, but not promote or provide the means with which the patient could end his or her own life. This includes not only assisting the patient to inject chemicals that will induce death, but also prescribing drugs and information about lethal doses, or administering a lethal dose of a drug to a patient to promote death (Figure 6-9). This is sometimes called **euthanasia**, or mercy-killing.

Case to Discuss: If a parent mentioned in passing that he or she would want the right to commit suicide in the event of a terminal illness, would you support that decision if the situation did in fact arise?

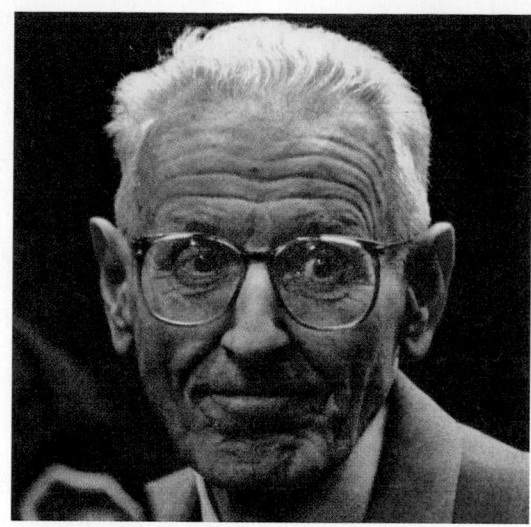

FIGURE 6-9   Dr. Jack Kevorkian, after being acquitted for numerous assisted suicides, was convicted in 1999 of second-degree murder and delivery of a controlled substance in the death of Thomas Youk, 52, who had amyotrophic lateral sclerosis (ALS or Lou Gehrig's disease). He will be eligible for parole in 6 years. (©AFB/CORBIS.)

Withholding or Withdrawing Life-Prolonging Treatment

A physician is committed to saving life and relieving suffering. Sometimes these two goals are incompatible, and a choice between them must be made. If possible, the patient should decide what treatment is given. Often the patient makes his or her wishes known to a responsible relative or other representative, in case the patient becomes incapacitated. Some patients wish to have a "do not resuscitate" (DNR) or "no code" order added to their charts. Usually such an order is desired so that no heroic measures are taken in a situation in which a patient would be unable or incompetent to make a decision. Advance directives are oral and/or written instructions for healthcare and usually are in the form of a living will or a durable power of attorney. Advance directives are strongly recommended by the AMA.

Patients of today are urged to create a living will. This is a document that states the wishes of the patient in case of terminal illness or an accident after which the patient cannot express his or her wishes. A durable power of attorney is a legal document that allows the patient to appoint someone who is trusted to make medical decisions for the patient in the event that the patient cannot make those decisions. This person is sometimes called a *healthcare proxy*. Federal law requires that patients be given information about advance directives by all facilities that participate in the Medicare and Medicaid programs.

Case to Discuss: How would a medical assistant handle the family of a patient who asks for advice about withdrawing life-prolonging treatment?

Quality of Life

Physicians must sometimes participate in or advise on decisions affecting the fate of a person whose prognosis is poor, such as a deformed newborn or a person of advanced age with many physical problems. The first thought may be the burden that the patient will be to the family or society in caring for this person. However, the AMA insists that the physician's primary consideration be what is best for the patient.

Case to Discuss: A mentally ill single woman who is institutionalized becomes pregnant and refuses to give up her maternal rights so that the child can be adopted. Even if she were to reconsider, what complications result if the child is born deaf and has a severe liver disorder? Should the child be fed and cared for by the hospital staff?

Clinical Trials and Investigation

Without **clinical trials** and investigation, no new drugs or procedures would be developed. However, all such investigation must follow a competently designed systematic program with due concern for the welfare, safety, and comfort of patients. The physician-patient relationship does exist in clinical investigation, and when treatment of the patient is involved, voluntary written consent must be obtained from the patient or the patient's legally authorized representative. Additional restrictions apply to minors or mentally incompetent adults. Physicians must show the same concern for the welfare and safety of the person involved in the clinical trials as they would if the person were a private patient.

Case to Discuss: If your brother were homosexual and wanted to participate in clinical trials for a vaccination against HIV, would you support his decision?

Cost of Healthcare Services

Concern for the quality of patient care should be the physician's first consideration. However, the physician should be conscious of costs and not provide or prescribe unnecessary services. Access to an adequate level of healthcare for all members of our society is now a moral expectation, but certainly not a right. Cost must be considered when providing these services, as well as the degree of benefit to the patient, the duration of the benefit, and the number of people who will benefit.

Case to Discuss: Should an 87-year-old patient with cardiovascular disease and stomach cancer have an expensive breast reconstruction surgery?

Organ Donation

Organ donation is not only considered ethical by the AMA but is encouraged when appropriate. However, it is considered unethical to participate in proceedings in which the donor receives payment, except reimbursement of expenses directly incurred in the removal of the donated organ. The rights of both the patient and the donor must be equally protected. In cases in which the donor has lost his or her life, the death must be certified by a physician other than the recipient's physician.

Some religions do not believe in transfusing blood, and cases in which such beliefs come to bear must be dealt with carefully. If the patient is a minor and the parents refuse the child a blood transfusion, some states would hold the parents liable for danger to or abuse of a child. However, the court system is reluctant to fight the parents over their religious beliefs and would intervene only in extreme circumstances.

Case to Discuss: A woman dies with a living will that states that she wishes her organs to be donated. Her mother, still living, disagrees with the decision and does not want her daughter's organs donated. What should health professionals do in this situation?

CRITICAL THINKING APPLICATION

- Monica has often thought about being an organ donor. She is very much in favor of organ donation because of her interest in the medical field. Her parents are very opposed to this because of their religious beliefs. How can Monica deal with this conflict within her family?
- If Monica dies before her parents do, how can she ensure that her wishes are carried out?

Capital Punishment

The CEJA does not consider participation in the act of capital punishment by a physician to be ethical. The physician may certify the death of the person but should not administer a lethal injection or induce death in any way. This conflicts with the physician's role as a healer, much in the same manner as physician-assisted suicide.

Case to Discuss: A very emotional patient, the parent of a child who was raped and killed, has been given the opportunity to attend the execution of the murderer. She expresses concerns about being able to cope with the memory of her daughter during the execution and asks you if you would attend in the same situation. What advice do you give the patient?

Ethical Issues Surrounding HIV

Being HIV positive creates a whole new world of ethical concerns for patients as well as those who support and care for them. When the HIV crisis first came to public attention, so many variables about the virus were unknown, and this created a wealth of misinformation. Those infected with the virus were often forced to leave their homes, were shunned in society, and faced rejection seemingly everywhere they turned, all because of fear of the illness (Figure 6-10).

Today clinical trials are underway for vaccinations against HIV, but clinical trials need volunteers for testing. Because vaccinations are often made of an attenuated or weakened strain of a virus, there are serious concerns as to who will receive the vaccination. Researchers have considered testing the vaccination in several Third World countries that have a high number of prostitutes and a thriving sex industry. These people, with no intentions of changing their lifestyle no matter the risks, may see vaccination trials as their chance of not contracting HIV. However, there is a question of the ethics of not submitting our own citizens to testing instead of those from disadvantaged countries.

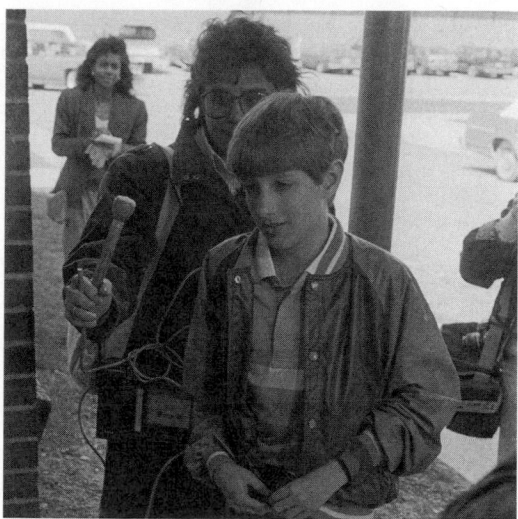

FIGURE 6-10   After a long court battle, Ryan White won the right to attend public school, despite his HIV status. (© Bettmann/CORBIS.)

Because of the discrimination practiced even today against people who are infected with HIV, there are problems with testing in some states that report the names of HIV-positive patients to various health departments and agencies. Although the stated intention is to ensure that these patients receive care, the accompanying effect is the risk of discriminatory practices. Some states use code systems called **unique identifiers** to assist in helping maintain the confidentiality of those getting tested for HIV. However, other states insist by statute that the names be reported. Some states require mandatory HIV testing for prisoners and those who have committed sex crimes. Insurance is a difficult issue when a person is infected with HIV, and some policies can be cancelled if HIV infection is discovered. This may prompt providers who want to treat patients infected with HIV to delay reporting the infection as long as possible, using other diagnoses regarding symptoms as opposed to the underlying cause of the patient's problems. All of these ethical issues are difficult to resolve, especially since currently there is no cure for HIV infection.

Ethics and the Human Genome

The mapping of the human **genome** has been in the news for several years. The genome project formally began in 1990 with the primary goal of identifying all of the approximately 30,000 genes present in the human body. Access to genetic information prompts many concerns and presents ethical, legal, and moral questions. Most of the major healthcare agencies and organizations in the United States and worldwide will be involved in the decisions made about this type of information, including the Centers for Disease Control and Prevention (CDC), National Institutes of Health (NIH), DHHS, Food and Drug Administration (FDA), Centers for Medicare and Medicaid Services (formerly HCFA), and many others. Experts will be needed to educate Congress, federal agencies, and state and local governments, because laws must be passed regarding the use of genetic information. The rapid pace of

science surpasses the ability of lawmakers to keep up, so the challenge ahead with regulation of the use of genetic information is a mammoth one.

The mapping of the human genome and the information provided have raised concerns about privacy and confidentiality issues: Who actually owns genetic information, and who will be allowed to control it? Logically, it would seem that the patient owns his or her own genetic information, but if that is so, then the patient should be able to control access to it. Also, decisions must be made on the fair use of genetic information. Employers, schools, courts, insurance companies, adoption agencies, and the military are just a few examples of organizations that could potentially misuse genetic information and discriminate against those whom they may wish to target for inclusion or exclusion. There are reproductive issues as well, and questions about the reliability of genetic testing.

Patients will have to be counseled thoroughly on the risks and limitations of genetic technology. The answers to many questions are uncertain. Should a parent be allowed to test a minor child for adult-onset diseases? Should testing be performed for diseases that have no cure? All of these issues need resolution before the widespread use of genetic information.

Other Ethical Issues

Interprofessional Relationships

If a medical assistant recognizes or suspects an error in a physician's orders, there is an ethical obligation to report this to the physician. Questioning a possible error is necessary, even if it means risking the displeasure of the physician or supervisor. It could save a life or prevent a lawsuit if there is an error.

Physicians often refer a patient to another physician for diagnosis and treatment when it is necessary. A physician should make these referrals only when confident that the patient will receive competent treatment.

Unless there are legal restrictions in the state, a physician in private practice is free to choose whom he or she will treat. Although private practitioners may refuse certain patients, they must treat those who have already been accepted in the practice, or face possible charges of neglect. This does not include referring a patient to another physician for a condition that is not within the scope of the original physician's practice.

A sports medicine physician must keep in mind that the professional responsibility at a sporting event is to protect the health and safety of the participants, with personal judgments being governed only by medical considerations.

In years past it was considered unethical for a physician to have any type of romantic relationship with nurses or assistants in the office or hospital. Although this is not as stringent a rule today, it is very wise to not fraternize with co-workers, especially subordinates, at the workplace.

Confidentiality

Confidentiality is one of the cardinal rules of the medical profession. It is completely unethical and unacceptable to divulge any information about a patient to any other person not directly related to the patient's care. The easiest places to breach confidentiality are in an elevator, break room, or lunch room. One never knows whose relative is behind the medical assistant, listening to conversations that are inappropriate. Breach of patient confidentiality is grounds for immediate termination from a healthcare facility or physician's office.

When minors request confidential services, physicians should encourage them to include their parents. However, if the minor does not wish to involve them and the law does not require otherwise, physicians should allow competent minors to consent to medical care and should not notify the parents without the minor patient's consent.

Confidentiality restrictions apply to information in patient records and charts, as well as what the medical assistant is told by the patient or patient's family (Figure 6-11). Never investigate a patient record strictly for curiosity. All information in the record must be kept in the strictest confidence. If records are computer based, accessing records for patients that do not fall directly under the medical assistant's realm of duty is also considered unethical. Never share information on patients with anyone outside the medical facility or office, including your own immediate family.

CRITICAL THINKING APPLICATION

- Susan, Delaney's birth mother, comes to the office for a check-up 6 weeks after the baby is born. Susan looks a little sad, and when Monica questions her, she asks how Delaney is doing. What should Monica tell her?
- How can the office protect itself from issues about confidentiality in this unusual adoption scenario?

Advertising

The only restrictions on advertising by physicians are those that specifically protect the public from deceptive practices. Standards regarding advertising and publicity have been liberalized over the years, but any advertisement or publicity must be true and not misleading. Tes-

timonials of patients, for instance, should not be used in advertising, because they are difficult to verify or measure by objective standards. Statements regarding the quality of medial services are highly subjective and difficult to verify.

Communications with the Media

Although information regarding some patients such as celebrities and politicians may be considered news, the physician cannot discuss any patient's condition with the press without authorization from the patient or the patient's legal representative. The physician may release only authorized information or that which is public knowledge. Certain kinds of news are a part of public records. This is known as news in the **public domain** and includes births, deaths, accidents, and police cases.

A medical assistant must be aware that only the physician is authorized to release information, and under no circumstances should the medical assistant violate the confidential nature of the physician-patient relationship. It is unethical even to certify or verify that the patient is under the physician's care without the patient's permission. Policy must be in place for every medical office as to how media inquiries should be handled and to whom they should be referred. Never voluntarily speak to the press without authorization from the physician.

Computers

The expanding uses of computer technology permit the accumulation of an unlimited amount of medical information. With the use of computers in the physician's office and the employment of computer service organizations, confidentiality becomes even more difficult to maintain. In general, all information must only be entered and accessed by authorized personnel, and a tracking system should be used to identify which employees access information. Breaches in computer policies should be considered a breach of patient confidentiality, and the consequences should be stringent enough to deter employees from accessing information to which they are not entitled (Figure 6-12). Information from the computer should only be disseminated to those who have a legitimate reason for needing the information.

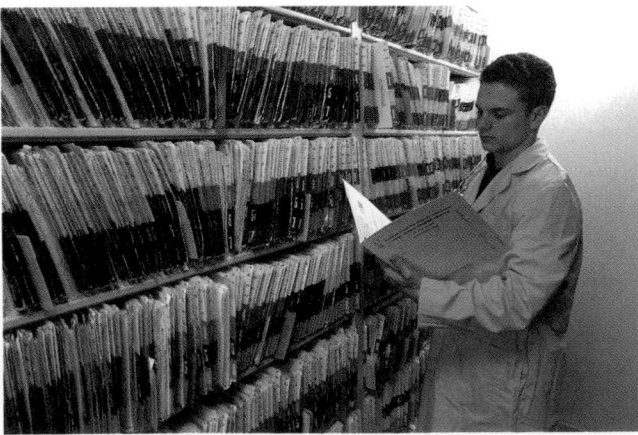

FIGURE 6-11 Confidentiality issues apply to all information about the patient, including what is charted and what is spoken between the patient and the medical assistant.

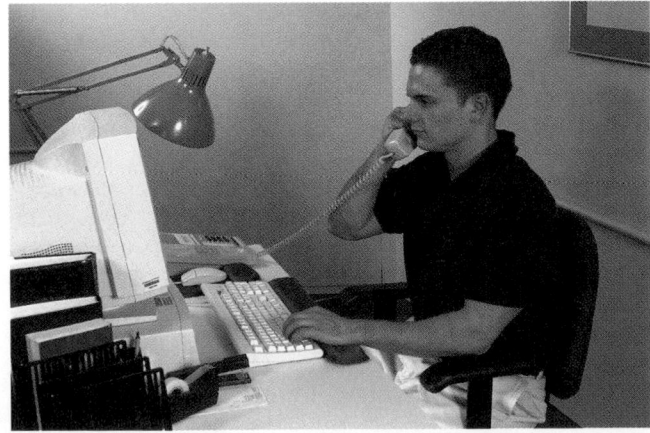

FIGURE 6-12 With the advent of advanced computer technology, a medical assistant must be particularly careful about using information about patients on the computer.

Fees and Charges

Charging or collecting an illegal or excessive fee is unethical. The medical assistant is responsible for keeping informed about current billing regulations and to see that they are conscientiously followed.

Requesting that payment be made at the time of treatment is entirely appropriate, and very common in today's medical offices. Often managed care patients are asked to remit their co-payment before seeing the physician on the day of their visit. If the patient is notified in advance, adding interest or other reasonable charges to delinquent accounts is also considered ethical. Most offices use a patient information booklet that provides a written reference of all policies and that is given to new patients on their first visit. A reasonable charge may be made for the cost of duplicating patient records.

Fee Splitting and Contingent Fees

If a physician accepts payment from another physician solely for the referral of a patient, both are guilty of an unethical practice called *fee splitting*. This practice, whether with another physician, a clinic, a laboratory, or a drug company, is unethical.

Although attorneys often accept a case on a contingent fee basis, it is unethical for a physician to engage in this practice. The fee in this case is contingent on a successful outcome, but a physician should never set his or her fee on the successful outcome of medical treatment. A physician's fee must always be based on the value of service provided to the patient.

Insurance Forms

Although physicians' offices in times past would willingly file the claim on all insurance policies for their patients, some have changed their policies to a payment up-front system and give patients the information needed to file the claim themselves. Many offices will still file at least one insurance claim for established patients but may charge for multiple or complex insurance filing. This practice is entirely ethical if in conformity with local custom.

Waiver of Insurance Co-payments

Physicians may opt to write off or waive co-payments to facilitate patient access to medical care. If access to care is directly threatened because the patient cannot make the co-payment, the physician may forgive the payment. However, routine waiver of the co-payments may violate the policies of some insurers, both public and private. Physicians should ensure that their policies on co-payments are consistent with applicable law and within legal boundaries of their contracts with insurers.

Professional Courtesy

Professional courtesy is defined as the provision of medical care to physician colleagues or their families and staff free of charge or at a reduced fee. This is a long-standing tradition, but certainly not an ethical requirement. Physicians make the decision as to who will receive professional courtesy in their offices, and this should be written into the office policy manual.

Appointment Charges

It is ethical for a physician to charge for a missed appointment or one that was not cancelled within a stated time if the patient has been fully advised in advance that such a charge may be made. Discretion should be used in applying such charges, however, since the patient may have encountered an emergency. Often adding a missed appointment charge to the bill of a patient who never cancels in advance will prompt a call in the future when the appointment cannot be kept.

Prescribing Drugs and Devices

The physician should not be influenced in the prescribing of drugs, devices, or appliances by a direct or indirect financial interest in the supplier. A physician may own or operate a pharmacy but generally may not ethically refer his or her patients to that pharmacy. Patients should enjoy the same freedom of choice in deciding who will fill their prescriptions as they do in choosing a physician.

Health Facility Ownership by a Physician

A physician may ethically own or have a financial interest in a for-profit or other health care facility, such as a free-standing clinic or health club. However, before admitting or referring a patient to that facility, the physician has an ethical obligation to reveal such ownership to the patient. In general, physicians should not refer patients to a health facility that is outside their office practice and at which they do not directly provide care or services.

Ghost Surgery

The substitution of another surgeon without the patient's consent is called *ghost surgery*. The patient has a right to choose his or her own physician or surgeon. To make a substitution without consulting the patient is deceitful and unethical.

Discipline Within Medicine

A physician should expose incompetent, corrupt, dishonest, or unethical conduct on the part of members of the profession, without fear of loss of favor. A physician may be subject to civil or criminal liability, including loss of license to practice medicine, for violation of government laws. Expulsion from membership is the maximum penalty that may be imposed by a medical society for violation of ethical standards.

Physicians and Infectious Disease

A physician who knows that he or she has an infectious disease should not engage in any activity that creates an identified risk of transmission to the patient. Simple colds and other minor illnesses will arise occasionally, but illnesses that would cause a significant risk to the patient should not be given a chance to cause infection.

Substance Abuse

It is unethical for a physician to practice medicine while under the influence of a controlled substance, alcohol, or other chemical agents that could impair the ability to properly care for the patient or perform procedures.

Closing Comments

The study of ethics requires much thought and honest appraisal of what the medical assistant believes. Sometimes **introspection** of this type is difficult. Often our beliefs are a result of our environment, upbringing, and other factors that have influenced our thinking and actions from the time we were small children to our current age. It is important that our belief system be one that we have created personally, not just a set of beliefs accepted from another source. Medical assistants should take a serious look at the thoughts and concepts that make up their own concepts of ethics. It is important to approach ethical decisions calmly, logically, and without haste.

Patient Education

Patients may not always understand the ethical standards that physicians and medical assistants adhere to. They may ask a medical assistant questions about their own health or the health of a fellow patient. Medical assistants must educate patients regarding the issues of confidentiality in such a way that the patient does not take offense, explaining that all patients deserve to have their medical and personal information kept private. Now more than ever, there are ethical obligations to privacy as well as legal ones. A medical assistant must be certain that all patients understand that they are entitled to confidential treatment of their records and that the facility is dedicated to that principle.

Legal and Ethical Issues

The prime objective of the medical profession is to render service to humanity, and this must be a medical assistant's first concern as well. The importance of respecting the confidentiality of information learned from or about patients in the course of employment cannot be overemphasized. It is unethical to reveal patient confidences to anyone, and this includes family, spouse, best friends, and other medical assistants. A medical assistant must never mention the names of patients outside the place of employment, because sometimes the doctor's specialty reveals the patient's reason for consultation.

Never discuss one patient's case with another patient. If curious patients ask questions about others, simply explain that medical assistants are obligated to keep all patient information confidential. This can be done in a tactful and kind manner. Patients who ask questions of a medical nature about his or her own case should be referred to the physician for information and instructions, unless the physician has authorized the medical assistant to provide this information. A medical assistant must

avoid giving advice of a personal or professional nature to the patient, because they tend to identify remarks made by any of the assistants as reflecting the advice of the physician. By avoiding these situations, medical assistants protect themselves, the physician, and the patient. Confidential papers, case histories, and even the appointment book should be kept out of sight of curious eyes.

Medical assistants have an ethical obligation to keep abreast of current developments that affect the practice of medicine and care of the patients. Membership in a professional organization provides access to continuing education for maintaining knowledge and skills pertaining to the performance of medical assisting.

In rare instances a medical assistant is faced with a situation in which the physician-employer's conduct appears to violate established ethical standards. Before making any judgments, the medical assistant must be absolutely sure of all the information and circumstances. If unethical conduct occurs, the medical assistant must then make his or her own decision about continued employment in the facility and whether the unethical behavior should be reported to law enforcement, the local medical society, or the hospital where the physician has been granted privileges. Would it be wise to remain in the office under the circumstances? Would it be better to seek other employment? Would remaining adversely affect future opportunities for employment with another physician?

These decisions are difficult, especially if the relationship and employment conditions have been favorable and congenial. An ethical medical assistant will not wish to participate in known substandard or unlawful practices, especially those that might be harmful to patients. Additionally, the medical assistant must never make inaccurate reports regarding unethical behavior, and should realize that some states can prosecute individuals who file a false report. Be absolutely certain of the facts before making such accusations against any health professional.

SUMMARY OF SCENARIO

Pregnancy is usually a joyous time, but Monica has learned that even such an anticipated event can bring ethical issues to light. She has realized that there are two or more sides to every situation and that she must be open and willing to look at all sides when making an ethical decision.

Medical assisting is a rewarding career, but sometimes the decisions that the medical professional is faced with making are quite difficult. Monica must learn to be nonjudgmental and not to inflict her opinions on her patients. They must make their own decisions regarding their health and emotional well-being, and the medical assistant should not influence their thinking unfairly.

Monica will continue to evaluate her own ideas and beliefs throughout her career as a medical assistant. Periodic self-evaluation is good for everyone, and she will grow emotionally from the experiences that patients bring about where ethical issues are concerned.

SUMMARY OF LEARNING OBJECTIVES

- Ethics are judgments of right and wrong or actions on issues that have implications of a moral right and wrong. Etiquette deals with courtesy, customs, and manners. Rights are claims that are made by a person or group on society, a group, or an individual. Although these terms have different definitions, the concepts are interrelated, and often all are involved in ethical questions.

- Ethical distress is a problem to which there is an obvious solution, but some type of barrier hinders the action that needs to be taken. An ethical dilemma is a situation in which there are two or more solutions, but in choosing one, something of value is lost in not choosing the other. A dilemma of justice involves allocation of benefits and how they are to be fairly distributed. Two or more authority figures, each with his or her idea of how to handle a certain situation, are the center of the locus of authority ethical problem. Only one of the authority figures can prevail. Often an ethical problem has several aspects and more than one type of problem is presented.

- Making an ethical decision is easier when approached logically and considered using a five-step process. First, one gathers relevant information; then identifies the type of problem. After determining the ethical approach to use, one should explore alternatives. Finally, all that is left is to complete the action and make the decision.

- Although healthcare professionals do not have to abide by the opinions of the CEJA, the Council's opinions are highly regarded, and many professionals practice in accordance with these opinions. Often providers will abide by the opinions to avoid controversy, but there are still many who openly oppose the decisions of the CEJA.

- Unique identifiers maintain the confidentiality of patients who are tested for HIV. Some individuals might hesitate to be tested if they were concerned that their name would be reported to various agencies. Using the unique identifiers, patients may have much more confidence that the chances of discrimination resulting from their HIV status are lessened.

- There are many ethical concerns regarding genetic testing. Many patients are concerned about how the information gained will be used and who will have access to the information. Questions arise regarding the ownership of the information. When negative information is found, other ethical problems arise that will need to be addressed. Knowledge of a person's genetic blueprint could lead to discrimination. There are countless issues that must be examined before the use of genetic information becomes widespread.

- Confidentiality is of major importance in the medical profession. The patient's privacy should be of prime concern to a medical assistant. It is a serious enough issue that a breach of patient confidentiality is sufficient reason for immediate termination of an employee. Because it is such a critical aspect of patient care, it is considered highly unethical to reveal any information about a patient to anyone else. All medical assistants are required and expected to uphold the confidentiality of the information with which they come into contact.

KEY INTERNET WEBSITES

- American Medical Association Council on Ethical and Judicial Affairs
  For active weblinks to each website visit
  http://evolve.elsevier.com/Kinn/

CHAPTER 7

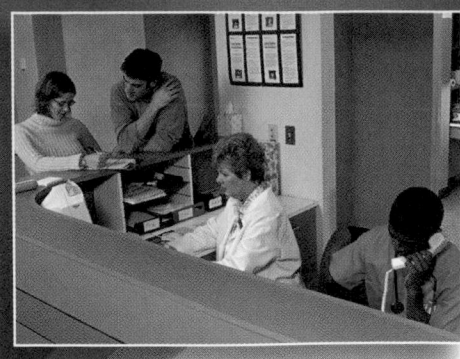

Scenario

Barbara Johnson is the new office manager for two neurologists in an urban area. Recently she was subpoenaed to appear in court with medical records to testify about a patient who was referred to one of the physicians for whom she works. Dr. Rebecca Patrick saw the patient several years ago; this patient has brought a medical professional liability case against a surgeon in another city. Barbara is considered the custodian of records and will take the records to court and answer questions about the information in the patient's chart.

One of Barbara's first priorities is to make certain that the office is operating in compliance with the legal regulations that affect the facility. She is knowledgeable about OSHA requirements, and because her father was an attorney, she is very familiar with legal issues.

Two of the employees Barbara supervises, Samantha and Lynda, are newly graduated from medical assisting school and are anxious to learn more about the statutes and laws that affect the physicians' office. Barbara is more than happy to share what she has learned with them. She is excited about her new job and eager to be a great success.

Medicine and Law

Learning Objectives

- Define and spell the terms listed in the vocabulary.
- Distinguish between an act, a statute, and an ordinance.
- Know the two types of law.
- Explain the three basic categories of criminal law.
- Distinguish which type of civil law deals with medical professional liability.
- Explain the four essential elements needed for a valid contract.
- Distinguish between interrogatories and depositions.
- List three things to remember when testifying in court.
- Discuss the advantages of arbitration.
- Differentiate among malfeasance, misfeasance, and nonfeasance.
- Explain the importance of informed consent.
- List several legal disclosures the physician must make.
- Explain the importance of the Health Insurance Portability and Accountability Act.
- Distinguish between OSHA and CLIA, explaining which is an actual agency.
- Discuss the three ways that a physician can obtain a license to practice medicine.
- Discuss the ways that a physician might lose a license to practice medicine.

National Curriculum Competencies

TRANSDISCIPLINARY COMPETENCIES

2a. Identify and respond to issues of confidentiality
2b. Perform within legal and ethical boundaries

Vocabulary

act The formal action of a legislative body; a decision or determination of a sovereign state, a legislative council, or a court of justice.

allegation A statement by a party to a legal action of what the party undertakes to prove, an assertion made without proof.

appeal A legal proceeding by which a case is brought before a higher court for review of the decision of a lower court.

appellate Having the power to review the judgment of another tribunal or body of jurisdiction, such as an appellate court.

arbitration The hearing and determination of a cause in controversy by a person or persons either chosen by the parties involved or appointed under statutory authority.

arbitrator A neutral person chosen to settle differences between two parties in a controversy.

assault An intentional, unlawful attempt of bodily injury to another by force.

assent To agree to something, especially after thoughtful consideration.

bailiff An officer of some U.S. courts usually serving as a messenger or usher, who keeps order at the request of the judge.

battery A willful and unlawful use of force or violence on the person of another.

Code of Federal Regulations (CFR) A coded delineation of the rules and regulations published in the Federal Register by the various departments and agencies of the federal government. The CFR is divided into 50 titles that represent broad subject areas, and then chapters that provide specific detail.

concurrently Occurring at the same time.

contributory negligence Statutes in some states that may prevent a party from recovering damages if he or she contributed in any way to the injury or condition.

damages Loss or harm resulting from injury to person, property, or reputation; compensation in money imposed by law for losses or injuries.

decedent A legal term for a deceased person.

docket A formal record of judicial proceedings; a list of legal causes to be tried.

due process A fundamental constitutional guarantee that all legal proceedings will be fair; that one will be given notice of the proceedings and given an opportunity to be heard before the government acts to take away life, liberty, or property; a constitutional guarantee that a law will not be unreasonable or arbitrary.

emancipated minor A person under legal age who is self-supporting and living apart from parents or guardian; a mature minor considered to possess a sufficient understanding of self-care and responsibility.

expert witness A person who provides testimony to a court as an expert in a certain field or subject to verify facts presented by one or both sides in a lawsuit, often compensated and used to refute or disprove the claims of one party.

felony A major crime, such as murder, rape, or burglary; punishable by a more stringent sentence than that given for a misdemeanor.

fine A sum imposed as punishment for an offense; a forfeiture or penalty paid to an injured party or the government in a civil or criminal action.

guardian ad litem Legal representative for a minor.

implied consent Presumed consent, such as when a patient offers an arm for a phlebotomy procedure.

informed consent A consent in which there is understanding of what treatment is to be undertaken and of the risks involved, why it should be done, and alternative methods of treatment available (including no treatment) and their attendant risks.

infraction Breaking the law; a minor offense of the rules.

judicial Of or relating to a judgment, the function of judging, the administration of justice, or the judiciary.

jurisdiction A power constitutionally conferred on a judge or magistrate to decide cases according to law and to carry sentence into execution; jurisdiction is original when it is conferred on the court in the first instance, called original jurisdiction; or it is appellate, which is when an appeal is given from the judgment of another court.

jurisprudence The science or philosophy of law; a system or body of law or the course of court decisions.

law A binding custom or practice of a community; a rule of conduct or action prescribed or formally recognized as binding or enforceable by a controlling authority.

liable Obligated according to law or equity; responsible for an act or circumstance.

libel A written defamatory statement or representation that conveys an unjustly unfavorable impression.

litigious Prone to engage in lawsuits.

manifestation Something that is easily understood or recognized by the mind.

misdemeanor A minor crime, as opposed to a felony, punishable by fine or imprisonment in a city or county jail rather than in a penitentiary.

municipal A court that sits in some cities and larger towns and that usually has civil and criminal jurisdiction over cases arising within the municipality.

negligence Failure to exercise the care that a prudent person usually exercises; implies inattention to one's duty or business; implies want of due or necessary diligence or care.

ordinance An authoritative decree or direction; a law set forth by a governmental authority, specifically a municipal regulation.

other potentially infectious material (OPIM) Substances or material other than blood that has the potential to carry infectious pathogens, such as body fluid, urine, semen, and others.

paraphrased A restatement of a text, passage, or work giving the meaning in another form.

perjured testimony The voluntary violation of an oath or vow either by swearing to what is untrue or by omission to do what has been promised under oath; false testimony.

precedence To surpass in rank, dignity, or importance; to be, go, or come ahead or in front of.

precedents A person or thing that serves as a model; something done or said that may serve as an example or rule to authorize or justify a subsequent act of the same kind.

preponderance of the evidence Evidence that is of greater weight or more convincing than the evidence offered in opposition to it; evidence that as a whole shows that the fact sought to be proven is more probable than not.

physician office laboratories (POLs) Laboratories owned by a private physician or corporation, such as the lab inside a physician's office or a free-standing laboratory.

prudent Marked by wisdom or judiciousness; shrewd in the management of practical affairs.

quackery The pretense of curing disease.

reasonable doubt Doubt based on reason and arising from evidence or lack of evidence; it is not doubt that is imagined or conjured up, but doubt that would cause reasonable persons to hesitate before acting.

relevant Having significant and demonstrable bearing on the matter at hand.

statute A law enacted by the legislative branch of a government.

stipulate To specify as a condition or requirement of an agreement or offer; to make an agreement or covenant to do or forbear something.

subpoena A writ or document commanding a person to appear in court under a penalty for failure to appear.

testimony A solemn declaration usually made orally by a witness under oath in response to interrogation by a lawyer or authorized public official.

Uniform Commercial Code (UCC) A unified set of rules covering many business transactions; it has been adopted in all 50 states, the District of Columbia, and most U.S. territories.

verdict The finding or decision of a jury on a matter submitted to it in trial.

Law is a fascinating subject. When law is applied to medicine, it can provoke interesting case studies and complex decisions. In today's **litigious** society, medical assistants, as well as physicians and other staff members, must take steps to protect themselves from lawsuits. Legal issues underlie many aspects of the provision of healthcare in a physician's office. Although the wording of statutes and regulations is often long and complicated, medical assistants must stay abreast of the rules governing medical facilities and do everything possible to remain in compliance with the standards and regulations for all organizations that oversee the medical industry.

Jurisprudence and the Classifications of Law

Jurisprudence, the science and philosophy of law, comes from the Latin words *juris*, which means "law, right, equity, or justice," and *prudentia*, which means "skill or good judgment."

Law is a custom or practice of a community. It is a rule of conduct or action prescribed or formally recognized as binding or enforceable by a controlling authority. Law is the system by which society gives order to our lives. The U.S. Constitution is the supreme law of the land, which takes **precedence** over federal statutes, court opinions, and state constitutions. However, within the states, the state constitution is the supreme law within the boundaries of that state, unless it conflicts with the U.S. Constitution. States cannot pass laws that conflict with the U.S. Constitution, nor can local governments pass laws that conflict with the state constitution.

A law enacted at the federal level, which must be passed by Congress, is called an **act. Statutes** are laws that have been enacted by state legislatures. Local governments create and enact **ordinances**. Much of our law is based on previous **judicial** and jury decisions, which are called **precedents**. Often judges and juries follow precedents when making a decision on a case before them. There are two basic categories of jurisprudence: criminal law and civil law.

Criminal Law

Criminal law governs violations of the law that are punishable as offenses against the state or government. Such offenses involve the welfare and safety of the public as a whole rather than of one individual. Criminal offenses are classified into three basic categories: misdemeanors, felonies, and treason.

Misdemeanors. A minor crime, as opposed to a felony, is called a **misdemeanor**. Such a crime is punishable by **fine** or imprisonment in a city or county jail rather than in a penitentiary. Misdemeanors vary from state to state and are often divided into subgroups or classes, such as class A, class B, or class C misdemeanors. In most states, the subgroups are divided from most serious offenses to lesser offenses. Some states have created a subcategory of misdemeanors for **infractions**, which are often called violations. Infractions are minor offenses, such as traffic tickets, which are punishable only by a fine.

Felonies. A felony is a major crime, such as murder, rape, or burglary, and is punishable by a more stringent sentence than that given for a misdemeanor. Federal law and most state statutes classify felonies as crimes punishable by imprisonment for more than 1 year, whereas misdemeanors are punishable by imprisonment for 1 year or less. Usually a convicted felon cannot vote, hold public office, or possess a firearm. Felonies are often divided into subgroups or degrees, such as first degree, second degree, and third degree. The first-degree offense is normally the most serious.

Treason. Treason, the most serious crime, is the offense of attempting to overthrow the government. High treason constitutes a serious threat to the stability or continuity of the government, such as an attempt to kill the president. The President of the United States has the right to declare an action against the United States to be an act of war, as opposed to an act of treason, which is considered a crime. For instance, although the terrorist attacks of September 11, 2001, were certainly a threat against the United States, they were declared acts of war.

Civil Law

Civil law is concerned with acts that are not criminal in nature, but those that involve relationships of individuals with other individuals, organizations, or government agencies. There are many types of civil law that address numerous issues. The three that most directly affect the medical profession include tort law, contract law, and administrative law.

Tort Law. Tort law provides a remedy for a person or group who has suffered harm from the wrongful acts of others. Four elements must be established in every tort action. First, the plaintiff must establish that the defendant was under a legal duty to act in a particular fashion. Second, the plaintiff must demonstrate that the defendant breached this duty by failing to conform his or her behavior accordingly. Third, the plaintiff must prove that the breach of the legal duty proximately caused some injury or damage. Fourth, the plaintiff must prove damages, the injury or loss suffered. Medical professional liability, or medical malpractice, falls into the category of tort law.

Contract Law. A contract is an agreement creating an obligation. Contract law touches our lives in many ways practically every day, but we usually do not give much thought to its influences. If a person parks a car in a parking garage for a monthly fee and signs a contract for a year, then begins parking elsewhere and refuses to pay the fee, the person may be **liable** for the fees for the duration of the entire contract. If damage occurs to the person's vehicle while it is parked in the garage, the garage may be responsible for reimbursement, if the contract does not **stipulate** otherwise. A contract does not have to be formalized in writing to be binding on the parties involved. Oral contracts are also valid in many states in most situations.

Administrative Law. Administrative law involves regulations set forth by governmental agencies. For example, the Internal Revenue Service (IRS) has thousands of regulations and codes, and the typical American does not understand all of them, which may result in errors when filing taxes. The laws that allow the IRS to collect taxes and pursue restitution are administrative laws. Other agencies that are involved with administrative law include the Social Security Administration, Immigration and Naturalization Service, and the Centers for Medicare and Medicaid Services (formerly the Health Care Financing Administration [HCFA]).

Anatomy of a Medical Professional Liability Lawsuit

A medical liability case often stems from a breach of trust or miscommunication between the physician and the patient. Even when the physician has made an error, often the level of trust between the physician and patient will determine whether a lawsuit will be pursued. First, the physician-patient relationship must be formed. Before discussing this relationship, it is important to understand what is necessary for a contract to be valid and enforceable.

There are four essential elements to a contract. First, there must be **manifestation** of **assent** or a "meeting of the minds." This element is proven by an "offer" and the "acceptance" of that offer. The parties to the contract must understand and agree on the intent of the contract. Second, the contract must involve legal subject matter. An obligation that requires an illegal action, such as a gambling contract, is not an enforceable contract. Third, both parties must have the legal capacity to enter into a contract. This means that the parties must be adults of sound mind, or an **emancipated minor**. Fourth, there must be some type of consideration. Consideration is an exchange of something of value, for example, money for the physician's time.

CRITICAL THINKING APPLICATION

Barbara works for Dr. Rebecca Patrick, who saw the patient bringing the lawsuit against the surgeon as a referral patient. Does Dr. Patrick have a contract with the patient, based on a physician-patient relationship? Why or why not?

The physician-patient relationship is generally held by courts to be a contractual relationship that is the result of three steps:

1. The physician invites an offer by establishing availability.
2. The patient accepts the invitation and makes an offer by arriving for or requesting treatment.
3. The physician accepts the offer by accepting the patient and undertaking treatment. The physician may explicitly accept the patient's offer or implicitly accept the offer by exercising their independent medical judgment on behalf of the patient.

Before accepting a patient, the physician is under no obligation, and no contract exists. However, once the physician has accepted the patient, an implied contract does exist (Figure 7-1). This implied contract assumes that the physician will treat the patient using reasonable care

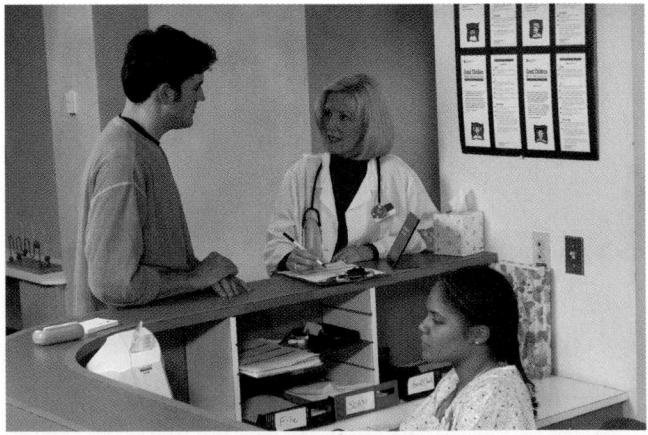

FIGURE 7-1 The physician-patient relationship is built on a strong foundation of trust, but it is also a contractual relationship.

and that the physician possesses a degree of knowledge, skill, and judgment that might be expected of any other physician in the same locality and under similar circumstances. It is extremely important that no express promise of a cure be made by anyone in the office, including the physician, because this would become a part of the contract.

The patient's responsibility in this agreement includes the liability of payment for services and a willingness to follow the advice of the physician. Most physician-patient contracts are implied contracts. Although many forms may be completed by the patient before being accepted by the physician, they do not in most cases constitute a formal contract for each specific visit to the physician.

CRITICAL THINKING APPLICATION

- If the patient does not pay for the services rendered by the physician, does this negate the physician-patient contract?
- How might Barbara, Samantha, and Lynda ensure that patients understand that they are expected to follow the advice of the physician?

After the physician-patient relationship has been established, the physician is obligated to attend the patient as long as attention is required, unless the physician or patient terminates the contract. When a physician terminates the contract, the patient must be given notice of the physician's intentions so that the patient has sufficient time to secure another physician. The physician may write a letter of withdrawal from medical care of the patient, and it should be delivered by certified mail, return receipt requested. A copy of the letter and the return receipt should be attached to the patient's chart and permanently retained.

To protect the physician against a lawsuit for abandonment, the details of the circumstances under which the physician is withdrawing from the case should be included in the patient's medical chart. The letter of withdrawal does not have to specify a reason for withdrawal unless the physician so chooses, but it should state the following:

- That professional care is being discontinued
- That the physician will provide copies of the patient's records to another physician on request
- That the patient should seek the attention of another physician as soon as possible

A patient who wishes to terminate the physician-patient relationship simply no longer seeks the physician for treatment. The patient does not have to inform the office; however, if this is done, the office manager or physician should follow up with a letter confirming notice that the patient has ended the relationship.

The Statute of Frauds

In 1677, a statute was adopted in England that was designed to reduce the occurrence of **perjured testimony** by providing that certain contracts could not be enforced if they depended on the testimony of witnesses alone and were not evidenced in writing. The provisions of this English statute have been closely followed by statutes adopted in all 50 states in the United States.

The promise to pay the debts of another person is an example of a contract that usually must be made in writing. If a third party who is not otherwise legally responsible for a patient's medical bills agrees to pay them, the agreement cannot be enforced unless it is in writing. Or, if a physician entered into an agreement to perform a series of treatments for a given sum, and this series covered a time span of more than 1 year, the contract would have to be in writing to be enforceable.

Preliminaries of Litigation

Once a patient has decided to file a lawsuit against a physician, the first step is usually to find an attorney who will accept the case. This may be a frustration to many patients: attorneys may not wish to initiate litigation against a physician. Like physicians, an attorney does not have to accept a case he or she does not wish to pursue, and this is often because the attorney does not see enough of a financial benefit from the time it would take to work on the case. Although this sounds a bit harsh, the attorney runs a business, as does a physician, and must make good business decisions as to how his or her time is spent and invested.

CRITICAL THINKING APPLICATION

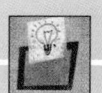

- For what reasons might a physician not wish to accept a patient?
- Must the physician treat every patient who attempts to make an appointment?
- How might Barbara tactfully explain that the physician will not accept the patient into treatment?

Lawsuits are filed in a variety of different courts, and different states have different types of courts at various levels. There are several branches of the state judiciary. At the local level, there are usually **municipal** courts. These are courts in a city or town that usually deal with ordinance violations. Municipal judges may issue search and arrest warrants. Some states also have justice of the peace courts, which have **jurisdiction** over many misdemeanors and some civil matters, as well as concurrent jurisdiction over some matters along with the municipal courts. The judges that preside over justice of the peace courts may also issue search warrants and arrest warrants. They often function as small claims courts, which the medical assistant may have contact with in cases of patients who do not pay their bills. Both municipal and justice of the peace courts are local trial courts with limited jurisdiction.

County courts are higher than municipal and justice of the peace courts. These courts handle misdemeanors and civil matters up to a certain monetary limit. District courts have unlimited jurisdiction in criminal and civil matters. They are the highest state courts, other than appellate courts. When one party of a lawsuit is dissatisfied with a lower court's decision, it has the right to

appeal to a higher court for review and possible reversal of the decision. Most states have an **appellate** court for both criminal and civil matters. The U.S. District Court handles federal matters of both a criminal and civil nature. States also have Supreme Courts that handle a limited number of appellate cases.

The U.S. Supreme Court has authority given by Article III, Section One of the Constitution, to ensure equal justice under the law (Figure 7-2). The Supreme Court interprets and guards the Constitution of the United States. There is one Chief Justice and eight Associate Justices who are appointed by the President and confirmed by the Congress. Approximately 7000 cases are on the **docket** per term, which runs from the first Monday in October to the first Monday of October in the next year.

CRITICAL THINKING APPLICATION

Samantha and Lynda are curious as to how Supreme Court decisions affect the individual physician's office. What Supreme Court decisions have affected the medical profession?

Preparing for Court

Medical professional liability suits are far from rare, and every physician faces the probability of being sued at least once during his or her career. When a suit is filed, preparation for court should start expeditiously. A medical assistant may be involved in preparing materials for court and scheduling or participating in depositions. The best advice for a medical assistant in this position is to remember to tell the truth. Attorneys will help to prepare the defense of the physician and the staff, but everyone should be truthful in the answers that are given to the court to avoid losing his or her credibility in the trial and to avoid charges of perjury (Figure 7-3).

Interrogatories

Before the trial, the physician may be requested to complete an interrogatory, which is a list of questions from each party to the other in the lawsuit. Answers to the interrogatory must be provided within a specified time, and the answers are considered to be given under oath. Only the parties named in the lawsuit may be questioned through interrogatories.

Depositions

A deposition is testimony taken from a party or witness to the litigation and is not limited to the parties named in the lawsuit. A witness who is not a party to the lawsuit may be summoned by **subpoena** for the deposition. The deposition is usually taken in an attorney's office in the presence of a court reporter and is taken under oath. The person giving the deposition is called the *deponent*. The transcribed deposition, once finished, is sent to the deponent for review, and the deponent is at liberty to request any necessary changes or corrections in the document.

CRITICAL THINKING APPLICATION

- Samantha and Lynda are anxious to hear about Barbara's experiences in testifying in court. She mentions that attorneys often advise witnesses to "answer the question, then be quiet." What might be meant by this advice?
- Discuss the phrase, "the truth, the whole truth, and nothing but the truth."

Subpoenas

A subpoena is a document issued by a court requiring a person to be in court at a specific time and place to testify as a witness in a lawsuit, either in a court proceeding or in a deposition. A *subpoena duces tecum* is a

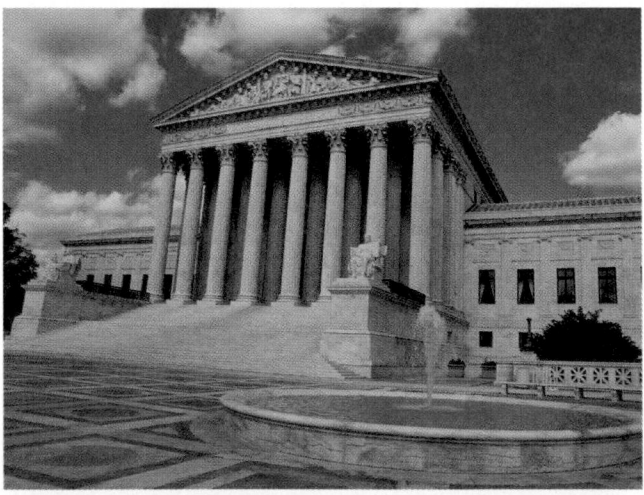

FIGURE 7-2 The U.S. Supreme Court. The Supreme Court decides cases that involve interpretation of the Constitution of the United States.

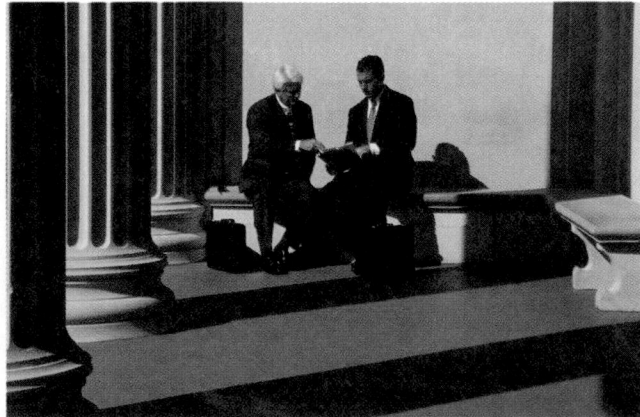

FIGURE 7-3 Preparation is of primary importance to the physician facing a medical professional liability case. A competent and experienced attorney is necessary to provide an adequate defense and present the physician's views to the court.

legally binding request to provide records or documents to appear in court and is usually issued to the person considered the custodian of the records. This may be the medical assistant or office manager. A fee may be demanded for the time spent in compiling the records and for photocopying charges, but this fee must be requested at the time the subpoena duces tecum is served, or it is considered to be waived. Physician approval must be obtained to release or copy any patient records. Original records should never be released under any circumstances.

Discovery

Discovery is the pretrial disclosure of pertinent facts or documents by one or both parties to a legal action or proceeding. Many states have extensive discovery statutes that require each side to reveal to the other the facts that they "discover" while investigating the case. Discovery is also considered the process of uncovering facts in a lawsuit before the court proceedings.

Presentation of evidence may be by **testimony**. A witness is called who has some information about an aspect of the case and is asked questions by one or both attorneys. The witness will not know about every part of the case, but something that the person knows will be **relevant** to the case.

Another type of evidence may be documentary evidence. This is any type of evidence brought before the court by document or display. It could be a patient's chart, or a letter, a lab result, or a photograph. All of these are usually entered into evidence and numbered for easy reference.

CRITICAL THINKING APPLICATION

Samantha wonders what she should do if she ever finds negative information during a medical professional malpractice case that might harm her employer's defense. What advice would you offer? Would it be considered an obligation or a choice to report the employer of wrongdoing?

Preparing Witnesses and Testifying

Attorneys will prepare witnesses who may be called to testify during the court proceedings. They will review the questions that will be asked and potential questions that the opposite side may present. The attorney will help the witness to clarify the answers that he or she gives so that they are sharp and succinct. One of the first rules that attorneys learn in law school is to never ask a question to which they do not already know the answer.

Witnesses should be certain that they know the exact location of the courthouse and to which floor and court-room they are to report. They should always be on time for a court appearance, because the judge and jury may frown on those appearing late. That frown may also include a fine or confinement in jail for contempt of court!

When called to testify, it is critical that the witness dress conservatively and in a manner that shows respect for the court. Normal business attire should be adequate, but if there is ever any doubt, consult the attorney.

If any documents are to be referenced while testifying, the witness should review the documents before the court appearance so that the needed information will be easy to locate and discuss. The witness should speak clearly and at a volume audible to the attorneys and parties to the suit, the judge, the jury, and the court reporter. The witness should always answer each question aloud, because the court reporter must record those answers and cannot specify that the witness "nodded yes" as a response to a question.

If a question is confusing, the witness should ask the attorney to restate or repeat it. Attorneys may ask the witness to speak up, but this should not be intimidating to the witness. If the witness does not know the answer to a question or does not recall, that should be stated clearly and confidently. Above all, the parties involved are expected to tell the truth and must be seen as credible witnesses (Figure 7-4). Lying under oath constitutes perjury, which carries stiff penalties. Listening is as important as speaking, so the witness should be sure to listen to the question, and answer it, elaborating only if the attorney asks for more details.

If an attorney lodges an objection to a question, the witness should be silent until the judge rules on the objection. The objection may be sustained or overruled. Sustaining the objection means that the judge agrees with the objection and will not allow the question stated in that manner. If the judge allows the question, he or she will overrule the objection. Then the witness will be allowed to answer. The witness should never display a combative or hostile attitude and should not make sarcastic remarks while testifying in court. This is the fastest way to show

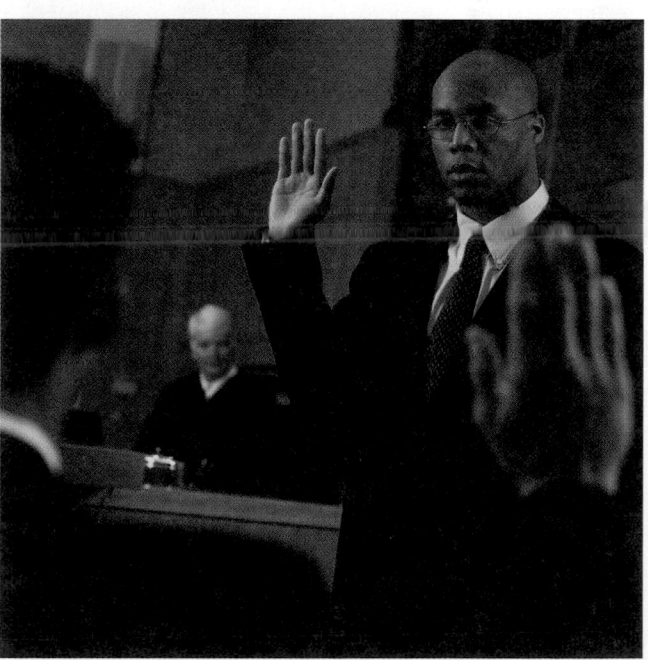

FIGURE 7-4 Witnesses must be credible and tell the truth on the stand in court to avoid charges of perjury.

disrespect for the judge, the jurors, and the court itself. No matter the circumstances, the court is no place to express discontent. The witness should be professional at all times and restrain inappropriate comments and belligerent behavior. Using "yes Sir" and "no Ma'am" is appropriate in the courtroom. Always address the judge as "your Honor."

Inside the Courtroom

It is beneficial to know the role of each person in a court of law (Figure 7-5). The person or body bringing the lawsuit to court is referred to by different terms, depending on what type of case is to be presented. In a criminal court, the government brings the case and is represented by a prosecutor. Legal documents will read, for example, "The State of Texas v. Robert Smith" in criminal cases. In this case, the fictitious Robert Smith is the defendant. In civil court, the person or group bringing the case to court is called the *plaintiff* (or *complainant* in some court systems), and the opposite party is called the *defendant* or *respondent*. A judge will preside over the case, providing instructions concerning the law to the jury, if a jury is present. If there is no jury, the judge decides the case. This is called a "bench trial." A *witness* is a person who gives testimony, knowing some pertinent information about the case (Figure 7-6). Often a court reporter takes notes of the proceedings, and a **bailiff** may be present, who assists in keeping order. All of these individuals should be treated with respect and courtesy.

Burden of Proof

In a criminal case, the burden of proof is on the prosecution, which must prove guilt beyond any **reasonable doubt**. Reasonable doubt is defined as the level of certainty a juror must have to find a defendant guilty of a crime. It is real doubt, based on reason and common

sense after careful and impartial consideration of all the evidence, or lack of evidence, in a case.

Civil cases must be proven by a **preponderance of the evidence**. This means that there must be a greater weight of evidence that points toward the defendant/respondent as being responsible for the act involved in the case.

To understand the difference between reasonable doubt and preponderance of the evidence, think of the scales of justice (Figure 7-7). For a case to be proven beyond a reasonable doubt, the scales should tip heavily toward either guilt or innocence. However, for a case to be proven by preponderance of the evidence, the scales need only tip slightly one way or the other.

To illustrate the difference in the standard of proof in criminal and civil cases, consider "The People of the State of California v. Orenthal James Simpson." In O.J. Simpson's criminal trial, although there was much circumstantial evidence, there was also enough doubt that the scales could not tip heavily toward a verdict of guilty, and Mr. Simpson was acquitted. But in the civil trial brought by family members of Nicole Brown Simpson and Ron Goldman after the criminal trial had ended, there was just enough evidence to tip the scales in favor of the families' claim that Mr. Simpson was somehow responsible for the deaths of Nicole and Ron. This is the equivalent to a preponderance of the evidence.

CRITICAL THINKING APPLICATION

The discussion of the burden of proof prompts Barbara, Samantha, and Lynda to discuss the case of O.J. Simpson. Discuss whether reasonable doubt existed in his criminal trial.

Outcome of the Case

Once both sides have presented their case to the judge or jury, usually they are given the opportunity to present a final summation of their case. After this is done, the jury retires to consider the **verdict**. This can take minutes, hours, days, or weeks. After the jury reaches a verdict, the judge may enter a judgment on that verdict or may disregard the verdict if the evidence does not support the jury's decision. The judge may also revise the verdict to comply with statutes, such as statutory limits on the amount of punitive damages. The final decision of the trial court is reflected in the judgment, signed by the judge.

Either side normally has the right to appeal the decision to a higher court. However, not all appellate courts are required to hear all cases. For instance, the U.S. Supreme Court chooses the cases that it hears each year, and it is restricted to cases that involve interpretation of the Constitution of the United States and how that interpretation affects the people it governs.

In criminal cases, when a person is found guilty of the crime with which he or she is charged, a sentencing date will be set at which the punishment will be announced. This is usually set a few weeks to a month after the verdict is announced.

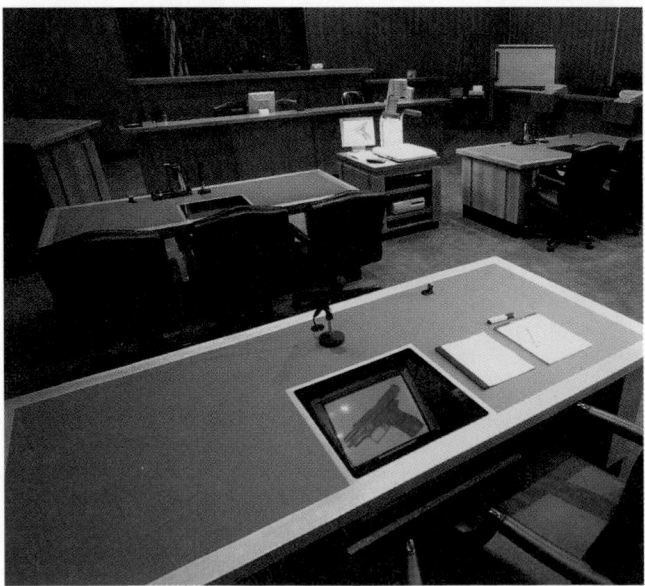

FIGURE 7-5 The inside of a typical U.S. courtroom.

HUMOR IN THE COURTROOM

Mary Louise Gilman has very possibly heard it all. As the editor of the *National Shorthand Reporter*, she collected enough courtroom bloopers to fill two books: "*Humor in the Court*" and "*More Humor in the Court.*" Here are a few examples!

Q: Were you acquainted with the deceased?
A: *Yes, Sir.*
Q: Before or after he died?

Q: What happened then?
A: *He told me, he says, "I have to kill you because you can identify me."*
Q: Did he kill you?
A: *No.*

Q: When he went, had you gone and had she, if she wanted to and were able, for the time being excluding all the restraints on her not to go, gone also, would he have brought you, meaning you and she, with him to the station?
A: *Objection. That question should be taken out and shot.*

Q: And lastly, Gary, all your responses must be oral. O.K.? What school do you go to?
A: *Oral.*
Q: How old are you?
A: *Oral.*

Q: ...and what did he do then?
A: *He came home, and next morning he was dead.*
Q: So when he woke up the next morning he was dead?

Q: ...any suggestions as to what prevented this from being a murder trial instead of an attempted murder trial?
A: *The victim lived.*

Q: What is your date of birth?
A: *July fifteenth.*
Q: What year?
A: *Every year.*

Q: This myasthenia gravis–does it affect your memory at all?
A: *Yes.*
Q: And in what ways does it affect your memory?
A: *I forget.*
Q: Can you give me an example of something you've forgotten?

Q: What was the first thing your husband said to you when he woke that morning?
A: *He said, "Where am I, Cathy?"*
Q: And why did that upset you?
A: *My name is Susan.*

Q: She had three children, correct?
A: *Yes.*
Q: How many were boys?
A: *None.*
Q: Were there any girls?

Q: Doctor, before you performed the autopsy, did you check for a pulse?
A: *No.*
Q: Did you check for a blood pressure?
A: *No.*
Q: Did you check for breathing?
A: *No.*
Q: So, then it is possible that the patient was alive when you began the autopsy?
A: *No.*
Q: How can you be sure, Doctor?
A: *Because his brain was sitting on my desk in a jar.*
Q: But could the patient have still been alive nevertheless?
A: *Yes, it is possible that he could have been alive and practicing law somewhere.*

FIGURE 7-6   Humor in the courtroom. (From Gilman M, editor: *More humor in the court*. Vienna, Vir, 1985, National Shorthand Reporters Association.)

Arbitration

Arbitration is an alternative to trial that uses a third party who has been selected because of the party's familiarity with or knowledge of the law or the issues involved to hear evidence and make a decision. Arbitration is common in modern business life. It is recognized by statute in the majority of the states and is usually available to the medical profession, affording an alternative method for resolving legal disputes between physician and patient. Many physicians and attorneys see arbitration as one way to solve the crisis of litigation in this country. Court battles can take years and be extremely expensive, and much of the money will revert to the attorneys involved in the case instead of the victors of the lawsuit.

In arbitration, the patient and the physician agree to submit the dispute to an **arbitrator** in an informal hearing. The arbitrator will render a legally binding decision based on very specific rules of arbitration. Arbitration applies essentially the same rights and the same measure of damages as a court. It is fair, less expensive, faster, and more confidential than court litigation.

The staff of each medical office should know whether arbitration statutes exist in the state where the office

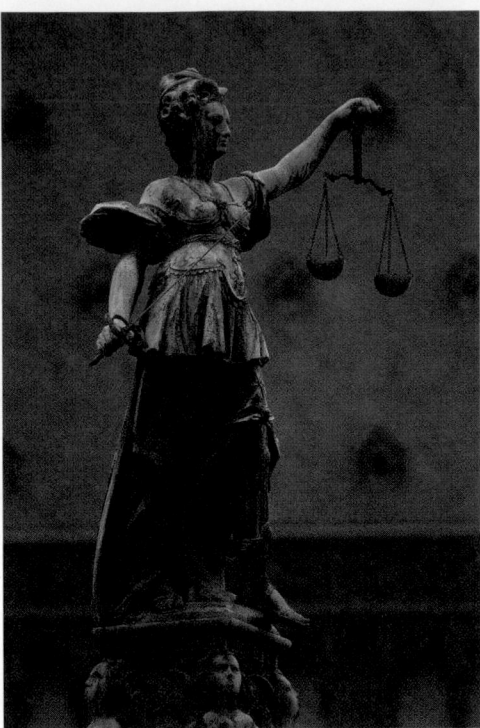

FIGURE 7-7 "Lady Justice." Justitia was the Roman goddess of justice and is the figure depicted in statues across the world, often holding both scales and a sword. Her scales imply the weighing of justice, and the blindfold represents the impartiality of justice.

conducts business. The state medical board or local medical society should be able to provide this information. An arbitration agreement is a contract and is subject to the judgment of the courts only as to the fairness of the agreement. The agreement is precisely worded by an attorney and should not be **paraphrased** when explaining it to a patient. Signing the agreement is a voluntary act by the patient, who has a grace period in which to revoke the agreement if he or she later decides against it. Likewise, a physician always has the option to decide not to care for a patient but must formally notify a patient if the decision is made to no longer render care.

If a physician elects to implement an arbitration agreement procedure with patients, every member of the physician's staff should know the details of the agreement, how and when the patient should sign up, and how to answer the patient's questions. The way that the program is presented to the patient and the willingness with which the office personnel answer the patient's questions will play a large part in whether courts will uphold the arbitration agreement as being fair and legal.

Both the patient and the physician have the opportunity to agree who will arbitrate the case, so that it does not favor one side over the other. By prior agreement, the arbitrator (or arbitrators) may be appointed by or from the American Arbitration Association, which is a neutral, private, nonprofit association dedicated to the advancement of out-of-court remedies. Its panels of arbitrators are made up of persons from business, the professions, and public interest groups.

Medical Professional Liability and Negligence

When injury results to a patient as a result of a physician's negligence, the patient may initiate a malpractice lawsuit to recover financial **damages**. However, experience has shown that the incidence of malpractice claims is directly related to the personal relationship and trust that exist between the physician and the patient. A deterioration of the physician-patient relationship is a common reason for the patient's decision to sue the physician for malpractice, even in situations where there is no real injury to the patient.

Medical professional liability, commonly called *medical malpractice*, is governed by the law of torts. The term *medical professional liability* encompasses all possible civil liability that can be incurred during the delivery of medical care. Medical professional liability is much more easily prevented than defended.

To understand medical malpractice, one must first understand the term **negligence**. Negligence, in general, implies inattention to one's duty or business, or the implication of a lack of necessary diligence or care. In medicine, negligence is defined as the performance of an act that a reasonable and **prudent** physician *would not* do or the failure to do an act that a reasonable and prudent physician *would* do. This, of course, also applies to any other healthcare professional. The standard of prudent care and conduct is not defined by law but would be left to the determination of a judge or jury, usually with the help of **expert witnesses** (Figure 7-8). Expert witnesses are members of the profession involved—in this case, medicine. To be considered an expert witness, a person usually belongs to a certifying or qualifying organization, against which the qualities of the defendant may be compared.

Professional negligence in medicine falls into one of three general classifications:

- *Malfeasance:* The performance of an act that is wholly wrongful and unlawful
- *Misfeasance:* The improper performance of a lawful act
- *Nonfeasance:* The failure to perform an act that should have been performed

A physician who performs an operation carelessly or fails to render care that should have been given may be found to have been negligent. Although a medical assistant acts as an agent of the physician in carrying out the majority of his or her duties, it is possible for the medical assistant to perform an act that can result in litigation.

For instance, if the medical assistant gives a patient the wrong medication or the wrong dosage of medication, both the physician and the medical assistant can be held liable for the error. Some states limit the scope of practice of medical assistants where medications are involved; however, if medical assistants are performing within the realm of duties for which they have received training and the physician is accepting responsibility for the actions of those in the medical office, they are usually allowed to dispense and administer medications unless prohibited by state law.

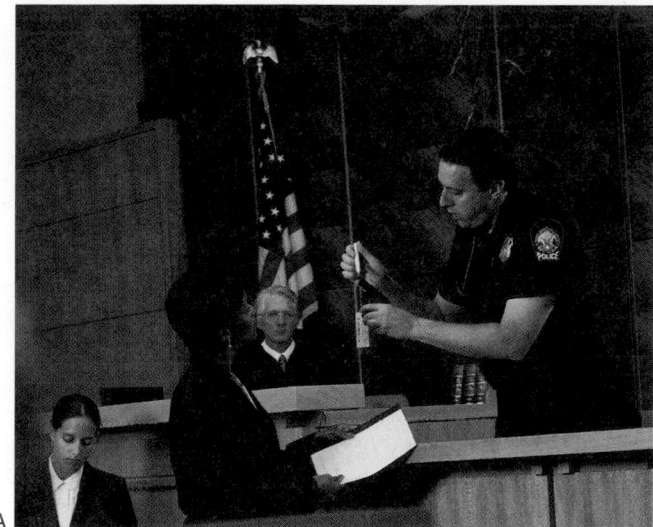
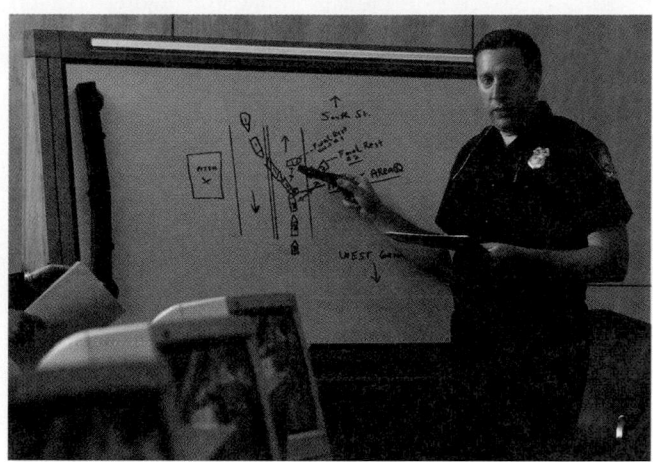

FIGURE 7-8   **A** and **B**, Expert witnesses help attorneys to prove or disprove the case in question by drawing on their experience with a given subject.

CRITICAL THINKING APPLICATION

Lynda is curious as to whether a physician is guilty of medical professional liability if he or she makes a mistake in diagnosing a patient. When might this be considered malpractice, and when might it not be considered malpractice?

What if the patient makes his or her condition worse? Is the physician then fully responsible? **Contributory negligence** exists when the patient contributes to his or her own condition and can lessen the damages that can be collected or even prevent them from being collected altogether.

The Four D's of Negligence

Negligence is not presumed—it must be proven. The Committee on Medicolegal Problems of the American Medical Association (AMA) has determined that patients must present evidence of four elements before negligence has been proven. These elements have become known as the Four *D*'s of Negligence:

1. *Duty.* Duty exists when the physician-patient relationship has been established. The patient has sought the assistance of the physician, and the physician has knowingly undertaken to provide the needed medical service.
2. *Dereliction:* Dereliction, or failure to perform a duty, is the second element required. There must be proof that the physician somehow neglected the duty to the patient.
3. *Direct cause:* There must be proof that the harm to the patient was directly caused by the physician's actions or failure to act and that the harm would not otherwise have occurred.
4. *Damages:* The patient must prove that a loss or harm has resulted from the actions of the physician.

If all four of these elements exist, then the patient may obtain a judgment against the physician in a medical professional liability case.

Types of Damages

There are several types of damages commonly seen in tort cases. They are nominal, punitive, compensatory, general, and special damages.

Nominal damages are small awards that are token compensations for the invasion of a legal right in which no actual injury was suffered. For instance, if an unauthorized medical facility employee accesses a patient's medical record and is discovered, but does not reveal any of the information in the record, the patient has not actually been harmed, but may be awarded nominal damages in a lawsuit for the invasion of the patient's privacy.

Punitive damages are designed to punish the party who committed the wrong in such a way to deter the repetition of the act, and are sometimes called exemplary damages. These damages were historically set so that the amounts would discourage intentional wrongdoings, misconduct, and outrageous behaviors. The amount of damages awarded would coincide in some percentage with the wealth of the defendant. Today there is much discussion of tort reform, which would place a cap on the amount of money that could be collected during personal injury litigation, including medical malpractice cases. Some have suggested a specific monetary figure, such as $500,000, as a limit on punitive damages, and others have suggested that plaintiffs be allowed to collect only up to three times the amount of compensatory damages.

CRITICAL THINKING APPLICATION

Samantha and Lynda disagree as to whether punitive damages should be awarded in medical professional liability cases. Samantha feels that nothing will compensate for certain losses, but Lynda feels that monetary compensation is reasonable when a loss has been suffered. Discuss both sides of the issue.

Compensatory damages are designed to compensate for any actual damages that are caused by the negligent person. They are intended to make the injured person "whole." Of course, nothing can substitute for the loss of an arm or a leg, for example, but compensatory damages help the patient or the patient's family recover from the loss.

General damages include compensation for pain and suffering, for loss of a bodily member or faculty, for disfigurement, or for other similar direct losses or injuries. The fact of the losses must be proven, but the monetary value does not.

Special damages are those injuries or losses that are not a necessary consequence of the physician's negligent act or omission. These may include the loss of earnings or costs of travel. Both the fact of these losses and the monetary value must be proven.

Standard of Care

If a physician were to be held legally responsible for every unsuccessful result occurring in the treatment of a patient, no person would undertake the responsibility of practicing medicine. The courts hold that a physician must do the following:

- Use reasonable care, attention, and diligence in the performance of professional services.
- Follow his or her best judgment in treating patients.
- Possess and exercise reasonable skill and care that are commonly possessed and exercised by other reputable physicians in the same type practice in the same or a similar locality.

Physicians who represent themselves as specialists must meet the standards of practice of their specialty. Whether or not they have met these requirements in treating a particular patient is generally a matter for the court to decide on the basis of testimony provided by an expert witness. Physicians are not required to possess extraordinary learning and skill, but they must keep abreast of medical developments and techniques, and they cannot experiment. They are also bound to advise their patients if they discover that the condition to be treated is one beyond their knowledge or technical skill.

In the worst of cases, a physician or medical facility may be faced with a wrongful death litigation. A wrongful death **allegation** is one in which the physician or medical facility is being blamed for the death of a patient as a result of error or inappropriate treatment. A wrongful death suit is usually brought by the family of the **decedent** against the physician or others involved with the patient.

A medical assistant should treat every chart touched as if it will end up in a court of law. Handwriting must be implicitly clear and legible, detailed, and leave absolutely no room for errors. Never mark out a mistake. Always draw one line through the error, then initial and date it. Nothing should be committed to memory. Remember, if it is not in the chart, it did not happen!

Consent

A physician must have consent to treat a patient, even though this consent is usually implied by virtue of the patient's appearance at the office for treatment. This **implied consent** is sufficient for common or simple procedures that are generally understood to involve little risk. A blood screen or taking vital signs are examples of procedures that usually involve implied consent. When more complex procedures are anticipated, the physician must obtain the patient's informed consent. A physician who fails to secure some formal expression of consent could be charged with the crime of **battery**.

The Health Insurance Portability and Accountability Act (HIPAA) of 1996 was designed for two major purposes. First, a standardization of electronic data exchange was sought in hopes that the efficiency of the healthcare system would be improved. Second, HIPAA was developed to protect health information and secure the contents of patient medical records. In the past, a section of the Health Insurance Claim Form (HCFA 1500) was reserved for the patient to authorize the release of medical information to the insurance company so that the claim could be evaluated and paid. Today, because of the influence of HIPAA, many medical offices are moving toward the use of a general consent form that is signed before the physician sees the patient. This form allows the physician to not only treat the patient, but also to use and submit health information to third parties for reimbursement.

Informed consent involves a deeper understanding of the patient's condition and a full explanation of the plan for treatment. Informed consent is not satisfied merely by having the patient sign a form. A discussion must occur during which the physician provides the patient or the patient's legal representative with enough information to decide whether to undergo the treatment or seek an alternative. After such discussion, the patient either consents or refuses to consent to the proposed therapy and signs a consent form. According to the AMA's standards for informed consent, the discussion should contain the following elements, at a minimum:

- The patient's diagnosis, if known
- The nature and purpose of a proposed treatment or procedure
- The risks and benefits of a proposed treatment or procedure
- Alternative treatments or procedures, regardless of the cost or the extent to which the treatment options are covered by health insurance
- The risks and benefits of the alternative treatment or procedure
- The risks and benefits of not receiving or undergoing a treatment or procedure

The discussion should be fully documented in the patient's medical record, and a copy of the signed form should be placed in the record. Treatment may not exceed the scope of the consent that the patient has given. Often the consent forms will be lengthy and mention excessive possibilities and complications. There may be language that attempts to be all-inclusive, such as "included, but not limited to" when risks are listed. It is wise to have an attorney review the forms that are used for informed consent, because those that are too broad or too specific can be detrimental to the physician in a medical professional liability case.

Patients cannot be forced to undergo any type of medical treatment or care. The ultimate decision regarding care must be left to the patient, and although medical professionals should disclose information to help the patient make a good, informed decision, the patient should never be persuaded to act in any manner or accept any treatment to which he or she does not agree. Should the patient decide not to undergo treatment that the physician feels is necessary, an informed refusal of treatment or care should be signed. This should be a statement similar to the informed consent, but will indicate that the patient has elected not to undergo treatment. Some physicians will discontinue all treatment if a patient does not participate in the care that the physician recommends. This document, once signed, should be added to the patient's medical record.

CRITICAL THINKING APPLICATION

Barbara stresses to Samantha and Lynda that there may be times in their professional career when a patient asks for their advice as to whether he or she should undergo a certain procedure or treatment. Barbara explains that patients often consider advice from the medical assistants in the office to be an extension of the physician's opinions. How might they handle such questions from patients?

Giving Consent to Medical Procedures. Mentally competent adults are certainly able to consent to medical procedures. However, if an act is unlawful, then the consent is invalid. For instance, if an abortion is performed in a state where abortion is considered illegal, then the consent to that procedure is null. Consent is also invalid if it is given by a person who is unauthorized to do so or if it is obtained by misrepresentation or fraud.

In an emergency, one may render aid or care to prevent loss of life or serious illness or injury. However, implied consent in this circumstance lasts only as long as the emergency exists, and formal consent must be obtained for further treatment as soon as the emergency has passed.

Physicians are sometimes reluctant to render aid in an emergency to someone who is not their patient for fear that they will later be charged with negligence or abandonment. In 1959, California passed the first Good Samaritan Act, which provides immunity from liability to volunteers at the scene of an accident for any civil damages as a result of rendering emergency care. Today, all 50 states have Good Samaritan statutes. As long as the emergency care is given in good faith and without gross negligence, and the healthcare worker only provides emergency care that he or she has been trained to provide, the likelihood of a successful lawsuit against that individual is very slim.

Adults who have been found by a court to be insane or incompetent usually cannot consent to medical treatment. Consent must be obtained from the guardian except in emergency situations.

Generally, when the patient is a minor, consent for surgery or treatment must be obtained from a parent, guardian, or **guardian ad litem**, except in an emergency requiring immediate treatment. If the parents are legally divorced or separated, consent should be obtained from the custodial parent, but if the child is visiting the second parent, consent may be obtained from that parent, because in this situation there is a temporary custody.

Consent is not required for minors in the following circumstances:

- When consent may be assumed, such as in a life-threatening situation
- When a certain treatment is required by law, such as a vaccination or x-ray evaluation for school entry or safety
- When a court order has been issued, as in a situation in which parents withhold consent for a necessary treatment because of religious reasons

In many states, treatment of sexually transmitted diseases, drug abuse, alcohol dependency, or pregnancy or providing birth control measures does not require parental consent.

Emancipation is defined by statute and varies from state to state. An emancipated minor is a person younger than the age of majority (usually 18 to 21 years) who meets one or more of the following conditions:

- Is married
- Is in the armed forces
- Is living separate and apart from parents or a legal guardian
- Is self-supporting

Some states include a minimum age for emancipation. Unless a statute declares otherwise, a minor who has the right to consent to treatment is entitled to the protection of his or her confidences, even from parents.

Statute of Limitations

A statute of limitations is a period of time after which a lawsuit cannot be filed. The statute of limitations varies from state to state and differs for various types of litigation. Many states have a 2-year statute of limitations for medical malpractice issues. However, in some instances, the statute of limitations may be extended because of a delay in the discovery of an injury. For example, a patient has surgery to replace a valve in the heart, and the surgery seems successful. Two years later, the patient obtains a routine echocardiogram and the physician discovers that the surgeon mistakenly replaced the aortic valve when the surgery was intended for the pulmonary valve. Although 2 years have already passed, the statute of limitations begins at the point of discovery of the injury, so the patient could now bring suit against the surgeon for the error.

Confidentiality

Confidentiality is one of the most sacred trusts that the patient places in the hands of the physician and his or her staff (Figure 7-9). Breach of patient confidentiality is grounds for immediate dismissal of a healthcare professional. The strictest care must be taken when handling patient records and discussing information about patients.

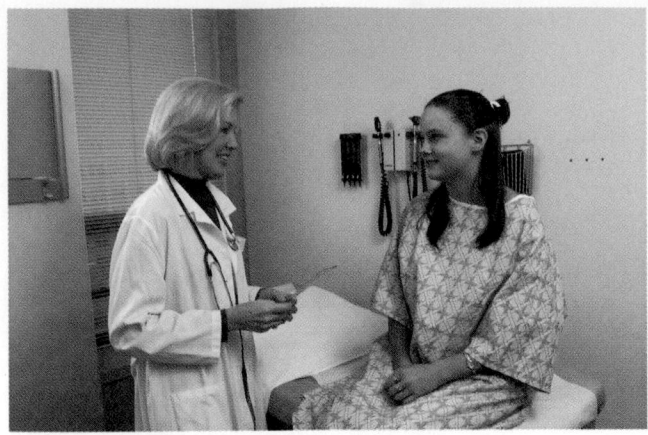

FIGURE 7-9 Patient confidentiality is the most important trust that exists between the physician and the patient.

There are many special cases in which patient confidentiality plays a vital role. A patient who is HIV positive may face discrimination if the information about his or her medical condition surfaces. Physicians who treat these patients may wish to take extra care when leaving phone messages or sending mail. Instead of leaving a message for a patient from "Dr. Watson's office," the medical assistant could say that the message is from "Terry Watson's office." This could indicate an attorney, accountant, or real estate broker. Curious co-workers or relatives may not grow as suspicious as they might if they were to encounter a message from a physician's office.

Patients who are receiving treatment for substance abuse are protected by federal statutes. Confidentiality is also of utmost importance to patients receiving treatment for mental health issues, sexually transmitted diseases, sexual **assault**, and any type of abuse.

Law and Medical Practice

Law affects the day-to-day practice of the physician. Some of the ways in which the medical assistant will encounter legal issues in the physician's offices are discussed in this section.

Legal Disclosure

The physician is charged with safeguarding patient confidences within the constraints of the law, but according to state laws, which vary somewhat throughout the nation, certain disclosures must be made. Frequently the medical assistant is involved with the responsibility for reporting these events.

Births and deaths must be reported. In some states, detailed information about stillbirths is required. Physicians must also report cases that may have been a result of violence, such as gunshot wounds, knife injuries, or poisonings. Any death from accidental, suspicious, or unexplained causes must also be reported. In some states, occupational diseases and injuries must be reported within specific time limits.

Sexually transmitted diseases are reportable in every state. All fifty states require that patients who have confirmed cases of acquired immunodeficiency syndrome (AIDS) be reported by name to the local health department. However, just over 30 states require that patients who are HIV positive be reported. Individuals are reported either by name or by unique identifiers. A continuing controversy exists as to whether the reporting prompts patients to receive care or deters patients in high-risk groups from seeking care.

Child abuse is a leading cause of death among children younger than 5 years of age, and health care professionals are required by law to report any suspected cases of child abuse. The report should be made as soon as evidence is discovered that gives the physician "cause to believe" that abuse or neglect has occurred. Even if the evidence is uncertain, the physician should report the evidence and allow the government to investigate and determine what action to take to protect the child. However, it is essential to make every attempt to ensure that the report is legitimate, because it could lead to the child's being removed from the home and placed in foster care. Cases of spousal and elder abuse are difficult, because the person being abused is often reluctant to report the situation for fear of further mistreatment. The law requires that suspected cases of abuse to children, elderly persons, or any others at risk be reported to the authorities.

Local health departments publish lists of diseases that are reportable as well as the method that should be used in reporting. Often this can be done by telephone or mail. Appropriate forms must be used for mail reporting, which are supplied by the health department or available on their websites. County and state health departments periodically issue bulletins that are sent to healthcare providers and provide information about disease outbreaks and various statistics. Local health departments should be consulted for specific procedures and reporting protocols.

Patient Self-Determination Act

The Patient Self-Determination Act of 1990 brought the term *advance directives* to the forefront of medical care. This act requires healthcare facilities to develop and maintain written procedures that ensure that all adult patients receive information about living wills, durable powers of attorney for healthcare, and advance directives. These documents place the decision-making power into the hands of the patient and the patient's family, providing them with written notification of their right to consent to or refuse medical treatment.

Patients' Bill of Rights

One of the most important contributions that President Clinton offered to America during his terms in office was his active pursuit of a Patients' Bill of Rights. Confidentiality of medical records, guaranteed access to emergency care and specialists, timely accessibility to healthcare, and an appellate process for those dissatisfied with the decisions made by healthcare providers are some of the rights that are proposed. One important aspect of this legislation deals with the rights of patients to sue their health maintenance organizations (HMOs).

Because it is a patient's right to understand his or her diagnosis, prognosis, and all aspects of care, one must take special care when dealing with a patient with whom there may be a language barrier. If the patient's ability to understand is limited, an interpreter may be needed to ensure that there is adequate communication from physician to patient.

Controlled Substances Act of 1970

On May 1, 1971, the Controlled Substances Act of 1970 became effective. In October 1973, a regulatory agency known as the Drug Enforcement Administration (DEA) became a part of the U.S. Department of Justice. The DEA works with local, state, federal, and international agencies and organizations to address and regulate the serious issues of drug use and abuse in the United States.

Before administering, prescribing, or dispensing any drugs, a physician is required to register with the regional office of the DEA. This registration is renewable every 3 years. If a physician works from more than one office, he or she must register each individual office. Regulations regarding the writing, telephoning, and refilling of prescriptions vary according to which schedule is involved.

Under the Controlled Substances Act, drugs are categorized into Schedules I, II, III, IV, and V. Drugs in Schedule I have the highest potential for abuse and addiction, and those in Schedule V have the least abuse potential.

Schedule I substances are those that have no accepted medical use in the United States. Examples include heroin and d-lysergic acid diethylamide (LSD). Only the physician who is involved in conducting research with such drugs is concerned with Schedule I substances.

Schedule II drugs have a high abuse potential, with severe risk of mental and physical dependence. They include certain narcotic, stimulant, and depressant drugs, such as opium, morphine, codeine, and methylphenidate (Ritalin). Controlled substances in Schedule II can be obtained only with a federal triplicate order form obtained from the DEA. A special inventory must be maintained on controlled substances and retained for 2 to 3 years, depending on state requirements. When a controlled substance is removed from inventory, it must be recorded. The record must show the date, the name of the drug, the dosage, and the name of the patient, physician, and employee involved. Schedule III, IV, and V substances do not require triplicate forms.

Schedule III substances have an abuse potential that is lesser than that of the first two schedules. They include compounds that contain limited quantities of certain narcotic drugs combined with nonnarcotic substances. Examples include acetaminophen (Tylenol) with codeine, hydrocodone, butalbital with aspirin and caffeine (Fiorinal), and several steroids.

Schedule IV substances have still less potential for abuse. Phenobarbital, diazepam (Valium), propoxyphene (Darvon and Darvocet), alprazolam (Xanax), chlordiazepoxide (Librium), and pentazocine lactate (Talwin) are examples.

Schedule V substances have less abuse potential than those in Schedule IV but still warrant control. They include preparations that contain moderate quantities of certain narcotics that may be found in cough medicines and antidiarrheal products.

The physician may call a prescription to the pharmacist, but the pharmacist must transcribe it in writing before filling it. With permission from the physician, the medical assistant may orally transmit a prescription for controlled substances only in Schedules III, IV, or V, and the dispensing pharmacist must put the prescription into writing before filling it. The medical assistant cannot under any circumstances orally transmit a prescription for a Schedule II drug.

Stored controlled substances must be kept in a locked cabinet or safe. Any loss of controlled drugs by theft must be reported to the regional office of the DEA at the time the theft is discovered. If a physician discovers that his or her DEA number is being used in the unauthorized prescribing of controlled substances, he or she should report the incident to the DEA, to the state regulatory agency, and to the local police authorities. This is especially important in the case of employees whose employment has been terminated and who are suspected of drug theft in the office. There have been numerous cases of retaliation by fired employees who report to the DEA exactly what they have actually taken, yet accuse the physician or other staff members of taking the controlled substances. This results in messy investigations and months of follow-up, so any suspected employee drug use or abuse should be documented and reported to the local authorities. Periodic drug testing of employees is one way to help prevent office drug abuse.

A physician who discontinues medical practice must return the registration certificate and any unused order forms and triplicate prescription pads to the nearest office of the DEA. The regional DEA office will advise the physician on the disposition of any controlled drugs still on hand.

CRITICAL THINKING APPLICATION

Barbara explains the importance of reporting any employee who is suspected of using drugs or taking drugs from the office. This may be difficult, since co-workers are often friendly and may hesitate to report such acts. Discuss ways to handle this situation.

Uniform Anatomical Gift Act

The Uniform Anatomical Gift Act was approved by the National Conference of Commissioners on Uniform State Laws in 1968. Although many states had passed laws before this time that permitted living persons to make a gift of their body or portions of it after death, the laws were so different from state to state that arrangements for a donation in one state might not be recognized in another. All states have adopted the Uniform Anatomical Gift Act or similar legislation.

Essentially, the model law for donation states the following:

- Any person of sound mind and 18 years of age or older may give all or any part of his or her body after death for research, transplantation, or placement in a tissue bank.
- A donor's valid statement of gift is paramount to the rights of others except when a state autopsy law may prevail.
- If a donor has not indicated an intent to donate during his or her lifetime, his or her survivors, in a specified order of priority, may do so.
- Physicians who accept organs or tissues, relying in good faith on the documents, are protected from lawsuits. The physician attending at the time of death, if acquainted with the donor's wishes, may dispose of the body under the Uniform Anatomical Gift Act.
- The time of death must be determined by a physician who is not involved in the transplantation, and the attending physician cannot be a member of the transplant team.
- The donor may revoke the gift, or the gift may be rejected by the proposed recipient.

The most important clause of the act permits the donation to be made by a will (without waiting for probate) or by other written or witnessed documents, such as a card designed to be carried by the person or a Uniform Donor Card (Figure 7-10). The Uniform Donor Card is considered a legal document in all 50 states. Many states now list donor preference on the driver's license as well.

The provisions of the Uniform Anatomical Gift Act are so designed that the offer is exercised only after death. Therefore donors should reveal their intentions to as many of their relatives and friends as possible and to their physician. Because the human body and its parts are not commodities in commerce, no money can be exchanged in making an anatomical donation itself. Fees are charged for performing the transplant and various procedures, but organs cannot be bought and sold. It is also important to note that family members should be prepared to receive the body of the person who has donated his or her entire body to research once the research facility has completed its study. This can often be a traumatic experience, rekindling the grief process once again, so the procedures and final disposition of the body should be decided at the time of the donation to avoid this difficult situation.

Health Insurance Portability and Accountability Act of 1996

HIPAA was signed into law on August 21, 1996, and all healthcare providers must be in compliance by April 2003. Its history began in the Clinton healthcare reform proposals. HIPAA was designed for several purposes, with many goals in mind. Limiting administrative costs of healthcare and privacy issues, as well as prevention of fraud and abuse, are of primary importance within the HIPAA regulations.

The use of electronic transmissions would ideally lower the administrative costs of providing healthcare, but this led to problems with privacy regarding health information. Therefore the law also had to provide security and confidentiality guarantees for the individual patient. Extensive privacy rules, including the use of unique identifiers, have shaped the law.

The final regulations regarding the privacy legislation sections of HIPAA were published in December 2000, after HCFA reviewed more than 50,000 comments and concerns on this important subject. All healthcare organizations that transmit any health information electronically must comply with HIPAA, and fines as well as prison terms can be imposed on those who do not comply with the regulations.

HIPAA will have a tremendous effect on the healthcare industry. All healthcare providers, clearinghouses, and health plans that use electronic information must comply with HIPAA regulations.

Occupational Safety and Health Act and the Bloodborne Pathogens Standard

In 1970, President Nixon signed the Occupational Safety and Health Act, which created what we know today as the Occupational Safety and Health Administration (OSHA). OSHA is a division of the U.S. Department of Labor, and since its creation workplace injuries, illnesses, and fatalities have been significantly reduced. OSHA's mission is to ensure workplace safety and a healthy environment within the workplace.

Although OSHA is commonly thought of as the regulatory agency that requires steel-toed boots and hard hats, the medical industry moved into the OSHA spotlight in the late 1980s, when the threat of HIV infection extended to healthcare workers. Hepatitis and other pathogens were already of concern to healthcare workers, but when HIV, the virus that causes AIDS, was identified, action was needed to better protect the individuals who cared for patients with these infectious diseases. OSHA's Final Ruling on Bloodborne Pathogens became fully effective in July 1992, and since that time, various additions have been made to update the regulations in light of new information learned about bloodborne pathogens.

The law requires medical facilities to comply with the Bloodborne Pathogens standard and to be able to prove

---

DONOR   DONOR CARD

I _____, have spoken to my family about organ and tissue donation. I wish to donate:
__ any needed organs and tissue
__ only the following organs and tissue: _____
The following people have witnessed my commitment to be a donor.
donor signature _____ date _____
witness _____
witness _____
next of kin _____ ph _____

FIGURE 7-10   Organ donation card.

that compliance to OSHA inspectors if necessary. The actual standard can be found in the 29 **Code of Federal Regulations (CFR)** 1910.1030. The following information details the legal requirements of the OSHA Standard as it pertains to the physician's office.

General Duty Clause. No law can cover every single situation that may arise in the course of daily living. Because of this, OSHA's general duty clause is a catch-all regulation that fits almost any situation not specified in any other section of the law. The general duty clause simply states that a workplace must be free of any hazard that might cause serious harm or death. For example, one breach of the general duty clause is the "failure of a facility to provide reasonable security procedures at a retail store." Although not a specific breach of any regulation, this fits nicely into the general duty clause.

OSHA Regulations as Performance-Based Standards. OSHA regulations are considered performance-based standards. This means that adequate compliance depends largely on what happens in the facility. For instance, the same regulations may not apply to two offices located right next to each other. Would it be possible that a family practitioner could be fined for not having sharps containers, and then the same OSHA inspector goes next door to a surgeon's office and does not fine the surgeon for not having sharps containers? It is possible if the surgeon does not perform any invasive, surgical, or any other procedures in the office that involve blood!

This is one reason that employees must be trained in their individual facilities. Even if training was done 1 month before a job change, the employee must be trained again in the new facility. Offices and procedures are different from place to place, and the employee must have adequate training to function successfully in the medical office.

OSHA inspectors can recommend fines when a facility is found to be out of compliance with an OSHA standard. One of the most common infractions is that the facility has an Exposure Control Plan in the facility but is not using it or following the procedures and policies set forth within it. This could lead to an inspector's declaring the facility to be *willfully negligent.* Willful negligence exists when "an employer representative was aware of the requirements of the [OSHA] Act, or the existence of an applicable standard or regulation, and was also aware that the condition or practice was in violation of those requirements, and did not abate the hazard." Fines for noncompliance can quadruple for willful negligence.

COMMON OSHA VIOLATIONS

- No eyewash facilities available
- No labeling or improper labeling of hazardous chemicals
- No MSDS for each hazardous chemical
- Storage of contaminated laboratory coats with clean ones

- Not communicating hazards to employees
- No documentation of initial employee training
- No documentation of annual employee training
- No annual hazard assessment performed
- Having an Exposure Control Plan but not following it
- No proof of destruction of hazardous waste
- No Emergency Action Plan in the facility
- No Written Exposure Control Plan
- OSHA Form 300A not posted during required period
- No records of hepatitis B vaccinations or declination forms

---

Exposure Control Plan. The Exposure Control Plan can be a part of the regular safety plan written for the medical facility or may be a stand-alone document, but it must cover all of the elements required by OSHA. This plan must be in writing and be reviewed annually, and there must be written documentation that the plan was reviewed and updated or revised, if needed. A hard copy must be provided to employees on their request within 15 working days, and the plan must be available at all times in the workplace.

The plan must delineate the tasks that employees perform where there is risk of blood exposure. It must also classify jobs within the facility according to the likelihood of exposures. For instance, some job duties would always expose the employee to blood or **other potentially infectious materials (OPIM)**, often on a daily basis. Some duties would only occasionally expose the employee, and other duties would never expose the employee to blood or OPIM. Employees must be told which category they are a part of, and what duties they will perform that could lead to exposures.

The Exposure Control Plan must contain a Waste Management section that details how waste is removed from the facility and destroyed. Most medical offices contract with companies that specialize in removing and destroying medical waste. The office must keep the receipts given by the company that prove that the waste was taken away from the facility and then incinerated or otherwise destroyed.

The plan must also contain a section on Hazardous Materials Communication, which explains what substances in the facility are hazardous and how to handle a spill or exposure to those products. Only the manufacturer of a chemical can determine whether it is hazardous, and Material Safety Data Sheets (MSDS) must be kept on almost all chemicals and reagents in the facility. Recent rulings have exempted some chemicals, but without the MSDS information, a medical assistant could not determine what type of health, reactivity, flammability, or other risks the chemical could have.

If the facility has equipment for x-ray studies, a Radiation Safety Plan must also be written and followed. All facilities should have an Emergency Action Plan in place, which provides procedures in case of tornadoes, fires, floods, or any other type of emergency that might occur in the office. This plan should contain floor plans of the facility, diagrams depicting the most efficient exits from the building, and the chain of command in an emergency. Diagrams with exit routes should be posted in every room of the medical office. At least annually, a hazard assessment must be performed on the entire facility. The hazard assessment is an inspection for problem areas in which the facility might be out of compliance. The facility must have documentation that the hazard assessment was done.

OSHA Recordkeeping Regulations. An injury or illness is considered to be work related when an event or exposure in the work environment contributed or caused the condition or significantly aggravated a preexisting condition. OSHA made several changes in the regulations concerning work-related injury recordkeeping to simplify forms, protect employee privacy, encourage employee involvement, and enable computer usage for meeting OSHA requirements. The revised rules took effect on January 1, 2002. Three basic forms are now used to keep records regarding injuries, accidents, and illnesses related to the workplace. The forms are as follows:

- *OSHA Form 300—Log of Work-Related Injuries and Illnesses* (Figure 7-11): Information is posted on form 300 regarding work-related deaths and every work-related injury or illness that involves loss of consciousness, restricted work activity or job transfer, days away from work, or medical treatment beyond first aid. An OSHA Form 301 (Injury and Illness Incident Report) should be completed for each entry on the log.
- *OSHA Form 300A—Summary of Work-Related Injuries and Illnesses* (Figure 7-12): Form 300A must be completed even if no injuries or illnesses occurred during the year that were work related. It must be posted in a common area for viewing by all employees, and provides the total number of accidents, illnesses, and injuries in the facility for the previous year. The length of time that this information must be posted has increased from 1 month to 3 months, specifically from February 1 to April 30 each year. An additional change is the certification of the form. A company executive must examine the document and certify that it is accurate.
- *OSHA Form 301—Injury and Illness Incident Report* (Figure 7-13): Form 301 is used to report what actually happened when an employee suffers a work-related injury or illness. This form, or an acceptable substitute, such as a state worker's compensation form, must be completed within 7 calendar days after notification of the illness or injury. The form should be completed as quickly as possible so that an exact recollection of events can be documented. Now that the new recordkeeping regulations have become effective, employees are guaranteed access to their OSHA 301 forms for the first time.

The log and summary forms must be kept on file for a minimum of 5 years. Only the Summary should be posted during the specified time period from February 1 to April 30 each year, reflecting information from the previous calendar year. The forms are not sent to OSHA unless specifically requested.

CRITICAL THINKING APPLICATION

Barbara quickly realizes that the office is using older versions of OSHA Forms 300 and 301. Where might she look or go to find updated information and copies of forms?

It is wise to keep a communication log of calls to OSHA in which questions were asked or information verified. Note the day and time called, the first and last name of the person spoken to, the person's title, and the question asked and response given. Take detailed notes while discussing the issue on the phone. This log could be invaluable if a question ever arises about a subject discussed with a local OSHA official. It may make the difference when an OSHA inspector suggests a hefty fine. If the medical facility can show documentation that a certain procedure was discussed with an OSHA official and decisions were made based on that discussion, the facility may have sufficient evidence that the law was considered and the facility did its best to comply.

Needlestick Safety and Prevention Act. An estimated 600,000 to 800,000 injuries occur annually among healthcare workers. One third of these injuries happen during the disposal process. In an effort to reduce these injuries that can lead to exposure to HIV, hepatitis B virus (HBV), or other bloodborne pathogens, OSHA revised its Bloodborne Pathogens standard to comply with the Needlestick Safety and Prevention Act, which became law on November 6, 2000. The new regulations became effective on April 18, 2001.

Employers are now required to involve employees in the selection of needle safety devices. The facility must be able to prove that consideration was given to various types of devices that promote needle safety, what led to the decision to choose the device currently in use, and which employees were involved in these decisions. A list should be kept of which employees contributed to the selection decisions. Minutes from meetings, copies of employee response forms, and the forms used to solicit input are good methods of proving that employees were involved in the selection process.

CRITICAL THINKING APPLICATION

Barbara needs input about the needle safety devices being used in the facility. Should she call a meeting of the entire office, or are there specific employees that should be present? If so, discuss who should have input in these decisions.

A needlestick and sharps injury log must also be kept in the medical facility. At a minimum, the log must include the following information:

OSHA's Form 300

Log of Work-Related Injuries and Illnesses

Year 20 05

U.S. Department of Labor

Occupational Safety and Health Administration

Form approved OMB no. 1218-0176

Attention: This form contains information relating to employee health and must be used in a manner that protects the confidentiality of employees to the extent possible while the information is being used for occupational safety and health purposes.

You must record information about every work-related death and about every work-related injury or illness that involves loss of consciousness, restricted work activity or job transfer, days away from work, or medical treatment beyond first aid. You must also record significant work-related injuries and illnesses that are diagnosed by a physician or licensed health care professional. You must also record work-related injuries and illnesses that meet any of the specific recording criteria listed in 29 CFR Part 1904.8 through 1904.12. Feel free to use two lines for a single case if you need to. You must complete an Injury and Illness Incident Report (OSHA Form 301) or equivalent form for each injury or illness recorded on this form. If you're not sure whether a case is recordable, call your local OSHA office for help.

Establishment name _____

City _____   State _____

Identify the person

(A) Case no.	(B) Employee's name	(C) Job title (e.g., Welder)

Describe the case

(D) Date of injury or onset of illness	(E) Where the event occurred (e.g., Loading dock north end)	(F) Describe injury or illness, parts of body affected, and object/substance that directly injured or made person ill (e.g., Second-degree burns on right forearm from acetylene torch)

Classify the case

Using these four categories, check ONLY the most serious result for each case:

(G) Death
(H) Days away from work
(I) Remained at work — Job transfer or restriction
(J) Remained at work — Other recordable cases

Enter the number of days the injured or ill worker was:

(K) On job transfer or restriction ____ days
(L) Away from work ____ days

Check the "injury" column or choose one type of illness:

(M)
(1) Injury
(2) Skin disorder
(3) Respiratory condition
(4) Poisoning
(5) All other illnesses

Page totals

Be sure to transfer these totals to the Summary page (Form 300A) before you post it.

Page ____ of ____

Public reporting burden for this collection of information is estimated to average 4 minutes per response, including time to review the instructions, search and gather the data needed, and complete and review the collection of information. Persons are not required to respond to the collection of information unless it displays a currently valid OMB control number. If you have any comments about these estimates or any other aspects of this data collection, contact: US Department of Labor, OSHA Office of Statistics, Room N-3644, 200 Constitution Avenue, NW, Washington, DC 20210. Do not send the completed forms to this office.

FIGURE 7-11   OSHA Form 300—Log of Work-Related Injuries and Illnesses. (Source: US Department of Labor, Occupational Safety and Health Administration.)

OSHA's Form 300A

Summary of Work-Related Injuries and Illnesses

Year 20___

U.S. Department of Labor
Occupational Safety and Health Administration

Form approved OMB no. 1218-0176

All establishments covered by Part 1904 must complete this Summary page, even if no work-related injuries or illnesses occurred during the year. Remember to review the Log to verify that the entries are complete and accurate before completing this summary.

Using the Log, count the individual entries you made for each category. Then write the totals below, making sure you've added the entries from every page of the Log. If you had no cases, write "0."

Employees, former employees, and their representatives have the right to review the OSHA Form 300 in its entirety. They also have limited access to the OSHA Form 301 or its equivalent. See 29 CFR Part 1904.35, in OSHA's recordkeeping rule, for further details on the access provisions for these forms.

Number of Cases

Total number of deaths	Total number of cases with days away from work	Total number of cases with job transfer or restriction	Total number of other recordable cases
___ (G)	___ (H)	___ (I)	___ (J)

Number of Days

Total number of days of job transfer or restriction	Total number of days away from work
___ (K)	___ (L)

Injury and Illness Types

Total number of . . .
(M)

(1) Injuries ___
(2) Skin disorders ___
(3) Respiratory conditions ___

(4) Poisonings ___
(5) All other illnesses ___

Post this Summary page from February 1 to April 30 of the year following the year covered by the form.

Public reporting burden for this collection of information is estimated to average 50 minutes per response, including time to review the instructions, search and gather the data needed, and complete and review the collection of information. Persons are not required to respond to the collection of information unless it displays a currently valid OMB control number. If you have any comments about these estimates or any other aspects of this data collection, contact: US Department of Labor, OSHA Office of Statistics, Room N-3644, 200 Constitution Avenue, NW, Washington, DC 20210. Do not send the completed forms to this office.

Establishment information

Your establishment name _____

Street _____

City _____ State ____ ZIP ____

Industry description (e.g., Manufacture of motor truck trailers) _____

Standard Industrial Classification (SIC), if known (e.g., SIC 3715) ____ ____

Employment information *(If you don't have these figures, see the Worksheet on the back of this page to estimate.)*

Annual average number of employees _____

Total hours worked by all employees last year _____

Sign here

Knowingly falsifying this document may result in a fine.

I certify that I have examined this document and that to the best of my knowledge the entries are true, accurate, and complete.

Company executive _____ Title _____

(___) _____ / ___ / ___
Phone Date

FIGURE 7-12 OSHA Form 300A—Summary of Work-Related Injuries and Illnesses. (Source: US Department of Labor, Occupational Safety and Health Administration.)

OSHA's Form 301
Injury and Illness Incident Report

U.S. Department of Labor
Occupational Safety and Health Administration

Form approved OMB no. 1218-0176

Attention: This form contains information relating to employee health and must be used in a manner that protects the confidentiality of employees to the extent possible while the information is being used for occupational safety and health purposes.

This *Injury and Illness Incident Report* is one of the first forms you must fill out when a recordable work-related injury or illness has occurred. Together with the *Log of Work-Related Injuries and Illnesses* and the accompanying *Summary*, these forms help the employer and OSHA develop a picture of the extent and severity of work-related incidents.

Within 7 calendar days after you receive information that a recordable work-related injury or illness has occurred, you must fill out this form or an equivalent. Some state workers' compensation, insurance, or other reports may be acceptable substitutes. To be considered an equivalent form, any substitute must contain all the information asked for on this form.

According to Public Law 91-596 and 29 CFR 1904, OSHA's recordkeeping rule, you must keep this form on file for 5 years following the year to which it pertains.

If you need additional copies of this form, you may photocopy and use as many as you need.

Completed by _____

Title _____

Phone (____) ____ - ____   Date ____ / ____ / ____

Information about the employee

1) Full name _____

2) Street _____
   City _____ State _____ ZIP _____

3) Date of birth ____ / ____ / ____

4) Date hired ____ / ____ / ____

5) ☐ Male
   ☐ Female

Information about the physician or other health care professional

6) Name of physician or other health care professional _____

7) If treatment was given away from the worksite, where was it given?
   Facility _____
   Street _____
   City _____ State _____ ZIP _____

8) Was employee treated in an emergency room?
   ☐ Yes
   ☐ No

9) Was employee hospitalized overnight as an in-patient?
   ☐ Yes
   ☐ No

Information about the case

10) Case number from the Log _____ (Transfer the case number from the Log after you record the case.)

11) Date of injury or illness ____ / ____ / ____

12) Time employee began work _____ AM / PM

13) Time of event _____ AM / PM ☐ Check if time cannot be determined

14) *What was the employee doing just before the incident occurred?* Describe the activity, as well as the tools, equipment, or material the employee was using. Be specific. *Examples:* "climbing a ladder while carrying roofing materials"; "spraying chlorine from hand sprayer"; "daily computer key-entry."

15) *What happened?* Tell us how the injury occurred. *Examples:* "When ladder slipped on wet floor, worker fell 20 feet"; "Worker was sprayed with chlorine when gasket broke during replacement"; "Worker developed soreness in wrist over time."

16) *What was the injury or illness?* Tell us the part of the body that was affected and how it was affected; be more specific than "hurt," "pain," or sore." *Examples:* "strained back"; "chemical burn, hand"; "carpal tunnel syndrome."

17) *What object or substance directly harmed the employee? Examples:* "concrete floor"; "chlorine"; "radial arm saw." *If this question does not apply to the incident, leave it blank.*

18) *If the employee died, when did death occur?* Date of death _____

Public reporting burden for this collection of information is estimated to average 22 minutes per response, including time for reviewing instructions, searching existing data sources, gathering and maintaining the data needed, and completing and reviewing the collection of information. Persons are not required to respond to the collection of information unless it displays a current valid OMB control number. If you have any comments about this estimate or any other aspects of this data collection, including suggestions for reducing this burden, contact: US Department of Labor, OSHA Office of Statistics, Room N-3644, 200 Constitution Avenue, NW, Washington, DC 20210. Do not send the completed forms to this office.

FIGURE 7-13 OSHA Form 301—Injury and Illness Incident Report. (Source: US Department of Labor, Occupational Safety and Health Administration.)

- Description of the incident
- The type and brand of device used when the incident took place
- Location of the incident

The regulations that took effect in 2001 require all needlestick and sharps injuries to be reported and documented, not just the ones that result in injury or illness.

OSHA Training Requirements. All employees, including full-time, part-time, and temporary employees with a risk of occupational exposure, must receive training within the facility in which they are employed at two very specific times. Initial training must be conducted before commencement of any work-related duties by a new employee. In addition, training must be conducted on an annual basis to update and inform employees on new regulations and procedures related to OSHA compliance. The initial training requirement is one of the most frequently breached regulations, yet is critical for the safety of the employee.

Training must include the following:

- Making accessible a copy of the regulatory text of the standard and explanation of its contents
- General discussion on bloodborne diseases and their transmission
- Universal precautions and body substance isolation
- The Exposure Control plan
- Engineering and work practice controls, including handling of needles and sharps
- Personal protective equipment
- Hepatitis B vaccine
- Response to emergencies involving blood
- Potential sources of infection and tasks that might preempt exposure
- Written schedules for cleaning
- Handling contaminated laundry
- How to handle exposure incidents and spills
- The postexposure evaluation and follow-up program
- Reading Materials Safety Data Sheets (MSDS), signs, labels, and color-coding (Figure 7-14), and locations of these items

There must be an opportunity for questions and answers, and the trainer must be knowledgeable in the subject matter. Documentation of the training sessions should be kept in each employee's personnel file or a special file for OSHA-related information.

CRITICAL THINKING APPLICATION

Barbara reviews the employee files and finds that neither Samantha nor Lynda received OSHA training when they were initially hired. How might Barbara rectify this and what documentation would be helpful?

Hepatitis B Vaccination. The hepatitis B vaccination series must be offered to employees at risk of occupational exposures at no cost to the employee. The employee cannot be asked to pay in advance for the vaccination and be reimbursed, nor can the employee be asked to put the vaccination series on his or her personal health insurance policy. It must be made available to the employee within 10 working days of initial hire or assignment. The vaccination series can be declined by the employee, who must sign a declination form. If at any time the employee decides to receive the vaccination series, this must still be offered at no cost. The employee does not have to offer a reason for the declination. Prescreening or postvaccination serological tests cannot be required.

The vaccination series is completed within a 6-month period. The second vaccination is given 1 month after the first, and the third 5 months after the second. Documentation should be provided to the employee for each vaccination received. Currently a booster dose of the hepatitis B vaccination is not required. However, if a routine booster is recommended by the U.S. Public Health Service in the future, it must be made available at no cost to employees.

CRITICAL THINKING APPLICATION

Lynda has not disclosed to anyone at the facility that she has had a case of hepatitis. Should she discuss this matter with Barbara? Is Lynda required to discuss this matter with Barbara? Is Lynda placing her patients at risk? If Lynda declines the hepatitis vaccination, must she explain why on the declination form?

Clinical Laboratory Improvement Act. The Clinical Laboratory Improvement Act (CLIA) was a result of the Congressional investigation of **physician office laboratories (POLs)** and the deficiencies in the quality of the services and results provided by these laboratories. A set of minimum standards for laboratories was established, which involved quality improvement in test procedures. Quality control and assurance, as well as personnel and proficiency testing, are of utmost importance to the facility complying with CLIA.

CLIA regulations set the minimum standard for laboratory practice and quality. Remember that CLIA is not a governmental agency, but a law. CLIA is enforced by the Department of Health and Human Services (DHHS). OSHA is a law (Occupational Safety and Health Act), but also an agency (Occupational Safety and Health Administration). This is an important difference between the two.

Some tests conducted in the laboratory are exempt from CLIA standards. These tests include the following:

- Nonautomated dipstick or tablet urinalysis
- Fecal occult blood
- Ovulation using visual color comparison
- Urine pregnancy using visual color comparison
- Erythrocyte sedimentation rate
- Hemoglobin by copper sulfate method
- Spun microhematocrit
- Blood glucose using certain devices cleared by the FDA for home use
- Specialized self-contained hemoglobin tests

Material Safety Data Sheets communicate hazards to employees about the products and chemicals used in the medical office. They also inform the employee as to what to do in case of an exposure. OSHA requires that MSDS sheets are kept on all hazardous chemicals, unless exempted. Only the manufacturer can determine if a product is hazardous. MSDS sheets can be obtained from either the manufacturer or the medical supply company from which the product was ordered. They must be provided after requested from the manufacturer within 30 days. Keep copies of requests to prove that an attempt has been made to obtain the MSDS information.

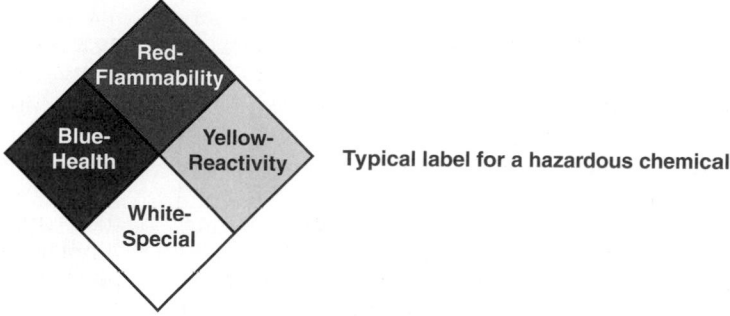

Typical label for a hazardous chemical

The appropriate number should be placed inside each box that applies in the figure above. Most offices use the National Fire Protection Association Rating System. Many MSDS sheets provide the labeling information on the sheet. Others must be read thoroughly to determine how the labels should be completed. If the MSDS says that a chemical has a "moderate to high" hazard, label it high. If it says "low to moderate," label it moderate. Never guess at the numbers used for the label—always consult the MSDS. If individual containers are labeled, the facility is said to always be out of compliance, because it is easy to miss a container that may have just arrived in a shipment. Many medical facilities place labels on a permanent fixture next to where the product is stored, but it must be permanently stored in that area.

Simple Rating Guide
0—no hazard
1—slight hazard
2—moderate hazard
3—high hazard
4—extreme hazard

NFPA Rating Summary					
Health (Blue)			**Reactivity (Yellow)**		
4	Danger	May be fatal on short exposure. Specialized protective equipment required.	4	Danger	Explosive material at room temperature.
3	Warning	Corrosive or toxic. Avoid skin contact or inhalation.	3	Danger	May be explosive if shocked, heated under confinement, or mixed with water.
2	Warning	May be harmful if inhaled or absorbed.	2	Warning	Unstable or may react violently if mixed with water.
1	Caution	May be irritating.	1	Caution	May react if heated or mixed with water but not violently.
0		No unusual hazard.	0	Stable	Not reactive when mixed with water.
Flammability (Red)			**Special Notice Key (White)**		
4	Danger	Flammable gas or extremely flammable liquid.	W		Water reactive.
3	Warning	Flammable liquid flash point below 100° F.	Oxy		Oxidizing agent.
2	Caution	Combustible liquid flash point of 100° to 200° F.			
1		Combustible if heated.			
0		Not combustible.			

FIGURE 7-14   Labeling and the National Fire Protection Association (NFPA) Rating System. (Courtesy the National Fire Protection Association.)

Offices that only perform these tests may obtain a certificate of waiver and will not be routinely inspected for CLIA compliance. Tests of moderate or high complexity must be performed by trained personnel with education and experience in the test areas in which they are working. A list of the moderate- and high-complexity procedures can be found in the July 26, 1993, issue of the Federal Register, and updates are periodically published that detail any changes in the list or regulations regarding testing procedures. Laboratories apply for a CLIA certificate through their local health departments and will be periodically inspected for compliance.

Physician Licensure and Registration

A graduate of a medical school must be licensed before beginning the practice of medicine. Licensure is regulated by state statutes through the Medical Practice Acts. It is important for a medical assistant to understand licensing and other laws and regulations that are intended to protect patients, physicians, medical assistants, and other healthcare workers.

Medical Practice Acts

Medical practice acts existed as early as colonial days. However, these acts were later repealed, and in the mid-nineteenth century practically none of the states had laws governing the practice of medicine. As one might expect, a rapid decline in professional standards followed. The general welfare of the people was endangered by medical **quackery** and inadequate care. By the beginning of the twentieth century, medical practice acts were established by statute and were again in effect in every state. The purpose of the medical practice acts is as follows:

- To define what is included in the practice of medicine within that state
- To govern the methods and requirements of licensure
- To establish the grounds for suspension or revocation of license

Licensure

A doctor of medicine (MD), doctor of osteopathy (DO), or doctor of chiropractic (DC) degree is conferred on graduation from medical or chiropractic school. The license to practice medicine or chiropractic is granted by a state board, frequently known as the State Board of Medical Examiners or Board of Registration. Licensure may be accomplished by examination, reciprocity, or endorsement.

Examination. Every state requires medical doctors to pass a written examination. The Federation of State Medical Boards and the National Board of Medical Examiners agreed in 1990 to establish a single licensing examination—the Federation Licensing Examination (FLEX)—for graduates of accredited medical schools. Medical graduates in the United States must pass either the FLEX examination, the U.S. Medical Licensing Examination (USMLE), or the National Board of Medical Examiners' Examination (NBME). Osteopathic physicians pass the National Board of Osteopathic Medical Examiners' Comprehensive Osteopathic Medical Licensing Examination (COMLEX).

Reciprocity. Some states grant the license to practice medicine by reciprocity; that is, they automatically recognize that the requirements of the state in which the license was granted meet the standards required by the second state.

Endorsement. Most graduates of medical schools in the United States have been licensed by endorsement of the National Board certificate. To explain in simpler terms, a state will offer a license to a physician based on the examinations taken to grant the license, not by virtue of the license granted from another state. Licensure by endorsement is granted on a case-by-case basis. Graduates who have not been licensed by endorsement are required to pass a state board examination.

In all states graduates of foreign medical schools who are seeking licensure by endorsement must meet the same requirements as graduates of medical schools in the United States, in addition to various other qualifying factors.

Exemptions. Some graduates may not wish to engage in the practice of medicine; their interests may lie in research or administration, or even in the practice of law with a special interest in medical liability. In such instances licensure is not required. Licensed physicians in the Armed Forces, Public Health Service, or Veterans Administration facilities need not be licensed in the state in which they are employed. However, the Department of Defense is encouraging states to require full licensure of military personnel.

Registration and Reregistration

After a license is granted, periodic reregistration is necessary annually or biennially. A physician can be **concurrently** registered in more than one state. The issuing body notifies the physician when reregistration is due. A medical assistant can aid the physician by being aware of when the registration fees are due, thus preventing a possible lapsing of the registration.

Many states require proof of continuing education besides payment of a registration fee. Continuing education units (CEUs) are granted to physicians for attending approved seminars, lectures, scientific meetings, and formal courses in accredited colleges and universities. A total of 50 hours per year is the average requirement for a license renewal. A medical assistant may be expected to help the physician arrange for completing the required units for license renewal.

Revocation or Suspension

Under certain conditions, the license to practice medicine may be revoked or suspended. Grounds for revocation or suspension of the license to practice medicine fall within one of three categories:

1. *Conviction of a crime:* This may include felonies such as murder, rape, larceny, and narcotic violations.
2. *Unprofessional conduct:* Failure to uphold the ethical standards of the medical profession may be indicated by betrayal of patient confidence, giving or receiving rebates, and excessive use of narcotics or alcohol.
3. *Personal or professional incapacity:* Such incapacity is difficult to label or prove. For example, advanced age or an injury may reduce the apparent capacity of some physicians. Certain illnesses can affect the memory or judgment necessary to practice medicine.

A physician studies many years to learn the profession before becoming licensed by the state to practice medicine. A medical assistant is not licensed to practice medicine and must never prescribe or attempt to diagnose a patient's ailment. This is the illegal practice of medicine. For this reason, a medical assistant must use great care in discussing the patient's complaints and treatment with them because patients identify the medical assistant's remarks as being the opinion of the physician.

Closing Comments

The majority of patients never entertain the thought of taking legal action against their physicians, and a medical assistant should not develop an attitude of skepticism. However, a medical assistant can play an important role in preventing medical claims.

Give scrupulous attention to the needs of each patient and avoid leaving them alone for long periods. This espccially applies to young children and elderly patients. Always avoid criticism of other physicians or healthcare facilities. Never give out any information about the patient without written consent and verify the identity of anyone asking for information about a patient.

Use discretion in phone and office conversations. One never knows who is standing just around the corner. Be aware of tone of voice and attitude during spoken conversations. Communicate office policies and procedures to patients clearly in advance of treatment whenever possible.

Keep accurate records that show exactly what was done to the patient and when it was done. Make no promises as to the outcome of treatment. Record cancelled and no-show appointments and record the facts if a patient discontinues treatment.

Check office equipment often to ensure that it is working properly. Keep drug samples and prescription pads out of sight. Never diagnose, prescribe, or offer a prognosis. Perform only the tasks for which you are trained and keep abreast of new findings and procedures in healthcare. Correctly follow all federal and state regulations.

Play a positive part in the prevention of medical liability claims. Take care of the patient in a compassionate and competent way, and malpractice will not be a frequent issue in the medical facility.

Patient Education

Perhaps the most important detail to remember with regard to patient education and law is patience. Many medical forms are complicated, and regulations change often. Patients are not usually as well educated as the medical assistant on matters concerning legal policies and procedures. Often patients become frustrated with the number of changes that they are expected to contend with, and they may unintentionally project this frustration onto the medical assistant. Remain calm and answer questions, offering as much assistance to the patient as possible.

Legal and Ethical Issues

Generally, the law holds that every person is liable for the consequences of his or her own negligence when another person is injured as a result. In some situations this liability also extends to the employer. Physicians may be held responsible for the mistakes of those who work in their healthcare facility, and sometimes they must pay damages for the negligent acts of their employees.

Under the doctrine of respondent superior, physicians are legally responsible for the acts of their employees when the employees are acting within the scope of their duties or employment. Physicians are also responsible for the acts of assistants who are not their own employees if they commit acts of negligence in the presence of the physician while under the physician's immediate supervision. *Respondeat superior* is a Latin term meaning "let the master answer." When physicians practice as partners, they are liable not only for their own acts and those of their partners, but also for the negligent acts of any agent or employee of the partnership. A medical assistant, while acting within the scope of the employment contract, is considered an agent of the employer.

Medical assistants who are guilty of negligence are liable for their own actions, but the injured party generally sues the physician, because there is a better chance of collecting damages. However, even an assistant who has no money can still be liable for any negligent action. This fact illustrates the continuing importance of exercising extreme care in performing all duties in the professional office.

SUMMARY OF SCENARIO

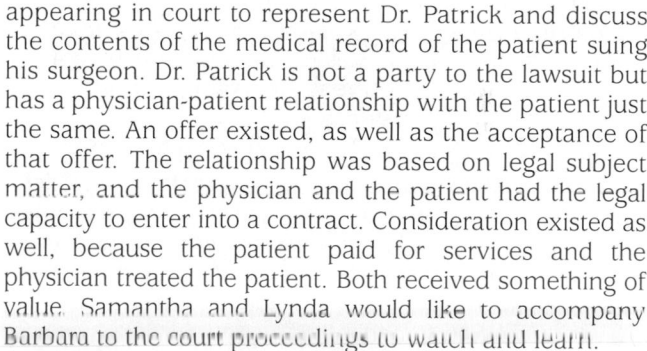

Barbara is enthusiastic about her new job and duties. She is confident about appearing in court to represent Dr. Patrick and discuss the contents of the medical record of the patient suing his surgeon. Dr. Patrick is not a party to the lawsuit but has a physician-patient relationship with the patient just the same. An offer existed, as well as the acceptance of that offer. The relationship was based on legal subject matter, and the physician and the patient had the legal capacity to enter into a contract. Consideration existed as well, because the patient paid for services and the physician treated the patient. Both received something of value. Samantha and Lynda would like to accompany Barbara to the court proceedings to watch and learn.

Even if a patient does not pay for treatment, a contract still exists. The physician may elect to terminate the physician-patient relationship if the patient does not pay, but the trust that the patient places in the physician can be considered a thing of value. Patients should understand their role in their treatment, and their responsibilities to the physician. Often this information is communicated in the patient policy brochure or may be verbally discussed with the patient. Physicians are not required to accept all patients; for instance, not all physicians deliver babies. Some physicians do not treat patients with worker's compensation claims. The physician does have the right to see the types of patients he or she wishes and is competent to treat but should never discriminate on the basis of race, sex, or any other protected status. A physician may not always be correct in his or her diagnoses, but this does not mean that the physician has committed malpractice. However, if expert witnesses feel that the physician should have made a different diagnosis based on the case, then the physician might be held liable for negligence. If an employee has information about a case that is damaging to the physician, he or she is ethically obligated to report the information, but rarely legally liable to speak up unless a law has been broken.

Samantha and Lynda have learned many new concepts about law from Barbara and are anxious to watch the court proceedings. They will learn more by seeing the actual process of law at work. Barbara looks forward to sharing more knowledge with the employees as they continue to work together.

SUMMARY OF LEARNING OBJECTIVES

- Different types of laws and regulations affect us, depending on the origination of the law. Acts are introduced at the federal level and must be passed by Congress. State legislative bodies develop statutes, and local governments create ordinances.

- Criminal law governs violations that are punishable as offenses against the state or government. Civil law is concerned with acts that are not criminal in nature, but those that involve individual relationships and relationships between others, groups, or government agencies.

- Misdemeanors are minor crimes, punishable by a fine or imprisonment in a city or county jail. Felonies are major crimes, such as rape, murder, or burglary. Most felonies carry punishment of imprisonment for at least one year, and they are divided into subgroups, usually first-, second-, and third-degree felonies. Treason is an attempt to overthrow the government. High treason constitutes a serious threat to the stability of the government, for example, an attempt on the life of the President.

- Tort law is the division of civil law that deals with medical professional liability. Tort law provides relief for those who have suffered harm from the actions of others. The plaintiff must establish duty, breach of duty, damages as a result of the breach of duty, and the extent of the damages suffered.

- Four elements are essential to a valid, legal contract: (1) there must be a "meeting of the minds" or manifestation of assent; (2) the contract must involve legal subject matter; (3) the parties to the contract must have the legal capacity to enter into a contract; and (4) some type of consideration must be offered.

- Interrogatories are lists of questions directed from each party of a lawsuit to the other. Interrogatories are answered under oath and only directed to the parties actually named in the lawsuit. Depositions, however, can be taken from any witness or party to the lawsuit. They are also taken under oath, and often witnesses are subpoenaed to offer a deposition.

- Testifying in court can sometimes be an intimidating experience, but good preparation beforehand will alleviate many anxieties. Discussing potential questions with the attorney will help prepare the witness for giving testimony. Always tell the truth to avoid charges of perjury. Speak clearly and distinctly and do not hesitate to ask the attorney to repeat a question. There is no harm in a brief pause to think about an answer. Dress conservatively, know the location and room of the court in advance, and always arrive on time. Credibility is critical in a medical professional liability trial.

- Arbitration is a popular alternative to court trials. It involves the use of a third party familiar with law or the issues at hand. It is recognized by statute in most states and provides a faster, confidential, fair, and less expensive resolution to a dispute.

- Malfeasance, misfeasance, and nonfeasance are types of negligence often involved in medical professional liability cases. Malfeasance is performing an act that is completely wrong or unlawful. Misfeasance, comparable to a mistake, is the improper performance of a lawful act. Nonfeasance is the failure to perform some act that should have been performed.

- Informed consent gives the patient a full understanding of the condition that has been diagnosed, including what could happen if the patient undergoes treatment, refuses treatment, or delays treatment. It provides the patient with information on the advantages and risks of a medical procedure and alternative treatments that the patient may wish to consider. Informed consent places the control in the hands of the patient, who is given the opportunity to make the decisions about his or her healthcare. Patients can never be forced to undergo any type of procedure or treatment.

- Several disclosures must be made by the physician with regard to a patient's health that do not require patient consent. Information about births and deaths, injuries or illnesses as a result of violence, accidental or suspicious deaths, sexually transmitted diseases, and any type of abuse are examples of legal disclosures that must be made by healthcare professionals.

- Passage of the Health Insurance Portability and Accountability Act of 1996 offered the healthcare profession extensive privacy rules and regulations concerning the electronic transfer of information. The Act also limited administrative costs by supporting the use of electronic transfer of information, and presented fraud and abuse prevention guidelines. The privacy issues that surround HIPAA, however, have been the most discussed and debated topics related to this law.

- The Occupational Safety and Health Administration is an agency and a division of the U.S. Department of Labor. More than 2300 employees work for OSHA, and the agency runs on an annual budget of approximately $443 million as of 2002. Twenty-six states have their own OSHA programs, which adds an additional 3100 employees. The Occupational Safety and Health Act of 1970 created this agency to ensure safety in the workplace. The Clinical Laboratory Improvement Act is a law that regulates the quality of services provided by laboratories. CLIA is enforced by the Department of Health and Human Services.

■ Physicians may receive a license to practice medicine through examination, reciprocity, or endorsement. FLEX, USMLE, and NBME are all designed for graduates of accredited medical schools. Some states recognize the requirements of another state in which a license was granted, and through reciprocity will give a physician a license to practice medicine. Endorsement is the method of obtaining a license by recognition of the passed examinations, instead of by virtue of the license obtained in another state. Most physicians in the United States are licensed by endorsement, because they take the examination after graduating from medical school

and this prompts the receipt of the license, after proper application and providing all required documentation. Practicing medicine without a license is illegal.

■ A physician may lose his or her license to practice medicine if convicted of a crime, found guilty of unprofessional conduct, or as a result of personal or professional incapacity. An arrest will not cause the physician to lose the license, since this is an allegation not yet proven in court. Unprofessional conduct is usually determined by local medical societies or other organizations, such as a hospital, with which the physician is affiliated.

KEY INTERNET WEBSITES

- American Medical Association
- Department of Health and Human Services
- Occupational Health and Safety Administration
- United States Supreme Court
  For active weblinks to each website visit
  http://evolve.elsevier.com/Kinn/

UNIT two

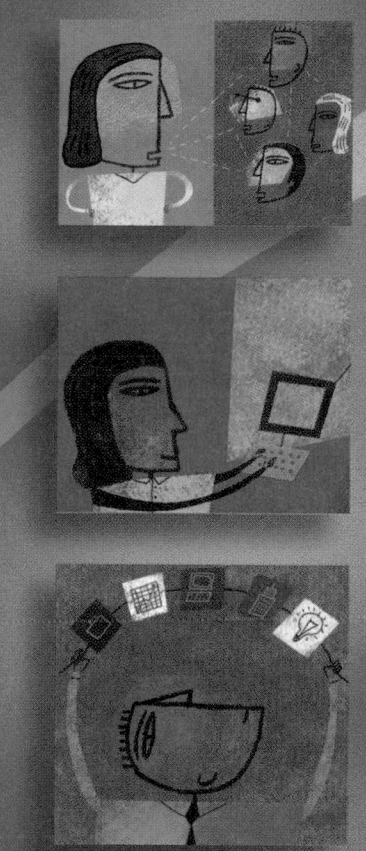

Administrative Medical Assisting

CHAPTER 8

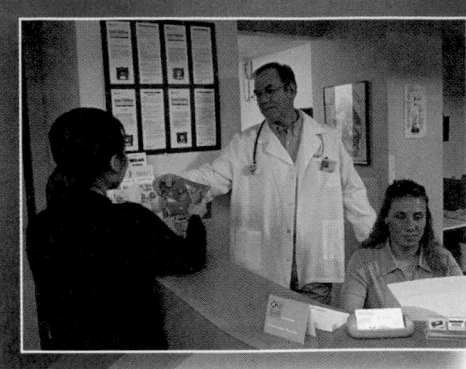

Scenario

Dr. Michael Bouchard is aware of the advantages of networking his office computers and having Internet access to meet the needs of his facility. Every day he sends and receives many important email messages to and from patients and colleagues. His staff members use the computer for communications and to access sources of online information. Patient tracking, accounting functions, and health information retrieval are immensely faster on a computer than with the use of a paper-based system. One other distinct advantage to Dr. Bouchard is the scheduling features of his software. Because the schedule is shared, everyone in the office knows the doctor's schedule and avoids double-booking and miscommunications. Dr. Bouchard sends his staff members for regular computer training so that all of them can use the computers in the best and most efficient ways possible.

Computers in the Medical Office

Learning Objectives

- Define and spell the terms listed in the vocabulary.
- List several ways that the computer can be effective in a medical office.
- Explain the basic functions that a computer performs.
- Explain the basic parts of a computer.
- List the three elements that differentiate microprocessors.
- Discuss the differences among various types of printers.
- Explain the importance of a motherboard.
- Explain and give examples of peripheral devices.
- List and discuss several types of file formats.
- Explain the concept of computer networking.
- Define the function of browsers.
- Discuss the importance of computer security.

National Curriculum Competencies

TRANSDISCIPLINARY COMPETENCIES

4c. Utilize computer software to maintain systems
Computer terminology and overview of
computer concepts
Knowledge of basic computer commands and
functions

Vocabulary

applications software Software programs designed to perform specific tasks.

artificial intelligence The aspect of computer science that deals with computers taking on the attributes of humans. One such example is expert systems, which are capable of making decisions, such as software that is designed to help a physician diagnose a patient, given a set of symptoms. Game-playing programs and programs that are designed to recognize human speech are other examples.

ASCII codes Acronym for American Standard Code for Information Interchange; a code representing English characters as numbers where each is given a number from 0 to 127.

backup Any type of storage of files to prevent their loss in the event of hard disk failure.

banners Advertisements often found on a web page that can be animated to attract the user's attention in hopes that he or she will click on the ad, be redirected to the advertiser's home page, and purchase from the site or gain information from the site.

bit The smallest unit of information inside the computer, represented by either the digit "0" or "1"; eight bits equal one byte.

byte A unit of data that contains eight binary digits, or bits.

cache A special high-speed storage that can either be a part of the computer's main memory or can be a separate storage device. One function of a cache is to store websites visited in the computer memory for faster recall the next time the website is requested.

CD burner A device that is capable of "writing" data onto a blank compact disk (CD) or copying data from one CD to a blank CD.

computer A machine that is designed to accept, store, process, and give out information.

cookies Messages sent to a web browser from a web server that identify users and can prepare custom web pages for them, possibly displaying their name on return to the site.

cursor A symbol appearing on the monitor that shows where the next character to be typed will appear.

cyberspace Describes the nonphysical space of the online world of computer networks in which communication takes place.

database A collection of related files that serves as a foundation for retrieving information.

device driver The program or commands given to a device connected to a computer that enable the device to function. For instance, a printer may come equipped with a software program that must be loaded onto the computer first, so that the printer will work.

digital subscriber line (DSL) High-speed, sophisticated modulation scheme that operates over existing copper telephone wiring systems; often referred to as "last-mile technologies," because DSL is used for connections from a telephone switching station to a home or office, and not from between switching stations.

digital versatile disk or digital video disk (DVD) An optical disk that holds approximately 28 times more information than a CD; a DVD is most commonly used to hold full-length movies. Compared with a CD, which holds approximately 600 megabytes, a DVD has the capacity to hold approximately 4.7 gigabytes.

disk A removable device with a magnetic surface that is capable of storing computer programs, stored in a hard plastic square; also called diskettes, and early versions were called "floppy disks."

disk drives Devices that load a program or data stored on a disk into the computer.

ecommerce An abbreviation for *electronic commerce*; used to describe the sale and purchase of goods and services over the Internet; doing business over the Internet.

email Communications transmitted via computer using a modem.

environment The state of a computer, usually determined by the programs that are running as well as hardware and software characteristics.

fax Abbreviation for *facsimile*; also, a document sent using a facsimile (fax) machine.

flash Animation technology often used on the opening page of a website to draw attention, excite, and impress the user.

font A design for a set of type characters; a combination of typeface, spacing, pitch, and other qualities. Fonts are named; examples include Times Roman, Arial, and Garamond.

format To magnetically create tracks on a disk where information will be stored, usually done by the manufacturer of the disk.

gigabyte Approximately 1 billion bytes; abbreviated GB.

hard copy The readable paper copy or printout of information.

HTML Acronym for HyperText Markup Language, which is the language used to create documents for use on the Internet.

HTTP Acronym for HyperText Transfer Protocol, which defines how messages are formatted and transmitted over the Internet. When a URL is entered into the computer, an HTTP command tells the web server to retrieve the requested web page.

hub A common connection point for devices in a network containing multiple ports, often used to connect segments of a LAN.

icon A picture, often on the desktop of a computer, that represents a program or an object. By clicking on the icon, the user is directed to the program.

input Information entered into and used by the computer.

Java A commonly used object-oriented high-level programming language that is well suited for the Internet.

megabyte Approximately 1 million bytes; abbreviated MB.

megahertz The measuring device for microprocessors, abbreviated MHz. A megahertz is 1 million cycles of electromagnetic currency alternation per second and is used as a unit of measure for the clock speed of computer microprocessors. The hertz is a unit of measure named after Heinrich Hertz, a German physicist.

MIDI Acronym for Musical Instrument Digital Interface; a MIDI interface allows computers to record and manipulate sound.

modem A device that allows information to be transmitted over telephone lines, at speeds measured in bits per second (bps); short for modulator-demodulator.

monochromatic Having or consisting of one color or hue.

multimedia The presentation of graphics, animation, video, sound, and text on a computer in an integrated way, or all at once. CD-ROMs are the most effective multimedia devices.

output Information that is processed by the computer and transmitted to a monitor, printer, or other device.

queries Requests for information from a database.

router A device used to connect any number of LANs, which communicate with other routers and determine the best route between any two hosts.

scanner Device that reads text or illustrations on a printed page and can translate the information on that page into a form that the computer can understand.

search engines Programs that search documents for keywords and return a list of documents containing those words.

server A computer or device on a network that manages shared network resources.

sound card Device that allows a computer to output sound through speakers that are connected to the main circuitry board, or motherboard.

switch In networks, a device that filters information between LAN segments and decreases overall network traffic and increases speed and bandwidth usage efficiency.

systems software The operating system and all utility programs that allow the computer to function and perform operations.

TCP/IP Acronym for Transmission Control Protocol/Internet Protocol; a suite of communications protocols used to connect users or hosts to the Internet.

telecommunication The science and technology of communication by transmission of information from one location to another via telephone, television, telegraph, or satellite.

URL Acronym for Uniform Resource Locator; specifies the global address of documents or information on the Internet. The URL provides the IP address and the domain name for the web page, such as *microsoft.com*.

virtual reality An artificial environment presented to a computer user that feels as if it were a real environment, often using special gloves, earphones, and goggles to enhance the experience.

Zip drive A small, portable disk drive that is primarily used for backing up information and archiving computer files. A 100-megabyte Zip disk will hold the equivalent of about 70 floppy disks.

Computers in the New Millennium

Nearly 60 years ago, in 1946, the first electronic computer (ENIAC) was completed after 2½ years in the making. It weighed 30 tons, required a space of 15,000 square feet, and cost more than $1 million. Since that time, a computer explosion has taken place, and today our lives are affected by computers on a daily basis. Personal computers, laptop or notebook computers, and even cell phones that send and receive **email** are commonplace. Our world is now one of enhanced **telecommunications**, where faster processing of information is both needed and expected. Most people venture into **cyberspace** on a daily basis, where a world of information is waiting with the simple click of a mouse!

For many years computers have been used in medical facilities, including physicians' offices. The development of software, the decrease in the cost of computer hardware, and the time savings that the computer brings to the office make it well worth the investment. Computers are now standard equipment in healthcare facilities (Figure 8-1). A medical assistant must have more than computer literacy—a good understanding of the way computers work and their capabilities is essential in a medical office.

Computers in the Medical Office

Getting Started

Even with some basic knowledge of computer components and of what computers can do, without hands-on knowledge, the beginner may have some initial fear of the unknown. However, the computer is only a machine that takes its direction from the person operating it. It will perform the tasks that it is told to do. A computer cannot really think or make decisions (yet); it will wait for commands that will prompt it to act. Dialog boxes appear that ask for input from the user. This is how the computer communicates with the person using it. Computers assist workers in medical offices in some of the following ways:

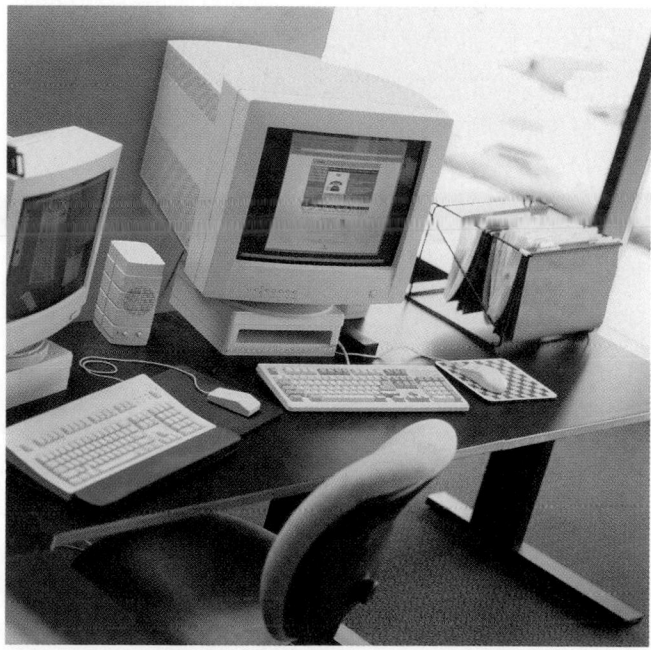

FIGURE 8-1 Computers are an invaluable tool for today's medical office.

- Performing repetitive tasks
- Reducing errors
- Speeding up production
- Recalling information on command
- Saving time
- Reducing paperwork and storage space
- Allowing for more creative and productive use of workers' time

The more familiar a medical assistant becomes with the computer, the better skilled he or she will become in its use. Occasionally errors will be made, and the computer may respond with an error message. However, the monitor screen normally indicates what to do next. The computer will usually allow the operator the opportunity to figure out the correct information and input that information into the computer. A help menu can always be accessed, or the instruction manual can be consulted; help lines and technical support are available as well when problems occur. The problem may be with the software, or with the computer itself. Usually it is fairly easy to determine which is causing the problem.

Rarely will the computer "break," although this is a common fear among new users. It is unlikely that records will be destroyed by accident; usually very specific commands are needed to delete stored information. However, a medical assistant must take care not to shut off the computer without saving the information that has been entered. By using a computer in the classroom and practicing at home or at a library, if possible, the medical assistant will gain familiarity with computer operation and confidence that it can be mastered. Mastery is accomplished only through practice.

With a knowledge of computer terms, the ability to follow step-by-step instructions, and reasonable expertise with a keyboard, a medical assistant can rapidly learn and use almost any computer system. Although the computers and the software may vary from facility to facility, basic computer operation is similar, and if the instructions given by the computer are carried out, the user should be successful in the tasks attempted.

Computer Basics

A **computer** is a machine that is designed to accept, store, process, and provide information (Figure 8-2). Computers serve the following basic functions:

- *Input:* **Input** includes any information that enters the computer. It can take a variety of forms, from commands that are entered from the keyboard to data from another computer or device, such as a scanner. The device that feeds data into a computer is called an *input device*, such as a mouse, scanner, or keyboard.
- *Processing:* Processing is the act of manipulating the data that are currently inside the computer to carry out a certain task.
- *Output:* **Output** is anything that exits the computer. Output can appear in many forms, such as binary numbers, characters, pictures, printed pages, or a simple image on the monitor. Output devices include monitors, speakers, and printers.
- *Storage:* The act of retaining data or applications is called storage. Data can be stored on disks, on CDs, or on separate drives, such as a **Zip drive**.

CRITICAL THINKING APPLICATION

Dr. Bouchard plans to send two of his employees to a training class on using a new software program designed to perform all computer functions needed for his practice. Although he can only send two employees, how can the others learn the system?

Would it be beneficial or detrimental to close the office for a day to educate the other employees about the system? What should the physician consider before losing a day of patient visits?

Parts of the Computer

A medical assistant must understand the function of the different parts of a computer. The physical pieces that can be touched and seen are called hardware. Computers

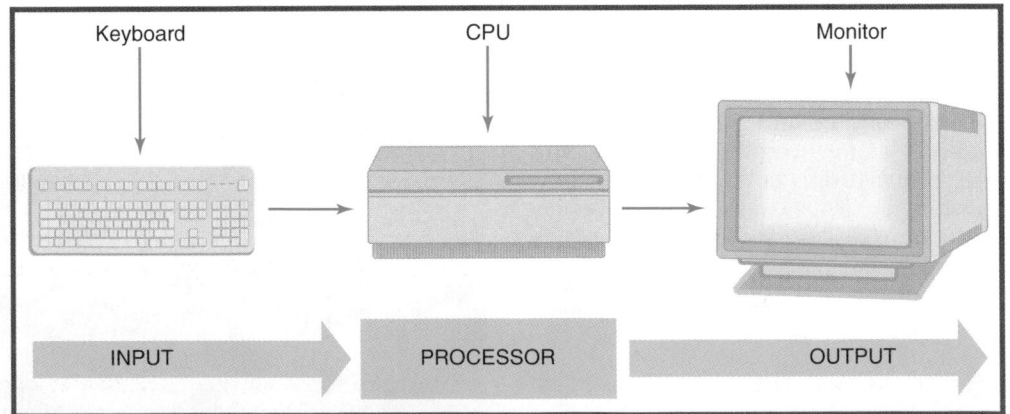

FIGURE 8-2 Input devices allow data to be entered into the computer, where they are processed; output is available in several different forms.

using Windows software have an option in the control panel for adding hardware. This shortcut makes adding new equipment easy and provides instruction all along the way. Hardware provides the medium on which software can be used. Most personal computers (PCs) have a microprocessor, monitor, keyboard, mouse, and printer.

Microprocessor

Inside the casing of the main computer hardware, the microprocessor is housed. The microprocessor is the central unit of the computer that contains the logic circuitry, which carries out the instructions of a computer's programs. It is considered the most important piece of hardware in a computer system. Microprocessors act as the brain of the computer and interpret instructions from a program. Microprocessors, sometimes called *central processing units*, are differentiated by three basic elements:

- *Bandwidth:* Bandwidth describes how much information can be sent over a connection at one time, or how many bits can be processed in one single instruction. **Bits,** short for binary digits, are the smallest pieces of information on the computer. Eight bits make up one **byte**.
- *Clock speed:* Clock speed determines how many instructions per second that the processor can handle. Clock speed is measured in **megahertz** (MHz). One megahertz equals 1 million cycles per second, so a processor that operates at 300 MHz executes 300 million cycles per second.
- *Instruction set:* The instruction set is the set of instructions that the microprocessor can execute.

The higher the bandwidth and clock speed, the faster and more powerful the microprocessor. For instance, a 32-bit microprocessor that runs at 50 MHz is more powerful than a 16-bit microprocessor that runs at 25 MHz.

A microprocessor contains memory consisting of electronic and magnetic cells, each of which contains information. There are two kinds of memory: read-only memory (ROM) and random access memory (RAM). ROM is internal memory that contains a portion of the operating system and computer language. This is sometimes known as *main memory*. Data that have been "burned" onto a ROM chip cannot be removed and can only be read, similar to a CD-ROM, unless the CD is a "rewriteable" type. With this permanent memory, much less information has to be transferred from a disk to start the computing process. ROM cannot be overwritten and is not erased when the power is shut off. RAM can be thought of as an internal scratch pad for the computer. It contains the program instructions and the data that are currently processing. RAM is normally erased when the power is shut off.

CRITICAL THINKING APPLICATION

A colleague of Dr. Bouchard's has mentioned that he knows about a website that has several software programs online that can be downloaded free of charge. Dr. Bouchard investigates the site and realizes the software has been pirated. What concerns could this cause if he uses the software in his office? What would happen if any of this software malfunctioned?

Monitor

A monitor, which looks very much like a television screen, is a device used to display computer-generated information. A few are **monochromatic,** but most monitors today are color, capable of being adjusted for brightness, sharpness, and other settings of the user's choice. Color monitors allow for a high quality display, and the more advanced models have resolutions capable of reproducing quality pictures good enough for viewing a **digital video disk** (DVD). By viewing the monitor, the user receives instant feedback on entries into the computer. Monitors are sometimes referred to as *displays* and are considered output devices.

Keyboard

For most computers, the keyboard is the primary text input device. Keyboards contain special function keys, such as the escape key, tab key, cursor movement keys, numeric keys, shift keys, and control keys. Additional function keys, numbered *F1* to *F12,* are used to perform specific word processing or other computer-related operations. Used alone, a function key may create bold print, underline, indent, or call up a help screen. Used in conjunction with the *Ctrl, Alt, or Shift* keys, the function keys can produce other desired results, such as activating the printer, inserting the current date into a document, retrieving a file, or moving a designated block of text.

Mouse

The mouse first became a widely used computer tool when Apple Computers made it a standard part of the Apple Macintosh computer. It resembles a mouse because of its shape and the cord, which attaches it to the microprocessor. The mouse is a pointing device with a ball on the bottom that is moved by rolling it on a flat table top or mouse pad. Some computers, especially laptops, have a built-in device called a *trackball* that is moved with the finger or thumb and serves the same function as a mouse. Other computers have a touchpad or a track-point that is manipulated to control the cursor. The **cursor** is a pointer or flat bar appearing on the monitor that shows where the next character will appear, which is the insertion point. The mouse allows the user to navigate around the screen quickly and click on links to access websites.

Printer

Printers are output devices. Documents appearing on the monitor may be directed to a printer to produce a printout or **hard copy** of a document. Many printers are bidirectional, which means they print both from left to right and from right to left. The type of printer used should depend on the job being performed.

Dot matrix printers are inexpensive and produce a moderate-quality hard copy. They form letters or shapes that they are directed to print by arranging patterns of dots on the paper. They operate faster than letter-quality machines, but the print lacks the clarity generally desired for a professional look.

Ink jet printers use an ink cartridge that feeds an array of nearly microscopic tubes, each of which has a heating element that is energized during the printing process. The ink cartridge may be black-and-white or color. Ink jet printers cost less than laser printers, but the ink cartridges they use are fairly expensive and increase the operating cost.

Laser printers use xerographic technology similar to that in photocopiers, so the laser printer is able to produce an almost limitless variety of forms and sizes as well as complex graphics. One disadvantage of ink jet and laser printers is that they are incapable of producing multiple copies with carbon sets or multicopy forms, which are often used by insurance companies for their filing forms.

Some printers today are multifunctional, serving as a printer, **fax, scanner,** and copier. Although these are excellent for home offices, they may not be the best investment for offices that will use these machines often during the day.

CRITICAL THINKING APPLICATION

Dr. Bouchard has asked his office manager to perform a cost comparison on a printer for three of the office computers. He prefers that they have scanning and fax capability. What are some of the features that the office manager will be interested in knowing about these machines?

Inside the Computer

Basic knowledge of the parts of a computer and their function will help a medical assistant to deal with minor technical issues and give him or her the ability to speak with technical support personnel with more ease.

Motherboard

A motherboard is the main circuit board for the computer, to which other devices can be attached. Usually it contains the processor, the memory, and other controllers and devices that allow the system to operate and function.

Disk Drives

Today's computers have various **disk drives** on which information can be stored or accessed. The hard disk or hard drive is a magnetic disk inside the computer that holds from approximately 10 **megabytes** to several hundred **gigabytes** of information (Figure 8-3). Application

software is normally saved to the hard disk and stored there on the computer for use when needed. This is commonly called the C drive.

Floppy disks or diskettes are normally used in the computer's A drive, although the drives can have different names or labels, depending on the brand of computer. Floppy disks were so named because the original $5\frac{1}{4}$-inch variety was housed in a soft plastic cover that would "flop" if waved up and down. The $3\frac{1}{2}$-inch diskettes are less frequently used now, because CDs have a higher capacity for holding information. However, diskettes are still in use and are easily portable.

CRITICAL THINKING APPLICATION

Dr. Bouchard mentions that he noticed CD-R disks on sale over the weekend. The price that he saw was $30 for 100 CD-Rs. One of the medical assistants noticed a 30-pack of CD-Rs for $9.99. Which is the better buy?

CD-ROM

Most of today's personal computers are equipped with CD-ROM drives, which allow the storage of data on a compact disc. CDs hold much more information than floppy disks. A single CD can store as much information as approximately 700 floppy disks, which is the equivalent of about 300,000 text pages (Figure 8-4). A CD-RW is one on which data can be written, erased, and rewritten. Computers that have a **CD burner,** or CD-R drive, can take information from one CD or another source and write it to another CD. The computer must also have software that enables the burner to work. Software that is installed on a computer to allow a hardware device to function is called a **device driver**.

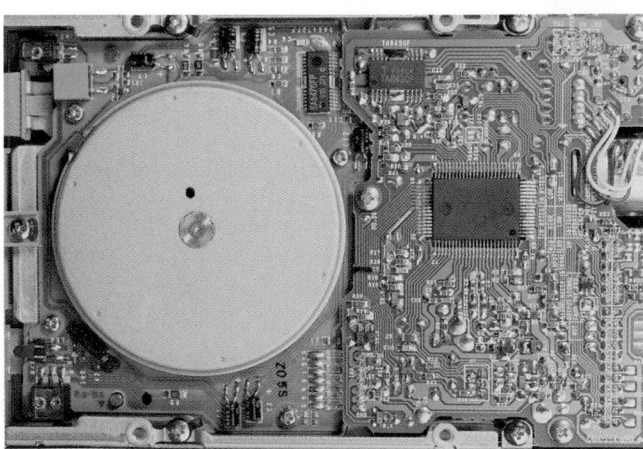

FIGURE 8-3 Hard drives store data and applications for fast and effective access and retrieval. Although a program installed on a hard drive can be removed, most programs are placed there for permanent use, such as Microsoft Office or Peachtree Accounting.

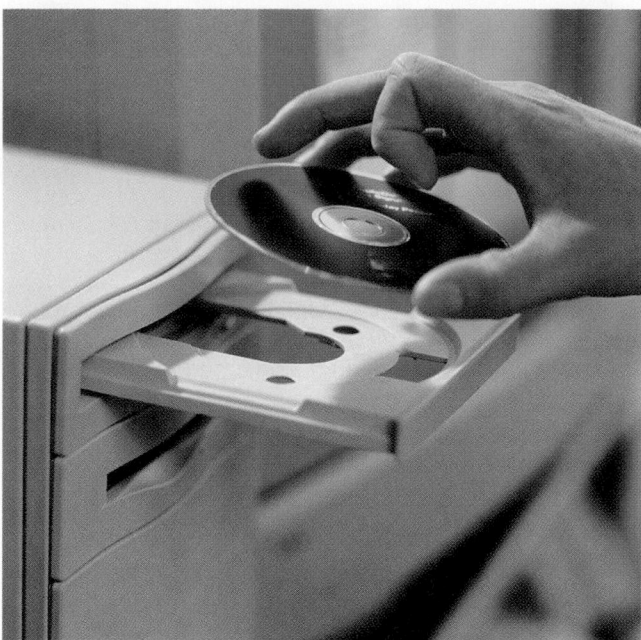

FIGURE 8-4 CD-ROMs allow the user to store and retrieve large amounts of information. Many computers are now equipped with CD-ROM burners, which allow copying of information from one CD to another, or from Internet files to CD-ROMs.

Expansion Boards

Expansion boards are devices that are inserted into a computer that give the computer added capabilities. For example, a **sound card** may be installed so that music or **MIDI** files can be heard from the unit. Other expansion boards are video adapters, internal modems, and graphics accelerators.

Software

Software encompasses the programs and utilities that are loaded onto or inside the computer and used to carry out the work performed by the machine. There are two types of software: systems software and applications software. **Systems software** serves as the operating system of the computer and allows it to run and carry out the functions that the computer performs. For instance, Windows XP, Linux, and the now somewhat antiquated DOS are all types of operating systems software. **Applications software** refers to the programs loaded onto the computer that carry out the work for the actual users of the computer. Examples of applications software are Microsoft Office, MediSoft, and Medical Manager. Applications programs are designed to perform specific tasks, such as word processing, billing, accounting, appointment setting, insurance form preparation, payroll, and **database** management. Many software applications are available for complete medical practice management.

Modems

A **modem,** short for modulator-demodulator, is a device over which data can be transmitted via telephone lines and other media, such as a coaxial cable. Modems can be internal or external. An internal modem is built or added to the inside of the computer casing. A cable modem operates over cable TV lines, and uses the coaxial cable to provide faster Internet access. **Digital subscriber line** (DSL) modems operate over phone lines like normal modems, but they use a different frequency; thus the telephone can be used while the computer is accessing the Internet. Often a filter is attached to the phone that removes other frequencies wherein the DSL is working, avoiding interference with the telephone line operation.

Speakers and Microphones

Some computers have external speakers to provide a higher quality sound from the computer. Many computers also have built-in speakers that provide a fair quality of sound. Microphones can be built-in or attached, so that the user can speak directly into the computer, even to someone on the other side of the world!

Peripheral Devices

Peripheral devices are those that are not essential to the operation of the computer. For instance, the computer will operate without a modem, although a modem is necessary to access the Internet. A mouse is even considered a peripheral device, because everything that the mouse can access can also be reached by certain buttons on the keyboard, although often multiple keys have to be pressed at once. This section discusses some of the peripheral devices in use today.

Scanner

Scanners read text, illustrations, or photos printed on paper and put them into a **format** that the computer can understand. Photographs can be placed into the scanner, saved on the computer, and then used in a document.

Digital Cameras

Digital cameras use a charge-coupled device (CCD) to convert light into electrical charges. Digital cameras do not use film. Light strikes the surface of a photosite inside the camera, and then filters add color and create the digital image. Many digital cameras can be attached directly to a computer and photos can be downloaded from the camera to the computer. Other cameras use a disk to put the pictures into the computer.

> **CRITICAL THINKING APPLICATION**
>
> How might a digital camera be of use to a physician in his or her medical practice? What care should be taken when using the camera with a patient?

Zip Drives

A Zip drive is a disk drive that has a very high storage capacity and is attached externally to a computer. It is usually used as a **backup** device for important data that should not be lost. Zip drives can hold between 100 and 250 megabytes of data and can even be stored somewhere other than the facility so that they are safe in case of fire or other destructive event.

Adding a Program to a Computer

Adding or loading a program onto a computer is relatively easy. Most programs today come in the form of a CD-ROM. The program will contain instructions as to how it should be loaded onto the computer. Watch the monitor for steps to complete and information concerning the user's preferences, then follow all of the directions given.

In a Windows **environment,** the control panel provides an option called *add/remove programs*. Once clicked, this will allow the program in the CD disk drive to be loaded onto the computer. At several points the computer may ask the user questions about his or her preferences for the program. Often the computer may need to be restarted after installation.

When removing a program from the computer, the "add/remove programs" **icon** should be accessed and directions followed for removal of the program. This may be the only way to completely remove the program from the computer system.

File Formats

A file is a collection of data. There are many types of files that are related to computers. A text file, for example, contains some type of text, which is the main body of printed words or written matter on a page. Often an extension exists at the end of the file name that designates what type of file the document is. A file named manual.com might indicate that the file is some type of command file. A few of the common file extensions include the following:

- *JPEG:* JPEG stands for Joint Photographic Experts Group and is a format often used for photographs.
- *GIF:* GIF stands for Graphics Interchange Format, which supports color and is often used for scanned images and illustrations rather than photographs.
- *DOC:* A file that includes the extension .doc is usually a file created by a word processor or word processing software, and stands for *document*.
- *TXT:* A text file usually has the extension .txt after its name. Characters in a text file are represented by their **ASCII codes**.
- *RTF:* RTF stands for Rich Text Format. This type of file combines ASCII codes with special commands that distinguish variations, such as a certain **font**.
- *BMP:* Bit-mapped graphics are indicated by the extension *.bmp*. These are compiled by a graphics image that is set in rows or columns of dots.

A medical assistant who is familiar with these types of files will be able to save and open them correctly and use the computer to the fullest advantage in the medical office.

Computer Networking

A network is a group of two or more computer systems that are linked together. There are several types of networks:

- *LAN:* A LAN is a Local-Area Network, or a computer network spanning a relatively small area. Most LANs are contained in a single building or group of buildings and are connected by a **router**, but LANs can be connected to other LANs even at a distance. A **hub** is a device that connects several computers or networks together, and a **switch** is designed to help the LAN run more efficiently by controlling local network traffic.
- *MAN:* MAN stands for Metropolitan-Area Network. A MAN spans an area that does not exceed a metropolitan area or city and connects several LANs together.
- *WAN:* A WAN is a Wide-Area Network, which spans a relatively large geographic area. Typically, a WAN consists of two or more LANs or MANs. These networks can be connected through public networks, such as a telephone system, or through leased lines or satellites. The largest WAN that exists is the Internet.
- *HAN:* A HAN is a Home-Area Network, which connects computers inside a user's home.
- *CAN:* A CAN is a Campus-Area Network, often used on college campuses and sometimes on military bases.

Servers

A **server** is important to the network, because it is the computer that manages the shared network resources. There are several types of servers. When many computers are connected to one printer, often a print server manages these printers. File servers are used for file storage, and database servers are used to process database **queries.** Some servers are considered to be dedicated servers, meaning they only perform tasks as a server, although a server may also operate as a normal computer.

Clients

A client is a computer that is configured to request access to resources from a server. Server applications, like access to the Internet, network printing, or email access, can run on a server and are accessed by the clients so that they can accomplish these tasks.

The Internet

The Internet is a global network that connects millions of computers together. This fascinating structure has made the world a smaller place (Figure 8-5). Through chat programs, one can talk with individuals literally on the other side of the world and be introduced to cultures that 20 years ago would never have been understood. Through web pages we can visit different parts of the world and learn and see many things that previously were impossible for the average person to experience. **Ecommerce** allows us to shop on the net, from the most exclusives shops in Beverly Hills to the corner grocery store. The Internet has changed the way we learn, do business, communicate, and entertain ourselves.

Each computer connected to the Internet is called a *host* and is independent of all the others. The users of each computer determine which services to make available to other users on the Internet. Often a company or organization also has an Intranet, which is a local network that uses Internet technology within a company or single location but does not have access to the Internet directly.

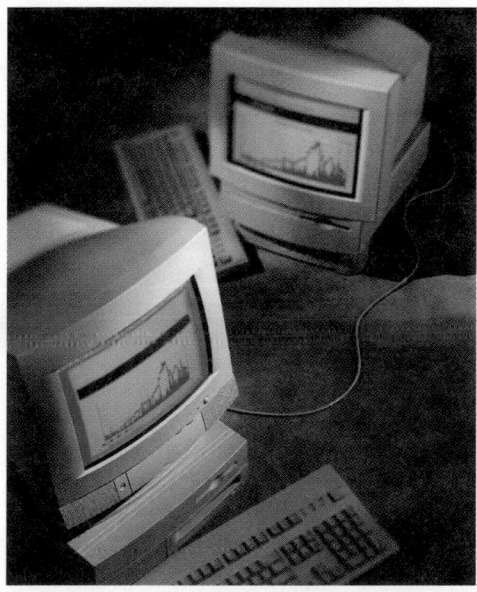

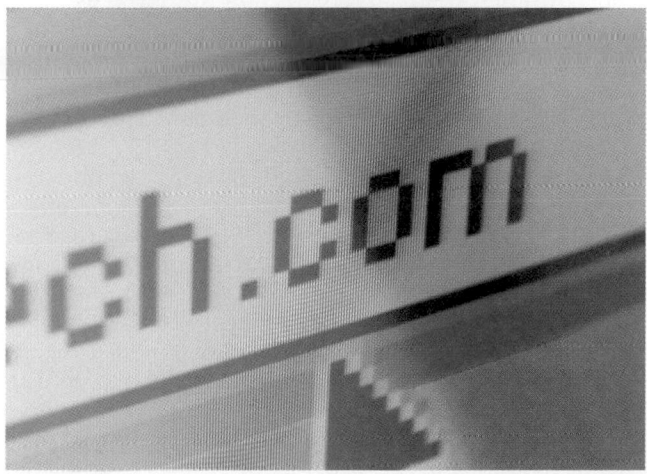

FIGURE 8-5 Computers in today's businesses can speak to each other from across the room or across the world.

Internet service providers (ISPs) are companies that provide access to the Internet. Examples include America Online, Mindspring, Verizon, Earthlink, and Yahoo. ISPs issue each user an IP (Internet Protocol) address, which is a unique identifier for that user's particular computer on a **TCP/IP** network. An IP address is a 32-bit number written as four numbers separated by a period. Each number can be zero to 255, so a valid IP address could be 10.145.32.254. Messages are defined and transmitted over the Internet when a **URL** is entered into the browser and an **HTTP** command tells the web server to retrieve the requested web page.

Domain names identify one or more IP addresses, such as *microsoft.com* or *ama-assn.org*. There are a limited number of top-level domains to which a domain name can be attached. Some of these top-level domains include .com (familiarly called *dot-com*) for commercial businesses; .org for organizations, usually nonprofit; .edu for educational institutions; .gov for government agencies; and .net for network organizations. Most Internet sites use a language called **HTML,** which was one of the first and is still one of the most popular languages used to create web pages. **Java** is another popular language used in website creation.

Many physicians and health organizations offer a website with information about their services. In today's data-driven society, this is an excellent way to educate the public about the services the organization offers and to provide all types of information to the audience that the organization wishes to reach. To obtain a domain name, one must pay a small fee to have the name registered and added to a central database, if the desired name is available. Companies such as *register.com* or *verisign.com* offer domain name registration services.

Websites often contain **banners,** which attract the eye of the user and tempt a click of the mouse, taking the user to a new website. They are similar to internet commercials. These sites usually contain advertisements or surveys and can track the number of times a user views the site. These views are called "hits." Banners and website home pages sometimes use **flash,** which is designed to grab the interest of the user with multimedia and encourage further exploration of a website.

Browsers

Web browsers are software applications that allow the user to locate and display web pages. The most commonly used browsers are Netscape Navigator and Microsoft Internet Explorer. These browsers are able to display graphics as well as text and can also present **multimedia** information, the quality of which is dependent on the computer system in use and the Internet connection speed. Browsers also have a bookmark capability that allows the user to mark a certain web page and then easily return to it by clicking on its link in a drop-down box in the browser's menu. The **cache** allows quick retrieval of previously viewed sites because the computer remembers and saves the information on the hard drive. **Cookies** store information about individual users, like screen names and passwords.

Browsers and other websites also contain **search engines.** These are programs in which a topic, word, or group of words can be entered, and the engine will search the Internet for matches. A listing of those matches will appear, and the user can click on each match to reference information and complete research. Information on just about any subject can be found through using search engines.

POPULAR SEARCH ENGINES

www.alltheweb.com	www.netscape.com
www.altavista.com	www.search.aol.com
www.excite.com	www.search.msn.com
www.google.com	www.webcrawler.com
www.hotbot.com	www.yahoo.com
www.lycos.com	

CRITICAL THINKING APPLICATION

Dr. Bouchard likes that all employees have Internet access at his office, but is still concerned that there will be occasional misuse of the computer. He does not want the staff to use the computer for personal business, but does not mind if they check their personal email on a break or at lunch. What are some reasonable policies for office Internet usage?

The Computer as a Co-Worker

The computer is a valuable tool in the medical office. It can assist in filing insurance claims by sending information from the computer in the office to the computers at the insurance company using a modem. Electronic processing of insurance claims not only saves time but also provides immediate information as to whether a claim will be accepted. Errors in coding or procedure are immediately evident, and many rejections can be avoided even before the claim is transmitted. Many insurance companies give preferential treatment to providers who file claims electronically.

The demographics about a patient will appear on computerized patient ledgers, listing name, address, telephone number, and insurance information. As services are rendered, charges are entered into the computer and payments will be displayed as well. This helps the medical facility to maintain an accurate balance of all patient accounts.

At the appropriate time each month, the computer can print a patient's billing statement, which shows detail of charges, payments, adjustments, and the current balance. Additionally, the computer can be programmed to age the accounts according to any criteria selected and to include this information on the billing statement. A series of collection letters can be developed and personalized for individual patients as they are needed.

Database software makes it possible to organize a large volume of information that can be used in a number of ways. One of the most practical uses is the organization of identifying information on each patient. The computer can also store clinical information about patients using much less space and with greater security than papers in a patient's chart. Access to records can be limited with passwords.

The computer has virtually replaced the appointment book in many medical offices today. Software for appointment-setting ranges from relatively simple programs to very sophisticated systems. An advantage to computer scheduling is that more than one person can access the system at one time, and the same information is available to all users.

Computers are even being used as marketing tools and virtual secretaries in some modern medical offices (Figures 8-6 and 8-7). Computers can be programmed to call all patients with appointments for the next day to remind them to visit the doctor, or perhaps call all patients due for a 6-month eye or dental examination. As a marketing tool, computers can be programmed to call all phone numbers in a certain area code with a prerecorded message about a new procedure available at the office or a new physician in the area. Although many individuals are annoyed at the telemarketing concept and being called by a computer, the success rate is good. Computers can call thousands upon thousands of phone numbers, relay a message, and track replies within a matter of hours. This could never be accomplished in the same time period by humans. These methods of using the computer open all kinds of doors for the medical practice of the future.

The medical office should routinely perform a file backup to be sure that valuable data can be retrieved in the event of a system failure. Many medical office software programs have an automatic backup function, but some must be done manually. It is wise to keep backup copies of the database and other critical documents off the premises in case of fire or other tragedy.

Computer Security

Patients are entitled to the utmost confidentiality with respect to their medical records and the release of any information of a personal nature. Computer technology allows the accumulation and storage of a vast amount of data that may be accessible to a variety of individuals, making it imperative that guidelines be set up for the protection of that data.

Encryption is the translation of data into a code that is not readily understood by most users. It is one effective way to achieve data security. To access or read an encrypted file, the user must have a password that enables the code to be decrypted. Once the code is decrypted, it is then useable by the application. Encrypted data are called *cipher text*.

Some individuals attempt to access information in a computer without the owner's consent. These people may intend to use the information just for fun or may have a malicious intent, such as to steal or corrupt the data. Although these people are commonly called *hackers,* computer enthusiasts insist that the correct term for

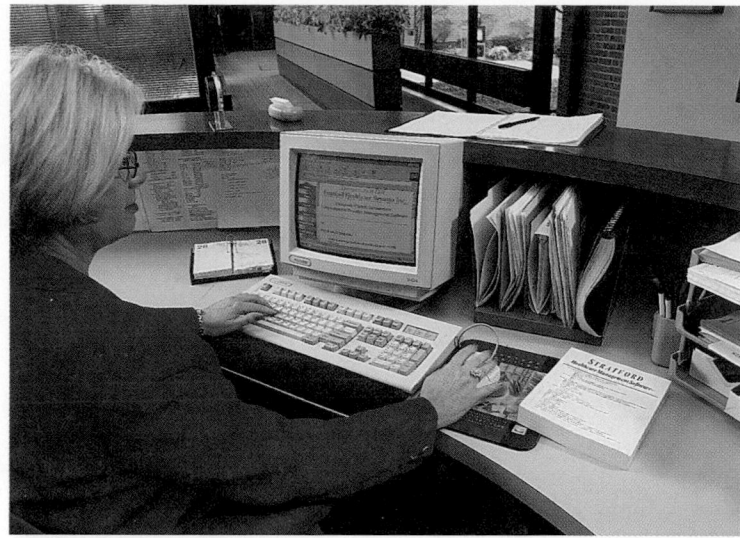

FIGURE 8-6   Computers assist the staff members and physicians of the medical office in numerous ways, making the office run in a more efficient manner.

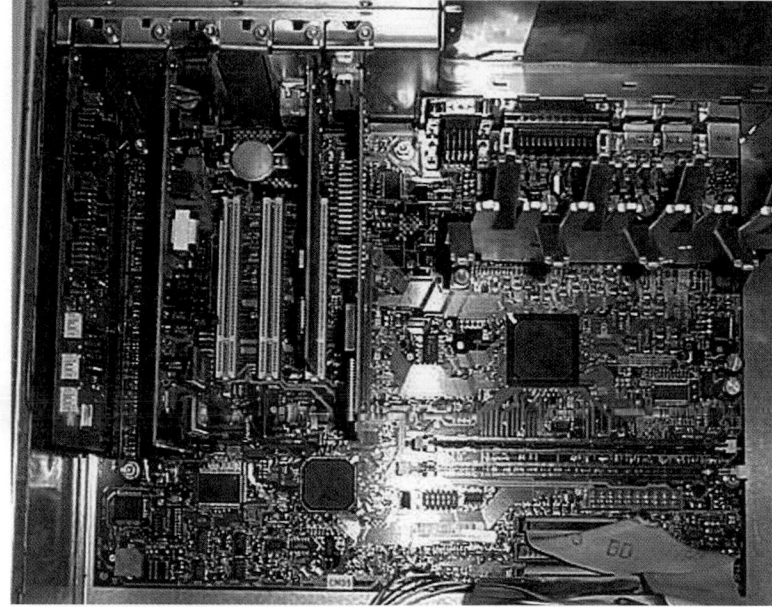

FIGURE 8-7   Inside a computer. Today's microprocessors are designed so that memory, additional drives, and other hardware can be easily added to the system.

individuals who break into computers with dishonorable intent is *crackers*. The term hacker originally simply described a person who enjoyed learning about using computers and becoming proficient in that use.

There are various ways to protect computers and data from unauthorized access. Firewalls are systems designed for just such a purpose and can be implemented into both the hardware and the software of the computer. Firewalls are often used to prevent individuals from accessing private networks. Each message sent and received is examined and the firewall blocks those that do not meet specific security criteria. Passwords, frequent password changes, and user logs also help protect data and the integrity of the database.

Viruses are programs or pieces of code that are loaded onto a computer, usually without the owner's knowledge, that can act like a physical virus in that they can make the computer "sick." Viruses can replicate themselves, copying themselves over and over again, and then be passed to other computers through emails, usually without the sender's knowing that a virus was passed along. Even simple viruses can quickly use all available memory and bring the system to a standstill; some can completely corrupt the computer's hard drive. More dangerous types of viruses can transmit over networks, bypassing security systems and destroying valuable data. This is why antivirus software is an important part of any computer system.

Electronic Signatures

A recently introduced convenience option is the electronic signature. Electronic signature programs are offered both as stand-alone products and as part of computerized medical record systems. After dictated reports are transcribed, a physician can use a password and personal identification number (PIN) to electronically "sign" the document by clicking on an icon after it has been reviewed for accuracy. Once the document has been signed, it cannot be altered—only addenda are allowed.

Computers and Ergonomics

The increased use of computers in the workplace has underscored the need to choose comfortable, safe furniture and equipment. Repetitive strain injury (RSI) accounts for the majority of work-related injury claims. This includes a number of conditions that are caused by repeatedly straining certain nerves, muscles, or tendons. Carpal tunnel syndrome is one example of RSI.

To avoid such injuries, office staff should use posture chairs that support the lumbar section of the back, with a correct angle of the knee and the feet resting on the floor. Of the many designs for keyboards available, one should be chosen that allows the correct angle at the elbow and the wrist to be held in a neutral position.

Eyestrain is another danger arising from continuous use of a computer. The monitor should be just below eye level and at an arm's length away. At least once each hour, the user should take a break from looking at the monitor.

Closing Comments

Computers should be thought of as additional workers in the office. A medical assistant who learns how best to use the computer and discovers as many of its capabilities as possible will be a valuable employee.

Read the manuals that accompany equipment and programs and try new applications for old procedures. Computers are designed to save time, so look for ways to make the day's workload lighter by taking full advantage of the computer.

The future promises more rapid technological advances, since computer equipment can become archaic in as short a time as 6 months after purchase. **Artificial intelligence,** voice recognition, **virtual reality,** and retinal scanning, seen mostly in the movies, will become commonplace in our homes and businesses. These tools will make the work environment even faster and more efficient, as the world becomes a smaller place.

Patient Education

The evolution of computers will continue to bring about changes in medical facilities of the future. Medical staffs will find themselves educating their patients about computer use, because there are numerous programs in development that will allow patients to "check in" once they arrive at the office and verify their identity. A medical assistant will need patience to instruct these procedures and assure the patients that these new methods will increase their security as well as the protection of their medical records.

With the growing number of medical databases online, physicians can now use information on the Internet to help educate their patients about the illnesses that they are facing. While consulting with the patient, with a few clicks of the mouse, the physician can print out excellent information, often that will assist the patient with referrals to help agencies and suggestions for better healthcare.

Legal and Ethical Issues

Concerns about confidentiality continue to be a top priority among patients, and some feel that computers are not as secure as paper-based record-keeping. However, computers can promote a higher degree of accuracy. Some physicians even use computers inside the treatment room to immediately record findings and diagnoses. Care must be taken to ensure that only authorized personnel can access computer-based patient information at all times.

SUMMARY OF SCENARIO

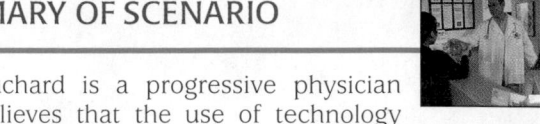

Dr. Bouchard is a progressive physician who believes that the use of technology will assist him in the care of his patients. He understands the need to train his staff and keep them up to date on the latest versions of their computer software. His willingness to close his office for staff-wide training demonstrates his commitment. He is cost conscious and looks for the best available equipment for the investment he is willing to make.

Dr. Bouchard often uses digital camera equipment to take "before" and "after" pictures of his patients, but only with their special written consent. He also uses the computer to send his patients a monthly email newsletter with health information and special news about the practice.

He monitors his staff's Internet usage but is reasonable about allowing them a small degree of personal access on breaks and at lunch.

He is very interested in new developments for healthcare facilities, such as those that will allow his patients to check in themselves and gain access to limited information about their own medical record. He has a vision that one day his patients will be able to download their statement or perhaps their child's immunization records from their home computers, reducing the staff's workload and providing instant access to some information for his patients. Insightful physicians like Dr. Bouchard will see the computer as a co-worker in the medical facility.

SUMMARY OF LEARNING OBJECTIVES

■ The computer can be an effective tool in the medical office. It performs repetitive tasks, reduces errors, speeds up production, recalls information on command, saves time, reduces paperwork, and allows for more creative and productive use of workers' time.

■ The computer performs four basic functions, which are input, processing, output, and storage. Input includes information that is put into the computer, and output is information that comes out of the computer. Processing is in-between, and is the actual manipulation of data. Storage is the retention of data inside the computer or on storage medium.

- There are several basic parts that make up a computer system. The microprocessor is the brains of the system that interprets the instructions given to it by an application program. The monitor allows the user to see immediate output on a screen, and printers allow the output to be printed to a hard copy. The keyboard and mouse serve as input devices.

- Three elements differentiate microprocessors. The bandwidth describes the amount of information that can be sent over a connection at one time, while the clock speed determines the number of instructions per second that the processor can handle. The instruction set is the instructions that the microprocessor can execute.

- There are three main types of printers in use in today's medical offices. Dot matrix printers produce output of moderate quality but are inexpensive. Ink jet printers use a cartridge and a heating element to produce an image on a page. A laser printer uses technology similar to a photocopier.

- The motherboard is the main connection board to which all other devices are connected inside the computer. It contains all of the essential wiring and expansion devices needed to operate the computer, as well as the battery that keeps the clock and calendar running when the computer is turned off.

- Peripheral devices, such as scanners, Zip drives, and other devices, are not necessary to the function of the computer but perform special functions.

- File format refers to the extension just after the file name, which describes the method used to save the file. This also helps to identify the type of file on the computer. For example, a JPEG file is often used for photographs, a GIF file is used for scanned illustrations or images, and a TXT file is usually specifically for text for a printed page.

- Computer networks are groups of two or more computers linked together. These networks can be local or cover a city or wide geographic area. Some are limited to a few buildings. Networks often share resources, such as printers.

- Browsers are software applications that allow a user to find information on the Internet. They are able to show graphics, and often multimedia, such as videos. The most commonly used browsers are Internet Explorer and Netscape Navigator.

- Computer security is critical, especially because confidential patient information is stored on computers in medical facilities. There are several ways to enhance computer security, such as the use of firewalls and antivirus programs. Restrictions as to who may log in and the use of passwords also will assist the facility to ensure that only authorized individuals have access to confidential information.

KEY INTERNET WEBSITES

- Webopedia—an Online Computer Dictionary
  For active weblinks to each website visit
  http://evolve.elsevier.com/Kinn/

CHAPTER 9

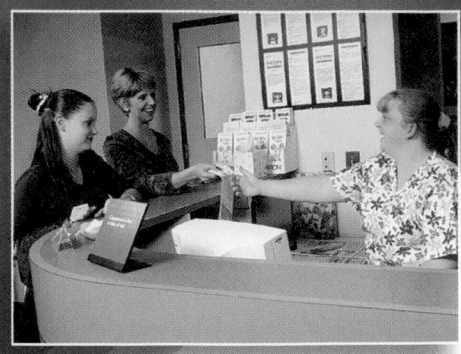

Scenario

Ashlynn McDowell is a recent graduate of a medical assisting program and has begun her first position as a receptionist in an obstetrician's office. It has been Ashlynn's lifelong goal to work with pregnant women, and she is determined to perform to the best of her abilities. However, Ashlynn has never held a job in a professional office. She knows that she will need to practice all of the skills she learned in school with regard to being an effective receptionist.

The physician Ashlynn works for, Dr. Stella Frank, is customer service oriented and wants her patients to feel special and well cared for. She insists that they be treated as important and that their concerns be taken seriously. Ashlynn is anxious to build trust with the patients and offer help to them with the problems they encounter. She knows that she will be required to speak clearly and distinctly and be adept at follow-up skills. She plans to dress professionally each day, so that she projects the right image to the patients with whom she comes in contact. Ashlynn will strive to be the type of employee who presents a willingness to learn, an ability to adapt, and a heart with compassion for the patient. She is a team player who sincerely wishes to cooperate with other staff members that might need her help.

Dr. Frank is pleased that she has found such an eager person to add to her staff and will provide assistance and guidance to her as she learns how to make her patients feel a part of her clinic family. Ashlynn's self-esteem has increased because she feels she is making a great contribution to healthcare.

Telephone Techniques

- Define and spell the terms listed in the vocabulary.
- Determine and discuss the source of incoming calls to a physician's office.
- Describe how one develops a pleasing telephone voice.
- Demonstrate the correct way to hold a telephone handset.
- Explain why courtesy is so important when speaking on the telephone.
- Discuss different ways to handle callers who wish to speak to the physician.
- List the seven items needed to take a telephone message correctly.
- Explain how angry callers might be handled.
- Discuss how the medical assistant should handle callers with a complaint.
- List several questions to ask when handling an emergency call.
- Discuss several useful sections of the introductory pages of the phone directory.
- Demonstrate the correct way to answer the telephone in the office.
- Demonstrate the correct way to accurately record a message and take a request for action.
- Demonstrate the most efficient way to call in a prescription or prescription refill to a pharmacy.

National Curriculum Competencies

TRANSDISCIPLINARY COMPETENCIES

1b. Recognize and respond to verbal communication
1d. Demonstrate telephone techniques

2a. Identify and respond to issues of confidentiality
3a. Explain general office policies
3e. Identify community resources

Vocabulary

clarity The quality or state of being clear.

competent Having adequate abilities or qualities; having the capacity to function or perform in a certain way.

cultivate To foster the growth of; to improve by labor, care, or study.

diction The choice of words especially with regard to clearness, correctness, or effectiveness.

enunciation Utterance of articulate, clear sounds.

inflection A change in pitch or loudness of the voice.

invariably Consistent; not changing or capable of change.

jargon The technical terminology or characteristic idiom of a particular group or special activity.

monotone A succession of syllables, words, or sentences in one unvaried key or pitch.

multitasking Performing multiple tasks at the same time.

pitch The property of a sound, especially a musical tone, that is determined by the frequency of the waves producing it; the highness or lowness of sound.

provider Individual or company that provides medical care and services to a patient or the public.

salutation An expression of greeting, goodwill, or courtesy by words or gestures.

screen Something that shields, protects, or hides; to select or eliminate through a screening process.

stat Medical abbreviation for immediately; at this moment.

tactful Having a keen sense of what to do or say to maintain good relations with others or to avoid offense.

tedious Tiresome because of length or dullness.

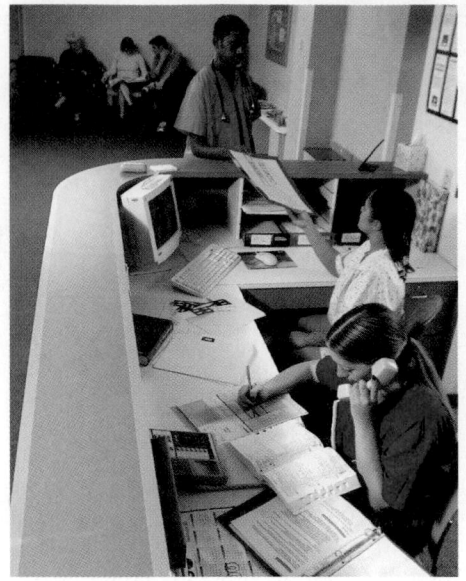

FIGURE 9-1 The telephone plays a vital role in the success of a medical practice.

Effective Use of the Telephone

Active Listening

Although great emphasis is placed on rules for speaking, the importance of active listening is often overlooked. The same attention should be given a telephone conversation that would be given a face-to-face conversation. Concentration is not always easy for a medical assistant who is juggling several duties at once in the medical office, so he or she must practice focusing on the call at hand. Effective active listening also provides vital information about the nature of the call—whether the caller is distressed and agitated or has a concern that needs to be addressed immediately.

Developing a Pleasing Telephone Voice

Individuals who call a physician's office should hear a pleasant, friendly voice when they are greeted. It is a common sales technique to be sure that the caller "hears a smile." Customer service is critical in today's medical offices, and this technique is quite useful for medical assistants, who are likely to be the caller's first point of contact with the practice. Be sure to enunciate words clearly, pronouncing them separately and distinctly. **Diction, pitch,** and **clarity** are important as well. Avoid speaking in a **monotone;** instead, use **inflection,** or a change in the pitch and loudness of the voice when speaking. This helps the speaker to emphasize certain points during the conversation.

When a telephone call is received from a stranger, one usually tries to visualize that person's appearance and perhaps will form an opinion of his or her personality. The caller may sound mature, somewhat worried, well educated, or frantic. As discussed in Chapter 5, communication is a two-way street, so the caller will be forming an impression of the person answering the phone at the

The telephone is the lifeline of a medical practice as well as a powerful public relations tool. The majority of patients who are seen in a medical facility make their initial appointments by telephone. When used appropriately, the telephone can help build a medical practice from its beginning and throughout its life (Figure 9-1). If used inappropriately, it can destroy even a flourishing practice. Medical assistants must remember that the voice on the other end of the line is that of the patient, and telephone calls can never be considered an interruption of the work day.

Most incoming calls are from these sources:
- Established patients calling for appointments or to ask questions
- Individuals reporting emergencies
- Other physicians who are making referrals
- Laboratories reporting vital information regarding a patient
- New patients making a first contact with the physician's office

same time. Sometimes these impressions are incorrect, but much can be assumed by what is heard on the telephone.

Always use a friendly and warm tone of voice and project confidence when speaking with patients. Be courteous and **tactful** and choose words carefully. Every caller should be made to feel that the medical assistant has time to attend to his or her wishes. A small mirror, placed near the telephone, will serve as a reminder to smile. If the medical assistant is rushed to pick up the telephone, he or she should wait a few seconds until able to answer graciously without seeming breathless or impatient.

Be alert and interested in the person who is calling. Always give full attention to the caller and do not allow distractions from the conversation. Build a pleasant, friendly image for the office. Talk naturally and avoid repetition of mechanical words or phrases, such as "uh huh" and "you know." Avoid the use of professional **jargon,** such as referring to *otalgia* when the patient is reporting an *earache*. Using correct grammar adds to the caller's favorable impression. Speak distinctly; clear pronunciation and **enunciation** are vital. Move the lips, tongue, and jaw freely. Talk directly into the mouthpiece. Never answer the telephone when eating, drinking, or chewing gum. A well-modulated voice carries best. Use a normal tone of voice, neither too loud nor too soft. Talk at a moderate rate, neither too quickly nor too slowly. Be expressive and vary the tone of voice. This will bring out the meaning of sentences and add color and vitality to what is said.

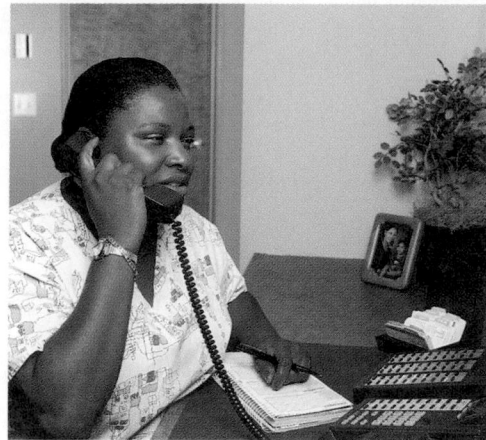

FIGURE 9-2   The handset should be held in the center, with the mouthpiece about 1 inch in front of the lips.

Speak directly into the telephone immediately after removing it from its cradle. When turning to face another part of the room, make sure the handset moves, too; otherwise, the voice will be lost. A medical assistant who speaks too fast, enunciates poorly, or fails to speak directly into the transmitter may not be easily understood by the person on the other end of the receiver.

Maintaining Confidentiality

Keep in mind that all communications in a healthcare facility are confidential. If others are nearby, use discretion when mentioning the name of the caller. Be careful about being overheard when repeating any symptoms or other information received by telephone. Never use a speaker phone to listen to voice mail or hold a phone conversation within the hearing range of others.

CRITICAL THINKING APPLICATION

Ashlynn has a tendency to speak a little fast in her normal conversations. How will she need to adjust as she is answering phones in the medical office? She is also a friendly person and enjoys talking on the phone. What precautions should she take so that this does not become an issue on the job?

CRITICAL THINKING APPLICATION

Ashlynn hears two employees speaking on the intercom in a derogatory manner about a patient who just left the office. How should she handle this situation? Who should Ashlynn report this activity to, if anyone, and why? What problems could be caused when staff members are overheard talking in this manner?

Holding the Telephone Handset Correctly

A medical assistant must develop professional telephone habits in the medical office and correct the more casual habits that are used at home. Consider how the handset is held. It should be placed so that the medical assistant's voice is relayed distinctly and accurately. Practice holding the handset around the middle, with the mouthpiece about 1 inch from the lips and directly in front of the teeth (Figure 9-2). Never hold it under the chin. Check the proper distance by taking the first two fingers and passing them through sideways in the space between the lips and the mouthpiece. If the fingers just squeeze through, then the lips are the correct distance from the telephone and the voice will go over the line as close to its natural tone as possible. When using a headset, speak directly into its mouthpiece, positioning it the same distance from the mouth as a regular telephone.

Thinking Ahead

It is always helpful to think ahead when there is an important call to make. Have the patient's chart or the bill in question at hand before dialing the phone. Write down a list of questions to ask or goals for the conversation. Keep the call short and simple, then free the line for other calls.

Most offices keep a list of frequently called phone numbers to offer patients for referrals. A list of local pharmacies and hospitals and their departments is also very helpful. All of these are time-savers that will help the medical assistant to better serve patients.

PROCEDURE 9-1

Answering the Telephone

GOAL: To answer the telephone in a physician's office in a professional manner and respond to a request for action.

EQUIPMENT AND SUPPLIES

- Telephone
- Message pad
- Pen or pencil
- Appointment book
- Notepad

PROCEDURAL STEPS

1 Answer the telephone by the third ring, speaking directly into the mouthpiece, which should be positioned one inch from the mouth.
Purpose: Answering promptly conveys interest in the caller. Proper positioning of the handset allows for audible tone and carries the voice well.

2 Speak distinctly with a pleasant tone and expression, at a moderate rate, and with sufficient volume for the calling party to understand every word.

3 Identify the office and/or physician and yourself.
Purpose: The caller will know that the correct number has been reached and the identity of the staff member.

4 Verify the identity of the caller.
Purpose: To confirm the origin of the call.

5 Triage the call, if necessary.
Purpose: To determine if the caller has an emergency and needs immediate attention, or a referral to the emergency department of a hospital.

6 Determine the needs of the caller, and provide the requested information or service, if possible. Provide the caller with excellent customer service. Be as helpful as possible.
Purpose: The medical assistant can handle many calls and conserve the time and energy of the physician or other staff members.

7 If unable to assist the caller, transfer the call to the appropriate person. Before transferring the call, provide the person to whom the call is being transferred with as much information as possible about the caller and his or her needs.
Purpose: To provide good customer service and be as helpful to the caller as possible.

8 Take a proper message for further action, if required.
Purpose: Not all calls can be responded to immediately.

9 Terminate the call in a pleasant manner and replace the receiver gently. Always allow the caller to hang up first.
Purpose: To promote good public relations, provide excellent customer service, and ensure that the caller has no further questions.

Techniques for Incoming Telephone Calls

Many incoming calls will be received in the medical office during the course of a single day. Each one deserves the medical assistant's complete and **competent** attention (Procedure 9-1).

Answering Promptly

Whenever possible, answer the telephone on the first ring, and always by the third ring. If the facility has several incoming lines or more than one telephone, it will sometimes be necessary to interrupt a conversation to answer another call. It is considered courteous to say, "Pardon me just a moment; the other line is ringing." Answer the second call and determine who is calling. If it is not an emergency, ask that person to hold while the first call is completed. Do not make the mistake of continuing with the second call while the first caller waits. Return to the first call as soon as possible and apologize briefly for the interruption.

Think of what would happen during a face-to-face conversation. A second person who approaches people involved in a conversation would not expect to interrupt and be heard at length. However, if the second call is an emergency, take a moment to return to the first line and alert the caller that he or she will have to be kept waiting or be called back.

Never answer a call by saying, "Please hold" without first finding out who is calling. It could be an emergency, and it is extremely discourteous. It takes only a moment to be polite, and this practice could save a life.

Keep the focus on the call. Attempting **multitasking** while answering the telephone will take attention away from the patient. Treat the phone call just as if the patient were standing in the office face-to-face.

Identifying the Facility

The response to an incoming call should be to first identify the facility and then the person answering the phone. Numerous telephone greetings can be used. Discuss which are best with the physician or office manager. Examples of telephone greetings include the following:

- "This is Dr. Frank's office, Miss McDowell speaking. How may I help you?"
- "Frank Maternal Health Clinic, this is Miss McDowell. How may I help you?"
- "Stella Frank's office, this is Miss McDowell. How may I help you?"

Some physicians avoid using the title "Doctor" so that they may protect their patient's confidentiality. For instance, if a physician needs to call and leave a message for a patient, that patient's curious co-workers might attempt to investigate what type of physician is being seen. Dropping the "Doctor" when leaving messages and when answering the telephone can be an effective means of protecting the patient's privacy.

Merely saying "Hello" is unsatisfactory. The caller will **invariably** ask if he or she has reached the physician's office, so time is wasted, and the opportunity to create a favorable impression of your facility has been lost.

The use of a **salutation** in telephone identification is optional. Sometimes the addition of "Good morning" or "Good afternoon" to the identification is awkward. A rising inflection or a questioning tone in your voice indicates interest and a willingness to assist and eliminates the need for an additional greeting.

When you have decided on the greeting to be used, practice it until you can say it easily and smoothly without having to think about what you are saying. It is critical that the greeting not be rushed so that all callers can easily understand exactly what is being communicated.

CRITICAL THINKING APPLICATION

Most offices dictate how the phone is to be answered. What should Ashlynn do if she is very uncomfortable with the way she is being asked to answer the phone? Who should ultimately make the decision as to how the phone is answered?

Identifying the Caller

If the caller does not identify himself or herself, ask who is calling. Repeat the caller's name by using it in the conversation as soon as possible. Name repetition assures the patient that he or she has been correctly identified and is pleasing to the patient. Try to use the person's name at least three times during the call, and remember other courteous expressions, such as "thank you," "please," and "you're welcome" as often as possible. However, if other patients are within the range of your voice, remember that the caller's privacy should be respected.

Occasionally a caller will refuse to identify himself or herself to the medical assistant and may be quite insistent on speaking with the physician. The individual could be a patient, and the medical assistant should make every attempt to identify the patient and assist his or her needs. Such callers may also be salespersons who are fully aware that if their identity is revealed, they will never get the opportunity to speak to the physician. These people may be firmly told, "Dr. Frank is busy with a patient and has asked that we take messages for her. If you will not leave a message, you may wish to write a letter to her and mark it 'personal.'"

Screening Incoming Calls

Most physicians expect the medical assistant to **screen** all telephone calls. The physician and office manager will provide guidance as to the type of calls that should be routed to the physician and those that he or she will want to return at a later time. The medical assistant should become familiar with their preferences and also use good judgment, much of which comes with experience, in deciding whether to put a call through to the physician (Figure 9-3).

If it is the policy of the office, put calls from other physicians through at once. If the physician is busy and cannot possibly come to the telephone, explain this briefly and politely and then say that the physician will return the call as soon as possible.

Many callers will ask, "Is the doctor in?" or "May I speak to the doctor?" Avoid answering this question with a simple "Yes" or "No" or by responding with the question, "Who is calling, please?" If the physician is not in, say so *before* asking the identity of the caller. Otherwise, the impression may be created that the physician is just not willing to talk with this person.

STAYING IN CONTROL OF CALLS

The Dartnell Corporation publishes a newsletter entitled "Effective Telephone Techniques" that is an excellent tool for building good customer relations while using the phone. One issue suggests ways to control calls and keep them from becoming too lengthy. Try the tips below to keep callers on track and make all phone time productive.

- Ask the caller, "How may I help you today?"
- If the caller becomes sidetracked, say "You were describing the pain in your side?"
- When making a call, get right to the purpose of it after the initial greeting by saying "I was calling you about..."
- Keep explanations short and direct.
- Type information directly into the database, if used, while speaking on the phone.
- Keep personal and friendly comments to a minimum, or only one per call.
- Once the business is concluded, say "If there are no other questions..." and bring the conversation to a close.

FIGURE 9-3 Several tips to stay in control of the telephone calls in the medical office.

If the physician is away from the office, the rule of offering assistance still holds. The medical assistant may say, "No, I am sorry, Dr. Frank is not in. May I take a message?" or "No, I am sorry, but Dr. Frank will be at the hospital most of the morning. May I ask her to return your call after 1 o'clock?"

If the physician is in and is available for telephone calls, a typical response would be, "Yes, Dr. Frank is in; may I say who is calling, please?"

When physicians prefer to keep telephone calls to a minimum, say, "Yes, Dr. Frank is here, but she is not free to come to the phone. May I take a message, please?" By responding in this way, the physician is not committed to taking the call.

During the time that a physician is examining a patient, he or she will not wish to be interrupted with a routine call. In such cases you might say, "Yes, Dr. Frank is in but is with a patient right now. May I help you?" or "Yes, Dr. Frank is in but is with a patient right now. Is there anything you would like me to ask her?"

Try to guard against being overprotective. A patient should be able to talk with the physician when necessary; but unless it is an emergency, the patient is probably willing to do so at the convenience of the physician. The medical assistant who answers the telephone acts as a screen, not a roadblock.

CRITICAL THINKING APPLICATION

Ashlynn answers the phone and a male pharmaceutical representative who has been visiting the clinic for several months is on the phone. She cheerfully greets him and asks if he is calling to make an appointment. He states that he wants to make an appointment with Ashlynn—for a date. How should she handle this call? What problems could arise if this were a patient and Ashlynn accepted the date?

Find out exactly how calls are to be handled when the physician is out of the office and under what circumstances he or she can be interrupted when the physician is on the premises. **Cultivate** a reputation for being helpful and reliable. Medical assistants will save the physician many interruptions if patients develop confidence in their ability to help them and have faith in their promises to take their messages and deliver them properly.

Minimizing Wait Time

When a call cannot be put through immediately, ask, "Would you prefer to wait, or shall I call you back when Dr. Frank is free?"

If the caller elects to wait, remember that waiting with a silent telephone can be irritating and **tedious**. The waiting time always seems long, no matter how brief it really is. Many of today's phones are equipped with timers that tell the caller exactly how long they have been waiting on hold. The longer they wait, the more irritated they may become. Let no more than 1 minute pass without breaking in with some reassuring comment. For instance: "I'm sorry, Dr. Frank is still busy."

If the wait is longer than expected, the caller may wish to reconsider and call back at another time or have the call returned. By going back on the line at frequent intervals, the caller has an opportunity to express such concerns. Ask the caller if he or she wishes to continue waiting. The medical assistant could say, "I'm sorry to keep you waiting so long, Ms. Hughes. Would you prefer to have me return your call when Dr. Frank is free?"

Try to give the caller some estimate of when he or she may expect the return call. In any event, be considerate and remember that irritation can be lessened each time the medical assistant returns to the call by saying, "Thank you for waiting, Ms. Hughes."

When it is necessary to leave the telephone and obtain information, ask the caller, "Will you please wait while I get the information?" Listen for a reply. If it will take longer than a few seconds to get the information, give some estimate of the time required and offer to call back. When returning to the telephone, always thank the caller for waiting. Requests that might require pulling the patient's chart from the files are best handled with a call back to the patient.

Remember that leaving a person on hold ties up one of the physician's telephone lines, and an emergency call could be coming through, or new patients might be attempting to call. The majority of phone calls that come in to a physician's office during the day are important, so the lines should be kept clear as much as possible.

Transferring a Call

Always identify the person who is calling when a call is transferred to the physician or another person in the facility. Always ask the patient's permission to place him or her on hold and to transfer the call. It is considered poor customer service to simply transfer the call to a co-worker's voice mail without warning the caller that the person is not available. Any person who refuses to give a name should not be put through unless the medical assistant has been specifically instructed to do so. If the person is not immediately available, ask the caller whether he or she would prefer to be put through to voice mail. Some callers simply believe their call will receive more attention if a human takes the message. If the caller insists, take a written message and deliver it to the proper person as soon as possible.

One very important skill that all medical assistants should learn is "who does what" in the medical facility. Knowing about the functions of the office and which person is responsible for which areas will make a significant difference in the customer service provided to the patient. To illustrate: suppose that the medical office employs one insurance receptionist, named Sarah, and three insurance billers. Opel handles names that begin with *A* through *G*, David handles names that begin with *H* through *P*, and Andrea handles names that begin with *Q* through *Z*. If a call comes to the office and the patient has an insurance question, the medical assistant could put the call through to Sarah. However, better customer service dictates that the medical assistant ask the name of the patient and put the call through to the person who handles that patient's particular claims. If the patient's name is Rebecca Whitehead, the medical assistant should call Andrea and ask if she may transfer Ms. Whitehead's call to her. The fewer times the caller is transferred, the happier the caller.

When the caller is a patient, the physician will probably need the patient's chart at hand during the conversation. If there is no concern about others hearing the conversation, the medical assistant can announce the caller's name on the intercom and tell the physician that the chart is on its way back to his or her office. Remember that it is vital to protect the patient's right to privacy. If there are others within hearing range, take the chart to the physician and say, "Dr. Frank, this patient is waiting on the telephone to speak with you."

Ending a Call

When a caller's requests have been satisfied, do not encourage inappropriate chatting or permit the call to monopolize your time unnecessarily. The telephone lines should be cleared for other calls. Allow the person who placed the call to hang up first, and be sure to thank him or her for calling. Close the conversation with some form of "good-bye" and replace the telephone on its cradle gently.

Taking a Telephone Message

Always have a pen or pencil in hand and a message pad nearby when answering the telephone. Several calls may be answered before there is an opportunity to relay a message or carry out a promise of action. The *written message* is vital (Procedure 9-2).

There are numerous types of message pads available today (Figure 9-4). An ordinary spiral-bound stenographer's notebook is inexpensive, sturdy, and well proportioned; lies flat on a desk; and can be filed for future reference if desired. Never use small scraps of paper for messages; they are too easily lost. Bear in mind that the message book should be kept indefinitely in the medical office, because it could be used as evidence in a court of law. Messages should also be added to the patient's chart once acted on, or at a minimum, noted in the chart.

Date the bottom of the first blank page in the notebook at the beginning of each day. This creates a permanent record that can be referred to later if the need arises. Check off each message in the log as it is delivered or taken care of. This creates a good reminder system.

A minimum of seven items are needed to take a telephone message correctly:
1. The name of the person to whom the call is directed
2. The name of the person calling
3. The caller's daytime and/or evening telephone number
4. The reason for the call
5. The action to be taken
6. The date and time of the call
7. The initials of the person taking the call

Messages that are to be transmitted to another person may be rewritten on individual message slips and delivered or posted on a message board later. Impression-sensitive message pads that provide a copy of each page ensure that no message will be forgotten and are the best way to keep track of messages. The nature of the message will determine whether it should be reported immediately. The person who completes the call must sign and date it. If the call is from a patient and relates in any way to the medical history, or if any instructions were given or queries answered, this information should be placed in the patient's chart. Message forms are available that have a self-adhesive backing and can be placed permanently in the patient's case history.

Taking Action on Telephone Messages

The message procedure is not complete until the necessary action has been taken. Notations on the memo pad should be carried over to the following day if they have not been completed, but this should be a rare occurrence. Do not trust to memory messages that were not attended to from previous days; always carry them forward in writing.

Make brief notations of patients' reactions while talking to them on the telephone. The physician does not require a character study, but it is helpful to know when a patient appears fearful, apprehensive, or nervous. If a patient shows such symptoms, it may be wise to consult with or transfer the call to the physician.

When the employer is talking to another physician about a referral, the medical assistant may be requested to take down a brief outline of the patient's case history while listening on the extension telephone. This information can be typewritten and incorporated with the patient's chart and handed to the physician before the patient is seen.

Retaining Telephone Records

Each office must develop a policy regarding retention of telephone message records. Many offices elect to keep message pads for the same period that the statute of limitations exists for medical professional liability cases. Remember, phone records would include telephone bills, especially those that detail long-distance charges. Keeping these records can be of assistance in proving any number of claims, including the number of times that patients called the office and the fact that calls to the patient were returned. Be sure that accurate telephone records are kept to ensure good patient care and customer service

Typical Incoming Calls

One reason for having a medical assistant answer incoming calls is to spare the physician unnecessary interruptions during visits with patients. Many calls relate to the administrative aspects of the office and can actually be better handled by the medical assistant. The policy regarding how calls are to be handled should be clearly set forth in the office procedures manual.

Some of the kinds of calls that can be handled by the medical assistant in most offices will be discussed next.

PROCEDURE 9-2

Taking a Telephone Message

GOAL: To take an accurate telephone message and follow up on the requests made by the caller.

EQUIPMENT AND SUPPLIES

- Telephone
- Message pad
- Pen or pencil
- Notepad

PROCEDURAL STEPS

1 Answer the telephone using the guidelines in Procedure 9-1.

Purpose: Answering promptly and courteously conveys interest in the caller and promotes good customer service.

2 Using a message pad or notepad, take the phone message, obtaining the following information:
- The name of the person to whom the call is directed
- The name of the person calling
- The caller's daytime and/or telephone number
- The reason for the call
- The action to be taken
- The date and time of the call
- The initials of the person taking the call

Purpose: Accurate information allows the staff member to address the caller's issues quickly and efficiently.

3 Repeat the information back to the caller after the message is recorded on the message pad.

Purpose: To verify that all information taken has been recorded accurately.

4 Provide the caller with an approximation of the time and date that he or she will be called back, if possible.

Purpose: To be considerate of the patient's time, and keep him or her from sitting next to the phone awaiting a call.

5 End the call and wait for the caller to hang up first.

6 Deliver the phone message to the appropriate person. Separate trays or slots for each staff member are helpful.

7 Follow up on important messages.

Purpose: To make certain that important issues are addressed in a timely manner.

8 Keep old message books for future reference. Carbonless copies will allow the facility to keep a permanent record of phone messages.

Purpose: To have a permanent source of messages in case a number is needed after the paper message has been discarded.

9 File pertinent phone messages in the patient's chart.

Purpose: To keep a permanent record of important information in the patient's chart.

New Patients and Return Appointments

Procedures for handling appointments for new patients and scheduling return appointments are discussed in the chapter on appointment scheduling. In general, provide excellent customer service to the caller. Remember that the routine questions that may be asked should be answered in a polite and cheerful manner. Follow the designated office procedure as to what information should be gathered and recorded when appointments are made.

Directions

Each office should have a clear set of directions written out that can be read to the caller when there is a request for directions. Prepare directions from various points in the area; for instance, one set would guide a patient who is coming from the north, and another set will be for a patient coming from the south. Place these directions close to the telephone so that all employees can access them easily. Not all employees live close to the clinic or are familiar with all areas, so the written set of directions will be helpful to all staff members and those who call the facility.

Inquiries About Bills

A patient may ask to speak with the physician about a recent bill. Ask the caller to hold for a moment while the ledger is pulled. If nothing irregular is found on the ledger, return to the telephone and say, "I have your account in front of me now. Perhaps I can answer your question." Most likely, the caller will have some simple inquiry, such as whether the insurance has paid, or may wish to delay making a payment until the next month. Not all patients realize that the medical assistant usually makes such decisions and is the best person with whom to discuss these matters.

A patient may have a question about a statement that was received in the mail. If billing matters are handled by another employee, tell the patient that you will transfer his or her call to the billing office. If you are responsible for billing, politely ask the patient to hold the line while you pull the patient ledger. When you return to the line, thank the patient for waiting and explain the charges carefully. If

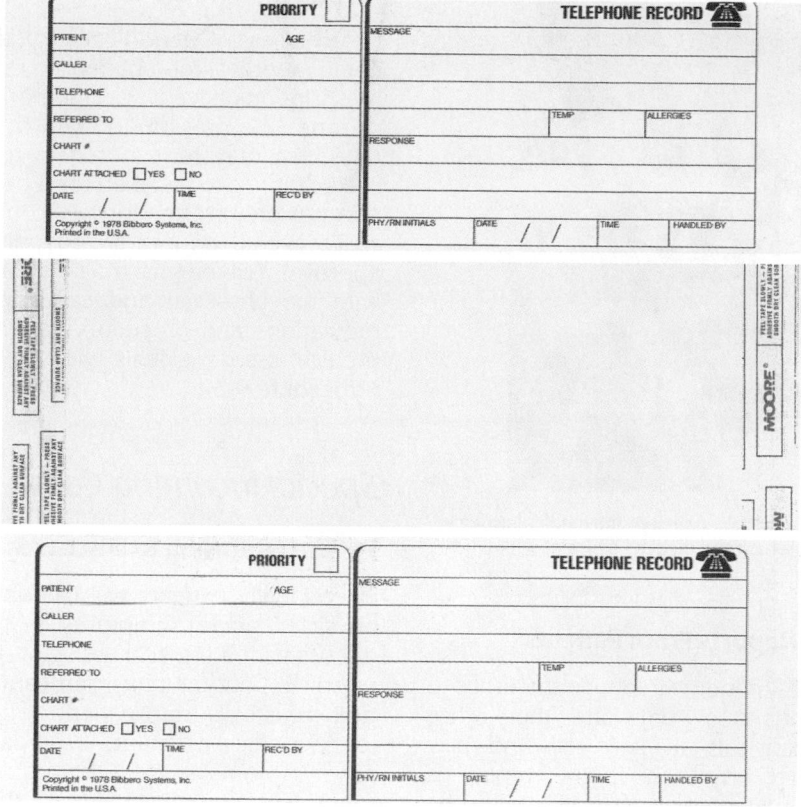

FIGURE 9-4   Phone message forms with self-adhesive backing make charting the call easier and more time efficient. (Courtesy Bibbero Systems, Inc., Petaluma, CA 94654.)

there is an error, apologize and say a corrected statement will be sent out at once. Always remember to thank the patient for calling. If patients are properly advised about charges at the time that services are rendered, the number of these calls will be considerably reduced.

Inquiries About Fees

Fees vary widely in each medical office, and it is very difficult to quote an exact fee before the patient is seen by the physician. However, a good range should be given to the patient as to what they should expect to pay, especially on the first visit. Asking a patient to just appear at the office without having any idea of the cost is unreasonable. Discuss with the physician or office manager what range should be quoted to the patient and then follow your quotes with the statement that the fees will vary, depending on the patient's condition and tests that the physician orders. If fees are regularly discussed on the telephone, write a suggested script in the policy manual. Do not be evasive. Have a schedule of fees available.

Participating Provider

Patients may call the office to inquire as to whether the physician is a participating **provider** with their particular insurance plan or managed care organization. The physician should keep a carefully updated list of which plans are valid. This is important, because insurance benefits vary for participating and nonparticipating providers.

Requests for Assistance With Insurance

In today's environment of managed care, copays, Medicaid, and Medicare, insurance claims will more than likely be completed and filed by the healthcare facility. Nevertheless, patients may call to inquire about their coverage or ask whether there has been any response to the filing of the claims. A medical assistant or member of the staff whose responsibility is the filing of insurance claims will have the knowledge to answer these inquiries (Figure 9-5). Be patient with these inquiries, because insurance is a difficult subject to understand, even for those who are trained and familiar with the various forms and procedures to use. Some patients, especially elderly ones, are quite confused when dealing with these insurance companies. Help them as much as possible so that they can collect the benefits to which they are entitled.

Radiology and Laboratory Reports

Laboratory and radiological findings may be telephoned to the physician's office on the day the procedures are performed, when their results are urgently needed. The medical assistant can take these reports and relay them to the physician. More often, the report is faxed to the physician if it is a **stat** report. Original reports will be delivered by mail for the permanent record. Some facilities are equipped to receive laboratory results directly from the laboratory by computer.

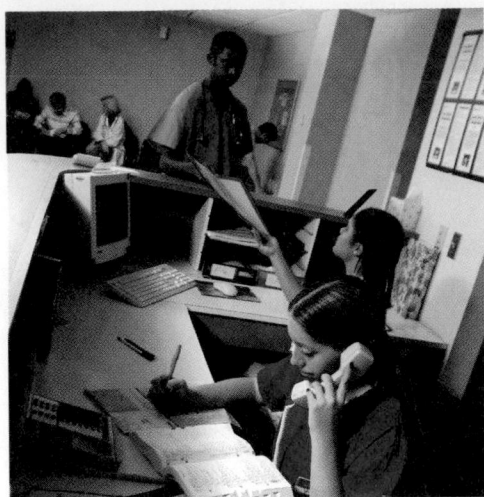

FIGURE 9-5 Many of the calls that come into the medical office are insurance questions, with which the medical assistant will assist the caller.

Satisfactory Progress Reports From Patients

Physicians sometimes ask patients to phone the office to report on their conditions a few days after their office visit. The medical assistant can take such calls and relay the information to the physician if the report is satisfactory. Assure the patient that you will inform the physician about the call.

Routine Reports From Hospitals and Other Sources

There may be routine calls from a hospital and other sources reporting a patient's progress. If it is only a normal reporting procedure, take the message carefully, make sure that the physician sees it and then place the message in the patient's medical record.

Office Administration Matters

Not all calls concern patients. There may be calls from the accountant or auditor or calls regarding banking procedures, office supplies, or office maintenance, most of which the medical assistant can handle or refer to the appropriate person. For some of these calls the medical assistant may need to gather additional information and return the call.

Requests for Referrals

Physicians who are liked and respected by their patients frequently will be called for referrals to other specialists. If the physician has furnished the medical assistant with a list of practitioners for this purpose, these inquiries can usually be handled without consulting the physician. However, the physician should always be informed of such requests.

Some managed care organizations require a physician referral before a patient may see a specialist. This referral should come from the physician, unless he or she has authorized automatic referrals. Handle these calls as quickly as possible so that the patient may make an appointment to see the referral physician.

Prescription Refills

Pharmacies will periodically call the physician's office to obtain approval for a patient to refill a prescription. Most prescriptions have a specific notation as to the number of times the prescription can be refilled. However, the physician may have noted in the chart that a certain medication is to be taken for 6 months, but the prescription was only written for 1 to 2 months. Any prescription refills should be authorized only with the physician's approval. Tell the pharmacist that you will have to check with the physician and call back. Be sure that state regulations and procedures are followed any time the medical assistant deals with prescription refills or calls (Procedure 9-3).

Special Incoming Calls

Patients Refusing to Discuss Symptoms

Occasionally patients will call and wish to talk with the physician about symptoms that they are reluctant to discuss with a medical assistant. Patients do have a right to privacy, but the physician cannot be expected to take numerous calls from patients who do not wish to speak to the medical assistant. If the patient refuses to discuss any symptoms, suggest that he or she make an appointment with the physician to discuss the problem in person.

Unsatisfactory Progress Reports

If a patient under treatment reports that he or she is still not feeling well or that the prescription the doctor provided is not helping, do not try to practice medicine by giving the patient medical advice. Make detailed notes about the patient's comments, then present them to the physician. He or she will make the decision as to whether the patient should return to the office or may make a medication change. Follow up with the patient and convey the physician's instructions.

Requests for Test Results

When the physician orders special tests for the patient, the patient may be told to call the office in a couple of days for the results. Never assume that the patient will call for results. It is ultimately the responsibility of the physician to notify the patient of test results. Be certain that the physician has seen the results and has given permission before sharing the results with the patient. Patients do not always understand that the medical assistant does not have the privilege of giving out information without the permission of the physician. If the result is unfavorable, the physician should be the one to inform the patient and give further instructions. This call must be handled tactfully; otherwise, the patient may feel as if the staff is concealing information.

Most physicians prefer that medical assistants only provide normal test results to the patients. However, the medical assistant may provide abnormal test results to the patient if authorized by the physician. For example, when a patient has a questionable Pap smear, the medical

PROCEDURE **9-3**

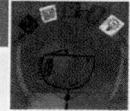

Calling the Pharmacy With New or Refill Prescriptions

GOAL: To call in an accurate prescription to the pharmacy for a patient in the most efficient manner.

EQUIPMENT AND SUPPLIES

- Prescription
- Notepad
- Patient chart
- Telephone

PROCEDURAL STEPS

1 Receive the call from the patient requesting a prescription, using appropriate telephone technique.

Purpose: To provide consistently good customer service when speaking with callers.

2 Obtain the following information from the patient:
- Patient's name
- Telephone number where he or she can be reached
- Patient's symptoms and current condition
- History of this condition
- Treatments the patient has tried
- Pharmacy name and telephone number

Purpose: To have the information the physician will need to make a determination as to whether a prescription will be called in for the patient, or whether he or she needs to come to the office to be seen by the doctor.

3 Write in the patient's chart the prescription that the physician wishes the patient to have. Be very careful to transcribe the information correctly. Read it back to the physician.

Purpose: To have a permanent record of the prescription in the chart, and make certain that the prescription is exactly what the physician wants the patient to take, eliminating errors in medication name and dosage.

4 If the prescription is a refill, give the physician the patient's chart with the message requesting a refill attached, along with the information in procedure step two as listed above.

Purpose: To have the patient's chart as reference and provide the physician with the information needed to determine if the medication requested should be refilled.

5 Note the comments that the physician writes in the chart. If the prescription is written or a refill is approved, call the patient's pharmacy and ask to speak to a member of the pharmacy staff.

6 Ask the pharmacy staff member to repeat the prescription back to you.

Purpose: To verify that the pharmacy staff member took the prescription down accurately.

7 Note the date and time that the prescription was called to the pharmacy in the chart.

Purpose: To provide a permanent record of the medication being called to the pharmacy, along with the correct dosage amounts and frequency of doses.

8 Call the patient to notify him or her that the prescription has been called in. Provide any information regarding the prescription doses, frequency, etc. that is requested by the physician. Tell the patient when to return to the office, if necessary. Ask the patient to write this information down.

Purpose: To inform the patient as to the dosage and frequency, so that if an error is made by the pharmacy, the patient will notice a discrepancy and the error can be corrected prior to taking any dosages of the medication.

---

assistant is usually the person who calls the patient with the results and further instructions from the physician. If the patient then has any questions about the test results, he or she must then be referred to the physician. The medical assistant will need good communication skills to relay information such as this without crossing the lines of practicing medicine without a license. HIV test results should never be given on the telephone, and the physician should always inform the patient when a HIV test returns as being positive.

Patients who call the office for results of tests must be appropriately identified before the results are given. Some offices use a special code that is written in the chart, and knowledge of this code or password gives the person access to the information. Make sure the right individual is on the line before offering test results. Especially be careful in situations in which the family includes a "Senior" and "Junior." If the medical assistant calls and asks for Robert Smith, the elder Mr. Smith may answer, whereas the younger Mr. Smith is the one who came to the office for tests. Awkward situations can be created when the office staff do not accurately identify the patient.

Requests for Information From Third Parties

The patient must give written permission before any member of the physician's staff can give information to third-party callers. This includes insurance companies, attorneys, relatives, neighbors, employers, and any other third party.

Complaints About Care or Fees

A medical assistant may be able to offer a satisfactory explanation to a patient who complains about the care he or she received or the fee charged. If a patient seems angry, offer to pull the chart, research the problem, and if needed, discuss it with the physician. Four magic words often calm the angry patient: "Let me help you." This reassures the patient that someone is willing to talk about the problem. However, if you are unable to appease the patient easily, the physician or office manager may prefer to talk directly to the patient.

Calls From the Physician's Family and Friends

Personal calls to the physician from family members or friends are handled in accordance with instructions from the physician. If the physician does not wish to take the calls, the medical assistant must tactfully tell the caller that the physician cannot be disturbed at that time.

Calls From Staff Members' Family and Friends

The telephone lines should never be burdened with an excess of personal calls to the staff. A call is necessary in emergencies, but staff members should never monopolize the telephone for personal business and conversations. Emergency calls could be coming through, and the lines must be clear. Keep these calls to an absolute minimum.

Handling Difficult Calls

Angry Callers

No matter how efficient you are on the telephone or how well liked your employer may be, sooner or later there will be an angry caller on the line. There may be a legitimate reason for the anger, or the caller's irritation may have resulted from a misunderstanding. It is a real challenge to handle such calls. First, take the required action—even if it is to say that the matter will be discussed with the physician as soon as possible and the patient will be called back later. If answers are not readily available, a friendly assurance that the situation is important and that every attempt will be made to find the answer quickly will usually calm the angry feelings.

The medical assistant may find that lowering the tone of voice and volume of speech may force the angry caller to do the same in order to hear. This method does not always work, but it is usually true that when dealing with an angry person, calm promotes calm. There are always those who will misread this method and become even angrier, thinking that their complaint is not being taken seriously. Human relations are so critical when dealing with other individuals, because the more skilled the medical assistant becomes, the better able he or she is to deal with multiple types of personalities.

Always avoid getting angry in response, and try to get to the root of the real problem. Express interest and understanding, take careful notes, and follow through with the problem to the most appropriate resolution. Never

"pass the buck" by saying, "That isn't my job," or "I am not the person who filed that insurance claim." No matter whose fault the problem is, it is best to deal with it and find a solution instead of placing blame.

> ### CRITICAL THINKING APPLICATION
>
> An angry caller raises his voice at Ashlynn over an issue that happened before she began to work at the facility. She suggests that he speak with the office manager, but he refuses and continues to berate Ashlynn. What choices does she have in this situation and should she simply hang up on the patient?

Aggressive Callers

Aggressive callers insist that they receive whatever action *they* feel is necessary, and they usually insist on action immediately. Treat these callers with a calm, poised attitude, but do not allow the caller's aggression to initiate inappropriate action. Reassure the caller that the concern being shared is valid and will receive the full attention of the right person. Explain when they can expect a response from the office, and be sure to follow up that the appropriate action was taken on the call.

Unauthorized Inquiry Calls

Some individuals call the physician's office requesting information to which they are not entitled. These callers must be told politely but firmly that such information cannot be provided to them because of privacy laws. Insistent callers should be referred to the office manager or physician.

Sales Calls

Sales calls are often thought of as an interruption to the physician's busy day, but some salespersons may have important information on products, equipment, or services that the office uses regularly. Do not completely disregard salespersons, but do not allow them to monopolize time or telephone lines, either. Keep these calls quick and to the point. Most professional salespersons realize that the physician's and the staff's time is extremely valuable and will respect this. Developing a good rapport with representatives ("reps") from the companies whose products are frequently used in the practice may result in discounted prices and first news of sales and promotions. In turn, these people rarely waste the time of office personnel.

Physician Shopping

Some calls will be from prospective patients seeking information about the office and the types of illnesses or conditions that the physician treats. Consider these callers to be future patients, or as those who may refer patients to the office. Always be polite and answer questions respectfully. Remember, even if the caller does not become a patient, he or she may share his or her impressions of the practice with another prospective patient.

Complaints

For callers with a complaint, use an approach similar to the one used with angry callers. Do not make an attempt to blame, and never argue with the patient. Find the source of the problem and then present the options to the caller as to how the situation can be resolved. It is very important to remember to treat callers in the same manner that one would wish to be treated. A complaint may seem small and insignificant to the office staff, but to the patient, it could be paramount. Provide good customer service to patients, and complaints will be few and far between.

Emergency Calls

Many emergency calls require judgment on the part of the person answering the phone in the medical practice. Good judgment comes from experience and proper training by the physician in what constitutes a real emergency in each type of practice and how such calls should be handled. If the physician is not immediately available, what should the staff do? The person answering the telephone should first determine whether the call is truly urgent.

If the physician is in, the call should probably be transferred immediately. All offices should have a written plan of action for the times that the physician is not physically present in the office to handle the call. The physician and medical assistant may also jointly develop typical questions to ask the caller to determine the validity and disposition of an emergency. Some examples of questions to ask would include the following:

- At what telephone number can you be reached?
- What are the chief symptoms?
- When did they start?
- Has this happened before?
- Are you alone?
- Do you have transportation?

If the call is such that an ambulance is dispatched, the policy in most offices is to stay on the line until the paramedics or police arrive on the scene.

Triage Guidelines

In the facility with multiple employees, the physician may designate one individual as the triage nurse or assistant. Within the environment of managed care, every physician would be wise to have a written telephone protocol for handling urgent situations and emergencies. The protocol should state that the employees are bound by the written guidelines and that any giving of advice by unauthorized personnel may be grounds for dismissal.

A special sheet of instructions listing specific medical emergencies such as chest pain, heavy bleeding, fainting, seizure, and poisoning should be posted by each telephone. The phone numbers for the nearest poison control center, hospital, and ambulance should be listed. Such calls should be routed to a physician immediately. Additional instructions should include what action to take if no physician is available (e.g., sending the patient to an emergency department or calling an ambulance or 911). Most offices have some means of constant contact with the physician, whether by pager, cell phone, or another method.

Getting the Information the Physician Needs

As the medical assistant gains experience and knows the physician better, he or she will begin to have a sense of the questions that the physician will have for patients that call the facility. For instance, the physician will be interested in how long the patient has had symptoms, what makes the symptoms better or worsens them, what remedies have been tried, what has worked and not worked, and other specifics about the condition the patient is experiencing. If the patient complains of painful urination, the medical assistant will learn to ask about pain in the back, blood in the urine and/or stool, and cramping. One way to learn about questions to ask is to listen to the physician carefully as he or she questions patients about their symptoms. This will help the medical assistant to learn more about signs and symptoms, and will enable him or her to be a better assistant to the physician.

Remember to always be "patient with your patients." Those who call the medical office for help are almost never at their best. When feeling ill, people are often short-tempered and even display poor manners. Some can be verbally abusive. Care for patients as if they were family members, and they will feel care and compassion in the medical facility.

Telephones in the Millennium

Voice Mail

Voice mail is widely used in today's business offices, because it affords an around-the-clock method for receiving patient messages. Yet it can prove frustrating to many who find themselves speaking to an electronic device more often than talking with a human being. Voice mail allows the caller to hear a recorded message that may also provide information about what to do in case of an emergency. Voice mail is similar to an answering machine and will record a caller's message that can later be retrieved. Often voice mail allows special temporary greetings when the user is away from the office. Keep patients happy by answering voice mail messages promptly.

Answering Machines

Answering machines do the same job as voice mail, but a machine is attached to the telephone rather than being an integral part of the office phone system. With the inexpensive cost of voice mail, most businesses have retired their answering machines and have chosen more modern methods of message-taking.

Answering Services

Because a physician's telephone is an all-important tool of the practice, there must be someone to answer it at all times—day and night, weekends and holidays. This presents no problem during weekdays, but nights and weekends require special attention. Most physicians subscribe to telephone answering services that provide round-the-clock coverage. Answering services normally provide an operator (rather than a recording device) to answer the phones, and this is often preferred over standard voice mail. There are two types of operator-answered services. With the first type, physician-subscribers leave messages with, or obtain patients' messages from, a service whose number appears in the local telephone directory after the physician's number, with a notation to call the second number after hours. This form of service is somewhat inconvenient for the patient but is far better than no coverage at all. In the second type, the answering service has a direct connection with the office telephone. When the telephone rings in the physician's office or at home, it also signals on the switchboard of the answering service. As long as the telephone is ringing, it will continue to signal at the answering service. If no one answers within a certain agreed-on number of rings, the answering service operator takes the call. This method provides continuous live telephone coverage.

Even during the day, such an answering service can function effectively. There may be times when the staff are assisting the physician and not available to answer the telephone. Not answering the telephone is extremely poor policy, so if the office has an agreement with the answering service, its operators will accept calls in such situations. With this direct-wire answering method, the operator answers the telephone in the same manner as the regular staff.

The answering service will greatly appreciate receiving a call every day from a member of the physician's staff before leaving the office with information as to where the physician will be during the evening or other special messages. The next morning, a staff member should call the service and ask for any messages they may have taken. Usually there will be messages from patients who called after office hours but whose calls were not urgent enough to merit an emergency call to the physician. An answering service can act as a buffer for the physician and help eliminate too frequent, unnecessary calls during the late evening or night hours.

Automatic Call Routing

In automatic call routing, a call is answered by an automated operator's message that presents a list of options, such as "If you are calling about your account, press 1; to make an appointment, press 2;" and so forth. The impersonal nature of automation does not lend itself well to answering the telephone in a private physician's office, but the medical assistant will encounter it frequently when placing outgoing calls.

Call Forwarding

Call forwarding allows the user to forward calls to another designated number, such as a cellular phone. Usually a code is entered, then the phone number to which the calls should be forwarded. This keeps the user from missing important calls when away from the main telephone.

Caller ID

Caller ID allows the user to see who is calling before picking up the handset to answer the phone. The caller's phone number and name appear on a screen, and the user can decide whether to take the call. If the user subscribes to call-waiting services, another benefit called *call-waiting caller ID* is often available. Call-waiting caller ID allows the user to see who is calling even when the user is already on the phone.

Cellular Phones

Considered a luxury item only 10 years ago, cellular (or cell) phones have become commonplace in today's world (Figure 9-6). Many people no longer have a home phone because of the expense of having two phones, and the cell phone is usually the better buy for the money. Several of the more popular cell phone companies offer free long-distance calls in the United States and may provide users free night and weekend minutes as a bonus. Some of today's advanced cell phones will even allow the user to access the Internet through the telephone, and the user can check email.

Pagers

The popularity of pagers has dwindled somewhat with the growth of cell phones. However, pagers are quite useful in reaching individuals to notify them that they are needed quickly. Physicians often carry pagers with them at all times.

Fax Machines

A fax machine can be a great time and labor saver in conveying patient information from physician to physician or from physician to hospital. It allows its user to send and receive copies of printed documents over telephone lines to other facilities that have fax machines (Figure 9-7). Most offices find this machine indispensable.

CELL PHONE RULES OF ETIQUETTE

1. *Hang Up and Drive:* Take care when using the phone and driving. It is best to pull over and talk on the phone instead of trying to manipulate the car and carry on a conversation.
2. *Turn Off the Phone at the Right Time:* Never leave the phone on during meetings or at public events like movies and formal dinners.
3. *Respect Personal Space:* Most people do not want to hear personal or business conversations while they are in line for a movie or eating dinner. Step away when speaking on the cell phone in public.
4. *The Phone Is Not a Human:* Nothing is more rude than having dinner with a friend and taking a casual call on the cell phone. Pay attention to the human and turn the phone off until later.
5. *Keep it Charged:* It is very frustrating to speak to someone on a cell phone who can not hear. Keeping the phone charged will cause less periods of static and more clarity when in use.

FIGURE 9-6 Etiquette rules for cellular phones.

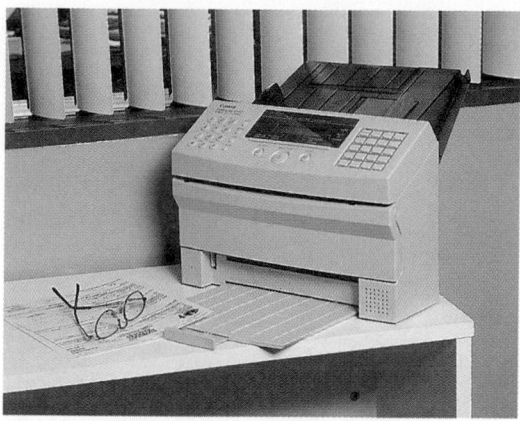

FIGURE 9-7 Fax machines allow the transfer of written data from one place to another with the simple dial of a telephone number.

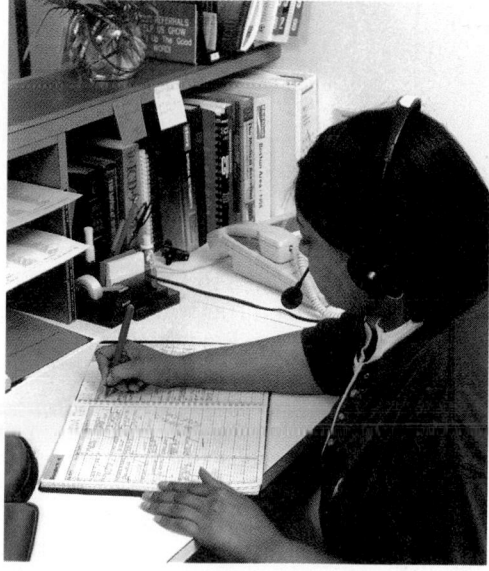

FIGURE 9-8 Using a headset helps the medical assistant keep hands free while using the telephone and is better ergonomically.

Unless precautions are taken to ensure security of information arriving by fax, there is the danger of loss of confidentiality. When sending sensitive material, it is wise to telephone ahead to alert the receiver that this information will be arriving so that the appropriate person will be on hand to receive it.

Headsets

In today's world of multitasking, the headset helps a medical assistant to keep hands free while speaking on the phone. A popular headset is a very lightweight plastic earphone and microphone combination that allows the wearer to move about the room and to have the hands free (Figure 9-8). One brand name is StarSet. Originally designed for astronauts, it weighs less than 1 ounce and is worn behind the ear or clipped to the wearer's glasses. The headset can be equipped with a cord up to 10 feet long for easy mobility. It also has an optional quick-disconnect feature that allows the user to separate the headset even during a call without breaking the connection.

Using Long Distance and Special Services

Long-distance calls are simple to place, usually inexpensive, and efficient. When information is needed in a hurry, it is much more expedient to telephone rather than wait for an exchange of letters. Before placing a long-distance call, have the correct number ready. This number often may be obtained from a letterhead or from other records. If you do not have the number, you may obtain directory assistance by dialing the area code of the party you are calling, followed by 555-1212. In some areas you must dial 1 before the area code. Directory assistance is now an automated service in many regions, and you will be asked for the name of the city and the person you are calling. There is often a charge for using directory assistance.

One alternative to directory assistance is using the Internet to find phone numbers. A search for the business or physician the medical assistant is looking for may yield the information needed. There are also Internet services that allow the user to call long distance, and sometimes even internationally, through the computer with absolutely no long-distance charges.

Time Zones

The continental United States is divided into four standard time zones: Pacific, Mountain, Central, and Eastern

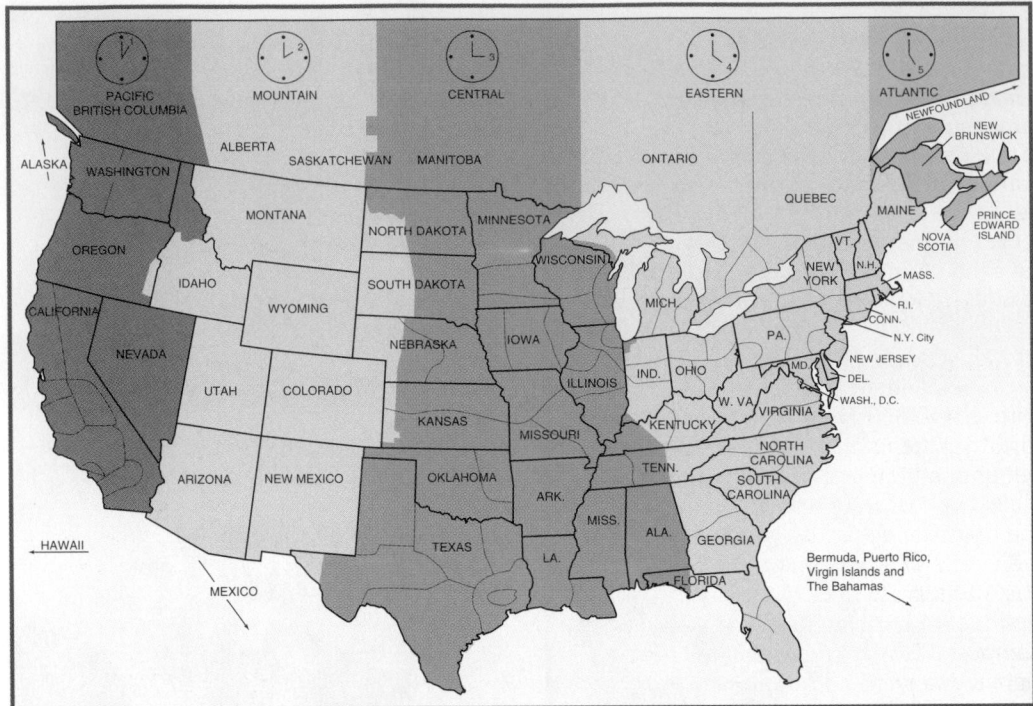

FIGURE 9-9   Time zones across the United States.

(Figure 9-9). When it is noon Pacific time, it is 3 PM Eastern time. When calling from San Francisco to New York, plan to make the call no later than 2 PM if the call is to a business or professional office. When it is 2 PM on the West Coast, it is 5 PM on the East Coast. Only Arizona, Hawaii, and a part of Indiana do not observe Daylight Saving Time.

International Service

International Direct Distance Dialing (IDDD) is available in many areas. International dialing codes are the same for all companies offering IDDD. Depending on your long-distance company, additional numbers or codes may preface the international access, country, and city codes. IDDD is still not available in all areas. If it is available, you may place international station-to-station calls by dialing in sequence:

1. International code 011
2. Country code
3. City code
4. Local telephone number
5. The pound sign (#) button if your telephone is Touch-Tone

After dialing any international code, allow at least 45 seconds for the ringing to start.

Wrong Numbers

One slip in direct distance dialing can mean a call to Los Angeles or New York instead of Dallas. If you reach a wrong long-distance number, be sure to obtain the name of the city and state that was called. Report this information promptly to the local operator, so the facility will

not be charged for the call. If you are cut off before terminating a call, report this as well. The operator will either reconnect the call or make an adjustment of the charge.

Conference Calls

Conference telephone service is of great value to the medical profession in notifying and explaining to a family how a patient is progressing. It has exceptional value in family conferences, at which a quick decision by the entire family regarding a patient's condition is required.

This service can connect from 3 to 14 points for a two-way conference in which each person can hear or talk to all others participating. Conference calls may be local or long distance. Charges are added for the number of places connected, the mileage, and the length of the conversation.

Conference calls can be set up by a normal long-distance operator or through conference call services. To schedule a call, contact either an operator or the calling service and relay the pertinent information about time, date, and the individuals who are to be included in the call. Many businesses have conference call capabilities on their phone or computer systems. Notify everyone participating in the call of the time, date, number to call, and subjects to discuss. If prior arrangements are made with all parties, there is a better chance of reaching everyone and having a successful conference.

Operator-Assisted Calls and Services

Operator-assisted calls include calls such as:
- Person-to-person
- Billing to a third party
- Collect calls

- Requests for time and charges
- Certain calls placed from hotels
- Credit for wrong numbers
- Conference calls
- Some international calls

There is an initial charge and a service charge for operator-assisted calls provided through most phone service providers.

Office Telephone Equipment Needs

Number and Placement of Telephones

Familiarity with a multiple-line telephone system is a must for medical assistants. Few healthcare facilities can get along with just one telephone line. Two incoming lines along with a private outgoing line with a separate number for the physician's exclusive use is the minimum recommended.

One medical assistant can handle no more than two incoming lines, so the addition of more lines may also involve additional staffing (Figure 9-10). If there is a staff member assigned solely to dealing with insurance and billing, a separate line and listing in the telephone directory for this service may considerably lessen the load on the main incoming lines.

Telephones should be placed where they are accessible but private. Rather than placing telephones in the examining rooms, many practices have a wall telephone placed near a stand-up desktop outside the examining room.

Some facilities also place a telephone in the reception room for the convenience of patients and to prevent their asking to use the facility's phones. However, recent trends suggest that a separate telephone line with a limited calling area for the convenience of patients who need to call out may be preferable. This telephone should not be in the reception room but in an area available to patients on request. It should be placed low enough for use by patients in wheelchairs. Wherever possible, other telephones should be placed on the wall to conserve desk space.

Equipment Selection

Selection of telephone equipment and services offers many options. The *six-button key set*, with several incoming lines, an intercom line, and a hold button, has been the standard business phone for decades. It is still being used in many offices. Lights within the buttons flash slowly for incoming calls and blink rapidly to remind of calls being held; a steady light indicates that the line is in use.

A popular modern system is the two-line speaker phone that has distinctive ringing and flashing indicators that reveal which line is receiving a call. It also has other features:

- Last number redial
- Volume control on the receiver, ringer, and speaker
- Memory for frequently dialed numbers
- Intercom paging

Another available feature, *ring back on hold*, allows the caller who dials a busy number to place it on hold. When the called line is free, the connection is completed and the caller is reminded.

Larger facilities tend to select small switchboard-type equipment. One system can start with as few as 2 lines and 6 extensions and expand to a maximum of 8 outside lines and 24 extensions.

Using a Telephone Directory

The primary purpose of the telephone directory, of course, is to provide lists of those who have telephones, their telephone numbers, and, in most cases, their addresses. Additionally, the directory is an aid in checking the spelling of names and in locating certain types of businesses through the yellow pages. Some directories are color coded, with residence listings on white pages, business numbers on pink pages, and business by categories and advertisements on yellow pages. Often, federal, state, county, and city government listings are included as blue pages. Directories are usually organized into three sections:

- Introductory pages
- Alphabetical pages (white pages)
- Yellow pages

The introductory pages are sometimes entirely overlooked by subscribers. This section precedes the white alphabetical pages and provides basic information concerning the telephone services in the area, including the following:

- Emergency services (fire, police, ambulance, and highway patrol)
- Service calls
- Dialing instructions for local and long-distance calls
- Area codes for some cities

The introductory pages may also include the following:

- A survival guide for newcomers to the community
- Community service numbers
- Prefix locations
- Rates
- International calling information
- Time zones

Government Listings

Some directories include ZIP code maps for the local area. Take a few moments to become familiar with the local directory; then use it frequently for getting information fast.

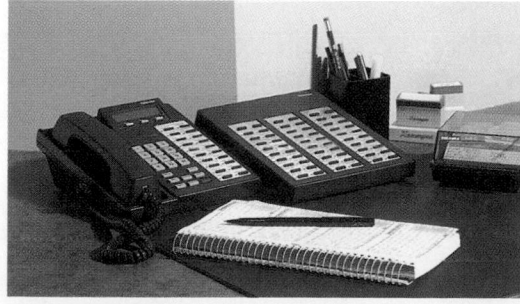

FIGURE 9-10 Multiline telephones allow numerous calls to come into the office at once. Each call deserves the same kind of attention and care from the medical assistant.

The white pages are an alphabetical listing of telephone subscribers with their telephone numbers and, in most cases, their addresses.

The yellow pages directory, sometimes published separately, contains listings for businesses arranged by the product or services they sell. Physicians are listed alphabetically, usually under the heading *Physicians and Surgeons*, and have the option of another listing by type of practice.

In some metropolitan areas, a street address telephone directory is published that is arranged by street address, followed by the name and telephone number of the person or business at that address.

Organizing a Personal Phone Directory

Organize telephone numbers in a tabbed 3- × 5-inch desktop file or a rotary file. Binders with clear sheet protectors also work well as personal phone directories. Emergency numbers might be typed on a colored card or flagged with a color tab. A personal directory of telephone numbers should include all the numbers that are frequently called.

Closing Comments

A telephone can be a tool to build a physician's practice, or one to break it apart. Medical assistants must become proficient in good telephone technique and must ensure that the caller hears compassion and patience in the voice of the medical assistant, even over the phone. A medical assistant must convey a genuine sense of caring for the patients that call the facility, just as if they were standing in the office face-to-face. By keeping this in mind, the medical assistant will play a major role in patient satisfaction, and the patients will find their medical care a pleasant process.

Patient Education

Today's telephone systems allow physicians to educate patients while they are on hold; recordings may be played that offer health information on subjects from *A* to *Z*. These messages can be professionally recorded or custom designed by the physician and staff. Special events may be announced, with the option to press a certain number for more information about the event.

Some phone directories offer listings of health information in the introductory pages. A patient may call a main number and then press a second number to reach the subject of his or her choice. Such features help to address the needs of today's more information-oriented consumers of health care, who have an interest in healthy lifestyles and in gaining useful information immediately.

Legal and Ethical Issues

The guidelines for medical confidentiality apply equally to telephone conversations, and care must be taken to ensure that no one overhears sensitive information. Use discretion when mentioning the name of a caller or a patient.

Placing and receiving personal phone calls should be avoided during work hours. This is a facet of professional behavior for the medical assistant and will probably be addressed in the office's employee procedures manual. The telephone is a business line and should be reserved for calls from patients or others conducting business with the office. The medical assistant should encourage friends and family to call him or her at home, so that all patient calls may get through to the office.

Telephone and message records may be brought into court as evidence, so be sure that all messages are complete and legible. Most offices should keep these records for at least the same amount of time as the statute of limitations in their state.

SUMMARY OF SCENARIO

Ashlynn is quickly becoming a part of the team at Dr. Frank's office and developing into a well-liked asset to the staff. She has learned to slow down when speaking on the phone and to adjust her volume and pitch, depending on the patient with whom she is speaking. Although she tends to be quite talkative, she is balancing just the right amount of friendly chat with the business at hand. Dr. Frank is very pleased with her performance.

Ashlynn takes care when she speaks to patients and others on the phone so that she does not breach confidentiality in any way. She has become comfortable with the way she is to answer the telephone. The pace of her speech and the wording are now a habit. Ashlynn is determined to maintain a professional relationship with all of the people related to her work environment. She is adept now at handling calls from angry patients and can maintain control with even the most aggressive callers. She shows much promise for a long and rewarding career in the medical field and is satisfied with the track her career is on at the present time. As she continues to settle into her position, she looks forward to learning more about efficiency and time management. Her good attitude and desire to learn will only enhance her performance at work and make her an employee worth promoting and of great value in the facility.

SUMMARY OF LEARNING OBJECTIVES

■ Incoming calls to a physician's office come from a wide variety of sources. Established or new patients may be calling to set appointments. Insurance companies may be seeking information about a claim. Hospitals, nursing facilities, or other healthcare units may need to report the progress of a patient. Laboratory results may be coming in for a patient who is very ill. Routine sales calls and telemarketing calls also come to the office, in addition to personal calls to the physician and staff members.

■ A pleasing telephone voice is one that is friendly and conveys a favorable impression of the physician's practice. Enunciate words and pronounce them clearly and distinctly. Vary the pitch of your voice, avoiding a monotonous or droning manner. Always be courteous and use tact.

■ The telephone handset should be held around the middle of the shaft, with the mouthpiece situated approximately 1 inch from the lips, in front of the teeth. Talk directly into the handset so the caller can clearly hear what is being said. Do not hold the mouthpiece beneath the chin, because the voice may not be heard clearly. Do not lean the head downward to hold the phone between the ear and the shoulder to avoid sore muscles and neck problems.

■ It is vital to be courteous to patients and other callers. First impressions are important, and a medical assistant's phone manner sets the tone for the caller's perception of the physician's practice. Customer service is important to today's physician, because many patients have choices among their healthcare providers as to which physician provides their care, and the attitude of staff members may play a large part in such a decision. Good customer care to patients means that they will not only continue to see the provider, but they will also refer other patients to the physician. This is one of the best ways to help a practice grow.

■ The physician's time is valuable but is also centered around his or her patients. It would be physically impossible for the physician to take all of the calls from those who wished to talk each day. Therefore the medical assistant must screen the physician's calls and make decisions about which ones should be put through to the physician. The medical assistant should offer to take a message and attempt to find out exactly what the caller's needs are and how they can be resolved. The patient should not feel that the physician is totally inaccessible, but must also understand that the patient in the office must have his or her full attention.

■ Seven distinct items are needed when taking a phone message, including the name of the person to whom the call should be directed and the name of the person calling. The caller's telephone number must be noted as well as the reason for the call. The medical assistant should describe the action to be taken. The date and time of the call should always be noted, as well as the initials of the person taking the call, so that if there is any question, that person can be identified and asked.

■ Never return anger when a caller is angry. Remain calm and speak in tones that are perhaps slightly quieter than those of the caller. This often prompts the caller to lower his or her tone of voice. Offer to help the angry person, and ask questions to gain control of the conversation, moving it toward solution. Do not argue with angry callers.

■ Callers who have a complaint should be handled in a similar way as angry callers. Remain calm and offer to help. Take a serious interest in what the caller has to say. Let the caller know that his or her concerns are important to the staff and the physician. Find the source of the problem and determine exactly what the caller wants or expects toward its resolution. Always follow up with complaints and be sure that they were resolved as much to the caller's satisfaction as possible.

■ Several questions should be asked when an emergency call comes to the medical office. First, obtain a phone number at which the caller can be reached in case there is a sudden disconnection. Ask about the chief symptoms and when they started. Find out if the patient has had similar symptoms in the past and what happened in that situation. Determine whether the patient is alone, has transportation, or needs an ambulance dispatched to the location. In cases of severe emergencies, do not hang up the phone until the ambulance or police arrive.

■ The introductory pages of the telephone book contain several sections of useful information, such as area codes, emergency service information, long-distance calling information, time zones, government listings, and community service numbers. It may be helpful to tear these pages out and place them in clear sheet protectors, then add them to a binder for easy reference.

KEY INTERNET WEBSITES

- The Dartnell Corporation
  For active weblinks to each website visit
  http://evolve.elsevier.com/Kinn/

CHAPTER 10

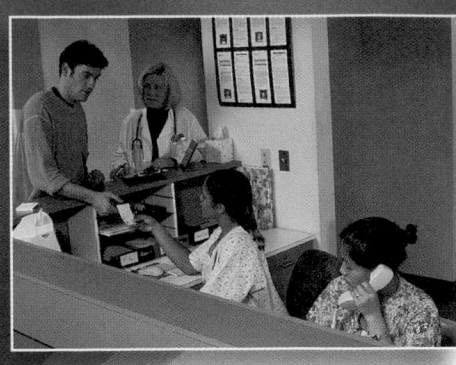

Scenario

Ramona West is the medical assistant in charge of scheduling appointments for Dr. Charlotte Brown. Ramona is an extremely organized person who thinks quickly and creatively. One of her professional goals is to ensure that the office stays on schedule throughout each day and that patient wait time is kept to an absolute minimum. She is fortunate that Dr. Brown is cooperative and time oriented, so they work well together to reach this common goal.

Ramona usually arrives at work at least 15 minutes early to begin her preparations for the day. She pulls patient charts each evening for the next day, so that they are easily accessible each morning. Throughout the course of her duties, she pays particular attention to the patients that arrive in the office. Ramona greets each patient by name. She often makes a short note in the patient chart about what events are happening in the life of each patient. With a quick glance, she remembers that a certain patient has a new granddaughter, or another patient just returned from a weeklong Caribbean cruise. Ramona uses this information to carry on a brief but cordial conversation with the patient. Patients appreciate that she goes the extra mile to remember something about them, and this promotes excellent patient relations.

Ramona leaves a little time in the morning and afternoon for emergency appointments. She calls to confirm patient appointments in advance or emails them, and this increases her show rate. Her friendly and caring attitude make her a favorite among the patients, and Dr. Brown is pleased with the relationship-building skills that Ramona has developed.

Scheduling Appointments

National Curriculum Competencies

ADMINISTRATIVE COMPETENCIES

1a. Schedule and manage appointments
1b. Schedule inpatient and outpatient admissions and procedures

TRANSDISCIPLINARY COMPETENCIES

1b. Recognize and respond to verbal communication
1d. Demonstrate telephone techniques
2d. Document appropriately
3a. Explain general office policies
3b. Instruct individuals according to their needs
4a. Utilize computer software to maintain office systems

Vocabulary

disruption An unexpected event that throws a plan into disorder; an interruption that prevents a system or process from continuing as usual or as expected.

established patients Patients who are returning to the office who have previously been seen by the physician.

expediency A means of achieving a particular end, as in a situation requiring haste or caution.

integral Essential; being an indispensable part of a whole.

interaction A two-way communication; mutual or reciprocal action or influence.

intermittent Coming and going at intervals; not continuous.

interval Space of time between events.

matrix Something in which a thing originates, develops, takes shape, or is contained; a base on which to build.

no-show A person who fails to keep an appointment without giving advance notice.

prerequisite Something that is necessary to an end or to carry out a function.

proficiency Competency as a result of training or practice.

socioeconomic Relating to a combination of social and economic factors.

triage Process of evaluating the urgency of medical need and prioritizing treatment.

The most valuable asset within a medical practice is the physician's time. The person responsible for scheduling this time must understand the practice, be familiar with the working habits of the physicians, and have clear guidelines for time management within the practice.

Appointment scheduling is the process that determines which patients will be seen by the physician, the dates and times of appointments, and how much time will be allotted to each patient based on his or her complaint, as well as the physician's availability. Time management involves the realization that there will always be unforeseen interruptions and delays. Most providers of medical care find that efficient scheduling of appointments is one of the most important factors in the success of the practice. There are many approaches to scheduling, and each facility must find what suits it best.

Guidelines for Appointment Scheduling

One of the most common complaints that patients have is the amount of money they pay for such short visits with the physician. A patient may say, "I only saw the doctor for 5 minutes and could not even remember all the questions I wanted to ask!" The patient must feel confident that the physician took enough time to understand his or her concerns. Well-planned scheduling and adherence to that schedule will allow the physician to do more than run in and out of examination rooms, leaving little time for the patient to talk with the physician.

Some medical offices stick to a strict schedule, with little room for maneuvering, whereas many are more flexible in scheduling to meet the needs of the patients and the providers. The key to good scheduling is organization and teamwork in the office. Without these, even the best-planned schedule will not succeed.

The person who is scheduling appointments must learn the physician's habits and desires. If the physician suggests scheduling patients every 15 minutes but always spends 20 to 25 minutes with a patient, the schedule must be adjusted. Talk with the physician and/or office manager and compromise so that the schedule is a workable one. Some physicians need prompting to end the patient visit and move to the next patient. The medical assistant who is assisting in the examination room can help the physician remain on schedule.

Guides for Scheduling

The scheduling system must be individualized to each specific practice. The following guidelines are general and can be applied to any practice, whether paper-based or computer-based. Three items must be considered when scheduling—patient need, physician preference and habits, and available facilities.

Patient Need

A major consideration in determining office hours and appointment times is the **socioeconomic** status of the area being served. The office staff should answer the following questions:

- Is the office located in a busy metropolitan area or a rural agricultural community?
- Are the patients young, middle-aged, or retirement age?
- Is the area more industrial or residential?
- What type of patients are seen?
- Are evening and weekend appointments essential for most of the patients served?

After these items are considered, the scheduler must allot time based on the patient needs for each individual office visit. These needs can be assessed by determining:

- What is the purpose of this visit?
- What is the age of the patient?
- Will the patient require the physician's time for the entire visit, or will another staff member perform all or part of the service?
- Is the patient a young mother who prefers to schedule her appointments while her children are at school?
- Does the patient object to traveling after dark?
- Is the patient a day worker who cannot take time off?
- Is the patient a child whose parents are both working during the day?

The office should make every attempt to meet the patient's needs, while balancing the physician's preferences and available facilities.

Physician Preferences and Habits

The preferences and habits of the physicians in the practice must be considered before a scheduling plan can be established and followed. Consider the following:

- Does the physician become restless if the reception room is not packed with waiting patients?
- Does the physician worry if even one patient is kept waiting?
- Is the physician methodical and careful about being in the facility when patient appointments are scheduled to begin?
- Is the physician habitually late?
- Does the physician move easily from one patient to another?
- Does the physician require a "break time" between a few patients?
- Would the physician rather see fewer patients and spend more time with each one, or schedule more patients each day?

All of these preferences and habits become an **integral** part of the scheduling process (Figure 10-1). Keep in mind that the physician cannot spend every moment of the day with patients. There are telephone calls to make and receive, reports to examine and dictate, meetings to attend, mail to answer, and many other business items that require the physician's attention. An experienced staff can handle many—but not all—of these tasks.

CRITICAL THINKING APPLICATION

Ramona has noticed that Dr. Brown is taking a little longer with patients than normal and that she is running consistently behind schedule by about 5 to 15 minutes. How can she help to rectify this situation?

Discuss ways of approaching the physician when he or she is the cause of the delays in the schedule. What opening remarks can the medical assistant use to start the discussion in a positive way?

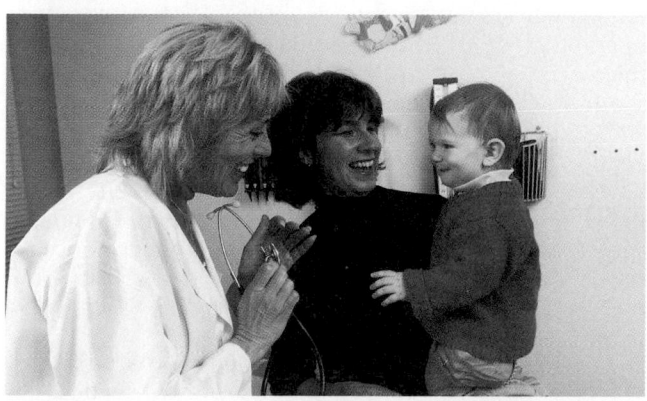

FIGURE 10-1 The habits and preferences of the physician must be considered when scheduling appointments for patients.

Available Facilities

There is no point in getting a patient into the office at a time when no facilities are available for the services needed. For example, suppose that in a two-physician office there is only one room that can be used for minor surgery. You would not schedule two patients requiring minor surgery for the same time block even though both doctors could be available. If there is only one electrocardiograph, you would not book two electrocardiograms at the same time. As the medical assistant gains **proficiency** in scheduling, patient needs will be paired with the available facilities, according to the physician's preference.

Selecting the Method of Appointment Scheduling

The two most common methods of appointment scheduling are using an appointment book and computer-based scheduling. There are advantages and disadvantages with each, and the physician's office should weigh the benefits and choose the method that best suits the physician and the staff.

Appointment Books

Office suppliers carry a variety of appointment book styles. There are certain basic features to consider when choosing an appointment book:

- The size should conform to the desk space available.
- It should be large enough to accommodate the practice.
- It should open flat for easy writing and reference.
- It should allow space for writing when, who, and why.

Some appointment books show an entire week at a glance, and many are color coded, with a special color for each day of the week (Figure 10-2). This is very helpful when the physician asks the patient to return, for instance, in 2 weeks. If Wednesdays are colored yellow, the medical assistant can flip quickly to the correct day and schedule the appointment. Multiple columns may be available to correspond with the number of doctors in a group practice, and the time can be divided according to their preferences.

Computer Scheduling

The computer has replaced the appointment book in many practices. Software for appointment scheduling ranges from relatively simple programs that merely display available and scheduled times to more sophisticated systems. Many programs can display such information as the length and type of appointment required and day or time preferences. The computer can then select the best appointment time based on the information entered into the computer.

The computer can also be used to keep track of future appointments. For example, when a patient calls and inquires about an appointment, the system can search

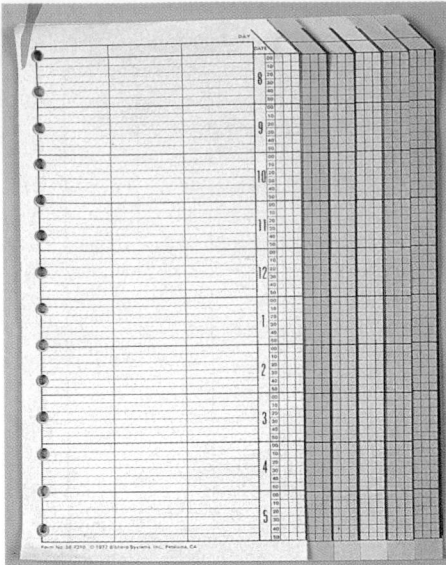

FIGURE 10-2   Color-coded appointment book pages help a medical assistant to flip to the right day of the right week quickly. Appointments for multiple physicians can be color-coded in the book.

by his or her name to find the time and date. Printouts can also run to show the physician's daily schedule, including the patients' names and telephone numbers and the reason for the visit. Multiple copies of these schedules can be made, according to the needs of the practice.

One advantage of computer scheduling is that more than one person can access the system at one time, and the information is available to all operators. The medical assistant can generate a hard copy of the next day's appointments before leaving each evening. In some facilities, employees still maintain an appointment book as a backup to computer scheduling.

Self-Scheduling

The future of appointment scheduling includes *self-scheduling*, which is a method by which a patient can log on to the Internet and view a facility's schedule, then schedule his or her own appointment (Figure 10-3). Software is available that will allow the patient to self-schedule through secure links to the physician's appointment book. The software or internet site for the physician's office should give the patient guidelines as to the amount of time needed for certain appointments, or should only allow a certain length of time to be self-scheduled, such as 15 minutes. These systems will reduce calls to the office and are available to the patient 24 hours a day. Some of these systems will also send an automatic email reminder to the patient the day before the appointment, requesting a reply to confirm. These systems are less frustrating to patients, who do not have to wait on hold to speak to the person who does scheduling for the office. Appointments that are more lengthy or complicated should be scheduled through the office staff.

Advance Preparation

Having chosen an appropriate method of appointment setting, some advance preparation should be done. This is sometimes called *establishing the* **matrix** (Procedure 10-1). Block off time slots when the physician is routinely not available to see patients, such as days off, holidays, time for hospital rounds, and meetings. In the space in which a patient's name would normally be placed, note the reason the time is blocked off. Always try to account for every time period in each day. The medical assistant should also make a note of social or family engagements to help the physician remember these obligations. Because time is a valuable commodity for the physician and the office staff, the schedule is the tool that assists in making certain that the day runs smoothly.

Types of Appointment Scheduling

Different types of appointment scheduling are used to meet the various needs of the medical facility, the providers, and the patients served. Several methods are discussed next. Some offices use a combination of methods to create the right mix of activity during the day.

Open Office Hours

Few healthcare facilities in metropolitan areas have open office hours with no scheduled appointments, but this system is still found in some rural areas, where the way of life is governed not so much by the clock as by the needs of the people in the area. Many freestanding emergency clinics also offer open office hours. With open office hours, the facility is open at given hours of the day or evening, and the patients are "scheduled" by the physician by mentioning to the patient that he or she should return "in a couple of weeks" for follow-up. At **intermittent** times the patients come in, knowing in advance they will be seen in the order of their arrival. Physicians who use this method say that it eliminates the annoyance of broken appointments and of the office running behind schedule. The open office hours method has also been referred to as *tidal wave scheduling*.

There can be many disadvantages to open office hours. The office may already be crowded when the physician arrives, resulting in an extremely long wait for some patients. Patients may arrive in waves throughout the day,

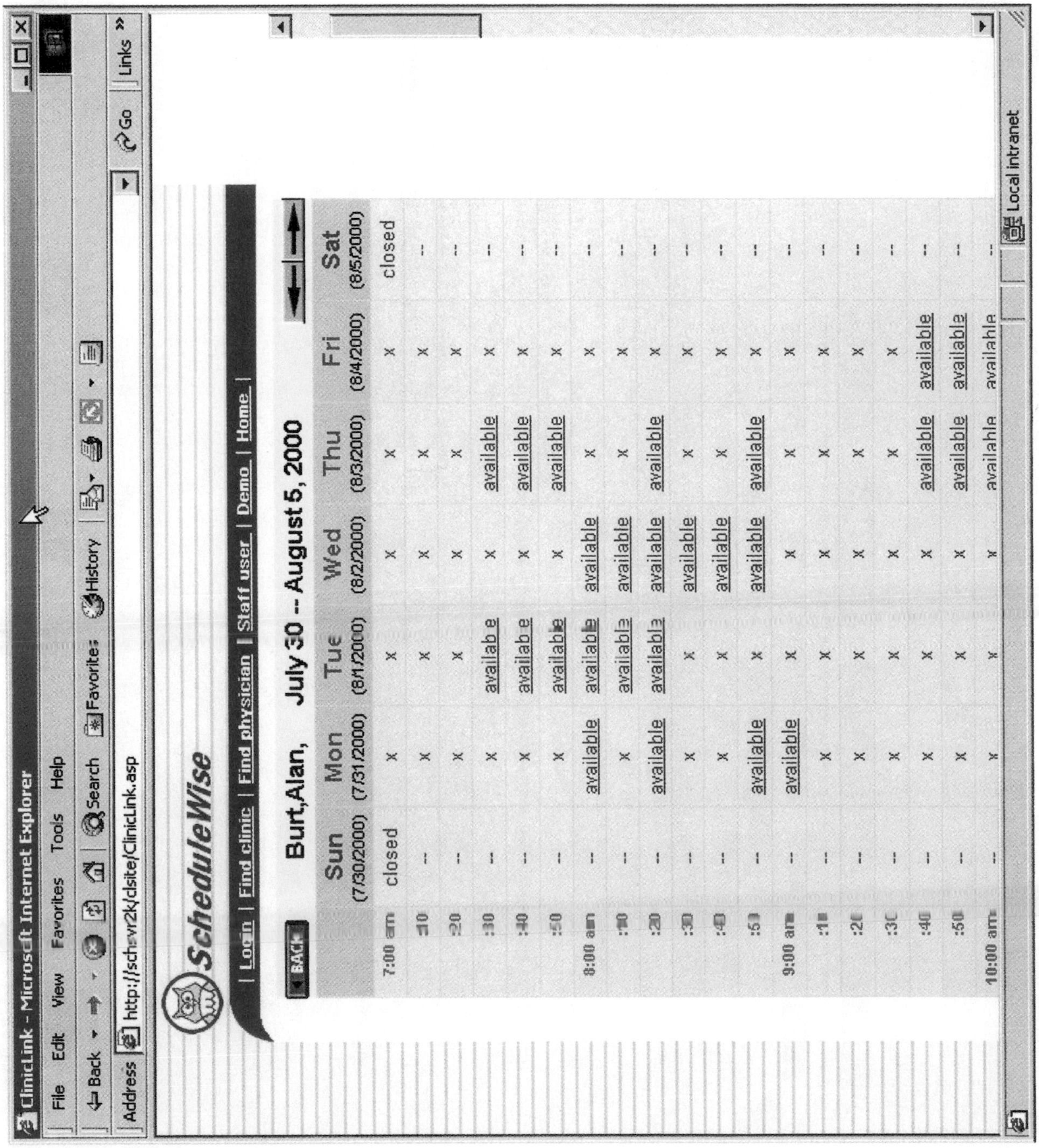

FIGURE 10-3 New computer scheduling programs allow patients to access the physician's schedule over the Internet and schedule their own appointments. *continued*

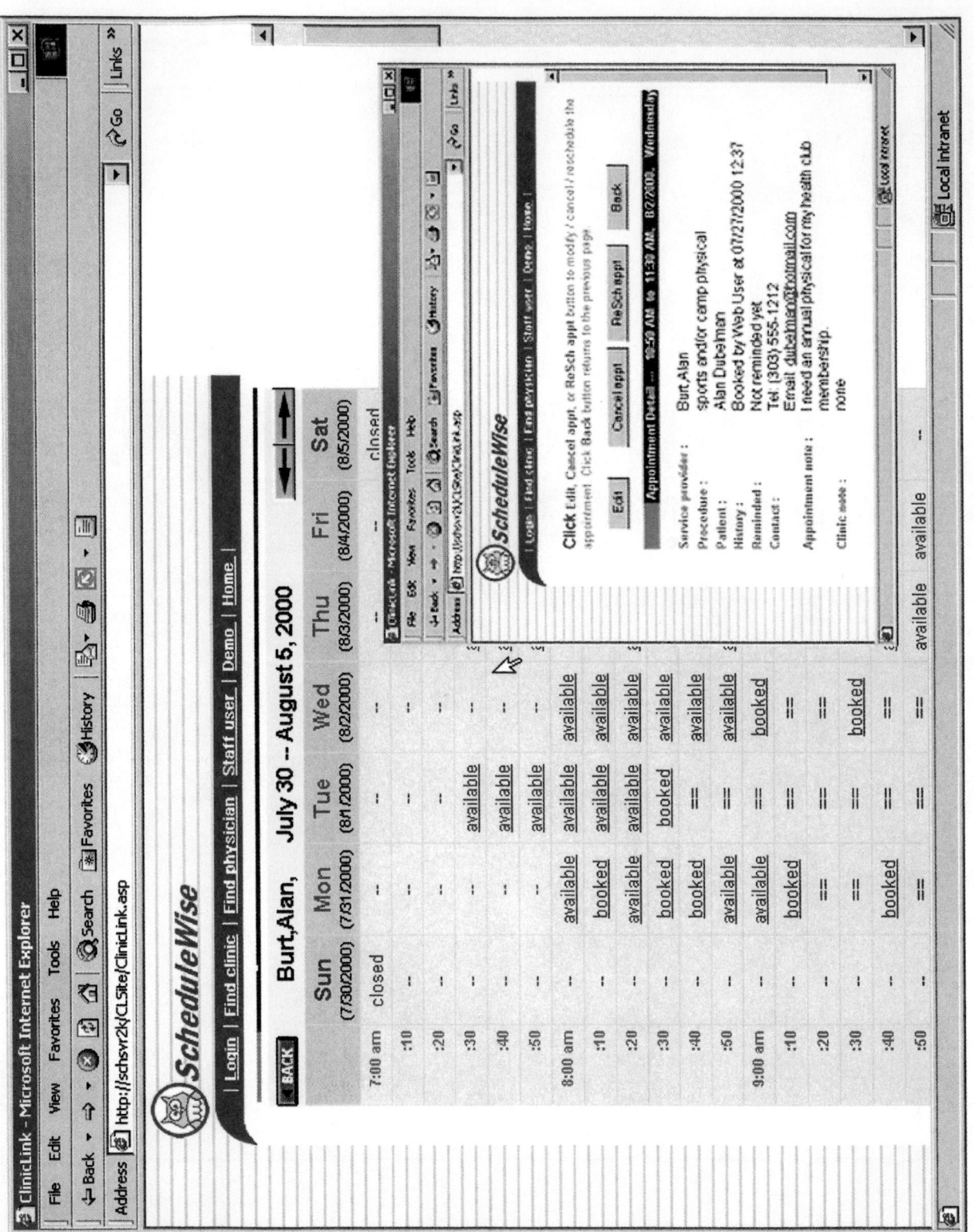

FIGURE 10-3—Cont'd For legend see previous page.

PROCEDURE 10-1

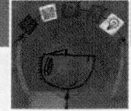

Preparing and Maintaining the Appointment Book

GOAL: To establish the matrix of the appointment page, arrange appointments for 1 day, and enter information according to office policy.

EQUIPMENT AND SUPPLIES

- Page from appointment book
- Office policy for office hours and doctors' availability
- Clerical supplies
- Calendar
- Description of patients to be scheduled

PROCEDURAL STEPS

1 Determine the hours that a physician will not be available.

Purpose: To block out those hours on the appointment page for the day.

2 Establish the matrix of the appointment page for the day.

Purpose: To leave available only those time slots that can be used for patient appointments.

3 Identify each patient's complaint.

Purpose: This information is necessary in allotting time and space for the appointment.

4 Consult guidelines to determine the length of time necessary for each patient.

5 Allot appointment time according to the complaint and facilities available.

6 Enter information in the appointment book.

Note: A telephone number must follow the patient's name. If the patient is new, add the letters *NP* (new patient) after his or her name.

7 Allow buffer time in the morning and afternoon.

Purpose: To allow the physician and staff a short rest period and catch-up time.

---

which causes parts of the day to be very busy and parts to be slow. This makes it difficult to get other office duties accomplished. Without planning, the facilities and staff can be overburdened.

Other types of practices that have open office hours include emergency centers, many of which are open 24 hours a day. Although called emergency centers, most of these facilities deal with general practice cases.

Scheduled Appointments

Studies have shown that practitioners are able to see more patients with less pressure when their appointments are scheduled. Unfortunately, the skill required for scheduling appointments is often not fully appreciated by the practitioner or office manager, resulting in the responsibility being delegated to the least qualified medical assistant. Although the skill and attitude of the assistant who manages the appointment schedule is very important, the ultimate success of the system lies in the cooperation of the physicians.

Flexible Office Hours

Most scheduling practices are carryovers from the days when expectant mothers of families with young children relied on one wage earner. Today families commonly have two working parents. As a result, many healthcare providers are turning to extended-day and flexible office hours. Staff hours are affected by these schedules, but this

flexibility works to the advantage of the employee and the employer. For instance, if a medical assistant has decided to continue his or her education, morning class hours become available if he or she agrees to work evening hours. Scheduling evening and weekend hours may increase the size of the practice because of the convenience offered to patients.

CRITICAL THINKING APPLICATION

Dr. Brown would like to implement evening appointments one night each week and open the office every other Saturday morning. She feels this will better serve her patients with children who have difficulty making daytime appointments. If this is her primary goal, should other types of patients be seen during these time slots? Why or why not?

Wave Scheduling

Many office schedules lack flexibility, and wave scheduling is an attempt to create short-term flexibility within each hour. Wave scheduling assumes that the actual time needed for all of the patients seen will average out over the course of the day. Instead of scheduling patients at each 20-minute interval, wave scheduling places three patients in the office at the same time, and they are seen in the order of their arrival. Thus, one person's late arrival will not disrupt the entire schedule.

Modified Wave Scheduling

There are several ways to modify the wave schedule. One method is to have two patients scheduled to come in at, for example, 10:00 AM, and a third at 10:30 AM. This hourly cycle is repeated throughout the day. Another application would have patients scheduled to arrive at given intervals during the first half of the hour, and none scheduled to arrive during the second half of the hour. Physicians can modify wave scheduling to best suit the clinic's needs.

Double Booking

Booking two patients to come in at the same time, both of whom are to be seen by the physician, is poor practice. Of course, if each appointment is expected to only take 5 minutes, there is no harm in telling both to come at the same time and reserving a 15-minute period for the two. This is simply one method of wave scheduling. However, if each patient requires 15 minutes, two will require 30 minutes. This must be reflected in the scheduling. It is not considered double booking if a patient comes to the office to receive a treatment by someone other than the physician, such as a patient receiving a physical therapy modality or an allergy injection.

Grouping Procedures

Another method of scheduling that appeals to many practitioners is the grouping or categorizing of procedures. For instance, an internist might reserve all morning appointments for complete physical examinations or well-baby visits. A surgeon might devote one day each week to seeing only referral patients. Obstetricians often schedule pregnant patients on different days than gynecology patients. The physician and staff can experiment with different groupings until the plan that works best for the practice eventually becomes evident. In applying a grouping system of appointments, the medical assistant may find it helpful to color-code the sections of the appointment book being reserved for designated procedures.

Advance Booking

Often appointments are made months in advance. When any appointment is made, an appointment card should be completed and given to the patient. All appointment cards should mention that patients must give 24 hours' notice if they are unable to keep the time reserved for them. Most offices have some type of confirmation procedures by which patients are called the day before to verify that they will keep the appointment.

Time Patterns

When booking appointments, a medical assistant should make it a policy to leave some open time during each day's schedule, so that if a patient calls with a special problem that is not an immediate emergency, there will be some time available to book the patient for at least a brief visit. It is also wise to keep one time slot available in the morning and afternoon specifically for emergencies. A busy physician will always be able to fill these open slots of time, and having them in the schedule will cause the least amount of **disruption** during the day. If possible, time should be set aside in the morning and afternoon for a break. Even 15 minutes will give the physician time to return calls from patients, verify prescription calls, or answer questions.

Studies have shown that in the average medical practice, Mondays and Fridays are the most hectic days of the week. Patients may have been waiting the whole weekend to call for an appointment and expect to be seen immediately on Monday. Similarly, toward the end of the week, small problems that could magnify if left unattended over the weekend may prompt the patient to be anxious to see the physician on Friday. Incorporating more buffer time on these 2 days may be worthwhile.

Patient Wait Time

Be conscious about the amount of time that the patient sits in the reception area. Ideally, the patient's name will be called to go to the examination room precisely at the scheduled appointment time (Figure 10-4). However, the scheduling has failed if the patient then waits in the back office for 30 minutes to see the physician. Make it clear to the patient whether he or she is free to leave the office when the physician has finished the examination. Some patients mistakenly wait in the room until told they are free to leave, when they could have left several minutes sooner.

If a patient has waited more than 15 minutes in the reception area, the medical assistant should briefly explain the delay and offer to reschedule the appointment. The longer patients sit and wait, the more anxious and frustrated they become. Remember, some patients are there to see the physician for test results or may be expecting a negative diagnosis. Do not make their visit more stressful by forcing them to wait for a long time.

Of course, some delays are unavoidable. The physician may be delayed as a result of unforeseen circumstances, or there could be a patient with an emergency. Occasion-

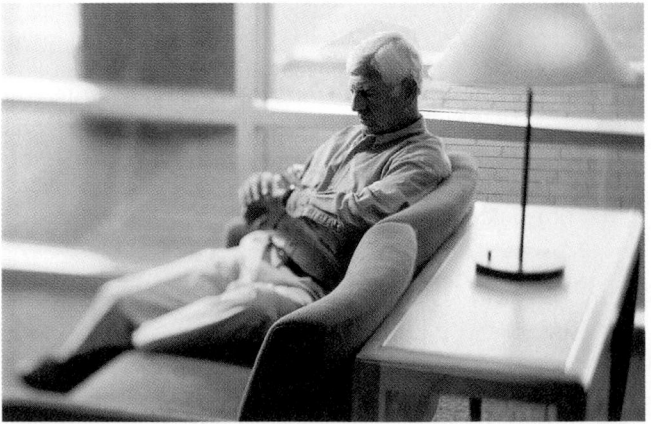

FIGURE 10-4 One of the most common patient complaints is the time spent in the reception area.

ally a physician becomes ill or must be unexpectedly absent from the office. Briefly explain the situation to the patient and allow him or her to decide whether to wait or reschedule. If a delay is forthcoming, attempt to call patients who may be en route to the office and inform them that there will be a delay. Again, offer to reschedule, or allow the patient to come in and wait to see the physician. Always ask for the patient's cell phone number for just such events.

CRITICAL THINKING APPLICATION

Ramona offers to reschedule patient appointments if the schedule ever falls more than 15 minutes behind. If a patient becomes belligerent about the delays, how can Ramona handle the situation in a professional manner?

Telephone Scheduling

It is just as important for a medical assistant to be pleasant and express a desire to be helpful on the telephone as it is when meeting face-to-face. This is especially true when making appointments, because the telephone contact may be the patient's first impression of the facility. Often the manner in which the booking is made makes more of an impact than the convenience of the appointment time.

Be especially considerate if the time requested for an appointment must be refused. Briefly explain why the time is not available and offer a substitute date and time. Comply with the patient's desires as much as possible and do not show any annoyance if the patient does not understand the scheduling process. Most people, however, understand the need for a well-managed office and are willing to cooperate.

Many offices offer the patient a choice when scheduling the appointment, and let the patient decide which option is best for him or her. For example, the following dialog might take place during the scheduling call:
- "Mrs. Thomas, Dr. Stern is available to see you in the office next Tuesday or Wednesday, January 6 or 7. Which day is better for you?"
  "I will be working on Wednesday, so I would like to come on Tuesday."
- "Do you prefer a morning or afternoon appointment?"
  "The afternoon is best for me."
- "Great. Would 1:30 or 3:30 be a better time?"
  "I can be there at 1:30."
- "Then Dr. Stern will see you at 1:30 next Tuesday, January 6. Thank you for calling, Mrs. Thomas. We'll see you then!"

These small courtesies will give patients the feeling that they are in control of their time. Always repeat the time to reinforce the appointment, and do not hesitate to ask the patient if he or she has a pen with which to jot down the time and date. While repeating the information to the patient, check the appointment book or computer screen to ensure that it was posted correctly.

Write legibly when using an appointment book. These records could be called to court, and the medical assistant must be able to read his or her own writing if asked to testify. Form the habit of entering the patient's daytime telephone number after every entry. It may become necessary to cancel or rearrange the schedule in a hurry, and many precious minutes can be saved if the telephone number is handy. Cell phone numbers are also quite useful when tracking down a patient quickly.

Scheduling Appointments for New Patients

Arranging the first appointment for a new patient requires time and attention to detail (Procedure 10-2). This first encounter provides the first impression of the office and may set the tone for all subsequent visits. Tact, courtesy, and professionalism are extremely important. During the conversation with the new patient, request preliminary information to assist in deciding how much time to allot for the visit on the appointment schedule. The physician may also expect the medical assistant to give general instructions to patients seeking care for specific complaints. For example, the patient may be required to bring a urine specimen or to make certain that laboratory tests are completed before the appointment. Some offices obtain enough information to build a patient chart before the office visit; others wait until the patient actually arrives to construct the chart.

After the necessary information has been recorded, offer the first available appointment to the patient. Whenever possible, offer the patient choices between two dates and times. Ask the patient if he or she knows the directions to the office, or offer the physical address for those who wish to obtain exact directions from one of the many Internet sites, such as Mapquest. Tell the patient whether there are any special parking conveniences and whether the office will provide a token or parking validation. The options that the patient will have for the first payment should also be discussed. If payment is expected immediately, inform the patient. The office staff should expect patient concerns about the amount of the first bill and address this issue in advance of the appointment so that there are no surprises or misunderstandings. Before ending the conversation, repeat the appointment date and time, then thank the patient for calling.

Some medical offices mail an information packet about their facility to new patients, especially if the appointment is several days away. With today's technology and the patient's email address, such information can also be sent via the Internet. This information should tell the patient about the nature of the practice, introduce the medical staff, and explain appointment policies and financial arrangements.

If another physician has referred the patient, the medical assistant may need to call the referring physician's office to obtain additional information before the patient's appointment. This information should be printed out and given to the attending physician in advance of the patient's arrival.

PROCEDURE 10-2

Scheduling a New Patient

GOAL: To schedule a new patient for a first office visit.

EQUIPMENT AND SUPPLIES

- Appointment book
- Scheduling guidelines
- Appointment card
- Telephone

PROCEDURAL STEPS

1 Obtain the patient's full name, birth date, address, and telephone number.
Note: Verify the spelling of the name.

2 Determine whether the patient was referred by another physician.
Purpose: You may need to request additional information from the referring physician, and your physician will want to send a consultation report.

3 Determine the patient's chief complaint and when the first symptoms occurred.
Purpose: To assist in determining the length of time needed for the appointment and the degree of urgency.

4 Search the appointment book for the first suitable appointment time and an alternate time.

5 Offer the patient a choice of these dates and times.
Purpose: Patients are better satisfied if they are given a choice.

6 Enter the mutually agreeable time in the appointment book followed by the patient's telephone number.
Note: Indicate that the patient is new by adding the letters *NP*.

7 If new patients are expected to pay at the time of the visit, explain this financial arrangement when the appointment is made.
Purpose: The patient will be aware of the payment policy and can come prepared to pay at the time of the visit.

8 Offer travel directions for reaching the office as well as parking instructions.
Purpose: To relieve any anxiety about being able to find the medical facility.

9 Repeat the day, date, and time of the appointment before saying good-bye to the patient.
Purpose: To verify the patient understands the date and time of the appointment.

Many offices call each patient the day before the appointment as a reminder and a courtesy. This can be a time-consuming procedure, but most patients appreciate this service, and it may open appointments for others if the original patient cannot keep the scheduled time slot. Email can also be programmed to send reminders to patients of their appointments the day before if the email address is obtained. This procedure can run automatically, taking no time away from the medical assistant's other duties.

Scheduling Appointments for Established Patients

In Person

Most return appointments for **established patients** are arranged when the patient is leaving the office. It is a good policy for all patients to stop by the front desk before leaving, in case there is any information needed from the patient or any outside scheduling to do. The patient's chart can be reviewed to see whether the physician ordered any laboratory tests or procedures, and these can be scheduled and discussed with the patient. When making a return appointment, follow the same procedures as scheduling any appointment by phone, offering the patient choices in the day and time slots. If a certain time is not available that the patient specifically requests, offer two alternatives. Always give the patient an appointment card and any necessary instructions at this time, along with a bright smile. Never forget to provide excellent customer service to the patient.

By Telephone

Usually it is only necessary to determine when the patient is required to return and then to find a suitable time on the schedule. Established patients do not usually need directions and parking information, unless the office has recently moved. If there has been a lengthy **interval** since the patient's last visit, the medical assistant should recheck certain information and enter any changes on the patient's chart. Be sure to ask whether insurance companies or benefits have changed, and it is always a good idea to verify the address and phone numbers of the patient. If an email address is not on file, obtain one for quick and easy notification of appointments and other events.

Scheduling Other Types of Appointments

There are other appointments that a medical assistant will make and that will appear on the appointment schedule, such as surgeries the physician will be performing at a hospital or other facility, hospital rounds and consultations, appointments and meetings, and even house calls if the physician performs them. The physician must also have time to get from one location to another, so driving time must be considered when arranging all appointments.

Surgeries

When scheduling a surgery, call the facility where the procedure will be performed as soon as the operation is planned. Most surgical departments and centers have a surgical secretary that makes these arrangements. Provide all necessary information as well as any special requests that the physician may have, such as the amount of blood to have available for the patient. The secretary may want all of the patient's insurance information and will certainly want a phone number so that the patient could be contacted before the surgery if necessary. Be sure that all of this information is handy before placing the call.

Some hospitals request that the patient complete a preadmittance form so that all records can be processed before the patient is admitted. In such cases it may be the medical assistant's responsibility to see that this is done. These are general guidelines only, because procedures will vary in different areas and hospitals.

Outside Visits

If the physician regularly makes house calls or visits patients in skilled nursing facilities, a special block of time will need to be reserved in the appointment schedule. The physician will need demographic information, such as addresses, room numbers, and the best route to each home or facility. Remember to allow for travel time. Although most physicians never make house calls because of the ease of seeing patients in the office, they may be necessary in certain situations. The physician's medical bag should always be prepared and well-stocked before he or she has to make any outside visits.

Outside Appointments

A medical assistant is often requested to arrange laboratory or radiography appointments for patients. Before calling the facility to schedule the appointment, be sure all necessary information is handy. When the patient is informed of the time and place for the appointment, relay any special instructions that may be necessary. Then, note these arrangements in the patient's chart. Some offices will make a reminder call to the patient, or a reminder email message can be sent.

Outpatient testing is common, because most physicians do not have extensive x-ray or laboratory equipment in their offices. MRIs, CT scans, numerous x-ray evaluations, ultrasonography, and simple blood tests all may need to be scheduled (Procedure 10-3). Provide the patient with the name, address, and phone number of the facility where the tests will be performed.

Some patients may require a series of appointments, such as at weekly intervals. Try to set up these appointments on the same day of each week at the same time of day. This considerably reduces the risk that the patient will forget an appointment.

In some cases, the medical assistant may be responsible for scheduling inpatient admissions or inpatient surgical procedures (Procedures 10-4 and 10-5). This is similar to scheduling outpatient testing, but the medical assistant must coordinate with the hospital instead of with an outside facility.

Special Circumstances

Late Patients

Probably every medical practice has a few patients who are habitually late for appointments. This seems to be a problem for which no cure has been found. Emergencies and small delays can happen to anyone, but a patient who constantly arrives late can place a strain on the practice. Such patients can be booked as the last appointment of the day. Then, if closing time arrives before the patient does, there is no obligation to wait. Some medical assistants tell the patient to come in 30 minutes before the appointment time that is actually scheduled. Make an attempt to work with patients who have occasional difficulties arriving on time, but do not allow the schedule to be constantly disrupted by late patients.

CRITICAL THINKING APPLICATION

Seth Jones is always late for his appointments. How might Ramona approach him about this? What can Ramona do to assist Mr. Jones in arriving for appointments on time?

Rescheduling Canceled Appointments

Changes sometimes must be made in the appointment schedule. Unexpected conflicts might arise that force a patient to change the appointment time. When rescheduling an appointment, be sure that the first appointment day and time is removed from the appointment book or database, and then set the new appointment. Otherwise, the patient will be expected in the office on 2 days, and time will be wasted with calls and follow-up, only to find out that the appointment was rescheduled.

Emergency Calls

Periodically, emergency or urgent calls will come to the office and an appointment will need to be scheduled. To some extent, all calls that come to the office go through a **triage** process, and emergencies are prioritized to evaluate

PROCEDURE 10-3

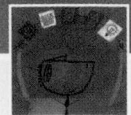

Scheduling Outpatient Admissions and Procedures

GOAL: To schedule a patient for outpatient admission or procedure within the time frame needed by the physician, confirm with the patient, and issue all required instructions.

EQUIPMENT AND SUPPLIES
- Diagnostic test order from physician
- Name, address, and telephone number of diagnostic facility
- Patient demographic information
- Patient chart
- Test preparation instructions
- Telephone
- Consent form

PROCEDURAL STEPS

1 Obtain an oral or written order from the physician for the exact procedure to be performed.
Purpose: To have a documented order for the procedure to be performed.

2 Precertify the procedure with the patient's insurance company, if necessary.
Purpose: To make certain that expected insurance benefits are valid and the procedure will be covered by the patient's insurance policy.

3 Determine the physician and patient availability.
Purpose: To be certain that the patient will be able to comply with the arrangements for the test and that the physician is available, if he or she must be present for the procedure. The urgency of the needed test results affects the time and date of the appointment needed.

4 Telephone the diagnostic facility and schedule the procedure or test.
- Order the specific test needed.
- Provide the patient's diagnosis.
- Establish the date and time.
- Give the name, age, address, and telephone number of the patient.
- Provide the demographic information for the patient, including insurance policy numbers and addresses for filing claims.

- Determine any special instructions for the patient or special anesthesia requirements.
- Notify the facility of any urgency for test results.

Purpose: To schedule the procedure or admission and provide needed information.

5 Notify the patient of the arrangements, including:
- Name, address, and telephone number of the diagnostic facility.
- Date and time to report for the test.
- Instructions concerning preparation for the test (e.g., eating restrictions, fluids, medications, enemas).
- Tell what preadmission testing will be necessary, if any.
- Ask the patient to repeat the instructions.

Purpose: To be certain that the patient understands the preparation necessary and the importance of keeping the appointment. If time permits, issue written instructions to the patient.

6 Have the physician review the consent form with the patient. The patient should sign the consent form and a copy should be placed in the chart. Note arrangements on the patient's chart.
Purpose: To make certain that the patient understands the risks, benefits, and alternatives to the procedure. To ensure follow-up on diagnosis and/or treatment.

7 Place reminder on the physician's tickler or desk calendar, if needed. Be sure the information is listed on the office schedule. Check the postsurgical status of the patient. Follow up if results are not received in a timely manner.
Purpose: To check whether the appointment was kept and a report was received from the testing facility.

---

the urgency of the need to see the physician. Triage is an extremely important function that requires experience and knowledge of signs and symptoms, as well as tact.

Emergencies may include emotional crises as well as the more obvious physical problems. Patients with emergencies should be seen the same day. The urgency of the call can be initially determined by having a list of questions prepared for reference with the help of the physician. The physician should determine what is con-

sidered urgent. The patient may need to be referred directly to the emergency department of a hospital, or the physician may want to see the patient that day in the office. In many cases, the caller will consider the situation more urgent than his or her responses to the medical questions may indicate. Skillful handling of these situations requires considerable tact. Maintaining a caring and reassuring response will frequently alleviate the fear evidenced by the caller.

PROCEDURE **10-4**

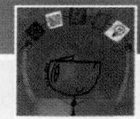

Scheduling Inpatient Admissions

GOAL: To schedule a patient for inpatient admission within the time frame needed by the physician, confirm with the patient, and issue all required instructions.

EQUIPMENT AND SUPPLIES

- Admission orders from physician
- Name, address, and telephone number of inpatient facility
- Patient demographic information
- Patient chart
- Any preparation instructions for the patient
- Telephone
- Admission packet for the patient

PROCEDURAL STEPS

1 Obtain an oral or written order from the physician for the admission.
   Purpose: To have a documented order for the admission.

2 Precertify the admission with the patient's insurance company, if necessary.
   Purpose: To make certain that expected insurance benefits are valid and the admission will be covered by the patient's insurance policy.

3 Determine the physician and patient availability if the admission is not an emergency.
   Purpose: To be certain that the patient will be able to comply with the arrangements for the admission and that the physician is available to care for the patient during the admission. The urgency of the admission affects the time and date of the appointment needed.

4 Telephone the diagnostic facility and schedule the admission.
   - Order any specific tests needed.
   - Provide the patient's admitting diagnosis.
   - Establish the date and time.
   - Convey the patient's room preferences.
   - Give the name, age, address, and telephone number of the patient.

   - Provide the demographic information for the patient, including insurance policy numbers and addresses for filing claims.
   - Determine any special instructions for the patient.
   - Notify the facility of any urgency for test results.
   Purpose: To schedule the admission and provide needed information.

5 Notify the patient of the arrangements, including:
   - Name, address, and telephone number of the facility.
   - Date and time to report for admission.
   - Instructions concerning preparation for any procedures, if necessary (e.g., eating restrictions, fluids, medications, enemas).
   - Tell what preadmission testing will be necessary, if any.
   - Ask the patient to repeat the instructions.
   Purpose: To be certain that the patient understands the preparation necessary and the importance of admittance. If it is your office policy to do so, give an admission packet to the patient that contains the orders and basic instructions for the admission.

6 Note arrangements and the admission on the patient's chart.
   Purpose: To ensure follow-up on diagnosis and/or treatment.

7 Place reminder on the physician's tickler or desk calendar, if needed. Be sure the information is listed on the office schedule. If the physician keeps a list of all inpatients, add the patient's name to that list.
   Purpose: To keep a record of the number of days the patient was seen in the hospital by the physician during rounds for insurance billing purposes.

Acutely Ill Patients

There is sometimes a fine line between an emergency patient and an acutely ill patient, but the latter should be seen as soon as possible. At the very least, let the physician decide whether an appointment should be made for another day. For example, a patient may report having had flu symptoms for several days and now has an elevated temperature. The physician will probably want more information before deciding whether the patient should be seen immediately or whether some other course of action is appropriate. The 15- to 20-minute breather time saved in the middle of the morning may rescue the schedule and provide the needed time for the patient. Escort these patients to the exam room upon their arrival if possible. Patients with symptoms of infection should be placed so as to prevent cross-contamination.

Physician Referrals

If another physician telephones and requests that a patient be seen today, most offices will honor that request if at all possible. It is important to keep a schedule that will not be intolerant of this type of request.

PROCEDURE **10-5**

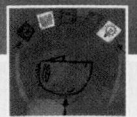

Scheduling Inpatient Surgical Procedures

GOAL: To schedule a patient for inpatient surgery within the time frame needed by the physician, confirm with the patient, and issue all required instructions.

EQUIPMENT AND SUPPLIES

- Orders from physician
- Name, address, and telephone number of inpatient facility
- Patient demographic information
- Patient chart
- Any preparation instructions for the patient
- Telephone
- Consent form

PROCEDURAL STEPS

1 Obtain an oral or written order from the physician for the admission.
Purpose: To have a documented order for the admission.

2 Precertify the admission with the patient's insurance company, if necessary.
Purpose: To make certain that expected insurance benefits are valid and the admission will be covered by the patient's insurance policy.

3 Determine the physician availability if the surgery is not an emergency. Another physician may be the surgeon. If this is the case, the surgery will need to be coordinated with his or her office as well.
Purpose: To be certain that the physician is available to care for the patient during the admission and the surgery. The urgency of the surgery affects the time and date of the appointment needed.

4 Telephone the hospital surgical department and schedule the procedure.
- Order any specific tests needed.
- Provide the patient's admitting diagnosis.
- Establish the date and time.
- Give the name, age, address, and telephone number of the patient.
- Provide the demographic information for the patient, including insurance policy numbers and addresses for filing claims.
- Determine any special instructions for the patient.
- Notify the facility of any urgency for the surgery.

Purpose: To schedule the surgery and provide needed information to the facility.

5 Notify the patient of the arrangements, if the patient is not already admitted to the hospital. Include:
- Name, address, and telephone number of the facility.
- Date and time to report for admission.
- Instructions concerning preparation for any procedures, if necessary (e.g., eating restrictions, fluids, medications, enemas).
- Tell what preadmission testing will be necessary, if any.
- Ask the patient to repeat the instructions.

Purpose: To be certain that the patient understands the preparation necessary and the importance of surgery. If it is your office policy to do so, give an admission packet to the patient that contains the orders and basic instructions for the surgery.

6 The physician should review the consent form with the patient. Have the patient sign a consent for the surgical procedure. Keep the original consent in the patient's chart and give a copy to the patient.
Purpose: To ensure that the patient understands the risks, benefits, and alternatives to the surgical procedure.

7 Note arrangements on the patient's chart.
Purpose: To ensure follow-up on diagnosis and/or treatment.

8 Place reminder on the physician's tickler or desk calendar, if needed. Be sure the information is listed on the office schedule. If the physician keeps a list of all inpatients, add the patient's name to that list. Follow up with the hospital after the procedure regarding the patient's condition as required by the physician.
Purpose: To check on the patient's status and keep a record of the number of days the patient was seen in the hospital by the physician during rounds for insurance billing purposes.

Patients Without Appointments

There must be a policy agreed on by the physician and then carried out by medical assistants for patients without appointments. A patient who requires immediate attention will most likely be accommodated into the schedule somehow. If the patient does not need immediate care, a brief visit with the physician and a scheduled appointment at a later time may be the answer. The medical assistant may simply have to turn down the request. Follow established office policy.

The medical assistant should always make it clear, even when accommodating patients without appointments, that the office runs on an appointment basis. Try to convey the message that appointments save not only the physician's time but also the patient's time. Emphasize that the physician is able to give the patient full attention and more time if an advance appointment is made.

Failed Appointments

Why do patients fail to keep appointments? Some are simply forgetful. Once this tendency is detected in a patient, form the habit of telephoning or emailing a reminder the day before the appointment, or send a postcard timed to arrive 1 or 2 days in advance.

A patient who has been pressed for a payment may stay away because of his or her inability to pay for medical services. Do not make the mistake of classifying all such patients as "deadbeats." Many have every desire to pay, but they cannot afford to and feel embarrassed about their situation, so they avoid their appointments.

If the office consistently runs behind schedule, some patients may not be willing to waste any time waiting to see the physician. Time is a valuable commodity for patients as well, and every effort must be made to get patients in at their appointment time and out quickly.

One other reason for failed appointments that is often overlooked is a patient's state of denial regarding his or her condition. For instance, if a patient has been recently diagnosed as HIV positive, he or she may avoid doctor appointments, because going to see the physician forces the patient to face the reality of the disease. Take special care with such patients, and if denial is suspected, discuss this with the physician, who may wish to refer the patient for counseling.

It is important to determine the reason for failed appointments and do whatever is possible to remedy the situation. Telephone the patient to be sure there is no misunderstanding. If the patient's health is such that medical care must continue, write a letter and explain this to the patient. Send the letter by certified mail, with return receipt requested. Keep the letter in the patient's chart for legal protection.

No-Show Policy

Some patients may not realize the importance of keeping their appointments. The patient who does not arrive for a scheduled appointment or reschedule it is called a **no-show**. A busy practice must have a very specific policy on appointment no-shows and enforce it effectively. The first time a patient fails to show, note the fact on the medical chart and/or ledger card. The second time, warn the patient, and if a third no-show occurs, consider dropping the patient by using the customary methods that provide legal protection for the physician.

The physician may wish to charge patients for not showing up or rescheduling the appointment. Be understanding whenever possible, but do not let a patient take advantage of the physician's time. The office policy manual must state that patients may be charged for missed appointments, especially if the time slot could not be filled with another patient. Many physicians do not press this issue, but it is an available tool if needed.

Recording the Failed Appointment

When a patient fails to keep an appointment, a notation should be made in the patient's chart as well as in the appointment book or database. If the patient is seriously ill, the physician should also be told about the failure to show. In some cases, it may be necessary to call or write the patient to remind that a missed appointment may have serious effects on the patient's health.

Increasing Appointment Show Rates

Everyone benefits from a full schedule of appointments that are kept. There are several ways to increase appointment show rates.

Appointment Cards

Most healthcare facilities use appointment cards to remind patients of scheduled appointments, as well as to eliminate misunderstandings about dates and times (Figure 10-5). Make a habit of reaching for an appointment card while writing an entry in the appointment book. After the date and time have been written on the card, double-check with the book to see that the entries agree.

Confirmation Calls

Patients who have made appointments in advance may appreciate a confirmation call to remind them that they have a time set aside to see the physician. Always note the phone number that the patient prefers the office use for such calls. Many individuals now have a home phone, cell phone, and work number; however, they may wish calls from the physician to go only to their home phone. The preferred phone number can be highlighted in the chart or on the computer. The office must use caution in making calls to patients because of the significance of privacy guidelines and standards. Some offices may wish to prepare a release form in which the patient grants the office staff permission to contact the patient. Many physicians insist that messages left on voice mail not mention the term "doctor" for confidentiality reasons. The medical assistant might say:

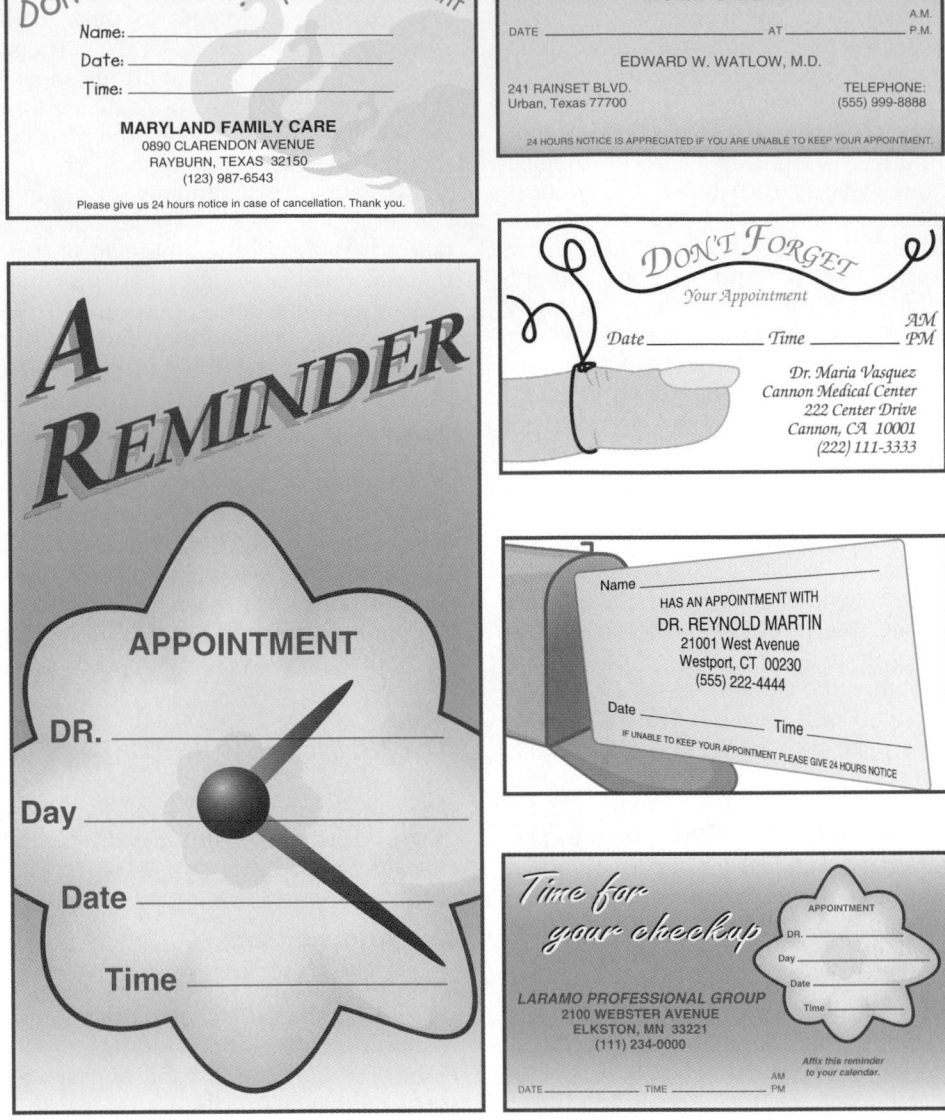

FIGURE 10-5 Examples of appointment cards.

"This is Pam at Robert Welch's office confirming your appointment tomorrow at 2:00 pm. Please call us if you cannot make the appointment. Our number is 555-212-0909. Thank you!"

Email Reminders

Many computer scheduling programs have the capacity to send an email to patients to remind them of appointments the day before. This is a great time-saver for the office staff, because no time is taken to perform this duty, other than the original scheduling of the appointment.

Mailed Reminders

Mailed reminder cards may be sent to patients by the office staff. This method is a bit time consuming, but worth the effort if the patients show for their appointments.

A patient who is due for an appointment but has not yet arranged a date and time may be sent a reminder. A simple way of handing this is to have a supply of postcards on hand, and while patients are still in the office, have them write their name and address on the postcard. Then place the card in a tickler file box under the date it is to be mailed.

Innovative Ideas

Knowing that time is valuable to patients as well as the physician, many of today's offices try to make the time spent at the office as productive as possible for the patient. Some reception areas are equipped with computers, televisions, and even video games and movies for children. Often a small desk with a phone will allow the patient to do a limited amount of work, if needed, while waiting to see the physician. Keeping the patient's needs in mind makes the patient less likely to break an appointment.

Handling Cancellations and Delays

When the Patient Cancels

Inevitably, some cancellations will occur. If a list is kept of patients with advance appointments who would like to come in sooner, the medical assistant can begin calling to try to get one of them in to fill the available opening. By placing a colored dot beside their names in the appointment book where the first appointment was made, the medical assistant can readily identify which patients to call to fill the vacancy.

When the Physician Is Delayed

There will be days when the physician is delayed in reaching the office. If there is advance notice of the delay, start calling patients with early appointments and suggest that they come later. If some patients have already arrived before the office learns of the delay, explain that an emergency has detained the physician.

Show concern for the patient but avoid being overly apologetic, which might imply some degree of guilt. Most patients realize that a physician has certain priorities. The patient who is in the office may be inconvenienced, but it is not a life-or-death matter. If this kind of situation occurs frequently, however, consider devising a different scheduling system.

When the Physician Is Called for Emergencies

Physicians are conscious of their responsibilities for responding to medical emergencies, and most patients will be sympathetic to such occurrences if the medical assistant takes the time to explain what has happened. The medical assistant may say:

> "Dr. Wright has been called away to answer an emergency. She asked me to tell you she is very sorry to keep you waiting. There will be at least a 1-hour delay."

Ask the patient:

> "Do you wish to wait? If it is inconvenient, I'll be glad to give you the first available appointment on another day. Or perhaps you'd like to have some coffee or do some shopping and return in an hour."

As quickly as possible, call the patients who are scheduled for a later hour. In many offices, especially those of obstetricians, surgeons, and general practitioners, it sometimes is necessary to cancel a whole day's appointments. For this reason, it is particularly important to have the daytime telephone number of each patient available so that the appointment can be rescheduled. If it is at all possible, cancel appointments *before* the patient arrives in the office to find that the physician is not available. The **expediency** of the office staff in contacting the patients who will be affected by an emergency will be most appreciated.

When the Physician is Ill or Out of Town

Physicians get ill, too, and the patients who are scheduled to be seen during the course of the physician's expected recovery period must be informed of this. They need not be told the nature of the illness. When the physician is called out of town for personal or professional reasons, the appointments will have to be canceled or rescheduled. It is customary to give the patient the name of another physician, or possibly a choice of several, who will be providing care during such absences. For security reasons, it is best to merely state that the doctor is unavailable. Stating over the telephone that the physician is out of town could lead to attempted burglary or other unauthorized intrusion of the premises.

Other Types of Appointments

There will be a wide range of other unscheduled callers with whom the physician will need to meet. Handle all of these individuals with care and courtesy.

Physicians

Another physician dropping in to the facility should be ushered in to see the physician as soon as possible, regardless of the appointment schedule. If the physician is seeing a patient, explain the situation and, if possible, take the visiting physician into a private room to wait. Then notify your employer as soon as possible. Visits from other physicians are usually brief and do not appreciably affect your schedule.

Pharmaceutical Representatives

Also known as *detail persons* or *reps*, representatives from pharmaceutical houses are frequent visitors to physicians' offices and are generally welcomed when the schedule permits. They are well trained and bring valuable information on new drugs to the physician. The medical assistant is often expected to screen such visitors and turn away those whose products would not be used in that practice. If the representative or the pharmaceutical company is unknown to the office, ask for a business card, then check with the physician, who will decide whether to see the caller.

Specialists usually limit their conferences with pharmaceutical representatives to their line of practice. The medical assistant, together with the physician, can prepare a list of the representatives with whom the physician is willing to spend time, and then let the list be the determining factor in future conferences. The medical assistant can say whether the physician will be available that day and give an estimate of the waiting time or suggest a later time at which to return. The caller can then make a decision regarding whether to wait or return later. The pharmaceutical representative is usually quite understanding and cooperative and is willing to wait patiently a long while for just a brief visit with the physician. The medical assistant should in turn treat the representative with courtesy, showing as much cooperation as possible.

In some cases, the representative will just leave literature or materials for the physician with the medical assistant. The detail person who is not on the calling list for a particular physician will also appreciate the saving in time by knowing this in advance. Most representatives say they would rather be told outright if the physician does not wish to see them than to be given some evasive reply.

Salespersons

Salespersons from medical, surgical, and office supply houses call regularly at physicians' offices. Sometimes they will want to see the physician, but the office manager or the medical assistant who is in charge of ordering supplies usually is able to handle these calls.

Unsolicited salespersons can sometimes present a problem in the professional office. If the physician does not wish to see such callers, the medical assistant must firmly but tactfully send them away. Suggest that they leave their literature and cards for the physician to study and say that the physician will contact them if further information is desired.

Miscellaneous Callers

From time to time, other callers appear in the medical office. Some are civic leaders seeking the physician's aid in community projects. Others may be church leaders, insurance representatives, solicitors for fund drives, and so forth. A general policy regarding seeing such callers should be established so that each incident does not require a separate discussion and decision.

Civic leaders should be treated with courtesy and consideration when they telephone or come into the office. Most physicians feel a responsibility to take an active part in community affairs, but no one can participate in all activities. The responsibility for accepting or refusing such community appointments is sometimes delegated to the office manager or medical assistant. In this event, one should use discretion and exercise great tact and courtesy. Turning away community leaders with a blunt refusal does not create good medical public relations.

When it is necessary to refuse requests for community projects, the medical assistant can explain that the physician is already participating in such community projects as, for example, the Boy Scouts, Girl Scouts, Kiwanis, and the Health Council and cannot accept additional responsibilities at this time. The practice of tact, courtesy, and consideration applies to every caller in the healthcare facility.

Planning for the Next Day

Before leaving at the end of the day, look over the appointments scheduled for the next day. Review the charts for scheduled patients. If laboratory tests or other procedures were scheduled on the patient's last visit, determine that the reports are available in the chart. If the patient is scheduled for specific procedures on this visit, make certain that everything that will be needed for the procedure is on hand and available. Planning can save many precious moments at the time of the patient visit.

Closing Comments

The person charged with the responsibility for scheduling appointments will have a huge impact on the efficiency of the medical office. A friendly and helpful attitude is a **prerequisite** for cordial **interaction** with patients and the ability to make compromises that will benefit both the physician and the patient. The office that runs smoothly and stays on schedule is an indication of professionalism and competence and will be greatly appreciated by all who come into contact with the medical office.

Patient Education

Providing patients with an information booklet about the office will help to acclimate them to the policies and procedures of the office. Many physicians compile an extensive booklet that even provides tips as to when the physician should be called immediately, listing symptoms and signs of emergencies.

Educating the patient regarding office policies will help the facility to run smoothly from day to day. All patients should be familiar with the policies about appointments. This leads to fewer misunderstandings and conflicts over bills that might include a charge for a missed appointment.

If the facility offers web-based appointment scheduling, patients will have to be taught how to use the system. A printed pamphlet or information sheet will be helpful in providing instruction to the patient. It would be wise to have a special phone number that patients could call who have problems with the scheduling system. Choose a program that is simple to use and easy to understand for best results.

Legal and Ethical Issues

The appointment schedule may be used as a legal record and could be brought by subpoena into a court of law. Be sure that all handwriting in the book is completely legible and that information is routinely collected in a consistent manner for each entry. Do not fail to note a no-show in the patient's chart as well as the appointment schedule. This is often helpful when a physician must prove that the patient did not follow medical advice or that the patient contributed to his or her poor condition by missing appointments. Old appointment schedules should be kept for a time equal to the statute of limitations in the state in which the practice exists.

SUMMARY OF SCENARIO

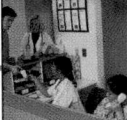

Ramona is an asset to the medical office, because her dedication and customer service skills help her to interact with patients in a positive way. She genuinely cares about the patients and makes every effort to meet their needs while following the preferences of her physician. She has found that her bright smile is a valuable tool to use when patients have been waiting and are growing restless.

Ramona cooperates with other staff members to get the patients seen as quickly as possible and minimize wait time. She is flexible and can change the order of the patients seen, if needed, to maximize the use of time and

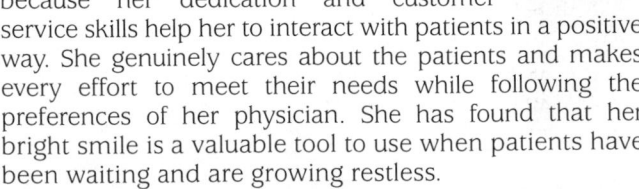

facilities in the office. Because she is so cheerful and friendly, patients do not seem to mind when she asks for their cooperation. She keeps current phone numbers and cell phone information so that she can notify a patient quickly if Dr. Brown is running behind schedule. Ramona's proficiency on the computer also is an asset, and she makes frequent use of email to take care of patient problems or rescheduling desires.

Because of the cooperation she receives from staff and patients alike, Ramona successfully runs an efficient office.

SUMMARY OF LEARNING OBJECTIVES

■ When scheduling appointments, a medical assistant must consider the patients' needs, the physician's preferences, and the available facilities. Make every attempt to schedule a patient at his or her most convenient time. This will help to avoid no-shows. The physician will outline preferences, which should be of high priority to the medical assistant. However, most physicians are flexible and will make adjustments according to the needs of the office. The availability of facilities within the office are perhaps the most inflexible. If a certain room or piece of equipment is being used for one patient, it usually cannot be used for another.

■ When choosing an appointment book, all of the needs of the office should be considered. If there are multiple physicians, the book should be arranged so that each physician is readily identified. Books that open flat on the surface of the desk are much easier to handle, but if there is not enough space to open the book entirely, another style might be better. The book should also provide enough space to write all of the patient information needed in the various time slots, such as the name, phone number, and reason for the visit.

■ Computerized scheduling programs are in demand today because they are easy to operate, simplifying scheduling appointments and making changes to the schedule. The computer can find the first available time much more quickly than scanning through an appointment book. Most programs can prepare reports and even notify patients automatically by email of the impending appointment. Web-based self-scheduling programs are becoming popular; these allow a patient to see the physician's available appointments and book his or her own date and time.

■ Self-scheduling would vastly reduce calls to the office, because a high number of everyday calls are requests to schedule appointments. Patients could make an appointment at midnight, if they desired.

■ Open office hours allow patients to come to the physician's office when it is convenient and wait in turn to see the physician. Scheduling specific appointments is the most popular method of seeing patients. Flexible office hours allow patients to see the physician during the evening and often on weekends. Many of today's medical offices have some flexible scheduling, because most families now consist of two working parents. Wave scheduling brings two or three patients to the office at the same time, and they are seen in the order of their arrival. This type of scheduling can be modified in many ways to suit the needs of the facility. Other scheduling methods include double booking and grouping of like procedures.

■ When the office is running 15 minutes behind schedule, the medical assistant should briefly explain the delay to the waiting patients and then offer to reschedule their appointments. Keep the patients informed of wait times until the schedule resumes.

■ Giving a patient a choice in appointment times to better meet his or her needs is a part of good customer service. Offering the patient a choice of 2 days, morning or afternoon, and two times helps to ensure that the patient will keep the appointment.

■ Because the appointment schedule might be called into a court of law, it is vital that the handwriting in the book be completely legible. Even if the book is 5 years old, the person charged with testifying in court should be able to clearly read all entries. Scribbled, messy handwriting implies incompetence and reflects on the practice.

■ Patients who are habitually late for appointments might be told to arrive 15 minutes before the time written in the book. Some offices book these patients as the last appointment of the day, so that if they do not arrive promptly, they do not see the physician. Usually talking with the patient and gaining an understanding of why the patient arrives late will improve the situation. The office can work with the patient to choose the best times that will result in a show appointment.

■ Some patients accidentally forget the appointment with the physician, and some are habitually careless about remembering their scheduled time. Small emergencies often come up, and in today's busy business world, some patients just cannot get away from their own offices or other obligations to visit the physician. In some cases patients do not keep appointments because they do not want to deal with a health issue confronting them.

KEY INTERNET WEBSITES

- Schedule Wise
  For active weblinks to each website visit
  http://evolve.elsevier.com/Kinn/

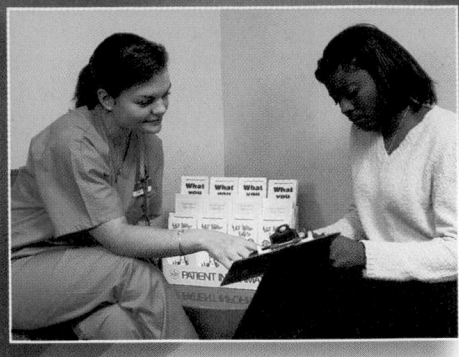

CHAPTER 11

Scenario

Most people enter the healthcare field for very specific reasons. One medical assistant, Georgina Robertson, recalls being in a serious car accident when she was about 6 years old, and as a result her vision was temporarily impaired. She remembers seeing a woman in a white uniform who offered words of comfort. She seemed to have a haze around her, which when combined with the lights, made her look as if she had wings. This vision of an "angel" never left her thoughts and led her into the medical field.

Today Georgina works for Dr. Stuart Wade, a cardiologist in a metropolitan city near Detroit. Georgina is a seasoned medical assistant, and she enjoys getting to know her patients. She makes notes on the chart that remind her of special events in the lives of the patients that visit Dr. Wade's office. The patients feel that she truly cares about them, aside from her duties at the clinic. Although she is efficient and time conscious, she always has a moment to share a warm smile or hear about a new grandchild. Georgina is a valued member of the medical team in her office. She is currently attending a state college in the evening hours, gaining credits toward her bachelor's degree. She plans to continue her education and perhaps apply to medical school one day.

Patient Reception and Processing

Learning Objectives

- Define and spell the terms listed in the vocabulary.
- Explain the purpose of the office mission statement.
- List several patient amenities and why these are important additions to the medical office.
- Describe how to prepare for patient arrivals.
- Explain why it is important to use the patient's name as often as possible.
- Discuss how the medical assistant may help the patient prepare for an examination.
- List and explain two methods of chart placement.
- Discuss how the medical assistant might deal with talkative patients.
- Explain how the medical assistant can recall closing duties.
- Discuss ways to make the patient feel at ease and comfortable in the medical office.
- Correctly prepare charts for registered patients who are scheduled.
- Demonstrate the correct way to register a new patient.

National Curriculum Competencies

TRANSDISCIPLINARY COMPETENCIES

2c. Establish and maintain the medical record
3b. Patient instruction

Vocabulary

amenity Something conducive to comfort, convenience, or enjoyment.

demographic The statistical characteristics of human populations (as in age or income) used especially to identify markets.

depleted To lessen markedly in quantity, content, power, or value.

fervent Exhibiting or marked by great intensity of feeling.

flagged Marked in some way as to remind or remember that specific action needs to be taken.

harmonious Marked by accord in sentiment or action; having the parts agreeably related.

immigrant A person who comes to a country to take up permanent residence.

intercom A two-way communication system with a microphone and loudspeaker at each station for localized use.

mnemonic A device, such as a sentence or rhyme, used as a memory aid (e.g., Roy G. Biv for remembering the colors of the spectrum: red-orange-yellow-green-blue-indigo-violet).

perception A quick, acute, and intuitive cognition; a capacity for comprehension.

phonetic Constituting an alteration of ordinary spelling that better represents the spoken language, that employs only characters of the regular alphabet, and that is used in a context of conventional spelling.

progress notes Notes used in the patient chart to track the progress and condition of the patient.

sequentially Of, relating to, or arranged in a sequence.

The patient reception area should be an inviting place in which patients feel comfortable. Visits to the physician can be times of great stress, so the office staff must do everything possible to make the experience pleasant for patients. A patient usually has a choice of healthcare providers and should be treated with excellent customer service. Good patient relations will result in referrals to the physician, and this helps the practice grow. When patients have a good experience with a physician, they are likely to tell others. When the office staff are committed to making the patient feel welcome and the focus is on care of the patient, the success of the practice is inevitable.

The Office Mission Statement

Healthcare providers often have a **fervent** reason for entering the medical field. One physician remembers the heritage his **immigrant** grandfather left in his heart. The physician has fond memories of his grandfather's pride and thankfulness for the opportunities he found in America, after coming to the United States with nothing but the clothes on his back. The grandfather's dream was to see his grandson become a physician, and that is exactly what he did. Even on the most trying days, he could step into his office and see the picture of his grandfather and find the strength and determination to care for his patients.

The office mission statement reflects this deep-seated desire by expressing the reasons for the existence of the practice (Figure 11-1). The physician may develop the mission statement alone or may consult the office staff for input. Many offices display the mission statement prominently in the reception area and on printed material, such as patient information booklets. Whatever the contents, each employee of the facility should be familiar with the statement and have a personal commitment to promoting the mission statement ideas in everyday practice.

The Reception Area

A first impression is lasting. Nowhere is this more important than in the healthcare facility, where the environment must appear orderly and faultlessly clean. The facility may be a physician's office, a hospital, a health maintenance organization, an insurance company, or one of the many other healthcare sources. No matter what facility is involved, the appearance of the reception room and the front desk, and a cordial greeting by the receptionist, influence a patient's **perception** of the entire facility and the care that he or she will receive.

The reception area is just that—a place to receive patients. The area should be planned for the patients' comfort, made as attractive and cheerful as possible, and kept clean and uncluttered (Figure 11-2). Often a medical assistant has the opportunity to assist in the design and decoration of this very important area.

WADE CARDIAC CLINIC MISSION STATEMENT

The mission of the Wade Cardiac Clinic is fourfold:

- The staff of the clinic promotes the highest standards of ethical medical practice.
- The physician and staff members commit to serving their patients with respect and courtesy.
- All staff members shall promote a healthy lifestyle and preventative measures for the patients that present to the clinic.
- The clinic will support medical patient education, scientific research and development, community service, and community health promotion.

It is our desire to give the best customer service to our patients and care for them as if they were members of our own families.

FIGURE 11-1 The mission statement should be presented to all employees early in their tenure, and the staff should strive to meet the mission every day.

Fresh, **harmonious** colors and cleanliness are the basis of an attractive room (Figure 11-3). Add comfortable furniture that is adequate to accommodate the peak load of patients seen each day and arrange it in conversational groups. Individual chairs are best (Figure 11-4); people sometimes prefer to stand rather than sit next to a stranger on a sofa. Provide good lighting, ventilation, and a regulated temperature for additional comfort, and the essentials are in place for an attractive reception area. A place to hang coats, rainwear, and umbrellas helps reduce reception room clutter. Professional designers can be consulted regarding reception room décor and improvements or when there is a problem area that inhibits office traffic.

Most physicians' offices are well supplied with recent magazines and pictorial travel books. Publications with short items of popular interest are favorites. Some offices have a book share program, where patients bring paperback books to the office and can trade them for another. The next time the office is visited, the paperback is returned and another can be taken. The reception room, incidentally, is not the place for the physician's professional journals.

A writing desk with writing paper in the reception area for the convenience of patients is a nice touch, as is restful music from a concealed speaker. A lighted aquarium or an educational display of some sort will enhance the attractiveness and individuality of the reception area of the professional practice. Patients are often interested in health-related brochures. The physician may also have a videotape or healthcare book library, which allows patients to check out items of interest to them.

Additions such as a television and VCR or DVD player will help the time pass much faster, especially in pediatric offices. Children enjoy Disney movies and cartoon programs, and these hold their interest until it is time to see the physician. A children's corner equipped with small-scale furniture and some playthings works well (Figure 11-5). Youngsters who might otherwise get into mischief are kept pleasantly occupied. Toys should be easily cleanable; plastic washable items are especially good. Take extra care to ensure that no toy has sharp corners that could injure a child and that there are no small parts that could be swallowed. In selecting toys, make certain that they will not stimulate the child toward noisy activity. And no rubber balls, unless there is time to chase them around the room!

Many of today's modern offices offer a computer for patient use while waiting to see the physician. This is a wonderful **amenity**, because the patient can make good use of his or her time while in the reception area. An amazing amount of work can be done just by checking office email, so providing Internet access to patients is also helpful. A telephone in the reception area is an asset and can be programmed by the phone company not to allow long-distance calls.

Periodically, take an objective look around the reception room. Could it use a little brightening or freshening up? Try to look at it as if you were seeing it for the first time. The receptionist is partly responsible for the appearance of the area by making certain that the room remains neat and orderly throughout the day. Check the temperature and lighting for comfort. Scan the room at various intervals during the day to ensure that the room is in order.

If the medical assistant's desk is in the reception area or in open view of the patients, it should be free of clutter. In particular, patients' charts and financial records should not be in sight. Computer monitors should not be in view of patients, to protect the confidentiality of records. Personal articles, coffee cups, and so forth should not be on the receptionist's desk.

Preparing for Patient Arrival

Advance preparation helps to make the day go smoothly and contributes toward a more relaxed atmosphere for all concerned. Some offices prepare for the next day on the evening before, whereas others prepare each morning. The office should be consistent and always perform the same routine.

Readying the Patient Charts

Pull the charts for the day (or the next day if this is done in the evenings), and check off the patient's name on a copy of the appointment schedule to be sure that all charts have been located and are ready (Figure 11-6). Occasionally

 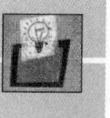

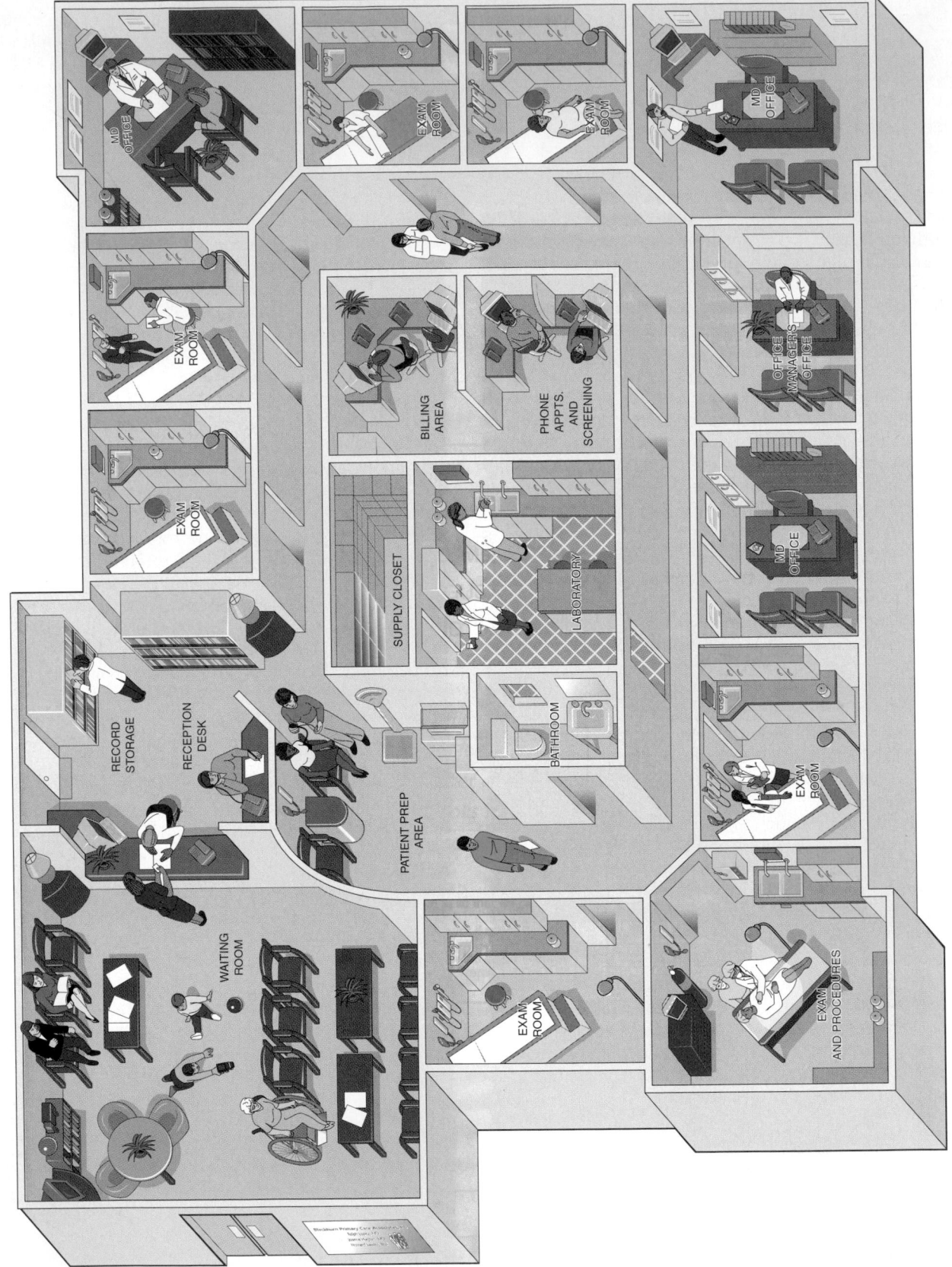

FIGURE 11-2   The medical office should be arranged so that the flow of traffic is conducive to the movement of patients throughout the office.

more than one patient may have the same or a similar name. Review each chart to verify that any recently received information, such as laboratory reports and radiograph readings, has been correctly entered, permanently attached to the chart, and that each chart is current (Procedure 11-1). Arrange the charts **sequentially** in the order the patients are scheduled to be seen. The medical assistant may be expected to place the charts of all the patients to be seen that day on the physician's desk, but it is more likely that the physician will prefer to receive a patient's chart just before seeing him or her. Be sure that there is enough space on the **progress notes** for the physician to write in the chart. A new sheet may need to be added.

Replenishing Supplies

Supplies at the reception desk need to be replenished regularly. Stationery, appointment cards, charge slips,

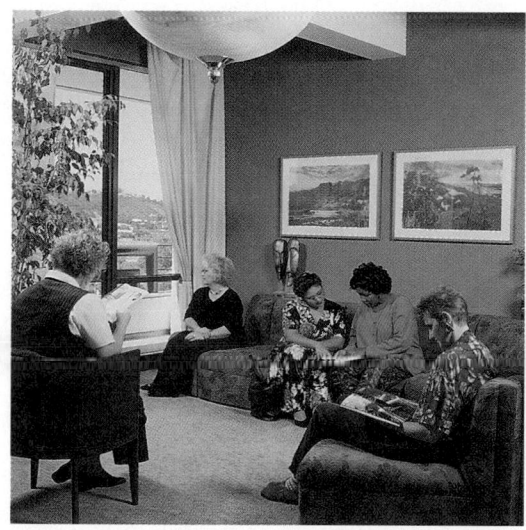

FIGURE 11-3   Patients appreciate cleanliness, restful colors, good ventilation, and light to read by when waiting in the reception area.

sharpened pencils, and any items likely to be needed during the day should be on hand when the day begins. Discovering that supplies are **depleted** during a busy day can seriously interrupt the flow of patient care. One person should be in charge of checking the inventory of supplies on a regular basis and ordering as necessary.

In a multiple-employee practice, a clinical assistant usually has the responsibility of checking clinical supplies and preparing the patient rooms. However, in a small practice there may be only one assistant in charge. Before patients start arriving, everything should be ready for the day so that the physician and medical assistant can give undivided attention to the patients' needs.

Greeting the Patient

Every patient has the right to expect courteous treatment in a physician's office. No matter what the patient's economic or social status may be, each individual who enters the reception room should receive a cordial, friendly greeting (Figure 11-7). Using a personal touch in receiving patients is important.

Patient Check-in

The reception desk is usually placed for a clear view of all visitors who come into the office. If there is only one medical assistant, it is sometimes impossible for each new caller to be welcomed personally. In this situation, some announcement system must be worked out. The patient who enters an empty reception room does not know whether to sit down, knock on the glass partition, or try to announce his or her presence in some way. A bell at the desk or window that the patient can ring is one solution. Sometimes a sign is placed in the reception room that reads, "Please sit comfortably. The receptionist will be with you shortly."

The receptionist should check the reception area each time he or she has been away from the desk to see if additional patients have arrived. These patients should

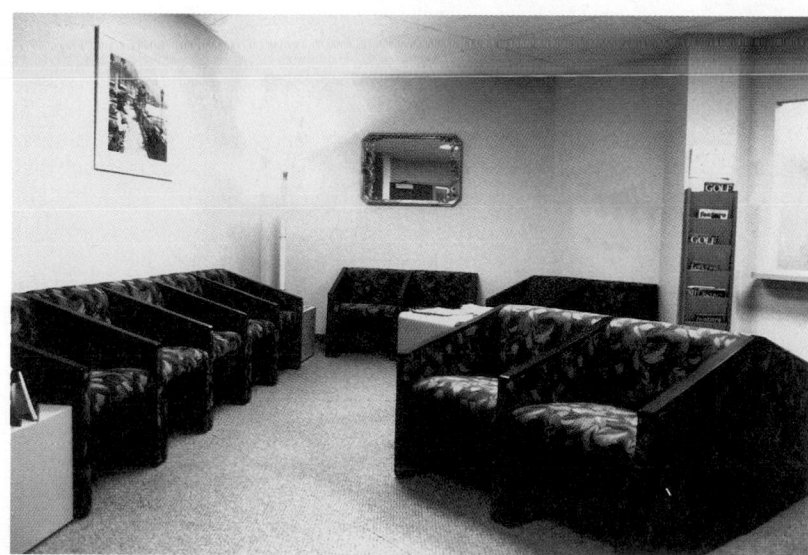

FIGURE 11-4   Patients tend to prefer individual seating. Comfortable seating helps patients relax and be at ease while waiting to see the physician. (Courtesy August Incorporated, Centerville, Ohio.)

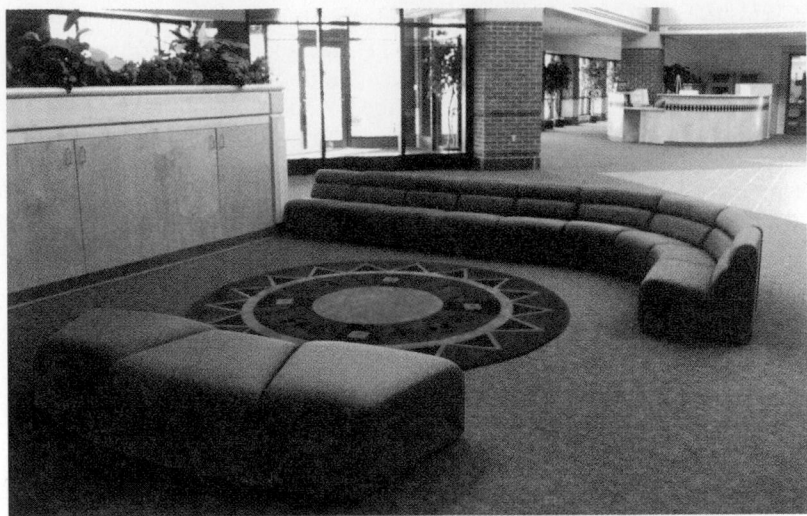

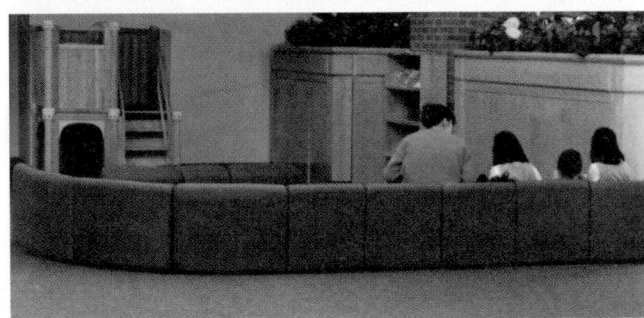

FIGURE 11-5 Furniture in a pediatrician's office should be durable and fun, child sized, and able to withstand the most active children. (Courtesy August Incorporated, Centerville, Ohio.)

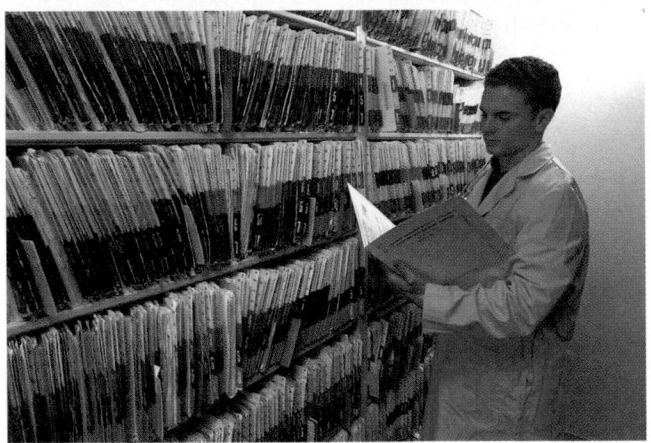

FIGURE 11-6 Charts should be pulled in advance for the patients arriving for appointments. Each chart should be checked to see whether it has adequate forms and is in good order for the physician's use.

also be greeted by name. The office staff should avoid having a sign-in register that stays at the patient reception window, because patient confidentiality is violated when others can read the register. It is preferable to hand the register to the patient if a sign-in sheet is used. Patients should not be expected to provide details of the reason for their visit in a public area. Remember to ask about the patient before asking about insurance.

CRITICAL THINKING APPLICATION

Everyone forgets someone's name on occasion. How might Georgina and her staff members remember names? What special tips or techniques assist in remembering names? Eventually a patient will come to the clinic whose name just cannot be recalled. How can the staff determine who the patient is without offending him or her?

Knowing the Patients

Cultivate the habit of greeting each patient immediately in a friendly, self-assured manner. Establish eye contact and smile while introducing yourself to the patient. For example, "Good morning, I'm Elizabeth Parr, Dr. Wade's medical assistant."

Patients like to be acknowledged when they arrive. All staff members should review the day's schedule in the morning to be prepared to greet patients by name and to know whether the patient is new or established (Figure 11-8). Learn how to pronounce each patient's name correctly, because incorrect pronunciations may offend and irritate some people. If the name is unusual, write the **phonetic** spelling on the record for reference. Using the patient's name often also ensures that the correct patient is being treated.

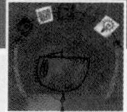

PROCEDURE 11-1

Preparing Charts for Scheduled Patients

GOAL: To prepare patient charts for the daily appointment schedule and have them ready for the physician before the patients' arrival.

EQUIPMENT AND SUPPLIES

- Appointment schedule for current date
- Patient files
- Clerical supplies (e.g., pen, tape, stapler)

PROCEDURAL STEPS

1 Review the appointment schedule.

2 Identify full name of each scheduled patient.

3 Pull patients' charts for files, checking each patient's name on your list as each is pulled.
Purpose: To determine that the correct charts have been pulled and that no charts have been omitted.

4 Review each chart.
Purpose: To reaffirm that:
- The correct patient chart has been pulled

- Any previously ordered tests have been performed
- The results of the tests have been mounted or entered in the chart
- Forms have been replenished inside the chart, such as progress notes, and so forth

5 Annotate the appointment list with any special concerns.
Purpose: To alert the physician regarding matters that should be checked or discussed with the patient.

6 Arrange the charts sequentially according to each patient's appointment.

7 Place the charts in the appropriate examination room or other specified location.

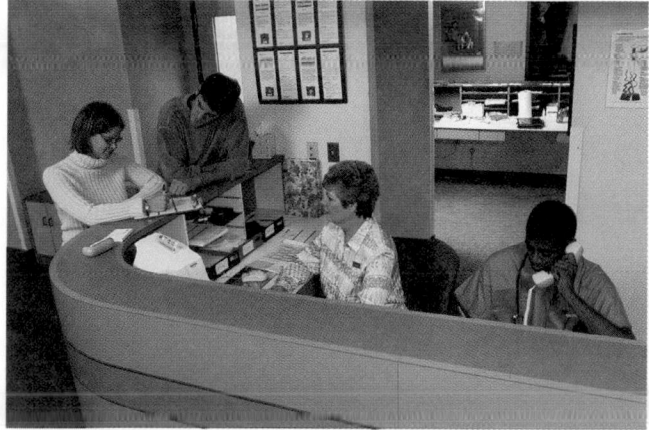

FIGURE 11-7 Greet all patients with a warm smile and assist them with forms they need to complete for the chart.

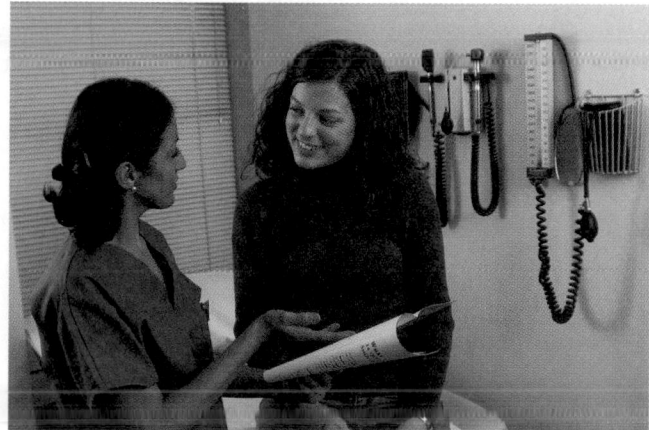

FIGURE 11-8 The medical assistant should develop a good relationship with the patient and be a caring advocate.

It is helpful to make brief notes in the chart about the current events in the patient's life. With this information, the medical assistant and the physician can read those notes before entering the examination room, and share a short dialog with patients at the beginning of their visits. An example follows:

Georgina:	Hello, Mrs. Williams, how are you today?
Mrs. Williams:	I am doing very well, Georgina, how are you?
Georgina:	I'm fine. How was the cruise you took with your husband last month?
Mrs. Williams:	It was wonderful! The water was the bluest I have seen!
Georgina:	You went to Grand Cayman and Cozumel, didn't you?
Mrs. Williams:	Yes, we did! I'm surprised you remember as many patients as you see each day!

This brief chat will confirm that the staff cares about the individual patients because they take an interest in their personal lives (Figure 11-9). Because the medical assistant or physician looked at the notes before entering the patient room, the patient assumes that the informa-

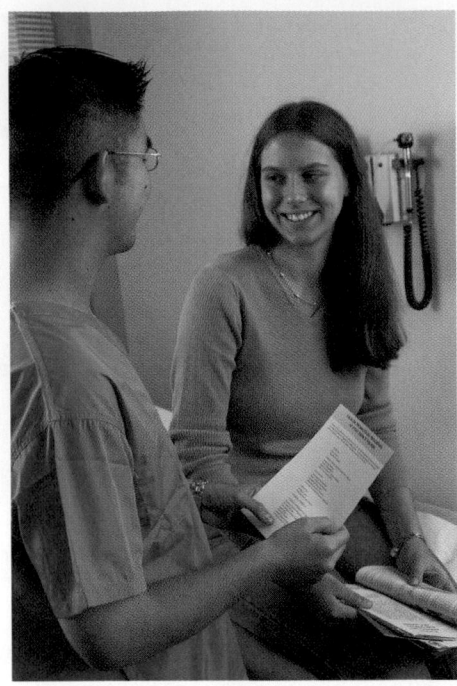

FIGURE 11-9 Patients appreciate being called by name and remembered from visit to visit.

tion is being recalled from memory, and that is an impressive customer service technique. Most patients appreciate the interest of the physician and the staff in their families, hobbies, and work.

Registration Procedures

Certain registration procedures are required on a patient's first visit to the facility (Procedure 11-2). Most physicians use a patient information form to gather **demographic** information about the patient. The form may be attached to a clipboard and handed to the patient with instructions to complete all parts of the form, with assurance that the assistant is ready and willing to answer any questions (Figure 11-10). The patient's name should appear prominently at the top of the form, followed by other pertinent facts in logical order. Most information sheets contain the following information:

- Patient's name and date of birth
- Responsible person's name
- Relationship to patient
- Address and telephone number
- Name, address, and telephone number of spouse
- Occupation

PROCEDURE 11-2

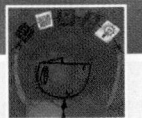

Registering a New Patient

GOAL: To complete a registration form for a new patient with information for credit and insurance claims, and to inform and orient the patient to the facility.

EQUIPMENT AND SUPPLIES

- Registration form
- Clerical supplies (pen, clipboard)
- Private conference area

PROCEDURAL STEPS

1 Determine whether the patient is new.

2 Obtain and record the necessary information:
- Full name, birth date, name of spouse (if married)
- Home address, telephone number (include ZIP and area codes)
- Occupation, name of employer, business address, telephone number
- Social Security number and driver's license number, if any
- Name of referring physician, if any
- Name and address of person responsible for payment
- Method of payment
- Health insurance information (photocopy both sides of insurance ID card)
- Name of primary carrier

- Type of coverage
- Group policy number
- Subscriber number
- Assignment of benefits, if required

Purpose: This information is necessary for credit and insurance claims.

3 Review the enter form and confirm patient eligibility for insurance coverage.

Purpose: To verify that the given information is complete and legible.

4 Determine that required referrals have been received, if applicable.

Purpose: Insurance coverage may not be valid without referral.

5 Explain medical and financial procedures to patients.

Purpose: The patient develops a comfort level and knows what to expect.

6 Collect co-payments or balance payment charges.

Purpose: Keeps accounts current and prevents the necessity of mailing statements.

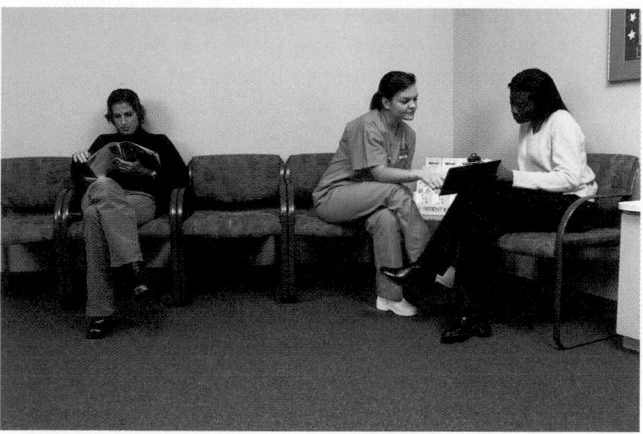

FIGURE 11-10   The medical assistant should take the time to explain forms that the patient does not understand and always be willing to answer questions.

- Place of employment
- Social Security number
- Driver's license number
- Nearest relative not living with patient, and his or her relationship
- Source of referral, if any

When the completed form is returned to the medical assistant, it must be checked carefully to verify that all the necessary information has been included.

Obtaining a Patient History

The personal and medical history, and the patient's family history, may be obtained by asking the patient to complete a questionnaire; the physician can augment this information during the patient interview. The experienced medical assistant may be expected to conduct the interview for the patient's personal and medical history, family history, and chief complaint. This is a very specialized procedure, and the interviewer must be specifically trained for the individual practice.

Consideration for Patients' Time

Once the preliminaries have been completed, the patient will expect to see the physician or practitioner at the appointed time. The medical assistant should get the patient in for treatment or consultation as near the appointment time as possible or explain any potential delay to the patient. All patients want to be kept informed about how long to expect to wait. Almost all patients will respond positively when the physician or the assistant comes to the reception area to apologize for any delay. Consideration for the patient's time is essential.

Most experts will agree that in a solo or small practice, there should seldom be more than three to five patients in the reception room. Wait time is one of the most frequently heard criticisms of the medical profession. The patient who complains about medical fees or the care received may actually be complaining about the long wait or discourteous service. Most patients are fearful and tense, but the medical assistant can often put them in a better frame of mind with just a friendly smile and a show of concern.

A crowded reception room is not always an indication of a physician's popularity. It may simply mean that the physician or the assistant is inefficient in scheduling patients. Business people, for example, who are in the habit of making the most of their time, are particularly displeased at what may appear to them to be inefficient scheduling of appointments. Any delay of longer than 10 to 15 minutes should be explained to the person waiting. Some personal attention, such as offering a drink of water, a cup of coffee, or a new magazine, may help to calm a patient who appears irritated with the delay. However, be sure that the patient is allowed caffeine before offering coffee. Be careful that the refreshment offered does not go against the physician's orders or would interfere with scheduled blood testing or other procedures.

Patients With Special Needs

Some patients will be physically challenged, some very ill, and some severely uncomfortable. There may be language or cultural barriers. Observe the patient's appearance and behavior. Is the patient pale or drawn looking? Do the eyes or voice reflect pain or discomfort? Find out how the patient is feeling before you suggest that he or she be seated to wait for the physician. The patient may need to lie down in a cool room or perhaps should be seen as an emergency.

The patient who is in a wheelchair or using a walker or crutches may need personal attention. Some patients may need help in disrobing even when a disability is not obvious. Ask if the patient needs assistance. The medical assistant must use good judgment in helping disabled patients, perhaps even bypassing some of the usual routines.

Escorting and Instructing the Patient

Sometimes we become so accustomed to our own surroundings that we forget that a stranger to the practice's environment may be confused or disoriented by all the hallways, doors, and rooms. Uncertainty creates anxiety. Take the time to personally escort the patient to the appropriate examination or treatment room (Figure 11-11). This is usually the responsibility of a clinical medical assistant. If a urine specimen is to be obtained, direct the patient to the rest room.

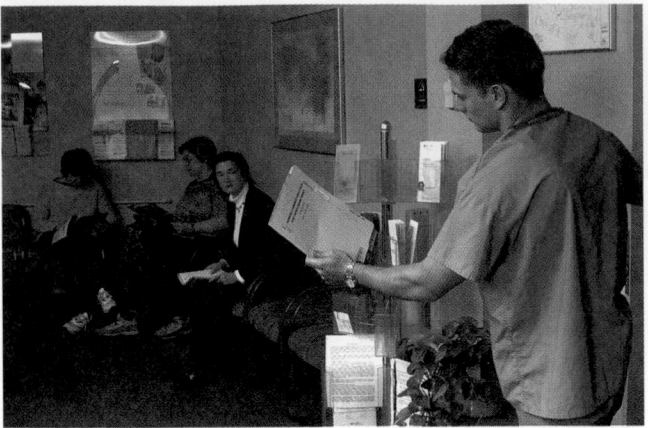

FIGURE 11-11   Pronounce the patient's name correctly and use it often. This promotes good customer service and pleases the patient.

If the patient is to disrobe, explain what garments, if any, can be left on, whether shoes are to be removed, that he or she must remove jewelry if an x-ray film is to be taken, and so forth. If a gown is to be worn, specify whether the opening should be in the front or back and tell the patient where he or she can hang up clothes if this is not obvious. An examination table should never be placed in such a position that the patient is exposed to passersby in the hallway if the door is opened. Imagine a patient ready for a Pap smear, facing the door as the physician enters! Allow patients a sense of modesty at all times and make all instructions crystal clear. Do not assume that patients will know what is expected of them. Be equally clear when the examination has been completed. Tell the patient whether he or she should go to the physician's office for consultation, or return to the reception area to wait, or whether he or she is free to check out with the front office and leave.

The medical assistant can help keep the schedule operating smoothly by immediately tidying each examination room and moving the next patient in so that the physician need have no idle moments waiting for a patient to be prepared. Try not to place a patient in an examination room just to clear out the reception area. It is especially inconsiderate to keep the patient waiting after being gowned, draped, and positioned on the examining table. A magazine rack on the wall of the treatment room is a welcome addition in some practices.

Chart Placement

Patient charts should never be left in the examination room to be picked up and read by a patient. This can cause misunderstandings because patients often do not know medical terms and abbreviations. Physicians have different methods of being signaled that a patient is ready to be seen. Often there are chart holders on the doors of the examination rooms, where the chart can be placed horizontally when the patient is ready to be seen. Then the physician can signal the medical assistant that he or she is finished examining the patient by placing the chart in an upright position on leaving the examination room.

Some offices have call systems, by which a physician can press a button to call the medical assistant for help with the examination. Today's physicians often prefer a second person in the room during examinations to avoid claims of sexual assault or harassment.

Other offices place patients in exam rooms in a certain order, and the physician knows, for instance, that when he or she has finished with the patient in room 1, the next patient will be waiting in room 2. The office should develop a method that allows the most efficient use of time while providing quality care to the patients.

Problem Situations

Talkative Patients

There can be certain problem patients in any professional office. Talkative patients, for example, take up far more of the physician's time than is justified. An alert medical assistant can usually spot this tendency during the initial interview. The patient's history can be **flagged** with a symbol to alert the physician. A prearranged agreement to contact the physician on the **intercom** at the end of the allotted time with the message that the next patient is waiting gives the physician an opportunity to conclude the interview. Once you have learned which patients take extra time, you can book them for the end of the day or simply allow more time for them.

> **CRITICAL THINKING APPLICATION**
>
> Georgina has one patient who insists on sitting close by her desk and attempting to chat the entire time she is waiting to see the physician. What is worse, she comes to her appointments at least an hour early. How might Georgina subtly deal with this patient?

Children

Children frequently present special management problems. It is sometimes advisable to escort younger patients into the treatment room without the parent. Of course, this should be at the discretion of the physician and must be with the permission of the parent. The physician cannot force the parent to leave the examination room by any means. Although this practice of separating children from their parents to treat their needs is not always feasible, it sometimes can be applied with great success. In some offices a token of the physician's friendship, such as a trinket or toy, is given to the child at the completion of the visit.

Angry Patients in the Reception Area

Every medical assistant at some time will be confronted by an angry patient. The anger may simply be a reflection of the patient's pain or fear of what the physician may discover on the examination. If possible, invite the patient into another room out of the reception area. Usually it is best to let the patient talk out his or her anger. A calm attitude on the part of the medical assistant, with a few remarks interjected in a low voice, will often pacify the patient. Under no circumstances should the assistant return the anger or become argumentative.

Patient Relatives

A patient will sometimes be accompanied by a relative or well-meaning friend who may become restless while waiting for the patient and attempt to discuss the patient's illness. The medical assistant should sidestep any discussion of a patient's medical care, except by direction of the physician. Also avoid a too casual attitude, such as "I'm sure there's nothing to worry about." A show of moderate concern and offering reassurance that "the patient is in good hands" usually takes care of the situation.

Patient Check-out

When the patient has been referred back to the front office for check-out, he or she should be greeted with a friendly smile and called by name. It is wise to form the habit of asking the patients if they have any questions once again. Then the chart must be checked to see when the physician wishes the patient to come back to the office. Most physicians will note this information on the encounter form. Make the return appointment, remembering the technique of giving the patient choices as to which day they wish to come, morning or afternoon, and specific time. Then ask the patient for their payment, using phrasing such as, "Your co-pay today is $15, Mrs. Williams. Will you be writing a check or would you like to charge this visit to your Visa?"

Be sure to thank the patient for coming, and wish him or her well as they leave the office (Figure 11-12).

The Friendly Farewell

As soon as the visit with the physician has been completed the medical assistant should be ready to take charge by assisting the patient in dressing, if necessary, and

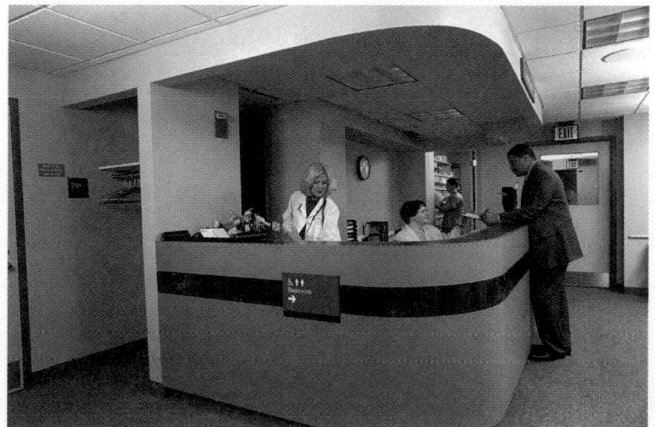

FIGURE 11-12 Always thank the patient for coming and wish him or her well.

by making sure that any questions that the patient may have are answered. In a small practice, this may be the responsibility of the administrative medical assistant.

If the patient has questions that the assistant can capably and ethically answer, the assistant should answer them clearly and note this on the patient's chart. Some questions can be answered only by the physician; in such cases the assistant can offer to get answers for the patient. Remember, patients view the medical assistant as an extension of the physician and the medical assistant must be very careful to avoid accusations of practicing medicine without a license.

The assistant can help convey a sense of caring by terminating the patient's visit cordially. If the patient is returning for another visit, the assistant can say something like "We'll see you next week." If it is the patient's last visit, a pleasant "I certainly hope you'll be feeling fine from now on" is appropriate. The assistant may wish to tell a patient on a last visit that he or she has been a fine patient and that it has been a pleasure to make his or her acquaintance. Whatever words of good-bye are chosen, all patients should leave the facility with the feeling that they have received top-quality care and were treated with friendliness, respect, and courtesy.

Leaving the Office for the Day

Each office should have a specific routine when it is time to leave the office for the day. Patient file cabinets must be locked and secure to help prevent breaches in patient confidentiality. Lab specimens may need to be placed in a lockbox outside the office for pickup. General housekeeping duties are often performed at the end of the day and certain reports may need to be generated for accounting purposes daily, weekly, or monthly. These are usually done at the close of the business day. The phones will usually need to be turned over to the answering service or voicemail.

Those responsible for closing the office should have a method in place for remembering each closing duty. For instance, if the medical assistant knows that five specific things must be done before leaving the office, it may help to devise a **mnemonic** device to jog the memory and ensure that each task is completed. For instance:

*L*eave lab specimens outside
*C*lose patient file cabinets
*L*ock safe
*L*ock file room door
*T*urn off lights
*S*et alarm

The mnemonic that the staff member remembers could be "*Loose cats leave lots to steal.*" The more nonsensical, the easier to remember. This trick can help the medical assistant recall every closing duty every day.

Closing Comments

A personal touch is vital to projecting a sense of care to the patients seen in the physician's office. Many medical offices are not concerned enough about the customer service aspect of the business. Patients talk about their experiences with their friends and relatives and may be an excellent source of referrals if they are treated with dignity and courtesy. If they have had a good experience, they will tell several people. If they have a poor experience, they tend to tell everyone they know! Be sure to have a part in each patient feeling a sense of satisfaction as they leave the office. All patients should feel that their time and money were well spent.

Patient Education

Offering a patient education center in the reception area is an effective way to provide up-to-date information about healthcare issues to patients. Brochures and information sheets can be displayed, and if the office is equipped with a VCR in the reception area, videotapes that deal with health topics can be available for viewing while the patient is waiting to see the physician.

Both the physician and the medical assistants caring for patients should ask if the patient has any questions during his or her visit to the office. Patients often complain that they did not have a chance to speak to the physician long enough to have their questions answered sufficiently. Be sure that this is not the case, and prompt the patient to ask about anything he or she is unclear on while the physician is still in the examination room.

Legal and Ethical Issues

A medical assistant must take care not to offer medical advice to a patient unless specifically instructed to do so by the physician. The patient sees the medical assistant as an extension of the physician and tends to weigh advice and comments by the medical assistant with the same validity as if they came from the physician. Provide only information that the physician has approved or is included in the office policy and procedure manuals.

When a patient complains, listen carefully and attempt to resolve the problem or assure the patient that the issue will be discussed with the appropriate staff member to find a solution. If someone other than the patient asks for information about the patient, refrain from discussion unless the patient or physician has authorized the release of information.

SUMMARY OF SCENARIO

Georgina is a person who truly makes a difference in the healthcare profession. She takes her role seriously as a patient advocate and strives to make her patients feel comfortable in her physician's office. She keeps the mission statement posted close to her desk and rereads it often to keep her focus clear. She shares the vision with the other staff members, who are supportive and in agreement with the purpose for which the office exists.

Dr. Wade promotes continuing medical education and encourages his staff members to participate in courses and seminars that will assist them in being more effective

patient advocates. The office sends birthday and Christmas cards to the patients in their database, and at their annual Christmas Party, the staff hand-signs each Christmas card. Georgina sends a monthly newsletter to the patients, some by mail and some by email, to keep the patients up to date on office policies and interesting health information. All of these activities indicate a strong caring attitude toward the patients. Georgina considers each one a customer of the clinic, and she is determined that they receive excellent customer service.

Wait times are at a minimum in Dr. Wade's office. Cell phone numbers and email addresses are gathered at registration and updated frequently so that the staff can quickly contact patients. Georgina offers new patients a form for evaluation of the office, so that they can provide input about the experience they had as a new patient. All of these efforts promote a trusting, caring relationship among physician, staff, and patients.

SUMMARY OF LEARNING OBJECTIVES

- The office mission statement is the philosophy of why the office exists. Often physicians develop the mission statement themselves, which outlines their vision and reasons for entering medical practice. Some physicians allow the office staff to assist in its development. All employees should become familiar with the mission statement and promote its ideas to all patients and visitors.

- Patient amenities include such things as a VCR, television, computer, telephone, and a desk where patients can sit and balance a checkbook or review work while away from the office. These features turn the time spent in the physician's office into productive minutes instead of wasteful ones.

- Some offices prepare for patient arrivals the evening before, and some in the morning. Patient charts must be pulled and should be reviewed, checking for completed laboratory tests, posting of results, and to ensure that there are ample progress notes for this visit. Rooms should be checked and inventoried to make certain there are enough supplies on hand and that they present a clean, neat appearance.

- People like hearing their own names; a better relationship is built between the staff and patients when the names are used often. Patients feel that the office staff care enough about them to acknowledge them, and this custom adds a personal touch.

- The medical assistant should escort the patient to the examination rooms and other areas of the office. Always tell the patient when to disrobe and exactly what should be removed. Offer to assist with disrobing if the patient needs extra help. Take care that the patient's purse or wallet is in a secure place. Be sure that doors do not open and expose the disrobed patient. Instruct the patient as to whether he or she may leave or should wait after seeing the physician. Ask whether the patient has any questions.

- Some medical offices place patient charts in a door file, which alerts the physician that the patient is ready to be seen. The chart may be placed horizontally or vertically, one placement meaning that the patient is ready for the physician, and the other meaning that the doctor is finished with the patient. Other offices place the charts in door files in a certain order. For example, if examination rooms 1, 2, and 3 are available, patients are seen in that order by the physician.

- Patients who are talkative may be lonely and enjoy the social interaction of their visits to the physician's office. Be as courteous as possible with talkative patients, expressing to them when necessary that another patient is waiting or the physician needs assistance. When said with a smile, most patients understand.

- Closing duties can be easily remembered by creating a mnemonic device, associating each duty with the first letter of each task, then making a nonsense sentence to prompt recollection of those duties. Lists posted close to the door will help, or developing a checklist of closing duties will help the medical assistant recall what to do before leaving for the day.

- The personal touch will help the patient to feel at home and comfortable in the office. An attractive reception area with various patient amenities will provide a warm atmosphere. Using the patient's name often and a gentle touch will impart a sense of caring as well.

KEY INTERNET WEBSITES

- August Incorporated
  For active weblinks to each website visit
  http://evolve.elsevier.com/Kinn/

CHAPTER 12

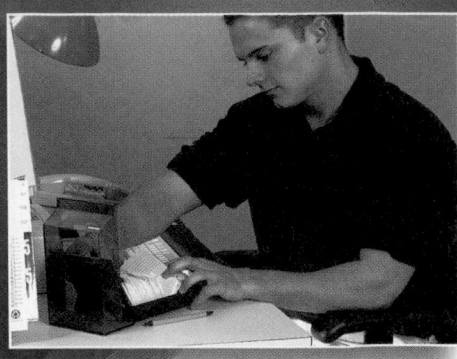

Scenario

Brandon Tipps is a medical assistant working with his father, Dr. Rick Tipps. Brandon has considered continuing his education to become a doctor, but he is not sure whether he would like to be a medical doctor, an osteopathic physician, or a chiropractor. He decided to spend his summer off from college working in his father's family practice so that he could get a close look at the inner workings of a physician's office.

Brandon assisted with every procedure in the clinic, including the administrative skills required in the front office. The staff has been overwhelmed with Brandon's ability to do any task, no matter how small, as if it was the most important task of the office. He continuously moves from employee to employee to ask what he can do to help. When the administrative medical assistant working in the front office, Darla Grover, was injured in a car accident and had to be off work for a while, Brandon stepped right in to her job and learned her duties quickly. His help meant that the office continued to run smoothly even with one employee absent for several weeks.

Brandon has an excellent command of the English language and types at speeds of about 60 wpm. He is organized and efficient, so he is able to handle the enormous amount of incoming and outgoing mail with very little assistance from the office manager. He is also able to answer phones and schedule appointments. He speaks clearly and is an expert at customer service. Many of Dr. Tipps' patients have come to know him during his time in the office. The patients and staff alike will certainly miss him once he returns to college.

Written Communications and Mail Processing

Learning Objectives

- Define and spell the terms listed in the vocabulary.
- Discuss the responsibility of the medical assistant with respect to equipment and supplies.
- List the four common sizes of letterhead stationery.
- Explain the various parts of speech.
- Name some of the essential references for the medical assistant's library.
- List several steps to complete before answering a business letter.
- Discuss the process of developing and the value of keeping a communications portfolio.
- Discuss the differences in the four letter styles.
- Explain the four standard parts of a business letter.
- List several ways to save money when mailing.
- Open, sort, and annotate incoming mail.
- Compose, proofread, and mail a business letter.
- Properly send a fax.

National Curriculum Competencies

COMMUNICATION COMPETENCIES

1a. Respond to and initiate written communication

OPERATIONAL COMPETENCIES

4a. Perform an inventory of supplies and equipment
4b. Utilize computer software to maintain office systems

Vocabulary

academic degree A title conferred by a college, university, or professional school on completion of a program of study.

annotating To furnish with notes, which are usually critical or explanatory.

archaic Of, relating to, or characteristic of an earlier or more primitive time.

archived To have filed or collected records or documents.

bond A durable, formal paper used for documents.

categorically Placed in a specific division of a system of classification.

clauses A group of words containing a subject and predicate and functioning as a member of a complex or compound sentence.

collect on delivery (COD) Method of payment used when an article or item is delivered and payment is expected before it is released.

concise Expressing much in brief form.

continuation pages The second and following pages of a letter.

curt Marked by rude or peremptory shortness.

disseminate To disperse throughout.

domestic mail Mail that is sent within the boundaries of the United States and its territories.

flush Directly abutting or immediately adjacent, as set even with an edge of a type page or column; having no indention.

girth A measure around a body or item.

grammar The study of the classes of words, their inflections, and their functions and relations in the sentence; a study of what is to be preferred and what avoided in inflection and syntax.

international mail Mail that is sent outside the boundaries of the United States and its territories.

intrinsic Belonging to the essential nature or constitution of a thing; indwelling, inward.

portfolio A set of pictures, drawings, documents, or photographs either bound in book form or loose in a folder.

ream A quantity of paper being 20 pounds or, variously, 480, 500, or 516 sheets.

recipient The receiver of some thing or item.

stationers Sellers of stationery.

substance number A number based on the weight of a ream of paper containing 500 sheets.

superfluous Exceeding what is sufficient or necessary.

watermark A marking in paper resulting from differences in thickness usually produced by the pressure of a projecting design in the mold or on a processing roll and visible when the paper is held up to the light.

Entrepreneur and co-founder of the Amway Corporation, Rich de Vos, believed in a simple principle regarding the many business papers that crossed his desk on a daily basis. He believed that each paper should be handled only once. Whatever the news, information, or action required, the paper should be dealt with immediately, and this resulted in the most efficient use of his time. This is an excellent concept that is beneficial in any business, including the medical office.

Correspondence and mail processing can consume a large part of the administrative medical assistant's day. Many physicians, when queried about the skills they most desire in an administrative assistant, have said that a person who can spell accurately and write a good letter is a valuable addition to the medical office. When a physician delegates the responsibility of composing letters or reports that have the potential to reflect positively or negatively on the practice, he or she is expressing confidence in the medical assistant.

Importance of Written Communications

Written communications offer the perfect opportunity for making a good impression on others, but they do not just happen. They require thought, preparation, skill, and a positive attitude. Written communications take many forms in the medical office. The medical assistant should be skilled in creating various forms of communication.

Written communications include original letters, memorandums, replies to inquiries, responses to requests for information, telephone messages, email, transcriptions, orders for supplies, instructions for patients, and a variety of other forms. These communications should be courteous to the reader, correct in content, and concise without being curt. Communication is truly an art as well as a skill. The ability to communicate effectively is extremely important to the administrative medical assistant who wishes to succeed and advance in his or her career.

CRITICAL THINKING APPLICATION

Brandon has just found a small backlog of correspondence that accumulated during the first 3 days that Darla was out of the office. A large amount of mail comes to the office each day. How can Brandon manage the daily mail and clear the pile of communications that accumulated over those 3 days?

Written Communication as a Public Relations Tool

Public relations involves "telling the organization's story." The public relations department or director of any organization exists to present a business in the best possible light and to communicate to the public and other interested parties all of the positive aspects of a business. With this understanding, it is easy to see why written communications are so important. These documents can present a professional image or a very poor image to the receiver. Although individual medical offices rarely employ public relations professionals, each member of the staff must be conscientious about the documents and materials that are present within and that leave the office. An envelope addressed carelessly or a patient information sheet that has been photocopied over and over insinuates that the office personnel are not concerned about the appearance of documents that leave the office. If the staff is careless in this respect, many patients will assume that the staff is careless with everything, including patient care!

Reflection on the Physician

Everything that happens in the medical office is a reflection on the physician or physicians who practice there. Letters with misspelled words or errors will give the reader a negative impression of the physician and the practice itself. Great care must be taken to ensure that each document in the office and sent from the office is well written and grammatically correct. Table 12-1 lists proofreader's marks, while Tables 12-2 and 12-3 list frequently misspelled and misused words.

Equipment and Supplies

To create a favorable impression with letters, the medical assistant must use good equipment and quality supplies. Whatever kind of equipment is available, it is the medical assistant's responsibility to know how to use it to the best advantage and to keep it in good working condition. If the equipment manual is available, study it and keep it handy for reference when problems occur. Know how to maintain equipment so that the effort made in composing the correspondence results in a quality appearance.

Equipment

Computers. Computers have made composing correspondence simple. Various letters and documents may be saved and reused time after time by changing the name and basic information contained within the text. Computers can add graphics to text, compute figures, and use multimedia in communications—all of which enhance the appearance and effectiveness of the document.

Word Processors. Word Processors are used mainly for letter writing and simple documents. The word processor has taken a backseat to today's desktop and notebook computers.

Typewriters. Most typewriters use correctable film ribbons that pass through the spool only one time. However, if the typewriter uses a cotton or silk ribbon that becomes lighter with use, be sure to change the ribbon before the resulting type impression becomes too light. The typewriter keys need to be cleaned frequently in typewriters that use a cotton ribbon. Typewriters, too, are all but **archaic** compared with the versatility of the computer.

Copiers. When a typewriter is used to compose a document, a copier may be used for making any necessary copies of the original. Here, too, maintain the copier so that copies are crisp and clear. The toner must be changed when needed and can be expensive. Multiple copies of documents are usually made on a copier rather than printed from the computer.

Scanners. Occasionally, documents are scanned and sent by email. Scanners provide high resolution and can produce images of written text and photos. Scanners are often used to create images so that older documents can be stored, much like the microfiche systems of the past.

Supplies

Stationery. The quality of paper unquestionably affects the reader's total impression of the communication. **Stationers** or printing companies are qualified to advise on the selection of paper, which can range from all-sulfite (a wood pulp) to all-cotton fiber (sometimes called *rag*). Letterhead paper is usually on **bond** with a 25% or higher cotton fiber content.

The weight of paper is described by a **substance number**. This number is based on the weight of a **ream** consisting of 500 sheets of 17 × 22-inch paper. The larger the substance number, the heavier the paper. If the ream weighs 24 pounds, the paper is referred to as *Sub 24* or *24-pound weight*. Letterhead stationery and matching envelopes are usually 16-, 20-, or 24-pound weight. This is often abbreviated as *16#, 20#,* or *24#.*

Sizes and Types of Letterhead Paper. Letterhead paper is available in four basic sizes:

Standard or letter	8½ × 11 inches
Monarch or executive	8¼ × 10½ inches
Baronial	5½ × 8½ inches
Legal	8½ × 14 inches

Standard letterhead is used for general business and professional correspondence. Monarch is often used by professional people for informal business and social correspondence. Baronial, which is a half-sheet of standard, is used for very short letters or memoranda. Legal, as its name indicates, is used for the lengthy documents presented in court or of a legal nature. Each size of letterhead should have its matching envelope.

Letterhead should be well designed and of a high-quality paper. The letter represents the sender, and the letterhead paper should be carefully chosen to promote the image that the sender wishes to convey. The paper itself makes a strong statement about the business or person it represents and can help the receiver form an impression of the professionalism of the business.

Bond paper has a felt side and a wire side. When a sheet of letterhead is picked up and held to the light, a design or letters can be read from the printed side. This design is called a **watermark** and is an indication of quality. The side from which the watermark can be read is the felt side of the paper and is the side on which printing or typing should be done. The watermark should always read across the page in the same direction as the typing.

Paper with a linen finish is so named because it is similar to fine cloth, with finely spaced lines crossing each other at right angles. Wove is a smooth paper that is normally inexpensive. Antique finish has a semismooth texture, and laid has a finish similar to that of corduroy. All of these paper finishes can make a very professional, impressive letterhead.

TABLE 12-1	Proofreader's Marks	
Proofreader's Mark	**Draft Copy**	**Finished Copy**
55⌈ Single space	55⌈ Read a good book / ⌊every day	Read a good book / every day
ds⌈ Double space	ds⌈ Where will you go / ⌊on your vacation?	Where will you go / on your vacation?
⧉ Indent two spaces	His address is / ⧉450 Newport Avenue	His address is / 450 Newport Avenue
⊙ Insert period	Mr⊙ Herbert Hoover	Mr. Herbert Hoover
⋀ Insert comma	Marysville⋀Indiana	Marysville, Indiana
⊙ Insert colon	Dear Mr. Adams⋀	Dear Mr. Adams:
;/ Insert semicolon	letter of March 6⋀your question	letter of March 6; your question
?/ Insert question mark	Will he come⋀	Will he come?
⋎ Insert apostrophe	the captains ship	the captain's ship
⋎⋎ Insert quotation marks	his remark⋀don't be late⋀	his remark, "don't be late"
=/ Insert hyphen	a one⋀time thing	a one-time thing
# Insert space	townhouse⋀	town house
⋀ Caret—to mark exact position of error	Insert caret to show error⋀#	Insert caret to show error
ꝑ Delete	ꝑ It may ~~not~~ be yours	It may be yours
◡ Close up	Cl◡ose	Close
ꝓ Delete and close up	Me◡erry Christmas	Merry Christmas
¶ Begin new paragraph	¶ At the time	At the time
no¶ No paragraph	no¶ This is correct	This is correct
// Align vertically	‖Ellen Peters / Alice Brown	Ellen Peters / Alice Brown
= Align horizontally	Dear Doctor ⟋Roberts	Dear Doctor Roberts
⌋ Move right	$10,000⌶	$10,000
⌐ Move left	⌐ Read a book	Read a book
⊓ Move up	⌐Move	Move
⊔ Move down	Move	Move
⌋⌐ Center	⌋$10,000⌐	$10,000
∿ Transpose	resile◡i◡nt	resilient
ⓢⓟ Spell out	③ years ago	three years ago
stet.... Let it stand	They were ~~very~~ sad	They were very sad
lc Lower case	It is a Big house	It is a big house
≡ Upper case	Robert birch	Robert Birch
sc Set in small capitals	Regional	REGIONAL
ital Set in italic	special	*special*
bf.... Set in bold	federal government	**federal government**
wf Wrong font	investment	investment
⋎3 Superscript	reference number 3⋎	reference number[3]
7⋀ Subscript	reference number 7⋀	reference number 7
⁀ Ligature Æ	ae⁀sop	æsop

TABLE 12-2	150 Frequently Misspelled or Misused English Words			
absence	corroborate	inimitable	persistent	ridiculous
accede	definitely	inoculate	personal	sacrilegious
accessible	description	insistent	personnel	seize
accommodate	desirable	irrelevant	possession	separate
achieve	despair	irresistible	precede	siege
affect	development	irritable	precedent	similar
agglutinate	dilemma	judgment	predictable	sizable
all right	disappear	labeled	predominant	stationary
altogether	disappoint	led	predominate	stationery
analyses (pl.)	disastrous	leisure	prerogative	subpoena
analysis (s.)	discreet	license	prevalent	succeed
analyze	discrete	liquefy	principal	suddenness
anoint	discriminate	maintenance	principle	superintendent
argument	dissatisfaction	maneuver	privilege	supersede
assistant	dissipate	miscellaneous	procedure	surprise
auxiliary	drunkenness	mischievous	proceed	tariff
balloon	ecstasy	misspell	professor	technique
believe	effect	necessary	pronunciation	thorough
benefited	eligible	newsstand	psychiatry	tranquility
brochure	embarrass	noticeable	psychology	transferred
bulletin	exceed	occasion	pursue	truly
category	exhilaration	occurrence	questionnaire	tyrannize
changeable	existence	oscillate	rearrange	unnecessary
clientele	February	paid	recede	until
committee	forty	pamphlet	receive	vacillate
comparative	grammar	panicky	recommend	vacuum
concede	grievous	parallel	referring	vicious
conscientious	height	paralyze	repetition	warrant
conscious	incidentally	pastime	rheumatism	Wednesday
coolly	indispensable	perseverance	rhythmical	weird

TABLE 12-3	Frequently Misspelled Medical Words			
abscess	defibrillator	intussusception	parietal	pruritus
additive	desiccate	ischemia	paroxysmal	psoriasis
aerosol	ecchymosis	ischium	pemphigus	pyrexia
agglutination	effusion	larynx	percussion	respiratory
albumin	epididymis	leukemia	perforation	rheumatic
anastomosis	epistaxis	malaise	pericardium	roentgenology
aneurysm	eustachian	malleus	perineum	sagittal
anteflexion	fissure	melena	peristalsis	sciatic
arrhythmia	flexure	mellitus	peritoneum	scirrhous
bilirubin	glaucoma	menstruation	petit mal	serous
bronchial	gonorrhea	metastasis	pharynx	sessile
cachexia	graafian	neurilemma	pituitary	sphincter
calcaneus	hemorrhage	neuron	plantar	sphygmomanometer
capillary	hemorrhoids	occlusion	pleura	squamous
cervical	homeostasis	optic chiasm	pleurisy	staphylococcus
chromosome	humerus	oscilloscope	pneumonia	suppuration
cirrhosis	idiosyncracy	osseous	polyp	trochanter
clavicle	ileum	palliative	prophylaxis	venous
curettage	ilium	parasite	prostate	wheal
cyanosis	infarction	parenteral	prosthesis	xiphoid

CRITICAL THINKING APPLICATION

Brandon realizes that his father's office does not have a method of inventory and supply ordering in place. The employees simply order more when they see that a certain supply is getting low, but there is no formal system. This often causes them to run out of certain supplies, especially stationery and envelopes. How might this issue be resolved?

Continuation Pages. The second and continuing pages of a letter are placed on plain bond that matches the letterhead in weight and fiber content. The stationery used for continuation pages should be an exact match to the letterhead, only without the letterhead printing. It is considered unprofessional to use different paper for the continuation pages.

Envelopes. Envelopes are usually made of the same paper as the letterhead stationery. Just as the continuation pages should be the same type of paper as the letterhead, so should the envelopes.

Envelopes also come in the following basic sizes:

- No. 10
- No. 6³/4
- Window

No. 10 envelopes are the general business size used for letter and legal stationery. No. 6³/4 envelopes and window envelopes are often used for statements.

Letter Styles

A business letter is usually arranged in one of three styles: block, modified block or standard, or modified block indented. A fourth style, called *simplified*, is occasionally used. The block and modified block styles are most commonly used in the physician's office.

Block Letter Style

When block letter style is used, all lines start **flush** with the left margin (Figure 12-1). This style is considered the most efficient but is less attractive on the page.

Modified Block Letter Style

The dateline, the complimentary closing, and the type-written signature all begin at the center when typing in modified block letter style. All other lines begin at the left margin (Figure 12-2).

Modified Block Letter Style With Indented Paragraphs

The modified block letter style with indented paragraphs is identical to the block style except that the first line of each paragraph is indented five spaces (Figure 12-3).

Simplified Letter Style

With the simplified letter style, all lines begin flush with the left margin (Figure 12-4). The salutation is

---

Elizabeth Blackwell, M.D.
223 Orange Avenue, N.W.
Cottonwood, UT 84121

January 26, 20—

Mr. Richard Fluege
3678 North Willow Avenue
Palm Beach, FL 33480

Dear Mr. Fluege:

Please send me full particulars on the professional suites you expect to offer for sale or rent in the Medical Arts Professional Annex.

In about six months, I will be ready to open my practice, and I am interested in locating in Florida. My preference is a street-level suite of approximately 2,000 square feet.

After I have had an opportunity to study the information you send me, I will write or telephone you if I have further questions.

Very truly yours,

Elizabeth Blackwell, M.D.

EB:mek

FIGURE 12-1 Block letter style.

MEDICAL ARTS PROFESSIONAL ANNEX
3678 North Willow Avenue
Palm Beach FL 33480

January 29, 20—

Elizabeth Blackwell, M.D.
223 Orange Avenue, N.W.
Cottonwood, UT 84121

Dear Doctor Blackwell:

We have two remaining street-level suites available for occupancy about July 1. These are marked on pages 3 and 4 of the enclosed descriptive brochure. If one of these suites appeals to you, we will be pleased to customize it for your practice.

Please feel free to call me collect at the number on the brochure for further discussion of your needs.

Sincerely yours,

Richard Fluege
Business Manager

RF:ab
Enclosure

FIGURE 12-2   Modified block letter style.

WILLIAM OSLER, M.D.
1000 South West Street
Park Ridge, NJ 07656

January 26, 20—

Robert Koch, M.D.
398 Main Street
Park Ridge, NJ 07656

Dear Doctor Koch:

Mrs. Elaine Norris

Thank you for referring your patient, Mrs. Elaine Norris, for consultation and care. She was examined in my office today.

FINDINGS: The patient complained of pain in the left lower quadrant and some abdominal tenderness. She had a temperature of 100.2 degrees.

RECOMMENDATIONS: The patient was placed on a soft, low-residue, bland diet, antibiotics, and bed rest for a few days. Upper and lower gastrointestinal x-rays will be performed next week.

TENTATIVE DIAGNOSIS: Diverticulitis of large bowel.

Mrs. Norris has been asked to return here for reevaluation in about ten days.

Sincerely yours,

William Osler, M.D.

WO:gm

FIGURE 12-3   Modified block letter style with indented paragraphs.

ROBERT KOCH, M.D.
398 Main Street
Park Ridge, NJ 07656

January 30, 20—

William Osler, M.D.
1000 South West Street
Park Ridge, NJ 07656

ANNABELLE ANDERSON

You will be pleased to know, Bill, that Mrs. Anderson is progressing nicely. Her wound is healing. Her temperature has returned to normal, and she is beginning to resume her usual activities.

Mrs. Anderson has an appointment to return here for one more visit next week. At that time, I will ask her to return to you for any further care.

ROBERT KOCH, M.D.

RK:hb

FIGURE 12-4 Simplified letter style.

replaced with an all-capital subject line on the third line below the inside address. The body of the letter begins on the third line below the subject line. The complimentary closing is omitted. An all-capital typewritten signature is entered on the fifth line below the body of the letter.

Types of Punctuation

Traditionally, the punctuation pattern is selected on the basis of letter style. Normal punctuation is always used within the body of a business letter. The other parts use either standard or open punctuation.

When standard punctuation is used, a colon is placed after the salutation, and a comma is placed after the complimentary closing. This is the punctuation pattern most commonly used. It is appropriate with the block or modified block letter styles.

When open punctuation is used, no punctuation is used at the end of any line outside the body of the letter unless that line ends with an abbreviation. This pattern is always used with the simplified letter style.

Spacing and Margins

Generally, a letter centered on a page is the most attractive. Accomplishing this is easy with today's computer programs, such as Microsoft Word or WordPerfect. Business letters are almost always single spaced. If a letter consists of only a few lines, double-space both the inside address and the message and indent the first line of each paragraph five spaces.

The first typed entry, which is the date, is usually placed on the third line below the letterhead or on line 13 if there is no letterhead. Continuation pages begin 1 inch from the top.

On standard letterhead, the side margins are usually $1^1/2$ to 1 inches on each side. The appearance of a very short letter is improved by increasing the width of all margins.

A 1-inch bottom margin is the minimum. This can be increased if the letter is to be carried over to a second page. Never use a second page to type only the complimentary closing and signature. Carry over a minimum of two lines of the body of the letter.

Parts of Letters

The structure of a letter and its placement on a page have been fairly well standardized into the following main parts:
- Heading
- Opening
- Body
- Closing

Heading

The heading includes the letterhead and the dateline. The printed letterhead is usually centered at the top of the page and includes the name of the physician or group and the address. It may include the telephone number and the medical specialty or specialties. In a group or corporate practice, the names of the physicians may also be listed. Occasionally, the heading also includes the name of an office manager.

The dateline consists of the name of the month written in full, followed by the day and year. The date should not be abbreviated, nor should ordinal numbers (e.g., 1st, 2nd, and 3rd) be used after the name of the month.

Opening

The opening consists of the inside address, the salutation, and the attention line, if there is one. The inside address has two or more lines, starts flush with the left margin, and contains at least the name of the individual or firm to whom the letter is addressed and the mailing address. When the letter is addressed to an individual, the name is preceded by a courtesy title, such as *Dr.*, *Mr.*, *Mrs.*, *Miss*, or *Ms*. When addressing a letter to a physician, omit the courtesy title and type the physician's name followed by his or her **academic degree**, such as *Rick P. Tipps, MD*. Do not use both a courtesy title and a degree that mean the same thing, as in *Dr. Rick P. Tipps, MD*.

CRITICAL THINKING APPLICATION

Brandon has noticed that some of the correspondence leaving the office is signed incorrectly, with "Dr. Rick P. Tipps, MD" in the typed signature line. This is an uncomfortable situation because Brandon realizes that the person who is typing the signature this way is the office manager.
- How might he approach her so that the mistake can be corrected?
- Is it wise to approach the office manager, or should Brandon go to his father? Why or why not?

The salutation is the letter writer's introductory greeting to the person being addressed. It is typed flush with the left margin on the second line below the last line of the address and is followed by a colon unless open punctuation is used. The words in the salutation vary depending on the degree of formality of the letter.

The attention line, if used, is placed on the second line below the inside address. If the name of the person for whom the letter is intended is known, that person's name is used in the inside address and he or she is addressed personally. If the letter is being addressed to a company or organization and directed to a division or department within the company, the division or department name is placed on the attention line.

Body

The body of a letter includes the subject line, if one is used, and the message. In medical office correspondence, the subject of a letter is frequently a patient. The patient's name is used as the subject line. Because the subject line is considered to be a part of the body of the letter, it is placed on the second line below the salutation. It may start flush with the left margin or at the point of indentation of indented paragraphs, or it may be centered. The word *subject*, followed by a colon, may be used or omitted entirely.

Begin typing the message on the second line below the subject line or on the second line below the salutation if there is no subject line. The first line of each paragraph may be indented five spaces or may start flush with the left margin, depending on the chosen letter style.

Closing

The closing includes the complimentary closing, the typed signature, the reference initials, and any special notations.

The complimentary closing is the writer's way of saying good-bye. It is placed on the second line below the last line of the body of the letter and is followed by a comma unless open punctuation is used. Only the first word is capitalized. The words used are determined by the degree of formality in the salutation. For example, if the salutation is *Dear Herb*, the closing might be *Cordially*, *Very truly yours*, or *Sincerely yours* with consistent punctuation. If the letter is addressed to a business, the complimentary closing most used is *Sincerely*.

A typewritten signature is a courtesy to the reader, especially if the name does not appear on the printed letterhead or if the personal signature is difficult or impossible to decipher. The typewritten signature is placed on the fourth line directly below the complimentary closing.

Reference initials that identify the typist are placed flush with the left margin on the second line below the typewritten signature. If the writer's name is included on the signature line, the writer's initials need not be included in the reference block unless desired. The writer's initials, if used, should precede the typist's initials and are separated by a colon or diagonal line. Examples include *mek*, *GB:mek*, or *GB/mek*.

Special notations are sometimes needed to indicate that enclosures are included with the letter or that copies of the letter are being distributed to others. If the letter indicates an enclosure, type the word *Enclosure* or *Enc.* on the first line below the reference initials. If there is more than one enclosure, specify the number (e.g., *Enclosures 3*). If copies are to be sent to others, type this notation in the same manner as the enclosure notation or after it if both notations are needed. The copy notation is usually written as *c:* or *copy to:* followed by the name or names of those to whom a copy will be sent. If the person to whom the letter is addressed is not to know that copies are being distributed to others, use the notation *bc:* for "blind copy" on all copies *except* the original. Place this notation either in the upper left of the letter at the margin or below the last notation at the lower left margin.

Postscripts

Although a postscript may sometimes be used to express an afterthought, it is often used to place emphasis on an idea or statement. Begin the postscript on the second line below the last special notation. Follow the style of the letter, indenting the first line if paragraphs were indented in the body of the letter or starting at the margin if indentation was not used in the letter.

Continuation Pages

If the letter requires one or more **continuation pages**, the heading of the second and subsequent pages must contain the following three items of information:
- The name of the addressee
- The page number
- The date

The heading should begin on the seventh line from the top of the page. Continuation of the body of the letter begins on the tenth line or the third line below the heading. There are three accepted forms for the continuation page heading, as shown below:

Rick P. Tipps, M.D.
Page 2
July 5, 2003

Rick P. Tipps, M.D.
Page 2
July 5, 2003
Subject: Susan Clemmons

Rick P. Tipps, M.D.   -2-   July 5, 2003

Signing the Letter

Some physicians prefer to compose and sign all letters that leave their offices. The majority are more than pleased to delegate to a competent assistant the responsibility of composing and signing letters of a business nature. Although not all authorities agree on the form to be followed, most recommend that a woman's typewritten signature includes a courtesy title (Miss, Mrs., or Ms.) and that the title not be enclosed in parentheses. It is not necessary to include the courtesy title in the handwritten signature.

In general, the physician signs all of the following:
- Letters that deal with medical advice to patients
- Letters to officers or committees of the medical society
- Referral and consultation reports to colleagues
- Medical reports to insurance companies
- Personal letters

The medical assistant usually composes and signs letters dealing with the following matters:
- Routine matters such as arranging or rescheduling appointments
- Orders for office supplies
- Notification to patients about surgery or hospital arrangements
- Collection of delinquent accounts
- Letters of solicitation

CRITICAL THINKING APPLICATION

One of the employees has brought an urgent letter to Brandon that his father neglected to sign before leaving the office for the day. The letter is to another physician reporting his findings on a referred patient. The employee asks Brandon to sign the letter. What should he do? What are some ways to resolve this situation, if the letter must leave in the mail today?

Writing Skills and Composing Tips

Business letters are much different than the social letters that the medical assistant may have written. Social letters tend to be long and chatty and do not necessarily follow any organized plan. Most business letters should be less than one page in length and carefully organized (Procedure 12-1). This takes practice and preparation.

The medical assistant should carefully read the letter to be answered. Make note of or underline any questions asked or materials requested. Then decide on the answers to the questions and verify the information. This is called **annotating**. Draft a reply, and then rewrite for clarity (Procedure 12-2). Keep most of the sentences short. Put only one idea in each sentence, and eliminate **superfluous** words. Be careful about using medical terms in correspondence with patients. Instead, use language that the reader will easily understand. Every person who writes letters develops his or her own personal style.

Most physicians conform to a highly professional and formal style in their dictation. The medical assistant who is given the responsibility of composing correspondence for the medical office should strive for the same degree of formality used by the physician. It would be inappropriate for the assistant to write in a breezy, informal style when acting as the representative of an employer who is more formal in his or her approach. The principal point to remember is that every letter produced in your office should project the image of the physician regardless of who composes or signs the letter.

Grammar Review

Good **grammar** is essential to writing effective, professional business letters. The medical assistant should have an understanding of the elements of acceptable grammar and writing skills.

Parts of Speech

Nouns. A noun is a person, place, or thing. Nouns can also be a thought, an idea, or a concept, as in *freedom* or *courage*. Common nouns name general persons, places, or things, such as *teacher* and *city*. Proper nouns are specific, such as *Mrs. Roberts* and *New York City*.

PROCEDURE 12-1

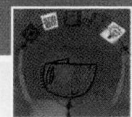

Composing Business Correspondence

GOAL: To compose a letter that will convey information in an accurate and concise manner, and that is easy to comprehend by the reader.

EQUIPMENT AND SUPPLIES

- Computer or word processor
- Word processing software
- Draft paper
- Letterhead
- Printer
- Pen or pencil
- Highlighter
- Envelope
- Correspondence to be answered
- Other pertinent information needed to compose a letter
- Electronic or hard cover dictionary and thesaurus
- Writer's handbook
- Portfolio

PROCEDURAL STEPS

1 Read through any correspondence to be answered and highlight the specific questions that should be addressed.

Purpose: To make certain that all of the issues raised in the correspondence are answered.

2 Make any necessary notes on the letter or a copy of the letter. A scrap sheet of paper may be used.

3 Prepare a draft of the letter using good grammatical skills and save it in the computer or word processor.

Purpose: To put the thoughts on paper for later revision and make the letter easy to understand for the reader.

4 Proofread a printed copy of the letter, using proofreader's marks to make corrections.

Purpose: To see the document as it will look once printed, and speed the process of writing by using proofreader's marks.

5 Make any necessary corrections.

6 Allow the physician or other interested parties to proofread the letter, if the medical assistant is not the person whose signature will appear at the bottom.

Purpose: To give the physician an opportunity to correct the letter and add additional thoughts, if desired.

7 Make any final changes, then print the letter on stationery. Allow the person whose name appears at the bottom to sign the letter.

8 Address the envelope using OCR guidelines and place the letter and any supporting documents inside. See Procedure 12-5 for using USPO OCR guidelines.

9 Mail the letter using correct postage.

Purpose: Using incorrect postage or guessing can delay the arrival time of the document.

Pronouns. Pronouns replace nouns and provide the writer with shortcuts so that proper nouns do not have to be constantly repeated. Pronouns include words such as *it, you, he, she, her, his, them, mine, you, yours, its, ours,* and *theirs.*

Verbs. Verbs are action words that express movement, such as *runs, drove,* or *type.* Linking verbs express a condition or state of being and include *am, are, was, be,* and *been.* Linking verbs also express the senses, as in *smell, hear, taste, touch, feel,* and *look.*

Adjectives. Adjectives are words that describe nouns and pronouns or may show which one, how many, and what kind of. *A, an,* and *the* are special types of adjectives called *articles.* Examples of adjectives include a *golden* sunset, a *mangy* dog, and a *crooked* nose.

Adverbs. Just as adjectives describe nouns, adverbs describe verbs, adjectives, or other adverbs. Adverbs specify when, where, to what extent, or how. Examples include *unusually* warm, *never* won, and *quite* cold.

Prepositions. Connecting words that show a relationship between nouns, pronouns, or other words in a sentence are called *prepositions.* Examples of prepositions include *by, from, of, to, in, at, with, into,* and *on.*

Conjunctions. Conjunctions join words or phrases. These helpful words include *and, or, nor,* and *but.*

Interjections. Interjections show strong feeling. They are often followed by an exclamation point and sometimes by a comma. *"Ouch! That really hurt!"* is a sentence that uses an interjection.

Making Sense of Sentences

Sentence structure is important when writing a professional letter or document. The medical assistant should know the basics of good sentence structure so that written documents will make sense and represent the medical facility and staff in a positive way.

PROCEDURE 12-2

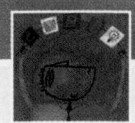

Proofreading Written Correspondence

GOAL: To compose a clearly written, grammatically correct business letter that is easily understood by the reader, and to eliminate spelling errors.

EQUIPMENT AND SUPPLIES

- Stationery
- Computer or typewriter
- Correspondence to be answered or notes

PROCEDURAL STEPS

1 Place the stationery into the printer or typewriter.

2 Scan through the letter to be answered or the notes about the correspondence to be written and highlight any questions that should be answered or points to be made.
Purpose: To ensure that the goals of the correspondence are fulfilled and no important points are omitted.

3 Write the letter using grammatical guidelines.

4 Print a draft copy of the letter. Read it carefully and highlight changes to be made or note any additions to be made. Use proofreader's marks.

Purpose: Seeing a hard copy of a letter is more conducive to finding errors and grammatical mistakes.

5 Revise the letter using the notes.

6 Read the letter once again on the screen. Complete spell and grammar checks if those tools are available on the computer.
Purpose: To locate any missed errors or misspelled words.

7 Print a final draft. Read the letter word for word and check once again for errors.

8 Have another person proofread especially important correspondence.
Purpose: Often another person can locate missed errors quickly.

9 Complete the final preparations for mailing the letter. Address the letter using guidelines for OCR and fast processing at the post office.

Types of Sentences. There are four basic sentence types, as follows: declarative, interrogatory, imperative, and exclamatory. Declarative sentences make a statement, whereas interrogatory sentences ask a question. Imperative sentences state a command or request. Exclamatory sentences express strong feeling. An example of each type is listed below.

Declarative	*She was the last person here.*
Interrogatory	*Are we going to the fair today?*
Imperative	*Clean your room before dinner.*
Exclamatory	*I am so excited for you!*

Sentence Structure. Sentences, when written correctly, follow certain patterns. There are three very basic patterns that are used in constructing sentences. These patterns are:
- Subject-predicate
- Subject-object
- Subject-complement

The subject of a sentence is usually a noun and is the word or group of words in a sentence that acts, is acted on, or is described by the verb. The predicate is the part of the sentence that contains the verb and tells what the subject is doing or experiencing or what is being done to the subject. The object is a noun, pronoun, or group of words functioning as a noun or pronoun that receives the action of the verb. The complement is a word or group of words in the predicate of a sentence that renames or describes a subject or object in that sentence.

Sentence Errors. Three main sentence errors plague most writers. These include the sentence fragment, the run-on sentence, and the comma splice.

A sentence fragment is an incomplete thought or a portion of a sentence that is punctuated as though it were a complete sentence. An example follows:

Although the doctor had seen the patient.

A run-on sentence contains independent **clauses** without a semicolon, comma, or conjunction between them. These sentences are also called *run-together* or *fused sentences*. An example follows:

The office was clean when the staff left on Friday the doors were locked.

A comma splice is a sentence in which a comma alone joins independent clauses. An example follows:

The storm grew worse, it began to snow.

More Types of Written Communications

There are many types of written communications other than a business letter. One of the most common types of written communication in the medical office is the telephone message. Seven items must be recorded when taking a phone message, including the following:

- The name of the person to whom the call is directed
- The name of the person calling
- The caller's daytime and/or cell phone number
- The reason for the call
- The action to be taken
- The date and time of the call
- The initials of the person taking the call

Email is a very popular way to send written communications in today's computer-literate society. Email messages can be saved, printed for the patient's chart, and **archived** for storage.

Faxes are another form of written communication. All faxes should have a cover sheet that states that the information contained within it is of a confidential nature and is intended only for the person to whom the fax was sent (Procedure 12-3).

Most offices **disseminate** various memorandums throughout the business week (Figure 12-5). These written documents must also be clear, concise, and grammatically correct.

CRITICAL THINKING APPLICATION

- Email is used more and more often to communicate with employees. Brandon has noticed that there are very few printed memos that circulate throughout the office. What are the advantages and disadvantages of communicating through email with employees?
- The office manager has given Brandon information to disseminate to all of the employees of the clinic. She did not specify whether to give out the memo by hand or by email but did state that the information was very important. Which would be the best method?

Personal Tools

Competent handling of written communications requires a basic knowledge of composition. A personal reference library that includes an up-to-date standard dictionary, a medical dictionary, a composition handbook, an English-language reference manual, and a thesaurus will be a tremendous help.

For those who have difficulty with spelling, keep a small loose-leaf indexed notebook or card index of words that are troublesome. When it is necessary to look up a word in the dictionary for spelling, record it in the notebook or card index for quick reference. The physician or a medical assistant who is familiar with the practice might compile a basic list of frequently used medical terms and abbreviations as a reference for the trainee.

PROCEDURE 12-3

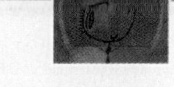

Preparing a FAX for Transmission

GOAL: To send a FAX from the medical office and ensure that it arrives at its destination in a confidential manner.

EQUIPMENT AND SUPPLIES
- FAX machine
- FAX cover sheet
- Correspondence to be sent

PROCEDURAL STEPS

1 Fill out a FAX cover sheet. Include the name of the person sending the FAX and that person's phone number. List the name of the person to receive the FAX and the FAX number where the document is being sent. Use cover sheets that contain a confidentiality statement.

Purpose: To identify a FAX that has been misdirected and to ensure that it goes to the right person when it arrives.

2 Note the number of pages that are being sent, including the cover page.

Purpose: To ensure that all pages are received.

3 Turn the last page upside down and write the fax number on the top of the document. Many machines require the documents to be in place prior to starting the fax. This allows the user to see the number without having to memorize it and make an error.

Purpose: To see the FAX number clearly once the pages have been placed in the FAX machine.

4 Follow the instructions for individual FAX machines.

5 Be sure the machine is set to provide a verification that the fax went through. Print the verification and attach it to the fax. Verify the arrival of critical FAX documents on the phone.

Purpose: To document that the fax arrived at its destination.

6 File the fax and verification sheet in the appropriate location.

Purpose: To maintain a record of information sent via FAX.

INTEROFFICE MEMORANDUM

TO   All Staff

FROM   Office Manager

DATE   December 1

SUBJECT   Holiday Schedule

Our entire facility will be closed on December 24, December 25, December 31, and January 1. The office will be on reduced staff during the days of December 26, 27, 28, 29, and 30. Assignments will be based on seniority of staff members. Please submit your preferences as soon as possible.

A

MEMO TO: George Walker

FROM: Stanley Barr

DATE: February 8

SUBJECT: Office rental

We are experiencing unexpectedly rapid growth in our business office and will soon need additional space for our increased number of employees. Do you have a larger facility available in this building? If so, I would like to hear from you regarding the location, square footage, and anticipated rental costs.

B

FIGURE 12-5 **A** and **B**, Examples of memoranda. Memos are intended to be short, specific, and to the point.

Developing a Portfolio

Letter composition can be sped up by developing a **portfolio** of sample letters to suit the various situations that frequently arise. As the physician approves letters, add them to the office portfolio. Suppose, for instance, a letter is needed for a patient who wishes to change an appointment. Compose a letter that is clear, concise, and courteous—and make an extra copy to place in the portfolio of letters. Alternatively, if using a computer, store the letter on a disk or on the computer's hard drive. If letters and other documents are stored on the hard drive, be sure to back the files up on disk or a zip drive. Do this each time a new kind of letter is written. Soon, the medical assistant will be able to select a letter from the portfolio and change it slightly to suit the current situation. This will make letter writing in the medical office quick and easy.

Mail Processing

Incoming Mail

Each day, a great variety of mail comes into the professional office and must be processed. Common items in the daily mail include the following:
- General correspondence
- Payments for services
- Bills for office purchases
- Insurance claim forms to be completed
- Laboratory reports
- Hospital reports
- Medical society mailings
- Professional journals
- Promotional literature and samples from pharmaceutical houses
- Advertisements

In large clinics and medical centers, the mail is opened by specially designated people in a central department to speed up this daily task. In the average medical office, however, a medical assistant opens the mail using the ordinary letter-opener method.

Opening the Mail

Before opening any mail, the medical assistant should have an agreement with the physician as to what procedure to follow regarding incoming mail—in other words, what letters should be opened and what pieces, if any, the physician prefers to open personally. For example, the physician may prefer to open any communications from an attorney or accountant, even when they are not marked *personal*. If there is any doubt in regard to opening an envelope, do not open the item and forward it to the person to whom it is addressed. Even a simple procedure such as opening the daily mail can be done with more efficiency if a good system is followed (Procedure 12-4).

Annotating

Annotating the mail is an additional service the medical assistant can perform. By reading each letter through, underlining the significant words and phrases, and noting

PROCEDURE 12-4

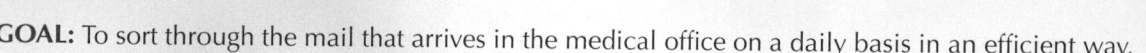

Opening the Daily Mail

GOAL: To sort through the mail that arrives in the medical office on a daily basis in an efficient way.

EQUIPMENT AND SUPPLIES

- Computer or word processor
- Draft paper
- Letterhead stationery
- Pen or pencil
- Highlighter
- Staple remover
- Paper clips
- Letter opener
- Stapler
- Transparent tape
- Date stamp

PROCEDURAL STEPS

1 Have a clear working space on the desk or countertop.

2 Sort the mail according to importance and urgency:

- Physician's personal mail
- Ordinary first-class mail
- Checks from insurance companies and patients
- Periodicals and newspapers
- All other pieces, including drug samples

3 Open the mail neatly and in an organized manner.

4 Stack the envelopes so that they are all facing in the same direction.

5 Pick up the top one and tap the envelope so that when you open it you will not cut the contents.

6 Open all envelopes along the top edge for easiest removal of contents.

7 Remove the contents of each envelope and hold the envelope to the light to see that nothing remains inside.

8 Make a note of the postmark when this is important.

9 Discard the envelope after you have checked to see that there is a return address on the message contained inside. Some offices make it a policy to attach the envelope to each piece of correspondence until it has received attention.

10 Date-stamp the letter and attach any enclosures.

11 If there is an enclosure notation at the bottom of the letter, ensure that the enclosure was included. If it is missing, indicate this on the notation by writing the word *no* and circling it. This may be as far as your employer will want you to proceed with handling the correspondence.

in the margin any action required, taking action on the mail is much easier. If the letter needs no reply, code it for filing at this time. A highlighter that does not photocopy may be used for annotating. When mail refers to previous correspondence, obtain this from the file and attach it or a copy. If the patient's chart is needed when replying to an inquiry, pull the chart and place it with the letter.

There should be a specific place for placing the opened and annotated mail in the medical office. This will probably be some area on the physician's or office manager's desk. After sorting, opening, and annotating the mail, place those items that the physician will wish to see in the established place, with the most important mail on top. Personal mail, of course, is to remain unopened. If a piece of personal mail addressed to the employer is opened in error, fold and replace it inside the envelope, and write across the outside *opened in error*, followed by the initials of the person who opened the mail. Use the same procedure with a piece of mail addressed to another office that may have been opened in error. In such cases, reseal the envelope with transparent tape and hand it to the mail carrier.

Responding to the Mail

In some offices, the physician and the medical assistant go over the mail together. Once the medical assistant gains confidence, he or she will find it easy to draft a reply to most inquiries. Usually, the physician is very pleased to delegate this responsibility, especially on matters that do not relate to patient care.

Letters of referral from other physicians should be carefully noted so that an answer may be sent after the patient has been seen and the physician can give a report. If considerable time may pass before such information can be sent, it is a courteous gesture to write a letter to the referring physician advising that a detailed report will follow. Some physicians send printed cards expressing thanks for referrals; others prefer to write thank-you letters to professional colleagues.

Mail Requiring Special Handling

Payment Receipts. Payments from patients and insurance companies will come to the office on a daily basis. All payments should be separated and recorded immediately in the day's receipts. If the patient requests a receipt, it should be mailed. Otherwise, the receipt may be placed in the patient's chart for delivery on a future office visit.

CRITICAL THINKING APPLICATION

Brandon notices that Mrs. Attaway, a widow and long-time patient of his father's, sent in a check for $125 for a bill. However, her insurance company had already paid $112 toward the bill. Brandon knows that Mrs. Attaway must be very careful with her money and has always paid her bills quickly. The policy of the office is to route the overpayment through the system, but refund checks are cut only once per month. What should Brandon do in this situation?

Insurance Information. Insurance information should be put in a predetermined place for handling by the billers. Documents relating to insurance should be passed to the appropriate person immediately to avoid delays and time limitations that might cause the claim to go unpaid.

Drug Samples. Sample drugs and related literature are usually delivered by pharmaceutical representatives, and may occasionally arrive in the mail. Determine from the physician what types of literature and samples should be saved. Most physicians keep pertinent new samples in a sample storage area, along with the accompanying literature for immediate reference. Other drug samples are **categorically** stored. Drugs should never be tossed into the trash.

Vacation Mail. When the physician is away from the office, it is generally the responsibility of a medical assistant to handle all mail. In this event, all pieces should be examined carefully. The medical assistant can then decide how to handle each piece based on the following questions:

- Is this important enough that I should phone or fax the physician?
- Shall I forward this for immediate attention?
- Shall I answer this myself or send a brief note to the correspondent, explaining that there will be a slight delay because the physician is out of the office?
- Can this wait for attention until the physician returns without appearing negligent?

If the medical assistant is unable to contact the physician or to forward important mail, he or she should always answer the sender immediately, explaining the delay and requesting cooperation. Instead of forwarding an original piece of mail and risking possible loss, make a copy for forwarding. Then, if the physician wishes the letter answered, notations can be made on the copy and returned without defacing the original letter.

When the physician is traveling from place to place, the envelope on each communication should be numbered consecutively. Doing this enables the physician to easily determine whether any mail has been lost or delayed. By keeping a record of each piece of mail sent out, with its corresponding number, anything that might be lost can be identified and remailed if necessary.

Correspondence not requiring immediate action that the medical assistant is unable to answer until the physician returns should be placed in a special folder marked *Requires Attention* and placed on top of other accumulated mail. Mail that the medical assistant can compose but that requires the physician's approval before mailing should be put into another special folder marked *For Approval*. When the physician returns, these letters can be rapidly checked and signed.

Any letters marked *Personal* may be acknowledged to the return address on the envelope. The brief acknowledgment should state that the physician is out of town for a certain length of time and will attend to the letter immediately on returning. This acknowledgment should also offer help in any way possible in the meantime.

Discard any mail that would ordinarily not be brought to the physician's attention. Some promotional literature falls into this category. Make certain that mailings from professional organizations are saved.

There may be rare periods when the entire facility is closed. In such cases, the post office can be contacted to hold mail until the facility reopens. The postal carrier cannot accept an oral request, so a formal request must be made. Never leave mail unattended to gather outside a mailbox or clutter up a doorway in a hall. Even mail slots may become filled or magazines may become stuck in them, causing important mail to pile up outside the slot. Far too much money and mail of a confidential nature are sent to physicians' offices to take chances on mail theft or destruction.

Outgoing Mail

Folding and Inserting Letters. Standard ways of folding and inserting letters are used so that the letter fits properly into the envelope and so that it can be easily removed without damage (Figure 12-6).

No. 10 Envelope. Bring the bottom third of the standard-sized letter up and make a crease. Fold the top of the letter down to within about $3/8$ inch of the creased edge and make a second crease. The second crease goes into the envelope first.

No. $6^3/4$ Envelope. For a standard-sized letter, bring the bottom edge up to within about $3/8$ inch of the top edge and make a crease. Then, folding from the right edge, make a fold a little less than one third of the width of the sheet and crease it. Folding from the left edge, bring the edge to within about $3/8$ inch of the previous crease. Insert the left creased edge into the envelope first.

Window Envelope. To fold a letter for insertion into a window envelope, bring the bottom third of the letter up and make a crease, then fold the top of the letter back to the crease you made before. The inside address should now be facing forward. This method is often followed for mailing statements.

Addressing the Envelope

Mailing Addresses. The U.S. Postal Service attempts to have all mail in standard-sized envelopes read, coded,

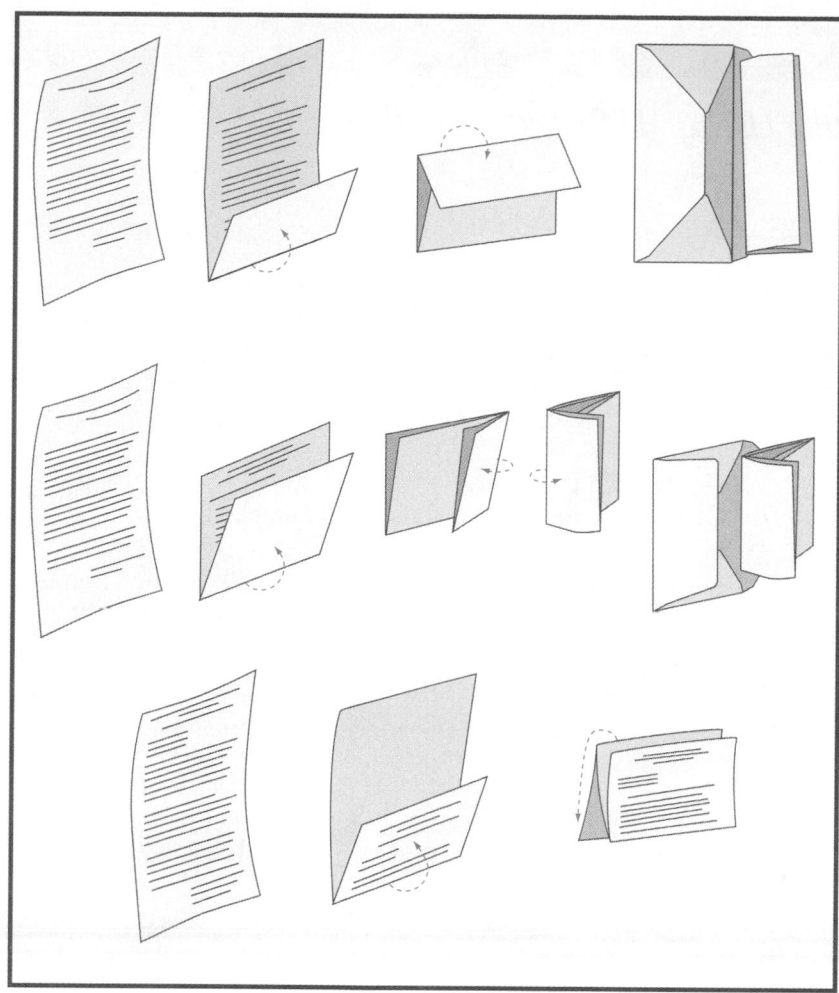

FIGURE 12-6 Correct methods of folding letters.

sorted, and canceled automatically at regional sorting stations where mail can be processed at a rate of 30,000 letters per hour. The success of automatic sorting depends on the cooperation of mailers in preparing envelopes in a format that can be read by automatic equipment (Procedure 12-5).

KEY POINTS FOR ADDRESSING ENVELOPES

- Use dark type on a light background; black on white is best.
- Do not use script or italic type; an electronic scanner cannot read these.
- Type all addresses in block format and in the area on the envelope that the scanner is programmed to read.
- Capitalize everything in the address.
- Eliminate all punctuation in the address.
- Use the standard two-letter state code instead of the spelled out name of the state.

- The last line of the address must contain the city, state code, and ZIP code, and it must not exceed 27 characters in length.
- The characters should be distributed so that they will not exceed the following limits:

Allowance for city name	13
Space between city name and state code	1
Allowance for state code	2
Space between state code and ZIP code	1
Space for basic ZIP code	5
Space for hyphen and four additional characters	5

If a city name contains more than 13 characters, you must use the approved code for that city as shown in the Abbreviations Section of the National Zip Code Directory.

MEDICAL ASSOCIATES INCORPORATED
4444 AVENIDA WILSHIRE
SAN CLEMENTE CA 92672-1500

HENRY B TURNER MD
PO BOX 845
JACKSONVILLE FL 32232-9950

PROCEDURE 12-5

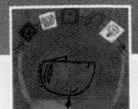

Addressing Outgoing Mail Using U.S. Post Office OCR Guidelines

GOAL: To correctly address business correspondence so that the mail arrives and is processed by the U.S. Post Office as efficiently as possible.

EQUIPMENT AND SUPPLIES

- Envelopes
- Computer or typewriter
- Correspondence

PROCEDURAL STEPS

1 Place the envelope into the printer or typewriter.

2 Enter the word processing program, such as Microsoft Word, and check the "Tools" section for envelopes. If this is not available in the word processing program, or a typewriter is being used, judge the area on the envelope that can be read by the optical character reader (OCR). The address block should start no higher than 2¾ inches from the bottom. Leave a bottom margin of at least ⅝ inch and left and right margins of at least 1 inch. Nothing should be written or printed below the address block or to the right of it.

Purpose: To ensure the correct placement of the address for accurate reading by the OCR.

3 Use dark type on a light background, no script or italics, and capitalize everything in the address.

Purpose: To ensure that the OCR can read the address.

4 Type the address in block format, using only approved abbreviations and eliminating all punctuation.

5 Type the city, state, and zip code on the last line of the address.

6 No line should have more than 27 total characters, including spaces.

7 Leave a ⅝-inch by 4¾-inch space blank in the bottom right corner of the envelope.

Purpose: To allow for bar code scanning (BCS).

8 Mail addressed to other countries includes the city and postal code on the third line, and the name of the country on a fourth line.

The Postal Service provides three special sets of abbreviations: (1) state names; (2) long names of cities, towns, and places; and (3) names of streets and roads and general terms, such as University or Institute. The information can be obtained from the Postal Service, or a program can be purchased for the computer. When these abbreviations are used, it is possible to limit the last line of any domestic address to 27 strokes. The next-to-last line in the address block should contain a street address or post office box number.

The address block should start no higher than 2³/₄ inches from the bottom. Leave a bottom margin of at least ⅝ inch and left and right margins of at least 1 inch. Nothing should be written or printed below the address block or to the right of it.

The regulations for addressing envelopes were developed mainly for volume mailers with computerized mailing lists (Figure 12-7). Some exceptions are acceptable to the Postal Service and its scanning equipment. For example, the traditional style of typing an address in lower case with initial capital letters is readable by the optical scanners. Also, if the ZIP code cannot fit on the line with the city and state, it can be placed on the line immediately below.

Return Addresses. Always place a complete return address on the envelope. The U.S. Postal Service will not deliver mail without postage. If there is no stamp on the envelope or if the stamp falls off and there is no return address, it will go to the dead letter office. There, the postal employees will open the mail in an attempt to identify the sender, but huge time delays may make the mail useless on delivery. If an address is found for the sender, the mail will be returned in an official envelope with a notice of postage due. If an address is not found for the sender, the mail is destroyed.

Notations. Any notations on the envelope directed toward the addressee, such as *Personal* or *Confidential*, should be typed and underlined on line 9 or on the third line below the return address, whichever is lower. Align it with the return address on the left edge of the envelope.

Any notations directed toward the postal service, such as *special delivery* or *certified mail*, should be typed in all capital letters on the upper right side of the envelope immediately below the stamp area. If an address contains an attention line, it should be typed above the organization line or on the line immediately above the street address or post office box number.

Sealing and Stamping Hints. Here's a suggestion for speeding up the sealing of a number of envelopes; at statement time, for example, many envelopes go into the mail at one time:

- Fan out unsealed envelopes, address side down, in groups of six to ten.

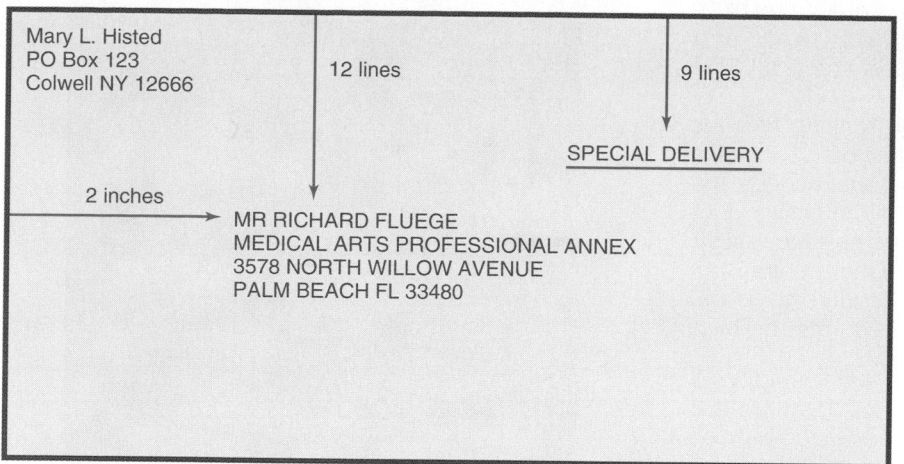

Placement of return address, mailing address, and mailing notation on 6 3/4 envelope

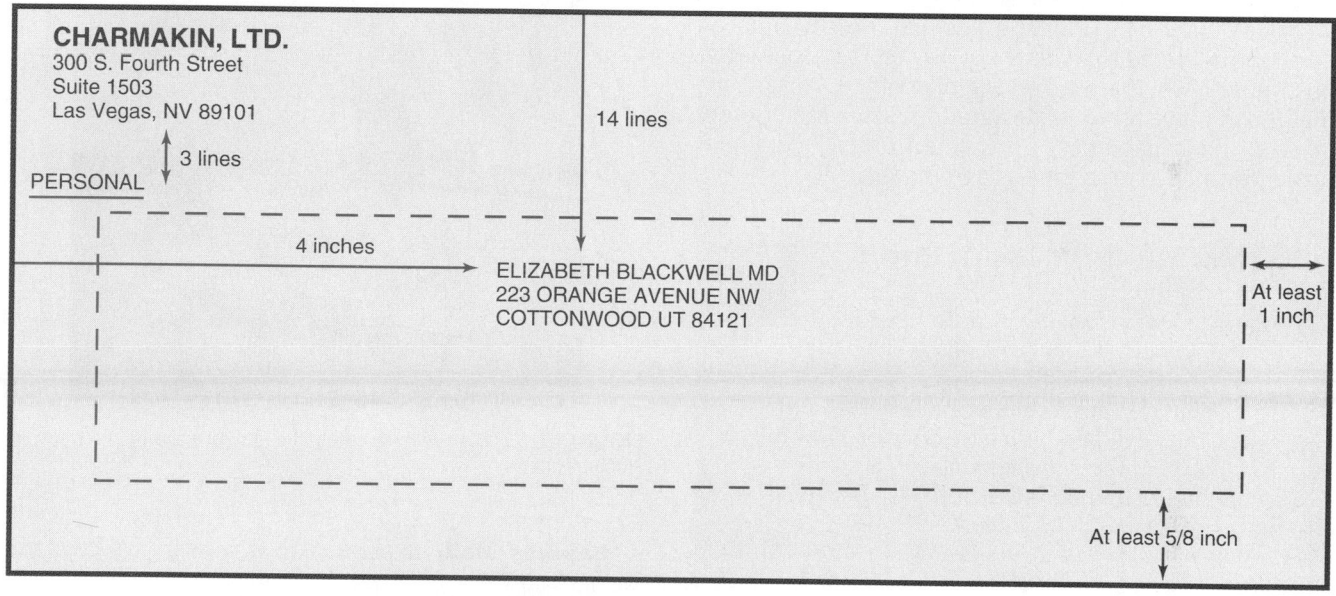

Placement of mailing address and Personal notation on No. 10 envelope

FIGURE 12-7   Addressing envelopes.

- Draw a damp sponge over the flaps, and starting with the lower piece, turn down the flaps and seal each one.

Do not use too much moisture because this may cause the glue to spread and several envelopes to stick together. A similar process simplifies stamping several letters at one time if not using a postage meter. If possible, purchase stamps by the roll. Tear off about ten stamps from the roll. Fanfold the stamps on the perforations so that they separate easily. Fan the envelopes address side up. Wet a strip of stamps with the sponge and, starting at one end of the fanned envelopes, attach the stamp at the end of the strip, tear it off, and proceed to the next envelope. Automated sealers and stampers are also available to make this procedure easier and more efficient.

Cost-Saving Mailing Procedures

Using ZIP Codes. The ZIP code is a very important part of an address, just as the area code is a very important part of a telephone number. ZIP codes start with the number 0 on the East Coast and gradually increase to number 9 on the West Coast and Hawaii.

The five-digit ZIP code was introduced in 1961. The first three digits identify a major city or distribution point, and all five digits identify an individual post office, zone of a city, or other delivery unit. The Postal Service later developed the nine-digit ZIP code, consisting of the original five digits followed by a hyphen and four additional digits that further identify the addressee's street location. The ZIP code is electronically transformed into a bar code. The office computer may have this capability. The Postal Code claims that the ZIP-plus-4, when used with the automated letter-sorting machinery, can eliminate 20 mail-handling steps and result in considerable savings. This saving is passed on to bulk mailers on mailings of 250 or more pieces that have typewritten addresses in machine-readable format along with the nine-digit ZIP code.

Presorting. Bulk mailers can get a discount on postage for presorting their mail. A discounted presort rate is charged on each piece that is part of a group of 10 or more pieces sorted to the same five-digit code or a group of 50 or more pieces sorted to the same first three-digit ZIP code.

Using Correct Postage. Although mailing fees are still one of our better bargains, the mailing costs for even a small office are a sizable item in the annual budget, and carelessness can cause them to soar. If the facility does not have a postage meter that dispenses postage exactly, then be sure that you are not putting too many stamps on your outgoing mail. Use an accurate postage scale and remember that only the first ounce requires the base rate; additional ounces are at a lower rate.

Getting Faster Mail Service

Postage Meters. The postage meter is the most efficient way of stamping the mail in a large business office (Figure 12-8). It can print postage onto adhesive strips that are then placed onto the envelopes or packages, or it can print the postage directly onto an envelope. Metered mail does not have to be canceled or postmarked when it reaches the post office. This means that it can move on to its destination faster. Meters vary in size and capabilities. Consult an office equipment dealer for information on postage meters.

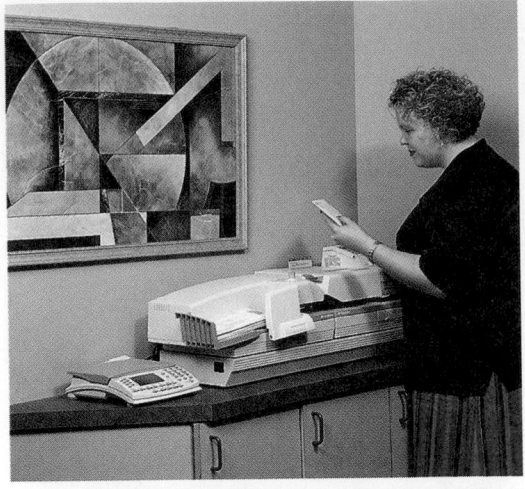

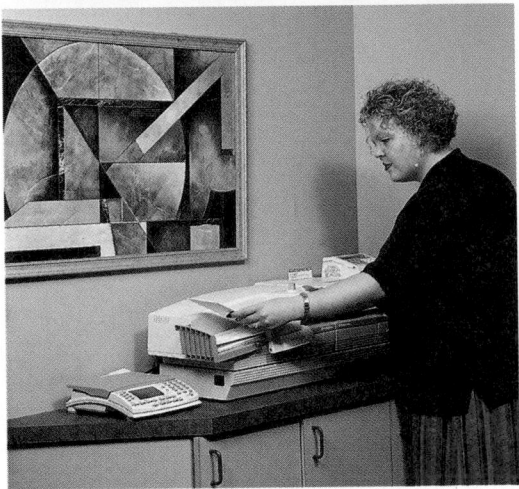

FIGURE 12-8   Postage meters help the mail processing run more efficiently.

CRITICAL THINKING APPLICATION

- Brandon knows that the mail processing would go much faster if the office invested in a postage meter. The office manager states that she has mentioned this to Brandon's father several times, but he did not purchase a meter. How might Brandon approach his father about this issue?
- What should Brandon do before discussing the postage meter with his father?

Mailing Practices. For large mailings, local letters should be separated from out-of-town letters. Letters or packages that need to be rushed should be taken directly to the post office for mailing. Others can be placed in street boxes or the building's mail chute for pickup. Packages should always be taken to a post office and weighed for proper postage. Place a letter tray on the desk or some other convenient place so that all outgoing mail is kept together until it is ready to leave the office.

Classifications of Mail

Mail is classified according to *type*, *weight*, and *destination*. The ounce and pound are the units of measurement. **Domestic mail** is that which is sent within the United States and its territories, and **International mail** is that which is sent outside the United States. Letters to distant points of the globe are in almost all cases sent by air and can be expected to reach their destination within a few days. The rates for international mail are based on increments of $\frac{1}{2}-1$ ounce. A table of rates can be obtained from the post office.

Express Mail. Express Mail is available 7 days per week, 365 days per year for items weighing up to 70 pounds and measuring 108 inches in combined length and **girth**. Service features include the following:
- Noon delivery between major business markets
- Merchandise and document reconstruction insurance
- Express mail shipping containers
- Shipment receipt
- Optional return receipt service
- Optional **collect-on-delivery (COD)** service
- Waiver of signature option
- Collection boxes
- Optional pickup service

First-Class Mail. First-class mail includes sealed or unsealed handwritten or typed material, such as letters, postal cards, postcards, and business reply mail. Postage for letters weighing 13 ounces or less is based on weight, in 1-ounce increments. Envelopes larger than the standard No. 10 business envelope should have the green diamond border to expedite first-class delivery.

Priority Mail. First-class mail weighing over 13 ounces is classified as Priority Mail, and the postage is calculated on the basis of weight and destination, with the maximum weight being 70 pounds.

Bound Printed Matter. Bound printed matter consists of advertising, promotional, directory, or editorial material (or any combination of such material). It must be securely bound by permanent fastenings such as staples, spiral binding, glue, or stitching, and cannot have the nature of personal correspondence. Loose-leaf binders and similar fastenings are not considered permanent.

Media Matter. Media matter is used for books, film, manuscripts, printed music, printed test materials, sound recordings, play scripts, printed educational charts, loose-leaf pages and binders consisting of medical information, videotapes, and computer recorded media such as CD-ROMs and diskettes. Media mail cannot contain advertising, and it cannot weigh over 70 pounds.

Special Services

Insured Mail. Insurance for coverage against loss or damage is available for Priority Mail, first-class mail, or parcel post.

Registered Mail. Mail of all classes, particularly that of unusually high value, can be additionally protected by registering it. The sender may request evidence of its delivery. Registering a piece of mail also helps to trace delivery, if necessary.

When sending a registered letter, it is necessary to go to the post office and fill in the required forms. All articles to be registered must be thoroughly sealed with U.S. Postal Service tape. Cellophane tape is not permitted. On receipt of the item, the **recipient** is required to sign a form that acknowledges delivery. A registered letter may be released to the person to whom it is addressed or to his or her agent. For an additional fee, a personal receipt may be requested (Figure 12-9). This ensures that the letter will be released only to the individual to whom it is addressed. Such pieces bear the label *To Addressee Only*.

Registered mail is accounted for by number from the time of mailing until the time of delivery and is transported separately from other mail under a special lock. In case of loss or damage, the customer may be reimbursed up to certain limits, provided that the value of the registered article has been declared at the time of mailing and that the appropriate fee has been paid.

Postal Money Orders. Postal money orders are a convenient way of mailing money, especially for the individual who does not have a personal checking account. They may be purchased in amounts as high as $700.

Special Delivery. Mail of any class that has been marked *special delivery* is charged at the special-delivery rate. Such pieces may be regular first- or second-class, registered, insured, or COD pieces. The special-delivery designation generally does not speed up the normal travel time between two cities but does ensure immediate delivery of the item when it arrives at the designated post office.

Special Handling. Third- and fourth-class mail sent by special handling receives the fastest service and ground transportation practicable—about the same as that for first-class mail. The special-handling fee is in addition to required postage and is determined according to weight. This fee does not include insurance or special delivery at the destination, but special delivery, if desired, is available at an added cost. If a parcel is sent by Priority Mail, special handling is of no additional advantage because it is already traveling at the greatest possible speed.

Certified Mail. Any piece of mail without **intrinsic** value and on which postage is paid at the first-class rate will be accepted as certified mail. Such items as contracts, deeds, mortgages, bank books, checks, passports, insurance policies, money orders, and birth certificates that are not themselves valuable but that would be difficult to duplicate if lost should be certified. Certified mail is also often used as an aid in debt collection.

Regular postage in addition to a certified mail fee must be affixed. For an additional fee, a receipt verifying delivery can be requested (Figure 12-10). Certified mail can be sent special delivery if the prescribed fees are paid. A record of delivery of certified mail is kept for 2 years at the post office of delivery; however, no record is kept at the post office of origin. Furthermore, this type of mail does not provide insurance coverage.

The medical assistant should keep a supply of certified mail forms and return receipts on hand. These may be obtained at any post office. Full instructions are included on the forms. Fees and postage may be paid using ordinary postage stamps, meter stamps, or permit imprints. Certified mail can be mailed at any post office, station, or branch or can be deposited in mail drops or in street letter boxes if specific instructions are followed.

Certificate of Mailing. If a sender needs proof of mailing but is not especially concerned with proof of receipt of an item, the most economic method is to obtain a certificate of mailing. Obtain this form at the post office and fill in the required information. Attach a stamp for the current fee and hand the form to the postal clerk along with the piece of mail. The clerk will postmark the receipt, initial it, and hand it back as acknowledgment of having received the piece of mail at the post office. This is sometimes used when mailing tax reports or other items that must be postmarked by a certain date.

Private Delivery Services

Not all mail is delivered by the U.S. Postal Service. Many private services pick up and deliver mail overnight. Among these are Federal Express, United Parcel Service, Emery, Airborne Express, and DHL. These services are highly advertised and competitive. All large cities and many smaller communities have centralized points where packages can be dropped off for the service of the sender's choice. Pickup service is also available in many communities.

CRITICAL THINKING APPLICATION

- The office has always used FedEx for sending packages. However, Brandon is curious as to whether FedEx offers the best rates. How might he gather this information?
- What should be considered when choosing a private delivery service?

Handling Special Situations

Forwarding and Obtaining a Changed Address.
By marking a piece of mail with the notation *Forwarding Service Requested*, the U.S. Post Office will forward mail to the new address if it is sent within 12 months of the change or if the receiver has left a forwarding order with the post office. At that time the forwarding order is expired unless the receiver requests that it be continued. Between 12 and 18 months, the piece will be returned to the sender with the new address noted. After 18 months, mail is usually returned with the reason for nondelivery noted. There is no charge for forwarding when priority or first-class mail is used.

If the mailer wants to know an addressee's new address, this service can be obtained from the post office by placing the words *Address Correction Requested* beneath the return address on the envelope. This can be hand-written, stamped, typewritten, or printed. The new address will be noted on a sticker and returned to the sender, and there is no charge for this if the item is sent priority or first-class mail. The post office charges a weighted fee for this service for standard mail and packages. If the envelope is marked *Change Service Requested*, the post office will dispose of the piece of mail and return a card to the sender showing the forwarding address of the addressee. If the piece was sent priority or first class, there

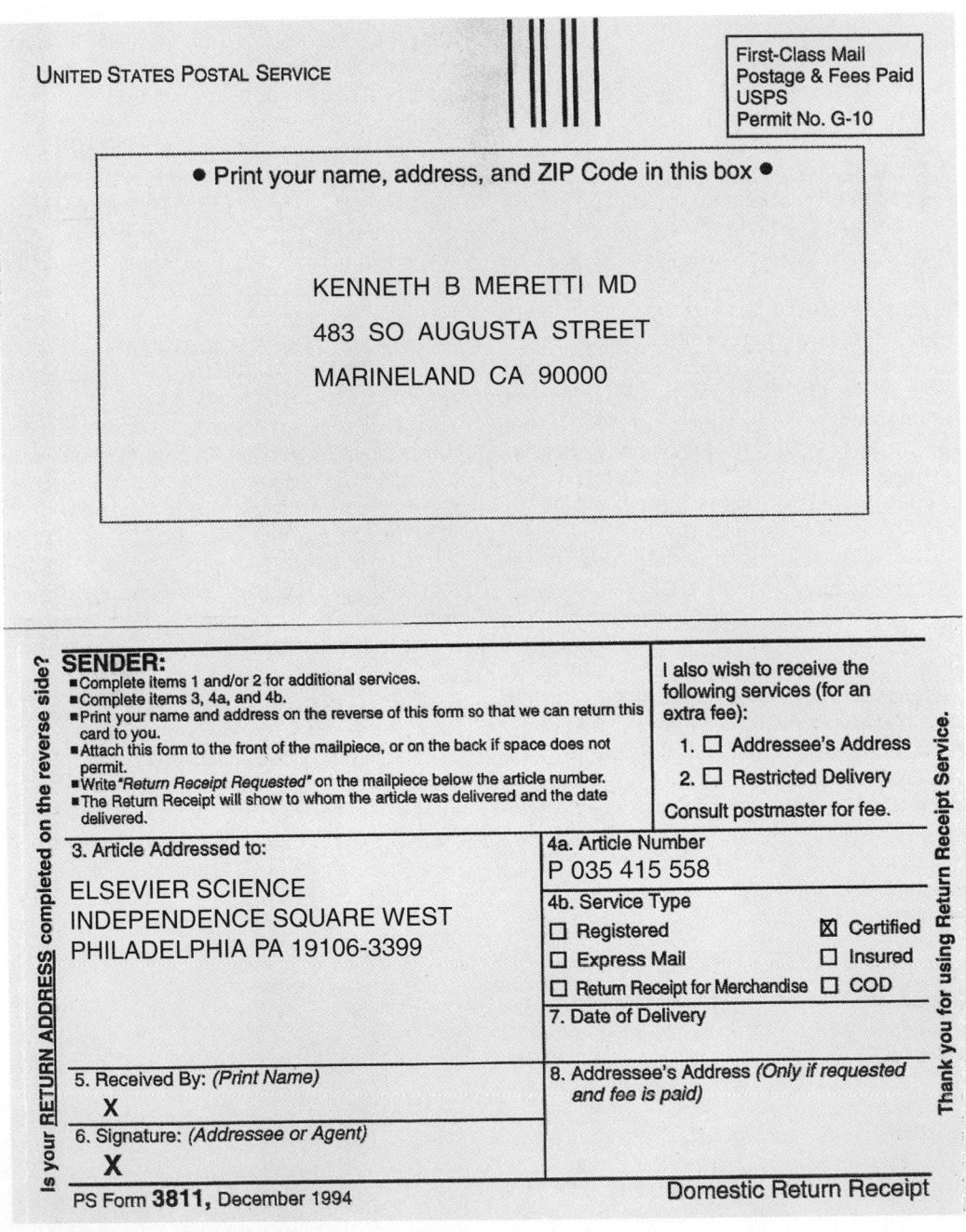

FIGURE 12-9   Delivery receipts for certified, registered, and insured mail. Attach to the back of the article, and endorse the front with the phrase *return receipt requested* adjacent to the article number.

FIGURE 12-9, Cont'd   For legend see opposite page.

is no charge for the service unless the notification is sent electronically, and then there is a small charge.

Recalling Mail. If a letter has been dropped in the mailbox by mistake, do not ask the mail collector to give it to you; he or she is not permitted to do so. However, mail can be recalled by making written application at the post office, together with an envelope addressed identically to the one being recalled. If the letter has already left the local post office, the postmaster, at the sender's expense, can notify the postmaster at the destination post office to return the letter. However, there is no guarantee that the letter will be retrieved.

Returned Mail. If a letter is returned to the sender after an attempt has been made to deliver it, it cannot be mailed again without new postage. It is best simply to prepare a new envelope with the correct address, affix the proper postage, and place in the mail.

When mail is returned to the medical office, be sure to correct the database, indicating that mail has been returned on a certain patient, so that postage is not wasted sending mail to that address again.

Tracing Lost Mail. Receipts issued by the post office, whether for money orders, registered mail, certified mail, or insured mail, should be retained until receipt of the item has been acknowledged. If, after an adequate time elapses, no acknowledgment of receipt

for such mailing arrives, notify the post office to trace the letter or package. Regular first-class mail is not easily traced, but the post office will make every attempt to find it for you. In tracing a lost letter or package, the post office requires that a special form be filled out; data from any original receipt should be written along with any other identifying information on this form.

Closing Comments

Remember that every letter sent from the medical office should project a professional image. Use neat handwriting when correspondence is not typed or generated on a computer. All of the office staff must be able to read items written years ago. It is worth the time and effort to brush up on English skills so that writing documents becomes as comfortable as setting an appointment or assisting in a procedure.

Patient Education

Medical offices often use brochures and printed material for the education of their patients. It is critical that these

P 268 875 363

US Postal Service
Receipt for Certified Mail
No Insurance Coverage Provided.
Do not use for International Mail *(See reverse)*

Sent to ELSEVIER SCIENCE	
Street & Number INDEPENDENCE SQUARE WEST	
Post Office, State, & ZIP Code PHILADELPHIA PA 19106-3399	
Postage	$
Certified Fee	
Special Delivery Fee	
Restricted Delivery Fee	
Return Receipt Showing to Whom & Date Delivered	
Return Receipt Showing to Whom, Date, & Addressee's Address	
TOTAL Postage & Fees	$
Postmark or Date	

PS Form **3800**, April 1995

Fold at line over top of envelope to the right of the return address

CERTIFIED

P 268 875 363

MAIL

FIGURE 12-10 Receipt for certified mail. Attach the bottom portion of the receipt to the top of the envelope, just to the right of the return address.

materials look professional and reflect a positive image for the physician and the facility. Be sure that copied material is clean without streaks and that it looks attractive to the eye. If the information is written by an office staff member, make certain that correct grammar is used and that several office members proofread the work for errors and proper use of the English language. It is wonderful to make a good first impression, but every impression in the medical office is an important one.

Legal and Ethical Issues

A copy should be kept of all communications leaving the office that relate to patient care. If any information is handwritten, it must be completely legible to the patient. Certainly, everyone should be able to read his or her own handwriting, even years later.

Since the appointment book is also considered a communications tool, the information entered by hand in the book must also be clear and easy to read. Take enough time to write legibly so that there is no confusion

when the document is referred to at a later date. In legal battles, all written documentation must be concise and must not promote questions about the content.

SUMMARY OF SCENARIO

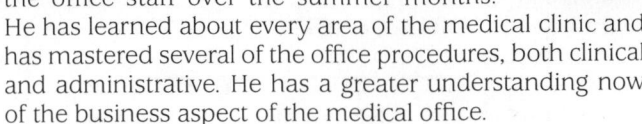

Brandon has been a tremendous help to the office staff over the summer months. He has learned about every area of the medical clinic and has mastered several of the office procedures, both clinical and administrative. He has a greater understanding now of the business aspect of the medical office.

His duties as a temporary administrative medical assistant have opened his eyes to the value and importance of the administrative personnel. He can easily see that from the receptionist to the scheduler to the insurance billers—all play a vital role in the smooth operation of the facility.

Toward the end of the summer, the office staff honored Brandon with a going-away party. He announced with a smile that he had decided, based on his experience in his father's family practice, that he wished to become a pediatrician. He expressed to the staff that he planned to hire them all away from his father! Then on a serious note, he thanked all the employees for their patience and for their willing spirit to let him learn from them. Everyone expects Brandon to be a complete success.

SUMMARY OF LEARNING OBJECTIVES

■ The medical assistant is responsible for making certain that equipment is in good working order. Warranties should always be mailed when new equipment is purchased, and the correct maintenance procedures should be followed to keep machines working at an optimal level. Supplies should be ordered before they run out, and prices should be compared to find the best quality for the best price available.

■ There are four basic sizes of letterhead stationery. Standard or letter stationery, which is most commonly used for business purposes, is $8\frac{1}{2} \times 11$ inches. Monarch or executive stationery is $8\frac{1}{4} \times 10\frac{1}{2}$ inches and is used for informal business correspondence. Baronial stationery is $5\frac{1}{2} \times 8\frac{1}{2}$ inches, whereas legal stationery is $8\frac{1}{2} \times 14$ inches.

■ The medical assistant should be familiar with the various parts of speech and the way to use them correctly in a sentence. Nouns name something, such as a person, place, or thing; pronouns are substitutes for nouns. Verbs are action words and express movement, a condition, or a state of being. Adjectives usually describe nouns, whereas adverbs usually describe verbs. Prepositions are connecting words, as are conjunctions. Interjections show strong feelings and are often followed by an exclamation point.

■ It is quite helpful to develop a personal tool collection that will assist the medical assistant with written communications in the medical office. An up-to-date dictionary, a medical dictionary, a composition handbook, an English-language reference manual, and a thesaurus will be valuable additions to the tool library.

■ Before any type of correspondence is answered, the piece should be read carefully. Often a highlighter is used for marking questions that must be answered, or notes may be written on the correspondence in pencil. A draft of the reply should be written first and then rewritten in its final draft.

■ Subsequent letters will be much easier to draft if the medical assistant develops a portfolio that contains sample letters and other types of communications. Once a letter is written, it can be saved on the computer hard drive or on a disk, or it can be printed and placed in a binder for easy viewing. If the letter is printed in a binder, it is wise to note on each example the file name as it is saved on the computer so that the document can be easily found again when needed. This is an excellent way to save time in the busy medical office.

■ Block is an efficient but less attractive letter style wherein all lines begin flush with the left margin of the paper. Modified block is similar, but some lines begin at the center of the page instead of the left margin. Modified block with indented paragraphs is identical to block style, with the exception of the indention of the paragraphs. Simplified letter style contains lines that begin flush at the left margin, but other items, such as the salutation and complimentary closing, are omitted.

■ The four standard parts of a business letter include the heading, the opening, the body, and the closing. The heading includes the letterhead and dateline, whereas the opening includes the inside address and any attention or salutation line. The body is the message of the document, and the closing is the signature, complimentary closing, reference initials, and special notations.

■ Money can be saved by consulting the post office when mailing, checking for better rates, and using ZIP codes. Consult a local post office when mailing in bulk to obtain the best rates.

KEY INTERNET WEBSITES

- Airborne Express
- DHL Worldwide Express
- Emery Forwarding
- Federal Express
- Merriam-Webster Online Dictionary
- United Parcel Service
- United States Post Office
  For active weblinks to each website visit
  http://evolve.elsevier.com/Kinn/

CHAPTER 13

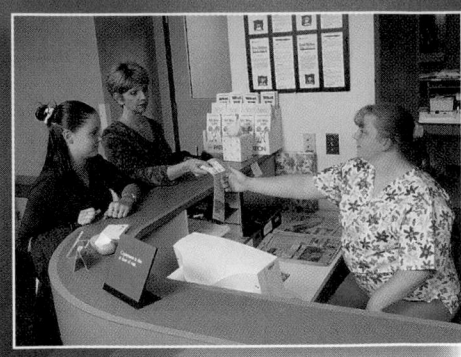

Scenario

Susan Beezler has just begun her career in the medical assisting profession. She is attending medical assisting school in the morning hours and works part-time for a family practitioner in the afternoons as a clerical/records assistant. Susan is eager to learn about medicine and looks forward to taking on more responsibility at the office.

The practice is growing swiftly and recently added a new physician, Dr. Alex Thomas. Dr. Thomas has enjoyed working with Susan and feels that her energy will be just what his patients need. He has taken a special interest in Susan and often lets her assist him with patients when her other duties allow.

Susan knows that although she is a beginner in the office, she will gain trust from her supervisors and patients as long as she projects a teachable attitude. She cheerfully performs filing and often does transcription for Dr. Thomas. The other staff members are pleased with her willing attitude to perform even the most mundane tasks. Her warm personality and caring way with patients ensure that she has a great chance at a long career in this medical office.

Susan enjoys sharing her experiences with the other students in her class. She is the only person who is currently working in the medical field, so the other students ask many questions about what Susan has experienced in the real world of medicine. She is very careful not to breach patient confidentiality as she discusses situations in general, never mentioning any patient names.

Susan feels a great sense of pride that she is already a member of the healthcare team and able to make a positive contribution to the lives of her patients.

Medical Records Management

National Curriculum Competencies

ADMINISTRATIVE COMPETENCIES

1c. Perform medical transcription
1d. Organize a patient's medical record
1e. File medical records

CLINICAL COMPETENCIES

4c. Obtain and record patient history

TRANSDISCIPLINARY COMPETENCIES

1c. Establish and maintain the medical record
1d. Document appropriately

Vocabulary

alphabetical filing Any system that arranges names or topics according to the sequence of the letters in the alphabet.

alphanumeric Systems made up of combinations of letters and numbers.

audit A formal examination of an organization's or individual's accounts or financial situation; a methodical examination and review.

augment To make greater, more numerous, larger, or more intense.

caption A heading, title, or subtitle under which records are filed.

chronological order Of, relating to, or arranged in or according to the order of time.

continuity of care Care that continues smoothly from one provider to another, so that the patient receives the most benefit and no interruption in care.

dictation The act or manner of uttering words to be transcribed.

direct filing system A filing system in which materials can be located without consulting an intermediary source of reference.

gleaned Gathered bit by bit (e.g., information or material); picked over in search of relevant material.

indirect filing system A filing system in which an intermediary source of reference, such as a card file, must be consulted to locate specific files.

microfilm A film bearing a photographic record on a reduced scale of printed or other graphic matter.

numeric filing The filing of records, correspondence, or cards by number.

objective information Information that is gathered by watching or observation of a patient.

obliteration Act of making undecipherable or imperceptible by obscuring or wearing away.

OUTfolder A folder used to provide space for the temporary filing of materials.

OUTguide A heavy guide that is used to replace a folder that has been temporarily moved from the filing space.

power of attorney A legal instrument authorizing one to act as the attorney or agent of the grantor.

pressboard A strong, highly glazed composition board resembling vulcanized fiber; heavy card stock.

procrastination To put off intentionally the doing of something that should be done.

provisional diagnosis A temporary diagnosis made prior to receiving all test results.

quality control An aggregate of activities designed to ensure adequate quality, especially in manufactured products or in the service industries.

requisites Something considered essential or necessary.

retention schedule A method or plan for retaining or keeping medical records, and their movement from active, to inactive, to closed filing.

shelf filing A system that uses open shelves rather than cabinets for storing records.

shingling A method of filing whereby one report is laid on top of the older report, resembling the shingles of a roof.

subjective information Information that is gained by questioning the patient or taken from a form.

tickler file A chronological file used as a reminder that something must be taken care of on a certain date.

transcription To make a written copy of, either in longhand or by machine.

vested Granted or endowed with a particular authority, right, or property; to have a special interest in.

A medical records management system is only as good as the ease of retrieval of the data in the files. Since the pace of the medical office is usually quite rapid, patient charts must be found quickly and also be functional, so that the information inside is easily obtainable.

There are few phrases more frustrating to the patient than "we cannot locate your chart." Patients have every right to question the competence of the medical care they are receiving if the office has problems simply finding a chart. Organization and adherence to set routines will help to assure that charts are accessible when they are needed.

Ownership of the Medical Record

Who actually owns the medical record? Patients often assume that because the information contained in the medical record is about them, the ownership of the record rightfully belongs to the patient. However, the owner of the physical medical record is the physician or medical facility, often called the "maker," that initiated and developed the record. The patient has the right of access to the information within but does not own the physical chart or other document pertaining to the record. The patient has a **vested** interest and thus has the right to demand confidentiality of all of the information placed in the chart.

The actual patient chart should never leave the medical facility from which it originated. Even the physician should refrain from taking the chart from the office to the hospital or nursing facility. If information from the chart is needed, copies can be placed in a file, and progress notes written on-site and returned to the original chart later. Patient charts should be kept in a locked room or locked filing cabinets when the office is closed.

CRITICAL THINKING APPLICATION

On Susan's third day at work, a man comes to the office and demands to see his mother's medical chart. Susan pulls the chart and sees an entry stating that the mother does not wish the son to have any information about her. What should Susan do in this situation? Are there any viable reasons why the son should have access to the mother's medical information?

Why Medical Records Are Important

Medical records exist for four basic reasons. First, the medical record assists the physician in providing the best possible medical care for the patient. The physician examines the patient and enters the findings on the patient's medical record. These findings are the clues to diagnosis. The physician may order many types of tests to confirm or **augment** the clinical findings. As the reports of these tests come in, the findings fall into place like the pieces of a jigsaw puzzle. Then, with the confirmation data to support the diagnosis, the physician can prescribe treatment and form an opinion about the patient's chances of recovery, assured that every resource has been used to arrive at a correct judgment. The medical record provides a complete history of all of the care given to the patient.

The medical record also provides critical information for others. By reading through the chart and discovering the methods used to treat the patient, healthcare professionals can provide a **continuity of care**. Each person knows what the patient has experienced and can provide continued care, even from one facility to another. For example, when a patient is transferred from a hospital to a skilled nursing facility, the information from the patient's hospital chart will help the nursing facility to better care for the patient. When patients move from place to place or caregivers change, copies of the pertinent chart information should move with the patient to provide this continuity of care.

The second reason for keeping medical records is to offer legal protection for those who provided care to the patient. A documented medical chart is excellent proof that certain procedures were performed or medical advice was given. An accurate chart is the foundation for legal defense in cases of medical professional liability. This is one reason that it is critical to write legibly in the chart and document exactly what happens to the patient. As we have emphasized throughout the book: "If it isn't charted, it didn't happen."

Third, medical records provide statistical information that is helpful to researchers. The patient's chart provides information about medications taken and the reactions to them. Medical records may be used to evaluate the effectiveness of certain kinds of treatment or to determine the incidence of a given disease. Often, physicians take part in drug studies that track adverse reactions and side effects. The effects of various treatments and procedures can also be tracked and statistics **gleaned** from the information gathered from patient charts. Correlation of such statistical information may result in a new outlook on some phases of medicine and can lead to revised techniques and treatments. The statistical data from medical records are also valuable in the preparation of scientific papers, books, and lectures.

Fourth, medical records are vital for financial reimbursement. The information in the medical chart supports claims for reimbursement and is required by most third-party payors.

Creating an Efficient Medical Record Management System

The medical record management system used in the medical office should provide an easy method for retrieving information. The files should be organized in an orderly fashion, and all of the information within the chart must be completely legible to the average reader. The information must also be accurate, and corrections should be made and documented properly. The wording in the chart should be easily understood and grammatically correct. An efficient method of adding documents to the chart must be in place, so that the physician or other provider always has the most up-to-date information.

Above all, the medical record management system must be one that works for the individual facility. Attempting to adopt a method used by another facility may not always be best. The system should be adapted to the facility and provider's needs.

Types of Records

The two major types of patient records include the paper-based medical record and the computer-based medical record. As computer technology advances, the paper-based medical record seems more and more inefficient. It is difficult to use a paper-based record for multiple purposes. In most cases, only one person can use the paper-based record at any given time, and the record is not available to others who need it when it is in use by a single person. Misfiled information is common, and the entire record can be misfiled as well. Data cannot be accessed easily for research and **quality control**, and in facilities with multiple departments, the information is difficult to share. The paper-based record is a good evidence of patient care, but it not nearly as useful in other capacities.

The computer-based medical record (also called the electronic health record) is much more efficient than the paper-based record. The book *Electronic Health Records: Changing the Vision** offers the following definition:

> An electronic health record is any information relating to the past, present, or future physical/mental health, or condition of an individual which resides in electronic systems used to capture, transmit, receive, store, retrieve, link, and manipulate multimedia data for the primary purpose of providing healthcare and health related services.

The computer-based medical record is a great improvement over the paper-based record, but it is not without its disadvantages. Patient confidentiality is critical and sometimes difficult to maintain with computer-based records. Many providers worry about computer malfunctions that would inhibit access to the record in an emergency.

Still, the advantages of the computer-based record seem to far outweigh the disadvantages. Information can

---

*Murphy GF, Hanken MA, Waters K: *Electronic health records: changing the vision*, Philadelphia, 1999, WB Saunders.

be accessed in a variety of physical locations, and more than one person can see the record at any given time. The patient database usually allows various types of statistical information to be recalled, which is a valuable tool. Patient information is available quickly in an emergency, even when the patient is not in his or her hometown. All of these advantages mean that the computer-based record will continue to be a key tool in the future.

CRITICAL THINKING APPLICATION

Some of the patients who visit Dr. Thomas have expressed concern that computer-based medical records may not be private enough. They are worried that unauthorized individuals could somehow access their information on the computer and somehow cause the patients harm. How might Susan alleviate the patients' fears? What disadvantages regarding confidentiality are associated with the computer-based patient record? Should a patient be allowed to decide whether his or her records will be kept by computer or by paper?

Organization of the Medical Record

Source-Oriented Records

The traditional patient record is source oriented; that is, observations and data are cataloged according to their source—physician, laboratory, radiology, nurse, technician—with no recording of a logical relationship between them. Forms and progress notes are filed in reverse **chronological order** (most recent on top) and filed in separate sections of the record by the type of form or service rendered—all laboratory reports together, all x-ray reports together, and so forth.

Problem-Oriented Medical Records

The problem-oriented medical record (POMR) is a radical departure from the traditional system of keeping patient records. It is sometimes referred to as the Weed system, because it was originated by Dr. Lawrence L. Weed, a professor of medicine at the University of Vermont's College of Medicine. The POMR is a record of clinical practice that divides medical action into four bases:

1. The *database* includes chief complaint, present illness, patient profile, review of systems, physical examination, and laboratory reports.
2. The *problem list* is a numbered and titled list of every problem the patient has that requires management or workup. This may include social and demographic troubles as well as strictly medical or surgical ones.
3. The *treatment plan* includes management, additional workups needed, and therapy. Each plan is titled and numbered with respect to the problem.
4. The *progress notes* include structured notes that are numbered to correspond with each problem number.

Several companies have developed file folders for the organization of patient data consistent with the problem-oriented medical record (Figure 13-1). The problem list is entered on the divider cover for laboratory reports. Special sections are provided for current major and chronic problems and for inactive major or chronic problems. The divider cover for progress notes is a chart for listing medications and other therapeutic modalities. Progress notes follow the SOAP approach. SOAP is an acronym for:

- Subjective impressions
- Objective clinical evidence
- Assessment or diagnosis
- Plans for further studies, treatment, or management

Some medical offices also used an "E" in the record, to represent "Evaluation." This section is used to record an assessment of the patient's understanding of and possible compliance with the treatment plan. As this is not used in every practice, the medical assistant may never see or use it to complete a patient record.

The POMR has the advantage of imposing order and organization on the information added to a patient's medical record. The records are more easily reviewed, and the likelihood of overlooking a problem is greatly reduced. The SOAP method essentially forces a rational approach to patient problems and assists in formulating a logical and orderly plan of patient care (Figure 13-2).

CRITICAL THINKING APPLICATION

Dr. Thomas wants Susan to thoroughly understand the SOAP method of charting. How would Susan explain each aspect of this method to a classmate? There are distinct differences between the SOAP method and the POMR. Help Susan distinguish between the two. Which method seems easier and more efficient to you?

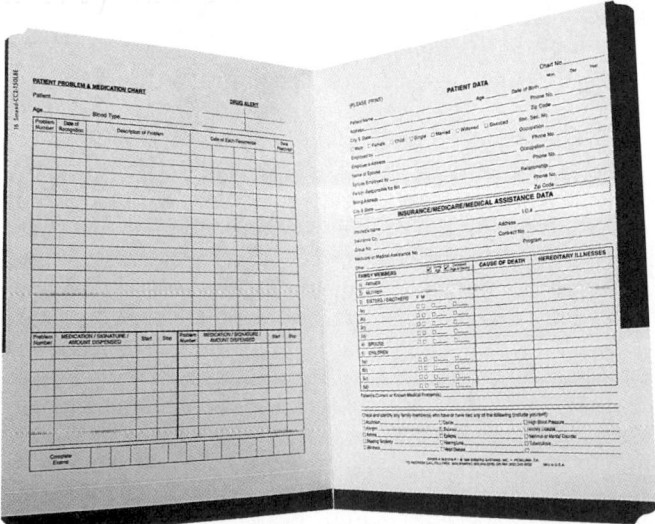

FIGURE 13-1 A chart designed for a problem-oriented medical record. Some charts are specifically adapted to the POMR. (Courtesy Bibbero Systems, Inc., Petaluma, Calif. 94954, (800) 242-2376, www.bibbero.com.)

OUTLINE FORMAT PROGRESS NOTES

Patient Name ___Fletcher, LeRoy___

Page ___1___

Prob. No. or Letter	DATE	**S** Subjective	**O** Objective	**A** Assess	**P** Plans
2	01/26/00	Patient complains of two days of severe high epigastric pain and burning, radiating through to the back. Pain accentuated after eating.			
			On examination there is extreme guarding and tenderness, high epigastric region. No rebound. Bowel sounds normal. BP 110/70		
				R/O gastric ulcer, pylorospasm.	
					To have upper gastrointestinal series. Start on Cimetidine, 300 mg. q.i.d. Eliminate coffee, alcohol, and aspirin. Return in two days.

Start each Progress Note (Subjective, Objective, Assessment and Plans) at the appropriate margin of the page. Write through the intervening columns to the right shaded column to create an outline form.

ANDRUS/CLINI-REC® PRIMARY CARE CHARTING SYSTEM FORM NO. 26-7115, ©1976 BIBBERO SYSTEMS, INC., PETALUMA, CA.

FIGURE 13-2 SOAP progress notes. The SOAP method keeps information organized and in a logical sequence. An actual progress note would include the physician's signature or initials after this entry. (Courtesy Bibbero Systems, Inc., Petaluma, Calif. 94954, (800) 242-2376, www.bibbero.com.)

Popularity of the POMR has continued to grow since its introduction in the 1960s, and it is especially advantageous in clinics, group practices, and hospitals, where more than one person must be able to find essential information in the chart.

Contents of the Complete Case History

The medical case history is the most important record in a physician's practice. For completeness, each patient's record should contain **subjective information** provided by the patient and **objective information** provided by the physician. If all entries are completed, the case history will stand the test of time. No branch of medicine is exempt from the necessity of keeping patient history records.

Subjective Information

Personal Demographics. The patient's case history begins with routine personal data, which the patient usually supplies on the first visit (Procedure 13-1). Most

patients are required to complete a patient information form (Figure 13-3). The basic facts needed are the following:

- Patient's full name, spelled correctly
- Names of parents if patient is a child
- Patient's sex
- Date of birth
- Marital status
- Name of spouse, if married
- Number of children, if any
- Home address and telephone number
- Occupation
- Name of employer
- Business address and telephone number
- Employment information for spouse
- Healthcare insurance information
- Source of referral
- Social Security number

Personal and Medical History. The personal and medical history, which is often obtained by having the patient complete a questionnaire, provides information about any past illnesses or surgical operations that the patient may have had and includes data about injuries or physical defects, whether congenital or acquired

---

PROCEDURE 13-1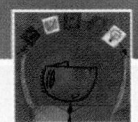

Initiating a Medical File for a New Patient

GOAL: To initiate a medical file for a new patient that will contain all the personal data necessary for a complete record and any other information required by the facility.

EQUIPMENT AND SUPPLIES

- Computer or typewriter
- Clerical supplies (pen, clipboard)
- Information on the agency's filing system
- Registration form
- File folder
- Label for folder
- ID card if using numeric system
- Cross-reference card
- Financial card
- Routing slip
- Private conference area

PROCEDURAL STEPS

1 Determine that the patient is new to the office.

2 Obtain and record the required personal data.
   Purpose: Complete information is necessary for credit and insurance claim processing.

3 Type the information onto the patient history form.

4 Review the entire form.
   Purpose: To confirm that the information is complete and correct.

5 Select a label and folder for the record
   Explanation: If color coding is used, a decision must be made regarding the appropriate color for the patient name.

6 Type the caption on the label and apply it to the folder.
   Explanation: Use the patient's name for alphabetical filing or appropriate number for numeric filing.

7 For a numeric filing system, prepare a cross-reference card and a patient ID number.
   Purpose: Numeric filing is an indirect system and requires a cross-reference to a patient's name for locating the chart. The patient will use the number of the ID card when arranging appointments or making inquiries.

8 Prepare the financial card, or place that patient's name in the computerized ledger.

9 Place the patient's history form and all other forms required by the agency into the prepared folder.

10 Clip an encounter form on the outside of the patient's folder.

Thank you for selecting our health care team!
To help us meet all your health care needs, please
fill out this form completely in ink. If you have any questions
or need assistance, please ask us - we will be happy to help.

Welcome

Patient # _____

Soc. Sec. # _____

Date _____

Patient Information (CONFIDENTIAL)

Name _____ Birth date _____ Home phone _____

Address _____ City _____ State _____ Zip _____

Check appropriate box: ☐ Minor ☐ Single ☐ Married ☐ Divorced ☐ Widowed ☐ Separated

If student, name of school/college _____ City _____ State ___ ☐ Full time ☐ Part time

Patient's or parent's employer _____ Work phone _____

Business address _____ City _____ State _____ Zip _____

Spouse or parent's name _____ Employer _____ Work phone _____

Whom may we thank for referring you? _____

Person to contact in case of emergency _____ Phone _____

Responsible Party

Name of person responsible for this account _____ Relationship to patient _____

Address _____ Home phone _____

Driver's license # _____ Birth date _____ Financial institution _____

Employer _____ Work phone _____ SSN# _____

Is this person currently a patient in our office? ☐ Yes ☐ No

Insurance Information

Name of insured _____ Relationship to patient _____

Birth date _____ Social Security # _____ Date employed _____

Name of employer _____ Union or local # _____ Work phone _____

Address of employer _____ City _____ State _____ Zip _____

Insurance company _____ Group # _____ Policy/ID # _____

Ins. co. address _____ City _____ State _____ Zip _____

How much is your deductible? _____ How much have you used? _____ Max. annual benefit _____

DO YOU HAVE ANY ADDITIONAL INSURANCE? ☐ Yes ☐ No   IF YES, COMPLETE THE FOLLOWING:

Name of insured _____ Relationship to patient _____

Birth date _____ Social Security # _____ Date employed _____

Name of employer _____ Union or local # _____ Work phone _____

Address of employer _____ City _____ State _____ Zip _____

Insurance company _____ Group # _____ Policy/ID # _____

Ins. co. address _____ City _____ State _____ Zip _____

How much is your deductible? _____ How much have you used? _____ Max. annual benefit _____

I authorize release of any information concerning my (or my child's) health care, advice and treatment provided for the purpose of
evaluating and administering claims for insurance benefits. I also hereby authorize payment of insurance benefits otherwise payable to me
directly to the doctor.

X _____ _____

Signature of patient or parent if minor   Date

FIGURE 13-3   The patient information form provides all of the information that the medical assistant needs to construct a patient chart.

(Figure 13-4). It also includes information about the patient's daily health habits.

The Patient's Family History. The family history comprises the physical condition of the various members of the patient's family, any past illnesses or diseases that individual members may have suffered, and a record of the causes of death. This information is important, because a hereditary pattern may be present in the case of certain diseases.

The Patient's Social History. The patient's social history includes information about the lifestyle the patient lives. If the patient drinks, how many drinks per day or

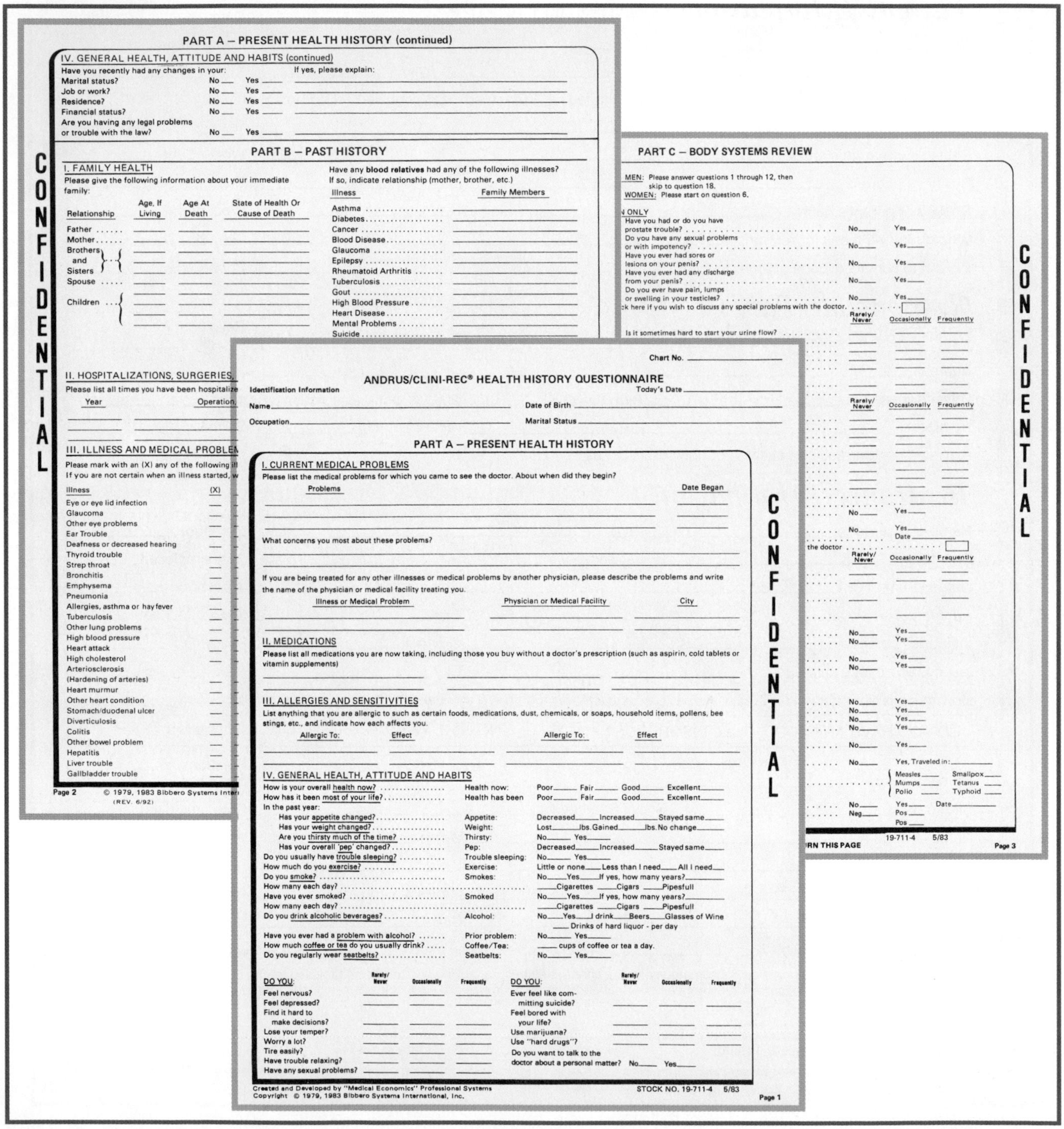

PART A – PRESENT HEALTH HISTORY (continued)

IV. GENERAL HEALTH, ATTITUDE AND HABITS (continued)

Have you recently had any changes in your: If yes, please explain:
Marital status? No___ Yes___
Job or work? No___ Yes___
Residence? No___ Yes___
Financial status? No___ Yes___
Are you having any legal problems or trouble with the law? No___ Yes___

PART B – PAST HISTORY

I. FAMILY HEALTH

Please give the following information about your immediate family:

Relationship | Age, If Living | Age At Death | State of Health Or Cause of Death
Father, Mother, Brothers and Sisters, Spouse, Children

Have any **blood relatives** had any of the following illnesses? If so, indicate relationship (mother, brother, etc.)

Illness | Family Members
Asthma, Diabetes, Cancer, Blood Disease, Glaucoma, Epilepsy, Rheumatoid Arthritis, Tuberculosis, Gout, High Blood Pressure, Heart Disease, Mental Problems, Suicide

II. HOSPITALIZATIONS, SURGERIES

III. ILLNESS AND MEDICAL PROBLEMS

Illness (X): Eye or eye lid infection, Glaucoma, Other eye problems, Ear Trouble, Deafness or decreased hearing, Thyroid trouble, Strep throat, Bronchitis, Emphysema, Pneumonia, Allergies, asthma or hay fever, Tuberculosis, Other lung problems, High blood pressure, Heart attack, High cholesterol, Arteriosclerosis (Hardening of arteries), Heart murmur, Other heart condition, Stomach/duodenal ulcer, Diverticulosis, Colitis, Other bowel problem, Hepatitis, Liver trouble, Gallbladder trouble

Page 2 © 1979, 1983 Bibbero Systems (REV. 6/92)

PART C – BODY SYSTEMS REVIEW

MEN: Please answer questions 1 through 12, then skip to question 18.
WOMEN: Please start on question 6.

CONFIDENTIAL

ANDRUS/CLINI-REC® HEALTH HISTORY QUESTIONNAIRE

Chart No. ______
Identification Information Today's Date ______
Name ______ Date of Birth ______
Occupation ______ Marital Status ______

PART A – PRESENT HEALTH HISTORY

I. CURRENT MEDICAL PROBLEMS

Please list the medical problems for which you came to see the doctor. About when did they begin?
Problems | Date Began

What concerns you most about these problems?

If you are being treated for any other illnesses or medical problems by another physician, please describe the problems and write the name of the physician or medical facility treating you.
Illness or Medical Problem | Physician or Medical Facility | City

II. MEDICATIONS

Please list all medications you are now taking, including those you buy without a doctor's prescription (such as aspirin, cold tablets or vitamin supplements)

III. ALLERGIES AND SENSITIVITIES

List anything that you are allergic to such as certain foods, medications, dust, chemicals, or soaps, household items, pollens, bee stings, etc., and indicate how each affects you.
Allergic To: | Effect | Allergic To: | Effect

IV. GENERAL HEALTH, ATTITUDE AND HABITS

How is your overall health now? Health now: Poor___ Fair___ Good___ Excellent___
How has it been most of your life? Health has been: Poor___ Fair___ Good___ Excellent___
In the past year:
Has your appetite changed? Appetite: Decreased___ Increased___ Stayed same___
Has your weight changed? Weight: Lost___ lbs. Gained___ lbs. No change___
Are you thirsty much of the time? Thirsty: No___ Yes___
Has your overall 'pep' changed? Pep: Decreased___ Increased___ Stayed same___
Do you usually have trouble sleeping? Trouble sleeping: No___ Yes___
How much do you exercise? Exercise: Little or none___ Less than I need___ All I need___
Do you smoke? Smokes: No___ Yes___ If yes, how many years?___
How many each day? ___Cigarettes ___Cigars ___Pipesfull
Have you ever smoked? Smoked: No___ Yes___ If yes, how many years?___
How many each day? ___Cigarettes ___Cigars ___Pipesfull
Do you drink alcoholic beverages? Alcohol: No___ Yes___ I drink___ Beers___ Glasses of Wine ___ Drinks of hard liquor - per day
Have you ever had a problem with alcohol? Prior problem: No___ Yes___
How much coffee or tea do you usually drink? Coffee/Tea: ___ cups of coffee or tea a day.
Do you regularly wear seatbelts? Seatbelts: No___ Yes___

DO YOU:	Rarely/Never	Occasionally	Frequently	DO YOU:	Rarely/Never	Occasionally	Frequently
Feel nervous?				Ever feel like committing suicide?			
Feel depressed?				Feel bored with your life?			
Find it hard to make decisions?				Use marijuana?			
Lose your temper?				Use "hard drugs"?			
Worry a lot?				Do you want to talk to the doctor about a personal matter? No___ Yes___			
Tire easily?							
Have trouble relaxing?							
Have any sexual problems?							

Created and Developed by "Medical Economics" Professional Systems
Copyright © 1979, 1983 Bibbero Systems International, Inc. STOCK NO. 19-711-4 5/83 Page 1

FIGURE 13-4 Database self-administered general health history questionnaire. Lengthy questionnaires should be completed by the patient before he or she is seen by the physician. Either mail the information to the patient in advance or ask the patient to come in early to complete the paperwork. (Courtesy Bibbero Systems, Inc., Petaluma, Calif. 94954, (800) 242-2376, www.bibbero.com.)

per week are consumed? If the patient uses cigarettes, how many packs a day are smoked? Drug use and even marital information can be considered the social history.

Patient's Chief Complaint. The patient's chief complaint is a concise account of the patient's symptoms, explained in the patient's own words. It should include the following:
- Nature and duration of pain, if any
- Time when the patient first noticed symptoms
- Patient's opinion as to the possible causes for the difficulties
- Remedies that the patient may have applied before seeing the physician
- Other medical treatment received for the same condition in the past

Objective Information

Objective findings, sometimes referred to as signs, become evident from the physician's examination of the patient.

Physical Examination and Findings and Laboratory and Radiology Reports. This section of the case history varies greatly with the specialty of the physician and the complaint of the patient. After the physician has examined the patient, the physical findings are recorded in the history (Figure 13-5). Results of other tests or requests for these tests are then recorded or, if they appear on separate sheets, attached to the history.

Diagnosis. The physician, on the basis of all evidence provided in the patient's past history, the physician's examination, and any supplementary tests, places the diagnosis of the patient's condition on the medical record. If there is some doubt, it may be termed **provisional diagnosis**.

Treatment Prescribed and Progress Notes. The physician's suggested treatment is listed after the diagnosis. Generally, instructions to the patient to return for follow-up treatment in a specific period of time are noted here as well (Procedure 13-2).

On each subsequent visit, the date must be entered on the chart and information about the patient's condition and the results of treatment added to the history, on the basis of the physician's observations. Notations of all medications prescribed or instructions given, as well as the patient's own progress report, should be placed in

the record. Any home visits are noted. If the patient is hospitalized, the name of the hospital, the reason for the admission, and the dates of admission and discharge are recorded. Much of this information may be obtained from the hospital discharge summary.

Condition at the Time of Termination of Treatment. When the treatment is terminated, the physician will record that information. For example:

August 18, 1999. Wound completely healed. Patient discharged.

Obtaining the History

The medical assistant usually secures the routine personal data. The personal and medical history and the patient's family history may be secured by asking the patient to complete a questionnaire, with the physician augmenting the information provided during the patient interview (see Procedure 25-1).

The Medical Assistant's Role. When the medical assistant is responsible for recording the patient's history, care must be exercised to ensure that the patient's answers are not heard by others in the reception room. If privacy is not possible, it is better to give the patient a form to fill out and then transfer this information to permanent records later. When privacy is available, the medical assistant may ask the patient questions and at the same time write or type the answers directly on the record. This method offers an opportunity to become better acquainted with the patient while completing the necessary records. In facilities where lengthy questionnaires are to be completed by the new patient, the questionnaire may be mailed to the patient with a request that it be completed and returned to the physician before the appointment. If the record is to be computerized, requesting the information ahead of time gives the office staff the opportunity to transfer information to the computer before the new patient's visit.

The patient's chief complaint may have been indicated to the medical assistant, but the physician will question the patient in more detail. Many practitioners write their own entries on the chart in longhand. Some may keyboard the findings direct into the computer. Others may dictate the material, either directly to the medical assistant or by using a recording device. If the material is dictated and typed, the physician should check each entry and then initial the entry to verify accuracy. For a chart to be admissible as evidence in court, the person dictating or writing the entries must be able to attest that they were true and correct at the time they were written. The best indication of that is the physician's signature or initials on the typed entry.

Making Additions to the Patient Record

As long as the patient is under the physician's care, the medical history is building. Each laboratory report, radiology report, and progress note is added to the record with

PROCEDURE 13-2

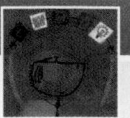

Preparing an Informed Consent for Treatment Form

GOAL: To adequately and completely inform the patient regarding the treatment or procedure that he or she is to receive, and provide legal protection for the facility and the provider.

EQUIPMENT AND SUPPLIES

- Pen
- Consent form

PROCEDURAL STEPS

1 After the physician provides the details of the procedure to be done, prepare the consent form. Be sure that the form addresses the following:
- The nature of the procedure or treatment.
- The risks and/or benefits of the procedure or treatment.
- Any reasonable alternatives to the procedure or treatment.
- The risks and/or benefits of each alternative.
- The risks and/or benefits of not performing the procedure or treatment.

Purpose: To make certain that the patient is fully informed about the procedure or treatment and the risks and/or benefits of having or not having it performed.

2 Personalize the form with the patient's name and any other demographic information that the form lists.

Purpose: To correctly identify the patient and the procedure.

3 Deliver the form to the physician for use as the patient is counseled about the procedure.

Purpose: To avoid charges of practicing medicine without a license. The physician should explain procedures, risks, benefits, alternatives, and answer all of the patient's questions.

4 Witness the signature of the patient on the form, if necessary. The physician will usually sign the form as well.

5 Provide a copy of the consent form to the patient.

Purpose: To make certain that the patient is fully informed regarding the procedure and has a copy of the information for his or her personal records.

6 Place the consent form in the patient's chart. The facility where the procedure is to be performed may require a copy.

Purpose: To maintain a permanent copy of the signed consent form.

7 Ask the patient if he or she has any questions about the procedure. Refer questions that the medical assistant cannot or should not answer to the physician. Be sure that all of the questions expressed by the patient are answered.

Purpose: To make certain that the patient is fully informed.

8 Provide information regarding the date and time for the procedure to the patient.

---

the latest information always on top (Procedure 13-3). Although each item is important, the most recent is usually of greatest significance to the patient's care. Again, the physician should read and initial each of these reports before it is placed in the record.

Laboratory Reports

Different colors of paper are often used for reporting different procedures. For example, urinalysis report forms may be yellow, blood count forms pink, and so forth. When laboratory slips are smaller than the history form, they should be placed on a standard $8\frac{1}{2} \times 11$-inch sheet of colored paper. Type or print the patient's name in the upper right corner, and then, with transparent tape, fasten the first report even with the bottom of the page. The second laboratory report will be taped or glued in place on top of and about $\frac{1}{2}$ inch above the first slip, allowing the date to show on the first report. By this method, called **shingling**, the latest report always appears on top (Figure 13-6). When checking previous reports, it

is necessary only to run a finger down the slips until the desired date is found; then flip up the slips above. Laboratory report carrier forms with adhesive strips may be purchased.

Radiology Reports

Radiology reports are usually typed on standard letter-size stationery. They are placed in the patient's history folder, with the most recent report on top. All radiology reports may be stapled together or kept behind a special divider in the chart.

Progress Notes

Reports on the patient's progress are continually being added to the case history. Each visit of the patient should be entered on the chart, with the date preceding any notations about the visit. The medical assistant can type or stamp the date on the chart when readying the charts for the patient's visits. Every instruction, pre-

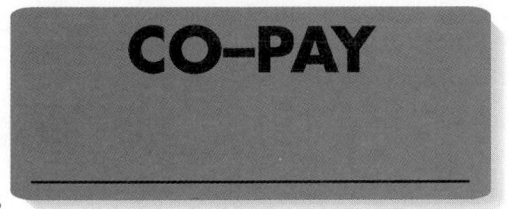

ALLERGIC: _____

_____

_____

A

CO-PAY

_____

B

ADVANCE DIRECTIVES

____ **Durable Power of Attorney for Healthcare**

____ **Living Will**

____ **Healthcare Surrogate**

C

FIGURE 13-5   A to C, Chart stickers. Information on stickers on the outside of the chart allows the physician and medical staff to quickly see important information about the patient. (Courtesy Bibbero Systems, Inc., Petaluma, Calif. 94954, (800) 242-2376, www.bibbero.com.)

PROCEDURE **13-3**

Adding Supplementary Items to Established Patient Files

GOAL: To add supplementary documents and progress notes to patient histories, observing standard steps in filing, while creating an orderly file that will facilitate ready reference to any item of information.

EQUIPMENT AND SUPPLIES

- Assorted correspondence, diagnostic reports, and progress notes
- Patient files
- Computer or typewriter
- Mending tape
- FILE stamp or pen
- Sorter
- Stapler

PROCEDURAL STEPS

1 Group all papers according to patients' names.
Purpose: Some related papers may require stapling.

2 Remove any staples or paper clips.
Purpose: Staples in the file folders are hazardous; paper clips are bulky and may become inadvertently attached to other materials.

4 Mend any damaged or torn records.

5 Attach any small items to standard-size paper.

Purpose: Small items are easily lost or misplaced in files.

6 Staple any related papers together.

7 Place your initials or FILE stamp in the upper left corner.
Purpose: To indicate that the document is released for filing.

8 Code the document by underlining or writing the patient's name in the upper right corner.
Purpose: To indicate where the document is to be filed.

9 Continue steps 2 through 7 until all documents have been conditioned, released, indexed, and coded.

10 Place all documents in the sorter in filing sequence.
Explanation: Sorter can be taken to file cabinet or shelf for placing documents in patient folders.

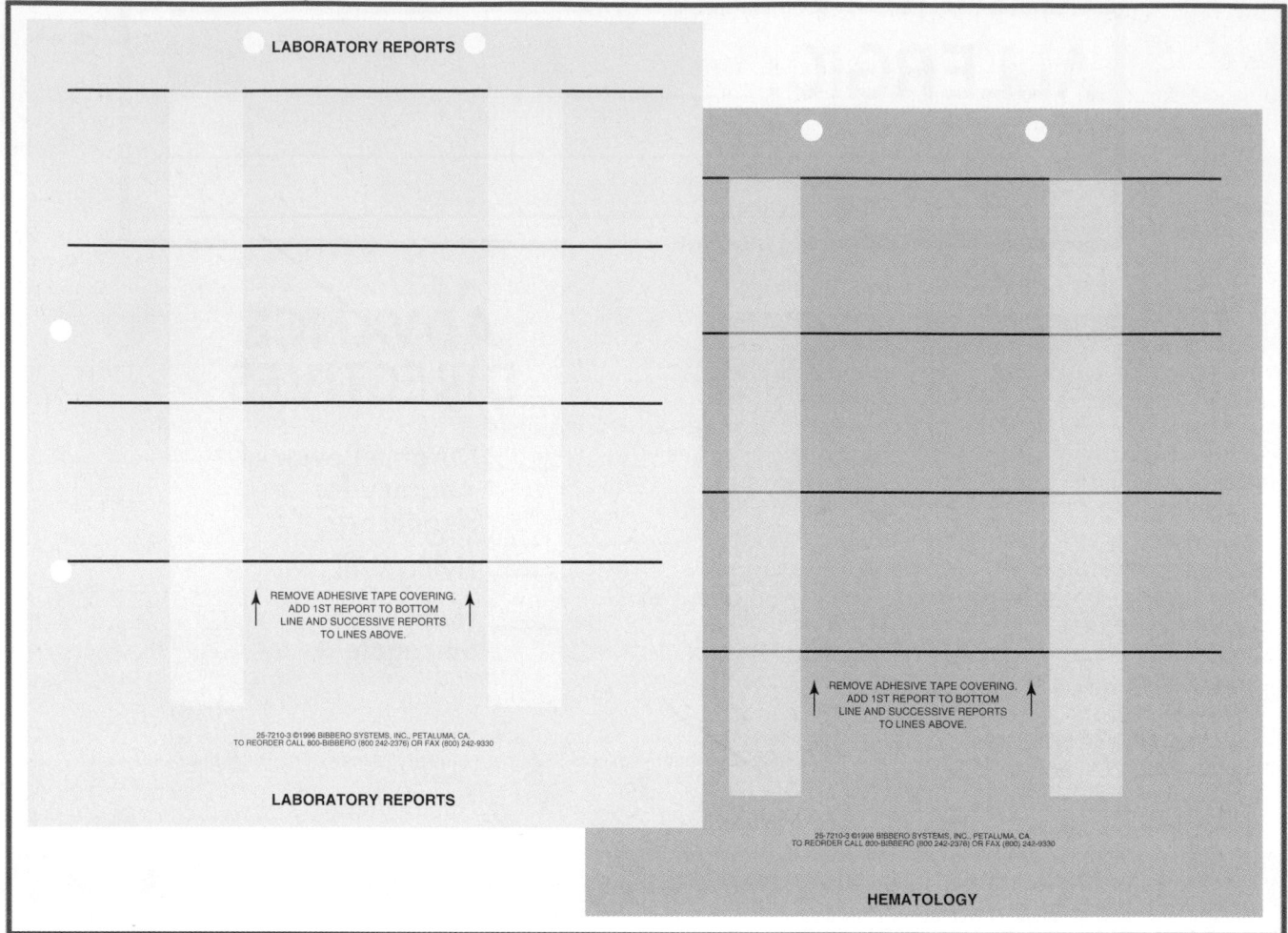

FIGURE 13-6 Shingled laboratory report forms. These forms make filing laboratory reports easy and provide a good adhesive so that the reports will not fall out of the chart if they are not standard size. (Courtesy Bibbero Systems, Inc., Petaluma, Calif. 94954, (800) 242-2376, www.bibbero.com.)

scription, or telephone call for advice should be entered with the correct date. It is always advisable to initial each entry, especially when several persons are handling and making entries on a patient's record. This aids in tracing entries about which there may be some question.

Making Corrections and Alteration of Medical Records

Sometimes it is necessary to make corrections on medical records. Erasing, correction fluid, or any other type of **obliteration** is never acceptable. To correct a handwritten entry, follow these three steps:
1. Draw a line through the error
2. Insert the correction above or immediately after the error.
3. In the margin, write correction or *Corr.*, the initial of the person correcting the entry, and the date.

Errors made while typing are corrected in the usual way. However, an error discovered in a typed entry at a later date is corrected in the same manner as described for a handwritten entry. Never attempt to alter medical records without using this specific correction procedure, because this alteration of records may indicate a fraudulent attempt to cover up a mistake made by a staff member or the physician. Do not hide errors. If the error could in any way affect the health and well-being of the patient, it must immediately be brought to the attention of the physician.

CRITICAL THINKING APPLICATION

Susan has been using an incorrect abbreviation for several weeks and is having a difficult time remembering the right abbreviation. After taking a call from Mrs. Johnston, she remembers that she used the incorrect abbreviation in her chart last week. When Susan pulls the chart, she notices that entries have been made after the ones that Susan made on Mrs. Johnston's last visit. How does Susan correct her error?

Keeping Records Current

One of the greatest dangers to good record keeping is **procrastination**. The record must be methodically kept current. It is the medical assistant's responsibility to see that this is done.

Case histories and reports may accumulate on the physician's or the medical assistant's desk during the day. After the last patient has gone, check each history to make certain that all necessary information has been recorded and that each entry is sufficiently clear for future understanding. Give the physician all extra reports, such as laboratory and radiology reports, to read and initial so that they may be filed in the patient's case history folder.

While the physician is reviewing these reports, pull the histories of any patients seen outside the office that day, as well as those of patients who have been given special instructions by telephone or for whom prescriptions were ordered. These entries are made in the same manner as for an office visit, but the type of call is explained in parentheses after the date.

A prescription pad, printed on no-smear, carbonless paper, is available for a timesaving, write-it-once system. By placing the prescription blank over the patient's record, the prescription is automatically copied on the record as it is written. Prescription carriers with adhesive strips are also available for the physician who uses duplicate prescription blanks (Figure 13-7).

The patient record should not leave the office. A physician's pocket call record can be used for outside calls, and the information can be transferred to the chart in the office (Figure 13-8). Notations should be made of any missed appointments or of refusals to cooperate with instructions as they occur.

After all records have been reviewed for the day, they should be placed in a file tray and locked away for the night if there is insufficient time to file them. Do not leave histories out in view at night, especially if the facility has a night cleaning service. On arrival the next morning, the medical assistant can index the histories for filing. Attach extra reports and information sheets. Always attach material to the chart permanently—do not simply drop forms into the folders. When this has been done, the records are ready for filing.

The physician may prefer to dictate progress notes rather than write them in longhand. At appropriate times during the day, everything is dictated: patient histories, physical examination findings, medications prescribed, follow-up findings, and summaries of telephone conversations. At the end of the day, the recorded information is given to the medical assistant for transcribing onto the records.

A great deal of time may be saved in transcribing these notes by using a continuous roll or pages of self-adhesive strips. When the transcription has been completed, the physician may wish to check the notes, underline important points, and initial each entry before returning the notes to the medical assistant for insertion into the charts to verify that they are correct in the event

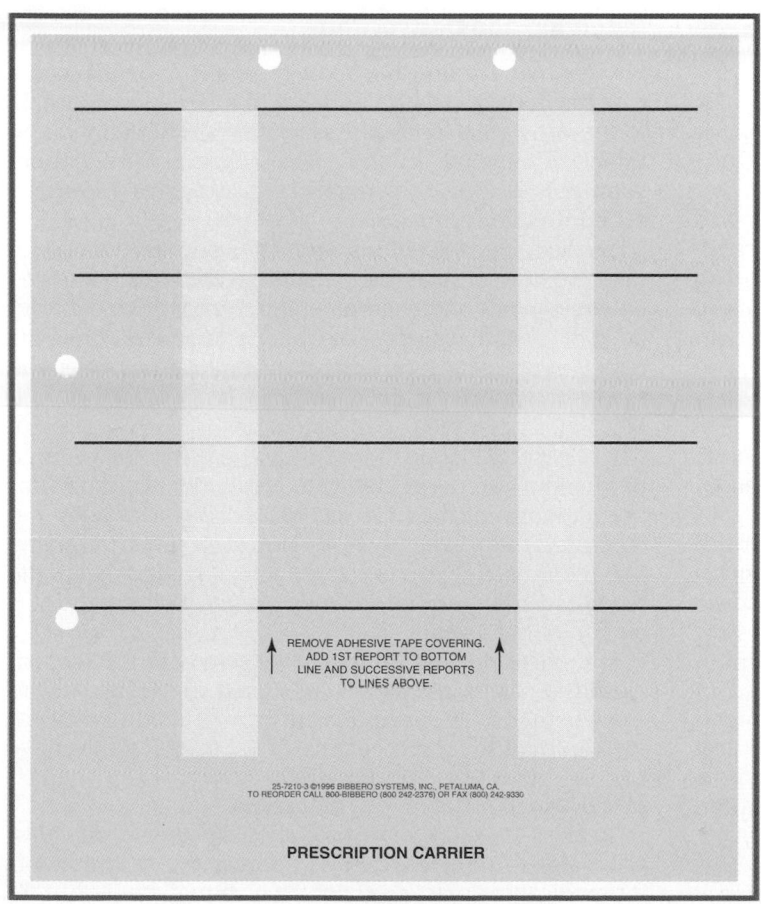

FIGURE 13-7 Filing copies of prescriptions. The self-adhesive on this form allows a copy of the prescription to be filed inside the patient's chart, and saves time over handwriting the information a second time. (Courtesy Bibbero Systems, Inc., Petaluma, Calif. 94954, (800) 242-2376, www.bibbero.com.)

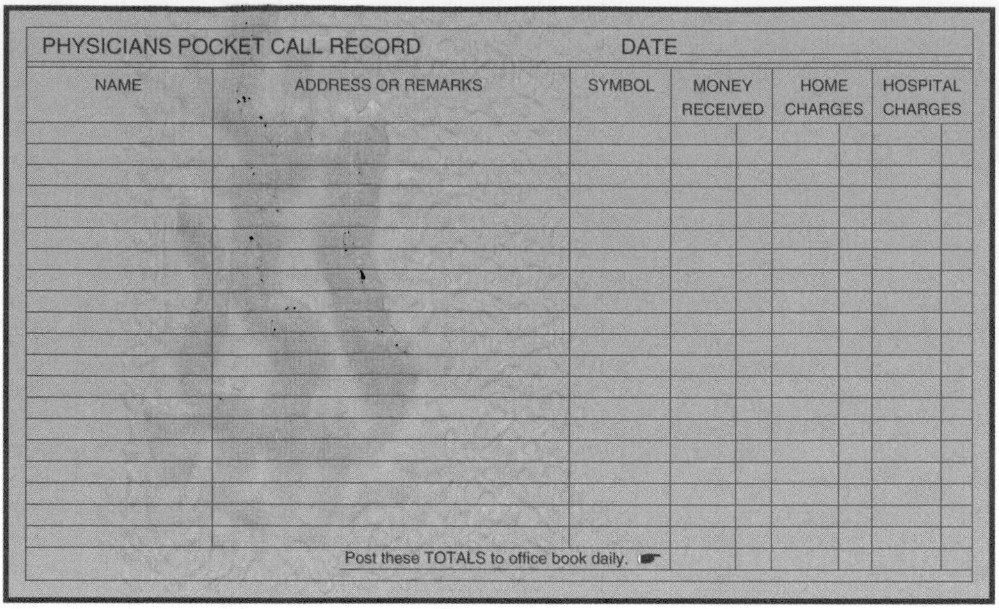

PHYSICIANS POCKET CALL RECORD		DATE					
NAME	ADDRESS OR REMARKS		SYMBOL	MONEY RECEIVED	HOME CHARGES	HOSPITAL CHARGES	
	Post these TOTALS to office book daily. ☞						

FIGURE 13-8 Physician pocket call record. The pocket call record may be used to record information about a patient seen away from the clinic, such as skilled nursing facility patients or hospital patients.

of **audit** or litigation. The use of self-adhesive strips saves removing the sheet from a chart that may be bound with metal fasteners, inserting the sheet into the typewriter, and putting the sheet back into the folder (Figure 13-9). It also simplifies the physician's part in checking and initialing the notes, because only the transcribed material is handled, not the bulky charts.

Transfer, Destruction, and Retention of Medical Records

Regular Transfer of Files

In most medical offices, records are filed according to three classifications:

- *Active files* are those of patients currently receiving treatment.
- *Inactive files* generally are those of patients whom the doctor has not seen for 6 months or longer. When such individuals return for care, their folders are replaced in the active file.
- *Closed files* are records of patients who have died, moved away, or otherwise terminated their relationship with the physician.

Some system must be established for regular transfer of files from active to inactive status or possibly destruction. The yearly expansion of charts and the file space available can influence the transfer period. Charts for patients who are currently hospitalized may be kept in a special section for quick reference, then placed in the regular active file when the patient is discharged from the hospital. In a surgical practice, there frequently is a specific date on which the patient is discharged from the physician's care and the notation made on the chart "Return prn" (for the Latin *pro re nata,* "as the occasion arises" or "when needed"). This record may safely be placed in the inactive file. In a general practice office, the outside of the folder may be stamped with the date of the visit each time the patient is seen. It will then be a simple matter to determine when the chart should be transferred to the inactive status. This is called the perpetual transfer method.

Retention and Destruction

Physicians have an obligation to retain patient records that may reasonably be of value to a patient, according to the American Medical Association (AMA) Council on Ethical and Judicial Affairs. There is no standard, nationwide rule to follow in establishing a records **retention schedule** at this time.

Medical considerations are the primary basis for deciding how long to retain medical records. For example, operative notes and chemotherapy records should always be part of the patient's chart. The laws regarding the retention of medical records vary from state to state, and many governmental programs, such as Medicare and Medicaid, have their own guidelines for records retention. These guidelines range anywhere from 3 years to permanent retention. When there is no restriction for the retention of medical records, it is best to keep the records for a 10-year period. However, when retaining the records of a minor, the facility should keep the records until the minor reaches the age of majority, plus an additional 3 years.

If a particular record no longer needs to be kept for medical reasons, the physician should check state law to see whether there is a requirement that records be kept for a minimum length of time (most states do not have such a provision). The time is measured from the last professional contact with the patient.

In all cases, medical records should be kept for at least as long as the length of time of the statute of limitations for medical malpractice claims, which may be 3 or more

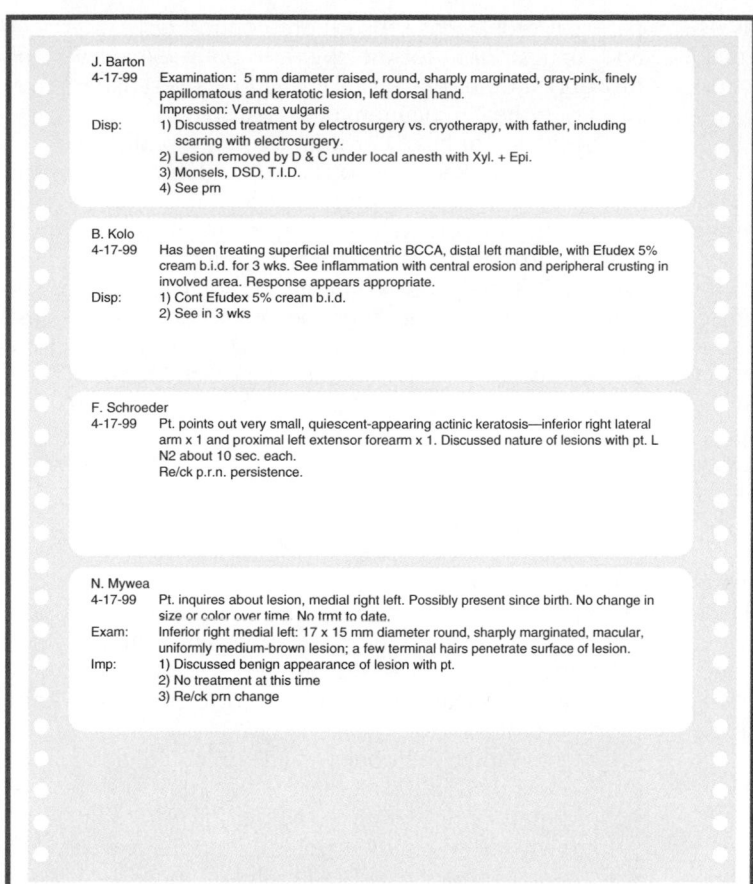

J. Barton
4-17-99   Examination: 5 mm diameter raised, round, sharply marginated, gray-pink, finely
           papillomatous and keratotic lesion, left dorsal hand.
           Impression: Verruca vulgaris
Disp: 1) Discussed treatment by electrosurgery vs. cryotherapy, with father, including
              scarring with electrosurgery.
           2) Lesion removed by D & C under local anesth with Xyl. + Epi.
           3) Monsels, DSD, T.I.D.
           4) See prn

B. Kolo
4-17-99   Has been treating superficial multicentric BCCA, distal left mandible, with Efudex 5%
           cream b.i.d. for 3 wks. See inflammation with central erosion and peripheral crusting in
           involved area. Response appears appropriate.
Disp: 1) Cont Efudex 5% cream b.i.d.
           2) See in 3 wks

F. Schroeder
4-17-99   Pt. points out very small, quiescent-appearing actinic keratosis—inferior right lateral
           arm x 1 and proximal left extensor forearm x 1. Discussed nature of lesions with pt. L
           N2 about 10 sec. each.
           Re/ck p.r.n. persistence.

N. Mywea
4-17-99   Pt. inquires about lesion, medial right left. Possibly present since birth. No change in
           size or color over time. No trmt to date.
Exam: Inferior right medial left: 17 x 15 mm diameter round, sharply marginated, macular,
           uniformly medium-brown lesion; a few terminal hairs penetrate surface of lesion.
Imp: 1) Discussed benign appearance of lesion with pt.
           2) No treatment at this time
           3) Re/ck prn change

A

FIGURE 13-9 **A** and **B**, Self-adhesive progress notes. Progress notes can be quickly filed into the chart when self-adhesive forms are used.

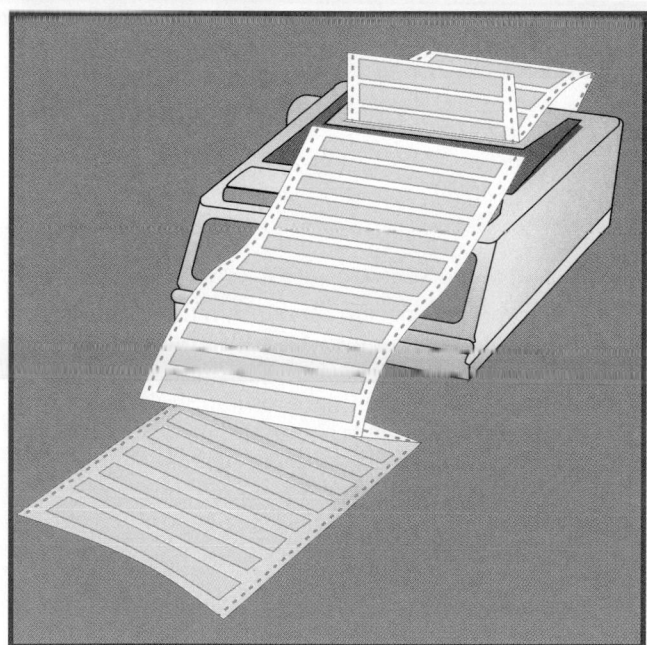

B

years, depending on the state law. In the case of a minor, the statute of limitations may not apply until the patient reaches the age of majority.

The records of any patient covered by Medicare or Medicaid must be kept at least 6 years. HIPAA recom-mends that records for patients who have died should be kept for at least 2 years.

Before discarding old records, patients should be given an opportunity to claim a copy of the records or have them sent to another physician, if it is feasible to give the patient that opportunity. To preserve confidentiality when discarding old records, the documents should be destroyed by shredding or through a professional document destruction service.

Protection of Records

Releasing original case histories to anyone outside the healthcare facility should be avoided. Instead, prepare a summary or photocopy the materials needed for reference and retain the original in the physician's office. With the facsimile machine becoming standard equipment in business facilities, as well as in many of our homes, the transfer of information is simplified and the records remain in safekeeping. Often only certain aspects of the record are requested by colleagues or others, and these can easily be supplied by faxing the required pages, observing precautions for confidentiality.

Occasions may arise when records are temporarily out of the office. Some physicians release case histories to their colleagues, or an original record may be subpoenaed by the court. In such instances, a colored **OUTfolder** should be inserted in the file in place of the regular folder and a notation made of the name, date, and to whom the record was released. Interim papers may be placed in the OUTfolder until the original is returned.

Long-Term Storage

Large healthcare facilities may find it advisable to microfilm records for storage. Another option is the transfer of paper records by laser beam onto optical disks. *Microfilm* and optical disk technology are both expensive and probably are not practical for any but a very large group practice or health maintenance organization.

Facilities that have computerized the patient records will be able to keep those records indefinitely on disk. Scanners can convert a paper record into an image on the computer screen resulting in an electronic medical record. Records can be scanned and stored in electronic format on writeable CD- or DVD-ROMs. The bulky paper files can then be put in storage or eliminated. There is no longer a need to fill hundreds of square feet of storage space or search through stack upon stack of storage file boxes for an inactive or closed file.

Releasing Medical Record Information

The medical facility must be extremely careful when releasing any type of medical information. The patient must sign a release for information to be given to any third party (Procedure 13-4).

Often a family member will call to inquire about a patient, but without the patient's specific request or release, no information may be given. Some offices have a "code" system whereby the patient gives the facility a code word, which must be used by a family member to receive medical information about the patient.

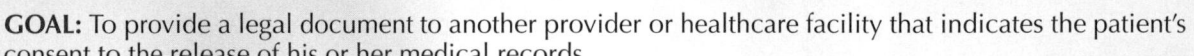

PROCEDURE 13-4

Preparing a Record Release Form

GOAL: To provide a legal document to another provider or healthcare facility that indicates the patient's consent to the release of his or her medical records.

EQUIPMENT AND SUPPLIES

- Medical record release form
- Pen
- Envelope

PROCEDURAL STEPS

1 Explain to the patient that a medical record release form will be necessary to obtain records from another provider. If the patient is having records sent to another provider, a release will also be required.

Purpose: To ensure the patient's understanding of the records release procedure and purposes.

2 Review the record release form with the patient and ask if the form is understood or if there are any questions about the form.

Purpose: To provide the opportunity for questions and to ensure the patient's understanding of the form.

3 Have the patient sign the form in the space indicated. If other demographic information is required, such as a social security number or other names used, complete that information as well.

Purpose: The patient must sign the form for records to be released by any medical facility.

4 Make a copy of the form for the file and then mail it to the appropriate facility. Note the date that the form was sent. Provide a copy to the patient if requested.

Purpose: To provide a record that the information or documents were actually requested on a certain date.

5 Follow-up to ensure that the requested records actually arrived.

Purpose: To make certain that the records needed by the physician to accurately and competently treat the patient are available in a timely manner.

```
┌─────────────────────────────────────────────────────────┐
│                RECORDS RELEASE AUTHORIZATION              │
│                                                           │
│  TO _____ │
│                        Doctor or Hospital                 │
│                                                           │
│  _____ │
│                          Address                          │
│  I HEREBY AUTHORIZE AND REQUEST YOU TO RELEASE TO:        │
│                                                           │
│                                                           │
│                                                           │
│  ALL RECORDS IN YOUR POSSESION CONCERNING _____  │
│                                                           │
│  _____ILLNESS AND/OR   │
│                                                           │
│  TREATMENT DURING THE PERIOD FROM _____TO _____.  │
│                                                           │
│  NAME _____ TEL. _____  │
│                                                           │
│  ADDRESS_____ │
│                                                           │
│  SIGNATURE _____ DATE _____ │
│                (If relative, state relationship)          │
│  WITNESS_____ DATE _____  │
│                                                           │
│      25-8104 © 1973 BIBBERO SYSTEMS, INC., PETALUMA,, CA. │
└─────────────────────────────────────────────────────────┘
```

FIGURE 13-10 Medical record release authorization. All requests for medical records should be in writing and the request should be kept in the patient chart. (Courtesy Bibbero Systems, Inc., Petaluma, Calif. 94954, (800) 242-2376, www.bibbero.com.)

Requests for medical information should be made in writing (Figure 13-10). It is unwise to accept a faxed request for medical information or a faxed release of information from a patient. Even requests from the patient's attorney or third-party payors must be cleared by the patient to receive information. Some attorneys may present a legal document called a **power of attorney**, which authorizes them to see the records. Still, this document is signed by the patient, so it is a release in itself.

CRITICAL THINKING APPLICATION

Susan has never seen a power of attorney and is curious about this type of document. How might she investigate and learn more about them? Who should Susan approach first for this information? The physician has an attorney that Susan has met once. Should she call him and ask about the document without notifying the physician? Why or why not?

Sometimes, the patient will want to view his or her own record. They certainly have a right to see this information, but some patients may not understand the terminology used in the record. A staff member should always remain with the patient who is viewing his or her medical records. Remember, the original medical record should never leave the medical facility.

When a release is presented to the office, only copy the records requested in the release. Do not provide additional information that is not requested. It is acceptable to charge reasonable copying fees to the person requesting the information.

Dictation and Transcription

Administrative medical assistants may find that transcribing **dictation** is one of the job requirements they perform periodically. **Transcription** can be performed from handwritten notes, such as those in shorthand, or from machine dictation. In a healthcare facility, the medical transcriptionist is a part of the team. Smooth operation of the facility may depend on the timely and accurate performance of assigned responsibilities, such as record documentation and the preparation of special reports.

The transcriptionist will find that *accuracy* and *speed* are primary **requisites,** as well as a strong grasp of medical knowledge, especially anatomy and physiology (Figure 13-11). Income depends on the transcriptionist's productivity, which may be measured by the number of pages, characters, or lines typed. The person who intends to do transcribing exclusively would do well to take a special course in transcription techniques. Certification is available through the American Association for Medical Transcriptionists.

Machine Transcription

Three stages of activity are involved in the process of dictation and transcription:

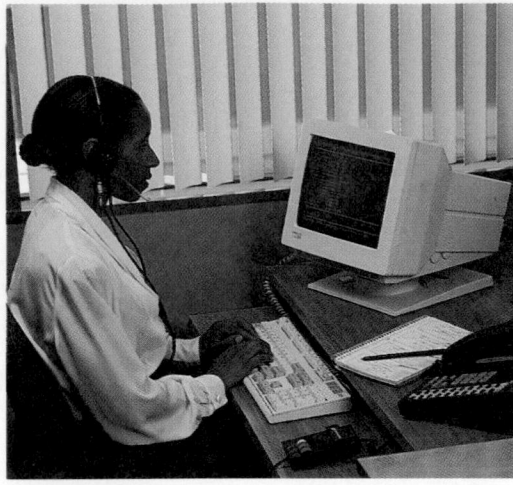

FIGURE 13-11 Medical transcriptionists must have excellent typing skills and good hearing. They must be accurate and use good grammatical skills while completing transcription duties.

- Dictating into a dictation unit
- Listening to what has been dictated
- Keyboarding the dictated text to a printed document using correct format and required punctuation

Dictation Unit

A dictation unit is used by the physician to record material to be typed. Dictation units vary in design and capabilities. A desktop dictation unit is common in an office setting. This may be a combination unit used for both dictation and transcription. Alternatively, a machine used only for dictation may remain at the physician's desk; a separate transcription unit, including headphones and a foot pedal, remains at the transcriptionist's station. A lightweight, portable, handheld dictation unit may be used for times when the physician wishes to dictate while traveling or attending meetings away from the office. Digital dictation machines are now available and are lightweight, portable, and hold more information than standard dictation recorders. Physicians in a larger setting may install transcribing equipment that they can access by telephone wherever they may be. Many hospitals have this arrangement. All produce a recording that the transcriptionist listens to while keyboarding the text.

CRITICAL THINKING APPLICATION

Susan would like to practice transcription skills at home, but she does not have a transcription unit. How could she do this without the proper equipment? Medical terminology is important to the medical assistant who does transcription. What are some ways Susan can improve her medical terminology skills?

Transcriber Unit

The unit operated by the transcriptionist may use magnetic tape, a cassette, or a disk. A desktop unit using mini-cassettes, microcassettes, or standard cassettes is typical in the physician's office.

There are many types and manufacturers of transcribing equipment, but most units contain certain standard features. Before using any equipment, the medical assistant should study the manufacturer's instruction manual. Most transcription units have a minimum of the following features:

- Stop and start control, with backup and fast-forward ability
- Speed control
- Volume control
- Tone control
- Indicator for locating special instructions and determining the document length

A beginning transcriptionist tends to listen to a few words, stop the machine, type those words, and then restart the transcriber unit. Through practice, the transcriptionist learns to coordinate keyboarding activity with listening skills and listen ahead, thereby retaining in memory more and more of the dictated material so that it becomes unnecessary to stop and start the machine for this purpose.

Keyboarding Unit

The most important piece of equipment for the transcriptionist is the typewriter or computer on which the printed text will be produced (Procedure 13-5). Many improvements have occurred within the past few years. Computers have attachable foot pedals and headphones that allow the medical assistant to perform transcription directly onto the unit. A variety of software programs are available to assist with transcription duties.

Filing Equipment

The vertical four-drawer steel filing cabinet, used with manila folders with the patient's name on the tab, was the traditional system of choice for years. The most popular system today is color coding on open shelves. There are also rotary, lateral, compactible, and automated files. Some records are kept in card or tray files. Regardless of the type or style of equipment, the best quality is always an economy. Some of the considerations in selecting filing equipment are as follows:

- Office space availability
- Structural considerations
- Cost of space and equipment
- Size, type, and volume of records
- Confidentiality requirements
- Retrieval speed
- Fire protection

Drawer Files

Drawer files should be full suspension; they should roll easily, close securely, and be equipped with a locking device. The best cabinets have a center trough at the bottom of each drawer with a rod for holding divider guides. Floor space of twice the depth of the drawer must

PROCEDURE 13-5

Transcribing a Machine-Dictated Letter Using a Computer or Word Processor

GOAL: To transcribe a machine-dictated letter into a mailable document without error or corrections, using a computer or word processor.

EQUIPMENT AND SUPPLIES

- Transcribing machine
- Word processor or computer with appropriate software
- Stationery
- Reference manual

PROCEDURAL STEPS

1 Assemble supplies.

2 Set up format for selected letter style.

3 Keyboard the text while listening to the dictated letter.

4 Edit the letter on the monitor.
   Purpose: The letter should be in mailable form before printing.

5 Execute a spell check.

6 Direct the letter to the printer.

---

be allowed so that the drawer can be pulled out to its full extent. A drawback of the vertical four-drawer files is that only one person can use a file cabinet at any given time. Filing is also slower because the drawer must be opened and closed each time a file is pulled or filed. Drawer files are relatively easy to move, but for safety reasons they should be bolted to the wall or to each other.

File drawers are heavy and can tip over, causing serious damage or injury unless reasonable care is observed. Open only one file drawer at a time and close it when the filing has been completed. A drawer left even slightly open can cause injury to a passerby.

Shelf Files

Shelf files should have doors to protect the contents. A popular type of shelf file has doors that slide back into the cabinet; the door from a lower shelf may be pulled out and used for work space. About 50% more material per square foot of floor space may be filed in shelf files when compared with the four-drawer file. Open shelf units hold files sideways and can go higher on the wall because there is no drawer to pull out (Figure 13-12). File retrieval is faster because several individuals can work simultaneously.

Open shelf units without doors are the most economical but offer little protection or confidentiality to the records. They are susceptible to water and fire damage. Shelf files are available in many attractive colors and can add a decorative note to the business office. Special storage or shelf space should be provided for x-ray films, if many films are stored.

Rotary Circular Files

Rotary circular files can hold a large volume of records. They save space and clerical motion. The files revolve

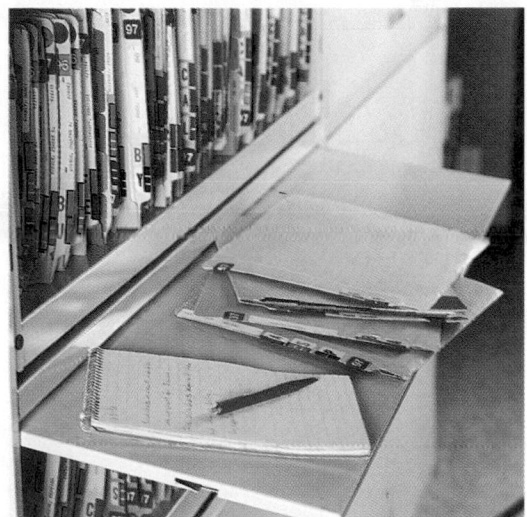

FIGURE 13-12 Open shelf filing is an efficient method, especially for color-coded filing systems. The shelf doors can often be used as workspace.

easily; some come with push-button controls. Several persons can work at one rotary file and use records at the same time. One disadvantage is that they afford less privacy and protection than files that can be closed and locked.

Lateral Files

Lateral files are good for personal files and are especially attractive for the physician's private office. They use more wall space than the vertical file but do not extend out into the room so far. The folders are filed sideways in the lateral file, left to right, instead of front to back as in a vertical file. Some have a pull-out drawer, as the vertical file does; others have doors that slide into the cabinet, exposing the filing space.

Compactible Files

The office with little space and a great volume of records might use compactible files, which are a variation of open shelf files. The files are mounted on tracks in the floor, and the units slide along the tracks so that access is gained to the needed records. They may be either automated or manual. One drawback is that not all records are available at the same time.

Automated Files

Automated files are very expensive initially and require more maintenance than do the other types of filing equipment. They will probably be found only in very large installations such as clinics or hospitals. These files bring the record to the operator instead of the operator going to the record. When the operator presses a button indicating the appropriate shelf, the shelf automatically moves into position in front of the operator for record retrieval. The automated or power file is fast and can store large amounts of records in a small amount of space. Only one person can use the unit at one time.

Card Files

Almost every office has some occasion to use a card file. This may be for patient ledgers, a patient index, library index, index of surgical tray setups, telephone numbers, or numerous other records. A good-quality steel box or tray is a sound investment.

Special Items

Metal framework is available that can convert a regular drawer file into suspension-folder equipment. The assistant with a great deal of filing may wish to purchase a portable filing shelf that fits on the side of an opened drawer and can be moved from place to place as needed. Another special filing item is a sorting file, which can be a great time saver. A portable file cart for the temporary filing of unbilled insurance claims may be quite useful. It may also be used for the preliminary sorting of charts to be refiled. This is sometimes called a *suspense file*.

Supplies

Divider Guides

Each file drawer or shelf should be equipped with plenty of dividers or guides. Some authorities recommend one guide for approximately each 1 1/2 inches of material, or every eight to ten folders. Guides should be of good-quality **pressboard** or strong plastic. Economy guides will soon become bent and frayed and have to be replaced. Divider guides have a protruding tab, which may be either an integral part of the card or may be made of metal or plastic. The guides reduce the area of search and serve as

supports for the folders. They are available in single, third, or fifth cut (one, three, or five different positions). The guide may have a projection at the bottom edge with a ring or hole through which a rod may go. This type of guide card is used in drawers that have a trough for the projection and a rod to hold the guides in place.

OUTguides

An **OUTguide** is a heavy guide that is used to replace a folder that has been temporarily removed (Figure 13-13). It should be of a distinctive color for quick detection. This makes refiling simpler and alerts the file clerk that a file is missing. Several colors may be used, each color designating the temporary location of the file. The OUTguide may have lines for recording information, or it may have a plastic pocket for inserting an information card.

Chart Covers of Folders

Most records to be filed are placed in covers or tabbed folders. The most commonly used is a general-purpose third-cut manila folder that may be expanded to 3/4 inch. These are available with a double-thickness reinforced tab that will greatly lengthen the life of the folder. Folders kept in drawers have tabs at the top; those kept on shelves have tabs at the side. There are many variations of folder styles obtainable for special purposes.

The vertical pocket, which is heavier weight than the general purpose folder, has a front that folds down for easy access to contents and is available with up to 3 1/2-inch expansion. These are used for bulky histories or correspondence.

Hanging or suspension folders are made of heavy stock and hang on metal rods from side to side of a drawer. They can be used only with files equipped with suspension equipment.

Binder folders have fasteners with which to bind papers within the folder. These offer some security for the papers but are time consuming in filing the materials.

The number of papers that will fit in one folder depends on the thickness of the papers. Near the bottom edge of most folders are one or more score marks, which should be used as the contents of the folders expand. If folders are refolded at these score marks, the danger of their bending and sliding under other folders is reduced, and a neater file results. Papers should never protrude from the folder edges, and they should always be inserted with their tops to the left. When papers start to ride up in any folder, the folder is overloaded.

Labels

The label is a necessary filing and finding device. Use labels to identify each shelf, drawer, divider guide, and folder. A label on the drawer or shelf identifies the nature of its contents. It should also indicate the range (alphabetical, numerical, or chronological) of the material filed in that space.

The label on the divider guide identifies the range of folder headings following that divider guide up to the next divider; for example, BaBo. The label on the folder

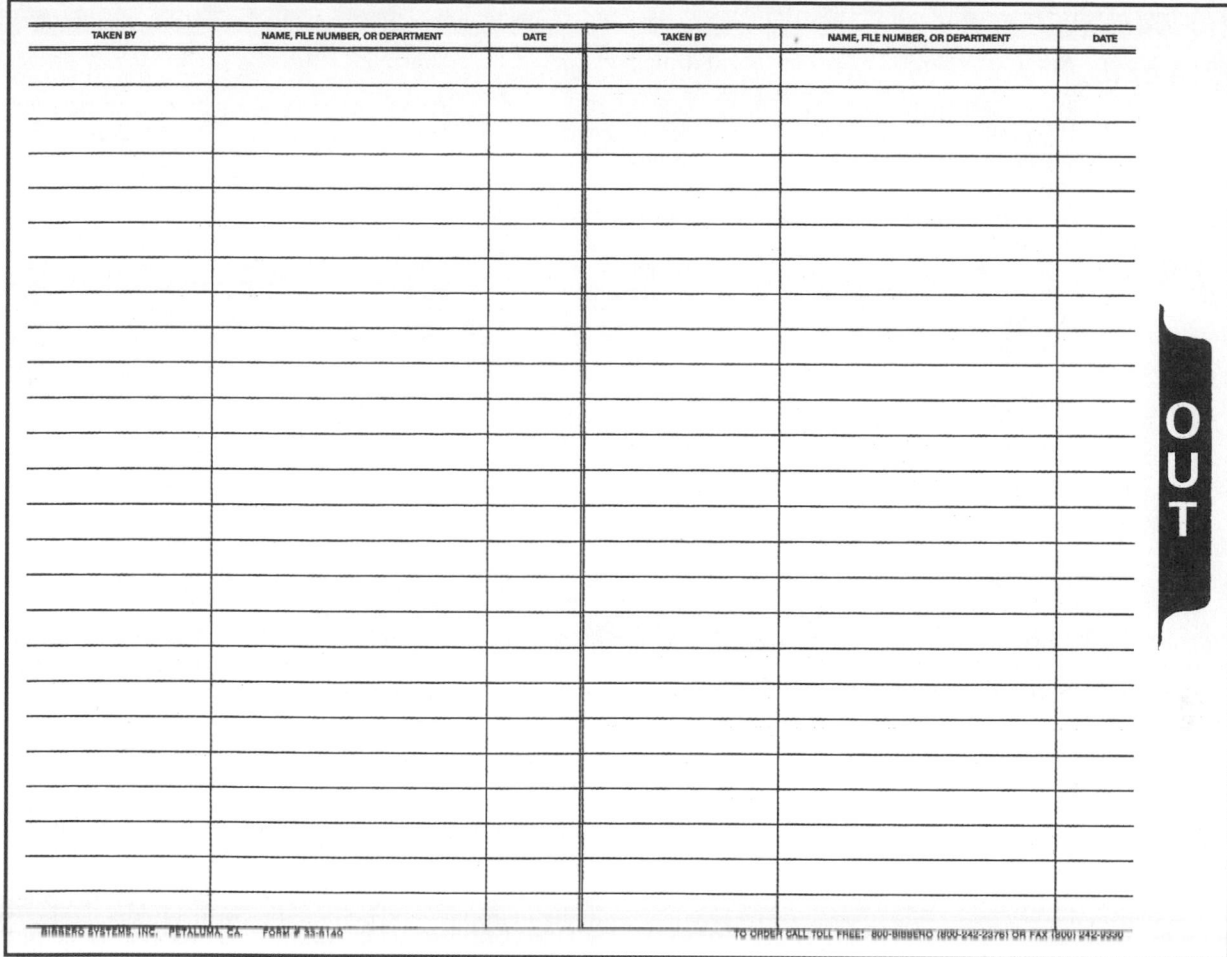

TAKEN BY	NAME, FILE NUMBER, OR DEPARTMENT	DATE	TAKEN BY	NAME, FILE NUMBER, OR DEPARTMENT	DATE

BIBBERO SYSTEMS, INC., PETALUMA, CA.   FORM # 33-8140

TO ORDER CALL TOLL FREE: 800-BIBBERO (800-242-2376) OR FAX (800) 242-9330

FIGURE 13-13   OUTguides provide tracking for files that are not in their proper location. The guide gives information as to where the file can be located. (Courtesy Bibbero Systems, Inc., Petaluma, Calif. 94954, (800) 242-2376, www.bibbero.com.)

identifies the content of that folder only. This may be the name of the patient, subject matter of correspondence, a business topic, or anything at all that needs to be filed. Label a folder when a new patient is seen or existing folders are full or when materials need to be transferred within the filing system.

Paper labels may be purchased in rolls of gummed tape; another type has adhesive backs that are peeled from a protective sheet. Labels are available in almost any size, shape, or color to meet the individual needs of any facility. Visit a stationer and study the catalogs to find the best product to meet the needs of the facility.

A narrow label applied to the front of the folder tab is the easiest to use and is satisfactory for folders kept in a drawer file. Labels for shelf filing should be identifiable from both front and back. Always type the label before separating it from the roll or protective sheet. Type the **caption** on the label in indexing order.

Filing Procedures

Filing of all materials involves five basic steps: conditioning, releasing, indexing and coding, sorting, and storing and filing.

Conditioning

Conditioning of papers involves (1) removing all pins, brads, and paper clips, (2) stapling related papers together, (3) attaching clippings or items smaller than page-size to a regular sheet of paper with rubber cement or tape, and (4) mending damaged records.

Releasing

The term *releasing* simply means that some mark is placed on the paper indicating that it is now ready for filing. This will usually be either the medical assistant's initials or a FILE stamp placed in the upper left corner.

Indexing and Coding

Indexing means deciding where to file the letter or paper, and coding means placing some indication of this decision on the paper (Table 13-1). This may be done by underlining the name or subject, if it appears on the paper, or writing the indexing subject or name in some conspicuous place. If there is more than one logical place to file the paper, the original is coded for the main location and a cross-reference sheet prepared, indicating this location and coded for the second

TABLE 13-1	Application of Indexing Rules			
Indexing Rule	Name	Unit 1	Unit 2	Unit 3
1	Robert F. Grinch	Grinch	Robert	F.
	R. Frank Grumman	Grumman	R.	Frank
2	J. Orville Smith	Smith	J.	Orville
	Jason O. Smith	Smith	Jason	O.
3	M. L. Saint-Vickery	Saint-Vickery	M.	L.
	Marie-Louise Taylor	Taylor	Marielouise	
4	Charles S. Anderson	Anderson	Charles	S.
	Anderson's Surgical Supply	Andersons	Surgical	Supply
5	Ah Hop Akee	Akee	Ah	Hop
6	Alice Delaney	Delaney	Alice	
	Chester K. DeLong	Delong	Chester	K.
7	Michael St. John	Stjohn	Michael	
8	Helen M. Maag	Maag	Helen	M.
	Frederick Mabry	Mabry	Frederick	
	James E. MacDonald	Macdonald	James	E.
9	Mrs. John L. Doe (Mary Jones)	Doe	Mary	Jones (Mrs John L.)
10	Prof. John J. Breck	Breck	John	J. (Prof.)
	Madame Sylvia	Madame	Sylvia	
	Sister Mary Catherine	Sister	Mary	Catherine
	Theodore Wilson, M.D.	Wilson	Theodore (M.D.)	
11	Lawrence W. Sloan, Jr.	Sloan	Lawrence	W. (Jr.)
	Lawrence W. Sloan, Sr.	Sloan	Lawrence	W. (Sr.)
12	The Moore Clinic	Moore	Clinic (The)	

location. Every paper placed in a patient's chart should have the date and name of the patient on it, usually in the upper right corner.

Sorting

Sorting is arranging the papers in filing sequence. Sort papers before going to the file cabinet or shelf. Do any necessary stapling of papers at the desk or filing table. Invest in a desktop sorter with a series of dividers between which papers are placed in filing sequence. One general-purpose sorter has six means of classification: alphabetical sections, numbers 1 to 31, days of the week, months of the year, numbers in groups of five, and space on the tabs for special captions to be taped when desired. In the preliminary sorting, place the papers in the appropriate division in the sorter. Then it is comparatively simple to arrange these groups into the proper sequence for filing.

Storing and Filing

In storing or filing papers in the folder, items should be placed face up, top edge to the left, with the most recent date to the front of the folder. Lift the folder 1 or 2 inches out of the drawer before inserting new material, so that the sheets can drop down completely into the folder. When refiling completed folders, arrange them in indexing order before going to the file cabinets.

Locating Misplaced Files

Unless files are promptly replaced after use, they may become lost. Papers may be misfiled, requiring a thor-ough search to find them. After a methodical and complete search through the proper folder, there are several places one may look for a misplaced paper: (1) in the folder in front of and behind the correct folder; (2) between the folders; (3) on the bottom of the file under all the folders; (4) in a folder of a patient with a similar name; or (5) in the sorter.

Indexing Rules

Indexing rules are fairly well standardized, based on current business practices. The Association of Records Managers and Administrators takes an active part in updating the rules. Some establishments adopt variations of these basic rules to accommodate their needs. In any case the practices need to be consistent within the system.

1. Last names of persons are considered first in filing; given name (first name), second; and middle name or initial, third. Compare the names beginning with the first letter of the name. When there is a letter that is different in the two names, that letter determines the order of filing. For example:

ab*e*
ab*i*
ab*m*
ab*x*
a*c*l
ac*m*
a*d*a
ad*e*
ad*i*

2. *Initials* precede a *name* beginning with the same letter. This illustrates the librarian's rule, "Nothing comes before something." For example:

> Smith, J.
> Smith, Jason

3. *Hyphenated personal names*. The hyphenated elements of a name, whether first name, middle name, or surname, are considered to be one unit. For example:

> Carlotta Freeman-Duque is filed as
> Freemanduque, Carlotta
> Cindy-Jean Green is filed as
> Green, Cindyjean

4. The apostrophe is disregarded in filing. For example:

> Andersons' Surgical Supply
> Andersons Surgical Supply

5. When indexing a foreign name and *cannot* distinguish the first and last name, index each part of the name in the order in which it is written:

> Cau Liu
> Talluri Devi

If you *can* make the distinction, you should use the last name as the first indexing unit:

> Liu, Jason

6. Names with prefixes are filed in the usual alphabetical order with the prefix being considered as part of the name. For example:

> von Schmidt is filed as Vonschmidt
> DeLong is filed as Delong
> LaFrance is filed as Lafrance

7. Abbreviated parts of a name are indexed as written if that is the form generally used by that person. For example:

> Ste. Marie is filed as Stemarie
> St. John is filed as Stjohn
> Wm. is filed as Wm
> Edw. is filed as Edw
> Jas. is filed as Jas

8. Mac and Mc are filed in their regular place in the alphabet:

> Maag
> Mabry
> *Mac*Donald
> Machado
> *Mac*Hale
> Maville
> *Mc*Aulay
> *Mc*Williams
> Meacham

If the files contain a great many names beginning with Mac or Mc, some offices file them as a separate letter of the alphabet for convenience.

9. The name of a married woman is indexed by her legal name (her husband's surname, her given name, and her middle name or maiden surname). For example:

> Doe, Mary Jones (Mrs. John L.)
> *not* Doe, Mrs. John L. (unless first name is unknown)

10. Titles, when followed by a complete name, may be used as the *last* filing unit if needed to distinguish from another identical name. For example:

> Mr. James D. Conley
> Conley James D Mr
> Dr. James D. Conley
> Conley James D Dr.

Titles without complete names are considered the *first* indexing unit:

> Madame Sylvia
> Sister Theresa

11. Terms of seniority, or professional or academic degree, are used only to distinguish from an identical name. For example:

> Theodore Wilson, PhD
> Theodore Wilson, Sr.
> Theodore Wilson, Jr.
> Theodore Wilson, MD

These examples would be filed in the following order:

> Theodore Wilson, Jr.
> Theodore Wilson, MD
> Theodore Wilson, PhD
> Theodore Wilson, Sr.

12. Articles such as *The* or *A* are disregarded in indexing:

Moore Clinic (The)

Filing Methods

The three basic methods of filing used in healthcare facilities are these:
- Alphabetical by name
- Numeric
- Subject

Patient charts are filed either alphabetically by name or by one of several numeric methods. Subject filing is used for business records, correspondence, and topical materials.

Alphabetical Filing

Alphabetical filing by name is the oldest, simplest, and most commonly used system. It is the system of choice for filing patient records in the majority of physicians' offices. If the medical assistant can find a word in the dictionary or a name in the telephone directory, then he or she already knows some of the rules.

The alphabetical system of filing is traditional and simple to set up, requiring only a file cabinet or shelf, folders, and some divider guides (Procedure 13-6). It is a **direct filing system**, in that the person filing need only know the name in order to find the desired file. Alphabetical filing does have some drawbacks:
- The correct spelling of the name must be known.
- As the number of files increases, more space is needed for each section of the alphabet. This results in periodic shifting of folders from drawer to drawer or shelf to shelf to allow for expansion.
- As the files expand, more time is required for filing or retrieving each folder because of the greater number of folders involved in the search. The time can be greatly reduced by color coding.

Numeric Filing

Some form of **numeric filing** combined with color and **shelf filing** is used by practically every large clinic or hospital. Management consultants differ in their recommendations; some recommend numeric filing only if there are more than 5000 charts, more than 10,000 charts, or in some cases more than 15,000 charts. Others recommend nothing but numeric filing. Numeric filing is an **indirect filing system**, requiring the use of an alphabetical cross-reference to find a given file. Some people object to this added step and overlook the advantages, which are that it:
- Allows unlimited expansion without periodic shifting of folders, and shelves are usually filled evenly.
- Provides additional confidentiality to the chart.

PROCEDURE **13-6**

Filing Medical Records and Documents Using the Alphabetical System

GOAL: To file records efficiently using an alphabetical system and ensure that the records can be easily and quickly retrieved.

EQUIPMENT AND SUPPLIES

- Medical records
- Physical filing equipment
- Cart to carry records, if needed
- Alphabetical file guide
- Staple remover
- Stapler

PROCEDURAL STEPS

1 Using alphabetical guidelines, place the records to be filed in alphabetical order. If a stack of documents is to be filed, place them in alphabetical order inside an alphabetical file guide or sorter. Use rules for filing documents alphabetically.
Purpose: To organize the filing process and file the record or document quickly without retracing steps and skipping from letter to letter.

2 Go to the filing storage equipment (shelves, cabinets, or drawers) and locate the spot in the alphabet for the first file.

3 Place the file in the cabinet or drawer in correct alphabetical order.

4 If adding a document to a file, place it on top so that the most recent information is seen first. This puts the information in the file in reverse chronological order.
Purpose: To provide access to the most pertinent and recent information.

5 Securely fasten documents to the chart. Do not just drop the documents inside the chart.
Purpose: To keep vital information from falling out of the chart and being lost.

6 Refile the chart in its proper place.

- Saves time in retrieving and refiling records quickly. One knows immediately that the number 978 falls between 977 and 979. By contrast, an alphabetical system, even with color coding, requires a longer search for the exact spot.

There are several types of numeric filing systems. In the straight or consecutive numeric system, patients are given consecutive numbers as they visit the practice. This is the simplest of the numeric systems and works well for files of up to 10,000 records. It is time consuming, and there is a greater chance for error when filing documents with five or more digits. Filing activity is greatest at the end of the numeric series.

In the terminal digit system, patients are also assigned consecutive numbers, but the digits in the number are usually separated into groups of twos or threes and are read in groups from right to left instead of from left to right. The records are filed backward in groups. For example, all files ending in 00 are grouped together first, then those ending in 01, etc. Next the files are grouped by their middle digits so that the 00 22s come before the 01 22s. Finally the files are arranged by their first digits, so that 01 00 22 precedes 02 00 22.

Middle-digit filing begins with the middle digits, followed by the first digit and finally by the terminal digits.

Some practices use the last four digits of each patient's Social Security number to file patient records. However, there is no legal requirement that every United States resident have a Social Security number, in which case a "pseudo number" would have to be issued.

Numeric filing requires more training, but once the system is mastered, fewer errors occur than with alphabetical filing (Procedure 13-7).

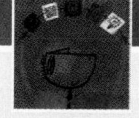

CRITICAL THINKING APPLICATION

Susan is unsure whether alphabetical or numeric filing is best in the medical office. What are some advantages and disadvantages of each method?

Subject Filing

Subject filing can be either alphabetical or **alphanumeric** (A 1-3, B 1-1, B1-2, and so on) and is used for general correspondence. The main difficulty with subject filing is indexing, or classifying—deciding where to file a document. Many papers require cross-referencing. All correspondence dealing with a particular subject is filed together. The papers within the folders are filed chronologically, the most recent on top. The subject headings are placed on the tabs of the folders and filed alphabetically.

Color Coding

When a color coding system is used, both filing and finding are easier, and misfiled folders are kept to a minimum (Procedure 13-8). The use of color visually

---

PROCEDURE **13-7**

Filing Medical Records and Documents Using the Numeric System

GOAL: To file records efficiently using a numeric system and ensure that the records can be easily and quickly retrieved.

EQUIPMENT AND SUPPLIES

- Medical records
- Physical filing equipment
- Cart to carry records, if needed
- Numeric file guide
- Staple remover
- Stapler
- Paper clips

PROCEDURAL STEPS

1 Using numeric guidelines, place the records to be filed in numeric order. If a stack of documents is to be filed, write the chart number on the document. Use rules for filing documents alphabetically.

Purpose: To organize the filing process and file the record or documents quickly without retracing steps and skipping from letter to letter.

2 Go to the filing storage equipment (shelves, cabinets, or drawers) and locate the numeric spot for the first file.

3 Place the file in the cabinet or drawer in correct numeric order.

4 If adding a document to a file, place it on top so that the most recent information is seen first. This puts the information in the file in reverse chronological order.

Purpose: To provide access to the most pertinent and recent information.

5 Securely fasten documents to the chart. Do not just drop the documents inside the chart.

Purpose: To keep vital information from falling out of the chart and being lost.

6 Refile the chart in its proper place.

restricts the area of search for a specific record. A misfiled chart is easily spotted even from a distance of several feet. In color coding, a specific color is selected to identify each letter of the alphabet. The application of the principle may be through using colored folders, adhesive colored identification labels, or various combinations of these. Any selection of colors may be used, and the division of the alphabet is determined by one's own needs. However, studies have shown that there is wide variation in the frequency with which different letters occur.

Alphabetical Color Coding. There are several ways of color coding files. One alphabetical system utilizes five different colored folders, with each color representing a segment of the alphabet. The *second* letter of the patient's last name determines the color.

As medicine continues to consolidate into larger facilities, with more patients under one management, the filing of patient charts becomes more complicated and color coding becomes more useful. Several color-coding systems use two sets of 13 colors—one set for letters A–M, and a second set of the same colors on a different background for the letters N–Z.

There are many ready-made systems available (e.g., Bibbero, Colwell, Kardex, Remington Rand, Smead, TAB, VisiRecord). Self-adhesive colored letter blocks with either two or three letters in the specific colors are supplied in rolls. The color blocks with the appropriate letter are placed on the index tab of the folder, along with the patient's full name. The letters are in pairs so that they can be seen from either side of the chart. Strong, easily differentiated colors are used, creating a band of color in the files that makes it easy to spot out-of-place folders (Figure 13-14).

Numeric Color Coding. Color coding is also used in numeric filing. Numbers 0 through 9 are each assigned a different color. In a terminal digit filing system, the colors for the last two numbers would be affixed to the tab. If the number 1 is red and 5 is yellow, all files with numbers ending in 15 form a red and yellow band. Usually a predetermined section of the number is color coded.

Other Color Coding Applications. There are many other ways to make color work for the efficient medical office. Small pressure-sensitive tabs in a variety of colors may be used to identify certain types of insured patients and other specific information. For example, a red tab over the edge of the folder may identify a patient on Medicaid, a blue tab may identify a CHAMPUS patient; a green tab may identify a workers' compensation patient; matching tabs may be attached to the insured's ledger card; research cases may be identified by a special color tab; and brightly colored labels on the outside of a patient chart can indicate certain health conditions, such as drug allergies. In a partnership practice, a different color folder or label may identify each physician's patients. Color can also be used to differentiate dates—one color for each month or year.

Business records may also utilize color coding. Main divider guide headings may be of one color, subheadings in a second color, and subdivisions in a third color. A fourth color might be used for personal items.

The use of color in filing is limited only by the imagination. One word of caution: Every person in the facility who uses the files must know the key to the coding, and the key should also be written in the facility's procedures manual.

PROCEDURE 13-8

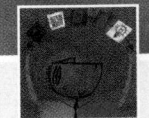

Color Coding Patient Charts

GOAL: To color code patient charts using the agency's established coding system to effectively facilitate filing and finding.

EQUIPMENT AND SUPPLIES

- List of patient charts to code
- File folders
- Information on agency's coding system
- Full range of color tabs

PROCEDURAL STEPS

1 Assemble patient charts.

2 Arrange charts in indexing order.
Purpose: When charts have been color coded, they will be in filing order.

3 Pick up the first chart and note the second letter of the patient's surname.

Explanation: For purpose of activity, the color coding system in the text will be used.

4 Choose a folder and/or caption label of the appropriate color.

5 Type patient's name on label in indexing order and apply to folder tab.
Purpose: To identify sequence of folder in filing system.

6 Repeat steps 4 and 5 until all charts have been coded.

7 Check entire group for any isolated color.
Purpose: If the order and color of the folders is correct, all charts of the same color within each letter of the alphabet will be grouped together.

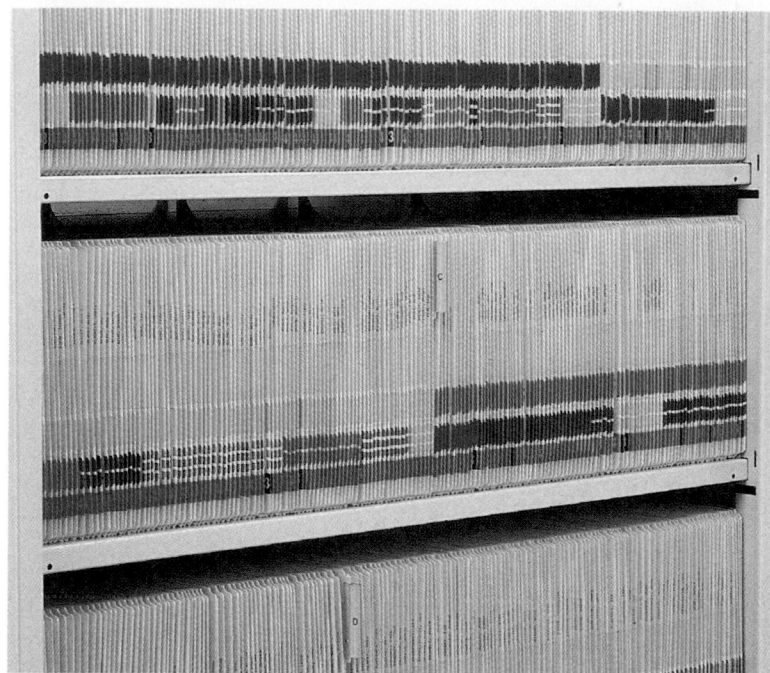

FIGURE 13-14   Color coding patient charts makes it easy to see a file that is misplaced. (Courtesy Bibbero Systems, Inc., Petaluma, Calif. 94954, (800) 242-2376, www.bibbero.com.)

Organization of Files

It is very difficult for a physician to study a disorganized history. Some systematic method must be followed in placing items in the patient folder. The content of the patient record has already been discussed. From the filing standpoint, it should be emphasized that when a patient record is not in actual use, there is only one place it should be—in the filing cabinet or shelf. Many precious hours can be lost in searching for misplaced or lost records that were carelessly left unfiled.

The patient's full name, in indexing order, should be typed on a label and attached to the folder tab. A strip of transparent tape can be placed on the label to prevent smudging if this is a problem. The patient's full name should also be typed on each sheet within the folder.

Health-Related Correspondence

Correspondence pertaining to patients' medical records should be filed with the case history. Other medical correspondence should probably be filed in a subject file.

General Correspondence

The physician's office operates as a business as well as a professional service. There will be correspondence of a general nature pertaining to the operation of the office. In all likelihood, a special drawer or shelf will be set aside for the general correspondence. The correspondence is indexed according to subject matter or names of correspondents. The guides in a subject file may appear in one, two, or three positions, depending on the number of headings, subheadings, and subdivisions.

Practice Management Files

The most active financial record is, of course, the patient ledger. In facilities that still use a manual system, this will be a card or vertical tray file, and the accounts will be arranged alphabetically by name. There will be at least two divisions:
- Active accounts
- Paid accounts

Miscellaneous Folder

Papers that do not warrant an individual folder are placed in a miscellaneous folder. Within the folder, all papers relating to one subject, or with one correspondent, are kept together in chronological order, the most recent on top, and then filed alphabetically with other miscellaneous material. Related materials may be stapled together. Never use paper clips for this purpose. When as many as five papers accumulate with one correspondent or subject, a separate folder should be prepared. Other business files include records of income and expense, financial statements, income and payroll tax records, canceled checks, and insurance policies. These papers may be filed chronologically.

Tickler or Follow-Up Files

The most frequently used follow-up method is that of a **tickler file**, so called because it tickles the memory that something needs to be done or followed up on a particular date. The tickler file is always a chronological arrangement. In its simplest form, it consists of notations on the daily calendar. If information, such as an x-ray report or laboratory report, is expected concerning a patient who has an appointment to come in, the medical assistant might make a note on the calendar or tickler file a day ahead to check on whether the report has arrived.

The tickler file is often a card file with 12 guides for the names of the months and 31 guides printed with numbers 1 through 31 for the days of the month. The guide for the current month, followed by the 31-day guides, is placed at the front of the file. Notations of actions to be taken are placed behind the guides for specific days of the current month. Notations for future months are placed behind the guide for that month. To be effective, the tickler file must be checked the first thing each day.

CRITICAL THINKING APPLICATION

Susan is responsible for checking the tickler file on a daily basis. What types of documents and duties might she find inside these files?

There are many ways to use the tickler file. It is a useful reminder for recurring events such as payments, meetings, and so forth. On the last day in each month, all the notations from behind the next month's guide are distributed among the daily numbered guides, and the guide for the month just completed is placed at the back of the file.

Transitory or Temporary File

Many papers are kept longer than necessary because no provision is made for segregating those that have a limited usefulness. This situation is avoided by having a *transitory* or *temporary* file. For example, if a medical assistant writes a letter requesting a reprint, the file copy is placed in the transitory folder. When the reprint is received, the file copy is destroyed. The transitory file is used for materials having no permanent value. The paper may be marked with a *T* and destroyed when the action is completed.

Closing Comments

Just like every aspect of the medical profession, advances in medical records management are occurring rapidly, allowing physicians and other caregivers to perform their duties in a more efficient and accurate way. A medical assistant must constantly be willing to learn and adapt to changes that result from legislation and technological strides. Because patients are fast becoming more computer literate, computers will become more generally accepted as a viable means of recording medical information. This is a positive change, because many patients and providers were not in favor of computer-based medical records when the concept was first presented to the general public.

Patient Education

The medical assistant should always explain any paperwork to the patient that he or she may be required to complete. Patients do not like to be told to simply "sign here." Take the time to explain any form that needs completion or a signature, so that the patient will understand the reason for collecting the information and the necessity of the information being available to the medical facility.

Many forms are similar, and patients may complain about answering the same questions on multiple forms. It can be frustrating for patients when they must list their address and phone numbers on each of several forms. Review and revise the forms used in the office often so that they are user-friendly for the office and patient alike.

Patients may need reassurance that each staff member in the physician's office is committed to complete patient confidentiality. Always be open to answering questions regarding the patient medical record.

Legal and Ethical Issues

The authority to release information from the medical record lies solely with the patient unless required by law by subpoena. Ownership of the record is often a subject of controversy. The record belongs to the physician; the information belongs to the patient.

When a medical record is used as evidence in a court case, the person who entered information in the chart must be able to read it, no matter how much time has lapsed since the entry was created. When a chart is corrected, the proper method must be followed and the record should never be obliterated.

Be sure to understand the laws concerning records retention. Records should be kept through the period of the statute of limitations, and possibly longer in certain situations. Take care with the medical chart, as it is the lifeline of patient care in the medical facility.

SUMMARY OF SCENARIO

Susan looks forward to attending her medical assisting classes each day and works diligently to perform to the best of her ability in the classroom. She strives to do well on each procedure check-off and each examination that she completes. Her instructors provide excellent feedback and appreciate her contributions to the classroom experience.

Susan has the attitude that everything she is allowed to do in the medical office is a learning tool. She regularly asks for additional responsibilities and is always ready to assist a co-worker. Dr. Thomas has recognized that she has the desire to learn, and he gives her many opportunities to glean more knowledge through the everyday activities in the office.

Although she is new to the medical profession, Susan learns quickly and thinks logically. She knows the rules and regulations regarding patient confidentiality and is always careful about the information she provides to those who request it. She is never hesitant about asking her office manager for guidance if she is unsure about any aspect of her duties. Susan is understanding and respectful when patients are concerned about their privacy. Her confidence and warm personality play a role in the trust that she earns from the patients at the clinic.

Susan is willing to admit when she has made an error and has sought advice from Dr. Thomas and her office manager when an error needed correction. Although filing is not one of her favorite duties, she can be counted on to give her best while completing this important task. She takes pride in her work and is efficient and accurate where medical records are concerned. When she is faced with a task that is new to her, she considers it a learning experience and seeks help when she is not completely certain about the way to handle a given situation.

Susan's co-workers are supportive and always willing to assist her as she learns to be the best medical assistant that she can possibly be. Her future as a professional medical assistant will certainly be laden with opportunity and advancement.

SUMMARY OF LEARNING OBJECTIVES

■ Several types of equipment and supplies are necessary when managing patient records. A variety of shelving units and filing containers are available. Open shelving allows the maximized use of color coded charts, which make finding misfiles quick and easy. Many file folder styles are available, and there are several types of forms to use within the patient charts. The preference of the physician and staff members who use these tools is important, as well as concerns such as cost and availability. A medical assistant should be conservative when ordering supplies and purchasing equipment, only ordering the number needed to save on office supply costs.

■ Five basic steps are involved in filing documents. The papers are conditioned, which is the preparatory stage for filing. Releasing the documents means that they are ready to be filed because they have been reviewed or read, and some type of mark is placed on the document to indicate this. Indexing involves the decision as to where the document should be filed, and coding is placing some type of mark on the paper relative to that decision. Sorting is placing the files in filing sequence. The last step is the actual filing and storing of the document.

■ Alphabetical filing is a simple and traditional filing system, whereby documents are filed in alphabetical order. Numeric filing systems use a number code to give order to the files. An alphanumeric system is a combination of the two.

■ Color coding is an excellent way to keep patient charts in order and swiftly locate those charts that have been misfiled. The medical assistant can tell at a glance when a chart is out of place. Color coding also makes retrieval of and refiling files quick and easy.

■ Medical records must be accurate primarily so that the right care can be given to the patient. The record also helps to provide continuity of care between providers, so that there is no lapse in treatment to the patient. The record serves as indication and proof in court that certain treatments and procedures were performed on the patient, so it can be excellent legal support if it is well maintained and accurate. Medical records also aid researchers with statistical information.

■ The physician owns the physical medical record, whereas the patient owns the information contained within.

■ The problem-oriented medical record categorizes each problem that a patient has and elaborates on the findings and treatment plan for all concerns. Detailed progress notes are kept for every individual problem. This method separates each of the patient's concerns and addresses them separately, whereas a traditional record may address all problems and concerns at one time. The problem-oriented medical record helps to assure that all individual problems are addressed.

■ Very simply, subjective information is provided by the patient, whereas objective information is provided by the physician or provider. Subjective information includes items such as the patient address, social security number, insurance information, and the patient's explanation of the condition he or she is experiencing. Objective information is obtained through the questions the physician asks and the observations made during the examination.

■ Correct procedures must be followed when making corrections to a patient chart. A single line should be drawn through the incorrect information, then initialed and dated. Some offices require a notation of "Corr." or "correction" on the chart as well. A medical assistant should never try to alter the medical record or cover up an error in charting.

KEY INTERNET WEBSITES

- American Health Information Management Association
- The Health Insurance Portability and Accountability Act
- The Informatics Review
- Professional Standards Review Council of America
  For active weblinks to each website visit
  http://evolve.elsevier.com/Kinn/

UNIT three

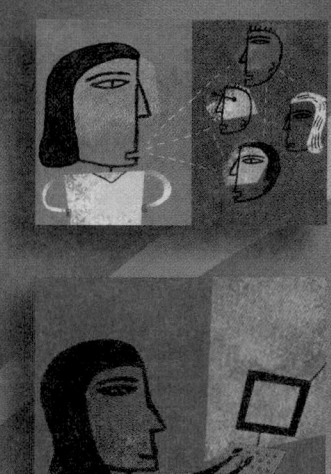

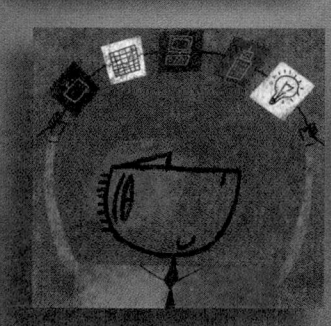

Financial Management

CHAPTER 14

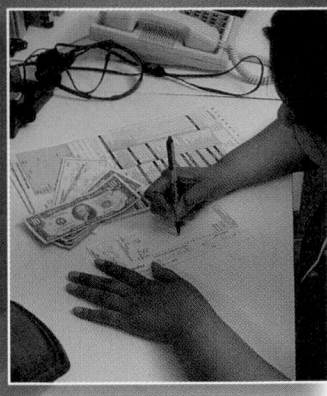

Scenario

Myra Morrison has worked for Dr. Jerry Wallace, an endocrinologist, for 3 years. She began as a receptionist, but she always had a knack for mathematics. This led Dr. Wallace to place her in charge of the accounting functions for the practice. When patients are ready to leave the clinic, Myra totals their bill and enters the charges and payments into the computerized ledger system. She also schedules their return appointments. Myra has learned quite a bit about medical insurance as well, so she can answer many of the patients' questions about their coverage and the benefits or exclusions of their insurance policies. There have been many cases in which she was able to decipher a confusing insurance claim and explain the reimbursement to the patient. Myra has a great attitude about assisting patients with insurance questions and does not hesitate to call the insurance company to ask questions on behalf of the patient. She provides the patients with exceptional customer service.

Myra knows that care must be taken when dealing with numerical transactions. Her handwriting is clear and legible, and she writes numbers the same way each time to avoid confusion and errors. She is able to use a manual pegboard but prefers the computer programs that do most of the work for her. Myra has some basic accounting background, so she can find errors easily and correct them. She even enjoys balancing the accounts on a daily basis to be sure all transactions were entered correctly.

Myra provides a valuable service to the patients that visit Dr. Wallace. She can always be counted on to follow up on any detail that needs attention. When patients call her for assistance, she takes no more than 24 hours to respond with the answers to their questions. She is a great patient advocate in the office. Some patients even tease her and ask her to balance their checkbooks! Myra is also willing to help any staff member with other duties whenever necessary. She is an enthusiastic team player who puts the patients first.

Professional Fees, Billing, and Collecting

Learning Objectives

- Define and spell the terms listed in the vocabulary.
- List three values that are considered in determining professional fees.
- Distinguish among the terms *usual*, *customary*, and *reasonable*.
- Discuss the value of estimates for patient treatment.
- Explain the concept of professional courtesy.
- Name the ways by which payment for medical services is accomplished.
- Explain why itemizing statements is important.
- Discuss why patients fail to pay accounts.
- Explain how to handle a "skip."
- Briefly explain some of the guidelines of telephone collecting.
- Explain professional fees to patients.
- Effectively use a pegboard system.
- Establish credit arrangements for patient payment.
- Prepare accurate monthly statements.
- Evaluate patient accounts for necessary collection procedures.

National Curriculum Competencies

2c. Post entries on a day sheet
2f. Perform billing and collecting procedures
3b. Post adjustments
3c. Process a credit balance

3d. Process refunds
3e. Post nonsufficient fund checks
3f. Post collection agency payments

Vocabulary

account A statement of transactions during a fiscal period and the resulting balance.

account balance The amount owed on an account.

accounts receivable ledger A record of the charges and payments posted on an account.

credit An entry on an account constituting an addition to a revenue, net worth, or liability account; the balance in a person's favor in an account.

debit An entry on an account constituting an addition to an expense or asset account or a deduction from a revenue, a net worth, or a liability account.

debit cards A card that looks like a credit card and by which money may be withdrawn or the cost of purchases paid directly from the holder's bank account without the payment of interest.

disbursements Funds paid out.

fee profile A compilation or average of physician fees over a given period of time.

fee schedule A compilation of preestablished fee allowances for given services or procedures.

fiscal agent An organization under contract to the government as well as some private plans to act as financial representatives in handling insurance claims from providers of health care; also referred to as fiscal intermediary.

guarantor A person who makes or gives a guarantee of payment for a bill.

instigate To goad or urge forward; to provoke.

medically indigent Able to take care of ordinary living expenses but not able to afford medical care.

payables The balance due to a creditor on an account.

pegboard system Also called the write-it-once system; a method of tracking patient accounts that allows the figures to be proved accurate through mathematical formulas.

posting Transferring or carrying from a book of original entry to a ledger; entering figures in an accounting system.

premium The consideration paid for a contract of insurance.

preponderance A superiority or excess in number or quantity; a majority.

professional courtesy Reduction or absence of fees to professional associates.

receipts Amounts paid on patient accounts.

receivables Total monies received on accounts.

third party payor Someone other than the patient, spouse, or parent who is responsible for paying all or part of the patient's medical costs.

transaction An exchange or transfer of goods, services, or funds.

The practice of medicine is a business as well as a profession, and the details of conducting the business aspects are often the responsibility of the medical assistant. Although service to the patient is the primary concern of the medical profession, a physician must charge and collect a fee for such services to continue providing medical care. The physician is one of many contributors in determining the amount of the fees. The medical assistant usually has the responsibility of informing the patient about financial matters, collecting the payment, and in some cases, making arrangements for deferred payment.

Why Patients Do Not Pay

Most patients truly want to pay the bills that they owe. However, there may be times that the patient experiences difficulties in meeting his or her obligations. The patient may have lost a job or insurance coverage. An emergency could arise that depletes finances. When patients are in a position in which they must choose between paying their medical bills or having electricity, the physician is often forced to wait for reimbursement for the services rendered. Although a few patients will absolutely refuse to pay for medical care they have received, most are honest and willing to pay but may need help with a payment plan. Terms can be arranged for collecting payment in full when both the office and the patient cooperate with each other. The medical assistant should attempt to work out a plan that the patient can abide by, and the patient should be expected to make promised payments.

How Fees Are Determined

Setting fees is no simple matter. The physician has three commodities to sell—time, judgment, and services. Yet the value of these commodities is never exactly the same to any two individuals. Medical care has little value except to the patient, and the value may not be consistent with his or her ability to pay. In every case, the physician must place an estimate on the value of the services. Such an arrangement is known as *fee for service*. This value may then be modified by other considerations.

Impact of Managed Care

An important consideration in today's atmosphere of managed care is the **preponderance** of patients who are enrolled in health maintenance organization (HMO) insurance contracts. Under managed care, the physician agrees to accept predetermined fees for specific procedures and services instead of the fee-for-service arrangement described in the preceding paragraph. The patient may be subject to a co-payment that is determined by the insurance contract and is collected at the time of service. A base capitation plan pays the provider a set amount for each patient enrolled that is meant to cover all of the person's healthcare expenses. Usually, capitation plans cover a group of individuals.

Prevailing Rate in the Community

One of the bases for determining charges on the fee-for-service basis is the economic level of the community. Different communities have different living scales, and this situation is reflected in medical fees as well. Consequently, the prevailing rate in the community—the average composite fee—must be taken into consideration by each physician. Strangely enough, fees that are too low drive patients away just as quickly as fees that are too high because the average person tends to judge worth of a product on its cost—low cost translates as low value.

Usual, Customary, and Reasonable Fees

Most insurance plans base their payments on what has become known as a *usual, customary, and reasonable (UCR) fee* for a given procedure.

- *Usual*—The physician's usual fee for a given service is the fee that an individual physician most frequently charges for the service.
- *Customary*—The customary fee is a range of the usual fees charged for the same service by physicians with similar training and experience practicing in the same geographical and socioeconomic area. There is now a growing tendency for fees to be determined by national trends rather than by local custom.
- *Reasonable*—The term *reasonable* usually applies to a service or procedure that is exceptionally difficult or complicated, requiring extraordinary time or effort on the part of the physician.

To illustrate, let us suppose that Dr. Wallace usually charges patients $100 for a first office visit. The usual fees charged for a first visit by other physicians in the same community with similar training and experience range from $75 to $125. Dr. Wallace's fee of $100 is within the customary range and would therefore be paid by an insurance plan that pays on a usual and customary basis. If, on the other hand, the range of usual fees in the community is from $60 to $85, the insurance plan would allow only the maximum within the range, or $85, to Dr. Wallace.

CRITICAL THINKING APPLICATION

Myra realizes that many of Dr. Wallace's patients are confused about insurance policies and are easily frustrated when payments are not as high as the patient thinks they should be. How can Myra help patients understand their policies better?

UCR rates were developed many years ago when indemnity plans were the most common type of health insurance coverage. However, since the majority of insurance plans today are some type of managed care, the UCR rates now are based on the prevailing managed care rate of payment in a region.

Fee Setting by Third Party Payors

The physician does not act alone in determining fees. A third party payor may provide the physician with a predetermined fee schedule that it will approve for payment. Some require preapproval of the fee before service is rendered. A third party payor may require precertification before it will pay for a specific service. Government programs such as Medicare and Medicaid have strict guidelines regarding reimbursement for fees and the raising of fees.

Physician's Fee Profile

The **fiscal agent**, or fiscal intermediary, for government-sponsored insurance programs as well as some private plans keeps a continuous record of the usual charges submitted for specific services by each physician. When these fees have been compiled and averaged over a given period, usually a year, the physician's **fee profile** is established. This fee profile is then used in determining the amount of third party liability for services under the program. One of the objections voiced by physicians is the lag between the time of a private fee increase and the time it is reflected in payments by an insurance carrier. It may be as long as 2 to 3 years.

Insurance Allowance

In some individual cases, the physician may not wish to charge the patient in addition to what will be allowed by the patient's insurance. This is often a professional courtesy for other healthcare professionals. The full fee should be quoted to the patient and charged to the account, with the understanding that after the insurance allowance has been received, the balance may be discounted. If a smaller fee is quoted and charged, the following problems may arise:

- The lower fee will alter the physician's fee profile.
- If it becomes necessary to bring suit for payment of the fee, only the reduced fee can be recovered.
- If the insurance allowance is paid on the basis of a certain percentage of the physician's fee and a lower fee is charged, the insurance allowance will be correspondingly lower.
- If the physician does this with many patients, the insurance company may take the position that the reduced fee is the physician's usual fee and base its payments accordingly. It may even be considered fraudulent in some instances.

Explaining Costs to Patients

It is natural for the patient, particularly one new to the practice, to wonder, "How much is this going to cost?" However, some patients may be reluctant to voice this concern. Do not wait for the patient to ask about the fees. It is the responsibility of the physician or the medical assistant to approach the subject if the patient does not do so (Procedure 14-1). Be prepared to discuss costs with any patient who is interested, and ask all patients if they have questions about the fees. A good way to open the discussion would be to ask the following:

"Mr. Willardson, do you have any questions about the costs of your operation? If you do, I'll be glad to review them."

In this preliminary discussion of fees, the physician or medical assistant must not sidestep the issue by saying,

PROCEDURE **14-1**

Explaining Professional Fees

GOAL: To explain the physician's fees so that the patient understands his or her obligations and rights for privacy.

EQUIPMENT AND SUPPLIES

- Patient's statement
- Copy of physician's fee schedule
- Quiet, private area where the patient feels free to ask questions

PROCEDURAL STEPS

1 Determine that the patient has the correct bill.
Purpose: To make certain that the bill belongs to this patient and that the insurance numbers, the address, and the telephone number are correct.

2 Examine the bill for possible errors.
Purpose: To demonstrate that the patient's concerns are important and that you are willing to make any necessary adjustments.

3 Refer to the fee schedule for services rendered.
Purpose: To explain how physicians determine their fees. If an error has occurred, correct it immediately with a sincere apology.

4 Explain itemized billing:
- Date of each service
- Type of service rendered
- Fee

Purpose: To make certain that the patient realizes the number and extent of the services rendered.

5 Display a professional attitude toward the patient.
Purpose: To reassure the patient that you have a thorough understanding of the fee schedule and show willingness to answer questions politely and completely.

6 Determine whether the patient has specific concerns that may hinder payment.
Purpose: To provide an opportunity for making special arrangements if needed.

7 Make appropriate arrangements for a discussion between the physician and patient if further explanation is necessary for resolution of the problem.

"*Don't worry about the bill; let's just get you well first.*" The patient may later complain about the bill because he or she misunderstood the complexity of the service.

Even in cases in which the physician quotes a fee, the medical assistant often has the responsibility of explaining the physician's fees to the patient. The medical assistant must know how fees are determined and why charges vary, as well as have a thorough knowledge of the physician's practice and policies to handle perplexing situations involving fees.

CRITICAL THINKING APPLICATION

Mr. Reynolds, one of Dr. Wallace's long-standing patients, continually complains about his insurance policies and the small payments made on his medical claims. He frequents the office at least twice a month for checkups and goes into a long speech about the problems with his insurance each time he stops to pay his bill at Myra's desk. He will continue complaining even when other patients come to pay their bills. How can Myra tactfully handle Mr. Reynolds and stop his complaints?

As the medical assistant's understanding of the practice increases, he or she can build respect for the physician's services by educating patients that money spent for medical care is an excellent investment in the future. It is a rare patient who understands the intricate procedures involved in diagnosis and treatment, especially when third party payors are involved. Be patient and understanding when questions arise in this area.

Advance Discussion of Fees

Advance fee discussions help the patient plan ahead for medical expenditures (Figure 14-1). Most patients want to pay their financial obligations but rightly insist on an accurate estimate of those obligations before they contract for purchase of goods or services. When a physician frankly discusses fees in advance with patients, even to the point of describing how a fee is established, misconceptions and complaints about overcharging and fee discrepancies are usually eliminated.

Explanation of Additional Costs

Explanations of medical costs should extend beyond the physician's own charges. For example, if a patient is to undergo surgery, the physician should also explain the costs of the operation, the anesthesiologist's and radiologist's charges, the laboratory fees, and the approximate hospital bill. The importance of calling in another physician for consultation should be explained to patients when consultation becomes necessary. It should be made

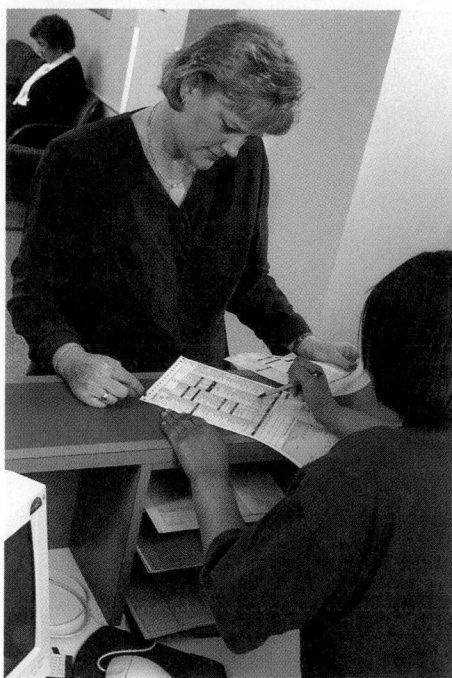

FIGURE 14-1   Taking a short amount of time to explain fees will often result in prompt payment for services.

clear, in advance, that there will be a separate bill submitted by the consulting physician. Patients do not always understand that the consultation is for the benefit of the patient, not the physician.

Estimates on Costs

Some physicians give patients an estimate of medical expenses before hospitalization. A few medical societies cooperatively develop estimate sheets or forms with local hospitals. Individual physicians occasionally work up their own estimate forms when a patient is embarking on long-term treatment. The physician should, however, emphasize that it is an estimate only and that the actual cost may vary somewhat.

Estimate slips should be prepared in duplicate so that the patient may have a copy and the original is retained in the patient's file. Duplicate estimate slips may help in the following ways:

- It may help to avoid forgetting that a fee was quoted.
- It may help eliminate the possibility of later misquoting the fee.
- It may help simplify collection by preventing misunderstanding and confusion over charges.

Guarantor's Ultimate Responsibility: The Bill

Patients must understand that the **guarantor** is the person ultimately responsible for the entire bill. The insurance policy is a contract between the policy holder and the insurance company or between a group of people (such as an employer) and a managed care organization. The actual physician is not a party to that contract. Therefore it is not the responsibility of the physician or staff to pursue insurance payment for the benefit of the patient. However, it is in the best interest of the staff to actively assist the patient if there are problems in securing payment for several reasons.

CRITICAL THINKING APPLICATION

- Madeline Amos has a 12-year-old diabetic son, Eric, who is Dr. Wallace's patient. Ms. Amos is divorced from her son's father, but the father is required to keep a medical insurance policy on the son. Myra knows that Ms. Amos has had numerous problems with the father. On a visit to the office, it is discovered that the insurance policy on the son has been cancelled. How does Myra explain this to Ms. Amos?
- What steps, if any, can be taken to assist Ms. Amos in paying her son's account?

First, the staff is almost always more knowledgeable about the insurance business than the patient. Many patients have never even read their insurance policies and have no idea as to what is or is not covered. Some patients expect the insurance to pay all costs simply because they are paying a high **premium**. The medical assistant may need to educate these patients about their policies and offer advice as to how the patients can effectively work with the insurance company to get answers to questions and make certain that they are receiving all of the benefits to which they are entitled.

Second, it is in the best interest of the staff to assist the patient in collecting from the insurance company so that the physician will be compensated for services rendered. Helping the patient in this area will usually result in the bill for care being paid. Another reason to actively assist the patient is that the medical assistant will gain knowledge about the insurance industry. The more experience the medical assistant has in working with third party payors, the more helpful he or she can be to the patients of the clinic. It is a good idea to keep a notebook with specific information about each type of policy that the office handles. This reference notebook will provide excellent guidance and suggestions for the medical assistant when working with a particular payor.

Always be sure to secure guarantors in writing. Most patient information sheets have a section that refers to the guarantor. There may be a statement that the guarantor signs indicating an agreement to pay the costs of medical care. States have varying statutes that deal with guarantors, so be sure that the office policies reflect compliance with those laws. It is especially important to secure a written agreement to pay for services when the care will be long term or when a costly treatment or surgical procedure must be done.

Encounter Forms

Encounter forms are the slips that are attached to charts while the patient is in the office; they are used for billing purposes. The encounter form provides information about the patient, such as the name, account number, and previous balance. Current charges and payments for the visit are added after the physician sees the patient. The physician can indicate on the encounter form when the patient should return to the clinic (Figure 14-2). The medical assistant then schedules an appointment and can even use the patient's copy of the encounter form to note the next appointment date and time.

The encounter form normally consists of three parts, with a white top sheet, a yellow sheet, and a pink sheet. The colors can vary, but usually the white copy is kept as a permanent record by the office, and the yellow and pink copies are given to the patient. The yellow copy is

LIC. # 999999	**JANE A. SMITH, M.D.**	TELEPHONE: (212) 555-4444
S.S. # 111-22-3333	*Reproductive Endocrinology*	FAX: (212) 555-4545
UPIN # A12365	123 FIRST AVENUE	
	ANYTOWN, N.Y. 22222	

PATIENT INFORMATION

PATIENT'S LAST NAME	FIRST	INITIAL	BIRTHDATE / /	SEX ☑FEMALE	TODAY'S DATE / /
ADDRESS	CITY	STATE	ZIP	RELATION TO SUBSCRIBER	REFERRING PHYSICIAN
SUBSCRIBER OR POLICYHOLDER			INSURANCE CARRIER		
ADDRESS	CITY	STATE	ZIP	INS. ID	COVERAGE CODE	GROUP

OTHER HEALTH COVERAGE? ☐ NO ☐ YES IDENTIFY — DISABILITY RELATED TO: ☐ IND. ☐ ACCIDENT ☐ PREGNANCY ☐ OTHER — DATE SYMPTOMS APPEARED, INCEPTION OF PREGNANCY, OR ACCIDENT OCCURRED: / /

ASSIGNMENT & RELEASE: I hereby assign my insurance benefits to be paid directly to the undersigned physician. I am financially responsible for non-covered services. I also authorize the physician to release any information required to process this claim.
SIGNED: (Patient, or Parent, if Minor)   DATE: / /

✔ DESCRIPTION	CODE	FEE	✔ DESCRIPTION	CODE	FEE	✔ DESCRIPTION	CODE	FEE
OFFICE VISIT			**OFFICE PROCEDURES**			**LABORATORY - IN OFFICE**		
New Patient			Sperm Wash	58323		Pregnancy Test	85160	
Consultation	99204		Cauterization of Cervix	57510		Urinalysis	81002	
Comprehensive	99205		Cervical Biopsy	57500		Stool Occult Blood	82270	
OFFICE VISIT			Endocervical Curettage	57505		Lyme Titer	86317	
Established Patient			Endometrial Biopsy	58100		Estradiol	82670	
Limited	99211		Office Endometrial Curettage	58102		Chemistry	80019	
Intermediate	99212		Post Coital Test	89300		CBC, pit., Diff.	85024	
Extended	99213		Artificial Insemination	58310		T3 Uptake	84479	
Comprehensive	99214		Pelvic Sonogram	76856		T4	84435	
Comprehensive	99215		Vulvar Biopsy	56600		TSH	84443	
SURGERY			Bilateral Mammogram	76091		ESR	85650	
D & C	58120		Unilateral Mammogram	76090		Pregnancy Test	84702	
Pregnancy Termination	59840		Breast Ultrasound	76645		FSH	83000	
Laparoscopy	56305		Abdominal Ultrasound	76700		Prolactin	84146	
Hysteroscopy	56351		Polypectomy	57500				
Laporotomy	49000							
Myomectomy	58140							
Hysterectomy	58150							

DIAGNOSIS: ICD-9

☐ Abortion, Incomplete 634.71	☐ Diabetes Mellitus 250.0	☐ Hyperthyroidism 242.9	☐ Pregnancy V22.2
☐ Abortion, Spontaneous ...634.90	☐ Dysmenorrhea 625.3	☐ Hypothyroidism 244.9	☐ Pregnancy Termination ...V72.4
☐ Alopecia 704.09	☐ Dyspareunia 625.0	☐ Infertility 628.9	☐ Premature Ovarian Failure .256.3
☐ Amenorrhea 626.0	☐ Dysuria 788.1	☐ Luteal Phase Insufficiency .628.8	☐ Premenopausal Menorrhagia .627.0
☐ Anemia 285.9	☐ Ectopic Pregnancy 633.9	☐ Menometrorrhagia 626.2	☐ Prolactinoma 253
☐ Anovulation 628.0	☐ Edema 782.3	☐ Menopausal Syndrome 627.2	☐ Prolapsed Uterus 618.1
☐ Atrophic Vaginitis 627.3	☐ Endometrial Hyperplasia .621.3	☐ Menorrhagia 626.2	☐ Rectocele 569.1
☐ Breast Cyst 610.1	☐ Endometriosis 617.0	☐ Monilial Vaginitis 112.1	☐ Thyroiditis 245.2
☐ Breast Mass 611.72	☐ Fatigue 780.7	☐ Obesity 278.0	☐ Trichomonas 131.0
☐ Breast Pain 611.71	☐ Fibrocystic Breast Disease .610.1	☐ Osteoarthritis 715.9	☐ Urinary Tract Infection 599.0
☐ Cervical Polyp 622.7	☐ Galactorrhea 676.6	☐ Osteopenia 733.9	☐ Uterine Fibroids 218.9
☐ Cervicitis 616.0	☐ Headache 784.0	☐ Osteoporosis 733.0	☐ Vasomotor Instability 780.2
☐ Condyloma 091.3	☐ Hemorrhoids 455.6	☐ Ovarian Cyst 620.2	☐ Vaginitis 616.1
☐ Cyclic Adrenal Hyperplasia .255.2	☐ Herpes 054.1	☐ Ovarian Insufficiency 256.3	☐ Vulvitis 616.1
☐ Cystocele 618.0	☐ Hypercholesterolemia 272.0	☐ Pelvic Pain 625.9	
☐ Cystitis 595.9	☐ Hyperprolactinemia 253.1	☐ Polycystic Ovary Syndrome 256.4	
	☐ Hypertension 401.9	☐ Postmenopausal Bleeding .627.1	

DIAGNOSIS: (IF NOT CHECKED ABOVE) — ADDITIONAL INFORMATION: — DOCTOR'S SIGNATURE

SERVICES PERFORMED AT: ☐ OFFICE ☐ University Hospital ☐ Day Surgery / University Hosp.
345 Second Avenue 678 Third Avenue
Anytown, N.Y. 23333 Anytown, N.Y. 23444

REFERRING PHYSICIAN:

ACCEPT ASSIGNMENT? ☐ YES ☐ NO

TOTAL TODAY'S FEE	
PREVIOUS BALANCE	
AMT. REC'D. TODAY	
NEW BALANCE	

INSTRUCTIONS TO PATIENT FOR FILING INSURANCE CLAIMS:
1. COMPLETE UPPER PORTION OF THIS FORM; SIGN AND DATE.
2. MAIL THIS FORM DIRECTLY TO YOUR INSURANCE COMPANY. YOU MAY ATTACH YOUR OWN INSURANCE COMPANY'S FORM IF YOU WISH, ALTHOUGH IT IS NOT NECESSARY.
PLEASE REMEMBER THAT PAYMENT IS YOUR OBLIGATION, REGARDLESS OF INSURANCE OR OTHER THIRD PARTY INVOLVEMENT.

INSUR-A-BILL ® BIBBERO SYSTEMS, INC. • PETALUMA, CA • © 5/95 (SB M-N)   (REV. 9/96)

FIGURE 14-2 An encounter form. The encounter form is used by the physician and staff to document what was done to the patient during an office visit and indicate when the physician wishes the patient to return. The copies of the form may be used to bill third party payors. (Courtesy Bibbero Systems, Inc., Petaluma, Calif. 94954, (800) 242-2376, www.bibbero.com.)

used by the patient for insurance billing (if not done by the office), and the pink copy is a receipt for the patient.

Encounter forms are sometimes designed to work with a **pegboard system** or may be available in continuous forms that can be placed in the printer for computer use. Encounter forms have been known by many aliases throughout the years; these include *superbills*, *charge slips*, and *multipurpose billing forms*.

Patient Account Transactions

A business **transaction** is the occurrence of an event or of a condition that must be recorded. For example, when a service is performed for which a charge is made, when a debtor makes a payment on account, when a piece of equipment is purchased, or when the monthly rent is paid, a business transaction has been completed.

Each of these examples is a transaction that must be recorded within the accounting system. The medical assistant will very likely encounter various other business transactions as he or she becomes more familiar with the individual needs of the employer's practice.

A patient's financial record is called an **account**. All of the patients' accounts together constitute the **accounts receivable ledger**. Account cards vary in design, but all will have at least three columns for entering figures. In the manual system these columns are as follows:

- *Debit column*—It is on the left, is used for entering charges, and is sometimes called the *charge column*.
- *Credit column*—It is to the right, is sometimes headed *Paid*, and is used for entering payments received.
- *Balance column*—It is on the far right and is used for recording the difference between the debit and the credit columns.

An *adjustment column* is available in some systems and is used for entering professional discounts, write-offs, disallowances by insurance companies, and any other adjustments. In a computer system, when a patient is called up by name or identification number, the patient's balance will appear. This is the individual patient's ledger.

Posting means the transfer of information from one record to another. Transactions are posted from the journal to the ledger; this is accomplished in one writing on the pegboard system. The **account balance** is normally a debit balance, which means that the charges exceed the payments on the account. A **debit** balance is entered by simply writing the correct figure in the balance column. A **credit** balance exists when payments exceed charges (e.g., when a patient pays in advance). This is common in obstetric practices.

Discounts are also credit entries and are entered in the adjustment column, or if there is no adjustment column, the discount is entered in the debit column and enclosed in parentheses. When the entry is made this way, it is recognized as a subtraction from the charges. When columns are totaled, any figure in red or in parentheses is always subtracted. **Receipts** are cash and checks taken in payment for professional services. **Receivables** are charges for which payment has not been received—amounts that are owing. **Disbursements** are cash amounts paid out. **Payables** are amounts owed to others but not yet paid.

Manual Posting

All charges and payments for professional services are posted to the ledger daily. The ledger then becomes a reliable source of information for answering all inquiries from patients about their accounts.

A separate account card or page is prepared for each patient at the time of the first visit or service. The heading of the account should include all information pertinent to collecting the account, such as the following:

- Name and address of person responsible for payment (the guarantor)
- Insurance identification
- Social Security number
- Home and business telephone numbers
- Name of employer
- Any special instructions for billing

Billing statements to the patient and the patient's insurance carrier are prepared from the ledger.

Computer Posting

The patient's name, date, diagnosis, and procedures are posted when the patient leaves the office. The database will retrieve the correct charges and post the charges on the computerized patient record and the accounts receivable ledger.

Write-It-Once, or Pegboard, System

The initial cost of materials for the pegboard system is slightly more than that for other accounting systems but is still moderate. The system is simple to operate, and training is included in most medical assisting programs.

The system gets its name from the lightweight aluminum or Masonite board with a row of pegs along the side or top that holds the forms in place. The accounting forms are perforated for alignment on the pegs. All of the forms used in any system must be compatible so that they may be aligned perfectly on the board. The pegboard system generates all the necessary financial records for each transaction with one writing, as follows:

- Encounter form
- Receipt
- Ledger card
- Journal entry

It may also include a statement and bank deposit slip.

The system provides current accounts receivable totals and a daily record of bank deposits and cash on hand, in addition to the record of income and expenses. The need for separate posting to patient accounts is eliminated, and the chance for error is decreased.

Using the Pegboard System

The pegboard system provides positive control over cash, collections, and receivables and ensures that every cent is accounted for and properly entered. It provides a record of every patient, every charge, and every payment, plus a daily recap of earnings—a running record of receivables and an audited summary of cash. The system requires a minimum of time. One writing allows a medical assistant to do the following:

- Enter a transaction on the day sheet.
- Give the patient a receipt for payment.
- Bring the patient's account up to date.
- Provide a current statement of account for the patient.
- Give the patient a notation of the next appointment.

All of these features communicate the money message to patients effectively and courteously and generate good financial records.

Gathering Required Materials. The pegboard may be of inexpensive Masonite construction with pegs down the left side, or it may be a more sophisticated aluminum sliding board that allows flexible positioning of materials. The basic pegboard forms follow:

- Day sheet (Figure 14-3)
- Patient ledger
- Encounter form

All of the forms must be compatible and are available from medical office supply companies. They may be customized to the practice, incorporating the usual services and procedure codes of the practice.

Preparing the Board. At the beginning of each day, place a new day sheet on the accounting board. Some systems have a sheet of clean carbon attached to the day sheet, others use special carbon with holes for the pegs, and some use NCR (no carbon required) paper. The carbon goes on top of the day sheet. Over the carbon, place the encounter form. The receipt has a carbonized writing line that should align with the first open writing line on the day sheet. If the slips are shingled, lay the entire bank of receipts over the pegs, with the top one aligned as mentioned. The remainder will be automatically in place. Receipts should be used in numerical order.

Pulling the Ledger Cards. If a great many patients are to be seen in a day, pull the ledger cards for all scheduled patients in the morning to save time (Figure 14-4). Keep the cards in the order in which the patients are scheduled to be seen.

Entering and Posting Transactions. As each patient arrives, insert the patient's ledger card under the first receipt, aligning the first available writing line of the card with the carbonized strip on the receipt. Enter the receipt number and date, the account balance in the space labeled *previous balance*, and the patient's name.

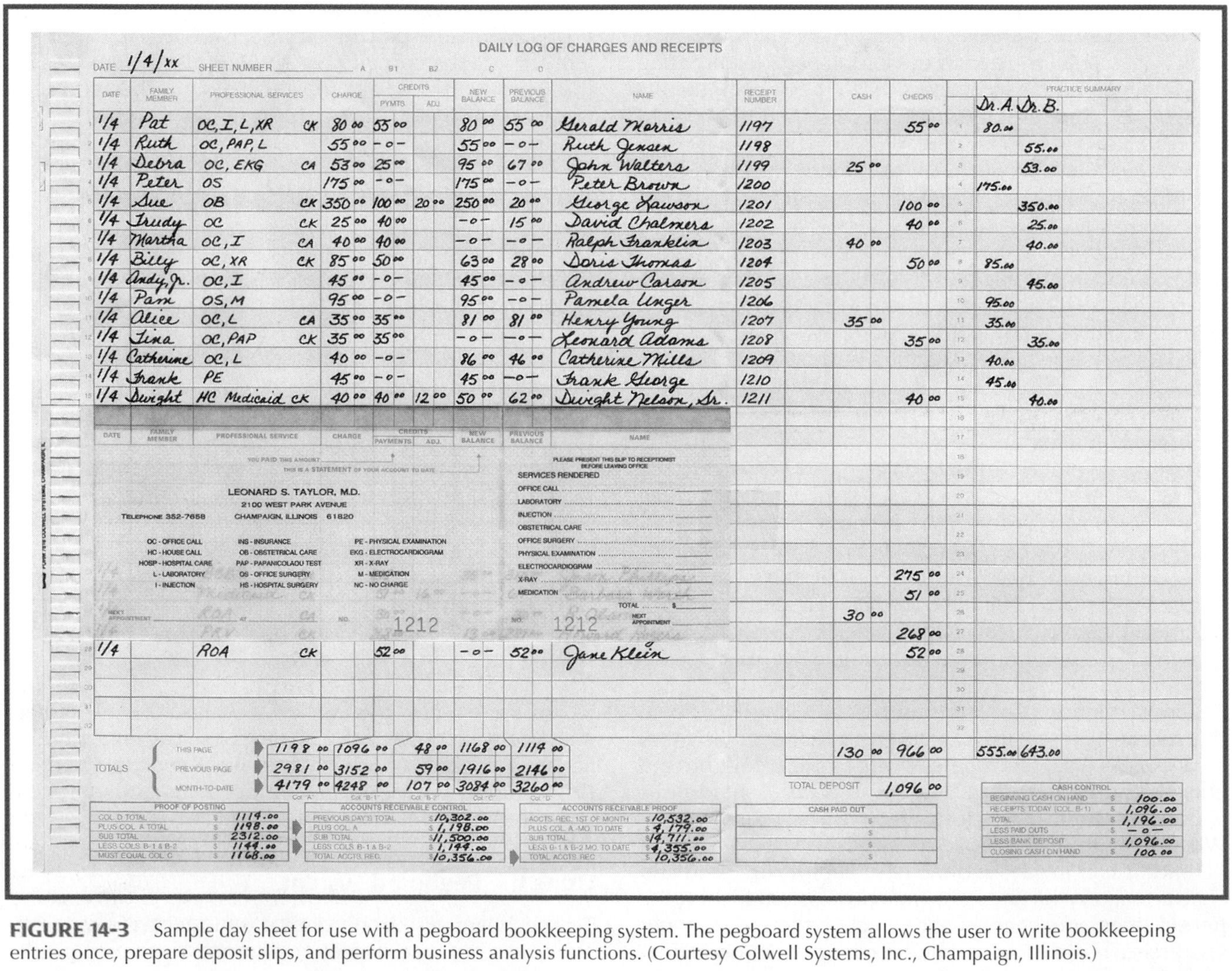

FIGURE 14-3 Sample day sheet for use with a pegboard bookkeeping system. The pegboard system allows the user to write bookkeeping entries once, prepare deposit slips, and perform business analysis functions. (Courtesy Colwell Systems, Inc., Champaign, Illinois.)

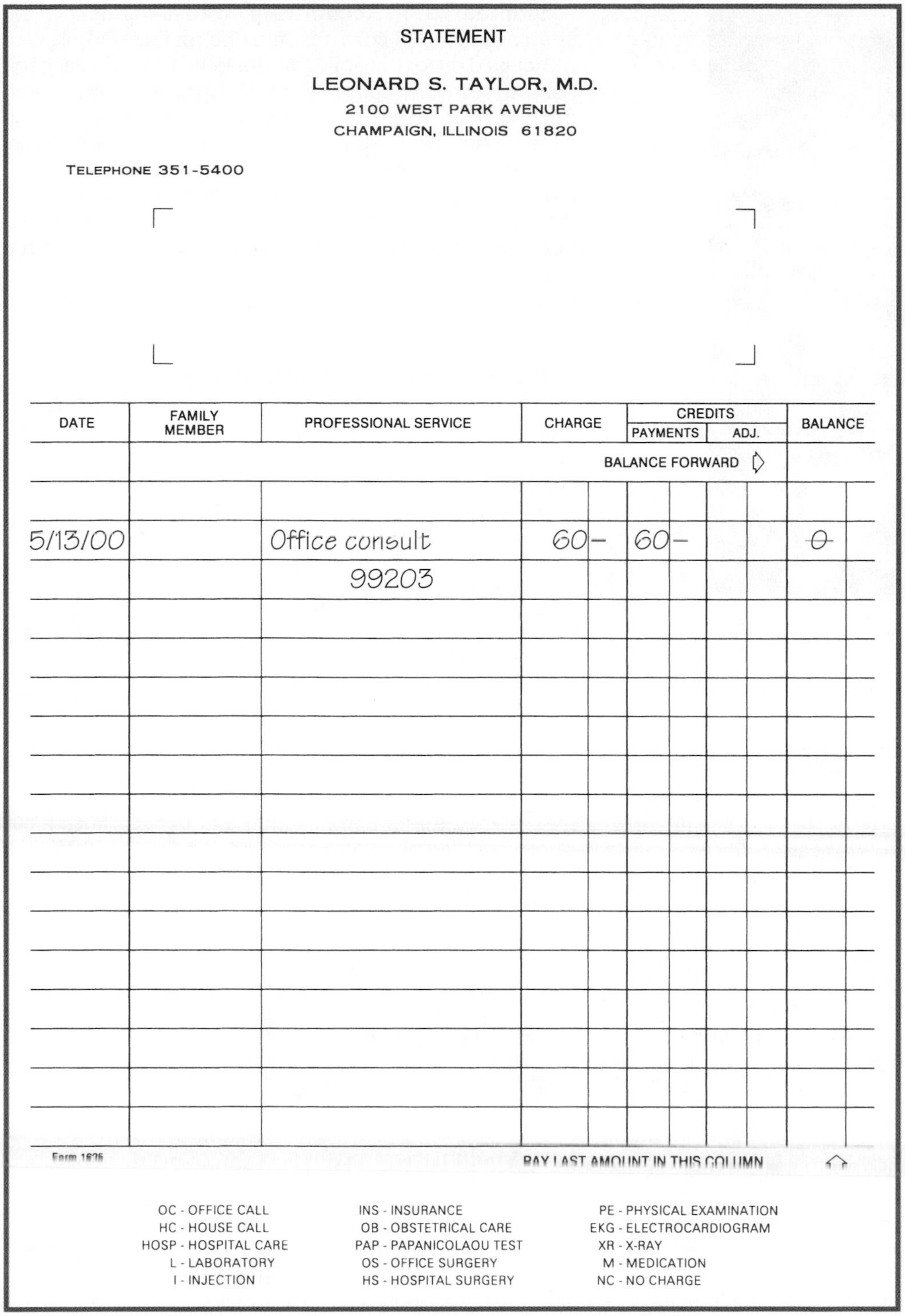

STATEMENT

LEONARD S. TAYLOR, M.D.
2100 WEST PARK AVENUE
CHAMPAIGN, ILLINOIS 61820

TELEPHONE 351-5400

DATE	FAMILY MEMBER	PROFESSIONAL SERVICE	CHARGE	CREDITS		BALANCE
				PAYMENTS	ADJ.	
		BALANCE FORWARD ▷				
5/13/00		Office consult	60—	60—		0
		99203				

Form 1825   PAY LAST AMOUNT IN THIS COLUMN

OC - OFFICE CALL	INS - INSURANCE	PE - PHYSICAL EXAMINATION
HC - HOUSE CALL	OB - OBSTETRICAL CARE	EKG - ELECTROCARDIOGRAM
HOSP - HOSPITAL CARE	PAP - PAPANICOLAOU TEST	XR - X-RAY
L - LABORATORY	OS - OFFICE SURGERY	M - MEDICATION
I - INJECTION	HS - HOSPITAL SURGERY	NC - NO CHARGE

FIGURE 14-4 Patient ledger card. A ledger card showing the charge and payment for an office consultation. (Courtesy Colwell Systems, Inc., Champaign, Illinois.)

The information recorded on the receipt is automatically posted to the ledger and the day sheet (Figure 14-5). The charge slip is then detached and clipped to the patient chart to be routed to the physician, who now has an opportunity to see how much the patient owes and can discuss the account in privacy, if desired.

After the service has been performed, the physician enters the service on the encounter form and asks the patient or the nurse to return it to the medical assistant. The assistant then has an opportunity to ask the patient whether this is to be a charge or cash transaction before completing the posting. Again, insert the ledger card under the proper receipt, checking the number that was previously entered to make sure the correct card is being used. Record the service by procedure code, post the charge from the fee schedule, enter any payment made, and write in the current balance (Procedure 14-2). If there is no balance, place a zero or a straight line in the balance column. If another appointment is required, enter the date and time at the bottom of the receipt.

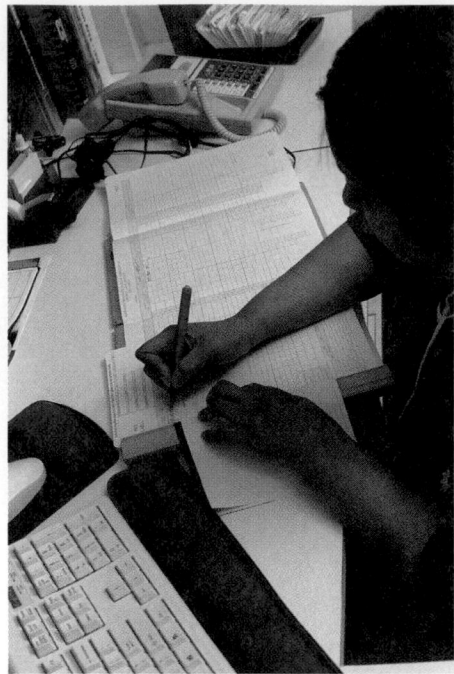

FIGURE 14-5   The pegboard system saves time by allowing several entries to be made at one time.

The transaction has now been posted to the journal and the ledger, and if payment was made by the patient, a receipt has been generated. The service receipt is given to the patient; no other receipt is necessary. The ledger card is ready for refiling.

File the encounter forms in numerical order for any internal audit. At the end of the month, the total of the encounter forms should equal the total of the charges recorded on the day sheets for the month (Figure 14-6).

Recording Other Payments and Charges. Payments will be received in the mail and may be brought in by patients some time after a service was performed. These payments are entered on the day sheet and the ledger card in the same manner as previously explained. Payments by mail do not require a receipt.

The physician may have daily charges for visits to patients in a hospital or convalescent facility. Enter these charges on the day sheet and ledger card only. Surgery fees are usually recorded as one entry that includes the surgery and aftercare.

CRITICAL THINKING APPLICATION

- Dr. Wallace sometimes forgets to write down information for billing when he goes to the hospital to check on his patients. Myra has a difficult time entering the charges for hospital visits because Dr. Wallace's records are not reliable in this area. How might Myra rectify this situation?
- How can Myra help Dr. Wallace to be more accurate in this area?

Summarizing Accounting Transactions. At the end of the day, all columns must be totaled and proved. Although all bookkeeping is done in ink, it is a good idea to write the totals in pencil until they have been proved. If an error is discovered, correct the entry in which it occurred. Do not attempt to erase or write over the incorrect entry. Simply draw one line through it and make a new entry on the first open writing line. Remember to reinsert the ledger card for these corrections. Also, if the entry included a receipt for the patient, make a new receipt and notify the patient of the correction.

Special Bookkeeping Entries

The following special entries are necessary occasionally and may be used with a pegboard or any other accounting system:

- Adjustments
- Credit balances
- Refunds
- Nonsufficient fund checks

Adjustments

At times, it is necessary to enter a credit adjustment. These could be for professional discounts, insurance disallowances, account write-offs, or payments that come to the office after the account has been placed for collections. If a patient or guarantor files bankruptcy, the charge will usually have to be adjusted off the books.

If the system has an adjustment column, enter them there. Otherwise, because the adjustment is actually a subtraction from the charge, enter it in the charge column with the figure enclosed in parentheses or circled and an explanation of the entry in the description column. When the column of figures is totaled, the circled figure is subtracted rather than added. The learner has a tendency to ignore the circled figures. This is incorrect—they must be subtracted.

Credit Balances

A credit balance occurs when a patient has paid in advance or there has been an overpayment or duplicate payment. For example, an overpayment occurs if the patient made a partial payment and later the insurance allowance was more than the remaining balance. The difference between the total amount of money received and the amount owed must be entered in the balance column and enclosed within parentheses or circled. This indicates a credit balance. Some credit balances are created when there has been an error in posting.

The credit balance is money owed to the patient. If the patient has paid in advance or wishes to leave the overpayment in the account in anticipation of future charges, care must be taken in figuring the balance on future transactions. Whereas normally a charge increases the balance, it will decrease a credit balance.

PROCEDURE 14-2

Posting Service Charges and Payments Using a Pegboard

GOAL: To post 1 day's charges and payments and compute the daily bookkeeping cycle using a pegboard.

EQUIPMENT AND SUPPLIES

- Pegboard
- Calculator
- Pen
- Day sheet
- Receipts
- Ledger cards
- Balances from previous day

PROCEDURAL STEPS

1 Prepare the board:
- Place a new day sheet on the board.
- Place a bank of receipts over the pegs, aligning the top receipt with the first open writing line on the day sheet.

2 Carry forward balances from the previous day.
Purpose: To keep all totals current.

3 Pull ledger cards for patient being seen that day.

4 Insert the ledger card under the first receipt, aligning the first available writing line of the card with the carbonized strip on the receipt.
Purpose: To ensure that one writing will correctly post the entry to receipt, ledger, and day sheet.

5 Enter the patient's name, the date, the receipt number, and any existing balance from the ledger card.

6 Detach the charge slip from the receipt and clip it to the patient's chart.
Purpose: The physician will indicate the service performed on the charge slip and return it to you.

7 Accept the returned charge slip at the end of the visit.

8 Enter the appropriate fee from the fee schedule.

9 Locate the receipt on the board with a number matching the charge slip.
Purpose: To make certain it is the correct receipt.

10 Reinsert the patient's ledger card under the receipt.

11 Write the service code number and fee on the receipt.

12 Accept the patient's payment and record the amount of payment and the new balance.
Purpose: To bring the patient's account up to date and provide a current statement for the patient.

13 Give the completed receipt to the patient.

14 Follow your agency's procedure for refilling the ledger card.

15 Repeat Steps 4 to 14 for each service of the day.

16 Total all columns of the day sheet at the end of the day.
Purpose: To determine total amount of the charges, receipts, and resulting balances for the day.

17 Write preliminary totals in pencil.
Purpose: To facilitate any necessary changes.

18 Complete proof of totals and enter totals in ink.

19 Enter figures for accounts receivable control.
Purpose: To complete daily accounting cycle.

Refunds

If a patient wishes to have an overpayment refunded, write a check for the amount due and enter the transaction on the day sheet. In most cases, the refund will result in a patient balance of zero.

CRITICAL THINKING APPLICATION

- Myra receives a phone call from a patient who says that she is due a refund, since her insurance company sent her an explanation of benefits for $654.00, and her balance was only $436. She demands an immediate refund, but Myra has not yet received the check. What should she do?
- Myra suspects that the check sent to pay on the account was an error. What should she do in this situation?

Nonsufficient Fund Checks

Sometimes, a patient sends in a check without having sufficient funds to cover it; this check is later deposited to the physician's account. The bank will return the check to

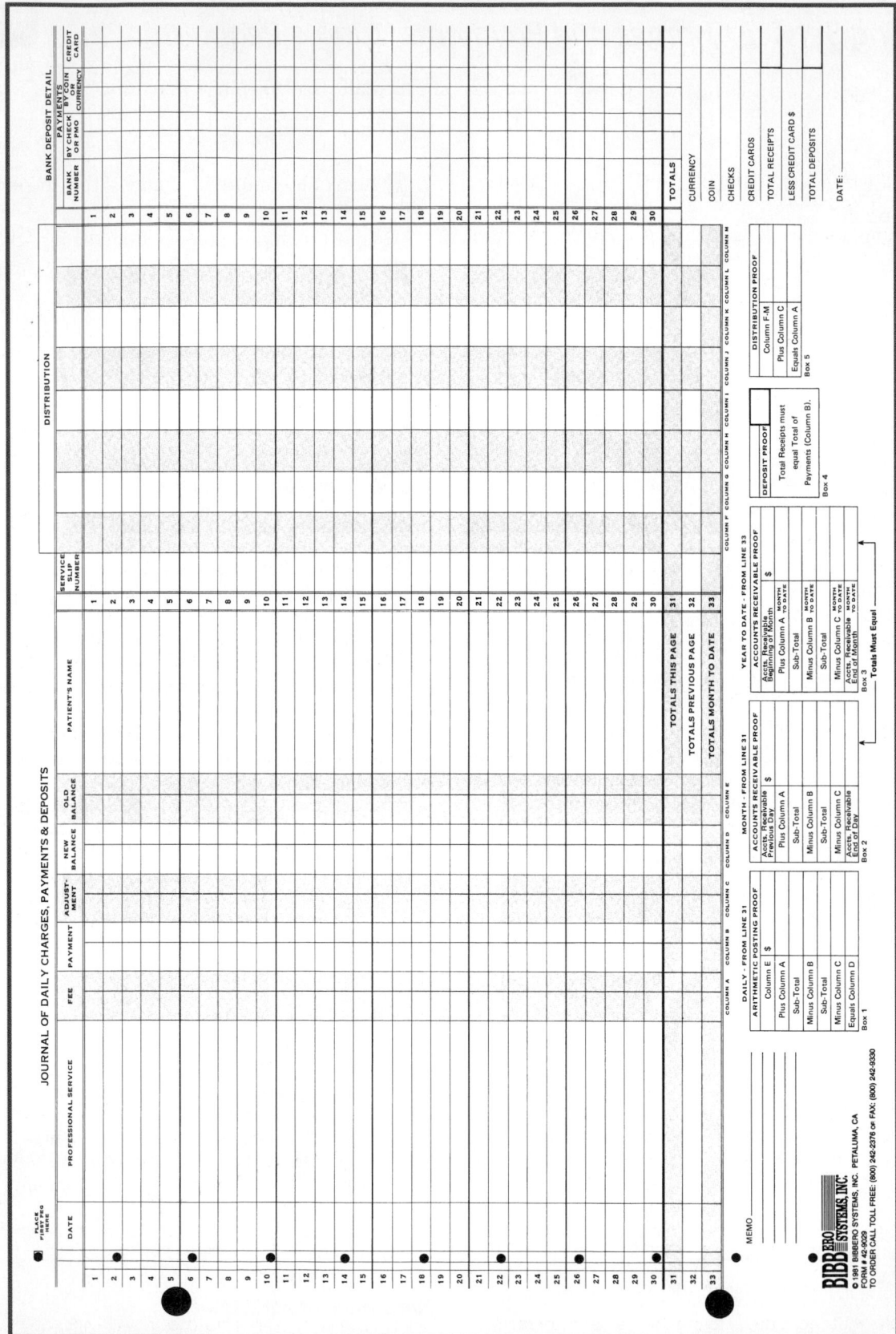

FIGURE 14-6 Sample day sheet used to log patient charges and receipts. (Courtesy Bibbero Systems, Inc., Petaluma, Calif. 94954, (800) 242-2376, www.bibbero.com.)

you marked NSF (*nonsufficient funds*). Two accounting functions must be performed. First, deduct the amount from the practice's checking account balance. Then add the amount back into the patient's account balance by entering the amount in the paid column in parentheses and increasing the balance by the same amount. Write a brief explanation of the transaction in the description column.

Balancing the Accounts Receivables and Accounts Receivables Control

The accounts receivable control is a daily summary of what remains unpaid on the accounts. Most offices also complete an end-of-day summary. These are integral parts of the office accounting system and are discussed in Chapter 23.

Paying for Medical Services and Treatment

The payment for medical services is accomplished in the following four ways:

1. Payment at the time of service
2. Internal billing when extension of credit is necessary
3. Internal insurance or other third party billing
4. Outside billing and collection assistance

Payment at the Time of Service

A large percentage of patients will have some type of health insurance for at least major items. Every practice in which there are patient visits should encourage time-of-service collection. It is especially important to collect co-payments and payment for office visits not covered by insurance. If patients get into the habit of paying their current charges before they leave the office, there are no further billing and bookkeeping expenses. If patients are informed when making an appointment that payment is expected at the time of service, they are not surprised when asked for payment at the end if the visit. Use a phrase, such as the following:

> "Your charge for today is $25.00. Will that be cash, check, or credit card?"

Many patients are hesitant to ask about charges and are unsure whether to offer to pay or to wait until asked. Make it easier for the patients by offering to accept their payments, because most people are prepared to pay small bills on a cash basis. If a patient requests to be billed, the medical assistant may say:

> "Our normal procedure is to pay at the time of service, unless other arrangements are made in advance."

Many offices accept credit cards for the convenience of their patients. **Debit cards** are now widely accepted for payment as well. Computers have made the electronic transfer of funds easy and convenient.

CRITICAL THINKING APPLICATION

- Mr. Page comes to Myra's desk to pay his account. His credit card is rejected, and a message comes back through the machine, saying that the card should be collected from the patient. How does Myra handle this situation?
- Mr. Page argues that he recently paid the balance of his account in full. What steps should Myra take in this case?

The medical assistant must believe that the physician and the facility have a right to charge for the services provided. Do not be embarrassed to ask for payment for the value of the service. When tact and good judgment are used in billing and collecting, patients appreciate the service they receive and the help the medical assistant provides. Give individual attention and personal consideration to each patient, and be courteous, showing a sincere desire to help the patient who has financial problems.

Billing After Extension of Credit

In some types of practice, particularly those involving large fees for surgery or long-term care, it becomes necessary to extend credit and establish a regular system of billing. This requires informing the patient of what the charges will be, what professional services these charges cover, and what the credit policy of the office is (Procedure 14-3).

Many practices do not have a true credit policy; thus each account continues to be evaluated individually. It is almost impossible to judge accounts objectively and equitably under such circumstances.

The physician and the staff should think through their situation, decide what they expect of patients with respect to payments, and how they will inform the patient. Although there will always be exceptions to any rule, there must be a rule, which should be in writing and conveyed to the patient at the outset of the relationship.

Some medical practices prepare an information booklet that includes the payment policy. New patients are given a copy of the booklet. Any patient who needs special consideration can be counseled by the medical assistant. The medical assistant who has the guidance and support of an established credit policy can perform with confidence when handling patient accounts. The credit policy must be fair and must address the following issues:

- Time when payment is due from patients
- Payment at the time of service
- Times when or if assignment of insurance benefits is accepted
- Completion of insurance forms by the office staff (or not)
- Billing procedures
- Collection protocol
- Length of time an account will be carried without payment
- Telephone collection protocol
- Use of a collection agency

PROCEDURE 14-3

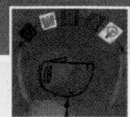

Making Credit Arrangements With a Patient

GOAL: To assist the patient in paying for services by making mutually beneficial credit arrangements according to established office policy.

EQUIPMENT AND SUPPLIES

- Patient's ledger
- Calendar
- Truth in Lending form
- Assignment of benefits form
- Patient's insurance form
- Private area for interview

PROCEDURAL STEPS

1 Answer all questions about credit thoroughly and kindly.

2 Inform the patient of the office policy regarding credit:

3 Payment at the time of first visit

4 Payment by bank card

5 Credit application
Purpose: To ensure complete understanding of mutual responsibilities.

6 Have the patient complete the credit application.
Purpose: To comply with office practices on the extension of credit.

7 Check the completed credit application.
Purpose: To confirm that all the necessary information is included.

8 Discuss with the patient the possible arrangements and ask the patient to decide which of those arrangements is most suitable.
Purpose: To ensure better compliance, which can be expected when the patient makes the choice.

9 Prepare the Truth in Lending form and have the patient sign it if the agreement requires more than four installments.
Purpose: To comply with Regulation Z.

10 Have the patient execute an assignment of insurance benefits.
Purpose: To comply with credit policy.

11 Make a copy of the patient's insurance card and have the patient sign a consent for release of the information to the insurance company.
Purpose: To ensure that a claim can be processed because consent for the release of information is necessary on most insurance forms.

12 Keep credit information confidential.

Installment Buying of Medical Services. Because installment buying is so much a part of our economic system today, the physician's office must be prepared to help patients budget for their medical care. Patients expect to use their credit resources and appreciate business-like assistance in establishing a payment plan. The medical profession has too long suffered a poor collection record because of its fear of appearing too commercial. The physician should be ready to arrange credit when medical bills will be high or when a patient for some reason is unable to pay at the time of service. In general, fees for routine office calls and small medical bills should be kept on a pay-as-you-go basis.

In recent years, companies have begun to offer credit or loans specifically for medical procedures. This is very popular for cosmetic surgeries. Offices that offer these types of procedures may wish to investigate these alternative financing services.

Truth in Lending Act. Regulation Z of the Truth in Lending Act, which is enforced by the Federal Trade Commission, requires that when there is a bilateral agreement between physician and patient to accept payment in more than four installments, the physician is required to provide disclosure of information regarding finance charges (Figure 14-7). Even if there are no finance charges

involved, the form must be completed stating this fact. The physician retains a copy of the form, and the original is given to the patient. Specific wording is required in the disclosure. Have the patient sign the agreement in your presence, because you must have proof of signing. The disclosure statement must be kept on file for 2 years. Although the disclosure statement is designed as protection for the debtor, it can be a good collection tool for the creditor.

It is recognized that physicians generally permit their patients to pay in installments, and as long as there is no specific agreement on the part of the physician for payment to be made in more than four installments and no finance charge is made, the account is not subject to the regulation. If the patient chooses to pay in installments instead of the full amount, this is considered a unilateral action. The physician, in accepting such payments, probably would not be subject to the provisions of the regulation. The physician's office, however, must be certain to bill for the full balance each time. If the statement is for only a partial payment, it then becomes a bilateral agreement and as such is subject to Regulation Z.

Helping patients budget their medical expenses is a rather new aspect of the business side of medical practice. However, it is a real service to patients and demonstrates

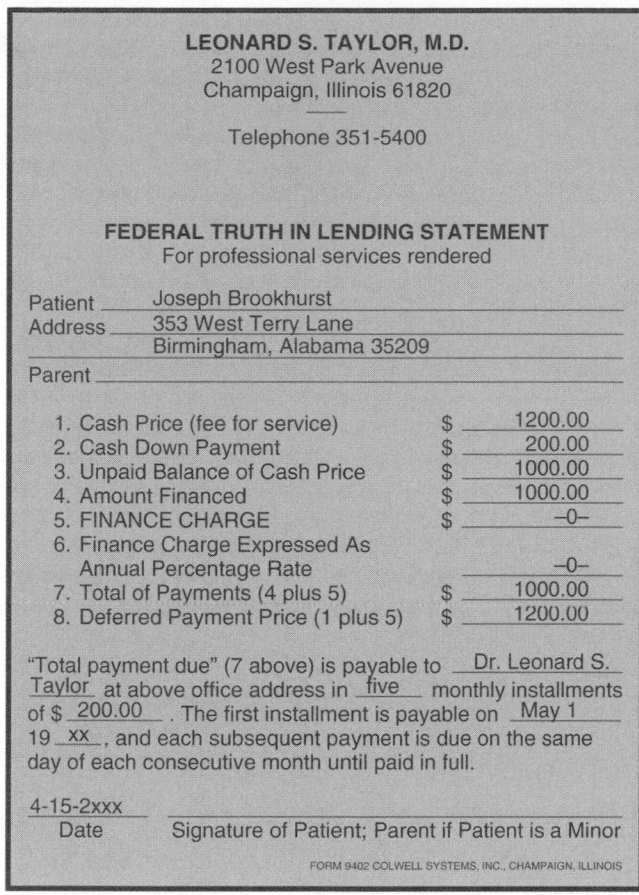

FIGURE 14-7   Disclosure statement. An example of a document for compliance with the Federal Truth In Lending Act. (Courtesy Colwell Systems, Inc., Champaign, Illinois.)

that the physician and the office staff are sincerely anxious to help patients pay their own way. It may also prevent many collection problems.

Confidentiality

Obtaining Credit Information. Credit information is confidential. It should be guarded as carefully as a confidential medical history and should be disclosed to no one. When asking for credit information from patients in the office, do so in a private area where others cannot overhear the conversation. A desk or table away from the reception area where a patient can sit in total privacy and complete a credit application is a great asset. Credit information is personal—it should be kept that way.

Credit Bureaus. Some physicians join a credit bureau, particularly in large cities where it is more difficult to gauge informally the patients' ability to pay. Credit bureaus gather credit information from many sources, pool it, and make it available to dues-paying bureau members. If the office receives a request for credit information about a patient, it is permissible to furnish it because the debtor, by giving the physician's name as a reference, has given implied consent; otherwise, the credit bureau would not have contacted the office. According to the Fair Credit Practices Act Amendments of 1975, the following information only can be given:

- When the account was opened
- How much the patient now owes

- What the highest amount of the account is at any time

You should avoid any reference to the following:

- Character
- Paying habits
- Credit rating

Billing Insurance or Other Third Parties

Insurance billing in the medical office is a courtesy to patients. Often, patients do not understand the policies and appreciate the assistance given by the medical office. Information on completing insurance forms and diagnostic and procedure coding is found in Chapters 15 through 18.

Independent Billing and Collection Services

Many healthcare facilities find it advantageous to refer their billing and collections to an independent billing service. The information related to services and fees is sent to the billing service on a daily or weekly basis. The servicing agent then handles all billing and collections, as well as any telephone inquiries. This system frees the regular office staff for more patient-oriented duties. An added advantage is that a person who is not connected with the patient care on a personal basis handles any dispute that may arise.

Internal Billing by the Account Manager

Billing Methods

In a practice with only a moderate number of accounts, the medical assistant handles the preparation and mailing of statements. This may be accomplished by using the following:

- A computer-generated statement
- An encounter form
- A typewritten statement
- A photocopied statement

The appearance of the statement carries a visual impact just as a letter does, so the statement heads should be carefully chosen and the typing clean and accurate. Statement heads are usually imprinted with the same information as the physician's letterhead. They should be of good quality and large enough to allow itemization of charges. Envelopes should be imprinted with *Address Correction Requested* under the return address to maintain up-to-date mailing lists. A self-addressed return envelope included with the statement encourages prompt payment. This is mainly for the convenience of patients who do not always have stationery available for sending a return payment or who are less likely to return a payment immediately if they must address an envelope.

Computer-Generated Statement. Patient accounts are generated and stored in the computer, and a statement can be produced whenever needed. The statement can show the service rendered on each date, the charge for each service, the date on which a claim was submitted to the insurance company, the date of payment, and the balance due from the patient. The computer may also be programmed to print messages on the statement, such as *Balance now 30 days past due* or a selection of other messages.

Encounter Form as a Bill. There are variations in style, but encounter forms are usually personalized for the practice. The form has space for all the elements required in submitting medical insurance claims, such as the following:

- Name and address of the patient
- Name of the insurance carrier
- Insurance identification number
- Brief description of each service by code number
- Fee for each service
- Place and date of service
- Diagnosis
- Physician's name and address
- Physician's signature

The encounter form can be used as a charge slip for office treatments if the physician checks the services performed at the completion of the visit and asks the patient to hand it to the medical assistant when leaving. Either the physician or the medical assistant may write in the amount of the fee. If a payment is made, it can be so indicated. Instructions to the patient for filing insurance claims are on the bottom left.

Statements. Statements must be correct and must include the patient's name and address as well as the balance owed. If statements are photocopied or microfilmed, special care must be taken that the ledger card is correct because it will be duplicated in the billing process.

Typewritten Statements. The use of continuous-form billing statements is a timesaver. The statements are printed in a roll with perforated edges for separation. The roll is fed into the typewriter for the first statement and remains until the last statement is typed, eliminating the time and energy necessary for inserting and removing each statement form from the typewriter.

Photocopied Statements. Coordinated ledger cards and copy paper are used in preparing photocopied statements. A perfect statement is ready for mailing in minimal time. Extra care must be used in posting the ledgers. A black pen should be used in making entries on the ledger card, because other ink colors do not reproduce well. Writing must be clear and legible. No personal notes should be made on the ledger cards unless there is something you wish conveyed to the patient. (It is possible to buy pencils with nonreproducible lead if you believe this is necessary for making collection entries.) Usually, a window envelope is used for mailing, which means that the name and address on the ledger must be neat, correct, and positioned correctly for the envelope window.

Internal Billing Procedures

Itemizing the First Statement. If the medical fee has been explained in advance, the monthly statement is merely a confirmation of what is owed, and there should be no misunderstanding. However, it is good business practice—and a courtesy to the patient—to itemize the charges. This is essential if the statement is to be used for billing the patient's insurance. Patients are entitled to an understanding of the physician's statement for medical services.

Itemizing statements is not difficult, and computerized statements usually automatically itemize the first statement. The simplest method is merely to allow space on the original statement, below the *For Professional Services* line, on which to list the separate charges for office visits, hospital calls, or treatments or tests performed in the medical facility.

Many physicians have devised their own itemized encounter forms, which are given to the patient when payment is made at the time of service or later mailed in a combination statement-reply envelope. The use of such charge slips simplifies the itemization procedure, because filling out the slips is usually just a matter of checking the procedures listed. Although the itemization of bills may seem tedious, the medical assistant will spend less time in explaining services provided, clearing up misunderstandings with patients, and following up on delinquent accounts by itemizing.

CRITICAL THINKING APPLICATION

Mrs. Deaton is frustrated because she claims she was never sent an itemized statement and now refuses to pay her account. Myra feels that this is a delay tactic, because she specifically recalls sending an itemized statement to the patient. How can this situation be remedied?

Time and Frequency of Billing

A regular system of mailing statements should be put into operation. Most people expect to receive statements from their creditors, and they plan their budgets around first-of-the-month bills received. Punctuality in billing encourages prompt payment.

Statements should be sent at least once each month. Some offices send bills immediately after treatment; others bill all patients on the same day each month. Mailing statements twice a month (e.g., half of the accounts on the tenth and the remaining half on the twenty-fifth) is also a common practice.

Once-a-Month Billing. If a monthly pattern is followed, bills should leave the office in time to reach the patient no later than the last day of each month and preferably before the twenty-fifth of the month. Planning ahead for the preparation of statements can lighten the burden of once-a-month billing (Procedure 14-4). The statement can be prepared at the time of service, postdated, and mailed at the end of the month.

Cycle Billing. Many physicians prefer to use the cycle billing system, which calls for the billing of certain portions of the accounts receivable at given times during the month instead of preparing all statements at the end of each month. Cycle billing is used in large businesses such as department stores, banks, and utility companies. Its many advantages include avoiding once-a-

PROCEDURE 14-4

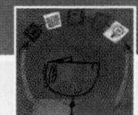

Preparing Monthly Billing Statements

GOAL: To process monthly statements and evaluate accounts for collection procedures in accordance with the agency's credit policy.

EQUIPMENT AND SUPPLIES

- Typewriter or computer
- Patient accounts
- Agency's credit policy
- Statement forms

PROCEDURAL STEPS

1 Assemble all accounts that have outstanding balances.

2 Separate accounts that need special attention in accordance with the agency's credit policy.

   Explanation: Routine statements should be prepared first, after which special attention can be given to delinquent accounts.

3 Prepare routine statements, including the following:

- Date the statement is prepared
- Name and address of the person responsible for payment
- Name of the patient, if different from the person responsible for payment
- Itemization of dates, services, and charges for the month
- Any unpaid balance carried forward (may or may not be itemized, depending on office policy)

4 Determine the action to be taken on accounts separated in Step 2.

5 Make a note of the necessary action on the ledger card (telephone call, collection letter series, small claims court, or assignment of collection agency).

   Purpose: To be used for guidance in executing an action and for later follow-up when necessary.

---

month peak workloads and stabilizing the cash flow. In a small office in which billing is done only once a month, the unexpected illness or absence of the medical assistant for any emergency can leave the physician in a financial bind if the statements do not go out.

The accounts are separated into fairly equal divisions, the number of divisions depending on how many times billing will be done during a month. For example, if the office expects to bill twice per month, divide the accounts into 2 equal groups; for weekly billing, divide into 4 groups, and for daily billing, divide into 20 groups.

Small alphabetical groups can be combined to keep the divisions nearly equal in the number of statements to prepare on each billing day. If the files are color coded, the medical assistant may wish to use the same alphabetical breakdown in billing. Regardless of constant changes in the individual accounts, the mailing dates for accounts in each section remain the same. A schedule for processing and mailing is thus established, and the workload is apportioned throughout the entire month.

Cycle billing allows the medical assistant to continue all routine duties each day, handling the statements on a day-to-day or weekly schedule rather than in one intensive period at the end of the month. This means that whole days need not be sacrificed from other duties to get statements in the mail. When the billing is spaced throughout the month, more time and consideration can be given to each statement, the itemization of bills is less burdensome, and the likelihood of error is decreased.

Patients generally accept the cycle billing system quickly, often with enthusiasm. However, if your office decides to change from a once-a-month billing system to a cycle billing system, patients should be notified in advance, and the new plan should be explained to them. To explain the new system to established patients, enclose a notice in each statement for 2 months before the transfer, describing the plan and indicating the future dates on which each patient will receive the bill.

Before a physician adopts the cycle billing system, particularly in a small community, several factors should be taken into consideration, such as the following:

- What is the general income level of the community, and how and when does the average patient get paid?
- Do local companies pay employees at various times during the month, or are most paychecks handed out at the beginning of the month?
- Would cycle billing benefit patients as well as the overall operation of the office?

Billing Third Party Payors. Collection problems may arise if the medical assistant fails to get the necessary insurance information, particularly Medicare and Medicaid information. In some instances, if the insurance forms are not completed correctly, the claim may be denied because of minor infractions such as failing to name the responsible party or omitting Social Security information, the policy number, or the group number.

Time limits must also be observed in billing third party payors. In cases of Medicare patients with a terminal illness, it may be best to accept assignment of benefits. If the physician does not take assignment, he or she may receive nothing because the family is not obligated to pay, and Medicare will not pay after a certain time or if the claim has not been correctly filed.

Billing Minors. Minors cannot be held responsible for payment of a bill unless they are emancipated. Bills for minors must be addressed to a parent or legal guardian. If a bill is addressed to a minor, the parent or parents could take the attitude that they are not responsible because they never received the bill.

If the parents are separated or divorced, the parent who brings the child in for treatment is responsible for payment. Whatever financial agreement exists between the parents is strictly their personal business and should not concern the medical office. The responsible parent should be so informed from the beginning.

If a minor appears in the office and requests treatment and you can ascertain that the person is legally emancipated, the minor is responsible for the bill. It may be wise to make a determination either with the business manager or with the physician as to whether your office wishes to treat this emancipated minor.

Care for Those Who Cannot Pay

The medical profession has traditionally accepted the responsibility of providing medical care for individuals unable to pay for these services. In spite of the increased scope of government-sponsored care for the **medically indigent**, physicians still donate thousands of dollars' worth of such medical services each year.

In many instances, medical care of the indigent is available through social service agencies. The medical assistant should learn about any local organizations and agencies that can aid the patient in obtaining the necessary assistance. The physician can provide only medical services. Other agencies must provide hospitalization, for example, or arrange for paying the costs of special therapy, rehabilitation, or medications. Unfortunately, there is still another segment of the population that consists of uninsured employees who are not eligible for public assistance, are not covered under a group policy, and cannot afford the high premiums for private medical insurance. Special attention must be given to helping these people arrange to pay their medical bills.

If a physician accepts a case for which a fee will not be paid, complete records must still be kept on the patient. The only deviation in procedure is that the financial record indicates no charge (n/c) in the debit column.

Fees in Hardship Cases

Sometimes a physician is faced with the problem of deciding whether to reduce or cancel a fee in a hardship case. Before adjusting or canceling a fee, the physician or the medical assistant should engage in a frank discussion of the patient's financial situation. Find out whether the patient is entitled to an insurance settlement of some kind. For instance, if the patient's injuries are the result of a car accident, there may be insurance through the automobile policy. Circumstances may qualify the patient for local or state public assistance, such as crime victim

assistance. If so, the assistant may direct the patient to the appropriate agency.

If the circumstances of hardship are known before the services are rendered, thorough discussion of what the fee will be and how it will be paid should take place at that time. The physician may suggest that a medically indigent patient seek care at a county hospital with public assistance. A physician should be free to choose his or her form of charity and not feel obligated to substantially reduce or cancel a fee when the circumstances are known in advance.

After the physician and patient have agreed on a fee, special circumstances may arise that create a hardship. If the physician then agrees to reduce the fee, the patient should be told that the reduction will be effective only after the adjusted amount is paid in full. For instance, if a fee of $500 is reduced to $350, the full amount of the $500 charge should appear on the ledger and when $350 has been received the remainder can be written off as an adjustment.

Pitfalls of Fee Adjustments

When a physician begins to reduce his or her fees, problems can arise. Patients may begin to expect that fees will be reduced in all circumstances. Patients may even doubt the competency of a physician who habitually reduces fees.

Great care should be taken in reducing the fee for care of a patient who dies. The physician's sympathy is with the family in such instances, but the physician's generosity in reducing a fee could be misinterpreted and result in a suit for malpractice. The family may suspect that the fee was reduced because the physician knows he or she made an error.

If the physician agrees to settle for a reduced fee in a situation in which the patient is disputing the fee, care should be taken to make certain the negotiations are without prejudice. By taking this precaution, the physician protects the right to collect the original sum should the patient refuse to pay the lowered fee. The offer of a discount therefore should be made in writing, with the insertion of the words "without prejudice" and a definite time limit for making payment stated. Prepare two copies of the agreement and have the signatures witnessed. Keep the original for the physician and give a copy to the patient.

A fee should never be reduced on the basis of a poor result or as a means of obtaining payment to avoid the use of a collection agency. A reduction for these reasons degrades the physician and the practice of medicine.

Professional Courtesy

Traditionally, physicians do not charge professional colleagues or their immediate dependents for medical care. Although the concept of **professional courtesy** is often attributed to Hippocrates, the foundations of professional courtesy today are derived from Thomas Percival's Code of 1803.

In some cases, giving professional courtesy represents the loss of a large amount of potential income. If there is a substantial outlay in the cost of materials, the professional colleague will probably wish to reimburse the physician for the materials used. Most physicians today subscribe to a health insurance plan. If the care they receive is covered by insurance, it is entirely ethical for the attending physician to accept the insurance benefits in payment for services.

If the services are frequent enough to involve a significant portion of the physician's professional time or if they extend over a long time, the physician may wish to charge on an adjusted basis. When professional courtesy has been offered and the recipient still insists on paying, the physician need not hesitate on ethical grounds to accept a fee for service.

Professional courtesy is often extended beyond fellow physicians and their dependents. Most physicians treat their own medical assistants, and often their families, without charge and grant discounts to nurses and medical assistants not in their direct employ. Student externs should never expect to be treated while serving in an externship capacity. Professional courtesy is sometimes extended to others in the healthcare field (e.g., pharmacists and dentists).

CRITICAL THINKING APPLICATION

Dr. Franklin has just finished seeing Dr. Wallace as a patient and insists to Myra that Dr. Wallace always extends him professional courtesy. This is not indicated on the ledger card, since several payments are shown on the record. Dr. Wallace has just left the office and is in an important meeting at the hospital. What should Myra do?

Collection Techniques

Sometimes, it becomes necessary to aggressively attempt to collect the balances that patients owe the physician (Procedure 14-5). Persuasive collection procedures include telephone calls, collection reminders and letters, and personal interviews.

Telephone Collection Calls

A telephone call at the right time, in the right manner, will be more successful than notes, a statement, or a collection letter. The personal contact of a telephone call will bring in more money than if a call is not made. In the absence of time to make calls, the collection letter is the next best avenue. If collections are a serious problem, it may pay to hire an extra person to do the telephoning. Written notification is a must before making a final demand for payment indicating that legal or collection proceedings will be started. There are no hard and fast rules for pursuing collections by telephone. Each case should be handled individually on the basis of the experience with the person involved.

GENERAL RULES TO FOLLOW IN TELEPHONE COLLECTIONS

What To Do

- Call the patient when it can be done with privacy.
- Call between 8 AM and 9 PM.
- Determine the identity of the persons with whom you are speaking. If you ask, "Is this Mrs. Noble?" and she answers, "Yes," it could be the patient's mother-in-law or daughter-in-law, who is also "Mrs. Noble." Use the person's full name.
- Be dignified and respectful. One can be friendly and formal at the same time.
- Ask the patient if it is a convenient time to talk. Unless you have the attention of the called party, there is little to be gained by continuing. If told that it is an inopportune time, ask for a specific time to call back, or get a promise for the patient to call the office at a specified time.
- After a brief greeting, state the purpose of the call. Make no apology for calling, but state the reason in a friendly, business-like way. The physician expects payment and the medical assistant is interested in helping the patient meet the financial obligation. Open the call with a phrase such as, "This is Alice, Dr. Wallace's financial secretary. I'm calling about your account." A well-placed pause at this point in the call sometimes gets an immediate response from the debtor in regard to the nonpayment.
- Assume a positive attitude. For example, convey the impression that the patient intended to pay and it is only a matter of working out some suitable arrangements.
- Keep the conversation brief and to the point, and avoid threats of any kind.
- Try to get a definite commitment payment of a certain amount by a certain date.
- Follow up on promises. This is best accomplished by a tickler file or a note on the calendar. If the payment does not arrive by the promised date, remind the patient with another call. If the medical assistant fails to do this, the whole effort has been wasted.

What Not To Do

- Do not call between 9 PM and 8 AM. To do so may be considered harassment.
- Do not make repeated telephone calls.
- Do not call the debtor's place of work if the employer prohibits personal calls.
- If a call is placed to the debtor at work and the person cannot take the call, leave a

GENERAL RULES TO FOLLOW IN TELEPHONE COLLECTIONS—Cont'd

message asking the debtor to "call Mrs. Black at 727-9238" without revealing the nature of the call; that is, do not state that the call is from "Dr. Wallace's office" or "Dr. Jones's medical assistant."
- Do not show hostility. An angry patient is a poor-paying patient. Insulted patients often do not pay at all.

Collection Letters or Reminders

Some consultants believe that a printed collection letter or reminder enclosed with a statement is more effective than a personal letter. Their attitude is that a patient may be embarrassed by a personal letter and feel that he or she has been singled out for attention. An impersonal printed message will probably encourage the debtor to send a payment. The printed form is a time saver and is recommended if a lack of time is contributing to poor collection follow-up. Standard printed forms are readily available, and the medical assistant can also design original forms.

Letters that are friendly requests for an explanation of why payment has not been made are still effective in

PROCEDURE 14-5

Aging Accounts Receivables

GOAL: To determine the age of accounts and decide what collection activity is needed.

EQUIPMENT AND SUPPLIES
- Patient ledger cards with a balance due
- Pen
- Computer
- Calculator

PROCEDURAL STEPS

1 Prompt the computer to compile a report on the age of accounts receivable. Many programs will have this report option that can be easily accessed.
Purpose: To determine which accounts have a balance due.

2 Divide the accounts into categories as listed below:
- 0–30 days old
- 30–60 days old
- 60–90 days old
- 90–120 days old
- Over 120 days old

Purpose: To determine how old the various accounts are and place the accounts into categories as to when the last payment was made.

3 If the computer program does not perform this function, manually pull all ledger cards that have a balance due and divide them into the categories listed above.

4 Examine the accounts to see which are awaiting an insurance payment. Action need not be taken if an insurance payment is expected and is not long overdue. Return those ledgers to the ledger tray.
Purpose: To avoid collection activity on accounts for which a payment is expected.

5 Follow the office procedure for collections on the accounts left. Collection reminder stickers may be placed on the statements sent to the patient, or a collection letter may be sent. Be sure that the stickers are inside the envelope, not on the outside.
Purpose: To prompt the patient to make a payment by pointing out the age of the account.

6 Call patients whose accounts are over 90 days old. Attempt to make payment arrangements with the patient.
Purpose: To attempt to collect from the patient or determine why the patient has not yet paid the account.

7 Send a collection letter to patients whose accounts are over 120 days old, if indicated, to encourage the patient to pay the account. If it is the office policy, mention that the account is in danger of being sent to a collection agency.
Purpose: To reach patients who are not available by telephone.

8 Add the total accounts receivable for each category and arrive at a figure outstanding for each. The physician may wish to have a report weekly or monthly on these figures.
Purpose: To have a current accounting of the amounts owed to the physician, and to double check the amount outstanding according to the pegboard system or computer software system.

9 Note any arrangements made with patients regarding payment of the accounts in the chart and/or on the ledger. Send a follow-up letter to remind the patients of their payment agreements.
Purpose: To document arrangements made and remind the patients of their obligation and promise to pay.

many cases. These letters should indicate that the physician is sincerely interested in the patient and wishes to help straighten out the financial obligations. The patient should be invited to visit the office to explain the reasons for nonpayment so that, if possible, special arrangements can be worked out. To give the patient an opportunity to save face, these letters can suggest that the patient may have overlooked previous statements.

On receipt of such a letter, most patients make some effort to explain their failure to make payment. If a patient really is having financial difficulties, the physician may be able to get public assistance for him or her. If it is a temporary financial embarrassment, the physician and the patient may together be able to work out a satisfactory installment plan for payment.

The medical assistant often is given a free hand in designing collection patterns and composing collection letters. Many medical assistants compose a series of collection letters, using model letters that they have found to be effective (Figure 14-8). Such a series usually includes at least five letters in varying degrees of forcefulness.

Sometimes, even the person with poor paying habits will pay the bill if treated with respect and consideration. The medical assistant should never go beyond the authority granted by the physician in pursuing collections. If there are questions about special collection problems, always check with the physician before proceeding. This is particularly important with patients whom you do not know personally (e.g., patients who the physician has seen in the hospital or at home and patients with no credit history). It is difficult to say whether pressing collections too hard loses more good will of patients than not pursuing collections diligently enough. The physician and the medical assistant together should agree on general collection policies as outlined earlier in this chapter, and then the policies should be followed. In all cases in which an account is to be assigned to a collection agency, be certain that the physician is aware of it.

Signing Collection Letters. In most medical offices, the medical assistant signs collection letters with the identification "Assistant to Dr. Brown" or "Financial Secretary" below the typewritten signature. Some physi-

---

1. Your account has always been paid promptly in the past, so this must be an oversight. Please accept this note as a friendly reminder of your account due in the amount of $ _____ .

2. Since your care in this office in March, we have had no word from you in regard to how you are feeling or your account due. If it is impossible for you to pay the full amount of $ _____ at this time, please call this office before June 15 so that satisfactory arrangements can be worked out.

3. Medical bills are payable at the time of service unless special credit arrangements are made. Please send your check in full or call this office before June 30.

4. If you have some question about your statement, we will be happy to answer it for you. If not, may we have a payment before the end of this month?

5. Unless some definite arrangement is made to reduce your balance of $ _____ , we can no longer carry your account on our books. Delinquent accounts are turned over to our collection agency on the 25th of the month.

6. **When a payment plan has been established, it can be reinforced by recognizing the first remittance with a letter of acknowledgment:**

   Thank you for the recent payment of $ _____ on your account. We are glad to cooperate with you in this arrangement for clearing your account. We will look for your next check at about the same time next month, and your final payment the following month.

7. **When a payment schedule has been arranged by a telephone call, it can be confirmed by letter.**

   As agreed upon in our telephone conversation today, we will expect you to mail a payment of $50 on February 10; $50 on March 10; and the balance on April 10. If some emergency should prevent your making one of these payments on time, please notify us immediately by telephone.

DO'S AND DON'TS

DO:

1. Individualize letters to suit the situation.

2. Design your early letters as mere reminders of debt.

3. Always imply that the patient has good intentions to pay, until lack of response over a period of time proves otherwise.

4. Send letters with a firmer tone only after you have sent one or two friendly reminders.

DON'T

1. Use the same collection letter for a patient with good paying habits as for one who is known to neglect financial obligations.

2. Place an overdue notice of any kind on a postcard or on the outside of an envelope. This is an **invasion of privacy.**

FIGURE 14-8 Suggestions for composing collection letters. Brief collection letters that ask patients to explain the lack of payment are often effective.

cians may wish to personally sign these communications, but generally the medical assistant who handles the accounts also signs the collection letters.

Personal Interviews

Personal interviews with patients can sometimes be more effective than a whole series of collection letters. By talking to a patient face to face, the medical assistant can come to an understanding of the problem more quickly and reach an agreement about future payment plans.

Occasionally, a patient may undergo a long course of treatment and yet make no attempt to pay anything on account. Perhaps such a patient is only waiting for the physician or the medical assistant to suggest that a payment be made. When there is advance knowledge that the patient will require extensive treatment, the matter of payment should be discussed early in the course of treatment, the credit policy explained, and some agreement reached as to a payment plan.

Because the fee for medical services is far more intangible than that of any commercial account, collection efforts must not be delayed too long. Any responsible, sincere patient will call or write the physician's office after receiving a second statement and explain the delay in payment or ask for a payment plan.

If it becomes necessary to refer the account to a collector, a good agency should have a 35% to 40% recovery rate with an account that is assigned within 4 or 5 months. This may drop to 25% if the account is held only a few more months. If recovery by the agency is greater than 40%, it may indicate that the collection effort by the medical assistant needs to be intensified.

The value of medical accounts diminishes in direct proportion to the length of time that has elapsed since service was rendered. Do not fight the law of diminishing returns. All collection activity is costly. Know when to stop and call on the services of a professional agency.

Special Collection Situations

Tracing "Skips." When a statement is returned marked *Moved—no forwarding address*, you may consider this account as a "skip." This generally is accepted as an indication that the patient is attempting to avoid liability for debts. Some so-called skips are innocent errors. The person may have been careless in not leaving a forwarding address, or the mistake may have occurred in the physician's office; the wrong name or address may have been placed on the statement. However, immediate action should be taken in regard to returned statements. Do not wait until the next billing time to attempt to trace the debtor.

SUGGESTIONS FOR TRACING SKIPS

- Examine the patient's original office registration card.
- Call the telephone number listed on the card. Occasionally a patient may move without leaving a forwarding address but will transfer the old telephone number. The new telephone number may be given when you call the old number.
- If you are unable to contact the individual by telephone, make a few discreet calls to the references listed on the registration card to get leads.
- Check the Internet to secure the names and telephone numbers of neighbors or the landlord, and contact these people to secure information about the debtor's whereabouts.
- Do not inform a third party that the person owes you money. Simply state that you are trying to locate or verify the location of the individual.
- Check the debtor's place of employment for information. If the person is a specialist in his or her field of work, the local union or similar organizations may be contacted. Although they may not give you the person's current address, they will relay the message that you are seeking to contact him or her. Often, people will be stirred into paying a bill if they think that their employer may learn of their payment failure.
- Do not communicate with a third party more than once. This is specifically forbidden by law (Public Law 95-109, Sec. 804) unless the third party requests the collector to do so.

The tracing of skips is a challenge to any medical assistant. A certified letter can be sent; by paying additional fees, you can ask the Postal Service to obtain a receipt including the address where the letter was delivered. The certified letter may be sent in a plain envelope so that the patient will not refuse to accept the letter because of the return address.

If all attempts fail, turn the account over to a collection agency without delay. Do not keep a skip account too long, because the trail may become so cold as time elapses that even collection experts will be unable to follow it.

Claims Against Estates. A bill owed by a deceased patient may be handled a little differently than regular bills. Courtesy dictates that a bill not be sent during the initial period of bereavement, but do not delay more than 30 days. The person responsible for settling the affairs of the estate will be assembling outstanding accounts and will expect to receive the medical bills along with all others. Address the statement using the following:

Estate of (name of patient)
c/o (spouse or next of kin, if known)
Patient's last known address

Do not address the statement to a relative unless you have a signed agreement that that person will be responsible. If for some reason the statement cannot be addressed as just suggested (e.g., if the patient was in a convalescent home and there is no name of a relative), seek information from the county seat in the county in which the estate is being settled.

A will is generally filed within 30 days of a death. A request to the Probate Department of the Superior Court, County Recorder's Office, will usually provide the name of the executor or administrator. The time limits for filing an estate claim are determined by the state in which the decedent resided.

After the name of the administrator or executor of the estate has been obtained, a duplicate itemized statement of the account should be sent to that person by certified mail, return receipt requested. If no response is received in 10 days, contact the executor or the county clerk where the estate is being settled and obtain forms for filing a claim against the estate. (Some states do not have special claim forms but will accept simple itemized statements.) This claim against the estate must be made within a certain length of time, varying from 2 to 36 months, depending on the state in which it is filed.

The executor of the estate will either accept or reject the claim and if it is accepted, will send an acknowledgment of the debt. Payment is often delayed because of the legal complications in settling an estate, but if the claim has been accepted, you will receive your money in due time. If the claim is rejected and there is full justification for claiming the bill, file a claim against the executor within a limited time, according to state laws. The time limit in such cases starts with the date on the letter of rejection that was sent in response to the original claim.

Because states have different time limits and statutes in regard to such matters, it is advisable for the medical assistant to contact the physician's attorney or the local court for the exact procedure to follow.

Bankruptcy. Bankruptcy laws were passed to secure equal distribution of the assets of an individual among the individual's creditors. Bankruptcy laws are federal and are applicable in all states. When notified that a patient has declared bankruptcy, do not send statements or make any attempt to collect on the account from the patient.

Chapter VII bankruptcy is usually a "no asset" situation. Because the physician's fee is an unsecured debt, there is little purpose in pursuing collection. Chapter XIII is known as *wage-earner bankruptcy*. Under Chapter XIII, the patient/debtor pays a fixed amount (agreed on by the court) to the trustee in bankruptcy. This is then passed on to the creditors. During this period, none of the creditors can attach the debtor's wages or otherwise attempt to collect the debt. It is sometimes beneficial to file a claim under Chapter XIII because small payments will be made by the debtor under the supervision of the court over a period of 3 years.

Using Outside Collection Assistance

When everything possible has been done internally to follow up on an outstanding account and the office has not received payment, the question arises as to what step to take next, as follows:

- Should the facility sue for the payment?
- Should the account be sent to a collection agency?
- Should the account be written off as a bad debt?

Before forcing an account, first consider the time element: Has the patient been given a fair chance to pay this bill? Have statements been sent regularly and used a systematic method of following the account? Ask if there might be a misunderstanding about the fee charged. Was the first statement fully itemized? A large unexplained bill may frighten a patient into making no payments at all because the whole balance looks too large.

If the correct registration forms to secure advance credit information were used, the medical assistant should know the financial abilities of the patient to pay. However, illness may have caused a loss of salary and resulted in temporary inability to pay. Try to thoroughly analyze the situation.

Could the patient have been dissatisfied with the care received? For some unknown reason, a patient may feel that he or she was not treated correctly. Perhaps the patient expected a complete cure too soon. Only an explanation of the condition, prognosis, and care can enlighten such patients, and this is best handled by the physician. If payment of a bill is pressed too hard and the patient is dissatisfied for some reason, a malpractice suit may be filed by the patient to seek retribution against the physician. The court can approve a period longer than 3 years in special cases, but cannot approve a period longer than 5 years.

Collecting Through the Court System

Making the Decision to Sue. Will a physician lose more good will by suing for a bill than by writing it off as a loss? One management official has related that, strangely enough, when a physician-client sued two patients for large amounts, the patients lost the cases, paid up, and were back in the office for treatment very shortly! However, most physicians believe it is unwise to resort to the court to collect medical bills unless there are extraordinary circumstances.

An account must be considered a 100% loss to the physician before legal proceedings are started. Remember to never threaten to **instigate** legal proceedings unless prepared to carry out the threat and have the physician's consent to issue such a warning. If the physician decides in favor of a lawsuit, investigate thoroughly before taking action. Litigation to collect a bill is generally in order when the following occur:

- The patient can afford to pay without hardship.
- The physician can produce office records that support the bill.
- The physician can justify the amount of the bill by comparing it with fee practices in the community.
- The patient's general condition after treatment is satisfactory.
- The persuasive powers of an ethical collection agency have been exhausted and the agency advises suing.
- The patient can be given ample warning of the physician's intention to sue.

- The defendant (whether a patient or a parent or legal guardian) is legally liable for the services rendered to the patient.
- The statute of limitations has ruled out any possible malpractice action.
- The physician is not bubbling over with indignation and is not in a negative frame of mind.

Small Claims Court. Many medical practices find the small claims court a satisfactory and inexpensive way to collect delinquent accounts. The law places a limit on the amount of debt for which relief may be sought in the small claims court. Because this varies from state to state (from $300 to $5000) and in some instances even within a state, this limit should be checked locally before seeking recovery in this manner.

Parties to small claims actions cannot be represented by an attorney at the trial but may send another person to court in their behalf to produce records supporting the claim. Physicians often send their bookkeeper or medical assistant with records of unpaid accounts to show the judge.

If the court awards a judgment for the amount owed, the plaintiff in small claims court may also recover the costs of the suit. For a very small investment in time and money, the physician who uses this method has done the following:

- Saved the time of a regular court action
- Had no attorney's fee to pay
- Not sacrificed the commission charged by a collection agency

After being awarded a judgment, the medical assistant must still collect the money. The only person in a small claims action who has the right of appeal is the defendant. An appeal by the defendant may have the judgment set aside. The plaintiff cannot file an appeal in a small claims action; the decision of the court is final.

The necessary papers for filing action and full instructions on the course to follow may be obtained from the clerk of the small claims court. The medical assistant who has never appeared in the court would probably be wise to attend once as a spectator to preview the procedure and feel more at ease when appearing for the physician.

A collection agency to which an account may have been assigned may not file or handle a small claims action. It must either sue in the regular municipal or justice court or attempt to collect the debt in some other manner.

Using a Collection Agency

The medical assistant should try every means possible to collect accounts before they become delinquent. As soon as the account is determined *uncollectible* through the office (i.e., the patient has failed to respond to the final letter or has failed to fulfill a second promise on payment), send the account to the collector without delay. Skips should be assigned immediately.

Even though collection by an agency will mean sacrificing from 40% to 60% of the amount owed, further delay will only reduce the chances of recovery by the professional collector. If the agency finds that the case deserves special consideration, it will seek the physician's advice before proceeding further.

Selecting a Collection Agency. There are a number of agencies either owned and operated as an integral part of the county medical society or operated separately from the medical society but supervised by the medical profession. These bureaus provide specialized medical collection services.

Another type of collection agency is a division of the local credit association, recognized by the National Retail Credit Association. If the local credit association does not maintain a collection department, it will be able to recommend a reputable one. A nationally recognized credit association has considerable responsibility and a high standard to maintain. These factors serve as monitors to its reliability.

The most common type of collection agency throughout the United States is the privately owned and operated agency. Many of these work with the local professional societies and strive to keep their work on a high ethical standard. Because a few bureaus are unethical and unscrupulous in their tactics, care should be taken to be sure that the one chosen is reliable and ethical. For the sake of comparison, many healthcare facilities use two or three agencies.

Responsibilities to the Collection Agency. When a reputable agency is selected, the medical assistant must be prepared to provide the agency with all the necessary data to enable it to begin prompt collection procedures on overdue accounts. The agency should receive the following:

- Full name of the debtor
- Name of the spouse
- Last known address
- Full amount of the debt
- Date of the last entry on account (debit or credit)
- Occupation of the debtor
- Business address
- Any other pertinent data

After an account has been released to a collection agency, the office makes no further collection attempts. Once the agency has begun its work, adhere to the following guidelines and procedures:

1. Send no more statements.
2. Mark the patient's ledger or stamp it so that everyone will know it is now in the hands of the collector.

3. Refer the patient to the collection agency if he or she contacts the office in regard to the account.
4. Promptly report any payments made directly to your office (a percentage of this payment is due the agency).
5. Call the agency if any information is obtained that will be of value in tracing or collecting the account.
6. Do not push the agency with frequent calls. The representatives of the agency will report regularly and will keep the office posted on collection progress.

Collection Agency Payments. If a patient sends a payment after the account has been turned over to a collection agency, the amount will need to be adjusted on the patient ledger. The collection agency will be due a percentage of the payment.

Closing Comments

Billing and collecting are critical duties in the medical office, and a responsible medical assistant is a great asset in this important area. Always maintain a positive attitude with the patients and guarantors. Remember that those who are ill or facing challenges are not always at their best and may not respond in a positive way to calls regarding their accounts. Make every attempt to work with each patient to develop a workable plan to clear their accounts.

Patient Education

Most patients are unaware of the actual coverage they have through their insurance policies. The medical assistant should encourage patients to read the entire policy so that they become familiar with its limitations and exclusions. Tell patients that when calling the company with questions, they should always write down the date, time, and name of the person with whom they spoke. Using email is helpful, because a record of the correspondence can be easily saved or printed. It is well worth the effort to make sure that patients have a general understanding of their health insurance coverage.

Often, patients do not dispute or question the company when a claim is rejected or not paid in the expected amount. Encourage them to call the company and question rejections if they do not understand why the claim was denied. Patients are paying for coverage and they should receive all of the benefits to which they are entitled.

Patients appreciate receiving an office-policy brochure or booklet that informs them about payment and credit options. The patient can use the printed booklet as a reference whenever questions arise, and its regular use by most patients will reduce the number of calls made to the office. Encourage patients to use the booklet. Helpful phone numbers or extensions, as well as instructions as to whom the patient should call for answers to questions at the medical facility, should be included.

Legal and Ethical Issues

A patient who has filed bankruptcy cannot be contacted or billed further. A threat to take collection action must be fulfilled or the creditor is in violation of the federal Fair Debt Collection Practices Act. Never say that the physician intends to take action if he or she does not plan to follow through.

The Federal Equal Credit Opportunity Act of 1977 bars discrimination in all areas of credit. If the physician agrees to extend credit to one credit-worthy patient, then the same arrangement must be offered to any other patient who requests it, as long as the patient is also credit worthy.

Since laws vary greatly from state to state, the medical assistant should review the statutes pertaining to billing and collecting in the area in which he or she lives. Develop a good understanding of what is required of the small business, such as a physician's office, in collecting fees and billing for amounts due. Remember that laws change often, and constantly update policies to reflect current statutes.

SUMMARY OF SCENARIO

Myra is a well-respected member of Dr. Wallace's office team. Her friendly attitude and flexibility make her a pleasure to interact with in the facility. She knows that there are only a few patients for whom she cannot work out some type of payment arrangements. She is professional in her dealings with those whom she contacts about outstanding accounts.

Dr. Wallace has noticed that more and more patients pay their accounts, and he attributes this to the care that Myra shows when working with them. She is never hesitant to ask for payment from the patient but is sensitive to their needs and struggles at the same time. She urges her patients to cooperate and make a good attempt to pay their accounts, and in return, Myra arranges a payment schedule that the patient can meet.

Myra's flexibility as an employee has paid off for Dr. Wallace several times. During a week-long period when the computer bookkeeping system was malfunctioning, Myra was able to retrieve information from her backup disks and use a pegboard system until the system was repaired. Her preparation allowed the office to continue operations without skipping a beat. Most patients did not even notice that the computer was not in use for the week.

Myra has also been able to fill in for other employees because of the versatility she gained from her medical assistant training. She has scheduled appointments and even assisted Dr. Wallace with minor office surgery. Myra feels that performing other duties is a nice change periodically, and she keeps her skills sharp. She has proved herself to be a valuable and efficient employee.

SUMMARY OF LEARNING OBJECTIVES

■ Medical services are valuable to the patient who receives them. The physician sets fees based on three commodities. The physician offers the patient his *time* and makes the most accurate *judgments* possible about the patient's medical condition. The *services* provided to the patient also figure into the fees that are set for various procedures.

■ Many third party payors use the UCR method of determining fees for procedures. The *usual* fee is what the physician normally charges for a given service. The *customary* fee is the range of fees charged by physicians who have similar experience in the same geographic area. Services or procedures that are exceptionally complicated and that require extra time deserve a *reasonable* fee and may be higher than the usual fee.

■ Providing estimates for medical care helps patients plan their finances when an illness or injury occurs. When estimates are provided, the possibility of later misquoting the fee is avoided. The office staff should keep a copy of the estimate in the patient's chart, which will help to avoid misunderstandings and confusion over charges.

■ Some physicians choose to extend professional courtesy to other physicians, medical professionals, and medical staff employees. This means that the physician either discounts or eliminates the charges for all or part of the services provided. The decision to offer professional courtesy should remain with the physician.

■ Payment for medical services is accomplished in several ways. Most physicians prefer that payment be received at the time of service. When the extension of credit is offered, internal billing is necessary. Some offices contract with external billing services. Often, patients have some type of insurance or managed care policy that pays at least a portion of the bill. When patients fail to meet their obligations, outside collection services may be used.

■ The first statement should always be itemized. This provides the patient and the guarantor with a record of each procedure and each charge. Insurance companies require itemized bills to reimburse the charges.

■ Rarely do patients not wish to meet their obligations by paying bills. Some do not have the money to pay for medical services, and if they do not have health insurance, it could be even more difficult to obtain medical care. The financial problem that the patient faces may be temporary, or it may be a long-standing situation. Only a few patients are actually unwilling to pay, so the medical assistant should work with the patient to develop a payment plan that the patient can meet.

■ Immediate action should be taken when the office classifies a patient as a "skip." Search the patient chart for all possible telephone numbers and call those that the patient has given. Do not reveal that the patient owes money. If it is necessary to leave a message, do not indicate that the call is from a physician's office. The employer may be called if the patient has not given specific permission not to call the place of business. Never communicate with a third party more than once unless invited to call back. A certified letter may be sent, and when address corrections are requested, the new address is often obtainable. Unless the skip is found quickly, the account is generally turned over to a collection agency.

■ When making collection calls to patients or guarantors, be sure to call within accepted calling hours, which are 8 AM to 9 PM. Be sure to correctly identify the person speaking, and always be respectful and courteous. State the purpose for the call, and keep the conversation business-like and professional. Keep a positive attitude, and convey to the patient that the call is to help devise a way that his or her obligations to the physician can be met. Never threaten the patient, and make every effort to get a commitment as to when payment can be expected. Most important, follow up on collection calls to ensure that patients send in the payment as promised.

KEY INTERNET WEBSITES

- Fair Credit Billing
- Fair Credit Reporting Act
- Federal Trade Commission
- Truth In Lending Act
  For active weblinks to each website visit
  http://evolve.elsevier.com/Kinn/

CHAPTER 15

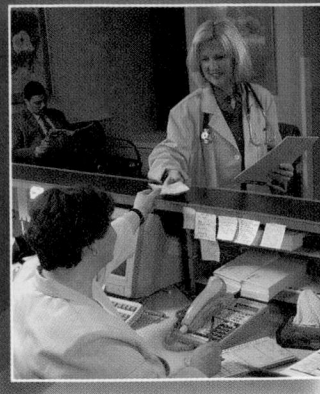

Scenario

Kay James has been an administrative assistant for Drs. Shuman & Taylor in their gastroenterology practice for the last two years. She simultaneously has been enrolled in the medical assistant program at her local college. As she has become quite knowledgeable, it is an appropriate decision for Kay to become more involved in ICD-9-CM and CPT coding.

When it comes to reimbursement, Kay is very aware of the legalities and importance of proper billing. Now she will use her experience and advance her position within the office. She knows that the practice is committed to compliance and feels assured that the patient charts are well documented so that her new task will be easier to carry out. Kay is hard working and looks forward to excelling in her new role as she is exposed to more aspects of becoming a medical assistant.

Basics of Diagnostic Coding

Brenda K. Burton
Carol A. Turiello

Learning Objectives

- Define and spell the terms listed in the vocabulary.
- Identify three purposes of ICD-9-CM.
- Explain the proper utilization of the ICD-9-CM.
- Understand and apply the basic coding rules in the use of the ICD-9-CM.
- Realize the Tabular List contains the most specific coding information.
- Comprehend and utilize instructional terms and symbols as defined in ICD-9-CM.
- Understand the use of V and E codes.
- Properly perform basic diagnostic coding.

National Curriculum Competencies

ADMINISTRATIVE COMPETENCIES

4e. Perform diagnostic coding

Vocabulary

ancillary diagnostic services Services that support patient diagnoses (e.g., laboratory or radiology services).

ancillary therapeutic services Services that support patient treatment (specialists or surgery).

"and" In the context of ICD-9-CM, the word "and" should be interpreted as "and/or."

"code also" When more than one code is necessary to fully identify a given condition, "code also" or "use additional code" is used.

"code if applicable" Notation meaning that the designated code may be principal if no casual condition is applicable or known.

coding Converting verbal or written descriptions into numerical and alphanumerical designations.

comorbidities Preexisting conditions that will, because of their presence with a specific principal diagnosis, cause an increase in length of **an inpatient** hospital stay by at least 1 day in approximately 75% of cases.

complications With respect to coding, conditions that arise during a hospital stay that prolong the length of stay by at least 1 day in approximately 75% of cases.

"diagnosis" The determination of the nature of a disease, injury, or congenital defect.

etiology The cause of the disorder; a claim may be classified according to etiology.

"excludes" Exclusion terms are always written in italics, and the word "excludes" is often enclosed in a box to draw particular attention to these instructions. Exclusion terms may apply to a chapter, a section, a category, or subcategory. The applicable code number usually follows the exclusion term.

"includes" This term appearing under a subdivision, such as a category (three-digit code) or two-digit procedure code, indicates that the code and title include these terms. Other terms also classified to that particular code and title are listed in the Alphabetic Indexes.

International Classification of Diseases, Ninth Revision, Clinical Modification **(ICD-9-CM)** System for classifying disease to facilitate collection of uniform and comparable health information, for statistical purposes and indexing medical records for data storage and retrieval.

International Classification of Diseases, Tenth Revision **(ICD-10)** System containing the greatest number of changes in ICD's history. To allow more specific reporting of disease and newly recognized conditions, the ICD-10 contains approximately 5500 more codes than ICD-9.

mandated Required by an authority or law.

"note" Notes are found in both the Alphabetic Index and the Tabular List as instructions or guides in classification assignments, defining category content or the use of subdivision codes.

"omit code" Term used primarily in Volume 3 **of the ICD-9-CM** when the procedure is the method of approach for an operation.

preexisting condition Physical condition of an insured person that existed before the issuance of the insurance policy.

primary diagnosis Initial identification of the condition or complaint that the patient expresses in the outpatient medical setting.

principal diagnosis That condition that after study is determined to be chiefly responsible for the patient's admission to the hospital.

"see" A direction given to the coder to look in another place. This term must always be followed and is found in the Alphabetic Index, Volumes 2 and 3.

"see also" A direction given to the coder to look elsewhere if the main term or subterm (or subterms) for that entry are not sufficient for coding the information. If a code number follows, "see also" is enclosed in parentheses. If there is no code number, "see also" is preceded by a dash.

"see category" A direction given to the coder to see a specific category (three-digit code). This must always be followed.

superbill A form on which to list procedures and ICD-9-CM codes most frequently used in a specific practice. The encounter is marked off on this form at the time of patient check out and utilized for billing purposes. This is usually called an encounter form.

"use additional code" This term appears only in volume 1 in those subdivisions in which the user should add further information by means of an additional code to give a more complete picture of the diagnosis. In some cases you will find "if desired" following the term. For the purpose of coding, the "if desired" phrase will not be used. When the term "use additional code...if desired" appears, you will disregard "if desired" and assign the appropriate additional code.

"with" In the context of ICD-9-CM, the terms "with," "with mention of," and "associated with" in a title dictate that both parts of the title be present in the statement of the diagnosis order to assign the particular code.

To facilitate accurate medical record-keeping and the processing of claims, it is essential to identify appropriate services and descriptions of diseases, injuries, and procedures. *The International Classification of Diseases, Ninth Revision, Clinical Modification* (ICD-9-CM) statistically classifies elements of a subject according to diseases, injuries, and operations.

For **coding** and reporting clinical information, the ICD-9-CM is used by healthcare providers, as required for participation in Medicare and Medicaid programs, in addition to its uses for tracking healthcare statistics. Practice management software and third party payers also recognize these codes.

Medical assistants are expected to adhere to ethical standards, only assigning and reporting codes that are clearly supported by concise documentation in the patient chart. When in doubt, a medical assistant should consult the attending healthcare provider for clarification. Maintaining and continually enhancing coding skills and keeping informed of changes in codes, guidelines, and regulations are necessary responsibilities for a coding professional.

The medical assistant, because of his or her involvement in both clinical and administrative aspects of the healthcare setting, is a key person in transitioning the verbal and written reasons for an encounter into the universally accepted numerical codes (ICD-9-CM).

Getting to Know ICD-9-CM

The Evolution of ICD Coding

The systematic classification of disease dates back to seventeenth century England. The classification of disease has progressed from the *International List of Causes of Death* in 1937, changing over the years to the *International Classification of Causes of Death*. In 1948, the list was revised yet again to become the first *International Classification of Disease* (ICD), published by the World Health Organization (WHO).

In 1979, the ICD-9-CM was published by the Department of Health and Human Services in the United States. The intention was to describe the clinical picture of the patient more precisely. Rather than just basic health statistical analysis, the term *clinical* emphasizes the modification's intent to better define morbidity data for indexing medical records, medical and ambulatory care, and review.

Since the passage of the Medicare Catastrophic Coverage Act of 1988, physicians have been required by law to submit **diagnosis** codes for Medicare reimbursement. The appropriate diagnosis is required when billing for services to Medicare beneficiaries.

Centers for Medicare and Medicaid Services (CMS), formerly known as the Health Care Financing Administration (HCFA), designated the coding system ICD-9-CM to be used by physicians.

Updates to the ICD-9-CM

The new ICD-9-CM numbers are published yearly; the responsibility for maintenance of the classification system is shared between the National Center for Health Statistics (NCHS) and CMS. The ICD-9-CM Coordination and Maintenance Committee is co-chaired by these organizations. The committee, meeting twice a year, was formed in 1985 to provide a public forum to discuss possible updates and revisions. The committee plays an advisory role, addressing suggestions. The public is welcome and encouraged to share their comments both before and at the meetings. The Director of NCHS and the Administrator for CMS make the final decisions after the December meeting, and the resultant revisions become effective October 1 of the following year.

Each year, before the October 1 effective date, the official code revisions (referred to as addenda) are published and made available to the public (Figure 15-1). The new codes and code extensions are published in the *Federal Register*.

ICD-10-CM. *The International Statistical Classification of Diseases and Related Health Problems, Tenth Revision* **(ICD-10)**, used to code and classify mortality data from death certificates, replaced the ICD-9-CM in 1999. The NCHS is the federal agency responsible for use of the ICD-10 in the United States. The NCHS has developed a clinical modification of the classification for

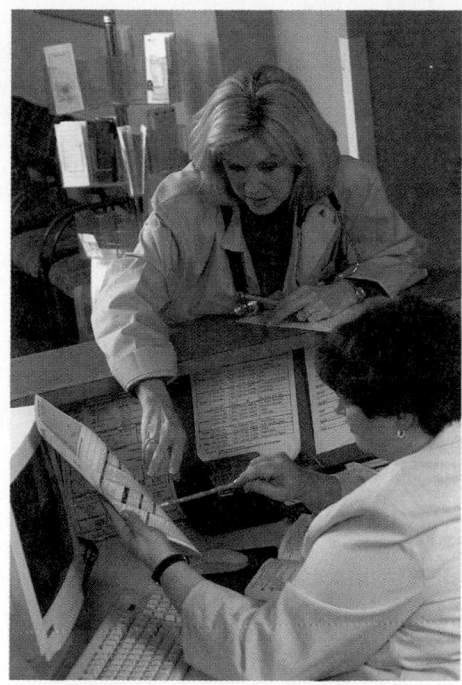

FIGURE 15-1   The team depends on the medical assistant to help keep them updated on coding changes.

morbidity purposes. The current draft of ICD-10-CM contains a significant increase in codes over those in ICD-9-CM.

The Health Insurance Portability and Accountability Act of 1996 (HIPAA), also known as the Kennedy-Kassebaum Act, includes "Standards for Electronic Transactions and Code Sets." HIPAA Transactions and Code Sets regulations were implemented to improve efficiency in healthcare delivery by standardizing electronic data interchange (EDI). Although there is currently no indication of when it will be released, ICD-10-CM is planned as the replacement for ICD-9-CM, Volumes 1 and 2. According to the Centers for Disease Control and Prevention (CDC):

> "There is not yet an anticipated implementation date for the ICD-10-CM. Implementation will be based on the process for adoption of standards under the Health Insurance Portability and Accountability Act of 1996. There will be a two year implementation window once the final notice to implement has been published in the Federal Register."

Additionally, of note, the draft version of ICD-CM-10 is now available for public viewing at: http://www.cdc.gov/nchs/about/otheract/icd9/icd10cm.htm.

CRITICAL THINKING APPLICATION

If Kay wanted to be prepared on behalf of the office by researching proposed changes or address concerns about ICD-9-CM coding issues, how would she best go about it?

Why Use ICD Codes?

In addition to the logistical layout of a standard system used in billing, some pertinent reasoning behind the utilization of ICD-9-CM codes would include the following:

- For data storage and retrieval
- To maximize reimbursement by accurate coding
- To shorten claims processing time
- To facilitate measurement of compliance with clinical guidelines

Compiling healthcare data also helps to measure the appropriateness and timeliness of medical care, enabling third party payers and providers to analyze payments for health services.

Format and Conventions of ICD-9-CM

The ICD-9-CM is published in various media, including book, CD, and downloadable file. It is ideal to have a printed book because of the limitations that an electronic format may present. This set comprises Volumes 1, 2, and 3.

Volume 1, Tabular List

Volume 1, containing 5 appendices and 17 chapters, is referred to as the Tabular List. This Volume classifies diseases and injuries according to **etiology** and organ system, dividing them into groups:

- Anatomical system type of condition
- Related groups of codes
- Three-digit codes (category codes)
- Fourth digit (subcategory codes)
- Fifth digit (subclassification codes)

Classifications of Sections and Structure of Chapters 1 Through 17. Each of the 17 chapters in Volume 1 is subdivided as follows:

- *Section:* A group of three-digit code numbers describing a general disease category
- *Category:* A three-digit code representing a specific disease within the section
- *Subcategory:* A further breakdown of the category, assigning a fourth digit
- *Subclassification:* Five-digit code giving the highest level of specificity to the disease state

> ### EXAMPLE OF THE CHAPTER STRUCTURE
>
> *Chapter:* Diseases of the Circulatory System
>   Chapter Seven (390-459)
> *Section:* Hypertensive Disease (401-405)
> *Category:* Hypertensive Heart Disease (402)
> *Subcategory:* Malignant (402.0)
> *Subclassification:* Without heart failure (402.00)

Volume 2, Alphabetic Index

Volume 2 contains an Alphabetic Index of disease and injury. This Volume contains more information than is contained in the Tabular List and is divided into three sections:

- Index of diseases
- Poison and external causes of adverse affects of drugs and other chemical substances
- Alphabetic Index of external cause of injury and poisoning

Volume 3, Procedures: Tabular List and Alphabetic Index

Volume 3 contains a tabular and alphabetic index of procedures. Unlike Volumes 1 and 2, it is not used in a physician's office but is primarily used in hospitals and other facilities to code the procedures performed in those settings. The procedure codes are two digits followed by a decimal and one or two additional digits.

Symbols, Abbreviations, Punctuations, and Notations

Symbols, abbreviations, punctuations, and notations appear in the listings to serve as instructional notes. Understanding their meaning and using their guidance is crucial to accurate coding. Many different publishers offer the ICD-9-CM, and there may be some differences in the symbols, notations, colors, or other reference marks used for convenience or to convey specific meaning. The medical assistant should be familiar with the manual in use in his or her office. Several examples are listed below.

Symbols

□	The lozenge symbol precedes a disease code when indicating that the content of a four-digit category has been moved or modified.
§	The section mark symbol is only used in the Tabular List of diseases and precedes a code denoting a footnote on the page.
•	The bullet symbol indicates a new entry.
▲	The triangle symbol indicates a revision in the Tabular List and a code change in the Alphabetic Index.
►◄	These symbols mark both the beginning and ending of new or revised text.
♀	Female diagnosis only.
♂	Male diagnosis only.
$\sqrt{4^{th}}$	Code requires a fourth digit.
$\sqrt{5^{th}}$	Code requires a fifth digit.

Abbreviations

NEC	Not elsewhere classifiable. The category number for the term including NEC is to be used only when the coder lacks the information necessary to code the term to a more specific category.
NOS	Not otherwise specified. This abbreviation is the equivalent of "unspecified."

Punctuation

[ ]	Brackets are used to enclose synonyms, alternative wordings, or explanatory phrases.
( )	Parentheses are used to enclose supplementary words, which may be present or absent in the statement of a disease or procedure without affecting the code number to which it is assigned.

:	Colons are used in the Tabular List after an incomplete term that needs one or more of the modifiers that follow to make it assignable to a given category.
{ }	Braces enclose a series of terms, each of which is modified by the statement appearing to the right of the brace.
Bold	Bold type is used for all codes and titles in the Tabular List.
Italics	Italic type is used for exclusion notes and to identify diagnosis that cannot be used as primary.

Notations

DEF	Appearing in blue indicates a definition of disease or a procedure term.
MSP	Identifies a specific trauma code that will alert the carrier that another carrier should be billed first. Medicare is to be billed second if payment from the first payer is not equal to or greater than what Medicare would reimburse.
PDx	Indicates a V code that can only be used as a primary diagnosis.
SDx	Indicates a V code that can only be used as a secondary diagnosis.

CRITICAL THINKING APPLICATION

It is Kay's responsibility to make sure the superbill and the practice management software contain valid, updated ICD-9-CM codes. How can she begin to prepare for the upcoming fiscal year during the last quarter of this fiscal year?

Steps in ICD Coding

As in other administrative duties, developing good coding habits starts in the beginning. Practicing coding as outlined below will assist the medical assistant to develop good coding habits and become an asset to the physician.

The following steps are always necessary to assign the appropriate ICD-9-CM code (Procedure 15-1):

1. Identify the key terms in the diagnostic statement, determining the main reason for the encounter (Figure 15-2). Keep in mind that the definitive diagnosis should be coded first. Some important points to remember:
   - Check documentation regarding a preexisting condition. Be sure this condition is currently being treated and not part of the past medical history.
   - *Never code conditions described as "rule out," "suspected," "probable," or "questionable."* (You do not want to give a patient a disease he or she does not have!)
   - If a patient requests that a different diagnosis be used that is not the correct or appropriate diagnosis for the visit, stating that his or her insurance company will not reimburse, you have a legal and ethical responsibility to code the diagnosis as documented in the patient's medical record.

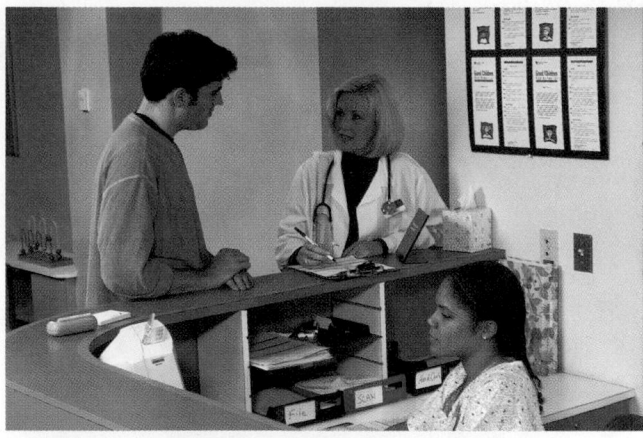

FIGURE 15-2 Coding begins with proper documentation of the patient's reason for visiting the physician.

   - If no definitive diagnosis is made, code the reason for the encounter.
2. Locate the diagnosis in the Alphabetic Index (Volume 2).
3. Read and understand any footnotes, symbols or instructions, following any cross-references, such as "**code also**."
4. Locate the diagnosis in the Tabular List.
5. Read and understand the inclusions and exclusions.
6. Make certain you include fourth and fifth digits when available, assigning to the highest level of specificity.
7. Assign the code, until all diagnosis elements are identified.
8. After assigning the code, double check to ensure accurate transfer from the book to the patient form and subsequent data entry.
9. Use the same process for secondary diagnoses and other conditions *addressed* during the encounter.

CODING EXAMPLE

A patient comes to the office with dehydration, nausea, and vomiting.
- Dehydration is the definitive diagnosis; the Alphabetic Index refers you to 276.5 in the tabular list
- 276.5—Volume depletion includes dehydration; it excludes hypovolemic shock
- Next code the signs and symptoms
- Nausea (see also Vomiting) with vomiting refers you to 787.01. This is a perfect example of why you need to read all the exclusions. If this patient were an infant, the code would be different.

The code for this adult patient would be:
- Dehydration 276.5
- Nausea and vomiting 787.01

Special Codes

In addition to the 17 chapters in Volume 1, two supplementary classifications are provided in ICD-9-CM. When

PROCEDURE 15-1

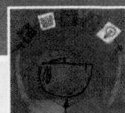

ICD-9-CM Coding

GOAL: To assign the proper ICD-9-CM code based on a medical documentation for auditing and billing purposes.

EQUIPMENT AND SUPPLIES

- Patient medical record
- Current ICD-9-CM code book
- Medical dictionary

Case Study:

Follow Up Visit

Name: Ms. Patient   ID: 3456

Date: 10/8/XX   DOB: 6/10/XX

This 82-year-old female was seen in the office 3 days ago with new onset CHF. She states she feels much better. She does note some small amount of leg edema but she feels this is significantly less than 3 days ago. She denies any chest pain in the last 3 days.

There has been no change in her History as noted in my note of 3 days ago.

On examination, her blood pressure is 150/70. Pulse is 72 and irregularly irregular. Her weight is 158 pounds, down 7 pounds in 3 days. HEENT examination reveals pupils to be equal, round, and reactive. Extraocular movements are intact. Conjunctiva pink. Neck is supple. No JVD. Carotids are 2 + bilaterally without bruits. Lungs are clear to auscultation and percussion. Cardiac examination reveals no heaves or thrills. There is a normal S1 and S2 with an irregularly irregular rhythm. There is a grade 2/6 systolic ejection murmur at the left sternal border and apex. The abdomen is soft, nontender, bowel sounds are present. The liver and spleen do not appear enlarged. Examination of her extremities reveals no edema, clubbing, or cyanosis. She is alert, oriented, with no focal motor deficits.

Impression: This pleasant 82-year-old woman has experienced a dramatic improvement in her CHF symptoms in the last 3 days. Her physical examination and CXR today reflect this improvement. At this time she is reluctant to undergo any further testing.

I will have her continue with the same medication, weigh herself daily, and return for follow-up in 2 weeks. Before she returns I will have her obtain a chemistry profile. She is instructed to call with any weight gain or chest pain.

PROCEDURAL STEPS

1 Identify the key term in the diagnostic statement.
   Purpose: To determine the definite diagnosis.

2 Locate the diagnosis in the Alphabetic Index.

3 Read and understand footnotes.
   Note: This includes any symbols, instructions, or cross-references.

4 Locate the diagnosis in the Tabular List.

5 Read and understand the inclusions and exclusions.

6 Make certain you include fourth and fifth digits where available.

7 Assign the code.
   Note: All diagnosis elements need to be identified. Double-check the code to ensure an accurate transfer to the patient form.

recording a code from these classifications, always write the alpha character first to distinguish the V or E code from a diagnosis code that has the same number of digits but no alphabetical character.

CRITICAL THINKING APPLICATION

Dr. Taylor has inadvertently circled the diagnosis for dysphagia on the patient's superbill. Kay assisted with the examination and knows the patient came in for rectal bleeding. What is the proper approach in correcting this code?

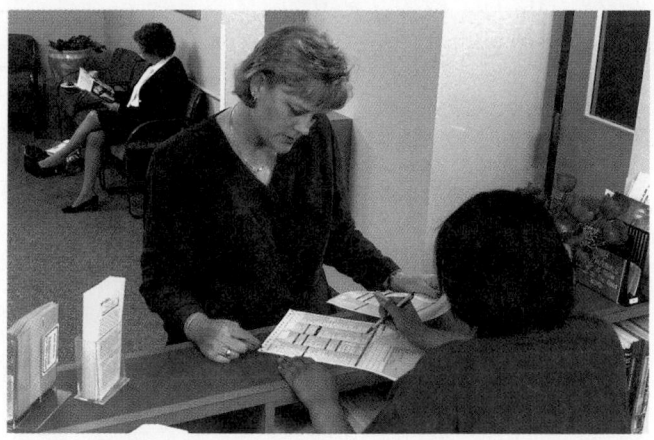

FIGURE 15-3   The encounter form is an important tool in gathering the diagnosis and symptoms needed for coding.

V Codes

The V code is used on occasions when the patient is not currently ill or to explain problems that influence his or her current illness or injury. The Supplementary Classification of Factors Influencing Health Status and Contact with Health Service (V Code, V01-V82) is used in cases such as preventive vaccination or chronic disease states such as dialysis for renal disease.

> Example: Exposure to rabies by rabid skunk
> Code as: Rabies V01.5

CRITICAL THINKING APPLICATION

If a patient presented with right lower quadrant pain and the physician simply wrote "R/O appendicitis" on the encounter form, how would Kay go about coding this?

CRITICAL THINKING APPLICATION

Mr. Smith has been a patient for several years and presents for a routine physical examination. Mr. Smith has Medicare as his primary insurance and asks Kay to list his long-standing hypertension as the reason for his visit, knowing that Medicare does not cover routine physicals. How should Kay handle this?

Appendices

The five appendices included in Volume 1, Tabular List, serve as a reference to the coder to provide additional information to futher define a diagnosis, classifying new drugs and to provide a quick reference for three-digit categories. The five appendices are as follows:

- *Morphology of Neoplasms:* The WHO established an adaptation of the ICD for Oncology (ICD-O). The morphology code numbers consist of five digits. The first four digits identify the histological type of neoplasm and the fifth digit indicates its behavior. M codes are used for statistical data only and are not used in physician billing. This section of the appendix is usually utilized by inpatient coders.
- *Glossary of Mental Disorders:* This glossary is an alphabetical listing of the psychiatric terminology that appears in Chapter 5, "Mental Disorders."
- *Classification of Drugs by AHFS List:* The adverse effect of drugs is coded according to the American Hospital Formulary Service (AHFS) list. The list is continuously revised and published under the direction of the American Society of Hospital Pharmacists (ASHP). This section is usually used by pharmacies.
- *Classification of Industrial Accidents According to Agency:* This appendix concerns the Statistics of Employment Injuries categorized by industrial agency. This section is usually used by government organizations, such as OSHA.
- *List of Three-Digit Categories:* This appendix is a breakdown of the chapters' categories; includes V and E codes.

E Codes

The E code is used to classify environmental causes of injury, poisoning, or other adverse effects on the body. Supplemental Classification of External Causes of Injuries and Poisoning (E Code, E800-E999).

> Example: Injury from butane explosion
> Code as: Accident caused by explosive material, explosive gases, Butane E923.2

Symptoms, Signs, and Ill-Defined Conditions (Chapter 16, 780-799)

Unlike the other chapters that contain diagnoses in Volume 1, Chapter 16 comprises symptoms, signs, and ill-defined conditions. If the terms "suspected," "suspicious," or "rule out" are used within the diagnosis, code the reason for the encounter. This could be the symptoms, signs, abnormal test results, or any other reason that the patient sought medical care (Figure 15-3). If there is any question about the reason for the encounter, check with the physician.

> Example: Rule out myocardial infarction
> Code as: Chief complaint: "chest pain"(central) 786.50

Maximizing Third Party Reimbursement

The most important aspect to remember with ICD-9-CM is to code the diagnosis to the highest level of specificity, linking the ICD-9-CM code to the Current Procedural Terminology (CPT) code. The CPT coding is further explained in Chapter 16.

Obtaining the correct reimbursement is important to the practice cash flow and depends on proper coding and billing techniques. Some other crucial points to remember when submitting diagnostic codes for claims are as follows:

- Use the current ICD-9-CM manual, staying informed of changes.
- Code accurately from documented information (Figure 15-4).
- Be sure diagnosis corresponds with symptoms and treatment.
- Review data entry to ensure no transposition of digits.
- Know insurance carriers' rules for submitting claims; for example, some insurance carriers allow only one or two codes per claim.
- Incomplete or inaccurate codes may result in insurance denial because of a lack of medical necessity.

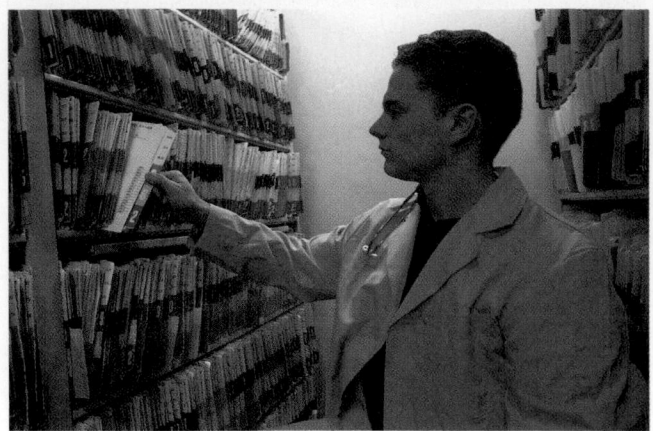

FIGURE 15-4 The patient's chart is used to support the diagnosis and can be accessed by authorized personnel should any questions arise.

the medical assistant realizes these codes are updated yearly, this makes them an asset in coding compliance.

Legal and Ethical Issues

Medical assistants are entrusted by the physician and practice that employs them. To this extent, a medical assistant must be responsible and knowledgeable to ensure that no fraud takes place in the coding and claims submission process.

The coding professional should not change codes or narratives in patient chart documentation to accommodate insurance reimbursement or policy coverage requirements. Deliberate misrepresentation may carry criminal and/or civil penalties.

CODING TIPS AND HINTS

- Always have a good medical dictionary.
- Use the most recent ICD manual and have your own copy.
- Make notes in your books.
- Do not code from the Alphabetic Index alone.
- Diagnoses are listed by first word, by a key word in a phrase, or by anatomical site involved.
- Avoid nonspecific codes.
- Be very careful when coding preexisting conditions.
- Make certain the documentation supports the diagnosis.
- Remember, inaccurate coding can lead to accusations of fraud and abuse.

SUMMARY OF SCENARIO

Kay has been very enthusiastic throughout her learning experiences at the practice. She knows that as time continues and she earns her certificate, she will enjoy being a medical assistant. As Kay progresses with diagnostic coding, she will also be able to help the physicians and nursing staff be attentive to details in documentation of the patient chart.

Although using the superbill to enter the codes for billing is an easy tool, knowing how to use the ICD-9-CM volumes is a necessary asset to ensure accurate coding when there is a question at checkout. Also, if additional information is requested by the insurance company to support a given diagnosis code, Kay can pull the patient's chart for research and documentation. Keeping in mind the aspect of maximum reimbursement, Kay will be knowledgeable in coding to the highest level of specificity.

Having access to the Internet will help Kay to be ready for new codes and to revise the superbill when needed. This will also be advantageous in an expedient revenue cycle.

Closing Comments

The medical assistant's knowledge of accurate diagnostic coding contributes to the legal and financial health of the practice. In most cases, ICD-9-CM codes are found on the provider's encounter form (or **superbill**) and/or in the practice management software. However, with literally thousands of current diagnostic codes, it may be necessary to code from the ICD-9-CM manual. Because

SUMMARY OF LEARNING OBJECTIVES

■ The medical assistant will become very comfortable with diagnostic coding with practice and patience. The ICD-9-CM is used to track healthcare statistics, as well as to facilitate accurate medical record keeping and ease in processing claims. Use of the ICD-9-CM is mandatory for participation in many federal, state, and private insurance programs.

■ Each of the three Volumes has a specific use. Start with the alphabetic list and then proceed to the tabular list when assigning a code. Only the inpatient coder uses Volume 3 of the ICD-9-CM.

■ Several basic coding rules exist that will assist the medical assistant in coding. Be sure that the most recent ICD-9-CM manual is being used, and keep a medical dictionary handy. As difficult codes are assigned, keep notes in the book for future reference. Proofread the claim and be sure that it makes good sense. Avoid nonspecific codes and use care when coding preexisting conditions.

■ Never code directly from the index. The tabular list contains the most specific information. Check and recheck the codes, making certain that the documentation supports the codes that are used on the claim.

■ The medical assistant should become familiar with all of the symbols used in the ICD-9-CM. Instructional codes should be read thoroughly and all directions followed while coding a claim.

■ E or V codes may help to clarify a code or explain the code further. V codes are used when the patient is not currently ill, but is being seen by health service professionals. This would include preventative visits to the physician or visits for vaccinations. E codes are used to explain that some external cause contributed to an adverse effect within the body.

KEY INTERNET WEBSITES

- American Academy of Professional Coders
- American Medical Association
- Centers for Medicare and Medicaid Services
- National Center for Health Statistics
- US Government Printing Office (to access *Federal Register*)
  For active weblinks to each website visit
  http://evolve.elsevier.com/Kinn/

REFERENCES

Fordney M: *Insurance handbook for the medical office*, ed 6. Philadelphia, 2002, WB Saunders.
ICD-9-CM easy coder, Montgomery, Ala, 2002, UnicorMed.
International classification of diseases, ninth revision, clinical modification (ICD-9-CM), volumes 1 and 2. Chicago, 2002, American Medical Association.

PROCEDURE 15-1

ANSWERS TO PROCEDURE 15-1

1 CHF

2 Congestion (heart) 428.0

3 None

4 428

5 Excludes:
Following cardiac surgery (429.4)
Rheumatic (398.91)
That complicating:
Abortion (634-638 with .7, 639.8)
Ectopic or molar pregnancy (639.8)
Labor or delivery (668.1, 669.4)

6 Code, if applicable, heart failure due to hypertension first (402.0-402.9, with fifth digit 1 or 404.0-404.9 with fifth digit 1 or 3),

7 428.9 Hearth failure, unspecified
Cardiac failure NOS
Heart failure NOS
Myocardial failure NOS
Weak heart

CHAPTER 16

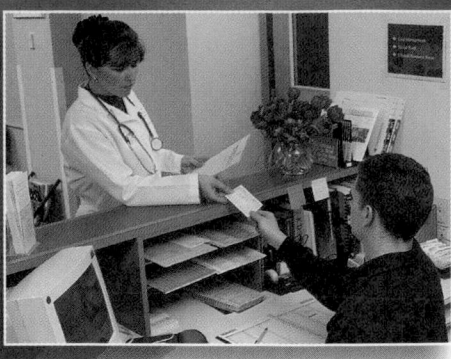

Scenario

As Kay James progresses in her education and continues as administrative assistant for Drs. Shuman and Taylor, she has enjoyed the challenges and has excelled on her diagnostic coding exams. She looks forward to being equally competent with procedural coding. Now, she is ready to move on to procedural coding. As with ICD-9-CM, Kay can rely on accurate record keeping within the practice to perform this task.

As she prepares to graduate from her medical assisting educational program, Kay is excited to receive her degree and continue to be an asset to the practice. She anticipates gaining more responsibility as her knowledge becomes more well rounded.

Basics of Procedural Coding

Brenda K. Burton
Carol A. Turiello

Learning Objectives

- Define and spell the terms listed in the vocabulary.
- Identify three purposes of the CPT.
- List the classifications of sections in the CPT.
- Explain the use of guidelines and where they are located.
- Discuss the importance of modifiers.
- Briefly explain the importance of correctly assigning evaluation and management codes.
- Define *upcoding* and explain why it must be avoided.
- Accurately assign a CPT code based on medical documentation.
- Explain the basic rules for CPT coding.

National Curriculum Competencies

4d. Perform procedural coding

Vocabulary

bundled codes Procedures or services that are grouped together and paid as one.

component A constituent part; a part of a larger group.

downcoding A change in code done by the insurance company that receives a claim resulting in a lesser reimbursement. The change will usually be the code closest to the one submitted on the claim, because the code does not match in some way to the specifications of the insurance company.

modifiers Code additions that explain circumstances that alter a service that has been provided and clarify exactly what was done to the patient.

morbidity The relative incidence of disease.

mortality The number of deaths in a given time or place.

revenue The total income produced by a given source.

unbundled codes Separating the components of a procedure and reporting them separately.

upcoding A deliberate increase in a CPT code to receive higher reimbursements.

utilization Related to the process of reviewing procedures and services for medical necessity.

As with diagnostic coding, accurate use of the CPT-4 is essential. The medical assistant facilitates accurate medical record keeping and the efficient processing of claims by using the CPT-4, which identifies appropriate procedures and services common to the physician's office. CPT-4 is used in the claims submission process to receive reimbursement from payors as well as to track physician productivity.

Medical assistants are expected to adhere to ethical standards when involved in all aspects of coding. Again, as with diagnostic coding, the medical assistant should consult the attending healthcare provider for clarification when a question arises. CPT codes must be maintained, following the changes in guidelines and regulations. Medical assistants, because of their involvement in both clinical and administrative aspects of the healthcare setting, are key persons in converting the verbal and written reasons for an encounter into the universally accepted numeric and alphanumeric codes of CPT-4.

Getting to Know the CPT-4

The Evolution of CPT Coding

Current Procedural Terminology was first published in 1966 by the American Medical Association. It was based on the California Relative Value Study, developed by the California Medical Society. Its primary purpose was to simplify the reporting of procedures and/or services provided by physicians. In 1992 the most significant change was made to CPT with the replacement of the office and hospital visit codes with the Evaluation and Management (E&M) codes, identifying key elements to be documented in the medical record. CPT has been revised three times; the edition in current use is CPT-4.

Updates to the CPT

CPT is updated every October by the AMA and published for the next calendar year. The CPT is available as a printed manual or as an electronic file. As with the ICD-9-CM, it is ideal to purchase the printed version to be certain you have the entire contents for easy reference. Because the practice of medicine is constantly changing and new procedures are being developed, the AMA encourages suggestions from physicians, medical societies, and organizations. Forms are available from the AMA CPT Editorial Research and Development Department and on the AMA website (given at the end of the chapter). These changes are found in Appendix B of the CPT manual.

Why Use the CPT?

Medicare and most commercial insurance companies use CPT to identify and classify claims for payment. Although its use is standard in physicians' practices, CPT is not recognized in some facility settings or under special guidelines within an insurance company.

Physicians' practices use CPT to:
- Submit claims for services and procedures
- Track **utilization** of services and procedures
- Measure physician productivity

CRITICAL THINKING APPLICATION

As Kay learns more about CPT codes, what will she find similar to what she learned with ICD-9-CM?

Format of the CPT

There are three levels of CPT:
- Level I codes are developed by the AMA and contained in the current CPT Manual. They are five-digit codes and two-digit modifiers.
- Level II codes, known as HCPCS, are national codes developed by CMS to describe medical services and supplies not covered in the CPT. They consist of alphabetic characters (A through V) and four digits. Modifiers are either alphanumerical or two letters (AA to VP).
- Level III codes are local codes. Unlike Level I and II, these codes are not common to all carriers. They are assigned by local Medicare carriers to describe new procedures that are not yet in Levels I and II. These codes start with a letter (W through Z) followed by four digits. Note: when the HIPAA standards for electronic transactions are implemented, Level III codes will no longer be recognized for reimbursement reporting.

Symbols

Symbols appear in the listings to serve as instructional notes. Understanding their meaning and using their guidance is crucial to accurate coding.

- New code
- ▲ Code revision
- + CPT add-on codes
- Ø Exempt from the use of modifier –51
- ►◄ Revised guidelines, cross-references, and explanations
- → With a circle around it refers to *CPT Assistant*
- * Surgical procedure only

Sections

Evaluation and Management (E&M). The E&M section appears in the front of the CPT Manual and must be thoroughly understood. There is the most room for error when coding in this section. Since all specialties bill these services and these codes constitute 65% of the total Medicare part B payments to physicians, it is extremely important to understand this section. A full section devoted to understanding E&M coding appears later in this chapter.

Anesthesia Codes. This section contains anesthesia and modifier codes plus the very specific physical status modifiers developed by the American Society of Anesthesiologists to rank patients by level of complexity. The modifiers range from P1 (normal healthy) through P6 (brain dead) patients whose organs are being removed for transplantation. There are also add-on codes (+) that explain difficult circumstances. These are located in the Anesthesia Guidelines found at the beginning of the section and also in the medicine section of the CPT-4.

Surgery. The surgery section is further divided into 18 subsections by specific type of surgery. General guidelines are found at the beginning of the section and apply to all subsections. The subsections have specific guidelines that apply to that particular area. The subsections are further divided into subheadings. One of the most important explanations in the general guidelines is the definition of the surgical package; it is essential to know exactly what is and is not included in the package. All surgeries have *global periods*. These range from 0 (the actual calendar day of the procedure) up to 90 days (starting the day before the surgery and continues for 90 days). These global periods cover normal "routine" care during that time. Complications, new problems, or other injuries are reported using modifiers.

Radiology. In addition to radiology (x-ray diagnostic procedures), this section includes nuclear medicine and diagnostic ultrasound. This section requires a written report from the radiologist to the physician that ordered the test.

Pathology and Laboratory. Codes in the pathology and laboratory section cover laboratory tests and services of pathologists. It is important to understand that some tests are grouped into panels. These panels give a clearer picture of problems with an organ or disease.

Medicine. The medicine section covers a multitude of services provided to patients ranging from immunization through testing that is not included in other sections to services provided by a psychiatrist or a physical therapist, and osteopathic manipulation to home healthcare.

Classifications of Sections

- *Section* is a general grouping of codes, such as surgery, medicine, laboratory or radiology. It is the largest grouping within CPT.
- *Subsection* better defines the section.
- *Subheading* further defines the subsection.
- *Category* directs you to the specific procedures in which you will find the correct code.

CLASSIFICATIONS OF SECTIONS

Example

Section: Surgery
  Subsection: Integumentary
    Subheading: Skin; subcutaneous and accessory structures
      Category: Incision and drainage of abscess, CPT code 10060*

*The * symbol indicates surgical procedure only.*

Guidelines at the beginning of each section of the CPT manual refer to the whole section; guidelines specific to the subsections are listed as Notes at the beginning of the subsection. A medical assistant needs to read and understand these guidelines. Each section is unique and has very specific requirements. Attempting to code services without a working knowledge of the guidelines can lead to improper coding and possibly loss of **revenue**.

Steps in CPT Coding

The following is a brief outline of the considerations you will use in CPT coding. (To assign a CPT code, see Procedure 16-1.)

1. Know the CPT code book; there are changes each year, so even if you have been coding for years, you need to read the *introduction, guidelines, and notes* (Figure 16-1).
2. Review all services and procedures performed on the day of the encounter. Include all medications administered and trays and equipment used.
3. Find the procedures and/or services in the index in the back of the CPT book. This will direct you to a code (not a page number!). The code you are looking for may be listed as a procedure, body system, service, or abbreviation (this will usually refer you to the full spelling).
4. Read the description in the code and also any related descriptions that follow a semicolon; this will lead you to the most accurate code.
5. If the service is an E&M code, identify and perform the following:
   - Whether this is a new or established patient
   - Whether this is a consultation
   - Where the service was performed

PROCEDURE 16-1

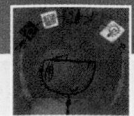

Assigning a CPT Code

GOAL: To assign the proper CPT codes based on medical documentation for auditing and billing purposes.

EQUIPMENT AND SUPPLIES
- Patient medical record
- Current CPT code book
- Medical dictionary

Case Study:

Initial Office Visit

Name: Mr. Patient   ID: 2345
Date: 3/28/XX   DOB: 9/12/XX

Mr. Patient is a 52-year-old white male who for the last 2 months has experienced moderate chest discomfort, radiating to his jaw when he shovels snow. The pain generally lasts about 5 minutes and is relieved with rest. He states he becomes short of breath when he experiences the chest discomfort.

The patient denies any chest pain or pressure at the present time. He is a diabetic and has been on insulin for the past 10 years. He has no known allergies.

His mother is living and well. His father was a diabetic and died when he was 40. The patient is not sure, but he thinks his father had a stroke. He has no brothers or sisters.

Mr. Patient is an electrical engineer and lives at home with his wife and two teenage children. He does not smoke and drinks an occasional beer.

Present medications: NPH insulin, multiple vitamins.

On physical examination: B/P 160/90. Pulse 90 and regular. Respiratory rate 20. Height 5'8". Weight 250 lbs. Face is somewhat flushed. Neck is supple. Carotid upstroke 2+ without bruits. No JVD. The lungs are clear. Heart sounds somewhat distant; S1, S2 regular; no systolic murmur appreciated. The abdomen is soft and nontender. The abdominal aorta is not palpable. Femoral and pedal pulses are strong. There is no lower extremity edema, no clubbing or cyanosis. No lymphadenopathy or scars noted. Heme negative brown stool. Prostate not enlarged.

ECG done today in my office shows NSR, rate 90. No ST-T abnormalities. The tracing is within normal limits. CXR—negative. Normal cardiac silhouette.

Given Mr. Patient's symptoms, diabetes, obesity, and probable family history, further work-up will include a fasting lipid profile and a nuclear stress test. After these tests, we can further discuss the possible need for a left heart catheterization.

- Review the documentation to determine the level of service
- Check to determine whether there is a reason to use a modifier

- Assign the five-digit CPT code

_____

PROCEDURE 16-1—Cont'd

PROCEDURAL STEPS

1 Identify if the patient is new or established.
   Note: Using the case described, assume that the key components for Mr. Patient's encounter with regard to evaluation and management are:
   • A detailed history
   • A detailed examination
   • Medical decision making of low complexity

2 Indicate where the patient is being seen.

3 Determine whether the visit is a consultation.

4 Determine whether the visit is due to illness or is a preventive medical service.

5 Determine the level of history.

6 Determine the level of examination.

7 Determine the level of medical decision making.

8 Assign the most accurate CPT code.

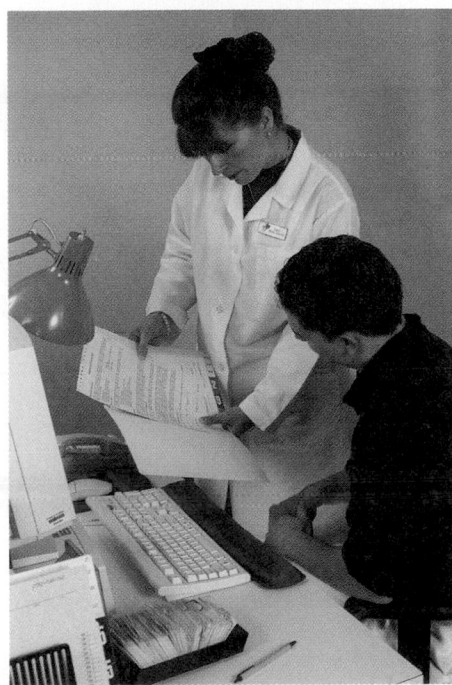

FIGURE 16-1 A medical assistant should always check with the healthcare provider when there is a question about which CPT code to use.

Modifiers

When used, **modifiers** explain circumstances that alter a service that has been provided. These circumstances do not change the basic meaning of the code but help clarify exactly what was done. It may be that the professional or technical component is being billed, more than one physician was involved in providing the service, a procedure had to be discontinued, and other circumstances. Modifiers can now be found in Appendix A of the CPT codebook.

Multiple Modifiers

Sometimes more than one modifier is needed. When this happens, the first modifier used is –99. This signals the person reviewing the claim that more than one modifier is being used.

Understanding Evaluation and Management

Factors Considered in E&M Coding

Type of Service. Services covered in the E&M section include, but are not limited to, physician encounters in all locations for "well" or "sick" visits, patient transport, case management services, preventative medicine services and prolonged services.

Place of Service. For payment purposes the place of service needs to match the type of service. The places of service are as follows:
   • Office (11)
   • Patient's home (12)
   • Inpatient hospital (21)
   • Outpatient hospital (22)
   • Emergency department (ED) hospital (23)
   • Ambulatory surgery center (ASC) (24)
   • Birthing center (25)
   • Skilled nursing facility (SNF) (31)
   • Nursing facility (32)
   • Custodial care facility (33)
   • Hospice (34)
   • Federally qualified health center (50)
   • Inpatient psychiatric facility (51)
   • Partial hospitalization, psychiatric facility (52)
   • Community mental health center (53)
   • Psychiatric residential treatment center (56)
   • Comprehensive inpatient rehabilitation facility (61)
   • Comprehensive outpatient rehabilitation facility (62)
   • End-stage renal disease treatment facility (65)
   • State or local public health clinic (71)
   • Rural health clinic (72)
   • Other unlisted facility (99)

Patient Status. Many of the CPT codes are classified by whether a patient is a new or established patient. A *new patient* is new to the practice or has not been seen by the specialty in group practice for more than 3 years. An *established patient* is one who has a continuing relationship with the practice and has been seen within the last 3 years.

Levels of E&M Services

Determining Factors. To understand the levels of history it is important to know the definition and components of the patient's history. The history relates to the patient's clinical picture and depends on the patient for answers to specific questions. The history is composed of the chief complaint, or reason the patient is being seen. This is usually in the patient's own words.

The *history of present illness* identifies the location, severity, timing, modifying factors, quality, duration, context and associated signs and symptoms relating to the chief complaint.

The *review of systems* has the patient answer questions about the following systems: constitutional, eyes, ear/nose /throat (ENT) and mouth, cardiac, gastrointestinal, musculoskeletal, endocrine, neurological, integumentary, psychiatric, genitourinary, allergic/immunologic, respiratory, and hematological/lymphatic.

The *past medical, family, and social history* is important, because patients' experiences with illness and surgery, whether they smoke, use illicit drugs and/or alcohol, if they are married, have children, where they live, and what diseases their blood relatives have had play an extremely important part in determining their risk factors for illness (Figure 16-2).

Now that it is understood what makes up the history, the various levels can be discussed.

- *Problem focused:* A problem-focused history concentrates on the chief complaint; it looks at the symptoms, severity, and duration of the problem. It usually does not include a review of systems (ROS) or family and social history.
- *Expanded problem focused:* The physician proceeds the same as for the problem-focused history but includes a review of the systems that relate to the chief complaint. Usually past, family, and social histories are not included.
- *Detailed:* The physician will document a more extensive history, ROS, and will document pertinent past, family, and social histories.
- *Comprehensive:* The physician will document responses to *all* of the components listed previously. A comprehensive history is usually taken during an initial visit with patients who have a significant history of illness.

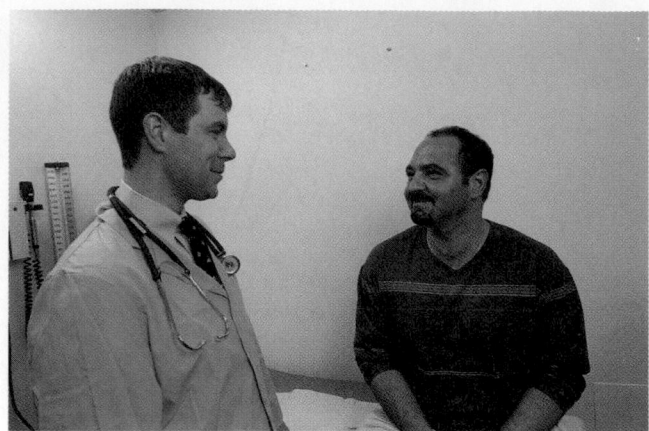

FIGURE 16-2 The medical assistant should document any history obtained from the patient.

Medical Decision Making. When a physician makes medical decisions, the decisions are based on many years of education and experience. To understand what goes into these decisions, the following guidelines have been developed.

NUMBER OF DIAGNOSES/MANAGEMENT OPTIONS. When we read the note the physician writes, we should be able to tell whether the patient's problem is minor or an established problem that is stable or getting worse or whether the patient has a new problem that the physician wants to watch or perhaps to order or perform more tests on.

AMOUNT AND COMPLEXITY OF DATA REVIEWED. The physician's note should tell us what laboratory tests, x-ray diagnostic procedures, and other tests have been ordered or reviewed.

RISK OF COMPLICATIONS AND MORBIDITY OR MORTALITY. There is often risk involved in medical care, either from the treatment given to the patient or from the lack of treatment and professional care. **Morbidity,** the relative incidence of disease, and **mortality,** which relates to the number of deaths from a given disease, are part of the assessment of risks made by the physician.

These three elements play a role in the complexity of the decision-making process used when treating a patient. The physician determines the level of care given to a patient, but must consider these three factors when choosing the E&M levels assigned to a patient on a given encounter. The physician cannot base the choice of E&M levels solely on the time spent with the patient. All elements must be considered when assigning the code. Usually, the physician circles this service code and other procedure codes on the encounter form as or just after the patient is seen in the office. Although a physician may allow the medical assistant to make notations on the encounter form, only the physician makes the decision as to which services and procedures are performed.

MEDICAL DECISION–MAKING COMPLEXITY LEVELS

- *Straightforward:* Minimal diagnosis/management options, minimal/none for the amount and complexity of data to be reviewed, and minimal risk to the patient of complications or death if untreated.

- *Low-complexity:* Limited number of diagnoses/management options, limited data to be reviewed, and low risk to the patient of complications or death if untreated.
- *Moderate-complexity:* Multiple diagnoses/management options, moderate amount and complexity of data to be reviewed, and moderate risk to the patient of complications or death if untreated.
- *High-complexity:* Extensive diagnoses/management options, extensive amount and complexity of data to be reviewed, and high risk to the patient for complications and/or death if the problem is untreated.

Examination. The examination is the objective part of the patient's visit (Figure 16-3). The physician examines the patient and makes notes referring to body areas and/or organ systems:

- *Body areas:* Head including face and neck, chest, including breasts and axillas, abdomen, genitourinary (GU), back, including spine and extremities.
- *Organ systems:* Constitutional, eyes, ears/nose/throat and mouth, cardiovascular, respiratory, gastrointestinal (GI), GU, musculoskeletal, skin, neurological, psychiatric, and hematological/lymphatic/immunologic.

The examination is divided into the following levels:

- *Problem-focused:* The examination is limited to the single body area or single system mentioned in the chief complaint.
- *Expanded problem-focused:* In addition to the limited body area or system, related body areas or organ systems are examined.
- *Detailed:* An extended examination is performed on the related body areas or organ systems.

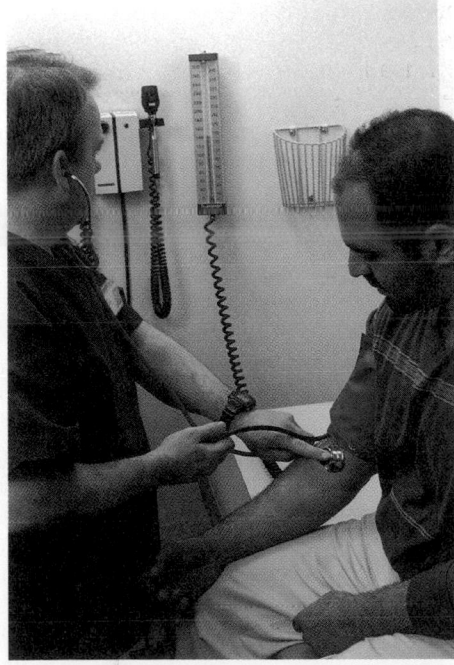

FIGURE 16-3 Examinations conducted by all members of the team are part of the documentation requirements for CPT coding.

- *Comprehensive:* A "complete" multisystem examination is performed.

Contributing Factors

Although the determining factors just discussed are the basis for E&M coding, there are circumstances in which other factors contribute to determining the level of service.

Counseling. Almost all E&M services contain a degree of counseling with the patient and/or the family. This is factored into the E&M code, and as long as this factor does not exceed 50% of the time spent with the patient, it is included in the E&M code.

Coordination of Care. Some patients need assistance in arranging for care beyond the visit or hospitalization. Some will need care in a skilled nursing facility or home health care. Others will need hospice care. The primary physician usually coordinates this care.

Nature of the Presenting Problem. The presenting problem is usually explained in the chief complaint. It can range from something as simple as a cold in an otherwise healthy patient to a life-threatening problem.

Time. CPT has provided assigned times for each of the CPT E&M codes. Time should not be the determining factor, *with one exception:* if more than 50% of the visit is spent counseling, *only time* determines the level of complexity.

> **PUTTING IT ALL TOGETHER TO DETERMINE THE CODE**
>
> - Determine whether the patient is new or established.
> - Where is the patient being seen—office, hospital, or other setting?
> - Is this a patient of the practice, or is someone requesting a consultation?
> - Is the patient "sick" or here for preventative medicine services?
> - Is the history problem-focused, expanded problem-focused, detailed, or comprehensive?
> - Is the examination problem-focused, expanded problem-focused, detailed, or comprehensive?
> - Is medical decision making straightforward, low, moderate, or high?
> - Pick the code.

CPT Coding Definitions

- **Bundled codes** describe procedures or services that are grouped together and paid as one. An example would be code 90700 Diphtheria, tetanus toxoids, and acellular pertussis vaccine for intramuscular use.

- **Unbundled codes** describe separating the components of a procedure and reporting them separately. To use the diphtheria example, if someone reports the three vaccines separately, it gives the impression that three injections rather than one were given.
- **Upcoding** is a deliberate increase in a CPT code to receive higher reimbursements. This is a target of CMS investigations and should never be done.
- **Downcoding** is usually done by the insurance companies if, on review, the examiner feels the documentation does not match the code description.

CRITICAL THINKING APPLICATION

If a patient was referred for epigastric pain and Dr. Shuman performed an ultrasound examination of the gallbladder, what would Kay need to consider to properly code this encounter?

CODING TIPS AND HINTS

- Always have the latest edition of CPT and HCPCS.
- Follow the CCI information quarterly.
- Never code something because it is "close" to the description; research it further.
- Review the guidelines and refer to them as part of your routine. It would be extremely difficult for any one person to know all the specific guidelines.
- Keep the lines of communication open with the physician and never hesitate to ask for clarification.
- Develop and use an audit sheet that you are comfortable with and do periodic code reviews. This may not be your responsibility, but understanding how a chart audit is done can help you in your coding responsibilities.
- Know the modifiers and use them when appropriate.
- Know abbreviations, especially for laboratory procedures.

Legal and Ethical Issues

Medical assistants must be responsible and remain knowledgeable about CPT to ensure that no fraud takes place in the coding and claims submission process. Medical assistants should also ensure that proper precautions are taken to avoid incorrect coding, data entry errors, and false claims submissions.

Codes or narratives should not be altered in patient chart documentation to increase insurance reimbursement or to accommodate policy coverage requirements. Deliberate misrepresentation may carry criminal and/or civil penalties.

SUMMARY OF SCENARIO

Kay enjoys working toward becoming a medical assistant. As Kay progresses with learning procedural coding, she envisions herself as becoming more well rounded in her knowledge of the practice's administrative operations.

The encounter form is a common document used to enter the procedure when a patient checks out, but knowing how to use the CPT manual is essential when notes must be coded from outpatient procedures performed by Dr. Shuman or Dr. Taylor. As with diagnostic coding, Kay can pull the patient chart for research and documentation if any questions arise about a claim. Kay knows that coding to the highest level of specificity will help in accuracy and obtaining maximum reimbursement.

Kay continues to use the Internet to network and research. She stays informed of the changes in procedural coding by ordering the CPT Manual each year.

SUMMARY OF LEARNING OBJECTIVES

- The CPT serves three basic purposes. First, it is used to submit claims to third-party payors for reimbursement. Second, the CPT is used to track utilization and ensure that the procedures performed relate to the patient diagnosis. Third, the CPT is a method of measuring physician productivity.

- The CPT contains several sections, including general groupings of codes; subsections, which better define the sections; subheadings, which make the subsection even more specific; and categories, where the actual code can be found.

- Guidelines are provided at the beginning of each section of the CPT and offer information about the codes in that particular section and specific coding instructions. Special circumstances for coding may be included. These should be read thoroughly and clearly understood before a medical assistant attempts any coding in that section.

- Modifiers are important, because they further clarify and explain a service that may have been difficult to perform or a complicated procedure. The modifier offers the payor a logical explanation for extra charges that were incurred because of the special circumstances. If these are not used, the provider may be paid a reduced amount of money.

The payor must be completely convinced that the amount charged is a fair amount for the procedure performed.

■ Most claims for services in a physician's office include an evaluation and management code. This code indicates how much time, decision making, and evaluation were employed by the physician as he or she examined the patient. Not all patient encounters take the same amount of time or use the same amount of decision-making ability. Therefore no physician should charge for 1 hour of time with the patient when only 15 minutes was spent. The evaluation and management codes clarify exactly what was needed to provide quality care to the patient.

■ Upcoding is assigning a code for a procedure that is deliberately "higher" than the actual code to increase the amount of reimbursement to the provider. Physicians sometimes upcode because they feel the amount of reimbursement is too low, but this practice can constitute fraud and must be avoided at all times.

KEY INTERNET WEBSITES

- American Academy of Professional Coders
- American Medical Association
- Centers for Medicare and Medicaid Services
- National Center for Health Statistics
- US Government Printing Office (to access *Federal Register*) For active weblinks to each website visit http://evolve.elsevier.com/Kinn/

REFERENCES

Fordney M: *Insurance handbook for the medical office*, ed 6. Philadelphia, 2002, WB Saunders.

Buck C: *Step-by-step medical coding*, ed 4. Philadelphia, 2002, WB Saunders.

CHAPTER 17

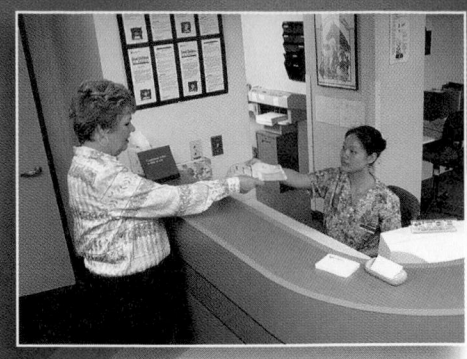

Scenario

The school where Kalene Umber receives her medical assistant training offers an optional job-shadowing module. For her assignment, she chose a nearby health center, where she observed the administrative responsibilities of the medical assistants employed in this multispecialty practice. Kalene found that some of the offices were organized and efficient, whereas others lacked a structured routine, especially in the insurance department. Kalene, a detail-oriented person who enjoyed her studies related to billing and coding, heard numerous comments from employees in the administrative area related to the volumes of work in the billing offices. Her office manager explained that the mountainous paperwork was created as a result of managed care requirements, rejected claims needing further research, and inconsistencies in the demands of the various insurance companies. Kalene agreed that keeping up with the requirements and regulations of the many third-party payors and government entitlement programs must be an overwhelming task. She concluded that billing and reimbursement are at the heart of the medical facility, and the correct completion of insurance claim forms is central to the success of the practice. She realized that becoming familiar with the complexities of the insurance claims process would be challenging, but through education, organization, and dedication, she was convinced that she could become a valuable employee and an advocate for the patients that needed her assistance in resolving issues related to their claims for reimbursement.

The Health Insurance Claim Form

Janet Beik
Alexandra P. Young

Learning Objectives

- Define and spell the terms listed in the vocabulary.
- Discuss the differences between paper claims and electronic claims.
- Differentiate between "clean" and "dirty" claims.
- Understand the guidelines for completing the CMS-1500 claim form.
- Explain how to complete each of the 33 blocks of the CMS-1500 claim form.
- List the OCR guidelines.
- Discuss methods of preventing claim rejections.
- Describe ways of checking the status of claims.

National Curriculum Competencies

ADMINISTRATIVE COMPETENCIES

4a. Apply managed care policies and procedures
4b. Apply third-party guidelines
4f. Complete insurance claim forms

TRANSDISCIPLINARY COMPETENCIES

1b. Recognize and respond to verbal communication
2a. Identify and respond to issues of confidentiality
2b. Perform within legal and ethical boundaries
2d. Document appropriately
3a. Explain general office policies
4c. Utilize computer software to maintain office systems

Vocabulary

assignment of benefits The transfer of the patient's legal right to collect benefits for medical expenses to the provider of those services, authorizing the payment to be sent directly to the provider.

audit trail The path left by a transaction when it has been completed, often referred to when tracking medical services used by patients or researching claims.

beneficiary Individual entitled to receive benefits from an insurance policy or program, or a governmental entitlement program offering healthcare benefits. Also called a *participant, subscriber, dependent, enrollee,* or *member.*

carrier As related to insurance, a company that assumes the risk of an insurance policy.

carrier-direct system A system for electronic data submission in which the medical facility has a computer system designed to transmit claims to a specific carrier directly, without first passing through a clearinghouse.

clean claim An insurance claim form that has been completed correctly (no errors or omissions) and can be processed and paid promptly if the claim meets the restrictions on covered services and items.

clearinghouse A centralized facility, sometimes called a *third-party administrator* (TPA), to whom insurance claims are transmitted. Clearinghouses separate, check, and redistribute claims electronically to various insurance carriers, and may offer additional services to the physician.

commercial insurance Plans (sometimes called *private insurance*) that reimburse the insured for expenses resulting from illness or injury according to a specific fee schedule as outlined in the insurance policy and on a fee-for-service basis.

digital signature A signature used for electronic claims; it consists of lines of text or a text box and is attached through a software application.

dingy claim A claim that is delayed because it cannot be processed, usually because the software used to transfer the claim or system changes make it incompatible with the receiving system.

dirty claim Claims that contain errors or omissions that cannot be processed or must be processed by hand because of OCR scanner rejection.

electronic claims Claims that are submitted to insurance processing facilities using a computerized medium, such as direct data entry, direct wire, dial-in telephone digital fax, or personal computer download/upload.

electronic data interchange The transfer of data back and forth between two or more entities using an electronic medium.

electronic signature A scanned signature or other such mark that is accepted as proof of approval and/or responsibility for the content of an electronic document.

employer identification number (EIN) The number used by the Internal Revenue Service that identifies a business or individual functioning as a business entity for income tax reporting.

fiscal intermediary An organization that contracts with the government to handle and mediate insurance claims from medical facilities, home health agencies, or providers of medical services or supplies.

incomplete claim A claim that is missing information and is returned to the provider for correction and resubmission.

insured An individual or organization who is covered by an insurance policy according to the policy terms, usually the individual or group who pays the premiums. Blue Cross/Blue Shield refers to this person or group as the *subscriber.*

invalid claim A claim that is incorrect in some manner or does not present a logical picture of the patient's situation.

Medigap A term sometimes applied to private insurance products that supplement Medicare insurance benefits.

national provider identifier (NPI) A lifetime number consisting of 10 digits that Medicare will use to replace the provider identification number (PIN) and the unique physician identification number (UPIN).

optical character recognition (OCR) The electronic scanning of printed items as images and use of special software to recognize these images (or characters) as ASCII text.

paper claims Hard copies of insurance claims that have been completed and sent by surface mail.

policyholder A person who pays a premium to an insurance company and in whose name the policy is written in exchange for the insurance protection provided by a policy of insurance, usually applicable to an automobile policy.

provider The company, individual, or group that provides medical services to a patient.

provider identification number (PIN) A number assigned to providers by carriers for use in submission of claims.

rejected claim A claim returned to the provider for clarification of any question and that must be corrected prior to resubmission.

third-party administrator An organization that processes claims and performs other business-related functions for a health plan.

third-party payor An entity that makes a payment on an obligation or debt but is not a party of the contract that created the debt.

unique provider identification number (UPIN) A number assigned by fiscal intermediaries to identify providers on claims for services.

universal claim form The form developed by the Health Care Financing Administration (HCFA) (now known as the Centers for Medicare and Medicaid Services [CMS]) and approved by the AMA for use in submitting all government-sponsored claims.

Medical insurance can be many things to many people. To some, it is a mound of paperwork. To others, it is a mass of confusion and regulations that seem to constantly change. But to a patient, medical insurance can quite literally be the difference between life and death. The lack of adequate and affordable healthcare is one of the most challenging issues faced by the government and the citizens of the United States. This makes health insurance a valuable benefit to most Americans. The enormous healthcare industry is the source of billions of dollars spent in this country each year. The leaders of the healthcare industry are constantly looking for ways to reduce costs and simplify the processes related to healthcare expense reimbursement.

The **universal claim form** (Figure 17-1), now called the CMS-1500 (formerly the HCFA-1500), was first developed in 1988 by the Health Care Financing Administration and approved by the American Medical Association Council on Medical Service for use in submitting Medicare claims. The CMS-1500 claim form answers the needs of healthcare insurers and can be downloaded along with detailed instructions on the CMS website.

The CMS-1500 form was renamed since HCFA became the Centers for Medicare and Medicaid Service on July 1, 2001. This governmental agency divides the former responsibilities of the Health Care Financing Administration into three entities, which are the Center for Medicare Management, the Center for Medicaid and State Operations, and the Center for Beneficiary Choices.

Because many changes will take place over the next several years, as healthcare facilities move into compliance with HIPAA regulations and more claims are submitted through **electronic data interchange**, medical assistants will need to stay abreast of the guidelines as they are released and implement those that are applicable to their individual facilities. Each facility should designate a person or persons to be responsible for implementation and continuous compliance with HIPAA.

Audit Trails

Electronic transactions leave behind a path or trail as they are processed, and this trail can be tracked or audited to provide a record. This record, called an **audit trail**, can be used to verify that information was processed correctly or to locate the source of an error. If an office uses a computerized accounting program and submits claims electronically, the task of keeping track of claims is simple, because the software is capable of printing out an "insurance aging report" by date, by patient name, or by carrier name. If **paper claims** are used, however, the medical assistant should establish a follow-up procedure for tracking insurance claims. This can be accomplished by using an insurance claims register or log (Figure 17-2). This document can be developed and updated with little effort using a spreadsheet software program.

Another method of tracking claims is a tickler file, also called a *suspense* or *follow-up file*. With this method, a copy of each insurance claim is filed chronologically, and the file is checked periodically for unprocessed (delinquent) claims. When the claim is paid, the copy is removed, and the information is posted on the patient's ledger card.

Delinquent claims remaining in the file after the normal contract time limits are pulled and then traced. If the claim has been denied, a letter may be sent to the insurance carrier's appeals department with a copy to the patient. (For more information on this topic, see Tracking Insurance Claims later in this chapter.)

Types of Claims

A medical assistant may submit insurance claims to a **third-party payor** or an insurance **carrier** either by hard copy (paper) or electronically. Most of today's computer software programs generate claims internally from the information that is entered into the database.

It is estimated that more than 6 billion insurance claims are filed every year—about 500 million per month. Of those claims, less than half are filed electronically. The remaining claims are still filed manually on a paper claim form. However, as the government and private insurers continue the migration toward time-saving electronic submissions, more claims will be submitted by electronic means. If a patient furnishes a different form from a **commercial insurance** company, it is usually acceptable to complete the CMS-1500 form and attach it to the commercial form for submission.

Paper

Paper claims often contain errors, which significantly lengthens payment turnaround time. About 30% to 35% of all paper claims are rejected because of typographical errors and errors of omission. Paper claims have advantages and disadvantages.

Advantages
- Documentation explaining unusual circumstances can be readily attached, if necessary and allowed.
- Start-up cost is minimal.
- Forms are readily available.
- Accepted by most third-party payors.

Disadvantages
- Completing forms is labor intensive.
- Costs of mailing, follow-up, and resubmission can become excessive.
- Greater chance for rejection.
- Cash flow is delayed because of slower reimbursements.
- Require a lot of storage space.

Electronic

Electronic claims processing reduces payment turnaround time by shortening the payment cycle and can reduce average error rates to less than 1% or 2%. Some insurance companies even waive the attachment requirements for many procedures when claims are submitted electronically. Some facilities use a **carrier-direct system**, in which claims are submitted directly to the specific carrier without first passing through a **clearinghouse**. There are also advantages and disadvantages to using electronic claims.

FIGURE 17-1 The CMS-1500 claim form.

Patient's Name Group/policy No.	Name of Insurance Company	Claim Submitted		Follow-Up		Claim Paid		Difference
		Date	Amount	Date	Date	Date	Amt	
Jones, Bob	BC/BS	1-7-03	319.37			2/28/03	294.82	24.55
Carson, David	BC	1-8-03	268.08	2-10-03	3-10-03			
Linden, Jan	Medicaid	1-9-03	146.15	2-10-03				
Paul, Emma	Medicare	1-10-03	96.28	2-10-03				
Cortez, Jose	Unicare	1-10-03	647.09	2-10-03				
Dimico, Joe	Tricare	2-1-03	134.78	3-10-03				
Coldman, Billy	Aetna	2-4-03	607.67	3-10-03				
Fritz, Renee	Travelers	2-10-03	564.55	3-10-03				
Wong, Chang	Prudential	2-15-03	1515.79					
Billings, Harry	Allstate	2-21-03	121.21					
Green, James	BC	2-24-03	124.99					

INSURANCE CLAIMS REGISTER Page No. _____

FIGURE 17-2 Insurance claims register.

Advantages

- Cost savings as a result of shortened preparation time.
- Cost savings in postage.
- Reduced claim rejection.
- Quicker payment turnaround time.
- Generation of claim status reports.

Disadvantages

- Computer hardware/software glitches and/or power outages that delay preparation or transmission.
- Issue of creating electronic attachments.
- Initial start-up is expensive.

Electronic claims can be submitted either directly to the carrier via modem, after being validated by the computer software program, or through a claims clearinghouse. A clearinghouse (also called a *third-party administrator*, or *TPA*) is a company that offers the healthcare **provider** (for a fee) the service of receiving claim transmissions, checking and preparing the claims for processing, consolidating claims so that one transmission can be sent to each carrier, and submitting claims in correct data format to the applicable insurance payor. Clearinghouses provide the following additional services:

- Audit claims to make sure all required fields are completed and data are correct.
- Report the number of claims submitted and the number of errors and their specifics.
- Forward claims to insurance carriers that accept electronic claims (Medicare, Medicaid, Blue Cross/Blue Shield, and others) or to another clearinghouse that may hold the contracts with specific payors.
- Keep provider offices updated as new carriers are added to the database.
- Generate informative statistical reports.

Typically with electronic claims processing, payments are received in half the time when compared with turnaround time for paper claims. Very soon after claims are transmitted, reports will be sent from the clearinghouse for tracking purposes, and the medical assistant will know in a very short time which claims have been rejected and which ones need additional information.

Whether the medical facility chooses to submit claims directly to the carrier or use the services of a clearinghouse, there is usually an "enrollment" process. Most government and many commercial carriers require enrollment so they can set up information about the medical office on their computer system. Some require a signed contract. The biggest obstacle in getting set up for electronic claims processing is the time it takes for approval from state, federal, and in some cases, commercial/HMO carriers. The only equipment requirements for electronic claims submission besides a computer are a modem and a working phone line. Clearinghouse services are not free, however. In addition to the set-up cost, many charge a nominal fee (usually less than a dollar) on a per-claim basis.

CRITICAL THINKING APPLICATION

Kalene is interested in learning more about filing claims electronically. In the medical facility where she is doing her externship, she has asked to work with Mrs. Leonard, who performs this procedure in the office. How can working closely with Mrs. Leonard benefit Kalene on this subject?

Claim Status

Obtaining timely and correct payment from third-party payors is a concern for many medical practices. Lost claims, delayed claims, and dirty claims result in healthcare providers waiting months for payment of professional services rendered. Most providers will agree that claim processing payment issues are at the heart of most provider-payor conflicts.

Clean Claims

A **clean claim** is one that has been filled out correctly, contains no missing data or errors, and has been submitted for payment within the time allowed by the insurer. Additionally, it has passed all claim edits and audits and can be processed and paid on the first submission.

Dirty Claims

If there are errors or omissions on claim forms, if they are improperly filled out, or if they are submitted after the time allowed by the third-party payor, claims are subsequently denied. Claims like these are known as **dirty claims**. The two main reasons for denial are (1) technical errors and (2) insurance policy coverage issues. Technical errors include typographical or mathematical errors and incorrect or incomplete information. Coverage issues are usually more complex and are not as readily resolved as technical errors. A common reason for rejection in this category is that a procedure listed on the claim is not a covered service or is involved with a preexisting condition.

Dingy Claims

A **dingy claim** results when the fiscal intermediary for Medicare cannot process a claim for a particular service or bill type, and the claim is put on hold until the necessary system changes are implemented and the claim can be paid correctly.

Incomplete Claims

An **incomplete claim** is missing some type of information.

Invalid Claims

An **invalid claim** is complete, but does not make logical sense or is incorrect in some way.

Rejected Claims

A *rejected claim* is one that has missing or incorrect information. **Rejected claims** subsequently require investigation, need further clarification, and/or possibly require answers or documentation for specific questions.

Denied Claims

Claims can be denied as the result of a technical error but are usually not paid because the medical service submitted is not covered under the policy, is an ineligible service, or must be applied to the deductible in accordance with the policy.

Rules for Completing the Health Insurance Claim Form

When the first appointment is made, the medical assistant should ask the patient for all pertinent insurance information. Much of this information is on the patient information form that is completed when the patient comes to the medical office for the initial visit and is inserted into the medical chart as well as entered into the computer's patient database. Additional information will have to be abstracted from the patient record for processing the insurance claim. Remember that the patient may not be the **beneficiary** of insurance reimbursement.

Patients should be asked during each visit whether their insurance information is complete and current. Many offices use a form that allows the patient to provide address and phone updates, as well as new insurance information. The use of sign-in sheets is now questionable, because such logs usually list all of the patients who visited the facility by name, and this violates privacy guidelines.

Health Insurance Claim Form Guidelines

A medical assistant can use the following general guidelines for completing a health insurance claim form:
- Photocopy the back and front of the patient's insurance card and place it in the medical record.
- If a patient has more than one insurance policy, it is important to get the name, address, group, and policy number for each company.
- Record the name of the subscriber if it is someone other than the patient.
- Obtain a signed authorization form for releasing information to the insurance carrier; for Medicare, obtain authorization to pay benefits directly to the physician (Figure 17-3).
- Complete all required blocks of the CMS-1500 claim form (Procedure 17-1).
- Proofread the form carefully.
- Make certain any necessary attachments are included with the completed form.
- Follow office policies and guidelines for claim review and signatures.
- Forward the original (red print) claim to the proper insurance carrier either by mail or electronically.
- If creating a paper claim, make a copy of the completed and signed claim form for the office records.
- Enter the appropriate information in the insurance log and record the insurance submission information on the patient's ledger (Figure 17-4).

Optical Scanning (OCR) Guidelines

Because many insurance carriers are using **optical character recognition (OCR)** scanners to transfer the information on claim forms to their computers' memories, the CMS-1500 claim form is printed in red ink. The reason for this is that the OCR process uses a red-bulb scanner, which causes the preprinted portion of the form to disappear or "drop out." The resulting image allows for "clean" recognition of the data inserted without the characters being obstructed by the lines and text of the form.

A medical assistant should use OCR scanning rules for completing the CMS-1500 form. Entries should be clear and sharp; carbon copies are not acceptable. A proportionally spaced 12-point font such as Courier works best. The following are additional guidelines:

ASSIGNMENT OF INSURANCE BENEFITS

I, the undersigned, represent that I have insurance coverage with and do hereby authorize
_____ to pay and assign directly to _____
(NAME OF COMPANY)   (NAME OF DOCTOR)

all surgical and/or medical benefits, if any, otherwise payable to me for services as described on the attached forms hereof, but not to exceed the charges for those services. I understand that I am financially responsible for all charges whether or not paid by said insurance. I hereby authorize said assignee to release all information necessary to secure the payment of said benefits.

Date _____   Signed _____

FIGURE 17-3   Assignment of benefits form.

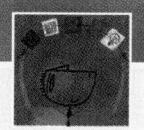

PROCEDURE **17-1**

Complete an Insurance Claim Form

GOAL: Accurately complete a CMS-1500 (formerly HCFA-1500) claim form.

EQUIPMENT AND SUPPLIES

- Patient information form
- Photocopy of patient's insurance ID card
- Encounter form
- Patient record
- Patient's ledger
- CMS-1500 form
- Typewriter or computer

PROCEDURAL STEPS

Patient/Insured Section

Block 1   Check the type of health insurance coverage applicable to the claim.

Block 1a   Enter the patient's insurance identification number or Medicare ID number exactly as it appears on his or her insurance card.

Block 2   Enter the patient's last name, first name, and middle initial following OCR guidelines.

Block 3   Enter the patient's birth date in MM DD YYYY format, and enter an "X" in the appropriate box for sex.

Block 4   For commercial and Blue Cross/Blue Shield claims, enter "SAME" if patient and insured (policyholder) are the same person. If the insured's name is different from the patient, enter the last name, first name, and middle initial in this block. If there is insurance primary to Medicare, list the name of the insured here. If Medicare is primary, leave blank. For CHAMPUS/TRICARE, enter the "sponsor's" name

Block 5   Enter the patient's street address on the first line, city and state on the second line, and the ZIP code and telephone number on the third line. Remember to use all capital letters and no punctuation.

Block 6   Check the appropriate box for the patient's relationship to insured. If Medicare is primary, leave blank.

Block 7   Enter the insured's address and telephone number, unless the insured and the patient are the same, in which case enter "SAME." Complete this item only when blocks 4 and 11 are completed. For Medicare and Medicaid, leave blank.

Block 8   Check the appropriate box for the patient's marital status and whether employed or a student.

Block 9   (Required if 11d is marked "yes.") If the patient has other medical insurance coverage, and he or she is not the insured, enter the insured's name, and complete boxes 9a through 9d. If there is no other insurance, leave 9a through 9d blank and proceed to block 10.

Block 9a   Enter the policy or group number of the insured's secondary insurance coverage. If the secondary policy is Medigap, enter the policy and/or group number preceded by MEDIGAP.

Block 9b   Enter the insured's birth date in MM DD YYYY format, and enter an "X" in the appropriate sex box.

Block 9c   Enter the name of the insured's employer or school, if applicable. Leave blank if a Medigap PayerID is entered in item 9d. Otherwise, enter the claims processing address of the Medigap insurer.

Block 9d   Enter the name of the secondary insurance plan or program. If the secondary insurer is a Medigap policy, enter the nine-digit PayerID number of the Medigap insurer. If there is no PayerID number, enter the Medigap insurance program or plan name.

Continued

PROCEDURE 17-1—cont'd

Block 10 Check the appropriate boxes in this section to identify whether the patient's condition was related to either his or her employment, auto accident, or other accident.

Block 10a Check "no" unless the illness, accident, or injury was the result of employment or occurred on the job or in the process of performing one's job.

Block 10b Check "no" unless the claim is related to an injury resulting from an automobile accident. In the case of an auto accident, enter the two-letter state code where the accident occurred.

Block 10c Enter an "X" in the appropriate box.

Block 10d This block is usually reserved for Medicaid as secondary payor claims. In some states, this block is used only if the patient is entitled to Medicaid. If this is the case, enter the patient's Medicaid number, preceded by MCD. For Medicare, leave blank. Some third-party payors want the word "ATTACHMENT(S)" entered into this field if there are attachments included with the claim.

Block 11 For commercial carriers, enter the group policy name/number from the patient's card. For BC/BS and Medicaid, leave blank. For insurance primary to Medicare, enter the insured's policy or group number. If Medicare is primary, the word "NONE" must appear in this block. By doing so indicates that Medicare is primary. NOTE: For a claim to be considered for Medicare Secondary Payer, a copy of the primary payor's explanation of benefits (EOB) must be included with the claim form.

Block 11a Enter the insured's birth date and sex if different from block 3. For Medicare and Medicaid, leave blank.

Block 11b Enter the employer's name if applicable. On Medicare claims, if there is a second policy and the insured's status is retired, enter the date of retirement preceded by the word "RETIRED."

Block 11c Enter the nine-digit PayerID number of the primary insurer. If no such number exists, enter the complete name of the primary payor's program or plan name.

Block 11d Check "no" if patient is covered by only one insurance policy. If the answer is "yes," give the name of the company and any other information available in block 9. For Medicare and Medicaid, leave blank.

Block 12 The patient or authorized person must sign and date this item unless a signature is on file. If this is the case, the words "SIGNATURE ON FILE" should be entered here. Leave blank on Medicaid claims.

Block 13 The patient or authorized person should sign and date this item if he or she agrees that benefits are to be paid directly to the provider. For Medicare supplements and cross-over claims, "SIGNATURE ON FILE" must also appear in this block. For Medicaid, leave blank.

Physician/Supplier Information

Block 14 Enter the date of the first symptom of the current illness, injury, or pregnancy in this block if one is documented in the chart notes or the date of the last menstrual cycle if the claim is related to pregnancy.

Block 15 Enter the date the patient was first treated for this condition. Leave blank for Medicare claims.

Block 16 Enter date(s) patient is unable to work in current occupation if it is a workers' compensation claim. Not required for most other carriers.

Block 17 Enter the name of the referring (or ordering) physician, if applicable.

Block 17a Enter the UPIN/NPI number of the referring/ordering physician listed in block 17.

Block 18 If the claim is for a related hospital stay, enter the dates of hospital admission and discharge. If the patient has not been discharged, leave the "to" box blank.

Block 19 This block is usually left blank. Some private payors insert the word "ATTACHMENT(S)" when specific documentation accompanies the claim.

Block 20 If laboratory procedures are listed on the claim in block 24, and these services were performed in the provider's facility, the "no" box is checked with an "X" or left blank. If lab work shown on the claim was done by an outside lab and billed to the provider, check the "yes" box, and enter the total amount of the charges. Leave this block blank if no lab tests were done.

Block 21 Enter the patient's diagnosis or diagnoses using ICD-9-CM code number(s), listing the primary diagnosis first. Up to four codes (in priority order) can be entered in block 21.

PROCEDURE **17-1—cont'd**

Block 22 Required only for replacement claims for Medicaid. Enter the appropriate 3-digit replacement code followed by the 17-digit transaction control number of the most current incorrectly paid claim.

Block 23 For private and commercial carriers and Medicaid, enter the 10-digit prior authorization number for those procedures requiring prior approval assigned by the peer review organization (PRO). Consult the specific guidelines for the payor to whom the claim is being submitted.

Block 24a The first date of service for the charge on this line should be placed in the "From" column. When a claim is for more than one day of the same service on a line item, the days must be in consecutive order. The last date of service is required in the "To" column. Enter the month, day, and year (in the MM DD YYYY format) for each procedure, service, or supply. When "from" and "to" dates are shown for a series of identical services, enter the number of days or units in 24G.

Block 24b Enter the appropriate place of service code.

Block 24c Enter the appropriate type of service code. NOTE: For private payors and Medicare, leave blank. All others, refer to specific guidelines.

Block 24d Enter the procedure, service, or supply code using appropriate five-digit CPT or HCPCS procedure code. Enter a two-position modifier when applicable.

Block 24e Link the procedure/service code back to the diagnosis code in block 21 by indicating the applicable number of the diagnosis code (1, 2, 3 or 4) to that line's procedure code.

Block 24f Enter the charge for each listed procedure, supply, and/or service.

Block 24g Enter the number of days or units. If only one service is performed, enter the number 1.

Block 24h Leave blank for all claims with the exception of certain Medicaid claims.

Block 24i For certain carriers, enter an "X" or "E" as appropriate if documentation indicates a medical emergency existed. Leave blank for Medicare claims.

Block 24j For commercial claims, BC/BS, Medicare, Medicaid, and TRICARE, leave blank. (Refer to specific third-party payor guidelines.)

Block 24k Enter the five-digit number that has been assigned when the provider was approved by the third-party payor. For Medicare, it is referred to as the "billing number." Blue Cross-Blue Shield and Medicaid have their own numbers. This is not the same as the UPIN number.

Block 25 Enter the provider's nine-digit Federal tax identification number and check the appropriate box in this field; or, in the case of an unincorporated practice or sole proprietorship, enter the provider's Social Security number.

Block 26 Enter the patient's account number as assigned by the provider's accounting system, if available. If you are submitting the claim electronically, you are required to provide a patient account number.

Block 27 Check the appropriate block to indicate whether the provider accepts assignment of benefits. If the supplier is a participating provider (PAR), assignment must be accepted for all covered charges. For nonPAR providers, this can be left blank. For Medicaid, check "yes."

Block 28 Total column 24f and enter the total charges in this field.

Block 29 Enter the total amount, if any, that has been paid by the patient. Leave blank if no payment has been made.

Block 30 Used when there is a secondary insurance. Enter the balance owing as indicated on the explanation of benefits (EOB).

Block 31 Enter the signature of the provider, or his or her representative and his or her initials, and the date the form was signed. The signature may be typed, stamped, or handwritten; however, the characters should not fall outside of the block.

Block 32 Enter the name and address of the facility where the services were performed if other than patient's home or physician's office. For Medicare, enter the name and address of the facility regardless of where services were provided.

Block 33 Enter the provider's billing name, address, zip code, and telephone number. Also, enter the billing number (from block 24k). Enter the Group NPI number, if the provider is a member of a group practice. Refer to specific third-party payor guidelines.

INSURANCE CLAIM REGISTER					
PATIENT	INSURANCE COMPANY	DATE FILED	AMOUNT BILLED	AMOUNT PAID	DIFFERENCE

FIGURE 17-4 Insurance log showing the date each claim was filed, the amount billed, the amount paid, and the difference that must be either discounted or billed to the patient.

- Use all uppercase letters.
- Omit all punctuation.
- Use the MM DD YYYY format (with a space between each set of digits) for all birth dates.
- Keep all entries within their respective boxes. "X's" must fall completely within the designated box. NOTE: If a computer software program is being used to generate forms, print a test pattern before printing the final form to ensure proper alignment. If a typewriter is being used, use the test strips on the right and left margins. To check horizontal alignment, type "X's" in both the left and right test patterns.
- For the following, substitute a blank space:
  - Dollar signs and decimal points in charges and ICD codes
  - Dashes preceding procedure code modifiers
  - Parentheses around telephone area codes
  - Hyphens in Social Security numbers
- Omit titles and other designations, such as Sr., Jr., II, or III, unless they appear on the ID card.
- When the charge is expressed in whole dollars, use two zeros in the "cents" column.
- If using a typewriter, do not use lift-off tape, correction tape, or correction fluid.
- Since photocopies of claims cannot be scanned, all resubmissions must be prepared using the original (red print) claim form.
- Do not include any handwritten data (other than signatures) on the forms.

- Do not staple anything to the form.
- Insert the name and address of the insurance company in the proper area in the top margin of the claim form.

Signatures on Health Insurance Claim Forms

A signature verifies that a person agrees with the statements in a document. On a health insurance claim form, there are spaces for the patient and/or **insured** to sign, as well as the provider. As with any document that is verified by signature, the text should be read thoroughly for accuracy prior to signing. The provider is ultimately responsible for the accuracy of the claim, but this does not release the individual who billed the claim from any liability.

Patient Signatures. The patient must sign the release of medical information authorization so that the provider can submit the claim for reimbursement. A signed authorization for a specific period of time may be used, in which case future claims during that time period can be noted "signature on file." Some patients may also sign a lifetime signature authorization, such as persons who are in a skilled nursing facility.

The patient may also sign the **assignment of benefits** block if he or she wants the payment to go directly to the provider. When the patient has already paid the provider, he or she may not sign this block so that the payment will come directly to the patient for reimbursement.

Provider Signatures. Providers may sign the insurance claim form by original signature or by signature stamp. They may also authorize an employee to sign the form, use a signature stamp, or use an **electronic signature** or **digital signature**. Providers who use billing services may offer this same type of authorization to the billing company that files claims on their behalf. Providers may also complete a certification letter for electronic claims once which serves the same purpose as an actual signature, when allowed by third-party payors and governmental entities.

The Health Insurance Claim Form

The CMS-1500 form is divided into two parts (see Figure 17-1). The top part of the form is the patient/insured section; the bottom half is the physician/supplier section. The name and address of the insurance company or government agency should appear in the upper right portion in the margin of the form. This information must be restricted to a 2-inch area just right of the bar code at the top (Figure 17-5).

When completing the CMS-1500 form, follow the guidelines that begin below. NOTE: Comments on filling out each individual block on the CMS-1500 form apply primarily to commercial, Medicare/Medicaid, and Blue Cross/Blue Shield claims.

CHAMPUS/TRICARE claims are similar to commercial claims, except where noted. To become proficient in completing forms for all major payors, a medical assistant should prepare a guidelines manual with detailed instructions on how each of the 33 blocks should be completed for each payor. Usually, claims guidelines can be obtained from the third-party payor. This manual should be updated periodically so that it remains current.

The following are general guidelines for completing the CMS-1500 claims forms.

Patient/Insured Section

Block 1 **Type of Insurance (required).** Check the type of health insurance coverage applicable to the claim. EXAMPLE: If the claim is primary for Medicare, check the Medicare box. If Medicare is secondary, check the "Other" box.

Block 1a **Insured's ID Number (required).** Enter the patient's insurance identification number or Medicare ID number exactly as it appears on his or her insurance card. For CHAMPUS/TRICARE, the sponsor's Social Security number is used.

Block 2 **Patient's Name (required).** Enter the patient's last name, first name, and middle initial following OCR guidelines.

Block 3 **Patient's Birth Date (required).** Enter the patient's birth date in MM DD YYYY format, and enter an "X" in the appropriate box for gender.

Block 4 **Insured's Name.** For commercial and Blue Cross/Blue Shield claims, enter "SAME" if patient and insured **(policyholder)** are the same person. If the insured's name is different from the patient, enter the last name, first name, and middle initial in this block. If there is insurance primary to Medicare, either through the patient or spouse's employment or any other source, list the name of the insured here. If Medicare is primary, leave blank. For CHAMPUS/TRICARE, enter the "sponsor's" name.

FIGURE 17-5 Correct placement of insurance company's address.

Block 5   **Patient's Address.** Enter the patient's street address on the first line, the city and state on the second line, and the ZIP code and telephone number on the third line. Remember to use all capital letters and no punctuation.

```
5. PATIENT'S ADDRESS (No., Street)

CITY                                    STATE

ZIP CODE            TELEPHONE (Include Area Code)
                         (    )
```

Block 6   **Patient's Relationship to Insured.** Check the appropriate box for the patient's relationship to the insured. If Medicare is primary, leave blank.

```
6. PATIENT RELATIONSHIP TO INSURED
   Self []  Spouse []  Child []  Other []
```

Block 7   **Insured's Address.** Enter the insured's address and telephone number, unless the insured and the patient are one and the same, in which case enter "SAME." Complete this item only when blocks 4 and 11 are completed. For Medicare and Medicaid, leave this blank.

```
7. INSURED'S ADDRESS (No., Street)

CITY                                    STATE

ZIP CODE            TELEPHONE (INCLUDE AREA CODE)
                         (    )
```

Block 8   **Patient Status.** Check the appropriate box for the patient's marital status and whether he or she is employed or a student.

```
8. PATIENT STATUS
   Single []   Married []   Other []

   Employed []  Full-Time []  Part-Time []
                Student       Student
```

Block 9   **Other Insured's Name (required if 11d is marked "yes").** If the patient has other medical insurance coverage, and he or she is not the insured, enter the insured's name and complete boxes 9a through 9d. If there is no other insurance, leave 9a through 9d blank and proceed to block 10.

Block 9a   **Other Insured's Policy or Group Number.** Enter the policy or group number of the insured's secondary insurance coverage. If the secondary policy is **Medigap**, enter the policy and/or group number preceded by "MEDIGAP."

Block 9b   **Other Insured's Date of Birth.** Enter the insured's birth date in MM DD YYYY format and enter an "X" in the appropriate sex box.

Block 9c   **Employer's Name or School Name (optional).** Enter the name of the insured's employer or school, if applicable. Leave blank if a Medigap Payer ID is entered in box 9d. Otherwise, enter the claims processing address of the Medigap insurer.

Block 9d   **Insurance Plan Name or Program Name.** Enter the name of the secondary insurance plan or program. If the secondary insurer is a Medigap policy, enter the nine-digit Payer ID number of the Medigap insurer. If there is no Payer ID number, enter the Medigap insurance program or plan name. (Medigap policies are identifiable by the numbers "99" in the seventh and eighth digits of the Payer ID.)

```
9. OTHER INSURED'S NAME (Last Name, First Name, Middle Initial)

a. OTHER INSURED'S POLICY OR GROUP NUMBER

b. OTHER INSURED'S DATE OF BIRTH          SEX
   MM   DD   YY                    M []      F []
c. EMPLOYER'S NAME OR SCHOOL NAME

d. INSURANCE PLAN NAME OR PROGRAM NAME
```

Block 10   **Is Patient's Condition Related to (required).** Check the appropriate boxes in this section to identify whether the patient's condition was related to his or her employment, an auto accident, or another accident. If any of the boxes in this block are checked "Yes," this may indicate that the patient's health insurance is not primary and that other insurance, such as workers' compensation or an automobile insurance policy, may be primary.

Block 10a   Check "No" unless the illness, accident, or injury was the result of employment or occurred on the job or in the process of performing one's job.

Block 10b   Check "No" unless the claim is for an injury resulting from an automobile accident. In the case of an auto accident, enter the two-letter state code where the accident occurred.

Block 10c   Enter an "X" in the appropriate box.

```
10. IS PATIENT'S CONDITION RELATED TO:

a. EMPLOYMENT? (CURRENT OR PREVIOUS)
          [] YES      [] NO
b. AUTO ACCIDENT?              PLACE (State)
          [] YES      [] NO    |___|
c. OTHER ACCIDENT?
          [] YES      [] NO
```

Block 10d   **Reserved for Local Use (optional).** This block is usually reserved for Medicaid as secondary payor claims. In some states, this block is used only if the patient is entitled to Medicaid. If this is the case, enter the patient's Medicaid number, preceded by "MCD." For Medicare, leave this blank. Some third-party payors want the word "Attachment(s)" entered into this field if there are attachments included with the claim.

10d. RESERVED FOR LOCAL USE

Block 11   **Insured's Policy or Group Number.** For commercial carriers, enter the group policy name/number from the patient's card. For Blue Cross/Blue Shield and Medicaid, leave this blank. For insurance primary to Medicare, enter the insured's policy or group number. If Medicare is primary, the word "NONE" must appear in this block. Doing so indicates that Medicare is primary. NOTE: For a claim to be considered for Medicare Secondary Payer, a copy of the primary payor's explanation of benefits (EOB) must be included with the claim form.

Block 11a   **Date of Birth.** Enter the insured's birth date and sex if different from block 3. For Medicare and Medicaid, leave this blank.

Block 11b   **Employer's Name.** Enter the employer's name if applicable. On Medicare claims, if there is a second policy and the insured's status is retired, enter the date of retirement, preceded by the word "RETIRED."

Block 11c   **Insurance Plan Name or Program Name (conditionally required).** Enter the nine-digit Payer ID number of the primary insurer. If no such number exists, enter the complete name of the primary payor's program or plan name.

Block 11d   **Is There Another Health Benefit Plan (required).** Check "No" if covered by only one insurance policy. If the answer is "Yes," give the name of the company and any other information available in block 9. For Medicare and Medicaid, leave this blank.

11. INSURED'S POLICY GROUP OR FECA NUMBER
a. INSURED'S DATE OF BIRTH   MM   DD   YY   SEX   M ☐   F ☐
b. EMPLOYER'S NAME OR SCHOOL NAME
c. INSURANCE PLAN NAME OR PROGRAM NAME
d. IS THERE ANOTHER HEALTH BENEFIT PLAN?   ☐ YES   ☐ NO   *If yes,* return to and complete item 9 a-d.

Block 12   **Patient's or Authorized Person's Signature (conditionally required).** The patient or authorized person must sign and date this item unless a signature is on file. If this is the case, the words "SIGNATURE ON FILE" or "SOF" should be entered here. Leave this blank on Medicaid claims.

READ BACK OF FORM BEFORE COMPLETING & SIGNING THIS FORM.
12. PATIENT'S OR AUTHORIZED PERSON'S SIGNATURE I authorize the release of any medical or other information necessary to process this claim. I also request payment of government benefits either to myself or to the party who accepts assignment below.
SIGNED _____   DATE _____

Block 13   **Insured's or Authorized Person's Signature.** As in block 12, the patient or authorized person should sign and date this item if he or she agrees that benefits are to be paid directly to the provider. For Medicare supplements and crossover claims, "SIGNATURE ON FILE" or "SOF" must also appear in this block. For Medicaid, leave this blank.

13. INSURED'S OR AUTHORIZED PERSON'S SIGNATURE I authorize payment of medical benefits to the undersigned physician or supplier for services described below.
SIGNED _____

CRITICAL THINKING APPLICATION

It is office policy to request that patients assign benefits when the patient does not pay for services immediately. One of the patients, Mr. Jones, seems hesitant to sign block 13 of the CMS-1500 form. How should Kalene explain the office policy to Mr. Jones?

Physician/Supplier Information

Block 14   **Date of Current Illness Injury (required on accident or medical emergency claims).** Enter the date of the first symptom of the current illness, injury, or pregnancy in this block if one is documented in the chart notes, or the date of the last menstrual cycle if the claim is related to pregnancy. Use caution here, because an incorrect date may indicate a preexisting condition, and the claim will be rejected.

14. DATE OF CURRENT: MM DD YY	ILLNESS (First symptom) OR INJURY (Accident) OR PREGNANCY(LMP)

Block 15   **Same or Similar Illness (optional).** Enter the date the patient was first treated for this condition. Leave this blank for Medicare claims.

> 15. IF PATIENT HAS HAD SAME OR SIMILAR ILLNESS.
> GIVE FIRST DATE   MM | DD | YY

Block 16 **Patient Unable to Work (optional).** Enter date(s) the patient is unable to work in his or her current occupation if it is a workers' compensation claim. Not required for most other carriers.

> 16. DATES PATIENT UNABLE TO WORK IN CURRENT OCCUPATION
>   MM | DD | YY   MM | DD | YY
> FROM   TO

Block 17 **Name of Referring Physician or Other Source (conditionally required).** Enter the name of the referring (or ordering) physician, if applicable. If the physician orders a test or procedure that is performed by an ancillary healthcare giver but the physician/source interprets the results, his or her **unique provider identification number (UPIN)** or **national provider identifier (NPI)** must be entered here, and the UPIN number entered in block 17a. EXAMPLE: If Dr. Smith orders an ECG, which is performed by the medical assistant but is interpreted by Dr. Smith, his name is entered into block 17 and his UPIN/NPI number in block 17a. This block is also required if billing for a consultation.

> 17. NAME OF REFERRING PHYSICIAN OR OTHER SOURCE

Block 17a **ID Number of Referring Physician (required if a referring physician is listed in block 17).** Enter the UPIN/NPI number of the referring/ordering physician listed in block 17.

> 17a. I.D. NUMBER OF REFERRING PHYSICIAN

Block 18 **Hospitalization Dates Related to Current Services (conditionally required).** If the claim is for a related hospital stay, enter the dates of hospital admission and discharge. If the patient has not been discharged, leave the "To" box blank.

> 18. HOSPITALIZATION DATES RELATED TO CURRENT SERVICES
>   MM | DD | YY   MM | DD | YY
> FROM   TO

Block 19 **Reserved for Local Use (not required).** This block is usually left blank. Some private payors insert the word

"Attachment(s)" when specific documentation accompanies the claim. There are circumstances on Medicare and/or Medicaid claims when information might be entered here. Check with the local fiscal intermediary or the guidelines of the individual third-party payor for details.

> 19. RESERVED FOR LOCAL USE

Block 20 **Outside Lab? (conditionally required).** If laboratory procedures are listed on the claim in block 24, and these services were performed in the provider's facility, the "NO" box in block 20 is checked with an "X" or left blank. If laboratory work shown on the claim was done by an outside laboratory and billed to the provider, check the "YES" box, and enter the total amount of the charges. Leave this block blank if no laboratory tests were performed.

> 20. OUTSIDE LAB? $ CHARGES
>   [ ] YES   [ ] NO

Block 21 **Diagnosis or Nature of Illness/Injury (required).** Enter the patient's diagnosis or diagnoses using ICD-9-CM codes, listing the primary diagnosis first, and code to the highest level of specificity. Up to four codes (in priority order) can be entered in block 21.

> 21. DIAGNOSIS OR NATURE OF ILLNESS OR INJURY. (RELATE ITEMS 1,2,3 OR 4 TO ITEM 24E BY LINE)
> 1. L___ . __   3. L___ . __
> 2. L___ . __   4. L___ . __

Block 22 **Medicaid Resubmission.** Required only for replacement claims for Medicaid. Enter the appropriate three-digit replacement code followed by the 17-digit transaction control number of the most current incorrectly paid claim.

> 22. MEDICAID RESUBMISSION
>   CODE   ORIGINAL REF. NO.

Block 23 **Prior Authorization Number.** This block can be completed in various ways. For private and commercial carriers and Medicaid, enter the 10-digit prior authorization number for those procedures requiring prior approval assigned by the peer review organization

(PRO). Consult the specific guidelines for the payor to whom the claim is being submitted.

23. PRIOR AUTHORIZATION NUMBER

Block 24a Date(s) of Service (required). The first date of service for the charge on this line should be placed in the "From" column. When a claim is for more than one day of the same service on a line item, the days must be in consecutive order. The last date of service is required in the "To" column. Enter the month, day, and year (in the MM DD YYYY format) for each procedure, service, or supply. When "From" and "To" dates are shown for a series of identical services, enter the number of days or units in block 24g.

Block 24b Place of Service (required). Enter the appropriate place of service code for the payor to which the claim is being submitted (Figure 17-6).

Block 24c Type of Service (if required). Enter the appropriate type of service code if required (Figure 17-7). NOTE: For private payors and Medicare, leave blank. For all others, refer to specific guidelines.

Block 24d Procedure Codes/Modifiers (required). Enter the procedure, service, or supply code using the appropriate five-digit CPT or HCPCS procedure code. Enter a two-position modifier when applicable. NOTE: If an unlisted procedure code is used (codes ending in –99), a complete description of the procedure must be given. Use a separate attachment to do this, if the carrier allows attachments.

Block 24e Diagnosis Code (required for multiple diagnoses). Link the procedure/service code back to the diagnosis code in block 21 by indicating the applicable number of diagnosis codes (1, 2, 3, or 4) to that line's procedure code.

Block 24f Charges (required). Enter the charge for each listed procedure, supply, and /or service.

Block 24g Days or Units (required). Enter the number of days or units. This field is normally used for multiple visits, units of supplies, anesthesia minutes, or oxygen volume. If only one service is performed, enter the number "1."

Block 24h EPSDT/Family Plan. Leave blank for all claims with the exception of certain Medicaid claims. (EPSDT is an acronym for "early and periodic screening diagnosis and treatment.") If this is applicable, enter the appropriate alpha referral code.

BLOCK 24B
PLACE OF SERVICE CODES

11 Doctor's office
12 Patient's home
21 Inpatient hospital
22 Outpatient hospital
23 Emergency department—hospital
24 Ambulatory surgical center
25 Birthing center
26 Military treatment facility/ uniformed service treatment facility
31 Skilled nursing facility (swing bed visits)
32 Nursing facility (intermediate/long-term care facilities)
33 Custodial care facility (domiciliary or rest home services)
34 Hospice (domiciliary or rest home services)
35 Adult living care facilities (residential care facility)
41 Ambulance–land
42 Ambulance–air or water
50 Federally qualified health center
51 Inpatient psychiatric facility
52 Psychiatric facility–partial hospitalization
53 Community mental health care (outpatient, twenty-four-hours-a-day services, admission screening, consultation, and educational services)
54 Intermediate care facility/mentally retarded
55 Residential substance abuse treatment facility
56 Psychiatric residential treatment center
60 Mass immunization center
61 Comprehensive inpatient rehabilitation facility
62 Comprehensive outpatient rehabilitation facility
65 End-stage renal disease treatment facility
71 State or local public health clinic
72 Rural health clinic
81 Independent laboratory
99 Other unlisted facility

FIGURE 17-6

Block 24i EMG (if applicable). For certain carriers, enter an "X" as appropriate if documentation indicates a medical emergency existed. Leave this blank for Medicare claims.

Block 24j Coordination of Benefits (COB) (if applicable). For commercial claims, Blue Cross/Blue Shield, Medicare, Medicaid, and TRICARE, leave blank. In some instances, the first two digits of the NPI number are entered in block 24j, with the remaining eight digits of the NPI in block 24k, including the two-digit location identifier. (Refer to specific third-party payor guidelines.)

Block 24k Reserved for Local Use. Enter the five-digit number assigned when the provider was approved by the third-party payor. For Medicare, it is referred to as the *billing number*. Blue Cross/Blue Shield and Medicaid have their own numbers. This is not the same as the UPIN number.

BLOCK 24C TYPE OF SERVICE CODES FOR MEDICAID, TRICARE, AND WORKERS' COMPENSATION

These codes should be selected depending on the procedure code used on each line. Codes may vary according to regions and claim administrators.

1 Medical care (e.g., evaluation and management services)
2 Surgery
3 Consultation
4 Diagnostic x-ray (e.g., ultrasound and nuclear testing)
5 Diagnostic laboratory
6 Radiation therapy
7 Anesthesia
8 Assistant at surgery
9 Other medical service (e.g., laboratory, venipuncture, handling of specimen)
0 Blood or packed red cells
A DME rental/purchase
B Drugs
C Ambulatory surgery
D Hospice
E Second opinion on elective surgery
F Maternity
G Dental
H Mental health care
I Ambulance
J Program for persons with disabilities
L Renal supply in home
M Alternate payment for maintenance
N Kidney donor
V Pneumococcal vaccine
Z Third opinion on elective surgery

FIGURE 17-7

24. A DATE(S) OF SERVICE From MM DD YY	To MM DD YY	B Place of Service	C Type of Service	D PROCEDURES, SERVICES, OR SUPPLIES (Explain Unusual Circumstances) CPT/HCPCS	MODIFIER	E DIAGNOSIS CODE	F $ CHARGES	G DAYS OR UNITS	H EPSDT Family Plan	I EMG	J COB	K RESERVED FOR LOCAL USE
1												
2												
3												
4												
5												
6												

Block 25 **Federal Tax ID Number (required).** Enter the provider's nine-digit federal tax identification number and check the appropriate box in this field; or, in the case of an unincorporated practice, enter the provider's Social Security number.

25. FEDERAL TAX I.D. NUMBER	SSN ☐ EIN ☐

Block 26 **Patient's Account No. (conditionally optional).** Enter the patient's account number as assigned by the provider's accounting system. If you are submitting the claim electronically, you are required to provide a patient account number.

26. PATIENT'S ACCOUNT NO.

Block 27 **Accept Assignment.** Check the appropriate box to indicate whether the provider accepts assignment of benefits. If the supplier is a *participating provider* (PAR), assignment must be accepted for all covered charges. For nonPAR providers, this can be left blank. For Medicaid, check "YES."

27. ACCEPT ASSIGNMENT?
(For govt. claims, see back)
☐ YES   ☐ NO

Block 28   **Total Charge (required).** Total column 24f and enter the total charges in this field.

28. TOTAL CHARGE
$

Block 29   **Amount Paid.** Enter the total amount, if any, that has been paid by the patient. Leave this blank if no payment has been made.

29. AMOUNT PAID
$

Block 30   **Balance Due.** Used when there is secondary insurance. Enter the balance owing as indicated on the explanation of benefits (EOB).

30. BALANCE DUE
$

Block 31   **Signature of Physician or Supplier Including Degrees or Credentials.** Enter the signature of the provider or representative, his or her initials, and the date the form was signed. The signature may be typed, stamped, or handwritten; however, the characters should not fall outside the block.

31. SIGNATURE OF PHYSICIAN OR SUPPLIER
INCLUDING DEGREES OR CREDENTIALS
(I certify that the statements on the reverse
apply to this bill and are made a part thereof.)

SIGNED   DATE

Block 32   **Name and Address of Facility Where Services Were Rendered.** Enter the name and address of the facility where the services were performed if other than the patient's home or physician's office.

32. NAME AND ADDRESS OF FACILITY WHERE SERVICES WERE
RENDERED (If other than home or office)

Block 33   **Physician's, Supplier's Billing Name, Address, Phone Number (required).** Enter the provider's billing name, address, ZIP code, and telephone number. (NOTE: A missing phone number may be cause for rejection.) Also enter the billing number

(from block 24k). Enter the group NPI number, including the two-digit location identifier, if the provider is a member of a group practice (although this is not required in most cases). (Refer to specific third-party payor guidelines.)

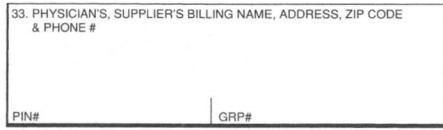

33. PHYSICIAN'S, SUPPLIER'S BILLING NAME, ADDRESS, ZIP CODE
& PHONE #

PIN#   GRP#

Appendix B lists and compares HCFA form requirements for each type of payor.

Preventing Claim Rejection

If a claim form is not sufficiently detailed, complete, and accurate, the insurance company may reject it.

Common Problems Areas

The following is a troubleshooting list of problem areas to check when proofreading claims:

- The patient's name, address, and ID number should be identical to the information printed on the insurance card.
- Patient's birth date and sex should correspond with the medical record.
- The word "NONE" should appear in block 11 if Medicare is the primary payor.
- The referring, consulting, or ordering provider's name and number should be entered in block 17 and 17a, if applicable.
- The physician's correct billing number should be entered in block 24k and again to the right of "PIN #" in block 33.
- The federal **employer identification number (EIN)** should be correct. (Often these numbers contain transpositions.)
- If services were rendered in a location other than the provider's office or the patient's home, the name and address of the facility should be entered in block 32.
- Accept assignment should be checked "Yes" if the physician is PAR.
- Be sure the diagnosis is not missing or incomplete.
- The diagnosis must be coded accurately and must correspond with the treatment.
- The patient must have authorized the release of information and the patient section completed accurately.
- Fees for each charge must be listed.
- The physician signature must be on the form in an accepted manner.

A medical assistant should be proactive rather than reactive when working with claim forms. He or she should make every effort possible to produce clean claims, rather than try to "fix" them after the fact.

The best way to avoid repeated claim rejections is to identify the reason for the rejection or denial. Everyone who has worked with medical insurance knows the process can be frustrating, because there are so many insurance companies, and each has its own requirements as to how the claim form should be completed. One way that a medical assistant might approach this challenge is by creating a "comparison chart" for the major payors. Keeping this chart handy for easy reference can minimize claim problems.

If a service is not covered because it is deemed medically unnecessary or unreasonable, but the Medicare patient still wishes to have the service, the patient should be required to sign an Advance Beneficiary Notice (ABN). This document means that the service cannot be claimed to Medicare, and if the notice is not signed in advance of the service taking place, the charges cannot be collected from the patient.

Medical assistants might consider the following items when creating a work-friendly routine for completing insurance claims:

- If possible, set aside a definite time for completing insurance claims.
- Have a central location for all insurance forms.
- Have readily available the necessary manuals, code books, and other references needed.
- Create a master list of codes most often used by the practice, including fourth and fifth digits, if appropriate. The list should be updated annually and never be considered a replacement for the coding manuals.
- Make it a practice to complete the forms as soon as possible after service is rendered, usually at the end of the day.
- Complete the forms by category (e.g., all Blue Cross, all Medicare)
- If using a computer billing program to print insurance forms, the computer will store insurance information on outstanding claims that can be printed in batches using the CMS-1500 forms. Adjust the printer so that the information prints correctly on the form.
- Transmit claims electronically whenever possible.

At times, a denied claim may involve policy issues beyond the control of the medical assistant. When this happens, he or she should contact the patient and discuss the problem. Normally, it is the patient's responsibility to resolve disputes regarding payment with the payor. The insurance policy is a contract between the company and the insured. However, the provider and those involved with the billing process in the medical facility should have a strong grasp for the types of claims and various insurers handled most often in the facility. If the medical assistant knows that the payor will deny the claims for any reason or that the benefits will not cover a service, the patient should be informed in advance and payment arrangements made.

It is often necessary to send a "tracer" to an insurance company to determine the status of a delinquent insurance claim (Figure 17-8). The accepted practice is to submit the tracer a day or two after the usual turnaround time of the payor.

Checking Claim Status

As mentioned earlier in this chapter, a duplicate copy of all submitted claims should be retained, and the medical assistant should establish some sort of structured routine for following up on pending claims. The Insurance Claim Register (see Figure 17-4), tickler files, and reports from the insurance database all help to keep track of paid and pending claims. The database can also generate an insurance aging report, which is useful in the follow-up of claims that have yet to be paid.

If claims are being submitted electronically either directly or through a clearinghouse, the medical assistant might allow 2 to 3 weeks before reimbursement is expected. For paper claims, allow an additional week or two to allow for necessary manual processing and mailing time. Time lengths between when a claim is submitted and when it is paid varies from payor to payor; however, an experienced medical assistant will soon become familiar with individual payment patterns of third-party payors and their claim turnaround times.

Complementary to a follow-up file, it is also a good idea to create an insurance log (Figure 17-9). An insurance log can be designed to track the status of each claim. By using this kind of tool, the medical assistant can easily see at a glance which claims are becoming delinquent and need follow-up. Any software with spreadsheet capabilities can easily accommodate this task.

Patient Education

The medical assistant needs to be well versed in completing CMS-1500 claim forms, and he or she should be able to explain confusing technical issues to patients in simple, understandable terms. Patients, especially

INSURANCE CLAIM TRACER

INSURANCE COMPANY NAME _____ DATE _____

ADDRESS: _____

PATIENT NAME _____ INSURED: _____

POLICY/CERTIFICATE NUMBER _____ GROUP NAME/NUMBER _____

EMPLOYER NAME AND ADDRESS: _____

DATE OF INITIAL CLAIM SUBMISSION _____ AMOUNT: _____

An inordinate amount of time has passed since submission of our original claim as described above. We have not received a request for additional information and still await payment of this assigned claim. Please review the attached duplicate and process for payment within seven (7) days.

If there is any difficulty with this claim, please check one of these below and return this letter to our office.

Claim pending because: _____
Payment of claim in process: _____
Payment made on claim: Date: _____ To whom: _____
Claim denied: (Reason) _____
Patient notified: Yes _____ No _____
Remarks: _____

Thank you for your assistance in this important matter. Please contact _____ in our office if you have any questions regarding this claim.

Office of: _____ M.D.

Address: _____
_____ TELEPHONE NUMBER: _____

FIGURE 17-8 Example of an insurance claim tracer. (Modified from Fordney M: *Insurance handbook for the medical office,* ed 7. Philadelphia, 2002, WB Saunders, p 266.)

General Physicians, Inc.
5515 Lake Dr.
Chicago, IL 00000

INSURANCE LOG

Patient's Name	Date of Service	Fee	Amt. Paid	Insurance Reimbursements		Amt. Due from Patient	Date	Amt. Reimbursed to Patient	Date	Current Balance
				Date	Amount					
Terry Holmes	2/5/03	$85	0	3/15/03	$75	$10	3/15			
	2/17/03	$30	30	3/30/03	$25	$5	3/30			
	3/24/03	$65	40	4/15/03	$32			$22	5/25/03	0

FIGURE 17-9 Example of an insurance log.

elderly ones, quickly become confused and frustrated over insurance issues—especially Medicare rules and regulations, which change nearly every year.

The medical assistant should attempt to keep patients fully informed of changes in insurance guidelines and patiently explain why some procedures and services are paid and others are not. It is the medical assistant's responsibility to become well acquainted with the various insurance plans used by the patients in their medical facility. When a claim is delayed or rejected, the medical assistant should make every effort to assist the patient or the insured to come to an acceptable resolution.

Whenever possible, the medical assistant must be able to explain insurance submission policies and patient financial responsibilities before the patient receives care. Signatures to authorize insurance billing, supplying information to insurance companies, and accepting assignments of benefits (if appropriate) should be obtained from all new patients.

Legal and Ethical Issues

The practice of medicine and the responsibilities of the medical assistant are greatly affected by the legislative process. It is extremely important to stay current on the laws that affect medicine, and in particular, the completion of the CMS-1500 claim form.

CRITICAL THINKING APPLICATION

An irate patient comes to the office and insists that his insurance claim was not filled out properly, because it was rejected by his insurance company. When she investigates, Kalene discovers that the reason for the rejection was that the insurance company considered the procedure "not medically necessary." What should she do? How can Kalene explain this situation to the patient?

The Health Insurance Portability and Accountability Act of 1996 (HIPAA), developed by the Centers for Medicare and Medicaid Services (CMS), is responsible for the implementation of various acts that protect individuals' health insurance and privacy standards. Medical assistants should familiarize themselves with this important insurance act.

Because of the emphasis on compliance in medical practices today, every medical office must create and implement a plan to identify potential compliance problems and correct them before a liability risk is incurred. It is mandated that all providers avoid fraud and abuse charges by following the regulations and guidelines provided by governmental entities and third-party payors.

SUMMARY OF SCENARIO

Kalene feels that she now has a better understanding of the insurance claims process. Before becoming a medical assisting student, she did not give much thought to what went on behind the scenes when she visited a medical office for her own personal healthcare. She now has a better grasp of what will be expected of her when she begins her career. No matter where she works and whether or not the office is computerized, organization, communication, dedication, and paying attention to detail head the list of requirements of becoming successful.

Kalene has asked for her instructor's help in developing a reference manual for the various third-party payors common to her area. She is looking forward to more hands-on experience in the medical office where she is doing her externship so she can gain as much knowledge as possible in every facet of medical assisting. She is also establishing positive relationships with the staff at her externship site. She feels the knowledge and expertise they share with her will do much to round out her education in the medical field in preparation for her career.

SUMMARY OF LEARNING OBJECTIVES

- For a better understanding of the medical insurance claims process, a medical assistant should familiarize himself or herself with the language and terms used in this area of administrative work.

- Insurance claims can be submitted in two forms: paper and electronic. There are advantages and disadvantages for both; however, electronic claims normally have fewer errors and historically are paid faster.

- Clean claims are those that can be processed and paid quickly; dirty claims contain errors and/or omissions that often result in rejection, thus greatly slowing down the reimbursement process.

- The insurance claim cycle begins when the patient first makes an appointment. The medical assistant should follow an established list of guidelines for CMS-1500 form completion, including obtaining a signed authorization to release information, and assign benefits, if applicable.

- There are 33 blocks in the CMS-1500 claim form and, except for a few blocks that ask for standard information, completion requirements vary from payor to payor. The medical assistant should familiarize himself or herself with each major payor's unique requirements in order to maximize reimbursement.

- Optical character recognition (OCR) scanning is the electronic transfer of information to data banks that simplify and speed up the claims process. Specific guidelines should be followed when completing claims to facilitate OCR scanning. A medical assistant should know and follow these guidelines precisely.

- Claim rejection and delay cost the medical facility time and money. Proven methods of preventing claim rejections should be established and adhered to.

- It is important to track claims once they are submitted. An insurance claim register, or log, can be created and used as one method of tracking claims. A routine should be established for claims follow-up.

KEY INTERNET WEBSITES

- American Association of Medical Assistants
- Centers for Medicare and Medicaid Services
- Electronic Claims Processing Facts
- Health Insurance Portability and Accountability Act
- Sunrise Services: electronic claims clearinghouse
  For active weblinks to each website visit
  http://evolve.elsevier.com/Kinn/

REFERENCES

Fordney M: *Insurance handbook for the medical office*, ed 7. Philadelphia, 2002, WB Saunders.

CHAPTER 18

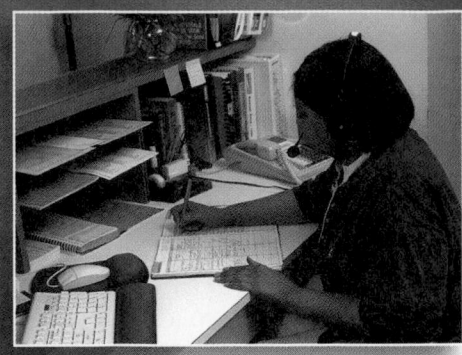

Scenario

The instructor in Beverly Studevant's administrative medical assistant class, Sandra Dickson, realizes that today's medical insurance can be challenging to understand. She asks Teresa Ward, a 25-year veteran in medical insurance billing and collecting, for assistance. Ms. Dickson knows that working with medical insurance can be quite rewarding, and experienced billers find the field financially rewarding as well. Ms. Ward agrees to come to class twice a week to work with Beverly and her classmates, answering their questions and helping them to see that medical insurance is not as complicated as it seems.

Ms. Ward shares her on-the-job experiences with Beverly and her classmates. Through a series of role-playing events, Ms. Ward acquaints the students with the guidelines of the various third-party payors. Beginning with simple case studies, Ms. Ward walks the students through the various stages of third-party reimbursement.

Beverly soon realizes that when insurance billing is broken down into manageable segments of information and applied to real life situations, it becomes an interesting task. Beverly feels almost like a detective as she follows up on claims and checks to ensure that the correct codes are used for diagnoses and procedures. She decides to investigate medical billing as a career and talks with Ms. Dickson about the possibility of performing her externship in a billing office.

Third-Party Reimbursement

Janet Beik
Alexandra P. Young

Learning Objectives

- Define and spell the terms listed in the vocabulary.
- Discuss the purpose of health insurance.
- Differentiate among the various types of insurance policies.
- Explain the numerous classifications of insurance benefits available.
- Demonstrate how insurance benefits are determined.
- Understand the healthcare reform efforts.
- Describe managed care, its history, and its effect on modern medicine.
- Differentiate among the different types of managed care options.
- List and discuss other major third-party payors.
- Interpret the procedure for verifying insurance benefits.
- Discuss the different types of fee schedules.
- Explain the procedure for tracking insurance claims.
- Obtain managed care referrals and precertifications.

National Curriculum Competencies

ADMINISTRATIVE COMPETENCIES

4a. Apply managed care policies and procedures
4b. Apply third-party guidelines
4c. Obtain managed care referrals and precertifications
4g. Use a physician's fee schedule

TRANSDISCIPLINARY COMPETENCIES

1b. Recognize and respond to verbal communication
1c. Recognize and respond to nonverbal communication
2a. Identify and respond to issues of confidentiality
2b. Perform within legal and ethical boundaries
3a. Explain general office policies

Vocabulary

allowed charge The maximum amount of money that many third-party payors allow for a specific procedure or service.

authorization A term used in managed care for an approved referral.

benefits The amount payable by an insurance company for a monetary loss to an individual insured by that company, under each coverage.

birthday rule Under law, when an individual is covered under two insurance policies, the insurance plan of the policyholder whose birthday comes first in the calendar year (month and day—not year) becomes the primary insurance.

capitation Payment method used by many managed care organizations wherein a fixed amount of money is reimbursed to the provider for patients enrolled during a specific period of time, no matter what services received or number of visits made.

Civilian Health and Medical Program of the Uniformed Services (CHAMPUS) A government-sponsored program wherein authorized dependents of military personnel receive medical care. This program is now referred to as TRICARE.

Civilian Health and Medical Program of the Veterans Administration (CHAMPVA) A health benefits program run by the Department of Veterans Affairs (VA) that helps eligible beneficiaries pay the cost of specific healthcare services/supplies.

coinsurance A policy provision frequently found in medical insurance whereby the policyholder and the insurance company share the cost of *covered* losses in a specified ratio (i.e., 80/20 means 80% is covered by the insurer and 20% by the insured).

coordination of benefits (COB) The mechanism used in group health insurance to designate the order in which multiple carriers are to pay benefits to prevent duplicate payments.

copayment A sum of money that is paid at the time of medical service; a form of coinsurance.

deductible A specific amount of money a patient must pay out-of-pocket before the insurance carrier begins paying. Usually this amount ranges from $100 to $500. This deductible amount is met on a yearly or per-incident basis.

dependents The spouse, children, and sometimes domestic partner or other individuals designated by the insured who are covered under a healthcare plan.

disability income insurance Insurance that provides periodic payments to replace income when an insured person is unable to work as a result of illness, injury, or disease.

effective date The date on which an insurance policy or plan takes effect so that benefits are payable.

exclusions Limitations on an insurance contract for which benefits are not payable.

fee for service An established schedule of fees set for services performed by providers and paid by the patient.

government plan An entitlement program or health-care plan that is sponsored and/or subsidized by the state or federal government, such as Medicaid and Medicare.

group policy Insurance written under a policy that covers a number of people under a single master contract issued to their employer or to an association with which they are affiliated.

guarantor The person who is responsible for paying a medical bill.

health insurance Protection in return for periodic *premium* payments, which provides reimbursement of expenses resulting from illness or injury. Includes these forms of insurance: accident, disability income, medical expense, and accidental death and dismemberment. Also known as *accident and health insurance* or *disability income insurance*.

Health Insurance Portability and Accountability Act (HIPAA) The Kassebaum-Kennedy Act designed to improve portability and continuity of health insurance coverage; to combat waste, fraud, and abuse in health insurance and healthcare delivery; to promote the use of medical savings accounts; to improve access to long-term care services and coverage; to simplify the administration of health insurance; and for other purposes.

health maintenance organization (HMO) An organization that provides a wide range of comprehensive healthcare services for a specified group at a fixed periodic payment. HMOs can be sponsored by the government, medical schools, hospitals, employers, labor unions, consumer groups, insurance companies, and hospital-medical plans.

indemnity plan Traditional health insurance plan that pays for all or a share of the cost of covered services, regardless of which physician, hospital, or other licensed healthcare provider is used. Policyholders of indemnity plans and their dependents choose when and where to get healthcare services.

individual policy An insurance policy designed specifically for the use of one person (and his or her dependents), not associated with the amenities of a group policy, namely higher premiums. Often called *personal insurance*.

managed care plans An umbrella term for all healthcare plans that provide healthcare in return for preset monthly payments and coordinated care through a defined network of primary care physicians and hospitals.

medical savings account A tax-deferred bank or savings account combined with a low-premium/high-deductible insurance policy, designed for individuals or families who choose to fund their own healthcare expenses and medical insurance.

medically indigent An individual who may be able to afford to pay for his or her normal daily living expenses but cannot afford adequate healthcare.

medically necessary Phrase indicating that the patient's symptoms and diagnosis justify or support specific medical services or procedures, as determined through a decision-making process used by third-party payors. Also known as *medical necessity*.

participating provider (PAR) A physician or other healthcare provider who enters into a contract with a specific insurance company or program, and by doing so, agrees to abide by certain rules and regulations set forth by that particular third-party payor.

policyholder The individual in whose name an insurance policy is written and who pays the premium; thus the "holder" of the policy.

premium The periodic (monthly, quarterly, or annual) payment of a specific sum of money to an insurance company for which the insurer, in return, agrees to provide certain benefits.

primary diagnosis The condition or chief complaint for which a patient is treated in an outpatient (physician's office or clinic) medical care setting.

principal diagnosis A condition established after study that is chiefly responsible for the admission of a patient to the hospital. Used in coding inpatient hospital insurance claims.

resource-based relative value system (RBRVS) A fee schedule designed to provide national uniform payment of Medicare benefits after being adjusted to reflect the differences in practice costs across geographic areas.

rider A special provision or group of provisions that may be added to a policy to expand or limit the benefits otherwise payable. It may increase or decrease benefits, waive a condition or coverage, or in any other way amend the original contract.

self-insured plan An insurance plan funded by an organization having a large enough employee base that they can afford to fund their own insurance program.

self-referral The act of a patient or insured individual who refers himself or herself to a specialist without requesting the referral to the primary provider, such as a woman seeking an annual gynecological examination. Managed care guidelines may require the patient to report the self-referral.

service benefit plan Plan that provides its benefits in the form of certain surgical and medical services rendered, rather than cash. A service benefit plan is not restricted to a fee schedule.

TRICARE See CHAMPUS.

utilization review A review of individual cases by a committee to make sure that services are medically necessary and to study how providers use medical care resources.

workers' compensation Insurance against liability imposed on certain employers to pay benefits and furnish care to employees who are injured and to pay benefits to dependents of employees killed in the course of or arising out of their employment.

The Purpose of Health Insurance

The purpose of **health insurance** is to help individuals and families offset the costs of medical care. Health insurance is defined as projection against financial losses resulting from sickness or accidental bodily injury. This protection provides payment of **benefits** for covered

sickness or injury. There are various types of health insurance, such as accident insurance, disability income insurance, medical expense insurance, and accidental death and dismemberment insurance.

Increasingly, the trend has been for health insurance policies to cover services that prevent illness or lead to early diagnosis. Health insurance normally covers **medically necessary** services and procedures; elective procedures (such as certain cosmetic surgeries) are usually not included under health insurance policies.

Cost of Coverage

In light of the rising costs of healthcare, to keep **premiums** in check, most insurance policies and programs do not pay all expenses resulting from accident or illness. A premium is the periodic (monthly, quarterly, or annual) payment of a specific sum of money to an insurance company for which the insurer agrees to provide certain benefits. Most policies do not begin to pay medical expenses immediately. The real cost to the individual at the time of treatment includes the following:

- Deductibles
- Copayment or coinsurance
- Costs for noncovered services

A **deductible** is an amount a **policyholder** agrees to pay out-of-pocket, per claim or per accident, toward the total amount of an insured loss before insurance coverage is effective. A deductible amount is stated in the insurance contract and normally ranges from $100 to $500. The higher the deductible, the lower the premium cost. Remember that the patient may not be the **guarantor** for the medical account. Be sure to verify who the guarantor is and obtain written documentation, if necessary, that this person agrees to be responsible for the account.

Coinsurance is a policy provision frequently found in medical insurance whereby the policyholder and the insurance company share the cost of *covered* losses in a specified ratio, such as 80/20 (80% by the insurer and 20% by the insured). Many plans now require a **copayment**, which is a type of coinsurance that is collected at the time of service. Copayments usually range from $10 to $25 for office visits but can vary according to the services rendered.

CRITICAL THINKING APPLICATION

Beverly notes that a patient, Mrs. Brent, underwent a covered procedure that cost $1000, which was the *allowable charge* of the insurance carrier. Mrs. Brent has a policy that provides coverage with a $250 deductible and an 80/20 coinsurance ratio. Mrs. Brent inquires how much of the total bill is her responsibility. How can Beverly calculate this? What would her response be to the patient? How can Beverly help the patient understand this complex information?

Under most circumstances, the deductible must only be paid one time per calendar year; however, some policies have a deductible per occurrence. The medical assistant should always verify the **effective date** on the patient's insurance card. It may be necessary to call the company to verify coverage and **exclusions**.

Some **managed care plans** require a copayment, which is a flat fee per office visit—from $5 to $20 or greater, depending on the charges. Any services or procedures that are not covered under the terms of the policy are the responsibility of the policyholder.

Coordination of Benefits (COB)

Coordination of benefits is a mechanism used in group health insurance to designate the order in which multiple carriers are to pay benefits and prevent duplicate payments. The purpose of COB provisions is to limit benefits to no more than 100% of the cost. If a plan does not have COB provisions, it becomes the primary payor and pays benefits first.

Laws establishing which payor is primary, including the **birthday rule**, were enacted in many states in January 1987. In the case of an employed person who is eligible for Medicare benefits, the employer's group plan is the primary carrier, and Medicare is secondary. However, because of the tremendous increase in health-care premiums in the last few years, a medical assistant might not encounter this phenomenon as much as in the past, because most couples and families are covered by only one policy. Still, some seniors work full-time and are also covered by Medicare benefits, so the medical assistant must be familiar with COB restrictions.

COB follows the rules of the plan that is the primary payor. If both plans have COB provisions, then:

- The policyholder's own plan is primary for that individual. There are some exceptions; for instance, the policyholder may have more than one policy or may be covered by another entity that is required to pay first, such as car insurance in the event of a motor vehicle accident. The primary coverage for **dependents** of the policyholder is determined by the birthday rule. The insurance plan of the policyholder whose birthday comes first in the calendar year (month and day—not year) provides primary coverage for each dependent.

The primary plan for dependents of legally separated or divorced parents is more complicated:

- The birthday rule is in effect if the parent who has custody of the dependent has not remarried. If the custodial parent has remarried, that parent's plan is primary for that dependent.
- If one parent has been decreed by the court to be the responsible party, that parent's policy is primary. This is not always the parent with legal custody of the child.
- If one of the plans originated in a state not having the COB law, the plan that did originate in a state having a COB law will determine the order of benefits.

All of this emphasizes the need to determine whether there is a birthday rule in the state in which the medical assistant is employed. To avoid complications and confusion later, it is important to establish primary and secondary payors before the patient is treated.

The Availability of Health Insurance

Health insurance is available to the majority of persons in this country through group, individual, or prepaid plans. In addition, many people are covered by government plans or entitlement programs. However, although health insurance might be available, it is not always affordable. A recent survey revealed that more than 46 million Americans—roughly 18% of the population—have no regular source for obtaining medical care, and lack of health insurance was a major obstacle.

Group Policies

Insurance written under a group policy covers a number of people under a single master contract issued to their employer or to an association with which they are affiliated. Group coverage usually provides greater benefits at lower premiums because of the large pool of people from whom premiums are collected. Physical examinations are normally not required and preexisting conditions are often waived. Often the employee shares the cost of coverage through payroll deductions.

Recently some smaller companies are finding themselves hard pressed to provide group coverage to their employees because of increasing premiums. Many have found it necessary to circumvent this problem by increasing deductibles and limiting eligibility to full-time workers only (over 30 hours per week). Congressional efforts have increased to find available and affordable health insurance for uninsured individuals, families, and people who lose their coverage as a result of job changes.

Individual Policies

Individuals who do not qualify for inclusion in a group or government-sponsored plan may apply to companies that offer individual policies—often called *personal insurance*. The applicant is normally required to fill out an extended health questionnaire and undergo a physical examination before acceptance. Unlike group policies, there is a risk that coverage may be denied, or the individual may have to accept a **rider**, or limitation, on benefits the policy will cover. Premiums are almost always higher with individual policies and often the benefits are less.

Government Plans

The federal government first became responsible for insuring a large group of people in 1956 with passage of Public Law 569. This law authorized dependents of military personnel to receive treatment by civilian physicians at the expense of the government. The program administering these benefits became the **Civilian Health and Medical Program of the Uniformed Services (CHAMPUS)**, which today is known as TRICARE (discussed in detail later in this chapter).

In 1965 the federal government provided for another group—the **medically indigent**—through a program that is still known as Medicaid. Title XIX of Public Law 89-97, under the Social Security Amendments of 1965, provided for agreements with states for assistance from the federal government to provide medical care for people meeting specific eligibility criteria.

On July 1, 1966, Medicare was established under the Social Security Administration as a national health insurance program for persons age 65 and older. The scope of coverage increased in 1973 to include Medicare coverage for disabled persons younger than age 65 receiving Social Security benefits, railroad retirees, and civil service retirees. This also included disabled workers of any age, disabled widows, disabled dependent widowers, adults disabled before age 18 whose parents are eligible or are retired on Social Security benefits, children and adults with end-stage renal disease, and living kidney donors (including all expenses related to the kidney transplant).

The passage of the Health Maintenance Organization Act in 1973 provided for federal aid to health insurance prepayment plans that met certain criteria. This brought about a rapid growth of the **health maintenance organization (HMO)**, which is an organization that provides comprehensive healthcare to an enrolled group for a fixed periodic payment. Some of these plans pay by **capitation**, which means that the provider is paid a fixed amount for each individual enrolled in the plan during a specified time period, regardless of the number of services provided to the patient. The provider still only collects the contracted rate, even if expenses cost much more than that rate for the time period.

Title VI of the Social Security Amendments Act of 1983 contained the prospective payment system (PPS) for hospitals, which was the beginning of the radical restructuring of the payment system to hospitals for Medicare inpatient services.

The most fundamental change in determining physicians' fees under Medicare since its inception was the **resource-based relative value scale (RBRVS)** reimbursement system put into effect in 1992.

Many large groups of people are covered by government plans or entitlement programs. A patient who is older than age 65 is covered by Part B of Medicare. A medically indigent patient may be eligible for Medicaid with or without Medicare. Dependents of military personnel are covered by **TRICARE** (formerly known as CHAMPUS); surviving spouses and dependent children of veterans who died as a result of service-related disabilities are covered by the **Civilian Health and Medical Program of the Veterans Administration (CHAMPVA)**.

Some wage earners are protected against the loss of wages and the cost of medical care resulting from an occupational accident, disease, or disability through **workers' compensation** insurance. An individual may collect benefits for health expenses from an automobile policy if the injury is related to a car accident or other such loss.

Self-Insured Plans

Many large companies or organizations have a big enough employee base that they choose to fund their own insurance program. This is called a **self-insured plan**. Technically, a self-funded plan is not insurance by true definition. The employer pays employee healthcare costs from the firm's own coffers. Recent surveys indicate about 40% of workers with employment-based health insurance are enrolled in plans that their employers self-insure. Usually benefits and premium costs under self-insured plans are similar to group plans. Self-funded plans tend to work best for companies that are large enough to offer good coverage, reasonable premium rates, and are able to pay large claims for expensive medical services. Often a third-party administrator (TPA) handles paperwork and claim payments for a self-insured group.

Medical Savings Account

In 1996 Congress made tax-free Medical Savings Accounts (MSAs) available to 750,000 American workers and their families. This is a type of self-insurance. Under a provision of the Kassebaum-Kennedy health insurance reform bill, small companies (with 50 or fewer employees), self-employed persons, and the uninsured can purchase health insurance policies and make tax-free deposits to an MSA. They can use their MSA money to pay small and routine healthcare expenses, reserving a high-deductible medical insurance policy to pay large, catastrophic expenses. Money that remains in the account at year's end earns tax-free interest. People can also elect to use MSA money to pay their health insurance premiums during a job change, which should reduce *job lock*, a situation in which people do not change jobs for fear of losing their health insurance.

There are both advantages and disadvantages to an MSA, and it is wise to investigate it thoroughly to learn its values and limitations.

Types of Insurance Benefits

An insurance package is tailored to the needs of each individual or group policy, and the combinations of benefits are limitless. A policy may contain one or any combination of the following benefits.

Hospitalization

Hospital coverage pays the cost of all or part of the insured person's hospital room and board and specific hospital services, such as the costs involved in having surgery in a hospital. Hospital insurance policies frequently set a maximum amount payable per day and a maximum number of days of hospital care. Some insurance companies require that the hospital be an accredited or a licensed hospital. Most hospital plans exclude admission for diagnostic studies.

Surgical

Surgical coverage pays all or part of a surgeon's fee; some plans also pay for an assistant surgeon. Surgery includes any incision or excision, removal of foreign bodies, aspiration, suturing, and reduction of fractures. Surgery may be accomplished in a hospital, physician's office, or elsewhere. The insurer frequently provides the subscriber with a surgical fee schedule that establishes the amount the insurer will pay for commonly performed procedures.

Basic Medical

Basic medical coverage pays all or part of a physician's fee for nonsurgical services, including hospital, home, and office visits. Usually there is a deductible amount payable by the patient as well as a copayment or coinsurance each time service is received. The insurance plan may include a provision for diagnostic laboratory, radiology, and pathology fees. Some medical plans do not cover routine physical examinations when the patient does not have a specific complaint or illness.

Major Medical

Major medical insurance (formerly called *catastrophic coverage*) provides protection against especially large medical bills resulting from catastrophic or prolonged illnesses. It may be a supplement to basic medical coverage or a comprehensive integrated program providing both basic and major medical protection. (For additional information on this topic, see the section on Disability Programs.)

Disability (Loss of Income) Protection

Weekly or monthly cash benefits are provided to employed policyholders who become unable to work as a result of an accident or illness. Many disability policies do not start payment until after a specified number of days or until a certain number of sick leave days have been used. Payment is made directly to the individual and is intended to replace lost income resulting from an illness or other disability. It is not intended for payment of specific medical bills, and it should not be confused with a regular insurance plan, entitlement program, or workers' compensation, in which compensation is provided for an employee who is injured on the job or cannot work as a result of a job-related illness or other disability.

Dental Care

Dental coverage is included in many *fringe benefit* packages. Some policies are based on a copayment and incentive program, in which preventive dental care (such as cleaning and x-ray films) is covered 100%, with most other coverage paid at 50%.

Vision Care

Vision care insurance may include reimbursement for all or a percentage of the cost for refraction, lenses, and frames.

Medicare Supplement

Many Medicare beneficiaries purchase a supplemental health insurance policy to help defray medical costs not covered, or only partially covered, by Medicare. Federal regulations now require that Medicare supplement contracts must be uniform in benefits to avoid confusion for the purchaser.

Special Risk Insurance

Special risk insurance protects a person in the event of a certain type of accident, such as an automobile or airplane crash, or for certain diseases, such as tuberculosis or cancer. There is usually a maximum benefit.

Liability Insurance

There are many types of liability insurance, including automobile, business, and homeowners' policies. Liability policies often include benefits for medical expenses payable to individuals who are injured in the insured person's home or car, without regard to the insured person's actual legal liability for the accident.

Life Insurance

Life insurance provides payment of a specified amount on an insured's death, either to his or her estate or to a designated beneficiary, or in the case of an endowment policy, to the policyholder at a specified date. Life insurance policies sometimes provide monthly cash benefits if the policyholder becomes permanently and totally disabled. Sometimes the proceeds from life insurance are used to meet the expenses of the insured person's last illness.

Long-Term Care Insurance

Long-term care insurance is a relatively new type that covers a continuum of broad-ranged maintenance and health services to chronically ill, disabled, or mentally retarded persons. Services may be provided on an inpatient (rehabilitation facility, nursing home, or mental hospital), outpatient, or at-home basis. The **Health Insurance Portability and Accountability Act (HIPAA)** of 1996 gives some federal income tax advantages to people who buy certain long-term care insurance policies.

How Benefits Are Determined

Insurance benefits may be determined and paid in one of several ways:
- By indemnity schedules
- By service benefit plans
- By determination of the usual, customary, and reasonable fee
- By relative value studies

Indemnity Schedules

Indemnity plans are traditional health insurance plans that pay for all or a share of the cost of covered services, regardless of which physician, hospital, or other licensed healthcare provider is used. Policyholders of indemnity plans and their dependents choose when and where to get healthcare services. In exchange for premiums that members pay, the indemnity plan reimburses members or the provider when claims are filed. The subscriber is often given a schedule of indemnities (fee schedule) when the policy is purchased, which explains the benefit payment amounts of the policy.

Indemnity plans typically have an annual deductible before the plan pays anything. Usually members also must pay a percentage of each charge—coinsurance. Most indemnity plans have an annual "out-of-pocket limit" on the amount members must pay for coinsurance payments. Because physicians and other providers are paid for each office visit, test, procedure, or other service they deliver, indemnity plans are often called **fee-for-service** plans.

This type of plan takes the major expense out of medical bills and helps keep premium costs down. The amount of premiums often determines the schedule of benefits. Indemnity benefits are usually paid to the person insured unless that person has authorized payment directly to the provider.

Service Benefit Plans

In a **service benefit plan** the insuring company agrees to pay for certain surgical or medical services without additional cost to the person insured. There is no set fee schedule.

In a service benefit plan, surgery with complications would warrant a higher fee than an uncomplicated procedure would. Premiums are sometimes higher for this type of coverage, but often payments are larger. Frequently payment of benefits is sent directly to the physician and is considered full payment for services rendered.

Usual, Customary, and Reasonable (UCR) Fee

Some insurance companies agree to pay on the basis of all or a percentage of the physician's usual, customary, and reasonable fee. Charges for a specific service are compared to a database of charges for the same service to other patients by the same type of physician, and to patients by other physicians performing same or similar services in the same geographic area. The insurance company determines whether the charge is usual, customary, and reasonable, and any amount over this **allowed charge** will not be paid.

Resource-Based Relative Value Scale

The RBRVS is one of the outcomes of the Medicare Physician Payment Reform that was enacted in the Omnibus Budget Reconciliation Act of 1989 (usually called *OBRA '89*). Since the beginning of Medicare, Part B of the program has paid physicians using a fee-for-service system based on customary, prevailing, and reasonable charges. The RBRVS, effective in 1992, changed this. The RBRVS consists of three parts:

1. Physician work
2. Charge-based professional liability expenses
3. Charge-based overhead

The physician work component includes the degree of effort invested by a physician in a particular service or procedure and the time it consumed. The professional liability and overhead components are computed by the Centers for Medicare and Medicaid Services (CMS).

The fee schedule is designed to provide national uniform payments after being adjusted to reflect the differences in practice costs across geographic areas. The fee schedule includes a conversion factor, which is a single national number applied to all services paid under the fee schedule. Conversion factors change according to Congressional enactment. (For more information on RBRVS, see the section on RBRVS under Fee Schedules.)

Healthcare Reform Efforts

Healthcare reform is not a new concept. It has recently been thrust to the forefront of the news since the advent of managed care. Changes in the way people in this country pay for healthcare began in the early 1900s, when Theodore Roosevelt made national health insurance one of the major issues during his 1912 presidential campaign.

In the middle of the twentieth century, it became apparent that some kind of taxpayer-funded healthcare program was needed for the growing elderly population. During President Lyndon Johnson's term in office, federal legislation in the form of Medicare for the aged and Medicaid for the indigent was enacted.

A variety of national health insurance plans were debated in Congress in the 1960s and 1970s. In 1973 Congress passed the Health Maintenance Organization (HMO) Act, which provided grants to employers who set up HMOs.

In the 1980s and 1990s politicians again proposed a variety of national health insurance plans. One such plan was known as "pay or play," because it would have forced employers to provide health insurance or pay into a national fund that would cover uninsured workers. A second plan, championed by President George Bush in 1991, would have provided tax breaks, vouchers, and other incentives to employers to extend health insurance benefits. A third proposal was based on the Canadian model of nationalized healthcare, which was opposed by most doctors and the insurance industry.

When President Bill Clinton took office in 1993, healthcare reform was a major issue on his platform. His proposals included a national health insurance program that would have ultimately provided coverage for most U.S. citizens, but the program was opposed by many insurance companies, medical entities, and small businesses.

In 1999 President Clinton and Congress struggled over the development of a "patient bill of rights" to protect people from service denials and other HMO limitations. Now many individual states have developed their own health insurance alternatives by using managed healthcare systems that monitor the type of services offered, setting fees for each service.

Efforts of healthcare reform continue today. Much activity is alive at the state level, where legislatures are gradually making changes in healthcare costs and delivery. A few states are enacting price control reform on prescription drugs, and many have granted patients greater rights relating to their health maintenance organizations—in some cases, the right to sue. Efforts are underway, and dedicated individuals and groups will make the difference in tomorrow's healthcare delivery methods.

CRITICAL THINKING APPLICATION

There is so much to learn in the medical insurance field, and everything keeps changing—almost on a daily basis. How can Beverly keep current on healthcare issues and reform? How can Beverly advise patients to keep abreast of the changes in their own personal healthcare coverage—such as Medicare?

The Advent of Managed Care

What is managed care? **Managed care** is an umbrella term for all healthcare plans that provide healthcare in return for preset scheduled payments and coordinated care through a defined network of physicians and hospitals. *Managed care* refers to healthcare plans that provide healthcare in return for scheduled payments and coordinate healthcare through a defined network of primary care physicians, hospitals, and other providers.

Under managed care, a medical group, such as an HMO or an independent practice association (IPA), is contracted to assume some of the responsibilities of the insurance company, such as claims processing, provider relations, member services, utilization review, and eligibility. A primary care physician (PCP) is usually selected by the patient (although not all managed care plans force the patient to choose a primary provider), and that physician manages all patient services. Managed care is essentially an attempt to lower healthcare costs in this country.

The History of Managed Care

Managed healthcare evolved in the 1970s in response to rising healthcare costs and national interest in new, cost-effective ways for providing access to quality healthcare. Membership in managed care plans is growing rapidly and is expanding into areas of the nation that previously did not have these types of healthcare delivery system models. An estimated 58 million Americans are enrolled in HMOs, and another 81 million are enrolled in other types of managed care plans. Managed healthcare plans may take many forms, ranging from staff/group model HMOs, to loose IPAs, to preferred provider organizations (PPOs).

The phenomenon of managed healthcare, however, is not new. The organization that is now Kaiser Permanente, one of the largest and best-known managed care systems in the nation, began during the Great Depression when an inventive young surgeon named Sidney R. Garfield looked at the thousands of men involved in building the Los Angeles Aqueduct and saw an opportunity. He borrowed money to build Contractors General Hospital, a 12-bed hospital in the middle of the Mojave Desert, 6 miles from a tiny town called Desert Center, and began treating sick and injured workers. But financing was difficult, and Dr. Garfield was having trouble getting insurance companies to pay his bills in a timely fashion. To compound matters, not all of the men had insurance.

Dr. Garfield refused to turn away any sick or injured worker, so he often was left with no payment at all for his services. In no time, the hospital's expenses far exceeded its income. This is when Harold Hatch entered the picture. He suggested that the insurance companies pay Dr. Garfield a fixed amount per day, per covered worker, up front. This "prepayment" idea solved the hospital's immediate money problems. Dr. Garfield also began emphasizing maintaining health and safety as opposed to merely treating injuries and sickness, which gave birth to "preventive" healthcare. For an additional nickel a day, workers could also receive coverage for non–job-related medical problems. Thousands of workers enrolled, and Dr. Garfield's hospital became a financial success.

Hearing of Dr. Garfield's success with the Southern California desert project, Henry Kaiser persuaded him to set up a similar plan for the workers on the Grand Coulee Dam and later for workers and their families at the shipyards in San Francisco and other Kaiser-managed facilities. At the peak of World War II, there were about 200,000 members in the plans. Health plans continued to grow and new ones opened across the country. Today the organization known as Kaiser Permanente serves nearly 9 million members.

The Health Maintenance Organization Act of 1973

Although managed care organizations have been in existence since the 1920s, it was not until the early 1970s that the federal government began to regulate managed care as a model of healthcare delivery. In 1973 Congress passed legislation creating federal standards and encouraging the expansion of HMOs. The Health Maintenance Organization Act of 1973 defined the characteristics of an HMO to include the following:

- An organized system for providing healthcare
- An agreed set of basic and supplemental health maintenance and treatment services
- A voluntary group of enrollees.

In 1976 Congress established the first specific federal requirement for Medicare contracts with HMOs and other managed care organizations. However, it was not until the 1980s that corporate America began to move its work force out of fee-for-service plans and into managed care arrangements. Corporate payments for health insurance benefits began to decline in the early 1990s.

The Effects of Managed Care on Modern Medicine

What impact has managed care had on healthcare costs? Managed care payors attempt to contain costs by limiting where patients can obtain services, from whom they receive these services, and what particular kinds of services they receive. Some managed care plans limit a patient's access to specialty care and simultaneously negotiate reduced payments to providers for services.

Managed care has been met with considerable controversy, and there are pros and cons that must be considered. It is important that medical assistants be well versed in the various types of managed care plans to fully understand their impact on healthcare costs.

Advantages of managed care include the following:
- Healthcare costs are usually contained.
- There are established fee schedules.
- Authorized services are usually paid.
- Most preventive medical treatment is covered.
- Patients' out-of-pocket expenses tend to be smaller than traditional insurance.

Disadvantages of managed care include the following:
- Access to specialized care and referrals can be limited.
- Physician choices in treatment of patients can be limited.
- The amount of paperwork may be increased.
- Treatment may be delayed because of preauthorization requirements.
- Reimbursement is historically less than that through traditional insurance.

Models of Managed Care

Health Maintenance Organizations

An HMO is an organization that provides healthcare in return for preset payments over a specified time period from its members. HMOs contract with healthcare providers (physicians, hospitals, and other health professionals), to provide services to plan members through a network of doctors, hospitals, and other healthcare professionals. HMO members must use these specific providers in order for their healthcare needs to be covered. Several types of HMOs are as follows:
- A *prepaid group practice model*, in which physicians form a group and contract with an HMO. These physicians' group practices are not owned by the HMO, but operate independently and contract with an HMO to provide medical treatment to enrolled members. Although the physicians work for a salary, it is paid by their own independent group, not by the administrators of the health plan.
- A *staff model*, in which the facility is owned by the HMO, and the health plan hires physicians directly and pays their salaries. Routine medical care is given by, or authorized by, the patient's PCP.
- An *independent practice association* is a closed-panel HMO. Instead of maintaining its own staff and clinic buildings, an IPA contracts with independently practicing physicians who continue to practice in their own offices. The IPA may pay each doctor a set amount per patient in advance (*capitation*), or fees charged for services to group members may be billed directly to the IPA rather than to the patient. Fees for services to nonmember patients are handled the same as any other fee for service. The physician may be contracted with several IPAs.

- An *exclusive provider organization* (EPO) combines features of HMOs (e.g., enrolled population, limited provider panel, gatekeepers, utilization management, capitated provider reimbursement, and authorization system) and PPOs (e.g., flexible benefit design, negotiated fees, and fee-for-service payments). It is referred to as "exclusive" because employers agree not to contract with any other plan. Members must choose medical care from network providers, with certain exceptions for emergency or out-of-area services. If a patient decides to seek care outside the network, he or she generally will not be reimbursed for the cost of treatment. Technically, many HMOs can be considered EPOs; however, EPOs are regulated under insurance statutes rather than federal and state HMO regulations.

Preferred Provider Organizations

The PPO model of managed healthcare preserves the fee-for-service concept that many physicians prefer. An insurer representing its clients contracts with a group of providers (physicians) who agree on a predetermined list of charges for all services including those for complex and usual procedures.

The care is not prepaid. Usually there are deductibles or coinsurance payments of 20% to 25% of the predetermined charge that the patient pays; the insurer pays the balance. A provider who joins a PPO does not need to alter the manner of providing care and continues to treat and bill the patients on a fee-for-service basis. When a patient covered under a PPO plan comes for treatment, the physician treats the patient and bills the PPO.

Technically, PPOs are not HMOs, but they do have more patient care management than regular indemnity insurance plans. PPOs furnish their subscribers with a list of member-providers from which subscribers can receive healthcare at PPO rates. Rates are quite often lower than those charged to non-PPO patients. If a patient goes to a physician who is not in the PPO network, the out-of-pocket cost is higher.

CRITICAL THINKING APPLICATION

The physicians in the practice in which Beverly is doing her externship are not members of a PPO that is well known in that geographic area. Many patients are confused when they have to pay a larger out-of-pocket fee for their medical services. How can Beverly explain the reason for larger out-of-pocket fees to nonmember patients?

More Third-Party Payors

Blue Cross and Blue Shield

Blue Cross and Blue Shield (BC/BS) is America's oldest and largest system of independent health insurers. It began in 1929 when an executive at Baylor University in Dallas came up with a plan for teachers to budget for their future hospital bills. The teachers paid $6 a year into a fund and were, in turn, guaranteed 21 days of free hospital care. Within 10 years the American Hospital Association officially embraced the concept of prepaid hospital care and symbolized their new program with a blue cross.

At the same time, workers in lumber camps in the Northwest developed a similar approach to deal with frequent logging accidents. Camp owners provided medical care for workers by paying physicians monthly fees for which a doctor would provide all the care the workers needed. Physicians formed groups, or medical service bureaus, which were linked to specific employers. The bureaus were identified with a blue shield, and they too quickly expanded in popularity.

Originally, Blue Cross plans were formed to cover the cost of hospital care, whereas Blue Shield plans were established to cover physicians' services. Today both brands represent the full spectrum of healthcare coverage. Now there are local Blue Cross plans operating in all 50 states, the District of Columbia, Canada, Puerto Rico, and Jamaica.

BC/BS no longer operates at the national level; plans are locally based, and they maintain their commitment to serving community needs. Each plan operates independently in its own service area, where it has the flexibility to respond to local healthcare needs. Plans can be organized as not-for-profit corporations or as for-profit companies, depending on the general business climate, their capital needs, and the regulatory environment.

BC/BS offers incentive contracts to healthcare providers. If the provider chooses to sign a member contract, he or she becomes a **participating provider (PAR)**. The healthcare provider then agrees to accept BC/BS reimbursement as payment in full for covered services. In turn, BC/BS agrees to reimburse providers directly and in a shorter time.

BC/BS identification cards carry the subscriber's name and identification number with a three-character alphabetical prefix. The letters are an important part of the number and must be included on the claim form.

MEDICAID

Title XIX of Public Law 89–97 under the Social Security Amendments of 1965 provides for agreements with states for assistance from the federal government in providing healthcare for the medically indigent. All states and the District of Columbia have Medicaid programs, but wide variations may exist among these programs.

The federal government provides basic funding to the state, after which the states individually elect whether to provide funds for extension of benefits. The state determines the type and extent of medical care that will be covered within the minimum requirements established by the federal government. Some local areas and states are developing HMOs that serve only patients who qualify for Medicaid.

A physician may accept or decline to treat Medicaid patients. The physician who does accept Medicaid

patients automatically agrees to accept Medicaid payment as payment in full for covered services. The patient cannot be billed for the difference between the Medicaid fee and the physician's normal fee. The patient can be billed for any services that are not covered by Medicaid. Eligibility for benefits is determined by the respective states.

Examples of individuals who qualify for benefits include the following:
- Persons receiving certain types of federal and state aid
- Persons who are medically needy
- Recipients of Aid to Families with Dependent Children
- Persons who receive Supplemental Security Income (SSI)
- For Qualified Medicare Beneficiaries (QMBs), Medicaid pays for Medicare Part B premiums, deductibles, and coinsurance for qualified low-income elderly
- Persons in institutions or other long-term care in nursing facilities and intermediate care facilities
- Medicaid purchase of COBRA coverage (low income persons who lose employer health insurance coverage)

A benefits identification card (BIC), which looks like a white credit card, or a sticker or label showing proof of eligibility is usually issued to the beneficiary. The BIC is verified by a point of service (POS) device similar to a credit card verification machine. The medical assistant must verify coverage each time the patient comes into the office before being seen if the state uses a BIC.

MEDICARE

Medicare is a federal health insurance program for:
- People 65 years of age and older
- People who are permanently disabled or blind
- People receiving dialysis for permanent kidney failure or who have had a kidney transplant

Medicare was developed in 1966 as a national health insurance program for the elderly. Before Medicare, only 50% of the nation's elderly had any health insurance. Today Medicare is the world's largest insurance program. It serves more than 38 million older and disabled Americans.

Medicare is administered by the CMS (formerly HCFA), a division of the Department of Health and Human Services (DHHS), and is based on laws enacted by Congress. Medicare has two parts, Part A and Part B.

Part A: Hospital Insurance. Retired people 65 years of age and older and people who receive monthly Social Security or railroad retirement checks are automatically enrolled for hospital insurance benefits and pay no premiums for this insurance. Part A covers:
- Inpatient hospital
- Skilled nursing facilities
- Home healthcare
- Hospice services

Part A is financed with special contributions deducted from employed individuals' salaries with matching contributions from their employers. These sums are collected, along with regular Social Security contributions, from wages and self-employment income earned during a person's working years. There is a deductible that a hospitalized patient must pay toward hospital expenses.

Medicare health insurance cards (Figure 18-1) identify whether a person has Part A alone or has both Part A and Part B insurance. A patient whose Medicare claim number ends in the letter *A* will have the same Social Security number and Medicare number. If a person has different Social Security numbers and Medicare numbers, the Medicare number ends in a *B* or a *D*. The letters after the Social Security number denote the patient's status, such as wage earner (A), widow (D), or other designations.

Part B: Medical Insurance. Persons who are eligible for Part A are also eligible for Part B, but they must apply for this coverage and pay a monthly premium. Some federal employees and former federal employees who are not eligible for Social Security benefits and Part A may still enroll in Part B. Certain disabled persons younger than age 65 years are also eligible. Part B covers:

- Outpatient hospital care
- Durable medical equipment
- Physicians' services
- Other medical services

A patient with Medicare Part B must meet an annual deductible before benefits become available, after which Medicare pays 80% of the *covered* benefits. Usually the physician *accepts assignment* of benefits for Medicare patients and is paid directly. In these cases the physician must accept the payment that Medicare allows and bills the patient for 20% of the charge allowed by Medicare. If the physician does not accept assignment, the patient must pay the entire bill (which cannot be greater than the limit set by Medicare for nonparticipating physicians), and the patient will receive a reimbursement check directly from Medicare.

Many Medicare enrollees also carry private supplemental insurance that pays the deductible and the 20% copayment not covered by Medicare.

TRICARE/CHAMPUS

TRICARE is the Department of Defense and military's comprehensive healthcare program for family members of active duty personnel, military retirees and their eligible family members under the age of 65, and survivors of all uniformed services. Before January 1994, this program was known as CHAMPUS, which stood for **Civilian Health and Medical Program of the Uniformed Services**, created in 1966 under Public Law 89-614.

The TRICARE program is managed by the military in partnership with civilian hospitals and clinics. It is designed to expand access to healthcare, ensure high-quality care, and promote medical readiness. All military hospitals and clinics are part of the TRICARE program and offer high-quality healthcare at low costs to plan users.

To be eligible for TRICARE, an individual must be a TRICARE/CHAMPVA recipient and entitled to retired, retainer, or equivalent pay and listed in the Defense Department's Defense Enrollment Eligible Reporting System (DEERS), which is a computerized data bank that lists all active and retired service members. Coverage is also available for a TRICARE-eligible spouse under age 65, and dependent, unmarried children under age 21 (23 if in college). Eligible spouses and children of active-duty service members may enroll as well as TRICARE-eligible widows, widowers, and ex-spouses (who have not remarried).

There are three choices under TRICARE:

- TRICARE Prime: The Department of Defense's managed care option, similar to a civilian HMO
- TRICARE Extra: A preferred provider network option
- TRICARE Standard: A traditional fee-for-service option formerly known as CHAMPUS

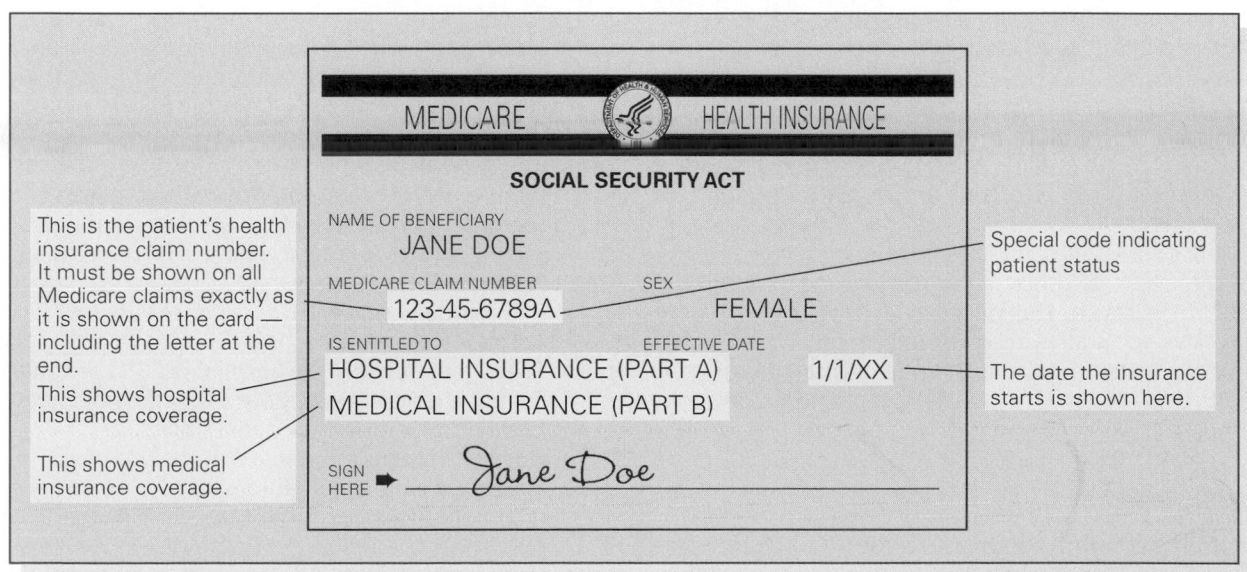

FIGURE 18-1 Medicare health insurance identification card. (From Fordney M: *Insurance handbook for the medical office*, ed 7. Philadelphia, 2002, WB Saunders, p 354.)

CHAMPVA

In 1973 a program similar to TRICARE/CHAMPUS was established for the spouses and dependent children of veterans suffering total, permanent, service-connected disabilities, and for surviving spouses and dependent children of veterans who had died as a result of service-related disabilities. This program, the **Civilian Health and Medical Program of the Veterans Administration (CHAMPVA)**, is a health benefits program in which the Department of Veterans Affairs (VA) shares with eligible beneficiaries the cost of certain healthcare services and supplies. The administration of CHAMPVA is centralized to VA's Health Administration Center (HAC) in Denver, Colorado.

After eligibility for CHAMPVA has been determined and identification cards are issued, the insured persons may obtain covered services and supplies from any provider who is appropriately licensed or certified to perform the services offered. Exceptions include certain mental health categories and free-standing ambulatory surgical centers.

Workers' Compensation

All state legislatures have passed workers' compensation laws to protect wage earners against the loss of wages and the cost of medical care resulting from occupational accident or disease. State laws differ as to the classes of employees included and the benefits provided.

No state's workers' compensation laws cover all employees. However, if a patient says that he or she was injured in the workplace or is suffering from a work-associated illness, the medical assistant should check with the patient's employer to verify the insurance coverage.

Compensation benefits include medical care benefits, weekly income replacement benefits for temporary disability, permanent disability settlements, and survivor benefits when applicable. The provider of service (e.g., doctor, hospital, therapist) accepts the workers' compensation payment as payment in full and does not bill the patient. Time limitations are set for the prompt reporting of workers' compensation cases. The employee is obligated to promptly notify the employer; the employer, in turn, must notify the insurance company and must refer the employee to a source of medical care.

In some states the employer and insurance company have the right to select the physician treating the patient. In essence, the purpose of workers' compensation laws is to provide prompt medical care to an injured or ill worker so that the person may be restored to health and return to full earning capacity in as short a time as possible.

Disability Programs

Disability income insurance is a form of health insurance that provides periodic payments to an individual to replace income (actual or presumed) when a sickness, injury, or disability (which is not a work-related condition) results in the insured being unable to work. A disability insurance policy can be obtained through employer-sponsored and/or government-funded programs, or private policies can be purchased through a commercial insurance company.

Mandated Programs. Several states require that employees be covered by nonindustrial disability (time loss) insurance. A small percentage (ranging from 0.3% to 1.2%) of the employee's salary may be deducted to cover the cost of this insurance. All regular employees, part-time or full-time, are covered until they retire.

Weekly benefits are based on the employee's salary and calculated using a predetermined formula. There is a waiting period before benefits begin (usually 7 days) and a time limit ranging from 26 to 52 weeks for benefits to continue.

Voluntary Programs. In states that do not have mandated disability insurance, employees or groups may solicit coverage from a commercial carrier.

Commercial Insurance

Many people are covered by health insurance issued by private (commercial) insurance companies. Physicians and medical societies control neither the premiums paid nor the benefits received from such policies. For traditional types of policies, payment is normally made to the subscriber unless the subscriber has authorized that payment be made directly to the physician.

Precertification and Preauthorization

Most insurance companies require precertification or preauthorization, usually within 24 hours, when a patient is going to be hospitalized or undergo certain procedures. Additionally, most managed care systems require preauthorization for a patient to be referred to a specialist or even for certain laboratory tests or other procedures.

It is necessary when a new patient makes an appointment to ask what type of insurance the patient has. If the patient belongs to an HMO, the medical assistant should check that plan contract for precertification or preauthorization requirements (Procedure 18-1). If you are not sure of the requirements, call the plan's contact number and keep a record of the requirements on a reference guide that you prepare with the following information:

- Plan name
- Address
- Telephone number (or numbers)
- Name and phone number of contact person
- Copayment amount or deductible
- Hospital benefits for inpatient and outpatient surgery
- Second opinion, preauthorization requirements, telephone number, and assistant surgeon with percentage
- Participating hospitals, radiology service providers, laboratories, and physicians

PROCEDURE **18-1**

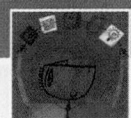

Obtaining Precertification

GOAL: Using the information in the case study, obtain precertification from a patient's HMO for requested services/procedures.

EQUIPMENT AND SUPPLIES

- Patient record
- Precertification form
- Patient's insurance information
- Telephone/FAX machine
- Pen/pencil

CASE STUDY

PATIENT NAME: Kasandra J. Schaffer 4444 Morning Glory Drive Creston, IL xxxxx	PATIENT NO. 54398 SS# XXX-22-3333
DATE OF VISIT: 9/22/XX	DATE OF BIRTH 11/21/XX

S. This elementary school teacher returns to the office today for follow-up of the course of treatment prescribed and testing from her initial visit one month ago. (See detailed H&P from 10/16/xx.) She reports no improvement. Her symptoms, including constant exhaustion, ringing in the ears, sinus problems, pain in the joints, sore throat, gastrointestinal "problems," and decreased libido persist. She reports she is keeping to her prescribed diet.

O. Vitals are within normal limits. HEENT: Negative; Heart RRR, Lungs CTA. Abdomen: Soft, nontender. Bowel sounds are normal. Initial testing, including blood, urine, stool and a mental status exam were all within normal limits. Results of these tests were reviewed with the patient.

A. The fact that all tests were negative and the fact that Kasandra has been suffering from the above symptoms for more than 6 months leads me to the diagnosis of chronic fatigue syndrome.

P. 1. Continue with lorazepam, 0.5 mg as needed for insomnia.
    2. Refer to Physical Therapy for strength/endurance training.
    3. Follow up in one month.

Ralph Lopez, MD/xx

FACT SHEET:

Insurance Carrier: John Deere HMO 1345 John Deere Road Moline, IL xxxxx	Phone/Fax: 555-222-3321 Group # 54JD Patient's ID No. 22-3333HMO

Patient's Employer: Creston School District

PCP: Ralph Lopez, MD (NPI#345 543 876)

Name of Health Care Provider to whom patient is being referred: Anton Moss, PT

Reason for request: 12 1-hour physical therapy sessions

Diagnosis Code: 780.71

Continued

PROCEDURE 18-1—cont'd

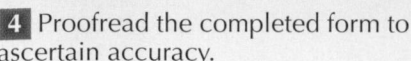

PROCEDURAL STEPS

1 Assemble the necessary documents and equipment.

2 Examine the patient record, and determine the service/procedure for which preauthorization is being requested, including the specialist's name and phone number, and the reason for the request.

   Purpose: To correctly complete the required form for gaining authorization from the patient's insurance carrier for the specified treatment.

3 Complete the referral form, providing all pertinent information requested.

4 Proofread the completed form to ascertain accuracy.

5 Role play the act of faxing the completed form to the patient's insurance carrier.

   Purpose: To inform the insurance carrier of the patient's medical condition; to request preauthorization for the requested treatment; to request a verification number; and to confirm the specific number of physical therapy sessions.

6 Place a copy of the completed form in the patient's medical record.

Utilization Management

Patient care review by healthcare professionals who do not provide the care is a necessary component of managed care to control costs. A **utilization review** committee reviews individual cases to make certain that medical care services are medically necessary and to study how providers use medical care resources. This committee reviews all physician referrals, emergency department visits, and urgent care. After review, this department will either approve or deny the referral, so it is important to submit exact documentation and precise statements. You will be able to contact this department directly; never refer a member or patient to this department.

Referrals and Authorizations

Managed care changes on a day-to-day basis. To compete within this market, some insurance companies have added a benefit that will allow a member or patient to self-refer (meaning an authorization is not required to see a specialist). Many plans for senior citizens now have a **self-referral** and a copayment as well as some other insurance coverage. Information on referrals and authorizations will apply if you are working for a primary care physician, an internist, a family practitioner, a general practitioner, a pediatrician, and sometimes an obstetrician or a gynecologist.

Referral is a term used in managed care when a patient is referred from a PCP to a specialist. When completing a referral form (Figure 18-2), it is imperative that all necessary information be included (Procedure 18-2). For example:

Referring physician ⇒ Specialist being referred to ⇒ Diagnosis ⇒ Treatment (medication ⇒ past and present) ⇒ Chart notes (if necessary) ⇒ Minor surgical procedures

If a referral is denied because of insufficient information or no medical necessity, the PCP's office will be notified. Some medical groups will notify both the PCP and the patient. When the PCP's office provides the medical group with the necessary information, the referral will be reviewed again.

A referral can take from a few minutes to a few days to be reviewed and approved or denied. There are three types of referrals:

1. A *regular* referral usually takes 3 to 10 working days for review and approval. This type of referral is used when a patient has not responded to a PCP's treatment and/or medication and the physician believes that the patient must see a specialist to continue treatment.
2. An *urgent* referral will usually take about 24 hours for approval. This type of referral is used when an urgent matter occurs and is not life threatening.
3. A *STAT* referral can be approved by telephone immediately after faxing it to the utilization review department. A STAT referral is used in an emergency situation as indicated by the physician, such as life or death situations, miscarriage, loss of limb, or other conditions of similar magnitude. Usually the physician will refer the patient by telephone and will fax the information with the referral afterward.

A regular referral is the most common and can be inconvenient for the patient. Most managed care plans require contacting the member services department to check the status of a referral. A cardinal rule is to never tell the patient that the referral has been approved unless you have a hard copy of the **authorization**. Authorization is a term used by managed care for an approved referral.

A referral becomes an authorization after it is reviewed by utilization management and/or the medical director and has been approved. When a referral is approved, the PCP's office will receive a copy of the authorization by mail or fax. Always review the authorization thoroughly. The patient will receive a letter with an authorization number and the approved services. The patient must present the authorization to the specialist's office

**MANAGED CARE PLAN
TREATMENT AUTHORIZATION REQUEST**

TO BE COMPLETED BY PRIMARY CARE PHYSICIAN
OR OUTSIDE PROVIDER

Health Net ☐   Met Life ☐
Pacificare ☐   Travelers ☐
Secure Horizons ☐   Pru Care ☐

Member No. _____

Patient Name: _____ Date: _____

M ____ F ____ Birthdate _____ Home telephone number _____

Address _____

Primary Care Physician _____ Provider ID# _____

Referring Physician _____ Provider ID# _____

Referred to _____ Address _____

_____ Office telephone no. _____

Diagnosis Code _____ Diagnosis _____

Diagnosis Code _____ Diagnosis _____

Treatment Plan: _____

Authorization requested for procedures/tests/visits:

Procedure Code _____ Description _____

Procedure Code _____ Description _____

Facility to be used: _____ Estimated length of stay _____

Office ☐   Outpatient ☐   Inpatient ☐   Other ☐

List of potential consultants (i.e., anesthetists, assistants, or medical/surgical):

_____

Physician s signature _____

TO BE COMPLETED BY PRIMARY CARE PHYSICIAN

PCP Recommendations: _____ PCP Initials _____

Date eligibility checked _____ Effective date _____

TO BE COMPLETED BY UTILIZATION MANAGEMENT

Authorized _____ Not authorized _____

Deferred _____ Modified _____

Authorization Request# _____

Comments: _____

FIGURE 18-2   Example of a referral form. (Modified from Fordney M: *Insurance handbook for the medical office*, ed 7. Philadelphia, 2002, WB Saunders, p 339.)

PROCEDURE 18-2

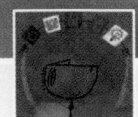

Obtaining a Managed Care Referral

GOAL: Using the information in the case study, accurately complete a referral form for the managed care patient.

EQUIPMENT AND SUPPLIES

- Patient record
- Referral form
- Patient's insurance information
- Pen/pencil

CASE STUDY

> PATIENT NAME: Calina V. Matucek   PATIENT NO. 5432
>
> DATE OF VISIT: 6/02/XX   DOB: 07/28/XX
>
> S. This 27-year-old female, an anthropology instructor at Bremmer College, comes to the clinic today complaining of fatigue, low-grade fever, stomach cramps, intermittent diarrhea, loss of appetite, and an erratic sleep pattern. She reports a 20-lb weight loss in the last two to three months. She is a vegetarian. Ms. Matucek was on an educational sabbatical to Indonesia at the onset of symptoms. She reports that while she was careful to drink bottled water, eating utensils were washed with untreated water. She was treated by a local doctor in Indonesia with an unknown drug (for suspected *Giardia lamblia*) and improved somewhat; however, the symptoms have returned. PFSH: See copy of form in chart.
>
> *ALLERGIES:* Penicillin and aspirin.
>
> O. Vital signs: T: 99.3; P: 84 and regular; R: 20. B/P: 114/74. Ht: 5 ft 8 in.; wt: 115 lb. HEENT: PERLA. Funduscopic: Benign. Sinuses: Nontender. Neck: Supple, no nodes or masses. Chest: Clear. COR: RRR without murmur. ABD: Somewhat guarded. Cranial nerves II-XII, sensory, motor, cerebellar grossly intact. Pt is pale and appears lethargic. Lab tests: See copies in chart of CBC w/automated diff and C&S taken at the ER on 6/04/xx.
>
> A. (1) Lambliasis, suspected
>   (2) Anemia, chronic, simple (probably due to the fact that she has been a vegetarian for approx. 10 years).
>
> P. Tylenol as directed for fever. An appointment has been scheduled with Gastroenterology on 6/12/xx.
>
>   Elwood P. Waxwood, MD/xx

Dr. Waxwood (phone 555-111-2222) is the primary care physician (PCP) in this case study, and Ms. Matucek is being referred to Terin B. McFlavin, Gastroenterologist (555-876-0987).

PROCEDURAL STEPS

1 Assemble the necessary documents and equipment.

2 Examine the patient record, and determine the service for which the patient is to be referred, including the specialist's name and phone number, and the reason for the referral.

Purpose: To correctly complete the required form for a PCP to refer a managed care patient to a specialist.

3 Role play with a partner the act of telephoning the patient's insurance carrier.

Purpose: To inform the insurance carrier of the patient's medical condition; to request authorization for the referral; to request a verification number; and to confirm the specific number of visits or length of treatment.

4 Complete the referral form, providing all information requested.

5 Proofread the completed form to ascertain accuracy.

6 Place a copy of the completed form in the patient's medical record.

receptionist on the day the services will be provided. An authorization provides the following information to both the PCP and the specialist:

1. An authorization number, which may be alphabetical, numeric, or alphanumeric.
2. The date on which it was received by utilization management, the date on which it was approved, and the expiration date.
   a. An authorization is good for 60 days.
   b. If services are provided after the expiration date, the services will be denied. If this happens, you need to contact utilization management or member services, ask for an extension, and answer a few questions. Sometimes you may have to involve the patient and/or the specialist's office.
   c. If the authorization expires and services have not been provided, you can request an extension. Utilization management will change the expiration date and will fax a copy to the PCP and specialist or will generate a new authorization with a new number.
3. A diagnosis code.
4. The name, address, and telephone number of the contracted specialist where services will be provided. Sometimes the PCP will refer the patient to a specialist but will not receive approval for that specialist and must get approval for another. Always be sure that any specialist to whom your physician refers patients is contracted with the same managed care plan as the PCP.
5. The comments section is the most critical area of a referral, because this area will designate what services are approved.
   a. The specified number of authorized visits to the specialist.
   b. An authorization may be issued for (1) evaluation only, (2) evaluation and treatment plan, (3) evaluation and biopsy, (4) evaluation and one injection, etc.
   c. Authorization for an evaluation only and/or treatment plan. When this authorization appears, the medical assistant must inform the patient that there will not be any treatment—only an evaluation and/or a treatment plan.

CRITICAL THINKING APPLICATION

Many private carriers and managed health plans have precertification or preauthorization requirements. How can Beverly explain the rationale of preapproval to inquiring patients?

Verification of Insurance Benefits

It is important to verify insurance benefits before providing services to patients. To verify benefits, the following steps should be taken:

1. When a patient calls for an appointment, identify what type of insurance the patient has or what managed care organization the patient belongs to.
2. When the patient arrives for the appointment, photocopy both sides of the patient's ID card (because copayments or amounts to be paid may appear on the back for hospital, office, and the emergency department).
3. Give the patient a letter to read and sign outlining the plan requirements and possible restrictions or noncovered items.
4. When referrals are required, explain the procedure to the patient so it is understood that without the referral, it is the patient's responsibility to pay for the physician's services.
5. Collect any copayments or deductibles.

Fee Schedules

A healthcare practitioner has three commodities to sell—time, judgment, and services. In every case, the healthcare practitioner must place an estimate on the value of these services. Fees for medical procedures and services differ from office to office based on the type of practice and the needs of the facility. The physician or physicians establishing the practice normally set the fees for procedures and services. In the past, most physicians worked on a *fee-for-service* basis (e.g., patients were charged for the provider's service based on each individual service performed).

In recent years third-party payors (particularly government and managed healthcare organizations) have greatly influenced what healthcare providers can charge by establishing what is referred to as the *allowable charge*. The allowable charge is the maximum that third-party payors will pay for a particular procedure or service.

When healthcare providers establish a fee schedule, there are other factors influencing what the charge for a particular procedure or service can be.

Relative Value Scale (RVS)

The RVS was pioneered by the California Medical Association in 1956 to help physicians establish rational, relative fees. Other states soon followed suit. Hundreds of the most commonly performed procedures were compiled, given procedure numbers similar to those in the AMA's Current Procedural Terminology (CPT) code list, and assigned a unit value. The assigned unit value represented the value of that procedure in relation to other procedures commonly performed. Although no monetary value was placed on the units, many insurance companies used the RVS to determine benefits by applying a conversion factor to assign a monetary value to the unit value. In 1978 the Federal Trade Commission (FTC) interpreted the California RVS as a fee-setting instrument and prohibited its publication and distribution. The FTC was attempting to make medical practice more competitive by ruling against the setting of fees and by encouraging physicians to advertise.

Resource-Based Relative Value Scale

As discussed earlier in this chapter, HCFA (now CMS) developed the first comprehensive RBRVS-based fee schedule, which was adopted by Medicare in 1992. The RBRVS-based fee schedule adjusts fees for differences in resources used to provide each service. The amount of resources required to perform a service is determined through the use of relative value units (RVUs) assigned to the CPT codes developed by the AMA. This system was implemented to standardize payment with an adjustment for overhead costs in different geographic areas. Since Medicare's introduction of RBRVS, most third-party payors have adopted similar approaches in developing their fees.

Tracking Insurance Claims

Chapter 17 discussed how a medical assistant should keep a log (or register) of insurance claims as they are received and processed. Forms should be date-stamped as they are received, and the information entered into the log. This log will enable the medical assistant to determine at a glance whether a claim form has been completed and mailed. In addition to keeping a log, it is also advisable to establish a routine for claims processing as follows:

- If possible, set aside a definite time for completing insurance claims.
- Have a central location for all insurance forms.
- Have all the necessary manuals, code books, and other needed references readily available.
- Create a master list of codes most often used by the practice, including fourth and fifth digits and/or modifiers, if appropriate.
- Make it a practice to complete the forms as soon as possible after services are rendered, usually at the end of the day.
- Use the CMS-1500 (formerly HCFA-1500) form as often as possible.
- Complete the forms by category (e.g., all Blue Cross, then all Medicare, and so on).
- If using a computer-billing program to print insurance forms, the computer will store insurance information on outstanding claims that can be printed in batches using the CMS-1500 form. Adjust the printer so the information lines up correctly on the form.
- Transmit claims electronically whenever possible.

Electronic Claims

A computerized medical practice uses the computer for processing claims electronically. This may be handled in several ways (e.g., transmitting data via modem, recording data on a computer disk and sending it to the payor or fiscal intermediary).

An obvious advantage of electronic billing is the amount of time saved with its use. The system interrupts the transmission of incomplete or incorrect data, giving the biller the opportunity for on-the-spot correction. The sender knows immediately whether the insurance company is accepting the claim. Another advantage of electronic billing is that it speeds up the date of payment, which results in an increase in cash flow to the practice.

Not all claims are suitable for electronic submission. For example, claims that are complicated and require a cover letter or those that require some kind of attachment must be sent on hard copy (paper) by mail or messenger.

Prospective Payment System

In April 1983, the Social Security Amendments Act of 1983 (Public Law 98-21) was signed into law. Title VI of this law contained the prospective payment system (PPS) for hospitals, which would begin the radical restructuring of the payment system to hospitals for Medicare inpatient services.

As identified by HCFA, now referred to as CMS, a major objective of the PPS was to establish the government as a prudent buyer of healthcare while maintaining beneficiaries' access to quality care. The prudent buyer objective was to be accomplished by paying Medicare providers a predetermined specific rate per discharge for diagnoses rather than on the basis of reasonable costs.

If a hospital does not contract with a regional office (RO), it is not eligible for payment from the Medicare program. The law provides authority to grant waivers from the PPS if a state has an approved hospital reimbursement control system. Additional criteria must be met by a state to receive approval and a waiver from the federal PPS.

Diagnosis-Related Groups (DRGs)

The DRG classification forms the basis for payment under the PPS. It is based on an average cost for treatment of a patient's condition, as opposed to the traditional method of payment based on actual costs incurred in the provision of care. Payment to the hospital of a DRG amount generally constitutes payment in full for services rendered to Medicare patients.

The DRG system, which classifies patients on the basis of diagnosis, was developed by Yale University researchers in the 1970s as a mechanism for utilization review. DRGs are derived from taking all possible diagnoses identified in the ICD-9-CM system, classifying them into 25 major diagnostic categories (MDCs) based on organ system, and further breaking them down into 495 distinct groupings, each of which is said to be medically meaningful. The principal diagnosis is the most critical factor in the assignment of DRGs. All diagnoses must reflect information contained in the patient's medical record.

To assign a case to a DRG, five pieces of information are necessary:

1. The patient's principal diagnosis and up to four complications or comorbidities
2. Treatment procedures performed
3. The patient's age

4. The patient's sex
5. The patient's discharge status

Hospital Coding

Chapters 15 and 16 discussed ICD-9, CPT, and HCPCS codes, which are used for diagnostic and procedural coding in physicians' offices and clinics. Hospitals use a slightly different coding approach. While hospitals do use CPT for coding procedures and volumes 1 and 2 of the ICD-9-CM manual for coding diagnoses on outpatient services, they use volume 3 of ICD-9-CM for coding inpatient services rather than CPT. This volume combines both the alphabetical and tabular lists for surgical and nonsurgical procedures and diagnostic procedures. Some publishers combine all three volumes into one manual, and others publish volume 3 as a separate book.

Another difference in hospital coding is that the patient's **principal diagnosis** is coded rather than the **primary diagnosis**. The principal diagnosis is that which is determined after study to be the major cause of the patient's hospital admission; a primary diagnosis (used in physicians' offices) is the condition considered to be the patient's major health problem. Another basic difference in inpatient diagnostic coding is that the insurance billing specialist codes all "rule out," "suspected," "likely," "questionable," "possible," or "still to be ruled out" situations as if one or more existed.

Finally, hospitals do not use the CMS-1500 claim form. They use the Uniform Bill (UB-92) claim form, also known as the CMS-1450 (Figure 18-3). For more information on hospital coding, refer to the reference listed at the end of this chapter.

HCPCS

Medicare carriers have since converted to CMS's (formerly HCFA's) Common Procedure Coding System (HCPCS, pronounced "Hic-Pics"). HCPCS, part of which is based on the current edition of CPT, is a five-digit alphanumeric coding system that can accommodate the addition of modifiers. There are three levels of codes assigned and maintained by most carriers:

1. Level I codes, which include 95% to 98% of all Medicare Part B procedural codes, and consist only of CPT codes (excluding those for anesthesiology, which is currently designated by surgery codes).
2. Level II codes, which are assigned by CMS (formerly HCFA) and are consistent nationwide. These codes are for physician and nonphysician services not contained in the CPT system. They are alphanumeric ranging from A0000 to V9999. These codes describe items such as drugs and durable medical equipment (DME).
3. Level III codes, which are assigned and maintained by each local fiscal intermediary. These codes represent services that are not included in the CPT system and are not common to all carriers. These codes range from W0000 to Z9999.

The Federal Register

The *Federal Register* is the official daily publication for rules, proposed rules, and notices of federal agencies and organizations, as well as Executive Orders and other Presidential documents. Publications are sponsored by the Office of the Federal Register (OFR) and produced by the Government Printing Office (GPO). The system was established to regulate complex social and economic issues after it was decided that agencies and the general public needed a centralized filing and publication system to keep track of rules and regulations.

Medical assistants can use the *Federal Register* for researching rules and regulations governing health insurance and coding. The *Federal Register* website is very user-friendly; just type in http://fr.cos.com/ to your computer's browser window, and your search engine will take you directly to their home page. From that point a search can be launched by topic, issue, or agency. Medical assistants may want to take a few minutes to browse this interesting website.

Patient Education

Understanding the ramifications of third-party reimbursement is challenging for a patient as well as a medical assistant. However, it is important that patients understand how their insurance works. Many, especially elderly persons, believe that if they have health insurance, all charges for their healthcare will be covered, and they don't always understand the intricacies of deductibles, copayments, medical necessity, and allowable charges.

One of the responsibilities of a medical assistant is to keep the patient informed and answer questions as they arise. Often medical facilities will provide informational brochures to their patients that explain how third-party reimbursement works, giving definitions of some of the more common terms used in the insurance claims process. If patients are well advised and comfortable with insurance facts before treatment begins, the medical experience will go more smoothly, and collection of fees not covered by their carrier will be easier. The medical assistant must use good communication skills, patience, and tact when discussing third-party reimbursement issues with patients.

CRITICAL THINKING APPLICATION

An elderly patient comes to the office complaining that Medicare did not pay her bill in full. "Medicare is supposed to pay 80% of all my medical bills," she insists. What information will Beverly need to get to the bottom of this problem? How will she explain it to this elderly patient in a way that she will understand?

Beverly notices that a new patient is a member of a PPO of which the physician in her office is not a member. How might Beverly explain this situation to the patient? How could she attempt to resolve it?

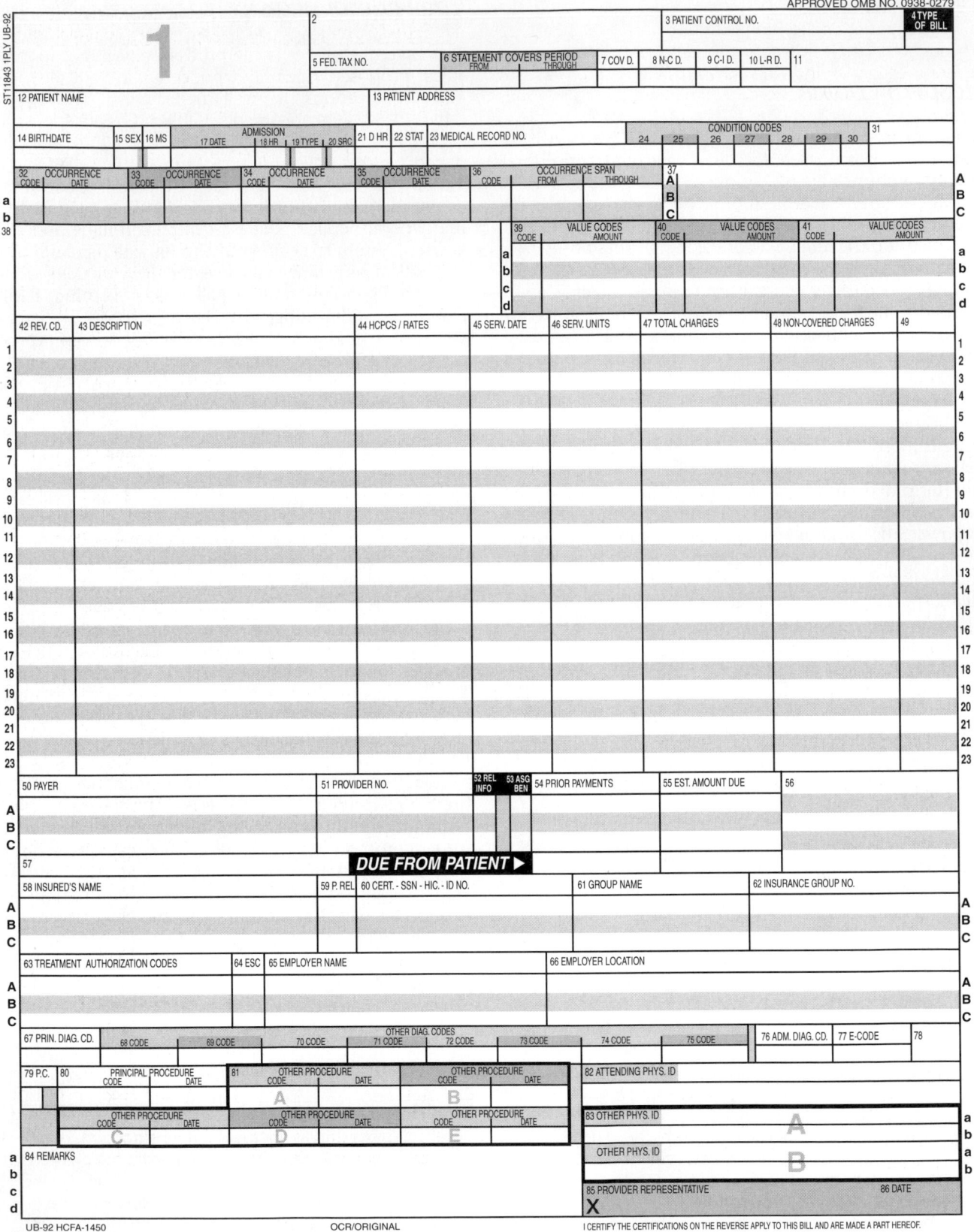

FIGURE 18-3 The UB-92 claim form. In the future, this form will be known as the CMS-1450 (UB-92).

Legal and Ethical Issues

Throughout their careers, medical assistants must remember that an individual's medical record is personal and private. Conversations between patients and their healthcare providers (and staff) are considered privileged communication. Nearly every day a medical assistant is in a position to read and hear information of a private medical nature, and both the caregiver and the patient expect that this information will not leave the medical office.

Unauthorized release of medical information carries over into the insurance claims processing area. Even though the patient expects the insurance form to be filled out and submitted for payment, this cannot be done without proper written release. This medical release form should be kept in the patient's chart, and it should be updated on a regular basis.

Managed care has often been criticized by the news media. Some types of managed care can create a physician-patient barrier that did not exist during the fee-for-service era. An extra effort in human relations by the medical assistant can help to overcome this barrier and put the patient at ease.

SUMMARY OF SCENARIO

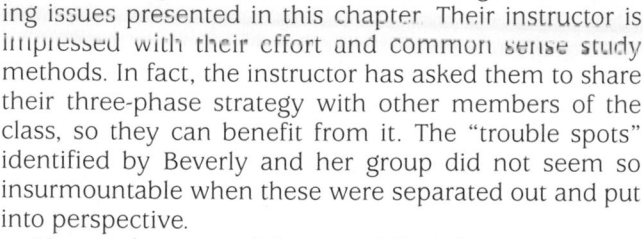

Beverly and her peers have their plan in place for being successful with the challenging issues presented in this chapter. Their instructor is impressed with their effort and common sense study methods. In fact, the instructor has asked them to share their three-phase strategy with other members of the class, so they can benefit from it. The "trouble spots" identified by Beverly and her group did not seem so insurmountable when these were separated out and put into perspective.

Managed care and how it differs from traditional indemnity insurance was one of the issues that needed additional study and discussion. The websites they researched shed light on the subject, and the students enjoyed "surfing the Web" for answers to their questions.

There is still a lot of information to digest in this chapter on third-party reimbursement, but Beverly is now much more comfortable with its concepts and no longer feels that understanding the various topics is impossible. A structured study routine coupled with group "brainstorming" and internet research proved to be a successful strategy. The coordination and teamwork involved in the group experience are valuable skills that can be transferred to the workplace once Beverly's career as a medical assistant begins.

SUMMARY OF LEARNING OBJECTIVES

- Medical assistants should have an understanding of the purpose of health insurance. This will help in the workplace not only by facilitating their knowledge of the subject, but also in educating patients. The trend for insurance policies to encourage preventive medicine can be appreciated.

- Insurance policies fall into many different categories and are available in many different forms. The ability to differentiate among the various types of insurance policies gives medical assistants a solid background in what is available on the market, what is included in each policy category, and the function of each. It is also important for medical assistants to understand and appreciate that there are still many people in this country that cannot afford and do not receive quality healthcare.

- Insurance packages are often tailored to the needs of each individual or group, and the ways to combine benefits are limitless. Health insurance policies normally contain a combination of the different benefits discussed in this chapter (e.g., surgical, basic medical, and major medical).

- Benefits are determined and paid in one of several ways: indemnity schedules, service benefit plans, determination of the UCR fee, and relative value studies. Medical assistants should become familiar with each of these methods and understand the ramifications of all.

- Healthcare has changed tremendously in recent years, and the cost of quality healthcare has skyrocketed. Efforts have been made in both the public and private sector to introduce various healthcare reform methods in order to contain these costs. Healthcare reform has had little success on a national level; however, state legislatures are beginning to pass laws that have brought improvement. Medical assistants should become well informed on the issues of healthcare reform and keep current by reading pertinent magazines and periodicals and paying close attention to news broadcasts.

- Managed care is a broad term used to describe a variety of health plans developed to provide healthcare services at lower costs. There is a lot of confusion as to what managed care entails. To fully understand managed care, a medical assistant must know its history and how it evolved. When the medical assistant is employed in a medical facility, he or she will undoubtedly be working with one or more managed care plans. Therefore it is important to know the various types (e.g., HMO, IPS, and PPO) and understand how each one functions. Managed care has had both positive and negative effects on modern medicine. The bottom line is to be well informed.

■ The maze of managed care options can create confusion in even the best-informed people. PPOs are another popular managed care option where physicians sign a contract with a PPO organization and agree to allow PPO members a discount for healthcare services. It may be difficult for medical assistants to become experts on every type of managed care; however, every medical assistant should research the ones that are the most common in his or her area of practice and concentrate on them.

■ Other major third-party payors the medical assistant should become familiar with are Blue Cross/Blue Shield, Medicaid, Medicare, CHAMPVA, TRICARE, and workers' compensation. Medicare is the largest third-party insurer in the country, making quality healthcare affordable for the elderly and select other groups. Medicaid is another government-sponsored healthcare plan for individuals who qualify for these benefits. Workers' compensation covers employees who are injured or who become ill as a result of accidents or adverse conditions in the workplace. Disability programs reimburse individuals for monetary losses incurred as a result of an inability to work for reasons other than those covered under workers' compensation.

■ Many problems can be prevented for both the patient and the medical office if the medical assistant develops and follows a procedure for verifying insurance benefits before services being rendered. This procedure includes gathering as much information as possible about the demographics of the patient and his or her insurance coverage. A pragmatic and tactful discussion with all new patients explaining the established policy that the medical office adheres to regarding the insurance claims process and the collection of fees not covered by their policy will pay off in the end.

■ It is important for the medical assistant, and patients alike, to realize that fees for medical procedures and services differ from office to office based on the type of practice and the needs of the facility. Until the advent of managed care, most physicians operated on a *fee-for-service* basis where the provider would render his or her services and charge accordingly. In recent years, government and managed care organizations have greatly influenced what healthcare providers can charge. Many third-party payors base reimbursements on what is referred to as the *allowable charge*. Other fee schedule types include the Relative Value Scale (RVS) and the resource-based relative value scale (RBRVS).

KEY INTERNET WEBSITES

- Blue Cross/Blue Shield
- Federal Register
- Kaiser Permanente
  For active weblinks to each website visit
  http://evolve.elsevier.com/Kinn/

REFERENCE

Fordney MT: *Insurance handbook for the medical office*, ed 7. Philadelphia, 2002, WB Saunders.

CHAPTER 19

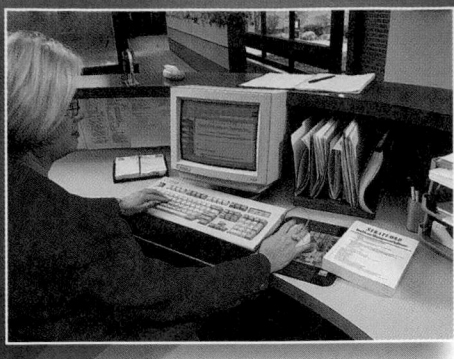

Scenario

Laura Anderson likes working with figures and has always been interested in bookkeeping. In high school she took all the bookkeeping and accounting courses that were offered, and during the summer months she helped out in the accounting department of the family business. In addition to her schooling and on-the-job experience, Laura wants to learn all she can about the financial transactions common to a medical practice. She is especially interested in electronic banking and all of the possibilities that it has to offer. Once her career in medical assisting is launched, Laura hopes to specialize in helping medical offices set up and run electronic banking systems.

Although Laura has had considerable bookkeeping experience, she realizes that there is still a lot to learn about the daily financial duties in a medical office, including accounts payable, working with the business checkbook, making deposits, reconciling bank statements, and many other banking responsibilities.

Taking on the bookkeeping functions of a medical office involves not only responsibilities to the physician and employer, but also to patients and the vendors from whom the medical office purchases supplies. Laura realizes that to perform well in her upcoming career as a medical assistant, she must learn all she can about the topics pertinent to her special interest areas and stay current with the rapidly changing world of finance.

Banking Services and Procedures

Janet Beik

Learning Objectives

- Define and spell the terms listed in the vocabulary.
- Explain how the Internet has changed traditional banking practices.
- State the four requirements of a negotiable instrument.
- Discuss the advantages of using checks.
- Identify the three most common types of bank accounts.
- Explain how you would handle mistakes made in preparing a check.
- List and discuss eight precautions to observe in accepting checks.
- Name and compare the four kinds of endorsements.
- Discuss the actions necessary when a deposited check is returned.
- Demonstrate the procedure for reconciling a bank statement.
- Correctly write checks for bill payment.
- Prepare a bank deposit and appropriate office documents.
- Accurately reconcile a bank statement with the office checking account.

National Curriculum Competencies

ADMINISTRATIVE COMPETENCIES

2a. Prepare a bank deposit
2b. Reconcile a bank statement
2g. Prepare a check

TRANSDISCIPLINARY COMPETENCIES

2b. Perform within legal and ethical boundaries

Vocabulary

bank reconciliation The process of proving that a bank statement and checkbook balance are in agreement.

clearinghouses Networks of banks that exchange checks with each other.

disbursements Money (funds) paid out.

drawee Bank or facility on whom a check is drawn or written.

drawer Person who writes a check.

e-banking Electronic banking via computer modem or over the Internet.

endorser Person who signs his or her name on the back of a check for the purpose of transferring title to another person.

holder Person presenting a check for payment.

m-banking Banking through the use of wireless devices, such as cellular phones and wireless Internet services.

maker (of a check) Any individual, corporation, or legal party who signs a check or any type of negotiable instrument.

negotiable Legally transferable to another party.

payee Person named on a draft or check as the recipient of the amount shown.

payor Person who writes a check in favor of the payee.

power of attorney A legal statement in which a person authorizes another person to act as his or her attorney or agent. The authority may be limited to the handling of specific procedures. The person authorized to act as the agent is known as the *attorney in fact*.

principal A capital sum of money due as a debt or used as a fund for which interest is either charged or paid.

Uniform Commercial Code (UCC) A series of laws (regulations), adopted by most states, that regulate the fields of sales of goods; commercial paper, such as checks; secured transactions in personal property; and particular aspects of banking, letters of credit, warehouse receipts, bills of lading, and investment securities.

Financial transactions in the professional office nearly always involve banking services and the use of checks. Therefore a medical assistant must understand the responsibilities involved in accepting payments, endorsing and depositing checks, writing checks, and regularly reconciling bank statements. Payments received in the medical office should be deposited as soon as possible—ideally, the same day. The medical assistant may very well be in charge of these financial responsibilities; therefore he or she must understand each transaction and what its function is.

Banking in the New Millennium

With the advent of the Internet, banking as we once knew it has changed. People once had to fight traffic and wait in line at crowded banks; today they can sit in the comfort of their own homes and do their banking on the computer at any time of day. It is now possible to conduct such electronic banking transactions as buying and selling shares, paying bills, and transferring funds between accounts. In addition, customers have access to information about stock market prices and news and historical analyses of shares, which makes buying or selling decisions easier.

In fact, it is no longer necessary to sit in front of a computer terminal to conduct banking transactions. Instead, customers can sit on a bus or a train or be waiting for a flight and still make their investments or carry out other bank services. All of this is possible by just turning on a mobile telephone.

Online Banking

Online banking is a means to perform banking services via the Internet. It is also called *PC banking, home banking, electronic banking,* **e-banking***,* or *Internet banking*. There are many facilities to choose from; most of them offer both basic and advanced services. Basic services usually include these:

- Checking account balances
- Transferring funds between accounts
- Paying bills electronically

Some of the advanced services that banks offer include the following:

- Applying for loans
- Downloading account information
- Trading stocks or mutual funds
- Viewing images of transactions (checks and deposits)

There are advantages and disadvantages to online banking. One of the most obvious advantages is the ability to bank at one's own convenience in one's own home or office at any time. This can save considerable time and expense, especially if banking must be done daily. Many people find online banking a convenient and comprehensive method for money management. Other advantages include ease of use, portability, and availability.

Disadvantages of e-banking include learning the software—it is less versatile than physical banking—and service options are often more limited. In addition, some experts believe that there may be a slight increase in risk as compared with conventional banking, although this has been debated by e-banking proponents. Forecasts show, however, that in spite of the disadvantages, banking via the Internet is becoming more popular, with an estimated 20% to 25% of homes and businesses using it.

The cost of online banking varies from bank to bank. Some charge a flat rate (from $5 to $10 per month), with varying fees for additional transactions.

Online Loans

Online lending is becoming more common as well. Loans are available for nearly anything consumers want to purchase—from homes and cars to small business loans and student loans for college tuition. Although online lending still has many loopholes, consumers can save time and money by comparison shopping the dozens of lenders available to find a good rate. Application forms can be downloaded for processing to initiate the process quickly, but the complicated loan process—especially for home mortgages—still requires coordination among many parties, and the sensitive financial and personal information needed for loan approval can raise online security concerns. Despite these issues, many people are "surfing the Web" for loans.

Online Convenience

Convenience is probably the number one reason people and businesses use the Internet for their financial services. There is no frenzied drive to the bank during rush hour, waiting in line, or working around the confines of banking hours. Online banking is available 24 hours a day, 7 days a week. In addition to Internet banking services, consumers can also pay bills online, without the delay of mailing. Credit card holders can check their balance and transaction status. Costly fees can be avoided for financial transactions left until the last minute, because online transactions can be accomplished in a matter of seconds. No need to wait and worry if the mail will get it there in time.

Customer-Oriented Banking

Americans are becoming more and more mobile. They want to conduct business and take care of personal concerns over cell phones on their way to and from work. In addition, the rapid pace of life requires rapid or "instant" solutions: people are buying take-out food at a record rate; some churches even offer drive-up services. It is no wonder that today's mobile consumers want the ability to conduct their financial transactions on the go, every day, at any time.

Banks no longer consider customers to be merely account numbers; to stay competitive, banks are being forced to look at the total customer picture. Some banks even offer a type of interactive voice response system that operates through speech recognition, allowing customers to conduct business through a combination of talking into the telephone and using the telephone keypad. The call centers of some banks employ live customer service personnel to answer questions and fulfill requests for all types of bank transactions.

Another customer-oriented innovation is mobile banking, or **m-banking**, which is emerging through the wireless technology market. Through the use of wireless devices such as cellular phones and wireless Internet services, customers can conduct a variety of financial transactions, set up alerts and notifications when bills are due, and make electronic transfers to pay these bills.

CRITICAL THINKING APPLICATION

Laura is excited about all of the possibilities available with e-banking and M-banking. Where can Laura learn more about electronic banking and its advantages and disadvantages compared with conventional banking?

Checks

A check is a bank draft or order to pay a certain sum of money payable on demand to a specified person or entity. The concept of writing and depositing checks as a method of conducting financial transactions dates back as far as the Roman Empire. Widespread check-writing didn't become popular, however, until the 1500s, when people in Holland began depositing excess cash with Dutch "cashiers," as a safer alternative than keeping money in their homes. These cashiers then paid the debts of the "depositors" on receipt of a written order. The word "check" was coined in England nearly 200 years later, when serial numbers were marked on these written orders of payment as a way to "check" on them. About 90% of all financial transactions in the United States are said to be effected by check.

A check is considered to be a **negotiable** instrument. For a check to be negotiable, it must:
- Be written and signed by a **maker**
- Contain a promise or order to pay a sum of money
- Be payable on demand or at a fixed future date
- Be payable to order or bearer

ADVANTAGES OF USING CHECKS

Using checks for the transfer of funds has many advantages:
- Checks are both safe and convenient, particularly for making payments by mail.
- Expenditures are quickly calculated.
- Specific payments can be easily located from the check record.
- A stop-payment order can protect the payor from loss due to stolen, lost, or incorrectly drawn checks.
- Checks provide a permanent reliable record of disbursements for tax purposes.
- The deposit record provides a summary of receipts.
- Checking accounts protect the money while on deposit.

Types of Checks

A medical assistant is probably familiar with the standard personal check, but there are many additional types of checks used in business transactions. He or she should also be familiar with other types of checks, which will be discussed next.

Bank Draft. A bank draft is a check drawn by a bank against funds deposited to its account in another bank.

Cashier's Check. A cashier's check is a bank's own check drawn on itself and signed by the bank cashier or other authorized official. It is also known as an *officer's* or *treasurer's check*. A cashier's check is obtained by paying the bank cashier the amount of the check, in cash or by personal check. Many banks charge a fee for this service. Cashier's checks are often issued to accommodate the savings account customer who does not maintain a checking account.

Certified Check. A certified check is the depositor's own check, on the face of which the bank has placed the word *certified* or accepted with the date and a bank official's signature. Because the bank deducts the amount of the check from the depositor's account at the time it certifies the check, the bank can guarantee that the amount is available. A certified check, like a cashier's check, can be used when an ordinary personal check might not be acceptable. If not used, a certified check should be redeposited promptly, so that the funds previously set aside are credited back to the depositor's account.

Limited Check. A check may be limited as to the amount written on it and as to the time during which it may be presented for payment—30, 60, or 90 days. The limited check is often used for payroll or insurance checks.

Money Order. Domestic money orders are sold by banks, some stores, and the United States Postal Service. Money orders are often used for paying bills by mail when an individual does not have a checking account. The maximum face value varies according to the source. International money orders may be purchased for limited amounts, indicated in U.S. dollars, for use in sending money abroad.

Traveler's Check. Traveler's checks are designed for persons traveling where personal checks may not be accepted or for use in situations in which it is inadvisable to carry large amounts of cash. Traveler's checks are usually printed in denominations of $10, $20, $50, and $100, and sometimes $500 and $1000. They require two signatures of the purchaser, one at the time of purchase and the other at the time of use. They are available at banks and some travel agencies. The use of traveler's checks is becoming less common, because major credit cards are widely accepted throughout the world.

Voucher Check. A voucher check has a detachable voucher form. The voucher portion is used to itemize or specify the purpose for which the check is drawn. It is used for the convenience of the **payor** and shows discounts and various other itemizations. This portion of the check is removed before presenting the check for payment and provides a record for the **payee** (Figure 19-1).

The Banking System

The Federal Reserve

Wanting to provide the nation with a safer, more flexible and stable monetary and financial system, Congress created the Federal Reserve in 1913 as the central bank of the United States. It consists of a seven-member Board of Governors with headquarters in Washington, D.C., and twelve Reserve Banks located in major cities throughout the country.

Figure 19-2 shows how the country is divided into the twelve regional Federal Reserve districts. For additional information on the Federal Reserve System and its regional banks, visit its website, listed at the end of this chapter.

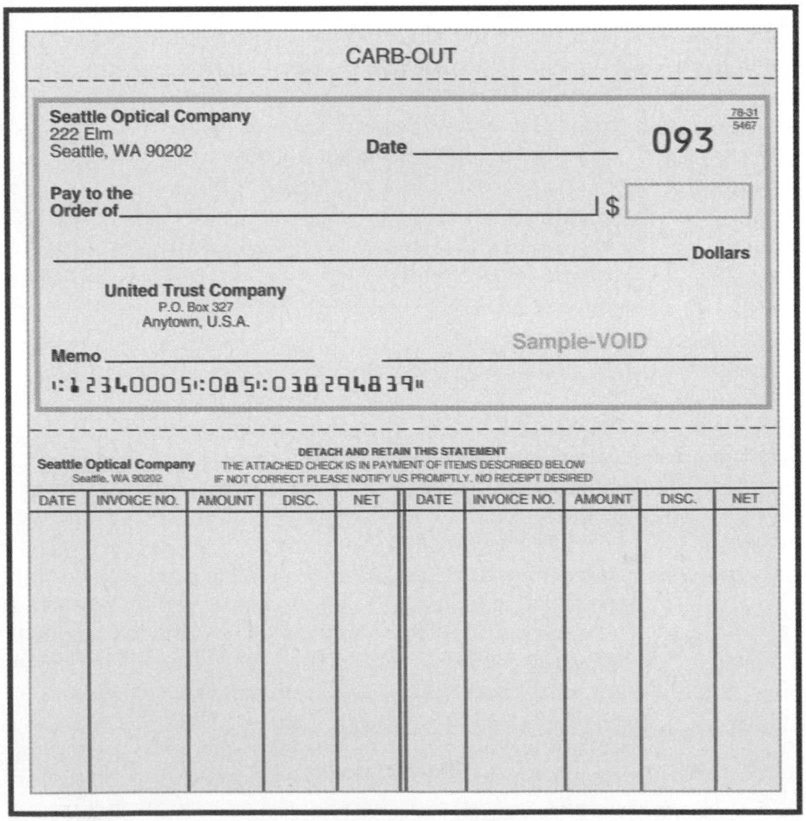
CARB-OUT

Seattle Optical Company
222 Elm
Seattle, WA 90202

Date ______ 093 78-31/5467

Pay to the Order of ______ $

______ Dollars

United Trust Company
P.O. Box 327
Anytown, U.S.A.

Memo ______ Sample-VOID

⑆123400005⑆085⑆038 294839⑈

DETACH AND RETAIN THIS STATEMENT

Seattle Optical Company
Seattle, WA 90202

THE ATTACHED CHECK IS IN PAYMENT OF ITEMS DESCRIBED BELOW
IF NOT CORRECT PLEASE NOTIFY US PROMPTLY. NO RECEIPT DESIRED

DATE	INVOICE NO.	AMOUNT	DISC.	NET	DATE	INVOICE NO.	AMOUNT	DISC.	NET

FIGURE 19-1 Page from a bank order book showing a sample voucher check.

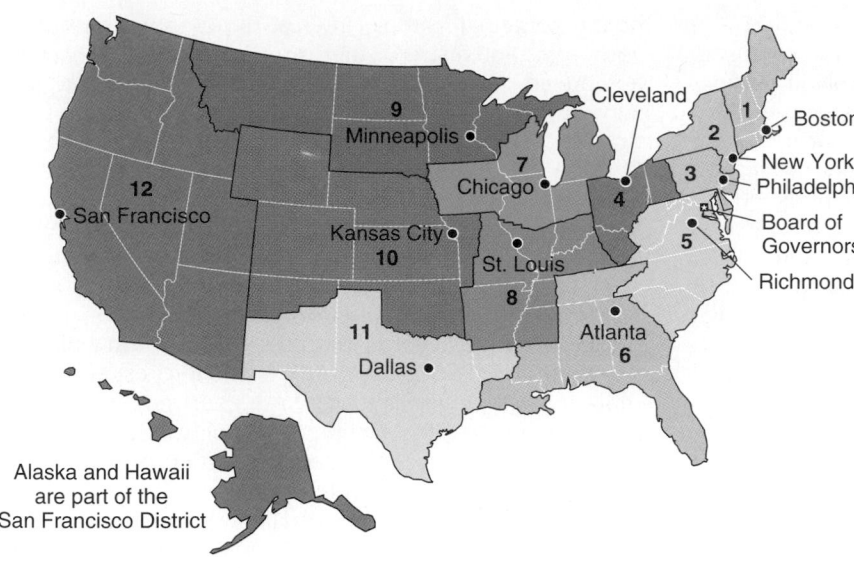

FIGURE 19-2   The twelve federal reserve districts.

Alaska and Hawaii are part of the San Francisco District

ABA Number

The ABA number is part of a coding system originated by the American Bankers Association. It appears in the upper right area of a printed check. The number is used as a simple way to identify the area where the bank on which the check is written is located and the particular bank within the area. The code number is expressed as a fraction (Figure 19-3), for example:

$$\frac{90\text{-}1822}{1222}$$

In the top part of the fraction, before the hyphen, the numbers 1 to 49 designate cities in which Federal Reserve banks are located or other key cities; the numbers from 50 to 99 refer to states or territories. The part of the number following the hyphen is a number issued to each bank for its own identification purposes. The ABA number is used in preparing deposit slips, to identify each check. The bottom part of the fraction includes the number of the Federal Reserve district in which the bank is located and other identifying information.

How Checks are Processed

When a check is presented for payment, the **drawee** (bank or facility on whom the check is drawn or written) pays the specified sum of money written on the face of the check to the **holder** (person presenting the check for payment). Checks received by the bank are turned over daily to a regional clearinghouse, which cancels each one by stamping, mechanically punching, or embossing them. The identifying code numbers, printed on the face of the check with magnetic ink, enables this "clearing" process to be accomplished quickly and efficiently. Checks due from and to all banks outside of a specific region are settled by means of computerized entries. The cancelled check is then either kept by the financial institution or returned to the **drawer** (person who wrote the check). Many banks no longer provide cancelled checks on a regular basis with the onset of internet banking services and most sophisticated computer systems. If the drawer needs proof of payment, a copy of the check can be requested from the bank if they are not returned in the monthly bank statement.

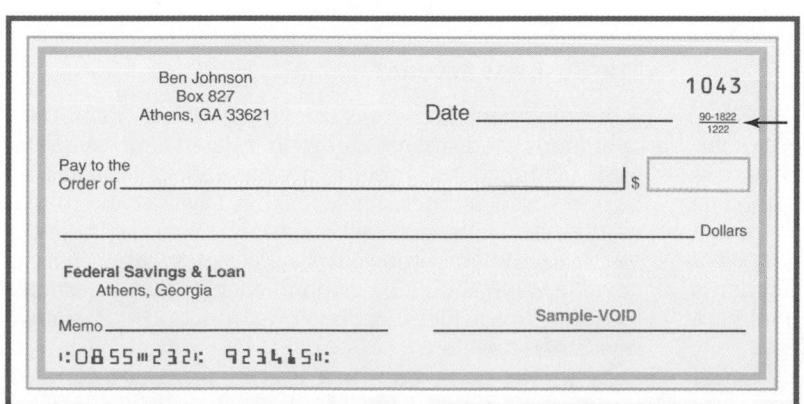

FIGURE 19-3   Sample check. The arrow indicates the American Bankers Association number.

Clearinghouses

As the use of checks grew, the system became confusing because so many different banks were involved. At first, messengers were used for collection; however, this involved a lot of traveling and carrying a lot of cash. Then, in a London coffee shop, a solution came about when two bank messengers discussing the shortcomings of the system realized they both had checks for each other. They decided to exchange them and save some time and effort. This practice evolved into a system of check *clearinghouses*—networks of banks that exchange checks with each other—that is still in use. Today banks in the United States can present checks to the Federal Reserve System or private clearinghouses for regional and national check collection.

Magnetic Ink Character Recognition (MICR)

Characters and numbers printed in magnetic ink are found at the bottom of checks. They represent a common machine language, readable by machines as well as by humans. When a check is deposited, the amount of the check can also be printed in magnetic ink below the signature. MICR identification facilitates processing through a high-speed machine that reads the characters, sorts the checks, and does the bookkeeping.

Bank Accounts

Common Types of Accounts

Checking Accounts. By placing an amount of money on deposit in a bank, a depositor can set up a checking account. Simply stated, a checking account is a bank account against which checks can be written. Many variations in checking accounts have been developed over the years. Instead of a straight, non–interest-bearing account, one might have an insured money market checking account, which bears interest at the daily money market rate if a certain minimum balance is retained. Most banks, however, do not offer interest-bearing checking accounts for businesses.

A physician often requires three different checking accounts:

1. An account for personal and family expenses
2. A separate checking account for office expenses
3. A high-yield interest-bearing account for funds reserved for paying insurance premiums, property taxes, and other seasonal expenses.

A medical assistant's use will probably be limited to the office checking account.

Savings Accounts. Money that is not needed for current expenses can be deposited in a savings account. In most cases, savings accounts earn interest on the amounts deposited; that is, the bank pays the depositor a certain percentage monthly or quarterly for the use of the money in the savings account. An ordinary savings account draws interest at the lowest prevailing rate and has no minimum balance requirement and no check-writing privileges.

Interest. Interest is a charge (or payment) in exchange for the use of money. It is usually figured as a percentage of the **principal**. Simple interest is computed annually; compound interest is figured on the principal as well as any previous interest that has been added to the original sum of money and can be computed using a variety of time increments—daily, monthly, quarterly, and so on. Certain checking accounts draw a small amount of interest—1% or 2% on the average daily balance. Savings accounts usually pay a higher rate of interest than a checking account—2% to 3%. However, these rates fluctuate with the financial market.

Money Market Savings Account. An insured money market savings account requires a minimum balance, anywhere from $500 to $5000; draws interest at money market rates (which is usually a higher percentage rate that a regular savings account); and allows the writing of a specified number of checks (frequently three) per month. There may be a minimum fee charged for each transaction. Such checks are usually written for transfer of funds to a checking account. Some businesses transfer excess funds from their business checking account to a money market account over the weekend or over an extended holiday period to draw interest on the funds (Figure 19-4).

Individual Retirement Accounts (IRAs). IRAs are a type of individual savings plan that are allowed special tax treatment at the federal and sometimes state level. This tax-favored status is what distinguishes an IRA from an ordinary savings account; however, you must follow specific rules to get the tax savings. IRA rules are stricter than those for ordinary savings accounts.

There are several different types of IRAs, such as traditional, Roth, and Education. IRAs are often used as a way to prepare for retirement for several reasons:

- Savings grows tax-deferred
- Tax deductions are realized for contributions (for traditional IRAs)
- Interest earned may not be taxed at withdrawal (for Roth IRAs)

IRAs come in all shapes and sizes. It is important to study and know the rules of each one before deciding which is best for an individual's needs.

CRITICAL THINKING APPLICATION

One of Laura's co-workers wants to open an account at her local bank. She knows Laura has more experience in this field than she, so she asks for her advice. How might Laura advise her on this?

The Business Account

A business bank account is used for business or company operations and managing cash related to day-to-day business functions. There is a wide variety available for businesses today, including checking, savings, and money market accounts, as well as other types of financial elements. When setting up a business account, careful consideration should be given to each of these elements to determine which account best meets the particular needs of a business.

What to Look For in a Business Account. Most businesses want "the most bang for their buck." In other

Statement of Account   14700 CT

014143759	R		1	12/20/02
Account Number	Type	Items	Page No.	Statement Date

001

Current Balance	Previous Statement Date	Previous Balance
2896.34	11/21/02	2886.59

ANSWERS TO YOUR BANKING QUESTIONS 24 HOURS A DAY,
7 DAYS A WEEK.   CALL ANSWERLINE TODAY

****   SUPER INSURED MONEY MARKET ACCOUNT   ****

YOUR OPENING BALANCE OF: 2,886.59

NO   DEPOSITS LISTED TOTALING: .00

- OTHER CREDITS -

12-20 SUPER INSURED MONEY MKT. INT. PAID   9.75

1   CREDITS LISTED TOTALING: 9.75

NO   CHECKS LISTED TOTALING: .00

NO   DEBITS LISTED TOTALING: .00

EQUALS YOUR ENDING BALANCE OF: 2,896.34

DAILY ACCOUNT BALANCES
DATE	BALANCE	DATE	BALANCE	DATE	BALANCE
12-20	2896.34				

- - - - - - - - - - - - - - - SUPER INSURED MONEY MARKET STATEMENT - - - - - - - - - - - - - - - -

DATE	COLLECTED BALANCE	INTEREST RATES	DATE	COLLECTED BALANCE	INTEREST RATES
11-22	2,886.59	04.40	11-25	2,886.59	04.40
11-26	2,886.59	04.40	11-27	2,886.59	04.40
12-02	2,886.59	04.40	12-03	2,886.59	04.40
12-04	2,886.59	04.15	12-05	2,886.59	04.15
12-06	2,886.59	04.15	12-09	2,886.59	04.15
12-10	2,886.59	04.15	12-11	2,886.59	04.15
12-12	2,886.59	04.15	12-13	2,886.59	04.15
12-16	2,886.59	04.15	12-17	2,886.59	04.15
12-18	2,886.59	04.15	12-19	2,886.59	04.15
12-20	2,886.59	04.15			04.15

FIGURE 19-4   Example of a money market account statement. This type of check-writing has limited privileges.

words, they want to have the most services possible for the least amount of money—just as individuals do with personal accounts. Some of the service components available for business accounts include the following:

- Business checking with interest, accruing interest with either checking or savings accounts
- Free checks and deposits, with a maintained minimum balance (which varies from bank to bank)
- Overdraft protection, accomplished by linking the account to a savings account or to a bank-issued credit or debit card
- Online banking

Perks for Businesses. Many financial institutions are offering perquisites ("perks") for businesses opening accounts at their facility by offering special features. These may include the following:

- Business Express: A computerized cash management system that allows access to account information by telephone.
- "Sweep" account: An account in which excess funds over a minimum balance are "swept" into a higher yielding interest-bearing investment account. Then, when the balance in the account drops below the minimum, funds are "swept" back into it automatically.
- Business checking with "special features": A customized bank account designed for businesses with low to moderate transaction volumes and limited cash balances. This service helps business owners manage their day-to-day business and/or personal finances.
- Cash management account: Combines a checking account with a money market fund and a brokerage account. All cash activities are summarized on one monthly statement. This is ideal for business owners who do not have time for managing their money and/or investments.
- Other special features offered to businesses by banks include automatic bill paying, payroll preparation, and timed business deposits.

Business Checks. The checkbook most widely used in the professional office is a ledger-type book with three checks per page and a perforated stub at the left end of the check (Figure 19-5).

Checks may be in a bound soft cover or punched for a ring binder. The checks and matching stubs are numbered in sequence and preprinted with the depositor's name and account number, along with any additional information, such as address and telephone number. Check quantities of 100 to 300 are usually ordered at one time, and the cost is charged against the account. Numbered deposit slips in separately bound books are also supplied to the depositor.

Computer-Generated Checks. Instead of ordering checks to be printed by the bank, personalized checks can be ordered from printing houses to fit your computer's financial software program (e.g., Quicken). Checks can be prepared on the computer in much the same manner as using a typewriter. The checks may have one or more copies that serve as the record of checks written.

One-Write Check Writing. A one-write system of writing checks can save time and minimize errors in medical office **disbursements**. The office with a pegboard bookkeeping system (see Chapter 14) may wish to include one-write check writing. By using a combination check-writing system, such as the one illustrated in Figure 19-6, one check and one record of checks drawn handle both bill paying and payroll check writing.

When the check is written, a permanent record is created through the carbonized line of the check onto the record of checks drawn and the employee's payroll record, including a record of all deductions. Space is provided for the payee's address, so that the check can be mailed in a window envelope. This not only saves time but also ensures that the check will go to the right address. Suppliers of basic pegboard systems can also provide a check-writing system such as the one described.

Bill Paying and Check Writing

Establishing a Bill-Paying System

A systematic plan should be established for the writing of checks and the paying of bills. Check writing usually is done on a specific day or days of each month. An exception sometimes arises when it is possible to realize a good discount if payment of a bill is made within a specified time, such as 10 days. Such discounts are usually indicated at the bottom of invoices or billing statements.

When a check is written in payment of a statement or invoice, it is good practice to write on the invoice the number of the check and the date it was paid. Then if any question arises about whether or when the bill was paid, you can readily locate the check stub. The handling and writing of checks must be done with extreme care (Procedure 19-1).

Designated Times. Rather than haphazardly paying bills as they are received in the office, the medical assistant should establish a routine for paying bills at designated times, such as on the fifteenth and thirtieth days of each month. Most vendors allow a 30-day cycle to elapse before adding on interest or late fees.

One method of handling accounts payable is to create a chronological "tickler file" with dividers for each pay cycle (e.g., the 10th of the month, the 20th, and the 30th). Behind each of the dividers, the invoices can be arranged alphabetically, if desired. When the date arrives, the medical assistant can pull all of the bills from that section and prepare the checks.

Paying Bills to Maximize Money. In establishing the procedure for accounts payable, a medical assistant should keep in mind that most vendors allow 30 days to pay. When each invoice is received, check the "terms," which are usually located at the top of the document. A few vendors offer a discount (normally 1% to 2%) if bills are paid within a shorter period of time. If the terms say "Net 30," this means the total amount of the bill is due within 30 days. Remember to allow a certain number of days (2 to 5, depending on where payment is to be sent) for mailing. If the business checking account is an interest-bearing one, do not pay bills before their due date. In this way, the funds in the account will continue to draw interest until it is time to write the check.

Also, if the practice has a weekly service, such as a laundry or cleaning service that bills several times a month, accumulate the invoices and issue only one check per month. Checks are costly, and some banks charge businesses a fee for each transaction.

Automatic Withdrawals and Deductions. Some routine bills that occur monthly or on a regular billing cycle, such as insurance premiums, rent payments, and utility bills, can be set up to be paid automatically through prior arrangements with the bank.

Online Bill-Paying. An online bill-paying account can be established with a bank or other business entity.

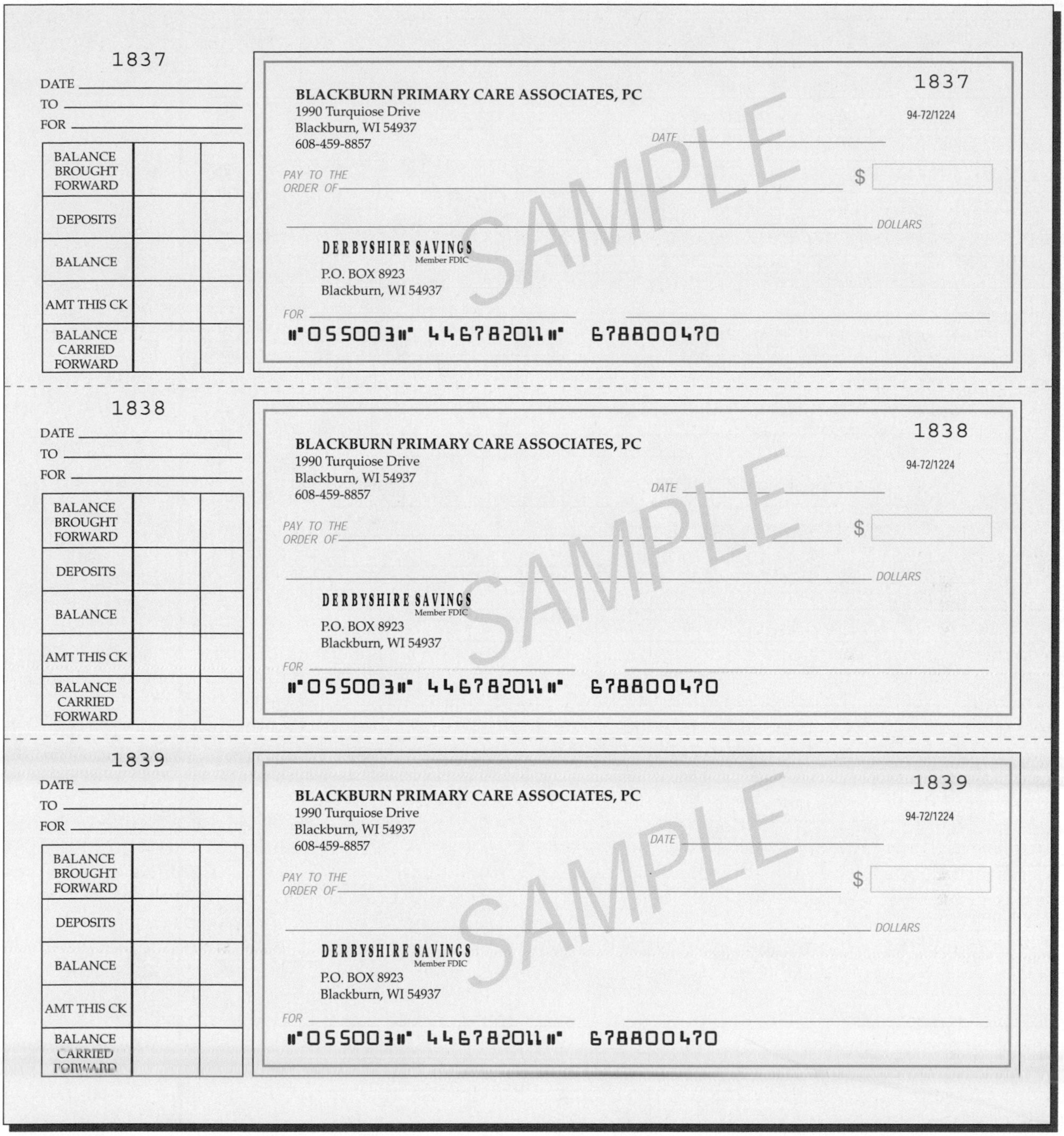

FIGURE 19-5   Example of business checks with stubs. (From Hunt SA: *Fundamentals of Medical Assisting*, Philadelphia, 2002, Saunders, p. 894.)

The bank then pays bills by automatically debiting the customer's account and crediting the merchant's account. More banks are offering this service; however, not all vendors accept electronic transfers in payment of bills. If a business decides to take advantage of online bill-paying, the options should be researched carefully, with consideration of the advantages and disadvantages involved.

Writing Checks

Instructions. Writing checks is a routine and basically simple function; however, there are certain guidelines to

follow that prevent potential problems. Figure 19-7 illustrates several correct methods to use when writing checks.

Figure 19-8 shows the correct method for writing a check for an amount less than a dollar (top). The check on the bottom illustrates an incorrect method of check writing. Note the incomplete name and space for altering (e.g., $6.00 could easily be changed to $26.00 or more, and 00 could be made into 88). When writing in the numerical amount of a check, begin as far to the left in the block as possible. When inserting the written amount of the check, again start as far to the left as possible, allowing

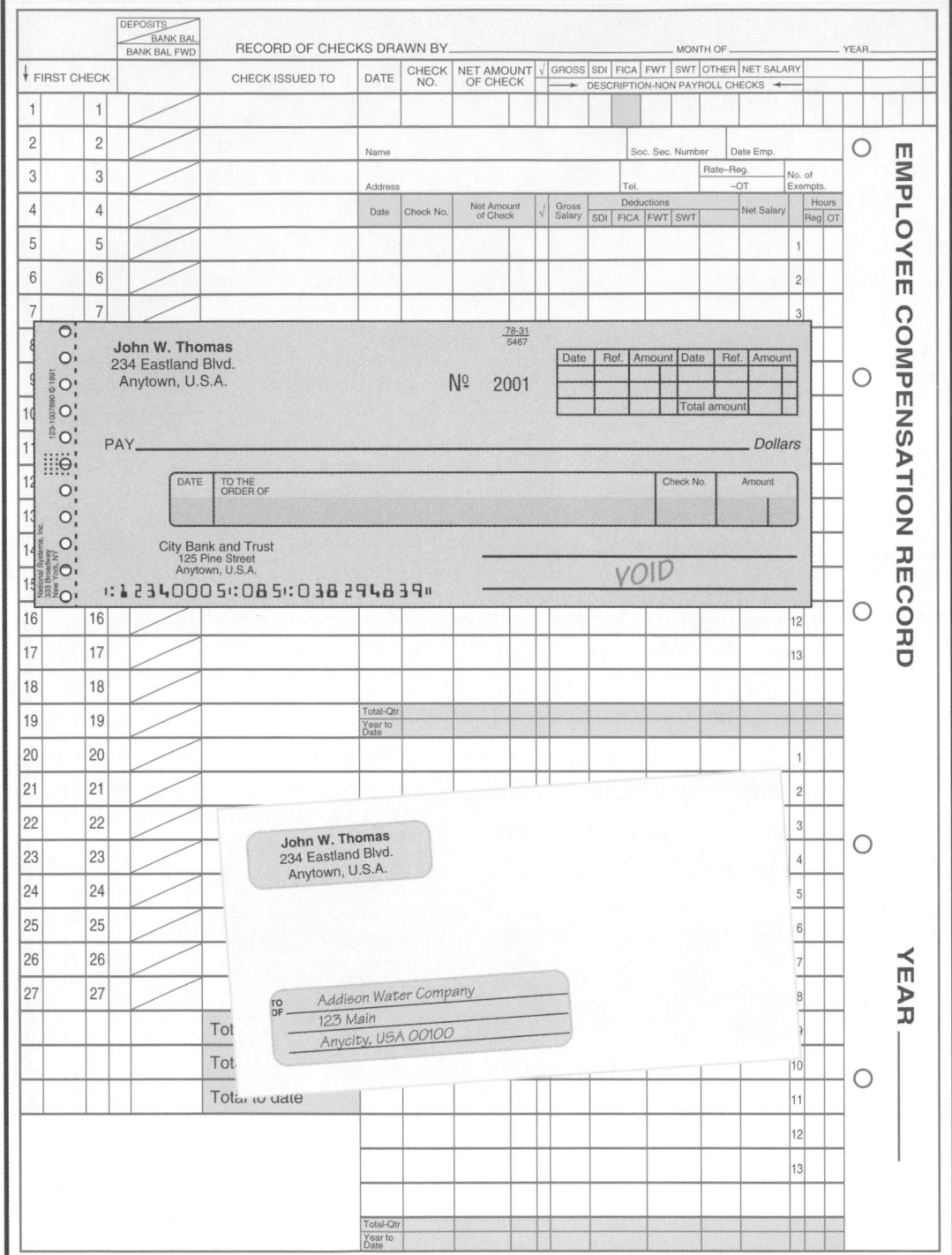

FIGURE 19-6
Pegboard system for check writing. (Courtesy Bibbero Systems, Inc., Petaluma, Calif. 94954, (800) 242-2376, www.bibbero.com.)

no space for added or altered words. Writing checks for less than a dollar is not recommended.

Checkbook Stubs. The check stub (the part that remains in the book after the check has been written and removed) is the depositor's own record of checks written, date, amount, payee, and purpose (Figure 19-9). It is important that the stub be completed before the check is written.

This prevents the possibility of writing a check and neglecting to complete the stub. If the stub is not completed and the check is sent out, you will have no record of the payee and the amount taken from the account until the cancelled check is returned at a later date. Consequently, you will be unable to balance the account or determine the amount on hand until the bank returns those cancelled checks. It is possible to get this information from the bank after the check has been cashed. There may be a charge for this service.

Signing Checks. After all checks have been written, place them along with the invoices or other verifying

PROCEDURE **19-1**

Writing Checks in Payment of Bills

GOAL: To correctly write checks for payment of bills.

EQUIPMENT AND SUPPLIES

- Checkbook
- Bills to be paid

PROCEDURAL STEPS

1 Locate the first bill to be paid. Before writing the check, fill out the stub or the place designated for recording expenditures. Include the date, name of payee, amount of check, the new balance to be carried forward, and usually, the purpose of the check.

Purpose: To prevent the possibility of delivering or mailing a check without entering the information in the checkbook.

2 Complete both the check and the stub with pen or typewriter.

Purpose: To avoid danger of alteration for any reason.

3 Date the check the day it is written (do not postdate).

4 Write the name of the payee after the printed words, "Pay to the Order of _____ " with the necessary information following. Do not use abbreviations unless so instructed.

5 Leave no space before the name and follow it with three dashes if there is space remaining.

6 Omit personal titles from the names of payees.

7 If a payee is receiving a check as an officer of an organization, the name of the office should follow the name. Example: "John F. Jones, Treasurer."

8 Start writing at the extreme left of each space. Leave no blank spaces. Keep the cents notation close to the dollars figure to prevent alteration.

9 Verify that the amount of the check is recorded correctly on the stub, in the box for the dollar ($) amount, and on the line where the amount is written in words.

10 If a check is written for an amount less than 1 dollar, the figures by the $ sign may be circled or enclosed in parentheses ($0.65) to emphasize the amount.

---

information on the physician's desk for signature. In some practices, the medical assistant who has charge of the financial matters is also allowed to sign the checks. This is accomplished by filing a **power of attorney** at the depositor's bank. The power of attorney may limit the check-signing authorization to a certain amount or to a limited time period.

Handling Corrections. Do not cross out, erase, or change any part of a check. Checks are printed on sensitized paper so that erasures are easily noticeable, and the bank has the right to refuse to pay on any check that has been altered. (See Figures 19-7 and 19-8 for examples of correct and incorrect check writing.) If a mistake is made, write the word "VOID" on the stub and the check, but do not throw out or destroy the check. It should be filed with the canceled checks so that it is available for auditing purposes.

Writing Cash Checks. A cash check is made payable to cash or bearer. Such checks are completely negotiable. Because these checks are easily cashed without positive identification, it is poor policy to write cash checks unless they are to be cashed at the time they are written. Some bank personnel may require that the person receiving the cash endorse the check. Many experts in the banking business advise their customers not to endorse a check written for cash or petty cash; often, if there is a problem, the person who endorses the check is liable. A medical assistant should never endorse a check written for cash or petty cash, as he or she is not a party in the transaction.

Mailing Checks. When checks are sent through the mail, the check should not be visible through the envelope. Either place the check within a letter or fold it into a plain sheet of paper. Checks may be folded at the right end to conceal the amount of money written. Make certain the envelopes are sealed before mailing, and the medical assistant should personally mail all checks as soon as possible after writing.

Special Problems With Checks

Special problems may arise when a check is written on nonexistent funds or when a payor wishes, for a legitimate reason, to prevent the payee from cashing a check.

Overdraws or Overdrafts. When a depositor draws a check for more than the amount on deposit in the account, the account becomes overdrawn. In most states, it is illegal to issue a check for more than the amount on deposit in the bank. Should this happen through error or oversight, the bank may refuse to honor the check and will return it to the bank that presented it for payment. Such a check is said to "bounce."

If a check is written by an established depositor, the bank may honor the check and notify the depositor that

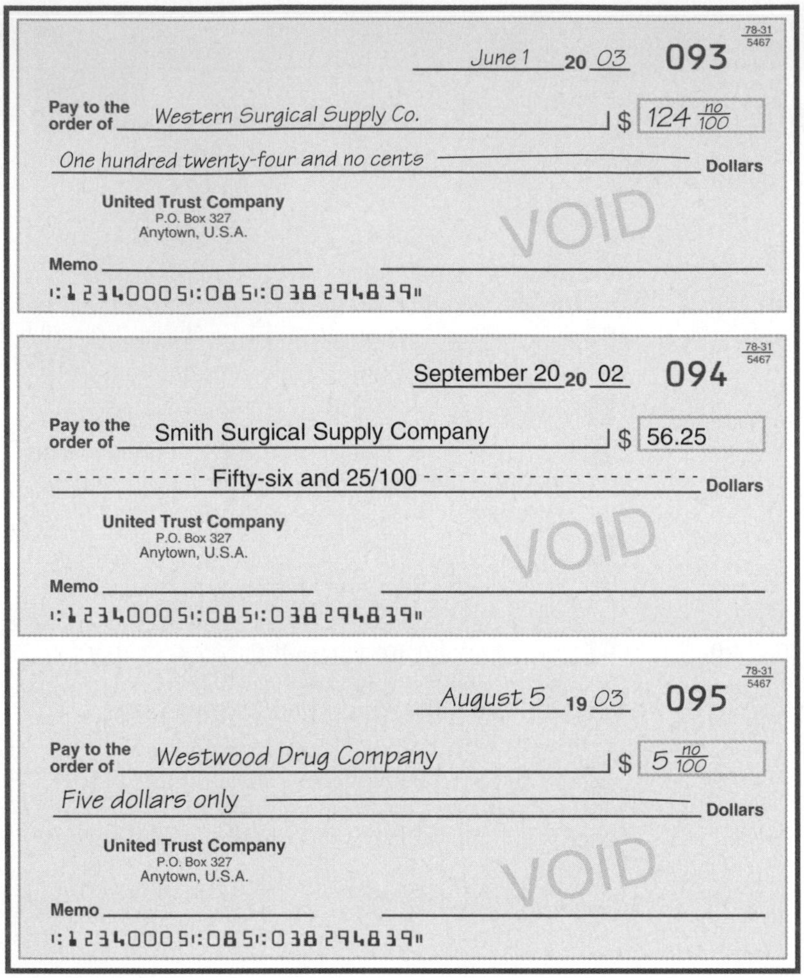

FIGURE 19-7 Correct methods of writing checks.

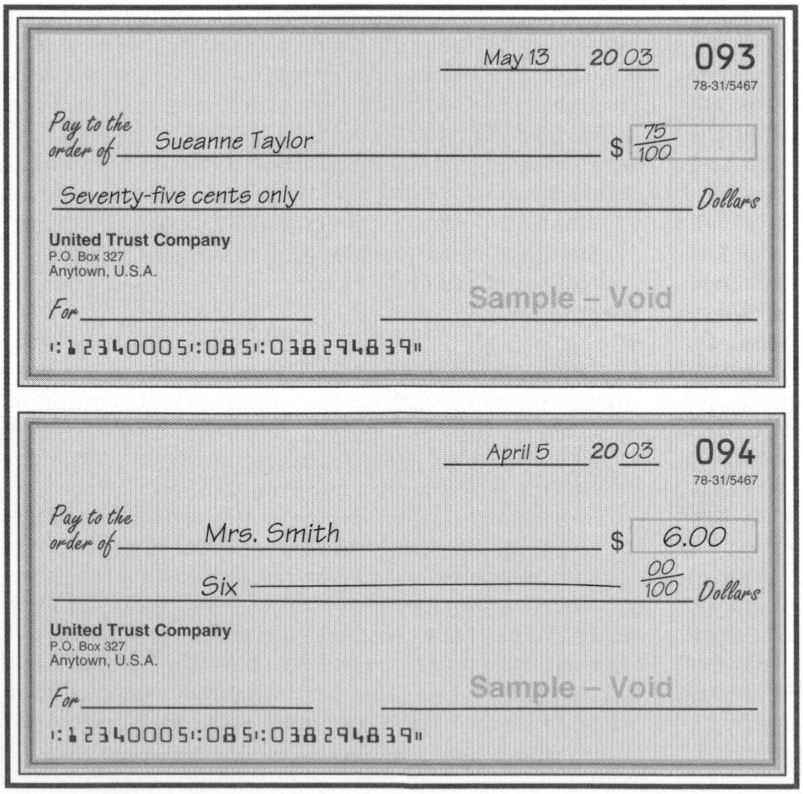

FIGURE 19-8 *Top,* Correct method of writing a check. *Bottom,* Incorrect method of writing a check, with incomplete name and space for altering (e.g., 6.00 could be made into 26.00 or more and 00 could be made into 88).

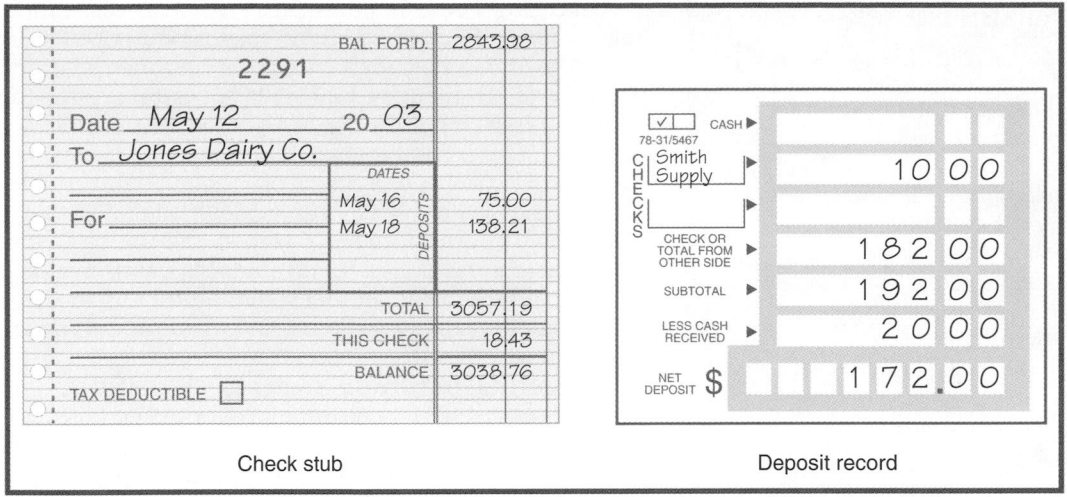

FIGURE 19-9 Methods of filling out a check stub.

the account is overdrawn. If the bank thus pays or covers the check, it issues an overdraft on the depositor's account. Considerable fees (from $10 to $25) are normally charged when an overdraft occurs.

Stop-Payments. A depositor or check writer who wishes to rescind the check has the right to request that the bank stop payment on it. Stop-payment orders should be used only in emergencies. Reasons for stop-payment requests are

- Loss of a check
- Disagreement about a purchase
- Disagreement about a payment

As with overdrafts, most banks charge a fee for stop payment orders.

Check Washing. Check washing is the fraudulent process of erasing or "washing out" the ink on a check with common household chemicals, such as bleach, benzene, or correction fluid. The person then rewrites the check to himself or herself, increasing the amount payable by hundreds and even thousands of dollars. It is estimated that check-washing fraud amounts to over $800 million a year in this country, and it is increasing at an alarming rate.

The National Check Fraud Center suggests the following to minimize the chance of check fraud:

- Ask your bank to advise your office when new books of checks are ready, then either pick them up or use a parcel delivery service to deliver them.
- Make sure cancelled checks are in a secured area, such as a bank lock box or a wall safe. Don't throw them in the trash.
- Check bank statements immediately after receiving them. If check fraud is not reported within 30 days

of receiving a monthly statement, the bank does not have to reimburse the loss (UCC Code 4-406).
- Print a return address on an envelope. A signature can be traced, duplicated, or forged.
- Don't discard credit card records or bills with trash.

For more information on how to avoid check fraud or what to do when fraud occurs, log onto the National Check Fraud Center's website, listed at the end of this chapter.

Accepting Checks

Precautions in Accepting Checks

A medical assistant is presented with checks for payment of physician's services on a daily basis. In most cases these are personal checks. Study the following Box for guidelines for accepting checks.

GUIDELINES FOR ACCEPTING CHECKS

- Scan the check carefully for the correct date, amount, and signature.
- Do not accept a check with corrections on it.
- If you do not know the person presenting a personal check, ask for identification and compare signatures.
- Accept an out-of-town check, government check, or payroll check only if you are well acquainted with the person presenting it and it does not exceed the amount of the payment.
- Acceptance of a third-party check is generally unwise. A third-party check is one made out to your patient by a party unknown to you. A check from the patient's health insurance carrier is an exception.
- When accepting a postal money order for payment, make certain it has only one

GUIDELINES FOR ACCEPTING CHECKS—cont'd

endorsement. Postal money orders with more than two endorsements will not be honored.

- Do not accept a check marked "Payment in Full" unless it does pay the account in full up to and including the date on which it is received. If a check so marked is less than the amount due, you will be unable to collect the balance on the account once you have accepted and deposited such a check. It is illegal for you to scratch out the words "Payment in Full."
- Accepting checks written for more than the amount due and returning cash for the difference between the amount of the check and the amount owed is poor policy. If the check is not honored by the bank, your office will suffer the loss not only of the amount of the check but also of the amount returned in cash.

Acknowledging Payment in Full

If payment in full is to be recognized in regard to a given check, the statement "Payment in Full to Date" must appear *on the back of the check*, above the endorsement, not on the face of the check. Canceled checks are a receipt for the maker of the check, not for the payee.

CRITICAL THINKING APPLICATION

A new patient wishes to pay for his services at the end of the office visit. The charge is $75. The patient writes the check out for $100 and asks Laura for $25 in currency in return. How should Laura handle the situation?

Returned Checks

Occasionally the bank may return a deposited check because of some irregularity, such as a missing signature or missing endorsement. More often, it is because the payor has insufficient funds on deposit to cover the check.

If a check is stamped "NSF," indicating *nonsufficient funds*, do not delay in contacting the person who gave you the check. If you are unable to contact the maker of a bad check, waste no time in tracking down all leads, such as referrals, numbers you obtained from credit cards, driver's license, and so forth. There are several places to which bad checks may be reported. Credit associations are often a great help when such problems arise. Turn the account over to a qualified collection agency if you do not succeed in collecting on the account yourself within a short time.

If a check is returned to your office marked "No Account" and it is a check that you had deposited promptly, you have obviously been swindled. This check should be given to the police, the local Better Business Bureau, or your collection agency.

Charging Fees. To cover their overhead costs, most banks currently charge both the payor and payee a fee of $15 to $30 dollars for a check that has been returned because of "insufficient funds." It is customary for the medical assistant to notify the person responsible for writing the check that it has been returned. Often the individual will have a plausible excuse and simply request that the check be "run through again." If this is the case, it is a wise practice to first call the bank and ask if there are sufficient funds to do this, thus avoiding additional time delay and fees. Some offices add these charges to the patient's account in an attempt to recoup the expense.

Collecting Returned Checks. There are several options available for collecting returned checks. As mentioned previously, the medical assistant might want to make an initial collection attempt by either telephoning or writing a letter to the patient. Many NSF problems can be cleared up quickly and easily using courtesy and tact, assuming that the situation was simply a mistake or oversight. If this method proves unsuccessful, the office might consider registering with a company that specializes in collecting bad checks. This can be done online or physically, using a local collection agency.

Additional methods of bad-debt collection are discussed in Chapter 14.

Legal Options. After all reasonable options for collecting NSF checks have been exhausted, a medical assistant may employ a collection method using the court system. Small claims court is a special court in which disputes are resolved inexpensively and quickly; it is a commonly used method that avoids costly attorney fees. Filing fees are in the $20 to $30 range, and there is usually a charge for having the papers served. There are restrictions, however. The amount for which the plaintiff (individual or company initiating the suit) can sue in a small claims lawsuit is limited to $5000. Other limitations vary from state to state. Contact the local Clerk of the District Court for the necessary forms and instructions in completing a small claims suit. For more information on filing small claims, refer to the government legal department's website, listed at the end of this chapter.

CRITICAL THINKING APPLICATION

When opening the mail, Laura notices a form from the bank with a check attached. It is a check from Elliott Benson, a new patient seen in the office the previous week, being returned for NSF. How should Laura handle this problem?

It is important that the medical assistant learn how to become "proactive" rather than "reactive" when it comes to problem patients. He or she should discuss fees with the patient on the first visit and gather all the financial and insurance information necessary to make a judgment as to whether the patient is able and willing to pay. An experienced medical assistant can often sense a "red flag" during this initial information-gathering process. If this happens, requesting payment in advance might be wise.

This practice should not be abused, however, and the medical assistant should follow the established office policy or discuss the matter with the office manager or physician when necessary.

Endorsements

An endorsement is a signature plus any other writing on the back of a check by which the **endorser** transfers all rights in the check to another party. Endorsements are made in ink, with either pen or rubber stamp, on the back of the check across the left (or perforated) end.

Why an Endorsement is Necessary

The Uniform Negotiable Instrument Act, applicable in all states, explains the need for an endorsement as follows:

> An instrument is negotiated when it is transferred from one person to another in such a manner as to pass title to another party. If payable to bearer, it is negotiated by delivery. If payable to order, it is negotiated by the endorsement of the holder completed by delivery.

The name of the last endorser of the check shows who last received the money. If a check is cashed for someone who did not endorse it and is returned for some reason, the bank will charge the check to the last endorser, not to the last person receiving the money. For this reason, it is not wise to cash a check made payable to another party without having the endorsement of the person who delivered the check to you for cashing.

Types of Endorsements

There are four principal kinds of endorsements. Blank and restrictive endorsements are the ones most commonly used.

Blank Endorsement. The payee signs only his or her name. This makes the check payable to the bearer. It is the simplest and most common type of endorsement on personal checks but should be used only when the check is to be cashed or deposited immediately.

Restrictive Endorsement. This specifies the purpose of the endorsement. A restrictive endorsement is used in preparing checks for deposit to the physician's checking account. An example is shown in Figure 19-10.

Special Endorsement. This endorsement includes words specifying the person to whom the endorser makes the check payable. For instance, a check naming Helen Barker as the payee may be endorsed to the physician by writing on the back of the check as follows:

> Pay to the order of
> Theodore F. Wilson, M.D.
> Helen Barker

The check is still negotiable but requires Dr. Wilson's signature or endorsement.

Qualified Endorsement. The effect of the endorsement is qualified by disclaiming or destroying any future liability of the endorser. Usually the words "without recourse" are written above by an attorney who accepts a check on behalf of a client but who has no personal claim in the transaction.

Methods of Endorsement

Stamp. As checks from patients and other sources arrive, they should be recorded on the ledger and immediately stamped with the restrictive endorsement "For Deposit Only." This is a safeguard against lost or stolen checks.

Any endorsement should agree exactly with the name on the face of the check. If the name of the payee is misspelled, it is usually necessary for the payee to endorse the check the way the name is spelled on the face, followed by the correctly spelled signature. The Uniform Commercial Code, Section 3-203, states:

> Where an instrument is made payable to a person under a misspelled name or one other than his own, he may endorse in that name or his own or both; but signature in both names may be required by a person paying or giving value for the instrument.

Most banks accept routine stamp endorsement that is restricted to deposit only, if the customer is well known and maintains an established account.

Signature. Some insurance checks or drafts require a personal signature endorsement; a stamped endorsement is not acceptable. This will be stated on the back of the check. In such cases, ask the payee to endorse the check, then stamp immediately below the signature the restrictive endorsement "For Deposit Only."

Making Deposits

The financial duties of a medical assistant include depositing checks and reconciling the bank statements with the checkbook. Checks should be deposited promptly, for these reasons:

- There is the possibility of a stop-payment order.
- The check may be lost, misplaced, or stolen.
- Delay may cause the check to be returned because of insufficient funds.
- The check may have a restricted time for cashing.
- It is a courtesy to the payor.

> Pay to the Order of
> Midwest National Bank
> Main Branch
> For Deposit Only
> CARLOS MACAULEY
> 301-012697

FIGURE 19-10   Example of a restrictive endorsement.

Preparing the Deposit

Deposit slips are itemized memoranda of cash or other funds that a depositor presents to the bank with the money to be credited to the account. All deposits must be accompanied by a deposit slip. A carbon or photocopy of the deposit slip should be kept on file (Procedure 19-2).

There are several types of deposit slips, sometimes called *deposit tickets*. The commercial slip is used for the office checking account. The deposit slips are printed with the number of the account in magnetic ink characters to correspond with the checks. Preprinted deposit slips are ordered along with the checks.

Some write-it-once accounting systems include a deposit slip that the bank will accept as the itemization if it is attached to the customer's numbered deposit slip. The deposit slip should be prepared before you go to the bank, with the money organized and ready to present to the bank teller.

Payment on patient accounts is generally made by check, but some payments are made in currency (paper money). Each type of fund is recorded separately on the deposit slip. The currency is usually listed first. Organize the currency so that all of the bills are facing in the same direction—for example, with the black-ink (portrait) side up. Place the largest-denomination bills on top.

Some banks prefer that checks be recorded individually by the ABA number; others use just the maker's name. If the checks are arranged alphabetically by the names of the patient accounts, with these names included on your office copy of the deposit slip, you will have a ready reference of checks deposited should a question arise regarding a patient's payment. Follow the procedure below for preparing a deposit slip (Figure 19-11):

1. List all checks on the back of the deposit slip.
2. Transfer the total to the front of the slip.
3. Enter the amount of the total deposit on the deposit slip stub.

Money orders, either postal, express, or others, are identified by "PO Money Order" or "Express MO." Remember that money orders cannot have more than two endorsements.

The deposit slip should be carefully totaled and the total entered in the checkbook. Any torn bills should be mended with transparent tape. Clip the currency together, and clip the checks in a separate packet. Then place the entire amount in a heavy envelope for taking to the bank. Deposit the currency and checks daily if possible.

Deposits by Mail

Depositing by mail saves time and is easily accomplished if the deposit consists of checks only. Banks usually supply their customers with special mailing deposit slips and envelopes on request (Figure 19-12).

Some mailing deposit slips have an attached portion that the bank will stamp and return to the customer as a receipt. Others may provide the customer with a receipt card that is sent along with the deposit each time for the bank's notation. The mailer shown in Figure 19-12 has a peel-off receipt for the depositor's records. Mailed deposits are prepared in the same manner as are regular deposits, but certain precautions should be observed.

PROCEDURE 19-2

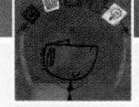

Preparing a Bank Deposit

GOAL: To prepare a bank deposit for the day's receipts and complete appropriate office records related to the deposit.

EQUIPMENT AND SUPPLIES
- Currency
- Six checks for deposit
- Deposit slip
- Endorsement stamp (optional)
- Typewriter
- Envelope

PROCEDURAL STEPS

1 Organize currency.
Purpose: To arrange currency in the best order for speedy and accurate presentation to the teller.

2 Total the currency and record the amount on the deposit slip.

3 Place restrictive endorsements on the checks, using an endorsement stamp or the typewriter.
Purpose: To transfer the title and protect checks from loss or theft.

4 List each check separately on the deposit slip by ABA number and its amount.

5 Total the amount of currency and checks and enter on the deposit slip.

6 Enter the amount of the deposit in the checkbook.
Purpose: To record the current balance in the account.

7 Prepare a copy of the deposit slip for the office record, including the names of the payors.
Purpose: For verification of checks deposited, if necessary.

8 Place the currency, checks, and deposit slip in an envelope for transporting to the bank.

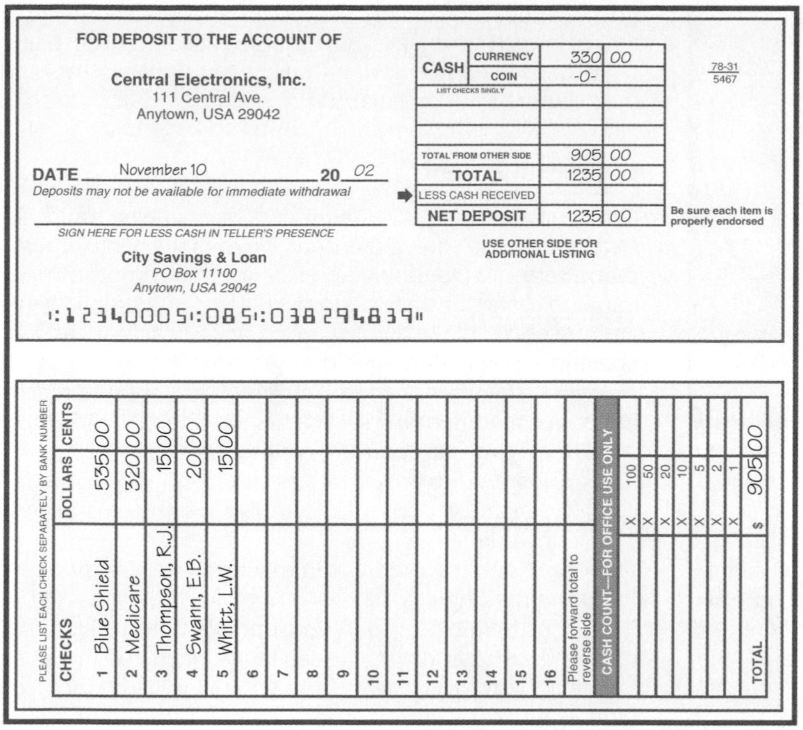

FOR DEPOSIT TO THE ACCOUNT OF

Central Electronics, Inc.
111 Central Ave.
Anytown, USA 29042

CASH	CURRENCY	330	00
	COIN	-0-	
LIST CHECKS SINGLY			

78-31
5467

DATE ___November 10___ 20_02_
Deposits may not be available for immediate withdrawal

TOTAL FROM OTHER SIDE	905	00
TOTAL	1235	00
LESS CASH RECEIVED		
NET DEPOSIT	1235	00

Be sure each item is properly endorsed

_____
SIGN HERE FOR LESS CASH IN TELLER'S PRESENCE

USE OTHER SIDE FOR
ADDITIONAL LISTING

City Savings & Loan
PO Box 11100
Anytown, USA 29042

⑆1234000⑆ ⑈08⑈ ⑆038 294839⑈

PLEASE LIST EACH CHECK SEPARATELY BY BANK NUMBER	CHECKS	DOLLARS	CENTS
	1 Blue Shield	535	00
	2 Medicare	320	00
	3 Thompson, R.J.	15	00
	4 Swann, E.B.	20	00
	5 Whitt, L.W.	15	00
	6		
	7		
	8		
	9		
	10		
	11		
	12		
	13		
	14		
	15		
	16		
	Please forward total to reverse side		
	TOTAL	$ 905	00

CASH COUNT—FOR OFFICE USE ONLY
× 100
× 50
× 20
× 10
× 5
× 2
× 1

FIGURE 19-11   Front and back of a deposit slip.

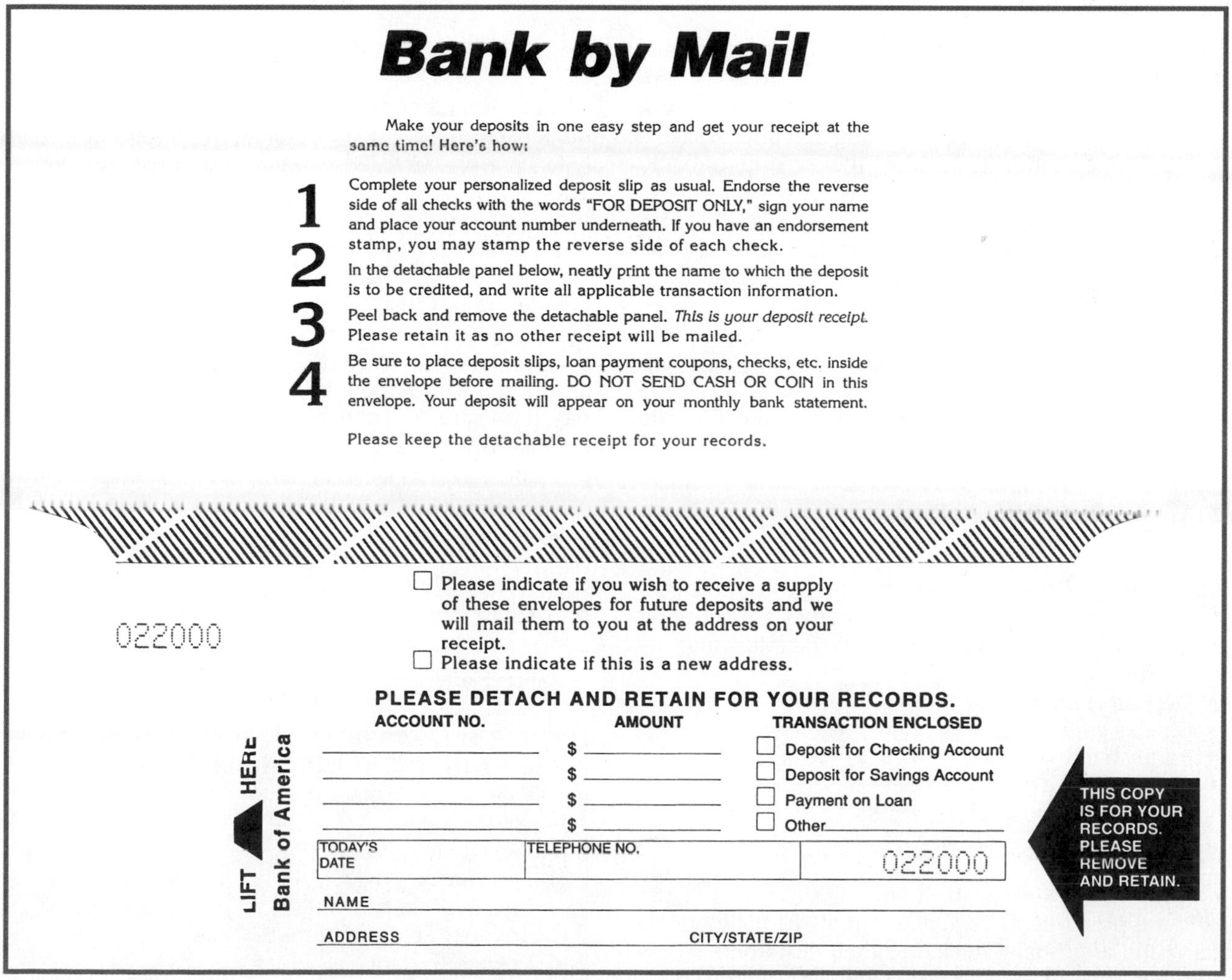

Bank by Mail

Make your deposits in one easy step and get your receipt at the same time! Here's how:

1 Complete your personalized deposit slip as usual. Endorse the reverse side of all checks with the words "FOR DEPOSIT ONLY," sign your name and place your account number underneath. If you have an endorsement stamp, you may stamp the reverse side of each check.

2 In the detachable panel below, neatly print the name to which the deposit is to be credited, and write all applicable transaction information.

3 Peel back and remove the detachable panel. _This is your deposit receipt._ Please retain it as no other receipt will be mailed.

4 Be sure to place deposit slips, loan payment coupons, checks, etc. inside the envelope before mailing. DO NOT SEND CASH OR COIN in this envelope. Your deposit will appear on your monthly bank statement.

Please keep the detachable receipt for your records.

022000

☐ Please indicate if you wish to receive a supply of these envelopes for future deposits and we will mail them to you at the address on your receipt.
☐ Please indicate if this is a new address.

PLEASE DETACH AND RETAIN FOR YOUR RECORDS.

ACCOUNT NO.	AMOUNT	TRANSACTION ENCLOSED
_____	$ _____	☐ Deposit for Checking Account
_____	$ _____	☐ Deposit for Savings Account
_____	$ _____	☐ Payment on Loan
_____	$ _____	☐ Other_____

LIFT ▲ HERE   Bank of America

| TODAY'S DATE | TELEPHONE NO. | 022000 |

NAME _____

ADDRESS _____   CITY/STATE/ZIP _____

THIS COPY
IS FOR YOUR
RECORDS.
PLEASE
REMOVE
AND RETAIN.

FIGURE 19-12   Example of a bank-by-mail deposit envelope. (Courtesy Valley Bank of Nevada, Las Vegas, Nev.)

DEPOSIT BY MAIL PRECAUTIONS

1. Do not send cash or currency by mail. If this is absolutely necessary, then send it by registered mail.
2. Use only a restrictive endorsement; use a deposit stamp or write the notation "For Deposit Only to the account of _____ ."
3. If you have not obtained mailing deposit slips or your bank does not provide them, make duplicate slips and mail them with your deposit. Ask the bank to stamp one copy and return it to you as a receipt.

Direct Deposits

Direct deposit is a plan in which payments are transferred, usually electronically, by a paying agency directly to the account of a recipient. Direct deposits are commonly used for paying salaries where paychecks are credited to employees' accounts—checking, savings, or any other type of account—at any financial institution.

Other Methods of Deposit

Advances in computer technology have allowed financial institutions to offer other methods of deposit to consumers and business customers. Some ATM machines will accept deposits, and there are checking accounts available that allow the customer to conduct the majority of banking services using the computer and ATM machines. These types of accounts may limit the amount of times the customer can use teller services without a fee.

Online banking allows customers to view their account, make transfers, order checks, pay bills, and perform numerous other transactions by simply logging on to the bank website and accessing the account with a password. Online banking is also an excellent way to research the checks that have cleared the bank and compute accurate bank balances.

Bank Statements and Reconciliation

A statement is periodically sent by the bank to the customer; it shows the status of the customer's account on a given date. This statement indicates the following:
- Beginning balance
- Deposits received
- Checks paid
- Bank charges
- Ending balance

Mailed Statements

Bank statements, similar to the one illustrated in Figure 19-13, are prepared at regular intervals (usually once a month) and are usually mailed to their customers. These statements may or may not include the accompanying cancelled checks, depending on bank policy and account type. The back of each page of the statement usually includes a reconciliation page so that the customer can determine what checks have still not cleared the bank, what deposits are not yet shown on the statement, and the accurate account balance.

Online Statements

Online statements, or e-statements, are an electronic version of a paper bank statement. Financial establishments that offer online banking services in an attempt to make banking easier for their customers claim that e-statements are a user-friendly way of viewing account balances and checking financial images online.

With e-statements, there's no need to continue receiving paper statements. The benefits include the following:
- Receiving statements quickly and easily
- Being able to save statements in an electronic file for examination and printing at the customer's convenience
- Keeping fees low by minimizing unnecessary paper and mailing costs

Various banks offer different options, and fees vary. If the medical assistant has been authorized to set up an online banking account with the financial institution used by the medical facility, he or she should visit the bank to discuss the details of what is involved.

Reconciling the Bank Statement

The bank statement balance and the customer's checkbook balance will usually be different, except in a relatively inactive account. The two balances must be reconciled. The reconciliation discloses any errors that may exist in the checkbook or, on rare occasions, in the bank statement (Figure 19-14).

The bank statement may include an entry for service charges that must be deducted from the checkbook balance. In all types of accounts, the bank may charge a fee for services. Usually in the case of an individual account, it is a flat fee; in a business account, the fee is based on services rendered. If the average or minimum balance is maintained at an established level, the bank may forego a service charge.

Most banks ask to be notified within a reasonable amount of time (e.g., 10 days) of any error found in the statement. The bank statement should be reconciled as soon as it is received. You will usually find a form to follow in carrying out this procedure on the back of the bank statement.

The reconciliation procedure may be put in a formula, as shown in the following box.

BANK STATEMENT RECONCILIATION FORMULA

Bank statement balance	$ _____
Less outstanding checks	$ _____
Plus deposits not shown	$ _____
Corrected Bank Statement Balance	$ _____
Checkbook balance	$ _____
Less any bank charges	$ _____
Corrected Checkbook Balance	$ _____

0821-402054

#821

|||||||||||||||||||||||||||||||||||||||||||||||||||||||

N
2

CALL (888) 555-2932
24 HOURS/DAY, 7 DAYS/WEEK
FOR ASSISTANCE WITH
YOUR ACCOUNT.

PAGE 1 OF 2   THIS STATEMENT COVERS: 6/22/02 THROUGH 7/22/02

INTEREST CHECKING
0821-402054

SUMMARY

PREVIOUS BALANCE	252.10		MINIMUM BALANCE	142.55
DEPOSITS	68.74+		AVERAGE BALANCE	220.00
INTEREST EARNED	.18+		ANNUAL PERCENTAGE	
WITHDRAWALS	109.55−		YIELD EARNED	.96%
CUSTOMER SERVICE CALLS	.00−			
INTERLINK/PURCHASE FEE	.00−		INTEREST EARNED 1994	2.23
MONTHLY CHECKING FEE				
AND OTHER CHARGES	.00−			

▶ **NEW BALANCE**   **211.47**

USE YOUR EXPRESS CARD TO MAKE UNLIMITED PURCHASES AT RETAILERS DISPLAYING
THE INTERLINK SYMBOL. (A $1 MONTHLY FEE MAY APPLY.)

TRY IT TODAY AT ARCO . . . MOBIL . . . LUCKY . . . RALPHS . . . SAFEWAY & MORE!

CHECKS AND WITHDRAWALS	CHECK	DATE PAID	AMOUNT	CHECK	DATE PAID	AMOUNT
	202	7/05	15.05	203	7/15	94.50

DEPOSITS				DATE POSTED	AMOUNT
	CUSTOMER DEPOSIT			7/22	68.74
	INTEREST PAYMENT THIS PERIOD			7/22	.18

BALANCE INFORMATION	DATE	BALANCE	DATE	BALANCE	DATE	BALANCE
	6/22	252.10	7/05	237.05	7/15	142.55
					7/22	211.47

24 HOUR CUSTOMER SERVICE

EACH ACCOUNT COMES WITH 3 COMPLIMENTARY CALLS PER STATEMENT PERIOD.

CALLS TO 24 HOUR CUSTOMER SERVICE THIS STATEMENT PERIOD: 0

INTEREST INFORMATION	FROM	THROUGH	INTEREST RATE	ANNUAL PERCENTAGE YIELD (APY)
	6/22	7/22	1.00%	1.01%

INTEREST RATE/APY AS OF 7/22/02 IF YOUR BALANCE IS

$ 0 - 4,999 . . . . .1.00%		1.01%
$ 5,000 - 9,999 . . . . .1.00%		1.01%
$ 10,000 AND OVER. 1.00%		1.01%

CALL 1-800-555-2932 IN CALIFORNIA ANYTIME FOR CURRENT RATES.

MEMBER FDIC

STATEMENT

FIGURE 19-13   Example of a regular checking account statement.

THIS WORKSHEET IS PROVIDED TO HELP YOU BALANCE YOUR ACCOUNT

1. Go through your register and mark each check, withdrawal, Express ATM transaction, payment, deposit or other credit listed on this statement. Be sure that your register shows any interest paid into your account, and any service charges, automatic payments, or Express Transfers withdrawn from your account during this statement period.

2. Using the chart below, list any outstanding checks, Express ATM withdrawals, payments or any other withdrawals (including any from previous months) that are listed in your register but are not shown on this statement.

3. Balance your account by filling in the spaces below.

ITEMS OUTSTANDING		
NUMBER	AMOUNT	
TOTAL	$	

ENTER

The NEW BALANCE shown on
this statement _ _ _ _ _ _ _ _ _ _ _ _ _ _ _ _ _ _ _ $_____

ADD

Any deposits listed in your register $_____
or transfers into your account $_____
which are not shown on this $_____
statement.   +$_____

TOTAL _ _ _ _ _ _ _ _ +$_____

CALCULATE THE SUBTOTAL _ _ _ _ _ _ _ _ _ $_____

SUBTRACT

The total outstanding checks and
withdrawals from the chart at left _ _ _ _ _ _ _ _ _ −$_____

CALCULATE THE ENDING BALANCE

This amount should be the same
as the current balance shown in
your check register _ _ _ _ _ _ _ _ _ _ _ _ _ _ _ $_____

FIGURE 19-14 Reverse side of a bank statement to be used for reconciling a checking account.

IF YOU SUSPECT ERRORS OR HAVE QUESTIONS ABOUT ELECTRONIC TRANSFERS

If you believe there is an error on your statement or Express ATM receipt, or if you need more information about a transaction listed on this statement or an Express ATM receipt, please contact us immediately. We are available 24 hours a day, seven days a week to assist you. Please call the telephone number printed on the front of this statement. Or, you may write to us at United Trust Company, P.O. Box 327, Anytown, USA.

1) Tell us your name and account number or Express card number.

2) As clearly as you can, describe the error or the transfer you are unsure about, and explain why you believe there is an error or why you need more information.

3) Tell us the dollar amount of the suspected error.

You must report the suspected error to us no later than 60 days after we sent you the first statement on which the problem appeared. We will investigate your question and will correct any error promptly. If our investigation takes longer than 10 business days (or 20 days in the case of electronic purchases), we will temporarily credit your account for the amount you believe is in error, so that you may have use of the money until the investigation is completed.

PROCEDURE 19-3

Reconciling a Bank Statement

GOAL: To reconcile a bank statement with the checking account.

EQUIPMENT AND SUPPLIES

- Ending balance of previous statement
- Current bank statement
- Canceled checks for current month
- Checkbook stubs
- Calculator
- Pen

PROCEDURAL STEPS

1 Compare the opening balance of the new statement with the closing balance of the previous statement.
  Purpose: To determine that the balances are in agreement.

2 Compare the canceled checks with the items on the statement.
  Purpose: To verify that they are your checks and that they are listed in the right amount.

3 Arrange the canceled checks in numerical order and compare with the checkbook stubs.

4 Place a checkmark (✓) on each stub for which a canceled check has been returned.
  Purpose: To locate any outstanding checks.

5 List and total the outstanding checks.

6 Verify that all previous outstanding checks have cleared.

7 Subtract the total of the outstanding checks from the bank statement balance.
  NOTE: Do not include any certified checks as outstanding because their amount has already been deducted from the account.

8 Add to the total in Step 7 any deposits made but not included in the bank statement.
  Purpose: To correct the credits in the bank statement balance.

9 Total any bank charges that appear on the bank statement and subtract them from the checkbook balance. Such charges may include service charges, automatic withdrawals or payments, and NSF checks.
  Purpose: To correct the checkbook balance.

10 If the checkbook balance and the statement balance do not agree, match the bank statement entries with the checkbook entries.

If the two *corrected balances* agree, you may stop there. If they do not agree, subtract the lesser figure from the greater figure; the difference will usually give you a clue to locating the error (Procedure 19-3).

QUESTIONS TO ASK IN SEARCHING FOR A POSSIBLE ERROR

- Is your arithmetic correct?
- Did you forget to include one of the outstanding checks?
- Did you fail to record a deposit or did you record it twice?

Signature Cards

When an account is first opened at a banking facility, the depositor will be required to affix his or her handwritten signature to a card, which is then kept on file at the bank. If a check comes through, and there is some suspicion that the depositor's signature has been forged, the bank personnel compare the signature on the check to the original one on the signature card.

In a business situation, as in a medical office, the physician often delegates the responsibility of paying bills to the medical assistant or other office staff. In this case, any staff member who has been authorized to sign the medical facility's checks must go to the bank and add his or her handwritten signature to the signature card. Only the people whose names appear on the signature card are authorized to sign checks, and it is the bank's responsibility to verify any questionable signatures.

Bonding

To protect their business establishments from embezzlement or other financial loss caused by employees who handle large sums of money, physicians often purchase fidelity bonds. Fidelity bonds reimburse the physician for any monetary loss caused by employees. There are three types of bonding methods:

- *Position-schedule bonding*, which covers a specific position rather than an individual, such as bookkeeper or receptionist
- *Blanket-position bonding*, which covers all employees
- *Personal bonding*, which covers specific individuals

For individuals to be bonded, a personal background investigation is normally necessary.

Patient Education

Medical assistants might want to encourage patients to pay for professional services rendered with a personal check because of the numerous benefits checks offer. If a patient attempts to pay for services with a third-party check (other than an insurance reimbursement), the medical assistant should tactfully explain why this is not a wise practice. Additionally, if a patient makes a mistake when writing a check, it is the responsibility of the medical assistant to point it out and request a new one, as corrections on the face of a check often render the check useless.

When a patient's check is returned from the bank marked "insufficient funds," the medical assistant should immediately call the patient and explain the problem, requesting that he or she correct the matter as soon as possible. It is important to remember, however, that most overdrafts are simply the result of mathematical errors or a delay in deposited funds being available for withdrawal. So the medical assistant should be patient and courteous when discussing NSF issues with patients. Patients need to know, however, that overdrafts are costly not only to them, but also to the medical facility.

Legal and Ethical Issues

If a mistake is made in preparing a check, do not destroy this check. Rather, write "VOID" across the face of the check, make a note on the check stub, and file the check with the cancelled checks for auditing purposes.

A stop-payment order may be placed with the bank in an emergency, such as a check being lost, or a disagreement about a purchase or payment.

Do not accept a check made payable to another party without having the endorsement of the person who gives the check to you. If the check is returned by the bank for any reason, the check will be charged to the last endorser, not the last person to receive the money.

SUMMARY OF SCENARIO

Laura has gained considerable knowledge through her experiences and work with the various aspects of the banking world. The goals she set for completing the assignments and competencies were accomplished in the time frame allowed by the instructor. She is comfortable now that she can readily apply this knowledge to whatever medical facility she works in.

Laura spent extra time outside of class exploring online banking and bill paying on the Internet and found a wealth of information available. Laura now plans to visit several banks in her area to see what kind of e-banking services they offer.

The versatility of the medical assistant's role and the variety of the opportunities available reinforce to Laura that she has made the right decision for her career choice.

SUMMARY OF LEARNING OBJECTIVES

■ The Internet has changed conventional banking as we know it, and it offers expansive opportunities without leaving home. As with everything, however, e-banking has both advantages and disadvantages, and it should be thoroughly researched before an online account is opened.

■ For an instrument (e.g., a check) to be "negotiable," it must meet certain criteria: (1) be written and signed by a maker, (2) contain a promise or order to pay a sum of money, (3) be payable on demand or at a fixed future date, and (4) be payable to order or bearer.

■ There are many advantages to using checks. These advantages include safety and convenience, quick calculation of expenditures, and a permanent record for tax purposes.

■ The three most common types of bank accounts are checking accounts, savings accounts, and money market savings accounts. Each one is slightly different, and each has its special uses.

■ Normally, when a mistake is made on a check, it should be marked "VOID" and a new check should be written. Some banks will accept minor errors if the maker initials the error. Erasures are not allowed, nor is the use of correction fluid.

■ List and discuss eight precautions to observe in accepting checks.

■ The four kinds of endorsements are (1) blank endorsement, in which the payee simply signs his or her name on the back of the check, (2) restrictive endorsement, which specifies which bank and what specific account the funds are to be deposited in, (3) special endorsement, which names a specific person as payee on the back of the check, and (4) qualified endorsement, which disclaims future liability. This type of endorsement is used when the person who accepts the check has no personal claim in the transaction.

■ When a deposited check is returned, the maker should be contacted immediately, informed of the situation, and asked to remedy the situation either by immediately depositing funds in his or her account to cover the check, or to pay the bill by alternative means—cash or money order.

■ The procedure for reconciling a bank statement is simple and straightforward; however, until it is done a few times, it can be confusing. Follow the formula listed in the box on p. 368. If the bank statement and checkbook do not balance, look for possible errors as listed in the box on p. 371.

KEY INTERNET WEBSITES

- The Federal Reserve System
- National Check Fraud Center
- State of California Department of Consumer Affairs (for information on small claims court)
  For active weblinks to each website visit
  http://evolve.elsevier.com/Kinn/

UNIT four

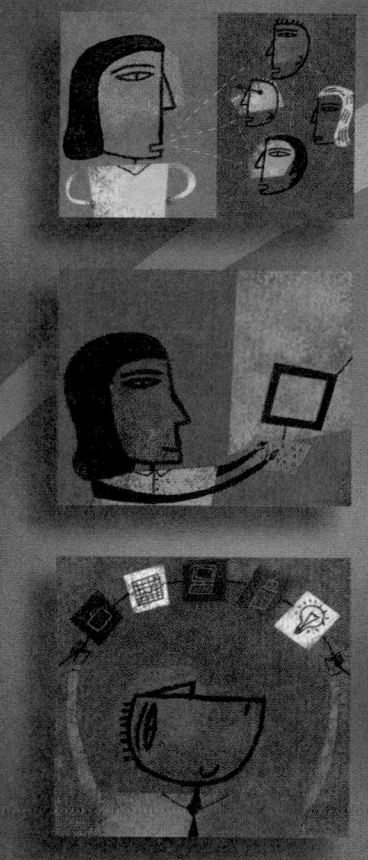

Medical Practice and Health Information Management

CHAPTER 20

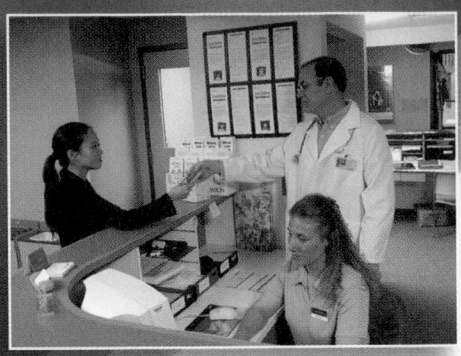

Scenario

Katherine Martinson is the office manager for Dr. Michael Bouchard, a family practitioner in a group practice located in a metropolitan area. The office usually carries a full schedule of patients each day. Katherine has been instrumental in the seamless operation of the practice. Before joining Dr. Bouchard, Katherine worked for a physician in the same group practice, Dr. Grant Bradley, who retired last year. She worked as an administrative medical assistant for 6 years before that. Her strength and ability to motivate employees led Dr. Bouchard to approach her about becoming his office manager once Dr. Bradley retired.

Katherine is the consummate professional but knows the importance of treating each employee as an individual. At weekly staff meetings, the employees offer input on the various procedures followed in the office. Katherine regularly counsels with the staff members, always asking for input as to how the office can function more effectively and implementing many of the suggestions in the day-to-day activities of the office. She knows that employees need to feel a part of the team, and by trying the procedures others suggest she validates them as an asset to the facility.

When there is a position available, Katherine is careful about whom she hires, always checking at least three references per applicant and verifying each place of employment. She trains each employee on every aspect of the job and keeps checklists that reflect the employee has been given instruction on certain skills.

Katherine makes sure that each person has the tools needed to do the job. She also explains overhead costs to employees and helps them to understand what is involved with the daily operation of the practice. With this information, the employees are more conservative about use of supplies and care of equipment. Major changes are presented to the entire staff, and although Dr. Bouchard has the final decision, he and Katherine seek the input of the staff, too. The cooperative attitude between management and the employees of the office provides a good atmosphere for teamwork, and Katherine and the physician are pleased with the results.

Medical Practice Management

National Curriculum Competencies

TRANSDISCIPLINARY COMPETENCIES

2d. Document appropriately

Vocabulary

affable Being pleasant and at ease in talking to others; characterized by ease and friendliness.

agenda A list or outline of things to be considered or done.

ancillary Subordinate; auxiliary.

appraisal To give an expert judgment of the value or merit of; judging as to quality.

blatant Completely obvious, conspicuous, or obtrusive, especially in a crass or offensive manner; brazen.

burnout Exhaustion of physical or emotional strength or motivation, usually as a result of prolonged stress or frustration.

chain of command A series of executive positions in order of authority.

circumvention To manage to get around, especially by ingenuity or stratagem.

cohesive The state of sticking together tightly; exhibiting or producing the cohesion.

disparaging Speak slightingly about, with a negative or degrading tone.

embezzlement Stealing from an employer; to appropriate goods, services, or funds for personal use without permission.

extrinsic External to a thing, its essential nature, or its original character.

impenetrable Incapable of being penetrated or pierced; not capable of being damaged or harmed.

incentives Something that incites or spurs to action; a reward or reason for performing a task.

insubordination Disobedient to authority.

intrinsic Originating or due to causes within a body, organ, or part.

mentor A trusted counselor or guide.

meticulous Marked by extreme or excessive care in the consideration or treatment of details.

micromanage To manage with great or excessive control or attention to details.

morale The mental and emotional condition, such as enthusiasm, confidence, or loyalty, of an individual or group with regard to the function or tasks at hand.

motivation The process of inciting a person to some action or behavior.

reprimands Criticisms for a fault; a severe or formal reproof.

retention To keep in possession or use; to keep in one's pay or service.

subordinate Submissive to or controlled by authority; placed in or occupying a lower class, rank, or position.

targeted Directed or used toward a target; directed toward a specific desire or position.

The management of a professional medical office can greatly influence the success of the operation. Good management will allow the physician to see and treat his or her patients in a functional environment with the confidence that the business side of the facility is operating as it should be. A well-managed office is not something that just happens. Great effort and strong teamwork are necessary to ensure that the day-to-day activities are carried out efficiently and that the many details that need attention are handled expeditiously.

Who's In Charge?

If there is only one medical assistant, that person must be able to assume many of the management responsibilities with cooperation from the physician. When there are two medical assistants, one administrative and one clinical, it is often the administrative medical assistant who is expected to assume the management duties. In the office with a larger staff, a line of authority must be established.

A facility with three or more employees should have one person designated as supervisor or office manager. This individual should have management skills and the ability to deal with personnel matters (Table 20-1). Other employees answer to the supervisor, and the supervisor answers to the physician or physicians. This sets up an orderly way for the office staff to consult with the physician regarding administrative or clinical problems, complaints, or grievances. It also allows the physician to check on the operation of the office, disseminate information on policy changes, and correct errors or grievances.

The career of medical assisting becomes more challenging with the passing years, and offers more opportunities for advancement. The recently graduated medical assistant, whose first position possibly was as a receptionist, may systematically be given more responsibilities and may eventually become the office manager of a large staff. There is a shortage in executive-level personnel, one of the most critical areas in healthcare. Specifically there is a need for individuals competent to develop and operate a health maintenance organization or prepaid group practice.

Management problems often can be avoided by carefully defining the areas of authority and responsibility of each employee. Many physicians say that friction between workers is their most common personnel problem. A definite **chain of command** must be established, and the physician must not undermine the supervisor's

TABLE 20-1	Qualities of an Effective Manager

- Uses good judgment
- Has good health
- Has the ability to organize
- Is willing to learn
- Possesses original ideas
- Has leadership ability
- Is fair with all employees
- Is flexible
- Has a sense of fairness
- Cares about employees
- Remains calm during crises
- Is open to constructive criticism
- Has good communication skills
- Uses good listening skills
- Is approachable

authority by **circumvention**. When employees know what is expected of them, they can plan both their daily and long-term work more effectively.

Duties of the Medical Office Manager

The duties carried out by medical office managers vary from place to place and practice to practice. Some physicians take on a much more active role in office management than others. The best management plan for the physician is to hire an office manager who is trustworthy and reliable, and then allow him or her to run the business aspects of the office. This frees the physician to concentrate on taking care of patients (Figure 20-1).

Some of the tasks performed by the medical office manager include:

- Preparing and updating policy and procedure manuals
- Developing job descriptions
- Recruiting new employees
- Orientation and training
- Performance and salary reviews
- Dismissal of employees
- Planning staff meetings
- Maintaining staff harmony
- Establishing work-flow guidelines

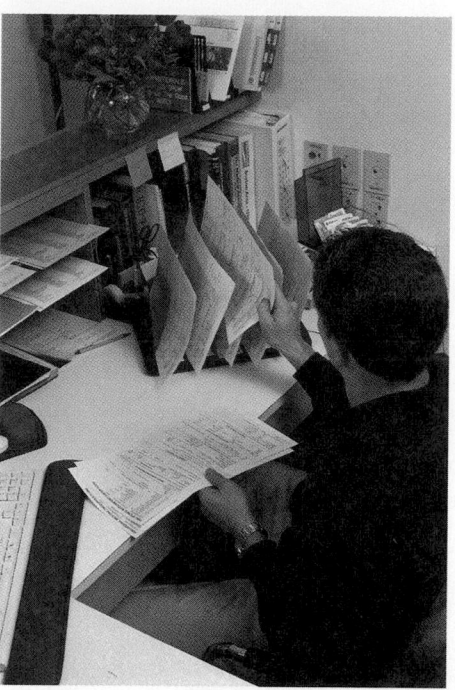

FIGURE 20-1   The office manager ensures that the medical facility runs smoothly so that the physician can concentrate on patient care.

PROCEDURE 20-1

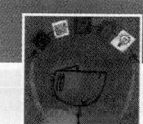

Making Travel Arrangements

GOAL: To make travel arrangements for the physician or another staff member.

EQUIPMENT AND SUPPLIES

- Travel plan
- Telephone
- Telephone directory
- Typewriter or computer
- Typing paper

PROCEDURAL STEPS

1 Verify the dates of the planned trip.
- Desired date and time of departure.
- Desired date and time of return.
- Preferred mode of transportation.
- Number in party.
- Preferred lodging and price range.
- Preferred ticketing method (electronic or paper).

2 Telephone a trusted travel agency to arrange for transportation and lodging reservations.

3 Arrange for traveler's checks, if desired.

4 Pick up tickets/e-receipts or arrange for delivery.

5 Check tickets to confirm conformance with the travel plan.

Purpose: To avoid any error due to misunderstanding and to verify compliance with requests.

6 Check to see that hotel and air reservations are confirmed.

7 Prepare an itinerary, including all the necessary information:
- Date and time of departure.
- Flight numbers or identifying information of other modes of travel.
- Mode of transportation to hotel(s).
- Name, address, and telephone number of hotel(s), with confirmation numbers if available.
- Name, address, and telephone number of travel agency.
- Date and time of return.

8 Place one copy of itinerary in the office file.
Purpose: It may be necessary to contact the traveler or to forward mail.

9 Give several copies of the itinerary to the traveler.
Purpose: The traveler may wish to have extra copies for family or friends.

- Improving office efficiency
- Supervising the purchase and care of equipment
- Educating patients
- Eliminating time-wasting tasks for the physician (Procedure 20-1)
- Marketing the practice
- Customer service

Office management can best be accomplished by developing a thorough office policy and procedure manual. This will be discussed later in the chapter.

The Power of Influence

Managers have a great deal of influence over the people they supervise. A successful manager must be interested in people and enjoy working with them on a daily basis. It is said that if one helps others get what they want in life, the individual usually gets what he or she wants as well. An effective manager discovers the motivation behind employees' drives to be a part of the profession in which they are employed, and then helps them achieve their individual goals. In turn, most employees are enthusiastic about working toward the facility's goals as productive team members.

Successful managers know that their employees should be encouraged to perform at optimal levels, and they are confident enough in their own skills to give credit to those employees who develop ideas and concepts for the team. These managers know how to let their employees help them "look good." A manager with a group of outstanding employees usually is looked upon as an effective leader.

CRITICAL THINKING APPLICATION

- When Katherine first began as Dr. Bouchard's office manager, she found several supportive employees, but a few were concerned about their new boss. How can a new manager help employees be at ease during the first few weeks?
- Katherine scheduled a time with each employee and asked the three things he or she liked best about the office and three things he or she liked the least. How does this help her to manage the office effectively?

The Manager as a Leader

Leaders nurture other people. They take the time to discover what makes people tick and then give them opportunities that will help them rise to new levels of responsibility. Leaders have a strong belief in people, and they express confidence in their abilities, seeing them as successes rather than failures. Often this belief exists before people prove themselves, and that provides motivation to reach their potential.

Perhaps most important, leaders listen to their people. Few things are more frustrating than an employee attempting to talk to a manager who is working on some project or typing on the computer. Listening involves eye contact and questions to ensure that the employee is understood. Being willing to take the time to listen is a step toward success as a manager.

Types of Leaders

There are three basic types of leaders today, including the charismatic leader, the transactional leader, and the transformational leader. Each has positive qualities and all can be successful in business.

Charismatic leaders have a special way of inspiring an unswerving allegiance and devotion from their followers. They encourage people to overcome great obstacles and buy into their vision for the organization or business. They also tend to trust their **subordinates** and earn trust in return.

Transactional leaders are structured and organized. They ensure that their subordinates understand their duties and roles. These leaders are fair and provide rewards when they have been earned. The transactional leader is hardworking, a planner, and strict about budgets and time frames.

Transformational leaders are innovative and able to bring about change in an organization. These leaders are relationship builders. They stress shared values and strive to create a common ground among team members. Transformational leaders are the most effective when an organization is experiencing change and reorganization.

Styles of Management

Some managers are democratic and willing to listen to employees. These managers are fair-minded and ask the opinions of the staff when making decisions. This is a contrast to the autocratic manager, who is more of a dictator, making demands and insisting tasks be done in a certain way—his or her way. The laissez-faire manager is easy-going and does not make a lot of demands on employees. This is a "go with the flow" manager who lets employees work on their own and does not **micromanage**.

Leading During Transitions and Change

Change is a part of the life of every person and every business. Most people are initially hesitant to face change and many people try to avoid it completely. However, a business cannot experience growth without change. The manager who is able to lead subordinates through periods of change will be a valuable asset to the organization. They will need guidance on maintaining focus on the tasks at hand. The manager should remain visible to the employees during times of change and communicate frequently with status reports and updates on policies and procedures.

The book *Who Moved My Cheese?* by Spencer Johnson, MD,* is one of the most innovative stories in recent years. Any manager or employee experiencing a time of change should study this simple, short book. The opening quotes A. J. Cronin, saying:

---

*Johnson S: *Who moved my cheese? An amazing way to deal with change in your work and in your life.* New York, 1988, The Putnam Publishing Group.

"Life is no straight and easy corridor along which we travel free and unhampered, but a maze of passages, through which we must seek our way, lost and confused, now and again checked in a blind alley. But always, if we have faith, a door will open for us, not perhaps one that we ourselves would ever have thought of, but one that will ultimately prove good for us."

Who Moved My Cheese? stresses several points about change that the good manager should remember, including:

- Change happens.
- Anticipate change.
- Monitor change.
- Adapt to change quickly.
- Move with the change.
- Enjoy change.
- Be ready to change again quickly and enjoy it again.

The simplicity of this advice does not diminish its truth. Change will happen in any person's job and personal life. Those who learn to adapt quickly and move forward will be the ones who survive the casualties of change.

The Role of Power

One definition of power is the ability to influence employees so that they carry out their directives. Leaders use many types of power.

Coercive power is manipulative, and the leader often makes threats or uses fear to accomplish goals. The fear of losing a job is one manipulation of power.

Granting rewards is a more positive use of power. When the leader is able to give employees some type of reward for a job well done, most strive to reach goals.

Expert power is a factor when the leader is knowledgeable about a subject. Employees respect leaders who know their job and how things should be done. Most people look up to a person who has a high degree of knowledge about a given subject. When working for someone who knows nothing about procedures or the services offered, employees frequently are frustrated.

Legitimate power is that of position or status. It does not really matter who the President of the United States is—the office itself carries the weight of power. Therefore the individual who serves as President holds legitimate power.

Referent power is granted from subordinates to those who lead by example. It is a power based on the admiration of the leader. Mentors, parents, and teachers are often the objects of referent power.

CRITICAL THINKING APPLICATION

- Katherine is a respected office manager in the facility where she works, but there are several other managers who are not as well liked. What makes a good office manager?
- Everyone has worked for at least one supervisor that they were not fond of. What traits make a poor office manager?

Abuse of Power and Authority

Unfortunately, many managers have the capacity to abuse the power they have. There are several ways to do this. A manager who puts up barriers and erects emotional walls with the employees will have difficulty forming a **cohesive** team. Some managers use other people as tools to get what they want, while others stick to their own level or stature, relating only to the inner circle of decision makers in the facility.

When there are no checks and balances in an organization, it is easy to abuse power. It is difficult to work with a manager who cannot look inside himself or herself and see mistakes. Some managers stress rules and conformity, leaving no gray areas where subordinates are concerned. Some show a false humility and pretend to care, but most employees can see right through this half-effort at a relationship. Others only hire "yes" people, who agree with everything that the manager says. All of these are abuses of power and indications of a poor manager.

The Power of Motivation

What motivates a person to reach a goal? In the list below, distinguish which motivators are effective in helping an individual reach goals:

- A challenge
- Money
- Praise
- Satisfaction
- Freedom
- Fear
- Family
- Insecurity
- Competition
- Fulfillment
- Integrity
- Honor
- Reputation
- Responsibility
- Prestige
- Needs
- Love

All of the motivators listed above could prompt an employee to action. There are two general types of motivation. **Intrinsic** motivation is internal or originates within someone. Intrinsic motivation is long term and can be a lifelong goal. **Extrinsic** motivation is external and more material in nature. Generally, extrinsic motivation is more short lived and less satisfying than intrinsic motivation.

CRITICAL THINKING APPLICATION

- Katherine knows that employees have different reasons and motivations for working. Some must work to help support their families, and others work simply because of a love for their field. How can Katherine discover her employees' motivations for working?
- How does this knowledge benefit the office manager?
- Can this knowledge help Katherine achieve her own goals?

Creating a Team Atmosphere

Teamwork is critical in the medical profession. In the physician's office the manager must promote an atmosphere in which the employees are willing to work together toward common goals. Low **morale** may exist in the office because of recent changes in policies or procedures, changes in staff or management, terminations of recent employees, lack of business, or any number of other reasons. The wise manager will take steps to constantly improve employee morale, including scheduling frequent meetings and keeping the employees abreast of changes and developments that affect them (Figure 20-2). Employees like to be kept "in the loop." Some managers attempt to shield employees from negative information, but this practice can cause rumors to circulate and make morale even worse.

Managers can improve morale by scheduling activities that involve the families of employees and making an obvious effort to include employees in various events. One of the most effective ways to improve employee morale is to communicate. Regular staff meetings are critical for good communication and smooth operation of the medical facility.

FIVE ESSENTIAL ELEMENTS OF A TEAM

- *Mutual accountability:* Each person on the team holds the others accountable for the success of the organization.
- *Common purpose and performance goals:* Short-term and intermediate goals must relate to the long-term goals of the group.
- *Small size:* Most successful teams have a small number of members, and fewer than 10 is optimum.
- *Common approach:* All of the team members must learn to work together toward the goal.
- *Complementary skills:* A variety of talent, skill, and ability are needed for a successful team.

From Katzenbach JR, Smith DK: Wisdom of teams: creating the high-performance organization. Boston, 1992, Harvard Business School Publishing.

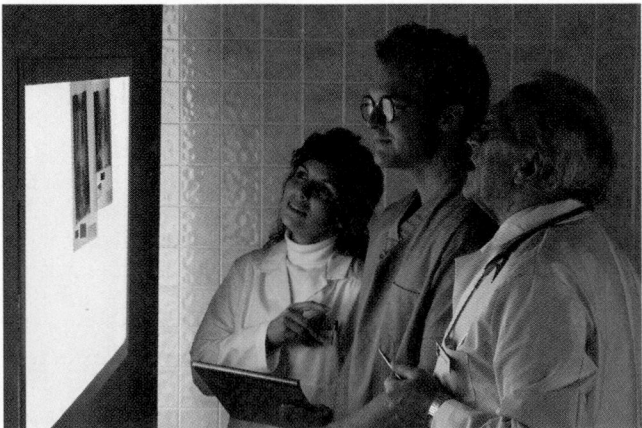

FIGURE 20-2 Communication is vital when building a team. Employees appreciate good communication with management. Sharing good and bad news openly with employees leads to fewer rumors and nervous workers.

Use of Incentives and Employee Recognition

The staff of the physician's office should feel satisfaction with the working conditions and atmosphere in the facility. The office manager plays a part in ensuring that this happens.

Incentives give the employees reason to perform over and above the level expected of them. For instance, if the staff meets or exceeds a goal that has been set, the physician may elect to provide tickets to a sports or entertainment event for the entire staff. A paid day off is always a great incentive for accomplishing a goal. Some physicians have an incentive program that is related to the collections for the office in a given period. These ideas provide a goal for the employees to work toward and an opportunity to expand their efforts as a team.

Recognition is a strong method of improving employee morale and encouraging outstanding performance. Certificates for peak performance in a given area are a great way to motivate employees. For instance, the office manager may decide to award a certificate each month to the employee who provides the best customer service. Patients could even be involved by allowing them to nominate employees for this honor. When an award is at stake, most employees will enjoy participating and striving toward the goals that have been set.

CRITICAL THINKING APPLICATION

- One of Katherine's employees, Jewel, is very sensitive about performing perfectly on the job. She is an excellent employee, but she does have a few weaknesses. However, she has received a lot of recognition for the good things she has done at work. Katherine still feels that she needs to discuss the areas where Jewel is performing weakly with her but knows that it will upset her. How might Katherine deal with this sticky situation?
- How can Katherine reassure Jewel that she is pleased with her overall performance?

Problem Employees

Occasionally, problem employees disrupt the flow of efficiency in the physician's office. Counseling these employees to find the source of their difficulties is the first step toward resolution. Many employees can be redirected to become productive staff members with a little patience and understanding on the part of the manager. However, some employees have negative attitudes that seem **impenetrable**.

The manager must never hesitate to counsel the employee who is not performing at the expected level, and this includes employees with attitude problems. A set regimen of counseling should be established. Many offices allow one verbal warning before written **reprimands** go into the employee files. If the manager does not make a habit of writing formal reprimands, there may be insufficient documentation of problems with the employee once the manager is ready to terminate him or her. Even small offenses, such as being tardy, should at least be noted in the employee's file. The manager should never be in a position that the termination of an employee cannot be justified by written documents.

Preventing Burnout

Burnout is defined as exhaustion of physical or emotional strength or motivation, usually as a result of prolonged stress or frustration. Medical professionals are particularly susceptible to burnout because of the intensity of their jobs. Even small decisions could affect the life of a patient. Therefore the office manager should take measures to help employees avoid burnout (Table 20-2).

Some of the causes of burnout include a stressful, disorganized home or work environment; poor human relations skills; a feeling of being out of control of one's life; excessive expectations from supervisors or family members; long work hours or time away from family and friends; and not being able to relax either at home or in the work environment.

Keeping the Management Relationship Professional

When people work together for an extended period, they often become **affable** and sometimes relationships develop into close friendships. This is a normal occurrence, but the office manager must be careful about becoming too close to his or her employees. When there is a friendly relationship, it is sometimes difficult to reprimand an employee when this is needed. Some employees will take advantage of a good relationship with the office manager and may begin to arrive late or call in sick more than usual. A healthy respect for each other must be maintained. The manager can have a good rapport with employees without becoming overly friendly, and this is the best policy. Some facilities have strict rules about fraternization with subordinates outside of the work facility. It is advisable to keep the relationship on a professional level at all times.

TABLE 20-2	Tips for Preventing Burnout

- Ask for help.
- Devote specific times for self-introspection or meditation.
- Understand what can be changed and what cannot be changed.
- Get some exercise.
- Organize and prioritize tasks.
- List tasks that are displeasing and delegate to others, if possible.
- Understand personal limitations.
- Take short vacations at least twice a year.
- Identify goals and try to perform only tasks that lead to reaching goals.
- Consider options, including changing jobs.
- Personalize work space with pictures and comforting items.
- Get a good understanding of a position and the stress involved before accepting it.

Selecting the Right Staff Members

The most important asset to any medical office is the staff that cares for the patients. From the doctor to the receptionist, all play a vital role in the well-being of those who visit the office. Selecting staff members that can be molded into a cohesive team is not an easy task. Care should be taken to choose employees who have the necessary skills and the right personality for the office. Never try to select employees who are all alike. A variety of personality types work better than several similar personalities.

Understanding the Needs of the Office

The office manager should discuss with the physician the type of employee needed when an opening arises. Ask what qualities he or she desires in the person who occupies that particular position and what tasks the person will be responsible for. Once the need has been established and the duties confirmed, the office manager can begin the recruiting process.

One of the most effective methods of finding new employees is through word of mouth. Ask other office managers, physicians, or medical professionals if they are aware of a person looking for employment who has the skills needed in the office. It is a good idea to keep a file of resumes that can be accessed when an opening exists in the office. Often the physician or office manager may know of a person working in another area of the clinic or perhaps in a nearby hospital who may be interested in a job change. Be careful in approaching a person who is already employed. There is no harm in asking if a person is interested, but if the reply is negative, do not pursue the issue further.

Employment agencies can be used to find staff members, but they may charge a fee for their services. The office manager may wish to contact a local medical assistant school to secure an extern. If the extern proves to be an asset to the office, then he or she may be offered the permanent position. Newspaper ads are another option for finding employees, but many resumes may be submitted from people who are not qualified, especially when the economy is not at its best. When creating an ad for the newspaper, list the basic requirements for the position. Briefly describe the office and location, and the personality type being sought. Some offices list a few of the benefits offered to attract applicants and may disclose a salary range as well.

Reviewing Resumes and Applications

Once several resumes or applications have been submitted, the office manager should set aside quiet time to review the documents. Place them into one of three stacks—stack one should contain resumes of individuals who will be called for an interview, stack two those of possible candidates but not the strongest, and stack three those of applicants who will not be called.

During this preliminary review process, look for several items. First, be sure the documents are neatly prepared and completely legible (Figure 20-3). The person hired will probably write in the patient charts, so this is a good opportunity to ensure that his or her handwriting can be read clearly. Second, look for gaps between positions. Be sure that any lengthy time of unemployment is explained. The application should be filled out completely, and no notations of "see resume" should be included. The application provides important information and an applicant who does not fill it out in its entirety might be classified as lazy and prone to taking shortcuts. Watch for inconsistencies or oversights, including information that seems incomplete. Also look for resumes that are **targeted** toward the job opening available in the clinic. Targeted resumes are written specifically for a certain position. With today's computer capabilities, job seekers can target their resumes for each job applied for, and this strategy tells the manager that the applicant has enough interest in the job to demonstrate that he or she meets the requirements.

Once the entire stack of documents has been reviewed and separated, return to the stack of potential interviews. Careful judgment and objectivity must be used in the search for an employee who is suitable for the practice. Before interviewing any applicant, the manager needs to know several details:

- What personal qualities and abilities must the applicant have?
- What responsibilities are involved with the position?
- What is the salary range that the physician is willing to offer?
- How soon the position will be open?

Once these facts are clear, the manager should review the final resumes and applications with the following questions in mind:

- Do the applicant's appearance and personal grooming meet the standards set forth in the policy manual?
- Has the applicant been employed previously? What duties were performed?
- If previously employed, how long was the applicant in the last position? Why did the applicant leave?
- What are the applicant's skills? Do these meet the requirements for the position as set forth in the office procedure manual?
- Does the applicant seem to accept and enjoy responsibility?
- What is the applicant's formal education? Is he or she registered or certified? If not, is the applicant interested in taking the examination?
- Is the applicant a member of a professional organization? Does he or she attend meetings?

Arranging the Personal Interview

If the applicant sent a letter asking for an interview, note whether the letter was correctly typed, included essential contact information, and whether he or she also provided an attractive resume. It is amazing how many resumes do not include a contact telephone number. By telephoning the applicant, there will be an opportunity to judge his or her telephone voice. The manager may wish to prescreen applicants with the telephone call, asking several questions about the person's education and experience. Because the employee probably will speak with patients on the telephone, clarity of speech will be important. Those who perform well during the prescreening should be scheduled for an interview.

CRITICAL THINKING APPLICATION

- Katherine was impressed with Carol Limpken's resume and application, but when scheduling an interview on the telephone she noticed that Carol's grammatical abilities were not as professional as Katherine would like. Should this influence Katherine's decision to hire Carol?
- Why is speech such an important issue in the medical office?

Set a time for the personal interview when the applicant can be given undivided attention. An applicant who is being considered for employment should have an opportunity to see the office when there is a fairly normal amount of activity. The prospective employee who is interviewed in a peaceful, quiet office on the physician's day out may not be prepared for the activity on a normal working day.

Before interviewing any applicant, be thoroughly familiar with the federal, state, and local fair employment practice laws affecting hiring practices. Both men and women receive protection from on-the-job discrimination, sexual harassment, mandatory lie detector tests, and unfair discharge. Title VII of the Civil Rights Act of 1964, as amended by the Equal Employment Opportunity Act of 1972, prohibits inquiries into an applicant's race, color, sex, religion, and national origin. Inquiries regarding medical history, arrest records, or previous drug use are also illegal. Most states have laws designed to protect the rights of job applicants, and these laws may impose additional restrictions.

If an application has not been submitted, have the applicant complete it at the time of the interview. The application form can serve as a check of the applicant's penmanship and thoroughness as well as become a permanent record if the individual is hired. Tell the candidate if the form should be completed in the applicant's own handwriting, and be sure to state this on the instructions. Check to see if the applicant was **meticulous** about following instructions and filling in all the blanks. This provides the manager with an indication of the individual's capacity for following directions.

APPLICATION FOR POSITION / Medical or Dental Office
AN EQUAL OPPORTUNITY EMPLOYER

(In answering questions, use extra blank sheet if necessary)

No employee, applicant, or candidate for promotion, training or other advantage shall be discriminated against (or given preference) because of race, color, religion, sex, age, physical handicap, veteran status, or national origin.

PLEASE READ CAREFULLY AND WRITE OR PRINT ANSWERS TO ALL QUESTIONS. DO NOT TYPE.

Date of Application

A. PERSONAL INFORMATION

Name - Last | First | Middle | Social Security No. | Area Code/Phone No. ( )

Present Address: - Street | (Apt #) | City | State | Zip | How Long At This Address?:

Previous Address: - Street | City | State | Zip | Person to notify in case of Emergency or Accident - Name:

From: | To: | Address: | Telephone:

B. EMPLOYMENT INFORMATION

For What Position Are You Applying?: | ☐ Full-Time ☐ Part-Time ☐ Either | Date Available For Employment?: | Wage/Salary Expectations:

List Hrs./Days You Prefer To Work | List Any Hrs./Days You Are Not Available: (Except for times required for religious practices or observances) | Can You Work Overtime, If Necessary? ☐ Yes ☐ No

Are You Employed Now?: ☐ Yes ☐ No | If So, May We Inquire Of Your Present Employer?: ☐ No ☐ Yes, If Yes: | Name Of Employer: | Phone Number: ( )

Have You Ever Been Bonded? ☐ Yes ☐ No | If Required For Position, Are You Bondable? ☐ Yes ☐ No ☐ Uncertain | Have You Applied For A Position With This Office Before? ☐ No ☐ Yes If Yes, When?:

Referred By / Or Where Did You Learn Of This Job?:

Can You, Upon Employment, Submit Verification Of Your Legal Right To Work In The United States?: ☐ Yes ☐ No Submit Proof That You Meet Legal Age Requirement For Employment? ☐ Yes ☐ No | Language(s) Applicant Speaks or Writes (If Use Of A Language Other Than English is Relevant To The Job For Which The Applicant Is Applying:

C. EDUCATIONAL HISTORY

Name & Address Of Schools Attended (Include Current)	Dates From	Thru	Highest Grade/Level Completed	Diploma/Degree(s) Obtained/Areas of Study
High School				
College				Degree/Major
Post Graduate				Degree/Major
Other				Course/Diploma/License/Certificate

Specific Training, Education, Or Experiences Which Will Assist You In The Job For Which You Have Applied.

Future Educational Plans

D. SPECIAL SKILLS

CHECK BELOW THE KINDS OF WORK YOU HAVE DONE:

☐ BLOOD COUNTS	☐ DENTAL ASSISTANT	☐ MEDICAL INSURANCE FORMS	☐ RECEPTIONIST
☐ BOOKKEEPING	☐ DENTAL HYGIENIST	☐ MEDICAL TERMINOLOGY	☐ TELEPHONES
☐ COLLECTIONS	☐ FILING	☐ MEDICAL TRANSCRIPTION	☐ TYPING
☐ COMPOSING LETTERS	☐ INJECTIONS	☐ NURSING	☐ STENOGRAPHY
☐ COMPUTER INPUT	☐ INSTRUMENT STERILIZATION	☐ PHLEBOTOMY (Draw Blood)	☐ URINALYSIS
OFFICE EQUIPMENT USED: ☐ COMPUTER	☐ DICTATING EQUIPMENT	☐ POSTING	☐ X-RAY
		☐ WORD PROCESSOR	☐ OTHER:

Other Kinds Of Tasks Performed Or Skills That May Be Applicable To Position: | Typing Speed | Shorthand Speed

ORDER # 72-110 • © 1976 BIBBERO SYSTEMS, INC. • PETALUMA, CA. • (REV. 1/95)
TO REORDER CALL TOLL FREE: (800) BIBBERO (800-242-2376) OR FAX (800) 242-9330   MFG IN U.S.A.

(PLEASE COMPLETE OTHER SIDE)

FIGURE 20-3 Application for employment. Candidates for jobs in the medical office should complete applications accurately, leaving no blanks or unanswered questions. (Courtesy Bibbero Systems, Inc., Petaluma, Calif., 94954, (800) 242-2376, www.bibbero.com.) *continued*

E. EMPLOYMENT RECORD

LIST MOST RECENT EMPLOYMENT FIRST   May We Contact Your Previous Employer(s) For A Reference? ☐ Yes ☐ No

1) Employer

Work Performed. Be Specific:

Address   Street   City   State   Zip Code

Phone Number
( )

Type of Business

Dates   Mo. Yr.   Mo. Yr.
From   To

Your Position

Hourly Rate/Salary
Starting   Final

Supervisor's Name

Reason For Leaving

2) Employer

Worked Performed. Be Specific:

Address   Street   City   State   Zip Code

Phone Number
( )

Type of Business

Dates   Mo. Yr.   Mo. Yr.
From   To

Your Position

Hourly Rate/Salary
Starting   Final

Supervisor's Name

Reason For Leaving

3) Employer

Worked Performed. Be Specific:

Address   Street   City   State   Zip Code

Phone Number
( )

Type of Business

Dates   Mo. Yr.   Mo. Yr.
From   To

Your Position

Hourly Rate/Salary
Starting   Final

Supervisor's Name

Reason For Leaving

F. REFERENCES — FRIENDS / ACQUAINTANCES NON-RELATED

(1)
Name   Address   Telephone Number   (☐ Work ☐ Home)   Occupation   Years Acquainted

(1)
Name   Address   Telephone Number   (☐ Work ☐ Home)   Occupation   Years Acquainted

Please Feel Free To Add Any Information Which You Feel Will Help Us Consider You For Employment

READ THE FOLLOWING CAREFULLY, THEN SIGN AND DATE THE APPLICATION

"I certify that all answers given by me on this application are true, correct and complete to the best of my knowledge. I acknowledge notice that the information contained in this application is subject to check. I agree that, if hired, my continued employment may be contingent upon the accuracy of that information. If employed, I further agree to comply with Company/Office rules and regulations."

Signature: _____   Date: _____

FIGURE 20-3—Cont'd   For legend see previous page.

The Interview

First make certain that the applicant feels at ease (Figure 20-4). Shake his or her hand and ask a few social questions before starting the interview. In general, follow good manners and see that the person to be interviewed is comfortable. Most people feel some butterflies in their stomach when interviewing, but the manager will get a better idea of the person's capabilities if he or she is relaxed and able to discuss strengths and background openly with the manager.

Begin with a few open-ended questions that cannot be answered with a simple "yes" or "no," such as "What were your duties during your last position?" When interviewing a recent graduate who does not have experience, ask questions such as, "What subject did you perform well in at school?" When speaking with the candidate, make a mental note of whether he or she displays essential personal qualities, such as the ability to converse easily, the capacity to listen, and a bright smile. The applicant should be interested enough in the position to ask intelligent questions and appear interested in the office and the physician's specialty.

Avoid inquiries that involve the applicant's privacy. The questions should be related to the available position and the applicant's ability to do the job. An interview is a two-way exchange of information between the applicant and the interviewer. If the applicant appears to be one who will receive serious consideration, explain what will be expected as an employee. Office policies regarding appearance, working hours, overtime, time off, and vacations may be discussed at this stage. Salary and other fringe benefits should be discussed once the manager is ready to offer the job. If the manager fails to mention these items, the applicant may be hesitant to inquire.

Some employers request a credit check before offering employment, especially if the individual will be handling practice finances. It can safely be assumed that one who is unable to handle personal financial affairs will be a poor risk in handling office finances.

Review the job description for the position being filled. The person being interviewed must understand the required duties and responsibilities of the job. Ask if the applicant has any questions, and close the interview on a positive note. Let the candidate know when a decision will be made and what further contact the office will initiate.

During the hiring proceedings, the manager may wish to invite the prospective employee to lunch with the staff or for coffee in the more relaxed atmosphere of the employee lounge. This presents an opportunity to discover whether the applicant's personality will mesh with the atmosphere of the office. Employees appreciate being asked their opinion on those who are potential team members.

An extensive list of interview questions can be found in Chapter 55.

Follow-Up Activities

When the interview is over, take a few moments immediately to rate the applicant. Jot down some notes so that the applicant will be remembered easily when the final decisions are being made as to who will be hired. Do not trust the impressions to memory, especially if several applicants have been interviewed. Never write harmful personal statements; instead, be objective and fair. Should the potential employee ever have cause to bring the physician to court for discrimination in hiring practices, there should be no **disparaging** information written down that would reflect in a negative way on the physician or office manager.

It is always advisable to carefully check all references and to follow through on any leads for information. It is best to use the telephone in checking references, because people are sometimes less than candid in a letter; furthermore, letter writing is time consuming and a reply may never be sent. If the email address for a reference is provided, this is an excellent way to check a reference, and the printed version may be added to the applicant's file.

Prepare a checklist before placing the call. When speaking with the person called, be sure to "listen between the lines." Note the tone of the replies to the questions. Do not ask questions that might incriminate the person answering them. The following questions are effective as an introduction:

1. When did (the applicant) work for you?
2. For how long?
3. What were the duties and responsibilities?
4. Did the employee assume responsibility well?

Some employers will provide information only on the date of hire, job title, and date of termination of the employment. Respect the company's policy and do not press for further information.

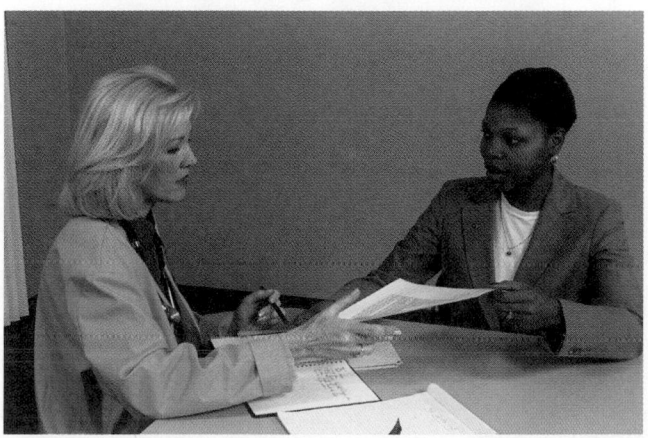

FIGURE 20-4   Put the applicant at ease. Job applicants perform at their peak when relaxed and calm.

CRITICAL THINKING APPLICATION

- While checking Carol's references, Katherine speaks to her last employer who makes the statement, "she is *not* eligible for rehire." The former employer placed strong emphasis on the word "not." All of Carol's other references were glowing. Should Katherine decide not to hire Carol on the basis of this employer's comment?
- How might Katherine find out more about the situation with the last employer?

Any person who is granted an interview should send a thank-you letter to the person who interviewed him or her. Watch the mail to see if any of the applicants perform this important follow-up task.

A second interview may be granted when the field is narrowed to two or three candidates. The physician may wish to participate in these interviews. Some offices conduct a group interview with several staff members present. Remember that these interviews become more and more stressful for the candidate, and the manager should expect some nervousness.

Making the Selection

When a decision has been reached to hire someone, it is best to bring the successful candidate back into the office to offer the position and negotiate the final details. Remember to notify all others who have interviewed for the position, so that they can look for other positions. They may have hesitated to accept other interviews, and it is unfair to keep individuals who are seeking employment hoping for a telephone call from the physician's office. Good etiquette requires dropping them a note or calling to say that the position is filled. Thank the individual for applying, and offer to keep his or her application on file. The office manager may wish to wait until the first-choice candidate has actually accepted the offer before notifying anyone else that the job has been filled. Don't expect the potential employee to answer the offer on the spot. Twenty-four hours is a reasonable time to consider the offer.

Orientation and Training—Critical Factors for Successful Employees

Recruitment does not end with the hiring. The orientation and training will help new employees to understand what is expected and to develop to their full potential (Figure 20-5). One of the most critical errors in bringing new staff members aboard is not providing them with a fair orientation and training period. The office manager should develop a checklist of the paperwork needed for newly hired staff and all of the information that should be covered with the new employee at the onset of the job.

Some managers assign a **mentor** to assist the new employee during the initial probationary period. This is a guide whom the new staff member can approach with questions and concerns (Figure 20-6). It is a good practice to use this type of "buddy" system, because the new person does not feel isolated and alone during the first few weeks on the job.

Acquaint the new employee with such aspects of the office as:

- Staff members and their names
- Physical environment and layout of the office
- Nature of the practice and specialty
- Types of patients seen in the office
- Office policies
- Long-range expectations

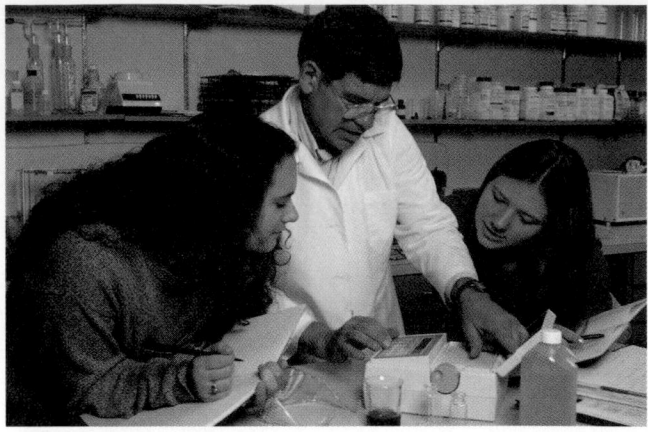

FIGURE 20-5 Training the employee well contributes greatly toward his or her success.

All new employees should be required to read the office policy and procedure manual. It is advisable for the manager to require the employee to sign a statement verifying that the manuals were read.

Be sure that all federal and state regulations are met where new employees are concerned. The Occupational Safety and Health Administration (OSHA) training must be provided to employees at risk of exposures before beginning any duties. Certain documents that verify the employee's right to work in the United States must be examined also. It is wise to insist on a fully completed personnel file before allowing the employee to work even 1 hour.

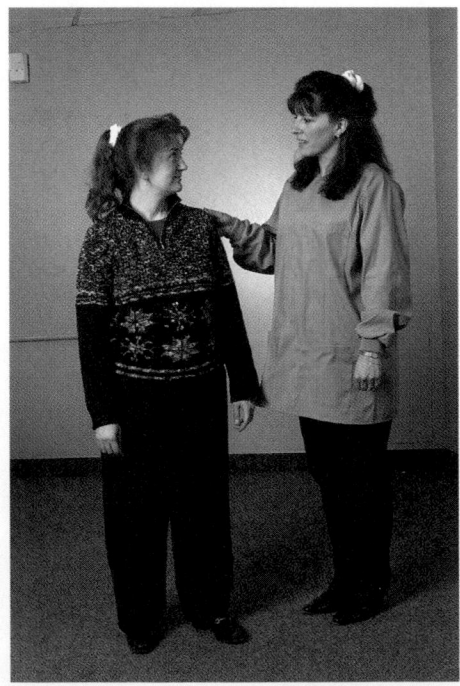

FIGURE 20-6 Mentors are valuable to the new employee. A mentor provides assistance to new employees who are learning their duties and growing accustomed to the medical office.

Job Descriptions

The job description is a tool designed to inform employees about the duties they are expected to perform. Well-written job descriptions list the essential functions of the job and reveal the chain of command that the employee should follow when questions or concerns arise. These documents provide a good guideline for employees so that they will understand exactly what is expected of them and what they are responsible for at work.

The job description should include a statement that says the employee must perform any additional duties as assigned by the supervisor. With this statement in place, the employee cannot say "that is not my job." All employees should be willing to pull together and assist with any tasks, but this statement gives added weight to assignments that are not specified in the written job description.

An effective manager understands the phrase "inspect what you expect." When duties are assigned, the manager should ensure that the tasks were completed correctly and in a timely manner. New employees should be monitored to make certain that their delegated tasks are getting done and getting done right. Without inspection, the manager cannot know that the new employee is meeting expectations. Once employees have earned a degree of trust, inspecting their work is not as necessary as in the beginning.

Staff Development Training

Continuous training and staff development are vital aspects of any medical office. Constant advancements and technological changes take place, and employees must be kept up to date on the changes. Meetings should be held at least quarterly to ensure that the staff is using the latest techniques and current regulations when dealing with issues that confront the medical facility.

Delegation of Duties

Delegating duties to subordinates allows managers to concentrate on the most critical aspects of their own jobs. Delegation also provides an opportunity for the employees to grow and learn new skills. Some managers are hesitant to assign duties to employees because they feel the tasks are too important not to complete themselves. However, this type of manager will soon be overrun with tasks and unable to complete them. Managers should place trust in employees who have earned it and allow them to prove their abilities.

Discover the strengths of individual employees and then assign them tasks that will use those strengths. If a medical assistant was hired to do administrative duties but is good with phlebotomy, encourage and allow the employee to assist with venipunctures whenever needed.

Using Performance Evaluations Effectively

A new employee should be granted a probationary period. Sixty to ninety days has been traditional, but many employers believe that 2 weeks is sufficient to determine whether the employee will be able to learn and adapt to the position.

A definite date for a performance review at the end of the probationary period should be set at the time of employment. This review should not be squeezed in between patient visits or be given a token few minutes at the end of a day. There should be ample time to relax and talk. At this time, tell the new employee how well expectations have been met and whether there are any deficiencies. Then give the employee an opportunity to ask questions. Sometimes an employee fails to perform because of never having been told what was expected. Although the probationary period does not always allow time to fully train an individual for a specific position, it is fair to assume that the potential for being a satisfactory employee can be judged at this time. Now is the time to talk out any problems and make suggestions for improvement.

The performance **appraisal** includes a judgment of both the quality and quantity of work, personal appearance, attitudes and team spirit, dependability, self-discipline, **motivation**, attendance, punctuality, and any other qualities essential to satisfactory performance of the job in question (Figure 20-7). The supervisor is responsible for ongoing performance appraisals of all employees, complimenting whenever possible and appropriate and offering helpful criticism when necessary. A formal performance appraisal at the end of the probationary period and at regular 6-month intervals thereafter, with a report to the physician employer, is helpful in the employee's salary review.

When negative information is to be relayed to the employee during a performance appraisal, sandwich the negative comment between two positive ones whenever possible. For instance, tell the employee:

"Jewel, you are a pro at greeting patients and making them feel at home. I would like to see you improve your time management skills, however, because I feel you are spending too much time with each individual patient. I must confess that they feel a part of the clinic family. Just watch the time and keep making them feel so welcome!"

Managers also may use the "feel, felt, found" approach when talking with employees about their performance. Consider the example below:

"Jewel, I feel the same way you do about the patients taking up a lot of our time. I know there are some that want to talk with us for hours, and I have felt the pressure of wanting to make them feel comfortable but having so much to do,

PERFORMANCE EVALUATION AND DEVELOPMENT PLAN
(OFFICE AND CLERICAL)

NAME: _____ DATE OF EVALUATION: _____

DATE OF HIRE: _____ DEPARTMENT: _____

JOB TITLE: _____ SUPERVISOR: _____

DATE APPOINTED THIS JOB: _____ MANAGER: _____

LAST REVIEW DATE: _____ LAST REVIEW RATING: _____

NEXT REVIEW DATE: _____ CURRENT REVIEW RATING: _____

PURPOSE

The purpose of this evaluation is to:

1. SET GOALS WITHIN SCOPE OF PRESENT JOB.
2. COMMUNICATE OPENLY ABOUT PERFORMANCE.
3. EVALUATE PAST PERFORMANCE.
4. DISCUSS FUTURE DEVELOPMENT PLANS FOR GROWTH.

INSTRUCTIONS

1. Supervisor to review form prior to completion. If specific items are not applicable they should be left blank.

2. Supervisor and employee to review job description prior to review.

3. In "COMMENTS" section supervisor may indicate which factors should be more heavily weighted in this particular evaluation.

4. Comments should be specific and job-related. All appropriate evaluation factors should be commented on to some degree.

I. POSITION OBJECTIVES AND MAJOR RESPONSIBILITIES. Summarize specific responsibilities of the job.

_____

_____

_____

II. ACCOMPLISHMENTS AND/OR IMPROVEMENTS. What specific accomplishments and/or improvements has employee made since last review with respect to set goals?

_____

_____

_____

PLEASE CONSIDER THE EMPLOYEE'S DEMONSTRATED PERFORMANCE AND MARK THE CIRCLE WHICH MOST CLOSELY DESCRIBES THAT PERFORMANCE.

4 - Performance consistently far exceeds expectations and requirements.
3 - Performance consistently exceeds normal expectations and job requirements.
2 - Performance consistently meets expectations and job requirements
1 - Performance usually meets expectations and minimum job requirements.
0 - Performance does not meet job requirements.

— CONTINUED, NEXT PAGE —

FORM # 72-119 © 1987 BIBBERO SYSTEMS, INC. PETALUMA, CA

TO REORDER CALL TOLL FREE:
800-BIBBERO /(800 242-2376) OR
FAX: (800) 242-9330 MFG IN U.S.A.

FIGURE 20-7 Performance evaluation and development plan. Performance evaluations should be considered tools that will help employees reach their personal goals and the goals of the organization. (Courtesy Bibbero Systems, Inc., Petaluma, Calif., 94954, (800) 242-2376, www.bibbero.com.)

7. <u>DEPENDABILITY:</u> CONSIDER ATTENDANCE, PUNCTUALITY, IDLE TIME AND RELIANCE WHICH CAN BE PLACED ON EMPLOYEE TO PERSEVERE AND CARRY THROUGH TO COMPLETION ALL ASSIGNED TASKS

    ◯ 0   ◯ 1   ◯ 2   ◯ 3   ◯ 4

_____

_____

_____

8. <u>COMPLIANCE WITH COMPANY POLICIES:</u> DOES THE EMPLOYEE COMPLY WITH RULES AND REGULATIONS WHICH APPLY TO SAFETY, FAIR EMPLOYMENT PRACTICES AND GENERAL ADMINISTRATIVE PROCEDURE.

    ◯ 0   ◯ 1   ◯ 2   ◯ 3   ◯ 4

_____

_____

_____

9. SPECIFIC PERFORMANCE	1	2	3	4	COMMENTS
A. Ability to handle scheduling:					
B. Willingness to work OT when necessary:					
C. Handling of calls and follow-up:					
D. Maintenance of equipment:					
E. Ability to handle patient complaints:					
F. Tact in dealing with patients:					
G. Speed (in specific technical procedures):					
H. Secretarial accuracy:					
I. Professional terminology:					
J. Assisting procedures:					
K. Laboratory techniques:					
L. X-ray techniques:					
M. Physical therapy:					
N. Collections:					
O. Medical Insurance:					
P. Bookkeeping:					

10. PERSONAL	1	2	3	4	COMMENTS
A. Grooming:					
B. Professional conduct:					
C. Energy, enthusiasm:					
D. Ability to handle stress:					

ADDITIONAL COMMENTS: _____

_____

_____

_____

_____

FORM # 72-119 © 1987 BIBBERO SYSTEMS, INC. PETALUMA, CA

FIGURE 20-7—Cont'd   For legend see previous page.

too. I have found that if I explain that I have a meeting or another patient to assist, they are very understanding and not offended. Perhaps you can try that approach, too."

Peer Evaluations

Some innovative companies use peer evaluations of employees to get a different view of the work performed by a worker. Asking co-workers to assist in the evaluation process can promote teamwork and cooperation. The rare employee will offer a poor evaluation because of a personal problem with another staff member but, for the most part, employees will provide fair, unbiased evaluations, knowing that they will also be evaluated when it is their turn.

360° evaluations are excellent tools for evaluating any employees, including managers. This evaluation usually consists of a questionnaire that is given to those who work closely with the employee, and they provide input regarding the performance of the person being evaluated.

Poor Evaluations Made Easier

No supervisor enjoys giving an evaluation that is not a positive one. It is difficult to know where to begin when the employee has not performed as expected or hoped. Perhaps the best way to open the conversation is to say, "This is not going to be a positive evaluation, and we have several items to discuss." The manager should have good documentation of the problems that led to the poor evaluation. If so, these can be reviewed with the employee with specific times, dates, and descriptions of incidents. If the manager does not document these issues, the conversation can become an argument and grow quite heated. Firm dates and times leave little room for defense and place the manager on the offensive.

CRITICAL THINKING APPLICATION

- While giving an evaluation on a particularly poor employee who Katherine plans to terminate, the employee begins screaming and accusing Katherine of discrimination and harassment. How should Katherine handle this situation?
- What are Katherine's options if the employee does not stop the inappropriate behavior?

Terminating Employees

The necessity for dismissing an employee is unpleasant at best, but if the ground rules are decided on in advance, written into the policy manual, and explained to all employees, the problem is partially solved. The policies must be applied equally and impartially to all. The final decision for dismissal probably will be made by the physician but may be based on the recommendation of the office manager or supervisor. The person who does the hiring should do the firing.

The probationary employee who does not prove satisfactory should be dismissed at the end of the probationary period, with tact and a full explanation of the reasons for dismissal. In all fairness, an individual should be told why the employment is ended and not be given weak excuses or untruths that do not help to correct deficiencies. If the manager is not straightforward in giving the reason for dismissal, the employee will not have the opportunity to grow and improve his or her performance.

An employee who has been in service for some time and is offering unsatisfactory performance should be warned and given an explanation of the specific improvements expected (Figure 20-8). If a second chance does not produce improvement in performance or attitude, then dismissal must follow. It should be done privately, with tact and consideration.

Most practice consultants believe that firing should come close to the end of the day, after all other employees have left, and that the break should be clean and immediate. If the office policy provides for 2 weeks' notice, the physician may wish to offer 2 weeks' pay, unless the circumstances that led to the dismissal were extremely **blatant**. A dismissed employee should never be allowed to train or influence a replacement.

The exit meeting should be planned just as carefully as the employment interview. Be honest with the employee. Discuss the employee's assets as well as liabilities and give the reasons for the termination. There is no need to dwell on the employee's deficiencies. These should have been thoroughly discussed at the warning interview, and the employee need only be told that the necessary improvements have not been made. Do listen to the employee's feedback, unless it becomes abusive. This may reveal some important administrative problems that need correction.

After dismissing an employee, do not leave that person in the office unattended. Request and get the office keys and any other equipment in the employee's possession before the dismissed employee leaves the building. Most states have strict payday laws that will not allow holding the final paycheck for any reason. Do not offer to give the employee a good reference unless it can be done sincerely.

Certain breaches of conduct, such as **embezzlement** and **insubordination** or violation of patient confidentiality, are grounds for immediate dismissal without warning.

Occasionally, an employee voluntarily terminates a job without giving a valid reason. The physician or office manager may wish to follow up with a letter to the former employee to seek out any problem that may have prompted the resignation.

CRITICAL THINKING APPLICATION

- Katherine has two employees who have never seemed to get along. One of the employees has a history of being vindictive and manipulative, but never in an obvious enough way for Katherine to have sufficient proof to reprimand her in writing. One day, this employee comes to Katherine's office to report that she saw the other employee, who has an exemplary record, taking drugs from the supply cabinet. How does Katherine react to this situation?
- What steps should Katherine take from here?

TERMINATION / REHIRE EVALUATION FORM

Employee Name__________________________ Social Security No.____________

Department __________________________ Title ______________

Termination Date ______________

Reason for Termination: ________Resigned ______Laid Off________Retired

Evaluation of Job Performance	Excellent	Very Good	Average	Poor	Unacceptable
Quality (accuracy, etc.)	☐	☐	☐	☐	☐
Quantity (productivity, consistency, etc.)	☐	☐	☐	☐	☐
Knowledge of Duties	☐	☐	☐	☐	☐
Reliability (absenteeism)	☐	☐	☐	☐	☐
Punctuality	☐	☐	☐	☐	☐
Ability to Cooperate with Co-workers	☐	☐	☐	☐	☐
Relationship with Patients	☐	☐	☐	☐	☐
Overall Attitude (willingness and commitment)	☐	☐	☐	☐	☐
Initiative	☐	☐	☐	☐	☐
Judgment	☐	☐	☐	☐	☐

Recommendation for Rehiring: ______________________________________

____

____

Comments:______________________________________

____

____

____

____

____

____

______________________________________ Date ______________

Supervisor's Signature

FORM # 72-123 PERSONNEL RECORDS ORGANIZING SYSTEMS • © 1987 BIBBERO SYSTEMS, INC. • PETALUMA, CA.
TO REORDER CALL TOLL FREE: (800) BIBBERO (800-242-2376) OR FAX (800) 242-9330 MFG IN U.S.A.

FIGURE 20-8 Termination form. Document the reasons for terminating employees and be sure that there is supporting documentation showing warnings and previous counseling efforts. (Courtesy Bibbero Systems, Inc., Petaluma, Calif., 94954, (800) 242-2376, www.bibbero.com.)

Fair Salaries and Raises

Medical office managers should recruit employees who will remain with the office for a long period of time. There are always situations when a part-time worker returns to college, or someone working during the summer months goes back to school. However, good employee **retention** is a goal to work toward.

In order to keep good employees, they must be paid a fair salary and will expect regular raises if they are performing as expected. The office manager can find information about salary comparisons on the Internet. Check the job duties and descriptions found on the web, and see if the salary that the medical facility is offering is comparable to other salaries for similar jobs in the area.

Merit raises are increases based on an employee's commendable performance. Cost of living increases are given when earned, usually after specific periods or annually, and are based on national statistics and trends. An employee who is being promoted may be awarded a salary increase, also. When the office pays a fair salary for the work being done, the physician will retain happy employees.

Staff Meetings

There must be some formal mechanism for keeping the office manager and other key employees current on the daily business affairs of the practice. One of the most common complaints from office personnel is that of being unable to discuss problems with the physician. The solution to this problem may be to hold regular staff meetings, which may be scheduled as frequently as weekly but should be no less often than quarterly (Figure 20-9). Some of the best ideas on improvement come from the office staff, and expressing ideas should be encouraged.

The simplest technique is to set aside a specific time for regular meetings at an hour when the most people can attend with the least disruption (Procedure 20-2). The meetings need not be long or overly formal, but to be effective they must be planned and organized. There must be a leader, and a secretary should be appointed to take notes. The effectiveness of the leader, a person who can balance firmness with fairness, is an important aspect of the meeting. This is usually either the physician or the office manager/supervisor. All members of the staff should be encouraged to submit ideas for discussion.

Draw up a simple **agenda** listing the issues to be discussed and prepare any supporting data needed for the meeting. There are many kinds of staff meetings. They may be purely informational, problem solving, or brainstorming. They may be work sessions for updating manuals, training seminars, or whatever is necessary to that individual practice. Or, meetings may be scheduled to discuss new ideas and any changes in office procedures. Some meetings are held simply to resolve specific problems. The staff meeting must not be allowed to deteriorate into a gripe session. Individual complaints should be handled privately.

The meeting must have a set agenda, with time for topics that need discussion on a regular basis, as well as time to handle any current problems. The agenda might be similar to that of any business meeting:

1. Reading of the last meeting's minutes
2. Discussion of any unfinished business
3. Discussion of any problems in the clinical area
4. Discussion of any problems in the administrative area
5. Discussion of any problems in common areas
6. Adjournment

Some physicians like to combine the staff meeting with a breakfast or lunch. The time or place is not important as long as it is neutral and meets the needs of the practice. Meetings should be conducted regularly, democratically, and without interruption. There must be follow-up to the items discussed; otherwise, the only result will be frustration and a reluctance to discuss problems at future meetings.

Seeing the Whole Picture

The office manager must keep a bird's-eye view on the office operations. He or she must look at the whole picture when difficulties arise. Remember, there are always two sides to every story, and there is usually truth intermingled with falsity. Do not form the habit of taking every word that an employee says as being 100% accurate. This is not meant to suggest that all employees are not truthful, but to encourage the office manager to look at all sides before making critical decisions.

See issues from the employees' point of view. Try to understand their perspective when dealing with everyday situations in the medical facility. Do not become closed-minded as a manager, unable to grasp what the employees see as important.

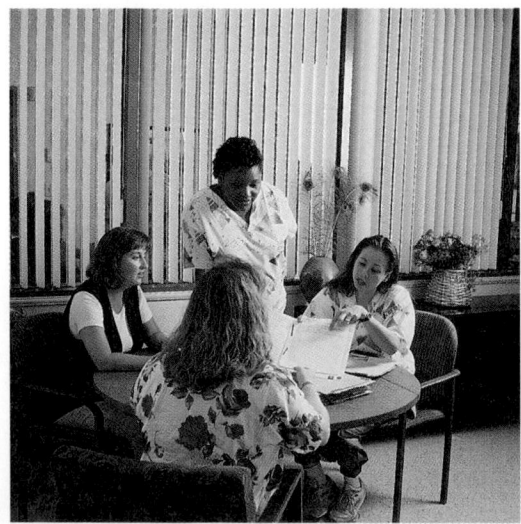

FIGURE 20-9 Periodic staff meetings are important tools for improving communication and resolving problems.

PROCEDURE **20-2**

Arranging a Group Meeting

GOAL: To plan and execute a productive meeting that will result in achieved goals.

EQUIPMENT AND SUPPLIES

- Meeting room
- Agenda
- Visual aids and equipment
- Handouts
- Stopwatch or clock
- Computer or word processor
- Paper
- List of items for the agenda

PROCEDURAL STEPS

1 Determine the purpose of the meeting and draft a list of the items to be discussed. Include the desired results of the meeting.

Purpose: To keep the focus on the issues at hand and make the meeting a productive one.

2 Determine where the meeting will be held, the time and date of the meeting, and the individuals who should attend.

Purpose: To have the demographic information about the meeting on hand prior to posting a notice. Only necessary staff members should attend, so that those not directly involved in the issues to be discussed will be allowed to continue their regular duties.

3 Send a memo, email, or letter to the individuals who should attend the meeting at least 10 days in advance, if possible. Send a copy to any supervisors who should be kept informed about the issues to be raised in the meeting.

Purpose: To allow for rescheduling if the key personnel cannot attend on the originally planned time and date. To keep managers informed of important details in areas for which they are ultimately responsible.

4 Be sure that the notice includes the following information:
- Date
- Time
- Place
- Directions, if not in a common meeting room or if away from the office
- Speakers and/or meeting topics
- Cost and registration information, if applicable

- List of items individuals should bring to the meeting

Purpose: To fully inform those who should attend the meeting of the demographic information and their responsibilities.

5 Finalize the list of items to discuss and place them in priority order.

Purpose: To keep the focus of the meeting on the issues at hand and to avoid discussion of nonrelated items. To make certain that the time spent in the meeting is productive for all involved.

6 Delegate any tasks that others can accomplish and follow-up to be sure that they fulfill their duties prior to the meeting.

Purpose: To ensure that all needed information and items are available for the meeting.

7 Assign a staff member the task of keeping notes and keeping time during the meeting.

Purpose: To have notes as to what happened so that a permanent record of what was discussed and the decisions that were made can be written after the meeting.

8 Make a list of all items that need to be taken to the meeting, including equipment such as microphones, projectors, screens, computers, disks containing presentations, etc.

Purpose: To be fully prepared and have all needed items in place during the meeting.

9 Compile the final agenda for the meeting.

10 On the meeting day, transport all items needed to the meeting room. Begin and end the meeting on time. Stay on track and follow the agenda.

Purpose: Following the plan and being considerate of the time that staff members devote to meetings will promote a positive attitude for meetings and will encourage group participation.

11 Follow-up whenever necessary on items discussed in the meetings. Distribute a synopsis of the meeting to all of the individuals who attended and keep a copy in a binder or folder.

Purpose: To have a permanent record of the meeting and items discussed and decided.

Other Office Manager Responsibilities

Patient Information Folder

Only a very small percentage of practices have a booklet that explains the information basic to the operational and service aspects of the practice. Yet, the physician and staff can easily compile a patient information folder cooperatively during a staff meeting. Experience has shown that if such a folder is given to every new patient, the number of incoming telephone calls can be reduced by an average of 20% to 30%. It also can reduce misunderstandings and forgotten instructions. The folder must of necessity be tailored to the specific practice.

The patient information folder should be an introduction to the practice and, if possible, mailed to a new patient before the first visit. A supply also may be left with referring physicians' offices to be given to patients coming to your office. It should be designed to fit easily into a No. 10 business envelope.

The cover should show the name of the practice, its location, and the practice logo, if there is one. Consider using a photo of the medical building for easy identification by the new patient, and a map to the office.

A statement of philosophy frequently is included in the introduction, followed by a description of the practice, such as in the example below:

> "The doctors and staff would like to welcome you to our office. We work as a team with the goal of providing prompt and thorough care of your problems. We are always working to improve our care and service in any way possible. Our practice is limited exclusively to the musculoskeletal system and its disorders. Therefore it is important for each patient to have a primary care physician such as a pediatrician, family physician, or internist to oversee the primary medical care for the entire patient. Our role is most effective as a consultant to your primary care physician."

Describe the office policy regarding appointments and cancellations, telephone calls, and the function of the answering service. If a separate business telephone line is available, be sure to include this information, as in the following example:

> "This office has two receptionists available to answer telephone calls during regular office hours. The office is very busy, and occasionally you will be asked to hold for a brief period. Please be patient with this. If you wish to speak to a doctor, your call usually will be returned during the next available break period or at the end of the office day. We receive many calls during the day, and it is unfair to the patients who have scheduled appointments to continually interrupt the doctor for telephone calls. Therefore the receptionist usually will take a message, and your call will be returned as soon as possible. Please inform the receptionist if your problem is urgent and she will let the doctor know this."

Describe any **ancillary** or laboratory services provided, how test results are reported, and your policy on prescription renewals. Patients need to know the provisions for emergency procedures: What hospitals does the practice use regularly? What is the night and weekend coverage? Hospitalization procedures and postoperative care and follow-up may also be included:

> "One of the doctors in the group is always on call for emergency situations. You may reach him by calling our office telephone number (714) 555-2323, and the answering service will put you in touch with the doctor on call at that time. Our doctors are on staff at St. Joseph Hospital (714) 555-3333 and, for children, Children's Hospital of Orange County (714) 555-4444. In case of emergency, call 911."

List all physicians in the practice; state their educational backgrounds, training, and board certifications; and define their specialties. List the names of key clinical and administrative staff members, such as registered nurses and nurse practitioners, medical assistants, the office manager, and the business manager. Provide the practice address, a map of how to get there, and information about the parking facilities.

Do not just stack these folders in the reception room for patients to pick up. Have the receptionist write the patient's name on the folder and hand it to the patient when he or she registers for the first appointment and suggest that the patient keep it for future reference.

Financial Policy Folder

A separate small folder covering the financial policies of the office can eliminate many questions and possible misunderstandings. Tailor the financial policy folder to the specific practice. Keep it small enough to fit into the billing envelope and send it out with the first monthly statement. If the practice sends out a welcome package before the patient's first visit, include the financial policy folder. Otherwise, present one at the first visit.

Spell out policies regarding billing and collection procedures, and make it clear that patients are responsible for the uninsured portion of the fees. If payment is expected at the time of service, put this in the folder. Keep the language simple and straightforward so that the message is clear:

> "We ask that our services be paid for at the time they are rendered. You will be provided with an encounter form so that you may bill your insurance company and be reimbursed for services paid at the time of your visit. Simply attach the encounter form to your insurance form and mail it to the insurance company. The appropriate diagnoses and charges will be on the encounter form. There is usually a greater charge for the initial visit, because this involves more time than follow-up visits. If you are sent to an outside office for laboratory testing or special x-rays, you will be billed separately from that office. We will be available to help if special circumstances arise involving difficulty with forms or receiving reimbursement. We will bill your insurance if you have a special situation such as surgery, prepaid health plans, Medicaid, CCS, or Senior Savers. We will complete disability papers as promptly as possible. However, you must obtain the necessary forms from your employer or the disability office."

The financial policy folder should also clearly state that the ultimate responsibility for payment lies with the patient.

Patient Instruction Sheets

In most medical offices there are patient procedures that occur over and over again. Instead of attempting to instruct a patient orally each time, why not develop clearly stated instruction sheets that can be reviewed with the patient and then give the patient the written instructions to take home? The following are suggestions for patient instruction sheets:

- Preparation for x-ray or laboratory tests
- Preoperative and postoperative instructions
- Diet sheets
- Performing an enema
- Dressing a wound
- Taking medications
- Using a cane, crutches, walker, or wheelchair
- Care of casts
- Exercise therapy

Moving a Practice

The thought of moving into a shiny new spacious office can be exciting. However, unless the move is planned in advance, moving day and the weeks that follow can be a nightmare.

Planning the New Quarters. Do some careful measuring to see how the furniture and equipment that will be moved will fit into the new quarters. If possible, draw the rooms to scale and show where each item is to be placed by the mover. Include the location of available electrical outlets in the floor plan. If new furniture, carpets, or equipment is needed, try to have them in place before moving day. Do not expect to have the new carpet installed the day of the move.

Establishing a Moving Date. Decide what day the move will take place and whether the office will close for 1 day or several. Select a mover and confirm the date. Patients must be notified of the move. As soon as the moving date is established, post a notice in the office and draw the patients' attention to it. Send announcement cards to the active patients. Many physicians place a notice in the local newspapers.

Notifying Utilities and Mailers. At least 60 days in advance of the move, start a change-of-address notification campaign. Notify publishers of journals and suppliers of catalogs. Cards for changes of address are available from the post office. Six weeks' notice generally is required on subscriptions, and postage due on forwarded journals can be very expensive. Notify the telephone company and utility companies well in advance so that there will be no break in service. File a change of address card with the local post office. Order stationery and business cards with the new address.

Packing. The moving company will supply packing cartons. Have each employee be responsible for packing and labeling the items from his or her own work area. Tag each carton with a number and keep a master list of what is in each numbered carton. This will help to find items that are needed. Also, if a carton should be lost or mislaid, a record of what was in it will be available. If time allows, just before moving is a good time to cull material from the files and discard old journals, supply catalogs, and any obsolete supplies or equipment.

Moving Day Strategy. Prepare a written outline of the moving day strategy, indicating each person's responsibility, and give each member of the office staff a copy. It may be wise to work in shifts to avoid confusion, but have one person stationed at the new address to direct the movers when they arrive.

Follow-Up. After the move, be sure to mention the new address when patients call for appointments. This often is neglected, especially after a few months have passed, and is very upsetting to the patient who tries to check in at the former address.

Closing a Practice

A medical practice may be closed because of retirement, death, a change in geographic location, or a change in profession. If the closing is unexpected, as in the case of sudden death of the physician, much of the burden falls on the staff. If the closing is voluntary and planned for, the physician may wish to consult an attorney or the local medical society for guidelines. The following information is useful in either event.

Advance Notice to Patients. The physician who anticipates retirement can begin cutting back the practice months in advance. Patients can be notified as they come in that the practice will be closing on a specified date and asked to begin arrangements for care from another physician. The physician also can ask that patients pay at the time of service, to minimize accounts receivable at the time of retirement.

Avoiding Abandonment Charge. To avoid a charge of abandonment, the physician should notify active patients by letter that the practice is being discontinued. The letter should be sent out at least 3 months in advance, if possible. If a patient has been discharged or has not been given care by the physician for at least 6 years, there is no obligation to send the notice.

Public Announcement. About 1 month after the physician begins telling patients of the closing, an announcement should be placed in a local newspaper, giving the closing date of the office, explaining any arrangements made for continuing care, and thanking patients for their support over the years.

Other Notices. Hospital affiliations should be informed early, particularly if the physician will be leaving the community. If the office space is being rented, be sure to notify the landlord in observance of the rental contract if there is one. Insurance carriers must be advised of the change. The state medical licensure board should be contacted. If the practice is incorporated, an attorney should be consulted about dissolving the corporation.

Patient Transfer and Patient Records. If another physician is taking over the practice, tell the patients about the new physician. However, be sure to explain that a patient's records will be transferred to the physician of his or her choice and that the request for transfer of records must be in writing. For convenience, the physician can have a form available that needs only the patient's signature.

Although the records belong to the physician, they can be transferred legally to another physician only with the consent of the patient. Any records not transferred should be stored, either in bulk or on microfilm or disk, until the statutes of limitations for malpractice and abandonment have run out.

Financial Concerns When a Practice Closes. Income tax returns and supporting documents should be kept for at least 3 years after the tax return was filed. Appoint someone to take care of any remaining outstanding accounts receivable.

Disposition of Controlled Substances. Check with the Drug Enforcement Administration (DEA) for current regulations on disposal of controlled substances and the physician's certificate of registration. Do not simply toss them out. The certificate will have to be sent to the DEA for cancellation, and then it will be returned. It may be necessary to produce an inventory of all controlled substances on hand when the practice is terminated, along with duplicate copies of the official order forms that were used to obtain them. Return any unused forms to the DEA. Do not use leftover prescription blanks for note pads. Burn or shred them to avoid misuse.

Professional Liability Insurance. The physician who is discontinuing active medical practice can safely drop the professional liability insurance. However, do not destroy any of the previous policies. Most professional liability claims are covered by the policy that was in effect at the time the alleged act of negligence took place. The suit may be filed many years later, and it is important that the old policy be available.

Furnishings and Equipment. Unfortunately, used office furniture and equipment do not bring much in the marketplace. If another physician is taking over the practice, the value of the furnishings and equipment can be negotiated. Many physicians donate their libraries to the local hospital and declare the gift as an income tax deduction. This is an item to check with the accountant.

A physician may reward loyal employees with severance pay. On average, this equals at least 1 month's salary plus prorated compensation for any unused vacation time. A letter of reference usually is offered.

There are many details to take care of in closing a medical practice. Contact the local medical society for further guidance.

Closing Comments

Successful office managers care about their employees and the vision for the office. They must be strong promoters of the office mission statement. The areas of authority and responsibility must be clearly defined to avoid management problems. A solid office policy and procedure manual will assist the office manager in running an efficient office.

Leadership is an important quality for any manager, and the medical office manager is no exception. The manager should develop good leadership skills, be fair and open-minded, and treat employees and patients as he or she would want to be treated. These actions will help to ensure a pleasant, productive working environment.

Patient Education

Educate patients about the policies and procedures in the office by providing patient information folders or brochures. When these documents are prepared and given to the patients formally, the patient is better informed and fewer calls will come to the office.

Legal and Ethical Issues

Office managers must stay abreast of current employment laws and regulations for all of the different agencies that govern the medical office. Joining an office manager's association will help the manager keep the office up to date and in compliance. Periodic checks on the websites of various organizations, such as OSHA, will help the manager to stay aware of the most recent changes in policies and rules.

Documentation is a critical aspect of the office manager's duties. The manager should keep detailed notes on the performance of employees and always discuss poor performance with employees. Never allow bad habits to go unmentioned. To the extent that it is possible, treat employees in a similar fashion and extend fairness to all.

SUMMARY OF SCENARIO

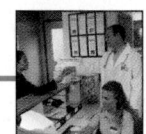

Katherine has made an impact on all of the staff members at Dr. Bouchard's office. She treats her employees well and is fair regarding office policies and procedures. Her subordinates appreciate her flexibility and professionalism as she deals with the many issues surrounding the operation of a medical office. Katherine treats the employees as team members, never speaking to them as if she were superior to them. She shares vital information with the staff so that they feel a part of the whole team, and feels that even some negative information should be related to the staff so that everyone is aware of the challenges the office faces. She makes good hiring decisions and firmly believes in a good orientation and training program. Dr. Bouchard has placed a great deal of trust in Katherine, and she has performed well, proving to be reliable in her position as office manager.

SUMMARY OF LEARNING OBJECTIVES

- Management is an important aspect of running a professional medical office. The physician counts on the office manager to run the business aspects of the office so that he or she can focus efforts on good patient care. A high degree of trust is placed with the office manager.

- A good office manager is fair and flexible. Good communications skills are necessary, as well as attention to details. The manager should care about the employees and have a sense of fairness. The ability to remain calm in a crisis is important, as is the use of good judgment and ability to organize tasks.

■ Charismatic leaders inspire allegiance and dedication while encouraging individuals to overcome great obstacles. The transactional leader is structured and organized, hardworking, and a planner. The transformational leader is excellent during times of transition and is effective at building relationships.

■ Power can be both a positive and negative entity. Power should not be used in a manipulative or coercive manner. Expert power is based upon a high degree of knowledge about a certain subject. Using rewards is one form of invoking power, and legitimate power is that of position or status. Referent power is granted from subordinates to those who lead by example.

■ Employees are motivated by various factors, including money, praise, insecurity, honor, prestige, needs, love, fear, satisfaction, and many others. The effective manager attempts to discover what motivates employees to do a good job.

■ Intrinsic motivation comes from within the employee. Extrinsic motivation has an outside source.

■ Asking for help, first and foremost, can prevent burnout. Managers often take on too many duties and do not delegate as much as they should. Exercise and rest help prevent burnout, as well as understanding one's own personal limitations. Focused goals are important and help keep the manager working toward the most critical tasks.

■ Resumes and applications should be reviewed for accuracy and completeness. Gaps in employment dates should be explained fully and the office manager should verify any references given. Documents should be legible and the information contained should be consistent without oversights.

■ The telephone voice of an applicant is important because most employees have occasion to answer the telephone while at work. The employee's voice should be clear and easily understandable. Good grammar skills must be used to reflect a professional image.

■ After interviewing a prospective candidate, the office manager should verify the facts on the resume and application and check several references. A comparison should be made between the candidates and the top two or three chosen for a possible second interview. It is wise to involve other staff members when choosing new employees for the office.

■ Mentors assist new employees by offering information regarding policies and procedures. The mentor can be a helpful advocate that the new employee can approach when there are questions about any aspect of the medical office.

■ Staff meetings may be held to relay information, solve a problem, or brainstorm ideas. Some meetings are designed as work sessions, while others may be scheduled to discuss new policies or changes in procedures.

KEY INTERNET WEBSITES

- 360° Evaluation
- Baudville Recognition—Putting Applause on Paper
- Panoramic Feedback
- Professional Association of Healthcare Office Management
- Salary Comparison and Calculator
- Successories
- Who Moved My Cheese?
  For active weblinks to each website visit
  http://evolve.elsevier.com/Kinn/

CHAPTER 21

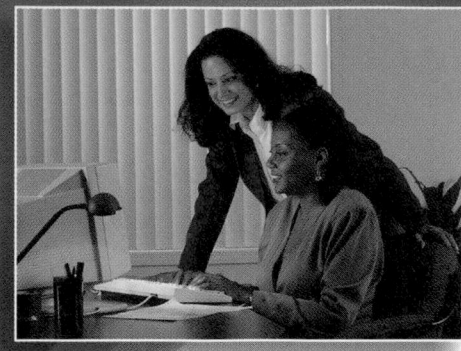

Scenario

Monica Ray is a medical assistant who is also pursuing a bachelor's degree in marketing. She has worked for Drs. Julie and Robert Todd for 2 years and, based upon her interest in marketing, the physicians have agreed to allow her to develop some new strategies for their obstetrics and gynecology office.

Monica is highly computer literate and can design web pages. She plans to incorporate several ideas she has seen on other physicians' websites, including a method of online scheduling. Monica is quite creative and she is excited about the challenge of providing such a service to the patients of the clinic.

Monica knows that planning is involved in any project, such as the facility's Internet presence. She plans to speak to every employee of the office to get input as to the design and content of the site. Patients will be able to provide her with additional suggestions as to what they would like to see, as well.

This new development for the office is just one way that Monica hopes to incorporate more formal customer service techniques. She plans to share the information she is learning in the classroom with the physicians and staff at the clinic. Monica and the doctors are fortunate that the staff is enthusiastic about these plans and eager to try new methods of customer service. The physicians plan to set specific goals with the help of the employees and to devise a reward system for reaching them. An exciting few months are ahead for this innovative group of medical professionals!

Medical Practice Marketing and Customer Service

Learning Objectives

- Define and spell the terms listed in the vocabulary.
- List the three steps to be followed when preparing to implement a medical marketing strategy.
- Explain the term *target market*.
- Discuss how suggestion boxes might help the medical facility to make improvements.
- List and discuss the "four p's" of marketing.
- Explain the five steps for developing a plan in marketing.
- Discuss how community involvement can make a difference in marketing efforts.
- Contrast the difference between advertising and public relations.
- Determine ways to promote a new practice.
- Discuss responses that help the medical assistant identify with the patient.
- Explain the concept of the internal customer.

Vocabulary

marketing The process or technique of promoting, selling, and distributing a product or service.

objectives Something toward which effort is directed; an aim, goal, or end of action.

outreach The process of using marketing and education strategies to reach and involve diverse audiences through the use of key messages and effective programs.

prosthetic The surgical or dental specialty concerned with the design, construction, and fitting of prostheses, which are artificial devices that replace missing parts of the body.

tangible Capable of being appraised at an actual or approximate value; capable of being precisely identified or realized by the mind.

target market A specific group of individuals to whom the marketing plan is focused.

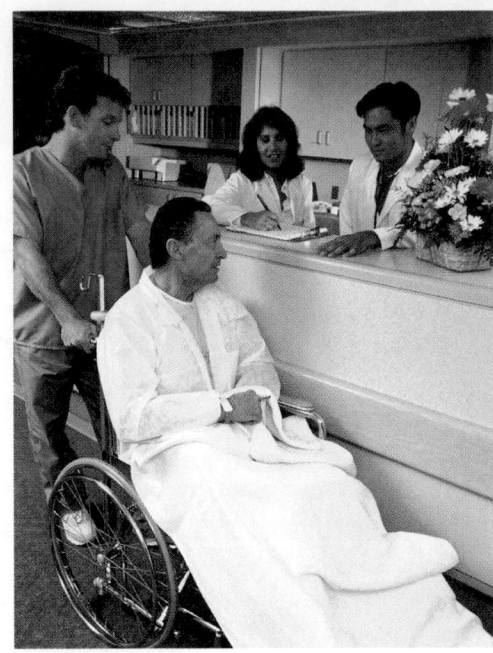

FIGURE 21-1 Friendly staff members are the best marketing tools. A smile is an excellent way to make patients feel welcome in the medical facility.

Each medical office should have a mission statement that defines the reason for the existence of the office. The physician's philosophy of medicine and reasons for pursing medicine as a career will greatly influence the mission statement. With this statement in place, the staff must develop goals that will assist them in meeting the mission. The goals can be met through a **marketing** and **outreach** plan for the practice and by providing excellent customer service to patients and visitors of the facility.

Developing Marketing Strategies

If a business is to grow, marketing strategies must be developed. A marketing strategy is designed to promote the services offered by the organization and encourage new business. Three steps are generally followed when preparing to implement or change medical marketing strategies:

- Evaluate what is being done now to increase patient flow.
- Decide what objectives are important and how meeting these objectives will be measured.
- Develop a plan with various means of marketing the practice and a specific methodology for implementing each phase.

Knowing the Target Market

During the strategic phase of developing a marketing plan, the physician and office manager must identify the **target market** for the services provided by the clinic. The target market is the group or groups of individuals that the office wishes to reach. Reaching the target market means that the specific groups are made aware of the clinic and what it has to offer. With managed care restrictions and regulations, competition for patients has become keen between physicians, and a facility that does not pursue growth runs a great risk of not surviving.

Several questions must be answered when discussing the target market. Consider the following:

- What specific outcomes do we hope to accomplish?
- What are the needs and desires of our target market?
- What are the characteristics of a typical member of the target market?
- How can the target market be reached in the most cost-effective ways?

Staff meetings are excellent times to brainstorm about reaching target markets. The staff can relate the needs of the patients who are currently coming to the medical office. If patients have made suggestions, they should be discussed and weighed as to which would most benefit the patient population of the facility (Figure 21-1).

CRITICAL THINKING APPLICATION

- Monica knows that the office has never attempted any formal marketing in the past. Because no one at her office is familiar with this task, who might she contact for advice and assistance?
- Even though her fellow staff members are not familiar with marketing, could they provide workable ideas?
- What are some ideas for marketing a medical practice?

CRITICAL THINKING APPLICATION

- What community resources could Monica seek as she is determining the target market of the practice?
- What information does she need to begin her search?

Suggestion boxes are a great way to solicit patient input. Ask patients for ideas as to how the clinic could operate in a smoother fashion and what additional services they would like to have. Check the suggestion box frequently. If the patient leaves his or her name on the suggestion form, it is a good customer service move to reward the patient for the suggestion. Mail the patient a coupon for a free lunch at a local restaurant or a free car wash at a local detailing shop. Involving other businesses in marketing efforts helps both attract new customers.

The "Four P's." The "four p's" of marketing include *p*roduct, *p*lacement, *p*rice, and *p*romotion. A physician's office offers medical services as a product. Some offices have **tangible** retail products that they also offer, such as vitamins or **prosthetic** devices. Placement involves the actual location of the medical office. It may be located in an urban area close to large neighborhoods of young professionals, or in a rural area with a few people living several miles apart. Placement can refer also to the setup of the office, the specific suite in a shopping strip where the office is located, or even the placement of retail objects on a shelf. Placement can greatly influence the traffic to the facility.

Price is simply the amount of money charged for goods and services provided. Promotion refers to the methods used to get the product or services to the consumers, or patients, in the case of the medical office.

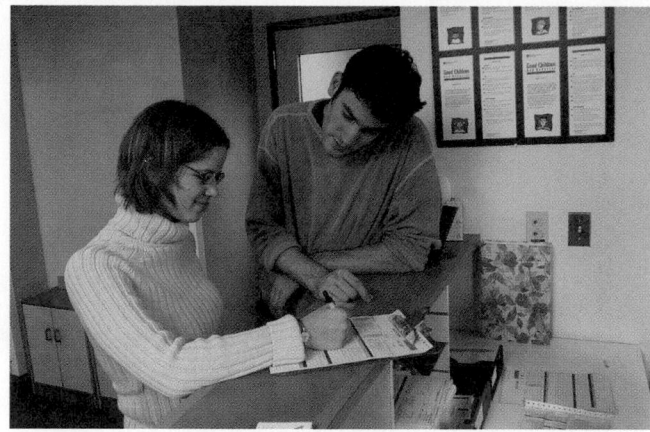

FIGURE 21-2   Offer services that are important in the geographical area of the office. College students may need to see a physician for minor illnesses, and they will appreciate offices that provide short office visits at a reasonable fee.

of other ideas that the physician would like to implement. They are:

1. Assessment
2. Research
3. Plan
4. Execution
5. Evaluation

Assessment is the phase of planning in which the problem or goals are reviewed. This is another excellent time for brainstorming. Research allows the physician or office manager to investigate the needs of the target market and then decide what the medical office can do to meet those needs. Planning the concept follows and, once a firm plan is in place, it is executed or carried out. Afterward, evaluate what went well and what problems occurred so that future efforts will be even more successful.

CRITICAL THINKING APPLICATION

- How can Monica investigate the charges for similar procedures at other clinics in her area?
- Why is this information important to Monica?

Deciding What Services to Offer. Once the physician and office manager have identified the target market, decisions can be made regarding what services should be offered to the patients. For instance, suppose the office is situated in a neighborhood of young families. There is a strong possibility that both parents work outside the home, so evening hours would be beneficial to these patients. The physician may decide to extend office hours to 8:00 PM twice a week and to open from 9:00 to 12:00 noon on Saturdays. If there are several schools in the area, particularly junior high and high schools, the physician may wish to offer a special price on sports physicals during the fall. Schools often require physicals, and if the physician offers them at a reasonable price, the entire family may decide to seek medical care from the physician.

If the office is located in a college town, the physician may wish to offer a special student rate for short office visits (Figure 21-2). If there are a number of senior citizens in the area, a senior citizen discount might be appropriate. Input from patients and staff members will be valuable in deciding what services to offer in the medical facility.

Developing a Plan

There are several specific planning steps that the facility may use for events, marketing strategies, and any number

Promoting the Practice

The physician and office manager should constantly watch for ways to promote the medical practice and keep its name in the public eye. Some of these methods are free of charge, and others will need detailed budgeting and planning.

Tapping into Free Resources

Many good promotional activities are relatively free to the physician. One of the most popular and beneficial to the physician is a professional website. If the physician or office staff has sufficient knowledge for website construction, then there is little or no cost to the doctor if one of the free website services is used.

Some newspapers offer an advice column wherein different types of professionals give general medical advice to those who write in with questions. Physicians volunteer to answer these questions in print and, in return, the office address, the office telephone number, and often the physicians' pictures are featured. This is an excellent way to generate patient calls and inform the public about the specialties and types of cases the physician handles.

CRITICAL THINKING APPLICATION

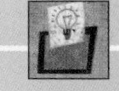

- Monica knows there are many opportunities and free resources in her area. Where should she begin to look?
- How might Monica's clinic partner with other businesses and services to provide excellent care and help each other at the same time?

Community Involvement

Getting involved in the local community is another way to promote a medical practice. Some physicians sponsor Little League Football, baseball teams, or bowling leagues. Some entire staffs participate in charity events and marathons, wearing t-shirts with the clinic name imprinted on the back.

The physician or staff may have specific charities that they support on an annual basis, or they may participate in United Way activities, which distribute funds to many different types of worthy organizations through payroll deductions and other gifts. Some medical facilities have volunteer programs in which employees receive recognition for participation in various activities. A good example includes blood donations. Many blood centers offer pins and recognition certificates for the number of pints of blood that volunteers donate. The office staff may set a goal to reach a certain number of donated pints in a year, and as recognition certificates are collected, the staff may wish to display them in a prominent place in the office. This is an indication to patients that the staff is concerned about the community and is volunteer minded. From a public relations standpoint, this is valuable to the medical office, because patients tend to expect medical professionals to be volunteer oriented.

Health fairs are a great avenue for promoting the services offered by the clinic, obtaining name recognition, and increasing public visibility. Some health fairs are huge, highly publicized events, while others are small, often held at a local shopping mall or grocery store. All of these events could be worthy projects for the physician and the medical office.

CRITICAL THINKING APPLICATION

- What community organizations might help Monica in her efforts to make the office an integral part of the community?
- What resources and community organizations are available in your area that would be good avenues for practice marketing and community service?

Advertising Plans and Agencies

Most physician offices do not use advertising agencies to promote their practices, but there are occasions when an agency might be useful (Figure 21-3). If a very special event is scheduled that needs extensive planning, then a public relations firm or advertising agency might be consulted. Unfortunately, the cost of these groups is usually high and beyond the reach of sole practitioners or small group practices. However, the investment may be well spent when an event is critical and attendance is important to its success.

There is a difference between advertising and public relations. Advertising could be defined as "creating or changing attitudes, beliefs, and perceptions by influencing people with purchased broadcast time, print space, or other forms of written and visual media." Broadcast time could be in the form of television commercials, radio broadcasts, or audiovisual aids. Print could be in a newspaper, magazine, or trade journal, while written and visual media may be a flier, brochure, or billboard. Public relations offerings are influential as well, using news broadcasts, radio reports, and magazine or newspaper articles to reach people. Most public relations efforts are free, but it is often difficult to get others interested enough in the activities the medical office is planning to warrant coverage.

Communication as a Marketing Tool

Many medical offices use communications tools to market the practice and improve customer service. Sending a monthly newsletter through mail or electronically provides health information and news about upcoming events. The newsletter can be very personalized for the office and might even include news about patients and the medical staff, as long as permission is obtained.

Sending birthday cards is an excellent public relations tool. Some offices sign the greetings at staff meetings and they are placed in a tickler file for the proper mailing date. Sending holiday greetings is another method of wishing patients well.

Automated call distribution is becoming a popular means of communicating with large numbers of people. A computer dials multiple numbers at the same time and plays a recorded message, which can be the actual physician reading a message. Although many people block such calls to their homes and an equal number hang up, the success rate of automatic call distribution is actually quite good.

Many individuals listen and respond to the calls, especially if they come from someone they know giving important information. For instance, if a medical clinic were planning to move to another part of the city, a program could be initiated to notify all patients with telephone numbers that the office will be moving after a certain date. The message could include the address of the new location, and even prompt patients to "press 1" if they need to schedule an appointment. The same principle could be applied to news about an upcoming health fair, a special seminar about a certain illness, or even an article that will be in the Sunday paper about the clinic.

FINDING A GOOD ADVERTISING AGENCY

1. *Define your objective in hiring an ad agency.* What do you want to achieve? What should be different after the agency goes to work for you? What kind of working relationship do you prefer?

2. *Check out sources.* Consider work you have seen or heard that has impressed you. Call friends and colleagues you trust and get their recommendations. Attend professional or trade association meetings, and talk to members who have used agencies before. Seek out their opinions, and note whose names come up often (both pro and con). Watch for articles about ad agencies in area papers, trade magazines, and related publications, such as chamber of commerce newsletters.

3. *Once you have a list of candidates, screen them by telephone.* Ask about their backgrounds, projects they have worked on, the results they have had, their fees, and anything else important to you. Then set up interviews with the three or four firms that impressed you the most.

4. *Interview the finalists.* Find out the following:
   - *Do they have experience working with your industry?* What is their track record when working with companies like yours? Do they understand your business and the nuances of what you do? If not, are they willing to research the information they need?
   - *Is there chemistry?* You can tell if there is a good "fit" with an ad agency. A good agency will express interest in getting to know you as an individual and learning more about your company. They will be good listeners and quick learners. They will make good suggestions and react quickly to your questions and opinions. They should demonstrate the ability to anticipate what is best for your business and be prepared to disagree with you if they feel you are on the wrong track.
   - *Do they show originality and creativity?* Based on the agency's previous work, do you feel these people understand how best to "sell" your product or service? If you operate a home healthcare agency, for example, you probably do not want an ad campaign that features technology over tenderness. Sensing your clientele, the agency should know enough about you to put together the appropriate message.
   - *Are they reliable and budget conscious?* No amount of chemistry and creativity can make up for a missed deadline or an estimate that is way off. Be sure the agency has not only the creative skills needed but also the time and commitment to devote to your needs. Whether you are the biggest or smallest client in their stable, you should be able to count on consistent attention to detail. Their staff should be available to answer your questions and be accountable for delays and expenses.

FIGURE 21-3   Selecting an advertising or public relations agency. (From Anderson L: Star makers. *Entrepreneurial magazine,* April 1997.)

Promoting a New Practice

Most physicians who open a new practice place an ad in local newspapers to announce the event. Usually a picture of the physician is included, and a map to the exact location may be available on the ad. Some physicians purchase clinics from others who are moving or retiring, but many will open a freestanding clinic in a new building, and the word about the new facility must be spread for the business to be a success.

Providing business cards for all employees is a good way to increase public knowledge about the facility. Some offices offer incentives for patient referrals from the staff or other patients, but the physician must ensure that there are no state statutes or ethical standards that prohibit this. The incentive could be a simple coffee cup with the clinic's logo on it or a book about a healthcare issue. Recognition is the important factor where referrals are concerned. A thank you card is the minimal acceptable "thanks" for patient referrals.

Some physicians hold an open house when the new facility opens. Often, those individuals who assisted with the business from its inception will attend the open house to lend support to the owners. Bankers, attorneys, accountants, and other physicians will often show their support by attending the open house. Pictures from this event should be placed on the facility's website or in the monthly newsletter.

Building a Practice Website

There are four basic steps involved in building a website for the medical practice. These steps include the following:
- Define the objectives of the website.
- Design the pages.

- Locate a web server where the pages can be uploaded.
- Upload the page to the web server.

Defining Objectives. When defining **objectives**, important decisions about specific goals must be considered. The physician and staff should discuss who the audience for the website will be and what will be included on the site. Most websites designed for physician offices and clinics are informational, developed mostly for patient and public use. Once the objectives are clearly defined, specific content can be written to place on the website.

Designing the Pages. Once the objectives are clear, begin developing ideas as to what the site will look like on the computer screen. Color choices, animation, and fonts will enhance the look that is being created and make a strong statement about the medical facility. The menus should be designed so that viewers can navigate easily through the site. Most users appreciate a means to go back to the page previously viewed and grow frustrated with sites that have an excessive number of pop-up boxes. Consistency is important, so it is a good idea to keep the same design theme on each page of the website.

The most important part of the website is the text. It has been said that every word in a book must add to the story, and this is a good way to look at the text in a website. Avoid repetition and remain clear about what is being communicated on the site. Headings and titles help to clarify the theme of each page. Use a spell checker before uploading the message and making it available for public viewing.

Photographs, graphics, music, and video can add fun to the website, but be careful not to overdo them. Graphics are often large files that take time to download. Most people will not wait more than about 10 seconds for a web page to load before clicking elsewhere. When designing web page graphics, remember that smaller is better. Graphics can be found by searching for "index of GIF files" or "GIF library." Once an appropriate file is found, it should be copied onto the hard drive by "right clicking" the graphic and selecting "save picture as." Music can be found by searching for "mid" or "midi." The search can even specify a certain singer, song, or composer. Always respect any copyrights that are designated on any file used. Many websites offer these files for free.

For a more professional-looking website, consider purchasing web development software, such as Macromedia's Dreamweaver or Microsoft's Front Page. These feature-rich products are fairly inexpensive and can help the medical assistant create very attractive, easy-to-maintain websites. Most products integrate tutorial and "help" features that explain how to use them.

Hyperlinks are words or graphics on a web page that, when clicked, take the viewer to another page or another website. To add a hyperlink, simply highlight the text field or graphic, select the hyperlink icon, and specify the destination address (uniform resource locator [URL]). Always specify the full URL.

The main page should always be assigned the file name "index.htm" or "default.htm." Other pages on the website can be assigned any name; however, keep the names short and avoid using special characters.

Locating a Web Server. At this point, the design of the website is complete, but the files reside on the computer hard drive, not on the Internet. Now the pages are ready to be uploaded, or published, to a web server that will allow them to be viewed on the Internet. The Internet service provider (ISP) that the office uses for email and online services may offer free web space to its customers. If not, there are a number of companies that will provide web space at no charge, but the user usually will be required to use banners on the site that advertise the ISP or other services. If no banner ads are desired, the medical facility may wish to use a paid provider. Some web hosting companies provide other services free of charge, like simple web page editors and email addresses.

Uploading the Website to the Web Server. When using a free web server, instructions and passwords will be sent to the user that describe how to upload files to the server. The password is necessary so that other people cannot alter the files. Copying the files from the local hard disk to the web server is a simple process. The hosting site will prompt the user for the name of the directory on the hard drive where the files are stored and for the names of the specific files to be uploaded. To avoid confusion, make certain that the files saved on the server have the same file names that were used on the hard drive.

Once all of the files have been uploaded, test the page on the web server and make certain that it functions properly and that all files have been uploaded correctly. It is also a good idea to test the page using a different computer to ensure that graphic files are being read from the server and not from the local hard drive.

Evaluating the Website. Include an email address where viewers of the website can interact with the creator with comments. This way problems with the site can be readily identified and corrected. It is also advisable to check the site every few days to make certain that it is functioning properly.

Counters often can be added to the website that will indicate how many people viewed it. This helpful tool will allow the medical facility to track how many people are viewing which pages.

Quality Customer Service in the Medical Practice

Treating the Patient as a Customer

The best way to increase the number of patients in a medical office is through word of mouth. When patients are satisfied with the treatment they receive, they will refer other patients to the physician. However, if they are dissatisfied, they will tell everyone they know!

Because patients often have a choice as to who provides their healthcare services, it is important that the physician's office become the patient's *first choice*. Some patients have such loyalty to a certain physician that even if their healthcare coverage would no longer pay for visits, they would continue to see that doctor. This happens because of the attitude of the physician and his or her office staff.

Helpful Attitudes. The physician and staff probably emote a helpful attitude in every contact with the patient. They sincerely ask, "How may I help you?" and then take steps to assist the patient in whatever way possible. Instead of pointing in the general direction of the radiology department, they take the patient there and introduce him or her to the receptionist. Instead of telling a patient on the telephone, "Ann handles the insurance billing—I'll transfer you to her," say, "One moment, Mrs. Brown, let me see if Ann is at her desk." Then place Mrs. Brown on hold, call Ann, and let her know that she has a call. Then return to Mrs. Brown and tell her that Ann is at her desk and transfer the call at that time. Be courteous and kind to every patient and visitor to the office. Good customer relations must be one of the primary goals of the medical facility. Patients count on the staff members to be reliable and available to help them to the best of their abilities.

CUSTOMER SERVICE AT NORDSTROMS

Use your good judgment in all situations. There will be no additional rules.

From the Nordstrom, Inc., Employee handbook. Courtesy Nordstrom, Inc.

Phrases that Undermine Successful Customer Service. There are several phrases that could be considered the "deadly sins" of customer service. These phrases should never be used when relating to patients and visitors:

- "I don't know."
- "I don't care."
- "I can't be bothered."
- "Ask someone else."
- "It's not my job."
- "It's not my fault."
- "I know that."
- "I'm right, you're wrong."

All of these phrases will give the patient or visitor a negative view of both the office and those who work in the facility.

Identifying with the Patient. Patients appreciate staff members who can identify with the problems they are facing. This is especially effective when a patient is upset or angry. For example, if a patient comes to the office complaining that charges were placed on his account for procedures that were not performed, the medical assistant may respond with a phrase similar to the following:

"Mr. Roberts, I understand that you are upset about these additional charges. I know I would be upset if I were billed for something I didn't receive. Let me help you though, by doing this . . . "

Identifying with the patient shows an understanding on the part of the staff member, no matter how upset the patient may be. Always acknowledge and restate the patient's concern. It proves that the medical assistant was listening and is interested in resolving the problem.

Remember, it costs much more to find new customers than to keep existing customers happy. Providing helpful, personal service impresses even the most difficult patient. To patients and visitors to the clinic, whomever they speak to represents the whole company. Perceptions and opinions will likely be formed based on experiences with only one person. Each individual employee must be aware that to the patient, each employee is the healthcare facility.

What Do the Patients Expect?

First, patients expect to be treated using the golden rule. They expect their concerns to be met with responsiveness, which means that the medical assistant should have a caring attitude. They also expect that the professionals in the medical office are knowledgeable about their field or specialty. An insurance biller should know more than just the basics of insurance filing. The office manager should have a certain degree of authority to handle problems and complaints. Patients also expect confidentiality and trust from the staff of the medical office. They expect an organized office that runs on schedule, and that if a staff member promises to do something, it is as good as done (Figure 21-4).

Remembering the Internal Customer

Most of us do not have problems figuring out who the external customers are in a medical practice. Patients, their families and friends, and visitors to the office are external customers. But who is the internal customer?

Internal customers are employees and staff members of the facility. Although they work for the business, they also are served by the business. If they are not pleased with the atmosphere of the medical facility, they are sure to look elsewhere for employment. Keeping the internal customer is just as important as keeping the external customer.

Closing Comments

Providing good customer service is a commitment that must be made by every employee of the medical facility, every single day. There will be times that the customer is not right, but he or she should be treated with dignity and respect at all times. Additionally, the expert customer service provider will have the knack for making the customer think he or she was right all along! The medical office is no exception to the requirements for providing good service to its patients, and doing so will result in an excellent reputation for the clinic, built by those who matter most—the patients.

Todd Family Medical Clinic

Julie Todd, M.D.   Robert Todd, M.D.
3343 Smithson Place
Dallas, Texas 75229

We are interested in the customer service you received today as a patient of our clinic. Please return this form by mail and help us evaluate our service to you!

Date of contact or visit: _____   Day of week: _____

Name of employees with which you made contact (if known):

How was this contact made?   ☐ by phone   ☐ by mail   ☐ in person

This is a (please check appropriate box)   ☐ complaint   ☐ comment

Description of situation:

Has the problem been resolved to your satisfaction, if any?   ☐ yes   ☐ no

If not, how can we resolve the problem?

Please rate the following based on your experience with our staff:

	Excellent	Good	Fair	Poor
Greeting to you by name	☐	☐	☐	☐
Familiarity with your account	☐	☐	☐	☐
Courtesy and willingness to help	☐	☐	☐	☐
Quickness in answering the phone	☐	☐	☐	☐
Time placed on hold	☐	☐	☐	☐
Quickness in locating your chart	☐	☐	☐	☐
All of your questions answered	☐	☐	☐	☐
Phone transfers kept to a minimum	☐	☐	☐	☐

Other suggestions and comments:

Name (optional): _____   Phone Number (optional): _____

FIGURE 21-4   Customer service evaluation form for the medical office. By using this form for patient feedback, the medical office manager can better assess patient expectations.

Patient Education

Endless opportunities for patient education exist through the practice's marketing and public relations efforts. Most physicians agree that a part of their obligation to the medical profession is to educate patients about healthcare issues. The public relations and practice's marketing staffs can work together to provide information to patients of the facility and to the general public.

Many physicians attend health fairs, where brochures and pamphlets can be distributed about conditions such as diabetes, heart disease, hypertension, and other disorders. Screenings for cholesterol and blood pressure checks are good ways to market a practice and gain new patients.

The medical assistant who knows how to build and maintain a simple website can be of great value to the physician. The practice website could provide opportunities for educating the patient, as well as special sections for upcoming events, an online newsletter, appointment setting, and even a separate patient education section. The website address should be included on stationery, business cards, and other documents used to promote the facility.

Legal and Ethical Issues

The physician must take care that patients do not use the information in brochures or on the practice website as medical advice or a substitute for the physician's counsel. When attaching links to other websites, be sure they are reputable. The patient may consider information on the practice's website to be an extension of the advice of the physician, so make sure that everything on the website is accurate.

The physician should review carefully all printed information that is used to promote the medical facility. Be sure that no misleading statements are included. A disclaimer should be used to remind patients that the information given in brochures and on websites is only general information. Patients should discuss specific medical issues with the physician.

SUMMARY OF SCENARIO

Monica knows that without growth, many businesses eventually fail. She is confident that with a simple marketing plan, the clinic will experience steady, continuous expansion. She has spoken to all of the office staff members and gained input from both employees and the patients of the clinic. Many offered excellent suggestions that Monica can incorporate into her marketing plan.

One of her first activities was to develop an annual calendar of special events and outreach efforts. A monthly newsletter and the practice website will be the main thrusts of her marketing plan. The newsletter will be available both in print and online. The patients in the office database who have email addresses will receive automatically a computer-generated email message containing a link that will take them directly to the online newsletter. Inside, patients will find health information and details about upcoming events.

Monica also planned one special activity for each month of the year. She scheduled a blood drive, a Christmas toy drive, and mini–health fair. Because both Dr. Julie and Dr. Robert Todd are dedicated to students who wish to pursue medicine, Monica even planned a career day for high school students interested in becoming physicians, inviting representatives from the medical school that the Todds attended. Because this is considered a public service, Monica was able to get press coverage on the local radio station and in the newspaper at no cost.

Monica visited a new restaurant located close to the office that serves heart-healthy dishes, met with the manager, and discussed ways that the two businesses could help each other. They decided to provide a "buy one entrée, get one free" coupon to patients who referred other patients to the clinic. In turn, Dr. Robert Todd agreed to hold his free nutrition seminars at the restaurant. This arrangement has proven to work well for both businesses.

Monica plans to track responses to each event to determine what efforts were the most effective. The website will allow her to count the number of times it is accessed, as well as which pages were the most popular within the website. She will keep the physicians informed and be open to their suggestions throughout the year. Monica is anxious to see results of her marketing efforts and feels confident of success.

SUMMARY OF LEARNING OBJECTIVES

■ When preparing to implement marketing strategies, first evaluate what currently is being done toward the marketing effort. Then, decide what the objectives of the marketing plan are and how they will be measured. Last, develop a specific plan and timeline for implementing each phase.

■ A target market is a very specific group of people or individuals that the medical facility wishes to serve. The geography where the individuals live, the lifestyle they are accustomed to, and the personality of the individuals all are ways to classify them into a specific target market. When identifying a target market ask, "Who is our patient?", "What does our patient want?", and "Why is it wanted?" These questions will help the medical facility to design a marketing plan to meet the needs of these individuals.

■ Suggestions from patients and employees should always be welcomed in the medical office. Often these people see the facility from a different point of view, and their suggestions can enhance the atmosphere and services that are offered.

■ A marketing plan must always address the "four p's," which are product, placement, price, and promotion. The product in a medical office would include the services, and any actual retail items that might be sold. Placement relates to the location of the office and its convenience to the patients, and the placement of retail items in the facility. Price represents the charges for goods and services, and promotion entails the ways in which the services are promoted to the general public and the target market.

■ When developing a marketing plan, the facility should first assess the efforts that have been made in the past and then research the results of those efforts. Next the plan is developed, which should include very specific steps for each aspect of the endeavor. After the plan is executed, the staff must evaluate its effectiveness and then determine whether the goals were met. The evaluation is important in planning future marketing strategies.

■ Involvement in the community is an excellent way to give to the medical profession and to remain in the public eye. These efforts can result in new patients for the facility. The public sees medical professionals as caring and compassionate, so volunteer activities reinforce this attitude and help to meet patient expectations.

■ Advertising is defined as a medium that creates or changes attitudes, beliefs, and perceptions through purchased broadcast time, printed material, or other forms of communication. Public relations are similar but rely more on news broadcasts or reports, magazine or newspaper articles, and radio reports to reach the audience.

■ The new medical practice can be promoted by placing an announcement in the newspaper about its opening. Some physicians hold an open house, inviting the public to visit the office. A website is an excellent promotional tool and should be listed on business cards and stationery. Community service and volunteer activities that mention the practice will also help to spread the word about the services that are available.

■ Identifying with the patient is an effective customer service tool. The medical assistant should express his or her understanding about the patient's concerns. Then, tell the patient that the situation can be resolved and how it will be resolved. Four magic words in customer service are, "Let me help you."

■ External customers are those who visit the facility, such as patients. However, staff members and employees are internal customers, who wish to derive a sense of satisfaction in working for the medical office. The internal customers are just as important as the external customers.

KEY INTERNET WEBSITES

- American Marketing Association
- Medical MultiMEDIA Group
- The Patient Education Institute
- United Way
  For active weblinks to each website visit
  http://evolve.elsevier.com/Kinn/

CHAPTER 22

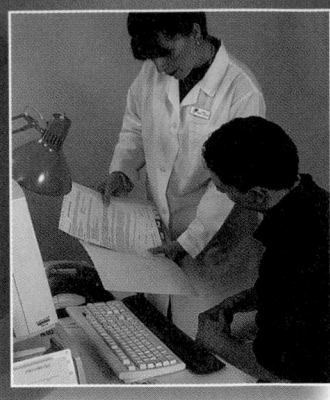

Scenario

Laura Kelly graduated from her medical assistant training 1 year ago and is now employed at a regional hospital in the quality assurance department as an administrative assistant. She enjoys working with statistics, is very detail oriented, has excellent computer skills, and is able to comprehend the lengthy regulatory text, such as that set forth in the Health Insurance Portability and Accountability Act (HIPAA) rules and guidelines. She has proven to be a valuable employee as the hospital has begun to comply with privacy laws.

Laura thought that quality assurance involved only patient satisfaction when she began working for the hospital. She has learned that this is just a small part of the total quality picture of the facility. The hospital has developed a patient questionnaire to solicit input from patients, and she enjoys talking with them about their experiences. Laura rarely encounters complaints, and she is proud to work for a medical facility that has practitioners who are concerned about giving exceptional care to patients. She now understands that there are many aspects to providing quality in a healthcare facility.

Laura also realizes that health information encompasses much more than the patient's chart. She knows that health statistics are vital to research and that physicians rely on statistical information when prescribing drugs, giving treatments, and performing other services. Providers frequently contact Laura to determine how many cases of a certain disease or disorder occurred at the hospital during a given period. The hospital database is very sophisticated and allows her to access many types of statistics quickly. Her office also monitors who enters the database and what information is accessed. This is one method of ensuring that privacy is maintained.

Laura has attended continuing education workshops that allow her to gain information that will help the staff to stay in compliance with the numerous regulations that govern the facility. She is eager to learn and assist her employers in keeping the hospital safe for all patients and visitors.

Health Information Management

Learning Objectives

- Define and spell the terms listed in the vocabulary.
- Describe several ways that health information is used.
- Contrast the nine characteristics of quality health data.
- Explain the four concerns of quality assurance.
- Discuss the importance of the HIPAA.
- Explain the functions of the National Center for Health Statistics (NCHS).
- Discuss the types of statistics kept by the NCHS.
- Define total quality management.
- Explain the function of Joint Commission on Accreditation of Healthcare Organizations (JCAHO).
- Discuss the importance of healthcare standards in medical facilities.

National Curriculum Competencies

2d. Document appropriately
2e. Perform risk management procedures

4a. Apply managed care policies and procedures
4b. Apply third party guidelines

Vocabulary

authenticated Proof of; with regard to medical records, it applies to a signature, initials, or computer keystroke by the maker of the record who verifies that the record is correct.

circumvent To manage to get around, especially by ingenuity or stratagem.

contraindication Something, as a symptom or condition, that makes a particular treatment or procedure inadvisable.

disparities Containing or made up of fundamentally different and often incongruous elements; markedly distinct in quality or character.

encrypt To convert from one system of communication to another; encode.

erroneous Containing or characterized by error or assumption.

gradient A change in response with distance from the stimulus.

nosocomial Originating or taking place in a hospital.

quality assurance Activities designed to increase the quality of a product or service through process or system changes that increase efficiency or effectiveness.

sentinel event An unexpected occurrence involving death or serious physical or psychologic injury, or the risk thereof.

standards Established by authority, custom, or general consent as a model or example; something set up and established by authority as a rule for the measure of quantity, weight, extent, value, or quality.

transpose To change the relative place or normal order of; to alter the sequence.

Prior to the 1990s, practitioners in the healthcare field were barely familiar with the term *health information management*. Today, it is a well-respected profession that employs thousands of individuals across the United States. As more medical facilities move toward computer-based medical records, more trained health information management professionals are needed. The medical assistant may wish to pursue employment in this growing field.

The health information management profession is supported by a national organization called the American Health Information Management Association. This association's House of Delegates developed a statement in 1994 that defines the profession. The statement reads:

"Health information management is the profession that focuses on healthcare data and the management of healthcare information resources. The profession addresses the nature, structure, and translation of data into usable forms of information for the advancement of health and healthcare of individuals and populations. Health information professionals collect, integrate, and analyze primary and secondary healthcare data; disseminate information; and manage information resources related to research, planning, provision, and evaluation of healthcare services."

Evolution of the Profession

In 1928, the American College of Surgeons realized that accurate medical records promoted good medical care. This desire for quality led to the establishment of the Association of Record Librarians of North America. Years later in 1970, the organization changed its name to the American Medical Record Association. Medical records professionals found employment in hospitals, health clinics, insurance companies, and other organizations that utilized medical records.

In 1991, the organization became known as the American Health Information Management Association. Advances in technology have brought the health information management profession from a paper environment into a highly sophisticated computer age, where physicians can access patient and statistical data in seconds.

CRITICAL THINKING APPLICATION

- Laura is eligible to join the American Health Information Management Association, and her employer will pay for her dues. How might joining this professional organization benefit Laura?
- How would the hospital benefit from Laura's membership in the organization?

The Use of Healthcare Data

Many people and various organizations use healthcare data in a multitude of ways (Figure 22-1). Primarily, healthcare data are used to plan care for patients and ensure that they receive continuity of care from one healthcare provider to another. However, the information provided through healthcare records is useful in other capacities.

For example, when a drug is being evaluated, statistics must be kept to help the manufacturers of the product determine its effectiveness. Information on side effects and other **contraindications** is reviewed and used to make the product safer and more marketable. Sometimes, the drug must be changed and then returned to clinical trials.

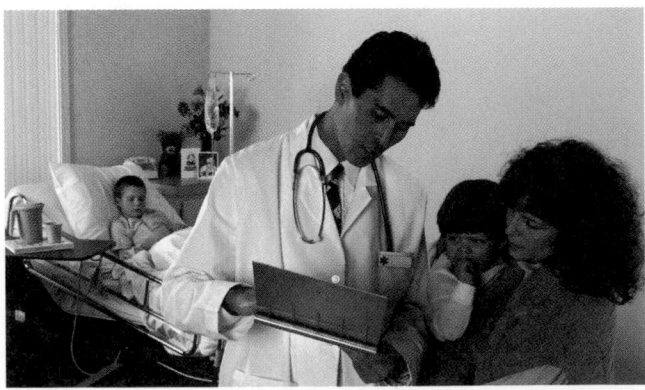

FIGURE 22-1   Physicians rely on health information to provide quality care to their patients.

Healthcare organizations gather information on the number of patients who enter the facility with the same diagnosis. This and other information helps them to plan what types of equipment will be needed to meet the needs of the patient population. For instance, if the geographic area where the facility is located contains a large number of patients with cardiac disease, a hospital may need to add a cardiac intensive care unit. If the facility is located in a neighborhood where there are many young families, the obstetrics and pediatrics departments may be expanded. Healthcare data and statistics guide planning for the needs of next week and for the next decade.

CRITICAL THINKING APPLICATION

- Laura has noticed that the hospital keeps extensive records on the admitting diagnosis and the discharge diagnosis. Why is this information important?
- If a certain physician is admitting numerous patients with the same diagnosis and is a family practitioner, what concerns might this raise for the facility?

Third-party payors use healthcare information to determine whether claims should be paid. The data provide proof that a certain procedure or treatment was medically necessary and therefore should be reimbursed (Figure 22-2). Government and regulatory agencies use data to make certain that healthcare facilities are in compliance with the various statutes and standards that govern them.

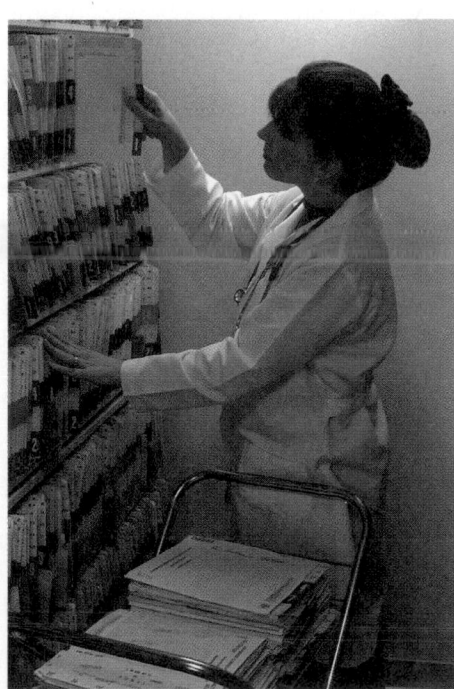

FIGURE 22-2 Healthcare providers often rely on statistics when treating their patients. Most statistical information is gleaned from patient charts.

Data also are used by facilities in determining whether quality healthcare is being provided to patients.

What Are Quality Data?

The information that is contained in a database is only as reliable as the person who entered it into the computer. Most database systems require information to be saved after it is entered by clicking an additional button. Without saving, the time and effort spent in entering the data have been wasted.

*Health Information: Management of a Strategic Resource** identifies nine characteristics of quality health data. These characteristics are validity, reliability, completeness, recognizability, timeliness, relevance, accessibility, security, and legality.

Validity

The validity of health data is synonymous with accuracy. Accuracy is one of the most important characteristics of data, whether in paper-based or computer-based records. Great care must be taken when characters are typed on the keyboard, so that letters or numbers are not **transposed.**

Reliability

The healthcare professional must be able to rely on the data presented. If a patient's medical chart is marked such that he or she has no allergies, the medical assistant must be able to trust that information and give an injection with the confidence that the patient is not allergic to the medication. Reliability also pertains to the degree to which the information in the database can be trusted.

Completeness

The information must not only be accurate, it must also be complete. If the medical assistant gives an injection yet fails to document it in the patient's chart, then the record is incomplete. If a computer system is designed to upload new information into the database every night and the system malfunctions, there is a strong possibility that the records contained within the system are incomplete, possibly missing vital information needed to care for the patient.

Recognizability

All users of health information must be able to interpret the data that are presented in the health record. The facility should have a consistent use of abbreviations so that no misunderstandings occur when reviewing a patient's chart.

*Abdelhak M, Grostick S, Hanken MA, Jacobs E: *Health information: management of a strategic resource*, ed 2. Philadelphia, 2001, WB Saunders.

Timeliness

Health data must be entered into the chart or database as soon as it happens. The medical assistant should never commit information to memory intending to enter it later. Reports from laboratories or medical tests also should be placed in the chart as soon as the information is reviewed by the physician, so that decisions made are supported by the latest information on the patient's condition.

Relevance

The information contained in the database must be relevant to be useful. Needless and meaningless statistics about patient treatments or drug interactions do not benefit providers and users of health information.

Accessibility

One of the advantages of a computer-based patient record is that it is accessible to multiple users at the same time. The facility must take care to provide access only to individuals who are authorized to view the records. The computer system should have a login capability, which prompts for a password. In addition, the system should keep records of who accesses information by time and date. Paper-based patient records should be returned to their proper place when they are not in use so that they will be accessible to all staff members.

Security

Although only certain employees are allowed to access health information, precautions must be taken to prohibit access to intruders. Firewalls are similar to filters that allow only certain types of data to enter or exit. Information can be **encrypted**, which means that it is changed into a code that can only be read once unencrypted. These precautions are necessary because of the sensitivity of patient information. Also, care must be taken to ensure that no one can change the information already contained in the record.

Legality

Many statutes govern medical records. The laws concerning record retention vary from state to state. Medical records cannot be altered but should be corrected according to accepted guidelines. The record must be completely legible and **authenticated** properly (Figure 22-3).

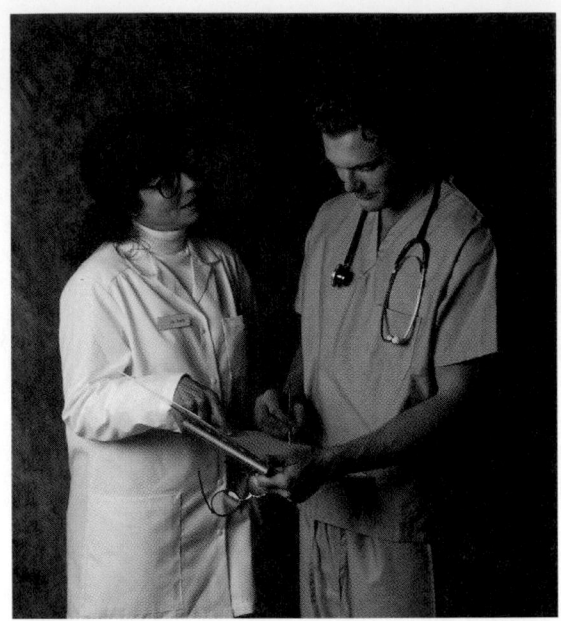

FIGURE 22-3 Physicians must authenticate medical records by initialing or signing their entries. Some computer systems automatically authenticate records.

The Challenges of Quality Assurance Problems

Many of the larger medical facilities today have entire departments that are devoted to **quality assurance**. Quality assurance is defined as the activities designed to increase the quality of a product or service through process or system changes that increase efficiency or effectiveness. Although many people assume that quality is determined solely by the patient, there is much more involved in quality assurance than just the patient's satisfaction with services rendered. Quality assurance also is concerned with the *overuse, underuse, misuse,* and *variations in use* of different healthcare services.

Healthcare services that are excessive and unnecessary cause costs to rise. Treatments and services that are overused include hysterectomies, tympanostomy tubes, and antibiotics. Medical studies have shown that up to 16% of all hysterectomies performed in 1993 were unnecessary and up to 23% of tympanostomy tube operations performed between 1991 and 1992 were unnecessary. Antibiotics are prescribed widely for common colds and acute bronchitis, but the drugs do not benefit these illnesses.

The underuse of services and treatments can be equally costly. Mammograms and cervical cancer screening tests can detect medical problems yet are not taken advantage of by enough at-risk patients (Figure 22-4). The use of beta blockers has been proven to reduce mortality in patients who have had heart attacks by as much as 43%, but often they are not prescribed for these patients. Diabetic patients should have their eyes checked regularly, but many do not. All of these are examples of the underuse of services that can affect the quality of healthcare.

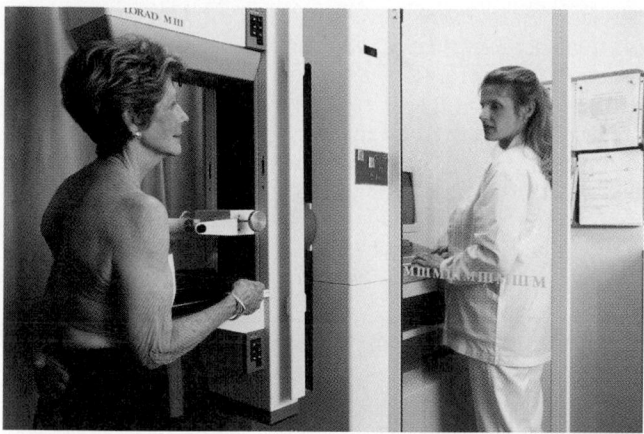

FIGURE 22-4 Healthcare professionals must encourage at-risk patients to have screening tests done, such as those for breast and cervical cancer.

CRITICAL THINKING APPLICATION

- How might a hospital employee encourage patients to have screening tests done, such as mammograms and for cervical cancer?
- What marketing strategies could Laura assist in developing that will result in more patients taking advantage of health screening opportunities?
- How do these services benefit the health facility?

Some healthcare services are misused. These errors can cause death, delay of correct diagnosis, unnecessary injuries, and increased healthcare costs. Examples of misuse can include laboratory tests that provide **erroneous** results. Medication errors can be fatal to patients or cause complications to the illnesses from which they are already suffering. Hospital injuries and **nosocomial** infections promote further complications. A study at the Harvard School of Public Health published in 1994 estimated that up to 180,000 needless deaths occurred each year as a result of preventable errors.

There are wide variations in services in different parts of the country. Discharge rates (which indicate that the patient left the hospital without expiring) are higher in some areas of the United States than others. Individuals who seek medical care are more conscientious and likely to seek health services in different geographic areas. All of these issues contribute to the concept of quality healthcare.

Health Insurance Portability and Accountability Act

As technology advanced and more health records became computerized, legislation dealing with privacy became imperative. HIPAA of 1996 was developed, in part, to help ensure the confidentiality of medical records. The statute, which became law in August of 1996, applies to those records that are created or maintained by healthcare providers, health plans, and healthcare clearinghouses that engage in certain electronic transactions.

The Office for Civil Rights, a division of the Health and Human Services Department, regulates HIPAA.

In August of 2002, the Department of Health and Human Services Secretary Tommy Thompson announced the final ruling relating to HIPAA's privacy act, which became effective April 14, 2003. Under the privacy rule:

- Patients must give specific authorization before entities covered by the regulation could use or disclose protected information in most nonroutine circumstances—such as releasing information to an employer or for use in marketing activities. Doctors, health plans, and other covered entities would be required to follow the rule's standards for the use and disclosure of personal health information.
- Covered entities generally will need to provide patients with written notice of their privacy practices and patients' privacy rights. The notice will contain information that could be useful to patients choosing a health plan, doctor, or other provider. Patients would generally be asked to sign or otherwise acknowledge receipt of the privacy notice from direct treatment providers.
- Pharmacies, health plans, and other covered entities must first obtain an individual's specific authorization before sending marketing materials. At the same time, the rule permits doctors and other covered entities to communicate freely with patients about treatment options and other health-related information, including disease management programs.
- Specifically, improvements to the final rule strengthen the marketing language to make clear that covered entities cannot use business associate agreements to **circumvent** the rule's marketing prohibition. The improvement explicitly prohibits pharmacies or other covered entities from selling personal medical information to a business that would market its products or services under a business associate agreement.
- Patients generally will be able to access their personal medical records and request changes to correct any errors. In addition, patients generally could request an accounting of nonroutine uses and disclosures of their health information.

Many healthcare organizations have concern about the costs of implementing and maintaining measures that will comply with the privacy regulations. However, the benefits of the act far outweigh the inconveniences of remaining in compliance. Patients have the right to expect complete confidentiality with regard to their health records (Figure 22-5).

CRITICAL THINKING APPLICATION

- Laura is concerned about the number of employees in her facility who are allowed to access patient information. For instance, all nurses have access to health information on all patients. Is this a good policy? Why or why not?
- Should all physicians have access to all patient records? Why or why not?

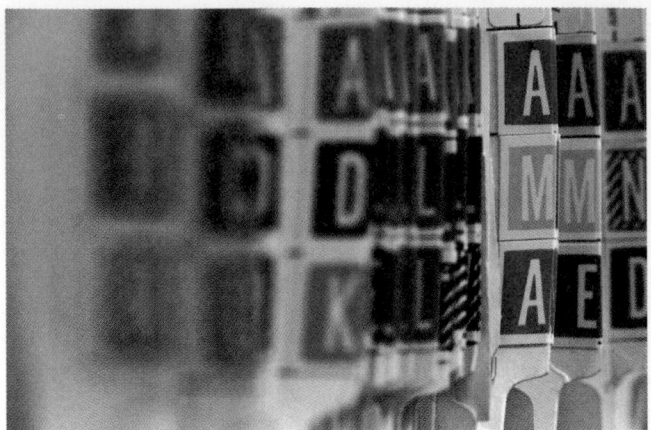

FIGURE 22-5 Patients must have the assurance that their medical records are only accessed by authorized individuals.

National Center for Health Statistics

The NCHS is a division of the Centers for Disease Control. The agency is the primary provider of health information statistics used to guide the actions and policies that relate to the health of the American public. The functions of the NCHS include:

- Documentation of the health status of the population and of important subgroups
- Identification of **disparities** in health status and use of healthcare by race, ethnicity, socioeconomic status (SES), region, and other population **gradients**
- Description of experiences with the healthcare system
- Monitoring of trends in health status and healthcare delivery
- Identification of health problems
- Support of biomedical and health services research
- Provision of information for making changes in public policies and programs
- Evaluation of the impact of health policies and programs

Statistics are of vital importance to many entities that are interested in the healthcare industry. Some of the available statistics through the NCHS are related to:

- Teenage pregnancy
- Incidence of HIV infection
- Alcohol and drug use
- Births
- Deaths
- Communicable diseases
- Infant health and mortality
- Leading causes of death
- Life expectancy
- Sexually transmitted diseases
- Suicide

Total Quality Management

Total quality management is management and control activities based on the leadership of top-level management, supported by the involvement of all employees and departments from planning and development to sales and service. These management and control activities focus on quality assurance. Qualities that satisfy the customer are built into products and services during the above processes.

For total quality management practices to be effective, all employees must make a commitment to provide patients with the best care possible. This includes top-level management as well as the staff members who work directly with the patients.

CRITICAL THINKING APPLICATION

- Laura has noticed that many employees are frustrated when confronted with quality assurance regulations. Often, they complain that the policies are a waste of time. How can Laura convince them that the regulations are important and foster cooperation from these people?
- Should adherence to quality assurance policies be a mandatory part of the employee's job description?

The Total Quality Management Concept. Much of the thrust of today's interest in total quality management originated from the teachings of W. Edwards Deming. Deming obtained a doctorate in mathematical physics from Yale University in 1928. He is perhaps best known for the work he did with Japanese managers and engineers regarding quality management. Deming compiled 14 points for managers to institute that were designed to place the emphasis on quality rather than quantity.

The following is an excerpt from Deming's book *Out of the Crisis** and briefly describes the Fourteen Points for Management.

- Create constancy of purpose toward improvement of product and service, with the aim to become competitive, to stay in business, and to provide jobs.
- Adopt the new philosophy. Western management must awaken to the challenge, must learn their responsibilities, and take on leadership for change.
- Cease dependence on inspection to achieve quality. Eliminate the need for inspection on a mass basis by building quality into the product or service in the first place.
- End the practice of awarding business on the basis of price tag. Instead, minimize total cost. Move toward a single supplier for any one item, on a long-term relationship of loyalty and trust.
- Constantly improve the system of production and service, to improve quality and productivity, and thus constantly decrease costs.
- Institute training on the job.
- Institute leadership. The aim of supervision should be to help people and machines and gadgets to do a better job. Supervision of management is in need of overhaul as well as supervision of production workers.

---

*Deming WE: *Out of the crisis.* Cambridge, Mass, 1986, Massachusetts Institute of Technology.

- Drive out fear, so that everyone may work effectively for the company.
- Break down barriers between departments. People must work as a team, to foresee problems of production and in use that may be encountered with the product or service.
- Eliminate slogans, exhortations, and targets for the work force asking for zero defects and new levels of productivity. Such exhortations only create adversarial relationships. Eliminate quotas and substitute leadership. Eliminate management by objective. Eliminate management by numbers and numerical goals. Substitute leadership.
- Remove barriers that rob the hourly worker of his right to pride of workmanship. The responsibility of supervisors must be changed from sheer numbers to quality.
- Remove barriers that rob people in management and in engineering of their right to pride of workmanship. This means the abolishment of the annual merit rating and of management by objective.
- Institute a vigorous program of education and self-improvement.
- Put everybody in the company to work to accomplish the transformation. The transformation is everybody's job.

Deming believed that these points would assist managers in bringing quality to the facility or business in which they were used (Figure 22-6). They are widely used in countless business and service organizations today.

Joint Commission on Accreditation of Healthcare Organizations

JCAHO is a nonprofit organization that assists healthcare facilities by providing accreditation services. The facilities participate in obtaining accreditation voluntarily, but over 17,000 healthcare facilities in the United States are accredited by and comply with JCAHO standards.

For many years, healthcare facilities were interested in meeting the minimum **standards** that would reflect quality healthcare. Recently, there has been a shift from simply meeting minimum standards to exceeding standards and providing optimal healthcare to patients (Figure 22-7). Standards are a set of criteria that the facility must adhere to and be able to prove their compliance.

Risk Management

A risk is any occurrence that could result in patient injury or any type of financial loss to the healthcare facility. The policies and procedures that facilities develop are designed to manage risk and prevent situations that can cause harm to persons or property for which the healthcare facility could be held liable.

Risk management programs in healthcare facilities should focus on financial loss prevention and reduce the possibility of negative publicity resulting from **sentinel events**. JCAHO defines a sentinel event as an "unexpected occurrence involving death or serious physical or psychological injury, or the risk thereof." Sentinel events must be investigated thoroughly and their contributing

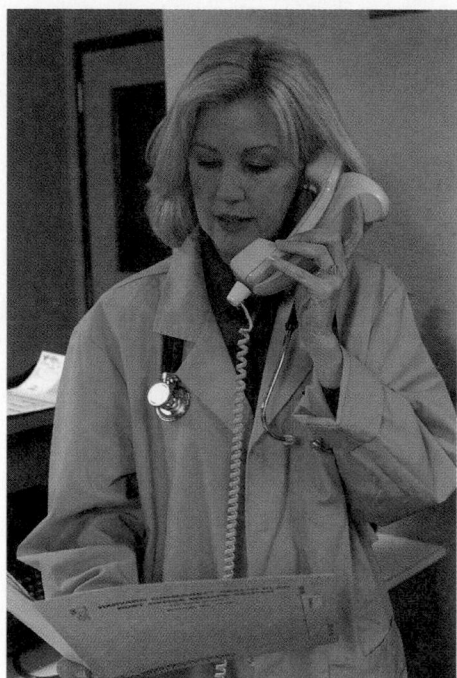

FIGURE 22-6 Quality management is a vital part of accreditation of healthcare organizations, and all physicians should be dedicated to providing optimal quality care to patients.

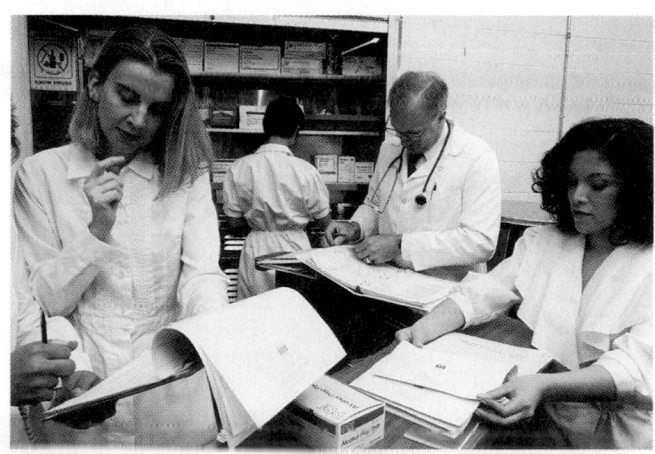

FIGURE 22-7 Accreditation of a healthcare facility takes teamwork and a commitment to quality assurance.

factors rectified so that they are avoided in the future. Records are kept of the sentinel events that happen in a facility, especially those that involve injury to patients.

Closing Comments

Health information management is a critical aspect of today's healthcare facility. Although regulations may seem stringent, the value of protecting the patient's privacy is immeasurable. Patients have the right to expect that their health information is kept confidential. The medical assistant should focus on meeting privacy guidelines and take great care when working with medical records and information.

Patient Education

HIPAA received a great deal of publicity. Patients had long been concerned about their rights to privacy regarding access to health information.

Many patients may have questions about HIPAA and the extent of their rights to limit access to their records. Be prepared to answer their questions or guide them to the right source for information.

Legal and Ethical Issues

The medical assistant must be familiar with the laws surrounding privacy issues and be able to guide patients as they have concerns. Seminars that will target the compliance issues that affect the physician's office often are available to the medical assistant. Most employers are willing to pay for such seminars so that the office can remain in strict compliance with legal issues. Remember that the medical profession is one of constant change. The medical assistant must have a positive attitude about the learning process, especially when new rules and regulations take effect.

SUMMARY OF SCENARIO

Laura is learning more about health information management each day that she goes to work. She has earned the respect of her supervisors, who often give her a lengthy, complicated document concerning regulations and ask her to read and summarize it for the staff. She has a knack for weeding out the actual requirements amid the excess of legalese.

Laura has developed good relationships with many of the staff physicians at the hospital. She has approached several of them about record authentication, and her bright personality helps to foster a sense of cooperation between the medical staff and the hospital staff. She has even begun to give coupons good for one lunch in the cafeteria when physicians form the habit of authenticating their records in a timely manner. The physicians appreciate the recognition for completing their duties on schedule.

Laura has given thought to continuing her education in the health management field and possibly gaining certification in this area. She knows that this will lend credibility to the knowledge that she has gained on the job. Her supervisors are pleased with her performance and know they can count on Laura to complete any task she is assigned on time with accurate results. Laura looks forward to a long career at the hospital and being of service to the patients and staff alike in the years to come.

SUMMARY OF LEARNING OBJECTIVES

- Both physicians and employees of medical facilities use health information in many ways. The information helps to ensure continuity of care from provider to provider. It assists manufacturers in determining side effects of drugs. It provides statistical information regarding primary and secondary diagnoses. Health information also helps the medical facility plan for future needs and capital equipment.

- There are nine characteristics of quality health data. Validity refers to the accuracy of the information, while reliability means that the information can be counted on to be accurate and medical decisions can be made based on the information. Completeness simply means that the information is available in its entirety, and recognizability refers to the data being understood by the users. Timely information allows the provider to make decisions based on the latest data about a patient or a treatment. Relevance refers to the usefulness of the health information, and accessibility means that the information is easily available to the provider when it is needed. Security encompasses the effort to keep unauthorized people from accessing health information. Legality refers to the correctness of the information and its authentication by the healthcare provider.

- Four concerns that surround quality assurance include the overuse, underuse, misuse, and variations in use of healthcare services. Overused services are excessive and cause cost increases. An example includes using the emergency room for nonemergencies. Underuse means that patients do not take advantage of many services they should be using, especially if they are at-risk patients. Misuse of services often reflects errors, such as lab errors or misdiagnoses. Variations in services simply means that in various parts of the country, individuals use services in different ways, which can influence the quality of care overall in the United States.

- HIPAA is a milestone in support of patient privacy issues. There are several facets of the act, but the most widely publicized sections deal with the right to patient privacy. The act will give a degree of control to patients and allow them information about who accesses their records. Patients must also give specific authorization for the use and dissemination of the information contained in the medical record.

- The NCHS is a part of the Centers for Disease Control. Health statistics are important, because they enable providers to better treat their patients. For instance, if a certain area has a high number of outbreaks of a particular disease, the physician may be better prepared to cope with patients with the symptoms of that disease, treating them faster and promoting a full recovery. Health statistics provide information about these types of issues. The NCHS helps to compile information such as the number of HIV infections, teen pregnancies, and other vital health data that is useful to medical professionals.

■ Some of the statistics kept by the NCHS include alcohol and drug use information, births, deaths, communicable diseases, infant health and mortality, and life expectancy.

■ Total quality management is management and control activities based on the leadership of top-level management, supported by the involvement of all employees and departments in an effort to provide quality assurance.

■ JCAHO is a nonprofit organization that offers accreditation services to healthcare facilities that wish to excel in healthcare services. Accreditation is voluntary; however, over 17,000 healthcare facilities in the United States are accredited by this agency.

■ Without strong healthcare standards, quality cannot exist. The focus of quality assurance has shifted in recent years from just meeting the minimum standards to providing optimal quality. People expect quality healthcare when they get treatment. Today's organizations that seek accreditation or focus their efforts on quality will exceed standards, not just meet them.

KEY INTERNET WEBSITES

- Agency for Healthcare Research and Quality
- Joint Commission on Accreditation of Healthcare Organizations
- National Center for Health Statistics
  For active weblinks to each website visit
  http://evolve.elsevier.com/Kinn/

CHAPTER 23

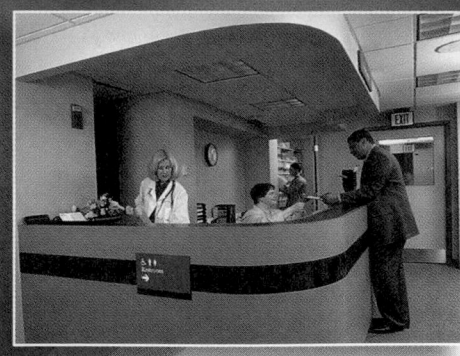

Scenario

Brenda Newman is the office manager for Dr. Susan Wilkins, a neurologist who is beginning her second year of practice. Dr. Wilkins is financially savvy and takes care with the money she has invested in her business. She encourages her employees to plan for the future, and offers them a retirement plan as well as opportunities for investing in mutual funds through payroll deduction. Her accountant, Grant Schmidt, assists Dr. Wilkins with the financial aspects of her practice, and is always willing to counsel the employees of the clinic about finances.

Mr. Schmidt has taught Brenda several methods of keeping track of the practice finances. Brenda is interested in learning more about general accounting rules and bookkeeping. She is able to perform computerized accounting duties and is also able to use a pegboard system. She is able to work with patients when they need to make payment arrangements, and has an excellent collection ratio.

Dr. Wilkins is cost conscious and does not order random supplies and equipment. Instead, she and Brenda plan the inventory for a 6-month period, and have needed to only order supplies every 6 months. By ordering in precise amounts, Dr. Wilkins saves money and uses the extra funds for staff development events and seminars. Each month, the budget is reviewed to ensure that the office is on track with expenses.

The team effort between Dr. Wilkins, Brenda, and Mr. Schmidt results in a balanced budget for the clinic, and subsequently the staff is able to enjoy more benefits and perks.

Management of Practice Finances

National Curriculum Competencies

2d. Perform accounts receivable procedures
2e. Perform accounts payable procedures
2h. Establish and maintain a petty cash fund

Vocabulary

accounts payable Debts incurred and not yet paid.

accounts receivable Amounts owed to the physician.

accounts receivable trial balance A method of determining that the journal and the ledger are in balance.

accrual basis of accounting Method of accounting in which income is recorded when earned, and expenses are recorded when incurred.

assets The entire property of a person, association, corporation, or estate applicable or subject to the payment of debts.

balance sheet A financial statement for a specific date that shows the total assets, liabilities, and capital of the business.

bookkeeping The recording of business and accounting transactions.

cash basis of accounting Method of accounting in which income is recorded when received, and expenses are recorded when paid.

cash flow statement A financial summary for a specific period that shows the beginning balance on hand, the receipts and disbursements during the period, and the balance on hand at the end of the period.

disbursements journal A summary of accounts paid out.

equities The money value of a property or of an interest in a property in excess of claims or liens against it.

fiscal year An accounting period of 12 months.

in balance The total ending balances of patient ledgers equal total of accounts receivable control.

invoice A paper describing a purchase and the amount due.

liabilities Something that is owed; a debt.

packing slip An itemized list of objects in a package.

petty cash fund A fund maintained to pay small unpredictable cash expenditures.

statement A request for payment.

statement of income and expense A summary of all income and expenses for a given period.

trial balance A method of checking the accuracy of accounts.

A physician's business records are the key to good management practice. The medical assistant who can keep accurate financial records and who will conduct the administrative side of the practice in a businesslike fashion is genuinely needed and appreciated.

Financial records that are complete, correct, and current are essential for:

- Prompt billing and collection procedures
- Professional financial planning
- Accurate reporting of income to federal and state agencies

What Is Accounting?

Accounting is a system of recording, classifying, and summarizing financial transactions. **Bookkeeping** is mainly the recording part of the accounting process. The book-

keeping must be done daily and is the responsibility of the administrative medical assistant in a small practice, and the office manager or financial manager in a larger practice.

Accounting Bases

There are two general bases, or methods, for accounting: the cash basis and the accrual basis. Most physicians use the **cash basis of accounting**, which means that charges for services are entered as income when payment is received, and expenses are recorded when they are paid. Merchants, on the other hand, generally use an **accrual basis of accounting**. Income is considered earned when services have been performed or goods have been sold, even though payment may not have been received. Expenses are recognized and recorded when incurred, even though they have not been paid.

Financial Summaries

The financial records of any business should at all times show:

- How much was earned in a given period
- How much was collected
- How much is owed
- The distribution of expenses incurred

From the daily entries, the accountant can prepare monthly and annual summaries that provide a basis for comparing any given period with another similar period. Periodic analyses of the financial records can result in improved business practices, better management of time, curtailment or elimination of unprofitable services, and better budgeting of expenses. With the appropriate software these analyses can be accomplished using the computer. The medical assistant may notice notations of AP/AR, which stand for **accounts payable** and **accounts receivable**.

CRITICAL THINKING APPLICATION

- Brenda has noticed several errors on encounter forms lately. These errors seem to be a result of not using a calculator when adding the charges once the patient checks out. Brenda has approached the person who assists the patients in this area, but has not seen any improvement in the errors. How might she convince the employee to follow precautions in adding charges?
- How might Mr. Schmidt educate the staff about the importance of accurate financial records?

The Cardinal Rules of Bookkeeping

There are many rules that apply to bookkeeping that the medical assistant must learn. First, use good penmanship so that the records are clearly legible, even years later. Use the same pen style and ink consistently. Keep columns of figures straight and write well-formed figures (a careless 9 may look like a 7; an open 0 may resemble a 6). Carry decimal points correctly.

Enter all charges and receipts immediately in the daily record or journal. Write a receipt in duplicate for any currency received (Figure 23-1). Writing receipts for checks is optional, but a consistent pattern should be followed. Post all charges and receipts to the patient ledger daily. Checks should be endorsed for deposit as soon as received. Verify that the total of the deposit plus the amount on hand equal the total to be accounted for in the daily journal. Petty cash funds should be used to pay for small unpredictable expenses. Pay all other expenses by check. A cancelled check is the best proof of payment. Bills should be paid before their due dates, after checking them for accuracy. Place date of payment and number of check on paid bills.

Do not erase, write over, or blot out figures. If an error is made, a straight line should be drawn through the incorrect figure and the correct figure written above it. Bookkeeping procedures are not complicated, but they do require concentration to avoid errors. There is no such thing as *almost* correct financial records. The books either balance or they do not balance. The bookkeeping is either right or wrong. This is not the place to be creative or take shortcuts.

The medical assistant should set aside a certain time each day for bookkeeping tasks, if possible. Do not attempt to work on financial records when busy attending patients or when there are other distractions.

Kinds of Financial Records

Daily Journal. The daily journal day sheet is the chronological record of the practice—the financial diary. All information regarding services rendered, charges, and receipts is first recorded in the daily journal. It is important that every transaction be recorded.

In addition to professional services rendered in and out of the office, there may be income from other sources, such as rentals, royalties, interest, and so forth.

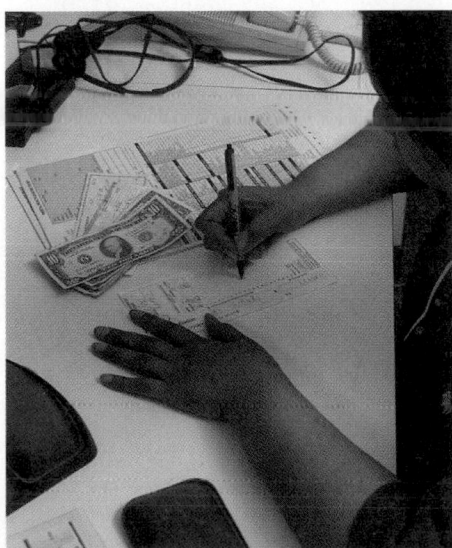

FIGURE 23-1 Accurate records reflect competency in the medical office. The medical assistant should use a calculator when adding figures and be careful not to transpose numbers.

Usually a special place is provided in the journal for such income. Any income that is not practice related should be recorded separately from patient receipts.

Checkbook. Receipts are usually deposited in the checking account, and a record of the deposit is entered in the journal and on the check stub. A copy of each deposit slip should be kept with the financial records. Bills are usually paid by check or online bill-paying services, and a record of the payment is entered on the check stub and in the disbursements section of the general journal.

CRITICAL THINKING APPLICATION

- Brenda has noticed two checks missing from the business checkbook. Dr. Wilkins is out of town for a week and unable to be contacted. How might Brenda determine where the checks are or to whom they were written?
- What steps can be taken to resolve the problem of not knowing the amount of a missing check?

Disbursements Journal

Manual Posting. In simplified accounting systems, the **disbursements journal** usually consists of a section at the bottom of each day sheet and a check register page at the end of each month, plus monthly and annual summaries. It must show:

- Every amount paid out
- Date and check number
- Purpose of payment

Computer Posting. Use the cash or check payments screen. Enter payment information and the computer can print the check, or enter information after the check has been manually prepared.

Petty Cash Records. A **petty cash fund** and voucher system should be established to take care of minor unpredictable expenditures such as postage due, parking fees, small contributions, emergency supplies, and miscellaneous small items. In the average facility, $25 to $50 is sufficient for the petty cash fund. If a larger sum is available, there is a tendency to pay too many bills out of petty cash instead of writing a check.

When the check for this fund is exchanged at the bank for small bills and coins, the money is placed in a cashbox or drawer that can be locked or kept in the safe at night. One person only should be in charge of the petty cash fund. This person must be able to account for the full amount of the fund at any time.

CRITICAL THINKING APPLICATION

- Brenda has noticed that on several occasions, employees have borrowed money from the petty cash fund. Is this an acceptable practice? Why or why not?
- How might Brenda keep an accounting of money taken from the petty cash drawer if she is not the person actually in control of it?

Payroll Records. The payroll record is an auxiliary disbursement record. A separate page or card for each employee, as well as a summary record, should be kept. This procedure is discussed in more detail later in this chapter.

Comparison of Common Bookkeeping Systems

Success in bookkeeping requires a thorough understanding of the system and what it is expected to accomplish. There are many variations in bookkeeping systems, from simple to complex, no one of which can meet the needs of every physician. The basic principles are the same for all; only the system of recording varies. The three most common systems found in the professional office are:

- Single-entry
- Double-entry
- Pegboard or write-it-once

An overview of the three systems is presented here. More detailed instruction for the pegboard system, the most widely used manual system in medical practices, is found in Chapter 14.

Single-Entry System

Single-entry bookkeeping is inexpensive, is simple to use, and requires very little training. It is the oldest and simplest of bookkeeping systems and includes at least three basic records:

- A general journal, also called a daily log, daybook, day sheet, daily journal, or charge journal.
- A cash payment journal, which in its simplest form is a checkbook.
- An accounts receivable ledger, which is a record of the amounts owed by all the patients. The accounts receivable ledger may be a bound book, a loose-leaf binder, a card file, or loose pages in a ledger tray.
- There may also be auxiliary records for petty cash and payroll records.

The records of charges and receipts are usually entered into a bound journal with a page for each day of the year, monthly summary pages, and an annual summary. Daily pages have columns for entering each transaction that show the patient's name, the service performed and the charge, any payments received, and the totals for charges and receipts. The daily totals are entered on the monthly summary, and the monthly totals are carried forward to the annual summary.

The same bound book may also have space for recording cash payments, or the checkbook may be the only cash payment journal. Monthly and annual summaries would be done from the checkbook.

The accounts receivable ledger usually consists of an account card for each patient on which are entered the charges and payments from the general journal. The patients' statements are prepared from these cards. In a single-entry system, each entry is made separately.

Although the single-entry system may satisfy the requirements for reporting to government agencies, it does have some drawbacks:

- Errors are not easily detected.
- There are no built-in controls.
- Periodic analyses are inadequate for financial planning.

The single-entry system was at one time widely used in healthcare facilities but has been largely replaced by more complete accounting systems.

Double-Entry System

Double-entry bookkeeping is also inexpensive but requires a trained and experienced bookkeeper or the regular services of an accountant. The transactions may be recorded manually or by computer. In addition to the basic journals used in a single-entry system, there may be numerous subsidiary journals. The system is based on the accounting equation:

Assets = Liabilities + Proprietorship (Capital)

Every transaction requires an entry on each side of the accounting equation, and the two sides must always be in balance. For this reason the system is called double-entry bookkeeping. It is the most complete of the three systems. An understanding of the basics of double-entry bookkeeping will help to clarify the principles of all systems.

Assets are the properties owned by a business, such as bank accounts, accounts receivable, buildings, equipment, and furniture. The rights to these assets are called **equities**. The equity of the owner is called *capital*, *proprietorship*, or *owner's equity*. The equities of the creditors to whom money is owed are called **liabilities**. The owner's equity or capital is what remains of the value of the assets after the creditor's equities or liabilities have been subtracted.

For example, if the physician purchased equipment for $1000, paid $250 down, and gave a promissory note for $750, the accounting equation would be:

$$\text{Assets} \quad \$1000 = \text{Liabilities} \quad \$750$$
$$+$$
$$\underline{} \quad \text{Capital} \quad \underline{250}$$
$$\$1000 \qquad\qquad \$1000$$

The total value of the asset is $1000. The owner's equity is $250, and the creditor's equity is $750. The accounting terms *capital*, *proprietorship*, *owner's equity*, and *net worth* are used interchangeably.

Few medical assistants are trained in accounting. If a double-entry system is used, a practice management consultant or the accountant who does most of the actual bookwork and reports usually sets it up. The medical assistant in this instance generally maintains only the daily journal, from which the accountant takes the figures once a month.

The double-entry system provides a more comprehensive picture of the practice and its effect on the physician's net worth. Errors show up readily, and there are many built-in accuracy controls; however, because of the time and skill required, it is not frequently used in the small practice.

Pegboard or Write-It-Once System

The pegboard is the most commonly used manual method of accounting in the physician's office. It is discussed at length in Chapter 14.

End-of-the-Day Summarizing

Most computer accounting systems will perform end-of-the-day summarizing automatically. If the office uses the pegboard system, the bottom of the day sheet has three sections to be completed that will show that the accounts have balanced for the day.

The first section is the proof of posting section, which deals with the transactions that occurred today on the day sheet. In the second section, the month-to-date accounts receivable proof, today's totals are being added to the month-to-date totals, and should balance to the penny. The last section is the year-to-date accounts receivable proof, which adds the accounts, including today's totals, to the year-to-date total.

Most systems also have a deposit ticket, which can be double-checked when adding the cash receipts and the checks. This is handy when preparing the day's deposit.

The totals at the bottom of the second and third sections must be an exact equal. When the end-of-the-day summarizing does not balance, the medical assistant should first check the addition of each column, both horizontally and vertically. This will result in finding most errors (Figure 23-2). Be sure that the instructions are followed to the letter. To avoid frustrating mistakes, it is best to use a calculator, even when adding small numbers.

Trial Balance of Accounts Receivable

A trial balance should be done once per month *after* all posting has been completed and *before* preparing the monthly statements. The purpose of a trial balance is to disclose any discrepancies between the journal and the ledger. It does not prove the accuracy of the accounts. For example, if a charge or payment was posted to the wrong account, or if the wrong amount was entered in the journal and then posted to the ledger, the totals would still "balance," but the accounts would not be accurate.

To begin, pull all the account cards that have a balance, enter each balance on the adding machine, and total the figures. This should equal the accounts receivable balance figure on the control. If there is no daily control, total all of the charges, all of the payments, and all of the adjustments for the month, and then do the computation illustrated below. The end-of-the-month accounts receivable figure must agree with the figure arrived at by adding all

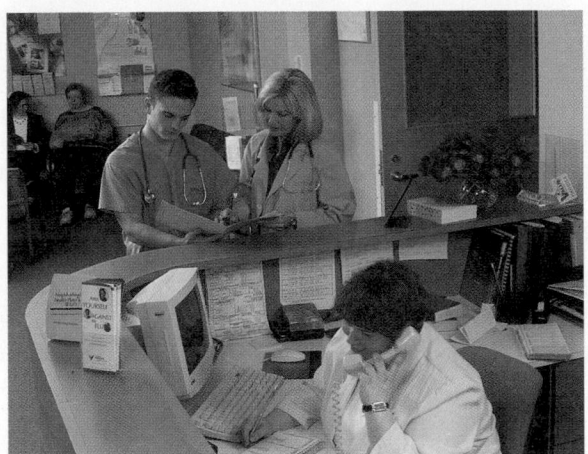

FIGURE 23-2 Ask the physician when unsure about financial information. When an unfamiliar statement arrives, check with the physician to be sure it should be paid.

the account card balances. The accounts are then said to be **in balance**. If the two totals do not agree, the error must be located.

Example of Balancing End-of-Month Accounts Receivable

Accounts receivable at first of month	$ _____
Plus total charges for month	$ _____
Subtotal	$ _____
Less total payments for month	$ _____
Subtotal	$ _____
Less total adjustments for month	$ _____
Accounts receivable at end of month	$ _____

Locating and Preventing Errors

After checking the tape and verifying that there is no error in calculation, the first step in locating an error in the trial balance is to find the difference between the two totals. Then search the daily journal pages and the account cards for an entry of the identical amount. Check each one found, and verify that it was posted correctly. Of course, there may be more than one error that adds up to this amount.

If there is only one error, and the amount of the error is divisible by 9, a figure may have been transposed. For example, if the difference is $81 (a number divisible by 9), the person who posted to the account may have written $209 instead of $290. If the amount of the error is divisible by 2, the amount may have been posted to the wrong column, reversing a debit and a credit.

A common error is made by entering the wrong amount in the previous balance column or in figuring the new balance. This kind of error will show up on the pegboard daily proof but could easily go undetected in the single-entry system. Carrying forward the wrong amount results in another common error total from one day to the next (e.g., carrying forward the beginning accounts receivable total rather than the ending accounts receivable total). There is always a chance of sliding a number, which means writing the first digit in the wrong column, such as writing 400 for 40 or 60 instead of 600.

Many bookkeepers avoid errors in the cents column by using a line (—) instead of writing two zeros when only even dollars are involved. For example, instead of writing $12.00, the bookkeeper will write $12.—. This eliminates the possibility of misreading zeros as other numbers. It also speeds the adding process when columns must be totaled.

If the medical assistant is unable to locate any numerical error, there is the possibility that an account card was lost or overlooked or was transferred as paid in full.

CRITICAL THINKING APPLICATION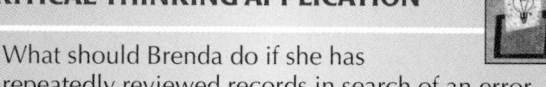

- What should Brenda do if she has repeatedly reviewed records in search of an error and is still unable to find it?
- Who should this be reported to?

Accounts Payable Procedures

Invoices and Statements

When an item is not paid for at the time of purchase, the vendor usually includes a **packing slip** with delivery of the merchandise. A packing slip describes the items enclosed. The vendor may also enclose an **invoice**. An invoice describes the items and shows the amount due. Always check to verify that the items listed on the packing slip and invoice are included in the delivery.

Invoices should be placed in a special folder until paid. The facility may be making more than one purchase from the same vendor during the month. Some vendors request that payment be made from the invoice; others expect to send a **statement** later. A statement is a request for payment.

Paying for Purchases

At the time of payment, compare the statement with the invoice to verify accuracy, fasten the statement and invoice together, write the date and check number on the statement, and place it in the paid file.

CRITICAL THINKING APPLICATION

- Brenda does not recall ordering a certain item from the office supply company. However, it was included in her last shipment and listed on the packing list. How can she recount whether the item was ordered?
- How would Brenda correct this problem if the item was in fact not ordered?

Recording Disbursements

Both the pegboard and the single-entry bookkeeping systems provide pages for recording disbursements. This is sometimes called a check register. On these pages, disbursements are distributed to specific expense accounts such as:

- Auto expense
- Dues and meetings
- Equipment
- Insurance
- Medical supplies
- Office expenses
- Printing, postage, and stationery
- Rent and maintenance
- Salaries
- Taxes and licenses
- Travel and entertainment
- Utilities
- Miscellaneous
- Personal withdrawals

Each check should be entered on the disbursement page, showing the date, the name of the company to which the check was written, the number and amount of the check, and the payment allocated to one or more of the expense accounts. It is important to separate personal expenditures from business expenses. Business expenses are tax deductible and are considered in determining net income from the practice, but personal expenditures are not. Although personal expenses are not deductible in determining net income from the practice, some qualify as personal deductions in computing personal income tax, so a careful accounting should be kept. Deductible expenses would include property taxes, interest paid out, contributions, and so forth.

Accounting for Petty Cash

The petty cash fund is a revolving fund (Procedure 23-1). It does not change in amount except to increase or decrease the established fund. To establish the petty cash fund, a check is written payable to Cash or Petty Cash and entered in the disbursements journal under Miscellaneous. This is the only time that the petty cash check is charged to Miscellaneous.

Each time the fund is replenished, the amount of the check is spread among the various accounts for which the money was used. This is determined from a record of expenditures. The headings of the columns should correspond to headings in the disbursements journal to which they will be posted.

A pad of petty cash vouchers is kept in or near the cash box. For every disbursement from the fund, the petty cashier should either have a receipt or prepare a voucher. The total of the petty cash vouchers and receipts plus the amount of cash in the box must always equal the original amount of the fund.

At the end of the month, or sooner if the fund is depleted, a check is written to Cash for replenishing the fund, but instead of being charged to Miscellaneous as previously, the amount of the check is divided among the various accounts affected.

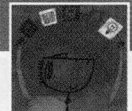

PROCEDURE 23-1

Accounting for Petty Cash

GOAL: To establish a petty cash fund, maintain an accurate record of expenditures for 1 month, and replenish the fund as necessary.

EQUIPMENT AND SUPPLIES

- Form for petty cash fund
- Pad of vouchers
- Disbursement journal
- Two checks
- List of petty cash expenditures

PROCEDURAL STEPS

1 Determine the amount needed in the petty cash fund.

2 Write a check in the determined amount.
Purpose: To establish a fund.

3 Record the beginning balance in the petty cash fund.

4 Post the amount to Miscellaneous on the disbursement record.
Purpose: To account for the original amount in the fund.

5 Prepare a petty cash voucher for each amount withdrawn from the fund.
Purpose: The vouchers will be used for internal audit.

6 Record each voucher in the petty cash record and enter the new balance.
Purpose: To record current balance and determine the need for replenishing the fund.

7 Write a check to replenish the fund as necessary.
Note: The total of the vouchers plus the fund balance must equal the beginning amount.

8 Total the expense columns and post to the appropriate accounts in the disbursement record.
Purpose: To record expenditures in the correct expense category.

9 Record the amount added to the fund.

10 Record the new balance in the petty cash fund.

Avoid the habit of borrowing from the petty cash fund. This admonition applies to the physician as well as to the medical assistant. If the physician requests cash from the fund, request a personal check or an office check in exchange for cash from the fund. It is also poor policy to use the petty cash fund for making change. In facilities where patients frequently pay with currency, a separate change fund should be kept.

Periodic Summaries

Financial summaries are compiled on monthly and annual bases. They may be prepared either by the medical assistant manually or on the computer or by the accountant. Common summary reports include:
- Statement of income and expense
- Cash flow statement
- Trial balance
- Accounts receivable trial balance and aging analysis
- Balance sheet

The **statement of income and expense** is also known as the profit and loss statement and covers a specific period. It lists all the income received and all expenses paid during the period. The total income is called gross income or earnings. The income after deduction of all expenses is the net income.

A **cash flow statement** starts with the amount of cash on hand at the beginning of the month (or for any specified period). It then lists the cash income and the cash disbursement made throughout the period, and concludes with a statement of the amount of cash remaining on hand at the end of the period.

A **trial balance** is necessary to determine that the books are in balance. All of the columns on the disbursements journal must be totaled at the end of the month. The combined totals of all the expense columns must be equal to the total of the checks written. If the figures do not balance, it is necessary to recheck every entry until an error is found.

The **accounts receivable trial balance** is done before sending out the monthly statements. First, record the total of the accounts receivable ledger at the end of the previous month; then add the charges for the current month and subtract the adjustments and the payments received. The remainder should equal the total of the accounts receivable ledger at the end of the current month.

The **balance sheet**, also known as a statement of financial condition, shows the financial picture of the practice on a specific date. Often, it is done only on an annual basis. The balance sheet is set up using the accounting equation:

Assets = Liabilities + Proprietorship

The title of the statement had its origin in the equality of the elements—the balance between the sum of the assets and the sum of the liabilities and proprietorship.

At the end of the accounting year, it is very simple to combine the monthly reports to compile the annual summaries. The annual summaries simplify the reporting of income for tax returns.

Payroll Records

Handling payroll records, whether for one employee or dozens of employees, involves frequent reporting activities (Procedure 23-2). Government regulations require the withholding of taxes from employees and payment of certain taxes due from both employees and employers. To comply with government regulations, complete records must be kept for every employee. All records of employment taxes must be kept for at least 4 years. These should be available for review by the Internal Revenue Service (IRS). Such records include the following:

- Social Security number of the employee
- Number of withholding allowances claimed
- Amount of gross salary
- All deductions for Social Security and Medicare taxes; federal, state, and city or other subdivision withholding taxes; state disability insurance; and state unemployment tax, where applicable

CRITICAL THINKING APPLICATION

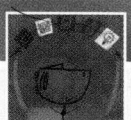

- Brenda hired a new employee on Friday, who reported to work on Monday. The new employee states that she cannot produce her Social Security card. Can Brenda allow the individual to work?
- Investigate the procedures for verifying a Social Security number.

Payroll Reporting Forms

Each employee and each employer must have a tax identification number. The Social Security number is the employee's tax identification number. Any person who does not have a Social Security number should apply for one, using Form SS-5 available from any Social Security Administration office.

The employer applies for a number for federal tax accounting purposes using Form SS-4, available at Social Security Administration offices. In states that require employer reports, a state employer number must also be obtained.

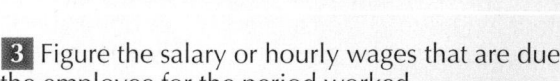

PROCEDURE **23-2**

Processing an Employee Payroll

GOAL: To process payroll and compensate employees, making deductions accurately.

EQUIPMENT AND SUPPLIES

- Checkbook
- Computer and payroll software, if applicable
- Pen
- Tax withholding tables
- Federal Employers Tax Guide

PROCEDURAL STEPS

1 Be sure that all information has been collected on the employees, including a copy of the Social Security card, a W-4 form, and an I-9 form.
Purpose: To make certain that the employee is eligible to work in the United States, and to determine what withholding amounts should be deducted from paychecks.

2 Review the time cards for all employees. Determine if any employees need counseling due to late arrivals or habitual absences.
Purpose: To address problem issues immediately and help to correct habits that can lead to employee termination.

3 Figure the salary or hourly wages that are due the employee for the period worked.
Purpose: To ascertain the amount owed to the employee.

4 Figure the deductions that must be taken from the paycheck. This usually includes, but is not limited to:

- Federal, state, and local taxes
- Social Security withholdings
- Medicare withholdings
- Other deductions, such as insurance, savings, and so forth
- Donations to organizations, such as the United Way

Purpose: To comply with federal, state, and local laws and deduct amounts for insurance, savings plans, and so forth.

5 Write the check for the balance due the employee. Most software programs can print the checks and explanations of deductions.

6 Have employees sign for their paychecks, if that is the policy of the office.

Before the end of the first pay period, the employee should complete an Employee's Withholding Allowance Certificate (Form W-4) showing the number of withholding allowances claimed (Figure 23-3). Otherwise, the employer must indicate withholding on the basis of a single person with no exemptions.

The employee should complete a new form when changes occur in marital status or in the number of allowances claimed. Each employee is entitled to one personal allowance and one for each qualified dependent. The employee may elect to take fewer or no allowances, in which case the tax withheld will be greater and a refund may be due when the employee's annual tax report is filed (Figure 23-4). If an employee claims more than 10 withholding allowances or an exemption from withholding and his or her wages would normally be more than $200 per week, the employer is required to send copies of these W-4 forms to the IRS.

A supply of all the necessary forms for filing federal returns, preprinted with the employer's name, will be furnished to an employer who has applied for an employer identification number. Extra forms may be obtained from the IRS office.

CRITICAL THINKING APPLICATION

- Mr. Schmidt has explained to Brenda that the more withholding deductions an employee claims, the less tax is taken from the paycheck. If Brenda's new employee wishes to claim seven deductions, and she only has three children and is single, could she do so legally?
- Why or why not?
- Why might it be risky to claim all of the deductions a person is legally entitled to?

Income Tax Withholding. Employers are required by law to withhold certain amounts from employees' earnings. These amounts must be reported and forwarded to the IRS to be applied toward payment of income tax. The amount to be withheld is based on the following:

- Total earnings of the employee
- Number of withholding allowances claimed
- Marital status of the employee
- Length of the pay period involved

The *Federal Employer's Tax Guide* includes tables to be used in determining the amount to be withheld. There is one table for single persons and unmarried heads of households and one for married persons. The tables cover monthly, semimonthly, biweekly, weekly, and daily or miscellaneous periods.

Employers Income Tax. The physician who is practicing as an individual is not subject to withholding tax but is expected to make an estimated tax payment four times a year. The accountant prepares four copies of Form 1040-S, Declaration of Estimated Tax for Individuals, for the ensuing year when the annual income tax return is prepared. The first form and the quarterly estimated tax for the next year are filed at the same time as the tax return. The remaining three forms, with the estimated tax due, must be filed on June 15, September 15, and January 15. It may be the business manager's responsibility to see that these returns are filed when due. The employer also contributes to Social Security and Medicare in the form of a self-employment tax.

Social Security, Medicare, and Income Tax Withholding. The Federal Insurance Contributions Act (FICA) provides for a federal system of old age, survivors, disability, and hospital insurance. The tax rate is reviewed frequently and is subject to change by Congress. As of 2001, the wage base for Social Security tax is $84,900 and the tax rate is 6.2% each for employers and employees. All wages are subject to the Medicare tax at a rate of 1.45% each for both employees and employers.

Quarterly Returns

Each quarter of the year, all employers who are subject to income tax withholding (including withholding on sick pay and supplemental unemployment benefits) of Social Security and Medicare taxes must file an Employer's Quarterly Federal Tax Return on or before the last day of the first month after the end of the quarter (Figure 23-5). Due dates for this return and full payment of the tax are April 30, July 31, October 31, and January 31. If deposits equaling full payment of taxes due have been made, the due date for the return is extended 10 days.

Annual Returns

The employer is required to furnish two copies of Form W-2, the Wage and Tax Statement, to each employee from whom income tax or Social Security tax has been withheld or from whom income tax would have been withheld if the employee had claimed no more than one withholding allowance. The forms should be given to employees by January 31. If employment ends before December 31, the employer may give the W-2 form to the terminated employee any time after employment ends. If the employee asks for Form W-2, the employer should give the employee the completed copies within 30 days of the request or the final wage payment, whichever is later.

Employers must file Form W-3, the Transmittal of Income and Tax Statement, annually to transmit wage and income tax withheld statements (Form W-2) to the Social Security Administration. These forms are processed by the Social Security Administration, which then furnishes the IRS with the income tax data that it needs from those forms. Form W-3 and its attachments must be filed separately from Form 941 on or before the last day of February after the calendar year for which the W-2 forms are prepared.

Federal Unemployment Tax

Employers also contribute under the Federal Unemployment Tax Act (FUTA). Generally, credit can be taken against the FUTA tax for amounts paid into a state unemployment fund up to a certain percentage. Employers are re-

Form W-4 (2002)

Purpose. Complete Form W-4 so your employer can withhold the correct Federal income tax from your pay. Because your tax situation may change, you may want to refigure your withholding each year.

Exemption from withholding. If you are exempt, complete only lines 1, 2, 3, 4, and 7 and sign the form to validate it. Your exemption for 2002 expires February 16, 2003. See **Pub. 505,** Tax Withholding and Estimated Tax.

Note: *You cannot claim exemption from withholding if* **(a)** *your income exceeds $750 and includes more than $250 of unearned income (e.g., interest and dividends) and* **(b)** *another person can claim you as a dependent on their tax return.*

Basic instructions. If you are not exempt, complete the **Personal Allowances Worksheet** below. The worksheets on page 2 adjust your withholding allowances based on itemized deductions, certain credits, adjustments to income, or two-earner/two-job situations. Complete all worksheets that apply. **However, you may claim fewer (or zero) allowances.**

Head of household. Generally, you may claim head of household filing status on your tax return only if you are unmarried and pay more than 50% of the costs of keeping up a home for yourself and your dependent(s) or other qualifying individuals. See line **E** below.

Tax credits. You can take projected tax credits into account in figuring your allowable number of withholding allowances. Credits for child or dependent care expenses and the child tax credit may be claimed using the **Personal Allowances Worksheet** below. See **Pub. 919,** How Do I Adjust My Tax Withholding? for information on converting your other credits into withholding allowances.

Nonwage income. If you have a large amount of nonwage income, such as interest or dividends, consider making estimated tax payments using **Form 1040-ES,** Estimated Tax for Individuals. Otherwise, you may owe additional tax.

Two earners/two jobs. If you have a working spouse or more than one job, figure the total number of allowances you are entitled to claim on all jobs using worksheets from only one Form W-4. Your withholding usually will be most accurate when all allowances are claimed on the Form W-4 for the highest paying job and zero allowances are claimed on the others.

Nonresident alien. If you are a nonresident alien, see **Instructions for Form 8233** before completing this Form W-4.

Check your withholding. After your Form W-4 takes effect, use Pub. 919 to see how the dollar amount you are having withheld compares to your projected total tax for 2002. See Pub. 919, especially if you used the **Two-Earner/Two-Job Worksheet** on page 2 and your earnings exceed $125,000 (Single) or $175,000 (Married).

Recent name change? If your name on line 1 differs from that shown on your social security card, call 1-800-772-1213 for a new social security card.

Personal Allowances Worksheet (Keep for your records.)

A Enter "1" for **yourself** if no one else can claim you as a dependent . . . . **A** _____

B Enter "1" if:
- You are single and have only one job; or
- You are married, have only one job, and your spouse does not work; or
- Your wages from a second job or your spouse's wages (or the total of both) are $1,000 or less.

B _____

C Enter "1" for your **spouse.** But, you may choose to enter "-0-" if you are married and have either a working spouse or more than one job. (Entering "-0-" may help you avoid having too little tax withheld.) . . . . **C** _____

D Enter number of **dependents** (other than your spouse or yourself) you will claim on your tax return . . . . **D** _____

E Enter "1" if you will file as **head of household** on your tax return (see conditions under **Head of household** above) . **E** _____

F Enter "1" if you have at least $1,500 of **child or dependent care expenses** for which you plan to claim a credit . . **F** _____

(**Note:** Do **not** include child support payments. See Pub. 503, *Child and Dependent Care Expenses,* for details.)

G **Child Tax Credit** (including additional child tax credit):
- If your total income will be between $15,000 and $42,000 ($20,000 and $65,000 if married), enter "1" for each eligible child plus **1 additional** if you have three to five eligible children or **2 additional** if you have six or more eligible children.
- If your total income will be between $42,000 and $80,000 ($65,000 and $115,000 if married), enter "1" if you have one or two eligible children, "2" if you have three eligible children, "3" if you have four eligible children, or "4" if you have five or more eligible children.

G _____

H Add lines A through G and enter total here. **Note:** *This may be different from the number of exemptions you claim on your tax return.* ▶ **H** _____

For accuracy, complete all worksheets that apply.
- If you plan to **itemize or claim adjustments to income** and want to reduce your withholding, see the **Deductions and Adjustments Worksheet** on page 2.
- If you have **more than one job** or are **married and you and your spouse both work** and the combined earnings from all jobs exceed $35,000, see the **Two-Earner/Two-Job Worksheet** on page 2 to avoid having too little tax withheld.
- If **neither** of the above situations applies, **stop here** and enter the number from line H on line 5 of Form W-4 below.

--------------------- **Cut here and give Form W-4 to your employer. Keep the top part for your records.** ---------------------

| Form **W-4** Department of the Treasury Internal Revenue Service | Employee's Withholding Allowance Certificate ▶ **For Privacy Act and Paperwork Reduction Act Notice, see page 2.** | OMB No. 1545-0010 2002 |

1 Type or print your first name and middle initial   Last name | **2** Your social security number

Home address (number and street or rural route) | **3** ☐ Single ☐ Married ☐ Married, but withhold at higher Single rate.
Note: *If married, but legally separated, or spouse is a nonresident alien, check the "Single" box.*

City or town, state, and ZIP code | **4** If your last name differs from that on your social security card, check here. You must call 1-800-772-1213 for a new card. ▶ ☐

5 Total number of allowances you are claiming (from line **H** above **or** from the applicable worksheet on page 2) | **5** _____

6 Additional amount, if any, you want withheld from each paycheck . . . . | **6** $ _____

7 I claim exemption from withholding for 2002, and I certify that I meet **both** of the following conditions for exemption:
- Last year I had a right to a refund of **all** Federal income tax withheld because I had **no** tax liability **and**
- This year I expect a refund of **all** Federal income tax withheld because I expect to have **no** tax liability.

If you meet both conditions, write "Exempt" here . . . . ▶ | **7** _____

Under penalties of perjury, I certify that I am entitled to the number of withholding allowances claimed on this certificate, or I am entitled to claim exempt status.

Employee's signature
(Form is not valid unless you sign it.) ▶ _____   **Date** ▶ _____

8 Employer's name and address (Employer: Complete lines 8 and 10 only if sending to the IRS.) | **9** Office code (optional) | **10** Employer identification number

Cat. No. 10220Q

FIGURE 23-3   IRS Form W-4: Employee's Withholding Allowance Certificate.

Form W-4 (2002)　　　　　　　　　　　　　　　　　　　　　　　　　　　　　　　　　　　　　Page **2**

Deductions and Adjustments Worksheet

Note:　*Use this worksheet only if you plan to itemize deductions, claim certain credits, or claim adjustments to income on your 2002 tax return.*

1　Enter an estimate of your 2002 itemized deductions. These include qualifying home mortgage interest, charitable contributions, state and local taxes, medical expenses in excess of 7.5% of your income, and miscellaneous deductions. (For 2002, you may have to reduce your itemized deductions if your income is over **$137,300** ($68,650 if married filing separately). See **Worksheet 3** in Pub. 919 for details.) . . .　**1**　$ _____

2　Enter:　{ $7,850 if married filing jointly or qualifying widow(er)　　　　　　　　}　. . .　**2**　$ _____
　　　　　 $6,900 if head of household
　　　　　 $4,700 if single
　　　　　 $3,925 if married filing separately

3　**Subtract** line 2 from line 1. If line 2 is greater than line 1, enter "-0-". . . . .　**3**　$ _____
4　Enter an estimate of your 2002 adjustments to income, including alimony, deductible IRA contributions, and student loan interest　**4**　$ _____
5　**Add** lines 3 and 4 and enter the total. Include any amount for credits from **Worksheet 7** in Pub. 919. .　**5**　$ _____
6　Enter an estimate of your 2002 nonwage income (such as dividends or interest) . . . .　**6**　$ _____
7　**Subtract** line 6 from line 5. Enter the result, but not less than "-0-" . . . .　**7**　$ _____
8　**Divide** the amount on line 7 by $3,000 and enter the result here. Drop any fraction . . . . .　**8**　_____
9　Enter the number from the **Personal Allowances Worksheet,** line H, page 1 . . . .　**9**　_____
10　**Add** lines 8 and 9 and enter the total here. If you plan to use the **Two-Earner/Two-Job Worksheet,** also enter this total on line 1 below. Otherwise, **stop here** and enter this total on Form W-4, line 5, page 1 .　**10**　_____

Two-Earner/Two-Job Worksheet

Note:　*Use this worksheet only if the instructions under line H on page 1 direct you here.*

1　Enter the number from line H, page 1 (or from line 10 above if you used the **Deductions and Adjustments Worksheet**)　**1**　_____
2　Find the number in **Table 1** below that applies to the **lowest** paying job and enter it here . . . . .　**2**　_____
3　If line 1 is **more than or equal to** line 2, subtract line 2 from line 1. Enter the result here (if zero, enter "-0-") and on Form W-4, line 5, page 1. **Do not** use the rest of this worksheet . . . .　**3**　_____

Note:　*If line 1 is **less than** line 2, enter "-0-" on Form W-4, line 5, page 1. Complete lines 4–9 below to calculate the additional withholding amount necessary to avoid a year end tax bill.*

4　Enter the number from line 2 of this worksheet . . . .　**4**　_____
5　Enter the number from line 1 of this worksheet . . . .　**5**　_____
6　**Subtract** line 5 from line 4 . . . .　**6**　_____
7　Find the amount in **Table 2** below that applies to the **highest** paying job and enter it here . . . . .　**7**　$ _____
8　**Multiply** line 7 by line 6 and enter the result here. This is the additional annual withholding needed . .　**8**　$ _____
9　Divide line 8 by the number of pay periods remaining in 2002. For example, divide by 26 if you are paid every two weeks and you complete this form in December 2001. Enter the result here and on Form W-4, line 6, page 1. This is the additional amount to be withheld from each paycheck . . . .　**9**　$ _____

Table 1: Two-Earner/Two-Job Worksheet

Married Filing Jointly				All Others			
If wages from **LOWEST** paying job are—	Enter on line 2 above	If wages from **LOWEST** paying job are—	Enter on line 2 above	If wages from **LOWEST** paying job are—	Enter on line 2 above	If wages from **LOWEST** paying job are—	Enter on line 2 above
$0 - $4,000	0	44,001 - 50,000	8	$0 - $6,000	0	75,001 - 95,000	8
4,001 - 9,000	1	50,001 - 55,000	9	6,001 - 11,000	1	95,001 - 110,000	9
9,001 - 15,000	2	55,001 - 65,000	10	11,001 - 17,000	2	110,001 and over	10
15,001 - 20,000	3	65,001 - 80,000	11	17,001 - 23,000	3		
20,001 - 25,000	4	80,001 - 95,000	12	23,001 - 28,000	4		
25,001 - 32,000	5	95,001 - 110,000	13	28,001 - 38,000	5		
32,001 - 38,000	6	110,001 - 125,000	14	38,001 - 55,000	6		
38,001 - 44,000	7	125,001 and over	15	55,001 - 75,000	7		

Table 2: Two-Earner/Two-Job Worksheet

Married Filing Jointly		All Others	
If wages from **HIGHEST** paying job are—	Enter on line 7 above	If wages from **HIGHEST** paying job are—	Enter on line 7 above
$0 - $50,000	$450	$0 - $30,000	$450
50,001 - 100,000	800	30,001 - 70,000	800
100,001 - 150,000	900	70,001 - 140,000	900
150,001 - 270,000	1,050	140,001 - 300,000	1,050
270,001 and over	1,150	300,001 and over	1,150

FIGURE 23-3—Cont'd　For legend see previous page.

SINGLE Persons—WEEKLY Payroll Period
(For Wages Paid in 2002)

If the wages are—		And the number of withholding allowances claimed is—										
At least	But less than	0	1	2	3	4	5	6	7	8	9	10
		The amount of income tax to be withheld is—										
$0	$55	$0	$0	$0	$0	$0	$0	$0	$0	$0	$0	$0
55	60	1	0	0	0	0	0	0	0	0	0	0
60	65	1	0	0	0	0	0	0	0	0	0	0
65	70	2	0	0	0	0	0	0	0	0	0	0
70	75	2	0	0	0	0	0	0	0	0	0	0
75	80	3	0	0	0	0	0	0	0	0	0	0
80	85	3	0	0	0	0	0	0	0	0	0	0
85	90	4	0	0	0	0	0	0	0	0	0	0
90	95	4	0	0	0	0	0	0	0	0	0	0
95	100	5	0	0	0	0	0	0	0	0	0	0
100	105	5	0	0	0	0	0	0	0	0	0	0
105	110	6	0	0	0	0	0	0	0	0	0	0
110	115	6	0	0	0	0	0	0	0	0	0	0
115	120	7	1	0	0	0	0	0	0	0	0	0
120	125	7	1	0	0	0	0	0	0	0	0	0
125	130	8	2	0	0	0	0	0	0	0	0	0
130	135	8	2	0	0	0	0	0	0	0	0	0
135	140	9	3	0	0	0	0	0	0	0	0	0
140	145	9	3	0	0	0	0	0	0	0	0	0
145	150	10	4	0	0	0	0	0	0	0	0	0
150	155	10	4	0	0	0	0	0	0	0	0	0
155	160	11	5	0	0	0	0	0	0	0	0	0
160	165	11	5	0	0	0	0	0	0	0	0	0
165	170	12	6	0	0	0	0	0	0	0	0	0
170	175	13	6	1	0	0	0	0	0	0	0	0
175	180	13	7	1	0	0	0	0	0	0	0	0
180	185	14	7	2	0	0	0	0	0	0	0	0
185	190	15	8	2	0	0	0	0	0	0	0	0
190	195	16	8	3	0	0	0	0	0	0	0	0
195	200	16	9	3	0	0	0	0	0	0	0	0
200	210	17	10	4	0	0	0	0	0	0	0	0
210	220	19	11	5	0	0	0	0	0	0	0	0
220	230	20	12	6	0	0	0	0	0	0	0	0
230	240	22	13	7	1	0	0	0	0	0	0	0
240	250	23	15	8	2	0	0	0	0	0	0	0
250	260	25	16	9	3	0	0	0	0	0	0	0
260	270	26	18	10	4	0	0	0	0	0	0	0
270	280	28	19	11	5	0	0	0	0	0	0	0
280	290	29	21	12	6	0	0	0	0	0	0	0
290	300	31	22	14	7	1	0	0	0	0	0	0
300	310	32	24	15	8	2	0	0	0	0	0	0
310	320	34	25	17	9	3	0	0	0	0	0	0
320	330	35	27	18	10	4	0	0	0	0	0	0
330	340	37	28	20	11	5	0	0	0	0	0	0
340	350	38	30	21	12	6	1	0	0	0	0	0
350	360	40	31	23	14	7	2	0	0	0	0	0
360	370	41	33	24	15	8	3	0	0	0	0	0
370	380	43	34	26	17	9	4	0	0	0	0	0
380	390	44	36	27	18	10	5	0	0	0	0	0
390	400	46	37	29	20	11	6	0	0	0	0	0
400	410	47	39	30	21	13	7	1	0	0	0	0
410	420	49	40	32	23	14	8	2	0	0	0	0
420	430	50	42	33	24	16	9	3	0	0	0	0
430	440	52	43	35	26	17	10	4	0	0	0	0
440	450	53	45	36	27	19	11	5	0	0	0	0
450	460	55	46	38	29	20	12	6	0	0	0	0
460	470	56	48	39	30	22	13	7	1	0	0	0
470	480	58	49	41	32	23	15	8	2	0	0	0
480	490	59	51	42	33	25	16	9	3	0	0	0
490	500	61	52	44	35	26	18	10	4	0	0	0
500	510	62	54	45	36	28	19	11	5	0	0	0
510	520	64	55	47	38	29	21	12	6	0	0	0
520	530	65	57	48	39	31	22	14	7	1	0	0
530	540	67	58	50	41	32	24	15	8	2	0	0
540	550	68	60	51	42	34	25	17	9	3	0	0
550	560	70	61	53	44	35	27	18	10	4	0	0
560	570	71	63	54	45	37	28	20	11	5	0	0
570	580	74	64	56	47	38	30	21	12	6	0	0
580	590	76	66	57	48	40	31	23	14	7	1	0
590	600	79	67	59	50	41	33	24	15	8	2	0

FIGURE 23-4   Pages from the 2002 Withholding Tax Table.

sponsible for paying the FUTA tax; it must not be deducted from employees' wages. For 1998 the FUTA tax was 6.2% of the first $7,000 in wages paid to each employee during the calendar year.

For deposit purposes, the FUTA tax is figured quarterly, and any amount due must be paid by the last day of the first month after the quarter ends. The formula for determining the amount due is set forth in the Federal Employer's Tax Guide.

An annual FUTA return must be filed on Form 940 on or before January 31 following the close of the calendar year for which the tax is due (Figure 23-6). Any tax still

MARRIED Persons—MONTHLY Payroll Period
(For Wages Paid in 2002)

If the wages are— At least	But less than	And the number of withholding allowances claimed is— 0	1	2	3	4	5	6	7	8	9	10
		The amount of income tax to be withheld is—										
$0	$540	$0	$0	$0	$0	$0	$0	$0	$0	$0	$0	$0
540	560	1	0	0	0	0	0	0	0	0	0	0
560	580	3	0	0	0	0	0	0	0	0	0	0
580	600	5	0	0	0	0	0	0	0	0	0	0
600	640	8	0	0	0	0	0	0	0	0	0	0
640	680	12	0	0	0	0	0	0	0	0	0	0
680	720	16	0	0	0	0	0	0	0	0	0	0
720	760	20	0	0	0	0	0	0	0	0	0	0
760	800	24	0	0	0	0	0	0	0	0	0	0
800	840	28	3	0	0	0	0	0	0	0	0	0
840	880	32	7	0	0	0	0	0	0	0	0	0
880	920	36	11	0	0	0	0	0	0	0	0	0
920	960	40	15	0	0	0	0	0	0	0	0	0
960	1,000	44	19	0	0	0	0	0	0	0	0	0
1,000	1,040	48	23	0	0	0	0	0	0	0	0	0
1,040	1,080	52	27	2	0	0	0	0	0	0	0	0
1,080	1,120	56	31	6	0	0	0	0	0	0	0	0
1,120	1,160	60	35	10	0	0	0	0	0	0	0	0
1,160	1,200	64	39	14	0	0	0	0	0	0	0	0
1,200	1,240	68	43	18	0	0	0	0	0	0	0	0
1,240	1,280	72	47	22	0	0	0	0	0	0	0	0
1,280	1,320	76	51	26	1	0	0	0	0	0	0	0
1,320	1,360	80	55	30	5	0	0	0	0	0	0	0
1,360	1,400	84	59	34	9	0	0	0	0	0	0	0
1,400	1,440	88	63	38	13	0	0	0	0	0	0	0
1,440	1,480	92	67	42	17	0	0	0	0	0	0	0
1,480	1,520	96	71	46	21	0	0	0	0	0	0	0
1,520	1,560	100	75	50	25	0	0	0	0	0	0	0
1,560	1,600	106	79	54	29	4	0	0	0	0	0	0
1,600	1,640	112	83	58	33	8	0	0	0	0	0	0
1,640	1,680	118	87	62	37	12	0	0	0	0	0	0
1,680	1,720	124	91	66	41	16	0	0	0	0	0	0
1,720	1,760	130	95	70	45	20	0	0	0	0	0	0
1,760	1,800	136	99	74	49	24	0	0	0	0	0	0
1,800	1,840	142	105	78	53	28	3	0	0	0	0	0
1,840	1,880	148	111	82	57	32	7	0	0	0	0	0
1,880	1,920	154	117	86	61	36	11	0	0	0	0	0
1,920	1,960	160	123	90	65	40	15	0	0	0	0	0
1,960	2,000	166	129	94	69	44	19	0	0	0	0	0
2,000	2,040	172	135	98	73	48	23	0	0	0	0	0
2,040	2,080	178	141	103	77	52	27	2	0	0	0	0
2,080	2,120	184	147	109	81	56	31	6	0	0	0	0
2,120	2,160	190	153	115	85	60	35	10	0	0	0	0
2,160	2,200	196	159	121	89	64	39	14	0	0	0	0
2,200	2,240	202	165	127	93	68	43	18	0	0	0	0
2,240	2,280	208	171	133	97	72	47	22	0	0	0	0
2,280	2,320	214	177	139	102	76	51	26	1	0	0	0
2,320	2,360	220	183	145	108	80	55	30	5	0	0	0
2,360	2,400	226	189	151	114	84	59	34	9	0	0	0
2,400	2,440	232	195	157	120	88	63	38	13	0	0	0
2,440	2,480	238	201	163	126	92	67	42	17	0	0	0
2,480	2,520	244	207	169	132	96	71	46	21	0	0	0
2,520	2,560	250	213	175	138	100	75	50	25	0	0	0
2,560	2,600	256	219	181	144	106	79	54	29	4	0	0
2,600	2,640	262	225	187	150	112	83	58	33	8	0	0
2,640	2,680	268	231	193	156	118	87	62	37	12	0	0
2,680	2,720	274	237	199	162	124	91	66	41	16	0	0
2,720	2,760	280	243	205	168	130	95	70	45	20	0	0
2,760	2,800	286	249	211	174	136	99	74	49	24	0	0
2,800	2,840	292	255	217	180	142	105	78	53	28	3	0
2,840	2,880	298	261	223	186	148	111	82	57	32	7	0
2,880	2,920	304	267	229	192	154	117	86	61	36	11	0
2,920	2,960	310	273	235	198	160	123	90	65	40	15	0
2,960	3,000	316	279	241	204	166	129	94	69	44	19	0
3,000	3,040	322	285	247	210	172	135	98	73	48	23	0
3,040	3,080	328	291	253	216	178	141	103	77	52	27	2
3,080	3,120	334	297	259	222	184	147	109	81	56	31	6
3,120	3,160	340	303	265	228	190	153	115	85	60	35	10
3,160	3,200	346	309	271	234	196	159	121	89	64	39	14
3,200	3,240	352	315	277	240	202	165	127	93	68	43	18

FIGURE 23-4—Cont'd   For legend see previous page.

due is payable with the return. Form 940 may be filed on or before February 10 following the close of the year, if all required deposits were made on time and if full payment of the tax due is deposited on or before January 31.

State Unemployment Taxes

All of the states and the District of Columbia have unemployment compensation laws. In most states, the tax is imposed only on the employer, but a few states require employers to withhold a percentage of wages for unem-

Form **941**
(Rev. January 2002)
Department of the Treasury
Internal Revenue Service (99)

Employer's Quarterly Federal Tax Return

▶ See separate instructions revised January 2002 for information on completing this return.

Please type or print.

OMB No. 1545-0029

Enter state code for state in which deposits were made **only** if different from state in address to the right ▶ (see page 2 of instructions).

Name (as distinguished from trade name)   Date quarter ended

Trade name, if any   Employer identification number

Address (number and street)   City, state, and ZIP code

| T |
| FF |
| FD |
| FP |
| I |
| T |

If address is different from prior return, check here ▶

IRS Use

| 1 1 | 1 1 | 1 1 | 1 1 | 1 1 | 1 | 2 | 3 3 | 3 3 | 3 3 | 3 3 | 4 4 | 4 | 5 5 | 5 |
| 6 | 7 | 8 8 | 8 8 | 8 8 | 8 8 | 9 9 | 9 9 | 10 | 10 | 10 | 10 | 10 | 10 | 10 | 10 |

If you do not have to file returns in the future, check here ▶ ☐   and enter date final wages paid ▶

If you are a seasonal employer, see **Seasonal employers** on page 1 of the instructions and check here ▶

1	Number of employees in the pay period that includes March 12th . ▶	1	
2	Total wages and tips, plus other compensation	**2**	
3	Total income tax withheld from wages, tips, and sick pay	**3**	
4	Adjustment of withheld income tax for preceding quarters of calendar year	**4**	
5	Adjusted total of income tax withheld (line 3 as adjusted by line 4—see instructions) .	**5**	
6	Taxable social security wages	**6a**	× 12.4% (.124) =	**6b**	
	Taxable social security tips	**6c**	× 12.4% (.124) =	**6d**	
7	Taxable Medicare wages and tips . . .	**7a**	× 2.9% (.029) =	**7b**	
8	Total social security and Medicare taxes (add lines 6b, 6d, and 7b). Check here if wages are not subject to social security and/or Medicare tax . . . . ▶ ☐	**8**	
9	Adjustment of social security and Medicare taxes (see instructions for required explanation) Sick Pay $_____ ± Fractions of Cents $_____ ± Other $_____ =	**9**	
10	Adjusted total of social security and Medicare taxes (line 8 as adjusted by line 9—see instructions)	**10**	
11	**Total taxes** (add lines 5 and 10)	**11**	
12	Advance earned income credit (EIC) payments made to employees	**12**	
13	Net taxes (subtract line 12 from line 11). **If $2,500 or more, this must equal line 17, column (d) below (or line D of Schedule B (Form 941))**	**13**	
14	Total deposits for quarter, including overpayment applied from a prior quarter	**14**	
15	**Balance due** (subtract line 14 from line 13). See instructions	**15**	

16 **Overpayment.** If line 14 is more than line 13, enter excess here ▶ $_____
and check if to be: ☐ Applied to next return **or** ☐ Refunded

● **All filers:** If line 13 is less than $2,500, you need not complete line 17 or Schedule B (Form 941).

● **Semiweekly schedule depositors:** Complete Schedule B (Form 941) and check here . . . . ▶ ☐

● **Monthly schedule depositors:** Complete line 17, columns (a) through (d), and check here . . . . ▶ ☐

17	**Monthly Summary of Federal Tax Liability.** Do not complete if you were a semiweekly schedule depositor.
(a) First month liability	**(b)** Second month liability	**(c)** Third month liability	**(d)** Total liability for quarter

Third Party Designee

Do you want to allow another person to discuss this return with the IRS (see separate instructions)?   ☐ **Yes.** Complete the following.   ☐ **No**

Designee's name ▶   Phone no. ▶ (   )   Personal identification number (PIN) ▶

Sign Here

Under penalties of perjury, I declare that I have examined this return, including accompanying schedules and statements, and to the best of my knowledge and belief, it is true, correct, and complete.

Signature ▶   Print Your Name and Title ▶   Date ▶

For Privacy Act and Paperwork Reduction Act Notice, see back of Payment Voucher.   Cat. No. 17001Z   Form **941** (Rev. 1-2002)

FIGURE 23-5   IRS Form 941: Employer's Quarterly Federal Tax Return.

Form 941
Payment Voucher

Purpose of Form

Complete Form 941-V if you are making a payment with **Form 941,** Employer's Quarterly Federal Tax Return. We will use the completed voucher to credit your payment more promptly and accurately, and to improve our service to you.

If you have your return prepared by a third party and make a payment with that return, please provide this payment voucher to the return preparer.

Making Payments With Form 941

Make payments with Form 941 only if:

1. Your net taxes for the quarter (line 13 on Form 941) are less than $2,500 and you are paying in full with a timely filed return or

2. You are a monthly schedule depositor making a payment in accordance with the **accuracy of deposits** rule. (See section 11 of **Circular E,** Employer's Tax Guide, for details.) This amount may be $2,500 or more.

Otherwise, you must deposit the amount at an authorized financial institution or by electronic funds transfer. (See section 11 of Circular E for deposit instructions.) Do not use the Form 941-V payment voucher to make Federal tax deposits.

Caution: *If you pay amounts with Form 941 that should have been deposited, you may be subject to a penalty. See Circular E.*

Specific Instructions

Box 1—Employer identification number (EIN). If you do not have an EIN, apply for one on **Form SS-4,** Application for Employer Identification Number, and write "Applied for" and the date you applied in this entry space.

Box 2—Amount paid. Enter the amount paid with Form 941.

Box 3—Tax period. Darken the capsule identifying the quarter for which the payment is made. Darken only one capsule.

Box 4—Name and address. Enter your name and address as shown on Form 941.

● Make your check or money order payable to the United States Treasury. Be sure to enter your EIN, "Form 941," and the tax period on your check or money order. Do not send cash. Please do not staple this voucher or your payment to the return or to each other.

● Detach the completed voucher and send it with your payment and Form 941 to the address provided on the back of Form 941.

▼ **Detach Here and Mail With Your Payment** ▼   Form **941-V** (2002)

Form 941-V

Department of the Treasury
Internal Revenue Service   (99)

Payment Voucher

▶ **Do not staple or attach this voucher to your payment.**

OMB No. 1545-0029

2002

1 Enter your employer identification number	2 **Enter the amount of the payment**	Dollars	Cents

3 Tax period	4 Enter your business name (individual name if sole proprietor)
◯ 1st Quarter ◯ 3rd Quarter	Enter your address
◯ 2nd Quarter ◯ 4th Quarter	Enter your city, state, and ZIP code

FIGURE 23-5—Cont'd   For legend see previous page.

ployment compensation benefits. An employer may be subject to federal unemployment tax and not subject to state unemployment tax. In some states, for instance, the employer with fewer than four employees is not subject to the state unemployment tax. The regulations for a specific state should be checked.

State Disability Insurance

Some states require that employees be covered by disability or sick-pay insurance. The employer may be required to withhold a certain amount from the employee's salary to pay for this insurance.

Form **940**

Department of the Treasury
Internal Revenue Service (99)

Employer's Annual Federal Unemployment (FUTA) Tax Return

▶ **See separate Instructions for Form 940 for information on completing this form.**

OMB No. 1545-0028

2001

T	
FF	
FD	
FP	
I	
T	

You must complete this section. ▶

Name (as distinguished from trade name)   Calendar year

Trade name, if any

Address and ZIP code   Employer identification number

A Are you required to pay unemployment contributions to only one state? (If "No," skip questions B and C) . ☐ Yes ☐ No

B Did you pay all state unemployment contributions by January 31, 2002? ((1) If you deposited your total FUTA tax when due, check "Yes" if you paid all state unemployment contributions by February 11, 2002. (2) If a 0% experience rate is granted, check "Yes." (3) If "No," skip question C.) . . . . ☐ Yes ☐ No

C Were all wages that were taxable for FUTA tax also taxable for your state's unemployment tax? . . . . . ☐ Yes ☐ No

If you answered "No" to any of these questions, you must file Form 940. If you answered "Yes" to all the questions, you may file Form 940-EZ, which is a simplified version of Form 940. (Successor employers see **Special credit for successor employers** on page 3 of the instructions.) You can get Form 940-EZ by calling 1-800-TAX-FORM (1-800-829-3676) or from the IRS Web Site at **www.irs.gov.**

If you will not have to file returns in the future, check here (see **Who Must File** in separate instructions), **and complete and sign the return** . . . . ▶ ☐

If this is an Amended Return, check here . . . . ▶ ☐

Part I Computation of Taxable Wages

1 Total payments (including payments shown on lines 2 and 3) during the calendar year for services of employees **1**

2 Exempt payments. (Explain all exempt payments, attaching additional sheets if necessary.) ▶ --- **2**

3 Payments of more than $7,000 for services. Enter only amounts over the first $7,000 paid to each employee. (See separate instructions.) Do not include any exempt payments from line 2. The $7,000 amount is the Federal wage base. Your state wage base may be different. **Do not use your state wage limitation**. **3**

4 Add lines 2 and 3 . . . . **4**

5 **Total taxable wages** (subtract line 4 from line 1) . . . . ▶ **5**

Be sure to complete both sides of this form, and sign in the space provided on the back.

For Privacy Act and Paperwork Reduction Act Notice, see separate instructions.   ▼ **DETACH HERE** ▼   Cat. No. 11234O   Form **940** (2001)

Form **940-V**

Department of the Treasury
Internal Revenue Service

Form 940 Payment Voucher

Use this voucher only when making a payment with your return.

OMB No. 1545-0028

2001

Complete boxes 1, 2, and 3. Do not send cash, and do not staple your payment to this voucher. Make your check or money order payable to the **"United States Treasury."** Be sure to enter your employer identification number, "Form 940," and "2001" on your payment.

1 Enter your employer identification number.

2 Enter the amount of your payment. ▶   Dollars   Cents

3 Enter your business name (individual name for sole proprietors).

Enter your address.

Enter your city, state, and ZIP code.

FIGURE 23-6   Employer's Annual Federal Unemployment Tax (FUTA) Return.

Form 940 (2001)   Page **2**

Part II   Tax Due or Refund

1	Gross FUTA tax. Multiply the wages from Part I, line 5, by .062						**1**	
2	Maximum credit. Multiply the wages from Part I, line 5, by .054 . .	**2**						
3	Computation of tentative credit (**Note:** *All taxpayers must complete the applicable columns.*)							

(a) Name of state	(b) State reporting number(s) as shown on employer's state contribution returns	(c) Taxable payroll (as defined in state act)	(d) State experience rate period		(e) State experience rate	(f) Contributions if rate had been 5.4% (col. (c) x .054)	(g) Contributions payable at experience rate (col. (c) x col. (e))	(h) Additional credit (col. (f) minus col.(g)) If 0 or less, enter -0-.	(i) Contributions paid to state by 940 due date
			From	To					

3a	Totals . . . ▶		
3b	**Total tentative credit** (add line 3a, columns (h) and (i) only—for late payments, also see the instructions for Part II, line 6) . . . . ▶	**3b**	
4			
5			
6	**Credit:** Enter the smaller of the amount from Part II, line 2 or line 3b; or the amount from the worksheet in the Part II, line 6 instructions	**6**	
7	**Total FUTA tax** (subtract line 6 from line 1). If the result is over $100, also complete Part III . .	**7**	
8	Total FUTA tax deposited for the year, including any overpayment applied from a prior year . .	**8**	
9	**Balance due** (subtract line 8 from line 7). Pay to the **"United States Treasury."** If you owe more than $100, see **Depositing FUTA Tax** on page 3 of the separate instructions . . . . . ▶	**9**	
10	**Overpayment** (subtract line 7 from line 8). Check if it is to be: ☐ **Applied to next return** or ☐ **Refunded** . . . . ▶	**10**	

Part III   Record of Quarterly Federal Unemployment Tax Liability (Do not include state liability.) **Complete only if** line 7 is over $100. See page 6 of the separate instructions.

Quarter	First (Jan. 1–Mar. 31)	Second (Apr. 1–June 30)	Third (July 1–Sept. 30)	Fourth (Oct. 1–Dec. 31)	Total for year
Liability for quarter					

Third Party Designee	Do you want to allow another person to discuss this return with the IRS (see instructions page 4)? ☐ **Yes.** Complete the following. ☐ **No**		
	Designee's name ▶	Phone no. ▶ ( )	Personal identification number (PIN) ▶

Under penalties of perjury, I declare that I have examined this return, including accompanying schedules and statements, and, to the best of my knowledge and belief, it is true, correct, and complete, and that no part of any payment made to a state unemployment fund claimed as a credit was, or is to be, deducted from the payments to employees.

Signature ▶   Title (Owner, etc.) ▶   Date ▶

✱   Form **940** (2001)

FIGURE 23-6—Cont'd   For legend see previous page.

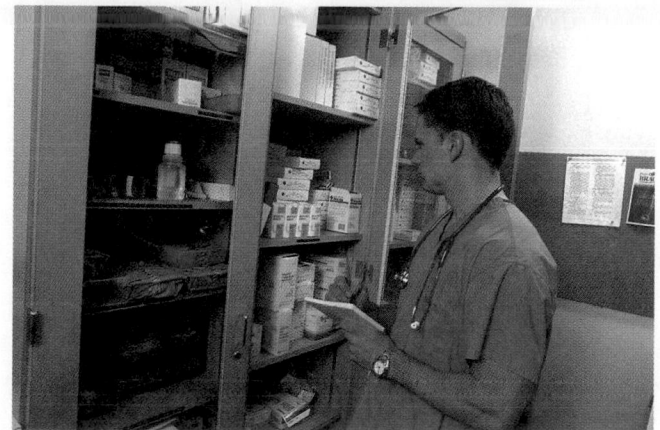

FIGURE 23-7   Inventory supplies and equipment before developing the annual budget. Once a good inventory has been completed, more accurate projections can be made for the expenses of the coming year.

Budgets

Growing businesses must develop budgets that help to plan finances over a certain period. Medical offices should compile a new budget before the beginning of each **fiscal year**. The best way to begin a budget is to look at the expenses from the previous year (Figure 23-7 and Procedures 23-3 and 23-4). These expenses should be divided into categories and then a total derived for each category. Each month should represent approximately $1/12$ of the total budget, not including large capital expenses.

Within the individual categories, examine expenses for those that could be eliminated or those that were underbudgeted. For example, if $3,345 was spent on office supplies and the budget was $3,000, either more money needs to be allotted for this category or cuts in spending are necessary. If $3,345 was spent and the budget was $4,000, the excess may be placed in another category for the next year.

PROCEDURE 23-3

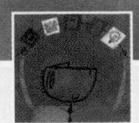

Establishing and Maintaining a Supply Inventory and Ordering System

GOAL: To establish an inventory of all expendable supplies in the physician's office and follow an efficient plan of order control using a card system.

EQUIPMENT AND SUPPLIES

- File box
- Inventory and order control cards
- List of supplies on hand
- Metal tabs
- Reorder tabs
- Pen or pencil

PROCEDURAL STEPS

1 Write the name of each item on a separate card (Figure 1*).

ORDER	(ITEM NAME)	3-ply Disposable Drape Sheets (white) 7459								ON ORDER
ORDER QUANTITY 300							REORDER POINT 100			
ORDER	QTY	REC'D	COST	PREPAID	ON ACCT	ORDER	QTY	REC'D	COST	PREPAID	ON ACCT
1/25	300	2/10	64.95	X							

INVENTORY COUNT

	JAN	FEB	MAR	APR	MAY	JUNE	JULY	AUG	SEPT	OCT	NOV	DEC
20 00	200											
20 00												

ORDER SOURCE

The Colwell Company

201 Kenyon Road

Champaign, IL 61820

UNIT PRICE

100 - $23.95

300 - $64.95

FORM 2450 COLWELL CO., CHAMPAIGN, ILLINOIS

Figure 1

Purpose: To establish a record of all items in inventory.

2 Write the amount of each item on hand in the space provided.
Purpose: To establish beginning inventory.

3 Place a reorder tag at the point where the supply should be replenished (Figure 2*).
Purpose: The tag will serve as an alert that supply is low.

4 Place a metal tab over the *order* section of the card.
Purpose: The metal tab will be a reminder to include this item in the next order.

5 When the order has been placed, note the date and quantity ordered and move the table to the *on order* section of the card.

6 When the order is received, note the date and quantity in the appropriate column, remove the tab, and refile the card.
Note: If the order is only partially filled, let the tab remain until the order is complete.

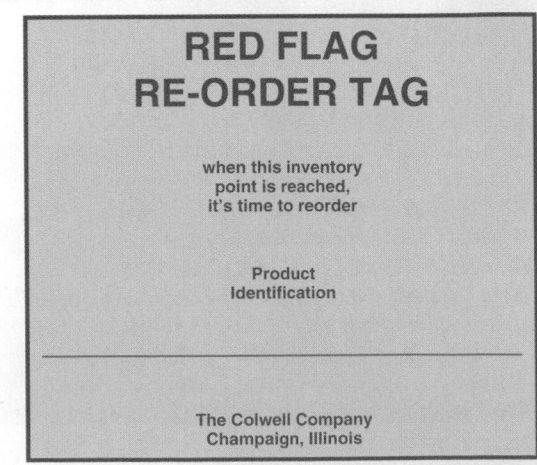

RED FLAG RE-ORDER TAG

when this inventory point is reached, it's time to reorder

Product Identification

The Colwell Company
Champaign, Illinois

Figure 2

*Courtesy of Colwell Systems, Champaign, Illinois.

PROCEDURE 23-4

Preparing a Purchase Order

GOAL: To prepare an accurate purchase order for supplies or equipment.

EQUIPMENT AND SUPPLIES

- List of current inventory
- Purchase order
- Pen
- Phone
- FAX machine

PROCEDURAL STEPS

1 Review the current inventory and determine what items need to be ordered.

Purpose: To determine what is needed so that the office will not be overstocked or understocked.

2 Complete the purchase order accurately, filling in all applicable spaces and blanks with the information requested.

Purpose: An accurately completed purchase order helps to eliminate mistakes in the order and in shipments.

3 List the items to be ordered, including quantity, item numbers, size, color, price, and extended price. Be sure that all applicable information is included.

Purpose: To help ensure accurate orders.

4 Provide the physician's signature, DEA certificate, and medical license when needed.

Purpose: Some items require these documents to verify that the physician is eligible to order them.

5 Call in, FAX, mail, or submit the order electronically to the vendor. Keep a copy for your records. Keep any verification provided that the order was received.

Purpose: To document exactly what was ordered on what date and provide proof that the order was received.

6 Note on the inventory which items are on order.

Purpose: To keep other staff members from preparing duplicate orders.

7 Keep a copy of the order in the appropriate place in the office filing system.

Purpose: To reference the order if needed and have a copy of the items ordered to compare with the packing list once the items arrive at the office.

CRITICAL THINKING APPLICATION

- Brenda has developed a preliminary budget. She realizes that several pieces of equipment need to be replaced in the coming year. However, Dr. Wilkins has expressed that she does not wish to make any capital purchases. How might Brenda approach Dr. Wilkins about the needed equipment?
- How might leasing equipment benefit the office? How can Brenda determine if this would be more or less expensive?

By monitoring expenses on a monthly basis, the physician can see if the facility is over budget, under budget, or right on target. Categories that have been overspent can be reconciled by taking funds from another category (for instance, category B) and adding them to the overspent category (category A). However, the amount taken must be subtracted from category B and added to category A. Those subtracted funds are no longer available in category B. Specific notes should be kept when categories are overspent, so that an adjustment may be made for the next fiscal year.

The following categories should be considered for the physician's operating budget:

- Insurance
- Rent
- Depreciation
- Loan payments
- Advertising/promotions
- Legal/accounting
- Miscellaneous expenses
- Supplies
- Salaries/wages
- Utilities
- Dues/subscriptions/fees
- Taxes
- Repairs/maintenance
- Medical equipment
- Administrative equipment
- Medication/pharmacy expenses

The physician should investigate whether leasing equipment might be a better option for the facility. Some leasing programs are very progressive and provide service contracts at no additional cost. Since depreciation costs are high, leasing might be the best answer to a new equipment need.

Insurance

Insurance coverage is one of the physician's major expenses. Almost every physician carries some type of malpractice insurance for protection against the cost of legal liabilities. Property and fire insurance are mandatory, and most physicians carry Workers' Compensation Insurance to cover employee injuries and accidents. The medical assistant may be asked to shop for the best insurance rates at the time of renewals.

Closing Comments

The physician will come to rely heavily on the person who manages the finances of the office. It is important that this individual keep information confidential. The entire staff must be conscious of the costs involved in operating a medical office and should adhere to their respective budgets as closely as possible. By being conservative, the physician may be willing to spend more money on pay increases and benefits to reward his or her employees.

Patient Education

There may be times when patients do not fully understand the costs involved in providing quality medical care. The medical assistant may need to educate the patient about the basic costs involved with the procedures that are performed in the office. Patients do not need a lengthy explanation, but may be set more at ease in knowing that the physician does not set his or her fees arbitrarily. The physician's office is a small business, like thousands of other small businesses, and should be able to pay its overhead and expenses.

Legal and Ethical Issues

The keeping of the financial records is a position of great trust and responsibility. Some physicians require the person placed in charge of the office finances to be bonded. This means that the facility has done a security check on an individual and the person was found worthy to be placed in a position of responsibility. A bond is issued by an entity on behalf of a second party, guaranteeing that the second party will fulfill an obligation or series of obligations to a third party. In the event that the obligations are not met, the third party will recover its losses via the bond.

Records must be accurate and completed on a daily basis. Daily journals should be kept indefinitely in support of tax returns.

SUMMARY OF SCENARIO

Brenda has learned much about the financial management of a physician's office. She is never hesitant to call the practice accountant, Mr. Schmidt, whenever a question arises. As she gains more experience, she understands the budgeting process, cost management, and the various methods of accounting practice.

There are many things that can affect the finances of a medical practice. However, the physician who is fairly conservative about spending and careful with investments should remain a stable part of the community's healthcare professionals. Dr. Wilkins lives by this philosophy and encourages her employees to manage money wisely, too. This attitude among all the staff members promotes a sense of teamwork and cooperation for the benefit of all.

SUMMARY OF LEARNING OBJECTIVES

- The financial records of any business should at all times show how much was earned in a given period, how much was collected, how much is owed, and the distribution of expenses incurred.

- Accounts payable refers to the amounts of money owed by a business and not yet paid, whereas accounts receivable refers to amounts owed to the business that are not yet paid.

- The three most common bookkeeping systems in use today are the single-entry system, double-entry system, and pegboard system. The single-entry method is the oldest accounting method, and utilizes a general journal, a cash payment journal, and an accounts receivable ledger. Payroll records and petty cash records may also be included. The double-entry system, which is more difficult to use than the single-entry system, requires an entry on each side of the accounting equation, and each side must always balance. The pegboard system requires a moderate initial investment to implement, but allows the user to perform several accounting functions at one time. It is often called the write-it-once system.

- A trial balance will reflect discrepancies between the journal and the ledger. It does not reveal errors in the individual accounts, but will show errors in the overall balances of accounts.

- The Internal Revenue Service requires that several employment records be kept for at least 4 years. These records include the Social Security number of the employee; the number of withholding allowances claimed; the amount of gross salary; all deductions for Social Security and Medicare taxes; federal, state, and city or other subdivision withholding taxes; state disability insurance; and state unemployment tax.

- Several deductions are taken from the employee's wages as required by law. These deductions are based on the total earnings of the employee, the number of withholding allowances claimed, the marital status of the employee, and the length of the pay period involved.

- There are five common reports used for accounting in the small business office: the statement of income and expense, the cash flow statement, the trial balance, the accounts receivable trial balance, and the balance sheet.

- The Employee's Withholding Allowance Certificate, or Form W-4, specifies the number of withholding allowances that the employee is claiming. The more allowances that are claimed, the less money that is taken from the employee's paycheck.

- The Federal Insurance Contributions Act requires that a certain amount of money be deducted from an employee's wages and designated for Medicare and Social Security programs. The current percentages are 1.45% for the Medicare contribution and 6.2% for Social Security. Both the employer and employee contribute these amounts.

- The physician's office must set a budget each fiscal year to prepare for all of the expenses that will be involved in running the office. Without a well-planned budget, the physician cannot control expenses. The expenditures from the past year should be evaluated when planning the new budget, paying particular attention to the expense categories that exceeded expected amounts.

KEY INTERNET WEBSITES

- Healthcare Financial Management Organization
  For active weblinks to each website visit
  http://evolve.elsevier.com/Kinn/

UNIT five

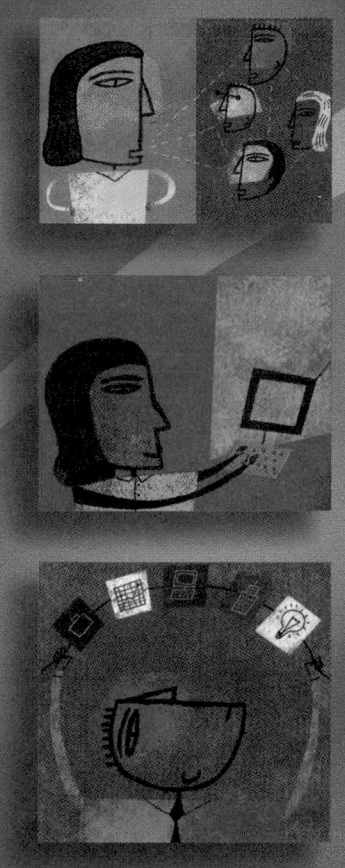

Fundamentals of Clinical Medical Assisting

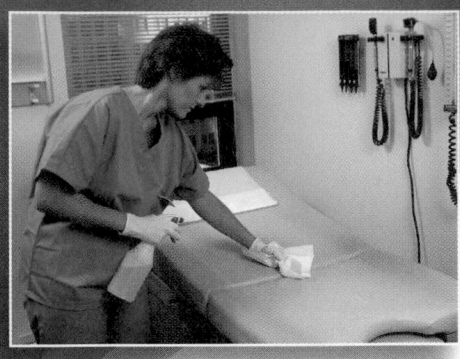

CHAPTER 24

Scenario

Rosa Lucia is a certified medical assistant working in a multi-physician pediatric practice. She is quite concerned about contracting an infectious disease while caring for her patients. Rosa learned about standard precautions while enrolled in her medical assistant program and now must implement that knowledge in the workplace.

Infection Control

Learning Objectives

- Define and spell the terms listed in the vocabulary.
- Recognize diseases caused by pathogenic microorganisms.
- Apply the chain of infection process to healthcare practice.
- Summarize the impact of the inflammatory response on the body's ability to defend itself against infection.
- Differentiate between humoral and cell-mediated immunity.
- Analyze the differences between acute, chronic, and latent disease processes.
- Compare virus and bacteria cell invasion.
- Specify potentially infectious bodily fluids.
- Integrate OSHA's requirement for a site-based Exposure Control Plan into office management procedures.
- Summarize the management of postexposure evaluation and follow-up.
- Explain the four major areas included in the OSHA Compliance Guidelines.
- Apply the concepts of medical and surgical asepsis to the healthcare setting.
- Differentiate among sanitization, disinfection, and sterilization procedures.
- Demonstrate the proper hand washing technique for medical asepsis.
- Demonstrate the correct procedure for sanitization of contaminated instruments.
- Apply patient education concepts to infection control.
- Discuss the legal and ethical concerns regarding medical asepsis and infection control.

National Curriculum Competencies

CLINICAL COMPETENCIES

1a. Perform hand washing
1d. Dispose of biohazardous materials
1e. Practice standard precautions

TRANSDISCIPLINARY COMPETENCIES

3d. Provide instruction for health maintenance and disease prevention

Vocabulary

anaphylaxis Exaggerated hypersensitivity reaction that, in severe cases, leads to vascular collapse, bronchospasm, and shock.

antibody Immunoglobulin produced by the immune system in response to bacteria, viruses, or other antigenic substances.

antigen Foreign substance that causes the production of a specific antibody.

antiseptic Pertaining to substances that inhibit the growth of microorganisms, such as alcohol and povidone-iodine solution (Betadine).

autoimmune Disturbance in the immune system in which the body reacts against its own tissue. Examples of autoimmune disorders include multiple sclerosis, rheumatoid arthritis, and systemic lupus erythematosus.

candidiasis Infection caused by a yeastlike fungus that typically affects the vaginal mucosa and skin.

coagulate Capable of being formed into clots.

contaminated Soiled with pathogens or infectious material; nonsterile.

disorder A disruption of normal system functions.

germicides Agents that destroy pathogenic organisms.

hereditary Pertaining to a characteristic, condition, or disease transmitted from parent to offspring on the DNA chain.

nosocomial infection Infection acquired during hospitalization or in a healthcare setting; often caused by *Escherichia coli*, hepatitis viruses, *Pseudomonas*, and *Staphylococcus* microorganisms.

palliative An agent that relieves or alleviates symptoms without curing the disease.

parenteral Injection or introduction of substances into the body through any route other than the digestive tract such as subcutaneous, intravenous, or intramuscular administration.

pathogenic Pertaining to disease-causing microorganisms.

pathophysiology Study of the biological and physical manifestations of disease as they are related to system abnormalities and physiological disturbances.

permeable To pass or soak through.

pyemia The presence of pus-forming organisms in the blood.

relapse The recurrence of the symptoms of a disease after apparent recovery.

remission The partial or complete disappearance of the clinical and subjective characteristics of a chronic or malignant disease.

rhinitis Inflammation of the mucous membranes of the nose.

spores Thick-walled reproductive cells formed within bacteria and capable of withstanding unfavorable environmental conditions.

tinea Any fungal skin disease that results in scaling, itching, and inflammation.

urticaria A skin eruption creating inflamed wheals; hives.

vector An animal, usually an insect or tick, that transmits the causative organisms of disease.

The concepts of disease transmission and the body's response to infection form the basis for understanding the importance of the first line of defense in preventing disease. Before we can assist in the prevention of disease, we have to look at methods we can use to minimize the chances of being a carrier of disease. One of the simplest ways of preventing the spread of disease is by washing your hands. As you continue through the remainder of this textbook, you will need to refer to the fundamental concepts of this chapter. Because of the need for infection control and the impact of OSHA guidelines on medical practice, every procedure begins and ends with hand washing. The concepts in this chapter are basic to all clinical practices and following them can lessen the transmission of disease, reduce the severity of disease, and might save the life of a patient or co-worker, or even your own life.

Disease

Disease is defined as any sustained, harmful alteration of the normal structure, function, or metabolism of an organism or cell. This pathological condition of the body presents a group of clinical signs, symptoms, and laboratory findings that set it apart as an abnormal entity, differing from other normal and pathological conditions. We recognize and categorize many different types of diseases: **hereditary** (genetic), drug-induced, **autoimmune**, degenerative, communicable, and infectious, to name only a few. Sometimes a specific disease may fit two or more categories.

Any disease caused by the growth of **pathogenic** microorganisms in the body falls into the category labeled infectious diseases. The entrance of a living microbe into the body is not disease, because until the infected cell or organism shows a harmful alteration of its structure, physiology, or biochemistry, disease is either not detected or not considered present. In fact, a living microbe may be ingested, injected, or inhaled and never cause disease in that person. An unaffected person, however, could still transmit the infection to another person. In this case, we call the unaffected person a *carrier*.

Microorganisms are almost everywhere. We carry them on our skin, in our bodies, and on our clothing. They are in ice, boiling water, the soil, and the air. The only places that are free of microorganisms are the insides of sterilized containers and in certain internal body organs and tissues. Organs and tissues that do not connect with the outside by means of mucus-lined membranes are, in the normal state, free from all living microorganisms.

The Chain of Infection

Infectious diseases can spread only if certain factors occur. These factors, or links, make up the chain of infection. Break the chain, and you break the infectious process (Figure 24-1).

The chain of infection starts with the *infectious agent*. There are five groups of potentially pathogenic microorganisms: viruses, bacteria, protozoa, fungi, and rick-

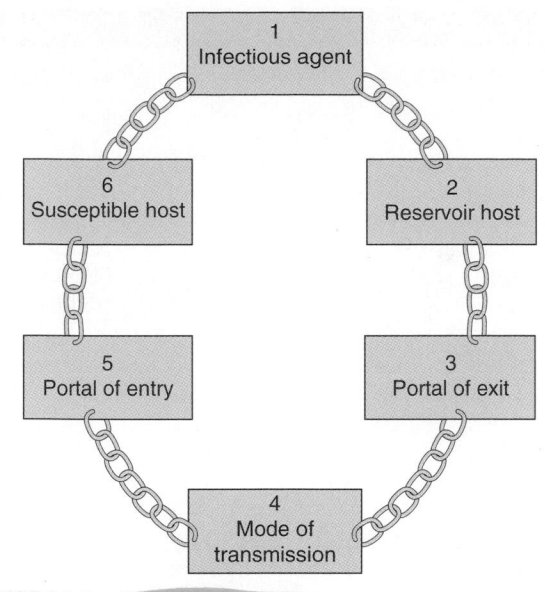

FIGURE 24-1   Chain of infection.

ettsia. Tables 24-1 through 24-4 identify and describe typical diseases caused by these pathogens, their mode of transmission, patient symptoms, and medical laboratory diagnostic procedures for each. Infection cannot occur without the presence of an infectious microorganism so the best way for healthcare workers to prevent the spread of disease is to use adequate infection control procedures such as consistent hand washing and the proper use of **antiseptics** as well as disinfection and sterilization methods.

The smallest of all pathogens, viruses, lead the list of important disease-causing agents. Viral microorganisms are intracellular parasites that take over the DNA of the invaded cell. Viral invasion may not cause significant immediate symptoms since host cells infected with viruses can produce a substance called *interferon*, which protects nearby cells. Antibiotics are unable to destroy viral invaders that enter a normal cell and multiply within the cell. Therefore the treatment for viral infections typically focuses on the relief of symptoms or **palliative** treatment. To counteract and destroy the virus invaders,

TABLE 24-1	Common Diseases Caused by Viruses					
Disease	**Organism**	**Description**	**Transmission**	**Symptoms**	**Specimens**	**Tests**
HIV-positive acquired immunodeficiency syndrome (AIDS)	HIV	DNA retrovirus	Contact with an infected person's blood and/or blood-contaminated body fluids, semen, CSF, synovial, and amniotic fluids	Weight loss, chronic fevers, lymphadenopathy, recurrent infections, oral lesions, Kaposi's sarcoma, *Pneumocystis carinii* pneumonia, candidiasis	Blood	HIV serologic tests; ELISA test; positive result to Western blot
Hepatitis A	HAV	RNA virus	Fecal-oral route; contact with carrier, contaminated food or water	Mild fever, malaise, nausea, headache, jaundice	Blood	IgM, IgG
Hepatitis B	HBV	DNA virus	Blood, body fluids, contaminated instruments	Dark urine, light stools, liver tenderness	Blood	HbsAg, anti-HBc, anti-HBs
Hepatitis Delta	HDV	RNA virus	Requires the presence of HBV	Jaundice, cirrhosis	Blood	Anti-HDV
Hepatitis C	HCV	RNA flavivirus	Blood transfusions, hemodialysis, IV drug users	Jaundice, chronic liver disease, cirrhosis, hepatocellular carcinoma	Blood	Transaminase levels, anti-HCV
Herpes simplex	HSV	Exhibits latency	Direct contact	Causes cold sores and genital herpes, painful papules and vesicles	Swab of vesicles	Culture and cytology
Chickenpox or shingles	Varicella zoster virus (VZV)	Exhibits latency, may cause shingles (herpes zoster) in patients with chickenpox in the past	Direct contact	Vesicles, pustules, fever, general malaise, painful area along nerve pathway with herpes zoster	Swab of vesicles	Culture and cytology, clinical diagnosis

TABLE 24-2	Common Diseases Caused by Cocci					
Disease	**Organism**	**Description**	**Transmission**	**Symptoms**	**Specimens**	**Tests**
Pneumonia	*Streptococcus pneumoniae*	Gram-positive cocci in pairs	Direct contact, droplets	Productive cough, fever, chest pain	Sputum; bronchoscopy secretions	Culture, Gram's stain
Strep throat	*Streptococcus pyogenes* (group A strep)	Gram-positive cocci in chains	Direct contact, droplets, fomites	Severe sore throat, fever, malaise	Direct swab	Direct agglutination; culture, white blood cell count and differential
Wound infection, abscesses, boils	*Staphylococcus aureus*	Gram-positive cocci in clusters	Direct contact, fomites, carriers; poor hand washing	Area red, warm, swollen; pus; pain; ulceration or sinus formation	Deep swab; aspirate of drainage	Culture and sensitivity (aerobic and anaerobic)
Staphylococcal food poisoning	*Staphylococcus aureus*	Gram-positive cocci in clusters	Poor hygiene and improper refrigeration of foods	Vomiting, abdominal cramps, diarrhea	Suspected food, stool	Culture
Toxic shock	*Staphylococcus aureus*	Gram-positive cocci in clusters	Use of absorbent packing materials (e.g., tampons, nasal packs)	Fever, headache, nausea, vomiting, delirium, low blood pressure	Swab, blood	Culture and serology
Gonorrhea	*Neisseria gonorrhoeae*	Gram-negative diplococci; intracellular in white blood cells	Sexually transmitted	*Females*: pelvic pain, discharge. May be asymptomatic *Male*: urethral discharge; pain on urination	Swab of cervix, urethra; rectal and pharyngeal swabs in homosexuals	Gram's stain; culture
Meningococcal meningitis	*Neisseria meningitidis*	Gram-negative diplococci	Respiratory tract secretions	High fever, headache, projectile vomiting, delirium, neck and back rigidity, convulsions, petechial rash	Nasopharyngeal swabs, cerebrospinal fluid, blood	Gram's stain; culture; cell counts and chemistries

interferon and the antiviral agents acyclovir (Zovirax), amantadine (Symmetrel), and zidovudine (Retrovir) may be prescribed.

Bacteria are tiny, primitive cells that produce diseases in a variety of ways. Pathogenic bacteria can secrete toxic substances that damage human tissues, act as parasites inside human cells, or form colonies in the body that disrupt normal human functions. Bacteria are classified according to their shape or *morphology* and include spherical-shaped (cocci), rod-shaped (bacilli), and spiral-shaped (spirilla) structures. Some bacteria can produce resistant forms called **spores** that make treatment difficult. When bacteria invade the body there are several ways to treat the patient. The most common approach is the use of antibiotics to destroy or inhibit the growth of the invader.

We all have *normal flora*, or nonpathogenic bacteria that reside in various body systems, especially the digestive tract, and provide protection from disease by competing for nutrients that pathogenic bacteria require to grow and multiply.

Protozoa are unicellular parasites that have the ability to replicate and multiply rapidly once inside the host. Examples of protozoa-related diseases include giardia, which is confined to the gastrointestinal tract, and malaria, which invades the blood system. Protozoa infections are frequently seen in tropical climates due to the need for **vectors** to transmit the disease. For example, the mosquito transmits malaria.

Fungi are a division of plants that may be unicellular or multicellular and includes such growths as mushrooms,

TABLE 24-3	Diseases Caused by Protozoa and Other Parasites			
Disease	**Organism**	**Transmission**	**Symptoms**	**Tests/Specimens**
Malaria	*Plasmodium* species (protozoa)	Bite of the *Anopheles* mosquito	Chills, fever (cyclic)	Blood: examination of stained film for parasites
Toxoplasmosis	*Toxoplasma gondii* (protozoa)	Fecal contamination (cat litter); congenitally	Febrile illness, rash; congenital: jaundice, enlarged liver and spleen, brain abnormalities	Skin test
Amebic dysentery	*Entamoeba histolytica* (protozoa)	Fecal contamination of food and water	Bloody diarrhea, cramping, fever	Stool for O & P
Giardiasis	*Giardia lamblia* (protozoa)	Common in intestinal tract opportunist; contaminated surface water	Asymptomatic to severe diarrhea and abdominal discomfort	Stool for O & P; intestinal biopsy; string test
Interstitial plasma cell pneumonia	*Pneumocystis carinii*	Widely prevalent in animals. Occurs in debilitated persons, immunosuppressed; commonly associated with acquired immunodeficiency syndrome	Pneumonia-like	Biopsy
Trichinosis	*Trichinella spiralis* (roundworm)	Ingestion of undercooked pork, bear meat	Nausea, fever, diarrhea, muscle pain and swelling, edema of face	Biopsy; blood tests
Tapeworm	*Taenia* species	Undercooked meats (beef and pork)	Abdominal discomfort, diarrhea, weight loss	Stool for O & P
	Diphyllobothrium latum	Undercooked fish; common among Norwegians, Japanese	As above; may become anemic	Stool for O & P
Pinworm	*Enterobius vermicularis* (roundworm)	Fecal-oral	Severe rectal itching, restlessness, insomnia	Scotch tape applied to perianal region for ova
Scabies	*Sarcoptes scabiei* (itch mite)	Direct contact; clothing, bedding	Nocturnal itching; skin burrows	Skin scrapings for parasites
Lice	*Pediculus humanus*; *Phthirus pubis* (crab)	Direct contact; clothing, bedding, furniture (can transmit other diseases via bite)	Intense itching; skin lesions	Finding adult lice or eggs (nits) on body or hair

O & P, Ova and parasites.

molds, and yeasts. Many forms are pathogenic and can cause such diseases as **candidiasis** and **tinea** infections. Fungi grow best in dark, moist environments. Treatment with antifungal agents includes the application of topical preparations for tinea infections, such as Lotrimin or Nizoral; vaginal suppositories for candidiasis, such as Monistat; or oral medications, such as Diflucan and nystatin. Fungal infections are also called *mycotic* infections.

Rickettsia are a group of microorganisms that have some of the characteristics of both bacteria and viruses. Like viruses, they are obligate parasites that require living host cells for growth but are larger than viruses and can be viewed by a regular microscope. Vectors such as fleas, ticks, and mites usually transmit pathogenic forms of rickettsia. Diseases caused by rickettsia can be treated with antibiotics and include Lyme disease and Rocky Mountain spotted fever, which are both transmitted by ticks.

The second link in the chain of infection is the *reservoir host*. Reservoir hosts may be people, insects, animals, water, food, or **contaminated** instruments. Most pathogens must gain entrance into a host or else they will die. The reservoir host supplies nutrition to the organism, allowing it to multiply. The pathogen either causes infection in the host or, in the case of vector-borne diseases, exits from the host in great enough numbers to cause disease in another host.

The chain of infection continues with the *means or portal of exit*. This is how the pathogen escapes the reservoir host. Exits include the mouth, nose, eyes, ears, intestines, urinary tract, reproductive tract, and open wounds. Again, the use of standard precautions such as latex gloves, masks, proper management of wounds, disposal of contaminated products, and hand washing all help control the ability of the infectious material to spread from one host to another.

TABLE 24-4	Selected Fungal Diseases			
Disease	Organism	Predisposing Conditions and Transmission	Symptoms	Tests/Specimens
Thrush (oral yeast); Candida (vaginal yeast)	Candida species (yeast)	Oral: during birth; other: following antibiotic therapy, oral birth control, severe diabetes	White, cheesy growth	Swab for KOH prep, culture
Athlete's foot, jock itch, ringworm (tinea)	Several species of dermatophytes (skin fungi)	Opportunist; direct contact; clothing; prolonged exposure to moist environment	Hair loss, thickening of skin, nails; itching; red, scaly patches	Skin scraping for KOH prep; skin, hair for culture
Histoplasmosis	Histoplasma capsulatum	Inhalation of dust contaminated with bird or bat droppings	Mild, flu-like to systemic	Serologic
Cryptococcosis	Cryptococcus neoformans	Contact with poultry droppings	Cough, fever, malaise; can become systemic	Sputum culture
Sporotrichosis	Sporothrix schenckii	Farmers, florists, people exposed to soil	Skin lesions that spread along lymphatics; can become systemic	Cerebrospinal fluid culture, India ink direct examination, scrapings; serologic

KOH, Potassium hydroxide.

After exiting the reservoir host, organisms spread by *transmission*. Transmission is either direct or indirect. *Direct transmission* occurs from contact with an infected person or with the discharges of an infected person, such as feces or urine. *Indirect transmission* occurs from *droplets* in the air expelled from coughing, speaking, or sneezing; vectors that harbor pathogens; contaminated food or drink; and contaminated objects (called *fomites*). Proper sanitation of water and food; utilizing sanitization, disinfection and sterilization procedures; and the use of **germicides**, such as Wavecide and Cidex, help control the transmission of pathogens.

The next step in the chain of infection is the *means or portal of entry*. This is how the transmitted pathogen gains entry into a new host. The means of entry, like the means of exit, may be the mouth, nose, eyes, intestines, urinary tract, reproductive tract, or an open wound. The first line of defense against pathogenic invasion is the intact integumentary system or skin, which serves as a mechanical barrier to infection. Anatomical defense mechanisms also include integumentary secretions, tears, cilia, mucous membranes, and the pH of body fluids. The body's second line of defense includes the inflammatory process and the immune system response. The immune system responds by producing **antibodies** specifically designed to combat the presence of a foreign substance or **antigen**. This process is called *humoral immunity*. The immune system also reacts at the cellular level with *cell-mediated immunity* by causing destruction of pathogenic cells at the site of invasion. An example of cell-mediated immunity is *phagocytosis* where specialized immune system cells called macrophages actually ingest and destroy pathogenic microbes.

If the host is a *susceptible host*, that is, one that is capable of supporting the growth of the infecting organism, the organism will multiply. Factors affecting host susceptibility include the location of entry, the dose of organisms, and the condition of the individual. If the conditions are right, the organisms reach infectious levels, the susceptible host becomes a reservoir *host*, and the cycle begins again.

Individuals who are effectively immunized against a disease, such as hepatitis B, are not susceptible to the disease even if exposed to the pathogen, because their immune systems have created antibodies to protect them. Besides immunization, other ways to decrease susceptibility to disease are proper nutrition and healthy lifestyles.

CRITICAL THINKING APPLICATION

Tommy Anderson, a 5-year-old patient, is seen in the office with an outbreak of impetigo. Rosa must apply the concepts of the chain of infection and infection control methods to teach Tommy and his mother how to prevent the spread of the infection to other members of the family. What procedures should she follow after Tommy's visit to prevent the spread of the infection to other patients, staff, and herself?

The Inflammatory Response

When trauma occurs to the body, it alerts protective mechanisms, and the body responds in a predictable manner, called *inflammation*. To defend itself, the body initiates specific responses that destroy and remove pathogenic organisms and their by-products or, if this is not possible, limit the extent of damage caused by pathogenic organisms and their by-products. This process characterizes the four classic symptoms of inflammation: redness, swelling or edema, pain, and heat.

Figure 24-2 details the inflammatory response. When the body is exposed to an infectious agent or a foreign sub-

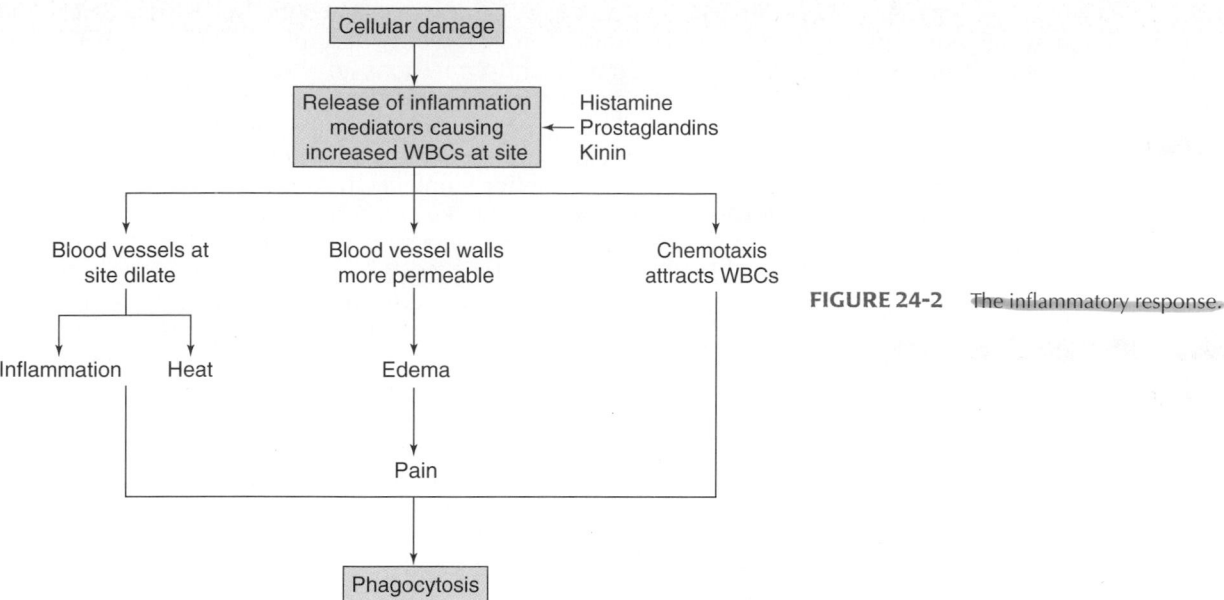

FIGURE 24-2 The inflammatory response.

stance, cellular damage occurs at the site. Inflammation mediators, histamine, prostaglandins, and kinins, are released and result in three different responses at the cellular level. All three actions are designed to increase the number of white blood cells (WBCs) at the injury site.

First, blood vessels at the site dilate, causing an increase in the local blood flow that results in redness or inflammation and heat. Blood vessel walls become more **permeable**, which assists in the release of WBCs to the site. The WBCs begin to form a fibrous capsule around the injury site to protect surrounding cells from the damage or the source of infection. Blood plasma also filters out of the more permeable vessel walls, resulting in *edema*, which puts pressure on the nerves and causes pain. Finally, *chemotaxis*, the release of chemical agents, occurs, attracting WBCs to the site. The increase in the number of WBCs at the site results in phagocytosis, or the engulfing and destruction of microorganisms and damaged cells. Destroyed pathogens, cells, and WBCs collect in the area and form a thick, white substance called *pus*.

If the pathogenic invasion is too great for localized control, the infection may collect in the body's lymph nodes, where more WBCs are present to help fight the battle. This causes swollen glands or *lymphadenopathy*. If the body is too weak or the number of pathogens is too great, the infection may spread to the bloodstream. A systemic infection, called *septicemia* or *blood poisoning*, may occur that could ultimately affect the entire body. Another term for septicemia is **pyemia**. Without appropriate medical intervention, death can occur.

CRITICAL THINKING APPLICATION

Rosa's next patient appears to have a localized inflammatory response to a splinter. What signs and symptoms should she expect the patient to exhibit?

Types of Infections

Acute Infection

Acute infections have a rapid onset of symptoms but last a relatively short time. The prodromal period is that time when the patient first exhibits vague, nonspecific symptoms of the disease. In an acute viral infection, the host cell typically dies within a period of hours or days. Symptoms appear after the tissue damage begins to occur. Usually, the virus can be isolated only shortly before or after the prodromal period. In most acute infections, such as the common cold, the body's defense mechanisms eliminate the virus within 2 to 3 weeks.

Chronic Infection

Infections that persist for a long period of time, sometimes for life, are called chronic infections. In the case of chronic viral hepatitis B, patients are asymptomatic but the virus is detectable with blood work and remains transmissible throughout their lives. Hepatitis B, or *serum hepatitis*, is transmitted by blood or blood products as well as all body fluids. It is a serious health hazard to medical personnel. All individuals employed in a healthcare setting should be immunized against hepatitis B.

Latent Infection

A latent infection is a persistent infection in which the symptoms cycle through periods of **relapse** and **remission**. Cold sores (oral herpes simplex) and *genital herpes* are latent viral infections. The virus first enters the body and causes the original lesion. It then lies dormant, in a nerve cell away from the surface, until a certain provocation (illness with fever, sunburn, or stress) causes the virus to leave the nerve cell and seek the surface again. Once the virus reaches the superficial tissues, it becomes detectable for a short time and causes another outbreak at the site. Another herpes virus, *herpes zoster*, causes *chickenpox*. This virus then may lie dormant along a nerve pathway and later erupt as the painful disease *shingles*.

Slow Infection

Slow infections progress over very long periods. These conditions include the degenerative neurological diseases, such as progressive Lyme disease or advanced syphilis.

OSHA Bloodborne Pathogen Standard

Chapter 7 introduced the role of the Occupational Safety and Health Administration (OSHA) in protecting patients and healthcare personnel from potentially harmful substances in the medical facility. Because of concern about the increasing prevalence of HIV and hepatitis B (HBV), in 1987 the Centers for Disease Control (today called the Centers for Disease Control and Prevention [CDC]) recommended a new approach to potentially infectious materials called *universal precautions*. The underlying concept of universal precautions was that since it is impossible for healthcare workers to know whether patients have an infectious **disorder**, all blood and certain body fluids must be treated as if they are known to be infectious for bloodborne pathogens. Therefore precautions should be implemented for all patients, regardless of knowledge of their individual health history. At the same time, utilization of universal precautions procedures protects patients from any bloodborne infection the healthcare worker may be carrying.

OSHA recognizes that employees face significant health risk as the result of occupational exposure to blood or other potentially infectious materials that may contain hepatitis B (HBV), hepatitis C (HCV), or the human immunodeficiency virus (HIV). In July 1992 OSHA began enforcing work practice controls to reduce or eliminate occupational exposure to bloodborne pathogens. Employers with workers who are at risk of occupational exposure to blood or other infectious materials must implement an Exposure Control Plan that details employee protection procedures. The plan must describe how an employer will use a combination of controls, including personal protective equipment, training, medical surveillance, hepatitis B immunizations, record keeping of occupational injuries, and labeling of hazardous materials. Engineering controls such as safer medical equipment, puncture-proof sharps containers, and shielded needle devices are recommended as the primary way to decrease or eliminate employee exposure. Employer failure to comply with the OSHA Bloodborne Pathogens Standard could result in a maximum penalty of $7000 for the first violation and up to $70,000 for repeated violations.

New Fundamentals

The CDC estimates that medical personnel sustain almost 600,000 exposure incidents annually from contaminated sharps. In response to the CDC's concern about employee risk, the U.S. Congress passed the Needlestick Safety and Prevention Act, which became effective in April 2001. Subsequently, revisions to the Bloodborne Pathogens Standard have included mandatory review and update of the Exposure Control Plan to reflect current changes in exposure reduction technology and making the plan accessible for employee use. In addition, employers are now required to keep a confidential sharps injury log that describes the device involved in the incident and the details of how and where the incident occurred. Employers must also make available to employees effective sharps management devices, such as syringes with sliding shields, needles that retract after use, and jet injection systems that do not require needles for **parenteral** administration. Parenteral exposure includes accidental needlesticks, occupation-related human bites, and exposure of potentially infectious material to nonintact skin, as in the presence of cuts and abrasions on employee hands.

The revised standard also clarifies the use of washing or flushing any exposed body area or mucous membrane immediately or as soon as possible after exposure to potentially infectious materials. This includes hand washing after the removal of gloves or other personal protective equipment. The best way to reduce occupational risk of infection is to follow the Pathogen Standards. Healthcare workers must take adequate nondiscriminatory precautions to protect themselves. Figure 24-3 summarizes OSHA standard precautions.

> ### ●POTENTIALLY INFECTIOUS FLUIDS ●
>
> - Cerebrospinal (CSF), synovial, pleural, pericardial, peritoneal, mucous, and amniotic fluids
> - Liquid or semiliquid blood
> - Vaginal and seminal secretions
> - Saliva in dental procedures
> - Body fluid visibly contaminated with blood
> - Unknown body fluid
> - Human tissue, including tissue culture, cells, or exudates
> - HIV has been isolated from CSF, synovial, and amniotic fluids, and hepatitis antigens have been detected in synovial, amniotic, and peritoneal fluids.
> - Items that are contaminated with any of the above potentially infectious materials require special handling.
> - Pus

Compliance Guidelines

Because the Pathogen Standards are written to cover employees working in all health fields, it is obvious that only some of the regulations apply to the ambulatory care setting. Safety and infection control fundamentals go beyond hand washing and the disease cycle. The information presented here is as it applies to the medical assistant profession.

OSHA STANDARD PRECAUTION HIGHLIGHTS

* Wash hands or flush any exposed area.
  Immediately after touching blood, body fluids, secretions, excretions, and contaminated items whether you have worn gloves or not.
  Immediately after you remove gloves
  Between patient contacts
  When necessary to prevent transfer of microorganisms

* Use plain soap for routine handwashing and an antimicrobial or antiseptic agent for specified situations.

* Wear clean, nonsterile gloves when touching blood, body fluids, secretions, excretions, mucous membranes, nonintact skin, and contaminated items.

* Change gloves between procedures on the same patient after exposure to potentially infective material.

* Remove gloves immediately after patient contact and wash your hands.

* Wear protective barrier equipment (e.g., mask, goggles, face shield, gown) to protect the mucous membranes of your eyes, nose, and mouth, and to avoid soiling your clothing when performing procedures that may generate splashes or sprays of blood, body fluids, secretions, or excretions.

* Care of linens and equipment that are contaminated with blood, body fluids, secretions, or excretions in a way that avoids skin and mucous membrane exposures, clothing contamination, and microorganism transfer to other patients and environments. Dispose of single-use items appropriately.

* Take precautions to avoid injuries before, during, and after any procedures using needles, scalpels, or other sharp instruments.

* Ensure that used needles are not recapped, purposely bent, broken, removed from disposable syringes, or otherwise manipulated by hand. Never direct the point of a needle toward any part of your body; instead use a one-handed "scoop" technique or a device designed for holding the needle sheath.

* Employers must supply current sharps management devices such as syringes with sliding shields.

* An up-to-date exposure control plan must be available.

* Employers must maintain a confidential record of sharps injuries.

* Place used disposable syringes and needles, scalpel blades, and other used sharps in a puncture-resistant container that is located as close as possible to the area of use.

* Use barrier devices (e.g., mouthpieces, resuscitation bags) as alternatives to mouth-to-mouth resuscitation.

FIGURE 24-3 OSHA standard precaution highlights. (From revision to OSHA's Bloodborne Pathogens Standard, April 2001.)

Barrier Protection. Medical assistants should routinely use appropriate barrier precautions when contact with blood or other body fluids is anticipated. Barrier protection, or personal protective equipment (PPE), includes specialized clothing or equipment such as latex gloves, face masks, face shields, protective glasses, laboratory coats, barrier gowns, mouthpieces, and resuscitation bags (Figure 24-4) that protect you from potentially infectious substances. The purpose of PPE is to prevent or minimize the entry of infectious material into your body.

Since implementation of universal precautions, the use of latex gloves is commonplace in healthcare facilities. As a result, there has also been an increase in allergic reactions associated with latex products. Hypersensitive reactions to latex gloves or the powder that lines them may be localized, with eruptions of **urticaria**, dermatitis, conjunctivitis, and **rhinitis**; or systemic, with asthmatic reactions or an **anaphylaxis** response. If you or a patient shows signs of sensitivity to latex, the healthcare provider is required to provide gloves made of nonallergenic materials as barrier devices.

Protective equipment must be used if there is any chance that you will be involved in any of the following activities:

* Touching a patient's blood and body fluids, mucous membranes, or skin that is not intact.
* Handling items and surfaces contaminated with blood and body fluids.
* Performing venipuncture, finger punctures, injections, and other vascular access procedures.
* Assisting with any surgical procedure. If a glove is torn or an injury occurs, the glove is removed and replaced with a new glove as soon as safety permits. The instrument involved in the incident is removed from the sterile field.

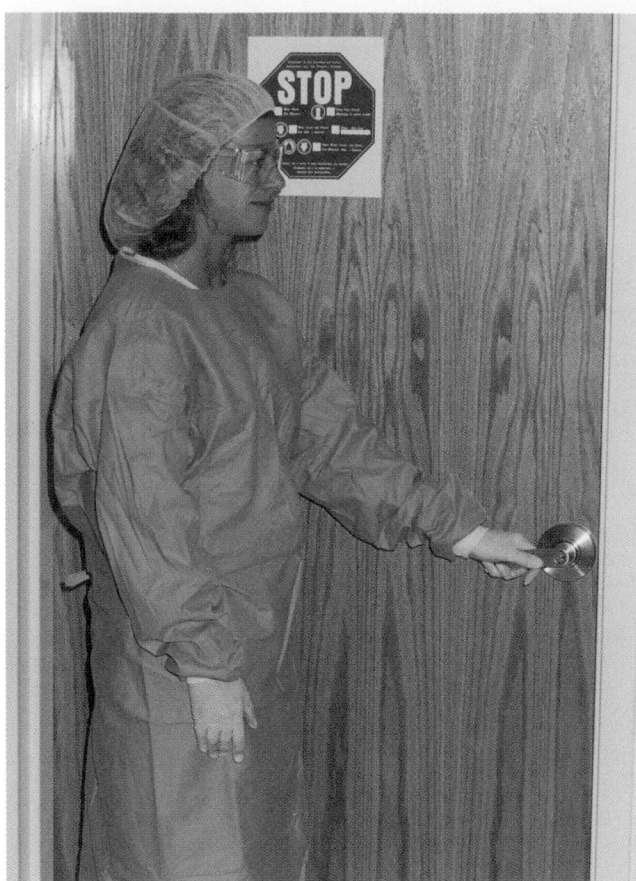

FIGURE 24-4 Barrier protection.

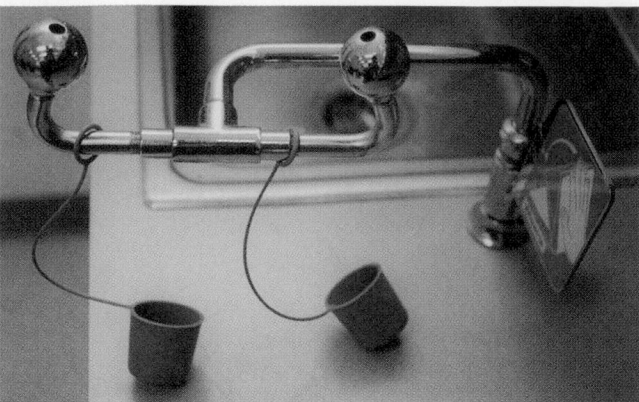

FIGURE 24-5 Eye washing unit.

Environment Protection. The environment protection section of the compliance guidelines covers controls to minimize the risk of occupational injury by isolating or removing any physical or mechanical health hazard in the medical workplace. Every medical assistant must adhere to these safety rules.

- Observe warning labels on biohazard containers and equipment.
- Minimize splashing, spraying, and spattering of drops of potentially infectious materials. Splattering of blood onto skin or mucous membranes is a proven mode of transmission of HBV.
- Bandage any breaks or lesions on your hands before gloving.
- If exposed body surfaces, such as the eyes, come in contact with body fluids, flush with water and/or scrub with soap and water as soon as possible (Figure 24-5).
- Contaminated needles and other sharps should not be recapped, bent, broken, or resheathed. Needle units are now required to have sliding shields or some other protective device for use after injection.
- Use hemostats to attach and remove scalpel blades from handles.
- Contaminated reusable sharps should not be stored or processed in a way that requires employees to reach by hand into the containers.
- Immediately after use, dispose of syringes and needles, scalpel blades, and other sharp items in a labeled, leakproof, puncture-resistant biohazard container. The container must be located as close as possible to the area where the instruments are used.
- All specimens must be placed in a container that prevents leakage during collection, handling, processing, storage, transport, and shipping. Avoid contaminating the outside of the container or the label with the specimen substance. If the outside is contaminated, the container should be disinfected. One method is using a 1:10 dilution of sodium hypochlorite (household chlorine bleach and water) and then placing the container in an impervious bag for transport. The container must have a biohazard label that alerts others it holds potentially infectious material. Gloves should be worn throughout this procedure.

- Handling, processing, and disposing of all specimens of blood and body fluids.
- Cleaning and decontaminating spills of blood or other body fluids.

 SAFETY ALERT *Gloves and gowns* contaminated with body fluid of any kind must be removed and placed in a designated area or biohazard container, and hands or any other exposed area must be washed or flushed as soon as possible. *Protective eyewear* must be made of safety glass and have side shields. Standard prescriptive eyeglasses are not considered effective. All face shields, goggles, and glasses with side shields are acceptable. All PPE must be removed before leaving the medical facility.

CRITICAL THINKING APPLICATION

Rosa is caring for an injured 3-year-old child with an open wound on his right knee. She puts on latex gloves to clean the wound and the mother demands to know why. How can she explain her actions?

- Mouth pipetting or the sucking of blood through tubing is prohibited.
- Contaminated test materials should be decontaminated before reprocessing or should be placed in impervious bags and disposed of according to policy.
- Equipment that has been contaminated with blood or body fluids should be decontaminated before being repaired in the office or transported to the manufacturer. There is no documented evidence of HIV transmission from contaminated environmental surfaces; however, surface contamination is a proven mode of transmission for HBV.
- Smoking, eating, drinking, applying cosmetics or lip balm, and handling contact lenses are prohibited in work areas where there is reasonable likelihood of contamination from bloodborne pathogens.
- Food and drink cannot be kept in refrigerators, freezers, shelves, or cabinets, or on countertops where blood or other potentially infectious materials could be present.

Housekeeping Controls. The OSHA Standard specifies certain housekeeping measures be followed to promote a work area that is clean and sanitary. One requirement is a posted schedule for cleaning and decontaminating each work area where exposure could occur. This documentation must be specific and include information on the surface cleaned, type of waste encountered, and procedures performed in the designated area.

- Work surfaces must be immediately decontaminated with a disinfectant (such as a 1:10 solution of sodium hypochlorite) after accidental spills of blood or body fluids and at the end of each procedure.
- Disinfection and decontamination of all reusable containers must be done on a routine basis.
- Sharps containers are to be maintained in an upright position to keep waste inside and as close as possible to the work usage area. Never attempt to reach inside a sharps container and do not overfill them. Replace containers on a routine basis and be certain that the lid is closed securely before preparing them for biohazard waste disposal.
- Never pick up spilled material or broken glassware with hands. Brooms, brushes, dustpans, and pickup tongs or forceps should be used and the material placed immediately into an impervious biohazard bag or container at the spill site (Figure 24-6). Use an absorbent professional biohazard spill preparation as directed to decontaminate the site.
- Handle soiled linen as little as possible and always while wearing gloves or other protective equipment. Linens soiled with blood or body fluids should be double bagged and transported in labeled, leakproof biohazard bags.
- Contaminated materials and/or infective waste are to be handled with extreme caution to prevent exposure. Biohazardous waste must be collected in impermeable red polyethylene or polypropylene biohazard-labeled bags or containers and sealed (Figure 24-7). This waste must be disposed of in accordance with all applicable federal, state, and local regulations. Disposal methods include treatment by heat, incineration, steam sterilization, chemical treatment, or other equivalent methods that render the waste inactive before it can be placed in a landfill.

CRITICAL THINKING APPLICATION

Using the techniques learned in Chapter 1, create a mind map that identifies the details of OSHA's Bloodborne Pathogens Standard.

Hepatitis B Vaccination. Hepatitis B vaccine must be available free of charge to all employees who are at risk for occupational exposure to bloodborne pathogens, whether they are full-time or part-time workers, within 10 days of starting employment. The vaccine is administered by intramuscular injection in 3 doses. The second injection is administered 4 weeks after the first and the third injection 6 months after the first.

Although the effectiveness rate of the vaccination is almost 96%, employees should have a blood titer drawn after completion of the injection cycle to determine whether they have created antibodies against the disease. If the employee did not respond to the first series or if the series was not completed, revaccination with a second 3-dose series is recommended. If antibodies still do not develop, no further vaccination is given.

Employees may decline the immunization process but must sign a declination form that is kept on file as a record of worker refusal. However, the employee may receive the vaccine at a future date free of charge.

Postexposure Follow-Up. If a worker is exposed through an accidental needlestick, a human bite, exposure to broken skin, or from a splash or splatter onto mucous membranes, such as the eyes, there are certain procedures that must be followed.

- Immediately, or as soon as possible after exposure, the worker should wash or flush the exposed area.
- The exposure incident must be immediately reported to the supervisor.
- The employee must immediately receive a confidential medical evaluation. All documentation related to the incident must remain confidential, not disclosed to any individual without the employee's express written permission, and kept for at least the duration of the worker's employment plus 30 years.
- An incident report must be filed that documents details surrounding the exposure incident, the route or type of exposure, and the identity, if known, of the source individual. The source individual is the person, living or dead, whose blood or potentially infectious material was the source of the occupational exposure.
- The exposed worker is tested for HBV and HIV if consent is given. If the employee refuses the tests but blood is drawn, the sample must be stored 90 days for the worker to decide whether screening is wanted.
- The source individual, if known and if consent is given, is also screened for HBV and HIV. Depending on state regulations, the employee may be told the results of the source individual's tests.

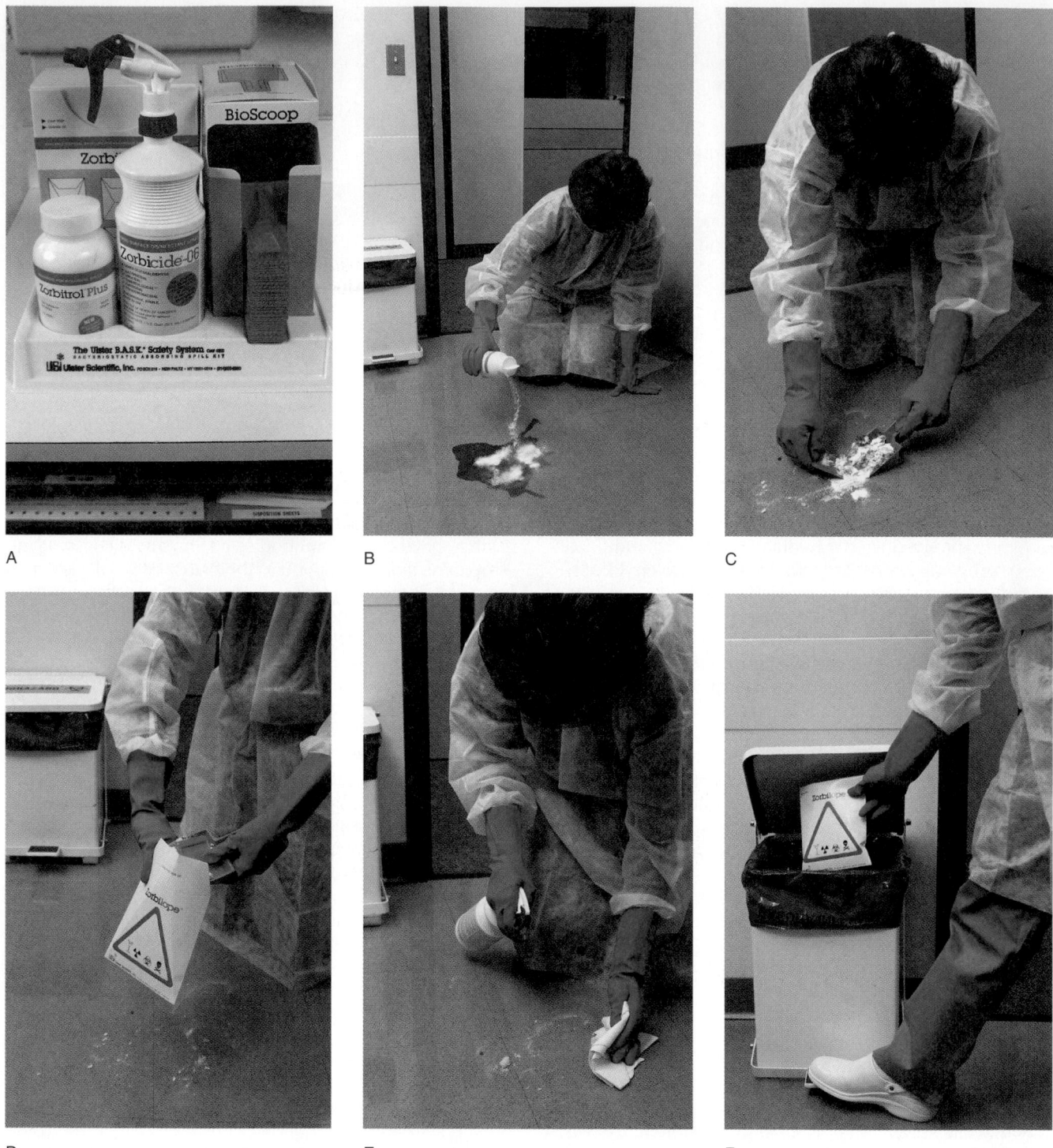

FIGURE 24-6   Cleaning spilled material. **A**, Clean-up kit with printed instructions. **B**, Sprinkle congealing powder over the spill. **C**, Scoop up spill. **D**, Place contents in bag. **E**, Wipe area thoroughly with germicide. **F**, Place all contaminated material in biohazard bag or container.

- If not vaccinated against HBV, the employee is offered vaccination. The physician may recommend administration of gamma globulin as a preventative measure. If so, it should be administered within 24 hours of the exposure.
- The injured employee must receive a copy of the healthcare provider's written opinion within 15 days of the completion of the evaluation.

- The exposed worker must receive health counseling regarding the risk of illness or other adverse outcomes of exposure and the potential for as well as consequences of transmission of the disease to family, patients, and others.

Because students are not considered employees and are attending an educational institution, OSHA standards do not apply. However, all healthcare students are at risk of

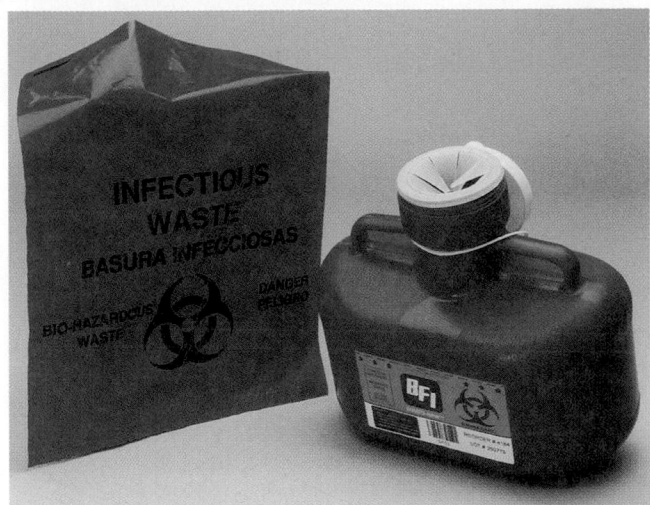

FIGURE 24-7   Biohazard bag and biohazard sharps container.

bloodborne pathogen exposure and should follow all OSHA guidelines designed to protect individuals from exposure.

A complete unabridged copy of OSHA's Bloodborne Pathogens Standard may be obtained at their website, www.osha.gov.

CRITICAL THINKING APPLICATION

Rosa's office has been especially busy today. While administering an injection to a frightened 6-year-old child, a co-worker has an accidental needlestick. She tells Rosa about the incident but does not know what to do. What steps should be taken to manage the situation?

Aseptic Techniques: Prevention of Disease Transmission

Asepsis means freedom from infection or infectious material. *Medical asepsis* is defined as the removal or destruction of disease-causing organisms *after they leave the body*. When we practice the principles of medical asepsis, we are directing our efforts at preventing reinfection of the patient or the cross-infection of other patients or ourselves. The goal is to eliminate or minimize pathogens by following OSHA's Bloodborne Pathogens Standard and disinfecting objects as soon as possible after contamination. This creates a healthcare environment that is as free of pathogens as possible.

Surgical asepsis is defined as the destruction of organisms *before they enter the body*. This technique is used for any procedure that invades the body's skin or tissues, such as surgery or injections. Any time the skin or mucous membrane is punctured, pierced, or incised (or will be during a procedure), surgical aseptic techniques are practiced.

Everything that comes into contact with the patient should be sterile, such as gowns, drapes, instruments, and the gloved hands of the surgical team. Minor surgery, urinary catheterizations, injections, and some specimen collections, such as blood collection and biopsies, are performed using surgical aseptic technique. This technique is presented in Chapter 54.

Because it is not possible to sterilize your hands, the goal of hand washing is to reduce skin bacteria by the use of mechanical friction, antimicrobial soaps, and warm running water. Normally there are two types of bacteria on your skin: *transient bacteria*, which are surface bacteria that are introduced by fomites and remain with you a short time, and *resident bacteria*, found under fingernails, in hair follicles, in the openings of the sebaceous glands, and in the deeper layers of the skin. The goal of thorough hand washing is to remove or decrease the numbers of transient bacteria on the surface of the skin, thus preventing transient bacteria from becoming resident bacteria.

The most effective barrier against infection is the unbroken skin. If the skin and mucous membranes are intact, medical asepsis can be practiced for most noninvasive (not penetrating through human tissues) procedures, such as pelvic and proctological examinations. Instruments and objects used in medical aseptic procedures must be decontaminated or sterilized before being used on another patient. Medical aseptic procedures may also include the use of gowns and masks, but these are not sterile and are worn to protect you more than the patient.

Hand Washing

Hands must be washed, using the correct technique, before and after each patient is examined or treated and also when stipulated in the Bloodborne Pathogens Guidelines. It is not necessary to do an extended scrub each time, but the first scrub in the morning should be extensive, lasting 2 to 4 minutes. Subsequent hand washing may be brief, lasting 1 to 2 minutes, unless your hands are excessively contaminated. A good antimicrobial soap with chlorhexidine, such as Hibiclens, which has antiseptic residual action that will last several hours, should be used. Each office sink should be equipped with a liquid soap dispenser. A water-soluble lotion may be rubbed into your hands after washing and drying them. Dry, cracked, chapped skin interrupts the skin's integrity and can result in transmission of disease.

Proper hand washing depends on two factors: running water and friction. Water should be warm, because water that is too hot or too cold will cause the skin to become chapped. Friction means the firm rubbing of all surfaces of the hands and wrists. Remember that your fingers have four sides and fingernails have two sides. For the medical hand wash, all jewelry except a plain wedding band is removed. A wristwatch may be left on if it can be moved up on the forearm away from the wrist area. Hands are washed under running water, with the fingertips pointing downward. Soap and friction are applied to the hands and wrists. Allow the water to wash away debris from the wrists down toward the fingertips (Procedure 24-1).

PROCEDURE **24-1**

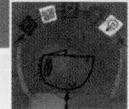

Performing Medical Aseptic Hand Washing

GOAL: To minimize the number of pathogens on your hands, thus reducing the risk of pathogenic transmission.

EQUIPMENT AND SUPPLIES

- Sink with running water
- Antimicrobial liquid soap in a dispenser (bar soap is not acceptable)
- Nail brush or orange stick
- Paper towels in a dispenser
- Water-based antimicrobial lotion

PROCEDURAL STEPS

1 Remove all jewelry except your wristwatch, which should be pulled up above your wrist or removed, and a plain gold wedding ring.

Purpose: Jewelry is capable of concealing microorganisms.

2 Turn on the faucet and regulate the water temperature to lukewarm.

Purpose: Water that is too hot can cause skin to become dry and chapped.

3 Allow your hands to become wet, apply soap, and lather using a circular motion with friction while holding your fingertips downward (Figure 1). Rub well between your fingers.

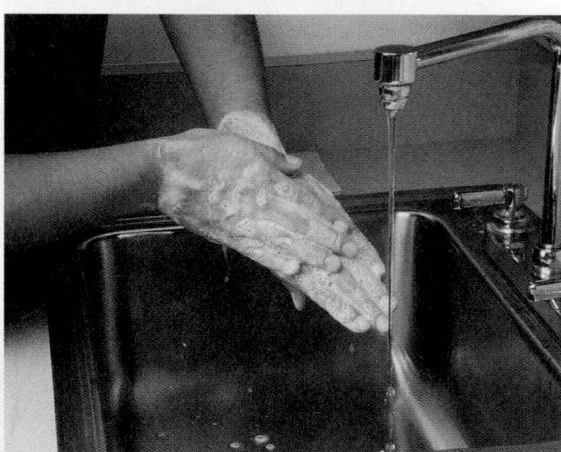

Figure 1

Purpose: Friction removes soil and contaminants from your hands and wrists.

If this is the first hand washing of the day, use a nail brush or an orange stick and thoroughly inspect and clean under every fingernail during step 3.

4 Rinse well, holding your hands so that the water flows from your wrists downward to your fingertips (Figure 2).

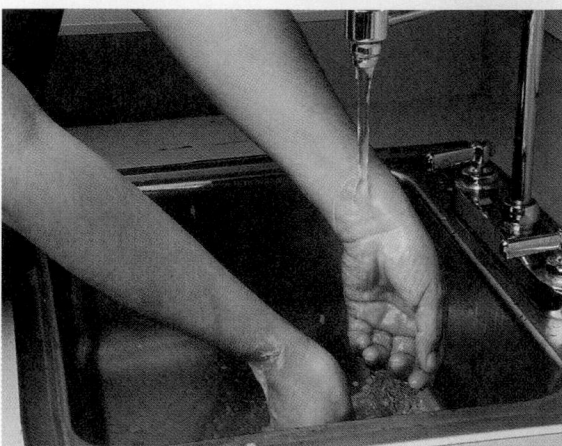

Figure 2

Purpose: Soil and contaminants will wash off your skin and down the drain.

5 Wet your hands again and repeat the scrubbing procedure using vigorous, circular motion over wrists and hands for at least 1 to 2 minutes.

Purpose: Time is required for friction and motion to eliminate all possible soil and contaminants.

6 Rinse your hands a second time, keeping fingers lower than your wrists.

Purpose: To ensure that the hands are really clean.

7 Dry your hands with paper towels. Do not touch the paper towel dispenser as you are obtaining towels (Figure 3).

Purpose: Touching the dispenser contaminates your hands, and you will need to start over.

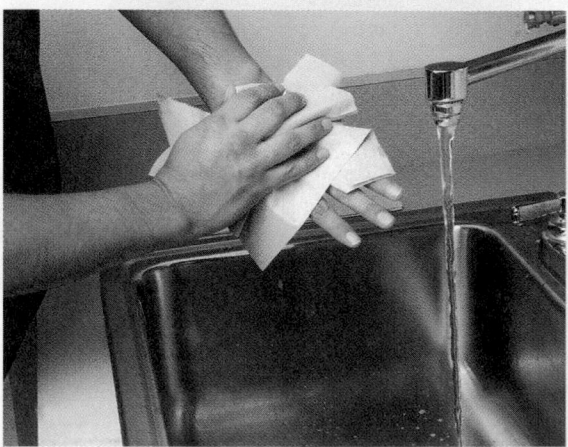

Figure 3

PROCEDURE 24-1—Cont'd

8 If faucets are not foot operated, turn off the water faucet with the paper towel (Figure 4).

Purpose: The faucet is dirty and will contaminate your clean hands.

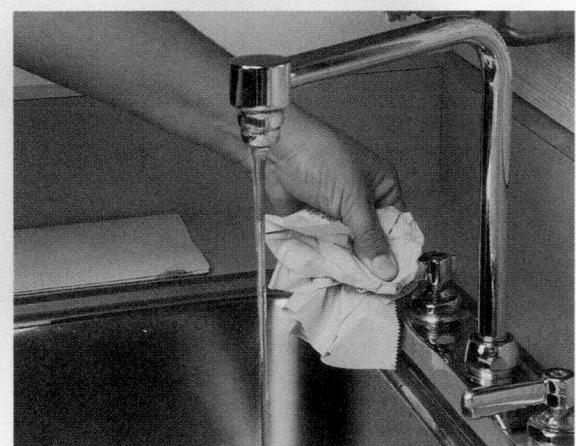

Figure 4

9 After completion of drying your hands and turning off faucets (if necessary), place used towels into a waste container.

Purpose: Always discard contaminated waste immediately to eliminate the source of infection.

10 Apply a water-based antibacterial hand lotion to prevent chapped or dry skin.

Purpose: Chapped skin eliminates the first line of defense against infectious organisms.

Remember, the goal of aseptic hand washing is to protect you from infection and prevent cross-contamination of microorganisms from one patient to another. Use this procedure after you finish with one patient and before you attend to another patient; after you finish handling one specimen and before you handle another specimen; before and after you use toilet facilities; whenever you touch something that causes your hands to become contaminated; when you arrive at work and before you leave the office; before and after eating; and at the end of the day.

Overview of CDC Hand Hygiene Guidelines. The Centers for Disease Control and Prevention recently released new recommendations for hand hygiene in healthcare settings. Hand hygiene is a term that applies to either hand washing, use of an antiseptic hand rub, or surgical hand antisepsis. Evidence suggests that hand antisepsis, the cleansing of hands with an antiseptic hand rub is more effective in reducing nosocomial infections than plain hand washing. *When using an alcohol-based hand rub, apply the product to the palm of one hand and rub the hands together, covering all surfaces of the hands and fingers, until the hands are dry. Follow the manufacturer's recommendations regarding the volume of product to use.*

- Continue to wash hands with soap and water whenever the hands are visibly soiled.
- Use an alcohol-based hand rub to routinely decontaminate the hands in the following clinical situations:
  - Before and after client contact.
  - After contact with body fluids or excretions, mucous membranes, nonintact skin, and wound dressings.
  - If moving from a contaminated-body site (rectal area or mouth) to a clean-body site (surgical wound, urinary meatus) during client care.
  - After contact with inanimate objects (including medical equipment) in the immediate vicinity of the client.
  - After removing gloves.
- Before eating and after using a restroom, wash hands with soap and water.
- Antimicrobial-impregnated wipes (i.e., towelettes) are not a substitute for using an alcohol-based hand rub or antimicrobial soap.

Sanitization

Instruments and other items used in office surgery, examination, or treatment must be carefully cleaned *before* proceeding with the steps of disinfection or sterilization. Sanitization is the cleansing process that decreases the number of microorganisms to a safe level as dictated in public health guidelines. This cleansing process removes debris such as blood and other body fluids from instruments or equipment. Blood and debris must be removed so that later disinfection with chemicals or sterilization with steam, heat, or gases can penetrate to all the instrument's surfaces (Procedure 24-2).

The medical assistant should always wear gloves, thick utility gloves if the instruments have sharp or pointed edges, while performing sanitization to prevent possible personal contamination of potentially infectious body fluids that may be present on the articles being cleaned (Procedure 24-3). The procedure should be completed immediately after use of the instruments in a separate workroom or area to avoid cross-contamination with clean instruments and equipment. If this is not possible, rinse the used items under cold water and then place them in a low-sudsing, rust-inhibiting, enzyme-containing, detergent solution. Never allow blood or other substances that can

PROCEDURE 24-2

Sanitization of Instruments

GOAL: To remove all contaminated matter from instruments in preparation for disinfection or sterilization.

EQUIPMENT AND SUPPLIES

- Sink with hot running water
- Sanitizing agent or low-sudsing soap with enzymatic action
- Utility gloves
- Brush
- Towels
- Appropriate waste container

PROCEDURAL STEPS

1 Put on utility gloves.
Purpose: To provide personal protection against potentially infectious matter and sharp instruments.

2 Separate sharp instruments from other instruments to be sanitized.
Purpose: To prevent possible self-injury.

3 Rinse the instruments under cold running water.
Purpose: To help remove debris and prevent coagulation of body fluids.

4 Open hinged instruments and scrub all grooves, crevices, and serrations with a brush.
Purpose: Microorganisms can hide under contaminants and not be destroyed by the disinfection process.

5 Rinse well with hot water.
Purpose: Hot water removes all soap and contaminant residue.

6 Towel dry all instruments thoroughly.
Purpose: Wet instruments can rust or become dull and also dilute disinfectant/sterilizing chemicals.

7 Remove utility gloves and wash hands thoroughly.
Purpose: To remove any possible contaminants.

8 Place sanitized instruments in designated area for disinfection or sterilization.
Purpose: Sanitized instruments must be removed from cleaning area to prevent possible cross-contamination.

---

coagulate to dry on an instrument. When you are ready to sanitize instruments, drain off the soak solution and rinse each instrument in cold, running water. Separate the sharp instruments from the others since other metal instruments may damage the cutting edges and the sharp instruments may injure the other instruments or you. Clean all the sharp instruments at one time, when you can concentrate on avoiding the dangers of injury to yourself. Open all hinges and scrub serrations and ratchets with a small scrub brush or toothbrush. Rinse the instruments in hot water, then check carefully for proper working order before they are disinfected or sterilized. The items should be hand dried with a towel to prevent spotting. Sanitization is a very important step, and it cannot be overlooked or done carelessly. The use of *disposable* instruments when working with human blood or giving injections minimizes the need for sanitization, disinfection, and sterilization.

Ultrasonic Sanitization. Sound waves can be used for sanitization of instruments by placing the instruments in a bath of ultrasonic cleaner and water. The sound vibrates and causes bubbling, thereby loosening the materials attached to the instruments. Ultrasonic cleaners are beneficial, since they do not damage even the most delicate instruments and workers do not run the risk of an accidental sharp injury.

Disinfection

Disinfection is the process of killing pathogenic organisms or of rendering them inactive. It is not always effective against spores, the tubercle bacilli, and certain viruses. Disinfectant chemicals may kill microbes within a short time but are usually very hard on the instruments. Some chemicals, such as Cidex, are effective enough to kill all organisms, but the usual immersion time for these sterilants is 10 or more hours. For equipment and countertop surfaces, the cheapest and most reliable method for disinfection is the use of a 1:10 bleach solution. It is an effective and noncaustic disinfectant that can be used to wipe laboratory countertops where human blood and other body-fluid samples are handled. It can also be used for soaking reusable rubber goods before sanitizing. In addition, bleach solution is used to disinfect dialysis equipment and is an effective disinfectant for surfaces that have come into contact with viruses, including HIV.

There are many types of disinfecting agents that have varying degrees of effectiveness. It is important to follow manufacturer's guidelines on how to properly use each product, as well as understand its advantages, disadvantages, and the possible sources of error.

Disinfection is very difficult to verify, because there are no convenient indicators to ensure destruction of the organisms. Even when the manufacturer's directions for chemical strength and immersion times are followed, there are six common errors that can cause chemicals to lose their effectiveness:

1. Instruments are not thoroughly sanitized, and attached organic matter inhibits or prevents the action of the disinfectant. No chemical can kill unless it

PROCEDURE **24-3**

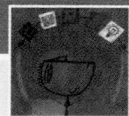

Removing Contaminated Latex Gloves

GOAL: To minimize pathogen exposure by aseptically removing and discarding contaminated gloves.

EQUIPMENT AND SUPPLIES

- Latex examination gloves
- Biohazard waste container

PROCEDURAL STEPS

1 With the dominant hand, grasp the glove of the opposite hand near the palm and begin removing the first glove (Figure 1). Arms should be extended from the body and hands pointed down.

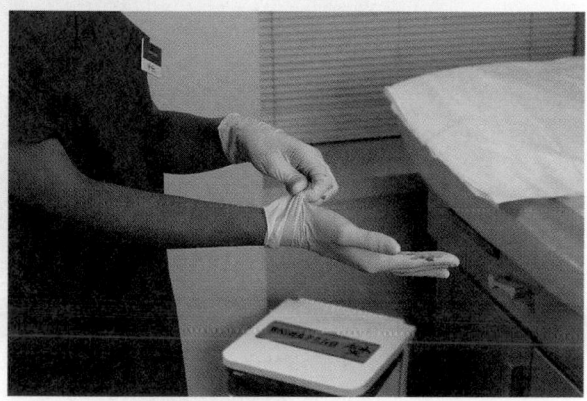

Figure 1

Purpose: Having the hands held down and away from the body helps avoid possible contamination.

2 Pull the glove inside out until you reach the fingers, holding the contaminated glove in the dominant gloved hand (Figure 2).

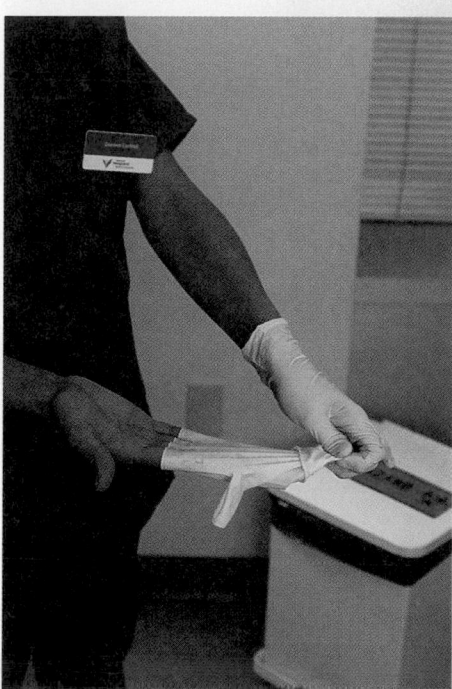

Figure 2

Purpose: Taking the glove off inside out prevents transmission of pathogens to a nongloved surface.

3 Insert the thumb of the nongloved hand inside the cuff of the remaining contaminated glove (Figure 3).

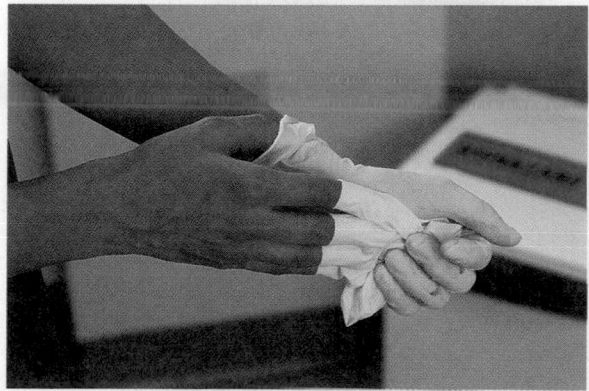

Figure 3

4 Pull the glove down the hand inside out over the contaminated glove being held, leaving the contaminated side of both gloves on the inside.

Purpose: The medical assistant is now protected from the contaminated surface of both gloves.

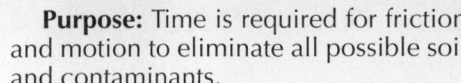

PROCEDURE 24-3—Cont'd

5 Properly dispose of the inside-out contaminated gloves in a biohazard waste container (Figure 4).

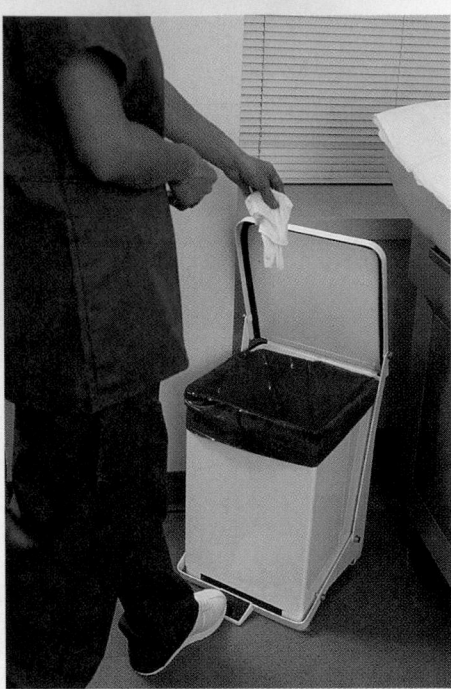

Figure 4

Purpose: Time is required for friction and motion to eliminate all possible soil and contaminants.

6 Perform a medical aseptic hand wash as described in Procedure 24-1.

Purpose: To minimize the number of pathogens on your hands, thus reducing the risk of pathogenic transmission.

---

reaches all instrument surfaces, therefore, complete sanitization is absolutely necessary.

2. Sanitized instruments are not dried, and the moisture on the instruments dilutes the disinfectant solution beyond the effective concentration.
3. A solution is left in an open container, and evaporation changes its concentration.
4. Solutions are not changed after the recommended period for use has expired.
5. The solutions are not prepared properly or not mixed properly before using.
6. The recommended manufacturer's temperature for use and storage is not maintained.

Alcohol is the most widely used antiseptic, but recent studies indicate that it is not as effective as other products in inhibiting the growth and reproduction of microorganisms on the skin surface. Isopropyl alcohol is an excellent fat solvent, which makes it good for cleansing the skin, but continued use leads to tissue breakdown. Other antiseptic chemicals, such as povidone-iodine solution (Betadine), are effective antimicrobial agents that are safe to use on patient skin.

Disinfection by Boiling (Moist Heat). Boiling (212°F or 100°C) kills most vegetative forms of pathogenic bacteria, but bacterial spores and some viruses associated with infectious hepatitis are resistant to temperatures of 212°F and less. No matter how much heat is applied or how vigorous the boil, water will reach only

212°F at sea level. The higher the elevation, the lower the temperature required to reach boiling (e.g., in Denver, Colorado, water boils at 202°F). This temperature is not high enough to kill spores and hepatitis viruses. Because of these limitations, *boiling does not sterilize* and is used for disinfection only. Boiling can be used to disinfect instruments, such as nasal or ear specula, that do not penetrate body tissues. An article must be boiled at a rolling (not vigorous) boil for at least 15 minutes to be adequately disinfected.

CRITICAL THINKING APPLICATION

Rosa is responsible for orienting the new medical assistant in the office on sanitization and disinfection procedures. Outline the important concepts and methods of each.

Sterilization

Sterilization, or the destruction of all microorganisms, is essential when conducting surgical asepsis. To ensure proper sterilization for aseptic procedures, an area should be set aside in each office for just this purpose. The area should be divided into two sections. One section is used for receiving contaminated materials. This area should have a sink as well as receiving basins, proper cleaning agents, brushes, sterilizer wrapping paper, sterilizer envelopes and tape, sterilizer indicators, disposable gloves, and designated biohazard waste containers. The other section should be reserved for receiving the sterile items after they are removed from the sterilizer. Clear, clean plastic bags in which to store sterile packs may be kept in the sterile area. Both areas should be spotlessly clean and well organized. Sterile technique will be addressed in Chapter 54.

Role of the Medical Assistant In Asepsis

Medical asepsis is one of the few procedures that directly affect the health of the patient, physician, and staff. The spread of pathogens in the ambulatory care setting can be controlled only through effective and consistent application of the Bloodborne Pathogens Standard and proper sanitization, disinfection, and sterilization of supplies, equipment, and work surfaces.

The medical assistant must develop an inner sense for aseptic procedures. It is important that these techniques be done on such a routine basis that they become an unbreakable habit. The use of disposable items is highly recommended in the control of the infection process. However, when disposable equipment is used, the assistant must follow recommended disposal guidelines.

Patient Education

The medical assistant should take every opportunity to educate his or her patient on the infection process and ways of preventing disease transmission. The best time to instruct your patient in aseptic techniques that can be used at home is while you are performing the aseptic procedure. For example:

- While hand washing, explain to the patient that this routine is part of daily hygiene and is particularly important for patients who are very young or old or who seem to get sick frequently. Discuss with the patient that hands should be washed before and after meals; after sneezing, coughing, or nose blowing; after using the bathroom; before and after changing a dressing; and after changing an infant's diaper.
- Explain to the patient how using disposable tissues to cover the nose and mouth when coughing or sneezing decreases the possibility of transmitting illness between household members.
- Discuss proper ways for disposing of used tissues, especially when one member of the household is suspected of having a communicable disease.
- Instruct the patient regarding the differences between sterile and clean dressings and bandages. Show him or her step by step how to change a dressing properly and then how to dispose of the contaminated items.

There are many ways that a medical assistant can help the patient. Here are a few more suggestions to educate and inform the patient about asepsis and infection control:

1. Set up an information table in the waiting room with take-home pamphlets and literature.
2. Mail a periodic newsletter to patients regarding infection control, especially during flu season.
3. Demonstrate and explain aseptic procedures to patients and/or family members, inviting them to participate.

Legal and Ethical Issues

A number of legal and ethical concerns are related to medical asepsis and infection control in the ambulatory care setting. Personal discipline is the primary concern in medical asepsis. Typically you are alone when performing a medical aseptic procedure, so if contamination occurs you are the only one who knows. If contamination occurs, it is your responsibility to start over again with clean supplies. One of the medical assistant's main responsibilities is to carry out disinfection and sterilization procedures with precision and total effectiveness. There is no room for compromise. Patients should have absolute assurance that they are being taken care of in an aseptic atmosphere and under aseptic conditions. This assurance is just as important for the protection of the physician and staff as it is for the patient. Allowing the physician to assume that the correct aseptic techniques have been employed in the preparation of equipment and allowing him or her to use contaminated equipment on a patient can result in possible malpractice. Honesty on the part of the medical assistant builds self-respect and contributes to professional achievement.

One of the primary reasons for performing aseptic procedures completely and effectively is to prevent the development of **nosocomial infections** in susceptible patients. These infections that are acquired in the health-care environment can be especially devastating to elderly or debilitated patients. Ignorance of the various aseptic techniques or carelessness can be dangerous and is inexcusable before the law.

More than 36 states have adopted Good Samaritan legislation, which protects bystanders and first responders from liability when they perform life saving procedures at the scene of an accident. If the individual acts in good faith, is not compensated, and performs techniques to the best of his or her knowledge, he or she is not liable for civil damages. However, because OSHA regulates employer responsibility for management of bloodborne pathogens, exposure at the scene of an accident will not be covered by employer postexposure incident policies. Therefore healthcare workers who volunteer their assistance in an emergency must enact bloodborne precautions as much as possible without expectation of medical follow-up at the workplace.

SUMMARY OF SCENARIO

Implementing standard precautions throughout daily practice is crucial to the welfare and protection of both the patient and the healthcare worker. Rosa must be sure to routinely wash hands, familiarize herself with the office's exposure control plan, utilize PPE when needed, follow appropriate procedures for cleaning up contaminated spills, and understand postexposure follow-up if there is an accidental exposure. In addition, Rosa must follow guidelines for sanitization, disinfection, and sterilization of appropriate instruments and equipment.

SUMMARY OF LEARNING OBJECTIVES

■ Pathogenic microorganisms are disease-causing microbes that fall into the categories of viruses, bacteria, protozoa, fungi, or rickettsiae. Tables 24-1 through 24-4 provide details on various diseases, their causative organisms, mode of transmission, typical patient symptoms, and the type of body specimen collected and tests performed to determine the diagnosis.

■ The chain of infection represents the method of infectious disease spread. It consists of the infectious agent and the reservoir host, continues with the means or portal of exit from the host, the mode of transmission, the means or portal of entry into a new host, and the presence of a susceptible host. To stop the spread of infection at least one of these links must be broken.

■ The inflammatory response is the body's reaction to the introduction of a foreign substance or antigen. It involves the release of inflammation mediators, which, through three separate actions, results in an increase of WBCs at the site of the injury.

■ The body's immune system operates on two different levels. Humoral immunity creates specific antibodies to combat antigens, and cell-mediated immunity attacks the source of the infection at the cellular level.

■ Acute diseases have a rapid onset and short duration; chronic diseases last over a long period, perhaps a lifetime; latent diseases cycle through relapse and remission phases.

■ Bacterial infections can be treated with antibiotics but viral infections, since they involve viral takeover of cellular DNA or RNA material, cannot be treated with antibiotics.

■ OSHA has designated certain body fluids, including cerebrospinal (CSF), synovial, pleural, pericardial, peritoneal, mucous, and amniotic fluids as potentially infectious for bloodborne pathogens. Blood, vaginal and seminal secretions, saliva, and human tissue are also in this category.

■ The Exposure Control Plan must be available for employee review and contain specifics on controls for bloodborne pathogens including PPE, training, hepatitis B immunization, record keeping, and the labeling and disposal of all biohazard waste.

■ Postexposure follow-up involves immediate cleansing of the site, examination of the source individual's and worker's blood, administration of prophylactic medications, health counseling, and confidential treatment of all medical records.

■ The OSHA Compliance Guidelines stipulate the management and implementation of barrier protection devices, environment protection, housekeeping controls, and administration of the hepatitis B immunization.

■ Medical asepsis involves the removal or destruction of pathogens, and surgical asepsis is the destruction of all microorganisms. Medical aseptic techniques are used to create an environment that is as free of pathogens as possible, whereas surgical asepsis, or sterile technique, is employed any time the patient's skin or mucous membranes are disrupted.

■ Sanitization is the cleaning of contaminated articles or surfaces to reduce the numbers of microorganisms; disinfection is the process of killing pathogenic organisms; and sterilization results in the destruction of all microorganisms.

■ A medical assistant must take every opportunity to teach patients about infection control and the potential danger of blood and body fluids. This includes demonstrating aseptic techniques, the proper management of infectious materials at home, and the importance of frequent and consistent hand washing.

■ A medical assistant is responsible for applying infection control procedures in all situations at all times in order to prevent cross-contamination and the development of nosocomial infections in patients.

KEY INTERNET WEBSITES

- Centers for Disease Control and Prevention
- Environmental Protection Agency
- National Institutes of Health
- Occupational Safety and Health Administration
- United States Public Health Service
  For active weblinks to each website visit
  http://evolve.elsevier.com/Kinn/

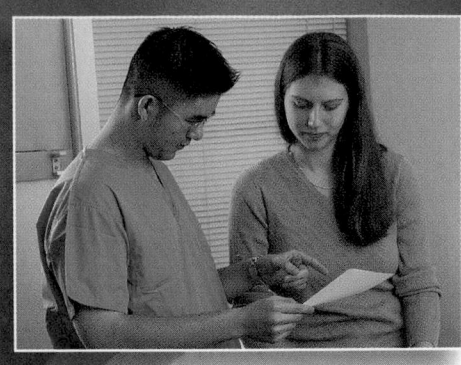

CHAPTER 25

Scenario

Chris Isaccson, CMA, works in an ambulatory care setting within the local hospital. He is responsible for initial patient interviews, taking medical histories, and documentation. Chris is having difficulty gathering the information needed from some of the clients. Patients do not always respond openly and honestly to him, and therefore the attending physician is not satisfied with his work. His supervisor is responsible for helping him improve his interview skills.

Patient Assessment

Learning Objectives

- Define and spell the terms listed in the vocabulary.
- Employ the components of holistic care in the patient assessment process.
- Describe the components of the patient's medical history.
- Define and apply the qualities of a helping relationship.
- Display sensitivity to diverse patient populations.
- Demonstrate therapeutic communications including the use of the linear communication model and active listening techniques.
- Recognize the importance of nonverbal communication when interacting with patients.
- Identify barriers to communication and their impact on patient assessment.
- Detect patient utilization of defense mechanisms and resultant barriers to therapeutic communication with a healthcare professional.
- Apply therapeutic communication techniques with patients across the lifespan.
- Demonstrate professional patient interview techniques.
- Integrate detailed information about the chief complaint into concise, accurate documentation methods.
- Use various medical record systems employed in the physician's office.
- Describe the connection between the interview process and implementation of patient education practices.
- Determine risk management strategies for the ambulatory care setting.
- Obtain a written medical history from a patient.

National Curriculum Competencies

CLINICAL COMPETENCIES

4a. Perform telephone and in-person screening
4c. Obtain and record patient history

TRANSDISCIPLINARY COMPETENCIES

1b. Recognize and respond to verbal communication
1c. Recognize and respond to nonverbal communication
2a. Identify and respond to issues of confidentiality
2c. Establish and maintain the medical record
2d. Document appropriately
2e. Perform risk management procedures

Vocabulary

biophysical Pertaining to the science dealing with the application of physical methods and theories to biologic problems.

chief complaint The reason for the patient's seeking medical care.

cognitive Pertaining to the operation of the mind process by which we become aware of perceiving, thinking, and remembering.

congruence The verbal expression of the message matches the sender's nonverbal body language.

diagnosis Concise technical description of the cause, nature, or manifestations of a condition or problem. *Initial:* Physician's temporary impression, sometimes called a *working diagnosis. Differentiated diagnosis:* comparison of two or more diseases with similar signs and symptoms. *Final:* Conclusion physician reaches after evaluating all findings, including laboratory and other test results.

familial Occurring in or affecting members of a family more than would be expected by chance.

present illness The chief complaint, written in chronological sequence, with dates of onset.

psychosocial Pertaining to a combination of psychological and social factors.

rapport Relationship of harmony and accord between the patient and the healthcare professional.

As medical professionals directly involved in gathering information from patients about their health status, medical assistants must remember that a healthy state is more than the absence of disease. The assessment process should be a reflection of the entire patient, not just a report about signs and symptoms. Lifestyles and environmental factors can create disease and therefore should be considered when we gather information about the **chief complaint**. Not just physical data but **cognitive**, **psychosocial**, and behavioral data are significant for the analysis of a patient's health status. This method of analyzing the development of disease is based on a holistic perspective. *Holistic patient care* recognizes that illness is the result of many factors, not just physical ones.

Assessment factors are a list of **biophysical** signs and symptoms. The first step in treating a disease process is for the physician to determine the patient's medical **diagnosis**. The identification of disease begins with the physician's *working* diagnosis, which he or she has determined through the patient's history, report of the chief complaint, and physical examination. Next the physician orders laboratory tests, diagnostic examinations, and/or a referral visit to another physician to substantiate or refute the working diagnosis. Once the test results are received, the *clinical* diagnosis is established. The patient is then treated, and after a period of time is reevaluated to see whether the clinical diagnosis has changed. If it has, the new diagnosis is called the *differentiated* diagnosis. The physician continues to evaluate the progress of the patient and order tests and/or alters treatment as needed.

However, patient care does not start with the physical examination; it begins when the patient makes first contact with the office. Even before the examination, the medical assistant has the opportunity to interact with the patient to ensure that he or she feels comfortable during the process and that all the necessary information is obtained.

Interviewing patients, assisting with examinations, and documentation are important responsibilities for a medical assistant. You must know the components and techniques for securing a medical history that will help the physician in the diagnosis and treatment of the patient. The more complete the medical history, the more efficient the physician's care and treatment will be.

Medical History

Collecting the History Information

When a new patient calls or comes in for an appointment, the patient is asked to complete a health history form. Besides being useful for diagnosing and treating the patient, the self-history allows the patient more participation in the process. The form may be mailed to the patient's home before the appointment or may be completed in the office during the first visit.

If you are responsible for taking a portion of the medical history, conduct the interview in a private area free from outside interference and beyond the hearing range of other patients (Figure 25-1). Patients will not talk freely where they may be overheard or interrupted. The interview room should be physically comfortable and conducive to confidential communications. Legally and ethically, the patient has the right to privacy, and access to the patient's medical record is permitted only to individuals directly involved in the patient's care. Listen to the patient. Do not express surprise or displeasure at any of the patient's statements. Remember, you are there not to pass judgment but to gather medical data. Document the information in an organized manner, exactly as given by the patient, without opinion or interpretation.

In some facilities the physician takes the medical history during the patient's initial visit. The physician will correlate

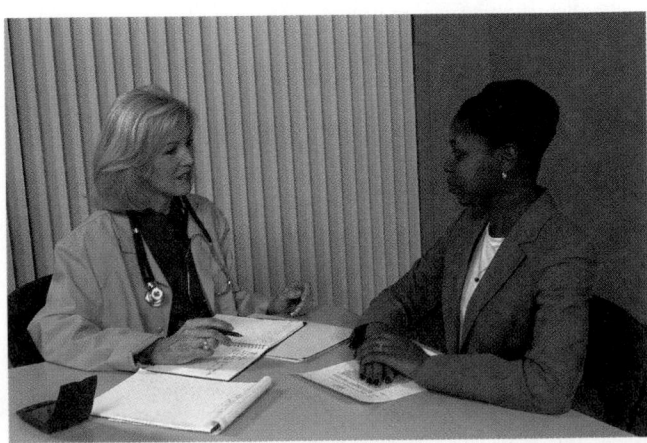

FIGURE 25-1 Private patient interview area.

the physical findings in the examination with the information in the history. The complete medical history and the physical examination form the foundation and starting point for all patient/physician contracts.

Components of the Medical History

Medical history forms may vary, depending on the physician's preference and the practice specialty. The most common medical history method includes these components:

1. *Database:* Record of the patient's name, address, date of birth, insurance information, personal data, history, physical examination, and initial laboratory findings. As new information is added, it becomes a part of this database.
2. *Past history (PH) or past medical history (PMH):* Summary of the patient's previous health. It includes dates and details regarding the patient's usual childhood diseases (UCD or UCHD), major illnesses, surgeries, allergies, accidents, and immunization record.
3. *Family history (FH):* Details regarding the patient's mother and father, their health, and, if deceased, the cause and age of death. Hereditary and/or **familial** diseases and disorders are recorded here and may include information about siblings and offspring. This information is important because certain diseases and disorders have familial and/or hereditary tendencies.
4. *Social history (SH):* Information regarding the patient's lifestyle, hobbies, entertainment preferences, education, occupation, use of tobacco and alcohol, sleeping habits, methods of exercise, diet, and sex life are noted in this section. This information assists the physician in planning treatment for the patient or in determining causative factors for disease. It also provides a holistic picture of the patient's health.
5. *Systems review (SR) or review of systems (ROS):* Guide to general health; tends to detect conditions other than those covered in the **present illness**. Often a patient may think certain health problems irrelevant and fail to mention them. These problems may help the physician in determining the cause of the disorder being presently explored. A system review is obtained by a logical sequence of questions regarding the state of health of body systems, beginning with the head and proceeding downward.

Understanding and Communicating With Patients

To provide quality patient care, we must communicate effectively with the patient and provide a warm, caring environment. Positive reactions and interactions with the patient are essential. As the patient progresses through the various levels of healthcare, all members of the medical team must exercise a variety of special skills to enhance the process. These skills are not all technical and medical. Many involve the art of caring for the patient as a human being; that is, consistently implementing

respectful patient care. Because medical care is of an extremely personal nature, a medical assistant must always remember that each patient is an individual with certain anxieties. These anxieties often cause people to act and react in different ways, making effective verbal and nonverbal communication with each patient absolutely essential.

Healthcare professionals accept the responsibility of developing helping relationships with their clients. The interpersonal nature of the patient–medical assistant relationship carries with it a certain amount of responsibility to detach your self-interest and focus on the needs of your patients. A medical assistant, simply by the way he or she treats and interacts with patients, can create either a positive or a negative patient response to care. You are usually the first person the patient communicates with and therefore you play a vital role in initiating therapeutic patient interactions.

Sensitivity to Diversity

Demonstrating respectful patient care is extremely important when working with a diverse patient population. *Empathy* is the key to creating a caring, therapeutic environment. Empathetic sensitivity to diversity first requires those interested in healthcare to examine their own values, beliefs, and actions. It is impossible to treat all patients with caring and respect until you first recognize and evaluate personal biases. There are many reasons why we think and act a certain way. The first step in understanding the process is to evaluate your individual *value system*. Why do you have certain attitudes or beliefs about the worth of individuals or things?

CRITICAL THINKING APPLICATION

What do you value most in life? What is important to you? What influences you to act in a certain way? Make a list of five "things" you value the most and share them with the class. Try to determine why you feel so strongly about those particular items.

Many different factors shape value system development. Value systems begin as learned beliefs and behaviors. Families, as well as cultural influences, shape the way we respond to a diverse society. To develop therapeutic relationships, you must recognize your own value system to determine whether it could affect your method of interaction. Other factors that influence reactions include socioeconomic and educational backgrounds. Whatever the history of value system development, preconceived ideas about people because of their race, religion, income level, ethnic origin, sexual orientation, or gender can cause serious trouble for the therapeutic relationship. It is impossible to treat your patients empathetically unless you can connect with them in some way. Personal biases, or prejudices, act as overwhelming barriers to the development of therapeutic relationships (Figure 25-2).

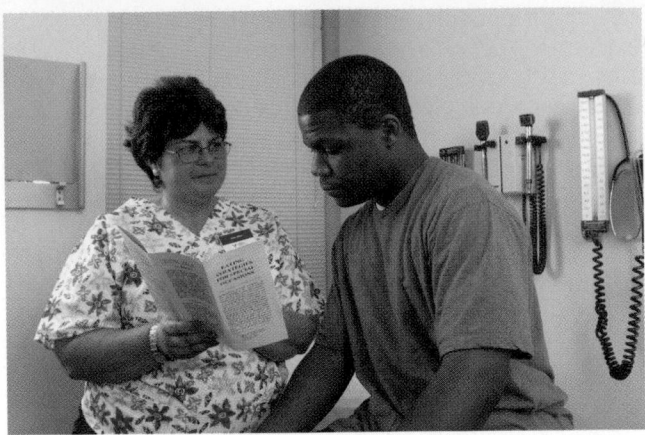

FIGURE 25-2 Respectful patient care.

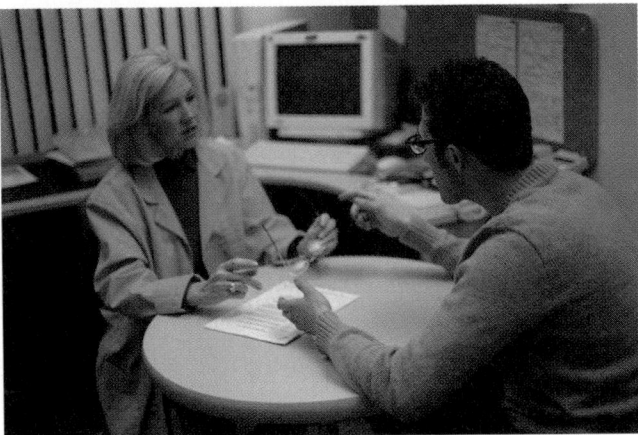

FIGURE 25-3 Active listening.

CRITICAL THINKING APPLICATION

Honestly evaluate your personal biases. What do you find unacceptable in people? Do you pre-judge an individual based on his or her affiliation with a particular group or because of a certain lifestyle decision? Do these biases create barriers to the development of therapeutic relationships? If so, how can you get beyond these barriers?

Therapeutic Techniques

Chapter 5 introduced the communication process. The linear communication model describes communication as an interactive process involving the sender of the message, the receiver, and the crucial component of feedback to confirm the reception of the message. All medical assistants must be effective communicators. You will play a vital role in collecting and documenting patient information. If your methods of collection or recording are faulty, it could seriously affect the quality of patient care.

Active Listening Techniques. Active listeners go beyond *hearing* the patient's message to concentrating, understanding, and *listening* to the main points in the discussion. Active listening techniques encourage patients to expand on and clarify the content and meaning of their messages. They are very useful communication tools to implement when a patient is agitated or upset, since these methods help patients clearly hear what they are saying.

There are three processes involved in active listening: *restatement*, *reflection*, and *clarification*. Restatement is simply paraphrasing, or repeating, the patient's statements with phrases such as "You are saying…" or "You are telling me the problem is…." Reflection involves repeating the main idea of the conversation while also identifying the feelings of the sender. For example, if the mother of a young patient is expressing frustration about her child's behavior, a reflective statement identifies that feeling with the response, "You sound frustrated about…." Or, if a new insulin-dependent diabetic patient exhibits anxiety about administering injections, an appropriate reflective statement recognizes the patient's feelings with "You are anxious about…." Reflective statements clearly demonstrate to patients that you are not only listening to their words, but you are also attending to their feelings. Therefore reflection is an excellent method of communicating concern to your patients. Finally, clarification seeks to summarize or simplify the sender's thoughts and feelings as well as resolve any confusion in the message. Questions or statements that begin with "Give me an example of…" or "Explain to me about…" help patients focus on the chief complaint as well as give you the opportunity to clear up any misconceptions before documenting patient information.

Listening is not a passive role in the communication process; it is active and demanding. You cannot be preoccupied with your own needs, or you will miss something important. For the time of the patient interview, no one is more important than this patient. Listen to the way things are said, the tone of the patient's voice, and even to what the patient is not saying out loud. Listening is probably the most effective communication technique available. It requires the medical assistant's complete attention and a great deal of energy (Figure 25-3).

Nonverbal Communication. Much of what we communicate to our patients is through the use of conscious or unconscious body language. Our nonverbal actions, such as gestures, facial expressions, and mannerisms, are learned behaviors that are greatly influenced by our family and cultural backgrounds. The body naturally expresses our true feelings; in fact, experts say that more than 90% of communication is nonverbal in nature. Most of the negative messages communicated through body language are unintentional; therefore, while conducting patient interviews, it is important to remember that nonverbal communication behaviors can seriously affect the therapeutic process.

The verbal messages you send are only part of the communication process. You have a specific context in mind when you send your words, but the receiver puts his or her own interpretations on them. The receiver attaches meaning determined by his or her past experiences, culture, self-concept, as well as the current physical and emotional state. Sometimes these messages and interpretations do not coincide. Feedback from the patient is crucial in determining the patient's understanding of the message. It takes mutual understanding by both the interviewer and the person being interviewed to have successful communication.

Observing your patient during the interview will foster mutual understanding. The purpose of observing nonverbal communication is to become sensitive to or aware of the feelings of others as conveyed by small bits of behavior, rather than words. This sensitivity enables you to adapt your behavior to these feelings, to consciously select your response, either verbal or nonverbal, and thereby have a favorable effect on others. The favorable effect may consist of providing emotional support, conveying that you care, defusing the other's fear or anger, or providing an invitation to release pent-up feelings by talking about the situation that aroused the feelings. Table 25-1 lists some patient nonverbal behaviors that may indicate anxiety, frustration, or fear.

You can do much to put a patient at ease through the tone of your voice. Facial expression and the ease and confidence of your movements demonstrate to the patient a sincere interest. Therapeutic use of space and touch are also important ways of sending nonverbal messages to your patients. You should establish eye contact, sit in a relaxed but attentive position, and avoid the use of furniture as a barrier between you and the patient. Give the patient your undivided attention and let your body language inform each patient that you are interested in his or her medical problems (Figure 25-4). The key to successful patient interaction is **congruence** between verbal and nonverbal messages. Although choosing the correct words is very important, only 7% of the message received is verbal, so to be seen as honest and sensitive to the needs of your patients you must be aware of your nonverbal behavior patterns. The nonverbal message the patient receives by the medical assistant's listening behavior should be, "You are a person of worth and I am interested in you as a unique person."

PREPARING THE APPROPRIATE ENVIRONMENT

Ensure Privacy

Make sure the room you are using is unoccupied for the entire time allowed for the interview. The patient needs to feel sure that no one can overhear the conversation or interrupt.

Prevent Interruptions

Inform your co-workers of the interview and ask them not to interrupt you during this time. You need to concentrate and to establish **rapport**. An interruption can destroy in seconds what you have spent many minutes building up.

Prepare Comfortable Surroundings

Conducting the interview in comfortable surroundings reduces patient anxiety. Keep the distance between you and the patient at 4 to 5 feet. Arrange chairs so you and the patient are comfortably seated at eye level and the desk or table does not act as a barrier between you.

Take Judicious Notes

Note-taking should be kept to a minimum while you try to focus your attention on the person. Note-taking during the interview has disadvantages, such as breaking eye contact and shifting your attention away from the patient, which diminishes the patient's sense of importance. However, it is important to write down pertinent details as you are interviewing, because you may forget important facts if you do not note them at the time of the discussion. With experience you will develop a personal type of shorthand that you can use during the interview process.

HELPFUL LISTENING GUIDELINES

Listen to the main points in the discussion.
Attend to both verbal and nonverbal
     messages.
Be patient and nonjudgmental.
Do not interrupt.
Never intimidate your patient.
Use active listening techniques: restatement,
     reflection, and clarification.

Environmental Factors. Before you meet with the patient, prepare the physical setting. The setting may be an examination room, the staff lounge, or an office. In any location, optimal conditions are important to have a smooth, productive interview.

TABLE 25-1	Nonverbal Communication Observations
Area Observed	**Observation**
Breathing patterns	Rapid respirations, sighing, shallow thoracic breathing
Eye patterns	No eye contact, side-to-side movement, looking down at hands
Hands	Tapping fingers, cracking knuckles, continuous movement, wet/sweaty palms
Arm placement	Folded across chest, wrapped around abdomen
Leg placement	Tension, crossed and/or tucked under, tapping foot, continuous movement

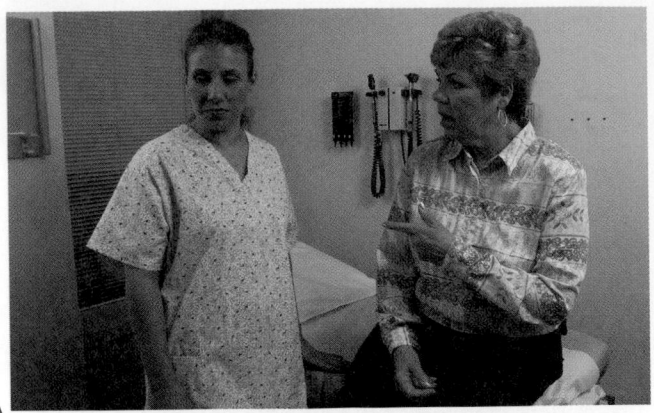

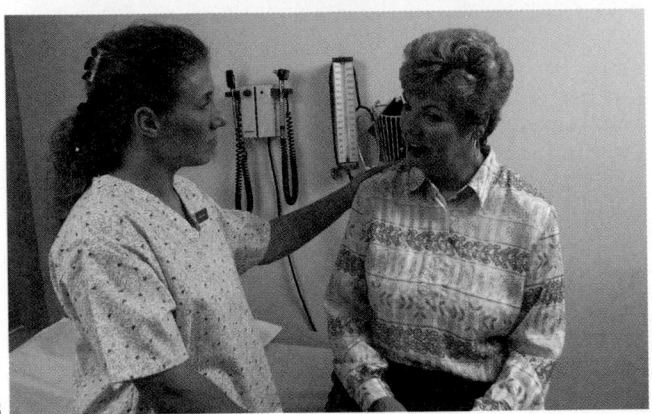

FIGURE 25-4 **A,** Ineffective nonverbal language. **B,** Therapeutic nonverbal language.

Open-Ended Questions. An open-ended question asks for general information. It states the topic to be discussed, but only in general terms. Use it to begin the interview, to introduce a new section of questions, whenever the person introduces a new topic, or to gather more details from the patient.

> What brings you to the doctor?
> How have you been getting along?
> You mentioned having dizzy spells. Tell me more about that.

This type of question encourages the patient to respond in a manner that is comfortable for him or her. It allows the patient to express himself or herself fully and provide details about the chief complaint.

Closed Questions. Direct or closed questions ask for specific information. This form of questioning limits the answer to one or two words, a yes or no in many cases. Use this form of question when you need confirmation of specific facts, such as when asking about past health problems.

> Do you have a headache?
> What is your birth date?
> Have you ever broken a bone?

Interviewing the Patient

The interview, or gathering the patient's medical history, is the first and most important part of data collection. The

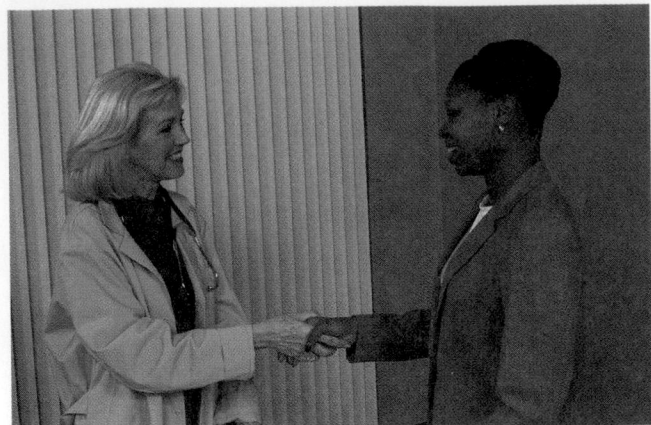

FIGURE 25-5 Greeting the patient.

medical history identifies patient health strengths and problems and is a bridge to the next step in data collection, the physical examination. At this point the individual knows everything about his or her own health state and you know nothing. Your skill in interviewing will glean the necessary information as well as build rapport for a successful working relationship.

Consider the interview as a form of *contract* between you and your patient. The contract consists of spoken and unspoken language and addresses what the patient needs and expects from the healthcare visit. The patient interview consists of three stages: the initiation or introduction, the body, and the closing.

The *initiation* of the interview is the time to introduce yourself and identify the patient as well as the purpose of the interview (Figure 25-5). If you are nervous about how to begin, remember to keep it short. The patient is probably nervous too and is anxious to get started. Address the patient, using his or her last name, and give the reason for the interview:

> Mr. Coleman, my name is Stacey and I am a certified medical assistant who works with Dr. Yang. I have some questions to ask you regarding your health history. Would you mind sharing this information with me?

After the brief introduction, move on to the body of the interview. This is when you use various therapeutic communication techniques to determine why the patient is seeking healthcare, the patient's perception of the problem, the characteristics of the problem, and the patient's expectations of care. During this time use active listening skills, meaningful silence, congruent verbal and nonverbal communication, and a combination of open and closed statements and questions to gather the details of the patient's history and current health problem (Table 25-2).

Conclude the interview by summarizing the results of your interaction. The *closing* of the interview should clarify the patient's chief complaint, the purpose of the health visit, and the patient's expectations of care. This is the patient's opportunity to add any additional details or to explain further the characteristics of their health problem.

TABLE 25-2	Therapeutic Communication Techniques
Technique	**Value**
Open-ended questions	Encourages patient to respond in a comfortable manner
Direct questions	Ask for specific information; usually reply is a yes or no answer
Listening	Nonverbally communicates your interest in the patient
Silence	Nonverbally communicates your acceptance of the patient
Establishing guidelines	Helps the patient to know what is expected
Acknowledgment	Shows the importance of the patient's role
Restating	Checks your interpretation of the patient's message for validation
Reflecting	Shows the patient the importance of his or her feelings
Summarizing	Helps patient to separate relevant from irrelevant material

Interview Barriers

In Chapter 5 we discussed barriers to communication. In this chapter we are going to look at the effect of communication blocks on the patient interview. Certain communication behaviors create nonproductive messages that may be misleading or restrict the patient's response.

Providing Unwarranted Assurance. Mrs. Miller says to you, "I know this lump is going to turn out to be cancer." The typical reply is almost automatic: "Don't worry, I'm sure everything will be fine." This type of answer indicates her anxiety is insignificant and denies her the opportunity to further discuss her fears. A reflective response, such as, "You are really worried about…" acknowledges her feelings as well as demonstrates empathy and a willingness to listen to her concerns.

Giving Advice. Mrs. Thompson has just finished talking to the doctor and she looks at you and says, "Dr. Rowe says I need surgery to get rid of these gallstones. I just don't know. What would you do?" If you give her an answer, you have shifted the accountability for decision-making from her to you, and she has not worked out her own solution. Does this woman really want to know what you would do? Probably not. You could respond to her question with, "Based on what the doctor told you, what do you think you should do?" or "Do you need further information to make your decision?"

Using Medical Terminology. You must adjust your vocabulary to the patient. The more the patient understands about what is happening and what the management of the problem will be, the better the outcome is. Misinterpreted communication is the most frequent error encountered in patient care. One of the biggest problems for the patient is in understanding medical terminology. Closely observe the patient's body language while receiving instructions or patient education. If the patient shows signs of not understanding the procedure, ask the patient to repeat back to you the information or instructions. This repeat-demonstration form of providing feedback ensures that the patient completely understands what is happening.

Leading Questions. During the interview, you ask the patient, "You don't smoke, do you?" By asking the patient questions in this manner, you indicate the preferred answer. To tell you that he or she does smoke would surely meet with your disapproval. Keep your questions positive. A better way of asking would be to say, "Have you ever smoked?" or "Do you use tobacco?"

Talking Too Much. Some medical assistants associate helpfulness with verbal overload. The patient may let the interviewer talk at the expense of his or her own need to express himself or herself. Always remember: when interviewing a patient you should listen more than you talk.

Defense Mechanisms. In Chapter 5 we discussed the impact of defense mechanisms on professional communications. Many individuals respond to anxiety-provoking situations by automatically relying on defense mechanisms. Since defense mechanisms are used consciously or unconsciously to block an emotionally painful experience, it is understandable why patients facing a traumatic diagnosis or a difficult treatment would need to protect themselves from the reality of the situation. The problem is, how can we ensure compliance with treatment if the patient is in denial, projecting feelings onto the healthcare worker, or repressing the need for treatment or diagnostic follow-up? The medical assistant needs to be sensitive to the use of defense mechanisms by patients and must consistently apply therapeutic communication techniques to patient interactions.

CRITICAL THINKING APPLICATION

Mr. Gonzales, a 48-year-old patient recently diagnosed with hypertension, did not show up today for his follow-up appointment. Chris calls to find out why he failed to keep the appointment, and the patient tells Chris he forgot to come, even though an appointment reminder call was made yesterday. He also tells Chris he has not been taking his medicine and does not understand why it is so important for him and his wife to meet with the dietitian. Is this patient exhibiting defense mechanisms? How should Chris manage the situation?

Communication Across the Lifespan

The key to effectively communicating with patients is using an age-specific approach. Given the age and developmental level of your patient, how can you best interact with him or her as well as with significant family members?

For example, Tasha is a 2-year-old patient scheduled for a physical examination. How can you best interact with the child and her father to ensure that the history phase of the visit is complete and accurate? Therapeutic use of nonverbal language is essential when interacting with children of all ages. Getting down on the child's level, establishing eye contact, and using a gentle but firm voice are ways of gaining the child's confidence and cooperation. Children fear the unknown, so it is important to explain all procedures with language the child understands. At the same time, the medical assistant needs to continue to communicate to the child's caregiver so he or she can contribute to the intake process (Figure 25-6). Some important guidelines to follow when conducting the health history of a child include the following:

- The environment should be safe and attractive.
- Do not keep children and their caregivers waiting any longer than necessary, since they become anxious and/or distracted quickly.
- Do not offer a choice unless the child can truly make one. If part of the treatment requires that the child receive an injection, asking her if she'd like her shot now will get an automatic "No." However, giving her a choice of stickers after the injection is appropriate.
- Praising the child during the examination helps decrease anxiety and increase self-esteem. When possible, direct questions toward the child so he or she feels part of the process.
- Involving the child in the examination by permitting him or her to manipulate the equipment may help relieve anxiety. If possible, use your imagination and make a game of the assessment or the procedure.
- A typical defense mechanism seen in sick or anxious children is regression. The child may refuse to leave mother's lap or may want to hold a favorite toy during the procedure as a comfort measure. Look for signs of anxiety such as thumb-sucking or rocking during the assessment.
- Listen to parents' concerns and respond truthfully to questions (Figure 25-7).

Older children may also display difficulty during the health visit (Figure 25-8). To help them gain a sense of control, they should be allowed to make certain decisions about treatment. For example, Heather, a 13-year-old diabetic patient, could be given the choice of having her father present during the visit. Or, if she requires an insulin injection, the adolescent could choose the site of the injection or perhaps administer the medication herself.

This would give the medical assistant an opportunity to observe her technique as well as permit Heather to exert her independence.

Privacy is also an important issue to consider with older children. During the physical examination, respect privacy by keeping body exposure to a minimum and adequately preparing the child for procedures and positions. In addition, older children want to know what is going on during the examination, what to expect, and what the findings mean, so it is important to keep them informed in a language they can understand. The child should always be encouraged to ask questions, which should be answered as completely and clearly as possible. Take every opportunity to teach your patients, regardless of their age, about their disease and significant wellness factors (Figure 25-9).

Patient education is extremely important when interacting with adult clients. Therefore using language they can understand and involving them in treatment decisions as much as possible are essential in developing a helping relationship with your older patients. Adults are bombarded by multiple responsibilities, so stress-related health problems are not unusual in this patient population.

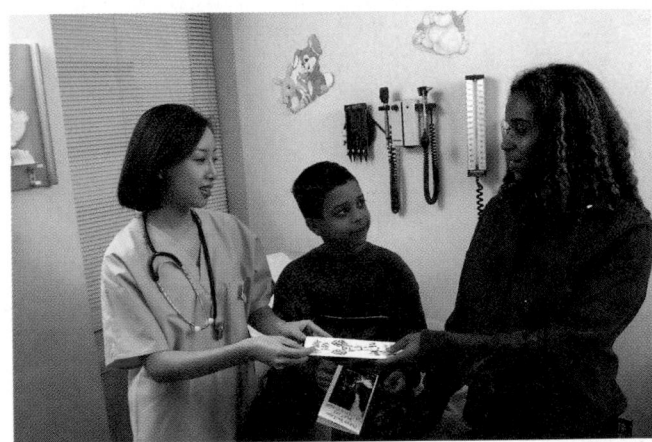

FIGURE 25-7 Responding to parental concerns.

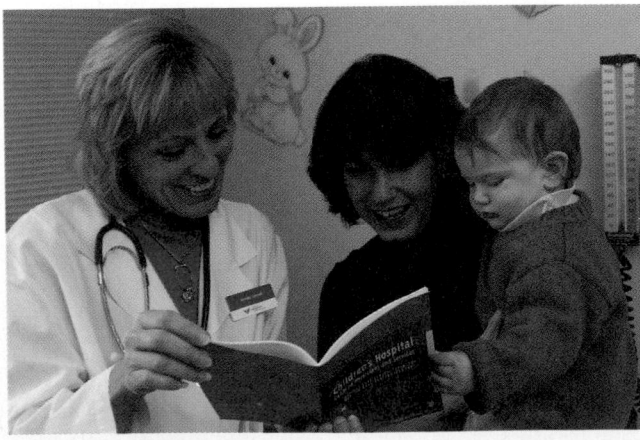

FIGURE 25-6 Interacting with a parent and child.

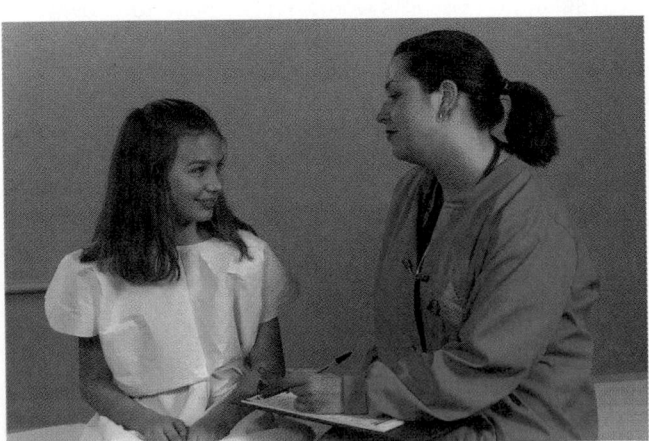

FIGURE 25-8 Interacting with a school-aged child.

Get to know your adult clients and emphasize preventive healthcare when possible (Figure 25-10). Specific communication techniques for therapeutic interactions with aging adults will be addressed in Chapter 45 (Procedure 25-1).

Assessing the Patient

After completion of the interview, the patient is escorted to an examination room and prepared for the physical examination, which is performed by the physician or healthcare professional such as a physician's assistant or nurse practitioner. The medical assistant's role in assisting with the physical examination will be discussed in detail in Chapter 29. During the examination the healthcare provider will methodically check all the body systems. As this examination is done, the physician is mentally comparing the patient's system with established norms for that system. When something deviates from the accepted normal range, it is documented in the patient's chart. Table 25-3 lists the systems of the body and the signs and symptoms that would be evaluated for each system. The usual examination begins with the top of the head

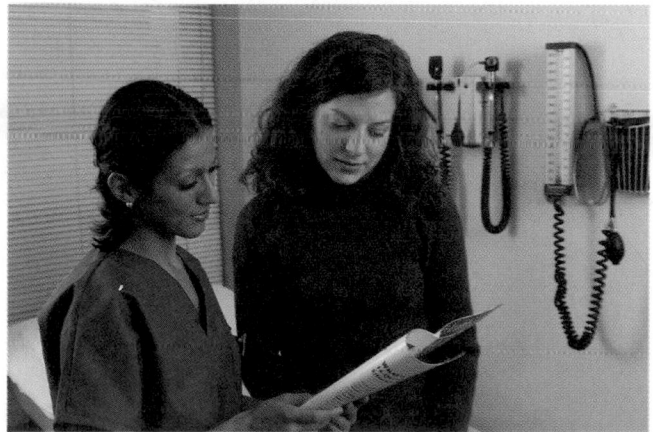

FIGURE 25-9   Interacting with an adolescent.

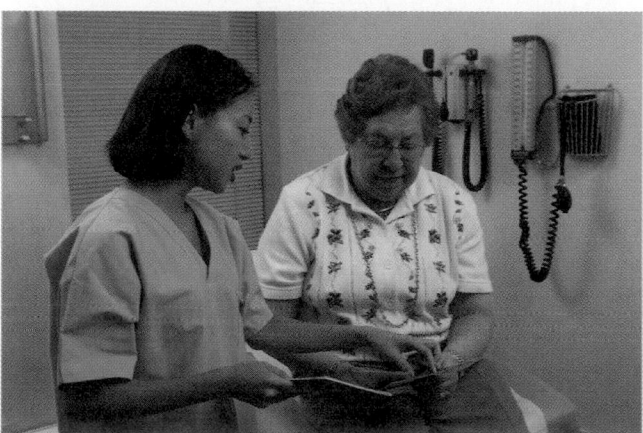

FIGURE 25-10   Adult patient education.

and progresses to the feet. However, depending on the specialty of the physician, the order may vary.

Signs and Symptoms

When the physician completes the examination, all of the signs and symptoms documented will be evaluated. To better understand the examination processes, it is important that you know the difference between a sign and a symptom.

Subjective findings, or *symptoms*, are perceptible only to the patient; they are what the patient *feels*. Only the patient feels an ache, pain, or dizziness, and only the patient can tell you it exists. The typical method of recording a complaint of pain is to quantify the pain by asking the patient, "On a scale of 1 to 10, with 1 being the least amount of pain and 10 being the greatest, how would you describe the pain?" Symptoms of the greatest significance in identifying a disease are called *cardinal symptoms*.

Objective findings, or *signs*, are perceptible to a person other than the patient, specifically the physician and the medical assistant. They are the signs that a physician detects when examining a patient. The physician feels, sees, or hears the signs that are often associated with a certain disease or abnormal condition. A mass that a physician feels in the patient's abdomen is an objective finding and a sign of an abnormal condition. The medical assistant obtains the patient's blood pressure, temperature, and pulse, which are also objective signs.

Other terms that require understanding are the words *functional* and *physical* (organic). When a condition or disease is functional, it is without organic cause; that is, the organ appears normal, but it is not functioning normally. An example of a functional problem would be if the patient has had repeated bouts of increased urinary albumin, but all tests on the kidney show a normal, healthy organ. A physical, or organic, disease or condition is one in which the abnormality can be seen or felt or clinically proven via laboratory or other diagnostic tests.

Documentation

The method used for charting may vary, depending on the healthcare provider's preference. However, regardless of the type of documentation used, certain charting procedures have been standardized to meet the necessary legalities of maintaining medical records accurately and concisely. Accurate and complete documentation is one of the primary responsibilities of a medical assistant (Figure 25-11).

CORRECT METHOD OF CHARTING

- Check the name on the record and be certain that the information being charted is recorded on the correct form on the correct patient's chart.

PROCEDURE **25-1**

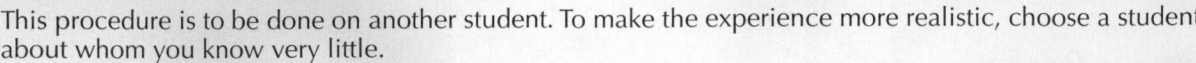

Obtaining a Medical History

This procedure is to be done on another student. To make the experience more realistic, choose a student about whom you know very little.

GOAL: To obtain an acceptable written background from the patient to help the physician determine the cause and effects of the present illness. This includes the chief complaint (CC), present illness (PI), past history (PH), family history (FH), and social history (SH).

EQUIPMENT AND SUPPLIES

- History form
- Two pens—a red pen for recording patient allergies and a black pen to meet legal documentation guidelines
- A quiet, private area

PROCEDURAL STEPS

1 Greet and identify the patient in a pleasant manner. Introduce yourself and explain your role.

Purpose: To make the patient feel comfortable and at ease.

2 Take the patient to a quiet, private area for the interview and explain to the patient why the information is needed.

Purpose: A quiet, private area is necessary to protect confidentiality and prevent interruptions. An informed patient is more cooperative and thus more likely to contribute useful information.

3 Complete the history form by using therapeutic communication techniques. Make sure that all medical terminology is adequately explained. A self-history may have been mailed to the patient before the visit. If so, review the self-history for completeness.

Purpose: Therapeutic communication techniques will assist the medical assistant in gathering complete information while the self-history is designed to save time and to involve the patient in the process.

4 Speak in a pleasant, distinct manner, remembering to maintain eye contact with your patient.

Purpose: Positive nonverbal behaviors create a friendly atmosphere.

5 Record the following statistical information on the patient information form:

    Patient's full name, including middle initial
    Address, including apartment number and ZIP code
    Marital status
    Sex (gender)
    Age and date of birth
    Telephone number for home and work
    Insurance information if not already available
    Employer's name, address, telephone number

6 Record the following medical history on the patient history (PH) form:

Chief complaint (CC)	Present illness
Past history	Family history
Social history	

Purpose: This is information that the physician needs to know to make an accurate assessment and diagnosis. The physician usually completes the review of systems (ROS) during the preexamination interview.

7 Ask about allergies to drugs and any other substances, and record any allergies in red ink on every page of the history form, on the front of the chart, and on each progress note page. Some practices apply allergy alert labels to the front of each chart.

Purpose: The presence of an allergy may alter medication and treatment procedures.

8 Record all information legibly and neatly and spell words correctly. Print rather than write in longhand. Do not erase, scribble, or use whiteout. If you make an error, draw a single line through the error, write "error" above it, add the correction, and initial and date the entry.

Purpose: To maintain a medical record that is understandable and defensible in a court of law.

9 Thank the patient for cooperating and direct him or her back to the reception area.

10 Review the record for errors before you pass it to the physician.

11 Use the information on the record to complete the patient's chart. Keep the information confidential.

Purpose: All information concerning the patient must remain in the office. This information may be legally and ethically discussed with only the physician.

Documentation Practice: Your patient's CC is dizziness for 2 weeks. She denies headaches, Hx of ear infections, or Hx of hypertension. Her BP is 172/94, T 97.6, P 88, R 22. Document pertinent patient findings using the SOAPE method.

S: _____

O: _____

_____

CORRECT METHOD OF CHARTING—Cont'd

- All charting is done in black ink. *Never use pencil.*
- Write in a clear, legible manner.
- When entering information on a patient's chart, sign the entry, including the appropriate initials after your name (e.g., CMA). The month, day, and year must precede the entry.
- All unusual complaints, symptoms, or reactions must be noted in detail. Include complete information regarding the *onset*, *duration*, and *frequency* of signs and symptoms.
- Describe objective data, such as the presence of a wound, using correct anatomical medical terminology.
- If the patient reports pain, the quality and intensity of the pain should be recorded using a pain scale of from 1 to 10.
- If patient comments are entered in the patient's own words, enclose them in quotation marks.
- Document a complete medication history, including both prescription and over-the-counter (OTC) medications taken on a regular basis, the last dose taken of the medication, the effectiveness of the medication, and any other pertinent details.
- Record details regarding a previous history of the current chief complaint (CC).
- Learn to be observant and to note anything that seems pertinent.
- Spelling, abbreviations, symbols, and terminology used must be accurate.
- Review your documentation immediately after completion so errors can be detected while the information is fresh in your mind.
- *Never* scribble, erase, or use whiteout on an error. For legal purposes it must be possible to read the corrected error.
- Correct the error by drawing one line through it. Write "error" above the corrected word or words and date and initial the correction. Then write in the correction.
- If details are omitted, add information by documenting after the last entry. Record "late entry," include date and time of note, and document the omitted information (see Figure 25-11).

Terminology

Medical terminology is a language system that is based on Latin and addresses processes occurring in specific body systems, procedures, diagnostics, and diseases. The system depends on the use of a suffix, which is defined first, a root word, and many times a prefix. If a word un-familiar to you is used, it is important to learn the meaning, correct spelling, pronunciation, and proper usage of the term. Learning medical terminology is an ongoing process of vocabulary building. Consistent use of a good medical dictionary is essential. To aid you in learning, a terminology glossary has been provided in the back of this textbook, and a vocabulary section appears at the beginning of each chapter. Because the physician communicates using the medical terminology system and documentation is completed in this form, it is essential that you become comfortable and familiar with medical terms and their correct usage.

Charting Methods

Problem-Oriented Medical Record. The problem-oriented medical record (POMR) method of medical record keeping introduces a logical sequence to recording the information obtained from the patient. It is based on the scientific method and was designed to solve a problem. The medical history and physical examination fit into a special format that clarifies each patient's problem. Each patient problem, or diagnosis, is defined and documented on a problem list sheet at the beginning of the chart. Therefore the POMR assists with the process of auditing the medical record. In addition, the system is designed for and easily adapted to computerized medical records systems. The POMR system includes four basic parts:

1. *Database:* Includes the patient's health history, physical examination, and the results of baseline laboratory and diagnostic procedures. This information allows the physician to compile a health problem list for the patient.
2. *Problem list:* A list of the identified patient problems kept in the front of the patient's chart. It is the table of contents or the index of the chart that defines patient health concerns, including diagnosis, treatment, and education needs. The problem list takes a holistic approach by including psychosocial as well as physical needs. Each problem entered here is numerically listed and dated and is supported by the database. The problems are then identified and referred to throughout progress note documentation by their assigned number. If over time an additional problem is identified, the information is added to the problem list. If the problem is resolved, the date of problem resolution is entered next to the problem.
3. *Plan:* A written plan for each problem identified on the problem list, outlining further studies, treatments, and patient education (Figure 25-12).
4. *Progress notes:* The first letter of each part of the progress note adds up to SOAPE; therefore, this portion of the POMR system is called the SOAP notes, (or SOAPE notes when evaluation is included) (Figure 25-13). Each progress note utilizes the following format:
   - *S* for *subjective* data, which is the purpose of the visit, with the patient's words in quotation marks, or a summary of the patient's statement regarding the chief complaint. If quotation marks are not used, the subjective entry typically starts with "Patient reports…" or "Patient c/o…." The medical

TABLE 25-3	Body System Assessment

Appearance

Body build, posture, and gait
Height and weight fluctuation
Hygiene and grooming
Emotional state and mood

Head and Neck

Size, shape, and contour of head
Hair and scalp
Palpation of neck, thyroid, trachea
Difficulty in swallowing
Change in voice, hoarseness

Eyes

Visual acuity and field
Inspection of eyelids and eyeballs
Pupillary reaction and eye movement
Inspection of internal eye structures
Measurement of ocular pressure

Nose

Size, shape, and symmetry
Deviated septum, nasal congestion
Sense of smell

Respiratory

Size and shape of chest
Phlegm, cough, sneezing, wheezing
Coughing of blood, asthma, emphysema
Upper respiratory tract infections

Gastrointestinal

Symmetry, tenderness, pain
Changes in appetite, nausea, vomiting
Jaundice, ulcers, gallstones
Change in bowel habits: diarrhea, constipation,
   hemorrhoids, stool color

Genitalia (Male)

Infertility, sterility, impotency
Testicular pain, penile discharge
Penile enlargement or discomfort
Erections, emissions, hernias
Prostate or testicular enlargement

Neurologic

Level of consciousness, headaches
Reflex reactions, general weakness
Speech changes, memory loss, seizures
Changes in balance, incoordination

Lymph Glands

Enlargement, tenderness
Female breasts: symmetry, lumps

Skin

Color, turgor, and tone
Lesions or scars
Temperature, rashes, itching
Moles, sores, lumps, acne

Arms and Legs

General appearance and symmetry
Palpation of arm muscles
Limitation of movement
Inspection of fingernails
Deformities, joint stiffness

Ears

Hearing deficits
Inspection of size, symmetry, placement
Discharge, ringing in the ears, infection

Mouth and Throat

Inspection of gums, teeth, tongue, pharynx
Bad breath, changes in salivation
Sense of taste

Cardiovascular

Shortness of breath, chest pain
Heart murmur, palpitations, night sweats
Cold hands, leg cramps, varicose veins
Hypertension, valvular disease

Urinary

Changes in urinary habits: hesitancy, urgency, frequency,
   night voiding, pain when voiding, loss of stream force
Kidney stones, urinary tract infections
Dribbling, incontinence

Genitalia (Female)

Menses regularity, flow, pain, duration
Premenstrual symptoms, menopause
Obstetric history, birth control method
Estrogen therapy, reproductive surgeries
Pain during intercourse, sterility

Legs and Feet

Symmetry, scars, bruises, lumps, swelling
Broken bones, deformity, sprains, strains
Gout, arthritis, osteoporosis
Inspection of toenails

Endocrine

Weight change, fatigue, bulging eyes
Increased thirst or hunger, neck swelling
Excessive sweating, heat/cold intolerance

assistant documents this information based on details gained from the patient interview.

- *O* for *objective* data, which includes anything that is observed or measurable, including vital signs (VS), the exact anatomical location of an injury, difficulty with gait, and so on. The medical assistant is responsible for documenting complete and accurate objective data about all patient signs.

- *A* for *assessment* of the problem, which is usually the physician's preliminary diagnosis or the cause of the patient's chief complaint.

- *P* for the *plan* of care is physician documentation of how the health problem will be managed, including diagnostic studies, treatments, and patient education.

- *E* for *evaluation* is the assessment of the patient's understanding of the treatment and ability to

Professional Medical Offices
1722 E. North Avenue Suite 109
Aloha, HI 99751

Patient Name _Gastrin, Eleanor C._ DOB _8/15/40_ Chart # _3361_
            Last   First   MI

Allergies _Iodine_

Date	Time	Progress Note
7/4/02	10 AM	c/o fever x 3 days. Productive cough.
		~~T-101, P-72, R-61~~ Error SW 7/4/02
		T-101, P-72, R-16 S. Watkins, CMA
7/4/02	10:20AM	Late entry
		Denies wheezing, SOB S. Watkins, CMA

FIGURE 25-11
Documentation correction.

PROGRESS SHEET

Date		Allergies _Penicillin_

Patient name: _Fiddleman, Fred D._

9-9-02	c/o Fever for past two days. Productive cough
	Difficulty in breathing. Possible pneumonia
	Order Chest x-ray
	Rx: Keflex 500 mg #24 Cap † bid
	Phenergan Syrup ℥ iv Sig: ℥ ii prn cough
	Return in one week M.D.

FIGURE 25-12 Initial plan for POMR progress notes.

comply with the treatment plan and diagnostics ordered. This is not used in every practice, and may not ever be put in the record by a medical assistant.

CRITICAL THINKING APPLICATION

Document the following scenario using the POMR method:

The patient c/o a sore throat with pain of 5 on a 1-10 scale and fever for 2 days. He has been taking OTCs for relief of symptoms. His VS are T 100.4, P 88, R 20. He also has an erythemic papular rash across his chest.

S: _____

O: _____

_____

_____

Source-Oriented Medical Record. The source-oriented medical record (SOMR) is the most common form of record keeping in physicians' office practices. The data in the chart are organized according to sections such as History and Physical (H&P), Progress Notes, Laboratory Results, Consultations, and so on. All information is filed in reverse chronological order, with the most recent report or progress note placed on top. Progress notes are made each time the patient is seen or contacted by telephone. Documentation in the progress notes is based on details surrounding the patient's chief complaint (CC) or treatment protocol. The primary disadvantage of the SOMR system is that it can be very time consuming to find a back entry regarding a particular problem or treatment.

Computerized Medical Record (CMR). Many ambulatory care settings, especially multipractice facilities and health maintenance organizations (HMOs), use computer systems that collect and file patient information as well as link offices together. These systems are usually designed for the particular type of needs of the practice but are often set up so that information can be directly entered into the patient's chart. The physician dictates the findings and a transcriptionist enters the information, or many physicians are now using Palm Pilot–type devices to directly download information into the patient's computerized file.

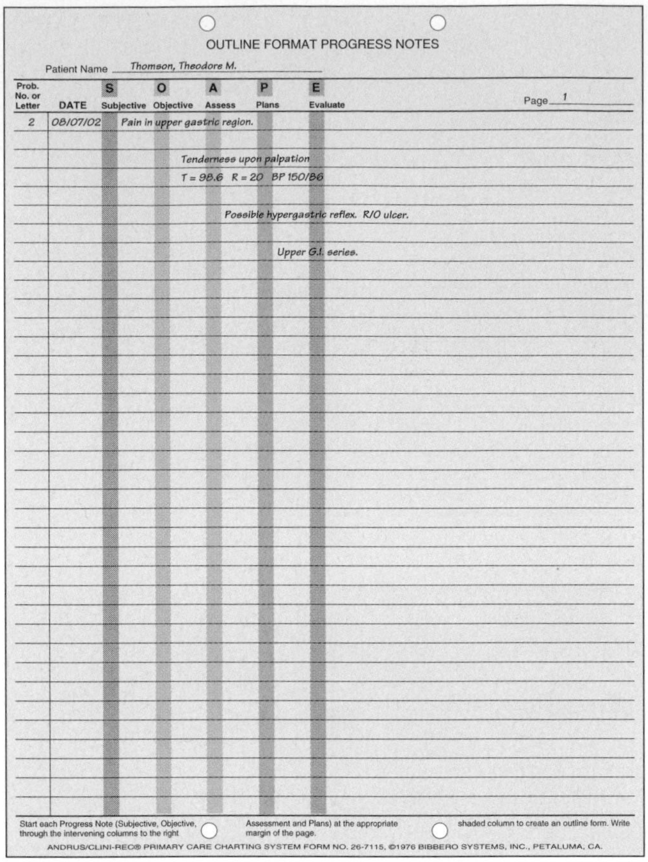

OUTLINE FORMAT PROGRESS NOTES

Patient Name Thomson, Theodore M.

Prob. No. or Letter	DATE	S Subjective	O Objective	A Assess	P Plans	E Evaluate	Page 1
2	08/07/02	Pain in upper gastric region.					
			Tenderness upon palpation				
			T = 98.6 R = 20 BP 150/86				
				Possible hypergastric reflex. R/O ulcer.			
					Upper G.I. series.		

Start each Progress Note (Subjective, Objective, through the intervening columns to the right.   Assessment and Plans) at the appropriate margin of the page.   shaded column to create an outline form. Write

ANDRUS/CLINI-REC® PRIMARY CARE CHARTING SYSTEM FORM NO. 26-7115, ©1976 BIBBERO SYSTEMS, INC., PETALUMA, CA.

FIGURE 25-13 Structured notes for the POMR system. (Courtesy Bibbero Systems, Petaluma, Calif.)

Patient Education

Finding time to conduct patient education in a busy healthcare practice can be challenging. Every opportunity to interact with patients should be considered a potential "teaching moment." The perfect time to begin the education process is during the initial patient interview, since this is when you will first become aware of patient lifestyle factors that may negatively impact wellness. Or, perhaps during the interview process the patient mentions a financial, social, or psychological problem that could be helped with referral to a community or hospital-based service. Your interactions with patients and implementation of therapeutic communication skills as well as interview techniques are crucial to the quality of care received in your practice.

Legal and Ethical Issues

The medical history is a confidential record that can be shared only with healthcare personnel who are directly involved in the care of the patient. Data provided to you by the patient or that you read in the patient's chart are confidential; you must not share any of this information with anyone. The consequences for disclosing private information to individuals not involved in the patient's

care can be very serious and can result in the loss of your job, court-imposed fines, and even imprisonment.

In addition to maintaining patient confidentiality, consistently implementing correct documentation procedures is crucial for medical practices. The medical chart is considered a legal record, and court cases can be won or lost based on the clarity and completeness of staff documentation. It is absolutely essential that medical assistants document all patient information in a factual, nonjudgmental manner. Physicians can find themselves in serious liability trouble, not because of poor practice, but because of administrative deficiencies and poor communications. *Risk management* practices focus on these problems as a way of reducing the chances of professional liability claims.

FACTORS THAT CONTRIBUTE TO SOUND RISK MANAGEMENT PRACTICES

- Periodic review or auditing of patient office records
- Consistent charting of accurate and complete clinical facts and test results
- Adequate office procedures for informing patients of test results as well as documenting this communication
- Appropriate use of abbreviations and legible recording on the patient chart as well as corrections made in the legally required manner
- Documentation that shows diagnostic tests have been received, reviewed by the attending physician, and filed in a timely manner
- Documented evidence of appropriate discharge and continuing care instructions

---

SUMMARY OF SCENARIO

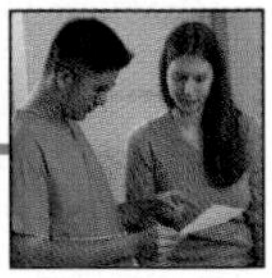

The office supervisor met with Chris and reviewed the essential techniques for gathering patient information. Therapeutic communication includes demonstrating respectful patient care, using active listening skills, observing nonverbal behaviors, and using a combination of both open and closed questions. Chris described the parts of the patient interview and recognized typical barriers to patient communication. Chris's workplace uses POMR documentation methods, so he reviewed the specifics of this type of record keeping with his supervisor. In conclusion, the significance of patient confidentiality was emphasized, and Chris agreed to work at implementing the techniques for therapeutic communications.

SUMMARY OF LEARNING OBJECTIVES

■ Holistic care includes assessing the patient's health status through the collection of physical, cognitive, psychosocial, and behavioral data.

■ The medical history consists of the patient's database, past medical history, family and social histories, and the review of systems.

■ Developing a professional helping relationship with patients is the responsibility of all healthcare workers. The helping relationship involves consistent application of respectful patient care that recognizes the impact of patient anxieties on interactions and responses to treatment.

■ Sensitivity to diverse populations includes the application of empathetic communications and an awareness of the impact of individual value systems and personal prejudices on patient interactions.

■ The linear communication model illustrates communication as an interactive process between the sender and receiver of the message with feedback a crucial part of the process. Active listening techniques, which include restatement, reflection, and clarification, help the medical assistant go beyond hearing the message to actually listening to and appropriately responding to the patient's main point.

■ Approximately 90% of patient interactions occur through nonverbal language. The key to successful patient interaction is congruence between verbal and nonverbal messages.

■ Certain communication styles can be misleading or restrict the patient's response. A medical assistant must be alert to using such faulty techniques as inappropriately providing reassurance, giving advice, using medical terminology without clarification, asking leading questions, and talking too much. These behaviors interfere with gathering complete data during the interview and are obstacles to developing rapport with your patient.

■ Patients use defense mechanisms to protect themselves in emotionally challenging situations. A medical assistant must consistently apply nonjudgmental therapeutic communication skills to maintain professional relationships.

■ Therapeutic communication techniques vary according to the age and developmental level of the patient. A medical assistant should be aware of how to interact most effectively with various age groups, including young children, adolescents, adults, elderly patients, and family members. Age-specific application of interview styles ensures clear communication between the health professional and the patient.

■ The patient interview is divided into the introduction, the body, and the summary or closing. Throughout the interview the medical assistant should use professional interview techniques, such as empathetic patient care, sensitivity to patient diversity, active listening skills, appropriate nonverbal communication, attention to the interview environment, avoidance of communication barriers, and framing questions and statements in an open or closed manner, depending on the information to be elicited.

■ The ability to document accurately and completely is an essential skill for all medical assistants. Documentation should describe the patient's chief complaint, describe all pertinent signs and symptoms, and demonstrate the correct use of medical terminology, with appropriate abbreviations. Any error in the medical record must be corrected according to legally approved methods.

■ There are three main forms of medical record systems. These include the POMR method, which uses SOAPE charting to define the patient's health problems. The most frequently used form of medical record keeping is the SOMR, which organizes patient data into specific sections. The CMR system compiles computer records for patient data.

■ The perfect time to initiate patient education is during the initial patient interview. A medical assistant should take advantage of every "teaching moment" to get to know his or her patients and promote patient wellness.

■ Risk management practices focus on reducing the chances of professional liability claims. Accurate and complete documentation on the patient's chart is crucial for successful risk management. In addition, maintaining strict confidentiality of patient information and factual, nonjudgmental, legible recording of patient data are essential to professional patient care.

KEY INTERNET WEBSITES

HOLISTIC CARE

- American Academy of Osteopathy
  For active weblinks to each website visit
  http://evolve.elsevier.com/Kinn/

CULTURAL DIVERSITY

- Jamarda Resources, Inc. – specializes in cultural diversity and educational products for healthcare providers.
  For active weblinks to each website visit
  http://evolve.elsevier.com/Kinn/

PATIENT'S BILL OF RIGHTS

- Patients Before Profits: the Patient's Bill of Rights.
  For active weblinks to each website visit
  http://evolve.elsevier.com/Kinn/

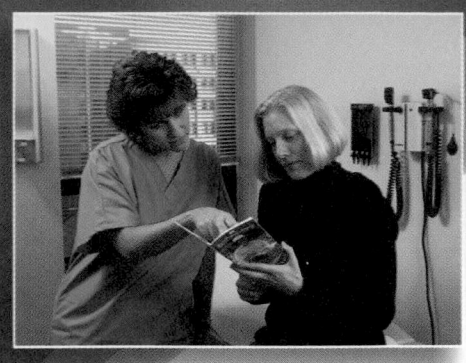

CHAPTER 26

Scenario

In a busy family-practice office, medical assistant Taylor DiSalvo is working with a patient, Mr. Sam Ignatio, 68 years old, who has just been diagnosed with insulin-dependent diabetes mellitus. Mr. Ignatio knows nothing about his disease or how to manage it; has never seen a glucometer and never handled needles; consumes a high-fat, high-carbohydrate diet; does not exercise on a regular basis; is 50 pounds overweight; has functional deafness in his left ear and decreased sound quality in his right ear; and shows early signs of diabetic-related vision loss. Taylor is responsible for overall management of Mr. Ignatio's patient teaching plan.

Where should Taylor begin? Mr. Ignatio is faced with a serious illness, and his future health depends on compliance with a wide range of lifestyle changes. How can Taylor make certain he understands the importance of following treatment and disease-monitoring guidelines? The methods Taylor chooses to teach this patient about his disease can have an impact on his eventual health outcome.

This chapter will help students recognize the individual learning needs of patients and provides guidelines for developing effective teaching approaches. The concepts in this chapter are basic to all patient education interventions, and following them can affect a patient's understanding of the disease process as well as his or her willingness to comply with physician-recommended disease management.

Patient Education

Learning Objectives

- Recognize the implications of the holistic healthcare model on patient education.
- Illustrate at least five guidelines for patient education that can affect overall patient wellness.
- Define six patient factors that have an impact on learning.
- Summarize education approaches for patients with language barriers.
- Determine potential barriers to patient learning.
- Implement a variety of teaching methods and strategies that are responsive to individual patient needs.
- Demonstrate the ability to develop an appropriate and effective patient teaching plan.
- Describe the role of the medical assistant in patient education.
- Integrate the legal and ethical implications of patient teaching into the ambulatory care setting.

National Curriculum Competencies

TRANSDISCIPLINARY COMPETENCIES

3b. Instruct individuals according to their needs
3d. Provide instruction for health maintenance and disease prevention
3e. Identify community resources

Patient Education and the Holistic Healthcare Model

Patient education should begin with the first contact between the patient and the healthcare team (Figure 26-1). A well-informed patient is more likely to comply with treatment and adopt a healthy lifestyle. However, informing a patient about his or her disease is only a portion of the health-teaching process. The key to successful health teaching is that patients actually implement teaching guidelines.

Decreases in hospital admissions and shorter hospital stays have resulted in the need for patients and families to assume responsibility for care that was once the responsibility of hospital staff. This means that those of us who work in ambulatory care settings have an even greater responsibility to meet the educational needs of our patients. To develop an effective teaching approach, we must implement a *holistic model* that considers not only the patient's physical state but also his or her emotional, social, psychological, economic, and spiritual needs. The holistic model suggests we look at patients and determine needs based on a complete view of their lives rather than just as an analysis of their specific diseases. It is our responsibility not only to teach patients about disease processes but also to help them implement related skills and changes in lifestyle to promote recovery and improve function.

GUIDELINES FOR PATIENT EDUCATION

- Provide knowledge and skills to promote recovery and health.
- Include family and significant others in education interventions.
- Encourage patient ownership and participation in the teaching process.
- Promote safe and appropriate use of medications and treatments.
- Encourage patient adaptation to healthy behaviors.
- Provide information on accessing community resources.

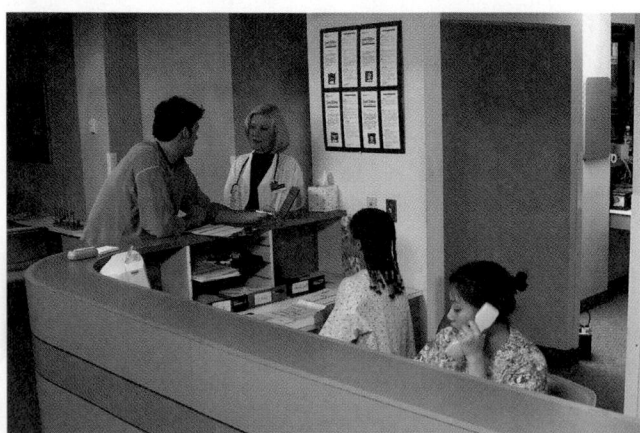

FIGURE 26-1   First contact with a patient.

Patient Factors that Affect Learning

There are many factors or patient characteristics that may affect the patient's ability to learn. Medical assistants must be aware of these factors to develop a patient education approach that best meets the needs of each patient. A summary of these factors follows.

Perception of Disease Versus Actual State of Disease. Patients respond to a particular diagnosis in many different ways. One of the predictors of how a patient will respond, and therefore how he or she will react to health education, is the patient's perception of the disease. Previous life experiences may greatly influence your patient's knowledge base and/or desire to learn about his or her disease. Does the patient recognize and accept the seriousness of the diagnosis? Or perhaps does your patient overreact to potential disease risks? Both of these responses will determine the patient's willingness to learn about the disease as well as compliance with treatment recommendations.

How do you think it will affect Taylor's patient education efforts if Mr. Ignatio does not consider diabetes a serious disease?

Patient Need for Information. The patient's perception of the impact of the disease on his or her general health will also determine the need for information about the disease. Does the patient express a desire to learn all he or she can about the disease, or does the patient resist or act indifferent to teaching efforts? One patient education guideline is to promote patient *ownership* of the learning process. To do this you may first have to persuade the patient that he or she does actually need to understand the disease before he or she can improve overall wellness.

What is the appropriate response if Mr. Ignatio tells Taylor his father was a diabetic and had to have both legs amputated because of the disease, so he doesn't think it matters if he manages his blood sugar—he will still have major health complications?

Patient Age and Developmental Level. Depending on the age of patients and/or their ability to understand information about their disease, you may need to adapt the teaching plan to meet their specific learning needs. For example, educating a 5-year-old insulin-dependent patient about diabetes management requires an approach that is different from the one used for 68-year-old Mr. Ignatio. Many times the key to patient understanding and compliance is the involvement of family members.

While conducting an assessment of Mr. Ignatio's diet, Taylor learns that his wife cooks all his meals and packs his lunch daily. What should Taylor do to make certain Mr. Ignatio's diet complies with diabetic recommendations?

Patient Mental and Emotional State. Even a well-planned teaching intervention can be ineffective if the patient is unable to pay attention because of anxiety, stress, anger, or denial (Figure 26-2). Frequently patients will use defense mechanisms to protect themselves from the reality of a serious illness. It is important that the medical assistant be sensitive to the mental state of the patient and adapt teaching interventions as needed.

Mr. Ignatio has just been told about his disease. He already shared that his father died of diabetes. Do you think he is able to pay attention to patient teaching about how to give his insulin injections? What should Taylor do to manage this problem?

Influence of Multicultural and Diversity Factors on Patient Education. Culture, family background, and religious beliefs influence patient actions. Working with patients from diverse backgrounds is an exciting challenge; however, for patient education to be successful it is essential that the medical assistant be aware of and sensitive to the impact of these factors on patient learning (Figure 26-3). Some questions you should consider when teaching a patient from a diverse background include the following:

- Is language an issue with your patient (Figure 26-4)? If the patient is unable to understand English verbally or read it correctly, do you have a substitute method for getting the information across?
- Does the patient's culture, ethnic background, or religion influence the way he or she perceives disease as well as the role of healthcare workers?
- What strategies or techniques might minimize patient education problems?
- Are there community resources that could facilitate patient learning?

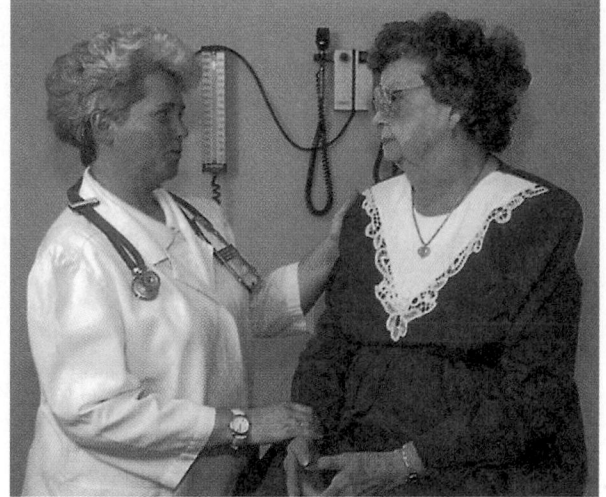

FIGURE 26-2   Demonstrating sensitivity to patient needs.

APPROACHES FOR PATIENTS WITH LANGUAGE BARRIERS

- Address the patient by his or her last name.
- Be courteous and use a formal approach to communication.
- Use gestures, tone of voice, facial expressions, and eye contact to emphasize appropriate parts of the discussion.
- Integrate pictures, handouts, models, and other aids that visually depict the material.
- Monitor the patient's body language, especially facial expression, for understanding or confusion.
- Use simple, everyday words as much as possible.
- Demonstrate all procedures and have the patient return the demonstration to check for understanding.
- Implement the teaching plan in small manageable steps.
- Give the patient written instructions for all procedures and treatments.
- Use an interpreter when appropriate, if available.

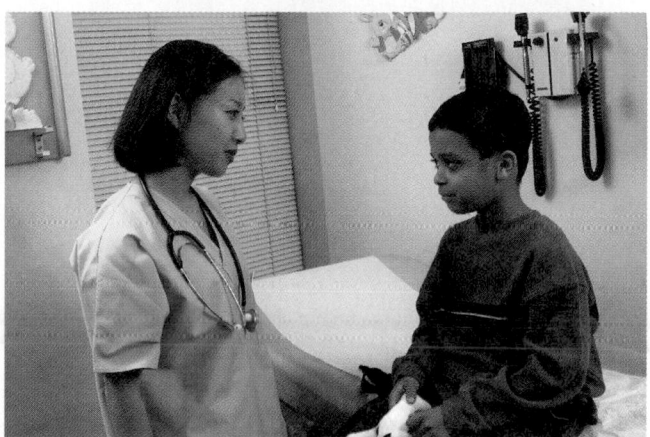

FIGURE 26-3   Considering diversity.

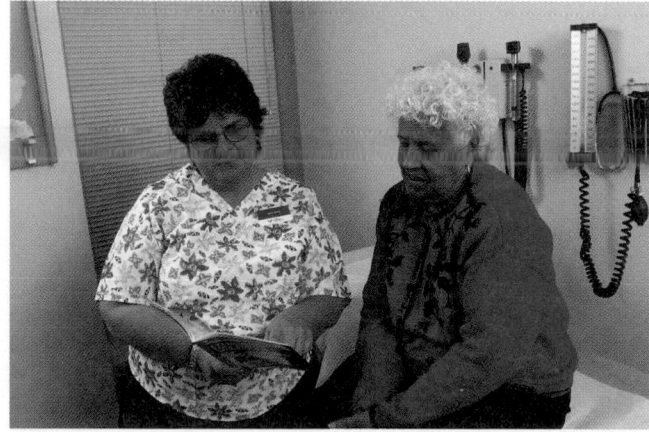

FIGURE 26-4   Managing language barriers.

Patient Learning Style. Chapter 1 presented information on individual learning styles that affect you as a student. These same factors will have an impact on your patient's learning preference. Some patients learn best from discussion or lecture, whereas others must think or reflect about the material before understanding it. Some patients can learn from observing; others must act or do something with the material to learn it. Start your teaching intervention by asking your patient how he or she prefers to learn new material and pattern your teaching interventions along those lines.

Mr. Ignatio tells Taylor that he could never learn things by listening to someone tell him what to do. What approach to learning would best meet his needs?

Impact of Physical Disabilities. The patient must first be assessed to determine whether he or she can adequately hear instructions, see written material, and manipulate any required treatment equipment. All teaching efforts are lost if disabilities interfere with a patient's capacity to understand information or to properly handle equipment (Figure 26-5). A hearing or speech impairment may require the use of sign language with supplemental written instructions. If the patient is unable to manipulate equipment because of a physical disability or vision problem, family or community resources may be necessary for the patient to manage his or her care.

Mr. Ignatio's physical assessment revealed hearing and vision problems. Is he able to understand verbal instructions clearly? Will he be able to draw up the correct amount of insulin? What can be done to adapt the teaching intervention to meet his needs?

CRITICAL THINKING APPLICATION

Implement the holistic education model to determine and respond to Mr. Ignatio's individual learning needs.

The Teaching Plan

What is it that patients need to know to manage their diseases appropriately? What is it about an individual patient that needs to be addressed for a teaching intervention to work? What are the immediate and long-term goals of patient education? What teaching materials or strategies should be used to meet the learning needs of the patient and also effectively relay the information? How can the teaching plan be implemented successfully? How does the medical assistant manage the limited time available for patient teaching? How do you know the patient is learning and actually implementing this knowledge into disease management? One of the most important aspects of patient teaching is to *be flexible* and to provide information about *what* patients want to know

when patients want to know it. These and other guidelines for developing an appropriate and effective teaching plan follow.

Assess Patient Learning Needs

Developing a teaching plan that works for each individual first requires an assessment of the patient as a learner and consideration of any characteristics that might affect the learning process. Many of these factors have already been addressed, such as the patient's learning preference, perception of the illness, age, background, multicultural influences, language barriers, and disabilities. The medical assistant must also consider what the patient already knows about the diagnosis and whether that knowledge includes misconceptions about the disease. The goal of the assessment process is to create a teaching plan that meets the needs of the patient to understand and manage his or her illness. The learning assessment therefore should consider what the patient needs to know, what the patient *wants* to know, and what can be done in the *time available* for learning.

Before developing a specific approach to patient education, a medical assistant must also consider potential barriers to learning besides those already presented, such as the presence of pain. If a patient is in acute distress, he or she will be unable to concentrate on the information. In this case the amount of material must be adjusted to meet the patient's immediate needs and time should be planned in the future for a more in-depth transfer of information.

Does Mr. Ignatio exhibit any potential barriers to learning about his disease?

POTENTIAL BARRIERS TO PATIENT LEARNING

Individual learning style
Age and developmental level
Use of defense mechanisms
Language
Motivation to learn
Physical limitations or disabilities
Emotional or mental state
Cultural or ethnic background
Pain
Time limitations

Determine Teaching Priorities

Once you have conducted an adequate assessment of your patient as a learner and you understand your patient's learning needs, the next question is, "Where do I start?" A patient such as Mr. Ignatio has a significant amount of information to learn before he can completely manage his disease. The volume of information might seem overwhelming, unless priorities are established. How do you know what material should be first? The first question to ask is, "What are the patient's immediate versus long-term needs?" What must this patient know

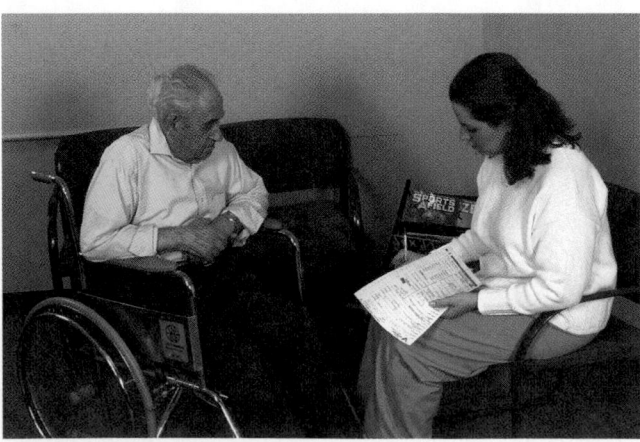

FIGURE 26-5   Assessing learning challenges.

today to do what he has to do to take care of himself, and what does he need to know overall about his illness to promote healthy behaviors?

Because the patient learning assessment told you what your patient knows about his or her disease, that is a good place to start. Confirm what the patient knows about the problem and attempt to correct any potential misconceptions. If you start with something the patient knows and understands, he or she will feel more competent and capable of managing new material. You should then go on to the new material the patient is most anxious about. If the patient is nervous or afraid about a particular item, he or she will be unable to pay attention to any other new material until the anxieties are addressed.

For example, if Mr. Ignatio is most concerned about giving himself injections, that is the first skill he should learn. Once he is confident about that particular part of treatment, he will be able to pay attention to diet and exercise recommendations. You should always begin with the basic details about the disease and add more information during each patient visit.

Every interaction with the patient is an opportunity to conduct health education. One of the major problems with delivering quality patient education in an ambulatory setting is the lack of time. Therefore a medical assistant must take advantage of every "teaching moment." That is, every time you interact with the patient, use it as an opportunity to assess the patient's current education needs and provide as much information or guidance as possible during the time available about that specific learning need (Figure 26-6).

Use the waiting room as a place for learning by providing up-to-date education materials on a wide variety of health issues. Many offices have video set-ups in the waiting room for patient education while he or she is waiting to be seen. These can be specific to the type of physician practice or can provide general health information.

Decide on Appropriate Teaching Materials

What teaching device would best meet the needs of your patient? A wide variety of patient education materials are available, and deciding which ones best meet your patient's needs depends on the patient's learning preference, individual characteristics, and lifestyle factors. Individualized instruction is the key to understanding and patient compliance; however, additional materials will help reinforce the information.

When possible, all patient instruction should include a handout or some type of printed material that reinforces information and can be used by the patient as a resource. Patient factors such as the use of defense mechanisms, emotional state, and language barriers can limit the patient's ability to comprehend and remember information. Printed information is needed to help the patient and the patient's family understand what is happening and what needs to be done to improve the patient's health (Figure 26-7). Informational flyers can be ordered from medical office suppliers, pharmaceutical company representatives, and health education companies. Many hospitals also offer free educational materials about diagnostic procedures, immunizations, and other disease-related topics. The ambulatory care setting where you are employed may also develop its own educational materials. Some guidelines to follow if you are responsible for developing or ordering educational supplies include the following:

- Material should be written using lay language at a sixth- to eighth-grade level to promote general patient understanding.
- Information should be well organized and clearly described.
- Check all material for accuracy.
- Should be in an appealing and professional format.
- Copies should be available in other languages when possible.

Other teaching materials include the use of videos or Internet sites to reinforce or expand knowledge. Both videos and Internet sites allow patient learning to be self-directed and self-paced. They also permit the patient to learn material in a nonstressful environment, which improves patient learning potential. Depending on the patient's age or access to the appropriate technology, using videos or referring the patient to healthcare sites on the Internet may help to develop patient ownership of the learning process and will provide excellent resources for

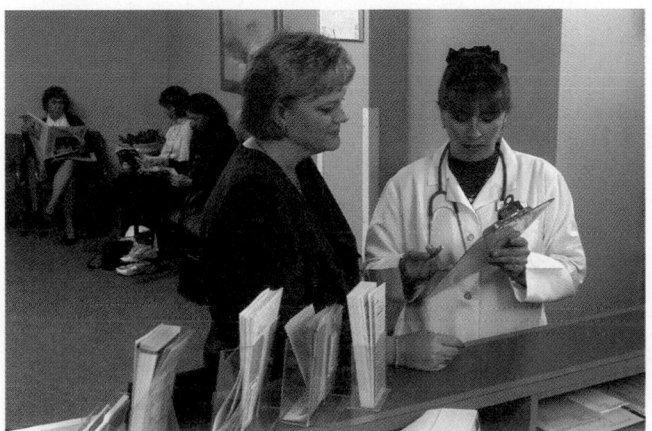

FIGURE 26-6   A teaching moment.

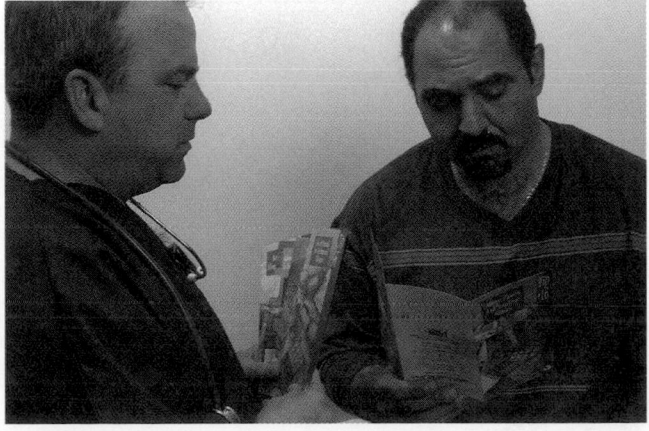

FIGURE 26-7   Reviewing printed information.

patient referral. However, using the Internet as a resource for patient education information has its drawbacks. It is important that the patient understand there is no oversight or control over information posted on the web; therefore some sites may offer information that is erroneous, out of date, or misleading. Provide patients with accurate, well-researched sites and/or be informed about what sites patients are accessing to make certain that recommendations support the physician's treatment protocol. At the end of the chapter there is a list of Internet sites that can be used for patient referral. See if you can add any to the collection.

Decide on Appropriate Teaching Methods

There are a variety of ways to get the message across to your patients. One of the best ways of managing a large amount of information in a short period is to use community resources to reinforce the message. Your local area provides a wide range of education services for your patients to help them better understand and manage their health problems, to promote wellness, and to provide support for treatment compliance. Hospitals and many community agencies and organizations provide patient education opportunities, support groups for specific problems or diseases, and learning materials. These same groups may help the patient by providing professional consultation for many topics including diet, exercise, and emotional support. It is important that a medical assistant be aware of the various resources available in the community for patient education and referral.

Based on your evaluation of Mr. Ignatio's learning needs, what community resources would help him and his family better understand and manage his disease?

Teaching patients specific skills is also an important component of health education. The best way to teach a patient how to accurately manipulate and operate medical equipment is to use demonstration/return demonstration of the skill (Figure 26-8). Using the exact piece of equipment the patient will be using at home, the medical assistant should first demonstrate to the patient how to perform the skill, ask for questions and explain further as needed, then have the patient return the demonstration before leaving the office. This allows the medical assistant to observe the patient performing the task and correct any mistakes or clarify any misconceptions before the patient has to use the equipment at home alone.

For some patients an effective method for monitoring health education is to have the patient keep a journal of his or her activities and response to treatment. For example, a patient who is trying to adapt to a new diet could record daily intake to get a better idea of whether he or she is following through with dietary recommendations. In the case of Mr. Ignatio, recording blood glucose levels from routine glucometer readings will reinforce the results of compliance with medication and diet therapies.

Another vital link to the success of patient education is family involvement. If the patient is being treated holistically, the family plays an integral role in patient wellness. Involving family members in patient education efforts provides support and understanding for the patient while managing family concerns about the patient's welfare. An educated family member can be an excellent resource for patient concerns as well as a vigilant reinforcer of healthy behaviors (Figure 26-9).

CRITICAL THINKING APPLICATION

The physician recommends that Mr. Ignatio start a 1200-calorie diabetic diet for weight reduction and blood glucose control, monitor glucometer readings three times per day, and start with three injections of insulin daily. After you consider various teaching methods, which strategies do you think would be most useful in helping Mr. Ignatio to learn about his disease and to implement the doctor's recommendations?

Implement the Teaching Plan

After you have completed the patient assessment, decided on teaching materials and methods that match your patient's characteristics and learning needs, and adapted the material and your approach for any potential barriers to learning, it is time to actually implement the plan. Conduct the lesson in a quiet area away from distractions.

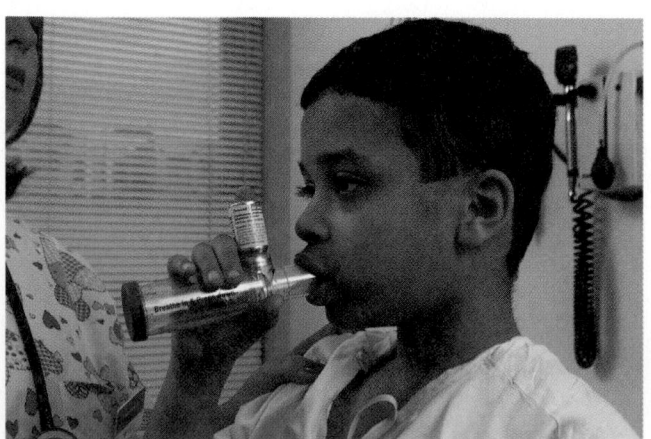

FIGURE 26-8 Demonstration/return demonstration.

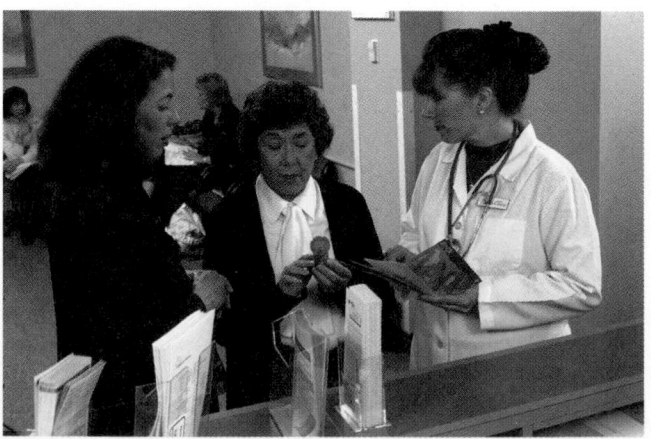

FIGURE 26-9 Family involvement in patient education.

You must assemble any equipment the patient will need. The patient should learn to handle and practice on the same type of equipment that will be used at home so there is no problem in transferring the skill. Time is always an issue in the ambulatory care setting, so it is important to present only the material or skill that is possible for the patient to master before the end of the appointment. Throughout the lesson, remember to maintain an adequate pace for learning—not too fast and not too slow—to optimize the patient's understanding.

One of the most important aspects of successful patient teaching is to consistently ask for feedback about the process (Figure 26-10). It also helps to restate, repeat, or rephrase the material to make certain patients understand the process. As patients provide correct feedback about what they are learning or demonstrate skills correctly, it is important to be positive about their progress. It also helps to summarize the material learned or the skills mastered at the end of each teaching intervention as a way of reviewing the material and clarifying important concepts.

The medical assistant should continue to evaluate the teaching plan throughout the process to make certain that the time was adequate for the patient to learn what was needed, that the patient was able to pay attention and understand the process, and that the patient learned and understood the information needed to care for himself or herself at home. In addition, plans should be made for what material will be covered during the patient's next visit. All of this information needs to be included in the progress note about the lesson. In addition, the medical assistant must document details regarding the material covered, the patient's competency or level of skill in learning treatment techniques, and any referral to community or hospital experts or education groups.

SUMMARY OF THE TEACHING PLAN

Conduct Patient Assessment.

- Consider pertinent patient factors.
- Identify barriers to learning.
- Prioritize patient information.
    Determine the patient's immediate and long-term needs.
- Decide on appropriate teaching materials and methods.

Prepare the Teaching Area and Assemble Necessary Equipment and Materials.

- Use supplies and equipment the patient will use at home.
- Provide positive feedback for correct display of skills.

Maintain Adequate Pace, Not Too Fast.

Repeatedly Ask for Patient Feedback to Confirm Understanding.

- Eliminate barriers to learning.
- Address immediate learning needs.

- Use repetition and rephrasing to promote understanding.

Summarize the Material Learned or Skill Mastered at the End of Each Teaching Interaction.

Outline a Plan for the Next Meeting.

Evaluate the Teaching Plan.

- Was there enough time to complete the lesson?
- Was the patient physically and psychologically ready for the information?
- Were the goals for the session reached?

Document the Teaching Intervention.

- Material covered
- Patient response or level of skill performance
- Plans for next session
- Community referrals

CRITICAL THINKING APPLICATION

Taylor DiSalvo has just completed the initial patient education session with Mr. Ignatio and his wife. Taylor used demonstration/return demonstration to teach him how to properly check his blood glucose levels with the glucometer he will be using at home. He also demonstrated how to draw up and administer an insulin injection. Taylor answered Mrs. Ignatio's questions about his diet but referred the couple to the dietitian at the hospital for further diet information. Taylor plans to review the skills practiced today at Mr. Ignatio's next appointment and continue the teaching intervention with the importance of checking feet daily for any signs of infection or open areas. Accurately and completely document Taylor's initial education intervention.

ROLE OF THE MEDICAL ASSISTANT AS PATIENT EDUCATOR

- Reinforce physician instructions and information.
- Encourage patients to take an active role in their health.
- Use each patient interaction as an opportunity to conduct health teaching.
- Keep information relevant to patient needs.
- Establish and maintain patient rapport.
- Communicate clearly.
- Be sensitive to patient learner factors.
- Modify the teaching plan as needed to best meet the needs of patients.

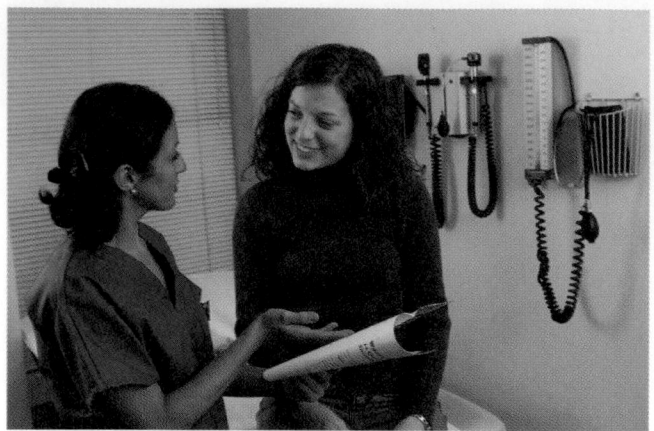

FIGURE 26-10 Patient feedback.

Legal and Ethical Issues

Providing adequate, correct, understandable information to patients is integral to the informed consent mandate within the Patient's Bill of Rights. All patients have the right to information before they agree to care. An extension of this concept is the right for patients to understand their disease process and manage their health. Another consideration from the Patient's Bill of Rights is the issue of patient confidentiality as it relates to patient education. When developing and implementing the teaching plan, designing teaching interventions and strategies, and referring patients for community assistance, a medical assistant must protect the patient's confidentiality.

Essential factors in risk management for the ambulatory care setting are conducting adequate patient education and follow-up. Integral to risk management is also the importance of completely and accurately documenting each patient education intervention. The patient's chart should clearly describe the education intervention, methods and materials used, the patient's response to the intervention, the date of each session, and the individual who conducted each intervention. Each documentation entry should completely describe the material covered and the patient's feedback regarding the information so there is no doubt the patient understood the information and was able to perform any related skills properly and adequately.

Teaching interventions should demonstrate sensitivity to multicultural factors and diverse populations. Meeting the needs of all patients without evidence of prejudice is a key risk management step.

SUMMARY OF SCENARIO

After interacting with Mr. Ignatio, Taylor realizes the significance as well as the complexity of educating patients in the ambulatory care setting. Despite the time constraints that are typical in this particular healthcare setting, patients must still learn how to manage their diseases and follow treatment guidelines. Approaching each patient as an individual

learner with particular needs and characteristics is crucial to ultimate success with a teaching plan. Using a holistic model, Taylor has considered all of the ramifications of diabetes mellitus on Mr. Ignatio's life and has made efforts to include family and community resources in the management of his disease.

SUMMARY OF LEARNING OBJECTIVES

- The holistic model suggests patient education should consider all aspects of patient life, including physical, psychological, emotional, social, economic, and spiritual needs.

- The guidelines for patient education include providing knowledge and skills that promote recovery and health; including family in education interventions; encouraging patient ownership of the education process; promoting safe use of medications and treatments; encouraging healthy behaviors; and providing information on how to access community resources.

- Patient factors that have an impact on learning include the patient's perception of disease versus the actual state of disease; the need for information; age and developmental level; mental and emotional state; the influence of multicultural and diversity factors; individual learning style; and the impact of physical disabilities on the education process.

- Education approaches for patients with language barriers include addressing the patient formally and courteously; using nonverbal language to promote understanding; integrating pictures or models that visualize the material; observing the patient for understanding or confusion; using simple lay language; demonstrating procedures; implementing teaching in small, manageable steps; providing written instructions; and utilizing an interpreter when available.

- Potential barriers to patient education include patient learning style; physical limitations; age and developmental level; emotional or mental state that interferes with learning; use of defense mechanisms; cultural or ethnic factors; language; the presence of pain; patient motivation to learn; and limited time for teaching.

- Teaching materials and methods that are effective include the use of printed materials, videos, and approved Internet sites to gather information; referral to community resources and experts; demonstration/return demonstration of medical skills; patient journals of events; and involving family members in the education process.

- The parts of the teaching plan include an assessment of learning needs; eliminating learning barriers; determining teaching priorities; using appropriate teaching materials and methods; gathering feedback repeatedly to ensure patient understanding; summarizing the material at the end of each education session; planning for the next meeting; evaluating the effectiveness of the session; and completely and accurately documenting the details of the teaching intervention.

■ The role of the medical assistant in patient education is to reinforce physician instructions and information by encouraging patients to take an active role in their health; using teaching moments effectively; keeping information relevant to the patient; establishing and maintaining patient rapport; communicating clearly; remaining aware of learning factors; and being flexible with the teaching plan.

■ Appropriate patient education reflects the Patient's Bill of Rights emphasis on patient confidentiality as well as informed consent. Risk management practices related to patient education include accurate and complete documentation of patient education sessions and sensitivity to the diverse needs of the patient.

KEY INTERNET WEBSITES

PATIENT RESOURCES

- American Cancer Society
- American Diabetes Association
- American Heart Association
- American Red Cross
- Information Center for Individuals with Disabilities
- Self Help for Hard of Hearing People
- The Wellness Community
  For active weblinks to each website visit
  http://evolve.elsevier.com/Kinn/

CHAPTER 27

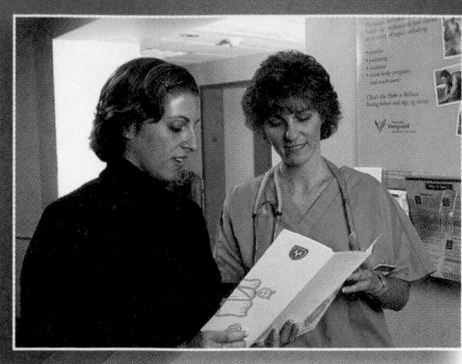

Scenario

Marcia Schwartz, CMA, is employed by an internal medicine practice in her hometown. She recognizes that many of the patients seen in the practice have diseases that are influenced by diet and lifestyle factors. She learned about the importance of good nutrition and wellness in her medical assistant program. In addition, Marcia has continued to attend workshops and read about current trends in nutrition, so she is prepared to provide assistance to her patients.

Nutrition and Health Promotion

Learning Objectives

- Define and spell the terms listed in the vocabulary.
- Describe the types and functions of dietary nutrients.
- Describe the role of carbohydrates, fats, and protein in the daily diet.
- Explain the need for vitamins and minerals in the diet.
- Apply Food Guide Pyramid guidelines to patient diet recommendations.
- Implement nutritional assessment techniques.
- Demonstrate the concepts of therapeutic nutrition.
- Interpret food labels and their application to healthy diets.
- Define the concepts of health promotion.
- Understand the role of the medical assistant in nutrition and health promotion.
- Determine and record a measurement of body fat.
- Accurately explain the nutritional labeling of food products to a patient.

National Curriculum Competencies

CLINICAL COMPETENCIES

4a. Perform telephone and in-person screening

TRANSDISCIPLINARY COMPETENCIES

2d. Document appropriately
3b. Instruct individuals according to their needs

3d. Provide instruction for health maintenance and disease prevention
3e. Identify community resources

Vocabulary

amino acids Organic compounds that form the chief constituents of protein and are used by the body to build and repair tissues.

cholesterol Substance produced by the liver and found in plant and animal fats that can produce fatty deposits or atherosclerotic plaques in the blood vessels.

deficiencies Conditions caused by a below-normal intake of a particular substance.

diabetes mellitus type 1 A disease in which the beta cells in the pancreas no longer produce insulin. Patients must rely on daily insulin administration to utilize glucose for energy and prevent complications.

diabetes mellitus type 2 A disease in which the body is unable to utilize glucose for energy as a result of either a lack of insulin production in the pancreas or resistance to insulin on the cellular level.

digestion Process of converting food into chemical substances that can be used by the body.

hydrogenated Combined with, treated with, or exposed to hydrogen.

obesity An excessive accumulation of body fat (usually defined as more than 20% above the recommended body weight).

osteoporosis Loss of bone density; lack of calcium intake is a major factor in its development.

registered dietitian Person with a minimum of a bachelor's degree in foods and nutrition who is concerned with the maintenance and promotion of health and the treatment of diseases through diet.

triglycerides Fatty acid and glycerol compounds that combine with a protein molecule to form high- and low-density lipoproteins.

turgor Resistance of the skin to being grasped between the fingers and released; refers to normal skin tension; is decreased in dehydration and increased with edema.

vertigo Dizziness; a sensation of faintness or an inability to maintain normal balance.

Good health is a state of emotional and physical well-being that is determined, to a large extent, by diet. A key to health promotion and disease prevention is sound nutrition. We are what we eat, since the food we consume is used to build and repair every part of our bodies. A well-nourished person is also better able than a poorly nourished individual to ward off infections. Consequently, a poor diet is directly related to multiple health problems.

HEALTH PROBLEMS RELATED TO POOR NUTRITION

Anemia: Low iron or folate intake

Cancer: High-fat, low-fiber diet (cancer of the colon, breast, or cervix)

Constipation: Low-fiber, inadequate fluids; high-fat diet; sedentary lifestyle

---

Diabetes: High-calorie, high-fat diet; obesity; sedentary lifestyle

Hypercholesterolemia: High-fat, low-fiber diet

Hypertension: High-calorie, high-fat diet; obesity

Osteoporosis: Low calcium intake; inadequate vitamin D or lack of sun exposure

---

The physician, the medical assistant, and the **registered dietitian** (RD) are all closely involved in the nutritive care of a patient. The physician prescribes the diet, and ideally the dietitian instructs the patient in how to follow it. If professional aid is not available, the medical assistant may be asked to discuss the diet with the patient, answer questions, and explain certain aspects of the modifications involved. Occasionally, patients may hesitate to ask the physician details about the diet, or questions may arise after the patient leaves the office. The medical assistant is the one the patient turns to for answers. Therefore you should be able to answer basic questions on normal nutrition and should have a fundamental knowledge of the diets that physicians prescribe most often.

There are many reasons that people eat the way they do. Encouraging patients to make significant lifestyle changes regarding their diets requires sensitivity to these reasons. The choices people make about what they eat are greatly influenced by their background and relationships. Every culture, religion, and ethnic group has its own beliefs and practices about food. For example, according to the Hindu religion, eating beef is forbidden. Certain Jewish practices govern the types and preparation of food. Food is also more than sustenance—it represents family and celebrations and has an entire psychological component that we must be aware of to care for each individual patient most effectively.

Nutrition and Dietetics

Nutrition refers to all the processes involved in the intake and utilization of nutrients. *Nutrients* are the organic and inorganic chemicals in food that supply the energy and raw materials for cellular activities. Nutrients include carbohydrates, fats, and proteins. *Metabolism* is the process in which nutrients are used at the cellular level for growth and energy production as well as excretion of waste. Metabolism occurs in two ways. *Anabolism* is the building phase in which smaller molecules, such as amino acids, are combined to form larger molecules, such as proteins. *Catabolism* is the breaking down phase in which larger molecules, such as glycogen, are converted into smaller glucose molecules for energy. **Digestion** is a combination of mechanical and chemical processes occurring in the mouth, stomach, and small intestine that result in reducing nutrients into absorbable forms including amino acids, fatty acids, glycerol, and glucose. Nutrients are absorbed in the small intestine and then carried by the bloodstream to all parts of the body.

The term *nutrition* is also used to indicate nutritional status, or the condition of the body resulting from the utilization of nutrients. Public interest in nutrition has increased in recent years owing to the growing concern about wellness and health promotion. *Dietetics* is the practical application of nutritional science to individuals. It is the combined science and art of feeding individuals or groups under different economic or health conditions according to the principles of nutrition and management. A registered dietitian's role is the promotion of good health through proper diet and the therapeutic use of diet in the treatment of disease.

Nutrients

To nurture life, the nutrients in food must perform one or more of three basic functions in the body: (1) providing a source of fuel or energy, (2) supplying nutrients to build and repair tissues, and (3) regulating metabolic processes. No one food supplies all the nutrients required; therefore a combination of different foods is necessary to promote health. With a little planning, it is possible to supply all the body's needs from a well-balanced diet. Dietary **deficiencies** result in undernourishment or malnourishment and may lead to a variety of diseases. Good nutrition is an important part of health promotion for all individuals but especially for pregnant women, young children, and the elderly.

The role of diet in supplying energy is crucial to body functions. Every action of the body, whether voluntary or involuntary, requires energy. Even when asleep, the body still needs a source of energy to keep vital organs functioning. *Basal metabolism* is the amount of energy needed to maintain essential body functions. The *basal metabolic rate* (BMR) is the amount of energy used by a fasting, resting individual to maintain vital functions. The rate is determined by the amount of oxygen used and is defined in units of heat energy called *calories* (cal). Because this unit represents a relatively small amount of energy and metabolism involves much larger quantities of energy, the large calorie (Cal), or *kilocalorie* (kcal), is commonly used. A *kilocalorie* is defined as the amount of heat required to raise the temperature of 1 kg of water 1° C. Of the seven food constituents (carbohydrates, proteins, fats, water, minerals, vitamins, and fiber), only carbohydrates, proteins, and fats are capable of furnishing the body with energy. The amount of energy, or kilocalories, needed by a given individual varies according to activity level, basal metabolic requirements, and the presence of disease. Most adults between 20 and 40 years of age require 1800 to 3300 kcal/day. A patient is generally said to be overweight or underweight when his or her present weight is compared with nutritional assessment standards. **Obesity** may be caused by excessive caloric intake in relation to the expenditure of calories, or because of certain endocrine imbalances.

One of the ways nutrients are categorized is by whether they are a required part of the diet or whether they can be anabolized in the body. An *essential* nutrient cannot be manufactured by the body and therefore must be part of the diet or a deficiency disease will occur. A *nonessential* nutrient can be created within the body and so does not need to be included in the diet.

Nutrient Components

Carbohydrates. Carbohydrates (CHO) are chemical organic compounds composed of carbon, hydrogen, and oxygen and are primarily plant products in origin. They are divided into three groups based on the complexity of their molecules: simple sugars, complex carbohydrates (starch), and dietary fiber. Each has a function in health and consists of many variations. With the exception of fiber, carbohydrates are easily digested and absorbed into the body. Simple sugars are quickly absorbed, whereas complex carbohydrates must be processed before they can be absorbed in the intestinal tract. Dietary fiber is indigestible and passes through the gastrointestinal tract unchanged.

The main function of carbohydrates is to supply fuel for energy as well as all basic cellular activities. To meet energy needs, carbohydrate is metabolized at a rate of 4 kcal/g. When digested, carbohydrate is converted into glucose, which is carried by the bloodstream to cells that need energy. A small amount of glucose is stored in the liver and muscles as *glycogen*. This stored glucose is available to supplement dietary supplies of carbohydrate. Excess amounts of carbohydrate are stored in the body as fat or *adipose* tissue. Carbohydrate is also needed to regulate protein and fat metabolism. As long as there are sufficient amounts of dietary carbohydrate available to meet the energy needs of the body, protein and fat are not needed to supply energy. This *protein-sparing* effect allows protein to be used for the repair and growth of tissues and prevents the build-up of waste materials from fat metabolism. In addition, the central nervous system (CNS) requires a constant minute-to-minute supply of glucose to function properly. Sustained low blood glucose levels can result in brain damage and death.

Dietary fiber is commonly called *roughage*. It is defined as the portion of the plant that cannot be digested or absorbed. However, fiber's inability to be digested makes it an important dietary asset. Fiber adds bulk to the intestinal tract that stimulates peristalsis and promotes regular bowel movements. It also combines with **cholesterol** in the intestine and is excreted through the bowel, thereby preventing absorption of cholesterol into the bloodstream. Water-soluble fiber found in oat bran, fruits, and vegetables helps to lower blood cholesterol levels. Insoluble fiber, which is found in whole grains and beans, helps prevent colon cancer and seems to reduce the risk of heart attack. The dietary recommendation for daily fiber intake is 25 to 40 g/1000 kcal, which is the equivalent of two large bowls of bran cereal or $1\frac{1}{2}$ cup of baked beans. Increasing fiber in the diet is not that difficult to do: three dried prunes contain 3 g of fiber; $\frac{1}{2}$ cup of peas about 4 g; $\frac{1}{2}$ cup of kidney beans 7 g; an apple with the skin 3.5 g; $\frac{1}{4}$ cup of raisins 3 g; and 3.5 ounces of air-popped popcorn, a whopping 15 g. Just keeping the skin on fruit and eating raw vegetables greatly increases the fiber content of the food.

CARBOHYDRATE CLASSES AND FOOD SOURCES

Complex Carbohydrates

Grains and grain products
Cereal, whole grain breads, pasta, rice, corn, barley
Potatoes, legumes, fruits, vegetables, seeds

Simple Sugars

Table sugar, molasses, milk, corn and maple syrup, honey, fruits, baked goods, candy

Fiber

Bran, oatmeal, whole-grain breads, beans, fruits, vegetables, seeds, dried fruit

CRITICAL THINKING APPLICATION

A patient, George Hawthorne, was recently diagnosed with hypertension and hypercholesterolemia, and has a family history of colon cancer. The physician recommends a high-fiber diet. Describe how Marcia should explain to Mr. Hawthorne the purpose of dietary fiber and give some examples of high-fiber foods.

Fats. Fats are the storage form of fuel used to back up carbohydrates as an available energy source. Fat is a much more concentrated form of fuel, producing 9 kcal/g of energy when metabolized. Dietary fats, or *lipids*, provide essential fatty acids and are needed for the absorption of fat-soluble vitamins. Fat gives food flavor and creates a feeling of *satiety* or satisfaction after eating. Adipose tissue, the stored form of fat in the body, supports and protects vital organs, insulates the body to help in the regulation of body temperature, and plays an important role in protecting nerve fibers as well as relaying nerve impulses.

Saturated and Unsaturated Fatty Acids. The main building blocks of fat are *fatty acids*, which can be either saturated or unsaturated. The chemical structure of a *saturated* fatty acid contains all the hydrogen possible and therefore is denser, heavier, and solid at room temperature. Examples of saturated fats are dairy products, eggs, lard, meat, and **hydrogenated** fats, such as margarine. Some fats, such as those in soft margarines, are partially hydrogenated. These fats are usually soft at room temperature. Most saturated fats come from animal sources. The main exceptions are coconut and palm oils, which are of plant origin but are exceptionally high in saturated fat.

The presence of trans fatty acids in food sources, especially in hydrogenated margarine products, is a new concern for health risks. Research indicates trans fats elevate serum lipid levels and inhibit the metabolism of essential fatty acids.

Unsaturated fatty acids can take on more hydrogen under the proper conditions and therefore are less heavy and less dense. If fatty acids have one unfilled hydrogen bond, the fat is called *monounsaturated*. Olives and olive oil, peanuts and peanut oil, canola oil, pecans, and avocados contain monounsaturated fats. *Polyunsaturated* fats, such as safflower, corn, cottonseed, and soy oils, have two or more unfilled hydrogen bonds. Unsaturated fats are found in plants and are usually liquid at room temperature.

FOOD SOURCES OF FAT

- Animal or saturated fats: Dairy products, meat, fish, eggs, coconut and palm oils
- Vegetable or unsaturated fats: Corn, olives, avocados, cottonseed, nuts, beans, olive and canola oils

Cholesterol. Cholesterol is a nonessential nutrient that plays a vital role in metabolic activities. It is only synthesized in animal tissue, so it is not found in plant foods. The primary food sources of cholesterol are egg yolks and organ meats, although all animal sources of food contain cholesterol. As a nonessential nutrient, it is also manufactured within the body, particularly in the liver.

The confusion between good and bad fat stems from the distinction between the fat in food and the fat in our bodies. The good fats in our diet are polyunsaturated and monounsaturated fats. The bad dietary fats are cholesterol, trans fats, and saturated fats. The fat in our bodies is divided into two *lipoprotein* categories. The good fats, or high-density lipoproteins (HDL), carry cholesterol from body tissues or the bloodstream to the liver for metabolism and excretion. The bad fats, or low-density lipoprotein (LDL) and very low–density lipoprotein (VLDL), carry cholesterol to the cells. LDL and VLDL form *atherosclerotic* plaques on arterial walls that frequently result in heart disease, hypertension, and strokes. However, serum LDL levels can often be successfully changed through diet. Using polyunsaturated and monounsaturated fat products reduces total serum cholesterol levels. In addition, using monounsaturated fats (olive, peanut, and canola oils) reduces LDL levels. Exercise is an important tool for lowering total serum cholesterol levels, increasing HDL levels, and decreasing **triglycerides**. The higher the serum level of HDL, the greater protection there is against cardiovascular disease. The normal HDL range is 30 to 80 mg/dl. A level below 30 indicates significant risk, while a value of 75 or greater provides protection and decreased risk of disease. Heart experts recommend an LDL level below 100 mg/dl and an HDL level of 60 mg/dl or greater (Table 27-1).

Another potential health risk from a high-fat diet is obesity. Too much fat in the diet is deposited in the body as stored adipose tissue. Currently fats make up 35% to 40% of the total calories in the American diet. Nutritionists and epidemiologists believe that decreasing dietary fat to 30%, with saturated fat making up no more than 10% of calories, would decrease the risk of developing cancer, atherosclerosis, hypertension, and heart disease.

TABLE 27-1	Recommendations for Total and LDL Cholesterol Levels					
	Total Cholesterol (mg/dl)			LDL Cholesterol (mg/dl)		
Age in years	Acceptable	Borderline	High	Acceptable	Borderline	High
2 to 20	< 170	170-199	> 200	< 110	110-129	> 130
> 20	< 200	200-239	> 240	< 130	130-159	> 160

DIETARY GUIDELINES FOR FAT CONSUMPTION

- Use only lean cuts and smaller portions of meat, trim visible fat.
- Substitute poultry and fish for red meat; remove poultry skin before eating.
- Avoid adding fat to the cooking process.
- Limit intake of organ meats and egg yolks.
- With elevated serum cholesterol, limit eggs to 2 to 3 per week, or use egg substitutes or egg whites only.
- Use low-fat or fat-free milk and milk products.
- Use low-fat or fat-free products.
- Choose liquid vegetable oils such as canola or olive oils.
- Limit use of margarines.

Beta-Carotene	Mixed Antioxidants
Apricots	Cloves
Broccoli	Green tea
Cantaloupe	Oregano
Carrots	Rice
Kale and	Rosemary
spinach	Sesame
Mustard greens	Thyme
Pumpkin	Wheat bran
Sweet potatoes	Wine
Winter squash	

BENEFITS OF OMEGA-3 FATTY ACIDS AND DIETARY FIBER

Omega-3 Fatty Acids

- Inhibit formation of VLDL
- Alter platelet activity to hinder formation of blood clots
- Increase antiinflammatory effects
- Sources: Seafood; marine oils from fatty fish (cod, salmon, mackerel)

Dietary Fiber

- Inhibits synthesis of cholesterol in the liver
- Clears LDL

Antioxidants. Cholesterol has been high on the list of dietary villains for years and has been thought to be a serious contributor to the development of heart disease. Recent studies indicate that the problem may not lie with the cholesterol itself, but in the way in which it reacts with oxygen, or the process of oxidation, in the bloodstream. Our bodies have developed mechanisms to protect us against toxins created by oxidation through utilization of antioxidant vitamins C and E and beta-carotene, but their amounts are not always sufficient. When there are enough antioxidants circulating in the blood, cholesterol is prevented from oxidizing. Without enough, the opposite is true, and damage to arteries begins. Therefore, in addition to lowering the cholesterol and saturated fat intake, increasing the dietary intake of antioxidants may prove to be of great help. Naturally occurring antioxidants are found in many fruits, vegetables, and certain seasonings.

FOODS CONTAINING ANTIOXIDANTS

Vitamin C	Vitamin E
Broccoli	Almonds
Cabbage	Chick peas
Cauliflower	Oatmeal
Grapefruit	Soy beans
Lemons	Sunflower
Oranges	seeds
Peppers	Wheat germ
Strawberries	
Tangerines	

CRITICAL THINKING APPLICATION

Mr. Hawthorne is attempting to control his hypercholesterolemia with diet and exercise. What recommendations regarding fat intake can Marcia make that will help him lower his total cholesterol and LDL levels as well as raise his HDL level?

Proteins. Proteins are very large, complex molecules. They are composed of units known as **amino acids**, which are the materials that our bodies use to build and repair tissues. There are 20 amino acids that are necessary for normal growth and maintenance of tissues. Of these, eight are essential amino acids that must be included in the diet, because humans do not have the enzymes necessary for their formation.

FUNCTIONS OF PROTEIN

- Builds and repairs body tissue
- Aids in the body's defense mechanisms against disease
- Regulates body secretions and fluids
- Provides energy

Proteins are classified according to whether they contain all essential amino acids in good proportion to one another. *Complete proteins* come from animal sources and contain a mixture of all eight essential amino acids. *Incomplete proteins* do not supply the body with all the essential amino acids. These are the vegetable proteins that must be used in specific combinations, because each is missing or extremely low in one or more of the essential amino acids.

PROTEIN FOOD SOURCES

Complete proteins: Meat, fish, poultry, eggs, and dairy products
Incomplete proteins: Whole grains, rice, soybeans or soy flour, nuts, and legumes

Fortunately, most foods have a mixture of proteins that supplement each other. Because there is little if any storage of amino acids in the body, it is important that a source of protein be included at each meal. Adult women need about 45 g of protein a day and men about 55 to 60 g. The average North American diet contains twice that amount. Excess protein is metabolized and some is excreted while the rest is stored as adipose tissue.

If incomplete proteins are the only source of protein in the diet, a food that is protein deficient in one amino acid should be eaten with one that is high in the same amino acid to get the needed mix of essential amino acids. Vegetarianism has become increasingly popular, and many different forms exist. Some vegetarians consume no red meats but will eat fish and poultry. *Lactoovovegetarians* eat primarily vegetable foods but also include eggs and/or dairy products in their diets. *Lactovegetarians* will consume milk and milk products in addition to vegetables but no other animal sources of food. *Vegans*, or strict vegetarians, consume no animal proteins at all, relying solely on vegetable foods for protein.

Those who eat some animal protein in the form of fish, eggs, and milk are generally not at risk nutritionally. However, vegans must include a variety of vegetable foods to ensure the nutritional adequacy of their diets. To supply sufficient protein, vegetables that complement each other must be eaten together to get the correct proportion of amino acids. This is customarily done in the diets of different cultures. For example, in Mexico, beans are combined with rice, and in Middle Eastern countries, wheat bread is combined with cheese.

EXAMPLES OF NUTRITIONALLY BALANCED INCOMPLETE PROTEIN COMBINATIONS

- Black beans and rice
- Peanut butter sandwich on whole-grain bread
- Split-pea soup with whole-grain bread
- Lentil soup and cornbread
- Sunflower seeds and navy bean soup

Vitamins (Micronutrients). Vitamins are organic substances that occur in minute quantities in plant and animal tissues and are essential for specific metabolic processes to proceed normally. Vitamins function as catalysts and help or allow metabolic reactions to proceed. Originally they were lettered or numbered as they were discovered. However, as they have been identified chemically, they have been given more specific names. In many cases their chemical names are as well known as their letter designations.

FUNCTIONS OF VITAMINS

- Regulate the synthesis of bones, skin, glands, nerves, brain, and blood
- Aid in the metabolism of protein, carbohydrates, and fats
- Prevent nutritional deficiency diseases
- Provide for good health at all ages

Vitamins are divided into two groups: *fat-soluble* (A, D, E, and K) and *water-soluble* (B complex and C). Some vitamins can be manufactured in the body. Vitamin A is produced from beta-carotene food sources such as carrots, pumpkin, and sweet potatoes. Ultraviolet light from the sun initiates the production of vitamin D in the skin. Vitamin K is created from intestinal bacteria.

Vitamins will not cure a disease or illness, other than one caused by the lack of that nutrient. For example, adding vitamin C to a patient's diet will not cure bleeding gums, unless the condition is specifically caused by a lack of ascorbic acid, the chemical name for vitamin C. It should also be noted that toxic symptoms from excessive ingestion of fat-soluble vitamins can occur, since they are capable of being stored in the body, compared with water-soluble vitamins, which are typically excreted in the urine. However, large intakes of some water-soluble vitamins may cause adverse effects. Table 27-2 contains complete information on vitamins. Nutrition experts agree that the greatest benefit from vitamins comes from their natural ingestion as part of the diet rather than in supplement form.

Extensive research is underway regarding the role vitamins play in disease prevention and treatment. Research indicates antioxidant vitamins (C, E, and A) can prevent cell membrane damage that leads to cancer

TABLE 27-2	Vitamin Facts						
Vitamin	U.S. RDA*	Best Sources	Functions	Deficiency Symptoms†	Toxic?	Processing Tips	Did You Know?
A (carotene)	5000 IU/day	Yellow or orange fruits and vegetables, green leafy vegetables, fortified oatmeal, liver, dairy products	Formation and maintenance of skin, hair, and mucous membranes; helps us see in dim light; bone and tooth growth.	Night blindness, dry and scaly skin, frequent fatigue	Yes, in high doses, but beta-carotene is nontoxic	Serve fruits and vegetables raw and keep covered and refrigerated. Steam veggies; broil, bake, or braise meats.	Low-fat and skim milks are often fortified with vitamin A, which is removed with the fat.
B₁ (thiamine)	1.5 mg/day	Fortified cereals and oatmeals, meats, rice and pasta, whole grains, liver	Helps body release energy from carbohydrates during metabolism; growth and muscle tone.	Heart irregularity, fatigue, nerve disorders, mental confusion	No, high doses are excreted by the kidneys.	Do not rinse rice or pasta before and after cooking. Cook in minimal water.	Pasta and breads made of refined flours have B₁ added because it is lost in the milling process.
B₂ (riboflavin)	1.7 mg/day	Whole grains, green leafy vegetables, organ meats, milk and eggs	Helps body release energy from protein, fat, and carbohydrates during metabolism.	Cracks in corners of mouth, rash, anemia	No toxic effects reported.	Store foods in containers that light cannot enter; cook vegetables in minimal water; roast or broil meats.	Most ready-to-eat cereals are fortified with 25% of the U.S. RDA for B₂.
B₆ (pyridoxine)	2 mg/day	Fish, poultry, lean meats, bananas, prunes, dried beans, whole grains, avocados	Helps build body tissue and aids in metabolism of protein.	Convulsions, dermatitis, muscular weakness, skin cracks, anemia	Long-term megadoses may cause nerve damage in hands and feet.	Serve fruits raw or cook for shortest time in little water; roast or broil meats.	Because B₆ aids in use of protein in the body, the need for B₆ increases with protein intake.
B₁₂ (cobalamin)	6 µg/day	Meats, milk products, seafood	Aids cell development, functioning of the nervous system, and the metabolism of protein and fat.	Anemia, nervousness, fatigue, and, in some cases, neuritis and brain degeneration	No toxic effects reported.	Roast or broil meat and fish.	Vegetarians who do not eat any animal products may need a supplement.
Biotin	0.3 mg/day	Cereal/grain products, yeast, legumes, liver	Involved in metabolism of protein, fats, and carbohydrates.	Nausea, vomiting, depression, hair loss, dry, scaly skin	No toxic effects reported.	Storage, processing, and cooking do not appear to affect this vitamin.	Biotin deficiency is extremely rare in the United States.
Folate (folacin, folic acid)	0.4 mg/day	Green leafy vegetables, organ meats, dried peas, beans, and lentils	Aids in genetic material development and involved in red blood cell production.	Gastrointestinal disorders, anemia, cracks on lips	Some evidence of toxicity in large doses.	Store vegetables in refrigerator and steam, boil, or simmer in minimal water.	Deficiencies can occur in premature infants and pregnant women.

Continued

TABLE 27-2	Vitamin Facts—cont'd						
Vitamin	U.S. RDA*	Best Sources	Functions	Deficiency Symptoms†	Toxic?	Processing Tips	Did You Know?
Niacin	20 mg/day	Meat, poultry, fish, enriched cereals, peanuts, potatoes, dairy products, eggs	Involved in carbohydrate, protein, and fat metabolism.	Skin disorders, diarrhea, indigestion, general fatigue	Nicotinic acid form should be taken only under physician's care.	Roast or broil beef, veal, lamb, and poultry. Cook potatoes in minimal water.	Niacin is formed in the body by converting an amino acid found in proteins.
Pantothenic acid	10 mg/day	Lean meats, whole grains, legumes, vegetables, fruits	Helps in the release of energy from fats and carbohydrates.	Fatigue, vomiting, stomach stress, infections, muscle cramps	No toxic effects reported.	Eat fruits and vegetables raw.	It is believed some pantothenic acid is produced in the gastrointestinal tract.
C (ascorbic acid)	60 mg/day	Citrus fruits, berries, and vegetables—especially peppers	Essential for structure of bones, cartilage, muscle, and blood vessels. Also helps maintain capillaries and gums and aids in absorption of iron.	Swollen or bleeding gums, slow wound healing, fatigue/depression, poor digestion	Intakes of 1 g or more can cause nausea, cramps, and diarrhea.	Do not store or soak fruits and vegetables in water. Refrigerate juices and store only 2 to 3 days.	Smokers may benefit from an increased intake of vitamin C.
D	400 IU/day	Fortified milk, sunlight, fish, eggs, butter, fortified margarine	Aids in bone and tooth formation; helps maintain heart action and nervous system.	In children: rickets and other bone deformities. In adults: calcium loss from bones.	High intakes may cause diarrhea and weight loss.	Storage, processing, and cooking do not appear to affect this vitamin.	Sunlight starts vitamin D production in the skin.
E	30 IU/day	Fortified and multi-grain cereals, nuts, wheat germ, vegetable oils, green leafy vegetables	Protects blood cells, body tissue, and essential fatty acids from harmful destruction in the body.	Muscular wasting, nerve damage, anemia, reproductive failure	Relatively nontoxic.	Store in air-tight containers away from light.	Most fortified cereals have 40% of the RDA.
K	*	Green leafy vegetables, fruit, dairy and grain products	Essential for blood clotting functions.	Bleeding disorders in newborns and those on blood-thinning medications	Not toxic as found in food.	Store in containers away from light.	Vitamin K is also formed by bacteria in the colon.

IU, International units; *mg*, milligrams; *μg*, micrograms.

*For adults and children older than 4.

†Many of the symptoms outlined under this heading can also be attributed to problems other than vitamin deficiency. If you have these symptoms and they persist, consult your physician.

*There is no U.S. RDA for vitamin K; however, the Recommended Dietary Allowance is 1 μg/kg of body weight.

Information for this chart was obtained from the Food and Drug Administration, the American Institute for Cancer Research, and the United States Department of Agriculture/Human Nutrition Information Service. Vitamins A, D, E, and K are fat soluble; the other vitamins in this table are water soluble.

and heart disease. Vitamins C and E also appear to protect against the development of cataracts. Vitamin E is recommended to help prevent blood clot formation and coronary heart disease. In addition, B vitamins may help lower LDL levels, and for women planning a pregnancy, folic acid is recommended to prevent neural tube defects.

Because vitamins and dietary supplements are regulated as food and not drugs, there are no standards or regulatory mechanisms for their production. Thus various brands differ in the amount of substance available, its quality, and its level of absorption. The U.S. Pharmacopoeia (USP), an independent organization that sets standards for drugs, recently developed standards for vitamins. It is recommended that consumers look for the USP label on products that adhere to these standards.

Minerals (Electrolytes). Minerals are required by the human body in relatively small amounts, but even so, they are absolutely essential for life (Table 27-3). Of the 19 or more that form the mineral composition of the body, at least 13 are needed to maintain a healthy state. Minerals must be supplied by the diet or from supplements. Recommended daily intakes have been established for 12 minerals. Minerals contribute to the body's water-electrolyte balance and acid-base balance and are essential components of enzymes. Minerals also help regulate muscular and nervous activities, blood clotting, and normal heart rhythm.

Minerals present in the largest amounts include sodium, potassium, calcium, chlorine, phosphorus, and magnesium. Those present in very small amounts, the *trace elements*, include iron, zinc, copper, selenium, chromium, manganese, iodine, and fluorine. The minerals that are needed only in trace amounts seem either to behave as part of hormone or enzyme systems or to work with vitamins in various metabolic reactions throughout the body. For example, iodine is part of the thyroid hormone *thyroxine*, and another hormone, *insulin*, has zinc as part of its structure. Cobalt, on the other hand, is an essential part of vitamin B_{12}.

Calcium, iodine, and iron are the minerals most frequently missing in the American diet. Some of the leading causes of disease-related mineral deficiencies include **osteoporosis** from lack of vitamin D and/or calcium as well as iron-deficiency anemia. Meanwhile, high sodium levels are associated with hypertension.

DAILY CALCIUM RECOMMENDATIONS

Age	Recommended Intake
1-3	500 mg
4-8	800 mg
9-18	1300 mg
19-50	1000 mg
51 and older	1200 mg

Water. Water is all too often overlooked when nutritional status is evaluated. The body is approximately 80% water and can survive longer without food than it can without water. Water is part of almost every vital body process.

FUNCTIONS OF WATER

- Plays a key role in the maintenance of body temperature
- Acts as a solvent and the medium for most biochemical reactions
- Acts as the vehicle for transport of substances such as nutrients, hormones, antibodies, and metabolic waste
- Acts as a lubricant for joints and mucous membranes

Water is lost daily from the body in urine, feces, sweat, and expiration. Extensive water losses from diarrhea, vomiting, burns, or perspiration can lead to electrolyte losses that result in life-threatening imbalances. Water is contained in almost all foods; however, a healthy diet should include about eight glasses of water a day.

The Food Guide Pyramid

In 1992, to reflect the new dietary guidelines that called for more consumption of grains and less consumption of meat, sweets, and fats, the Food Guide Pyramid was introduced by the United States Department of Agriculture (USDA) (Figure 27-1). The pyramid is divided into six sections. The largest sections are the foods that should be consumed in the largest quantities. The grain group, the largest section, was placed at the bottom of the pyramid, with foods high in fat and simple sugars placed at the top to emphasize the difference in importance between the two substances in the diet. The Food Guide Pyramid shows how the proportions of each basic food group contribute to a balanced diet.

Two symbols, a circle and a triangle, are used on the pyramid. The circle indicates fat that occurs naturally or is added, and the triangle indicates sugar that is added. These symbols show how fat and sugar can occur naturally or be added to foods in the five basic food groups.

Explaining this food pyramid to patients will encourage healthful eating habits. Many patients have never been educated in nutrition and do not know how to plan a healthy diet for themselves or their families. Good nutrition is a balance between carbohydrates, protein, vitamins, minerals, fiber, and water, with limited amounts of fat, sodium, sugar, and alcohol. Calorie intake must be balanced with energy output in order to maintain a healthy body weight. The USDA is currently reassessing the pyramid to ensure that people understand what foods fall into the various categories and the number of recommended daily servings. Table 27-4 explains the number of servings and samples of foods for each serving for the six sections.

TABLE 27-3	Minerals		
Functions	**Sources**	**Deficiency Symptoms**	**Toxicity Symptoms**
Mineral and Elemental Symbol: Calcium (Ca^{2+})			
Helps muscles to contract and relax, thereby helping to regulate heartbeat Plays a role in the normal functioning of the nervous system Aids in blood coagulation and the functioning of some enzymes Helps build strong bones and teeth May help prevent hypertension	Primarily found in milk and milk products; also found in dark green, leafy vegetables, tofu and other soy products, sardines, salmon with bones, and hard water	Poor bone growth and tooth development, leading to stunted growth and increased risk of dental caries, rickets (bowing of legs) in children, osteomalacia (soft bones) and osteoporosis (brittle bones) in adults, poor blood clotting, and possible hypertension	Kidney stones
Mineral and Elemental Symbol: Chloride (Cl$^-$)			
Involved in the maintenance of fluid and acid-base balance Provides an acid medium, in the form of hydrochloric acid, for activation of gastric enzymes	Major source is table salt (sodium chloride); also found in fish and vegetables	Disturbances in acid-base balance, with possible growth retardation, psychomotor defects, and memory loss	Disturbances in acid-base balance
Mineral and Elemental Symbol: Magnesium (Mg^{2+})			
Helps build strong bones and teeth Activates many enzymes Participates in protein synthesis and lipid metabolism Helps regulate heartbeat	Raw, dark green vegetables, nuts and soybeans, whole grains and wheat bran, bananas and apricots, seafoods and coffee, tea, cocoa, and hard water	Rare but in disease states may lead to central nervous system problems (confusion, apathy, hallucinations, poor memory) and neuromuscular problems (muscle weakness, cramps, tremor, cardiac arrhythmia)	Drowsiness, weakness, and lethargy and in severe toxicity skeletal paralysis, central nervous system depression, respiratory depression, and ultimately coma and death
Mineral and Elemental Symbol: Phosphorus (PO$_4$)			
Helps build strong bones and teeth Present in the nuclei of all cells Helps in the oxidation of fats and carbohydrates (energy metabolism) Aids in maintaining the body's acid-base balance	Milk and milk products, eggs, meats, legumes, whole grains, soft drinks (used to make the "fizz")	Rare but with malabsorption can cause anorexia, weakness, stiff joints, and fragile bones	Hypocalcemic tetany (muscle spasms)
Mineral and Elemental Symbol: Potassium (K$^+$)			
Plays a key role in fluid and acid-base balance Transmits nerve impulses and helps control muscle contractions and promotes regular hearbeat Needed for enzyme reactions	Apricots, bananas, oranges, grapefruit, raisins, green beans, broccoli, carrots, greens, potatoes, meats, milk and milk products, peanut butter and legumes, molasses, coffee, tea, cocoa	May cause impaired growth, hypertension, bone fragility, central nervous system changes, renal hypertrophy, diminished heart rate, and death	Hyperkalemia (excess potassium in the blood) with cardiac function disturbances
Mineral and Elemental Symbol: Sodium (Na$^+$)			
Plays a key role in the maintenance of acid-base balance Transmits nerve impulses and helps control muscle contractions Regulates cell membrane permeability	Salt (sodium chloride) is the major dietary source; minor sources occur naturally in foods such as milk and milk products and several vegetables	Hyponatremia (too little sodium in the blood)	May cause hypertension, which can lead to cardiovascular diseases and renal (kidney) disease; in the form of salt tablets, can cause gastric irritation

TABLE 27-3	Minerals—cont'd		
Functions	**Sources**	**Deficiency Symptoms**	**Toxicity Symptoms**
Mineral and Elemental Symbol: Chromium (Cr^{3+})			
Activates several enzymes Enhances the removal of glucose from the blood	Liver and other meats, whole grains, cheese, legumes, and brewer's yeast	Weight loss, abnormalities of the central nervous system, and possible aggravation of diabetes mellitus	Inhibited insulin activity
Mineral and Elemental Symbol: Copper (Cu^{2+})			
Aids in the production and survival of red blood cells Part of many enzymes involved in respiration Plays a role in normal lipid metabolism	Shellfish—especially oysters—liver, nuts and seeds, raisins, whole grains, and chocolate	Anemia, central nervous system problems, abnormal electrocardiograms, bone fragility, impaired immune response; may be a factor in failure to thrive in premature infants	In Wilson's disease and Huntington's chorea (both hereditary diseases), copper accumulation causes neuron and liver cell damage
Mineral and Elemental Symbol: Fluorine (F^-)			
Helps the formation of solid bones and teeth, thereby reducing incidence of dental caries, and may help prevent osteoporosis	Fluoridated water (and foods cooked in fluoridated water), fish, tea, gelatin	Increased susceptibility to dental caries	Fluorosis and mottling of teeth
Mineral and Elemental Symbol: Iodine (I^-)			
Helps regulate energy metabolism through being part of thyroid hormones Essential for normal cell functioning, helps to keep skin, hair, and nails healthy	Primarily from iodized salt, also found in saltwater fish, seaweed products, vegetables grown in iodine-rich soils	Goiter, cretinism in infants born to iodine-deficient mothers, with accompanying mental retardation and diffuse central nervous system abnormalities	Little toxic effect in individuals with normal thyroid gland functioning
Mineral and Elemental Symbol: Iron (Fe^{3+})			
Essential to the formation of hemoglobin, which is important for tissue respiration and ultimately growth and development Part of several enzymes and proteins in the body	Heme sources: organ meats—especially liver, red meats, and other meats Nonheme sources: iron-fortified cereals, dark green leafy vegetables, legumes, whole grains, blackstrap molasses, dried fruit, and foods cooked in iron pans	Iron-deficiency anemia and possible alterations that impair behavior	Idiopathic hemochromatosis, which can lead to cirrhosis, diabetes mellitus, skin pigmentation, arthralgias (joint pain), and cardiomyopathy
Mineral and Elemental Symbol: Manganese (Mn^{2+})			
Needed for normal bone structure, reproduction, normal functioning of cells and the central nervous system A component of some enzymes	Nuts, whole grains, vegetables and fruits, coffee, tea, cocoa, and egg yolks	None observed in humans	Iron-deficiency anemia through inhibiting effect on iron absorption; pulmonary changes, anorexia, apathy, impotence, headaches, leg cramps, and speech impairment; in advanced stages of toxicity resembles Parkinson's disease
Mineral and Elemental Symbol: Selenium (Se)			
Part of an enzyme system Acts as an antioxidant with vitamin E to protect the cell from oxygen	Protein-rich foods (meat, eggs, milk), whole grains, seafood, liver and other meats, egg yolks, and garlic	Keshan disease (a human cardiomyopathy) and Kashin-Bek disease (an endemic human osteoarthropathy)	Physical defects of the fingernails and toenails and hair loss

Continued

TABLE 27-3	Minerals—cont'd		
Functions	**Sources**	**Deficiency Symptoms**	**Toxicity Symptoms**
Mineral and Elemental Symbol: Zinc (Zn^{2+})			
Plays a role in protein synthesis Essential for normal growth and sexual development, wound healing, immune function, cell division and differentiation, and smell acuity	Whole grains, wheat germ, crabmeat, oyster, liver and other meats, brewer's yeast	Depressed immune function, poor growth, dwarfism, impaired skeletal growth and delayed sexual maturation, acrodermatitis	Severe anemia, nausea, vomiting, abdominal cramps, diarrhea, fever, hypocupremia (low blood serum copper), malaise, fatigue

From Poleman CM, Peckenpaugh NJ: *Nutrition essentials and diet therapy*, ed 6, Philadelphia, WB Saunders, 1991, pp 128-129. Data from Garrison RH, Somer E: *The nutrition desk reference*, New Canaan, Conn, Keats Publishing, 1985; and Griffeth HW: *Complete guide to vitamins, minerals and supplements*, Tucson, Fisher Books, 1988.

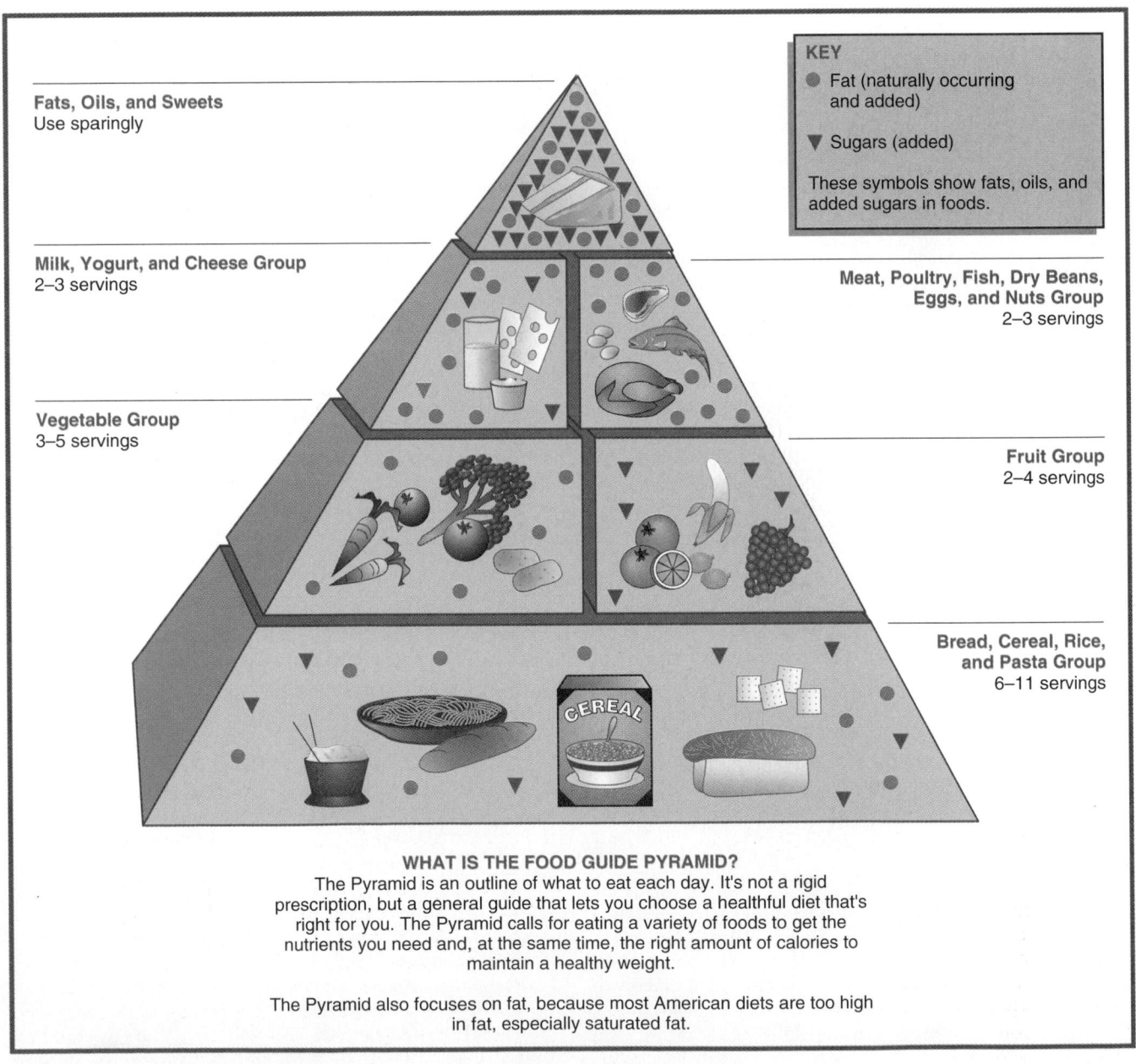

WHAT IS THE FOOD GUIDE PYRAMID?
The Pyramid is an outline of what to eat each day. It's not a rigid prescription, but a general guide that lets you choose a healthful diet that's right for you. The Pyramid calls for eating a variety of foods to get the nutrients you need and, at the same time, the right amount of calories to maintain a healthy weight.

The Pyramid also focuses on fat, because most American diets are too high in fat, especially saturated fat.

FIGURE 27-1 Food Guide Pyramid. (From U.S. Department of Agriculture.)

TABLE 27-4	Food Guide Pyramid Facts	
Nutrient Category	**Number of Servings/Day**	**Examples of Single Servings**
Fats, oils, and sweets	Use sparingly; limit sweets to a few servings/week	• No more than one small serving/day
Milk, yogurt, and cheese	Ages 2-6 years and adults under 50, two servings; 7- to 20-year-olds and adults over 50, three servings	• 1 cup milk or yogurt • 1½ oz natural cheese • 2 oz processed cheese
Meat, poultry, fish, dry beans, nuts	Ages 2-6, most women, and older adults, two servings (total 5 oz); older children, teen girls, active women, most men, two servings (6 oz); teen boys and active men, three servings (7 oz)	• 2-3 oz cooked lean meat, poultry, or fish (size of deck of cards) • 1 cup cooked dry beans • ¼ cup tofu, 2½ oz soyburger, 1 egg • 2 tbl peanut butter or ⅓ cup nuts (each counts as 1 oz of lean meat)
Vegetable group	Ages 2-6, most women, and older adults, three servings of different vegetables; older children, teen girls, active women, most men, four servings; teen boys and active men, five servings	• 1 cup raw leafy vegetables (spinach or lettuce) • ¾ cup of other vegetables, cooked or raw • ¼ cup vegetable juice
Fruit group	Ages 2-6, most women, and older adults, two servings; older children, teen girls, active women, most men, three servings; teen boys and active men, four servings	• 1 medium fruit (apple, banana, orange, pear, etc.) • ¼ cup chopped, cooked, canned fruit • ¾ cup fruit juice
Bread, cereal, rice, and pasta	Ages 2-6, most women, and older adults, six servings; older children, teen girls, active women, most men, nine servings; teen boys and active men, 11 servings	• 1 slice bread • 1 cup cereal • ½ cup cooked cereal, rice, pasta

Nutritional Status Assessment

During the physician's examination of the patient, he or she assesses the patient's nutritional status. The physician considers the patient's age; height and weight; overall health status; recent changes in weight; diet and exercise habits; and lifestyle, culture, and educational background. In addition to this information, the physician may check the patient's skin **turgor**, assess the percentage of body fat, and calculate the body mass index.

Body Fat Measurement

The location of body fat is very important. Studies conducted in the United States and in Sweden indicate that the body has two different fat stores: one at the hips and the other in the abdomen. Fat at the hips is more common in women and is used to store energy for special purposes, such as during pregnancy and breastfeeding. Abdominal fat seems to be more dangerous to overall health. The waist and hips of the patient are measured and correlated with the waist-to-hip ratio (the bigger the belly, the higher the ratio). Normal ratios are less than 0.75 in women and are 0.9 to 0.95 in men.

At the physician's request, the medical assistant may be asked to perform body fat measurements on a patient. The percentage of body fat may be an indicator of overall health as well as risk for cardiovascular disease. Body fat can be measured by several methods. The most conclusive, although inconvenient in general medical practice, is body density measurement, which is obtained with the patient submerged under water to obtain the weight of the body when completely submerged. Another method is through the use of a specialized scale that gives the weight and body fat percentage while the patient stands on it. A reliable method of measuring body fat uses a specially designed caliper to measure the thickness of a fold of tissue in three areas: the triceps, the subscapular, and the suprailiac regions (Procedure 27-1).

Calculating Body Mass Index

To determine how healthy the patient's weight level is the physician may want you to calculate the patient's body mass index (BMI). The BMI is the relationship of weight to height and is now considered a more accurate predictor of weight-related health risks than traditional height/weight charts, since it provides a good estimate of the degree of body fat. There are two methods for determining a patient's BMI. The nomogram in Figure 27-2 can be implemented using the patient's weight in kilograms or pounds and the height in centimeters or inches. To practice using the nomogram, angle the edge of a piece of paper or a ruler from your weight (on the left) to your height (on the right). Then read the BMI where the edge crosses the centerline. The BMI can also be calculated mathematically by dividing the weight in pounds by the square of the height in feet. Individuals with BMIs between 19 and 22 are thought to live the longest. Death rates are significantly higher for people with indexes of 25 and above. If the risk is anything other than acceptable, it may indicate a need for dietary modifications. This will have to be decided by the physician when all of the information on the patient is evaluated.

PROCEDURE **27-1**

Determining Fat-Fold Measurements

GOAL: To accurately determine and record a measurement of body fat.

EQUIPMENT AND SUPPLIES

- Fat-fold body calipers
- Pencil and paper

PROCEDURAL STEPS

1 Read the directions for the caliper before you begin.

2 Gather the equipment and supplies needed to complete the procedure and wash hands.

3 Identify the patient.
    Purpose: To make sure that you have the right patient.

4 Explain the procedure to the patient.
    Purpose: To provide assurance to the patient and education about the fat measurement procedure.

5 Using the triceps of the upper arm, grasp the skinfold with the thumb and index finger. Make sure that the fold is at a parallel angle by keeping the thumb and index finger in line with one another. Be sure you do not grasp muscle tissue or pinch too tightly (Figure 1).

Purpose: Best site to start with because it is the easiest to obtain.

6 Place calipers over the fold and measure.

7 Record the measurement.

8 Grasp the subscapular region located beneath the shoulder blade and obtain your second measurement (Figure 2).

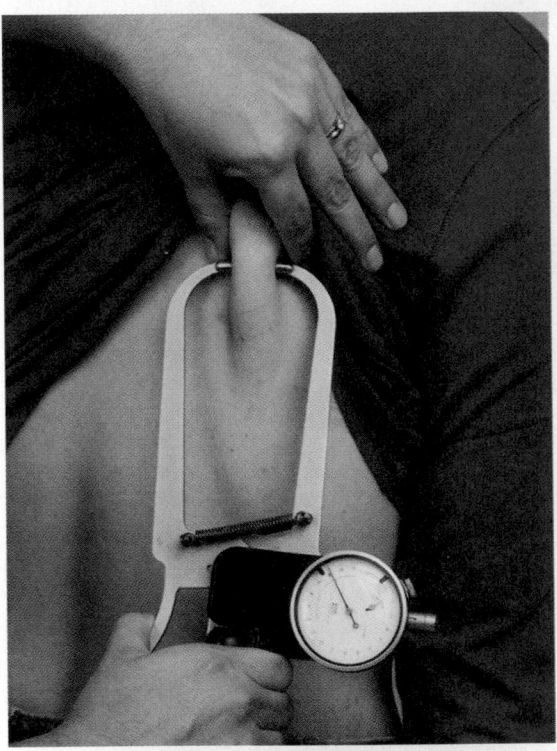

Figure 2

9 Record the measurement.

10 Using the suprailiac area located posteriorly and immediately superior to the fanning of the hip bone, obtain your third measurement (Figure 3).

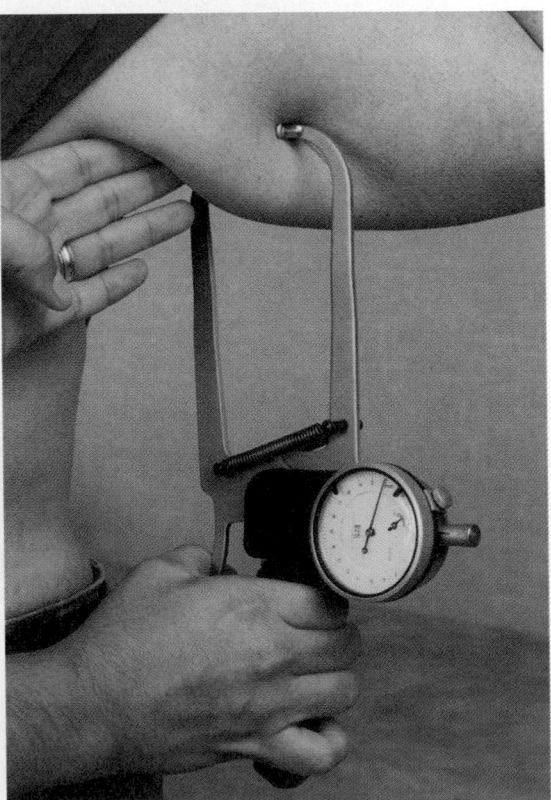

Figure 1

PROCEDURE 27-1—Cont'd

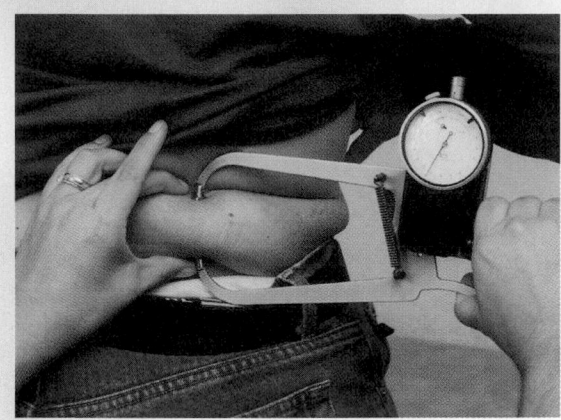

Figure 3

11 Record the measurement.

12 Determine total percent of body fat using Table 27-5.

13 Record the calculations in the patient's medical record.
   Purpose: A procedure is not completed until it is recorded.

14 Disinfect equipment and return to its proper place.

15 Wash your hands.
   Purpose: Infection control.

TABLE 27-5	Body Fat Classification			
Classification	Triceps	Scapular	Abdomen	Total
Male				
Lean <7%	<7 mm	<8 mm	<10 mm	<25 mm
Acceptable 7%-15%	7-13 mm	8-15 mm	10-20 mm	25-48 mm
Overfat >15%	>13 mm	>15 mm	>20 mm	>48 mm
Female				
Lean <12%	<90 mm	<7 mm	<7 mm	<23 mm
Acceptable 12%-25%	9-17 mm	7-14 mm	7-15 mm	23-46 mm
Overfat >25%	>17 mm	>14 mm	>15 mm	>46 mm

INDICATIONS ASSOCIATED WITH BMI RANGES

- Between 19 and 25 is a healthy weight range
- Between 25 and 30 is considered overweight
- Anything over 30 is considered obese

CRITICAL THINKING APPLICATION

The physician encourages Mr. Hawthorne to lose weight to lower his at-risk BMI index of 29. Explain how Marcia should teach Mr. Hawthorne about the importance of his BMI, how it is measured, and how he can calculate his index at home.

Therapeutic Nutrition

Although a majority of patients are treated medically without the use of a therapeutic diet, there are some illnesses and diseases that can be cured and patients whose recovery can be facilitated by the use of a special diet. For example, patients with hypertension, hypercholesterolemia, certain gastrointestinal diseases, and **diabetes mellitus types 1 and 2** all benefit from a therapeutically planned diet. It is important to take into consideration the patient's lifestyle, cultural influences, and background to ensure cooperation.

Modifying a Diet

The normal diet can be modified with regard to the following features (or combination thereof) to create a therapeutic diet:

- Consistency
- Caloric level
- Levels of one or more nutrients
- Bulk or fiber content
- Spiciness
- Levels of specific foods

In general, the normal diet is modified by restricting foods that are sources of the nutrient involved in the disease process. Except for the nutrient in question, the recommended daily allowances can usually be met. However, if several restrictions are ordered for the same patient, a nutrient supplement may be necessary.

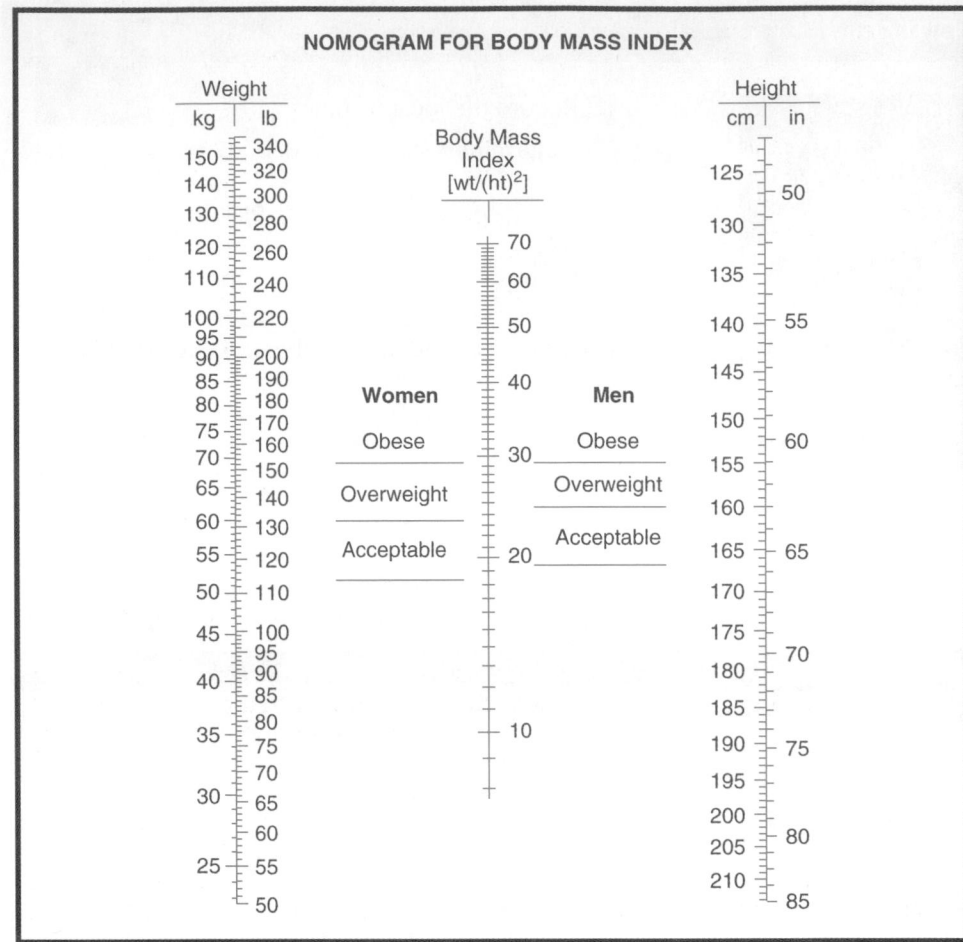

FIGURE 27-2 Nomogram for body mass index.

Soft or Light Diet. When a soft or light diet is prescribed, foods with roughage are eliminated (no raw fruits or vegetables). No strongly flavored or gas-forming vegetables are allowed (onions, beans, broccoli, and cauliflower). In many cases, spices are limited. Often this diet is used after surgery to place less strain on the gastrointestinal system or for patients with certain gastrointestinal disorders.

Mechanical Soft Diet. A mechanical soft diet is a regular diet in which the food is chopped, ground, or pureed, depending on the degree of texture change required. No foods or spices are restricted. This diet may be used after dental or oral surgery or for patients who have difficulty chewing or swallowing.

Liquid Diet. There are two types of liquid diets. A clear liquid diet includes only broth soups, tea, and gelatin. In some cases, apple juice and cranberry juice may be allowed. A full liquid diet includes all foods allowed on a clear liquid diet plus milk, custards, strained cream soups, refined cereals, eggnog, milkshakes, and all juices. This diet may be indicated as part of the preparation process for diagnostic testing or for the first several days after major surgery.

Bland Diet. A bland diet restricts the dietary components that are classified as gastrointestinal irritants. Such a diet limits any foods that are chemically irritating (e.g., caffeine, pepper, chili, nutmeg, and alcohol) or mechanically irritating (e.g., high-fiber foods). No fried foods or highly concentrated sweets are allowed. Gas-forming vegetables belonging to the onion and cabbage family are also eliminated. A bland diet is commonly used for problems occurring in the gastrointestinal tract. Such a diet should supply sufficient nutrients for the individual to meet the recommended daily allowances, unless fruits and vegetables are eliminated.

Elimination Diet. Diets that modify the levels of specific foods are most frequently used to treat allergies of various kinds. There are two basic elimination regimens. A simple elimination diet removes only one or two foods that are suspected of causing the allergy. The Rowe elimination diet involves a more extensive program. Using this method, the basic diet consists of a few hypoallergenic foods such as rice cereal, apples, pears, carrots, sweet potatoes, lamb, and milk substitutes. If no allergic reaction is observed, single food–family groups are added slowly in periods of about 10 days. In children the most common allergies are to chocolate, wheat, eggs, and milk. In some cases it may be difficult to meet the recommended daily allowances for all nutrients. When this situation occurs, supplements should be ordered.

High- or Low-Fiber Diet. The amount of bulk or fiber in the diet is either increased or decreased, depending on the specific disorder of the colon or large bowel. In either case foods high in cellulose are considered to be high in fiber, because the body does not digest this carbohydrate well and a residue is left in the colon. In some instances a low-residue diet is distinguished from a low-fiber diet. In this case a low-fiber diet eliminates those foods with a high cellulose content, and a low-residue diet restricts milk, in addition to fiber content. Either diet should supply all the nutrients needed; however, if milk is restricted drastically, the calcium level must be watched carefully. Low-fiber diets are prescribed for patients with certain gastrointestinal disorders such as diverticulitis. High-fiber diets are recommended for patients with hyper-cholesterolemia or diabetes mellitus, and to prevent certain forms of cancer.

AMERICAN CANCER SOCIETY NUTRITIONAL GUIDELINES

- Increase intake of high-fiber foods such as fruits, vegetables, and whole-grain cereals.
- Eat plenty of dark green and deep yellow fruits and vegetables.
- Eat plenty of broccoli, cabbage, Brussels sprouts, kohlrabi, and cauliflower.
- Moderate use of salt-cured, smoked, and nitrite-cured foods, such as bacon and smoked sausage.
- Decrease total fat intake.
- Avoid obesity.
- Moderate use of alcoholic beverages.

Diabetic Diet. The specific diet for a diabetic patient is determined by the individual's health needs. The basic goal of managing the disease is to maintain consistent control of blood glucose levels. When developing a diabetic diet plan, the physician or registered dietitian must consider additional factors such as weight control methods and individual patient preferences and lifestyle factors. General guidelines for a healthy diabetic diet include:

- Five servings of dark-colored fruits and vegetables and six of whole grains each day
- Two weekly servings of fatty fish (salmon, cod, mackerel)
- Complex carbohydrates that are high in fiber, such as whole grains
- Monounsaturated fats (olive and canola oil)
- Daily serving of nuts, seeds, or legumes
- Fish or soy over poultry or other meat
- Avoid fad diets, especially those with high-protein, low-carbohydrate foods
- Reduce salt intake
- Avoid saturated fats (animal fat) and trans fats

Traditionally, the diabetic diet has been based on exchange lists, which include foods grouped according to similar calorie, carbohydrate, protein, and fat content. The objective of the exchange lists is to achieve the proper balance of carbohydrates, proteins, and fats while maintaining healthy weight and blood glucose levels. Menus are developed based on the food groupings and the optimal number of daily calories needed to meet the patient's needs. Foods can be substituted for each other within an exchange list but not between lists. You can get a copy of the exchange list by contacting the American Diabetes Association. Table 27-6 lists the number of exchanges per day allowed within certain calorie-restricted diabetic diets.

All carbohydrates will raise blood glucose levels to a similar degree. In general, 1 g of carbohydrate raises the blood sugar of someone who weighs 200 pounds by 3 points and for someone who weighs 150 pounds, by 4 points. However, not all carbohydrates raise the blood glucose level at the same *rate*. Choosing a carbohydrate that takes longer to affect blood glucose levels helps control the hyperglycemic peaks associated with the complications of diabetes mellitus. A new rating system, the *glycemic index* of foods, may help solve this problem. The glycemic index places carbohydrate foods on a scale from

TABLE 27-6	Diabetic Diet Exchanges per Day				
	No. of Exchanges or Servings in Each Group				
Exchange Groups and Serving Sizes	**1,200***	**1,500***	**1,800***	**2,000***	**2,200***
Starch/breads: One exchange equals 1 oz of bread and ½ cup cooked cereal, grain, or pasta	5	8	10	11	13
Meat and cheese: One exchange equals 1 oz. High fat exchanges should be used no more than 3 times/wk.	4	5	7	8	8
Vegetables: One exchange equals ½ cup cooked, 1 cup raw, and ½ cup juice	2	3	3	4	4
Fruits and sugar: No more than 10% of total daily CHO; each exchange equals 15 g CHO	3	3	3	3	3
Milk products: One exchange equals 1 cup or 8 oz; skim and very low fat milk products are recommended	2	2	2	2	2
Fats: One exchange equals 1 tsp of fat	3	3	3	4	5

CHO, Carbohydrate.
*Number of calories in the prescribed diabetic diet.

slowest to fastest effects on blood glucose levels. One of the scales is based on 100 glycemic units that is equivalent to the number of units in a glucose tablet. The glycemic index of foods helps diabetics understand the impact of different carbohydrates on blood glucose levels but must be accompanied by a dietary plan that considers the nutritional guidelines for all foods.

Heart Healthy Diet. The goals of a heart healthy diet are to eat foods that reduce overall cholesterol levels, decrease LDL, increase HDL, and keep blood pressure within normal limits. Other factors that must be considered for patients at risk for heart disease are the presence of obesity and exercise levels. Obesity is associated with elevated lipid levels, so weight management, when a factor, must be part of the patient's dietary plan. In addition, researchers report that an aerobic exercise program must be included for cholesterol levels to be maintained at healthy levels. Table 27-7 lists some of the recommended foods for a heart healthy diet.

GLYCEMIC INDEX OF SOME FOODS BASED ON 100

Honey	91	Oatmeal cookies	57
Puffed rice	90	Potato chips	56
White potato	87	Oatmeal	53
Corn chips	72	Sweet potato	50
White rice	72	Spaghetti	38
Whole-wheat bread	72	Yogurt	38
Shredded wheat	70	Milk	34
Brown rice	66	Kidney beans	33
Refined sugar	64	Fructose	22
Rye bread	64	Soy beans	14

CRITICAL THINKING APPLICATION

Ms. Rashad's blood pressure at this visit was 182/94. She is concerned about lowering her blood pressure and potential risks for heart disease. What facts should Marcia share with her about heart healthy diets that will help her understand the importance of nutrition in overall wellness?

CRITICAL THINKING APPLICATION

Samantha Rashad was recently diagnosed with diabetes mellitus type 2. She has met with the dietitian, but she has some questions about her 1200-calorie diabetic diet. The goal of her treatment is to maintain blood glucose levels within normal range, but also to help her lose weight. Based on Marcia's knowledge of the components of a healthy diet, what recommendations can she make to Ms. Rashad?

Reading Food Labels

In 1995 the USDA required that all food products carry a nutritional fact label (Figure 27-3). These labels are usually on the back of the package and are a source of nutrition information and facts on the nutrients within the labeled can or package. When planning or implementing a designated diet, the food label can be used as a valuable source of information (Procedure 27-2).

TABLE 27-7	Recommended Foods for a Heart Healthy Diet	
Food Category	**Healthy Choice**	**Decrease or Eliminate**
Fats & oils	*Monounsaturated fats:* canola & olive oils *Polyunsaturated fats:* sunflower, soy, corn, & sesame	*Saturated fats:* cream, lard, butter, margarine, dressings, & mayonnaise
Milk & milk products	Skim, low-fat, fat-free, or 1% milk-fat products	Whole, condensed, & evaporated milk; cream, half-and-half, & whipped topping
Cheese	Low or non-fat hard cheese, low-fat cottage cheese, part-skim ricotta, or other cheeses	All whole milk cheeses, cheese foods and spreads, creamed cheeses, & processed cheese
Breads	Any whole-grain bread, muffin, roll, pita, or cracker	White flour products, croissants, sweet or buttered rolls, and doughnuts, etc.
Cereals	Any whole-grain cereal that is low in fat, sugar, & sodium but high in fiber	Granola or other cereals with palm or coconut oils
Vegetables	Dark green leafy vegetables, boiled or baked potatoes, & low-sodium soups & juices	Deep-fried vegetables, canned products high in sodium, & pickled vegetables
Fruits	All fresh or frozen fruits & juices without added sugar & dried fruit	Coconut, fruits canned in syrup, & dried fruits with sodium preservatives
Fish	Fresh or frozen fish, clams, scallops, & lobster	Fried, smoked, or salted fish; oil-packed canned fish, sardines, anchovies, oysters, & crab
Meat	Chicken & turkey, remove skin & trim fat; lean & extra lean beef, veal, pork, & lamb	Goose & duck; organ meats; decrease all good & choice cuts of beef & eliminate prime cuts; fried & processed meats

REQUIRED CONTENTS OF A FOOD LABEL

- Front of the label shows any special health claims
- Individual serving size and number of servings per container
- Total calories per serving and calories derived from fat content
- Percentage of daily value (percentage of daily nutrient requirements in serving)
- Gram totals for total fat, cholesterol, sodium, total carbohydrate, and protein
- Total fat is broken down into a gram total and daily percentage for saturated fat
- Total carbohydrate is broken down into dietary fiber and sugars
- Daily value percentages for vitamins A and C, calcium, and iron
- Recommended daily amounts (RDA) for each nutrient
- Ingredients listed in order of importance

How to Use Label Information

Start with serving size information, which is listed in both household and metric units. The amount of each nutrient in the food is expressed in two ways: in terms of weight per serving and as a percentage of the daily value. By using the percentage of daily values, you can determine whether a food contributes a lot or a little of a particular nutrient. However, if you eat more or less than the serving size on the label, you will need to adjust the amounts of nutrients accordingly. Keep in mind that the percentage of daily values is based on the amount of food usually eaten in 1 day. The goal is to choose foods that total 100% of your daily nutrition needs.

The ingredient list also can help you learn more about the foods you eat. Ingredients are listed in descending order of weight. That helps you get an idea of the proportion of an ingredient in a food (Figure 27-4). Artificial colors have to be named in the ingredient list; they no longer can be stated as color added. This is an important item for individuals with food allergies or certain specialized diets. In addition, the total percentage of juice in juice drinks must be declared so that you can see exactly how much juice is in the product.

The front label is where manufacturers often place statements describing the nutritional qualities of their product. The government has set strict conditions under which statements such as "low fat," "cholesterol free," and "good source of fiber" can be used as part of the front label. The Food and Drug Administration (FDA) permits claims linking a nutrient or food to the risk of a disease or health-related condition, but only those health claims that are supported by scientific evidence are allowed.

NUTRITION FACTS

Serving size 1¼ cup (30 g)
Servings per container about 16

Amount per serving	Cereal	Cereal with ½ cup skim milk
Calories	110	160
Calories from fat	0	0

	% Daily value**	
Total fat 0 g*	0%	0%
Saturated fat 0 g	0%	1%
Cholesterol 0 mg	0%	1%
Sodium 270 mg	11%	14%
Total carbohydrate 26 g	9%	11%
Dietary fiber less than 1 g	0%	0%
Sugars 3 g		
Other carbohydrate 22 g		
Protein 2 g		

Vitamin A	0%	6%
Vitamin C	10%	10%
Calcium	0%	15%
Iron	50%	50%
Thiamin	25%	25%
Niacin	25%	25%
Vitamin B$_6$	25%	25%
Folate	25%	25%
Vitamin B$_{12}$	25%	30%

*Amount in cereal. One half cup skim milk contributes an additional 40 calories, less than 5 mg cholesterol, 65 mg sodium, 6 g total carbohydrate (6 g sugars) and 4 g protein.
**Percent daily values are based on a 2,000 calorie diet. Your daily values may be higher or lower depending on your calorie needs:

	Calories:	2000	2500
Total fat	Less than	65 g	80 g
Saturated fat	Less than	20 g	25 g
Cholesterol	Less than	300 mg	300 mg
Sodium	Less than	2400 mg	2400 mg
Total carbohydrate		300 g	375 g
Dietary fiber		25 g	30 g

Calories per gram:
Fat 9 • Carbohydrate 4 • Protein 4

FIGURE 27-3   Nutritional facts label.

REGULATED NUTRITIONAL CLAIMS FOR FOOD LABELS

- Light: One third fewer calories than in the regular product
- Fresh: Raw; never frozen, processed, or preserved
- Calorie-free: Less than 5 calories per serving
- Sugar-free: Less than 0.5 g of sugar per serving
- Sodium-free: Less than 5 mg of sodium per serving
- Fat-free: Less than 0.5 g of fat per serving

REGULATED NUTRITIONAL CLAIMS FOR FOOD LABELS—cont'd

- Cholesterol-free: Less than 2 mg of cholesterol per serving
- Saturated fat–free: Less than 2 g of saturated fat per serving
- High: Provides more than 20% of the recommended daily consumption of the nutrient, as in *high-fiber*
- Lean: Cooked meat or poultry with less than 10.5 g of fat, of which less than 3.5 g is saturated fat
- Extra lean: Cooked meat or poultry with less than 4.9 g of fat, of which less than 1.8 g is saturated fat
- Low-sodium: Less than 140 mg of sodium
- Low-calorie: Less than 40 calories
- Low-fat: 3 g or less of fat
- Low saturated fat: 1 g or less of saturated fat and not more than 15% of calories from saturated fat
- Low cholesterol: 20 mg or less of cholesterol and 2 g or less of saturated fat

From U.S. Food and Drug Administration.

Organic Foods Production Act

In 1990 the USDA proposed that rules be established regarding the labeling of food that was organically grown. Since then the USDA has been working on establishing regulations to validate the fast-growing organic food industry. These regulations state that food labeled "organic" must have been grown without the use of any chemical pesticides, herbicides, or fertilizers. It also prohibits the use of hormones in seed preparation.

In addition to the rules that regulate the growing of fruits and vegetables, there are also regulations for meat, poultry, and milk. As with plants, the use of all hormones is prohibited during any phase of the animal's growth or in the preparation of the product for consumption. Therefore milk that carries the organic label has no added vitamins or chemicals.

Foodborne Diseases

Eating or drinking contaminated food can result in a foodborne disease. There are many different types of bacteria, viruses, and parasites that can contaminate food but the most common are *Escherichia coli 0157:H7, Salmonella,* and *Campylobacter*. Patients may present with a variety of symptoms but the first are typically gastrointestinal—nausea, vomiting, stomach pain, and/or diarrhea. There

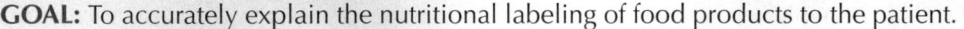

PROCEDURE 27-2

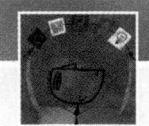

Teaching the Patient to Read Food Labels

GOAL: To accurately explain the nutritional labeling of food products to the patient.

EQUIPMENT AND SUPPLIES

- One each of four bars: Snickers, Twix, Healthy Choice, Fat-Free Fruit Bar
- Pencil and paper

PROCEDURAL STEPS

1 Explain what you are going to talk about to the patient. Be sure to include reasons why food labels are a valuable source of nutritional information in diet planning.

2 Using the labels on each bar, point out the nutritional information according to the guidelines in the text.
  Purpose: Using actual labels assists in learning and reinforces practical application.

3 Give the patient the pencil and paper to write down the serving size of each type of candy bar.
  Purpose: Writing something down helps memory retention.

4 Compare similarities and differences together.
  Purpose: Comparing the results reinforces learning.

5 Next, have the patient write down the total caloric amount for each product serving.
  Purpose: To reinforce impact of high-calorie snacks on overall nutritional health.

6 Compare similarities and differences.

7 Write down the percentage of total, saturated, and unsaturated fats.
  Purpose: To review importance of low-fat diet and role of saturated fat in disease.

8 Compare similarities and differences.

9 Together, analyze the nutritional level of each.

10 Discuss any new information that was learned.
  Purpose: Important to gather feedback regarding the learning experience to clarify learning as needed.

11 Ask the patient if he or she will use this information when shopping and how it will be implemented into nutritional planning.
  Purpose: Role-play implementation of information to determine level of learning.

INGREDIENT LABEL

INGREDIENTS: COOKED WHITE RICE, WATER, COOKED CHICKEN TENDERLOINS, GREEN BEANS, CARROTS, RED PEPPERS, BROWN SUGAR. CONTAINS LESS THAN 2% OF MODIFIED FOOD STARCH, MUSTARD (VINEGAR, MUSTARD SEED, SALT, SPICES, TURMERIC), DIJON MUSTARD (WATER, MUSTARD SEED, DISTILLED VINEGAR, SALT, WHITE WINE, CITRIC ACID, TARTARIC ACID, SPICES), HONEY, MALTODEXTRIN (FROM CORN), SALT, EGG YOLK SOLIDS, SODIUM PHOSPHATE, VINEGAR POWDER (MALTODEXTRIN, MODIFIED FOOD STARCH, VINEGAR SOLIDS), XANTHAN GUM FLAVORS, SPICES, LEMON JUICE CONCENTRATE

FIGURE 27-4 Ingredient label. (Courtesy Weight Watchers International, Inc.)

is usually a delay of several hours to days after ingestion of the contaminated substance before symptoms begin. This is the *incubation period*, when the microbes are attaching to the intestinal walls and beginning to multiply. Diagnosis is confirmed with laboratory tests, the most frequent being a stool sample. However, more sophisticated tests may be needed to diagnose viral pathogens. Treatment depends on patient symptoms but if there is severe diarrhea and vomiting one of the biggest concerns is dehydration, especially with young children and older adults. In this case, replacing fluid and electrolytes is the most important part of care. Other treatments include the use of antidiarrheal medications and drugs that coat the gastrointestinal tract, such as Pepto-Bismol. When doing phone triage with patients having gastrointestinal symptoms, these are some of the items to consider:

Fever of 38.6°C (101.5°F) and above

Diarrhea longer than 3 days

Prolonged vomiting

Blood in the stools

Signs of dehydration: Decrease in urination, dry mouth, **vertigo**

Eating Disorders

Eating disorders are defined as any eating behavior pattern that can lead to a health problem. The two problems that cause the most serious health risks are *anorexia nervosa* and *bulimia*. These disorders can damage all of the body systems and cause death. Although 90% of reported cases occur in adolescent and young adult women, the incidence in males is increasing.

Anorexia nervosa is characterized by self-induced starvation. Anorexic individuals are typically adolescents when first diagnosed and tend to be perfectionists who are extremely sensitive to failure and any criticism. They use avoidance of food as a way of controlling their feelings and fear becoming grossly overweight if they allow themselves to eat. As a result, they lose an excessive amount of weight, usually 15% to 60% of their normal body weight, resulting in extreme malnourishment. They can die without medical intervention. If necessary, patients are fed intravenously or by nasogastric tube feedings to establish an immediate level of nourishment to the body

systems. Patients suffering from anorexia nervosa have a significantly distorted body image and require psychotherapy to alleviate depression, to deal with their emotional issues, and for assistance in forming a positive self-image.

Bulimia is more common than anorexia and is characterized by cycles of binging and purging. This behavior pattern usually begins in adolescence when an individual who is slightly overweight diets but fails to achieve the expected results. Psychologically the person believes that self-worth is related to being thin. Usually the pattern begins with some form of stress that upsets the individual who then turns to food for consolation. Intake during a binge period can reach as high as 20,000 calories. The eating binge is followed by self-induced punishment in the form of vomiting, using laxatives and enemas, excessive exercise, and food abstinence. Most individuals with bulimia have normal or above-normal body weight, but their weight can vary as much as 10 pounds during binging and purging cycles. Treatment programs are a combination of medication, psychotherapy, and nutritional counseling. The goal is to establish healthy eating patterns and to develop an improved self-image.

CRITICAL THINKING APPLICATION

A close friend of Marcia's sister is visiting at their home, and she hears the friend tell her sister that she is using Ex-Lax after every meal and secretly exercising for 3 hours at night after the rest of the family is asleep. She is 5 feet 6 inches tall and determined not to weigh over 100 pounds at graduation. What should Marcia do?

Obesity

Overweight and obesity affect 55% of the American population. Obese individuals are at risk for a wide range of health problems, including hypertension, diabetes mellitus type 2, coronary heart disease, stroke, gallbladder disease, osteoarthritis, sleep apnea, and certain types of cancer. The physician's assessment of patients with weight problems may include evaluation of the BMI and/or the patient's waist-to-hip ratio as well as the presence or risks of conditions associated with obesity. Research evidence indicates the risk for cardiovascular disease rises significantly if the BMI is over 25, and risk of death increases if the BMI is 30 and above. In addition, as BMI levels increase, so do the risks for hypertension and hypercholesterolemia.

GUIDELINES FOR MANAGING PATIENTS WHO ARE OVERWEIGHT OR OBESE

- Engage in 30 minutes of moderate physical activity every day.
- Reduce dietary fat as well as total calories.

GUIDELINES FOR MANAGING PATIENTS WHO ARE OVERWEIGHT OR OBESE—cont'd

- Initial goal to reduce body weight by 10% over a 6-month period.
- Attempt changes in lifestyle for at least 6 months before using prescribed weight loss drugs.
- Weight loss surgery is an alternative for certain patients with chronic, severe obesity.

BENEFITS OF EXERCISE

Increases self-esteem
Improves mood
Boosts energy
Strengthens heart
Strengthens muscles
Burns calories
Improves cholesterol levels
Relieves stress
Prevents bone loss
Decreases risk of some cancers

Health Promotion

The concept of health promotion includes such aspects as adequate nutrition, a healthy environment, ongoing health education, and an overall attempt to prevent disease and maintain optimum wellness. Wellness goes beyond the absence of disease to a state of moving toward fitness, stress management, and maximizing individual potential. Health promotion employs immunizations, appropriate personal hygiene, environmental sanitation standards, protection against occupational hazards, nutritious diets, and periodic health screenings and examinations to safeguard patients and promote wellness.

The medical assistant plays a key role in assisting the physician in many of these procedures. The medical assistant can work as an *advocate* by interacting with local social service agencies or insurance companies on behalf of the patient. The medical assistant also plays an important role in scheduling and assisting the physician with health screenings and physical examinations as well as assisting with health teaching.

For the remainder of this chapter we will discuss components of wellness that all medical assistants should promote.

Exercise

Exercise is defined as physical exertion for the maintenance or improvement of health or for the correction of a physical handicap. Exercise improves cardiorespiratory endurance; maintains musculoskeletal health by improving or maintaining strength, flexibility, and bone integrity; and relieves stress. Although most Americans say they know about the benefits of exercise, only 20% to 25% of adults exercise enough to gain significant health benefits. Twenty-five percent are not active at all, and nearly half of all American youths 12 to 21 years of age are not vigorously active on a regular basis.

A well-balanced diet is only half of the fitness equation; to ensure good health, adequate exercise and sufficient rest form the other half of the equation. As with special diets, exercise programs must be approved for each individual by the physician. It is the physician who determines the patient's exercise needs and tolerance levels to safeguard the patient from overexertion and potential injury.

Many forms of exercise are available. Some patients may find that it is best to go to a gym and develop a formal program of physical fitness. Others may purchase home exercise equipment so they can exercise in privacy. Many feel just getting out in the fresh air and walking is the best form of exercise. All of these are acceptable, because all have one thing in common: physical activity. Each individual should find the outlet that brings enjoyment and enrichment to his or her life. It is not the form of exercise that is important, but the participation in physical activity that promotes wellness.

If you are working with a patient who cannot engage in a full physical exercise program, you can suggest range of motion exercises. These exercise patterns are designed to improve circulation and promote muscle tone by putting each joint through its full range. Patients with disabilities such as partial paralysis, arthritis, bursitis, and musculoskeletal deformities may be helped with these exercises. Range of motion exercises will be presented in Chapter 40.

CRITICAL THINKING APPLICATION

The physician tells Mr. Hawthorne he must exercise to maintain a healthy lifestyle. What can Marcia tell him about the benefits of exercise and possible methods that might help him follow through with the physician's recommendation?

Stress Management

Stress stimulates the fight-or-flight response that physically prepares us to either fight off a stressor or run away from it. Unfortunately, most of the stress we experience on a daily basis is not something we can either physically battle or effectively run away from. Therefore the stress response can lead to multiple health problems if it is not therapeutically managed. The stress response results in the release of epinephrine (adrenaline), which increases the heart and respiratory rates, slows down peristalsis, increases blood supply to the skeletal muscles while decreasing blood to the periphery, causes overall muscular tension, and raises the blood pressure. If stress is permitted to build without release, multiple health problems can occur, some of which can lead to chronic disorders.

STRESS-RELATED HEALTH PROBLEMS

Muscular tension	Anxiety
Headaches	Hypertension
Gastric discomfort	Back pain
	Heart disease
Diarrhea	Gastrointestinal disorders
Fatigue	Autoimmune disorders
Insomnia	
Depression	

STRESS MANAGEMENT STRATEGIES

- Engaging in regular aerobic exercise
- Practicing time management
- Talking it over with someone you trust
- Practicing assertiveness
- Using relaxation and visualization exercises
- Avoiding caffeine and cigarettes, eating well, getting enough sleep
- Making time for yourself

Health Screening

Routine physical examinations and health screenings are important components of health promotion. The patient scheduled for a physical examination should have a health history completed or updated and should be weighed; blood pressure, temperature, pulse, and respirations recorded; and any complaints documented on the chart. Assisting with the physical examination will be covered in Chapter 29. The physician may order the following studies as part of the health screening process:

Tuberculin skin test
Papanicolaou (Pap) smear
Prostate-specific antigen (PSA) levels
Hemoccult test after age 50
Colonoscopy/sigmoidoscopy every 3 to 5 years after age 50
Mammogram yearly after age 50
Urinalysis
Serum cholesterol
Chest x-ray films
Electrocardiogram (ECG)

Patient Education

The medical assistant may be called on to discuss a diet plan with a patient, so it is extremely important to have a thorough knowledge of diet therapy. The patient must understand the diet and the rationale behind its use. If the patient feels uneasy or questions are unanswered, he or she may be less motivated to follow a diet plan. You can be a valuable asset to the physician, the dietitian, and the patient when implementing a specific diet.

When talking to patients about a diet, the medical assistant may find the following helpful:

- Use charts and diagrams to illustrate diets.
- Consider the patient's dietary likes and dislikes.
- Remember that ethnic and cultural foods are important.
- Encourage the patient to play an active role in the learning process.
- Suggest local support groups that can help in diet maintenance.

You can also play a vital role in health promotion by making sure that patients are scheduled for annual examinations and that they follow up with the physician's recommendations for dietary changes, exercise programs, stress management approaches, and health screening procedures. The medical assistant is the link between the patient and the physician as well as between the patient and available community resources.

Legal and Ethical Issues

Always remember that you are not a physician, nor are you a dietitian. Follow the physician's instructions, and if the patient has a question for which you are not sure of the answer, *always* ask the physician for his or her advice in handling the question. If your workplace employs a registered dietitian, refer questions involving meal patterns and food selection changes to him or her. When seeking advice in the field of nutrition and exercise programs, direct patients to someone who is a qualified expert. Use community resources as needed.

SUMMARY OF SCENARIO

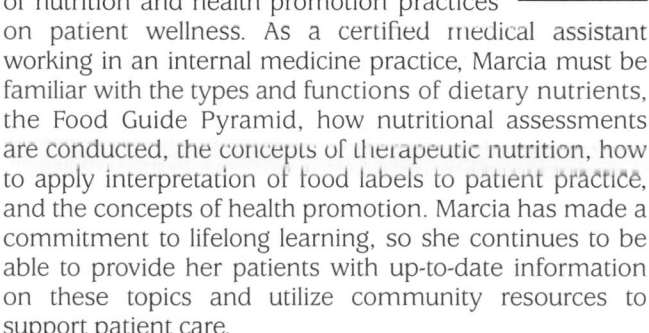

This chapter has emphasized the influences of nutrition and health promotion practices on patient wellness. As a certified medical assistant working in an internal medicine practice, Marcia must be familiar with the types and functions of dietary nutrients, the Food Guide Pyramid, how nutritional assessments are conducted, the concepts of therapeutic nutrition, how to apply interpretation of food labels to patient practice, and the concepts of health promotion. Marcia has made a commitment to lifelong learning, so she continues to be able to provide her patients with up-to-date information on these topics and utilize community resources to support patient care.

SUMMARY OF LEARNING OBJECTIVES

- Nutrients consist of carbohydrates, fats, proteins, vitamins, minerals, and water. Their primary functions are to provide the body with energy, protection, and insulation; build and repair tissues; and regulate metabolic processes.

- The primary function of carbohydrates is to provide the body with a ready source of energy.

Dietary fiber plays an important role in maintaining regularity and helping to prevent cancer and heart disease. Dietary fat provides essential fatty acids and is needed for the absorption of fat-soluble vitamins. Adipose tissue helps protect the organs of the body, insulates, and serves as a concentrated form of stored energy. Protein builds and repairs tissue and assists with metabolic functions.

- Vitamins are essential for metabolic functions and are classified as either fat- or water-soluble. They regulate the synthesis of body tissues as well as aid in the metabolism of nutrients. Vitamins also play a vital role in disease prevention. Minerals help maintain electrolytes and acid-base balance as well as regulate muscular action and nervous activities throughout the body.

- The Food Guide Pyramid was developed by the government as a visual representation of dietary guidelines. The pyramid is divided into six sections and depicts how the proportions of each basic food group contribute to a balanced diet.

- The physician's assessment of the patient's nutritional status includes an evaluation of the patient's current health and lifestyle habits as well as body fat measurements. Body fat can be measured as a waist-to-hip ratio, using calipers to measure fat-folds, or calculating the BMI.

- Therapeutic nutrition uses various diets to help treat or prevent disease. There are many ways diets can be modified, including changes in consistency and taste, monitoring caloric levels, altering amounts and types of specific nutrients, and managing the fiber content of foods. Two examples of diet therapies are the diabetic diet and the heart healthy diet, both of which can have a significant impact on patient wellness.

- The federal government requires all food manufacturers to follow certain guidelines when labeling packages. Labels provide facts on the nutritional value of foods. The food label can be a valuable tool in patient compliance with specialized diets.

■ Health promotion considers all aspects of patient care, including the concepts of general wellness, adequate nutrition, environmental health and safety, health education needs, and disease prevention. The components of health promotion include exercise, stress management, regular physical examinations, and health screening.

■ A medical assistant plays a key role in nutrition and health promotion, serving as a patient advocate and liaison between the patient and community resources. It is important for the medical assistant to understand various implications of nutrition and specific diets so he or she is capable of answering patient questions and thereby promoting compliance with treatment.

KEY INTERNET WEBSITES

- American Diabetes Association
- American Dietetic Association
- American Heart Association
- U.S. Department of Agriculture
  For active weblinks to each website visit
  http://evolve.elsevier.com/Kinn/

CHAPTER 28

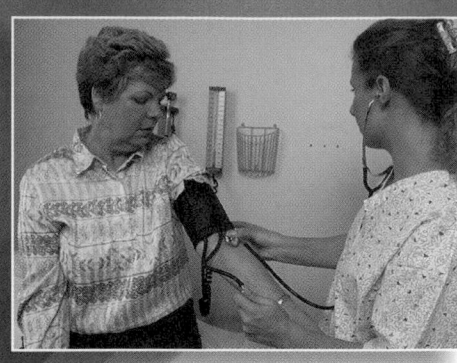

Scenario

Dr. Susan Xu is part of a multi-physician primary care practice. Each physician in the practice has a medical assistant who works directly with him or her. Carlos Ricci, CMA, is Dr. Xu's assistant. Carlos graduated from a medical assistant program 3 years ago and enjoys the variety of patients seen in Dr. Xu's practice. One of Carlos' responsibilities is to accurately monitor and record each patient's vital signs before the patient is seen by Dr. Xu.

Vital Signs

National Curriculum Competencies

CLINICAL COMPETENCIES

4b. Obtain vital signs

Vocabulary

apnea Absence or cessation of breathing.

arrhythmia Irregular heart rhythm.

bounding pulse Pulse that feels full because of increased power of cardiac contractions or as a result of increased blood volume.

bradycardia A slow heartbeat; a pulse below 60 beats per minute.

bradypnea Respirations that are regular in rhythm but slower than normal in rate.

cerumen A waxy secretion in the ear canal; commonly called *ear wax*.

COPD Chronic obstructive pulmonary disease; a progressive and irreversible lung condition that results in diminished lung capacity.

diurnal rhythm Patterns of activity or behavior that follow day-night cycles.

dyspnea Difficult or painful breathing.

elastic pulse Pulse with regular alterations of weak and strong beats without changes in cycle.

essential hypertension Elevated blood pressure of unknown cause that develops for no apparent reason; sometimes called *primary hypertension*.

febrile Pertaining to an elevated body temperature.

homeostasis Internal adaptation and change in response to environmental factors.

hyperlipidemia Excess of fats or lipids in the blood plasma.

hyperpnea Increase in the depth of breathing.

hypertension High blood pressure (systolic pressure consistently above 140 mm Hg and diastolic pressure above 90 mm Hg).

hyperventilation Abnormally prolonged and deep breathing usually associated with acute anxiety or emotional tension.

hypotension Blood pressure that is below normal (systolic pressure below 90 mm Hg and diastolic pressure below 50 mm Hg).

intermittent pulse Pulse in which beats are occasionally skipped.

irregular pulse Pulse that varies in force and frequency.

orthopnea Individual must sit or stand to breathe comfortably.

orthostatic (postural) hypotension Temporary fall in blood pressure when a person rapidly changes from a recumbent position to a standing position.

otitis externa Inflammation or infection of the external auditory canal.

pulse deficit The radial pulse is less than the apical pulse; may indicate peripheral vascular abnormality.

pulse pressure Difference between the systolic and the diastolic blood pressures (more than 30 points or less than 50 points is considered normal).

rales Abnormal or crackling breath sounds during inspiration.

remittent fever Fever in which temperature fluctuates greatly but never falls to the normal level.

rhonchi Abnormal rumbling sounds on expiration that indicate airway obstruction by thick secretions or spasms.

secondary hypertension Elevated blood pressure resulting from another condition.

sinus arrhythmia Irregular heartbeat originating in the sinoatrial node (pacemaker).

spirometer Instrument that measures the volume of inhaled and exhaled air.

stertorous Strenuous respiratory effort that has a snoring sound.

syncope Fainting; a brief lapse in consciousness.

tachycardia Rapid but regular heart rate exceeding 100 beats per minute.

tachypnea Respirations that are rapid and shallow; hyperventilation.

thready pulse Pulse that is scarcely perceptible.

unequal pulses Pulse in which the beats vary in intensity.

vertigo Dizziness.

Measurement of vital signs is an important aspect of almost every patient visit to the medical office. These signs are the human body's indicators of internal **homeostasis** and represent the general state of health of the patient. Because the medical assistant is chiefly responsible for obtaining these measurements, it is imperative to have confidence in the theoretical and practical applications of vital sign measurement. A medical assistant who understands the principles of and the reasons for these measurements will become a valuable asset to any medical office.

Accuracy is essential. A change in one or more of the patient's vital signs may indicate a change in general health. Variations may indicate the presence or disappearance of a disease process and therefore may suggest a need for a change in the treatment plan. Although the medical assistant obtains vital signs routinely, it is not a routine task. These findings are crucial to a correct diagnosis, and should never be measured with indifference or casualness. In addition to accurate measurement, care must be taken when charting the findings on the patient's medical record.

The *vital signs* are the patient's temperature, pulse, respiration, and blood pressure. These four signs are abbreviated *TPR* and *BP* and may be referred to as *cardinal signs*. It is a medical assistant's duty to understand the significance of the vital signs and to accurately measure and record them. Anthropometric measurements are not considered vital signs but are usually obtained at the same time as the vital signs. These measurements include height, weight, and other body measurements, such as fat composition and head and chest circumference.

Factors That May Influence Vital Signs

The vital signs are influenced by many factors, both physical and emotional. A patient may have consumed a hot or cold beverage just before the examination or may be angry or afraid of what the physician may find. For example, a patient has been asked to return to have a repeat Papanicolaou (PAP) smear because the first one showed the presence of unidentifiable cells. The medical assistant measures her blood pressure and finds it to be significantly elevated when compared with previous readings. It is possible, even probable, that this individual is anxious and apprehensive about the test results. What temperature reading might be expected on a patient who could not find a parking place and had to walk 4 blocks to the office and knew he would be late for his appointment? If you said it would be elevated, you are right. Certainly, this patient would have an increase in his metabolism because of the physical exercise, and as a result, his temperature would be elevated along with his pulse, respirations, and blood pressure.

Most patients, for one reason or another, are apprehensive during an office visit. These emotions may alter the vital signs, and the medical assistant must help the patient relax before taking any readings. It sometimes is necessary to obtain measurements a second time, after the patient is calmer or more comfortable. For a better picture of the patient's vital signs, the medical assistant may be asked to record the vital signs twice: at the beginning of the visit and just before the patient leaves the office. Table 28-1 lists the normal ranges of vital signs for various age groups of patients.

Temperature

Physiology

Body temperature is defined as the balance between the heat lost and the heat produced by the body. It is measured in degrees. The process of chemical and physical change within our bodies that produces heat is called *metabolism*. Body temperature is a result of this process. Examples of the factors that may elevate body temperature include respiration, muscle activity, emotional changes, and reproductive activities. Temperature elevation may also be caused by external factors, such as the temperature of the environment.

In illness, an individual's metabolic activity is increased; this causes internal heat production to increase, which in turn increases body temperature. The increase in

body temperature is thought to be the body's defensive reaction, because heat inhibits the growth of some bacteria and viruses.

When a fever is present, superficial blood vessels (near the surface of the skin) constrict. The small papillary muscles at the base of hair follicles also constrict and create goose bumps. Chills and shivering may follow, causing internal heat to be produced. As this process repeats itself, more heat is produced, and the body temperature becomes elevated or increases above normal levels. When more heat is lost than is produced, the opposite effect occurs, and body temperature drops below normal levels.

A variation from the patient's average range of body temperature may be the first warning of an illness or change in the patient's present condition. The body temperature is regulated by the hypothalamus. Average body temperature varies from person to person and is at different levels at different times in each person. This **diurnal rhythm** in a healthy person varies from 97.6° F to 99° F (36.4° C to 37.3° C); the average daily temperature is 98.6° F. The body temperature is lowest in the morning and highest in the late afternoon. In children, teething may cause a slight elevation in temperature but should not be the cause of a fever.

Fever

Infection, either bacterial or viral, is the most common cause of fever in both children and adults. It is unusual for infants to develop **febrile** illnesses during the first 3 months of life, but if one is present it is usually very serious. However, fever in young children is very common and accounts for an estimated 26% of office visits. Fevers are classified according to the 24-hour pattern they follow. The three most commonly seen patterns include the following:

1. *Continuous* fever rises and falls only slightly during a 24-hour period. It remains above the patient's average normal range and is called continuous because that is exactly what the pattern shows.
2. *Intermittent* fever comes and goes, or it spikes and then returns into the average range.
3. *Remittent* fever has great fluctuation but never gets back into the average range. It is a constant fever with fluctuating levels and thus is remittent.

TABLE 28-1	Normal Ranges for Vital Signs		
Age Group	Pulse	Respirations	Blood Pressure (mm Hg)
Newborn	120-160	30-50	60-96/30-62
Toddlers (1-3 yr)	90-140	20-30	78-112/48-78
Preschool (4-6 yr)	80-110	18-26	78-112/50-82
School age (7-11 yr)	75-110	16-22	85-114/52-85
Adolescent (12-16 yr)	60-100	14-20	94-136/58-88
Adult	60-110	12-20	100-140/60-90

TEMPERATURES THAT ARE CONSIDERED FEBRILE (elevated)

- Rectal or *aural* (ear) temperatures over 100.4° F (38° C)
- Oral temperatures over 99.5° F (37.5° C)
- Axillary temperatures over 98.6° F (37° C)
- *Fever of unknown origin* (FUO) is a fever over 100.9° F (38.3° C) for 3 weeks in adults and 1 week in children without a known diagnosis

CRITICAL THINKING APPLICATION

The mother of a 3-year-old calls the office to report that the child had an axillary temperature of 101° F at 9 AM this morning. The schedule is very full today, so Carlos has to decide whether the child should be seen today or first thing tomorrow. When should Carlos make the appointment?

Temperature Readings

A clinical thermometer is used to measure body temperature and is calibrated in either the Fahrenheit or the Celsius scale. The Fahrenheit (F) scale has been used most frequently in the United States to measure body temperature, but hospitals and many ambulatory care settings often use the Celsius scale. The formulas for conversion from one system to the other are as follows:

$$C = (F - 32) \times {}^{5}/_{9}$$
$$F = 9 \times C + 32 \div 5$$

CRITICAL THINKING APPLICATION

Using the formulas given, convert the following temperatures from one system to the other.
99° F = _____ ° C   102° F = _____ ° C
40° C = _____ ° F   45° C = _____ ° F

The thermometer is placed under the tongue, in the rectum, in the ear, or in the axilla, because large blood vessels are near the surface at these points. The average temperature values for these four sites, based on a statistical survey, are shown in Table 28-2.

Rectal temperatures, when measured accurately, are approximately 1° F or 0.6° C higher than oral readings. Axillary temperatures are approximately 1° F or 0.6° C lower than accurate oral readings. Rectal readings are close to the core body temperature because the mucous membrane lining with which the thermometer comes in contact is not exposed to the air; thus it does not vary as does the mucous membrane of the mouth or the skin of the axilla. However, the tympanic (ear) measurement is considered the *most accurate*, because it records the temperature of the blood that is closest to the hypothalamus and therefore reflects a true measure of the core body temperature. It is also fastest, least invasive, and easiest to perform.

TABLE 28-2	Average Temperature Values	
Site	Fahrenheit Scale (degrees)	Celsius Scale (degrees)
Oral mouth	98.6	37
Rectal butt-anal	99.6	37.6
Axillary under arm	97.6	36.4
Tympanic ear	98.6	37

When obtaining temperatures using the oral method of measurement, you do not have to indicate it when documenting the reading. However, in the patient's chart you do record an *R* for rectal, *T* for tympanic, and *A* for axillary readings to clarify the temperature site. It is impossible to accurately measure an oral temperature in a young child, because the technique requires that the patient keep his or her mouth closed. For young children the tympanic thermometer should be used if possible; if not, either a rectal or axillary temperature can be obtained.

Types of Thermometers and Their Use

Digital. Digital thermometers are battery operated and are available in both Fahrenheit and Celsius scales. One type of digital thermometer is a unit equipped with two probes: a blue one for oral use and a red one for rectal use only. Disposable covers fit snugly over the probes and are easily and quickly removed by pushing in the colored end of the probe. The instrument sounds an audible "beep" when the process is completed (between 10 and 60 seconds), and the reading appears on an LED screen on the face of the instrument (Procedure 28-1). Because the only part of the instrument that comes in contact with the patient is the probe, and that is sheathed, the risk of cross-infection is greatly reduced. Another type resembles the old mercury thermometers that OSHA no longer permits in healthcare facilities. These thermometers also have a digital screen where the temperature is read and should always be covered by a disposable sheath (Figure 28-1).

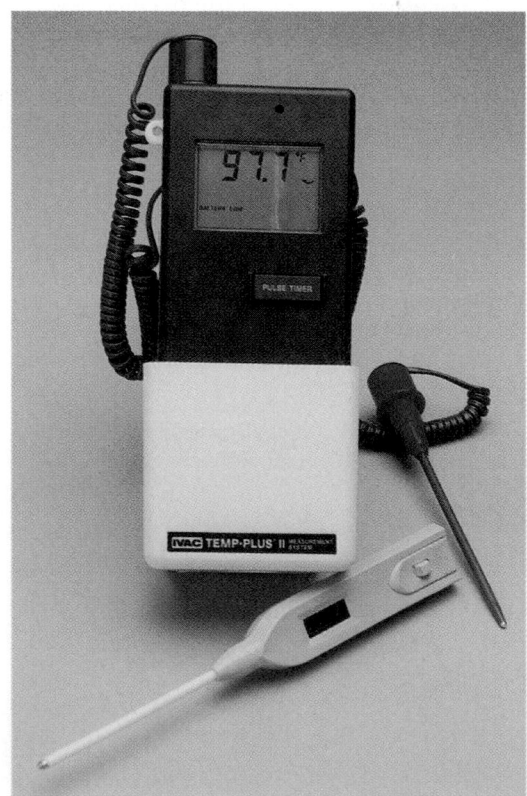

FIGURE 28-1 Digital thermometers.

PROCEDURE **28-1**

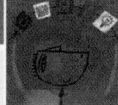

Obtaining an Oral Temperature Using a Digital Thermometer

GOAL: To accurately determine and record a patient's temperature using a digital thermometer.

EQUIPMENT AND SUPPLIES

- Digital thermometer
- Probe covers
- Biohazard waste container

PROCEDURAL STEPS

1 Wash your hands and assemble equipment and supplies.
    Purpose: Infection control.

2 Identify your patient and explain the procedure. Be sure that the patient has not eaten, drunk fluids, smoked, or exercised during the 30 minutes before the temperature is measured.
    Purpose: Identification of the patient prevents errors, and explanations are a means of gaining implied consent and patient cooperation. The temperature will be inaccurate if food or fluids have been ingested or the patient has exercised within 30 minutes.

3 Prepare the probe for use as described in package directions (Figure 1). Make certain probe covers are *always* used.

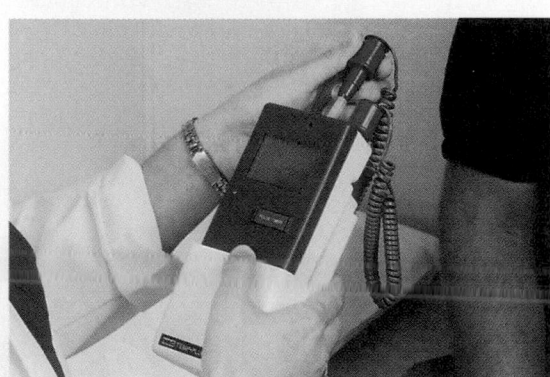

Figure 1

    Purpose: Infection control.

4 Place the probe under the patient's tongue (Figure 2) and instruct the patient to close the mouth tightly (Figure 3). Assist the patient by holding the probe end.

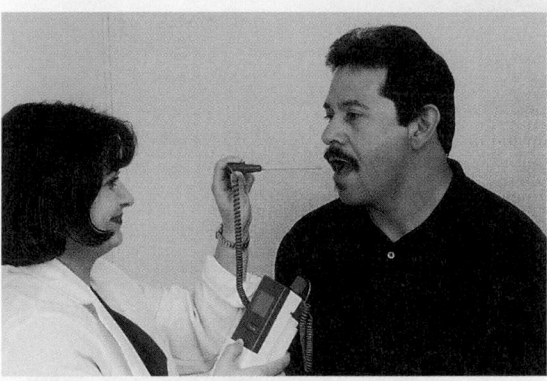

Figure 2

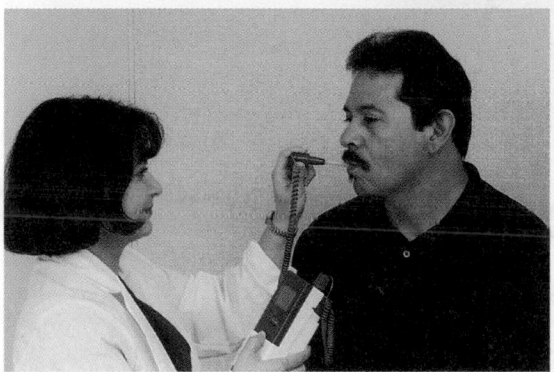

Figure 3

    Purpose: Air seeping into the mouth interferes with an accurate body temperature reading.

5 When the "beep" is heard, remove the probe from the patient's mouth and immediately eject the probe cover into the appropriate waste container.
    Purpose: The probe cover is contaminated and must be placed in a biohazard waste container.

6 Note the reading in the LED window of the processing unit you are holding (Figure 4).

Continued

PROCEDURE **28-1—Cont'd**

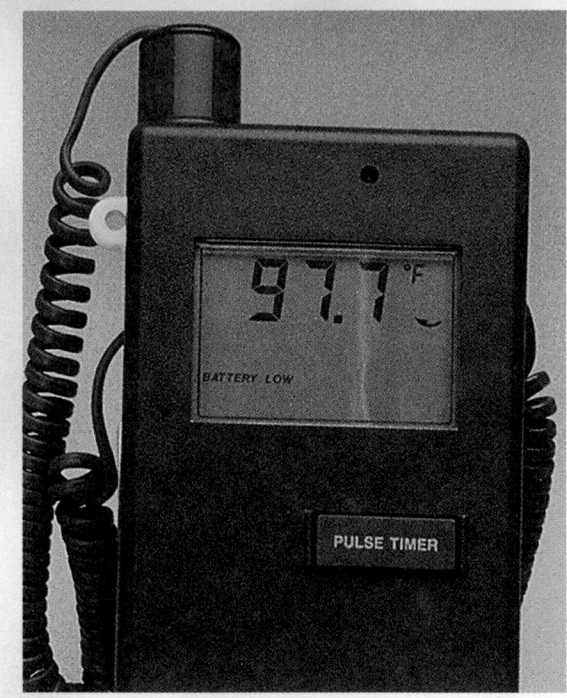

Figure 4

7 Record the reading on the patient's medical record (e.g., T = 97.7°).

Purpose: Procedures that are not recorded are considered not done.

8 Wash your hands and disinfect the equipment as indicated.

Purpose: Infection control and standard precautions.

See Appendix E for a charting example.

An oral temperature should not be taken if the patient has recently had something hot or cold to eat or drink or has just smoked.

Tympanic. The tympanic membrane of the ear can also be used for quick, accurate, and safe assessments of patient temperatures. It shares the blood supply that reaches the hypothalamus, which is the brain's temperature regulator. The ear canal is a protected cavity, so the aural temperature is not affected by factors such as an open mouth, hot or cold drinks, or even a stuffy nose. In addition, the covered probe is designed to bounce an infrared signal off the eardrum without touching it, so the risk of spreading communicable diseases during temperature measurement is greatly reduced.

The tympanic measurement system consists of a hand-held processor unit equipped with a tympanic

PROCEDURE **28-2**

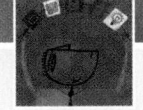

Obtaining an Aural Temperature Using the Tympanic Thermometer

GOAL: To accurately determine and record a patient's temperature using a tympanic thermometer.

EQUIPMENT AND SUPPLIES

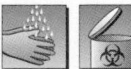

- Tympanic thermometer
- Disposable probe covers
- Biohazard waste container

PROCEDURAL STEPS

1 Wash your hands.
Purpose: Infection control.

2 Gather the necessary equipment and supplies.

3 Identify your patient and explain the procedure.
Purpose: Identification of the patient prevents errors, and explanations are a means of gaining implied consent and patient cooperation.

4 Place a disposable probe cover on the probe (Figure 1).

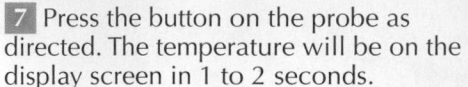

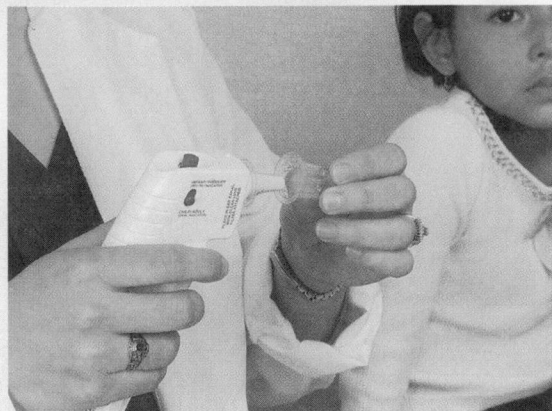

Figure 1

Purpose: To ensure a clean surface and prevent cross-contamination.

5 Follow the package directions to start the thermometer.

6 Insert the probe into the ear canal far enough to seal the opening. Do not apply pressure (Figure 2).

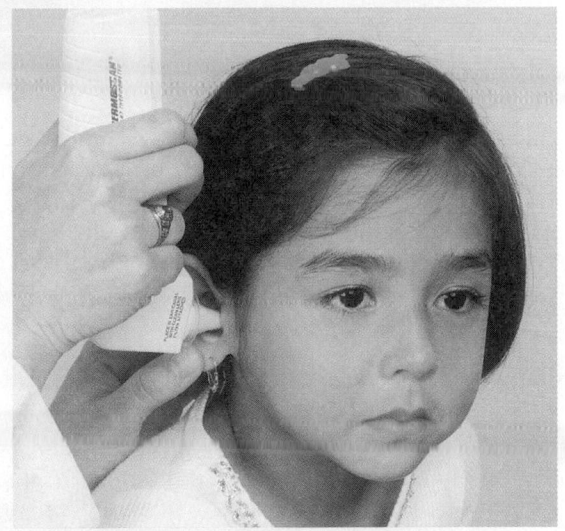

Figure 2

7 Press the button on the probe as directed. The temperature will be on the display screen in 1 to 2 seconds.

8 Remove the probe, note the reading (Figure 3), and discard the probe cover without touching it.

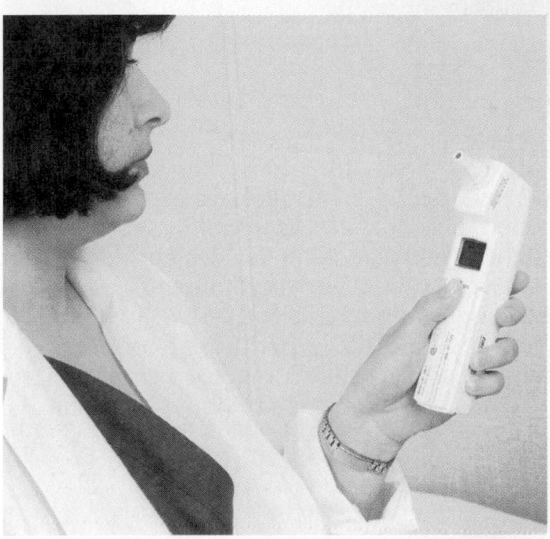

Figure 3

Purpose: The probe cover will be contaminated and must be disposed of in a biohazard waste container.

9 Wash your hands and disinfect the equipment if indicated.

Purpose: Infection control.

10 Record the temperature results (e.g., T = 98.6° [T]) on the patient's medical record.

Purpose: Procedures that are not recorded are considered not done.

See Appendix E for a charting example.

probe that is covered with a disposable speculum when being used (Figure 28-2). When the probe is placed into the ear canal, it gently seals the external opening of the canal, and the infrared energy emitted by the tympanic membrane is gathered. This signal is then digitized by the processor unit and shown on the display screen. Accurate readings are obtained in less than 2 seconds (Procedure 28-2). The speed and patient comfort of the tympanic thermometer have greatly influenced its popularity. This unit should not be used (1) if the patient has bilateral **otitis externa**, because the procedure would be uncomfortable for the patient, or (2) if impacted **cerumen** is present in both ears, because the reading may be inaccurate.

Disposable. Disposable thermometers (those that are used only once) are also available for obtaining body temperatures. They are frequently used in the home on small children. The reading is obtained by a heat-sensitive material that changes color according to the elevation of body temperature. There are two types of disposable thermometers that are frequently used by parents of young children. One type is placed on the child's forehead (Figure 28-3, *A*); the other is placed under the tongue (Figure 28-3, *B*). Although both types are fairly reliable, the

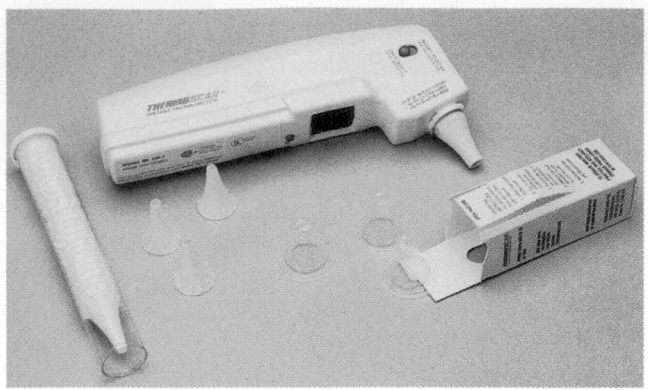

FIGURE 28-2 Tympanic thermometer.

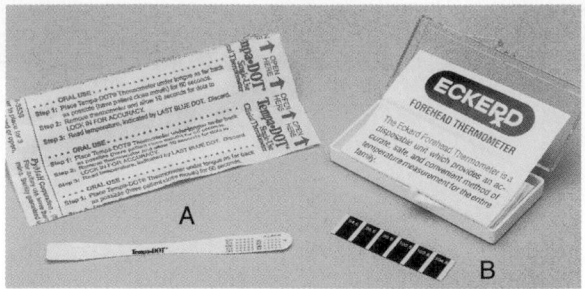

FIGURE 28-3 **A**, Tempa-Dot disposable oral strip thermometer. **B**, Eckerd forehead disposable thermometer. (**A** Courtesy Tempa-Dot, Sommerville, NJ; **B** Courtesy Eckerd, San Jose, Calif.)

temperature-sensing materials have expiration dates that are often overlooked. Disposable thermometers are considered good screening devices but not as accurate as the digital or tympanic thermometers.

Axillary. Studies indicate that axillary temperatures are very accurate when performed correctly. Axillary temperatures take more time to register the correct body temperature, but the method is safe, simple, and easily accessible (Procedure 28-3). When taking an axillary temperature using a digital thermometer, one should use the oral (blue) probe with a disposable probe cover. Because tympanic thermometers are relatively expensive, the axillary method may be a viable way for parents of young children to get accurate temperature readings without having to use the rectal method.

Rectal. Although the best method for measuring patient temperature is with the tympanic thermometer,

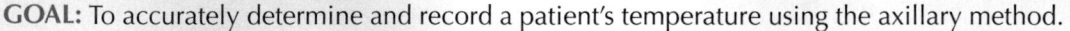

PROCEDURE 28-3

Obtaining an Axillary Temperature

GOAL: To accurately determine and record a patient's temperature using the axillary method.

EQUIPMENT AND SUPPLIES

- Digital unit
- Thermometer sheath or probe cover
- Supply of tissues
- Biohazard waste container

PROCEDURAL STEPS

1 Wash your hands.
Purpose: Infection control.

2 Gather equipment and supplies.

3 Introduce yourself, identify your patient, and explain the procedure.
Purpose: Identification of the patient prevents errors, and explanations are a means of gaining implied consent and patient cooperation.

4 Prepare the thermometer or digital unit in same manner as for oral use.

5 Remove the patient's clothing and gown the patient as needed to access axillary region.

6 Pat the patient's axillary area dry if needed.
Purpose: To ensure an accurate reading. Do not rub the area, because this may cause an elevated reading.

7 Cover the thermometer or probe and place the tip into the center of the armpit, pointing the stem to the upper chest, making sure the thermometer is touching only skin, not clothing.
Purpose: This location offers the most accurate axillary reading, and contact with clothing will alter the reading.

8 Instruct the patient to hold the arm snugly across the chest or abdomen until the thermometer beeps.
Purpose: Prevents air from leaking in and interfering with the temperature reading.

9 Remove the thermometer, note the digital reading, and dispose of the cover in the biohazard waste container.

10 Disinfect the thermometer if indicated.

11 Wash your hands.

12 Record the axillary temperature on the patient's medical record (e.g., T = 97.6° [A]).
Purpose: Procedures that are not recorded are considered not done.

See Appendix E for a charting example.

PROCEDURE **28-4**

Obtaining Rectal Temperature

GOAL: To accurately determine and record a patient's temperature using the rectal method.

EQUIPMENT AND SUPPLIES

- Digital thermometer for rectal use
- Thermometer sheath or probe cover
- Lubricant
- A supply of tissues
- Nonsterile gloves
- Biohazard waste container

PROCEDURAL STEPS

1 Wash your hands.
Purpose: Infection control.

2 Gather equipment and supplies.

3 Introduce yourself, identify your patient, and explain the procedure.
Purpose: Identification of the patient prevents errors, and explanations are a means of gaining implied consent and patient cooperation.

4 Remove the patient's clothing from the waist down and drape as needed.
Purpose: Protects patient privacy; ensures comfort and warmth.

5 Place an adult patient in Sims' position.
Purpose: This position will make the insertion of the probe easier and more comfortable for the patient.

6 Prepare thermometer using a sheath or probe cover on the *red* probe in the digital unit.
Purpose: Covering prevents cross-contamination.

7 Put on gloves.
Purpose: When there is a possible exposure to body fluid, standard precautions must be followed.

8 Lubricate the probe tip and insert into the rectum past the sphincter.
Purpose: Lubrication allows for easier insertion and more comfort for the patient.

9 Hold the thermometer in place until a beep is heard.
Purpose: Because of normal peristaltic movement, the probe will not stay in place unless it is held.

10 Remove the thermometer and note the reading on the LED window. Offer tissues to the patient.

11 Remove the sheath or probe cover and your gloves and discard into the appropriate biohazard waste container.
Purpose: Properly dispose of all contaminated material.

12 Wash your hands.

13 Assist the patient with positioning and dressing as needed.

14 Record the temperature with (R), which indicates a rectal temperature (e.g., T = 99.6° [R]).
Purpose: Procedures that are not recorded are considered not done.

See Appendix E for a charting example.

---

the rectal method may be used for newborns; when the axillary method cannot be used; or when a tympanic thermometer is not available and the patient has breathing difficulties, is uncooperative, or is unconscious. The procedure is the same as for the oral method, except the red probe must be used, covered with a disposable shield, and lubricated with a water-soluble jelly (Procedure 28-4). Stay with the patient. Adults should be kept in the prone or Sims' position, with their toes pointed inward, until the thermometer is removed. Place an infant in the supine position. Hold the legs straight up with one hand and hold the thermometer in place with the other (Figure 28-4). Alternatively, restrain a small child in the prone position with one hand at the buttocks and hold the thermometer in place with the other. You must *never* leave the thermometer in an infant or child unless you or the parent is holding onto the thermometer and the child's feet.

CRITICAL THINKING APPLICATION

How would the medical assistant handle a patient or adapt temperature-taking techniques in the following scenarios?
- A patient who is continuously talking with the thermometer in his or her mouth
- A 7-year-old child with bilateral otitis externa
- A 3-month-old infant when a tympanic thermometer is not available
- A 46-year-old patient with a severe asthma attack
- A 72-year-old patient with bilateral impacted cerumen
- A 28-year-old patient who just smoked a cigarette

Cleaning Thermometers

Digital. The digital unit or individual thermometers should be routinely cleaned with disinfectant. When

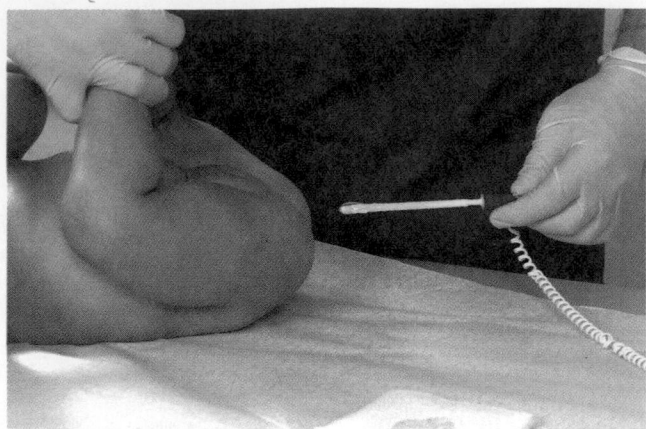

FIGURE 28-4 Infant rectal temperature.

ejecting the probe shield or removing the sheath, be careful not to contaminate the probe or the processing unit. If there is a chance that a patient's body fluids touched the unit, wipe it with disinfectant before returning it to the storage area. Oral and rectal probes should be cared for in the same manner.

Tympanic. Cleaning the tympanic unit follows the same guidelines as for the digital unit. When using the device on a small child, be conscious of what the child touches. If the processing unit is touched, be sure to clean it after use. However, be careful not to get the tip of the probe surface wet, and *always* use probe covers, because disinfectant can ruin the probe surface.

Disposable. Always discard a disposable thermometer in the appropriate waste container immediately after use to avoid contamination and the spread of pathogens to other patients. If you are instructing a parent in the use of a disposable thermometer at home, be sure to emphasize that it should be discarded immediately.

Pulse

Pulse reflects the palpable beat of the arteries as they expand with the beat of the heart. With every beat, the heart pumps an amount of blood, known as the *stroke volume*, into the aorta. Every artery throughout our entire body has a pulse beat, but it is impossible for us to measure all of them. When pulse is measured, an artery that is close to the body surface that can be pushed against a bone is used. Palpating the peripheral pulse gives the rate and rhythm of the heartbeat, as well as local data on the condition of the artery.

Pulse Sites

A pulse rate may be counted any place where an artery is near the surface of the body and the vessel can be pressed against a bone. The most common sites that are used to feel this rhythmic throbbing are at the following arteries: temporal, carotid, apical, brachial, radial, femoral, popliteal, and dorsalis pedis (Figure 28-5).

The *temporal* pulse is located at the temple area of the skull, parallel and lateral to the eyes (Figure 28-6). It

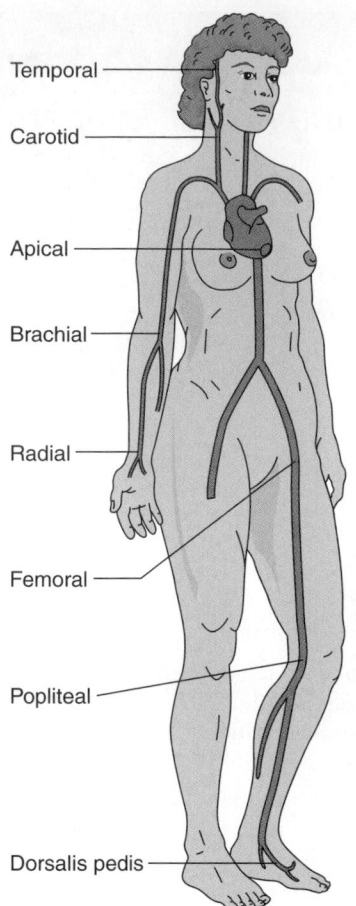

FIGURE 28-5 Pulse sites.

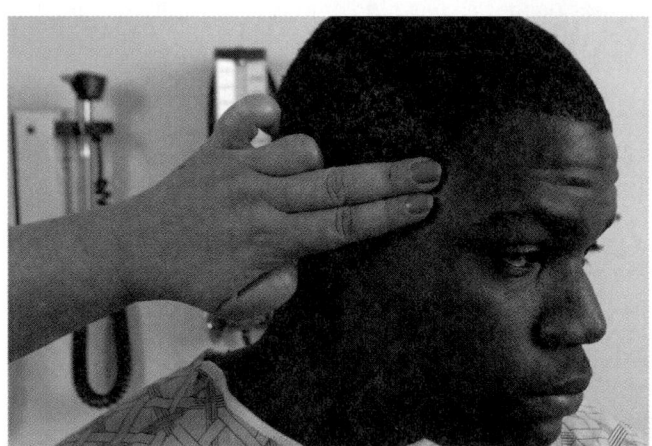

FIGURE 28-6 Temporal pulse.

is seldom used as a pulse site but may be used as a pressure point to assist in controlling bleeding from a head injury.

The *carotid* artery is located between the larynx and the sternocleidomastoid muscle in the front and to the side of the neck (Figure 28-7). It is most frequently used in emergencies and during cardiopulmonary resuscitation. It can be felt by pushing the muscle to the side and pressing against the larynx.

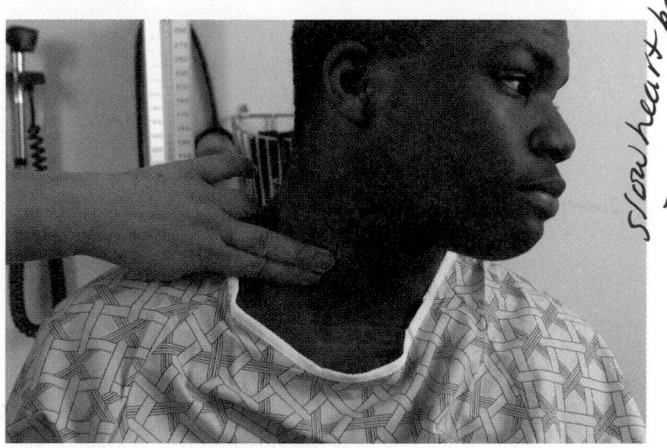

slow heart beat

FIGURE 28-7   Carotid pulse.

The *apical* heart rate, or the heartbeat at the apex of the heart, is heard with a stethoscope. It is often used for infants and young children or in adults if the radial pulse is difficult to feel or is irregular. An apical count may be requested if the patient is taking cardiac drugs or has either **bradycardia** or **tachycardia**. To determine the presence of a **pulse deficit**, the physician may listen to the apical beat while the medical assistant counts the pulse at another site. The apex of the heart is located in the left fifth intercostal space on the midclavicular line, that is, between the fifth and sixth ribs on a line with the midpoint of the left clavicle. The stethoscope is placed just below the left nipple between the fifth and sixth ribs. The pulse should be counted for 1 full minute, and documented with an *AP* beside the recorded count (Procedure 28-5).

Fast heart beat

The *brachial* pulse is felt at the inner (antecubital) aspect of the elbow. It is the artery felt and heard when taking a blood pressure (Figure 28-8). It can also be felt

To check a pulse → 15 sec × 4 . 30 sec × 2

PROCEDURE 28-5

Obtaining an Apical Pulse

GOAL: To assess the patient's apical heart rate.

EQUIPMENT AND SUPPLIES

- Watch with a second hand
- Stethoscope
- Alcohol wipes
- Patient gown

PROCEDURAL STEPS

1 Wash your hands and clean the stethoscope earpieces with alcohol swabs.
   Purpose: Infection control and standard precautions.

2 Introduce yourself, identify your patient, and explain the procedure.
   Purpose: Identification of the patient prevents errors, and explanations are a means of gaining implied consent and patient cooperation.

3 Assist the patient in disrobing from the waist up and provide the patient with a gown, open to the front.
   Purpose: To expose the chest and provide for patient privacy and warmth.

4 The patient should be either sitting or in a supine position.
   Purpose: Easier access to apical site at the apex of the heart.

5 Place the stethoscope just below the left nipple in the intercostal space between the fifth and sixth ribs (Figure 1).

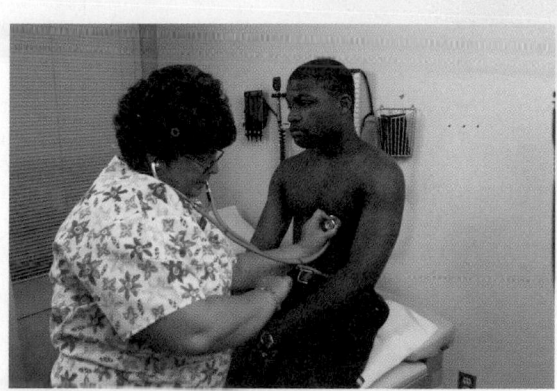

Figure 1

6 Listen carefully for the heartbeat.

7 Count the pulse for one full minute. Note any irregularities in rhythm and volume.
   Purpose: The apical pulse is *always* measured for 1 full minute to determine the most accurate reading.

8 Assist the patient to sit up and dress.

9 Wash your hands.

10 Record the pulse in the patient chart as AP (e.g., AP = 96) and record any arrhythmias.

See Appendix E for a charting example.

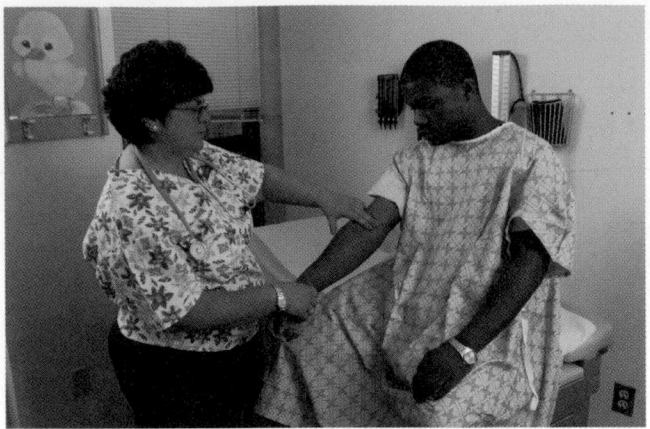

FIGURE 28-8 Brachial pulse.

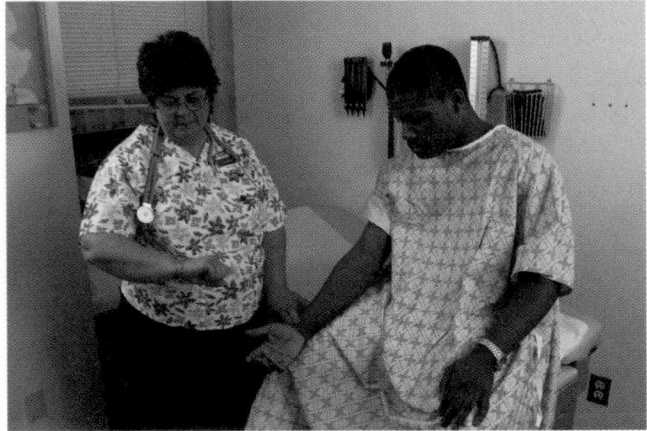

FIGURE 28-9 Radial pulse.

in the groove between the biceps and triceps muscles on the inner surface of the mid-upper arm.

The *radial* artery is the most frequently used site for counting the pulse rate. It is best found on the thumb side of the wrist, 1 inch above the base of the thumb (Figure 28-9).

The *femoral* pulse is located at the site where the femoral artery passes through the groin. One must press deeply below the inguinal ligament to palpate this pulse.

The *popliteal* pulse is found at the back of the knee. The patient must be in a recumbent position, with the knee slightly flexed. The popliteal artery is deep and difficult to feel. This artery is palpated and listened to with the stethoscope when a leg blood pressure reading is necessary.

The *dorsalis pedis (pedal)* artery is felt on the top of the foot, just slightly lateral to the midline, beside the extensor tendon of the great toe. This pulse may be congenitally absent in some patients. A good pulse rate at this site is an indicator of normal lower limb circulation and arterial sufficiency.

Characteristics of Pulse

When you are measuring a pulse, there are four important characteristics to note: (1) rate, (2) rhythm, (3) volume of the pulse, and (4) condition of the arterial wall. These characteristics depend on the size and elasticity of the artery, the strength of the contraction of the heart, and the tissues surrounding the artery. A patient's pulse may reveal valuable information about the cardiovascular system.

Rate. The pulse rate is a measure of the number of heartbeats felt from the pulsing of an artery. When the heart contracts, pressure throughout the arteries increases and the arteries expand. When the heart relaxes, arterial pressure decreases and the arteries relax. Each contraction and relaxation of the heart muscle is a heartbeat, and each resulting expansion and relaxation of the arteries is the pulse rate. Normally heartbeat (rate) and pulse rate are the same. The rate of the pulse is the number of beats (pulsations) that occur in 1 minute. Because the body must balance heat loss by increasing circulation (a faster heart rate), the pulse rate is proportionate to the size of the body. The smaller the body, the greater the heat loss and the faster the heart must pump to compensate. Therefore, infants and children normally have a faster pulse than do adults; as the aging process progresses, the pulse rate decreases.

Pulse rates normally vary as a result of a person's age, body size, gender, and health status. The rate is affected by an individual's activities, psychological state, and certain medications and is usually faster in women (70 to 80 beats per minute) than in men (60 to 70 beats per minute). Children tend to have more rapid pulse rates than adults do. When a person is sitting, the rate is more rapid than when lying down, and it increases when an individual stands or walks or runs. During sleep or rest, the pulse rate may drop as low as 45 to 50 beats per minute. Well-conditioned athletes tend to have pulse rates of 50 to 60 beats per minute.

Rhythm. The rhythm is the time between each pulse beat. Normal rhythm pattern has an even tempo, indicating that the time intervals between the beats are of equal duration. Abnormal rhythm, or **arrhythmia,** is described according to the rhythm pattern that is detected. An **intermittent pulse** occurs in all normal individuals and may be more noticeable during exercise or after drinking a beverage containing caffeine. One irregularity commonly found in children and young adults is **sinus arrhythmia,** in which the heart rate varies with the respiratory cycle, speeding up at the peak of inspiration and slowing to normal with expiration. If there are frequently skipped beats or if the beats are markedly irregular, the physician should be advised, because this may indicate heart disease. If an irregular rhythm is detected, the apical pulse should be measured for a full minute and recorded for the physician's review.

Volume. The volume or force of the pulse refers to the strength of the beat and is described as **bounding** or full; strong or normal; and **thready** or weak. The force of the heartbeat and the condition of the arterial wall, whether it is hard or soft, influences the volume. It is possible for the pulse to vary only in intensity and otherwise be perfectly regular. This condition can also indicate heart disease. The pulse force is recorded using a three-point scale.

THREE-POINT SCALE FOR MEASURING PULSE VOLUME

- 3 + = Full, bounding
- 2 + = Normal pulse
- 1 + = Weak, thready

Vessel Elasticity. As the vessel is palpated through the skin, the condition of the arterial wall must also be evaluated. Normally the wall would be described as being springy, resilient, and elastic. Abnormal findings include hard, ropelike, knotty, or wiry-feeling vessels, or any combination of these.

Determining Pulse Rate

Radial, Brachial, and Apical. The patient should be in a comfortable position, with the artery to be used at the same level as or lower than the heart (Procedure 28-6). The limb should be well supported and relaxed. The patient may be lying down or sitting. As with all pulse readings, the pads of the first three fingers are placed over the artery. Push until the strongest pulsation is felt. The pulse should be counted for 1 full minute. The 15- or 30-second interval is found to be less accurate than

---

PROCEDURE 28-6

Assessing the Patient's Pulse

GOAL: To determine and record a patient's pulse rate, rhythm, volume, and vessel elasticity.

EQUIPMENT AND SUPPLIES
- Watch with a second hand

PROCEDURAL STEPS

1 Wash your hands.
Purpose: Infection control.

2 Introduce yourself, identify your patient, and explain the procedure.
Purpose: Identification of the patient prevents errors, and explanations are a means of gaining implied consent and patient cooperation.

3 Place the patient's arm in a relaxed position, palm downward.
Purpose: The patient's radial artery is more easily palpated when the patient is relaxed and in this position.

4 Gently grasp the palm side of the patient's wrist with your first three fingertips approximately 1 inch above the base of the thumb (Figure 1).

Purpose: This position puts your fingertips directly over the artery. Press firmly, but if you press too hard, you will occlude the artery and feel nothing.

5 Count the beats for 1 full minute, using a watch with a second hand.
Purpose: Counting for 1 full minute allows you to obtain an accurate count, including any irregularities in rhythm and volume.

6 Wash your hands.
Purpose: Infection control.

7 Record the count and any irregularities on the patient's medical record (e.g., P = 72). Pulse is usually recorded immediately after temperature.
Purpose: Procedures that are not recorded are considered not done.

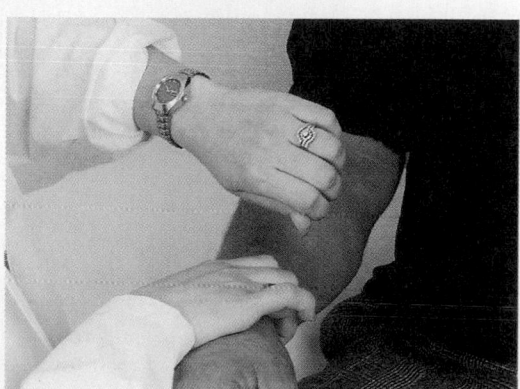

Figure 1

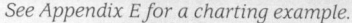

See Appendix E for a charting example.

the longer interval. Using shorter intervals invites error, because you often will be unable to evaluate the quality of the pulse rhythm.

Variations from the normal quality, such as an arrhythmia or a pulse that is thready, **elastic,** intermittent, **irregular,** bounding, or **unequal,** are noted and recorded. Some pulses are more difficult to feel than others, and the correct pressures to be used for each patient and site require practice and experience.

Both the medical assistant and the patient should be in relaxed positions. The sensitivity in your counting fingers is greatly reduced if you are in an awkward position. Too much pressure obliterates the patient's pulse, and too little pressure prevents detection of irregularities or of all of the beats. Record the number of beats in 1 minute. Assess the pulse, including rate, rhythm, volume, and elasticity. If the pulse rate is counted at any site other than the radial, the site should be recorded along with a notation of the site used.

CRITICAL THINKING APPLICATION

Mrs. Arnez has a documented thready, soft pulse. What site should Carlos use to measure the pulse?

Femoral, Popliteal, and Pedal. Pulses in the lower extremities may be difficult to find and equally difficult to hear. A Doppler unit, which is an ultrasound unit that magnifies the pulsation, may be used to locate and count these pulses accurately (Figure 28-10). This unit is battery operated and can be attached to a stethoscope so only you hear the beat, or it can be set so that both you and your patient can hear the pulsations.

Respiration

Physiology

The purpose of respiration is to provide for the exchange of oxygen and carbon dioxide among the atmosphere, the blood, and the body cells. Oxygen is taken into the body

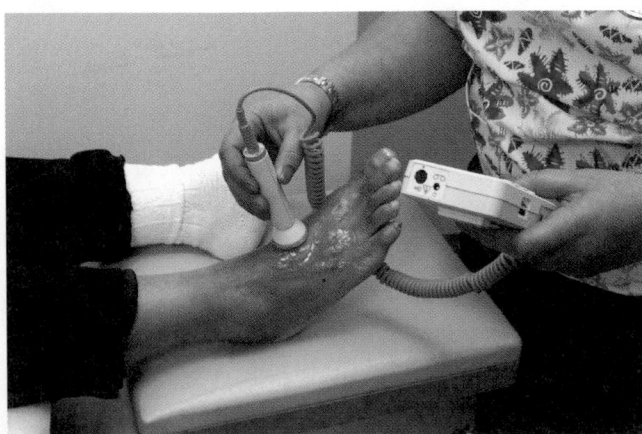

FIGURE 28-10 Doppler ultrasound unit measuring pedal pulse.

to be used for life-sustaining body processes, and carbon dioxide is released as a waste product.

One complete inspiration and expiration is called a *respiration.* During the inspiration phase, the diaphragm contracts, causing the lungs to expand and fill with air. During the expiration phase, the diaphragm returns to its normal, elevated position, causing the lungs to expel the waste air back into the atmosphere.

Respiration is both internal and external. *External respiration* is the exchange of oxygen and carbon dioxide in the lungs. *Internal respiration* occurs at the cellular level, when the oxygen in the bloodstream is utilized and the cells release carbon dioxide as a waste product to be transported back to the lungs for exhalation.

When there is a build-up of carbon dioxide in the blood, a message is sent to the medulla oblongata, which is located in the brain between the top of the spine and the brainstem. This respiratory control center then sends a message that triggers respiration. Therefore, respiration is controlled by the involuntary nervous system; this means we breathe automatically. Because a person can control respiration to a certain extent, it is also a voluntary body function. However, breathing is ultimately under the control of the medulla oblongata, which is why we can hold our breath only for a given length of time. Once the blood carbon dioxide level increases to the point at which cells become oxygen starved, a stimulus is sent and breathing begins involuntarily.

Characteristics of Respirations

Normally a person's breathing is relaxed, automatic, and silent. When determining the respiratory rate of a patient, you must note three important characteristics: (1) rate, (2) rhythm, and (3) depth.

Rate. The *rate* of respiration is the number of respirations per minute and is described as *normal, rapid,* or *slow.* Figure 28-11 shows sample rate patterns

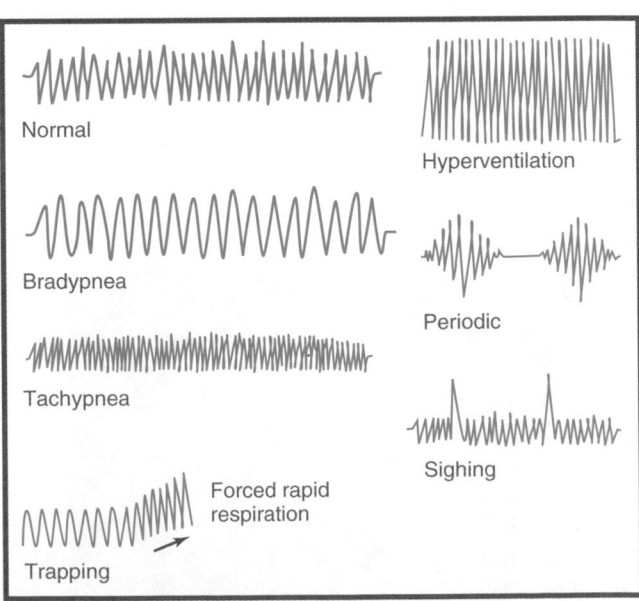

FIGURE 28-11 Respiration rate patterns, called spirograms, which are recorded using a spirometer.

as recorded using a **spirometer. Dyspnea** occurs in patients with pneumonia, asthma, or **COPD**. It also occurs after physical exertion or at very high altitudes. Other alterations in breathing are **bradypnea, apnea, tachypnea,** and **hyperpnea**. Hyperpnea is usually accompanied by **hyperventilation** and is often found in emotional conditions. **Orthopnea** frequently occurs in patients with congestive heart failure (CHF) and COPD. Typically there is a fairly constant ratio of four pulse beats to one respiration. As a rule, both pulse and respiration rates respond to exercise or emotional upsets.

Rhythm. *Rhythm* refers to the breathing pattern. A regular breathing pattern is normal in adults; however, the breathing pattern for infants is irregular. Automatic interruptions, such as sighing, are also considered normal.

Depth. The *depth* of respiration refers to the amount of air being inhaled and exhaled. When a patient is at rest, normal respirations have a consistent depth, which can be noted as you watch the rise and fall of the chest. Rapid, shallow breathing at rest occurs in some disease states, such as asthma and emphysema.

Normally no noticeable breath sounds occur during the breathing process; the exception is snoring. Noticeable breath sounds are a symptom of certain diseases, such as pneumonia and pulmonary edema. The descriptive characteristics for breath sounds are represented by the use of specific terminology (e.g., **rales, rhonchi,** and **stertorous**). These terms should be used when documenting abnormal breath sounds on the patient's medical record.

When an individual cannot inspire enough oxygen to supply all of the body's cells with oxygenated blood, the normal skin coloring, particularly around the mouth and the nail beds, turns a bluish, dusky color. This coloration, which represents the increased level of carbon dioxide present in the blood, is called *cyanosis*.

Counting Respirations

Because most people are unaware of their breathing, do not mention that you will be counting the respirations (Procedure 28-7). The respiratory rate is easily controlled, and patients self-consciously alter their breathing rates when they are being watched. Therefore, count the respirations while appearing to count the pulse. Keep your eyes alternately on the patient's chest and your watch while you are counting the pulse rate, and then, without removing your fingers from the pulse site, determine the respiration rate. It may be easier to count the respirations first, because that number is not as hard to remember (Figure 28-12). If the patient is lying supine, the arm may be crossed over the chest so the respirations can be felt with the rise and fall of the chest. Count the respirations for 30 seconds and multiply the number by 2. Avoid using the 15-second interval, because this can vary by a factor of +4 or −4, which is significant when dealing with such a small number. Note any variation or irregularity in the rate. Record the respiration count on the medical record.

PROCEDURE 28-7

Determining Respirations

GOAL: To determine and record a patient's respirations. Remember that the respiration count may be altered if the patient is aware that you are counting his or her breaths. Respirations are typically counted immediately after taking the pulse.

EQUIPMENT AND SUPPLIES

- Watch with a second hand

PROCEDURAL STEPS

1 Wash your hands.
   Purpose: Infection control.

2 Identify your patient.
   Purpose: Identification of the patient prevents errors.

3 The patient's arm will be in the same position as when counting the pulse. If having difficulty noticing breathing, place the arm across the chest to pick up movement.
   Purpose: This position allows you to feel or visualize the rise and fall of the chest wall.

4 Count the respirations for 30 seconds, using a watch with a second hand, and multiply by 2.
   Purpose: Counting for 30 seconds allows you to obtain an accurate count and determine any irregularities in rhythm or depth or unusual breathing patterns.

5 Release the patient's wrist.

6 Wash your hands.
   Purpose: Infection control.

7 Record the respirations on the patient's medical record after the pulse recording (e.g., R = 18).
   Purpose: Procedures that are not recorded are considered not done.

See Appendix E for a charting example.

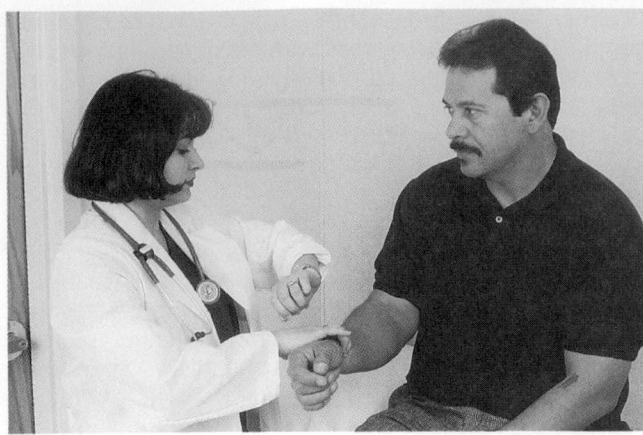

FIGURE 28-12 Hand position when counting respirations. The hands should be left in place as if still counting the patient's pulse.

CRITICAL THINKING APPLICATION

Tina Anderson, a 36-year-old obese patient, is wearing a heavy knit sweater and Carlos needs to obtain a respiration count. How should he handle the situation?

Blood Pressure

Blood pressure is a reflection of the pressure of the blood against the walls of the arteries. Each time the ventricles contract, blood is pushed out of the heart and into the aorta and pulmonary artery, exerting pressure on the walls of the arteries. There are actually two blood pressure readings: the *systolic* pressure is the highest pressure level that occurs when the heart is contracting and the pulse beat is felt, and the *diastolic* pressure is the lowest pressure level when the heart is relaxed and no pulse beat is felt. Systole (heart contraction) and diastole (heart relaxation) together make up the cardiac cycle. The difference between the systolic and diastolic pressures is the **pulse pressure.**

Blood pressure is read in millimeters of mercury, abbreviated *mm Hg*. However, the abbreviations do not have to be included when you document the reading on the patient's medical record. Blood pressure is recorded as a fraction, with the systolic reading the numerator (top) and the diastolic reading the denominator (bottom) (e.g., 130/80).

Factors Affecting Blood Pressure

The physiological factors that determine the blood pressure include blood volume, peripheral resistance created by blood viscosity, vessel elasticity, and the condition of the heart muscle and the arterial walls.

Volume is the amount of blood in the arteries. An increased blood volume increases the blood pressure, and a decreased blood volume decreases blood pressure. If a hemorrhage occurs, the blood volume drops, and so does the blood pressure.

Peripheral resistance of blood vessels refers to the relationship of the *lumen* or diameter of the vessel and the amount of blood flowing through it. The smaller the lumen, the greater the resistance to blood flow. Blood pressure is high with a small lumen and low with a large lumen. Vessels affected by fatty cholesterol deposits called *atherosclerotic plaques* become narrower over time, resulting in higher blood pressure levels.

Vessel elasticity is a vessel's capability to expand and contract to supply the body with a steady flow of blood. With age, lifestyle factors, or the presence of arteriosclerosis, vessel elasticity may decrease, causing the arterial walls to become firm and resistant; as a result, blood pressure will increase.

The condition of the heart muscle, or myocardium, is of primary importance to the volume of blood flowing through the body. A strong, forceful contraction empties the heart and tends to keep blood pressure within normal limits. If the myocardium becomes weak, blood pressure begins to increase in an attempt to maintain the necessary level of oxygen and nutrients needed by the body.

Evaluating Blood Pressure

When a patient's blood pressure (BP) is being tracked, frequent readings should be taken about the same time of day and by the same person. A person is said to have **essential** (primary) **hypertension** if the systolic pressure is greater than 140 mm Hg and diastolic pressure is greater than 90 mm Hg for two or more readings taken at each of two or more visits. Essential hypertension is the most common type of hypertension. **Secondary hypertension** is caused by another underlying pathological condition, such as renal disease, complications of pregnancy, endocrine imbalances, obesity, arteriosclerosis, atherosclerosis, and brain injuries. Temporary hypertension may occur with stress, pain, exercise, and exhaustion. Many patients experience *white-coat hypertension:* their blood pressure becomes elevated in the medical environment, although it is normal away from the healthcare facility.

Hypertension has been called the silent killer, because it frequently has no symptoms and individuals may go for long periods without knowing that they have a problem. Often hypertension is discovered during the medical treatment of another problem. Symptoms may include blurred vision, chest pain or *angina*, **vertigo,** dyspnea, fatigue, headaches, flushing, nosebleeds or epistaxis, and palpitations. Long-term, untreated hypertension is a major cause of strokes.

HYPERTENSION FACTS

- 50 million Americans have hypertension that requires treatment.
- Prevalence increases with age.
- There is a higher incidence of hypertension in blacks than in any other race.

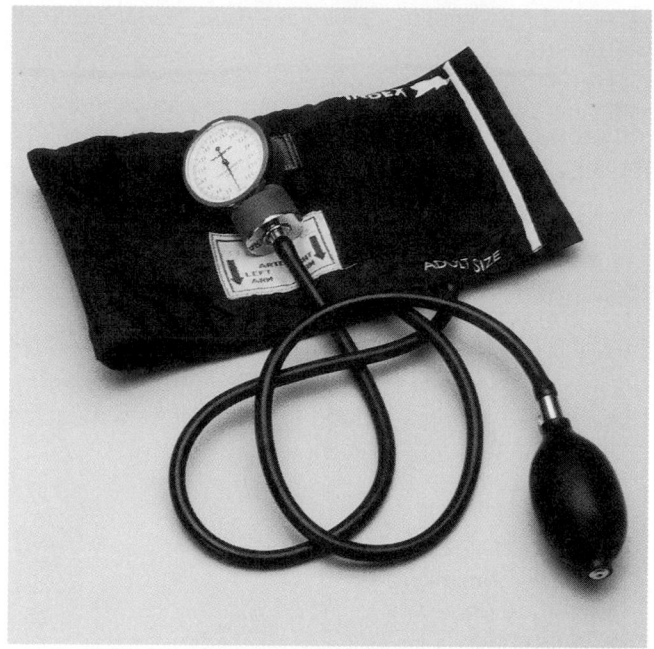

A

Hypotension is abnormally low blood pressure and may be caused by emotional or traumatic shock; hemorrhage; central nervous system disorders; and chronic wasting diseases. Persistent readings of 90/60 mm Hg or below are usually considered hypotensive. **Orthostatic (postural) hypotension** can cause patients to experience vertigo or **syncope.** Some medications can cause orthostatic hypotension.

CRITICAL THINKING APPLICATION

Mr. Samuel Long is a 43-year-old patient who was recently diagnosed with essential hypertension. What should Carlos discuss with Mr. Long to emphasize the dangers of his disease and to educate him about possible lifestyle modifications he needs to initiate to improve his health? Are there any community resources that might help Mr. Long and his family effectively manage his disease?

Measuring Blood Pressure

The instrument used to measure blood pressure is called the sphygmomanometer. The term *manometer* refers to an instrument used to measure the pressure of a liquid or a gas. *Sphygmo* means pulse. Thus, sphygmomanometer means an instrument used for measuring blood pressure in the arteries. The instrument consists of an inflatable cuff, an inflation bulb with a control valve, and a pressure gauge. The blood pressure mechanism consists of an aneroid dial attached to an inflatable cuff (Figure 28-13, *A*) or a floor model with a large angled face (Figure 28-13, *B*).

Sphygmomanometers are delicately calibrated instruments and must be handled carefully. They should be recalibrated regularly and checked for accuracy, either by you or by a medical supply dealer. The needle on the aneroid dial sphygmomanometer should rest within the small square or circle at the bottom of the dial. The dial can be calibrated by connecting it to a calibrated manometer. Pump both manometers to 250 mm Hg and

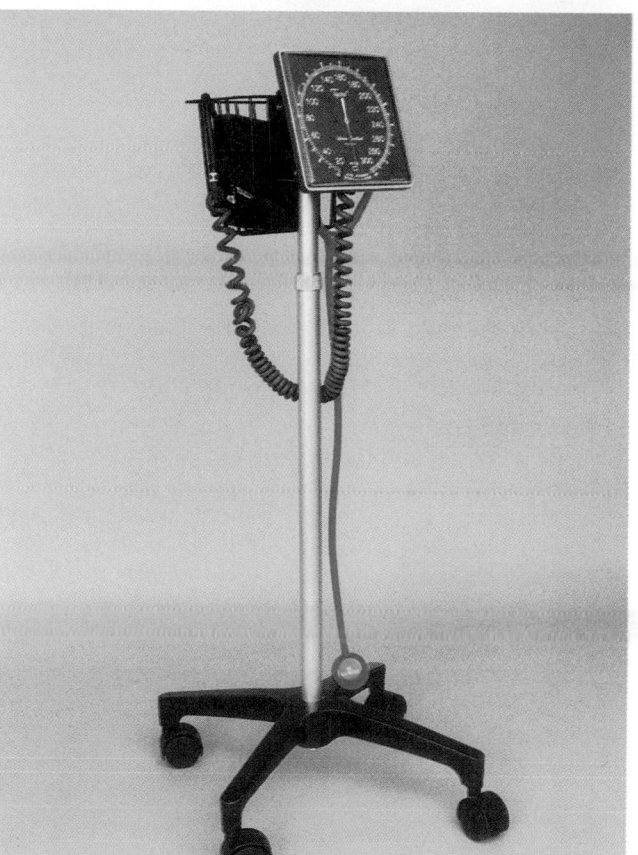

B

FIGURE 28-13   A, Aneroid dial system, with inflatable cuff. **B,** Aneroid floor model, with a large slanted face.

record readings on both machines at least four different times as the pressure is released. A correctly calibrated mechanism has no more than a 3-mm Hg difference between the two readings at any time during the deflation period. If the sphygmomanometer is not correctly calibrated, the patient's blood pressure reading will be inaccurate.

The sphygmomanometer must be used with a stethoscope. The objective of the procedure is to use the inflatable cuff to obliterate (cause to disappear) circulation through an artery. The stethoscope is placed over the artery just below the cuff, and then the cuff is slowly deflated to allow the blood to flow again. As blood flow resumes, cardiac cycle sounds are heard through the stethoscope, and gauge readings are taken when the first (systolic) and the last (diastolic) sounds are heard (Procedure 28-8).

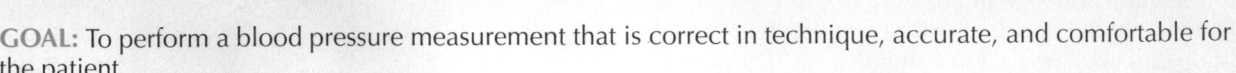

PROCEDURE 28-8

Determining a Patient's Blood Pressure

GOAL: To perform a blood pressure measurement that is correct in technique, accurate, and comfortable for the patient.

EQUIPMENT AND SUPPLIES

- Sphygmomanometer
- Stethoscope
- Antiseptic wipes

PROCEDURAL STEPS

1 Wash your hands.
Purpose: Infection control.

2 Assemble the equipment and supplies needed. Clean the earpieces of the stethoscope with alcohol swabs.
Purpose: Standard Precautions.

3 Introduce yourself, identify the patient, and explain the procedure.
Purpose: Identification of the patient prevents errors, and explanations are a means of gaining implied consent and patient cooperation.

4 Seat the patient in a comfortable position with legs uncrossed and the arm resting at heart level on the lap or a table.
Purpose: To promote patient relaxation and ensure obtaining a true reading. Crossed legs may increase the blood pressure and the arm above the heart level may cause an inaccurate reading.

5 Determine the correct cuff size (Figure 1).

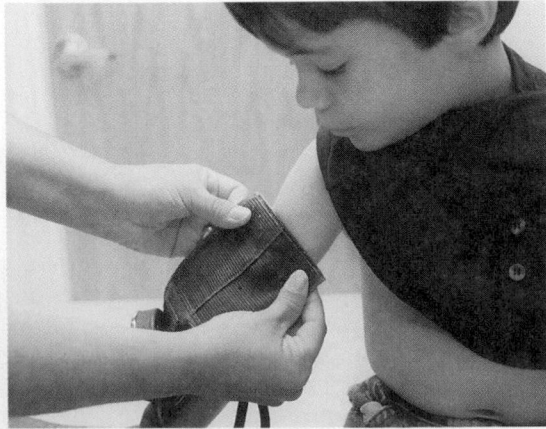

Figure 1

Purpose: An incorrect cuff size prevents accurate measurement of blood pressure.

6 Roll up the sleeve to about 5 inches above the elbow, or have the patient remove his or her arm from the sleeve.
Purpose: Tight clothing interferes with an accurate reading.

7 Palpate the brachial artery at the antecubital space in both arms. If one arm has a stronger pulse, use that arm. If the pulses are equal, select the right arm (Figure 2).

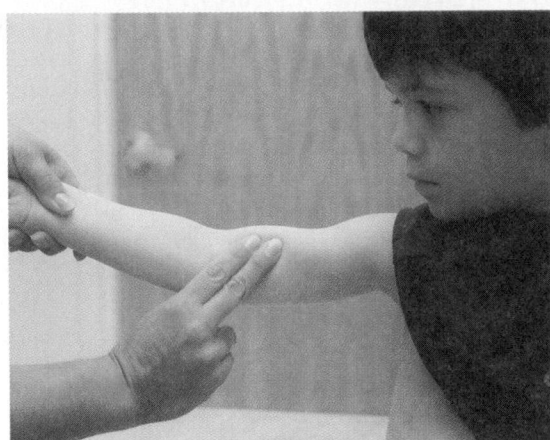

Figure 2

Purpose: A stronger pulse is easier to measure; the right arm is the universal arm of choice.

8 Center the cuff bladder over the brachial artery, with the connecting tube away from the patient's body and the tube to the bulb close to the body (Figure 3).

PROCEDURE **28-8—Cont'd**

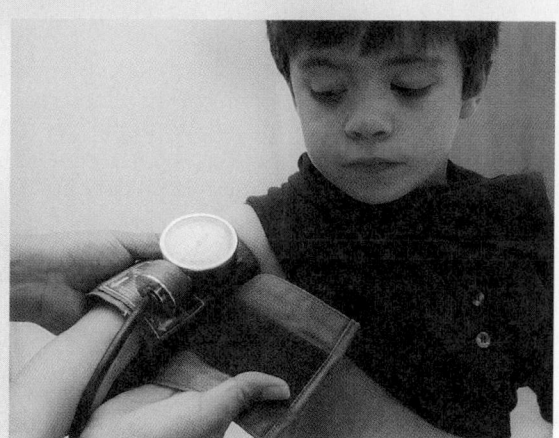

Figure 3

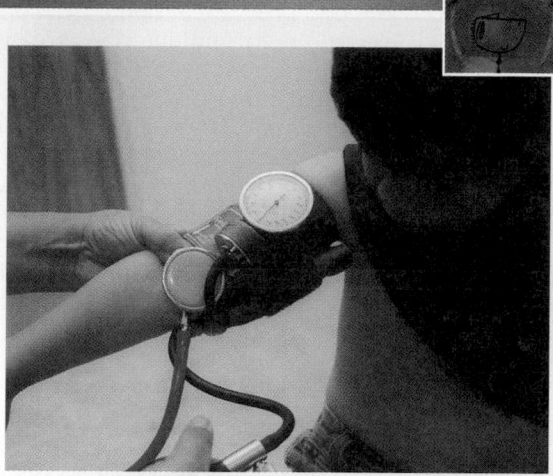

Figure 4

Purpose: Pressure must be applied directly over the artery for an accurate reading.

9 Place the lower edge of the cuff about 1 inch above the palpable brachial pulse, normally located in the natural crease of the inner elbow, and wrap it snugly and smoothly.

Purpose: This helps ensure an accurate reading. The cuff should be high enough on the arm that the stethoscope does not touch it so cuff sounds do not interfere with listening to the blood pressure sounds.

10 Position the gauge of the sphygmomanometer so that it is at eye level.

Purpose: The dial is calibrated for reading in this position.

11 Measure the patient's brachial pulse and mentally add 40 mm Hg to the reading.

Purpose: To determine the inflation level needed to find phase I of the Korotkoff sounds.

12 Insert the earpieces of the stethoscope turned down and forward into your ears.

Purpose: With the earpieces in this position, the openings follow the anatomic line of the ear canal and the blood pressure will be accurately heard.

13 Place the stethoscope bell over the palpated brachial artery firmly enough to obtain a seal, but not so tightly that you constrict the artery.

Purpose: The bell magnifies the low-pitch sounds better than the diaphragm and also forms a better seal.

14 Close the valve, and squeeze the bulb to inflate the cuff at a rapid but smooth rate to 20 mm above the palpated pulse level, which was previously determined in step 12 (Figure 4).

15 Open the valve slightly and deflate the cuff at the constant rate of 2 mm Hg per second.

Purpose: Careful, slow release allows you to listen to all of the sounds.

16 Listen throughout the entire deflation until the sounds have stopped for at least 10 mm Hg.

17 Remove the stethoscope from your ears, and record the systolic and diastolic readings as BP systolic/diastolic (e.g., BP 120/80).

18 If you are uncertain of your reading, release the air from the cuff, wait 1 to 2 minutes, then repeat the process. It is advisable to have the patient gently wiggle his or her fingers during the waiting period.

Purpose: This waiting time allows circulatory congestion to dissipate. NOTE: It is recommended that the blood pressure be checked and recorded in each arm during the initial assessment of the patient and then periodically after that for patients with hypertension.

19 Remove the cuff from the patient's arm and return it to its proper storage area. Clean the earpieces of the stethoscope with alcohol and return it to storage.

20 Wash your hands.

Purpose: Infection control.

Addendum: The physician may direct the medical assistant to record patient blood pressure in two different positions to determine the presence of *orthostatic hypotension.* To perform this skill:

1. Measure and record the patient's blood pressure (as detailed earlier) while the patient is either supine or sitting.
2. Leave the cuff in place.
3. Have the patient stand, and immediately measure the blood pressure again.
4. Record the second blood pressure as well as any patient symptoms, such as complaints of (c/o) vertigo or light-headedness.

See Appendix E for a charting example.

Blood pressure cuffs and stethoscopes are available in drug stores and retail stores for patients to use to measure their own blood pressure at home. These units can be aneroid, electronic, or computerized sphygmomanometers (Figure 28-14). If you have patients who are monitoring their pressures at home, be sure that they understand the mechanics of accurately obtaining a reading. It is best to have the patient bring his or her equipment to the office and demonstrate its use. While the patient is showing you the home equipment, you will have an ideal time to check technique and calibration, and answer any questions the patient might have regarding the use of the equipment. This is also a good opportunity to reinforce treatment plans, such as medication, diet, and exercise.

Heart Sounds

There are two basic heart sounds produced by the functioning of the heart during the cardiac cycle. The first sound, produced at systole (contraction), is dull, firm, and prolonged and is heard as a *lubb sound*. The second sound, produced at diastole (relaxation), is shorter and sharper and is heard as a *dupp* sound. Therefore *lubb-dupp* is the sound of one heartbeat.

Korotkoff sounds are the sounds heard during the measurement of the blood pressure. These sounds are produced by the vibrations of the arterial wall when it is compressed by the blood pressure cuff. The sounds were first discovered and classified into five distinct phases by Nikolai Sergeyevich Korotkoff, a Russian neurologist.

Phase I. Phase I is the first sound heard as the cuff deflates. The blood is resurging into the patient's artery and can be heard quite clearly as a sharp, tapping sound. Note the gauge reading when this first sound is heard. Record this as the systolic pressure.

Phase II. As the cuff deflates, even more blood flows through the artery. The movement of the blood makes a swishing sound. If you do not follow proper procedure in inflating the cuff, you may not hear these sounds because of their soft quality. Occasionally blood pressure sounds completely disappear during this phase. The loss of the sounds and their reappearance later is called the *auscultatory gap*. The silence may continue as the needle falls another 30 mm Hg. Auscultatory gaps occur particularly in hypertension and certain heart diseases, so if you notice such a gap, be certain to report it to the physician.

Phase III. A great deal of blood is now pushing down into the artery. The distinct, sharp tapping sounds return and continue rhythmically. If you do not inflate the cuff enough, you will miss the first two phases completely and you will incorrectly interpret the beginning of phase III as the systolic blood pressure (phase I).

Phase IV. At this point, the blood is flowing easily. The sound changes to a soft tapping, which becomes muffled and begins to grow fainter. Occasionally these sounds continue to zero. This may occur in children, in patients of any age after exercise or with a fever, or in pregnant patients if anemia is present. The American Heart Association recommends that the beginning of phase IV be recorded as the diastolic reading for a child.

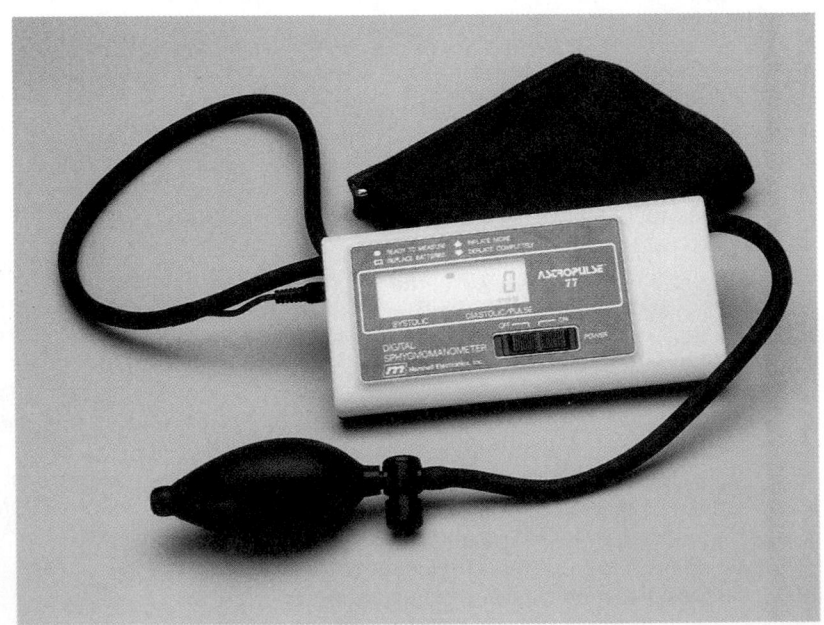

FIGURE 28-14 Personal blood pressure systems. **A,** Home system finger cuff. **B,** Digital blood pressure home system arm cuff.

Some physicians call the change at phase IV the *fading sound* and want it recorded between the systolic and the diastolic recordings (e.g., 120/84/70, with the 84 representing the gauge reading when the sounds of phase III have ended and those of phase IV are beginning). Other physicians consider phase IV the true diastolic pressure.

Phase V. All sounds disappear in this phase. Note the gauge reading when the last sound is heard. Record this as the diastolic pressure. ~~diastole~~

Palpatory Method

The systolic pressure may be checked by feeling the radial pulse rather than hearing it with the stethoscope. Place the cuff in the usual position and palpate the radial pulse, noting the rate and rhythm. Inflate the cuff until the pulse disappears, and then add 30 mm Hg more of inflation to get above the systolic pressure. Do not remove your fingers from the pulse or change the pressure of your fingers. Now, slowly release the pressure in the cuff and wait for the pulse to be felt again. Note the reading on the gauge and record the first pulse felt as the systolic pressure. The blood pressure is recorded as 52/P, with *P* indicating the systolic reading was palpated. The diastolic and the Korotkoff phases cannot be determined by this method. This method can be very useful in times of a medical emergency, such as shock, when the patient's blood pressure cannot be auscultated.

COMMON CAUSES OF ERRORS IN BLOOD PRESSURE READINGS

1. The limb being used is not at the same level as the heart.
2. The rubber bladder in the cuff has not been completely deflated before starting or retaking a reading.
3. The pressure is released too rapidly, resulting in an inaccurate reading.
4. The patient is nervous, uncomfortable, or too anxious, which may cause a reading higher than the patient's actual blood pressure.
5. The patient drank coffee or smoked cigarettes within 30 minutes of the elevation.
6. The cuff is improperly applied.
7. The cuff is too large or too small, too loose or too tight.
8. The cuff is not placed around the arm smoothly.
9. The bladder is not centered over the artery or it bulges out from the cover.
10. Failing to wait 1 to 2 minutes between measurements.
11. Defective instruments:
    a. Air leaks in the valve
    b. Air leaks in the bladder
    c. Aneroid needle that is not calibrated to zero

OSHA GUIDELINES FOR MEASURING VITAL SIGNS

- Wash your hands before and after each procedure.
- Always use protective disposable sheaths on all forms of thermometers.
- Immediately disinfect any equipment that has become contaminated during the procedure.
- Wear gloves when taking a rectal temperature.
- Wear gloves if the potential exists of contacting any open areas or body fluids.
- When caring for a patient with a known respiratory infectious disorder, such as tuberculosis, use protective clothing, including a face shield/mask as indicated.
- Dispose of all contaminated material, including thermometer covers, gloves, and disinfectant swabs, in the proper biohazard waste containers.

CRITICAL THINKING APPLICATION

Vital signs are documented with temperature (T) first, pulse (P) second, and respirations (R) last, with the blood pressure recorded after the TPR. Correctly document the following vital signs:

1. Oral temperature of 101.2°, apical pulse of 90, respirations 22, and orthostatic blood pressure of 138/88 supine and 110/70 standing.
2. Tympanic temperature of 36.8°, radial pulse of 66, respirations 18, and bilateral blood pressure of 128/76 in the left arm and 132/80 in the right arm.
3. Rectal temperature of 37.4°, pulse of 88, respirations 16, and blood pressure 106/60.
4. Axillary temperature of 97.7°, carotid pulse of 58, respirations 24, and palpated blood pressure of 62.

Anthropometric Measurement

Anthropometry is the science that deals with the measurement of the size, weight, and proportions of the human body. These measurements are often included in the initial measurement of vital signs. Because they are indicators of the state of health and well-being of a patient, the measurements of height and weight are discussed as part of the vital signs. Other measurements are discussed when pertinent in the specialty chapters.

Measuring Weight and Height

A patient's weight and height can be helpful in diagnosis, and the medical assistant must determine these readings with accuracy and empathy (Procedure 28-9). Weight and height are often routinely measured in many medical settings as the patient is being escorted to the exam-

PROCEDURE **28-9**

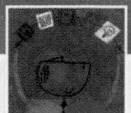

Measuring a Patient's Weight and Height

GOAL: To accurately weigh and measure a patient as part of the physical assessment procedure. NOTE: Be sure the scale is located in an area away from traffic to maintain patient privacy.

EQUIPMENT AND SUPPLIES

• Balance scale with a measuring bar

PROCEDURAL STEPS

1 Wash your hands.
Purpose: Infection control.

2 Identify your patient and explain the procedure.
Purpose: Identification of the patient prevents errors, and explanations are a means of gaining implied consent and patient cooperation.

3 If the patient is to remove his or her shoes for weighing, place a paper towel on the scale platform. The patient may be given disposable slippers to wear.

4 Check to see that the balance bar pointer floats in the middle of the balance frame when all weights are at zero.
Purpose: A floating pointer indicates that the scale is properly adjusted and in balance.

5 Help the patient onto the scale. Make certain that the female patient is not holding a purse and that the male patient has removed any heavy objects from pockets.

6 Move the large weight into the groove closest to the estimated weight of the patient. The grooves are calibrated in 50-lb increments. If you choose a groove that is more than the patient's weight, the pointer will immediately tilt to the bottom of the balance frame. You then must move it back one groove (Figure 1).

7 While the patient is standing still, slide the small upper weight to the right along the pound markers until the pointer balances in the middle of the balance frame.
Purpose: The pointer will float between the bottom and the top of the frame when both lower and upper weights together balance the scale with the patient's weight.

8 Leave the weights in place.

9 Ask the patient to stand up straight and to look straight ahead. On some scales the patient may need to turn with the back to the scale.

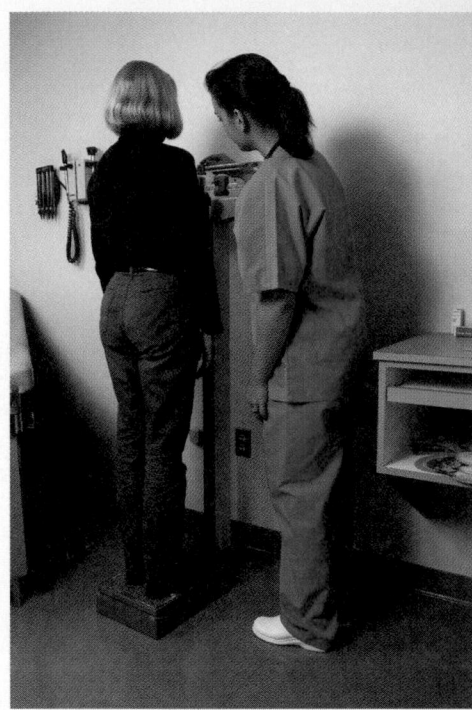

Figure 1

10 Adjust the height bar so that it just touches the top of the patient's head (Figure 2).

11 Leave the elevation bar set but fold down the horizontal bar.
Purpose: Maintain the height recording while protecting the patient from possible injury.

12 Assist the patient off the scale. Make certain that all items removed for weighing are given back to the patient.

13 Read the weight scale. Add the numbers at the markers of the large and the small weights and record the total to the nearest pound on the patient's medical record (e.g., Wt: 136½).

14 Record the height. Read the marker at the movable point of the ruler and record the measurement to the nearest quarter inch on the patient's medical record (e.g., Ht: 64¼).

PROCEDURE **28-9—Cont'd**

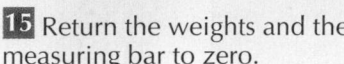

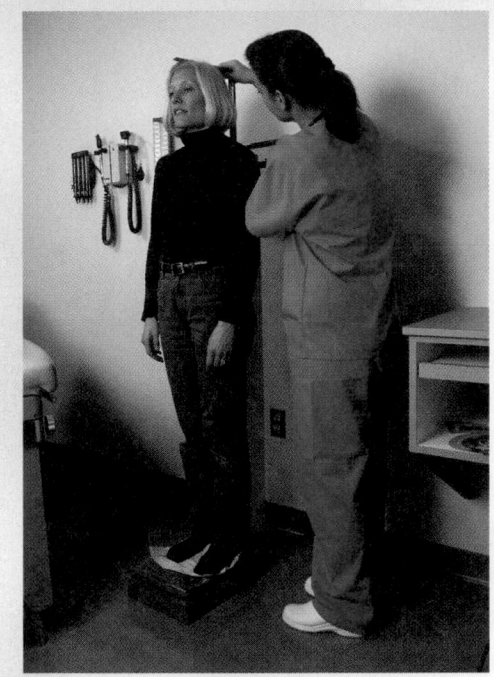

Figure 2

15 Return the weights and the measuring bar to zero.

16 Wash your hands.

17 Record the results on the patient's medical record.

See Appendix E for a charting example.

ination room. If this is the patient's first visit, the anthropometric measurements will be written in the baseline information and used as reference data in future visits when or as needed.

There are certain medical specialties and specific medical problems that may require continuous monitoring of weight. Hormone disorders (e.g., diabetes), growth patterns (seen in children), and eating disorders (e.g., obesity and bulimia) necessitate accurate weight checks as part of every medical visit. In addition, maternity patients and heart patients with fluid retention also need weight monitoring. Some scales are calibrated in kilograms, whereas others are in pounds. When it is necessary to convert a weight, use the formulas under Conversion Formulas.

CONVERSION FORMULAS

To convert kilograms to pounds:
  1 kg = 2.2 lb
  Multiply the number of kilograms by 2.2.
  EXAMPLE: If a patient weighs 68 kg, multiply
    68 by 2.2 = 149.6 lb.
To convert pounds to kilograms:
  1 lb = 0.45 kg
  Multiply the number of pounds by 0.45 *or*
    divide the number of pounds by 2.2 kg.
  EXAMPLE: If a patient weighs 120 lb, multiply
    120 by 0.45 = 54 kg *or* divide 120 by
    2.2 = 54.5 kg.

CRITICAL THINKING APPLICATION

*   A patient weighs 87 kg; how many pounds does he weigh?
*   A patient weighs 148 lb; how many kilograms does she weigh?

Weight. Some patients are sensitive or secretive about their body weight, so the scale should be located in an area that provides privacy from staff and other patients. Your manner and approach are very important in keeping patients from feeling embarrassed or shy. It is not necessary to remove shoes and clothing if patients are consistently weighed and measured with them on. Although the exact weight and height may not be determined, changes in the patient's weight and height can be detected and analyzed. As explained in Chapter 27, healthcare specialists are depending more on body mass index (BMI) ratios rather than traditional height and weight tables, but there still must be an accurate measurement of height and weight to accurately determine BMI. If patients are unstable, assist them onto the scale and to balance themselves. A walker can be placed over the scale for the patient to use as hand support when getting on or off or to balance on the scale (Figure 28-15).

If the physician prescribes weight measurement at home, make certain that the patient understands the importance of weighing himself or herself each day at the same time in clothing of similar weight. Body weight may vary considerably from early morning to late afternoon.

Teach the patient how to record the weight on a graphic record and how to make any other important notations.

Height. Height can be measured in inches or in centimeters. Measurement is easily accomplished by moving the parallel bar attached to the ruler on the scale. Height measurements used in pediatrics are discussed in Chapter 35.

CRITICAL THINKING APPLICATION

Mrs. Johnson is being seen for the first time by Dr. Xu. In what order should Carlos take her vital signs and her anthropometric measurements? Should the blood pressure be measured in both arms, with the patient both sitting and standing? What is the rationale?

THE ROLE OF THE MEDICAL ASSISTANT IN OBTAINING VITAL SIGNS

- Monitoring vital signs is a key responsibility of the medical assistant.
- It is crucial to correctly measure and describe all facets of each vital sign.
- The medical assistant must accurately and clearly document this information.
- The medical assistant should take advantage of all opportunities to answer questions and help the patient understand the significance of healthy vital signs.
- Patient privacy must be maintained throughout all procedures.
- Family members or caregivers should be included in patient care and education as indicated.
- Community resources should be used to promote holistic patient care.
- The medical assistant should be sensitive to cultural and ethnic factors that may affect patient compliance with physician recommendations, such as diet, exercise, weight control, and the use of medication.

Patient Education

All patients should know how to use a thermometer safely and accurately and the preferred site based on age and other patient factors. Because many types of temperature reading equipment are sold, ask the patient what type of equipment he or she uses at home to obtain temperature readings. Inexpensive digital models have greatly simplified home temperature taking.

To teach a patient how to assess the pulse rate, familiarize the patient with counting the beats and how to determine the rate, rhythm, and regularity of the beat. Use diagrams to teach pulse points and have the patient measure your pulse to assess the patient's accuracy and to provide any needed assistance.

If a patient is to keep track of respirations, a family member or helper will need to do this for the patient.

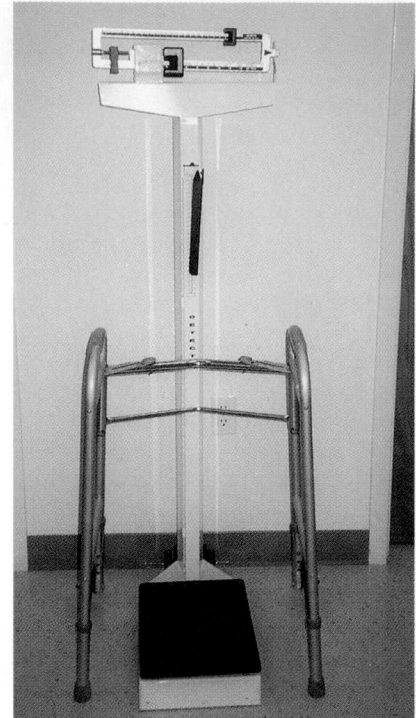

FIGURE 28-15 Walker over a scale to aid the patient in balancing.

The patient and all caregivers should also be taught self-assessment of impending complications as well as preventive breathing exercises.

Monitoring blood pressure at home has become very common. Suggest that the patient bring his or her equipment to the office and practice with it. In this way, you can be certain that the patient is using the equipment correctly and is hearing the systolic and diastolic beats using his or her own stethoscope and sphygmomanometer and recording the results accurately in a record book. One of the most common problems in hearing blood pressure accurately is in the placement of the earpieces in the ears. Patients frequently have the earpieces pointing backward instead of forward. This simple correction may eliminate the patient's problem in using home equipment.

Weight management can be a trying and emotional experience for a patient. Understanding how weight is affected by the time of day, by a particular activity, or by the type of scale used can help the patient to maintain a positive attitude. Have an assortment of weight management literature available for the patient to take home and use community resources when indicated to help the patient with weight-related issues (see Chapter 27 for further details).

Legal and Ethical Issues

A medical assistant must remember that as the physician's agent, he or she plays an important role in preventing legal claims against the physician and the medical office. A medical assistant must always function within the legal boundaries of the profession. When obtaining vital signs, carefully select your response to a patient who asks about the results. Patients should be told the results *only* when the physician has given the assistant consent to do so. Even when the physician has given consent, remember that you are never to diagnose; that is, you are never to evaluate or give an opinion of what the results may mean. For example, if a patient asks, "Is my blood pressure better?" you might reply, "The reading is 160/90 today." You have not said that it is worse, the same, or better but have informed the patient of the current blood pressure reading.

Always be very accurate in transcribing results onto the patient's medical record. If the results are incorrectly recorded, there is a chance that the patient will be incorrectly diagnosed or treated. This can result in legal action that may implicate you. A careless attitude toward the assessment of vital signs and toward documentation can lead to possible legal entanglement.

In every procedure in this chapter there is a reminder to record the test results. If there is no entry, the assumption is that it was not done. Cultivate sensitivity toward proper conduct and performance so that you can protect yourself and your physician-employer.

SUMMARY OF SCENARIO

Carlos recognizes the importance of measuring and recording patient vital signs and anthropometric measurements. Dr. Xu relies on Carlos to accurately provide this information. Carlos has never let these procedures become routine or done without thought, since the patient's vital signs are a reflection of his or her health status. In addition, Carlos is sensitive to the need for safeguarding patient privacy. He was concerned about privacy and confidentiality when first hired by Dr. Xu when he discovered the patient scale in the hall next to the waiting room. After discussing this with the office manager, the scale was moved to an examination room so patients could be weighed in privacy. Carlos continues to care for the patients in the practice while providing valuable assistance to Dr. Xu in her busy primary care practice.

SUMMARY OF LEARNING OBJECTIVES

■ The normal ranges for vital signs are summarized in Tables 28-1 and 28-2. The normal pulse, respiratory rate, and blood pressure averages vary according to age while temperature values vary according to the method.

■ There are multiple factors that affect the body temperature, including exercise, the environment, reproductive activities, anxiety, stress, anger, and disease.

■ The patient's temperature can be measured orally with a digital thermometer, in the ear using an aural thermometer, rectally, and in the axillary region.

■ The pulse rate reflects the number of times the heart contracts over a period of 1 minute. The pulse volume is the amount of force placed on the arterial walls when the heart beats; the rhythm of the pulse is the length of time between each beat.

■ When taking the pulse, the medical assistant should monitor and record the pulse rate, noting whether the rhythm is regular or arrhythmic, and if the volume is bounding, normal, or thready. Another quality that should be observed is the way the artery feels: is it soft and flexible or hard and ropelike?

■ The respiratory rate varies according to age, condition of the pulmonary system, psychological state, and the presence of disease. Several terms were discussed that indicate an abnormality in respirations: bradypnea, tachypnea, hyperpnea, dyspnea, and orthopnea.

■ The best way to obtain an accurate respiratory count is to count the number of respirations in a 30-second period and multiply by 2. This should be done immediately after taking the patient's pulse, while still holding the pulse point, and without warning the patient, because the patient may inadvertently alter the respiratory rate if he or she is aware you are counting breaths.

■ Physiological factors that affect blood pressure include the amount or volume of blood in circulation; the condition of the blood vessels, including the presence of atherosclerosis and arteriosclerosis; the degree of blood viscosity; and the strength of the myocardium.

■ The cause of essential hypertension is unknown; it is diagnosed when a patient has a systolic reading greater than 140 mm Hg two or more times and a diastolic reading greater than 90 mm Hg two or more times at each of two or more visits. This is the most common type of hypertension and may be discovered during a regular health visit. Secondary hypertension is caused by another underlying condition, such as renal disease, pregnancy, or congenital heart defects.

■ Patient weight and height are anthropometric measurements that are recorded during the initial patient visit and periodically after that, depending on patient needs and physician preference. The scale should be in a private location. Variations in weight may indicate physical or emotional disorders, including diabetes, CHF, hormone abnormalities, depression, and eating disorders.

■ Patient education regarding vital signs includes confirming the ability of the patient to monitor vital signs at home as needed, providing assistance in working home equipment systems, and confirming understanding of the need to comply with physician recommendations.

■ Legal and ethical implications for the medical assistant include following physician guidelines with patient disclosure, accurate monitoring and recording of vital signs, and consistently being alert to inaccurate readings or potential carelessness.

CHAPTER 29

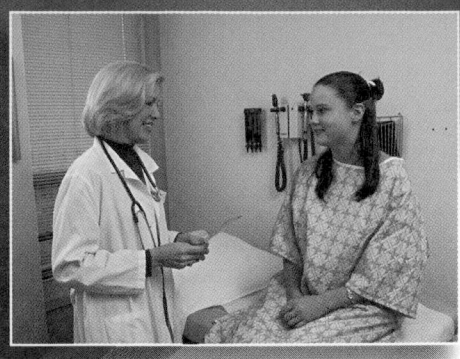

Scenario

Felicia Grand, a newly hired certified medical assistant (CMA), is working for Dr. Anna Kosto. Dr. Kosto is part of a busy multiphysician primary care practice. One of Felicia's chief responsibilities is to assist Dr. Kosto with physical examinations. Her duties include preparing and maintaining the examination room and equipment as well as preparing the patient for specific physical examinations.

Assisting With the Primary Physical Examination

Learning Objectives

- Define and spell the terms listed in the vocabulary.
- Describe the structural development of the human body.
- Identify the 11 body systems and the major organs or units in each.
- Recognize 10 instruments typically used during a physical examination.
- Describe the six methods of examination and give an example for each.
- Outline the basic principles of properly draping a patient for examination.
- Explain eight positions that may be used in examinations.
- Describe proper body mechanics.
- Outline the sequence of a routine physical examination.
- Summarize the role of the medical assistant in the physical examination process.
- Determine the role of patient education during the physical examination.
- Discuss the legal and ethical implications of the physical examination.
- Prepare the examination room and instruments for a physical examination.
- Position and drape a patient in six different examining positions while remaining mindful of patient privacy and comfort.
- Demonstrate proper body mechanics in transferring a patient from a chair to the examination table and back.
- Assist in the physical examination of a patient, correctly completing each step of the procedure in the proper sequence.

National Curriculum Competencies

CLINICAL COMPETENCIES

4d. Prepare and maintain examination and treatment area

4e. Prepare patient for and assist with routine and specialty examinations

Vocabulary

bruit Abnormal sound or murmur heard on auscultation of an organ, vessel, or gland.

emphysema Pathological accumulation of air in the tissues or organs; in the lungs, the bronchioles become plugged with mucus and lose elasticity.

manipulation Moving or exercising a body part by an externally applied force.

murmur Abnormal sound heard when auscultating the heart that may or may not have a pathological origin.

nodule Small lump, lesion, or swelling felt when palpating the skin.

sclera White part of the eye that forms the orb.

transillumination Inspection of a cavity or organ by passing light through its walls.

trauma Physical injury or wound caused by an external force or violence.

uremia Toxic renal condition characterized by an excess of urea, creatinine, and other nitrogenous end-products in the blood.

The human body is so complex that it is hard to imagine that science will ever entirely unravel its mysteries. Imagine billions of microscopic parts, each with its own functioning identity yet all working together in a systematic, organized manner for the perfect harmony of the entire organism. To promote health maintenance, healthcare professionals must understand how the body is put together, what role each part plays, how each part functions, and what happens to the body when disease occurs.

Anatomy and Physiology

Anatomy is the study of how the body is shaped and structured. It encompasses a wide range of subjects, including (1) structural development, (2) levels of organization, (3) relationships between microscopic parts, and (4) the interrelationship of structure and function.

Physiology is the study of body functions. This field is also subdivided into areas of study; some physiologists spend their entire lives studying only one function, such as how cells work, or how a single organ, such as the small intestine, is interrelated in function with the stomach and the large intestine.

It is almost impossible to separate these two sciences, because one continuously influences the other. Function affects structure, and structure affects function; for example, an infant has the ability to suck effortlessly because of the lack of teeth in its mouth. Once teeth appear, sucking becomes more tiresome, and the child now begins to chew and bite. Phenomena in structure and function affect the interrelationship of all body systems.

Structural Development

Cells. The basic unit of life is the cell. Cells determine the functional and structural characteristics of the entire body. Cells come in a variety of shapes and sizes and perform a vast array of functions. It is estimated that the human body is composed of about 100 trillion living, functioning cells.

Tissue. When cells with similar structure and function are placed together, they form tissues. The study of tissues is known as histology. All of the body tissues are grouped into four types. Listed below are the types of tissues distributed throughout the body and where they are located.

- Epithelial: Skin, glands, lining of body cavities and organs; classified as *squamous* (flat), *cuboidal* (square), or *columnar* (long and narrow). Epithelial cells are arranged in a single layer called *simple epithelium*, or in many layers called *stratified epithelium*.
- Connective: Supports and binds other body tissues; types include bone, cartilage, adipose, ligaments, tendons, blood, and lymph.
- Muscle: Produces movement; classified as either skeletal, cardiac, or smooth muscle.
- Nervous: Conducts nerve impulses; made up of neurons and supportive structures called *neuroglial* cells.

Organs. An *organ* is composed of two or more types of tissue bound together to form a more complex structure for a common purpose or function. An organ may have one or many functions and may be considered a unit in one or several systems.

Systems. A body *system* is composed of several organs and their associated structures. These structures work together to perform a specific function within the body. There are 11 systems in the human body. Each system has specific units within it, and each performs specific functions.

Table 29-1 summarizes the body systems and their primary organs.

TABLE 29-1	Body System Organization
Body System	**Systems, Organs, and Structures**
Integumentary	Skin, sweat glands, sebaceous glands, ceruminous glands, hair, nails
Musculoskeletal	Bones, joints, muscles, tendons, ligaments, cartilage
Nervous	Brain, spinal cord, nerves
Special senses	Eye, ear
Gastrointestinal	Mouth, pharynx, esophagus, stomach, small intestine, large intestine, liver, gallbladder, pancreas, anus
Cardiovascular	Heart, arteries, veins
Respiratory	Nose, pharynx, larynx, trachea, lungs
Endocrine	Pituitary, pineal, thyroid, thymus, pancreas, adrenal, parathyroid, ovaries, testes
Lymphatic and hematic	Lymph, spleen, tonsils, thymus, white blood cells, red blood cells, platelets, plasma
Urinary	Kidneys, ureters, bladder, urethra
Reproductive	Ovaries, fallopian tubes, uterus, vagina, mammary glands, testes, vas deferens, prostate gland, penis

Primary Care Physician

Primary care physicians (PCPs) treat patients of all ages for a broad range of diseases and complaints. A PCP is qualified to provide continuing healthcare for the entire family, from birth to old age. Within the healthcare system of today, many health insurance programs have converted to the primary care referral system. This means that most patients are required to have a PCP as their gatekeeper in personal healthcare. In this role, the PCP must first be contacted before the patient can be referred to specialty physicians for care.

The PCP evaluates a patient's total healthcare needs, provides personal medical care within one or more fields of medicine, and refers the patient to a specialist when an advanced or serious condition warrants additional expertise. The medical assistant's clinical responsibilities in the primary care office encompass assisting with patients who may have problems in any of the body systems and with procedures in all age groups. With such a diversified scope of practice, the physician and medical assistant must work as a team to use their time efficiently and still provide for the needs of the patients.

Physical Examination

The purpose of a physical examination is to determine the overall state of well-being of the patient. All major organs and all body systems are checked during a physical examination. As the physician examines the entire body the findings are interpreted, and by the time the examination is completed, the physician will have formed an initial diagnosis regarding the patient's condition. Frequently laboratory and other diagnostic tests are ordered to supplement the physician's initial diagnosis. The results of these tests are used to refine the patient's diagnosis, to aid the physician in planning treatment for the patient, in maintaining drug therapy, or in evaluating the patient's progress.

Preparing for the Physical Examination

The Medical Assistant's Role in the Physical Examination. Assessment of the patient begins with the first contact to the office. Before the examination, the medical assistant has the opportunity to interact with and react to the patient to ensure that he or she feels comfortable during the examination process and that all the necessary information is obtained.

Room preparation includes stocking and checking the room to be sure that it is clean, supplies are readily available, equipment is operational, and the room is both private and comfortable. Drapes, gowns, and any other patient supplies are arranged and ready for use. Instruments and equipment needed for the examination are prepared and properly covered. Expiration dates must be checked on all packages and supplies on a regular basis. The examination room should contain all required materials for standard precautions, including latex gloves, a sink with an antibacterial hand-washing agent, paper towels, biohazard waste containers, sharps containers, and impervious gowns and face guards. In addition, the room should be well lit and a comfortable temperature for the patient during the physical examination. Between patients, all potentially contaminated surfaces, including the examination table, should be cleaned with an appropriate disinfectant and supplies restocked as necessary (Figure 29-1).

Patient preparation includes checking the medical record for completeness and making certain that any needed consent forms are signed; gathering insurance information as needed; obtaining any specimens such as urine and blood; determining height, weight, and vital signs; conducting the initial investigation into the reason for the visit; documenting patient data; answering patient questions; and helping the patient physically prepare (removing clothing and gowning). Throughout this entire sequence of events, the medical assistant offers explanations of what he or she is doing to the patient and maintains patient confidentiality.

Assisting the physician includes handing the physician the instruments and equipment as requested; positioning and draping the patient during the different phases of the examination; providing supplies as needed; conducting follow-up diagnostic procedures, such as an electrocardiogram (ECG), eye or ear screening, and phlebotomy; documenting pertinent information; and acting as an advocate for the patient.

SKILLS AND RESPONSIBILITIES

A medical assistant's duties can be divided into three areas:
- Preparation and maintenance of the examination room and equipment
- Preparation of the patient
- Assisting the physician

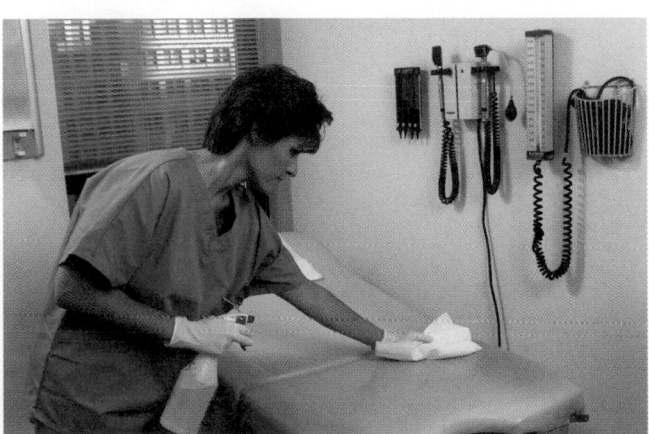

FIGURE 29-1   Disinfecting examination table.

CRITICAL THINKING APPLICATION

Felicia's first patient for the day is Harry Garcia, a 51-year-old truck driver who is scheduled for a complete physical examination. Mr. Garcia's insurance has changed since his last visit. The physician ordered an ECG to be performed and a complete blood panel to be drawn before the physical. What does Felicia need to complete before Dr. Kosto sees the patient?

Instruments and Equipment Needed for the Physical Examination. The instruments typically used during the physical examination are displayed in Figure 29-2. They enable the physician to see, feel, and listen to parts of the body. All equipment must be in good working order, properly disinfected, and readily available for the physician's use during the examination. The instruments most frequently used for the physical examination are described in the following paragraphs.

Nasal Speculum. A nasal speculum is a stainless-steel instrument used to inspect the lining of the nose, nasal membranes, and internal septum (Figure 29-3). When the handles of the nasal speculum are squeezed, the tips spread apart to dilate the nostrils, allowing the physician to visualize the internal aspects. An otoscope with a special attachment may also be used for nasal visualization.

Ophthalmoscope. An ophthalmoscope is used to inspect the inner structures of the eye. It has a stainless-steel handle containing batteries, onto which a head is attached. The head is equipped with a light and magnifying lenses and an opening through which the eye is viewed. Examination rooms are usually equipped with wall-mounted electrical units for the ophthalmoscope, otoscope, disposable speculums, and sphygmomanometer (Figure 29-4).

Otoscope. An otoscope is used to examine the external auditory canal and tympanic membrane. It has a stainless-steel handle containing batteries, onto which a head is fastened. The head contains a light that is focused through a magnifying lens and disposable ear speculum.

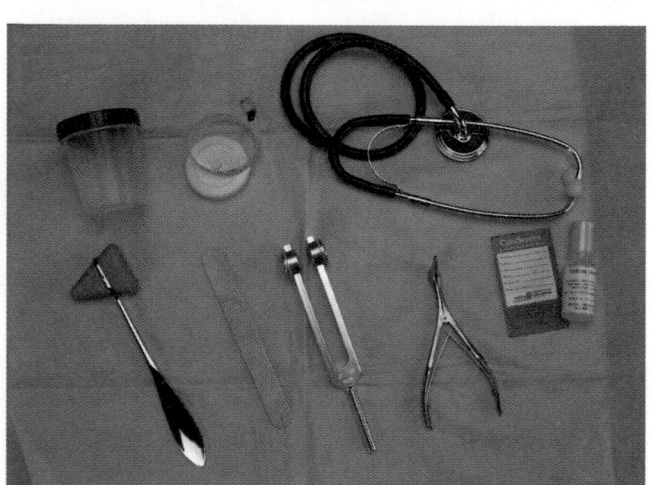

FIGURE 29-2 Instruments for the physical examination.

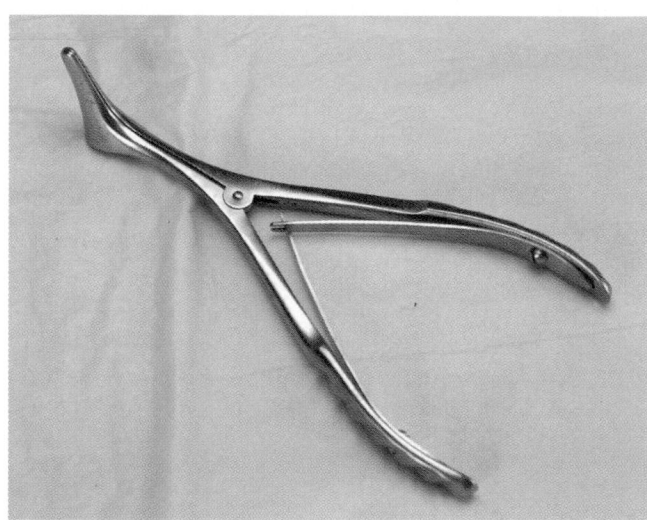

FIGURE 29-3 Nasal speculum.

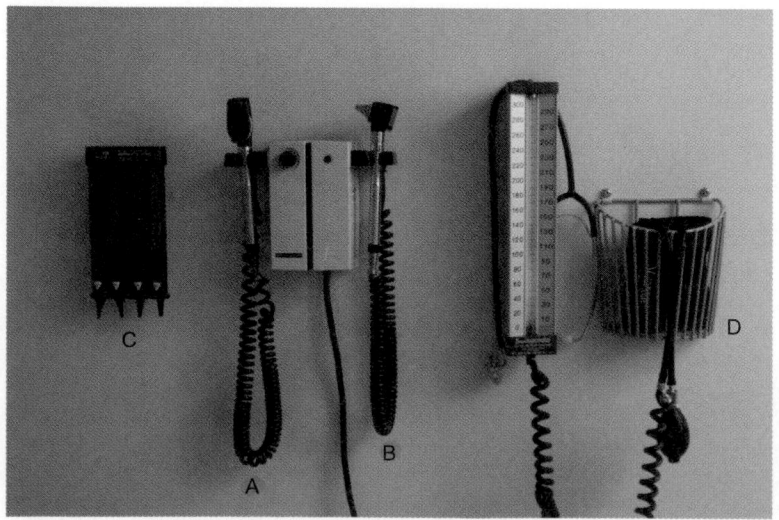

FIGURE 29-4 Examination room wall unit. **A,** Ophthalmoscope. **B,** Otoscope. **C,** Disposable speculums. **D,** Sphygmomanometer.

Tongue Depressor. A tongue depressor is a flat, wooden blade used to hold down the tongue when examining the throat (Figure 29-5).

Reflex Hammer. A reflex hammer is sometimes called a *percussion hammer*. This stainless-steel instrument has a hard rubber head used to test neurological reflexes of the knee and elbow when the tendons are struck (Figure 29-6).

Tuning Fork. Tuning forks come in different sizes, and each size produces a different pitch level (Figure 29-7, *A*). A tuning fork is used to check a patient's auditory acuity (Figure 29-7, *B*) and to test bone vibration (Figure 29-7, *C*). This aluminium instrument consists of a handle and two prongs that produce a humming sound when the physician strikes the prongs against his or her hand.

Stethoscope. A stethoscope is a listening device used when auscultating certain areas of the body, particularly the heart and lungs. This instrument comes in many shapes and sizes. All have two earpieces that are connected to flexible rubber or vinyl tubing (Figure 29-8). At the distal end of the tubing is a diaphragm or bell (many have both) that when placed securely on the patient's skin enables the physician to hear internal body sounds.

Gloves. Disposable latex gloves protect the healthcare worker and the patient from microorganisms. Under standard precautions, gloves are to be worn whenever there is a possibility of contact with all body fluids, broken skin or wounds, or contaminated items.

Tape Measure. A tape measure is a flexible ribbon ruler usually printed in inches and feet on one side and in centimeters and meters on the opposite side (Figure 29-9). Measurement is used to assess length and head circumference in infants, wound size, and so on.

Additional Supplies. Gauze squares, cotton balls, glass slides, cotton-tipped applicators, and laboratory request forms should be easily accessible for use during the examination.

Assisting With the Physical Examination

Methods of Examination. Examinations are performed as both a routine confirmation of the absence of illness and a means of diagnosing disease. Six methods of examining the human body are used by healthcare providers. All six methods are part of a complete physical examination.

Inspection. During inspection the examiner uses observation to detect significant physical features or objective data. This method of examination focuses on the patient's general appearance (the general state of health, including posture, mannerisms, and grooming) to more detailed observations, including body contour, gait, symmetry, visible injuries and deformities, tremors, rashes, and color changes.

Palpation. In palpation the examiner uses the sense of touch (Figure 29-10, *A*). A part of the body is felt with the hand to determine its condition or the condition of an underlying organ. Palpation may include touching the skin or a firmer exploration of the abdomen for underlying masses. This technique involves a wide range of perceptions: temperature, vibrations, consistency, form, size, rigidity, elasticity, moisture, texture, position, and contour. Palpation is performed with one hand, both hands (bimanual), one finger (digital), the fingertips, or the palmar aspect of the hand. A pelvic examination is done bimanually, whereas an anal examination is performed digitally. Do not confuse palpation with *palpitation*, which is a throbbing pulsation felt in the chest.

Percussion. Percussion involves tapping or striking the body, usually with the fingers or a small hammer, to elicit sounds or vibratory sensations. Percussion aids in the determination of the position, size, and density of an underlying organ or cavity. The effect of percussion is both heard and felt by the examiner. It is helpful in determining the amount of air or solid matter in an underlying organ or cavity. The two basic methods of percussion are *direct* and *indirect*. Direct (immediate) percussion is performed by striking the body with a finger. Indirect (mediate) percussion is used more frequently and is done by the physician placing his or her own fingers on the area and then striking the placed fingers with a finger of the other hand (Figure 29-10, *B*). Both a sound and a sense of vibration are evident here. The examiner quantifies the sounds in terms of pitch, quality, duration, and resonance.

Auscultation. In auscultation the examiner uses a stethoscope to listen to sounds arising from the body (not the sound produced by the physician, as in percussion,

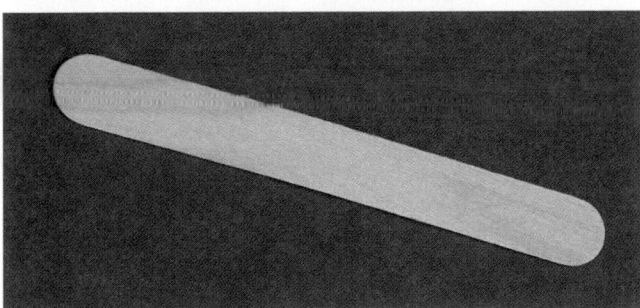

FIGURE 29-5 Disposable tongue depressor.

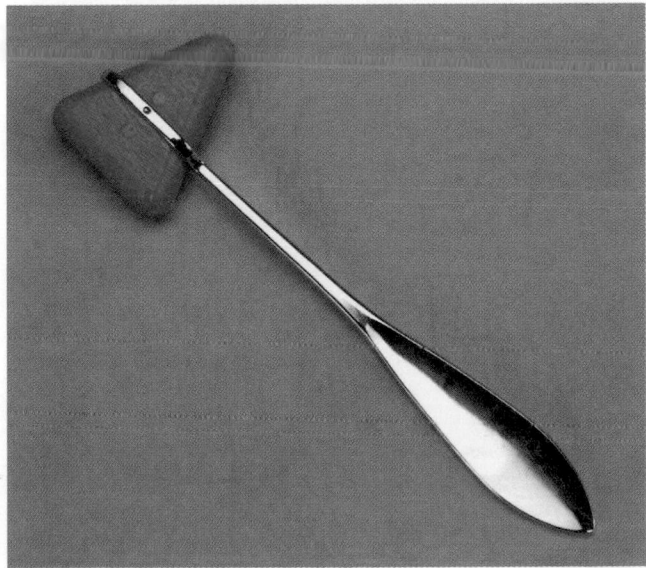

FIGURE 29-6 Reflex hammer.

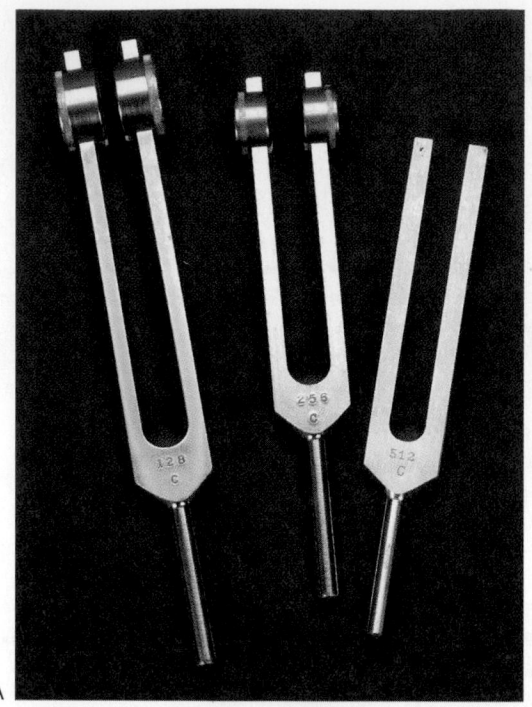

A

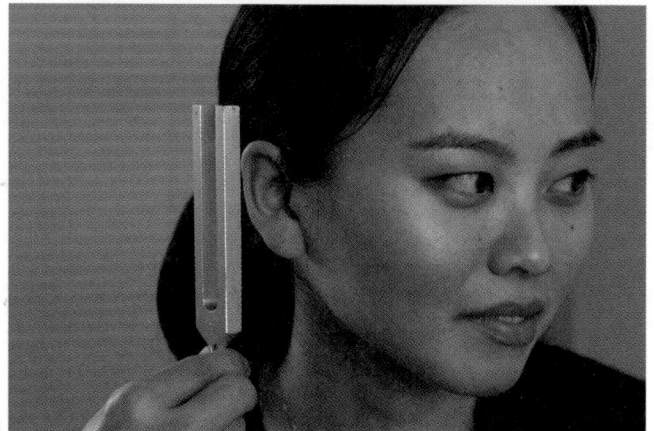

B

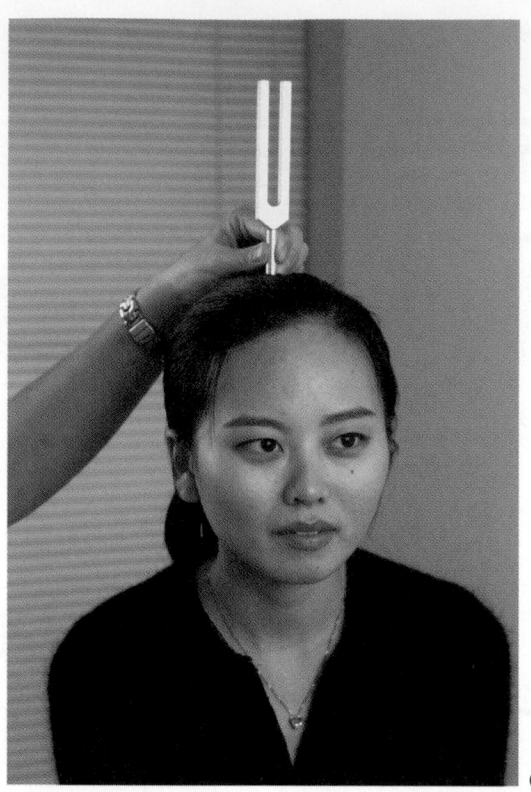

C

FIGURE 29-7 **A,** Tuning forks. **B,** Sound vibration test. **C,** Bone vibration test using parietal suture line.

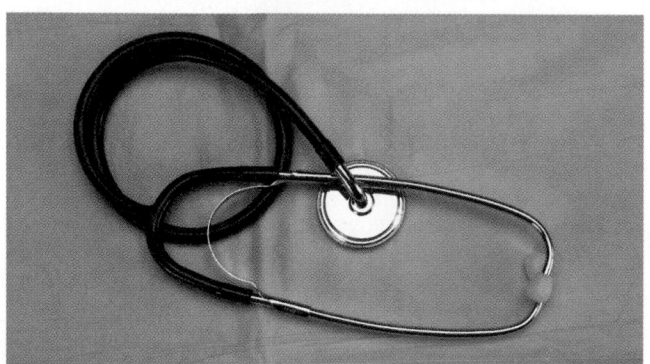

FIGURE 29-8 Stethoscope.

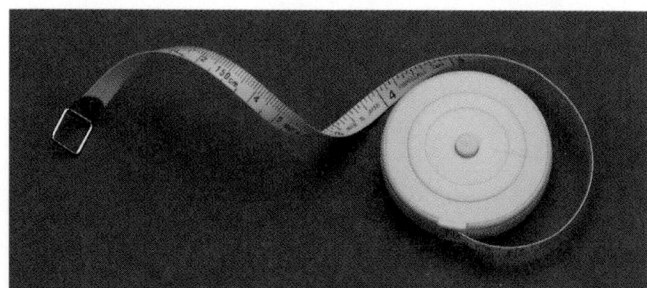

FIGURE 29-9 Tape measure.

but sounds that originate within the patient's body). Auscultation is a difficult method of examination, because the physician must distinguish between a normal and an abnormal sound (Figure 29-10, C). It is particularly useful

in evaluating sounds originating in the lungs, heart, and abdomen, such as a **murmur**, a **bruit**, and bowel sounds.

Mensuration. Mensuration is the process of measuring. Measurements are recorded of the patient's height and weight, the length and diameter of an extremity, the extent of flexion or extension of an extremity, the uterus

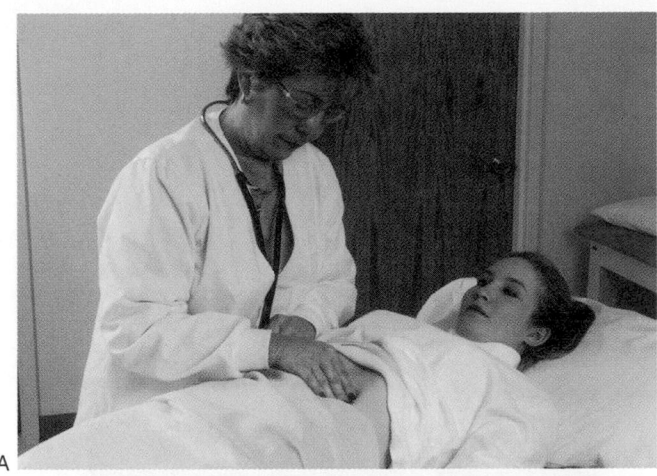

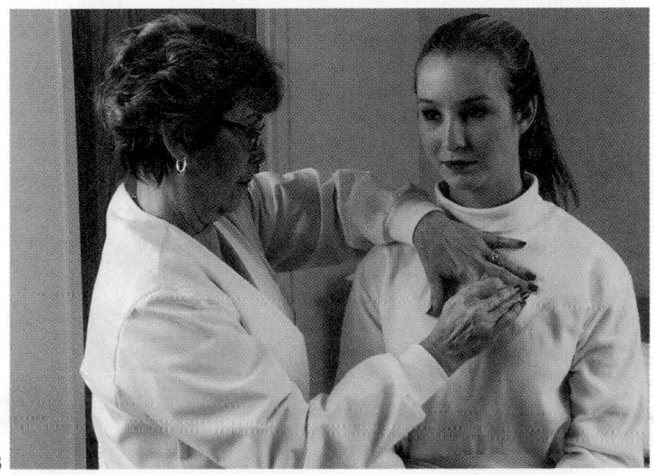

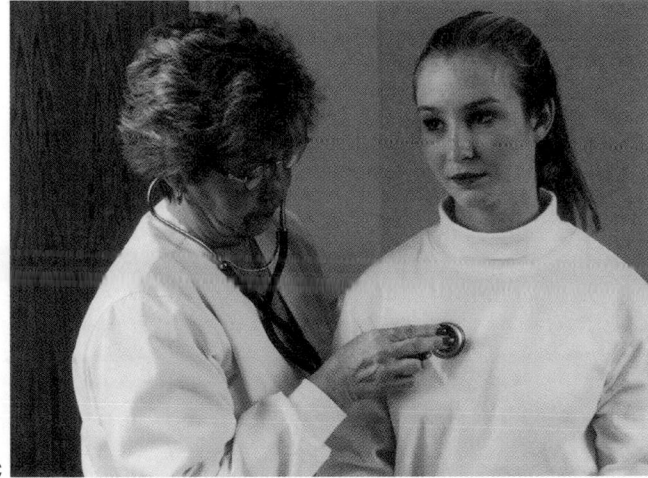

FIGURE 29-10   **A,** Demonstration of palpation. **B,** Demonstration of percussion. **C,** Demonstration of auscultation.

during pregnancy, the size and depth of a wound, or the pressure of a grip. Measurements are taken using a flexible tape measure or a circular wound measurement device and are usually recorded in centimeters.

Manipulation. Manipulation is the forceful, passive movement of a joint to determine the range of extension or flexion of a part of the body. Manipulation may or may not be grouped with palpation. It is usually considered

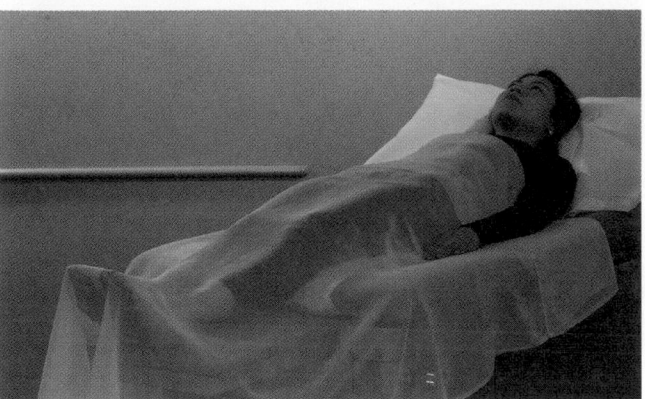

FIGURE 29-11   Patient in supine position.

separate from the four standard methods of examination (inspection, palpation, percussion, and auscultation) and is grouped with mensuration, especially by an orthopedist or a neurologist. Insurance and industrial reports often request this information in detail. For example, a patient involved in a work-related accident that caused joint damage may have to perform assisted range of motion exercises to the joint, with subsequent measurements of joint flexion and extension.

Positioning and Draping for Physical Examinations.   A variety of patient positions are used to facilitate a physical examination. The medical assistant instructs the patient about, and assists the patient into, these positions with as much ease and modesty as possible and helps the patient to maintain the position during the examination with as little discomfort as possible.

Draping with an examination sheet protects the patient from embarrassment and keeps the patient warm. However, the sheet must be positioned so that it allows complete visibility for the examiner and does not interfere with the examination. During the general examination, each part of the body is exposed one portion at a time. For gynecological and rectal examinations, the sheet is positioned on the diagonal across the patient. The following positions are used for medical examinations.

Supine (Horizontal Recumbent). In the supine position the patient lies flat, with the face upward and the lower legs supported by the extended foot rest (Figure 29-11). This position is used for the examination of the frontal portion of the body, including the heart, breasts, and abdominal organs. The patient's gown should be open down the front and the drape placed over any exposed area that is not being examined.

Dorsal Recumbent. In the dorsal recumbent position the patient lies face upward, with the weight distributed primarily to the surface of the back. This is accomplished by flexing the knees so that the feet are flat on the table. This position relieves muscle tension in the abdomen and is used for examination and/or inspection of the rectal, vaginal, and perineal areas. This position can be used for digital examinations of the vagina and rectum but is not used if an instrument such as a speculum is needed. To ensure the patient's privacy, it is important to keep the patient completely draped, with the drape at an angle, until the physician is present (Figure 29-12).

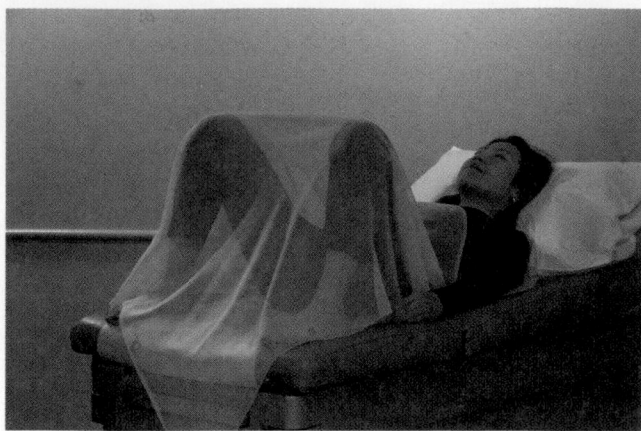

FIGURE 29-12   Patient in dorsal recumbent position.

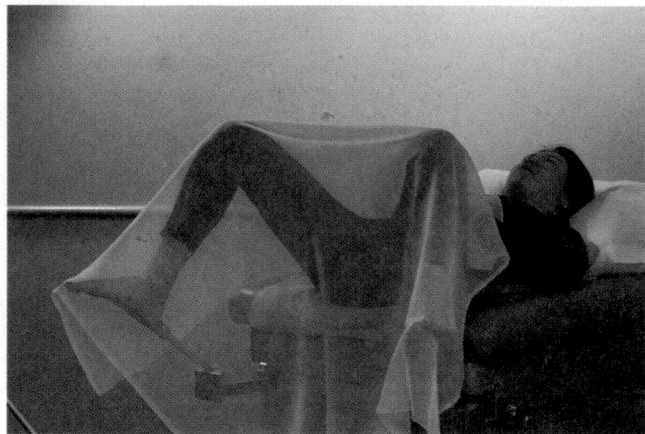

FIGURE 29-13   Patient in lithotomy position.

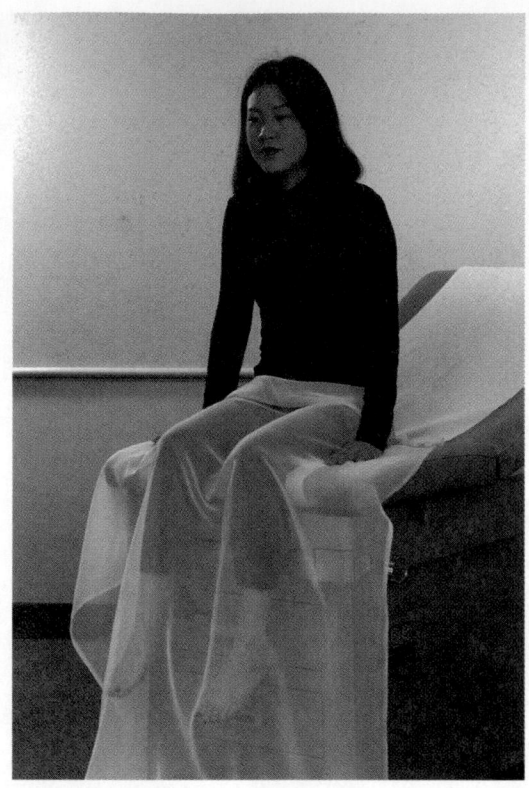

FIGURE 29-14   Patient in Fowler's position.

Lithotomy. For the lithotomy position the patient is placed on the back, with the knees sharply flexed, the arms placed at the sides or folded over the chest, and the buttocks to the edge of the table. The feet are supported in table stirrups. The stirrups should be placed wide apart and somewhat away from the table. If the heels are too close to the buttocks, the possibility of leg cramps is increased, and it is more difficult for the patient to relax the abdominal muscles. Make certain that the stirrups are locked in place. A drape is placed at an angle over the patient's abdomen and knees. The drape should be large enough to cover the breasts if the patient is not wearing a gown. The drape must be long enough to cover the knees and touch the ankles and wide enough to prevent the sides of the thighs from being exposed. The physician will lift the drape away from the pubic area when the examination begins (Figure 29-13). The lithotomy position is primarily used for vaginal examinations that require the use of a speculum and for Pap smears.

Fowler's. In Fowler's position the patient sits on the examination table with the head of the table elevated 90 degrees or simply sits at the edge of the table. This position is useful for examinations and treatments of the head, neck, and chest or for patients who find it difficult to

breathe lying down. The drape will vary according to the exposure of the patient (Figure 29-14).

Semi-Fowler's. The semi-Fowler's position is a modification of Fowler's position. Instead of the head of the table at a full 90-degree angle, it is lowered to a 45-degree angle. This position is useful for postsurgical examinations, patients with breathing disorders, and when the patient has an elevated temperature or is suffering from head trauma or pain (Figure 29-15). The drape and/or gown should cover the entire patient from the nipple line down.

Prone. The patient lies face down on the table, on the ventral surface of the body. This is the opposite of the supine position and is another one of the recumbent positions. The drape should cover from the middle of the back to below the knees, with the gown open to the back. The drape on a female patient should extend high enough to cover her breasts if she is to be turned over to the dorsal recumbent position during the examination (Figure 29-16). This position is used for examinations of the back and for certain surgical procedures.

Sims'. The Sims' position is sometimes called the *lateral* position. The patient is placed on the left side; the left arm and shoulder are drawn back behind the body so that the body's weight is predominantly on the chest. The right arm is flexed upward for support. The left leg is slightly flexed, and the buttocks are pulled to the edge of the table. The right leg is sharply flexed upward. The drape extends at an angle from under the arms to below the knees. The physician can raise a small portion of the sheet from the back of the patient to sufficiently expose the rectum. The remaining portion of the sheet

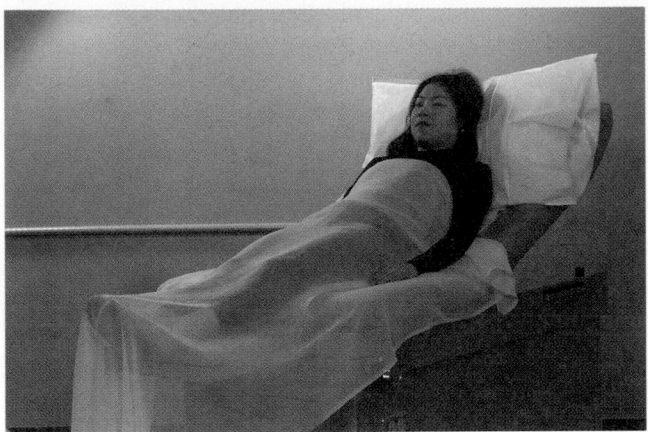

FIGURE 29-15   Patient in semi-Fowler's position.

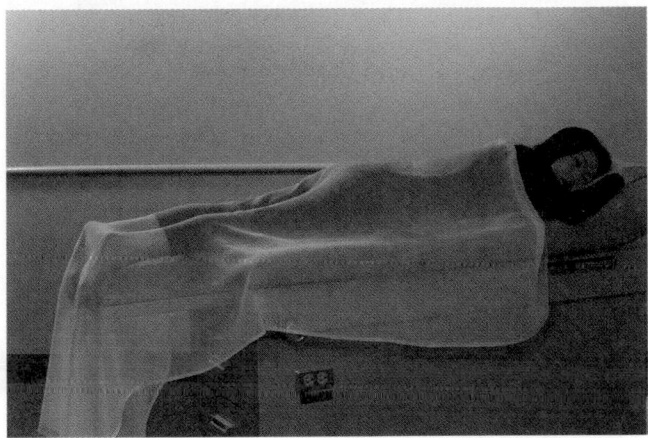

FIGURE 29-16   Patient in prone position.

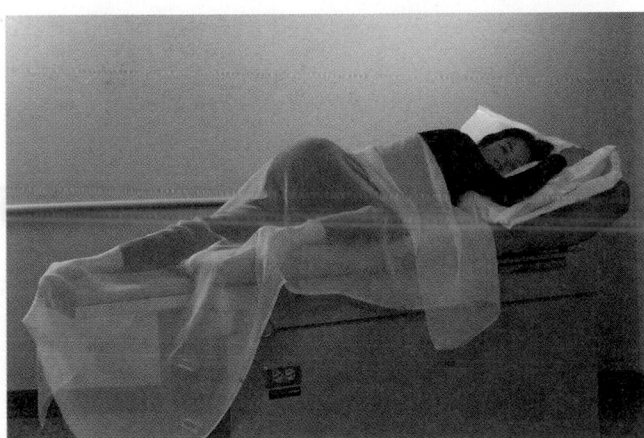

FIGURE 29-17   Patient in Sims' position.

covers the patient's chest area and thighs. This position is used for rectal examinations, rectal thermometer readings, instillation of rectal medications, and perineal and some pelvic examinations (Figure 29-17).

Knee-Chest. The patient rests on the knees and the chest with the head turned to one side. The arms can be placed under the head for support and comfort or bent and at the sides of the table near the head. The thighs are

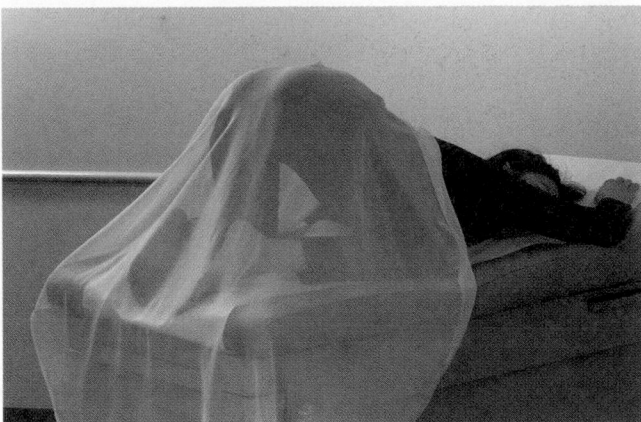

FIGURE 29-18   Patient in knee-chest position.

perpendicular to the table and are slightly separated. The buttocks extend up into the air, and the back should be straight. The patient will need assistance to do the knee-chest position correctly. It is difficult for most patients to maintain this position, so they should not be placed into it until the point in the examination that it is required. The medical assistant must remain with the patient for assistance and support the entire time that the knee-chest position is needed. If the correct knee-chest position cannot be obtained, the patient may have to be placed in a knee-elbow position. This position puts less strain on the patient and is easier to maintain. These positions are used for proctological examinations and sigmoid, rectal, and occasionally vaginal examinations. The patient's gown should open in the back, with a fenestrated (opening) drape or a single sheet draped at an angle over the patient's back at the sacral area (Figure 29-18).

Trendelenburg. The patient is supine on a table that has been raised at the lower end about 30 degrees. This places the patient's head lower than the legs. The patient's legs are then flexed over the end of the table. This position is sometimes used in cases of shock or low blood pressure. It is also a position for abdominal surgery, because the abdominal viscera gravitate upward and out of the way of the surgical procedure. A drape is placed over the patient, covering from the underarms to below the knees. This is not a position that is used routinely in the ambulatory care setting (Figure 29-19).

CRITICAL THINKING APPLICATION

Determine the correct patient position and method of gowning and draping for the following examinations:
- Instillation of a rectal suppository
- An annual Papanicolaou (Pap) smear
- Examination of the back
- Patient with dyspnea
- Breast examination
- Patient going into shock

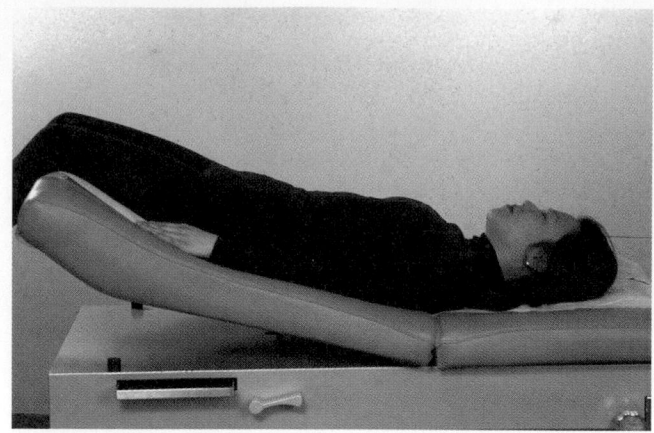

FIGURE 29-19 Patient in Trendelenburg position.

Principles of Body Mechanics

Proper body mechanics should be used consistently throughout the work environment when sitting or standing, lifting or carrying objects, pushing or pulling, or transferring patients. Without consistent application of correct anatomical alignment, it is very easy for injuries, especially lower back injuries, to occur (Figures 29-20 and 29-21).

Proper body alignment begins with good posture. Maintaining posture requires a combination of muscle efforts. Good posture keeps the spine balanced and aligned while sitting and standing.

Avoid twisting or turning; instead, move the feet to face the object needed. This will avert undue strain on the lumbar region. Do not cross the legs while sitting, because it interferes with circulation to the legs and feet. When sitting, keep the popliteal area (behind the knees) free from the edge of the chair. Pressure in this area interferes with circulation and may cause damage to

nerves in the area. Do a mental check of posture on a regular basis. Hold the head erect, with the face forward and chin slightly up, contract the abdominal muscles up and in, shoulders relaxed and back, feet pointing forward and slightly apart, and weight evenly distributed to both legs, with the knees slightly bent. Always be on alert for potential injuries that may result from poor body mechanics.

SAFE LIFTING TECHNIQUES

- Always get help if the load is too heavy.
- Do not reach for items. Clear barriers out of the way and get as close as possible to what needs to be lifted.
- Bend at the knees with the feet shoulder-width apart and *keep the back straight*. Use leg muscles to lift (see Figure 29-20).
- Keep the weight as close as possible to the body when carrying a heavy item (see Figure 29-21).
- Move feet in the direction of the lift. *Do not twist or turn on fixed feet.*
- Bend knees while keeping the back straight when lowering an item at the completion of the lift.
- If there is a choice, push a heavy item rather than pulling it.

Transferring a Patient

Frequently patients need assistance to move from a chair to the examination table or back again. There are multiple ways to transfer patients, but all should focus on correct body mechanics. If the patient is in a wheelchair, move

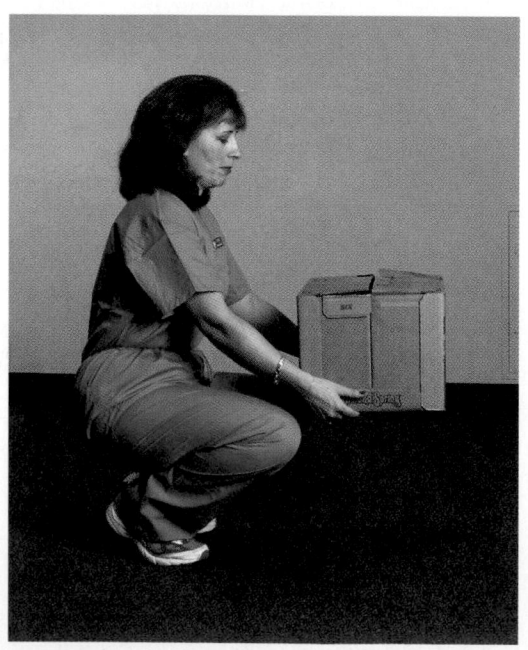
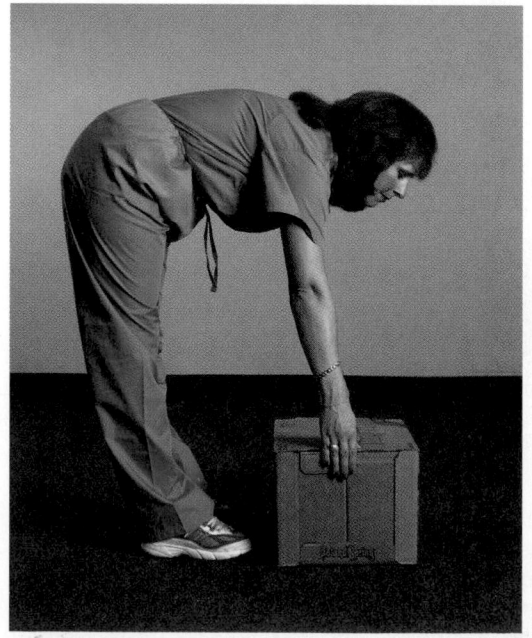

FIGURE 29-20 **A,** Proper lifting technique. **B,** Improper lifting technique.

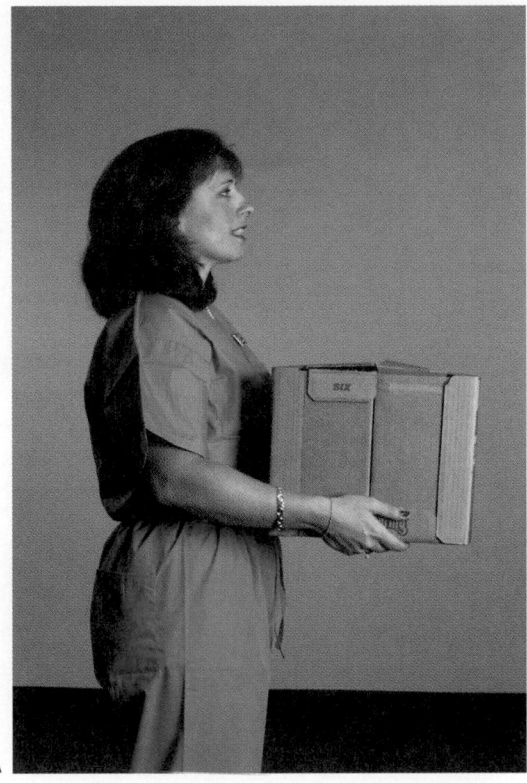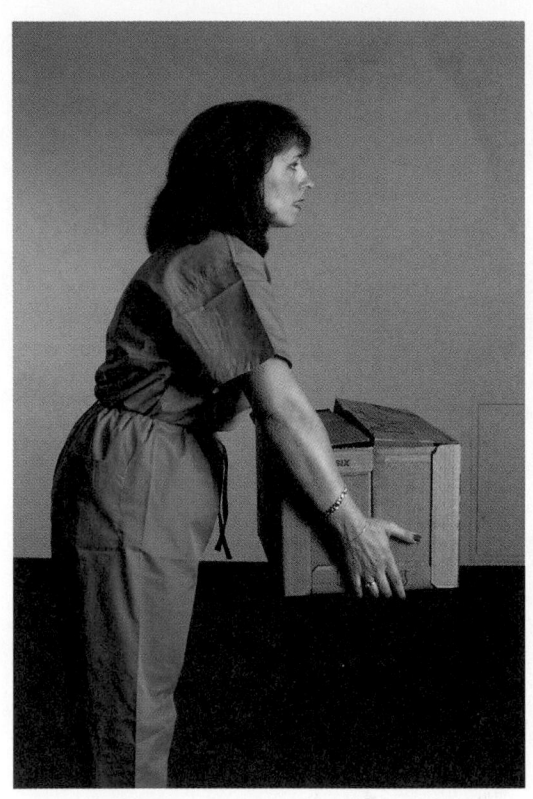

FIGURE 29-21   **A,** Carrying item close to body. **B,** Improper carrying technique.

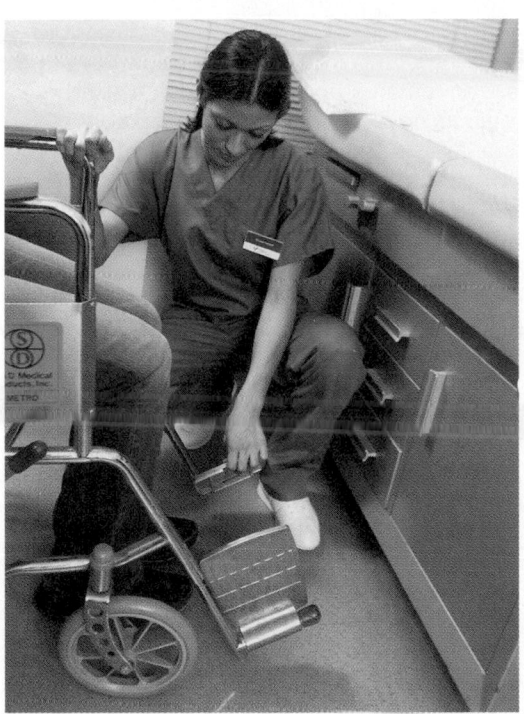

FIGURE 29-22   Wheels locked and foot rests elevated.

the chair close to the examination table, lock the wheels, and lift the foot rests out of the way (Figure 29-22). Explain the procedure to the patient and ask for his or her assistance.

If one side of the patient is stronger than the other, always provide support on the strong side. Place a step stool in front of the wheelchair near the examination table. Support the patient close to your body on the strong side, with one hand under the axillary region and the other either grasping the patient's hand or holding the forearm. When bending, *always bend at the knees and maintain the back's three natural curves, allowing the leg muscles to help in lifting*. Give the patient a signal and lift as the patient assists. Have the patient step up onto the stool with the strong leg and pivot (Figure 29-23). Ease the patient down onto the table, bending your knees while keeping your back aligned. Make sure the patient is comfortable and safely positioned on the table (Figure 29-24). It may be necessary to remain with the patient until the examination is completed to ensure patient safety. If the physician prefers that the patient be in a supine position, place one arm across the patient's shoulders and the other under the knees and smoothly lower the upper body to the table while raising the legs. Use the same pivoting techniques with proper body mechanics to help transfer the patient from the examination table back to the locked wheelchair. If the patient must hold on to you, have him or her hold your waist or shoulders, not your neck.

Examination Sequence

The physical examination sequence is fairly standard; however, variations may occur, depending on the physician's specialty, the medical necessity for the examination, and the physician's preference. There is much the medical assistant can do to facilitate the quality of patient care and the physician's schedule. A successful medical

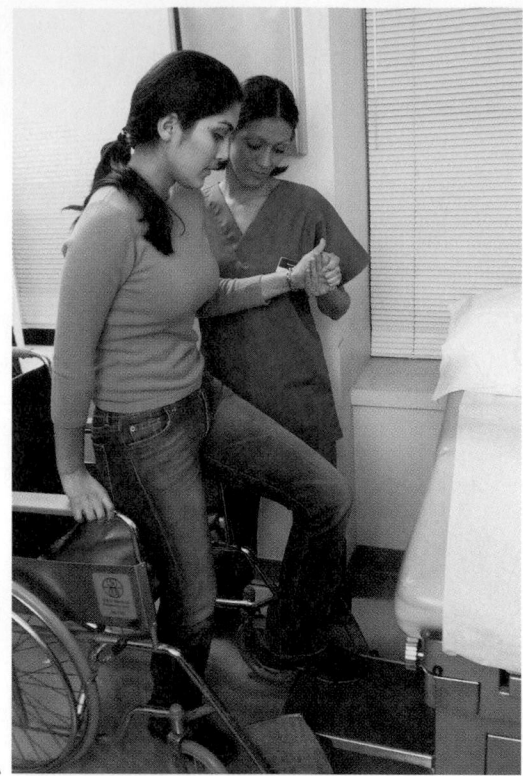

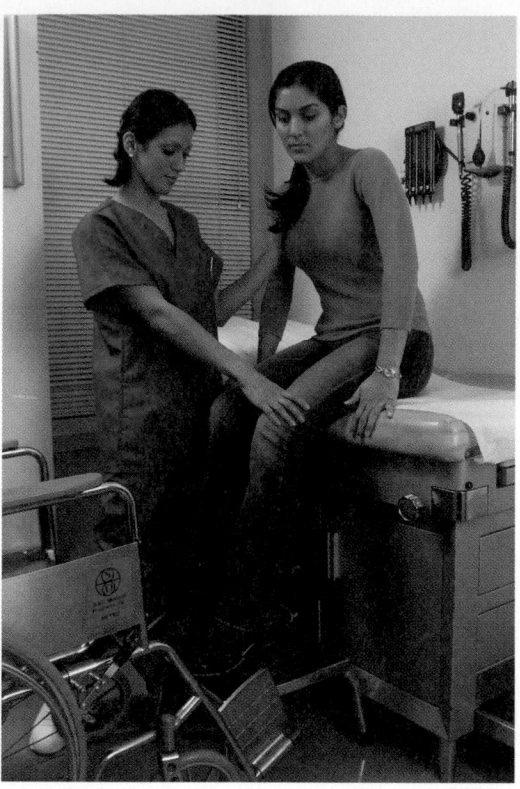

FIGURE 29-24   Sitting on table with support.

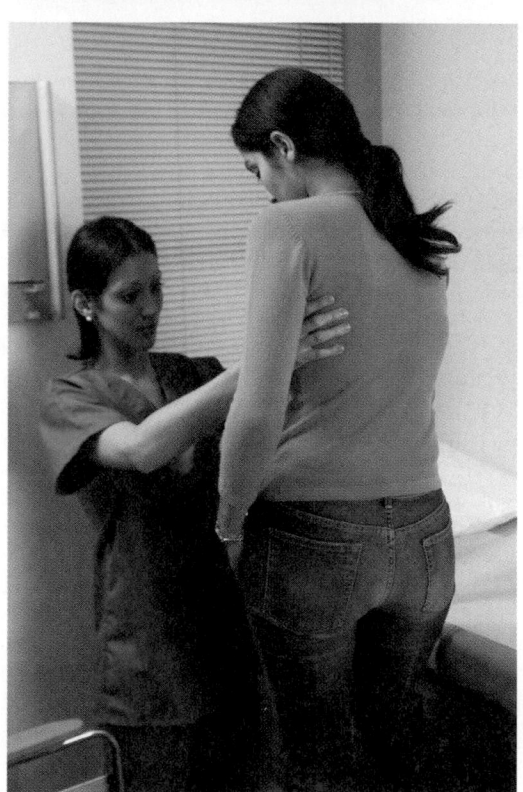

FIGURE 29-23   **A,** Strong side support. **B,** Pivot with support.

assistant develops a routine that is organized yet flexible enough to adjust to individual needs.

Give the patient a brief explanation of the examination process. Patients are more cooperative and less anxious if they understand what is expected of them. Assemble all the instruments needed for the examination. As the physician proceeds with the examination, make sure the patient remains unexposed by adjusting the drapes and gown as needed. In every examination, the medical assistant assists the physician by handing him or her the correct instruments and supplies needed.

A female assistant in the room during the examination of a female patient can avert potential lawsuits. If the physician is male, a female medical assistant must remain with a female patient throughout the examination unless the physician excuses the medical assistant from the room.

When the physician begins the examination, the medical assistant should keep conversation to a minimum and remain inconspicuous. The examination usually starts with the patient seated on the examining table. If the physician uses reflected light, the light source should be behind the patient's right shoulder. If illuminated instruments are used, then the standard overhead lights are sufficient. Be careful not to shine a light directly into the patient's eyes. Turning on lights while they are directed away from the patient and then carefully moving the light toward the area to be examined can accomplish this.

Presenting Appearance (General Appearance)

The physical examination starts with observations about the patient's appearance. Either of the terms *presenting appearance* or *general appearance* may be used on the medical record. These terms note whether the patient appears well and in good health (e.g., the patient may appear disoriented or in distress, well or undernourished, or may answer questions with ease or confusion).

The patient's *gait* (i.e., the manner or style of walking) often provides important information. The patient may limp, walk with the feet wide apart, exhibit a shuffle step, or have difficulty in maintaining his or her balance. In addition to gait, the patient's entire body movements are observed for possible muscle actions that the physician deems unusual. Posture is also observed for indications of pain, stiffness, or difficulty with limb movement. If the medical assistant notes any of these observations or the patient reports any complaints, these should be recorded in the patient's chart while the medical assistant is documenting the vital signs before the physician begins the examination.

Nutrition and Stature

The patient's height and weight are measured by the medical assistant before the examination begins. During the examination, the physician notes the body build and proportions. Any *gross* (immediately obvious) deformities are recorded. Sometimes abnormalities in height or body proportion may be caused by hormonal imbalances.

Speech

Speech may reveal a pathological condition. Some basic speech defects are *aphonia,* the inability to speak because of a loss of the voice, commonly seen with severe laryngitis or overuse of the voice; *aphasia,* the loss of expression through speech, writing, or sign resulting from injury or disease of the brain centers; and *dysphasia,* a lack of coordination and failure to arrange words in proper order, usually caused by a brain lesion. *Motor aphasia* occurs when the patient knows what she or he wants to say but cannot use muscles properly to speak such as in slurred or incoherent speech after a cerebrovascular accident (CVA). *Sensory aphasia* is when the patient pronounces the words easily but uses them inaccurately, such as in jumbled speech.

Breath Odors

Breath odors may or may not be diagnostic, although they are often associated with poor oral hygiene or dental care. Acidosis will give the strong odor of acetone, which is sweet and fruity, and may result from diabetes mellitus, starvation, or renal disease. A musty odor is usually associated with liver disease, and the odor of ammonia may be found in cases of uremia.

Skin

The condition of the skin can be a good reflection of the patient's nutritional status and hydration level. If dehydration is suspected, skin *turgor* is checked by pinching the skin on the posterior surface of the hands. The tissue is then observed to see how quickly it returns to the normal location. A delay indicates there is a decrease in tissue fluid, confirming the diagnosis of dehydration. Extreme dryness, scaling, extended wound healing, or frequent breaks in the skin may indicate systemic disease.

Fingernails and toenails often give some indication of a person's health. Brittle, grooved, or lined nails may indicate either local infection or systemic disease. *Clubbing* of the fingertips is associated with some congenital heart or lung diseases. *Spooning* of the nail is seen in some patients with severe *iron-deficiency anemia. Beau's lines* appear after an acute illness but will grow out and disappear. The PCP may refer the patient with skin disorders to a dermatologist for diagnosis and treatment.

Reflexes

The patient's reflexes are checked with the patient in the high Fowler's and supine positions. While the patient is sitting, the biceps are checked with the patient's arm flexed and supported by the examiner. The knee jerk (patellar reflex) and the ankle jerk (Achilles reflex) are checked using tapotement (a tapping or percussing movement) with either the fingers or the reflex hammer. The plantar reflexes (Babinski and Chaddock reflexes) are tested with the patient in either an upright or supine position.

Head

Once the physician makes overall observations of the patient's general condition, the physical examination typically begins with the head and face and moves downward toward the feet. The face reflects the patient's state and tells the physician a great deal about how the patient handles stress and illness. The skull, scalp, and face are palpated for size, shape, and symmetry. The distribution or the lack of hair and the hair texture may indicate hormonal changes. Excessive hair, especially facial hair in females, indicates a hormonal imbalance. As the head is examined, the physician assesses possible **nodules**, masses, or signs of **trauma**.

Neck

The neck is examined for *range of motion* (ROM) by having the patient move the head in various directions. The thyroid gland is given special attention for symmetry, size, and texture. The physician manually palpates the thyroid area, and the patient is asked to swallow several times. The physician palpates the thyroid gland both anteriorly and posteriorly. The carotid artery is palpated and auscultated for possible bruit. The lymph nodes are palpated. *Lymphadenopathy* (enlarged lymph nodes) is usually present if there is infection in the face, head, or neck.

Eyes

The pupils are checked for reaction by shining a light into the eye. If the pupils constrict equally and smoothly to the light stimulus the physician will document "PEARL" (which means the pupils are equal and respond to light). The **sclera** is checked for color, which ranges from white to pale yellow. The movements of the eyes are tested by having the patient follow the physician's finger. If the movement is within average range, it is written as "extraocular movement (EOM) intact." The physician uses the ophthalmoscope to examine the interior of the eye, including the retina and the intraocular vessels. Some diseases, such as diabetes mellitus, cause damage to the blood vessels of the retina.

Ears

The ears are examined with the use of the otoscope. The external ear is first checked for inflammation of the external auditory canal or the presence of ear wax (cerumen). The tympanic membrane (eardrum) is examined and should appear pearly gray. Scars appearing on the eardrum are frequently the result of earlier, chronic ear infections or perforations. The color of the eardrum is important to the diagnosis, because it may indicate fluids such as blood or pus behind the eardrum in the middle ear. The patient may be asked to swallow several times to observe movement of the tympanic membrane, which occurs on pressure changes in the eustachian tube. The eustachian tube equalizes air pressure between the middle ear and the throat. The ability of the tympanic membrane to move is crucial to the hearing process.

Mouth and Throat

The mouth, or oral cavity, is usually thought of in terms of oral hygiene and dental care. Dental hygiene includes the condition of the teeth, how the patient cares for the teeth and gums, and whether the teeth of the upper and lower jaws meet properly (occlude) for chewing. Healthy gums are pale pink, glossy, and smooth and do not bleed when pressure from a tongue depressor is applied. The palatine tonsils are usually visible. The physician may use a tongue depressor and a piece of gauze to grasp the tongue for careful examination of it. The floor of the mouth is examined by both inspection and palpation for enlarged lymph nodes, salivary gland function, and ulcerations. The insides of the cheeks are also examined for any abnormal marks or color.

Nose and Sinuses

The mucosa of the nasal cavity is examined for color and texture. The sinus meatus cannot be seen, but the frontal and maxillary sinuses may be examined by firm palpation over the area and by **transillumination**.

When disorders in the eyes, ears, nose, and throat are observed, and the physician believes that the condition warrants the attention of a specialist, the patient is referred to an ophthalmologist or an otorhinolaryngologist (ear, nose, and throat specialist).

Chest

While the patient is still in the sitting position, the chest, heart, lungs, and breasts are examined. The chest is examined for symmetric expansion. A tape measure may be used, especially if there is a variation between the upper and lower chest expansion. A patient with a history of **emphysema** may have a barrel-shaped chest.

With the stethoscope to the patient's back, the examiner listens to the lung sounds. The patient is asked to take deep and regular breaths. This may produce slight dizziness, but the patient should be assured that it is only the result of the deep respirations and will rapidly pass. The physician notes the types of respirations and the presence of lung sounds in all fields.

Because it takes considerable concentration to interpret heart sounds, the physician must have complete silence when listening to the patient's heart. The heart is examined using a stethoscope from both the anterior and posterior approaches to the patient. Further examination may include auscultation on the left, lateral side. In cases of heart disease, the physician may spend an extended period of time listening to heart sounds. If chest or heart abnormalities are found, the physician orders further diagnostic tests, including blood analysis, x-ray evaluation, and an electrocardiogram (ECG). Once the results of these studies are analyzed, the physician may refer the patient to a cardiologist for the heart or a pulmonologist or respiratory care specialist for a breathing disorder.

Breast and Testicular Examinations

A careful breast examination is part of the examination of every female, whether or not the patient is symptomatic. The patient is examined both visually and by palpation in high Fowler's position and then again in the supine position. Breast cancer is the most common malignancy occurring in women, and early detection is the key to successful treatment. This is a good opportunity to discuss and reinforce the consistent use of monthly self-breast examination (SBE). This technique is presented in Chapter 38. For male patients who have reached puberty or are 15 years of age or older, the physician will perform a testicular examination. The technique is presented in Chapter 37.

Abdomen

The patient is lowered to the dorsal recumbent position, and the drape is lowered to the pubic hair line. The gown is raised to just under the breasts. The physician stands to the patient's right side if at all possible. The patient's arms may be placed at the side, or the hands may be crossed over the chest or under the head. Relaxation of the abdominal muscles is absolutely essential for the abdominal examination. It sometimes helps to place a small pillow under the patient's head and knees to increase comfort and relieve muscular tension. The physician auscultates the abdomen in all quadrants to confirm the presence of complete bowel sounds and palpates the abdomen for any abnormalities.

Rectum

The rectal examination usually follows the abdominal examination or may be part of the examination of the male and female genitalia. The patient's comfort and dignity are vital. For this part of the examination, the physician needs examination gloves and lubricating jelly. Some physicians prefer to use an anoscope. The examination light must be directed at the perineal area during the examination.

Hemoccult test specimens are often collected at the time of the digital rectal examination. If this is a procedure that the physician performs, be sure to include the necessary collection folder with the examination equipment.

The specialty for disorders and diseases of the stomach and small intestine is gastroenterology; proctology is the specialty of the large intestine and rectum. These are discussed in Chapter 36. See Procedure 29-1 for assisting with the physical examination.

The Role of the Medical Assistant

The physical examination establishes a baseline from which a patient's healthcare is determined. The examination should never be considered routine. Each patient's needs are special, and the medical assistant must be prepared to assist when needed. Throughout the procedure the medical assistant must treat the patient with respect and guard individual privacy as much as possible.

The primary role of the medical assistant regarding the physical examination is to have the room, equipment, and supplies stocked and ready; the patient prepared, with vital signs, height, and weight measured and recorded; documentation completed on the patient's chief complaint or reported data; and the patient properly gowned and in position for the examination. During the examination the medical assistant should be prepared to hand the physician needed equipment or assist in any other way necessary. After the examination is completed, the medical assistant should provide assistance to the patient as needed; complete any diagnostic procedures ordered by the physician; assist in the patient's discharge; answer patient questions or complete patient education; and disinfect and restock the room for the next patient.

CRITICAL THINKING APPLICATION

Alice Greenbaum is a 68-year-old patient of Dr. Kosto's who is scheduled for an annual physical examination, including a breast check and Pap smear. Mrs. Greenbaum appears anxious about the examination and asks Felicia if the gynecological examination is necessary. How should Felicia manage this patient? What could she do to ease the patient's fears and prepare her for the examination?

Patient Education

To improve the overall health status of individuals and to enlist the patient as an ally in the examination process, the medical assistant can educate the patient in many different ways. Patient education contributes to the patient's holistic care. The physical examination process is an excellent time for the medical assistant to assess the

need for patient education. This assessment should be performed to identify the best way to meet the needs of the patient. When identifying these needs, consider the following:

- The information that the patient needs to know
- How to convey the information so that the patient will understand
- How the patient will use the information once he or she has it

Develop a plan to teach the patient. Think about the different modalities available, such as pamphlets, pictures, films, demonstrations, and community resources. The more interesting the information, the more fun it is to teach the patient, and the more enjoyment the patient will get out of learning. The medical assistant should always review teaching plans with the physician and follow the physician's direction in patient education. Chapter 26 offers details on how to create an effective patient education intervention.

CRITICAL THINKING APPLICATION

Dr. Kosto serves as the PCP in the area for residents of group homes for the developmentally delayed. Jimmy Cosgrove, a 38-year-old patient who is severely retarded, is being seen today for an abdominal postsurgical visit. Felicia is responsible for preparing the patient for the examination as well as educating Jimmy's caregiver on how to assist in his recovery. Describe how Felicia should prepare the patient and the room and develop a teaching plan that meets the needs of the patient and his caregiver.

Legal and Ethical Issues

The medical assistant must recognize that a legal and ethical contract exists between the patient and the physician. As the physician's employee, the medical assistant is part of that contract. Information gained during the physical examination is confidential and must remain that way. The medical assistant must uphold ethical responsibilities as written in the AAMA Code of Ethics: to render service, respect confidential information, and uphold the honor and high principles of the profession.

SUMMARY OF SCENARIO

As a new medical assistant, Felicia Grand has a great deal of responsibility when it comes to assisting with physical examinations. She must prepare the room for the particular examination ordered and also prepare and care for the patient during the procedure. Preparing the room includes making sure appropriate supplies and equipment are readily available, as well as planning for the privacy of the patient during the examination. Each examination is different, just as each patient has his or her own set of

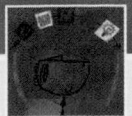

Preparing For and Assisting With the Physical Examination

GOAL: To help the physician examine patients by preparing the necessary equipment and ensuring patient safety and comfort during the examination.

EQUIPMENT AND SUPPLIES

- Stethoscope
- Ophthalmoscope
- Scale
- Tongue depressor
- Cotton balls
- Examination light
- Percussion hammer
- Lubricating gel
- Examination gloves
- Sphygmomanometer
- Otoscope
- Tape measure
- Gauze sponges
- Pen light
- Nasal speculum
- Tuning fork
- Biohazard container
- Laboratory request forms

- Specimen bottles/glass slides
- Patient gown
- Drapes
- Thermometer
- Cotton-tipped applicators

PROCEDURAL STEPS

1 Prepare the examining room according to acceptable medical aseptic rules.

Purpose: Room must be aseptically clean to prevent spread of infection.

2 Wash your hands.

Purpose: Infection control.

3 Locate the instruments for the procedure. Set them out in sequence.

Purpose: Promotes time management and ensures that all needed equipment and supplies are ready.

4 Identify the patient and determine whether the patient understands the procedure. If the patient does not understand, explain what to expect.

Purpose: To promote patient cooperation during the examination.

5 Review the medical history with the patient and investigate the purpose of the visit.

Purpose: Verifies that all information is current and complete.

6 Measure and record the patient's vital signs, height, and weight.

Purpose: To gather data needed before the examination begins.

7 Instruct the patient on how to collect the urine specimen, and hand the patient the properly labeled specimen container (see Chapter 49). Obtain any blood samples that are required (see Chapter 50). Obtain resting ECG if ordered (see Chapter 46).

Purpose: To obtain all specimens and tests as ordered by the physician.

8 Hand the patient a gown and drape. Instruct the patient on how to put the gown on. Help the patient with undressing as needed; however, most patients prefer to undress in privacy.

Purpose: To assist the patient in preparing for the examination.

9 Assist the patient in sitting on the narrow end of the examination table; place the drape over the patient's lap and legs. If the patient is elderly, confused, or feeling faint or dizzy, DO NOT leave him or her alone.

Purpose: To provide for the patient's warmth and modesty and to prevent a fall and injury.

10 Advise the physician that the patient is ready.

11 Assist during the examination by handing the physician each instrument as it is needed and by positioning and draping the patient.

12 When the physician has completed the examination, allow the patient to rest for a moment, then help the patient from the table. Assist with dressing, if necessary. Use proper body mechanics if assistance in transfer is needed.

Purpose: Ensure patient's stability and safety.

13 Record the necessary notes on the patient's chart and forward it to the physician for further notations.

14 Return to the patient and ask him or her if there are any questions. Give the patient any final instructions, and schedule tests as ordered by the physician and/or the next appointment.

Purpose: To clarify directions, eliminate any misunderstandings, and allow the patient to discuss any concerns. If there are misunderstandings or concerns beyond your scope of experience or skill, arrange for the physician to speak with the patient again.

15 Put on gloves and dispose of used supplies and linens in designated waste containers. Clean tabletop surfaces with disinfectant. Disinfect all equipment.

Purpose: Prevent cross-contamination with any potential infectious materials.

16 Remove gloves and discard them in the biohazard waste container and wash hands.

Purpose: Infection control.

17 Replace used supplies and prepare room for next patient.

needs. It is Felicia's responsibility to make sure the examination runs smoothly for the physician and to support the patient throughout the process.

SUMMARY OF LEARNING OBJECTIVES

- The human body is made up of trillions of microscopic cells that perform particular functions. When cells with similar structures and functions combine, tissues are formed. There are four types of tissues in the body: epithelial, connective, muscular, and nervous. A combination of two or more types of tissues creates an organ, while a number of organs joined together form a body system.

- Table 29-1 summarizes the 11 body systems and their primary organs.

- Instruments and supplies that are typically used in the physical examination include the nasal speculum, ophthalmoscope, otoscope, tongue depressor, reflex hammer, various tuning forks, stethoscope, sphygmomanometer, examination gloves, and tape measure.

- Methods of examination include inspection, palpation, percussion, auscultation, mensuration, and manipulation.

- Draping a patient for the physical examination requires constant attention to maintaining the privacy of the patient throughout the process while assisting the physician with exposure of the area being examined. The general rule is to cover all exposed body parts until the point in time during the examination when the physician must evaluate that particular area.

- The position assumed by the patient during the examination depends on the part of the body that is being examined. Possible patient positions include supine, dorsal recumbent, lithotomy, Fowler's, semi-Fowler's, prone, Sims', knee-chest, and Trendelenburg.

- Proper body mechanics must be applied throughout the work environment to prevent work-related injuries. Good body mechanics principles include maintaining balanced posture, moving feet in the direction of the lift to avoid twisting, carrying items close to the body, bending the knees while maintaining the back's three natural curves when lifting, using leg muscles to help lift, pushing a heavy item rather than pulling, and always getting help if the load is too heavy.

- The examination sequence is dependent on the type of examination and physician preference. The physician typically begins the examination by noting the patient's general health appearance, nutrition status, speech, breath odor, skin condition, and reflexes. The physician then begins the physical examination, starting at the head and working the way down through the body to the rectum. Any abnormalities are noted and may be further investigated with diagnostic tools after the examination is completed.

- The role of the medical assistant during the physical examination involves attention to the individual needs of the patient as well as assisting the physician with the procedure. This includes preparing the room and supplies, preparing the patient, documenting pertinent patient information, and assisting the physician throughout the process. After the examination is completed, the medical assistant should provide assistance to the patient as needed, complete diagnostic procedures as ordered, and disinfect and restock the examination room for the next patient.

- Before, during, and after the physical examination are excellent times to provide appropriate patient education. The medical assistant should clarify or reinforce any information provided by the physician as well as take advantage of "teaching moments" to promote patient well being.

- The medical assistant is part of the legal contract established between the patient and physician that begins at the time of the first visit to the ambulatory care facility. Maintaining confidentiality and providing respectful service are crucial to the integrity of that patient contract.

UNIT six

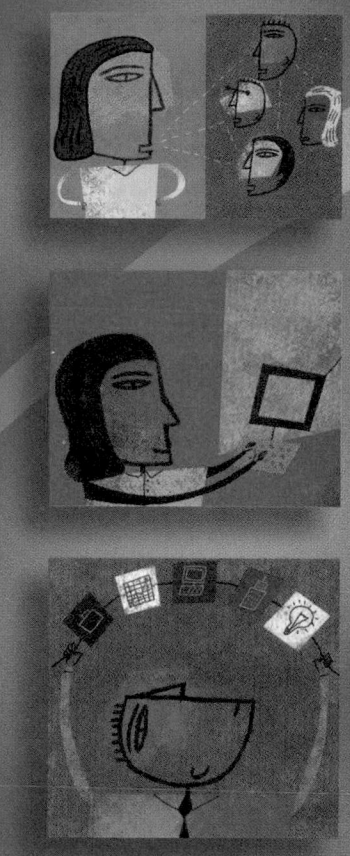

Assisting With Medications

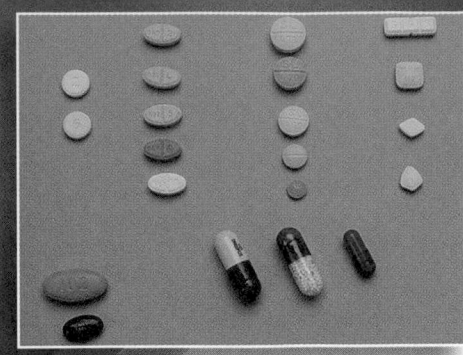

CHAPTER 30

Scenario

Kathy Augustino was hired recently to work for a primary care physician in her hometown. Her responsibilities include administering medications to a wide range of patients. To correctly and safely give patients medications in the ambulatory setting, she must understand the basic principles of pharmacology.

Principles of
Pharmacology

Learning Objectives

- Define and spell the terms listed in the vocabulary.
- Distinguish among the government agencies that regulate drugs in the United States.
- Cite the Drug Enforcement Administration (DEA) regulations for the management of controlled or regulated substances.
- List the DEA regulations for prescription drugs under each of the five schedules of the Controlled Substance Act.
- Differentiate a drug's chemical name, generic name, and trade name.
- Describe the use of drug reference materials.
- Summarize the clinical uses of drugs.
- Cite safety measures for the use of over-the-counter drugs.
- Diagram the parts of a prescription.
- Demonstrate the ability to accurately transcribe a prescription.
- Relate the principles of pharmacokinetics to drug usage.
- Describe factors affecting drug action.
- Differentiate between the therapeutic classifications of medications.
- Identify the legal ramifications of medication management for a medical assistant in an ambulatory care setting.

National Curriculum Competencies

CLINICAL COMPETENCIES

4g. Apply pharmacology principles to prepare and administer oral and parenteral medications
4h. Maintain medication and immunization records

Vocabulary

colloidal Pertaining to a gluelike substance.

enteric-coated Drug formulation in which tablets are coated with a special compound that does not dissolve until the tablet is exposed to the fluids of the small intestine.

generic Drugs that are not protected by trademark.

lumen Space within a vessel or tube.

over-the-counter drugs Medications sold without a prescription.

parenteral Denoting any medication route other than the gastrointestinal (oral).

Pharmacology is the broad science of the origin, nature, chemistry, effects, and uses of drugs. *Clinical pharmacology* comprises the study of the biological effects of a drug on a patient when used as a medical treatment, and the actions of a drug in the body over time, including the rate at which body tissues absorb a drug; where a drug is distributed or localized in the tissues; the route by which a drug is excreted; and *toxicity*, which is a drug's poisonous effect.

Medical assistants need to have a general understanding of the types of drugs that are available as well as their uses. For every medication administered, a medical assistant must understand the drug's action, typical side effects, route of administration and recommended dose, and individual patient factors that can alter the drug's effect and elimination. Drugs are constantly being developed and released for patient treatment; therefore medical assistants must continually update their knowledge of specific drugs used in the ambulatory care setting. Correct management of drug administration and patient education are crucial factors in providing safe drug therapy for all patients.

Government Regulation

Several federal agencies combine forces to regulate, safeguard, and manage the development and use of medications in the United States. The Food and Drug Administration (FDA), a division of the Department of Health and Human Services, regulates the development and sale of all prescription and **over-the-counter (OTC) drugs**. Pharmaceutical companies developing new medications must first gain FDA approval before the drugs can be sold to consumers. This approval process begins with toxicity testing in laboratory animals and progresses to the use of *clinical trials*, which involve human volunteers participating in controlled studies of the use of the drug. Only 1 of 10 new drugs ever reaches the clinical testing phase. If the drug is found to have an acceptable benefit-to-risk ratio, meaning it is effective without causing an unacceptable level of harm to the user, then the FDA approves the medication for release.

The original manufacturer of the drug is awarded copyright protection on that particular chemical compound

for 17 years. Therefore other pharmaceutical companies are unable to produce generic copies of the drug until the 17-year period is over. Besides approving new drugs for the marketplace, the FDA is also responsible for establishing standards for their purity and strength while being manufactured and ensuring that generic brands are effective and safe.

STANDARDS FOR DRUG MANUFACTURERS

- Identify every drug by a particular color, form, shape, size, and label.
- Produce every dose at the same tested strength.
- Produce the exact formula approved by the FDA.
- Use ingredients that are free from contaminants and of the highest quality.

OTHER FEDERAL AGENCIES INVOLVED IN THE REGULATION OF DRUGS

- Drug Enforcement Administration (DEA)— law enforcement agency responsible for the control of narcotic and drug abuse, the illegal sale of dangerous substances, and drug abuse prevention through public education.
- Federal Trade Commission (FTC)—regulates OTC advertising.

Controlled Substances

The Drug Enforcement Administration (DEA) was established in 1973 as part of the Department of Justice to enforce federal laws regarding the use of illegal drugs. According to the federal Controlled Substances Act (CSA), a drug or other substance that has potential for illegal use and abuse must be placed on the controlled substance list. Any new medication that has a similar action to a drug already on the controlled list is also considered one that has potential for abuse.

Most controlled drugs provide significant assistance to patients in need of their particular actions; however, certain guidelines must be followed to comply with the storage, record keeping, and security of controlled substances. In addition, federal law requires that all medical personnel, including medical assistants, share the responsibility of managing controlled substances on-site. Precautions must be taken to monitor the drug use of patients, protect prescription pads, maintain the records required by law, and report any known or suspected drug diversion or theft.

Based on guidelines set forth in the CSA, controlled substances are divided into five sections according to their addictive abilities and degree of abuse. The classifications range from Schedule I drugs, which are illegal and cannot be prescribed, to Schedule V, which have the least potential for addiction and abuse.

Every medical practice should have a copy of the controlled substances regulations. A medical assistant may secure this list from a regional office of the DEA. It is also important to be on the DEA's mailing list to receive updates as drugs are added, deleted, or moved from one schedule to another.

Table 30-1 summarizes the classification of controlled substances.

CRITICAL THINKING APPLICATION

Kathy is responsible for orienting a new medical assistant to the practice. Summarize the important points about government regulation of controlled substances that she should include in the orientation.

Regulation of Controlled Substances

There are specific CSA regulations governing the record keeping, physician registration, and inventory of controlled substances. Complete and accurate records must be maintained on the purchase and management of scheduled drugs in the ambulatory care setting. These records must be kept separate from the patient chart for 2 years and be readily available for inspection by the DEA at all times. Every time a controlled substance is dispensed and administered in the office, documentation of that process includes the number of doses of the drug on-site both before and after the medication is dispensed. Medical practices that dispense and administer controlled substances on-site have forms developed for this purpose. Any discrepancy in the count of the amount of medication available must be documented and co-signed by two employees.

Each physician who prescribes or who has controlled substances on-site must register with the DEA for a Controlled Substance Registration Certificate and will receive a specific DEA registration number that must be included on all controlled substance prescriptions. The certificate is renewable every 3 years and is specific to a particular site of practice. Therefore, if the physician dispenses or prescribes scheduled drugs at more than one site, a DEA registration number must be obtained for each site.

TABLE 30-1	Classification of Controlled Substances	
Schedule	**Guidelines**	**Drug Examples**
I	No accepted medical use High potential for abuse Possession of these drugs is illegal	Heroin, lysergic acid diethylamide (LSD), marijuana, methaqualone (Quaalude), mescaline, peyote, amphetamine variations
II	Accepted for medical use but with severe restrictions High potential for abuse May cause severe psychological or physical dependence	Opium, morphine, methadone, cocaine, amphetamine, cannabis, barbiturates, methylphenidate (Ritalin), oxycodone HCl (Percodan), hydromorphone HCl (Dilaudid), meperidine HCl (Demerol), codeine
III	Accepted for medical use Potential for abuse less than I or II May cause moderate to low physical dependence or high psychological dependence Includes combination drugs that contain limited amounts of narcotics or stimulants	Paregoric, acetaminophen/codeine (Tylenol with codeine), benzphetamine, suppositories with barbiturates, anabolic steroids, including testosterone
IV	Accepted for medical use Low potential for abuse May cause limited physical or psychological dependence in comparison to schedule III drugs Includes minor tranquilizers and hypnotics	Meprobamate (Equanil), chlordiazepoxide (Librium), diazepam (Valium), flurazepam (Dalmane), chloral hydrate, propoxyphene napsylate (Darvon), pentazocine lactate (Talwin), alprazolam (Xanax), triazolam (Halcion), temazepam (Restoril), chlorazepate dipotassium (Tranxene), lorazepam (Ativan), zolpidem tartrate (Ambien)
V	Accepted for medical use Low potential for abuse May cause limited physical or psychological dependence in comparison to schedule IV drugs Includes drug mixtures containing limited amounts of narcotics	Cough medicines containing codeine; kaolin/pectin belladonna alkaloids (Donnagel), diphenoxylate w/atropine (Lomotil), buprenorphine

All controlled substances must be stored in a safe or immovable locked cabinet. Prescription forms should be kept out of areas that are used by patients and preferably secured in an area that prohibits unauthorized or illegal use. DEA Prescription Form 222 and the state triplicate forms also need to be kept in a locked area.

Many ambulatory practices no longer keep controlled substances on-site. However, if there is a loss of drugs, it must be reported to the regional DEA office and local law enforcement authorities immediately. If a controlled substance is damaged or must be disposed of (e.g., a pill falls to the floor during dispensing), two employees must be present to witness the medication being flushed down the sink or toilet, and both must document the procedure on the controlled substance inventory form used by that office. If a large quantity of scheduled drugs must be disposed of, the local DEA office should be contacted for guidance.

Individual states may also regulate controlled substances; therefore it is essential that a medical assistant know his or her state's legal requirements.

There are specific guidelines for prescription orders of controlled substances. These include the following:

- Must be written in ink or typed.
- Must include the date prescribed; the name and address of the patient; and the name, address, and DEA number of the physician.
- Amount prescribed must be written out (ten rather than 10), usually for small quantities of the drug.
- Must be manually signed by the physician, although the medical assistant can prepare the prescription for the physician signature.
- Drugs in Schedules II, III, and IV must bear this label: *Federal law prohibits the transfer of this drug to any person other than the patient for whom it is prescribed.*

There are also specific rules, depending on the designated schedule of the prescribed controlled substance. Symbols C-II, C-III, C-IV, and C-V are used to indicate the specific schedule:

- Schedule II (C-II) prescriptions:
  1. Must be written unless an absolute emergency exists that requires a telephone prescription order. The amount in the phone order is limited to that needed during the emergency, and the physician must deliver a written prescription to the pharmacy within 72 hours.
  2. Cannot be refilled.
  3. Certain states require the use of multiple-copy prescriptions.
- Schedule III (C-III) and IV (C-IV) prescriptions:
  1. May be oral or written.
  2. May be refilled up to five times within 6 months of the original order.
- Schedule V (C-V) prescriptions:
  1. May be oral or written.
  2. May be refilled up to five times within 6 months of the original order.
  3. Depending on the state, may be dispensed by the pharmacist without a prescription.

CRITICAL THINKING APPLICATION

Kathy is responsible for maintaining the inventory of the controlled substances in the office. While checking the supply of meperidine she notices the expiration date of the medication is today. She must dispose of the remaining two pills. According to DEA regulations, how should she dispose of the medication?

Drug Abuse

Any drug, from aspirin to alcohol, may be misused or abused. Today there is a tremendous increase in the use of illegal and legal drugs. Treatment programs are available throughout the United States for people from all walks of life. Programs include detoxification, rehabilitation, and long-term rehabilitation maintenance.

Medical assistants may encounter patients who are misusing or abusing drugs. It is important to be alert to the symptoms of drug dependence and to notify the physician when you suspect a patient, or a co-worker, of having a problem with drug or alcohol dependency.

Drug misuse is the improper use of common drugs that can lead to dependence or toxicity. Examples of persons with chronic dependencies include people who cannot have a bowel movement unless they take a laxative; those who have used nasal decongestants for so long that they cannot breathe without the use of nasal sprays; or those who take so many antacids that they suffer systemic metabolic alkalosis.

Drug abuse is the continuous or periodic self-administration of a drug that could result in addiction (physical dependence). *Drug dependency* is the inability to function unless under the influence of a substance. *Psychological dependency* is the compulsive craving for the effects of a substance. *Habituation* is a mild form of psychological dependency, such as to caffeine. *Physical dependency*, or addiction, is a person's need to use a substance continuously to be able to function and to avoid physical discomfort. This type of dependency occurs when abused substances produce biochemical changes, usually in the nervous system tissues. Discontinuing a substance that causes physical dependency results in withdrawal symptoms. Withdrawal symptoms may be mild or potentially serious, resulting in convulsions and possibly death.

Regardless of the type of drug abused, it will have two effects on the person: acute and chronic. The acute effect is what the person feels when *intoxicated*, or directly under the influence of a particular substance. Chronic effects include the temporary or permanent physical and mental changes that result from long-term abuse.

The medical assistant is often called on to answer patient questions concerning drug abuse. The medical assistant should read and keep up to date on drug-related issues. Pamphlets and agency referral names should be available for patients. Patient concerns and questions regarding drug abuse should also be conveyed to the physician.

THE MEDICAL ASSISTANT'S ROLE IN PREVENTION OF DRUG ABUSE

- Carefully monitor patients who repeatedly call for prescription refills of controlled substances.
- Request medical records for patients who report previously being prescribed scheduled drugs.
- Keep prescription blanks in a safe place away from patient treatment areas and minimize the number of prescription pads in use at any given time.
- Never use prescription pads for notepads and never use preprinted or presigned forms.
- Keep only a limited supply of controlled substances on hand.
- Maintain complete and accurate records of controlled substances that are dispensed on-site as well as those prescribed. Include specific documentation in the patient chart for all prescribed controlled substances.

Drug Names

A single drug may have up to three names: chemical, generic, and trade. The chemical name represents the drug's exact formula. For example, the chemical name of the analgesic acetaminophen is *N*-(4-hydroxyphenyl). Acetaminophen is the generic name, and one of its trade names is Tylenol. All drugs have a **generic** or nonproprietary (official) name assigned to them. This name is much simpler than the chemical name, and it is not protected by copyright. The trade or brand name is assigned by the manufacturer and is protected by copyright. The use of generic names is encouraged over trade names to avoid confusion. Drugs are also classified by their use. For example, Advil is a brand name of the generic drug ibuprofen, which is classified as an analgesic and an antiinflammatory agent.

Approaches to Studying Pharmacology

A pharmaceutical glossary could be a book in itself. Many terms are combinations of the condition to be treated, with the prefix *anti* (e.g., antianginal, antianxiety, antiarrhythmic, anticoagulant, anticonvulsant, antidiarrheal). Notice how these names emphasize the drug's effect (use) rather than its action in the body. More recent classifications, such as *parasympathomimetic* and *cholinesterase inhibitors*, describe the pharmacological action rather than the therapeutic use. However, both viewpoints are necessary for a more complete understanding of drugs

and what they do in the human body. No one can remember all there is to know about clinical pharmacology. The number of new drugs being introduced into use far exceeds the number of older drugs being replaced or discontinued. The number of drugs available for clinical use grows beyond the ability to learn all there is to know about each medication. Therefore it is essential that a medical assistant understand how to use pharmacology resource books as references.

Reference Materials

Reference books that are updated annually or periodically should be available for easy reference at all medical facilities. Most references list drug information in the following sequence:

1. *Action:* How the drug provides the therapeutic results in the body or the use of the drug.
2. *Indication:* The conditions for which the drug is used.
3. *Contraindications:* Conditions that make the administration of a drug improper or undesirable.
4. *Precautions:* Actions necessary because of special conditions of the patient, drug, or environment that need to be considered for the drug to be successful or not harmful. The pregnancy risk category is included in this section as well as precautions for nursing mothers (Table 30-2).
5. *Adverse reactions:* Commonly observed side effects on a tissue or organ system other than the one being sought by the administration of a medication. Adverse reactions include *hypersensitivity* which causes an allergic reaction to the drug; *idio-*

TABLE 30-2	Pregnancy Risk Categories
Category of Risk	**Category Description**
A	Remote risk Controlled studies in women have failed to demonstrate risk to fetus.
B	Slightly more risk than A Animal studies show no risk but controlled human studies have not been done *or* animal studies show risk, but controlled studies in women have shown no risk.
C	Greater risk than B Animal studies have shown risk, but no controlled human studies have been done *or* no studies have been done in animals or women.
D	Proven risk of fetal harm Human studies show proof of fetal damage, but the potential benefits of use during pregnancy may make its use acceptable.
X	Proven risk of fetal harm Studies in women or animals show definite risk of fetal abnormality. Risks outweigh any possible benefit.

syncrasy, or unexplained, unusual response to the drug; psychological dependence or *habituation* to the drug; or *physical dependence* to the compound causing withdrawal symptoms in the patient if the medication is removed.

6. *Dosage and administration:* The usual route, dosage, and timing for administering the drug.

7. *How supplied:* Description of how the medication is packaged and specifics on how it should be administered.

Package Inserts. Every drug package contains an insert describing all the significant aspects of using the drug, including information on the chemical formulation of the drug and clinical studies. The information on the inserts is controlled by the FDA and is an excellent quick reference on new medications in the ambulatory setting.

Physicians' Desk Reference. *Physicians' Desk Reference* (PDR) is published annually by Thomson Medical Economics Company, Inc. (Oradell, NJ). For physicians who subscribe to *Medical Economics* magazine, a PDR is provided free. Copies can be purchased through the publisher or in local bookstores. Supplements are published throughout the year. This reference contains information on approximately 2500 drugs, and the product descriptions are identical to the package inserts. The drug manufacturers pay for this space, so the PDR could be called the yellow pages of the drug industry. The PDR is the most commonly used drug reference book and should be available in all healthcare settings.

The book's sections are color-coded and cross-referenced for easy use. The various sections allow you to begin searching for information concerning a drug from any starting point. You can start with the usage, classification, generic name, manufacturer's name, or trade name of a drug, or what the drug looks like. There is a special photographic section for visual product identification. Once you know which drug you want to study, the product information section lists the actual package insert information alphabetically, first by the manufacturer, then by the brand name.

There is also a separate PDR volume published annually for nonprescription drugs and dietary supplements.

U.S. Pharmacopeia/National Formulary. The *U.S. Pharmacopeia/National Formulary* (USP/NF) is the official source of drug standards for the United States. The *Pharmacopeia* was combined with the *National Formulary*, which lists the chemical formulas for all accepted drugs. This combined reference lists and describes all the approved medications in the United States that are considered useful and therapeutic in the practice of medicine. Single drugs rather than combined products (compound mixtures) are listed. If a drug name is the same as the official name in this volume, the drug will have the initials *USP* after it (e.g., digitoxin, USP).

Learning About Drugs

The study of pharmacology is difficult at best. However, there are a few ways you can make it easier.

First, take opportunities to observe the use of drugs in patient care. Studying about atorvastatin calcium (Lipitor) becomes more meaningful when you see how its lipid-lowering action actually affects a patient's blood cholesterol level.

Second, concentrate on the most important drugs in each classification. As you expand your knowledge to other drugs in each classification, you will easily understand new drugs by noting the similarities and differences between them and the basic, important drugs you studied first.

Third, learn about a drug's primary action and use and then expand your knowledge to its other actions and uses. Soon you will be able to name the drug that is usually indicated for a particular condition. Then, by knowing a drug's secondary effects, you will be able to understand what side effects are likely to occur during the use of the drug. More important, you will be aware of the contraindications for the drug (conditions that make the use of the drug improper or undesirable). Knowledge of the drug's actions will also enable you to predict what *toxic* reactions could occur from overdose.

TERMINOLOGY DESCRIBING DRUG USES

diagnostic Helps determine the cause of a particular health problem (e.g., injecting antigen serum for allergy testing).

palliative Indicates that the drug does not cure but provides relief from pain or symptoms related to the disorder (e.g., the use of an antihistamine for allergic symptoms).

prophylaxis Prevents the occurrence of a condition (e.g., vaccines prevent the occurrence of specific infectious diseases).

replacement Provides patients with substances needed to maintain health (e.g., insulin for patients with diabetes).

therapeutic Drugs used to treat the disorder and cure it (e.g., antibiotics cure bacterial infections).

Dispensing Drugs

There are two methods of dispensing drugs: over-the-counter and by prescription. OTC drugs are available to the public for self-medication without a prescription. These drugs have been approved by the FDA for general consumer use, but patients on prescription drugs should keep their healthcare providers informed about their OTC drug use.

A medical assistant who is directly involved in patient care should have an understanding of some basic facts regarding OTC drugs. Today patients are better informed about their personal healthcare and want to be active participants in healthcare decisions. They need facts to make informed choices when using OTC preparations. Most OTC preparations are safe if used as directed on the package; however, patient education contributes greatly to the safe and correct use of OTCs. Patients should be encouraged to do the following when choosing or using an OTC:

- Carefully read the package label and insert for use guidelines.
- Take only the recommended dose.
- Monitor the expiration date and discard when appropriate.
- Never combine an OTC with a prescription drug without the knowledge of the physician.
- Recognize that many OTC drugs are contraindicated in pregnancy, nursing mothers, and young children, and in the presence of certain diseases.
- Check with the pharmacist for questions or concerns.

The number of prescription drugs that have been granted OTC status is constantly increasing, and as the list of OTC drugs increases, so does the need for consumer education. Many OTC medications affect the safety and effectiveness of prescription drugs, so gathering a complete and accurate pattern of the use of OTCs should be part of every visit the patient makes to the physician.

Prescription Drugs. Federal law makes drugs that are dangerous, powerful, or habit-forming illegal to use except under a physician's order. A *prescription* is an order written by the physician for the compounding or dispensing and administration of drugs to a particular patient. Sometimes an order may be written for the medical assistant on the patient's medical record; however, most often it is a written order on a prescription blank for the pharmacist to fill. A prescription must be signed by the physician or the order cannot be carried out (Procedure 30-1). If the medical assistant is requested to

---

PROCEDURE 30-1

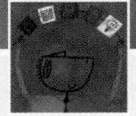

Preparing a Prescription for the Physician's Signature

GOAL: To accurately prepare a prescription for the physician's signature using appropriate abbreviations and prescription format.

EQUIPMENT AND SUPPLIES

- Prescription pad
- Drug reference materials if needed
- Black pen
- Patient chart

PROCEDURAL STEPS

1 Refer to the physician's written order for the prescription. If the physician gives a verbal order to write a prescription, write down the order and review it with the physician for accuracy.

Purpose: To ensure accuracy in writing the ordered medication.

2 If unfamiliar with the medication, look up the drug in a drug reference book (such as the PDR).

Purpose: The medical assistant should be familiar with the details about the drug, including correct spelling, how it is dispensed, strength, recommended dose, storage guidelines, drug-to-drug interactions, and possible side effects to make sure the transcription is correct and to be prepared to answer the patient's questions about the medication.

3 Ask the patient about drug allergies.

Purpose: The patient should be asked about drug allergies each time a medication is prescribed or dispensed, since these can change over time.

4 Using a prescription pad that has the physician's name, address, telephone number, and DEA registration number preprinted on the slip, begin to transcribe the physician order.

5 Record the patient's name, address, and date on which the prescription is being written.

6 Next to the ℞, write in legible handwriting the name of the drug (correctly spelled), the dosage form (such as tablet, capsule, and so forth, using correct abbreviations), and the strength ordered. For example, if the physician orders Lipitor, 40 mg tablets, by mouth, one tablet at bedtime, then the first line of the prescription should read: Lipitor 40 mg tabs. This is the *inscription*.

7 On the next line write *Disp*. This is the *subscription*, which includes directions to the pharmacist on the amount to be dispensed and the form of the drug. For the Lipitor order, the subscription would read: Disp: #30.

8 Next comes the *signature*. This includes directions for the patient, such as how and when to take the medicine, and is usually preceded by the symbol *Sig*. For the Lipitor order the signature would read: Sig: T̄ tab po hs.

9 The physician tells you the patient can get three refills of the prescription, so this information should be added at the bottom of the prescription.

10 The physician must sign the prescription before it is given to the patient.

11 Document on the patient's chart the medication order and any pertinent details, including patient education and refill information.

Purpose: All patient education should be documented for future reference, and the details about the prescription as well as refill information must be included for future prescriptions and/or refill orders.

phone in a prescription to the pharmacy for the physician, all of the pertinent information must be written down and reviewed by the physician for accuracy before the call is made. A note is also made in the patient's chart that a medication order was phoned in to the pharmacy, with all of the pertinent information about the order included (see Procedure 9-3).

Table 30-3 lists the top 50 prescribed drugs in the United States in 2001. Appropriate medical terminology and abbreviations are used to complete the prescription.

TABLE 30-3	Top 50 Prescribed Drugs in the United States in 2001	
Brand Name	**Generic Name**	**Classification By Use**
Hydrocodone w/APAP	Hydrocodone w/APAP	Analgesic/antitussive
Lipitor	Atorvastatin calcium	Lipid-lowering agent
Premarin	Conjugated estrogens	Estrogen: hormone replacement therapy
Tenormin	Atenolol	Beta-blocker: antihypertensive and treatment of myocardial infarction
Synthroid	Levothyroxine	Thyroid replacement hormone
Zithromax	Azithromycin	Antibiotic
Furosemide	Furosemide	Diuretic
Amoxicillin	Amoxicillin	Antibiotic
Norvasc	Amlodipine	Calcium channel blocker: antihypertensive and treatment of myocardial infarction
Xanax	Alprazolam	Antianxiety/hypnotic
Albuterol Aerosol	Albuterol	Bronchodilator
Claritin	Loratadine	Antihistamine
Hydrochlorothiazide	Hydrochlorothiazide	Diuretic/antihypertensive
Prilosec	Omeprazole	Inhibits gastric acid secretion
Zoloft	Sertraline	Antidepressant
Paxil	Paroxetine	Antidepressant
Dyazide	Triamterene/HCTZ	Diuretic/antihypertensive
Prevacid	Lansoprazole	Inhibits gastric secretion
Celebrex	Celecoxib	Antiarthritic
Zocor	Simvastatin	Lipid-lowering agent
Keflex	Cephalexin	Antibiotic
Glucophage	Metformin	Oral antihyperglycemic
Vioxx	Rofecoxib	Osteoarthritic agent
Zestril	Lisinopril	Antihypertensive/treatment of heart failure and acute myocardial infarction
Augmentin	Amoxicillin/clavulanate	Antibiotic
Propoxyphene N/APAP	Propoxyphene N/APAP	Analgesic
Prempro	Conjugated estrogens	Estrogen: hormone replacement therapy
Prednisone	Prednisone	Steroid: antiinflammatory
Ortho Tri-Cyclen	Norgestimate/ethinyl Estradiol	Oral contraceptive
Tylenol/Codeine	Acetaminophen/codeine	Analgesic
Zyrtec	Cetirizine	Seasonal allergic rhinitis
Allegra	Fexofenadine	Antihistamine
Levoxyl	Levothyroxine	Thyroid hormone replacement
Trimox	Amoxicillin	Antibiotic
Metoprolol Tartrate	Metoprolol	Beta-blocker/antihypertensive and antianginal
Ativan	Lorazepam	Antianxiety
Toprol-XL	Metoprolol	Beta-blocker, extended release
Prozac	Fluoxetine	Antidepressant
Ambien	Zolpidem	Hypnotic
Celexa	Citalopram	Antidepressant
Elavil	Amitriptyline	Antidepressant
Fosamax	Alendronate	Osteoporosis
Accupril	Quinapril	Antihypertensive/heart failure
Viagra	Sildenafil citrate	Erectile dysfunction
Pravachol	Pravastatin	Lipid-lowering agent
Naproxen	Naproxen	NSAID/arthritis
Neurontin	Gabapentin	Partial seizure disorders
Coumadin	Warfarin	Anticoagulant
Cipro	Ciprofloxacin	Antibiotic
Verapamil HCL	Verapamil	Calcium channel blocker/antiarrhythmic

Data furnished by National Data Corporation from www.rxlist.com.

The more common terms and abbreviations are listed in Table 30-4.

CRITICAL THINKING APPLICATION

Dr. Simon requests that Kathy write out the following prescription for his signature. "Take Lipitor 20 mg tablets daily at bedtime. Dispense 4 weeks' worth and may be refilled 2 times." How would Kathy write the prescription using the correct form as well as medical terminology and abbreviations?

SIX PARTS OF A PRESCRIPTION (FIGURE 30-1)

Superscription: Patient's name and address, the date, and the symbol ℞ (for the Latin *recipe*, meaning "take").
Inscription: Main part of the prescription; name of the drug, dosage form, and strength.

Subscription: Directions for the pharmacist; size of each dose, amount to be dispensed, and the form of the drug, such as tablets or capsules.
Signature: Directions for the patient; usually preceded by the symbol *Sig:* (for the Latin *signa*, meaning "mark"). This is where the physician indicates what instructions are to be put on the label to tell the patient how, when, and in what quantities to use the medication.
Refill information: May be regulated by federal law if the drug is a controlled substance; must write number of times refill allowed on the script.
Physician's signature: Must include the manual signature of the physician and the DEA number when indicated.

Drug Interactions With the Body

Pharmacology is the study of drugs, their *desired effect*, and what happens to a drug while it is in the body.

TABLE 30-4 | Common Prescription Abbreviations

Abbreviation	Meaning	Abbreviation	Meaning	Abbreviation	Meaning
aa	of each	MTD	maximum tolerated dose	sub-q	subcutaneous
ac	before meals	NPO	nothing by mouth	s̄s̄	one-half
ad lib	as desired	noct	at night	stat	immediately
agit	shake, stir	N/S	normal saline	tid	three times a day
am	morning	O₂	oxygen	tinct	tincture
amp	ampule	OD	overdose	TO	telephone order
au	each ear	OD	right eye	tus	cough
ad	right ear	OS	left eye	U	unit
as	left ear	OU	both eyes	vag	vagina
aq	water	OTC	over-the-counter (drugs)	ves	bladder
bid	twice a day	pc	after meals	VO	verbal order
c̄	with	PL	placebo	W/O	water in oil
cap	capsule	pm	afternoon	cm	centimeter
DC	discontinue	PMI	patient medication instruction	mcg, µg	microgram
DEA	Drug Enforcement Administration	po	by mouth	mg	milligram
dil	dilute	pr	per rectum	Gm, g	gram
disp	dispense	pulv	powder	kg	kilogram
ext	extract	q	every	cc	cubic centimeter
FDA	Food and Drug Administration	qd	every day	ml	milliliter
fl	fluid	qh	every hour	L	liter
h	hour	q2h	every 2 hours	gr	grain
hs	at bedtime	q3h	every 3 hours	dr	dram
inj	injection	q4h	every 4 hours	oz	ounce
IM	intramuscular	qid	four times a day	lb	pound
ID	intradermal	qm	every morning	♏	minim
IV	intravenous	qn	every night	gtt	drops
med	medicine	qod	every other day	t, tsp	teaspoon
meq	milliequivalent	qs	quantity sufficient	T, tbs	tablespoon
MLD	minimum lethal dose	R	rectal	C	cup, Celsius
mn	midnight	℞	"take thou"	pt	pint
MO	mineral oil	S, Sig	give the following directions	qt	quart
MOM	milk of magnesia	s̄	without	gal	gallon
MS	morphine sulfate	SC	subcutaneous	F	Fahrenheit

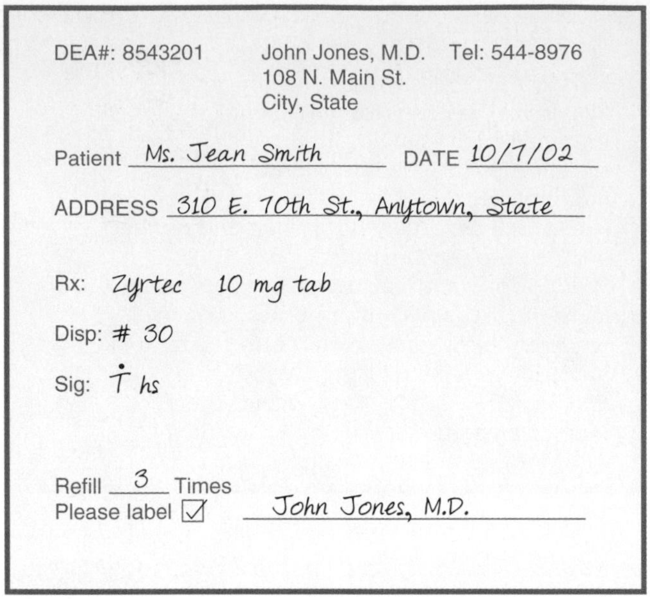

DEA#: 8543201   John Jones, M.D.   Tel: 544-8976
                       108 N. Main St.
                       City, State

Patient _Ms. Jean Smith_   DATE _10/7/02_

ADDRESS _310 E. 10th St., Anytown, State_

Rx: Zyrtec   10 mg tab

Disp: # 30

Sig: Ṫ hs

Refill _3_ Times
Please label ☑   _John Jones, M.D._

FIGURE 30-1   A sample prescription.

Different patients may react to the same dose of a drug in very different ways and the same patient may react to the same dose of a drug differently at various times. Therefore, of primary concern for management of medications is the effectiveness of drugs and their safety. *Pharmacokinetics* is the study of the movement of drugs throughout the body. There are four basic actions that occur when a drug is taken: absorption, distribution, metabolism, and excretion. By knowing what happens to the drug in the body, we can know the *onset* of a drug's activity (beginning), when the action is likely to peak, the minimum amount of drug needed (therapeutic dose), and the *duration* of a particular drug's activity. All these facts help the physician determine the appropriate dosage form, amount, route, and frequency of administration of a medication for a given patient.

PHARMACOKINETIC TERMS

absorption How a drug is absorbed into the body's circulating fluids, which depends on the route by which it is administered
distribution How a drug is transported from the site of administration to the various points in the body
metabolism How the drug is inactivated, including the time it takes for a drug to be detoxified and broken down into by-products
excretion The route by which a drug is excreted, or eliminated, from the body and the amount of time such a process requires

---

Drug Absorption

What happens to a drug from the time it is administered until it reaches the bloodstream is the first factor in determining the route of drug administration. The rate at which drugs are absorbed is dependent upon many factors including the drug's ability to be dissolved, the concentration of the dose, and the route of administration. An important point to remember is that no matter where a drug is absorbed, it can have one of two actions on the body: *local* (restricted to one spot or part; not general) or *systemic* (affecting the body as a whole). However, most drugs are used for their systemic effects. Even when drugs are used for local purposes, we know that no drug remains truly localized in the body. Any chemical that comes into contact with even the most superficial surface, such as the skin, has the potential to be absorbed into the bloodstream and to circulate to other tissues and organs.

Oral Route. Oral medications are convenient, safe, and relatively inexpensive. However, drugs that can be destroyed in any way by the digestive tract must be given by injection. Insulin and heparin are examples of drugs that are destroyed by the digestive process. Injection of medications leads to rapid absorption into the bloodstream but this increases the danger of overdose or possible infection. Most oral medications are absorbed by the small intestine, but a few are absorbed more rapidly in the stomach. After absorption into the bloodstream from the small intestine, drugs are carried to the liver. In this organ, much of the drug's potency is inactivated before it circulates to the tissues. This inactivation by the liver often makes it necessary to administer higher dosages orally than when given by injection.

Food slows the absorption of drugs. Therefore many medications are best prescribed 1 hour before or 2 hours after the ingestion of food. Food may also bind the drugs to it or in some other way destroy a drug. Tetracyclines, for example, are destroyed by milk products and antacids containing calcium salts. Therefore patients receiving tetracycline should be advised not to eat dairy products or take liquid or solid forms of antacids.

The stomach acids present during digestion alone may destroy certain drugs. Because some drugs are destroyed by the components of the digestive tract or irritate the empty lining of the stomach, many oral drugs are **enteric-coated** to keep them intact for passage into the small intestine or to prevent gastric irritation or vomiting.

Some drugs are not affected by the digestive processes but cannot be absorbed through the intestinal walls into the bloodstream. For example, neomycin has no therapeutic effect when taken orally (unless it is used to sterilize the bowel before bowel surgery). Other drugs may be unable to cross the bowel mucosa because of their poor solubility in lipids (fats), or they are inactivated by the pH of the gastrointestinal tract.

It is important to remember these absorption factors when administering medication by the oral route. If a patient has previously responded to a drug but is no longer responding, it may be important to question the patient's food-medication cycle. It could be that the patient is no longer taking the medication on an empty stomach as directed.

Parenteral Route. **Parenteral** refers to the administration of drugs by injection. The parenteral route results in the fastest action, because the medication is administered directly into the bloodstream or in tissues with a rich blood supply. However, there are several factors that determine the effectiveness and rate of absorption of injected medications.

The absorption of a drug in an aqueous (water) solution is faster in an area with more blood vessels. Therefore drugs deposited in the muscle will be absorbed faster than drugs given subcutaneously. The *intramuscular* (IM) route is chosen in an emergency for fast action or when larger amounts of the medication must be absorbed. The *subcutaneous* (SC) route is chosen when a slower, prolonged effect is desired.

A second way that parenteral drug absorption may be controlled is physically. A drug's absorption may be quickened by hand massage after injection. Absorption may also be slowed by pharmaceutical preparation of the drug in a physical form that slows absorption. These methods include suspending the drug in a solution that prolongs absorption, such as **colloidal** substances, fatty substances (oil), or insoluble salts or esters. Drugs suspended in these substances slowly dissolve in the tissues over a long time, and the patient can be spared costly, frequent, and sometimes painful injections. Penicillin G is suspended with procaine (hydrochloride) salts for this purpose. In addition, local anesthetics are sometimes mixed with epinephrine to keep the anesthetics and their effects in an area longer since epinephrine (adrenalin) constricts the blood vessels at the site thus retarding circulation and absorption.

The third parenteral route is *intravenous* (IV), which injects the medication directly into the vein. Because of the dangers of intravenous administration, only those members of the medical team who are licensed to do so may inject medication intravenously.

 SAFETY ALERT A medical assistant is not licensed to perform the intravenous administration of medications to patients. Because intravenous administration is so dangerous, medications given intravenously are usually administered in small doses through an intravenous infusion (IV drip) to monitor the effects in the body.

Other forms of parenteral routes include *intradermal* injection, which is below the skin but superficial to the subcutaneous tissues. This route is used mostly for allergy testing and skin testing. *Intrathecal*, or *intraspinal*, injections are used for spinal anesthesia and administering certain medications into the spinal column. *Intraarticular* or *intralesional* injections are used for administering corticosteroids into joints and lesions or anticancer drugs into cancerous tumors.

Mucous Membrane Absorption. Drugs may be absorbed by the mucous membranes of the mouth, throat, nose, eyes, rectum, vagina, and respiratory and urinary tracts. Some applications have a local effect, such as nasal sprays, eye drops, and rectal suppositories for constipation. Others have a systemic effect, such as a rectal suppository to control vomiting or a nitroglycerin tablet dissolved under the tongue (sublingual) to dilate the blood vessels and relieve the pain of angina pectoris. *Inhalation* is used to concentrate drugs locally in the lower respiratory passages or to produce systemic effects, such as general anesthesia.

Topical Absorption. Topical routes include the application of medications to the skin, eyes, and ears. Drugs in ointments, creams, lotions, and aerosols can be applied for the treatment of skin itching, inflammation, or other discomforts and for the treatment of skin infections with antibiotics. Nitroglycerin (for angina) is a drug that can be absorbed through the skin via a dermal patch, which releases it systemically.

Drug Distribution

Once a drug is absorbed, it must be transported by the circulatory system to the area where it will have its effect. In the bloodstream, drugs can attach to plasma proteins and then be freed to pass from the blood into the site of action. Drugs are then carried through the fluids into the cells of the tissues and organs. The amount of blood supply to a part affects the speed with which drugs reach certain tissues.

The *blood-brain barrier* is a functional barrier between the brain cells and the capillaries circulating blood through the brain. This barrier determines which substances can cross. For the substances that can, it regulates the degree and rate of their absorption into the brain tissue. The general anesthetic thiopental (Pentothal) is able to cross the blood-brain barrier immediately and produces sleep within seconds, whereas other sleep-producing drugs, such as the barbiturates, cross slowly and may take as long as 30 minutes to 1 hour to produce the same effect. The presence of the blood-brain barrier is a mixed blessing. It provides a physical barrier that protects the brain from potentially dangerous chemicals but at the same time makes it very difficult to treat central nervous system (CNS) disorders.

Drug Action

There are multiple theories that explain why drugs act the way they do. Drugs are believed to combine with body chemicals on the cell surface or within the cell itself. Correct cells are chosen because a particular drug has a *specific affinity* for a particular cell. The specific cell recipient is called a *receptor*, and the drug that has the affinity for it and produces a functional change in the cell is called the *agonist*. Not all drugs that bind to specific cells cause a functional change in the cell. These drugs act as an *antagonist* to the natural process and work by *blocking* a sequence of biochemical events.

Some drugs are believed to act by affecting the enzyme functions of the body. Drugs attach to enzyme substances and rob the enzymes from cells. As a result, the enzyme products needed for normal cellular function are not supplied, and the cell fails to function properly.

Certain antiinfective drugs have a *selected toxicity* for pathogens or parasites that have invaded the body. Penicillin and sulfonamides work because they poison, or interfere with the life processes of, bacteria without affecting the life processes of normal human cells. Research scientists continue to look for differences between cancer cells and normal cells to enable them to apply the principle of selected toxicity in cancer treatment. Only recently have anticancer drugs been produced that are selective and therefore not toxic to human cells.

Both drugs that have a selective affinity for cells and those that bind with enzymes can be counteracted by administering large amounts of the natural substances with which the drugs compete. This process is known as administering an *antidote* to a drug that may be acting as a poison. An antidote, such as Narcan, can be administered if a patient receives too much anesthesia or has taken a drug overdose.

Some drugs alter the function of a cell by affecting the physical properties of the cell membrane rather than altering the biochemical processes within the cell itself. This is especially true of drugs, such as anesthetics and alcohol, that affect nerve cells. A change in the cell membrane alters the permeability of the membrane, which in turn changes the flow of ions in and out of the cells. This change in ion flow alters the polarity (opposite effects at two extremities, the two extremities being inside and outside the cell membrane) on which nerve pulses are conducted and produces general sleep or stupor.

Drug Metabolism

After the drug is absorbed, distributed, and used, it is then metabolized for excretion. During metabolism the drug is converted into harmless by-products. These by-products are then more easily eliminated by the kidneys. Most drugs are broken down by the enzyme activity of the liver. The ability to break down the chemical components of a drug varies among individuals. Factors that determine this ability include age, the presence of other drugs, and liver disease. In some patients receiving long-term drug therapy, a drug may overstimulate the enzyme activity of the liver. This results in a too rapid destruction of the drug, and the patient has to take larger and larger doses for the drug to be effective. This situation is called *tolerance*.

Drug Excretion

The kidneys are the most important route for the elimination of drugs. Most drugs are filtered out of the blood circulating through the kidneys, broken down into harmless particles, and then excreted in the urine. Because the kidneys are so important in the elimination of drugs from the body, drug therapy must be carefully monitored in patients with kidney disease or malfunction. Drugs are also eliminated through the sweat glands and saliva and in bile. Exhalation, another mechanism for drug elimination, is the basis for measuring alcohol concentrations in the blood by the breathalyzer test. Drugs may be eliminated through the milk glands of a lactating mother, which means a woman breastfeeding a child has to be extremely careful about taking medications.

The combination of metabolism and excretion decreases the amount of drug in the body at any given time. The *half-life* of a drug is the time required for the amount of drug in the body to be decreased by 50%. Some drugs have extremely short half-lives (only minutes), whereas others can take days to leave the body. The amount of drug that is lost during one half-life depends upon how much drug is present. The half-life of a drug is used by the physician to determine the time of medication administration, or the dosage intervals. The shorter the half-life of the drug, the closer together the times in which it should be administered. If the next dose of the drug is not given within the half-life, then blood levels will drop and the patient will not receive adequate therapeutic effects from the treatment.

Factors That Affect Drug Action

As stated earlier, different people react to the same dose of medication in different ways, and the same patient can react to the same dose of the same drug differently on various occasions. The following factors are important in determining the correct medication for a patient.

Body Weight

A person's weight has a direct relationship with the effects of medication. Basically, the same dosage has less effect on a patient who weighs more and a greater effect on a person who weighs less. Manufacturers of adult medications calculate dosages based on a normal adult weight (approximately 150 pounds). Sometimes the physician will adjust the dosage to better suit the patient's body size. Pediatric medications are designed for the body weight or body surface area of children. If adult medications are used for children, the correct dosage must be calculated and adjusted for the child's body weight (see Chapter 31).

Age

The greatest effect of age on the body's response to a drug occurs in newborns and in elderly individuals. This usually is because of immature or deteriorating body systems. In addition, both groups are particularly sensitive to drugs that affect the central nervous system and are at risk for developing toxic drug levels. Dosage calculations for these two groups must be carefully decided, and therapy usually begins with very small doses. Chapter 45 discusses the use of medication in an aging patient in more detail.

Sex

Drugs may affect men and women differently. As previously mentioned, a pregnant woman has to be extremely cautious when taking medications to avoid damage to the developing fetus. In addition, some drugs have side effects that can stimulate uterine contractions, causing premature labor and delivery. Intramuscular medications are absorbed faster by men. Because women have a higher body fat content and a musculature with less blood supply, intramuscular drugs remain in their tissues longer than in men's tissues.

Time of Day

Diurnal means during the day or time of light. Diurnal body rhythms play an important part in the effects of some drugs. Sedatives given in the morning will not be as effective as when administered before bedtime, because the CNS is more stimulated and more resistant to the effects of the drug. Corticosteroid administration is preferred in the morning, because this best mimics the body's natural pattern of corticosteroid production and elimination.

Pathological Factors

Patients may adversely respond to drugs in the presence of liver or kidney disease, because the body will not be able to detoxify and excrete chemicals properly. Drugs may also produce pathological conditions of the liver or kidney, and patients may need monitoring. In patients with liver or kidney disease, some drugs may cause unconsciousness or death. Reactions in patients with other diseases or disorders may be quite different from the expected response. Therefore a thorough medical history of the patient must always be taken before administering medications. Even temporary pain and fever may alter the expected effect of a drug.

Immune Responses

The presence of a drug can stimulate a patient's immune response, and the patient will develop antibodies to a particular chemical. If the same drug is again administered, the patient will have an allergic reaction to the drug, ranging from a mild reaction to anaphylaxis, which is a serious respiratory and circulatory emergency. The group of drugs that most commonly causes allergic responses is antibiotics.

Psychological Factors

People may respond differently to a drug because of the way they feel about the drug. If a patient believes in the therapy, even a *placebo* (sugar pill or sterile water thought to be a drug) may help or bring about relief. A patient's personality can affect whether he or she will be co-operative in following the directions for a particular drug, and a patient's negative mind-set, or mental attitude, can reduce an expected response to a drug.

Tolerance

Tolerance is the phenomenon of reduced responsiveness to a drug. *Acquired tolerance* occurs after taking a particular drug for a period of time. *Cross-tolerance* occurs when a patient acquires a tolerance to one drug and becomes resistant to other similar drugs. *Physical dependence* often accompanies tolerance. The body becomes so adapted to the presence of the drug that it cannot function properly without it. To withdraw the drug is to throw the body out of its equilibrium, causing withdrawal symptoms.

Accumulation

When a drug is taken too frequently to allow for proper elimination, it accumulates in the tissues. The result is a more intense effect and a longer duration. Accumulation can cause overdose and/or toxic effects. Proper dosage

and timing of administration are the best prevention of drug accumulation.

Idiosyncrasy

Occasionally, a person reacts to a drug in a manner that is unexpected and peculiar to that individual only. An idiosyncratic response may manifest in many different ways, such as a hypnotic drug keeping a person awake, acting as a stimulant to this person rather than as a depressant. Usually these reactions cannot be explained.

Drug-Drug Interactions

Special care must be taken with patients who are taking more than one drug on a regular basis. One drug may increase or decrease the effects of another or cause untoward side effects to occur. To safeguard patients from potentially negative drug interactions, it is important to record a complete list at each visit of all the drugs the patient is taking, including OTCs. It is also a good idea to advise patients to fill prescriptions at the same pharmacy, because the pharmacist can use a computer program to check for potential drug interactions.

CRITICAL THINKING APPLICATION

Sylvia Kramer is a 72-year-old patient of Dr. Simon's who calls today and asks Kathy about how she should be taking her heart medicine, diltiazem HCl (Cardizem). Mrs. Kramer is a diabetic patient with hypertension and a history of heart disease. She also is overweight, has the potential for kidney disease, and takes a number of other prescriptions. What factors may have an impact on the potential effect of Mrs. Kramer's medication? What does Kathy need to tell her about Cardizem?

TERMS RELATED TO DRUG INTERACTIONS

antagonism The action of one drug decreases the intensity or shortens the duration of action of another drug. This occurs when certain antibiotics, including tetracycline, impair the absorption of birth control pills (BCPs), which results in a decrease of their effectiveness. Therefore, women taking oral contraceptives should use alternative methods of protection when taking tetracycline.

synergism One drug increases the intensity or prolongs the action of another drug. This can have a positive effect, as in using two different antibiotics to treat an infection, or a negative effect when two drugs lower the blood pressure to dangerous levels.

potentiation A form of synergism when the action of one of the drugs is increased by the presence of another drug. In this case, the two drugs have different actions, but one increases the effect of the other.

Classifications of Drug Actions

Clinical pharmacology is a complex subject. To make the subject easier, drugs are classified according to their actions on the body (e.g., diuretics or emetics). Drugs may also be classified according to the body system that they affect (e.g., drugs acting on the cardiovascular system). The following is a glossary of terms describing some basic drug actions. As you read some of the examples, remember that a drug classified as one type of agent may have other uses and actions on other systems of the body. For example, a drug classified as a diuretic may also be an antihypertensive drug, and a vasodilator may also be a respiratory antispasmodic. It takes time to understand not only the basic classification of a particular drug but also the many secondary uses and effects the drug has on the human body.

These are just a few examples of the different classifications of medications. Remember to research and review all medications before their administration.

Examples of Drug Classifications

Adrenergic

Action: Constricts blood vessels, narrows the **lumen** of a vessel
Examples: Epinephrine: Phenylephrine (Neo-Synephrine)
Primary use: Stops superficial bleeding; raises and sustains blood pressure; relieves nasal congestion

Analgesic

Action: Lessens the sensory function of the brain
Examples: Nonnarcotic: Aspirin; acetaminophen (Tylenol); ibuprofen (Advil, Motrin); narcotic: Meperidine (Demerol); hydrocodone (Vicodin); propoxyphene (Darvon)
Primary use: Pain relief

Anesthetic

Action: Produces insensibility to pain or the sensation of pain
Examples: Bupivacaine (Marcaine); lidocaine (Xylocaine)
Primary use: Local or general anesthesia

Antianxiety

Action: Reduces anxiety and tension
Examples: Chlordiazepoxide (Librium); diazepam (Valium); alprazolam (Xanax)
Primary use: Produces calmness and releases muscle tension

Antibiotic

Action: Kills or inhibits the growth of microorganisms
Examples: Cefaclor (Ceclor); tetracycline (Acromycin); amoxicillin (Augmentin)
Primary use: Treatment of bacterial invasions and infections

Anticholinergic

Action: Parasympathetic blocking agent; reduces spasm in smooth muscle
Examples: Scopolamine; atropine sulfate
Primary use: Dry secretions

Anticoagulants

Action: Delays or blocks the clotting of blood
Examples: Heparin; warfarin sodium (Coumadin)
Primary use: Treatment of blood clots

Antidepressant

Action: Treats depression
Examples: Fluoxetine (Prozac); imipramine pamoate (Tofranil); amitriptyline (Elavil)
Primary use: Mood elevator

Antiemetic

Action: Acts on hypothalamus center in the brain
Examples: Prochlorperazine (Compazine); trimethobenzamide (Tigan); metoclopramide (Reglan)
Primary use: Prevents and relieves nausea and vomiting

Antiepileptic (anticonvulsant)

Action: Reduces excessive stimulation of the brain
Examples: Phenytoin (Dilantin); phenobarbital; carbamazepine (Tegretol)
Primary use: Treatment of epilepsy and other convulsive disorders

Antifungal

Action: Slows or retards the multiplication of fungi
Examples: Miconazole (Monistat); nystatin (Mycostatin); amphotericin B
Primary use: Treatment of systemic or local fungal infections

Antihistamine

Action: Counteracts the effects of histamine by blocking action in tissues; may be used to inhibit gastric secretions
Examples: Brompheniramine maleate (Dimetane); chlorpheniramine (Chlor-Trimeton); diphenhydramine (Benadryl); promethazine (Phenergan); cimetidine (Tagamet); ranitidine (Zantac)
Primary use: Relief of allergies; prevention of gastric ulcers

Antihypertensive

Action: Blocks nerve impulses that cause arteries to constrict; slows heart rate, decreasing its contractility; restricts the hormone aldosterone in the blood
Examples: Atenolol (Tenormin); doxazosin mesylate (Cardura); metoprolol (Lopressor); methyldopa (Aldomet)
Primary use: Reduces and controls blood pressure

Antiinflammatory

Action: Acts as an antiinflammatory or anti-rheumatic

Examples: Nonsteroidal (NSAIDs): Ibuprofen (Advil, Motrin); naproxen (Naprosyn); steroidal: Dexamethasone (Decadron); prednisone (Cortisone)

Primary use: Treatment of arthritis and other inflammatory disorders

Antineoplastic

Action: Inhibits the development of and destroys cancerous cells

Examples: Interferon alfa-2a (Roferon-A); hydroxyurea (Hydrea); cyclophosphamide (Cytoxan); fluorouracil (Adrucil)

Primary use: Cancer chemotherapy

Antispasmodic

Action: Relieves or prevents spasms from musculoskeletal injury or inflammation

Examples: Methocarbamol (Robaxin); carisoprodol (Soma)

Primary use: Treatment of sports injuries

Antitussive (cough suppressant)

Action: Inhibits the cough center

Examples: Narcotic: Codeine sulfate; nonnarcotic: Dextromethorphan (Romilar, Robitussin DM)

Primary use: Temporarily suppresses a nonproductive cough; reduces the thickness of secretions

Bronchodilator

Action: Relaxes the smooth muscle of the bronchi

Examples: Aminophylline (Aminophyllin); theophylline (Theo-Dur); epinephrine (Adrenalin, Sus-Phrine); albuterol (Ventolin, Proventil); isoproterenol (Isuprel)

Primary use: Treatment of asthma, bronchospasm; promotes bronchodilation

Cathartic (laxative)

Action: Increases peristaltic activity of the large intestine

Examples: Magnesium hydroxide (Milk of Magnesia); bisacodyl (Dulcolax); casanthranol (Peri-Colace); psyllium hydrophilic muciloid (Metamucil)

Primary use: Increases and hastens bowel evacuation (defecation)

Contraceptive

Action: Inhibits conception

Examples: Medroxyprogesterone acetate (Depo-Provera); norgestrel (Ovrett); ethinyl estradiol and ethynodiol diacetate (Demulen 1/35)

Primary use: Family planning

Decongestant

Action: Relieves local congestion in the tissues

Examples: Ephedrine or phenylephrine (Neo-Synephrine); pseudoephedrine (Sudafed); oxymetazoline (Afrin)

Primary use: Relief of nasal and sinus congestion caused by common cold, hay fever, or upper respiratory tract disorders

Diuretic

Action: Inhibits the reabsorption of sodium and chloride in the kidneys

Examples: Hydrochlorothiazide (Dyazide, Esidrix, HydroDiuril); furosemide (Lasix); triamterene (Dyrenium)

Primary use: Increases urinary output, decreases blood pressure

Expectorant

Action: Increases secretions and mucus from the bronchial tubes

Examples: Diphenhydramine (Benylin); guaifenesin guaiacolate (Fenesin, Robitussin)

Primary use: Upper respiratory tract congestion

Hemostatic

Action: Controls bleeding; a blood coagulant

Examples: Phytonadione, vitamin K (Konakion); absorbable hemostatic agents, such as Gelfoam and Surgicel, are applied directly to a wound

Primary use: Control of acute or chronic blood-clotting disorder; formation of absorbable, artificial clot

Hypnotic (sedative)

Action: Induces sleep and lessens the activity of the brain

Examples: Secobarbital (Seconal); flurazepam (Dalmane); tamazepam (Restoril)

Primary use: Insomnia; lower doses sedate

Hormone replacement

Action: Replaces or compensates hormone deficiency

Examples: Insulin (Humulin); levothyroxine sodium (Synthroid); estrogen (Premarin)

Primary use: Maintenance of adequate hormone levels

Miotic

Action: Causes the pupil of the eye to contract

Examples: Carbachol (Isopto Carbachol); isoflurophate (Floropryl); pilocarpine (Isopto Carpine)

Primary use: Counteracts pupil dilation

Mydriatic (anticholinergic)

Action: Dilates the pupil of the eye

Examples: Atropine sulfate (Isopto Atropine)

Primary use: Ophthalmological examinations

Narcotic

Action: Depresses the central nervous system and causes insensibility or stupor

Examples: Natural narcotics: Opium group (codeine phosphate, morphine sulfate); synthetic narcotics: Meperidine (Demerol), methadone (Dolophine), and propoxyphene HCl (Darvon)

Primary use: Pain relief

Sympathetic blocking agent

Action: Blocks certain functions of the adrenergic nervous system

Examples: Propranolol (Inderal); metaprolol (Lopressor); phentolamine (Regitine); prazosin (Minipress)

Primary use: Treatment of cardiovascular conditions

Patient Education

It is important for the patient to be aware of the effects a drug may have and should have on his or her system. The medical assistant plays an important role in helping patients understand their medications, promoting compliance with treatment, and preventing complications. The following items should be considered when interviewing a patient and documenting on the patient chart:

1. Ask the patient if she is pregnant.
2. Preassess the patient for any adverse effects, such as allergy or drug-to-drug or drug-to-food interactions.
3. Observe the patient for any adverse effects for a minimum of 20 minutes after the administration of a medication in the office and inform the patient of possible adverse reactions to the medication that may occur at home.
4. Discuss with the patient how and when the prescribed drug is to be taken and if there are any special storage precautions.
5. Reassess that the patient is taking the medication properly.
6. Provide comfort, encouragement, and guidance to patients to ensure their understanding, safety, and cooperation while being on drug therapy.
7. Answer any questions asked. Remember if you are not certain of the answer, consult the prescribing physician.

Legal and Ethical Issues

The medical assistant plays a key role in the management of controlled substances in the ambulatory care setting. It is important that all rules regarding the record keeping, inventory, prescribing, dispensing, and documentation of scheduled drugs be followed according to state and federal regulations. The medical assistant may be responsible for filing for the initial DEA registration as well as the certification renewal. He or she should contact the DEA for instructions. Each DEA number is specific to a site, so multiple practice locations will require a DEA number for each facility.

Accurate and complete documentation is also essential for correct management of patient medications. Each time the patient is prescribed or administered a medication complete details must be included in the patient chart. Failure to do so could result in a serious error that could potentially harm the patient and result in litigation.

SUMMARY OF SCENARIO

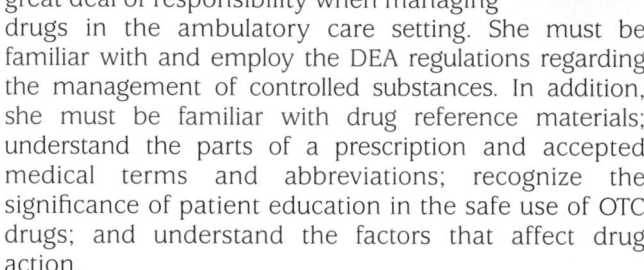

Medical assistant Kathy Augustino has a great deal of responsibility when managing drugs in the ambulatory care setting. She must be familiar with and employ the DEA regulations regarding the management of controlled substances. In addition, she must be familiar with drug reference materials; understand the parts of a prescription and accepted medical terms and abbreviations; recognize the significance of patient education in the safe use of OTC drugs; and understand the factors that affect drug action.

SUMMARY OF LEARNING OBJECTIVES

- Several federal agencies combine forces to regulate drugs in the United States. The FDA regulates the development and sale of all prescription and OTC drugs; the DEA enforces laws designed to control drug abuse and also educates the public about drug abuse prevention; the FTC regulates OTC advertisement.

- DEA regulations for the management of controlled substances include specific record-keeping guidelines; physician registration; and the inventory, storage, and disposal of controlled substances.

- Prescriptions written for controlled substances must comply with both state and federal regulations. The prescription must include details about the patient; information about the physician, including the DEA number; and the amount of drug written out; and the prescription must be manually signed by the physician. Orders for Schedule II drugs cannot be phoned in, except in an absolute emergency, and cannot be refilled. Schedule III, IV, and V drugs may be prescribed by phone and refilled up to five times in a 6-month period. In some states, Schedule V drugs can be dispensed by the pharmacist without a physician prescription.

- A single drug may have as many as three names: chemical, generic, and trade. The chemical name is the drug's formula; the generic or official name is assigned to the drug and may reflect the chemical name; the trade or brand name is the name given the compound by the developing pharmaceutical company and is protected by copyright for 17 years.

- Using drug reference materials is crucial to the safe administration of medications. Most drug reference books supply the action, indication, contra-indications, precautions, adverse reactions, dosage, administration guidelines, and method of packaging. The most frequently used drug reference guide is the PDR, but package inserts can also be used.

■ The clinical uses of drugs include therapeutic or curative; palliative drugs to relieve symptoms; pro-phylactic medications that prevent the occurrence of a condition; diagnostic drugs to help determine disease cause; and replacement drugs that provide substances that are normally occurring in the body.

■ OTC drugs may interfere or interact with pre-scription drugs. Some safety measures for the use of OTC drugs include carefully reading directions, taking only the recommended dose, discarding when expired, informing the physician of OTC use, and being aware of OTC contraindications in certain conditions.

■ The parts of a prescription include the super-scription, inscription, subscription, signature, refill information, and the physician's signature. A pre-scription must also provide the patient's name and address and the date the drug is prescribed.

■ Pharmacokinetics includes absorption, which de-pends on the route of administration (oral, parenteral, mucous membrane, or topical); distribution through the bloodstream; metabolism in the liver; and excretion primarily through the kidneys.

■ Multiple factors affect drug action, including weight, age, sex, diurnal rhythms, pathological fac-tors, immune responses, psychological factors, tolerance, accumulation, idiosyncrasy, and drug-to-drug interactions.

■ The chapter included multiple examples of drugs and their classifications. Drugs are generally classified according to their actions on the body or according to the body system they affect. Drugs may have multiple actions and therefore multiple classifications.

■ The legal responsibilities of medication manage-ment include compliance with DEA regulations regarding controlled substances as well as main-taining complete and accurate documentation on all medications administered and prescribed for each patient.

KEY INTERNET WEBSITES

- Drug Enforcement Administration
- National Community Pharmacists Association
- National Data Corporation
- Rx List: The Internet Drug Index
  For active weblinks to each website visit
  http://evolve.elsevier.com/Kinn/

CHAPTER 31

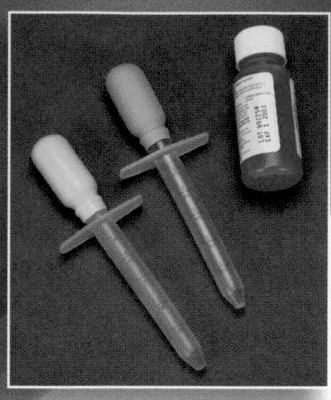

Scenario

Heather Izacco, a recent graduate from a medical assistant program in the area, has just been hired by a local cardiologist, Dr. Angio. One of her responsibilities will be to administer medications under the supervision of Dr. Angio. Heather is confident about her ability to administer the medicine but is unsure of her accuracy in pharmacology math. Heather never did well in math at school and had a difficult time calculating accurate doses and converting between math systems. Her supervisor, Mrs. Allison, suggests Heather review the math section of her textbook at home and be prepared to work out some sample problems next week.

Pharmacology Math

National Curriculum Competencies

CLINICAL COMPETENCIES

4g. Apply pharmacology principles to prepare and administer oral and parenteral medications

Vocabulary

nomogram A graph on which variables are plotted so that a particular value can be read on the appropriate line.

stat Immediately.

unit dose Method of preparing individual doses of medications by the pharmacy.

It is a medical assistant's responsibility to be absolutely certain that the medication prepared and administered to a patient is exactly what is ordered by the physician. Although many times drugs are delivered by the pharmacy or supplied by pharmaceutical representatives in **unit dose** packs, the dosage ordered may differ from the dose on hand. In this case, the medical assistant must be prepared to accurately calculate the correct dose before dispensing and administering the medication. There is never a margin of error in drug calculations, because even a minor mistake may result in serious complications for the patient. Therefore the medical assistant must take meticulous care in calculating all drug dosages.

If the dosage ordered by the physician is different from the dosage on hand, there are three basic steps the medical assistant must complete for accurate calculation of the prescribed dose:

1. Based on the type of system printed on the label, determine whether the physician's order is in the same mathematical system of measurement. If the systems vary (the order is in teaspoons but the label states the medication is prepared in milliliters), then accurately convert the order so that it matches the system used on the label.
2. Perform the calculation in equation form, using the appropriate formula.
3. Check your answer for accuracy and ask someone you trust to confirm your calculations.

All three of these steps must be completed before the medication is dispensed and administered. Confirm your calculations with the physician if you have any doubt of their accuracy.

Drug Labels

The first step in safely calculating drug dosage is to accurately read the label of the drug on hand to determine whether the physician's order and the packaged drug are in the same system of measurement. To do this, a medical assistant must understand some of the basic terms used on drug labels.

- *Strength:* The potency of the drug stated as a percentage of drug in the solution (2% epinephrine), as a solid weight (grams, milligrams, pounds, grains), or as a millequivalent or unit.
- *Dosage:* The size or amount of the drug available in the drug package. This could be in milliliters, teaspoons, or the number of tablets. For example,

the label may read "Imitrex, 6 mg/0.5 ml," which means that there are 6 mg of the drug in each 0.5 ml.
- *Solute:* The pure drug that is dissolved in a liquid to form a solution.
- *Solvent or diluent:* The liquid, which is usually sterile water or sterile saline, that dissolves the solute.

Systems of Measurement

Sometimes the physician will order a medication in a strength that is totally different from the one on the label of the vial or bottle. For example, the physician may order 1 gr (grain) of a drug, but the available dosage form is in milligrams. Before the medical assistant can use the ratio and proportion formulas to arrive at the amount to administer, he or she first must convert to one system or the other. The best way is to convert to the measurement system that is on the label (what is available), because that is the system the medical assistant will have to use to dispense the drug. There are three different systems of measurement for medications: the metric system, the apothecary system, and the household system.

The Metric System

The *metric system* of weights and measures is now used throughout the world as the primary system for weight (mass), capacity (volume), and length (area). In the United States the metric system is used for scientific work, including most pharmaceuticals. However, some medication forms still use the older apothecary system, which necessitates learning the two systems and the relationships (conversions) between the two.

The metric system of weights and measures is a decimal system, which means that it uses base 10. Each higher measure is 10 times the measure at hand; each lower measure is $1/10$ the measure. The fraction is always written as a decimal, and the number precedes the letters designating the actual measure. Thus $1\frac{1}{2}$ liters would be written 1.5 L (Table 31-1). The cubic centimeter (cc) and the milliliter (ml) are interchangeable. In the metric system, 1 cc is a measurement of area, and an area this size holds exactly 1 ml or $1/1000$ of a liter of fluid. The milliliter measures the *amount* of the medication, or the volume to be given orally or injected. The gram (g) measures the weight, or *strength*, of a solid medication

TABLE 31-1	Abbreviations and Symbols for Selected Weights and Measures		
Apothecary System		**Metric System**	
ℳ Min (M)	minim	g	gram
℈ scr	scruple	L	liter
ℨ dr	dram	cc	cubic centimeter
fl ℨ f dr	fluid dram	ml	milliliter
℥ oz	ounce		
fl ℥ fl oz	fluid ounce		
O pt	pint		
C gal	gallon		
	gr	grain	

such as a tablet, powder, or topical preparation. The units of measurement in the metric system are based on their prefixes, with *kilo-* meaning 1000 and *milli-* meaning 0.001. The prefixes mean the same whether used to measure volume or weight.

Conversions within the metric system may be necessary if the physician orders a unit that is different from the one on the label. Units within the metric system are converted by moving the decimal point in multiples of 10. When going from larger to smaller units of measurement, as in converting grams to milligrams, the answer will be a larger number, so the decimal point is moved to the *right*. Therefore 0.35 g = 350 mg. When smaller units of measurement are converted to a larger one, the answer will be a smaller number, so the decimal point is moved to the *left*. For example, 150 ml = 0.15 L. The following equivalents can be used to make conversions within the metric system.

1 kg = 1000 g	1 kl = 1000 L
1 g = 1000 mg	1 L = 1000 ml
1 mg = 1000 µg	1 ml = 1000 µl
1 dg = 0.1 g or ¹/₁₀ g	1 dl = 0.1 L or ¹/₁₀ L
1 cg = 0.01 g or ¹/₁₀₀ g	1 cl = 0.01 L or ¹/₁₀₀ L
1 mg = 0.001 g or ¹/₁₀₀₀ g	1 ml = 0.001 L or ¹/₁₀₀₀ L

CRITICAL THINKING APPLICATION

The first problems Heather reviewed were conversions within the metric system. Yesterday Dr. Angio ordered 0.45 L of a drug, but the label gave the contents in milliliters. How many milliliters should Heather have given?

The Apothecary System

With the *apothecary system*, the basic unit of weight for a solid medication is the grain, and the basic unit of volume for a liquid medication is the minim. As in the metric system, these two units are related: the grain is based on the weight of a single grain of wheat, and the minim is the volume of water that weighs 1 grain (gr). Either Roman or Arabic numerals may be used, but it is not proper to use them together in the same prescription. Either symbols or abbreviations are used; for example, one and a half drams might be written 3iss or dr 1¹/₂. The number follows the symbol or abbreviation. Table 31-2 compares the units of weight and volume in the metric and the apothecary systems. Fluid ounces (oz) is used to differentiate liquids from solid weight.

TABLE 31-2	Approximate Equivalents for Some Commonly Used Measures					
				Liquid Measure		
Grains	Grams	Milligrams	Apothecary		Metric (ml [cc])	
15	1.0	1000	1	quart	1000	ml (cc)
10	0.6	600	1	pint	500	ml
7¹/₂	0.5	500	8	fl oz	250	ml
5	0.3	300	7	fl oz	200	ml
4¹/₂	0.25	250	3.5	fl oz	100	ml
3	0.2	200	1	fl oz	30	ml
2	0.12	120	4	fl dr	15	ml
1¹/₂	0.1	100	2.5	fl dr	10	ml
1	0.06	60	2	fl dr	8	ml
³/₄	0.050	50	1	fl dr	4	ml
¹/₂	0.030	30	45	M	3	ml
³/₈	0.025	25	30	M	2	ml
¹/₄	0.015	15	15	M	1	ml
¹/₆	0.010	10	12	M	0.75	ml
¹/₈	0.008	8	10	M	0.6	ml
¹/₁₀	0.006	6	8	M	0.5	ml
¹/₁₂	0.005	5	5	M	0.3	ml
¹/₂₀	0.003	3	4	M	0.25	ml
¹/₃₀	0.002	2	3	M	0.2	ml
¹/₆₀	0.001	1	1.5	M	0.1	ml
¹/₁₀₀	0.0006	0.6	1	M	0.06	ml
¹/₁₂₀	0.0005	0.5	0.75	M	0.05	ml
¹/₁₅₀	0.0004	0.4	0.5	M	0.03	ml
¹/₂₀₀	0.0003	0.3				
¹/₂₅₀	0.00025	0.25				
¹/₃₀₀	0.0002	0.2				
¹/₄₀₀	0.00015	0.15				
¹/₅₀₀	0.00012	0.12				
¹/₆₀₀	0.0001	0.1				

Weight conversions: 1 lb = 0.45 kg; 1 kg = 2.2 lb; 10 lb = 4.5 kg; 10 kg = 22 lb; 30.0 g = 1 oz; 15.0 g = 4 d; 7.5 g = 2 d; 4 g = 1 d; 4 g = 60 grains.

Domestic equivalents: 1 teaspoon = 5 ml (cc) = 1 fl d; 1 tablespoon = 15 ml = 0.5 fl oz; 1 measuring cup = 250 ml = 8 fl oz; 4 measuring cups = 1000 ml = 1 quart.

Household Measurements

The household system is used in most American homes. This system of measurement is important for a patient at home who has no knowledge of the metric or apothecary systems; however, household measurements are not precisely accurate, so they should never be used in the medical setting. Nevertheless, a medical assistant must understand the conversions between medical and household measurements so the patient can be instructed on how to most accurately measure the medication at home.

The basic measure of weight in the household system is the pound (lb); the basic measure of volume is the drop (gtt). The household drop is equal to an apothecary minim, so these two systems are sometimes easily interchangeable. Both the household and the apothecary systems use the terms *dram* and *ounce* as units of measurement, so always be sure which system you are using. Medications are not measured in household weights, but many prescriptions contain directions using the household measurements of volume. Liquid oral medications are taken by the drop, teaspoon, or tablespoon and are supplied in bottles labeled in ounces or pints. Tables 31-3 and 31-4 show the household system of measurement (note that there are some apothecary and metric equivalents).

Conversions Between Systems of Measurement

Medication orders may need to be converted from one system to another if the order is written in one system and the drug label is in another. Using the conversions in Table 31-2, it is possible to directly convert many measurements or choose an equivalent and mathematically convert the order to the system on the drug label. The conversion is calculated by either multiplication or division. For example, if the physician orders 30 grains of the drug but the label is in gram units, to convert grains to grams the table tells us 15 gr = 1.0 g.

$$30 \div 15 = 2$$
$$2 \times 1.0\ g = 2.0\ g$$

Conversions between units of measurements can also be done using the following formula. The "Drug Have" is the amount or strength (unit of measurement of the drug) that is on the label. The "Wanted" is the amount or strength of the drug ordered by the physician.

$$\text{Drug Have} \times \frac{\text{Wanted}}{\text{Have}} = \text{Unit wanted in new system}$$
$$\text{(conversion)}$$

Using the same example, to convert 30 grains to milligrams:

$$30\ gr \times \frac{1.0\ g}{15\ gr} = \text{Unit wanted}$$

Cross-multiply the problem and the gr unit cancels out to give:

$$2 \times \frac{1.0\ g}{1} = 2.0\ g$$

Calculating Drug Dosages for Administration

The correct dosage of a medication may depend on the patient's age, weight, or state of health or on what other drugs the patient may be taking. Often, the physician will order a medication in a dosage that is different from that of the medications in stock. The difference may be in the system of measurement, the strength, or the form. There are formulas and mathematical tables of conversion for calculating the correct dosage of medication to be administered. It is helpful to look at how the correct calculation is arrived at, one step at a time.

Mathematical Equivalents

You may need to review some basics of arithmetic before you begin to tackle drug calculations. You must thoroughly understand the addition, subtraction, multiplication, and division of fractions and decimals, the relationship of decimals and fractions, and how they are converted from one to the other. In addition, you need to review how decimals and percentages are converted back and forth. Table 31-5 provides some examples of these relationships.

The table shows that a fraction is, in another sense, a ratio. For example, 1/4 (a fraction) is the same as the ratio 1:4 (one to four). If there is one apple and four oranges, then the number of apples that you have is 1/4 the

TABLE 31-3	Common Household Measures
60 drops*	1 teaspoon
1 dash	Less than 1/8 teaspoon
3 teaspoons	1 tablespoon
2 tablespoons	1 ounce
4 ounces	1 juice glass
6 ounces	1 teacup
8 ounces	1 glass or cup
16 tablespoons or 8 ounces	1 measuring cup
2 cups	1 pint
2 pints	1 quart
4 quarts	1 gallon

*Drop (gtt) = Approximate liquid measure, depending on kind of liquid measured and the size of the opening from which it is dropped.

TABLE 31-4	Household Equivalents			
60 gtt	=	1 t or tsp		
3 t or tsp	=	1 T		
180 gtt	=	1 T	=	1/2 oz
2 T	=	1 oz	=	6 t or tsp
360 gtt	=	2 T		
1 oz	=	30 cc or 30 ml		
6 oz	=	1 tcp		
8 oz	=	1 C or 1 glass		
2 C	=	1 pt	=	16 oz
2 pt	=	1 qt	=	32 oz
4 C	=	1 qt	=	32 oz
4 qt	=	1 gal	=	128 oz

TABLE 31-5	Mathematical Equivalents		
Percentage	Decimal	Fraction	Ratio
25	0.25	$^1/_4$	1:4
50	0.5	$^1/_2$	1:2
60	0.6	$^3/_5$ ($^6/_{10}$)	3:5
0.5	0.005	$^1/_{200}$	1:200
0.1	0.001	$^1/_{1000}$	1:1000
85	0.85	$^{17}/_{20}$	17:20
1	0.01	$^1/_{100}$	1:100

number of oranges, and the ratio of apples to oranges is 1:4. Now, divide the numerator 1 by the denominator 4 (a fraction is also an automatic division problem waiting to be solved):

$$4\overline{)1.00}^{\,0.25}$$

The act of dividing a fraction results in a decimal number. Decimal numbers can then be converted to percentages by moving the decimal two spaces to the right:

0.25 = 25.0%, commonly written 25%

Using the example of apples and oranges, you can see that 1 is 0.25, or 25%, of 4. Therefore the number of apples is 0.25, or 25%, of the number of oranges. If you need to review any of these concepts, please stop now and practice these steps of arithmetic.

Ratio and Proportion

Ratio is one way of expressing a fraction, or division problem, and shows the relationship of the numerator to the denominator. The comparison of two ratios is called a *proportion*. A proportion is written as follows:

$$\frac{4}{16} = \frac{1}{4} \text{ or } 4:16 = 1:4$$

This is read as 4 divided by 16 equals 1 divided by 4, or 4 is to 16 as 1 is to 4. The physician's order for a medication may be a ratio different from that of the medication that is in stock. To determine the correct proportion for administration, we must compare the ordered ratio with the available ratio (what is in stock).

The preceding proportion example has all the answers in it; there is nothing to solve. In calculating dosages, mathematical proportions are used, but with one element unknown. We must solve for that unknown, or *x*. For example:

$$\frac{4}{16} = \frac{1}{x}$$

Always in a proportion, we solve the problem by *cross-multiplication*. Do not confuse this with plain multiplication. If you see an equal sign (=) between two fractions, that indicates this is an equation to be *cross-multiplied*.

$$4 \times x = 16 \times 1$$

Therefore:

$$4x = 16$$

We know what $4x$ equals, but next we must find what $1x$, or x, equals. To find the value of x, we must find a way to leave x (or $1x$) alone on one side of the equation. We can change $4x$ to $1x$ by dividing the number 4 by itself:

$$4x \div 4 = 1x$$

But what we do on one side of an equation, we must do on the other side, or the equation will not be equal anymore. Therefore we divide 16 by 4:

$$16 \div 4 = 4$$

Therefore $x = 4$ and $\frac{4}{16} = \frac{1}{4}$

Calculating Dosages

For calculating dosages, a standard set of formulas is used (Procedures 31-1 to 31-4). These formulas use the *strength* (potency) and *dosage unit* (amount) of the drug. If the drug label reads "5 gr/tab," the strength is 5 grains and the dosage unit is 1 tablet. In liquids, the drug strength is called the *solute*, which is dissolved in a liquid called the *solvent*. Therefore, if a vial of injectable material reads "500 mg/ml," there are 500 mg (strength) of drug in every milliliter (amount) of liquid.

We can use these two examples and the proportion formula previously reviewed to work out two problems: (1) filling a syringe and (2) administering tablets.

Problem 1
Order: Give 250 mg of a drug.
Available: A vial marked 500 mg/ml.
Standard formula:

$$\frac{\text{Available strength}}{\text{Ordered strength}} = \frac{\text{Available amount}}{\text{Amount to give}}$$

Problem: Given the strength of the drug needed, the amount of fluid to be withdrawn must be determined.

Set up a proportion with the three known quantities: (1) the strength of the drug in the vial, (2) the unit of fluid in which that strength is contained, and (3) the strength of the drug the physician wishes to be administered to the patient.

Apply the problem to the standard formula:

$$\frac{500 \text{ mg}}{250 \text{ mg}} = \frac{1 \text{ ml}}{x \text{ ml}}$$

$$500 \times x = 250 \times 1$$

$$500x = 250$$

$$\frac{500x}{500} = \frac{250}{500}$$

$$x = {}^1/_2 \text{ ml} = 0.5 \text{ ml}$$

Solution: Administer 0.5 ml of the drug.

Problem 2
Order: Give 10 gr (grains) of a drug.
Available: A bottle with tablets labeled 5 gr each.

PROCEDURE 31-1

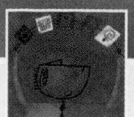

Calculating the Correct Dosage for Administration

GOAL: To calculate the correct dosage amount and choose the correct equipment when the physician orders 2.4 million IU of penicillin G benzathine (Bicillin) administered to a patient.

EQUIPMENT AND SUPPLIES

- Premixed syringes of Bicillin in the following two strengths are available:
  - 0.6 million IU/syringe
  - 1.2 million IU/syringe

PROCEDURAL STEPS

1 Read the order in quiet surroundings to make sure that you fully understand it.

2 Write out the order.

3 Examine the drug labels to see what strengths and amounts are available.

4 Write down the standard formula.

Standard formula:

$$\frac{\text{Available strength}}{\text{Ordered strength}} = \frac{\text{Available amount}}{\text{Amount to give}}$$

Problem: Given the strength of the drug needed, the number of tablets to be administered must be determined.

Set up a proportion with the three known quantities: (1) the strength of the drug in each tablet, (2) the unit amount that is one tablet, and (3) the strength of the drug the physician wishes to be administered to the patient.

Apply the problem to the standard formula:

$$\frac{5 \text{ gr}}{10 \text{ gr}} = \frac{1 \text{ tablet}}{x \text{ (number of tablets)}}$$

$$5 \times x = 10 \times 1$$

$$5x = 10$$

$$\frac{5x}{5} = \frac{10}{5}$$

$$x = 2 \text{ tablets}$$

Solution: Administer 2 tablets.

Use the *standard formula* for any type of calculation. You may be using strengths that are measured in international units (IU), as with penicillin; grams; milligrams; grains; or percentages. The forms in which drugs may be prepared include cubic centimeters (cc) or milliliters (ml), minims, drops, drams, ounces, pints, gallons (for making up diluted stock solutions from concentrated solutions, such as with alcohol and hydrogen peroxide), or spoonfuls.

Purpose: To eliminate the chances of error, orders should never be carried out unless the calculations are completed in writing.

5 Rewrite the formula, replacing the unknown values with the known quantities. The unknown x will be the amount of the drug to give.

6 Work the proportion problem by cross-multiplying to solve for x.

7 State your answer by filling in the blanks, as follows:

To administer 2.4 million IU of Bicillin, I would select _____ of the premixed syringes labeled _____.

Follow the steps previously shown, and, above all, discipline yourself to write down each step with complete calculations. This is the only way to ensure maximum accuracy and the safety of your patients. If you have difficulty with the calculation, or the answer does not seem quite right, ask the physician to check your calculation. A double check is always preferred.

CRITICAL THINKING APPLICATION

At work the next day Dr. Angio orders Heather to administer Acetaminophen Elixir 70 mg **stat** to a 6-year-old patient with a fever of 102.6° F. Heather checks the label of the Acetaminophen Elixir in the drug cabinet and discovers the bottle contains 120 mg per 5 ml in a 100 ml bottle. Using the standard formula presented earlier, how many milliliters should the child receive? If Heather is concerned about her calculation, what should she do?

Pediatric Dose

Calculating Dosage

Pediatric dosages are different from those in other age groups because of multiple factors, including differences in absorption and drug metabolism. However, the most important factor in determining pediatric dosage is body weight. A medical assistant must be especially careful in calculating dosages for children, because even a minor miscalculation may be dangerous.

Calculating the Correct Dosage for Administration Using Two Systems of Measurement

GOAL: To choose the correct system of measurement and calculate the correct dosage amount when the physician orders 120 mg of a drug to be administered to a patient. (Tablet label reads 1 gr each.)

EQUIPMENT AND SUPPLIES

- Tablets labeled 1 gr (grain) each
- Standard mathematical formula:
$$\frac{\text{Available strength}}{\text{Ordered strength}} = \frac{\text{Available amount}}{\text{Amount to give}}$$
- Conversion equivalent: 1 gr = 60 mg

PROCEDURAL STEPS

1 Read the order in quiet surroundings to make sure that you fully understand it.

2 Write out the order.

3 Examine the drug labels to see what strengths and amounts are available.

4 Convert the ordered system of measurement to the system of measurement on the label using the conversion formula.

$$\text{Drug Have} \times \frac{\text{Wanted}}{\text{Have}} = \text{Unit wanted in new system}$$
$$(\text{conversion})$$

5 Write down the standard formula.
Purpose: To eliminate the chances of error, orders should never be carried out unless the calculations are completed in writing.

6 Rewrite the formula, replacing the unknown values with the known quantities and using the system of measurement on the label. The unknown x will be the amount of the drug to give (amount to give).

7 Work the proportion problem by cross-multiplying to solve for x.

8 State your answer by filling in the blank, as follows:
To administer 120 mg of a drug from tablets labeled 1 gr (grain) each, give _____ tablet(s).

Calculating the Correct Pediatric Dosage When Only an Adult Medication Is Available

GOAL: To calculate the correct dosage amount for a 90-pound child using Clark's rule when the adult dosage is 250 mg.

EQUIPMENT AND SUPPLIES

- Adult dosage 250 mg/ml
- Clark's rule:
$$\text{Pediatric dose} = \frac{\text{Child's weight in lbs}}{150} \times \text{Adult dose}$$
- Standard mathematical formula:
$$\frac{\text{Available strength}}{\text{Ordered strength}} = \frac{\text{Available amount}}{\text{Amount to give}}$$

PROCEDURAL STEPS

1 Read the order in quiet surroundings to make sure that you fully understand it.

2 Write out the order.

3 Examine the drug labels to see what strengths and amounts are available.

4 Write down Clark's rule.
Purpose: To eliminate the chances of error, orders should never be carried out unless the calculations are completed in writing.

5 Using Clark's rule, replace the unknown values with the known quantities. The unknown x will be the pediatric strength ordered (pediatric dose).

6 Write down the standard formula.
Purpose: To eliminate the chances of error, orders should never be carried out unless the calculations are completed in writing.

7 Rewrite the formula, replacing the unknown values with the available quantities and the pediatric strength just determined. The unknown x will be the amount of the drug to give (amount to give).

8 Work the proportion problem by cross-multiplying to solve for x.

9 State your answer by filling in the blank, as follows:
To administer an adult medication labeled 250 mg/ml to a 90-pound child, give _____ ml.

PROCEDURE **31-4**

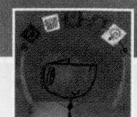

Calculating the Correct Dosage for Administration Using Body Weight

GOAL: To calculate correct dosage by using body weight method.
Ordered: Zovirax capsules 5 mg/kg every 8 hours for 7 days for a patient who has a diagnosis of herpes zoster. The patient weighs 176 pounds. The capsules are labeled 200 mg = 1 capsule.
Weight conversion: 2.2 lb = 1 kg

EQUIPMENT AND SUPPLIES

- Capsules labeled 200 mg/kg
- Balance scale
- Formula for conversion of pounds to kilograms
- Standard math formula:
$$\frac{\text{Available strength}}{\text{Ordered strength}} = \frac{\text{Available amount}}{\text{Amount to give}}$$
- Paper and pencil

PROCEDURAL STEPS

1 Read the order in quiet surroundings to make sure that you fully understand it.

2 Write out the order.

3 Examine the drug label to check the strength and amount.

4 Convert the patient's weight from pounds to kilograms.

176 lb ÷ 2.2 lb/kg = 80 kg

80 kg × 5 mg = 400 mg of acyclovir (Zovirax) every 8 hours for 7 days

5 Write down the standard formula.
Purpose: To eliminate the chances of error.

6 Rewrite the formula, replacing the unknown values with the known quantities. The unknown *x* will be the amount of the drug to give.

7 Work the problem by cross-multiplying to solve for *x*.

8 State your answer by filling in the blank as follows:

To administer 5 mg/kg of body weight of acyclovir (Zovirax) from capsules labeled 200 mg each, I would give _____ capsule(s).

Fried's Law

Calculation by Fried's law is for children younger than 1 year of age and is based on the age of the child in months compared with a child $12\frac{1}{2}$ years old. The calculation assumes that an adult dose would be appropriate for a child $12\frac{1}{2}$ years old (150 months).

$$\text{Pediatric dose} = \frac{\text{Child's age in months}}{150 \text{ months}} \times \text{Adult dose}$$

Young's Rule

Young's rule is for children older than 1 year of age.

$$\text{Pediatric dose} = \frac{\text{Child's age in years}}{\text{Child's age in years} + 12} \times \text{Adult dose}$$

Clark's Rule

Clark's rule is based on the weight of the child. This system is much more accurate than other pediatric methods, because children of any age can vary greatly in size and body weight. Clark's rule uses 150 pounds (70 kg) as the average adult weight and assumes that the child's dose is proportionately less. The formula is as follows:

$$\text{Pediatric dose} = \frac{\text{Child's weight in pounds}}{150 \text{ pounds}} \times \text{Adult dose}$$

West's Nomogram

West's nomogram uses a calculation of the body surface area of infants and young children to determine the pediatric dose. Many physicians use the **nomogram** as a quick reference for pediatric doses (Figure 31-1).

$$\text{Pediatric dose} = \frac{\text{Body surface area (BSA) of child in m}^2}{1.7 \text{ m}^2 \text{ (average adult BSA)}} \times \text{Adult dose}$$

Reconstituting Powdered Injectable Medications

Some medications are packaged as crystals or powder (*solute*) in a vial that must be mixed with sterile isotonic saline or sterile distilled water (*solvent*) to form a solution before it can be injected. In this case it is essential to carefully read the label directions to determine how much sterile solvent must be added to the solute to create a particular dosage strength.

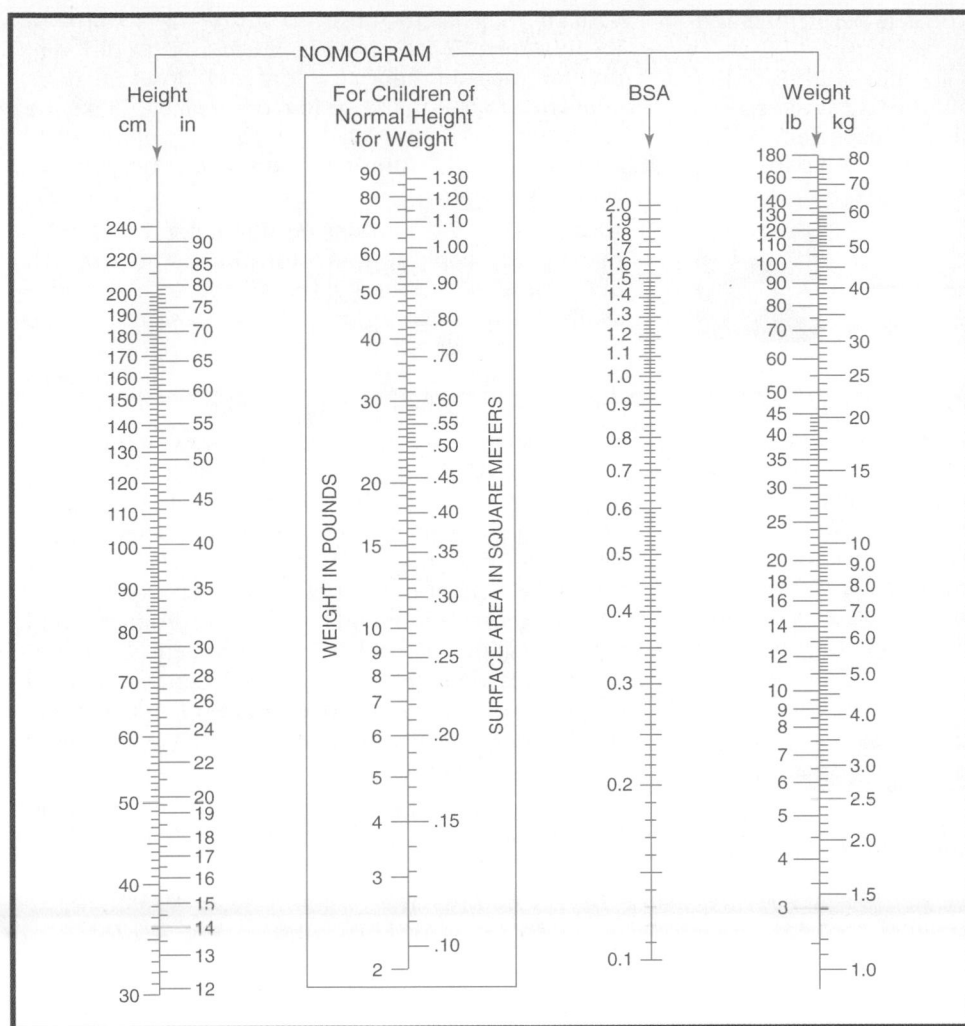

FIGURE 31-1 West's nomogram for estimation of body surface area. (From Behrman RE, Kliegman R, Jenson HB, editors: *Nelson textbook of pediatrics*, ed. 16. Philadelphia, 2000, WB Saunders.)

Example

The physician orders 500 mg of a drug.

The label reads "Add 5.5 ml sterile water to make 250 mg/ml; total volume of available solution will be 6 ml."

First: Inject 5.5 ml of sterile water into the vial of medication. Rotate the vial between the hands to mix the solutes and solvent. The total volume in the vial is now 6 ml.

Second: According to the label, every milliliter in the vial contains 250 mg of the drug.

Third: Label the vial with the date and time of reconstitution, because according to the particular drug guidelines, once the medication is mixed it must be discarded in a short period of time.

Fourth: Calculate the number of milliliters to withdraw from the vial to fulfill the physician's order for 500 mg of the drug using the standard formula.

$$\frac{\text{Available strength}}{\text{Ordered strength}} = \frac{\text{Available amount}}{\text{Amount to give}}$$

$$\frac{250 \text{ mg}}{500 \text{ mg}} = \frac{1 \text{ ml}}{x}$$

$$250x = 500$$

$$x = 500 \div 250$$

$$x = 2 \text{ ml}$$

Answer: To administer 500 mg from a vial labeled "250 mg/ml," administer 2 ml of medication.

Legal and Ethical Issues

A medical assistant who is responsible for medication administration must have complete mastery in calculating dosages, whether the prescribed dosage is for a child or an adult. If there is ever any doubt about the accuracy of a calculation, the medical assistant should always have a trusted colleague or the physician check the calculations.

The medical assistant who prepares and administers medications is ethically and legally responsible for his or her own actions. Laws vary from state to state; therefore it is essential that the medical assistant become familiar with the laws in the state of employment before giving medications. Legislation in some states gives physicians broad authority to delegate responsibility for giving medications. In this case, the medical assistant acts as the "agent" of the physician. The assistant is responsible and accountable for the acts performed and may be subject to penalties.

Regardless of the differences in state authorization laws, the courts will not permit the carelessness of healthcare workers to go unpunished, especially when such actions result in harm to or death of the patient.

SUMMARY OF SCENARIO

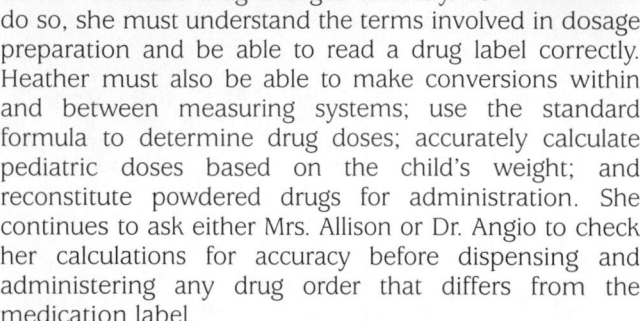

Heather recognizes how important it is to be able to calculate drug dosages correctly. To do so, she must understand the terms involved in dosage preparation and be able to read a drug label correctly. Heather must also be able to make conversions within and between measuring systems; use the standard formula to determine drug doses; accurately calculate pediatric doses based on the child's weight; and reconstitute powdered drugs for administration. She continues to ask either Mrs. Allison or Dr. Angio to check her calculations for accuracy before dispensing and administering any drug order that differs from the medication label.

SUMMARY OF LEARNING OBJECTIVES

■ Verifying the accuracy of calculations is essential before dispensing and administering all medications. First, the medical assistant must check the drug label with the physician's order to verify the systems of measurement. If the physician's order is in a different unit of measurement, the ordered dose must be converted to match the system on the label. Next, the calculation is completed using the appropriate formula. Finally, the calculation is checked for accuracy.

■ Drug label terms must be understood to implement pharmacology math formulas. The strength of the drug is its potency; the dosage is the amount available in the drug package; the solute is the crystal or powdered form of the drug; the solvent is the sterile liquid that is combined in the vial with the solute to create the drug solution.

■ There are three systems of measurement for drugs. The metric system is based on units of 10. The liter is a measure of the liquid volume of a drug, and the gram is a measure of the weight or strength. Units within the metric system are converted by moving the decimal point in multiples of 10. The apothecary system measures liquid volume in minims and weight in grains. Household measurements are based on pounds and drops. Table 31-2 can be used to convert from one system of measurement to another, or drug measurements can be converted by using the conversion formula.

■ The correct dose of an ordered drug can be calculated by using basic arithmetic involving fractions and ratios and proportions. The standard formula for calculating drug dosage uses the information about the drug's strength and amount (which is on the label) and the strength of the drug ordered, with the unknown (x) being the answer sought. The only way to gain confidence in using the standard formula is to practice dosage calculation frequently until you become comfortable with the math.

■ The medical assistant must be especially vigilant in calculating pediatric doses since even a minor error may be dangerous to a child. West's nomogram can be used to determine the pediatric dose if the child's height and weight are known. However, the most accurate method for determining a pediatric dose is Clark's rule, which is based on the child's weight.

■ In reconstituting powdered injectable medications, the medical assistant must add a particular amount of solvent (as recommended on the drug label) to a vial of powdered or crystalloid medication. Once the

solute and solvent are combined and mixed in the vial, a solution of medication is formed; the strength is based on equivalents printed on the drug label. Once the medication is mixed, it is important for the medical assistant to carefully read the label to determine how much of the drug must be withdrawn to equal the physician's order. This process frequently requires the use of the standard conversion formula to determine the accurate dose for administration.

■ A medical assistant who prepares, dispenses, and administers medications is ethically and legally responsible for his or her own actions. If there is any doubt regarding the accuracy of calculations, it is absolutely essential that the medical assistant have the physician or another trusted employee review the math before the medication is dispensed and administered. It is important for medical assistants to be aware of state laws that monitor medication administration by allied health workers.

ANSWERS TO PROCEDURES

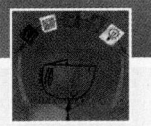

PROCEDURE 31-1: To administer 2.4 million IU of penicillin G benzathine (Bicillin), select two of the premixed syringes labeled 1.2 million IU per syringe.

PROCEDURE 31-2: To administer 120 mg of a drug from tablets labeled 1 gr each, give 2 tablets.

PROCEDURE 31-3: To administer an adult medication labeled 250 mg/ml to a 90-pound child, give 150 mg/ml.

PROCEDURE 31-4: To administer acyclovir (Zovirax), 5 mg/kg of body weight from capsules labeled 200 mg each, give a patient weighing 176 pounds 2 capsules (400 mg).

CHAPTER 32

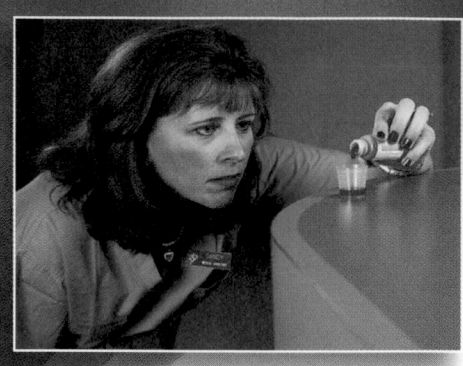

Scenario

Dr. Carla Thau just opened a new primary care office in the community. She is in the process of hiring office staff, and Dorothy Gaston, CMA, is being interviewed for a clinical assisting position. One of Dr. Thau's chief concerns is that the medical assistant working in the clinical area be familiar with medications and competent with their administration. Her primary concern is the safety of her patients, so she requires the individual hired to practice appropriate safety precautions for medication administration as well as to demonstrate his or her ability in dispensing and administering oral, topical, and parenteral drugs.

Administering Medications

Learning Objectives

- Define and spell the terms listed in the vocabulary.
- Apply safety precautions to the management of medication administration in the ambulatory healthcare setting.
- Summarize patient assessment factors that have an impact on medication administration.
- Outline safety guidelines for specific patient populations.
- Perform documentation of medication administration.
- Identify various drug forms and their administration guidelines.
- Specify parenteral equipment including details regarding needles and syringes.
- Employ OSHA guidelines in the management of parenteral administration.
- Describe and demonstrate parenteral administration types and locations.
- Recognize the role of the medical assistant in patient education for drug administration.
- Assess legal and ethical issues in drug administration in the ambulatory care setting.

National Curriculum Competencies

CLINICAL COMPETENCIES

4a. Perform telephone and in-person screening
4g. Apply pharmacology principles to prepare and administer oral and parenteral medications
4h. Maintain medication and immunization records

TRANSDISCIPLINARY COMPETENCIES

2d. Document appropriately
3c. Instruct and demonstrate the use and care of patient equipment

Vocabulary

bevel Angled tip of a needle.

bronchoconstriction Narrowing of the bronchiole tubes.

edema Abnormal accumulation of fluid in the interstitial spaces of tissues.

enteric coated A coating added to an oral medication that resists the effects of stomach juices; designed so medicine is absorbed in the small intestine.

hermetically sealed Sealed so no air is allowed to enter.

hypotension Low blood pressure.

immunotherapy Administering repeated injections of diluted extracts of the substance that causes an allergy; also called *desensitization*.

induration An abnormally hard, inflamed area.

loading dose Administering a double dose for the first dose of the medication; usually done with antibiotic therapy so that therapeutic blood levels are reached quickly.

meniscus The curved formation of liquids in a container.

polyuria Excretion of an unusually large amount of urine.

scored Tablet is manufactured with an indentation for division through the center.

vasodilation Increase in the diameter of a blood vessel.

viscosity The quality of being thick and of lacking the capability of easy movement.

volatile An explosive substance's capacity to vaporize at a low temperature.

wheal Localized area of edema or a raised lesion.

In previous medication chapters you learned about general pharmacology principles and pharmacology math. In this chapter you will learn about safety factors in drug administration, documentation guidelines, and the forms of medications and how they are administered. It is important to remember that medications have the potential to cause serious harm to the patient. Therefore the process of dispensing and administering medication orders must always be treated with great care. Each member of the healthcare team involved in medication administration must be constantly vigilant to prevent errors and deliver quality patient care.

No matter what types of medications are to be administered, the order must come from the physician. If the physician delegates drug administration to the medical assistant, it must be allowable under state laws. Every state has a medical practice act that defines whether a medical assistant can administer drugs under the supervision of a physician. Some states allow medical assistants to administer only certain types of medications; some prohibit medical assistants from giving injections. Information concerning the scope of practice for medical assistants in your particular state should be obtained from your local government or medical society. You should know what the law states and how your duties fit into that law.

Safety in Drug Administration

To ensure patient safety in drug administration, there are certain procedures that the medical assistant must perform every time a medication is ordered. First, it is absolutely essential that the medical assistant understand the physician's order. This means that the order can be clearly read and the physician has answered any questions regarding the medication, dose, strength, or route of administration. Once the order is clarified, it is the medical assistant's responsibility to look up the drug in a pharmacology reference, such as the *Physicians' Desk Reference* (PDR) (see Chapter 30), because a medication should never be given until its purpose, possible side effects, precautions, and recommended dose are known. After the medical assistant learns about the drug ordered, it is time to dispense and administer the medication. Safeguarding the patient during this process involves using the "seven rights" of proper drug administration:

1. *The right patient*. The easiest way to make sure the medication is being given to the patient ordered is to ask the patient his or her name or call the patient by name before administering the drug.

2. *The right drug*. This begins with clarifying the physician's order if needed. *Every* time a drug is dispensed, the label must be checked *three* times to confirm the right drug, dose, and strength. Compare the physician's written order with the label when:
   - Taking the medication from the storage area
   - Just before dispensing the medication from the container
   - When replacing the container to storage or before discarding the used container

3. *The right dose*. If the dose ordered does not match the dose available, perform appropriate pharmacology math procedures to determine the accurate dose. *Remember to have calculations checked if there is any doubt about the dose accuracy.*

4. *The right route*. Check the physician's order to clarify the route of administration, whether it is oral, mucous membrane, or parenteral. Patient assessment includes determining whether this is an appropriate route for that particular patient.

5. *The right time*. In the ambulatory care setting, most medications are ordered *stat*. However, it is important to check the physician's order to clarify the time of administration and refer to this information when looking up the drug to clarify any patient questions about home administration of the drug.

6. *The right technique*. A medical assistant must be familiar with the proper techniques for all routes of administration. If there are any doubts about the ability to administer a particular drug, always ask for help.

7. *The right documentation*. Immediately after giving the drug to the patient, document the date and time of administration; the drug's name, strength, dose,

and route of administration; any patient reactions to the medication; and details of patient education regarding the drug. For parenteral medications, the site of injection should be inspected before administration for scarring, altered pigmentation, or any other indication there might be a problem with medication absorption. The exact site of administration must be charted. If the patient calls in for a prescription refill, document all pertinent information on the patient chart as well.

ADDITIONAL SAFETY STEPS FOR MEDICATION ADMINISTRATION

- Prepare medications in a quiet, well-lit area.
- Pay close attention to all the steps involved in dispensing drugs.
- *Never* substitute a drug or drug strength. Consult the physician for any discrepancy between the medication ordered and the medication available.
- Store medications as ordered on the package and return containers to the proper storage area immediately after dispensing the dose.
- *The person who administers the medication is responsible for any drug errors.* Never administer a medication you have not personally prepared.
- If ordered to prepare a medication for the physician to administer, place the container with the dispensed drug so the physician can perform the seven rights.
- The physician should write every medication order before the medication is dispensed.
- Routinely check expiration dates when doing the seven rights. Properly discard expired drugs.
- Discard medications with damaged labels.
- If a medication is not administered after it is dispensed, discard it rather than return it to the container.
- Patients should be observed for 20 to 30 minutes after a medication is administered for untoward effects. Any reactions must be reported to the physician and documented on the patient's chart.

CRITICAL THINKING APPLICATION

Dr. Thau asks Dorothy what safety precautions she would routinely follow when administering a dose of omeprazole (Prilosec). Based on the information you have learned about safe drug administration, what steps should Dorothy follow in dispensing and administering the ordered medication?

Patient Assessment Factors

Although medications may be given only under the direct order and supervision of the physician, the medical assistant is part of the assessment and problem-solving processes in the care of the patient. In medicine, assessment never ends, and never is it the responsibility of just one person. A physician gives the order to administer medication to a patient based on a medical assessment, but you also must continue to assess the patient and the patient's environment as you follow through with the order. The physician depends on the medical assistant to be alert to changes or new information that could result in a condition or consequence that would make the use of a drug improper or undesirable. Before giving any medication, you should assess the patient, the drug, and the environment.

Drug therapy should be based on a holistic approach to patient treatment. The patient is more than a particular disease. There are many factors that may have an impact on the patient's compliance with drug treatment as well as the safety and effectiveness of medication therapy. The first step in holistic medication treatment is collecting a complete and accurate history. This includes gathering details regarding the patient's health history, current and past use of both prescription and over-the-counter (OTC) drugs, and any negative responses to drugs, especially drug *allergies*. Every time a patient is seen in the office, he or she should be asked about drug allergies. Most medical practices have a specific place on the patient's chart to document drug allergies, such as in red ink in the upper right corner of each documentation sheet, as well as a special label on the front of the patient's chart. It is crucial that the physician have accurate information regarding drug allergies to avoid serious complications and possibly death.

Patient assessment does not end with the administration of the drug. Observe patients carefully for drug reactions that may follow the use of injectable medications. Patients receiving penicillin (a drug with a high incidence of allergic response) or **immunotherapy** must remain in the office for 20 to 30 minutes in case of acute anaphylactic reaction. Acute anaphylactic reaction can result in respiratory failure and circulatory collapse within minutes if not reversed with epinephrine. Lesser allergic reactions include hives, swelling, and itching. An antihistamine, such as diphenhydramine (Benadryl), may need to be administered if these reactions occur.

Because patient factors such as age, weight, and height may be used to determine the correct therapeutic dose, accurate recordings of this information should be documented on the chart. As discussed in Chapter 30, chronic conditions, especially liver and kidney disease, may affect the body's ability to metabolize and excrete medications. Therefore a complete and accurate history is crucial to patient safety.

Besides the patient's physical state, other holistic factors also play a role in successful drug therapy. The patient must be able to understand the drug regimen, may need sufficient family support to follow treatment guidelines, and must be able to afford the ordered medication. Unless these criteria can be met, the patient may be unable to follow through with treatment protocol. It is important that the medical assistant investigate these issues and offer appropriate community support, if available, to help the patient maintain proper drug therapy.

Approaches to Special Patient Populations. Pregnant and breastfeeding women must be especially careful in taking OTC and prescription drugs, because medications are known to cross the placenta and may affect the developing fetus. A pregnant woman should not take *any* medication without the knowledge and approval of her physician. As discussed in Chapter 30, the Food and Drug Administration (FDA) has determined five pregnancy risk categories of drugs. The medical assistant should be familiar with the specific drug category before administering any medication to a pregnant woman. Besides passing through the placenta, medications are also transferred through breast milk. Therefore similar precautions must be used when the physician prescribes medications to a lactating mother.

As discussed in Chapter 31, special precautions must be followed when determining the correct dose of medication for children. Pediatric doses are primarily determined by the child's weight; therefore it is important to measure and record accurate weights on all children at each office visit. The way in which a child's body manages drug absorption, distribution, metabolism, and excretion is different from that of an adult's body, so these factors are taken into consideration when the physician prescribes a medication.

subcutaneous fat, which may affect the route of administration of some medications, especially parenteral sites. In addition, many elderly people have accompanying chronic diseases, such as circulatory, liver, or kidney disease, that may impact the distribution, metabolism, and excretion of medications. Many geriatric patients receive multiple medications, which increases the risk of drug contraindications and interactions. A holistic approach to aging patients should include a nutritional evaluation, because a poor diet may have an impact on the effect of the drug. Another very real concern for aging patients is the cost of drug therapy. Many patients on fixed incomes may not be able to afford the ordered drug but hesitate to inform the physician of this problem. It may be up to the medical assistant to ask the patient about his or her ability to pay for the ordered medication.

SUGGESTIONS FOR SUCCESSFUL MEDICATION ADMINISTRATION TO CHILDREN

- Explain why the medication is needed and how it will make them feel.
- Attempt to gain cooperation by getting down on their level and using a soft but firm voice.
- When possible, offer choices of care, such as, "Would you like your medicine in your leg or in your arm?"
- Divert the child to relieve stressful moments.
- If the child refuses to cooperate, get help as needed to restrain the child so the medication can be given safely.
- Encourage parents to participate as much as possible and make sure both the parent and child (if age appropriate) understand the ordered drug therapy.
- Offer a "treat," such as a sticker, at the end of the visit.

GUIDELINES FOR ADMINISTRATION OF MEDICATION TO GERIATRIC PATIENTS

- Educate the patient and family on the purpose of the drug; the time, dose, and route of administration; and common side effects. Instructions should be written clearly for home reference.
- If the patient has difficulty swallowing the medication, either crush (if allowed) or mix the medication in applesauce or pudding.
- Encourage the patient to drink plenty of fluids (at least eight glasses of water per day) while taking the medication.
- Reinforce the patient should take the medication as prescribed, not to skip doses or double doses.
- Request that patients bring to every physician visit all of the medications they are currently taking in their labeled containers, including OTCs, so a current medication record can be accurately maintained on the patient's chart.
- If patients are taking multiple medications, suggest the use of daily or weekly medication dispensers. These can be purchased in drugstores and restocked by family members on a weekly basis.
- Encourage patients not to share or "save" medications. All leftover medications should be discarded to avoid use beyond the expiration date.

Aging people are also more sensitive to the effects of medications, so certain factors must be considered when prescribing and administering drugs to this population group. The metabolic rate typically slows with the aging process, resulting in an increased susceptibility to a build up of chemicals in the body that may lead to toxic conditions. Part of the normal aging process is loss of

CRITICAL THINKING APPLICATION

Dr. Thau serves both pediatric and geriatric patients. Summarize key items Dorothy should consider when administering medications to these specialty patient population groups.

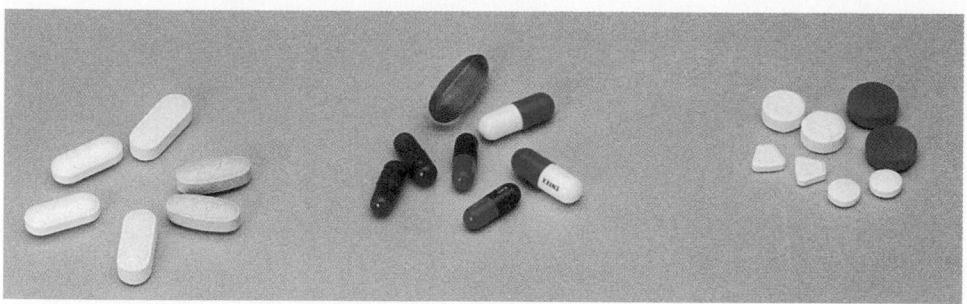

FIGURE 32-1 *Left to right,* Caplets, capsules, and tablets.

Assessment of the Patient's Environment

The patient's surroundings could determine an order's inappropriateness. The patient may become hysterical or uncooperative about receiving the medication, or the patient's family may protest the use of the drug. Administration of certain medications requires the presence of the physician. For example, due to the risk of anaphylactic shock, allergy injections should not be given unless the physician is present. In addition, the environment must be safe for drug administration. Be certain that the patient is comfortable and protected from further injury. If a patient is to receive an injection, take care to place the patient in a position that best exposes the site and protects the patient from injury in case he or she faints or has a drug reaction. If the patient is to take an oral medication with water, be certain that he or she is seated in a position that will prevent choking. Because any medication is potentially dangerous to a patient, emergency drugs must be readily available to counteract any adverse effects that might occur immediately after the administration of a medication. Emergency drugs should be in injectable form for rapid effect. Typically, emergency carts include adrenergics, such as epinephrine; anticholinergics, such as atropine; bronchodilators; and histamine blockers. The pharmaceutical management of emergencies is discussed in Chapter 33.

Drug Forms and Administration

As discussed in Chapter 30, the chosen route of drug administration determines the rate and intensity of the drug's effect. A drug prepared for one route but administered by another route may not have any effect at all and is potentially dangerous. Each route requires different dosage forms.

Solid Oral Dosage Forms

The basic forms for oral dosage are tablets, capsules, and lozenges (troches). Figure 32-1 depicts typical caplets, capsules, and tablets. Tablets are compressed powders or granules that, when wet, break apart in the stomach—or in the mouth if they are not swallowed quickly. Tablets may be *sugar* coated to taste better, or **enteric coated**, such as Ecotrin, to protect the stomach mucosa. Buffered tablets are also designed to prevent stomach irritation by combining the drug with a buffering agent that decreases the amount of acidity in the compound. Buffered or

enteric-coated tablets should never be crushed or dissolved. Only **scored** tablets can be cut in half. This is accomplished with a pill cutter, as shown in Figure 32-2.

Some tablets are coated with a volatile liquid that is meant to dissolve in the mouth, such as an antacid tablet. Caplets are tablets that are oblong, like capsules.

Capsules are gelatin coated and dissolve in the stomach, or they may be coated with substances that protect them from the acid action of the stomach. Timed- or sustained-release (SR) capsules or spansules are designed to dissolve at different rates over a period of time, to reduce the number of times a patient has to take a medication. These drugs should never be crushed or dissolved, because this would negate their timed-release action. Another form of oral mediation, lozenges or troches, are flattened disks that are dissolved in the mouth for coating the throat.

Liquid Oral Dosage Forms

Many liquid forms of medication are available. They differ mainly in the type of substance used to dissolve the drug: water, oils, or alcohol.

Solutions are drug substances contained in a homogeneous mixture with a liquid. Liquid forms include the following:

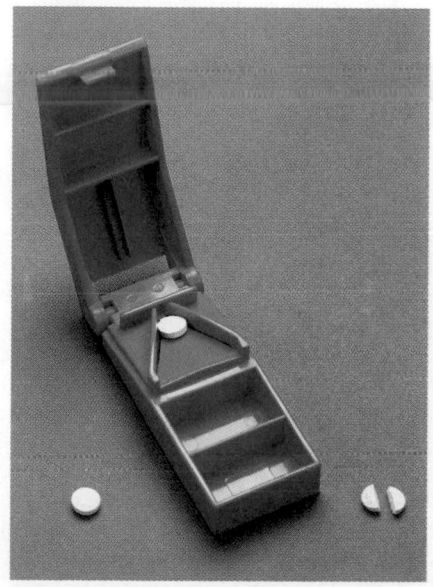

FIGURE 32-2 Pill cutter.

- *Syrups:* A syrup is a solution of sugar and water, usually containing flavoring and medicinal substances. Cough syrups are the most common.
- *Aromatic waters:* Aromatic waters are aqueous solutions containing **volatile** oils, such as oil of spearmint, peppermint, or clove.
- *Liquors:* Liquors are solutions that contain a nonvolatile material, such as alcohol, as the solute.

Suspensions are insoluble drug substances contained in a liquid. Examples include the following:

- *Emulsions:* An emulsion is a mixture of oil and water that improves the taste of otherwise distasteful products, such as cod liver oil.
- *Gels and magmas:* Gels and magmas consist of minerals suspended in water. Minerals settle; therefore products containing minerals must be shaken before use. Milk of magnesia is an example.

A drug substance can be mixed with alcohol to enhance the drug's properties. Examples include the following:

- *Fluid extracts:* Fluid extracts are combinations of alcohol and vegetable products that are more potent than tinctures. For example, belladonna fluid extract has a higher percentage of the powdered belladonna leaf than does tincture of belladonna.
- *Tinctures:* A tincture is an alcoholic preparation of a soluble drug or chemical substance, usually from plant sources. An example is tincture of belladonna. Examples of less potent tinctures are tincture of benzoin and tincture of iodine, which are applied externally.
- *Extracts:* Extracts are very concentrated combinations of vegetable products and alcohol or ether that are evaporated until a syrupy liquid, solid mass, or powder is formed. Extracts are many times stronger than the crude drug itself.
- *Elixirs:* An elixir is an aromatic, alcoholic, sweetened preparation. Elixir of phenobarbital is one example; the alcoholic cough medicines, terpin hydrate with codeine and plain elixir of codeine, are two more. Elixirs differ from tinctures in that they are sweetened. They should be used with caution in patients with diabetes or a history of alcohol abuse. Some pediatric medications retain the name of elixir, although they no longer contain alcohol.

Oral Administration. If the drug is not intended to coat the oral cavity or throat, oral medications should be taken with enough water to transport the drug to the stomach. Make certain that the patient is able to swallow the medication. It may be helpful to place the medication on the back part of the tongue. Liquid medications are ideal for children. Solid drugs should not be administered to children until they reach the age at which they can safely swallow a solid drug form without the danger of aspirating the drug. Oral syringes are an ideal way to give liquid medications to children, because there is less likelihood of spilling the medication (Figure 32-3). Liquid medications, especially those that stain the teeth, can be taken through a straw. If the patient has been vomiting or is nauseated, an alternative route of administration might be necessary. Always remain with the patient until all of the medication has been swallowed. Procedure 32-1 outlines how to dispense and administer oral medications.

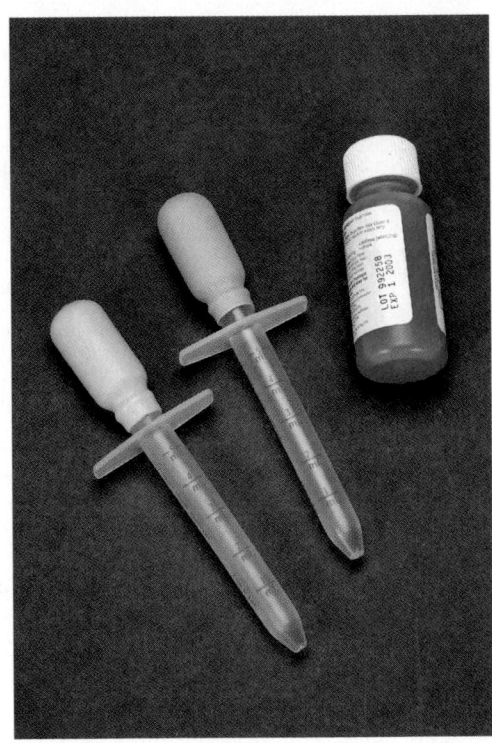

FIGURE 32-3   Sample oral syringes.

Mucous Membrane Forms

Some mucous membranes are selected for their ability to absorb medication for a systemic effect. The most commonly used areas are the gums, cheeks (buccal), under the tongue (sublingual), rectum, and the respiratory mucosa (inhalation). Nasal, ophthalmic, rectal, and vaginal preparations may also be applied to these mucous membranes for their localized effects. Inhalation drugs will be discussed in Chapter 43.

Rectal Administration. The rectal mucosa provides rapid absorption of a drug, even though the surface of the rectum is small. Drugs are absorbed directly into the bloodstream, without being altered as they would be by

PROCEDURE **32-1**

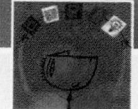

Dispensing and Administering Oral Medications

GOAL: To safely dispense and administer an oral medication to a patient.

EQUIPMENT AND SUPPLIES

- Container of ordered medication
- Medication cup
- Written physician order, including the drug name, strength, dose, and route

PROCEDURAL STEPS

1 Read the order and clarify any questions with the physician.

2 If you are unfamiliar with the drug, refer to the PDR or the package insert to determine the purpose of the drug, common side effects, typical dose, and any pertinent precautions or contraindications. Use the "seven rights" to prevent errors.

3 Perform calculations needed to match the physician's order. Confirm the answer with the physician if there are any questions.

4 Dispense medication in a well-lit, quiet area.
Purpose: To avoid distractions and possible errors.

5 Wash your hands.

6 Compare the order with the label on the container of medicine when you remove it from storage. Check the expiration date on the container and dispose of the medication if it has expired.
Purpose: To check the medication the first of three times.

7 Compare the order with the label on the container of medicine just before dispensing the ordered dose. Make certain that the strength on the label matches the order or that you dispense the correctly calculated dose.
Purpose: To check the medication the second of three times.

TO DISPENSE SOLID ORAL MEDICATIONS

8 Gently tap the prescribed dose into the lid of the medication container. Avoid touching the inside of the lid as well as the medication.
Purpose: Touching the medication or the inside of the container will contaminate the drug.

9 Empty the medication in the container lid into a medicine cup.

TO DISPENSE LIQUID ORAL PREPARATIONS

10 Shake medication well if required.

11 When pouring liquid medications the label should be held in the palm of the hand.

Purpose: To protect the label from medication spills. The medication must be discarded if unable to clearly read the drug label.

12 Place the medicine cup on a flat surface and, at eye level, pour the medication to the prescribed dose mark on the medicine cup (Figure 1).

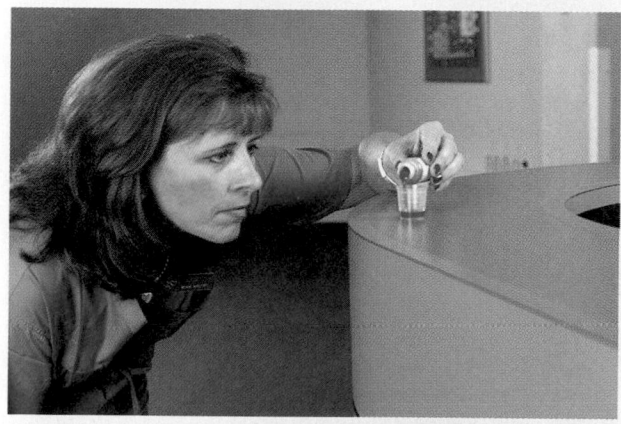

Figure 1

Purpose: At eye level the base of the **meniscus** is where the prescribed dose should be measured.

FOR BOTH SOLID AND LIQUID ORAL MEDICATIONS

13 Recap the container and compare the label and the physician order before replacing the container in storage.
Purpose: To check the medication the third of three times.

14 Transport the medication to the patient.

15 Greet and identify the patient by name.
Purpose: To be sure that you have the right patient.

16 Mention the name of the drug, why it is being given, and ask the patient if she or he has any allergies to the medication.
Purpose: To educate the patient on drug treatment and verify the patient is not allergic to the prescribed medication.

17 If needed, help the patient into a sitting position.

18 Administer the medication with water for tablets, capsules, or caplets. If the patient is receiving liquid medication, offer water after the medication is taken if appropriate. Make sure the patient swallows the entire dose.

PROCEDURE 32-1—Cont'd

19 Conduct patient education on the purpose of the drug, typical side effects, as well as dosage and storage recommendations. Refer to the physician to clarify information if needed.

Purpose: To ensure compliance with home drug therapy and to monitor for side effects.

20 The patient must remain in the office for 20 to 30 minutes after drug administration as a precaution against untoward effects.

21 If the patient experiences any discomfort after taking a medication, the physician should be notified immediately and the incident documented completely and accurately.

22 Wash your hands.

23 Document the administration of the drug, including the date and time; the drug name, dose, strength, and route of administration; any patient side effects; and patient education conducted about the drug.

See Appendix E for a charting example.

---

the digestive processes and without irritation to the patient's gastric mucosa. Rectal medications are useful if the patient is nauseated, vomiting, or unconscious. Manufacturers supply rectal medications in the form of gelatin or cocoa butter–based suppositories, which melt in the warmth of the rectum and release the medication, or in the form of enemas (Figure 32-4). Suppositories may be used to soften the stool or stimulate evacuation of the bowel; enemas are used to cleanse and evacuate the bowel.

The best time to administer a rectal drug intended for a systemic effect is after a bowel movement or enema. The patient should be cautioned to remain lying down for 20 to 30 minutes to prevent accidental evacuation of the drug by a bowel movement or elimination of the enema. Of course, suppositories intended to treat constipation are administered to bring about bowel evacuation. The patient should be instructed to insert the suppository about 2 inches above the rectal sphincter muscles; a little mineral oil or vegetable oil may be used as a lubricant. If suppositories are individually wrapped in foil, make certain the patient knows that the foil is the wrapper and is not part of the treatment.

Vaginal Administration. Vaginal suppositories, tablets, creams, and fluid solutions are used to treat local infections. Irrigating solutions (douches) may be used as antiinfective treatments. Creams and foams are available as local contraceptives. Vaginal instillation is most effective if the patient remains lying down; many preparations are therefore intended to be used at bedtime. The patient may need to wear a pad to absorb drainage. Solid suppositories and tablets may be lubricated or moistened with water and inserted by hand or with an applicator. Creams are instilled with applicators. Prepackaged, disposable irrigation kits are available for douching.

When instructing patients, confirm that the patient can differentiate the urinary meatus from the vaginal orifice and the rectum. Mistakes could result in vaginal infections or in damage or infection to the urinary tract. A simple drawing and explanation may be required.

Oral Administration. Mouth and throat agents come in the form of sprays, swabs, sublingual tablets, and buccal tablets. The mouth and throat membranes may be treated locally with antiseptics for oral hygiene and local infections, with anesthetics for relief of pain, and with astringents that form a protective film over the mucous membranes. The patient may have to gargle, or the area may be painted or sprayed. To paint or spray the throat, first look for the area of inflammation to be treated. Otherwise, the part needing treatment may be missed entirely. Avoid touching the posterior pharynx (back of the throat); this causes gagging and possibly vomiting.

Sublingual (SL) tablets are placed under the tongue, where they are rapidly absorbed into the bloodstream by the rich supply of capillaries. Sublingual absorption is systemic and bypasses the acids in the stomach. Nitroglycerin, used for treating the chest pains of angina pectoris, may be administered sublingually. Patients should not chew or swallow sublingual medications. The patient should be instructed not to smoke, eat, or drink immediately before administration of these drugs. *Buccal* tablets are placed between the cheek and the upper molars and are also quickly absorbed by the oral capillaries.

Nasal Administration. Nose drops, nasal sprays, and tampons are used for their localized effect, but, like the inhalation drugs, they may spill over into the bloodstream, causing a change in the heart rate, an increase in blood pressure, or central nervous system stimulation. Nasal

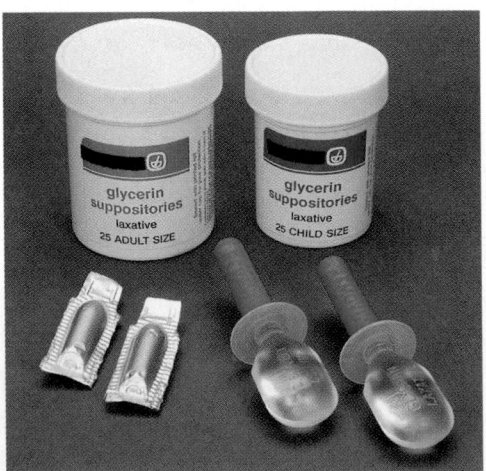

FIGURE 32-4 Sample rectal suppositories.

medications are commonly used for blocked nasal passages (decongestants) and nosebleeds (hemostatics). Instillation of nasal medications will be covered in Chapter 34. Nasal decongestant sprays are often misused by patients. Be sure to teach the patient not to exceed the amount or frequency ordered by the physician. If too much is used, these drugs can dry the mucosa and make congestion worse.

Topical Forms

Topical drugs are usually local in their effect, because most drugs applied to the skin are not designed for systemic effect. Skin medication forms include lotions, liniments, ointments, and transdermal patches. The medical assistant should wear gloves when applying any topical treatment to prevent self-administration of the drug.

Lotions. Often used to control itching, lotions are applied by dabbing with a soft cloth, cotton ball, or tongue blade. Calamine is an example. Some lotions are used to relieve congestion and pain in muscles and joints. After applying the lotion, the area may be covered with a thick cloth to retain heat. However, the therapeutic value of these preparations is controversial. Many believe that the effects of musculoskeletal lotions are limited to the skin surface where the medication is applied.

Liniments. Liniments (emulsions) have a higher portion of oil than do lotions, and volatile active ingredients may be added. Liniments are often used to protect dried, cracked, or fissured skin.

Ointments. Ointments are semisolid medications containing bases such as petrolatum and lanolin, or non greasy bases. Ointments are applied to dry, scaly areas with little or no hair and can exert a prolonged effect. They are used in small amounts and are applied with firm strokes to avoid increasing itchiness. Ointments that stain clothing should be covered. An ointment should be removed from a jar or tube with a tongue blade to prevent contamination of the remaining medication.

Transdermal Patches. Certain medications can be absorbed slowly through the skin to create a constant, time-released systemic effect (Figure 32-5). The nitroglycerin patch is particularly useful for patients with frequent attacks of angina. Hormone patches, mainly estrogen, can also be absorbed slowly through the skin, providing the needed hormonal levels to women. With dermal patches, drugs can be administered in a time-released manner for up to 3 days. The date and time the patch was applied should be written on the patch as well as documented in the patient's record.

- Rotate sites to prevent skin irritation. Follow package insert directions on where to apply the patch, avoiding scars and areas with a great deal of body hair.
- Keep the old patch on for 30 minutes after applying the new patch to maintain blood levels of the medication.
- Dispose of used patches appropriately, because the old patch may still contain some of the medication.

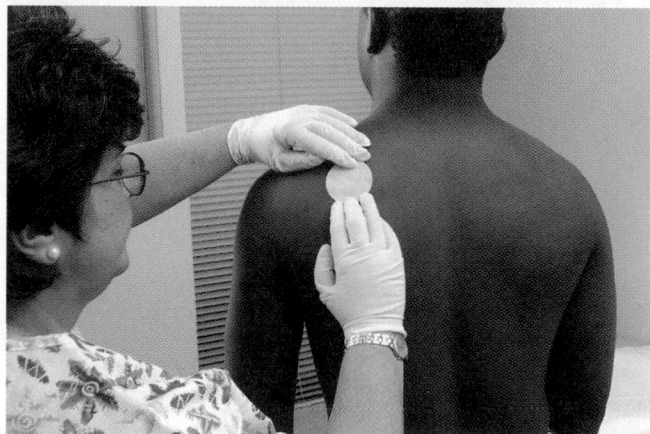

FIGURE 32-5 Transdermal patch.

Parenteral Medication Forms

Injectable medications must be sterile and in liquid form. The medications may come in an ampule, a single-dose vial, or a multidose vial (Figure 32-6). The drug is usually in a solution that is minimally irritating to human tissues, such as physiological saline solution or sterile water, and may contain a preservative or a small amount of antibiotic to prevent bacterial growth in the vial. All injectable medications are dated. Before use, check the expiration date and examine the solution for possible deterioration. If the medication is discolored or there is any sediment on the bottom of the vial, the vial should be discarded. A parenteral medication is administered with a sterile syringe and needle. Occupational Safety and Health Administration (OSHA) guidelines must be followed when using any sharp—including all types of needles—because every needle used on a patient is contaminated with blood and body fluids. A medical assistant must wear disposable gloves when administering parenteral injections, immediately dispose of the needle/syringe unit into a sharps container after use, and never recap or bend needles. *always*

Ampule. An ampule is a small **hermetically sealed** glass flask, usually containing a single dose of medication. Ampules have a neck with a scored weak point that is broken just before use (see Figure 32-6, *A*). Procedure 32-2 explains the special technique required for opening an ampule of medication and withdrawing medication for administration.

PATIENT TEACHING RECOMMENDATIONS FOR TRANSDERMAL PATCHES

- The patient may shower with the patch in place.
- If the patch is to remain on for 24 hours, apply a new patch at the same time every day.

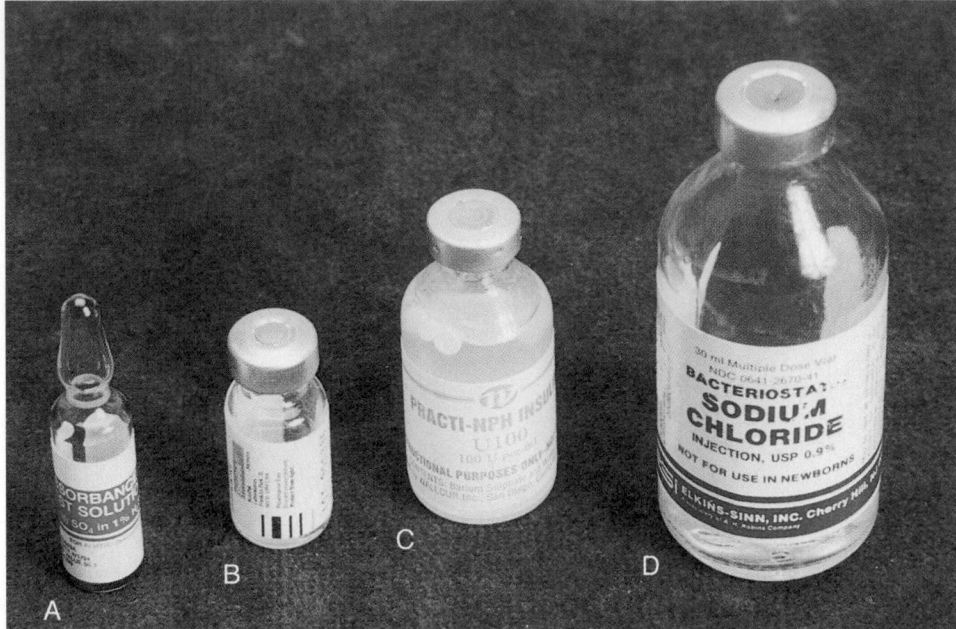

FIGURE 32-6 **A**, Ampule. **B**, Single-dose vial. **C** and **D**, Multidose vials.

PROCEDURE **32-2**

Filling a Syringe Using an Ampule

GOAL: To correctly and safely remove medication for administration from a glass ampule.

EQUIPMENT AND SUPPLIES

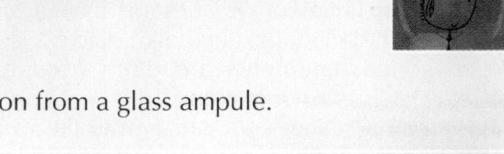

- Syringe/needle unit
- Filter needle
- Sterile gauze squares
- Sharps container
- Biohazard waste container
- Medication ampule
- Physician order
- Alcohol squares
- Disposable gloves

PROCEDURAL STEPS

1 Review physician's medication order for clarity. If unfamiliar with the drug, look it up in a reference book.

Purpose: The medical assistant should never dispense or administer a drug without making sure the physician order is legible and the details of the drug are known.

2 Wash hands and assemble equipment.

3 Perform medication label and physician order check when removing the ampule from storage. Check the expiration date on the ampule.

Purpose: To complete the first check of the order.

4 Gently tap the top of the ampule with your fingers to settle all the medication to the bottom portion of the flask (Figure 1).

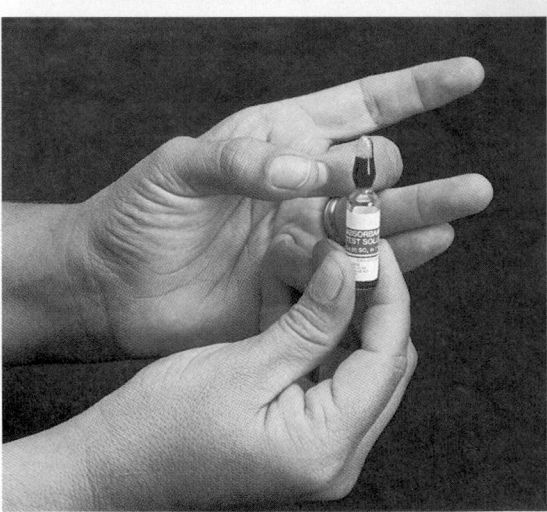

Figure 1

5 Thoroughly disinfect the neck of the ampule with alcohol squares. Check the label against the order a second time.

Purpose: Disinfection is done to prevent possible contamination of the medication.

6 Wrap the top of the ampule with a gauze square to protect yourself from the glass. Hold the covered ampule between your thumb and finger, in front of you and above waist level (Figure 2).

PROCEDURE 32-2—Cont'd

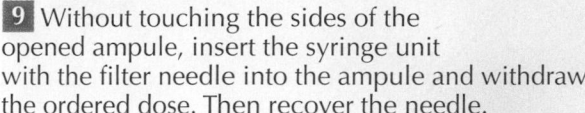

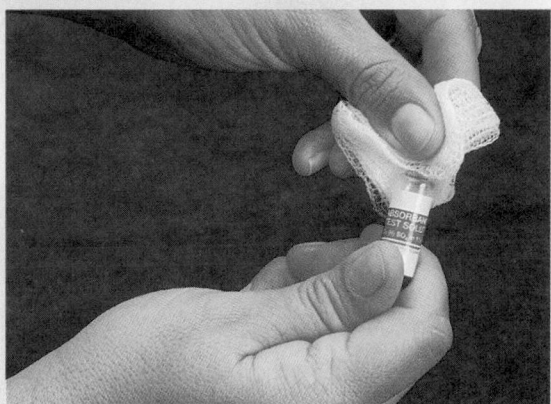

Figure 2

Purpose: To protect your fingers and maintain eye contact with the medication ampule at all times.

7 Push the top of the ampule away from your body to break the neck. You will hear a pop because the ampule is vacuum sealed. The glass is designed not to shatter, and the medication will not spill out. Dispose of the glass top in the sharps container.

8 Open the sterile syringe/needle unit. Touching the needle covers only, unscrew the needle from the syringe, place it on the counter, and attach the sterile filter needle.

Purpose: Must maintain the sterility of the unit, so only touch the needle covers. The filter needle is needed to withdraw the medication from the

ampule to prevent the accidental aspiration of glass fragments into the injection unit.

9 Without touching the sides of the opened ampule, insert the syringe unit with the filter needle into the ampule and withdraw the ordered dose. Then recover the needle.

10 Before discarding the ampule in the sharps container, check the physician order against the label one more time to complete the three label checks.

11 Change the filter needle, safeguarding the sterility of the injection unit, for an appropriate length and gauge needle based on the physician ordered route of administration and patient characteristics. Discard the used filter needle into the sharps container.

Purpose: A new needle is applied to prevent the possible injection of glass particles on or inside the filter needle.

12 Dispose of used alcohol and gauze squares.

13 Transport ordered medication in the injection unit to the patient. Identify the patient. Apply gloves and administer the medication as ordered. Discard the used syringe unit into a sharps container in the patient room. Remove gloves and discard in biohazard waste container and wash hands.

14 Answer patient questions and document the procedure in the patient chart.

Single-Dose Vial. A single-dose vial is a small bottle with a rubber stopper through which you insert a sterile needle to withdraw the single dose of medication inside. Before a sterile syringe and needle unit can be introduced into the solution, the rubber stopper must be wiped in a circular motion with alcohol or another suitable disinfectant.

Multidose Vial. A multidose vial is a bottle with a rubber stopper that contains enough medication for multiple injections. Because multidose vials are used more than once, extreme caution must be taken every time a needle is inserted into the medication to protect the medication from contamination, which could cause very serious infections in future patients. If at any time you feel that an error has been made or you suspect possible contamination, discard the vial. Never return unused medication to the vial. Learn to withdraw fluids to the correct mark. If you have more medication than you need in the syringe, eject the excess after you remove the unit from the vial. Vials are vacuum sealed. Each time you withdraw medication from a vial, you must first replace the portion of withdrawn medication

with the same portion of air. Not enough replaced air will make it difficult to withdraw the medication; too much replaced air will increase the pressure within the vial and force the medication into the syringe without your having to pull back on the plunger.

Prefilled Syringe. A prefilled syringe is a sterile, disposable syringe and needle unit packaged by the manufacturer with a single dose of medication that is ready to administer.

Cartridge Injection System. A cartridge injection system is a prefilled syringe and needle that is loaded into a metal or plastic cartridge (Figure 32-7). The same cartridge loader can be used repeatedly.

Parenteral Medication Equipment

Syringes and needles are manufactured in countless varieties for specific purposes and sometimes for specific medications. For example, there is a special syringe for insulin. Hypodermic needles are manufactured in many lengths and widths, depending on the depth needed, the **viscosity** of the medication to be injected, the ordered

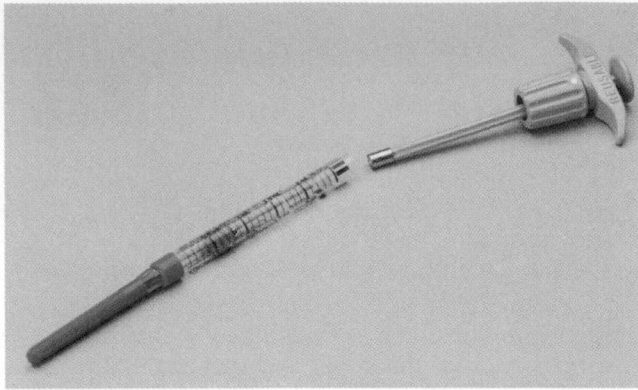

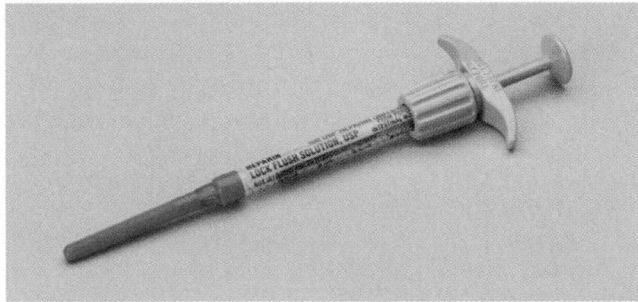

FIGURE 32-7 The Tubex injector system with disposable sterile medication cartridge.

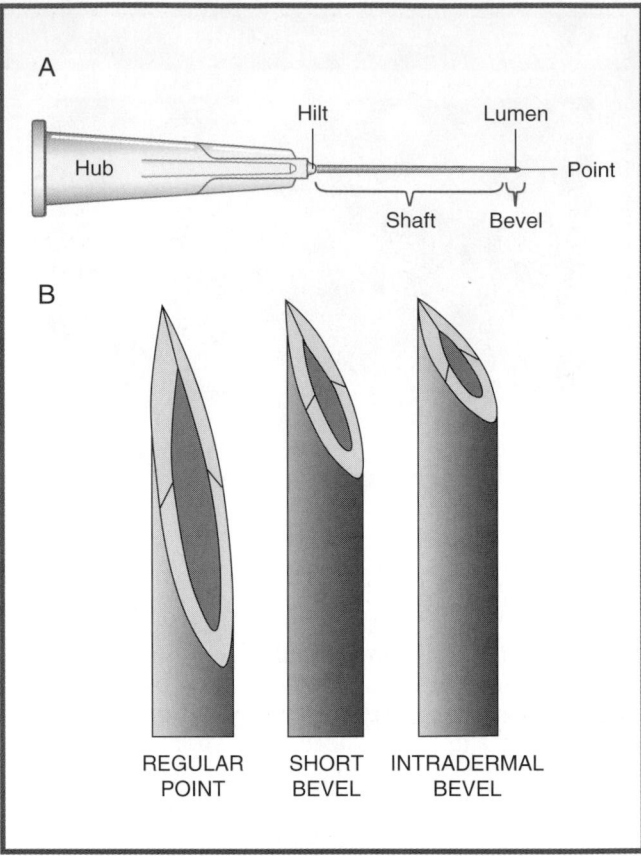

FIGURE 32-8 **A**, The construction of a hypodermic needle. **B**, Needle points. (**A** From Bonewit-West K: *Clinical procedures for medical assistants*, ed. 5. Philadelphia, 2000, WB Saunders.)

route of administration, and patient characteristics. Needles may be purchased separately or as part of a needle-syringe unit. Figure 32-8 shows the construction of a needle and the three common types of **bevel** points. Needles are measured for length from where the cannula/shaft joins the hub to the tip of the (needle) point.

Needle Gauge. The diameter or lumen size of a needle is called its *gauge*, and needle gauges range in size from 14 (the largest) to 28 (the smallest). *The larger the gauge number, the smaller the diameter of the needle.* The smallest gauges (27 to 28) are used for intradermal injections when a very small opening is desired. These fine needle widths leave a small amount of medication just below the surface of the skin, with a minimum amount of injury. Gauges 25 and 26 are commonly used for subcutaneous injections. With a medication that is in an aqueous solution and is easily injected through a small opening, these two gauges cause minimal tissue damage, and the patient experiences less pain. Larger needles (gauges 20 to 23) are usually necessary for intramuscular injections when the medication is thick, such as penicillin, or the length of the needle requires the extra support of a thicker gauge. A patient cannot feel the difference between a 20- and a 22-gauge needle. In fact, the medication is not forced as strongly into the tissues with the larger 20-gauge needle as with the 22-gauge one, and the patient actually experiences less pain. Needles larger than 20-gauge are not used for drug therapy. They are mostly used for venipuncture, blood donations, and blood transfusions.

Needle Length. The choices of needle lengths vary from 3/8 inch to 4 inches, depending on the area of the body to be injected and the route (depth) used. Intradermal injections require only the short 3/8-inch

needle. Needles that are 1/2 or 5/8 inch long are used for subcutaneous injections. Longer needles are necessary for depositing drugs intramuscularly. The choice of a 1-inch, 1 1/2-inch, 2-inch, 2 1/2-inch or 3-inch length depends on both the muscle being used and the size of the patient.

Syringes. Figure 32-9 illustrates the construction of a 3.0-ml and a 5.0-ml syringe. The parts of a syringe are its barrel, a calibrated scale (or scales), plunger, and tip. *Regular* syringes that hold up to 3.0 ml are usually calibrated with two scales: ml (cc) and minims. Larger *regular* syringes are calibrated in milliliters only. The *tuberculin* syringe is used for small quantities of drug, because it holds only up to 1.0 ml of injectable material. The *insulin* syringe is calibrated in units specifically for diabetic use. Insulin syringes are calibrated to hold either 50 U or 100 U of insulin. The type of calibration chosen depends on the total amount of insulin that is to be injected in one dose.

Disposable syringe and needle units are packaged in either sealed, rigid plastic containers or in peel-apart paper wrappers. Both individual needles and syringe-needle units are color coded for easy identification (Figure 32-10). Table 32-1 summarizes the needle and syringe sizes used for injections. With the establishment of standard precautions and the danger of needlesticks, syringes with retractable needle covers have been developed and must be made available to employees as an OSHA safeguard against

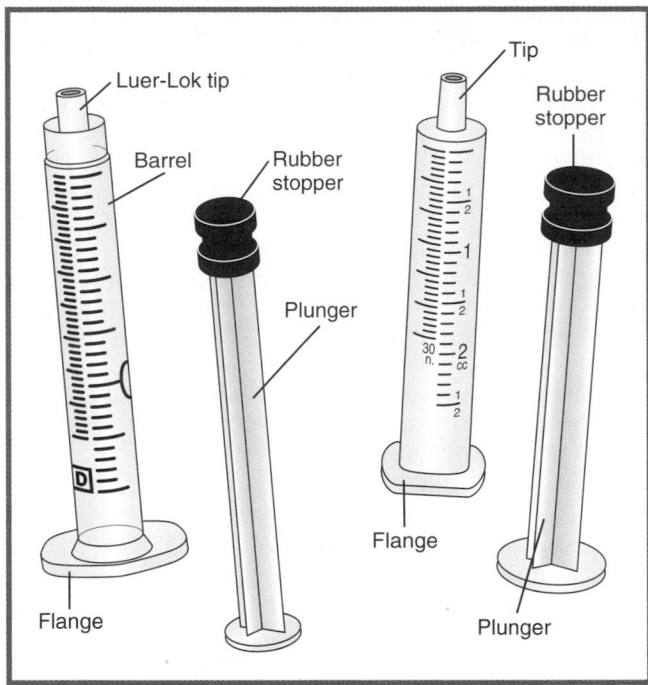

FIGURE 32-9 Parts of a syringe.

themselves injections that do not require needle disposal. One of the possible answers is the injector pen. There are different types available, depending on the amount of medication to be dispensed per injection and the type of medication being used. Administering insulin away from home has become easier with the development of the Nova Pen (Figure 32-11). It contains a predetermined type and amount of insulin that can be injected by the diabetic patient with minimal preparation.

In addition, there are EpiPens available that are automatic injector systems that contain a dose of epinephrine (Figure 32-12). These must be prescribed by the physician and come packaged with the correct dose for either an adult (0.3 mg of epinephrine) or child (0.15 mg of epinephrine). They are carried as a safety precaution by individuals who have anaphylactic reactions to such allergens as bee stings or certain types of foods. Anaphylactic reactions can be fatal if not treated immediately, so patients or their family members should be educated on the signs and symptoms of anaphylaxis and how to manage the EpiPen administration.

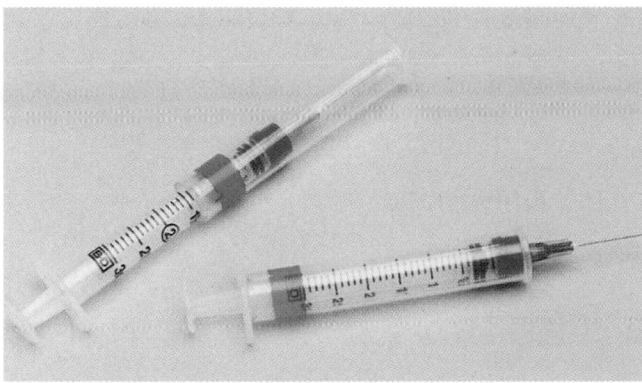

FIGURE 32-10 Disposable syringe with retractable needle cover.

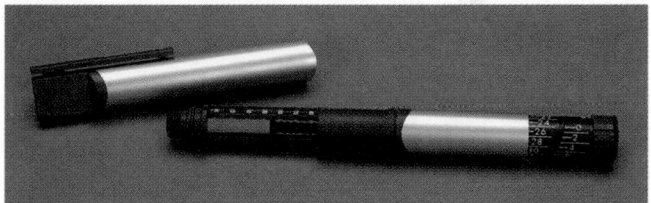

FIGURE 32-11 Nova Pen.

accidental needlesticks. A sample of one type of retractable needle cover is seen in Figure 32-10.

Specialty Syringe Units. With all of the concerns regarding needlesticks, proper disposal of needles, and cross-contamination of individuals through needle misuse, there are now devices available for patients who must give

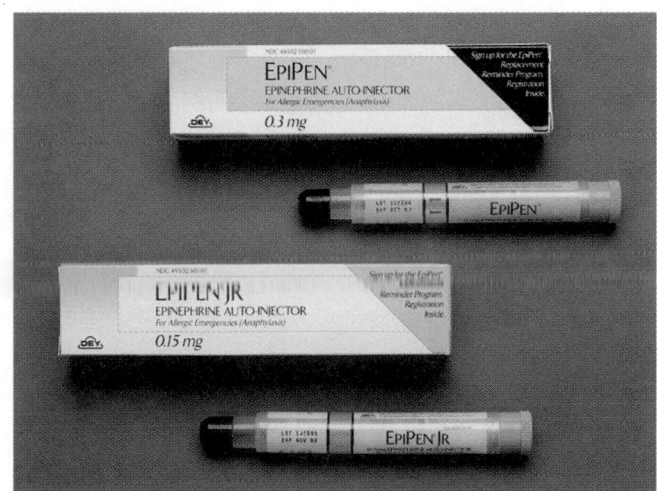

FIGURE 32-12 EpiPen prepackaged autoinjector.

TABLE 32-1	Needle and Syringe Sizes for Injections		
Route	**Gauge**	**Length (inches)**	**Syringe**
Intradermal	27-28	$3/8$	1 ml tuberculin
Subcutaneous	25-26	$1/2$, $5/8$	2 ml; tuberculin; insulin
Intramuscular	20-23	1-3	2-5 ml

The steps for EpiPen injection are quite simple:

1. Pull back the gray end of the autoinjector. This sets the device for use.
2. The injector can go through clothing, so firmly press the black tip on the outer aspect of the thigh and hold in place for 10 seconds. The injector automatically administers the prepackaged dose.
3. Remove the EpiPen and massage the injection area for a few minutes to promote absorption of the epinephrine.
4. The patient should still call a physician or go to the emergency department of a nearby hospital for follow-up care.
5. It is important that patients or family members periodically check the expiration date of the auto-injector device. If the device is near its expiration date, another prescription should be filled and the old unused device discarded. To be of service in an emergency, the EpiPen must be readily available at all times.

SIGNS AND SYMPTOMS OF AN ANAPHYLACTIC REACTION

- **Hypotension** resulting from systemic **vasodilation**
- Hives
- Difficulty breathing due to **bronchoconstriction**
- Difficulty swallowing due to **edema**
- Vomiting and diarrhea

Parenteral Administration

With practice, giving medications by injection will become easy and even automatic, but a medical assistant must always follow the physician's orders, the three order and label checks while dispensing the medication, and the seven rights throughout the procedure.

Develop techniques that provide maximum safety and comfort for the patient. Injections are least painful when the needle is inserted swiftly, the medication is injected slowly, and the needle is removed quickly. Remember that the same aseptic conditions necessary for minor surgery are necessary whenever you penetrate the protective skin barrier.

Injections are not given near bones or blood vessels. Injections should never be given in an area where there is scar tissue, a change in skin pigmentation or texture, or excess tissue growth, such as a mole or a wart. The point of injection should be as far as possible from any major nerve, and the site selected should be capable of holding the amount of medication that is injected.

Make certain that all materials are ready for use. Many offices have a central room where medications are prepared. The medication is then taken to the waiting patient in another room. Handling medication administration in this way has many advantages, but care must be taken that the syringe and needle unit are transported with sterile technique. After a syringe is filled, the cap is replaced for transport to the patient. Never transport more than one injection at a time, unless two or more are for the same patient or unless you have a special medication tray that has a named position for each syringe. Never combine two medications in a single syringe unless specifically ordered to do so by the physician. If you are preparing a medication for the physician to give, place the vial or empty ampule beside the filled syringe. This shows what medication is in the syringe and offers a double check (Procedure 32-3).

INTERACTION WITH A PATIENT WHEN GIVING AN INJECTION

1. Use a professional approach and tell the patient what you are going to do.
2. Small talk can keep the patient's mind off the procedure.
3. Never tell a patient that it will not hurt; you may destroy your credibility.
4. Make the patient as comfortable as possible, and allow for privacy.
5. Never allow the patient to stand during the procedure.
6. Keep the equipment out of the patient's sight as much as possible.
7. Wear gloves and other blood and body fluid protection barriers.
8. Immediately dispose of the contaminated needle in a sharps container.
9. *NEVER* recap a contaminated needle, but use retractable needle covers when they are available.
10. Wash your hands before and after the procedure.

Intradermal Injections. Intradermal (ID) injections are given *within the skin layers* (Figure 32-13 and Procedure 32-4). The ID site is used for allergy testing and tuberculin screening. One method of tuberculin screening is the tine test, which is administered with individually packaged disposable sterile stamps with four or six prongs on the end that have been treated with tuberculin solution (Procedure 32-5). The tine test, however, is not as accurate as the Mantoux (purified protein derivative [PPD]) intradermal screening test. With the Mantoux test, a 0.1 ml solution of PPD is injected into the intradermal layers. The site is then monitored after 48 to 72 hours. The result is considered positive if the **induration** is more than 10 mm in diameter. Patients may either be given a postcard with pictures having accurate measurements of indurations that can be sent back to the office, or they may be instructed to return to the office after the specified period for the staff to read the results (see Procedure 32-4, Figure 1).

PROCEDURE 32-3

Filling a Syringe Using a Vial

GOAL: To fill a syringe from a multidose vial, using sterile technique.

EQUIPMENT AND SUPPLIES

- Multidose vial containing the material to be injected
- Alcohol wipes
- Sterile needle and syringe unit
- Written order, including the drug name, strength, and route

PROCEDURAL STEPS

1 Wash your hands.

2 Read the order and choose the correct vial of medication.

Purpose: To check the medication the first of three times.

3 Choose the correct syringe and needle size, depending on the site and the quantity of medication to be injected (Figure 1).

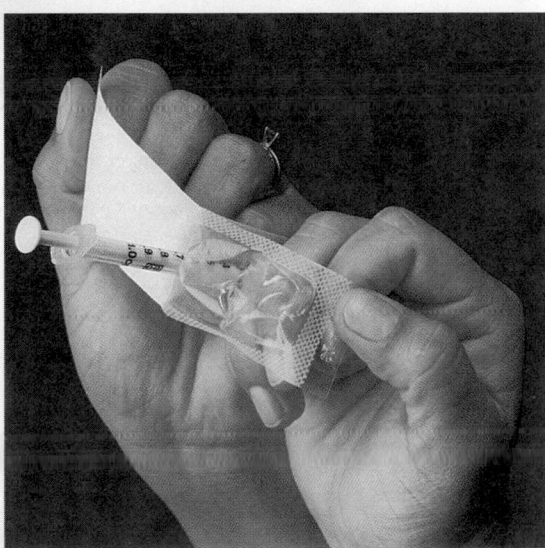

Figure 1

4 Compare the order with both the name of the drug on the vial of medication and the amount to be withdrawn in the syringe.

Purpose: To check the medication the second of three times.

5 Gently agitate the medication by rolling the vial between your palms (Figure 2).

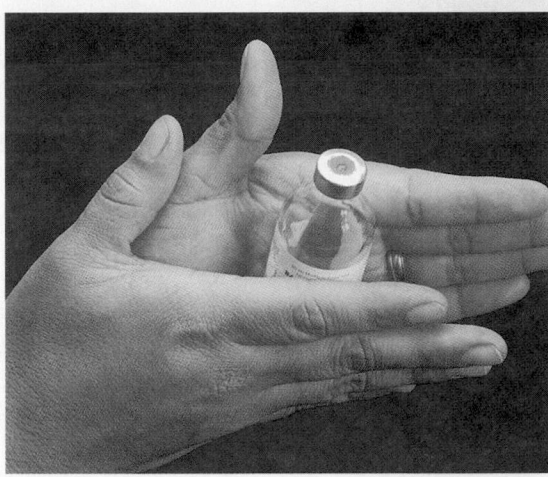

Figure 2

Purpose: To mix any medication that may have settled.

6 Check the quality of the medication and the expiration date.

Purpose: Dispose of the medication if it appears contaminated or is outdated.

7 Cleanse the rubber stopper of the vial with the alcohol wipe, using a circular motion (Figure 3). Place the vial on a secure flat surface, leaving the alcohol swab over the rubber stopper.

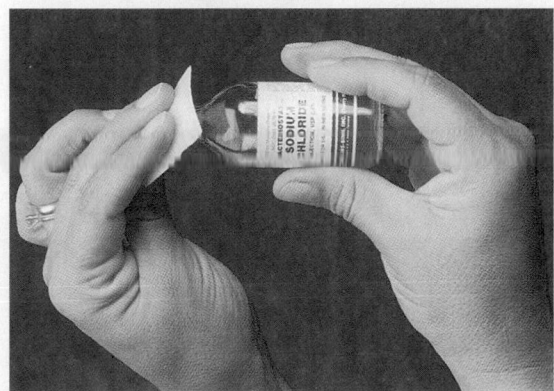

Figure 3

8 Grasp the syringe plunger and draw up an amount of air equal to the amount of medication ordered.

Purpose: Not enough replaced air will make it difficult to withdraw the medication; too much replaced air will force the medication into the syringe without pulling on the plunger to withdraw it.

PROCEDURE 32-3—Cont'd

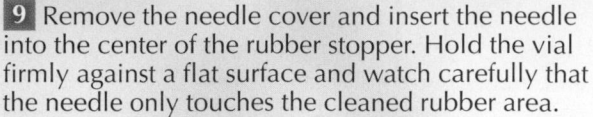

9 Remove the needle cover and insert the needle into the center of the rubber stopper. Hold the vial firmly against a flat surface and watch carefully that the needle only touches the cleaned rubber area.

10 Inject the aspirated air in the syringe into the vial.

11 Pick the vial and syringe unit up and invert it. Slowly pull back on the plunger with the unit at eye level until the proper amount of medication is withdrawn.

Purpose: Withdrawing medication rapidly will cause air bubbles to form in the syringe.

12 While the needle is still in the vial, check that there are no air bubbles in the syringe.

Purpose: Air bubbles displace medication, and the patient will not receive the proper amount of medication.

13 If there are air bubbles, slip the fingers holding the vial down to grasp the vial and syringe as a single unit.

Purpose: This frees your dominant hand.

14 With your free hand, tap the syringe until the air bubbles dislodge and float into the tip of the syringe.

15 Gently expel these tiny air bubbles through the needle, then continue withdrawing the medication.

16 Withdraw the needle from the vial, and replace the cover over the needle without the needle touching the sides.

17 Return the medication to the shelf or the refrigerator, checking that you have the correct drug and dosage.

Purpose: This is the third of the three drug label and order checks.

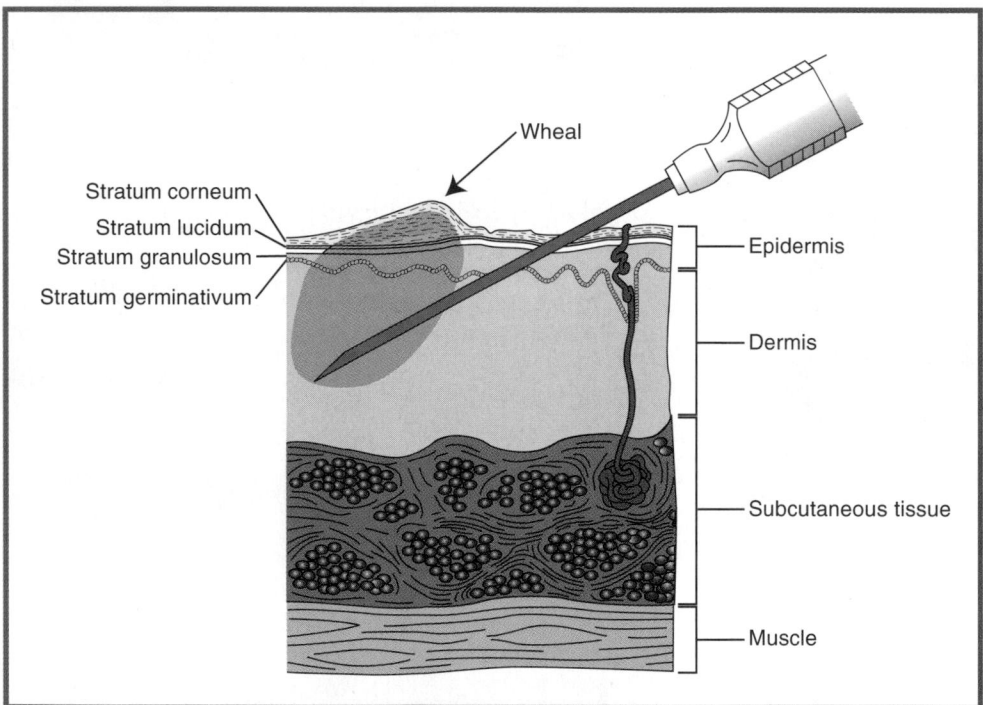

FIGURE 32-13 The intradermal injection is administered just under the epidermis. The drug is dispersed in an area where many nerves are present; thus, it causes momentary burning or stinging. Minute amounts of medication are injected. This method is used to test for allergies, drug sensitivities, and susceptibility to some diseases.

CRITICAL THINKING APPLICATION

Dorothy is ordered to give her first Mantoux test since being hired by Dr. Thau. Document below the details that Dorothy should include on the patient's chart. She administered 0.1 ml of purified protein derivative by ID injection into the patient's right mid-forearm and instructed the patient on how to read the results of the test and send the accompanying postcard back into the office.

When an ID injection is correctly administered, a small **wheal** is raised on the skin. A 3/8-inch, 27- or 28-gauge needle is used for ID injections. The angle of insertion is 15 degrees, almost parallel to the skin surface. The best site for injection is the center of the anterior forearm, but the upper chest and back are frequently used for allergy testing (Figure 32-14). Allergy testing will be discussed in Chapter 35.

Subcutaneous Injections. Subcutaneous injections (SC) are given just under the skin, into the fatty areolar layer called *adipose tissue* (Figure 32-15 and Procedure 32-6). Smaller doses of less irritating drugs are given by this method. The angle of insertion is 45 degrees;

PROCEDURE 32-4

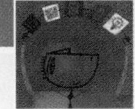

Giving an Intradermal Injection

GOAL: To inject 0.1 ml of purified protein derivative (PPD) to perform a Mantoux test as ordered by the physician.

EQUIPMENT AND SUPPLIES

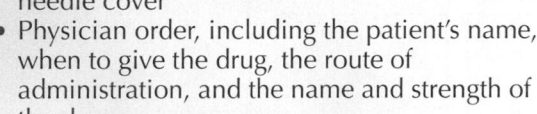

- Vial of tuberculin PPD
- Alcohol wipes
- 27-gauge, ⅜-inch sterile needle and syringe unit with retractable needle cover
- Physician order, including the patient's name, when to give the drug, the route of administration, and the name and strength of the drug
- Disposable gloves
- Gauze squares
- Sharps container

PROCEDURAL STEPS

1 Wash your hands. Follow standard precautions. Don nonsterile gloves.

2 Select the correct medication from the shelf or the refrigerator.
   Purpose: Some medications must be refrigerated.

3 Read the label to be sure that you have the right drug and the right strength. Perform the three label and order checks as the medication is dispensed.
   Purpose: Confirm that the medication label matches the physician's order. One medication may be manufactured and prepackaged in different strengths; for instance, an allergen may be available in 1:1000, 1:100, or 1:10 dilutions.

4 Warm refrigerated medications by gently rolling the container between your palms.

5 Prepare the syringe as described in Procedure 32-3, withdrawing the right dose.

6 Transport the medication to the patient.

7 Greet and identify the patient by name.
   Purpose: To be sure that you have the right patient.

8 Apply gloves and position the patient comfortably.

9 Locate the antecubital space, then find a site several fingerwidths down the anterior aspect of the forearm. Avoid any scarred, discolored, or pigmented areas.

10 Cleanse the patient's skin with an alcohol wipe using a circular motion, moving from the center outward.

11 Allow the antiseptic to dry.

12 Remove the cap from the needle.

13 With the thumb and first two fingers of your nondominant hand, stretch the skin of the forearm apart and taut.
   Purpose: Stretching the skin facilitates the insertion of the needle with minimal discomfort to the patient.

14 Grasp the syringe between the thumb and first two fingers of your dominant hand, palm down, with the needle bevel upward. Hold the syringe close to the plunger end.

15 At a 15-degree angle, carefully insert the needle through the skin just until the bevel point is under the skin surface.

16 Slowly and steadily inject the medication by depressing the plunger with your little finger. A wheal should appear.
   Purpose: A rapid injection may force the substance through to the surface.

17 After administering all of the medication, withdraw the needle.

18 Immediately slide the retractable cover over the contaminated needle and dispose of the syringe unit into a sharps container.

19 Do not massage but you may blot the area with a cotton ball or gauze square.
   Purpose: Massaging will disturb the wheal and interfere with intended results.

20 Make sure that your patient is comfortable and safe.

21 Observe the patient for any adverse reaction.

22 Dispose of the gloves in the biohazard container and wash your hands.

23 Record the procedure and any reactions that occurred at the site of the injection on the patient's medical record. Include the exact site of the injection
   Purpose: A procedure is not considered done until it is recorded. The exact site must be known to monitor reactions to the PPD in 48 to 72 hours.

24 Tell the patient when to return to the office for any reaction to be read, or give the patient a postcard to be completed and returned.
   Purpose: Patient education must be done to get intended results.

Continued

PROCEDURE **32-4—Cont'd**

READING THE MANTOUX TEST RESULTS

25 Apply latex gloves; using good lighting and with the patient's arm slightly flexed, measure the induration at the site of the injection.

Purpose: A positive Mantoux reaction occurs if the induration is inflamed, raised, and larger than 10 mm (Figure 1). Further diagnostic tests are ordered to either rule out or confirm the diagnosis of tuberculosis. These will be discussed in Chapter 43.

26 Discard the gloves in the biohazard waste container and wash your hands.

27 Document the results of the Mantoux test in the patient chart, including a complete description of the size of the induration, if any, and the appearance of the test site.

See Appendix E for a charting example.

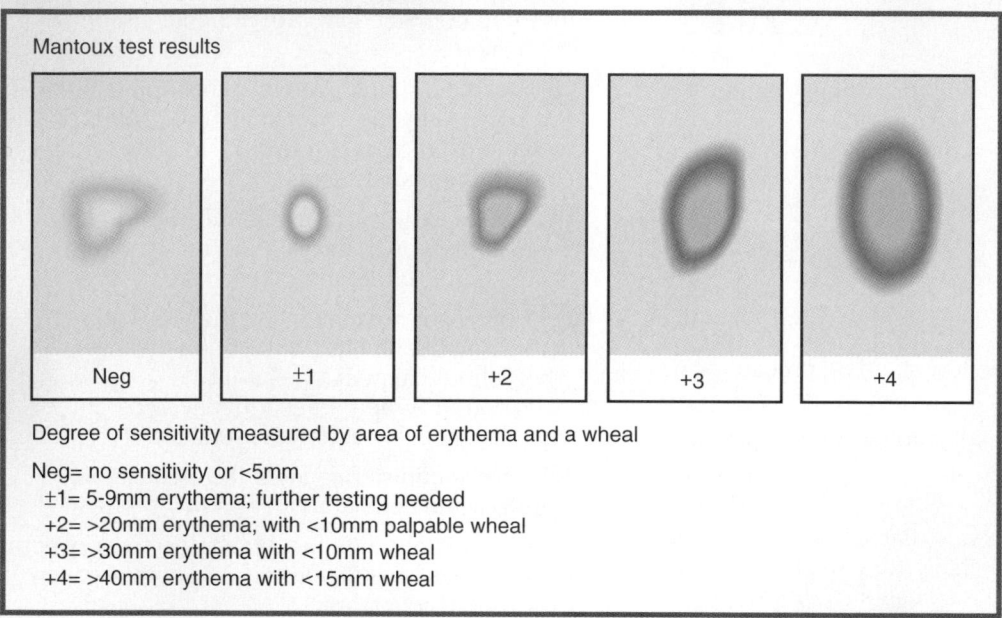

Mantoux test results

| Neg | ±1 | +2 | +3 | +4 |

Degree of sensitivity measured by area of erythema and a wheal

Neg= no sensitivity or <5mm
±1= 5-9mm erythema; further testing needed
+2= >20mm erythema; with <10mm palpable wheal
+3= >30mm erythema with <10mm wheal
+4= >40mm erythema with <15mm wheal

Figure 1

however, heparin and insulin are usually administered at a 90-degree angle. The posterior upper arm is the typical injection site, however, the abdomen, thigh, and upper back may be used (Figure 32-16). When multiple or frequent injections are ordered, such as routine insulin injections, the sites must be rotated to prevent tissue damage and problems with absorption of the medication. It is best to keep a rotation record (Figure 32-17).

INSULIN ADMINISTRATION GUIDELINES

- Typically more than one type of insulin is ordered for immediate administration. Check labels carefully and follow office policy in mixing insulins in the same syringe.
- Insulin is always ordered in unit amounts. Use the appropriate insulin syringe, either 50 U or 100 U, depending on the total amount of insulin ordered.

- Insulin should be stored in the refrigerator and gently rotated between hands to warm before dispensing.
- Do not massage the site after injection.

Intramuscular Injections. Intramuscular (IM) injections are given into the muscle when (1) drugs will irritate the subcutaneous tissues, (2) a more rapid absorption is desired, or (3) the volume of the medication to be injected is large. The angle of insertion is 90 degrees (Figure 32-18), and the preferred sites are the *gluteus medius, vastus lateralis, deltoid, and ventrogluteal* muscles of the adult (Figure 32-19) and the *vastus lateralis* of the infant and child. It is important to select a needle that is long enough so that the medication is not deposited into the upper adipose (fatty) tissue by error. Fatty tissue does not absorb medications well, and the medication may remain at the site of the injection. Be certain to select needles that are long enough, especially for obese patients. The recommended gauge is 20- to 23-gauge, and the length of the needle could be from 1 to 3 inches, depending on the size of the patient.

PROCEDURE 32-5

Administering a Tuberculin Tine Test

GOAL: To perform a tuberculin tine test.

EQUIPMENT AND SUPPLIES

- Tuberculin tine test stamp
- Alcohol wipe
- Disposable gloves
- Sharps container
- Physician's order

PROCEDURAL STEPS

1 Wash your hands. Follow standard precautions.

2 Greet the patient and verify patient name.

3 Explain the procedure.

4 Position the patient to reduce strain on the forearm. Use the same site as described in Procedure 32-4.

5 Cleanse the site with the alcohol wipe in a circular fashion from the inside outward. Allow alcohol to dry. Glove with disposable nonsterile gloves.

6 Pull the site taut with the nondominant thumb and fingers.

7 Press the prongs of the tine firmly against the cleansed area for 1 to 2 seconds (Figure 1*).

8 Immediately discard the stamp into the sharps container.

9 Do not massage the area.

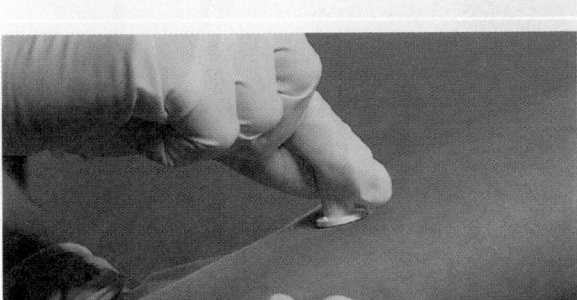

Figure 1

10 Dispose of the gloves in the biohazard container and wash your hands.

11 Observe the patient for untoward reactions and document the procedure, including the name of the test, time of administration, exact site of administration, and any patient complaints.

12 Instruct the patient to return to the office in 48 to 72 hours to have the results read, or explain how to read results at home.

See Appendix E for a charting example.
*Figure from Bonewit-West K: *Clinical procedures for medical assistants*, ed. 5. Philadelphia, 2000, WB Saunders.

In adults, the deltoid region can hold up to 2 ml of medication, whereas the vastus lateralis and gluteal sites can contain up to 5 ml. Infants and children should be given no more than 2 ml in the vastus lateralis or ventrogluteal sites.

When locating a site for an IM injection, expose the site so that you are able to visualize and palpate the landmarks correctly. Table 32-2 lists the sites as well as the criteria for choosing one site over another (Procedure 32-7).

Deltoid Site. The deltoid muscle, the muscular cap of the shoulder, is located at the top of the upper arm. The muscle mass is somewhat limited, so it cannot hold a large volume of medication. This triangular muscle is located between the acromion and deltoid tuberosities and the injection site is approximately two fingerbreadths below the acromial process (Figure 32-20). The major nerves and blood vessels located in the posterior portion of the arm must be avoided. Aqueous medications are most appropriate here, for example, vitamin B_{12}.

If frequent injections are ordered, rotate the site and alternate the right and left arm. The deltoid site is acceptable for adults and older children, but it should not be used when the muscle is small or underdeveloped. For a small arm, you may need only a 25-gauge $5/8$-inch needle; the 23-gauge 1-inch needle is most often used for an average-sized arm. The patient may be seated or lying down. When injecting, expose the entire shoulder rather than rolling up the sleeve. Grasp the muscle and stretch the skin before injecting the medication.

Vastus Lateralis (Thigh) Site. The vastus lateralis muscle is part of the *quadriceps group* of the thigh. It is one of the body's largest muscles, and because it is developed at birth, it is considered the safest IM injection site for infants. Many experts believe that as a site for adult IM injections, the vastus lateralis is better than either the deltoid or the dorsogluteal sites, because there are fewer major nerves and blood vessels in the vastus lateralis. The vastus lateralis muscle fills the midportion of the upper, outer thigh. In an adult, it can be located from one hand's width below the proximal end of the *greater trochanter* to one hand's width above the top of

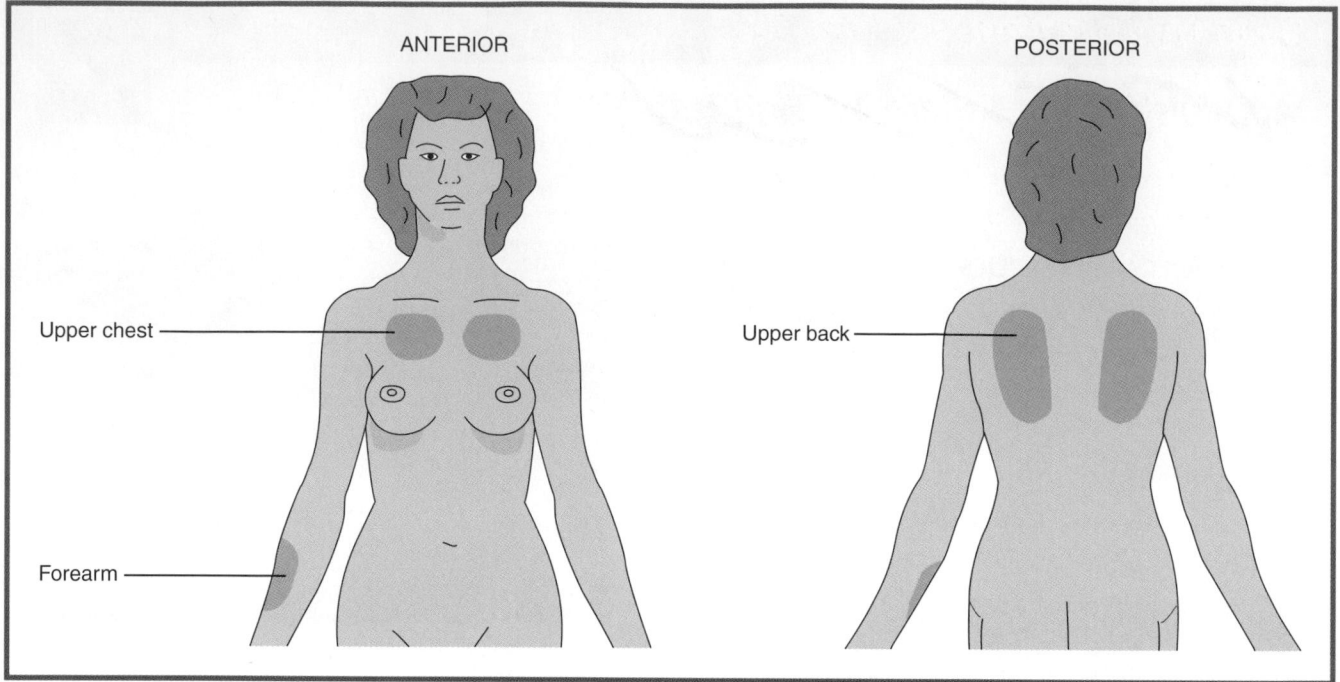

ANTERIOR   POSTERIOR

Upper chest —

Forearm —

Upper back —

FIGURE 32-14 Sites recommended for intradermal injections.

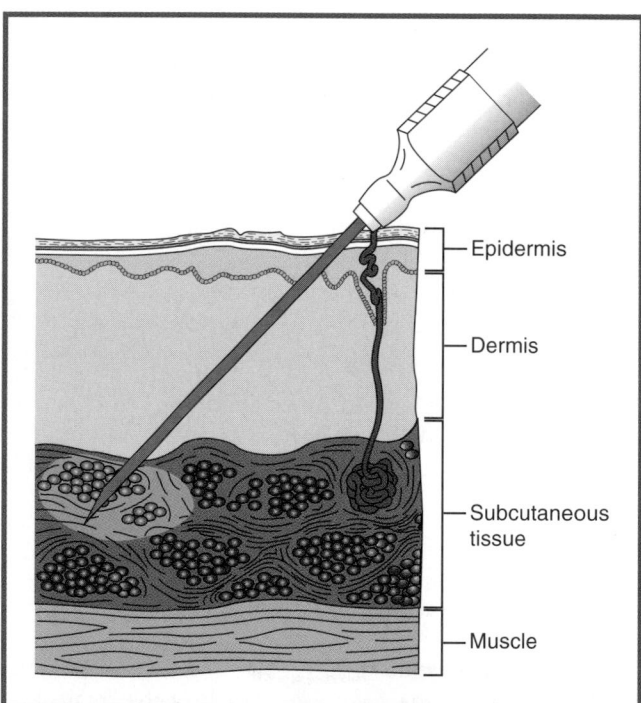

— Epidermis

— Dermis

— Subcutaneous tissue

— Muscle

FIGURE 32-15 The subcutaneous injection is administered with a 25- or 26-gauge, ½- or ⅝-inch needle. The method is used for small amounts of nonirritating medications in aqueous solution. It is injected at a 45-degree angle (at a 90-degree angle for insulin and heparin). The most common site is the posterior upper arm.

the *patella* (knee cap), or the mid-third of the upper outer leg.

Injecting infants and small children requires some special considerations. The choice of a site is based on muscular development, as well as the absence of major nerves and blood vessels. As mentioned above, the most popular site for IM injection in children and infants is the vastus lateralis muscle. Other sites are avoided for the following reasons:

- Infants do not have well-developed deltoid muscles.
- The sciatic nerve, located near the dorsogluteal site, is proportionately larger in the infant.
- The gluteus medius is not well developed until the child is walking.

The best policy is to ask the physician to show you just where to inject. Any site selected for infants and children has a greater margin for error, because the muscles are smaller than the muscles of adults.

Infants should be restrained by another assistant or the parent to avoid injury. If the child is old enough to understand, be honest and explain that the injection may sting for a minute, but that it is important to hold very still. Obtain assistance when giving an injection to an uncooperative child.

The recommended site for vastus lateralis injections in infants and children is below the greater trochanter of the femur but within the upper lateral quadrant of the thigh. When using the vastus lateralis site in an adult, the needle should be injected at a 90-degree angle, but with infants and children the needle should be injected at a 45-degree angle, with the needle point directed toward the feet. An adult patient may sit or lie supine, but it is easier to locate the vastus lateralis in pediatric patients with the child lying down.

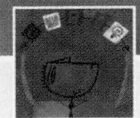

Giving a Subcutaneous Injection

GOAL: To inject 0.5 ml of medication into the subcutaneous tissue using a 25-gauge, ⅝-inch needle and syringe of correct size and type, as directed by the physician.

EQUIPMENT AND SUPPLIES

- A vial or ampule containing the medication to be injected
- Alcohol wipes
- Gauze squares or cotton balls
- A sterile needle and syringe unit with retractable needle cover
- Disposable gloves
- Sharps container
- A written order, including the patient's name, when to give the drug, the route of administration, and the name and strength of the drug

PROCEDURAL STEPS

1 Wash your hands. Follow standard precautions.

2 Select the correct medication from the shelf or the refrigerator.

Purpose: Some medications must be refrigerated or stored under special conditions.

3 Read the label to be sure that you have the right drug and the right strength. Perform the three label and order checks while dispensing the medication and the seven rights. Perform any necessary dose calculations.

Purpose: To promote safety and accuracy in drug therapy. One medication may be manufactured and prepackaged in different strengths. For instance, a particular drug may be available in vials of both 250 mg/ml and 500 mg/ml.

4 Warm refrigerated medications by gently rolling the container between your palms.

5 Prepare the syringe, withdrawing the right dose.

6 Transport the medication to the patient.

7 Greet and identify the patient by name.

Purpose: To be sure that you have the right patient.

8 Position the patient comfortably.

9 Expose the site.

10 Apply gloves and cleanse the patient's skin with the antiseptic sponge, using a circular motion, moving outward from the center.

11 Remove the cap from the needle.

12 With the thumb and fingers of your nondominant hand, grasp the tissue of the posterior upper arm.

13 Hold the syringe between the thumb and the first two fingers of your dominant hand, and with one swift movement, insert the entire needle up to the hub at a 45-degree angle.

Purpose: The depth of the injection is determined by the choice of needle length, not by how far you insert the needle. Once the needle is at the tissue layer, do not move the needle while injecting the medication.

14 Aspirate (except when administering heparin or insulin) by withdrawing the plunger slightly to be sure that no blood enters the syringe.

Purpose: Blood in the syringe means that the needle is in a blood vessel and not in the subcutaneous tissue. You must not inject a subcutaneous medication intravenously.

15 If blood appears, immediately withdraw the unit without injecting the medication and dispose of it in the sharps container. Compress the injection site with an alcohol swab or gauze bandage.

Purpose: To minimize bleeding and bruising.

16 Begin again with step 1.

17 If no blood appears in the syringe, push in the plunger slowly and steadily until all medication has been administered.

Purpose: A rapid injection may damage the tissues and be uncomfortable for the patient.

18 Place the gauze square next to the needle and withdraw it at the same angle of insertion. Immediately slide the retractable needle cover over the contaminated needle.

19 Gently massage the site with the gauze square (do not massage insulin or heparin injections).

Purpose: Massage helps to increase absorption and to decrease pain.

20 Discard the needle and syringe into the sharps container.

21 Make sure that your patient is comfortable and safe.

22 Dispose of the gloves in the biohazard waste and wash your hands.

23 Observe the patient for any adverse reaction. You may need to keep the patient under observation for 20 to 30 minutes.

24 Record the drug administration on the patient's medical record including the exact injection site, and on the required DEA record if the medication is a controlled substance.

Purpose: A procedure is not considered done until it is recorded.

See Appendix E for a charting example.

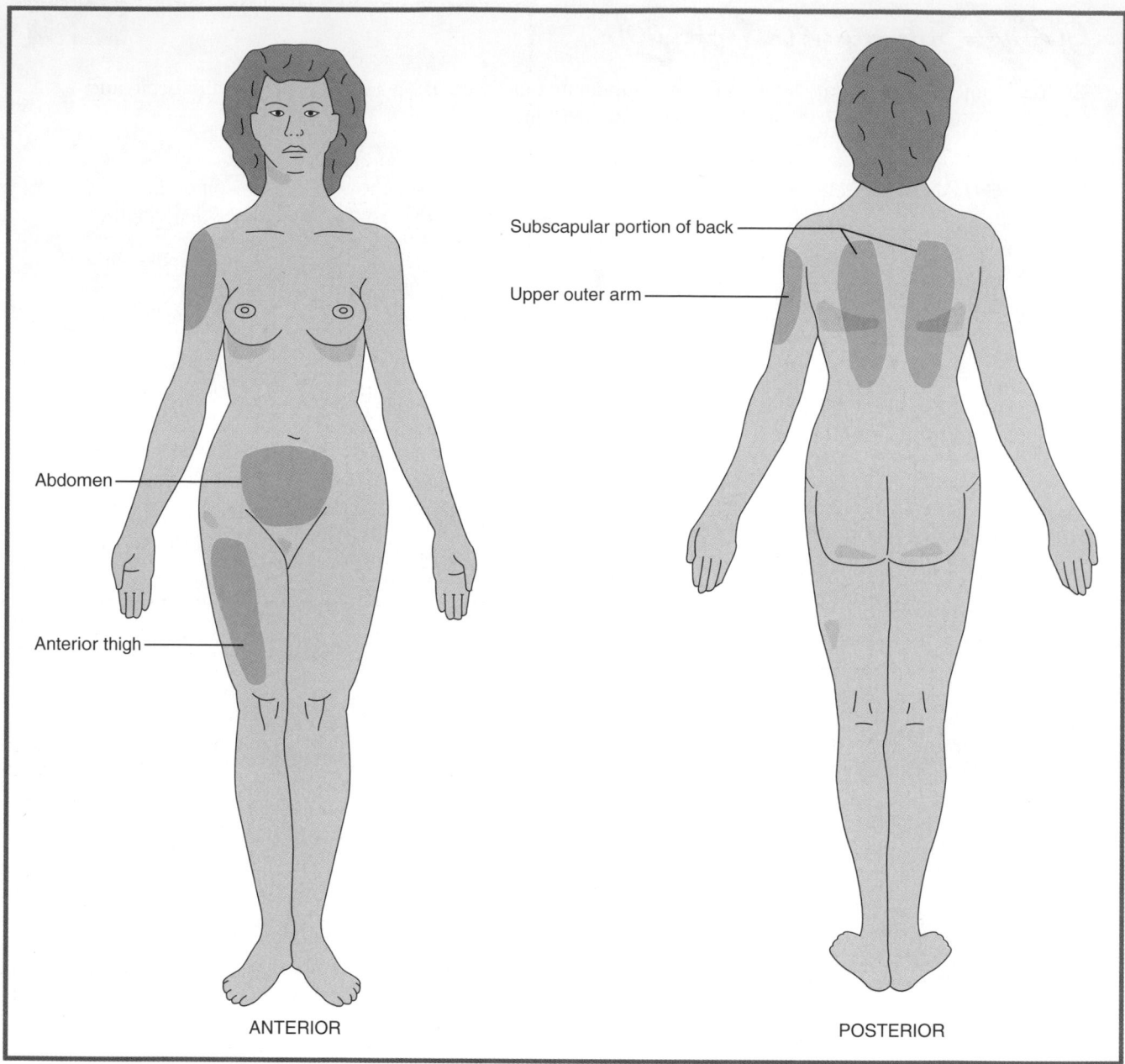

FIGURE 32-16 Areas of the body commonly used for subcutaneous injections.

CRITICAL THINKING APPLICATION

Dr. Thau wants to make certain that Dorothy is comfortable with the procedure for administering IM injections to infants. She orders Dorothy to give the first dose of the *Haemophilus influenzae* type B (Hib) vaccine to a 2-month-old infant in the office today for a well-baby check up. Dorothy administers the injection in the right vastus lateralis. Describe exactly where the injection was given and document the information Dorothy should include on the child's record.

Dorsogluteal (Gluteus Medius) Site. The dorsogluteal region is the traditional site for deep IM injections. However, complications from sciatic nerve injury are frequent enough that experts are suggesting that use of this site be

Back view

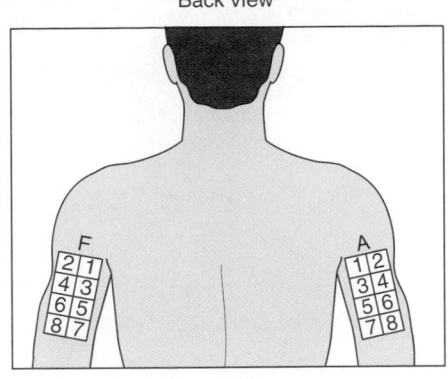

Front view

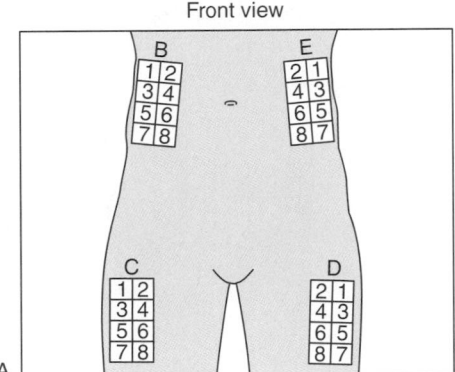

INJECTION LOG

	SITE		1	2	3	4	5	6	7	8
	Right arm	A								
	Right abdomen	B								
	Right Thigh	C								
	Left Thigh	D								
	Left abdomen	E								
B	Left arm	F								

FIGURE 32-17   **A**, Rotation sites for insulin injections.
B, Rotation log.

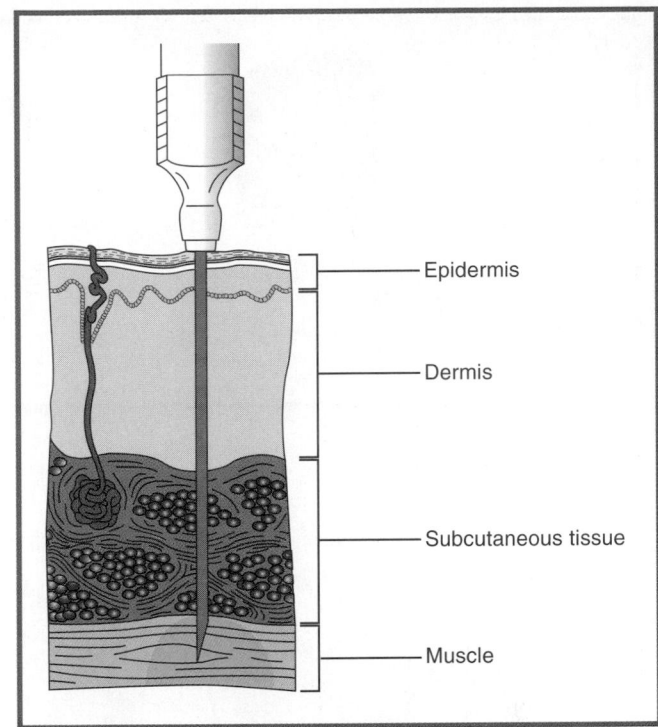

FIGURE 32-18   Anatomic illustration of the intramuscular injection. Note that the needle is inserted at a 90-degree angle and deposits the medication into the large central part of the muscle.

abandoned and replaced with the vastus lateralis and ventrogluteal sites. Regardless, the dorsogluteal site continues to be popular, and it is still acceptable for adults if care is taken to locate the exact site. It is recommended that this site *not* be used for pediatric patients.

The patient should lie in the Sims' position with the bottom leg straight and the top leg slightly bent. To locate the site, put the palm of your hand on the greater trochanter of the femur and point your fingers toward the posterior iliac spine. Palpate these bony prominences to make certain that you are at the correct site, and draw an imaginary line between these two anatomical markings. The injection is made into the gluteus medius muscle above the imaginary line (Figure 32-21).

Some medications for injection are packaged in vials as sterile powders or crystals that must be mixed with sterile water or saline before they can be administered. This process was discussed in Chapter 31; the amount of solvent to be added to the dry form of the drug (solute) depends on the physician's order and the label directions. After calculating the correct amount of liquid that must be added to the dry form of the drug to create the dose ordered by the physician, follow the guidelines in Procedure 32-8 to prepare the drug and administer it to the patient.

Ventrogluteal (Gluteus Medius) Site. Although considered safe, the ventrogluteal region is not used as frequently as the others previously discussed. This technique uses a larger mass of the gluteus medius muscle than when using the dorsogluteal site. The area is free of major nerves and blood vessels, and it is considered safe for both infants and adults (Figure 32-22). All types of intramuscular medications can be injected here, including thick, oily preparations.

To locate the site, position the patient in the Sims' position and place the palm of your hand on the greater trochanter, pointing your index finger toward the anterior iliac spine. Spread your middle finger back as far as possible from your index finger forming a triangular injection area. For a child, you will need a 1-inch needle, whereas in an obese adult patient, you may need a $2^1/_2$-inch needle to reach the depth of the muscle.

Z-Track Intramuscular Injection. Some intramuscular medications are irritating to the skin and subcutaneous tissues. The injection must be given in such a way as to prevent any leakage back from the deep muscle into the upper subcutaneous layers. The **Z**-track

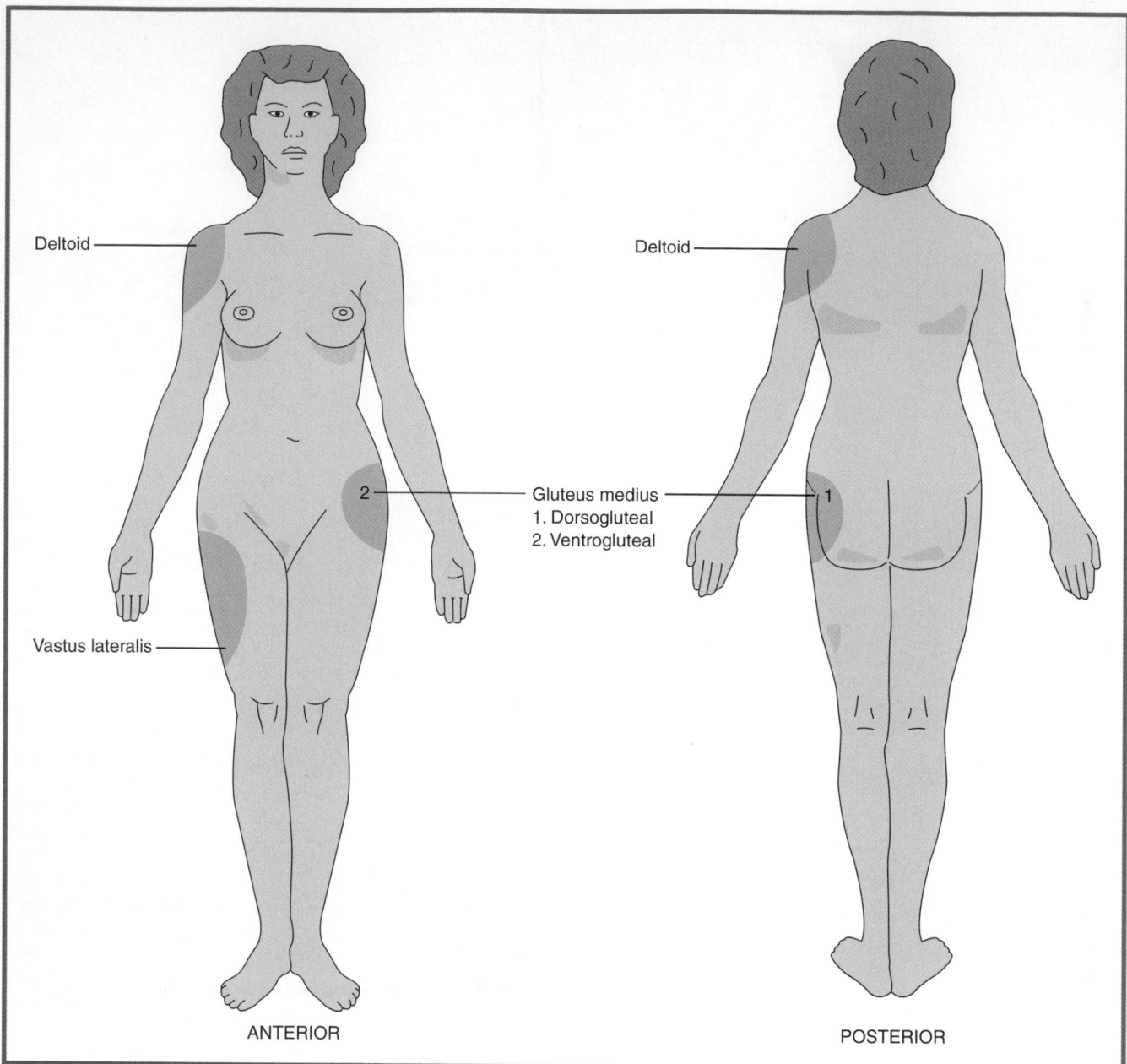

FIGURE 32-19 The muscles commonly used for intramuscular injection.

TABLE 32-2	Types of Injections		
Method	**Drug Amount**	**Sites**	**Examples**
Intramuscular	Adult, 1-2 ml	Deltoid	Epinephrine (Adrenalin)
	Adult, 2-5 ml	Vastus lateralis	Penicillin
		Dorsogluteal, ventrogluteal	Meperidine (Demerol)
	Child, 1-2 ml	Vastus lateralis, ventrogluteal	Penicillin
Intramuscular, **Z**-track	As above	Dorsogluteal, ventrogluteal	Irritating drugs
Subcutaneous	Adult, 0.1-2.0 ml	Upper outer arm	Insulin
		Thigh	Vaccines
		Abdomen	Toxoids
	Child, 0.5 ml	Upper outer arm	Vaccines
		Thigh, abdomen	Toxoids
Intradermal	Adult and child, 0.1 ml	Forearm	Tuberculin test, skin tests

PROCEDURE 32-7

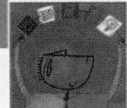

Giving an Intramuscular Injection

GOAL: To inject 2 ml of medication into the muscle, using a 22-gauge, 1½-inch needle and 3-ml syringe, as directed by the physician.

EQUIPMENT AND SUPPLIES

- A vial or ampule containing the ordered medication
- Alcohol wipes
- Cotton ball
- Sterile needle and syringe unit with retractable needle cover
- Disposable gloves
- Sharps container
- Written order, including the patient's name, when to give the drug, the route of administration, and the name and strength of the drug

PROCEDURAL STEPS

1 Wash your hands. Follow standard precautions.

2 Select the correct medication from the shelf or the refrigerator.

3 Read the label to be sure that you have the right drug and the right strength.

    Purpose: To perform the first of three drug label/order checks; one medication may be manufactured and prepackaged in different strengths; for instance, a particular drug may be available in vials of both 250 mg/ml and 500 mg/ml.

4 Warm refrigerated medications by gently rolling between your palms.

5 Calculate the correct dose if needed and continue with the three label checks while drawing the medication into the syringe.

6 Transport the medication to the patient.

7 Greet and identify the patient by name.

    Purpose: To be sure that you have the right patient.

8 Help the patient into an upright sitting position.

9 Apply gloves and expose the deltoid site. The mid-deltoid site is located approximately two to three fingerwidths below the acromial process.

10 Cleanse the patient's skin with the alcohol wipe using a circular motion, moving outward from the center (Figure 1).

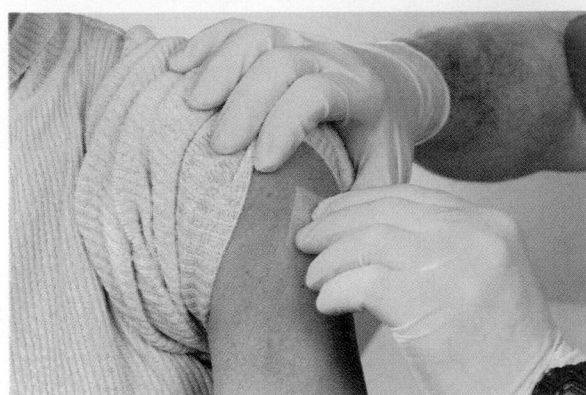

Figure 1

11 Remove the needle cover and with the thumb and first two fingers of your nondominant hand, spread the skin tightly. (At the deltoid, vastus lateralis, or rectus femoris sites, pinching of the tissue is also acceptable, as in Figure 2.)

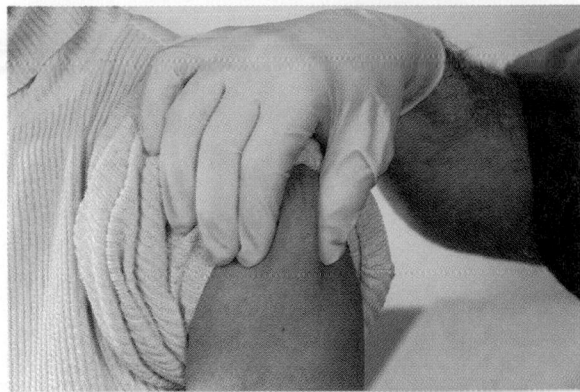

Figure 2

12 Grasp the syringe as you would a dart, and with one swift movement, insert the entire needle up to the hub, at a 90-degree angle into the muscle (Figure 3).

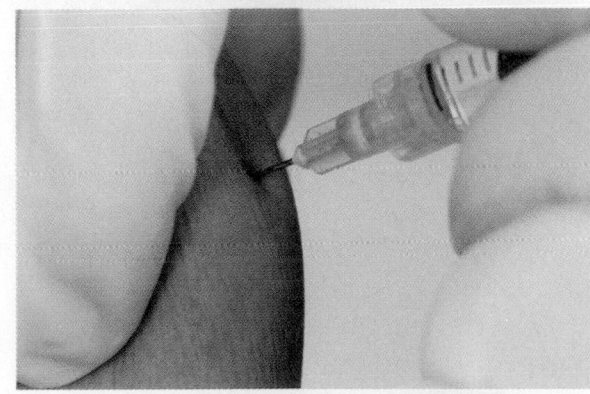

Figure 3

PROCEDURE 32-7—Cont'd

Purpose: The depth of the injection is determined by the choice of needle length, not by how far you insert the needle. Once the needle is at the tissue layer, do not move the needle while injecting the medication. Being in as far as the hub helps to keep the needle in one place.

13 Aspirate: Withdraw the plunger slightly to be sure that no blood enters the syringe.

Purpose: Blood in the syringe means that the needle is in a blood vessel and is not in the muscle tissue. You may *not* administer an intramuscular medication by the intravenous route.

14 If blood appears, immediately withdraw the syringe, discard it in the sharps container, and compress the injection site with the sponge.

15 Begin again with step 1.

16 If no blood appears in the syringe, push in the plunger slowly and steadily until all medication has been administered.

Purpose: A rapid injection is uncomfortable for the patient.

17 Place the cotton ball next to the needle and apply counter pressure to the area while you withdraw the needle at the same angle of insertion. Immediately slide the retractable cover over the contaminated needle and discard the syringe unit into the sharps container.

18 Gently massage the site with the cotton ball.

Purpose: Massage helps to increase absorption and to decrease pain.

19 Make sure that your patient is comfortable and safe.

20 Observe the patient for any adverse reaction. You may need to keep the patient under observation for 20 to 30 minutes.

21 Dispose of the gloves in the biohazard waste and wash your hands.

22 Record the drug administration on the patient's medical record, and on the required DEA record if the medication is a controlled substance.

Purpose: A procedure is not considered done until it is recorded.

See Appendix E for a charting example.

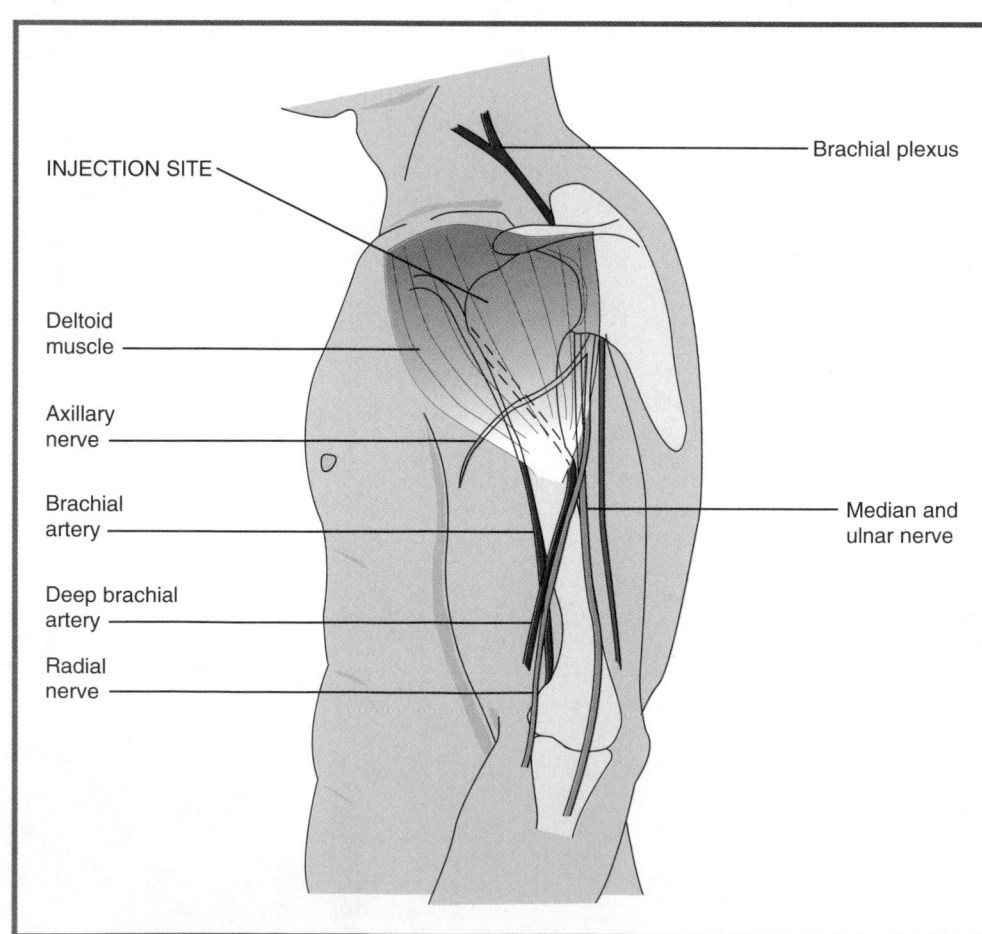

INJECTION SITE

Deltoid muscle

Axillary nerve

Brachial artery

Deep brachial artery

Radial nerve

Brachial plexus

Median and ulnar nerve

FIGURE 32-20 The deltoid muscle intramuscular site. This site is not recommended for infants, because the muscle is not well developed until later in childhood.

method displaces the upper tissue laterally before the needle is inserted.

The medication is prepared according to safety guidelines and gloves are donned. The skin is pushed to one side and cleaned as described for IM injections. Then the needle is injected and the medication is slowly released into the deep muscular tissue (Procedure 32-9). After the needle is withdrawn, the tissue is released, so that the needle track is to the side of where the medication was deposited into the muscle. This process prevents a direct pathway to the surface for the medication, thus protecting the subcutaneous and surface tissues from the irritating effects of the drug.

The medications for which **Z**-track injection is appropriate require a large muscle mass, so they should only be injected into the dorsogluteal site. Because the medication is so irritating to the tissues, the needle should be changed after drawing up the medication from the vial, and before drug administration to the patient.

Many medications that require the **Z**-track method should not be massaged after injection since massaging will encourage the spread of the medication. Use alternate sides for multiple or frequent injections to prevent tissue damage.

Patient Education

It is extremely important that a patient be instructed about how to take a medication and why he or she is taking it. Ideally, the patient is informed by the physician, but the medical assistant should be prepared to reinforce the physician's information to the patient or explain parts of the information that the patient did not understand. When a patient does not understand the need for the medication or the directions regarding how to take it, there is a greater risk that the medication will be taken incorrectly. As a result, the physician's orders will not be carried out, and the desired therapeutic effect will not be achieved. The patient should fully understand the type of medication, its route of administration, its desired effect, and the side effects that need to be reported if they occur.

If the patient receives medication in the physician's office, he or she should understand the expected results or possible side effects. For example, if a patient is given a diuretic in the office, he or she needs to know what the immediate effect is going to be. This helps the patient to understand the urgency and **polyuria** that will occur within a relatively brief period. When a pain medication is given, the patient should have full knowledge, so that the possibility of personal injury can be avoided.

The medical assistant should instruct the patient to take all of the medication prescribed. Many times, if a prescription is not completed, the treatment objectives may not be achieved. Patients should also be instructed to take their medication in the time sequence prescribed. This keeps the optimal level of the drug circulating in the bloodstream.

When sample medications are dispensed in the office to the patient, the package contains inserts that can be helpful in educating the patient. If there are certain parts of the inserts that the patient should review, highlight this information for quick reference. If the physician has specific written instructions for the patient to follow, read over the form with the patient before giving it to him or her to take home. Always remember that the more the patient knows and understands about how to take the medication and why it is prescribed, the greater the chances are that the drug treatment will be successful.

This would also be a good time to suggest that the patient check the status of medications at home. The National Association of Retail Druggists recommends that the medicine cabinet be checked once a month to determine the age and quality of medications. At that time the patient should dispose of any medications falling under the following guidelines:

1. Medicines for past illnesses
2. Any expired medicines, unidentified medications, or medications that are more than 2 years old

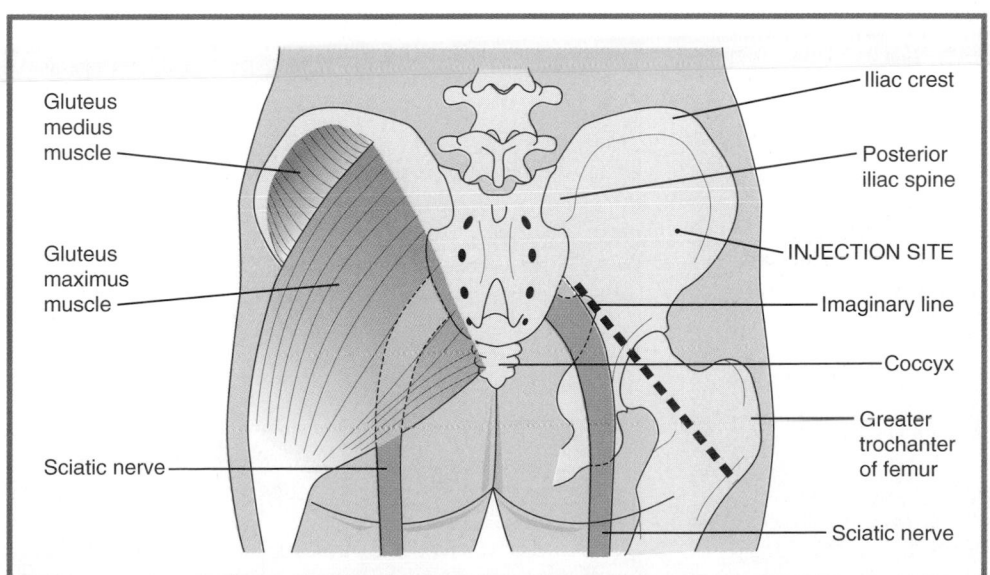

FIGURE 32-21 The dorsogluteal (gluteus medius) site is still preferred by many physicians.

Gluteus medius muscle
Gluteus maximus muscle
Sciatic nerve
Iliac crest
Posterior iliac spine
INJECTION SITE
Imaginary line
Coccyx
Greater trochanter of femur
Sciatic nerve

PROCEDURE 32-8

Reconstituting a Powdered Drug for Administration

GOAL: To reconstitute a powdered drug for intramuscular injection as ordered by the physician.

EQUIPMENT AND SUPPLIES

- Vial containing the ordered powdered medication
- Diluent: Sterile saline
- Alcohol wipes
- Cotton ball
- Two sterile needle and syringe units
- Disposable gloves
- Sharps container
- Written order, including the patient's name, when to give the drug, the route of administration, and the name and strength of the drug

PROCEDURAL STEPS

1 Wash your hands. Follow standard precautions.

2 Select the correct vial of powdered medication from the shelf and the recommended diluent for reconstitution. Perform the three drug label and physician order checks during preparation and the seven rights throughout the procedure.

3 Read the label to determine the correct amount of diluent to add to create the dose ordered by the physician. (Refer to Chapter 31 for assistance with calculations.) Calculate the correct dose, if needed, and continue with the three label checks.

4 Remove the tops from each vial and clean each with an alcohol wipe. Leave the wipes in place on top of each vial.

5 Grasp the syringe plunger and draw up the amount of air equal to the amount of diluent needed to reconstitute the drug.

Purpose: Not enough replaced air will make it difficult to withdraw the diluent; too much replaced air will force the diluent into the syringe without pulling on the plunger to withdraw it.

6 Remove the needle cover and insert the needle into the center of the rubber stopper of the diluent. Hold the vial firmly against a flat surface and watch carefully that the needle only touches the cleaned rubber area.

7 Inject the aspirated air in the syringe into the diluent vial.

8 Invert the diluent vial and aspirate the calculated or recommended amount of diluent.

9 Remove the needle from the diluent vial and inject the diluent into the drug vial. Remove the needle and discard it into the sharps container.

10 Roll the vial with the drug and diluent mixture between the palms of your hands to mix it thoroughly. Do not shake the vial unless directed to do so on the drug label. When the medication is completely mixed there is no residue or crystals on the bottom of the vial.

11 Aspirate air into the second syringe unit that is equal to the calculated amount of medication to be administered.

12 Inject the air into the mixed drug vial, invert the vial, and withdraw the ordered amount of medication.

13 Proceed as outlined in steps 6 to 22 in Procedure 32-7.

---

3. Hydrogen peroxide that no longer bubbles or has changed color, ointments or salves that have separated or are crumbly, vinegar-smelling aspirins, antiseptic solutions that are cloudy or have a solid residue on the bottom, and any medicine of uncertain quality

The Association also suggests the following:

1. Keep medicines stored away from light, heat, air, and moisture.
2. Use medicine from the original container until it is completely used or expired.
3. Do not combine medicines from several containers.
4. Keep medicine locked away from children.
5. Make sure that child-proof medicine caps are used properly.

Legal and Ethical Issues

A medical assistant must be extremely knowledgeable when administering medications in the physician's office. Follow all physician orders exactly as written. If you have a question about the order, ask for clarification before you proceed. It is advisable to give a medication only after the order is written in the patient's chart. This helps eliminate errors and possible omissions in medication therapy.

Legal responsibilities include the prevention of error by carefully following safe practice procedures in pouring and administering drugs. Always implement the seven rights and perform the three drug order and label checks when dispensing and administering medications. Anyone

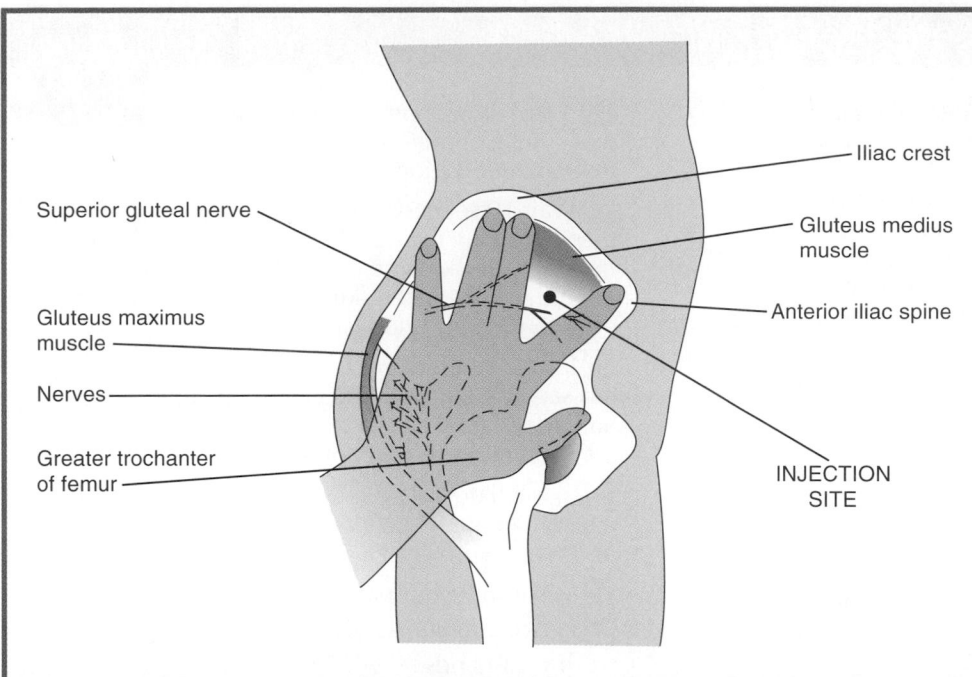

Iliac crest

Superior gluteal nerve

Gluteus medius muscle

Gluteus maximus muscle

Anterior iliac spine

Nerves

Greater trochanter of femur

INJECTION SITE

FIGURE 32-22 The ventrogluteal site can be used for most intramuscular injections.

PROCEDURE 32-9

Giving a Z-Track Intramuscular Injection

GOAL: To inject 1 ml of medication into the muscle using a 23-gauge, 2-inch needle and 3-ml syringe and the Z-track method, as directed by the physician.

EQUIPMENT AND SUPPLIES

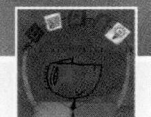

- Vial containing the ordered medication
- Alcohol wipes
- Cotton ball
- Disposable gloves
- Sharps container
- Sterile needle and syringe unit with retractable needle cover
- Written order, including the patient's name, when to give the drug, the route of administration, and the name and strength of the drug

PROCEDURAL STEPS

1 Wash your hands. Follow standard precautions.

2 Select the correct medication from the shelf or the refrigerator.

3 Perform the three order and label checks as well as the seven rights.

4 Warm refrigerated medications by gently rolling the container between your palms.

5 Prepare the syringe, calculating the right dose.

6 Replace the needle cover and give a slight turn to loosen the needle. Secure a new needle, still in its sheath, to the tip of the syringe. Discard the contaminated needle.

Purpose: The needle that was used to withdraw the medication is covered with a substance irritating to the skin and subcutaneous tissues.

7 Transport the medication to the patient.

8 Greet and identify the patient by name.

Purpose: To be sure that you have the right patient.

9 Position the patient comfortably in the Sims' position.

10 Expose the site and apply gloves.

11 Cleanse the patient's skin with the alcohol wipe, using a circular motion, moving outward from the center. Make sure to clean the actual area of injection.

12 Remove the needle cover.

13 Push the skin to one side and hold it firmly in place. If the skin is slippery, use a dry gauze sponge to hold the skin in place.

Purpose: Displacing the skin prevents irritating medications from leaking back to the surface.

PROCEDURE 32-9—Cont'd

14 Grasp the syringe as you would a dart, and with one swift movement, insert the entire needle up to the hub, at a 90-degree angle into the muscle.

Purpose: The depth of the injection is determined by the choice of needle length, not by how far you insert the needle. Once the needle is at the tissue layer, do not move the needle while injecting the medication. Being in as far as the hub helps to keep the needle in one place.

15 Aspirate: Withdraw the plunger slightly to be sure that no blood enters the syringe.

Purpose: Blood in the syringe means that the needle is in a blood vessel and not in the muscle tissue. You may *not* administer an intramuscular medication by the intravenous route.

16 If blood appears, immediately withdraw the syringe, dispose of the syringe unit in the sharps container, and compress the injection site with a gauze square or cotton ball.

Purpose: To minimize bleeding and bruising.

17 Begin again with step 1.

Purpose: Blood is now mixed with the medication, and the medication is considered contaminated. Blood may interact with the drug and may be irritating to the intramuscular tissues.

18 If no blood appears in the syringe, push in the plunger slowly and steadily until all medication has been administered.

19 Wait 10 seconds for medication to be dispersed, then withdraw the needle at the same angle of insertion. At the same time the needle is withdrawn, release the displaced skin to prevent the tracking of medication to the surface.

20 If the manufacturer recommends it, gently massage the site with the gauze square or cotton ball. Many medications requiring Z-track administration should not be massaged.

21 Immediately slide retractable needle cover over the contaminated needle and dispose of the needle and syringe unit into a sharps container.

22 Make sure your patient is comfortable and safe.

23 Dispose of gloves in the biohazard waste and wash your hands.

24 Observe the patient for any adverse reaction. You may need to keep the patient under observation for 20 to 30 minutes.

25 Record the drug administration on the patient's medical record, including the exact site of injection.

See Appendix E for a charting example.

administering a drug must know the possible serious complications related to the drug and be alert for side effects. The medical assistant must demonstrate compliance with individual state laws governing medications and their administration. Precise charting of the administration of medications as well as the management of prescriptions cannot be overemphasized.

The administration of drugs also involves ethical principles. *The patient always comes first.* With that foremost in mind, never risk giving an incorrect medication. There is no such thing as a small error, because any mistake may result in serious harm or possible death. If an error is made, it must be reported immediately to the physician so that measures can be taken to help the patient. It is difficult to admit that a mistake has been made, but it is *absolutely necessary*. For that reason, be sure to double-check your calculations with a co-worker or the physician before dispensing the drug. If a mistake is made, it must be completely documented, including the details of the error, to whom the error was reported, any action taken, and subsequent observations of the patient.

SUMMARY OF SCENARIO

Dorothy understands the importance of careful management of medications. Because of her concern for patient safety, she asks Dr. Thau to check all of her calculations and refers to the physician if she has any questions about medication orders or patient education. Since Dr. Thau is a primary care physician, it is important for Dorothy to understand the factors that affect the administration of medication to all age groups of patients. She routinely employs the standard three label checks when dispensing medications and implements the seven rights throughout medication administration procedures.

Dorothy also recognizes the importance of complete and accurate documentation of medications, whether they are administered in the physician's office or as a prescription order. In addition, she consistently applies the rules of standard precautions when preparing and administering parenteral medications.

SUMMARY OF LEARNING OBJECTIVES

■ Safety precautions in the management of medication administration should be consistently applied. Safe drug administration includes understanding the physician order, looking up the drug if it is unknown, and utilizing the three label checks and the seven rights every time a drug order is completed.

■ Patient assessment factors that affect medication administration include the continual evaluation of the patient's physical condition as well as such holistic factors as the impact of the patient's history, an accurate list of drug allergies, the patient's ability to understand the drug regimen and to be able to afford the treatment, as well as special patient factors based on age, weight, and condition.

■ Precautions in medication administration must be employed with pregnant and lactating women since drugs can pass through the placenta into the developing fetus as well as into the breast milk. Administration of drugs to pediatric patients is usually based on the weight of the child. Special precautions must be used, because the absorption, distribution, metabolism, and excretion of drugs are different in a child's body than in an adult's. Children also require a special approach for drug administration to be successful. Geriatric patients are more sensitive to the effects of medications because of altered metabolic rates, loss of subcutaneous fat, and accompanying chronic diseases. Aging patients are more likely to be taking more than one medication, so drug interactions are a potential problem. A holistic approach to medication management in aging patients includes a nutritional assessment, investigation into the cost of drug therapy, and adapted patient education methods.

■ Drugs are packaged in a variety of forms, with a variety of administration guidelines. Oral medications include both solid and liquid preparations; mucous membrane medications are absorbed rectally, vaginally, orally, nasally, or topically through the skin. Each form of medication has specific guidelines for administration, but all require the consistent use of the three label checks and the seven rights.

■ Parenteral medications are manufactured in either ampules or single-dose or multidose vials. The ordered route of administration, drug characteristics, and individual patient factors determine the correct gauge and length of needle needed for administration. The appropriate syringe is determined by the type of medication ordered and the amount of drug to be administered. Specialty syringe units, such as the Nova Pen and the EpiPen, are designed for the quick administration of certain medications.

■ OSHA guidelines include using syringe units with retractable needle covers; wearing disposable, nonsterile gloves and other appropriate protective gear when administering any medication that involves coming into contact with blood or body fluids; never recapping a contaminated needle and immediately discarding it into a sharps container; disposing of contaminated nonsharp materials in biohazard containers; disinfecting contaminated work areas; and washing hands before and after procedures.

■ Parenteral routes of administration include intradermal (ID), subcutaneous (SC), and a variety of intramuscular (IM) sites. The type of medication, the physician's order, and the unique characteristics of individual patients determine the route and site of administration. Each requires specific administration practices, which are described in Procedures 32-2 through 32-9.

■ Patient education is absolutely crucial to the correct administration of medication by patients at home. The patient should understand the purpose of the drug; the time, frequency, and amount of the dose; any special storage requirements; and the typical side effects that occur. The more the patient knows and understands about how to take the medication and why it is prescribed, the greater the chances that the drug treatment will be successful.

■ The medical assistant must be extremely knowledgeable when preparing and administering medications in the physician's office. If there are any questions about the order, ask for clarification before proceeding. Legal responsibilities include the prevention of error by carefully following safe practice procedures in pouring and administering drugs. The medical assistant must comply with individual state laws governing medications and their administration. Precise charting of the administration of medications as well as the management of prescriptions cannot be overemphasized.

UNIT seven

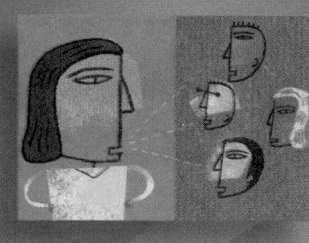

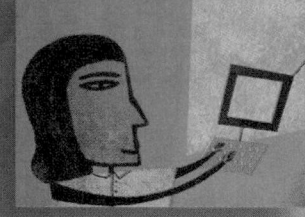

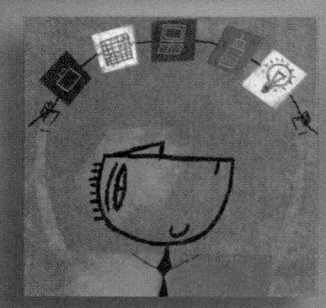

Assisting With Medical Specialties

CHAPTER 33

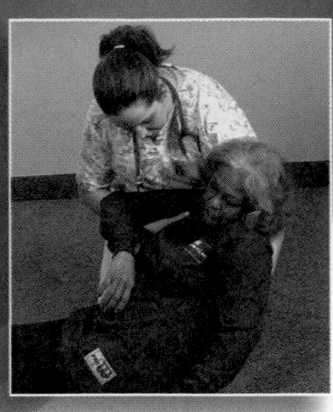

Scenario

Cheryl Skurka, CMA, has been working for Dr. Peter Bendt for about 6 months. During that time a number of patient emergencies have occurred in the office, and even more potentially serious problems have been managed by the phone screening staff. Cheryl is concerned that she is not prepared to assist with emergencies in the ambulatory care setting. Cheryl decides to ask Dr. Bendt for assistance, and he suggests she work with the experienced screening staff to learn how to manage phone calls from patients calling for assistance.

Assisting With Medical Emergencies

Learning Objectives

- Define and spell the terms listed in the vocabulary.
- Describe the medical assistant's responsibilities in an emergency.
- Identify supplies and equipment for emergency situations.
- Summarize the general rules for managing emergencies.
- Demonstrate screening techniques and documentation guidelines for ambulatory care emergencies.
- Determine appropriate action and documentation procedures for common ambulatory care emergencies.
- Recognize and respond to life-threatening emergencies in the ambulatory care setting.
- Identify and assist a patient with an obstructed airway.
- Apply patient education concepts to medical emergencies.
- Discuss the legal and ethical concerns regarding medical emergencies.
- Provide rescue breathing and perform adult CPR.
- Assist a patient with an obstructed airway.
- Demonstrate the use of an automated external defibrillator.
- Administer oxygen through a nasal cannula to a patient in respiratory distress.
- Assist and monitor a patient who has fainted.
- Control a hemorrhagic wound.

National Curriculum Competencies

CLINICAL COMPETENCIES

4i. Obtain CPR certification and first aid training

TRANSDISCIPLINARY COMPETENCIES

1d. Demonstrate telephone techniques

Vocabulary

asystole The absence of a heartbeat.

cyanosis Blue color of the mucous membranes and body extremities caused by lack of oxygen.

dyspnea Difficult or painful breathing.

ecchymosis A hemorrhagic skin discoloration commonly called bruising.

emetic A substance that causes vomiting.

fibrillation Rapid, random, ineffective contractions of the heart.

hematuria Blood in the urine.

mediastinum Space in the center of the chest under the sternum.

myocardium The muscular lining of the heart.

necrosis Pertaining to the death of cells or tissue.

photophobia Visual sensitivity to light.

polydipsia Excessive thirst.

polyuria Excreting large amounts of urine.

transient ischemic attack Temporary neurological symptoms because of a gradual or partial occlusion of a cerebral blood vessel.

First aid is defined as the immediate care given to a person who has been injured or has suddenly taken ill. It includes well-chosen words of encouragement, a willingness to help, a promotion of confidence by the demonstration of competence, and the performance of temporary physical care to alleviate pain or a life-threatening situation. Knowledge of first aid and related skills can often mean the difference between life and death, temporary and permanent disability, and rapid recovery and long-term hospitalization.

Frequently a medical assistant may be responsible for initiating first aid in the office and continuing to administer first aid until the physician or trained medical team arrives. Every medical assistant should successfully complete a course in cardiopulmonary resuscitation (CPR) and continue to hold a current CPR card as long as employed (see Procedure 33-2). Basic knowledge of CPR and life-support skills needs to be updated on a regular basis because of changes in procedures as new techniques are developed. For example, just recently both the Red Cross and the American Heart Association recommended the inclusion of automated external defibrillator (AED) training for all healthcare workers (see Procedure 33-1). Medical assistants need to be consistently trained on current emergency approaches and should encourage their local professional chapters to offer workshops on the management of emergencies in the ambulatory care setting.

THE MEDICAL ASSISTANT'S ROLE IN PERFORMING EMERGENCY PROCEDURES

1. Perform only the emergency procedures in which you are trained.
2. If an emergency occurs in the office, notify the physician.
3. If a physician cannot be located, contact the local EMS team.

Medical assistants are not responsible for diagnosing emergencies but are expected to make decisions on the management of emergencies based on their medical knowledge and training. If there is any doubt about how to manage a particular situation or emergency phone call, refer to the physician, office manager, or a more experienced member of the healthcare team.

Making the Facility Accident-Proof

Usually it is the medical assistant's responsibility to make the office as accident-proof as possible by keeping cupboard doors and drawers closed, wiping up spills immediately, and picking up dropped objects. All medications should be kept out of sight; dangerous drugs should be kept in locked cupboards. If there are children in the office, all sharp objects and potentially toxic substances must be kept out of reach. A medical assistant should never leave a seriously ill patient or a restless, depressed, or unconscious patient unattended.

Planning Ahead

Every healthcare facility should have a policy with specific procedures for the management of emergencies on site. When starting a new job, part of the orientation process is to review the site's policy and procedures manual. Be sure to clarify any questions you may have about how emergencies are managed in that particular facility.

Staff members should discuss possible emergencies that may occur and have an emergency action plan for rapid, systematic intervention. For instance, local industries may present unique problems that call for very specialized care. Plan for these, and ask the physician's advice on what procedures to follow and what supplies to have on hand. If there are several employees, each should be assigned specific duties. Organization and planning make the difference between systematic care for the patient and complete chaos.

Using Community Emergency Services

Most communities have an emergency medical services (EMS) system. This system includes an efficient communications network, such as the emergency telephone number 911, well-trained rescue personnel, properly equipped ambulances, an emergency facility that is open 24 hours a day to provide advanced life support, and hospital intensive care for the victims.

There are more than 300 poison control centers in the United States ready to provide emergency information for treating victims of poisonings. Many of the centers have toll-free lines. Every office is required to post a list of local emergency numbers. This list should be in plain sight and should be known to all office personnel. Include on the list

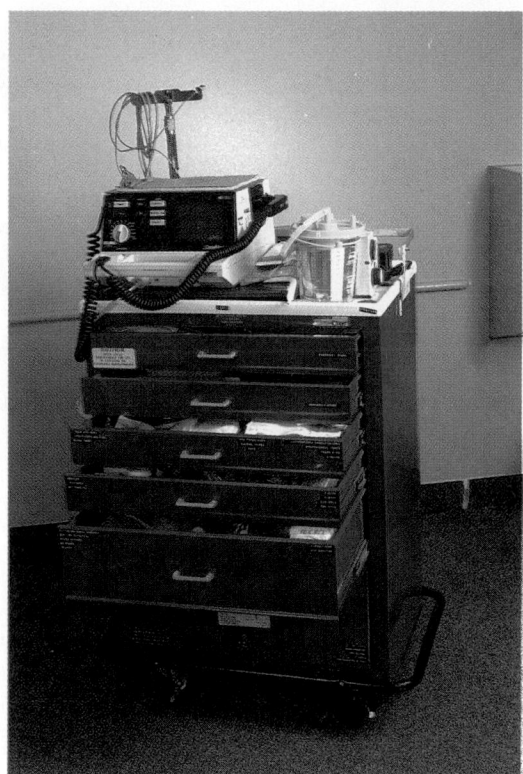

FIGURE 33-1   Office emergency cart with defibrillator. Drawers are marked for easy retrieval of emergency supplies.

the local EMS system, poison control center, ambulance and rescue squad, fire department, and police department numbers.

Supplies and Equipment for Emergencies

Emergency Supplies

Emergency supplies consist of a properly equipped "crash cart" or bag of first aid items needed for a variety of emergencies (Figure 33-1). The contents will vary to some degree, according to the type of emergencies each office encounters. Emergency supplies should be kept in an easily accessible place that is known to all personnel in the office, with inventories of supplies completed on a regular basis. Medication and sterile supplies expiration dates must be checked either weekly or monthly, including the status of available oxygen tanks and related supplies, and the cart should be replenished with fresh supplies after every use.

BASIC EMERGENCY SUPPLIES

Equipment

Adhesive tape in 1- and 2-inch widths
Airways—variety types and sizes

Alcohol wipes
Ambu-bag with assorted sizes of facial masks
Antimicrobial skin ointment
Cotton balls and cotton swabs
CPR masks—both adult and pediatric
Defibrillator
Elastic bandages in 2- and 3-inch widths
Flashlight with batteries
Gauze pads, 2 × 2- and 4 × 4-inch widths and roller bandage—both sterile and nonsterile
Gloves, sterile and nonsterile, in multiple sizes
Hot and cold packs (instant type)
Intravenous catheters, tubing, solutions (variety of types), and tourniquet
Personal protective equipment (PPE), including impervious gowns, splash-guards or goggles, and booties
Portable oxygen tank with regulator and mask
Scissors
Sharps container
Sphygmomanometer—both pediatric and adult regular and large sizes
Splints—various sizes
Sterile dressings—miscellaneous sizes, including two abdominal pads
Steristrips or suturing material
Suction machine and catheters
Syringes and needles in assorted sizes and gauges
Venipuncture supplies and butterfly units

Medications

Activated charcoal, bottle of 30 to 50 g
Amobarbital (Amytal)
Apomorphine
Antihistamine, injectable and oral
Atropine
Dextrose
Diazepam (Valium)
Digoxin (Lanoxin), injectable
Epinephrine (Adrenalin), injectable
Furosemide (Lasix)
Glucagon and/or glucose tablets
Ipecac syrup
Isoproterenol (Isuprel), aerosol inhaler and injectable
Lidocaine (Xylocaine), injectable
Metaraminol (Aramine)
Nitroglycerine tablets
Phenobarbital, injectable
Sodium bicarbonate, injectable
Sterile water for injection

Emergency pharmaceutical supplies should include certain basic drugs. These include epinephrine, which has multiple uses in emergency situations. As a vasoconstrictor, it controls hemorrhage, relaxes the bronchioles to relieve acute asthma attacks, and is an emergency heart stimulant used to treat shock. Epinephrine should be in a ready-to-use cartridge syringe and needle unit. These are supplied in 1.0-ml cartridges.

Other drugs used are atropine, digoxin (Lanoxin), and lidocaine (Xylocaine). Atropine decreases secretions, increases respiration and heart rate, and is a smooth muscle relaxant. It dilates the pupils and is a general cerebral stimulant. Atropine relieves gastrointestinal cramps and hypermotility and may also be used to relieve pain locally. Digoxin is used to treat congestive heart failure (CHF) and is good for emergency use because it has a relatively rapid action. Lidocaine is used intravenously to decrease heart arrhythmia and as both a local and topical anesthetic.

Apomorphine is a fast-acting and effective **emetic** and is used in cases of poisoning when a stomach pump cannot be employed. Syrup of ipecac is also an emetic and one that many physicians recommend be kept on hand in the home for use in emergencies.

Antihistamines are used in the treatment of allergic reactions and anaphylaxis. Isoproterenol, an antispasmodic, is used for bronchial spasms, and is also a cardiac stimulant. Some trade names for this product are Isuprel, Medihaler-Iso, and Norisodrine.

Other medications that may be found in a crash cart are metaraminol (Aramine) (50%, in a prefilled syringe), for severe shock; amobarbital sodium (Amytal) and diazepam (Valium), for convulsions and as sedatives; and furosemide (Lasix), for CHF. Glucagon is primarily used to counteract severe hypoglycemic reactions in diabetic patients taking insulin.

Defibrillators

A medical assistant may be required to assist the team with defibrillation of emergency patients. Defibrillation is indicated when a patient has no pulse and is in ventricular **fibrillation**. Defibrillators are devices that send an electrical current through the **myocardium** by means of hand-held paddles or self-adhesive pads applied to the chest. This electrical shock causes momentary **asystole**, giving the heart's natural pacemaker an opportunity to resume the heart rate at a normal rhythm. The automated external defibrillator (AED) has a computerized system that analyzes a cardiac rhythm and delivers voice-prompt instructions on how to operate the device (Figure 33-2 and Procedure 33-1). The AED uses self-adhesive pads that record and monitor the cardiac rhythm, and the device instructs the rescuer when to deliver the electrical charge. The apex-anterior position is the most commonly used paddle position, with the anterior (sternum) paddle or pads placed to the right of the upper sternum and the apex one to the left of the patient's left nipple at the left midaxillary line (Figure 33-3). For defibrillating a female patient, the apex paddle or pad is placed either next to or underneath the left breast.

General Rules for Emergencies

There are two types of emergencies that a medical assistant will face in the ambulatory care setting: office emergencies and home emergencies. Common office emergencies and their management will be discussed later in this chapter. Besides dealing with actual emergency situations on-site, a medical assistant is frequently the first person to interact with patients facing potential emergencies at home. It is estimated that one third of the telephone calls received in a physician's office are for some type of problem that requires attention. An immediate decision must be made on how to manage that problem—either with home care advice, scheduling an appointment, or in extreme emergencies, notifying EMS. When faced with an emergency, either on the phone or in the facility, the medical assistant should follow some general rules:

1. It is most important to stay calm. Reassure the patient and make him or her as comfortable as possible.
2. Assess the situation to determine the nature of the emergency. Decide whether the need is immediate. This decision requires calm judgment and medical knowledge.
3. Obtain as much information as possible to determine the appropriate action.
4. Immediately refer any concerns to the office supervisor or physician.

Telephone Triage Screening

Every time the phone rings in a healthcare setting, there could be a potential life or death situation on the other end of the line. One of the most important tasks performed by medical assistants every day is answering the phones and managing patient needs efficiently and appropriately. *Triage* is the process of sorting patients, in this case patient phone calls, according to the patients' need for care. There are emergency action principles that serve as a guide for managing emergency phone calls in the ambulatory care setting.

- If the patient's situation is life threatening, activate EMS/911.
  - *Never put the caller with a life-threatening emergency on hold, and always be the last to hang up.*
  - Remain on the line until help arrives and you have talked to EMS personnel.
- Immediately record the name of the caller and that of the patient, location, and phone number in case the connection is lost.
- If you are unsure how to manage the emergency situation, contact the physician.
- If the patient is referred to an emergency department or emergency room (ED or ER), call the emergency department to notify them of the patient's arrival and make a follow-up call to determine the patient's condition.
- Gather as much information as possible about what is wrong with the patient and when the problem started. Obtain details regarding the patient's condition including:
  - Level of consciousness: Alert, responsive, lethargic, or confused? Did the patient lose consciousness at any time? If so, how long?
  - Character of respirations (and pulse if the caller is able to determine this): Normal, rapid, shallow, or difficult?

PROCEDURE **33-1**

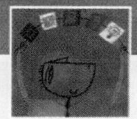

Using an Automated External Defibrillator (AED)

GOAL: To defibrillate adult victims with cardiac arrest. The majority of adult victims in sudden cardiac arrest are in ventricular fibrillation. Survival rates for victims with ventricular fibrillation are as high as 90% when defibrillation occurs within the first minute of collapse. Survival rates for cardiac arrest caused by ventricular fibrillation decrease by 7% to 10% with every minute that defibrillation does not occur.

EQUIPMENT AND SUPPLIES

- Practice AED
- Approved mannequin

PROCEDURAL STEPS (To be performed on an approved mannequin only.)

AED arrives after CPR has been started and two cycles of compressions and breaths have been completed.

1 Place the AED near the victim's left ear. Turn the AED on.

2 Attach electrode pads as pictured on the AED. Place electrodes at the sternum and apex of the heart. Make sure pads have complete contact with the victim's chest and they do not overlap (see Figure 33-3).

3 All rescuers must clear away from the victim. Press the ANALYZE button. The AED will analyze the victim's coronary status, will announce if the victim is going to be shocked, and automatically charges the electrodes (Figure 1*).

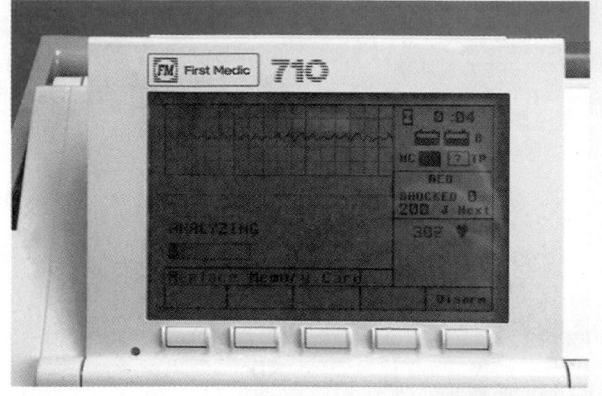

Figure 1

4 All rescuers must clear away from the victim. Press the SHOCK button if the machine is not automated. May repeat one to two more analyze-shock cycles.

5 If the machine gives the "no shock indicated" signal, assess the victim. Check the carotid pulse and breathing status and keep the AED attached until emergency medical services arrives.

*From Aehlert B: *ACLS quick review study guide,* ed 2. St Louis, 2001, Mosby.

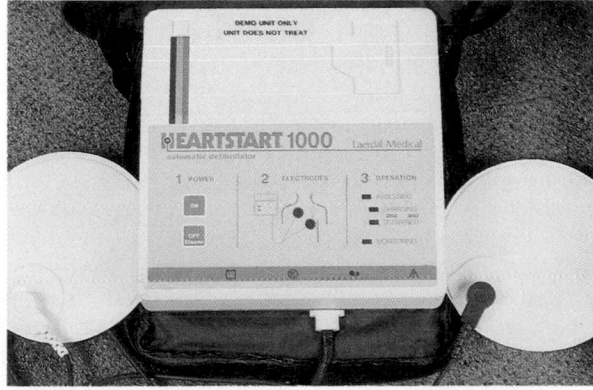

FIGURE 33-2 Fully automated external defibrillator. (From Aehlert B: *ACLS quick review study guide,* ed 2. St Louis, 2001, Mosby.)

- Is there bleeding? If so, how much, from where?
- Is there a suspected head or neck injury? If so, has the patient been moved? Is there a suspected fracture? Where?
- Does the patient have a history of this problem?
- Any other symptoms, such as fever, vomiting, diarrhea, or pain?
- Details regarding what has been done for the patient:
  - Medication: What, when? Dose, effectiveness?
- Thoroughly document the information gathered and any actions taken, including notification of EMS, whether the patient was sent to the emergency department or an appointment was scheduled, all home care recommendations, and whether the physician was notified and when.

Based on the outcome of the telephone interaction, a decision is made about when the practitioner will see the

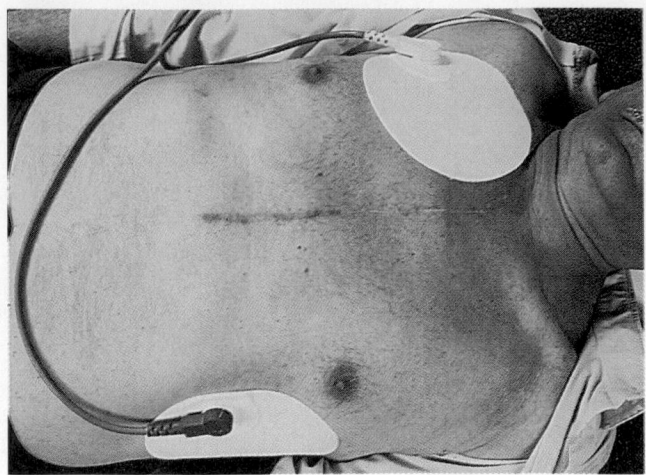

FIGURE 33-3   Connect the adhesive pads to the AED cables, and then apply the pads to the patient's chest at the upper-right sternal border and the lower-left ribs over the cardiac apex. (From Aehlert B: *ACLS quick review study guide*, ed 2. St Louis, 2001, Mosby.)

2. Allergies, current medications, and pertinent health history
3. Name of any person with the patient
4. Vital signs and chief complaint
5. Sequence of events, beginning with how the problem occurred, any changes in the patient's overall condition, and any observations made regarding the patient's condition
6. Details regarding procedures or techniques performed on the patient

patient. Emergency calls require either activation of EMS or immediate attention as soon as the patient arrives. Urgent calls require a same-day appointment if the patient has an acute condition or is in severe discomfort. This would include a young child with a high fever or a patient complaining of moderate to severe abdominal pain. The new patient will have to be worked into the day's schedule, which may cause a delay in currently scheduled appointments. Patients with other less urgent problems can be scheduled for appointments within the next 3 to 4 days.

> ### CRITICAL THINKING APPLICATION
>
> Cheryl is working with the phone triage staff when they receive a call from the mother of a 5-year-old patient; the mother reports that her son fell and cut his arm. What type of information should Cheryl gather about the injury? How should the incident be documented?

Management of On-Site Emergencies

An emergency can occur at any time to anyone. *Always follow standard precautions.* When an emergency occurs, it is impossible to determine the level of infection. All body fluids must be considered infectious, and the appropriate precautions must be employed. If the situation is life threatening, activate EMS and stay with the patient until you are relieved by the EMS provider or the physician.

> ### DOCUMENTATION OF AN ON-SITE EMERGENCY
>
> 1. Patient's name, address, age, and health insurance information

> ### CRITICAL THINKING APPLICATION
>
> Cheryl is working the front desk when a patient comes into the office limping and says she fell in the parking lot and hurt her ankle. Role-play the situation with a classmate and make a list of at least 10 questions Cheryl should ask the patient.

Life-Threatening Emergencies

If a patient in the facility exhibits any signs of nonresponsiveness, the clinician must be brought to the patient immediately. If there is no clinician in the facility, EMS should be activated. Even in situations in which a physician is present, the physician may order you to call 911 for immediate emergency care. Before beginning assessment of the patient, *put on gloves*, because any emergency situation may necessitate exposure to blood or body fluids.

Nonresponsive Patient

If the patient is nonresponsive, the physician must be notified immediately. The physician may instruct the medical assistant to activate EMS.

Caring for a patient who is nonresponsive first requires assessing the patient's respirations to determine the presence of breathing. Position the patient on the back and apply the head tilt–chin lift movement to open the airway. If there is a suspected head or neck injury, the neck should be manipulated as little as possible, so open the airway with the jaw thrust maneuver. Both of these actions relieve possible obstruction of the trachea by the tongue. Check for breathing by looking for a rise in the chest and either listening or feeling for air exchange (Figure 33-4). Breathing may suddenly cease for a variety of reasons, including shock, disease, and trauma. If no breaths are detected, artificial ventilation must be started immediately since death may occur within 4 to 6 minutes. There should be barrier devices on hand for artificial respirations (Figure 33-5) and should be used if rescue breaths are required (Procedure 33-2).

After giving the patient two slow breaths, check for cardiac circulation at the carotid pulse in the adult and

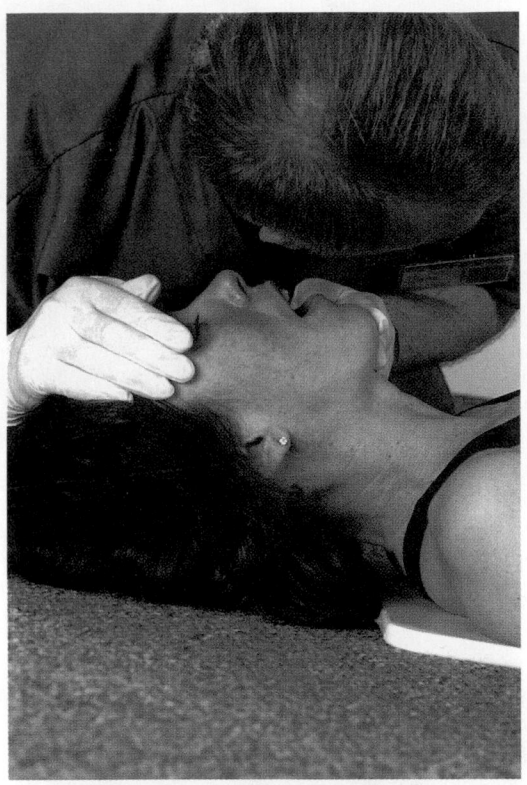

FIGURE 33-4   Checking for breathing in an unconscious patient.

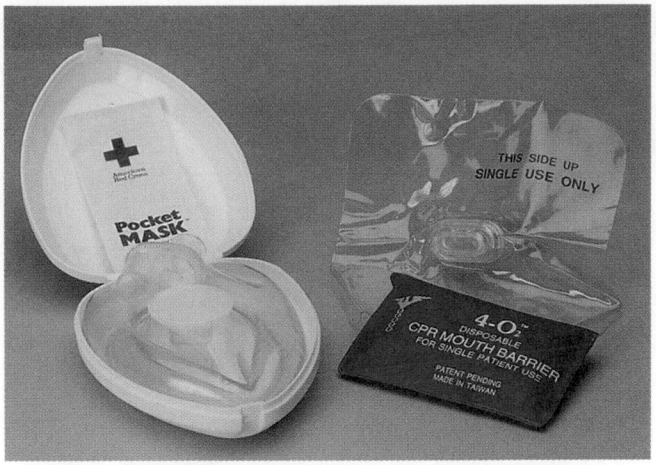

FIGURE 33-5   CPR mouth barriers.

child or the brachial pulse in the infant (Figure 33-6). If the pulse is present, continue ventilating the lungs every 5 seconds in the adult or one breath every 3 seconds in a child or infant. If the pulse is absent, begin cycles of chest compressions followed by two slow breaths.

When both breathing and pulse stop, the victim has suffered sudden death. There are many causes of sudden death, including heart disease, choking, drowning, poisoning, suffocation, electrocution, and smoke inhalation. CPR

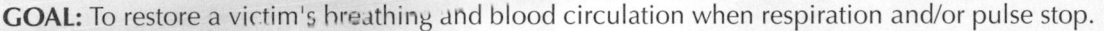

PROCEDURE **33-2**

Performing Adult Rescue Breathing and One-Rescuer CPR

GOAL: To restore a victim's breathing and blood circulation when respiration and/or pulse stop.

EQUIPMENT AND SUPPLIES

- Disposable gloves
- CPR ventilator mask
- Approved mannequin

PROCEDURAL STEPS (To be performed on an approved mannequin only.)

1 Establish unresponsiveness. Tap the victim and ask, "Are you OK?" Wait for victim to respond.

Purpose: To determine whether the victim is conscious.

2 Activate the emergency response system. Put on gloves and get ventilator mask.

Purpose: As soon as it is determined that an adult victim requires emergency care, immediately activate EMS. Most adults with sudden, nontraumatic cardiac arrest are in ventricular fibrillation. The time from collapse to defibrillation is the single most important predictor of survival.

3 Tilt the victim's head and lift the chin. Look, listen, and feel for signs of breathing. Place your ear

over the mouth and listen for breathing. Watch the rising and falling of the chest for evidence of breathing (Figure 1*).

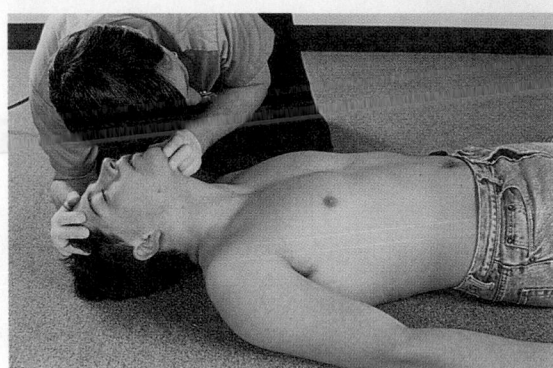

Figure 1

Purpose: To open the airway and determine if the victim is breathing.

4 If breathing is absent or inadequate, place the ventilator mask over the victim's mouth and give

PROCEDURE 33-2—Cont'd

two slow breaths (2 seconds per breath), holding the ventilator mask tightly against the face while tilting the victim's chin back to open the airway (Figure 2*). Allow time for exhalation between breaths.

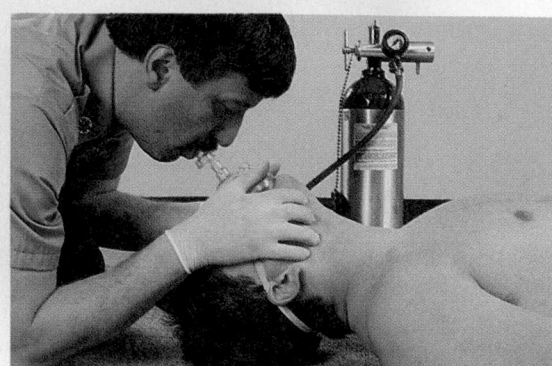

Figure 2

Purpose: The chin must be tilted back to open the airway and an airtight seal must be present so that air cannot escape around the mask.

5 Check the carotid pulse. If a pulse is present, continue rescue breathing (one breath every 5 seconds, about 10 to 12 breaths per minute). If no signs of circulation are present, begin cycles of 15 chest compressions (at a rate of about 100 compressions per minute) followed by two slow breaths (Figure 3*).

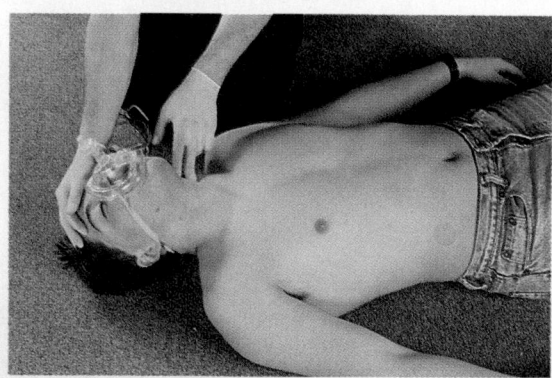

Figure 3

6 Kneel at the victim's side opposite the chest. Move your fingers up the ribs to the point where the sternum and the ribs join. Your middle fingers should fit into the area and your index finger should be next to it across the sternum.

7 Place the heel of your hand on the chest midline over the sternum, just above your index finger (Figure 4*).

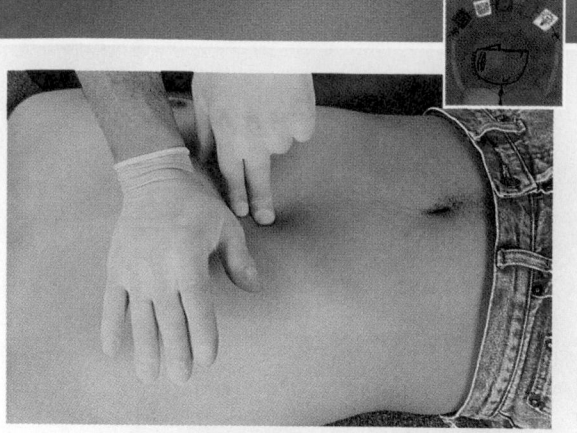

Figure 4

8 Place your other hand on top of your first hand and lift your fingers upward off of the chest (Figure 5*).

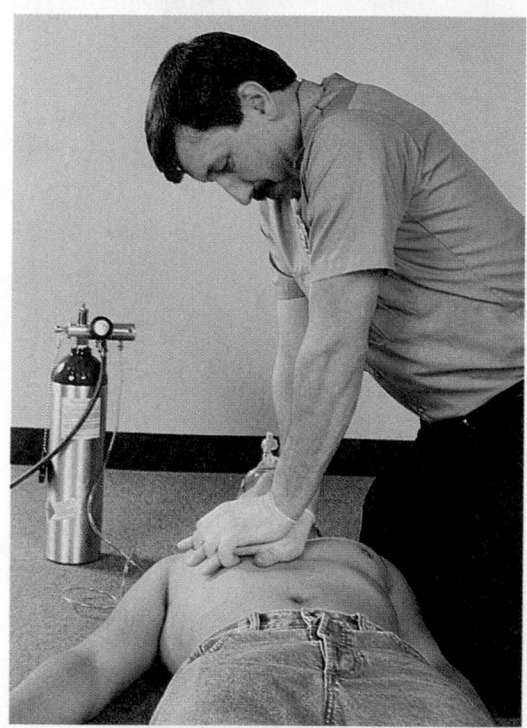

Figure 5

Purpose: This position gives you the most control, allowing you to avoid injuring the victim's ribs as you compress the chest.

9 Bring your shoulders directly over the victim's sternum as you compress downward, and keep your arms straight.

10 Depress the sternum 1½ to 2 inches for an adult victim. Relax the pressure on the sternum after each compression but *do not remove your hands* from the victim's sternum.

Purpose: The depth of compression is needed to circulate blood through the heart. Movement of the hands may cause injury to the victim.

PROCEDURE 33-2—Cont'd

11 After performing 15 compressions (at a rate of about 100 compressions per minute), open the airway and give two slow breaths.

12 After four cycles of compressions and breaths (15:2 ratio, about 1 minute) recheck breathing and carotid pulse. If there is a pulse but no breathing, continue rescue breathing (one breath every 5 seconds, about 10 to 12 breaths per minute) and reevaluate the victim's breathing and pulse every few minutes. If there are no signs of circulation, continue 15:2 cycles of compressions and ventilations, starting with chest compressions. Continue giving CPR until EMS relieves you.

13 Remove gloves and the ventilator mask valve and dispose in the biohazard container. Disinfect the ventilator mask per manufacturer recommendations. Wash hands.

14 Document the procedure and patient condition.

---

*From Henry M, Stapleton E: *EMT prehospital care*, ed 2. Philadelphia, 1997, WB Saunders.

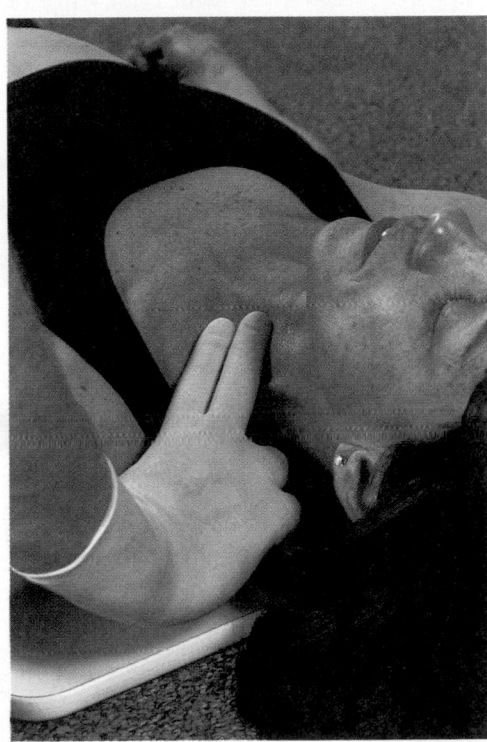
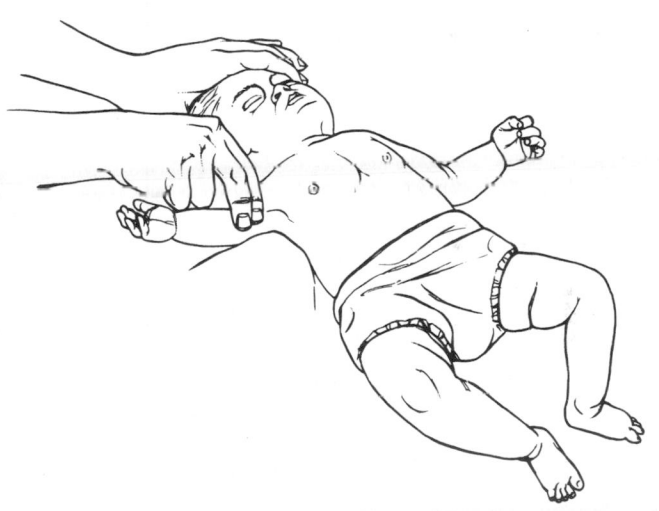

FIGURE 33-6 **A,** In an adult, check for carotid pulse. **B,** In an infant, check for brachial pulse.

---

must be started immediately in an attempt to prevent death or permanent damage to body organs, especially the brain. After four cycles of compressions and ventilations in the adult patient, recheck the pulse. If there are no signs of circulation, continue CPR until help arrives. If there is a pulse but no breathing, continue rescue breathing and occasionally monitor the pulse until help arrives.

Refer to the American Red Cross *Standard First Aid Manual* or *American Heart Association CPR Manual*, or the organizations' websites listed at the end of this chapter, for specific procedures and precautions in the management of respiratory and cardiac emergencies. As stated earlier, all healthcare professionals must have a current certification in CPR.

Heart Emergencies

Chest pain or *angina* can be associated with heart and lung disease, as well as a few other conditions. It can be quite serious; a patient with chest pain is treated as a cardiac emergency until a physician has ruled this out. The patient is often sweating and may have a gray, ashen appearance. The lips and fingernails may be blue, which is a sign of **cyanosis** (Figure 33-7). Frequently the patient will clutch the chest in pain. This pain may radiate from the **mediastinum** down the left arm and up the left side of the neck. The pulse may be rapid and weak and the patient often complains of nausea.

If a patient presents with any of these symptoms, report this to the clinician immediately. If the physician is not available, activate EMS. Use a wheelchair to move the

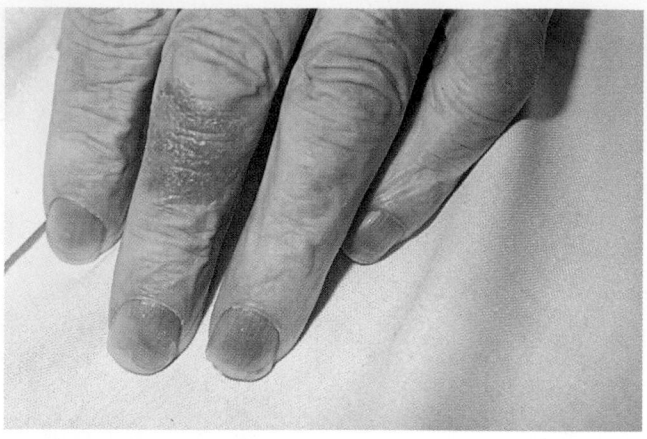

FIGURE 33-7 Cyanosis of nail beds. (From Henry MC, Stapleton ER: *EMT prehospital care*, ed 2. Philadelphia, 1997, WB Saunders.)

patient to an examination room. Breathing will be easier if the patient's head is slightly elevated or in Fowler's position. Keep the patient quiet and warm. Loosen all tight clothing. Take vital signs, including both apical and radial pulses. The physician may order oxygen started on the patient to relieve **dyspnea** (Procedure 33-3). Bring the emergency cart into the room and open the medication drawer so the physician is able to quickly prepare the medications needed. This may be epinephrine (Adrenalin), atropine, digitalis, calcium chloride, or morphine.

If the patient is conscious, ask about any medication that he or she has recently taken or is carrying. If the patient has an established heart disorder, the patient may be carrying nitroglycerin tablets. Nitroglycerin tablets are administered sublingually and may be given with the patient's consent (Figure 33-8). If the physician is in the office or is on the way, connect the patient to the electrocardiograph and record a few tracings. It may be necessary to start mouth-to-mouth resuscitation if there is no evidence of breathing. If chest pain progresses to cardiac arrest and loss of circulation, CPR must be performed.

PROCEDURE 33-3

Administering Oxygen

GOAL: To provide oxygen for a patient in respiratory distress.

EQUIPMENT AND SUPPLIES

- Portable oxygen tank
- Pressure regulator
- Flow meter
- Nasal cannula with connecting tubing

PROCEDURAL STEPS

1 Gather equipment and wash hands.

2 Identify the patient and explain the procedure.
Purpose: Patients must be taught to apply the nasal cannula with a nasal prong in each nostril and the tab resting above the upper lip. Patients who will be using oxygen at home need to be taught how to open the oxygen tank and to avoid open flames and not to smoke when oxygen is in use, since it is combustible.

3 Check the pressure gauge on the tank to determine the amount of oxygen in the tank.

4 If necessary, open the cylinder on the tank one full counterclockwise turn and attach the cannula tubing to the flow meter.

5 Adjust the administration of the oxygen according to the physician's order. Check to make sure the oxygen is flowing through the cannula.

6 Insert the cannula tips into the nostrils and adjust the tubing around the back of the patient's ears (Figure 1).

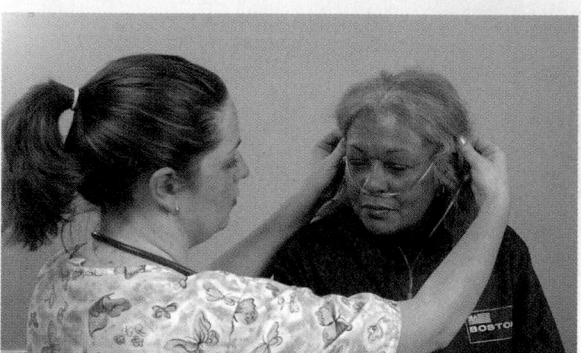

Figure 1

7 Make sure the patient is comfortable and answer any questions.

8 Wash hands.

9 Document the procedure, including the number of liters of oxygen being administered and the patient's condition. Continue to monitor the patient throughout the procedure and document any changes in condition.

See Appendix E for a charting example.

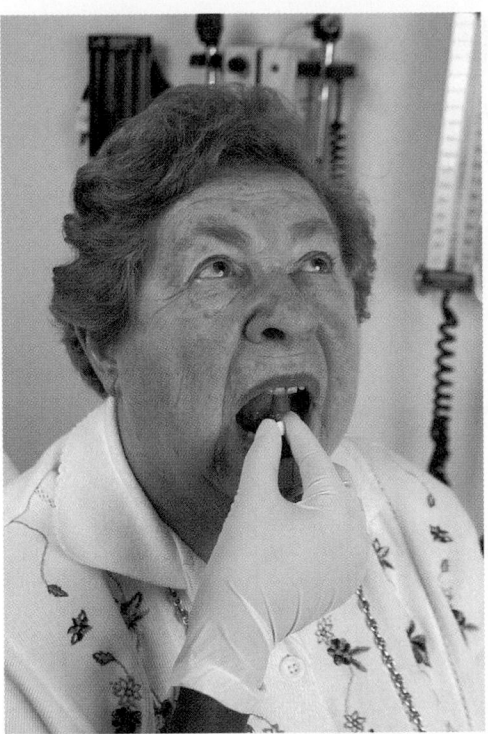

FIGURE 33-8 Nitroglycerin is administered beneath patient's tongue.

Signs of a Heart Attack. A heart attack, or *myocardial infarction*, is usually caused by a blockage of the coronary arteries that decreases the amount of blood being delivered to the myocardium. The most common signal of a heart attack is an uncomfortable pressure, squeezing, fullness, or pain in the center of the chest. This may spread to the shoulder, neck, jaw, or arms. The pain may not be severe. Other symptoms include sweating (*diaphoresis*), nausea or indigestion, shortness of breath (SOB), cold and clammy skin, and a feeling of weakness (*general malaise*).

SYMPTOMS OF HEART ATTACK IN WOMEN

Recent studies have revealed that women may experience different symptoms than the indicators traditionally cited for heart attack. These include the following:

- Back pain or aching and throbbing in the biceps or forearms
- Shortness of breath (SOB)
- Clammy perspiration
- Dizziness (*vertigo*)—unexplained lightheadedness or *syncopal* episodes
- Edema—especially of the ankles and/or lower legs
- Fluttering heartbeat or tachycardia
- Gastric upset
- Feeling of heaviness or fullness in the mediastinum

CRITICAL THINKING APPLICATION

Samantha Amos tells Cheryl when she enters the office that she has not been feeling well lately. She complains of aching in her arms, difficulty breathing, occasional dizziness, and swollen feet. Mrs. Amos does not have a history of heart disease. What should Cheryl do?

Choking

Choking is usually caused by a foreign object, often a bolus of food, lodged in the upper airway. The victim may clutch the neck between the thumb and index finger (Figure 33-9). This universal distress signal should be viewed as a sign that the victim needs help. If the victim has good air exchange or only partial airway obstruction and can speak, cough, or breathe, do not interfere but encourage the patient to continue coughing until the object is expelled. Monitor the patient for signs of respiratory distress, such as pallor and cyanosis. If the patient has a pronounced wheeze or a very weak cough, he or she has a partial airway obstruction with poor air exchange and may need help. If the patient is unable to speak, breathe, or cough, a complete airway obstruction exists and quick action must be taken to clear the airway. With a complete obstruction the patient will eventually lose consciousness from lack of oxygen to the brain. This condition may lead to respiratory and cardiac arrest. If the object is not removed, the victim may die within 4 to 6 minutes (Procedure 33-4).

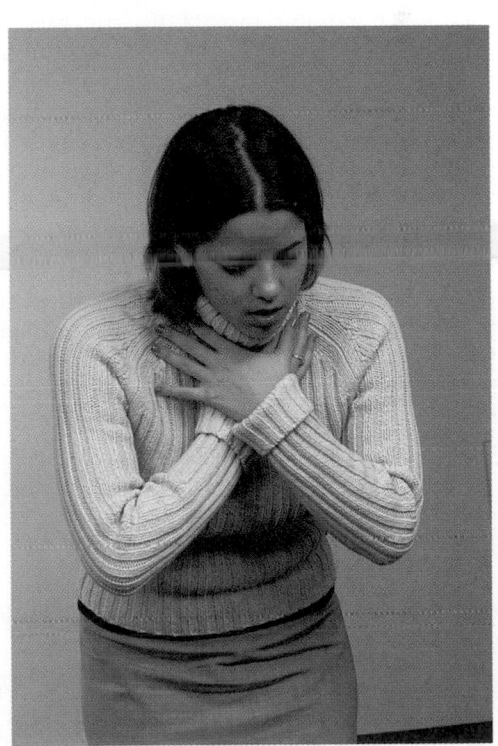

FIGURE 33-9 Universal sign of choking.

PROCEDURE **33-4**

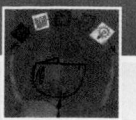

Responding to an Adult With an Obstructed Airway

GOAL: To remove an airway obstruction and restore ventilation.

EQUIPMENT AND SUPPLIES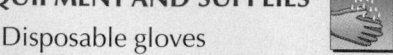

- Disposable gloves
- Ventilation mask (for unconscious victim)
- Approved mannequin to practice unconscious foreign body airway obstruction (FBAO)

PROCEDURAL STEPS (Unconscious maneuver to be performed on an approved mannequin only.)

1 Ask "Are you choking?" If victim indicates yes, ask "Can you speak?" If unable to speak, tell the victim you are going to help.
   Purpose: If the victim is unable to speak, is coughing weakly, and/or is wheezing, there is an obstructed airway with poor air exchange and the obstruction must be removed before respiratory arrest occurs.

2 Stand behind the victim with feet slightly apart.
   Purpose: With an obstructed airway, the victim may lose consciousness at any time. The rescuer must be prepared to safely lower the unconscious victim to the floor.

3 Reach around the victim's abdomen and place an index finger into the victim's navel or at the level of the belt buckle. Make a fist of the opposite hand (do not tuck the thumb into the fist) and place the thumb side of the fist against the victim's abdomen above the navel. If the victim is pregnant, place the fist above the enlarged uterus. If the victim is obese, it may be necessary to place the fist higher in the abdomen. It may be necessary to perform chest thrusts on a victim who is pregnant or obese.
   Purpose: The fist should be placed in the soft tissue of the abdomen to avoid injury to the sternum or rib cage.

4 Place the opposite hand over the fist and give abdominal thrusts in a quick upward movement (Figure 1).
   Purpose: Abdominal contents pushing against the diaphragm force trapped air out of the lungs and with it the obstruction.

5 Repeat the abdominal thrusts until the object is expelled or the victim becomes unresponsive.

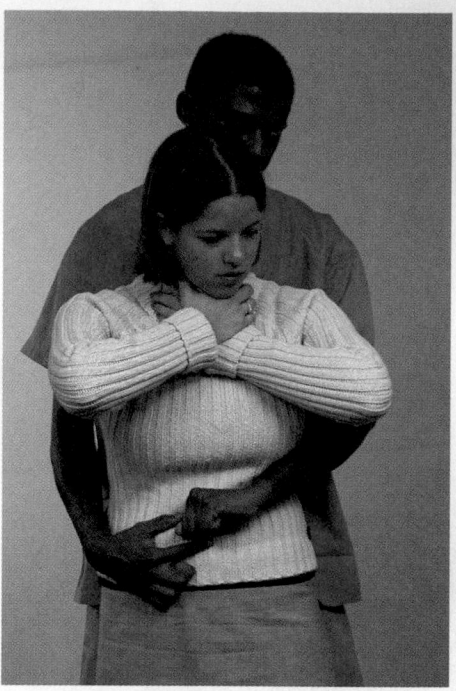

Figure 1

UNRESPONSIVE VICTIM

6 Activate the emergency response system.
   Purpose: If the obstruction is not relieved, the victim may go into respiratory arrest, which can lead to cardiac arrest.

7 Put on gloves if available and get ventilation mask. Open the victim's mouth and perform a finger sweep to determine if the foreign object is in the mouth and to remove it (Figure 2).

PROCEDURE 33-4—Cont'd

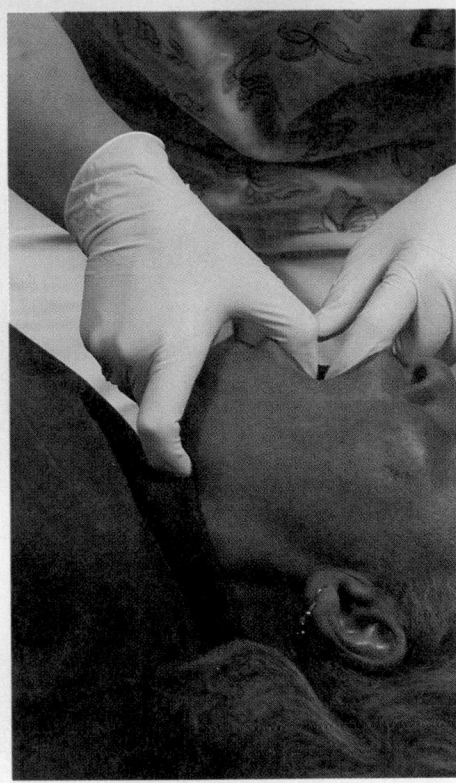

Figure 2

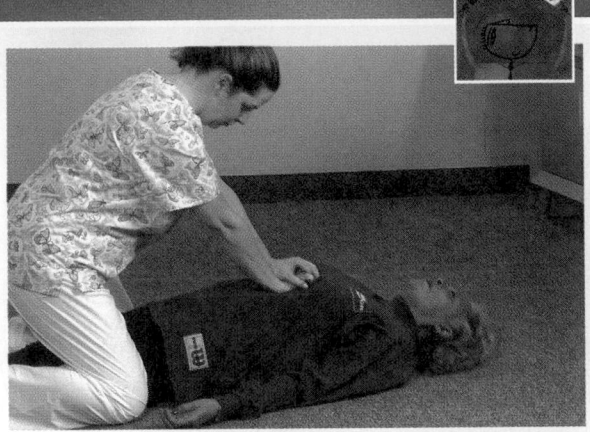

Figure 3

8 Open the airway with a head-tilt, jaw-thrust maneuver and attempt to ventilate using the barrier device with two slow breaths. If breaths do not go in (chest does not rise), retilt the head and try to ventilate again.

Purpose: If breaths do not go in, retilt the head to make sure that the airway is open.

9 If ventilation is unsuccessful, move to the victim's feet and kneel across the victim's thighs. Place the heel of one hand above the navel but below the xiphoid process of the sternum. Place the other hand on top of the first, with the fingers elevated off of the abdomen. Administer five abdominal thrusts (Figure 3).

10 Move back beside the head of the victim and repeat the finger sweep. If the obstruction is not found, continue cycles of two rescue breaths, five abdominal thrusts, and finger sweep until either the obstruction is removed or EMS arrives.

11 If the obstruction is removed, assess the victim for breathing and circulation. If a pulse is present, but there is no breathing, begin rescue breathing. If there is no pulse, begin CPR.

Purpose: The obstruction must be removed before air can be administered into the lungs for distribution to the body.

12 Once either patient is stabilized or EMS has taken over care, remove gloves and the ventilator mask valve and dispose in the biohazard container. Disinfect the ventilator mask per manufacturer recommendations. Wash hands.

13 Document the procedure and patient condition.

See Appendix E for a charting example.

The procedure for removal of a foreign airway obstruction is exactly the same for a child, *except* never perform a blind finger sweep on an unconscious child, because this may push a foreign body deeper into the airway. After administering the five abdominal thrusts, open the mouth and look for the obstruction. If the object is visible, remove it from the child's mouth and assess vital signs. If the object is not visible, administer two rescue breaths and repeat the series until the object is dislodged or help arrives.

To dislodge a foreign object from the airway of an infant, place the baby face down over your forearm and across your thigh. The head should be lower than the trunk, and you should support the head and neck of the baby with one hand. Using the heel of your other hand, deliver four blows to the back, between the infant's shoulder blades (Figure 33-10, *A*). Turn the infant to his or her back, with the head lower than the trunk. Using two fingers, deliver four thrusts to the midsternal area at the infant's nipple line (Figure 33-10, *B*). Examine the infant's mouth, and if the object is visible, pluck it out with your fingertips, but never perform a finger sweep on an infant. A baby's oral cavity is too small for a finger sweep; such an action may only lodge the obstruction farther into the

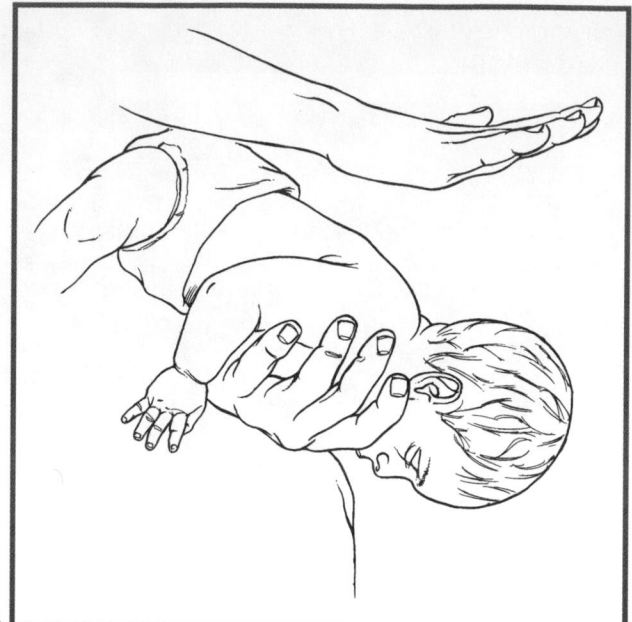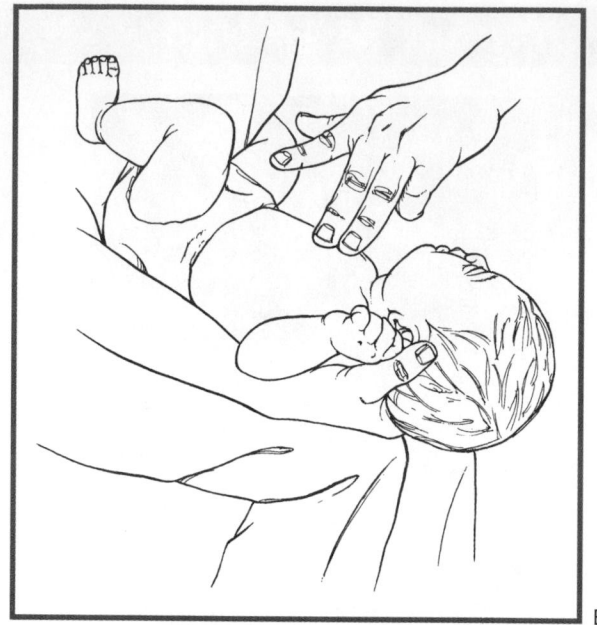

FIGURE 33-10 **A**, Back blows are administered to an infant supported on the arm and thigh. **B**, Chest thrusts are administered in the same position as for cardiac compressions. (From Henry MC, Stapleton ER: *EMT prehospital care,* ed 2. Philadelphia, 1997, WB Saunders.)

airway. If the obstruction is not visible, administer two rescue breaths by covering both the baby's nose and mouth with your mouth. Repeat the sequence until the foreign body is expelled or help arrives.

It is possible to perform the abdominal thrust maneuver on yourself if you are choking and there is no one nearby to help you. Press your fist into your upper abdomen with quick upward thrusts or lean forward and press the abdomen quickly against a firm object, such as the back of a chair.

Cerebrovascular Accident (Stroke)

A cerebrovascular accident (CVA), or stroke, is a disorder of the cerebral blood vessels that results in an impairment of the blood supply to part of the brain. This interruption in normal circulation of blood through the brain leads to some degree of neurological damage, either temporary or permanent, depending on the severity of the oxygen deprivation to the brain cells.

A minor stroke or **transient ischemic attack** (TIA) usually does not cause unconsciousness, and symptoms depend on the location of the circulatory problem in the brain as well as the amount of brain damage. TIA symptoms are temporary and may include headache, confusion, vertigo, ringing in the ears (*tinnitus*), temporary paralysis or weakness of one side of the body, transient limb weakness, slurred speech, and vision problems. TIA episodes indicate the patient is at risk for a major stroke.

Symptoms of a major stroke include unconsciousness, paralysis on one side of the body, difficulty in breathing and swallowing, loss of bladder and bowel control, unequal pupil size, and slurring of speech.

The patient who has suffered a major stroke should be protected against any further injury. Notify the physician and/or activate EMS. Keep the patient lying down and lightly covered. Maintain an open airway. Position the head so that any secretions will drain from the side of the mouth to prevent choking. Do not give the patient anything to eat or drink. Vital signs should be measured at regular intervals and recorded for the physician.

CRITICAL THINKING APPLICATION

Thomas Antonio, a 67-year-old patient, calls to report that when he woke up this morning the left side of his face was drooping and he had difficulty seeing out of his left eye. The symptoms went away in about 2 hours and he is feeling fine now. There are not any openings in the schedule for 2 days. When should Cheryl make Mr. Antonio an appointment? What questions should Cheryl ask Mr. Antonio?

Shock

Shock is a state of collapse resulting from failure of the circulatory system to deliver enough oxygenated blood to the body's vital organs. An injury, hemorrhage, infection, anesthesia, drug overdose, burns, pain, fear, or emotional stress causes this physiological reaction. Shock may be immediate or delayed, may be mild or severe, and is potentially fatal. There are many different types of shock, but the signs and symptoms are universal. The most common indicators of shock are a pale, gray, or cyanotic appearance; moist but cool skin; dilated pupils; weak and rapid pulse; marked hypotension; shallow and rapid respirations; lethargy or restlessness; and extreme thirst.

TYPES AND CAUSES OF SHOCK

Anaphylactic—a severe allergic reaction
Insulin—overdose of insulin causing severe
  hypoglycemia
Psychogenic or mental—excessive fear, joy,
  anger, or emotional stress
Hypovolemic—excessive loss of blood
Cardiogenic—myocardial infarction,
  pulmonary embolism, or severe CHF
Neurogenic—dilation of blood vessels
  resulting from brain or spinal cord injuries
Septic—systemic infection

If a patient exhibits signs of shock, ensure an open airway and check for breathing and circulation. Place the patient supine with the legs elevated to return the blood from the legs to the vital organs. Loosen all tight clothing and cover the patient with a blanket for warmth. Do not move the patient unnecessarily. Fluids may be given by mouth if the patient is alert. Because shock can develop into a life-threatening situation, it is advisable to administer only basic first aid care and to have the patient transported to the hospital.

Common Office Emergencies

The remainder of the chapter highlights typical emergencies seen either in the ambulatory care setting or in telephone triage situations. Table 33-1 summarizes common emergencies, the questions that should be asked, and possible home care advice.

Fainting (Syncope)

Fainting or *syncope* is a common emergency problem. Syncope is usually caused by a transient loss of blood flow to the brain, such as a sudden drop in blood pressure, which results in a temporary loss of consciousness. It can occur without warning, or the patient may appear pale; may feel cold, weak, dizzy, or nauseated; and may have numbness of the extremities before the incident. The greatest danger to the patient is an injury from falling during the attack. Therefore, if the patient presents with syncopal symptoms, immediately place the patient in a supine position. Loosen all tight clothing and maintain an open airway. Apply a cold washcloth to the forehead. Measure the patient's pulse, respiration rate, and blood pressure and report the findings to the physician. Keep the patient in a supine position for at least 10 minutes after consciousness has been regained. A complete patient history helps diagnose the possible causes of the attack, such as history of heart disease or diabetes. Document the entire episode and the patient's recovery time (Procedure 33-5).

If the patient does not recover quickly, the physician may activate EMS for transportation to the hospital. Syncope might be a brief episode in the development of a serious underlying illness, such as an abnormal heart rhythm, that may increase in severity or lead to sudden cardiac death.

Poisoning

Accidental poisonings result in the largest number of deaths in children in the United States. All poisonings are considered medical emergencies. Poisoning can occur by mouth, absorption, inhalation, or injection. Over-the-counter medications such as acetaminophen, detergents and bleach, plants, cough and cold medicines, and vitamins cause the majority of poison cases seen in young children. Other typical household poisons include drain cleaners, turpentine, kerosene, furniture polish, and paints (Figure 33-11). Signs and symptoms of poisoning vary greatly and include burns on the hands and mouth, stains on the victim's clothing, open bottles of medicines or chemicals, changes in skin color, nausea or stomach cramps, shallow breathing, convulsions, heavy perspiration, dizziness or drowsiness, and unconsciousness.

WHAT TO ASK WHEN A POISONING IS REPORTED

- The name of the poison taken and any information on the label
- How much was taken
- How long ago the poison was taken
- Whether vomiting has occurred
- Any pertinent symptoms, such as difficulty breathing or an altered state of consciousness
- The name, weight, and age of the victim
- Any first aid given

Instruct the caller *not* to hang up and *not* to leave the victim unattended. Call the local poison control center and forward all directions to the caller. Syrup of ipecac, which will cause vomiting within 15 to 20 minutes, should only be used if ordered by the physician or poison control center, because some substances can cause damage when vomited. Do not induce vomiting if the victim is stuporous, unconscious, or having a convulsion because of the risk of aspiration. If syrup of ipecac is recommended, give 2 teaspoons to infants 9 to 12 months old after the child drinks about 4 ounces of warm water. For a child 1 to 4 years old, administer 1 tablespoon after the child drinks 4 to 8 ounces of warm water. If the patient is to be seen by the physician or sent to the hospital, tell the caller to bring the container of poison or sample of vomitus with them so the chemical contents of the substance can be verified.

CRITICAL THINKING APPLICATION

A young mother calls in a panic to report her 18-month-old daughter swallowed at least half a bottle of cough syrup. The child is fussy and very sleepy, and the mother wants to give her ipecac immediately. What should Cheryl do?

TABLE 33-1	Telephone Triage Approach	
Emergency Situation	**Triage/Screening Questions**	**Home Care Advice**
Syncope	Was the patient injured?	Does not necessarily indicate a serious disease. If injured from a fall, the patient may need to be treated.
	Does the patient have a history of heart disease, seizures, or diabetes?	The patient should get up very slowly to prevent a recurrence, take it easy, and drink plenty of fluids.
		If the patient is to be seen, someone should accompany him or her to the clinician's practice.
Animal bites	What kind of animal (pet or wild)?	The health department or police should be notified.
	How severe is the injury?	
	Where are the bites?	Every effort must be made to locate the animal and monitor its health.
	When did the bite occur?	If the skin is not broken, wash well and observe for signs of infection.
Insect bites and stings	Does the patient have a history of anaphylactic reaction to insect stings?	If there is a history of anaphylaxis and the patient has an EpiPen, it should be administered immediately and EMS notified.
	Does the patient have difficulty breathing, have a widespread rash, or have trouble swallowing?	Activate EMS if the patient is having systemic symptoms.
		An antihistamine (Benadryl) relieves local pruritus.
Asthma	Does the patient show signs of cyanosis?	If a patient with asthma is unable to speak in sentences, has poor color, and is struggling to breathe even after inhaler use, he or she should be seen immediately or EMS should be activated.
	Has the patient used the prescribed inhalers?	
Burns	Where are the burns located, and what caused them?	Activate EMS for burns on the face, hands, feet, and perineum or those caused by electricity or a chemical, or burns associated with inhalation.
	Are there signs of shock (moist clammy skin, altered consciousness, rapid breathing and pulse)?	Activate EMS if there are signs of shock.
		The patient must receive a tetanus shot if it has been more than 10 years since the last one.
	Are there signs of infection (foul odor, cloudy drainage) in a burn more than 2 days old?	Schedule an urgent appointment if signs of infection are reported.
Wounds	Is the bleeding steady or pulsating?	Pulsating bleeding usually indicates arterial damage; activate EMS.
	How and when did the injury occur?	If the injury was caused by a powerful force, other injuries may exist.
	Does the patient have any bleeding disorders or is the patient on anticoagulant drugs?	Patient taking anticoagulants, with diabetes or anemia; schedule an urgent appointment.
	Is the wound open and deep?	A gaping, deep wound requires sutures.
Head injury	Did the patient pass out or have a seizure? Is the patient confused, vomiting, or is there clear drainage from nose or ears?	If the answer is "yes" to any of these symptoms, EMS should be activated.

PROCEDURE **33-5**

Caring for a Patient Who Has Fainted

GOAL: To provide emergency care for and assessment of a patient who has fainted.

EQUIPMENT AND SUPPLIES

- Sphygmomanometer
- Stethoscope
- Watch with second hand
- Blanket
- Foot stool or box
- Physician may order oxygen:
  - Portable oxygen tank
  - Pressure regulator
  - Flow meter
  - Nasal cannula with connecting tubing

PROCEDURAL STEPS

1 If warning is given that the patient feels faint, have the patient lower the head to the knees to increase blood supply to the brain (Figure 1*). If this does not stop the episode, either have the patient lie down on the examination table or lower the patient to the floor. If the patient collapses to the floor when fainting, treat with caution due to possible head or neck injuries.

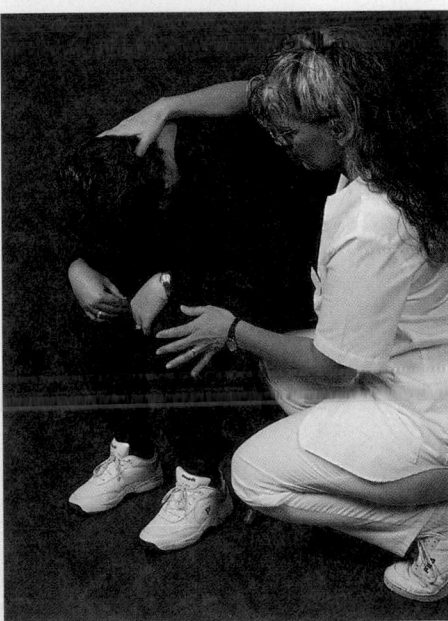

Figure 1

2 Immediately notify the physician of the patient's condition and assess the patient for life-threatening emergencies such as respiratory or cardiac arrest. If the patient is breathing and has a pulse, monitor the patient's vital signs.

3 Loosen any tight clothing and keep the patient warm, applying a blanket if needed.

4 If there is no concern about a head or neck injury, elevate the patient's legs above the level of the heart (Figure 2*).

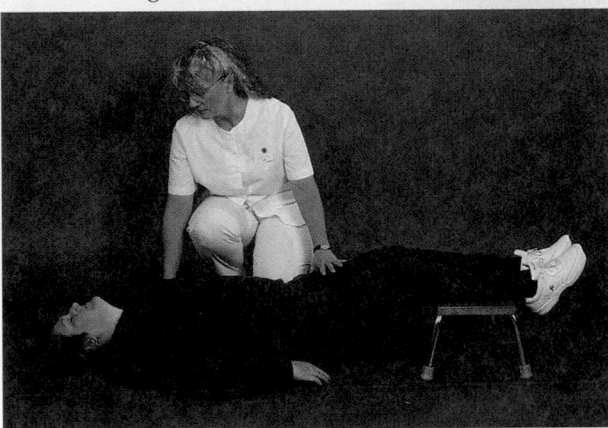

Figure 2

Purpose: Elevating the legs will assist with venous blood return to the heart. This may relieve symptoms of fainting by elevating the blood pressure and increasing blood flow to vital organs.

5 Continue to monitor vital signs and apply oxygen via nasal cannula if ordered by the physician.

6 If vital signs are unstable or the patient does not respond quickly, activate emergency medical services.

Purpose: Fainting may be a sign of a life-threatening problem.

7 If the patient vomits, roll the patient on his or her side to avoid aspiration of vomitus into the lungs.

8 Once the patient has completely recovered, assist the patient into a sitting position. *Do not* leave the patient unattended on the examination table.

9 Document the incident including a description of the episode, patient symptoms, vital signs, length of time, and any complaints. If oxygen was administered, document the number of liters and length of administration.

See Appendix E for a charting example.
*Figures from Bonewit-West K: *Clinical procedures for medical assistants*, ed 5. Philadelphia, 2000, WB Saunders.

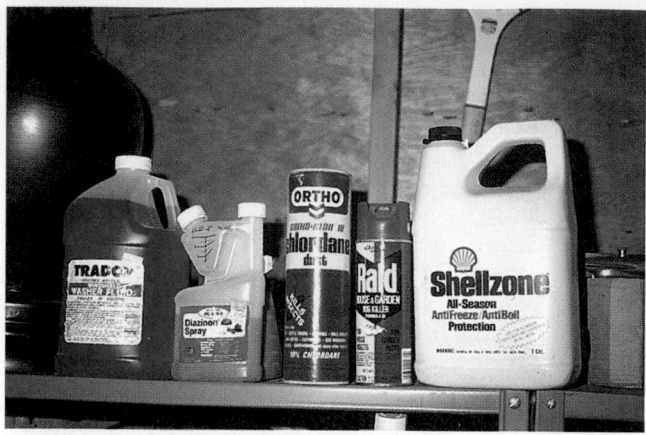

FIGURE 33-11 Hazardous household materials. (From Henry MC, Stapleton ER: *EMT prehospital care*, ed 2. Philadelphia, 1997, WB Saunders.)

Animal Bites

Potential complications from animal bites include rabies, tetanus, and local skin infections. Any animal bite that is extensive or deep should be seen by a physician. Human infection with rabies is rare, but if the bite occurs from a domestic animal, it is recommended that the animal be kept quarantined and under observation for 10 days to monitor for signs of the disease. The animal should not be killed, because a positive rabies identification is almost impossible to make if the animal has been dead for a period of time. If the bite is from a bat, raccoon, or any other wild animal, the animal is assumed to be rabid and the patient must undergo a series of rabies vaccine injections. Local skin infections can be prevented by immediately cleansing the area with antimicrobial soap and water. If the bite (including human) breaks the skin, the patient's tetanus immunization status must be checked and, if needed, a booster or the entire four-dose tetanus series must be administered.

Insect Bites and Stings

The bite or sting of an insect can be irritating and painful because of the chemical material injected from the insect, but it usually is not serious. Typical symptoms—inflammation, itching (*pruritus*), and edema—are local and confined to the area of the bite. Rarely, a severe allergic reaction occurs, which is a potentially dangerous situation that can lead to anaphylaxis. Signs and symptoms of a generalized reaction include a dry cough, feeling of tightening in the throat or chest, swelling or itching around the eyes, widespread hives, wheezing, dyspnea, and hypotension. Difficulty in talking is a sign of edema in the throat. In this situation, there is the possibility of imminent complete airway obstruction. This is a sign of a true emergency. Epinephrine and oxygen should be ready for immediate administration on the physician's orders. Antihistamines may be used, as well as corticosteroids, but the action of these agents is considerably slower than that of epinephrine. If the patient develops acute anaphylactic shock, death may occur within 1 hour unless medical intervention is initiated.

If the stinger is still lodged in the skin, scrape it off with a dull knife or fingernail. Be careful not to squeeze the stinger, because that will inject more venom into the skin. Apply ice in a towel or a plastic bag around the area to relieve the pain and slow the absorption of the venom. Calamine lotion or hydrocortisone cream may be applied to relieve itching. If the patient has a history of allergies, especially to insect venom, he or she should have access to an EpiPen injection system and use it immediately after the sting occurs and be transported to the nearest hospital for immediate care.

TICK REMOVAL

Ticks can cause a number of diseases, including Rocky Mountain spotted fever and Lyme disease. They embed their heads in the skin to obtain blood and should be removed intact by the following method:
- Grasp the body of the tick with tweezers and pull steadily and gently.
- Do not apply a match or cigarette to the area.
- If the entire tick is not removed, an office appointment must be made.

Asthma Attacks

Asthma is a condition characterized by expiratory wheezing, coughing, a feeling of tightness in the chest, and shortness of breath. During an asthma attack two different physiological responses occur. The lining of the respiratory tract becomes inflamed, edematous, and produces mucus, which results in a narrowing of the air passages. At the same time, bronchospasms occur that also constrict the airways. Attacks vary greatly between patients, and treatment must be individualized to minimize or eliminate chronic symptoms. (Treatment of asthma will be addressed in Chapter 43.) If the patient has been prescribed an inhaler, it should be used at the first indication of symptoms.

Seizures

Seizures may be idiopathic or may result from trauma, injury, or metabolic alterations, such as hypoglycemia or hypocalcemia. A *febrile* seizure is transient and occurs with a rapid rise in fever over 101.8° F (38.8° C). Febrile seizures occur in children between 6 months and 5 years of age. There are many different types of seizures, but they all are caused by a disruption in the electrical activity of the brain. The different types of seizures will be discussed in Chapter 41.

If a patient suffers a grand mal seizure, which involves uncontrolled muscular contractions, the most important factor is protecting the patient from possible injury. Clear anything from the area around the patient that could cause accidental injury and observe the patient until the seizure ends. Do *not* place anything in the patient's mouth, because it may damage the teeth or tongue. Do *not* hold the patient down, because that may result in muscle and bone injuries. If the patient remains unconscious after the seizure has subsided, position the patient in a side-lying position to maintain an open airway and to allow drainage of excess saliva. After the seizure is over, let the patient rest or sleep, but never leave the patient alone. Follow the physician's directives and assist in every way that you can. If the physician is not in the office, check the protocol section in the office procedure manual.

Call 911 for emergency assistance if the following occurs:

- The patient has not regained consciousness within 10 to 15 minutes.
- The seizure does not stop within a few minutes.
- The patient begins a second seizure immediately after the primary one.
- The patient is pregnant.
- There are signs of head trauma.
- The patient is a known diabetic.
- The seizure was triggered by a high fever in a child.

Abdominal Pain

Abdominal pain is a symptom caused by many different problems and may range from acute discomfort to life-threatening complications. The clinician should see every patient who reports abdominal pain; the question is how soon the patient should be seen. A patient with acute onset of severe and persistent abdominal pain, especially when this is accompanied by fever, should receive medical attention as soon as possible. There are a variety of causes for abdominal pain including intestinal infections, appendicitis, ectopic pregnancy, inflammation, hemorrhage, obstruction, and tumors.

Treatment in the ambulatory care setting varies with the cause of the pain:

- Keep the patient warm and quiet.
- Have an emesis basin available.
- Administer nothing by mouth (NPO).
- Do not apply heat to the abdomen unless so instructed by the physician.
- Check and record the patient's vital signs and follow the physician's directives.

TRIAGE/SCREENING GUIDELINES FOR URGENT PATIENT APPOINTMENT FOR ABDOMINAL PAIN

- Symptoms related to shock
- Severe, constant pain or waves of pain
- Bloody or tarry stools
- Fever greater than 101° F
- Pregnancy or a missed menstrual period
- Continuous vomiting or severe constipation
- Urinary symptoms such as frequency or **hematuria**
- Chest pain, SOB, or continuous cough
- Serious illness such as diabetes, heart disease, or cancer

Sprains and Strains

Sprains are tears of the ligaments that support a joint, and strains are injuries to a muscle and its tendons. Both injuries may also cause damage to blood vessels and surrounding nerve tissue. With a sprain the victim develops edema and **ecchymosis** around the injury, and any movement of the joint, especially a twisting one, results in pain. There usually is no swelling or discoloration with a strain and only mild tenderness unless the injured muscle or tendon is used. Tendon strains and ligament sprains take several weeks to heal, whereas muscle tears usually heal in 1 to 2 weeks, because muscle has such a rich blood supply. Details regarding orthopedic injuries will be discussed in Chapter 40. These injuries are treated by elevating the affected area, applying mild compression, and rapidly applying ice. Swelling will be reduced if the ice is applied within 20 to 30 minutes of the injury. After 24 to 36 hours, alternately applying mild heat and ice is usually indicated. The patient may be advised to immobilize the part.

Fractures

A fracture is a break or crack in a bone and can result from trauma or disease. Fractures are very painful, and the patient will have difficulty moving the injured part of the body. When a patient with a fracture is brought into the office, the medical assistant should make the patient as comfortable as possible. Place the patient in a position that does not place strain on the area. Notify the physician immediately and proceed according to the orders given. Emergency treatment for fractures includes preventing movement of the injured part through splinting, elevation of the affected extremity, application of ice, and control of any bleeding. If a patient with an open fracture is seen in the ambulatory care setting, he or she should be transported to the emergency department.

Burns

Burns are among the most frequent causes of injuries in the United States. Burn injuries can result from flame, heat, scalds, electricity, chemicals, or radiation. The skin surface may be reddened, blistered, or charred. The depth and extent of burns are the major determinants in classifying the severity of a burn. The extent of the pain is directly proportional to the extent of the surface area burned, as well as the depth and nature of the burn.

To triage a burn injury, it is necessary to understand what caused the burn, its location and approximate size, the depth of the burn, and whether any additional injuries also occurred. The percentage of the body surface area burned can be estimated using the Rule of Nines (Figure 33-12). Partial-thickness burns over 15% of the total body surface and full-thickness burns of less than 2% can be treated in the ambulatory care setting if the patient can be seen immediately. Patients with larger body surface area involvement or other complications should be immediately transported to a hospital, preferably one with a burn unit. A complete description of burns and their management is given in Chapter 35.

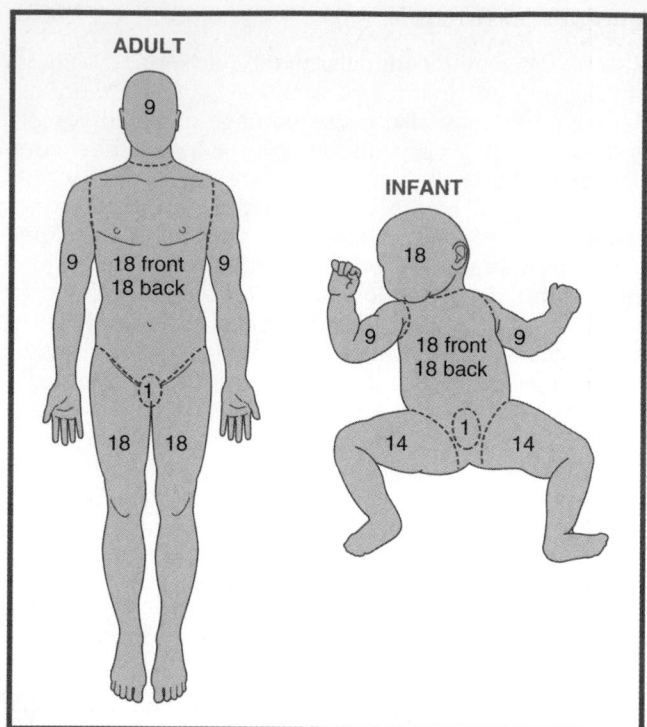

FIGURE 33-12 Rule of Nines classification of burns.

Lacerations

Lacerations are a common presentation in a primary care physician's office. A lacerated wound displays a jagged or irregular tearing of the tissues. The severity depends on the mechanism, site, and extent of the injury and the presence of foreign bodies or contamination in the wound. The injury that caused the laceration may also have caused damage to blood vessels, nerves, bones, joints, and organs within the body cavities.

When the patient arrives at the facility, apply gloves and notify the physician immediately. Have the patient lie down. Cover the injured area with a sterile dressing; use a dressing that is thick enough to absorb the bleeding (Procedure 33-6). Reassure the patient and explain your actions as much as possible. Ask the patient when he or she received the last tetanus inoculation and record the date in the patient's record. If it has been more than 10 years, the physician will probably want a booster injection given.

Wounds that are not bleeding severely and that do not involve deep tissue damage should be cleansed with antimicrobial soap and water to remove bacteria and other foreign matter. If the laceration is extremely dirty, the physician may want the area irrigated with a sterile normal saline solution.

A butterfly closure strip may be used over small lacerations to hold the edges together. If the wound is superficial and has straight edges, it may be closed with a microporous tape, which eliminates the discomfort of suturing and suture removal. After the clinician has completed patient care, apply sterile absorbent gauze directly to the wound. The dressing selected may vary in size and thickness according to the wound. Various

wound dressings and techniques for their application will be discussed in Chapter 54.

Figure 33-13 shows a patient handout from an emergency department on potential danger signs as well as instructions for follow-up care. Patient education forms should be printed in different languages for non–English-speaking patients.

Nosebleeds (Epistaxis)

Nosebleed, or *epistaxis*, is a hemorrhage that usually results from the rupture of small vessels within the nose. Nosebleeds can be caused by injury, disease, hypertension, strenuous activity, high altitudes, exposure to cold, overuse of anticoagulant medications such as aspirin, or nasal recreational drug use. Bleeding from the anterior nostril area is usually venous while that in the posterior region is usually arterial and more difficult to stop. Treatment of epistaxis varies according to the amount of bleeding and the presence of other conditions or the use of anticoagulant medications.

If the bleeding is mild to moderate and from one side of the nose, the patient should sit up, lean forward, and apply direct pressure to the affected nostril by pinching the nose. Continue constant pressure for 10 to 15 minutes to allow clotting to take place. Repeat if bleeding cannot be controlled, insert a clean pad of gauze into the nostril, and notify the physician. If the physician is not available, proceed with standard EMS protocols. Bleeding that is bilateral and continuous or in a patient with a bleeding disorder or on anticoagulant therapy should be considered a medical emergency.

Head Injuries

The severity of a head injury can vary greatly. The history of the injury—details on what and how it happened—is vital to determining management. With a head injury, the patient may appear normal; may experience dizziness, severe headache, mental confusion, or memory loss; or may even be unconscious. The loss of consciousness may be brief or prolonged; it may appear immediately or may be delayed. The victim may experience vomiting; loss of bladder and bowel control; and bleeding from the nose, mouth, or ears. The pupils of the eyes may be unequal and non-reactive to light.

All head injuries must be considered serious. Notify the physician or contact EMS immediately. If there is evidence of neck injury, stabilize the neck and do not attempt to move the victim. Do not administer anything by mouth. Keep the patient warm and quiet. Watch the pupils of the eyes, and record any changes. Obtain vital signs and record the extent and duration of any unconsciousness. If the patient is at home or is sent home after physician assessment, he or she should be watched closely for 24 hours after the injury for any change in mental status.

Foreign Bodies in the Eye

The eye is a delicate organ whose unique structure demands special handling. This kind of emergency is most uncomfortable, and it is often extremely difficult

PROCEDURE **33-6**

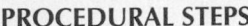

Controlling Bleeding

GOAL: To stop hemorrhaging from an open wound.

EQUIPMENT AND SUPPLIES

- Gloves, sterile if available
- Appropriate personal protective equipment according to OSHA guidelines including:
  - Impermeable gown
  - Goggles
  - Impermeable mask
- Sterile dressings
- Bandaging material
- Biohazard waste container

PROCEDURAL STEPS

1 Wash hands and apply appropriate personal protective equipment.
Purpose: To meet OSHA standard precautions.

2 Assemble equipment and supplies.

3 Apply several layers of sterile dressing material directly to the wound and exert pressure.
Purpose: Direct pressure to the wound will slow down or stop bleeding. Sterile supplies are needed to prevent wound infection.

4 Wrap the wound with bandage material. Add more dressing and bandaging material if bleeding continues.

5 If bleeding persists and the wound is located on an extremity, elevate the extremity above the level of the heart. Notify the physician immediately if bleeding cannot be controlled.

6 If bleeding still continues, apply pressure to the appropriate artery. If bleeding is in the arm, apply pressure to the brachial artery by squeezing the inner aspect of the upper mid-arm. If bleeding is in the leg, apply pressure to the femoral artery on the affected side by pushing with the heel of the hand into the femoral crease at the groin. *If bleeding cannot be controlled, it may be necessary to activate the emergency medical system.*

7 Once the bleeding is controlled and the patient is stabilized, dispose of contaminated materials into the biohazard waste container.

8 Disinfect the area, remove gloves, and dispose into biohazard waste.

9 Wash hands.

10 Document the incident including the details of the wound, when and how it occurred, patient symptoms, vital signs, physician treatment, and the patient's current condition.

---

to keep the patient from rubbing the eye. Tell the patient not to touch the eye in any way. If the physician has given prior permission, apply a few drops of ophthalmic topical anesthetic in the eye to relieve the patient's pain. The patient should be placed in a darkened room to wait for the physician, because **photophobia** is common with eye irritations. If there is a contusion and swelling, cold, wet compresses will help. Ask the patient to close both eyes and cover them with eye pads until the physician arrives. The physician may order an eye irrigation to remove the object. Unless the foreign object is clearly visible, do not attempt to search for it or to remove it.

Heat and Cold Injuries

Exposure to extremes in temperature can cause minor to severe injuries. Heat injuries occur most often on humid, hot days and result in cramps, heat exhaustion, or heat stroke. Heat-related muscle cramps are the initial sign of a heat-related emergency while *heat exhaustion* is a more serious condition. Patients with heat exhaustion appear flushed and report headaches, nausea, vertigo, and weak-

ness. *Heat stroke*, the most dangerous form of heat-related injury, results in a shutdown of body systems. Patients with heat stroke have red, hot, dry skin; altered levels of consciousness; tachycardia; and rapid, shallow breathing. This is a true medical emergency. If heat-related problems are recognized in the early stages and adequately treated, the patient does not usually develop heat stroke. Management of heat-related illnesses includes getting the person out of the heat; loosening clothing or removing perspiration-soaked clothing; and giving the person cool drinks if he or she is alert. An effective way to lower the victim's temperature is to apply cool, wet cloths and to fan the moist skin so evaporation occurs and heat is released from the body.

There are two types of cold-related injuries: frostbite and hypothermia. *Frostbite*, which is the actual freezing of tissue, occurs when the skin temperature falls to a range of 14° to 25° F. Prolonged exposure of the skin to cold causes damage similar to a burn. The tissue may appear gray or white, swollen, have clear blisters, or in full-thickness frostbite, show signs of tissue **necrosis**, including blackened areas and severe deformity. The more advanced

LACERATIONS

What you need to know . . .

It is important to prevent infection and to allow your cut to heal. Call your doctor or return to him or her immediately if any of the "danger signs" occur.

Return for recheck in _____ days
Return for suture removal in _____ days

Danger signs to watch for . . .

1. Increasing pain, swelling, redness, and warmth in the injured area.
2. Pus in or around the cut.
3. Fever greater than 100°F (38°C).
4. Blood soaking through the dressing.

If any of these signs occur, contact your doctor or return to the Emergency Department.

What to do at home . . .

1. Take all medicines exactly as directed.
2. Raise the injured area above your heart level for 1 to 2 days.
3. Keep the wound and bandage clean and dry. For cuts on the face, a bandage is often not necessary. All finger dressings must be changed within 24 hours.
4. Remove the bandage/dressing in 24 hours.
5. After 24 hours, you may shower or bathe. Begin cleaning the wound with clear water twice each day to remove crusting and scabbing. Then apply ointment (Polysporin).
6. Prevent sunburn. Use a sunscreen for 6 months (e.g., Pre-Sun or Eclipse).
7. If you have a private doctor or are a member of an HMO (e.g., Kaiser), you should call for an appointment for your recheck and suture removal. If you can't get an appointment, you are welcome to return here to complete your care.

Please remember . . .

1. The exam and treatment you have just received are not intended to provide complete medical care. You need to call your doctor to schedule a follow-up visit.

2. The X-rays or E.C.G. taken today will be reviewed by a specialist. If there is any change in your diagnosis, we will contact you.

FIGURE 33-13 Educational materials about lacerations for home care of a wound.

the frostbite, the more serious the tissue damage, and the more likely the body part will be lost. There is no feeling in tissue that is frozen, but as thawing occurs, the patient reports itching, tingling, and burning pain. Mild frostbite can be managed by applying constant warmth to the affected areas either by immersing the area in warm water (no warmer than 105° F) or wrapping it in warm, dry clothing. Friction should never be used, because this would increase tissue damage. If blisters have formed or if there is evidence of full-thickness frostbite, the patient should be transported to the nearest emergency room.

Hypothermia is a medical emergency that may result in death unless the patient receives immediate assistance. Systemic hypothermia is a core body temperature of less than 95° F, preferably taken with an Ototemp (tympanic thermometer). Symptoms of hypothermia include shivering, numbness, apathy, and loss of consciousness. If hypothermia is suspected, activate EMS and care for any life-threatening conditions until help arrives. Remove the victim's wet clothing and wrap the victim in blankets while moving him or her to a warm place. If the victim is alert, give warm liquids and apply heating pads (using a barrier to avoid burns) to help slowly warm the core body temperature.

Dehydration

A person dehydrates when he or she excretes more water than is taken in. Dehydration can be a very serious health emergency, leading to convulsions, coma, and even death. Infants, young children, and older adult patients are at greatest risk for developing serious complications from dehydration. Severe dehydration may be caused by excessive heat loss, vomiting, diarrhea, or lack of fluid intake. Symptoms include vertigo; dark yellow urine or no urine output for 8 to 10 hours; extreme thirst; lethargy or confusion; and abdominal or muscle cramps. If the patient exhibits any of these symptoms and is not able to retain fluids, schedule an urgent appointment or referral to the emergency department. Replacing lost fluids is vital, so the patient should be encouraged to drink water, tea, sports drinks, fruit juice, or Pedialyte.

Diabetic Emergencies

Diabetes mellitus will be covered in Chapter 42. The disease is caused by either a malfunction in the production of insulin in the pancreas or an inability of the cells to use insulin. Insulin is required on the cellular level so that glucose can be used for energy. Two different diabetic emergencies are caused by either *hyperglycemia* (high blood glucose levels) or *hypoglycemia* (low blood glucose levels).

Insulin shock is caused by severe hypoglycemia, because the diabetic patient either has taken too much insulin, has not eaten enough food, or has exercised an unusual amount. Symptoms have a rapid onset and include tachycardia, profuse sweating (*diaphoresis*), headache, irritability, vertigo, fatigue, hunger, seizures, and coma. It is important to provide glucose immediately, preferably in the form of glucose tablets, because they have a known concentrated quantity of glucose.

Diabetic coma results from severe hyperglycemia, because the body is not producing enough insulin, or may be caused by ingestion of too much food, stress or trauma, or an infection. Symptoms of impending diabetic coma develop slower than those from insulin shock; these include general malaise, dry mouth, **polyuria**, **polydipsia**, nausea, vomiting, SOB, and acetone- or "fruity"-smelling breath. If the patient or a caregiver when calling for an appointment reports these symptoms, notify the physician immediately, because the patient would typically be admitted to the hospital.

In an emergency situation, if a patient who has been diagnosed with diabetes mellitus exhibits signs and symptoms of a diabetic emergency, the patient should be given glucose. If the problem is caused by insulin shock (hypoglycemia), the patient will improve quickly after receiving glucose; if it is caused by diabetic coma (hyperglycemia), a small amount of added glucose will not affect the patient's condition, and he or she will need to be transported to the hospital regardless.

Patient Education

Emergencies can occur in the home, while on vacation, or in the physician's office. Patients need to learn how to handle emergency situations both by example and through instruction. The medical assistant must remain calm, triage the situation, call for help, and be prepared to administer appropriate first aid intervention. Brochures regarding home safety are also invaluable.

All patients, even children, should understand how to contact emergency medical services. This is especially important for families with members who have chronic diseases that are potentially life-threatening, such as heart conditions, severe allergic reactions, and asthma. Patients should be encouraged to post emergency numbers, such as the local EMS number, poison control center, and number of their primary care physician, next to the telephone. Families with young children need to "child-proof" their homes, being especially careful to keep potentially poisonous substances stored where children cannot get into them. "Mr. Yuk" stickers placed on poisonous containers can be an excellent educational tool for young children.

Remember to keep your American Red Cross and American Heart Association certifications current. Take advantage of community workshops to maintain and extend your skills. Post a list of community safety work-shops in an area where it can be seen by patients, and encourage them to attend. Your participation in emergency care workshops and your encouragement to have others participate may help to save lives.

Legal and Ethical Issues

Most states have enacted Good Samaritan laws to encourage healthcare professionals to provide medical assistance at the scene of an accident without fear of being sued for negligence. These statutes vary greatly, but all have the intent of protecting the caregiver. It is helpful for the medical assistant to understand the legal responsibilities and the rights of the caregiver. A physician or other healthcare professional is not legally obligated to give emergency care at the site of an accident, regardless of the ethical and moral considerations. Legal liability is limited to gross neglect of the victim or willfully causing further injury to the victim. As a caregiver, you are required to act as a reasonable person and cannot be held liable for personal injury resulting from an act of omission. The Good Samaritan statutes provide for the evaluation of the caregiver's judgment but are *only in effect at the site of an emergency*, not at your place of employment.

If you have never been trained in CPR, you cannot be expected to perform the procedure at the emergency site. However, in many states, a healthcare provider with CPR training and skills who is present at the scene can be declared negligent if cardiac arrest occurs and he or she does not administer CPR to the victim.

If the victim is conscious or if a member of his or her immediate family is present, obtain a verbal consent for the emergency care procedure before you begin. Consent is implied if the patient is unconscious and no family member is present.

Many types of emergencies can be handled in the physician's office. In an emergency situation, decisions that must be made quickly can determine whether the patient lives. A medical assistant must be prepared to act calmly and efficiently in emergency situations.

SUMMARY OF SCENARIO

Cheryl has learned through her work with the triage team and involvement in emergency care situations in the office how important it is to gather complete information about emergency situations as well as to act calmly and knowledgeably when managing all patient problems. She knows she must maintain her certification in CPR and continue to participate in workshops on emergency care to be prepared for the wide variety of patient problems seen in the ambulatory care setting. Working with the triage team has also reinforced the need to document all interactions on the telephone as well as during patient visits. Cheryl will continue to refer to the triage team or Dr. Bendt when she has questions, but she feels more confident in managing emergency situations at work.

SUMMARY OF LEARNING OBJECTIVES

- A medical assistant should be familiar with the healthcare facility's policy and procedures on the management of emergencies and maintain certification in CPR. Perform only the procedures in which you are trained, always notify the physician or activate EMS if the physician is unavailable. The medical assistant must make sure the facility is accident proof to prevent patient injuries on site, participate in planning for emergency situations, and post emergency telephone numbers for reference during an emergency.

- A physician's office must have a centrally located crash cart or emergency bag for all emergency supplies, equipment, and medication. This material must be consistently inventoried and maintained. The chapter provided a detailed list of materials that should be readily available for an on-site emergency, including a defibrillator if indicated by the physician's practice.

- Managing emergencies requires a calm, efficient approach to the situation. Assess the nature of the emergency and determine whether EMS should be activated or whether the patient requires an immediate or urgent appointment. Gather as many details as possible about the situation and refer to the physician when in doubt.

- Telephone screening is one of a medical assistant's most important tasks. Emergency action principles should be used to determine the level of a patient's emergency. These include determining whether the situation is life threatening and obtaining contact information about the patient as well as all pertinent information regarding the injury and patient signs and symptoms. This information must be shared with the physician, and all details must be documented on the patient's chart.

- Always follow standard precautions when caring for a patient with a medical emergency. Documentation of emergency treatment should include information about the patient; vital signs; allergies, current medications, and pertinent health history; the patient's chief complaint; the sequence of events, including any changes in the patient's condition since the incident; and any physician's orders and procedures performed.

- Life-threatening emergencies require immediate assessment, referral to the physician, and, if the physician is not present, activation of EMS. While waiting for assistance, determine the presence of breathing and circulation. Administer rescue breaths or CPR if this is indicated. Depending on the patient's signs and symptoms, monitor the patient for signs of a heart attack; administer the Heimlich maneuver if there is an obstructed airway; evaluate for signs of a CVA; and assess for shock. Ask for assistance when indicated and perform appropriate skills based on the patient's presenting condition.

- Common ambulatory care emergencies require an assessment, either by phone or on-site, of the patient's current condition and need for a physician's evaluation. Typical emergencies seen in a healthcare facility include syncope, accidental poisoning, animal bites, insect stings, asthma attacks, seizure activity, abdominal pain, orthopedic injuries, burns, lacerations, epistaxis, head and eye injuries, heat and cold injuries, dehydration, and diabetic emergencies. Each of these situations requires the medical assistant to calmly gather pertinent information from the patient and follow through with the facility's policy and physician orders on management of the emergency.

■ Patients should know how to contact emergency personnel, and families with young children should have poison control telephone numbers posted. Educating patients about how to care for minor emergencies at home is an important part of telephone triage in the ambulatory care setting. Encouraging patients to participate in community safety workshops and becoming CPR certified may help them to avoid emergencies as well as save lives.

■ Good Samaritan laws vary from state to state but are designed to protect any individual, whether a healthcare professional or lay person, from liability if he or she provides assistance at the site of an emergency. The law does not require a medically trained person to act, but if emergency care is given in a reasonable and responsible manner, the healthcare worker is protected from being sued for negligence. This protection, however, does not extend into the workplace.

KEY INTERNET WEBSITES

- American Heart Association
- American Red Cross
  For active weblinks to each website visit
  http://evolve.elsevier.com/Kinn/

CHAPTER 34

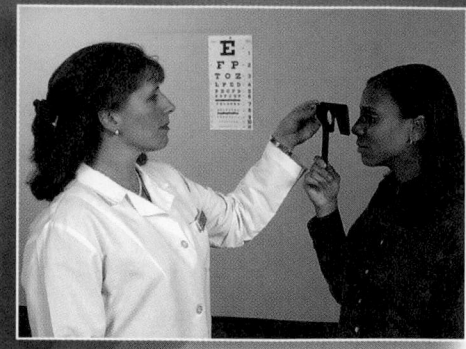

Scenario

Kim Tau, CMA, works in an outpatient clinic that specializes in the diagnosis and treatment of eye and ear disorders. Kim has been asked by her supervisor to help orient Amy Ling to the practice. Amy recently graduated from a medical assistant program and is familiar with basic eye and ear procedures but has many questions regarding her responsibilities at the clinic.

Assisting in Ophthalmology and Otolaryngology

Learning Objectives

- Define and spell the terms listed in the vocabulary.
- Explain the differences among an ophthalmologist, optometrist, and optician.
- Identify the anatomical structures of the eye.
- Describe how vision occurs.
- Differentiate among the major types of refractive errors.
- Summarize typical disorders of the eye.
- Define the various diagnostic procedures for the eye.
- Illustrate the purpose of eye irrigations and the instillation of medication.
- Identify the structures and explain the functions of the external, middle, and internal ear.
- Describe the conditions that can lead to deafness, including conductive, neurogenic, and congenital hearing losses.
- Define the major disorders of the ear, including otitis, impacted cerumen, and Ménière's disease.
- Explain the various otic diagnostic procedures.
- Identify the purpose of ear irrigations and instillation of ear medication.
- Summarize the nose and throat examination.
- Describe the effect of sensory loss on patient education.
- Conduct a vision acuity test using the Snellen chart.
- Assess color acuity.
- Properly irrigate a patient's eyes.
- Accurately instill eye medication.
- Accurately measure hearing acuity of a patient using an audiometer.
- Demonstrate ear irrigations.
- Accurately instill otic drops.
- Perform a throat culture.
- Accurately measure hearing acuity of a patient.

National Curriculum Competencies

CLINICAL COMPETENCIES

4e. Prepare patient for and assist with routine and specialty examinations

Vocabulary

accommodation Adjustment of the eye for seeing various sizes of objects at different distances.

amblyopia Reduction or dimness of vision with no apparent organic cause; often referred to as lazy eye syndrome.

audiologist An allied health care professional specializing in evaluation of hearing function, detection of hearing impairment, and determination of the anatomical site of impairment.

cones Structures found in the retina that make the perception of color possible.

fovea centralis A small pit in the center of the retina that is considered the center of clearest vision.

miotic Any substance or medication that causes constriction of the pupil.

optic disc Region at the back of the eye at which the optic nerve meets the retina; considered the blind spot of the eye, because it contains only nerve fibers and no rods or cones and thus is insensitive to light.

optic nerve Second cranial nerve that carries impulses for the sense of sight.

otosclerosis Formation of spongy bone in the labyrinth of the ear, often causing the auditory ossicles to become fixed and unable to vibrate when sound enters the ears.

ototoxic A substance or medication that damages the eighth cranial nerve or the organs of hearing and balance.

photophobia Abnormal sensitivity to light.

psoriasis Usually chronic, recurrent skin disease marked by bright red patches covered with silvery scales.

rods Structures located in the retina of the eye and forming the light-sensitive elements.

seborrhea Excessive discharge of sebum from the sebaceous glands forming greasy scales or cheesy plugs on the body.

A medical assistant is responsible for performing a wide variety of procedures in an ophthalmology or otorhinolaryngology practice. First, the anatomy and physiology of the eyes, ears, nose, and throat must be learned. Once there is an understanding of how these specialty sensory organs function, it is possible to master the skills needed to be a valuable asset to the physician.

The conditions covered in this chapter are those that are most frequently seen in the ambulatory care setting. There are many subspecialty areas for medical assistants to enter within the eye, ear, nose, and throat medical practice arena. Learning the fundamental procedures now provides a base on which to build the advanced techniques that will be needed if you choose to concentrate your expertise in these areas.

Examination of the Eye

Ophthalmology is the science of the eye and its disorders and diseases. A physician who specializes in the diagnosis and treatment of the disorders and diseases of the eye is an ophthalmologist. An optometrist is trained and licensed to examine the eyes and treat visual defects through corrective lenses and eye exercises. An optician receives training in filling prescriptions for corrective lenses, grinding the lenses, and fitting the eyewear. The optometrist and the optician are not medical doctors.

Anatomy and Physiology of the Eye

The eyes are the smallest yet most detailed and complex organs of the body. They are located within a bony *orbit* or cavity within the skull. This bony orbit provides protection and support to the eye. Only about one sixth of the eye lies outside this orbit. The eyelid assists in protecting the eye from physical trauma. The eyebrows help to keep irritants out of the eyes. The eyelashes line the margins of the eyelids and help trap foreign particles.

The *conjunctiva* is a thin mucous membrane that lines the eyelid and covers the outside of the eyeball, except for the centralmost portion, which is covered by the *cornea*. The mucus secreted from the conjunctiva helps to keep the eye moist. The eye blinks every 2 to 3 seconds. Blinking causes the *lacrimal gland*, which is located in the superior outer portion of the upper eyelid, to secrete tears. Tears move across the eyes, cleansing and moistening, and drain into the lacrimal canals in the medial corner of the eye. The tears then drain into the nasal cavity through the nasolacrimal duct. Thus, when you cry, the excess tears ultimately empty into your nose, producing a watery nasal discharge.

Eyeball. The eyeball consists of three layers. The outermost layer is the white, opaque *sclera* and the transparent cornea. The sclera is a tough, fibrous lining that protects all of the eyeball lying within the orbit, and the transparent cornea covers the exposed one sixth and serves as a clear window that allows light to enter the eye. The cornea also *refracts* or changes the direction of light rays after they enter the eye (Figure 34-1). The cornea was one of the first organs to be transplanted, and now corneal transplants are a common procedure. Long-term success after corneal implant surgery is excellent.

The *choroid* is the posterior portion of the middle layer of the eye. It is the vascular layer of the eye containing many blood vessels that supply nutrients to the outer layers of the *retina*. The choroid also contains a brown pigment that absorbs excess light rays that could interfere with vision. In the anterior part of this layer, the choroid creates the *iris* and the *ciliary body*. The iris is the colored portion of the eye. It is doughnut shaped, with the opening of the *pupil* in the center. The iris contains muscles that regulate the size of the pupil according to the intensity of the light, becoming smaller in bright light and opening wider in dim light. The ciliary body contains the *ciliary muscle*, which regulates the shape of the lens and also the *ciliary processes*, which secrete aqueous humor.

The inner layer of the eye includes the retina in the posterior portion and the lens in the anterior portion. It is in the retina where the **rods** and **cones**, **optic nerve**, **optic disc**, and **fovea centralis** are located. The delicate tissue of the retina is composed of light-sensitive neurons

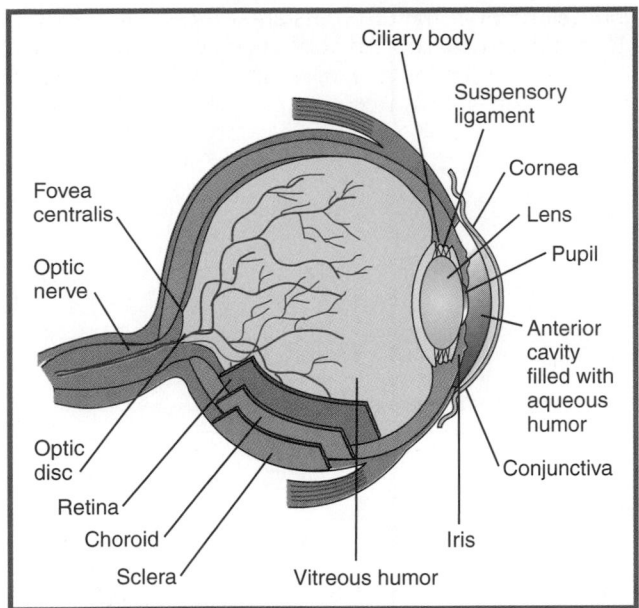

FIGURE 34-1   Anatomy of the eye.

TABLE 34-1	Functions of the Major Parts of the Eye
Structure	**Function**
Sclera	External protection
Cornea	Light refraction
Choroid	Blood supply
Iris	Light absorption and regulation of pupillary width
Ciliary body	Secretion of vitreous fluid; changes the shape of the lens
Lens	Light refraction
Retinal layer	Light receptor that transforms optic signals into nerve impulses
Rods	Means of distinguishing light from dark and of perceiving shape and movement
Cones	Color vision
Central fovea	Area of sharpest vision
Macula lutea	Blind spot
External ocular muscles	Movement of the globe
Optical nerve (cranial nerve II)	Transmission of visual information to the brain
Lacrimal glands	Secretion of tears
Eyelid	Eye protection

Modified from Damjanov I: *Pathology for the health-related professions.* Philadelphia, 1996, WB Saunders.

that convert light into impulses. These impulses travel to the brain by means of the optic nerve, and the brain converts them into a visual picture. The lens is a transparent, biconvex body that helps focus light after it passes through the cornea. The lens and the ciliary body divide the eye into two cavities. The posterior cavity is between the lens and the retina and contains the transparent, gel-like *vitreous humor.* The anterior cavity is between the cornea and the lens and is filled with *aqueous humor,* produced by the ciliary processes. Aqueous humor provides nutrients to the lens and cornea, because they do not have blood vessels.

Vision. Vision requires light and depends on the proper functioning of all parts of the eye (Table 34-1). A visual impulse begins with the passage of light through the cornea, where it is refracted and then passes through the aqueous humor and pupil into the lens. The ciliary muscle adjusts the curvature of the lens to again refract the light rays so they pass into the retina, triggering the photoreceptor cells of the rods and cones. At this point, the light energy is converted into an electrical impulse that is sent through the optic nerve to the visual cortex of the occipital lobe of the brain where interpretation occurs.

Disorders of the Eye

Refractive Errors. Four major types of refractive errors result when the eye is unable to focus light effectively on the retina. Refraction refers to the ability of the lens of the eye to bend parallel light rays coming into the eye so the rays are focused on the retina. An error of refraction means that the light rays are not being refracted or bent properly and thus do not focus correctly on the retina. Defects in the shape of the eyeball may cause a refractive error. Most refractive errors can be corrected by wearing corrective lenses (Figure 34-2).

Hyperopia (Farsightedness). When light enters the eye and focuses behind the retina, the person has hyperopia. This disorder is caused by an eyeball that is too short from the anterior to posterior wall. A hyperopic person has difficulty seeing objects close up, at reading or working level. A convex-shaped corrective lens aids the eye's internal lens to place objects on the retina and secure a sharp, detailed image.

Myopia (Nearsightedness). Myopia occurs when light rays entering the eye focus in front of the retina, causing objects at a distance to appear blurry and dull. Objects viewed at reading or working level can be seen clearly. In this disorder the eyeball is elongated from the anterior to the posterior walls and the image cannot be sharpened by the internal lens of the eye. A concave corrective lens is used to focus the light rays on the retina.

Presbyopia. As people age, most experience a decrease in the elasticity of the internal lens of the eye. This often causes vision changes after 40 years of age. The condition is characterized by a decrease in the ability to see at reading level. A combination corrective lens, known as a bifocal lens or progressive lens correction, is used to focus both distal and proximal objects directly on the retina.

Astigmatism. Astigmatism is an irregular focusing of the light rays entering the eye. This is usually caused by the cornea or the lens not being a smooth sphere but instead having an irregular shape or having wavy lines in it. This causes the light rays to be unevenly or diffusely focused on the retina, and images appear clear in the center but blurry around the perimeter. It is like attempting to focus on objects seen through a wavy piece of window glass.

Signs and Symptoms of Refractive Errors. Refractive errors in vision can lead to squinting, frequent rubbing of

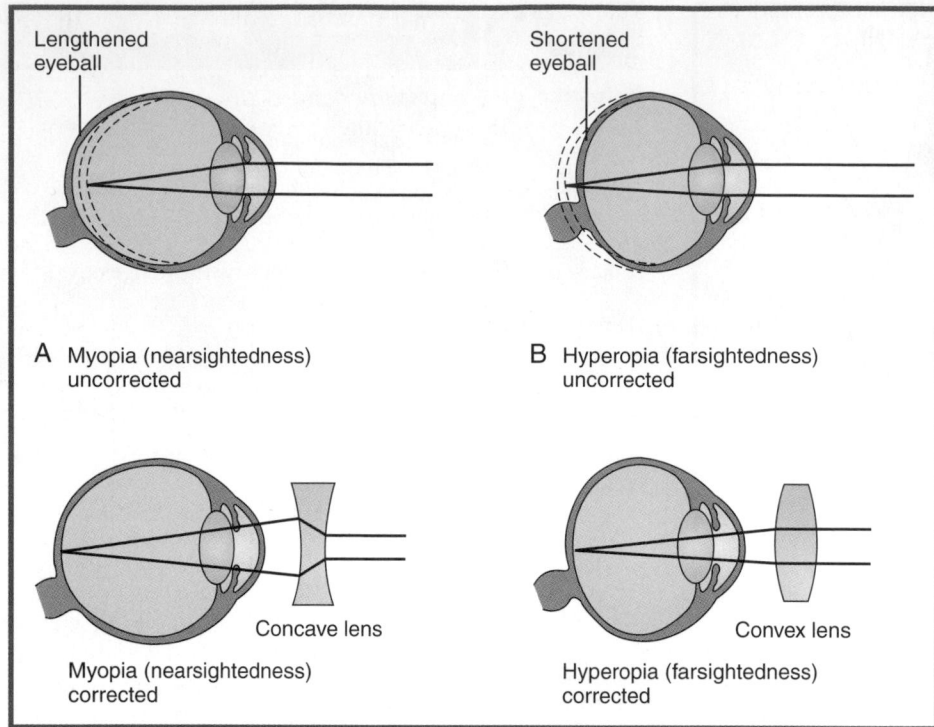

A Myopia (nearsightedness) uncorrected

B Hyperopia (farsightedness) uncorrected

Concave lens

Myopia (nearsightedness) corrected

Convex lens

Hyperopia (farsightedness) corrected

FIGURE 34-2 Errors in refraction. **A**, Myopia. **B**, Hyperopia.

the eyes, and headaches. The individual notices blurring of vision and/or fading of words at reading level. Some refractive errors are familial in nature.

Treatment of Refractive Errors. Eyeglasses and contact lenses are the traditional treatments for visual acuity problems caused by refractive errors. However, surgical procedures are now available to correct problems with the shape of the lens. One of these procedures, radial keratotomy, can correct myopia. Incisions are made in the cornea to alter the refraction of light through the eye and focus it directly on the retina. The surgery is performed on an outpatient basis, requiring only a short stay in the facility, and has minimal complications.

CRITICAL THINKING APPLICATION

Amy is assisting Dr. Hanser with visual acuity examinations when he asks her if she understands the etiology of refractive errors. Amy asks Kim over lunch what the different refractive disorders are and why they occur. What information should Kim include in the answer?

Strabismus. Strabismus is failure of the eyes to track together, which means both eyes do not look in the same direction at the same time. Adult development of strabismus is caused by a condition or disease elsewhere in the body, such as diabetes mellitus, muscular dystrophy, hypertension, or a head injury. In children, it is caused by weakness in the muscles that control eye movement. If it appears in infancy or childhood, it is most commonly associated with **amblyopia**. Amblyopia is often correctable until approximately 7 years of age or until the

retina is fully developed. Treatment involves the child wearing a patch over the unaffected eye so that the muscles of the "lazy" eye are strengthened. The main symptom in all age groups is *diplopia* (double vision).

Nystagmus. A constant, involuntary movement of one or both eyes is called *nystagmus*. The eye movement can be in any direction and is accompanied by blurred vision. It may be caused by a brain tumor, an inner ear lesion, or multiple sclerosis, or can be acquired from alcohol or drug abuse. A child born with the condition, congenital nystagmus, typically has multiple congenital abnormalities. A patient with the signs and symptoms of nystagmus should first have a neurological evaluation to determine the cause of the disorder. Treatment is based on the underlying cause of the condition, but children with congenital nystagmus will probably have it for the rest of their lives.

Infections of the Eye. There are many acute disorders of the eye that are frequently seen in the ophthalmology office. These include the following:

*   *Hordeolum* (stye): A localized purulent infection of a sebaceous gland of the eyelid; area is inflamed, swollen, and painful; usually caused by a staphylococcal infection; treated with warm compresses and either topical or systemic antibiotics.
*   *Chalazion:* A small cyst resulting from the blockage of a meibomian gland that lubricates the margins of the eyelid; can become infected, inflamed, swollen, and painful; may disappear spontaneously or may need to be surgically removed.
*   *Keratitis:* Inflammation of the cornea of the eye resulting in superficial ulcerations; caused by the herpes simplex virus, bacteria, or fungi, or may develop as a result of corneal trauma, such as intense light; symptoms include inflammation,

tearing, pain, and **photophobia**; it is treated with ophthalmic ointments and eyedrops and the use of an eye patch.

- *Conjunctivitis:* Inflammation of the conjunctiva; caused by irritation, allergy, or bacterial infection; bacterial conjunctivitis (pinkeye) is highly contagious and produces a purulent discharge; symptoms include inflammation, swelling and itching of the sclera, photophobia, and tearing; bacterial infections are treated with antibiotic ophthalmic preparations.
- *Blepharitis:* Inflammation of the glands and lash follicles along the margins of the eyelids; symptoms include itching and inflammation along the eyelash margins; may be caused by a staphylococcal infection, allergies, or irritation; treated with antibiotic ophthalmic ointment.

Disorders of the Eyeball

Corneal Abrasion. The cornea is the transparent outer covering of the eye and is prone to abrasion because of its location. Symptoms include pain, inflammation, tearing, and photophobia. It is usually caused by a foreign body in the eye or by direct trauma such as from contact lenses that fit poorly or are dirty. A corneal ulcer may also form and could become infected.

Diagnosis is based on patient signs and symptoms but can be confirmed with the use of a fluorescein stain, which makes the abrasions more visible. If the abrasions are caused by a foreign body, it must be removed first, and then the eye is treated with antibiotic ophthalmic ointment to prevent infection. Because corneal abrasions and ulcers can be quite painful, the patient usually feels better if the affected eye is covered with a dressing or patch until it heals.

Cataract. A cataract is a cloudy or opaque area in the normally clear lens of the eye that blocks the light into the retina, causing impaired vision. This condition may result from injury to the eye, exposure to extreme heat or radiation, or inherited factors. However, the majority of cataracts develop slowly and progressively as a result of the natural aging deterioration of the lens of the eye. With advanced cataracts the pupil of the eye appears white or gray.

Blurred and dimmed vision are the first symptoms of a cataract. The patient may need a brighter reading light or must hold objects closer to the eyes for better viewing. The continued clouding of the lens may cause diplopia. The patient also needs frequent changes of eyeglass prescription.

When the patient's vision becomes distorted or appears to be deteriorating, the ophthalmologist performs a simple penlight or slitlamp examination to confirm the diagnosis. The only known effective treatment is surgical removal of the lens. This is performed as an outpatient procedure in the ophthalmologist's office or clinic. After the eye is anesthetized, the inner portions of the lens—the nucleus and cortex—are removed. The capsule is retained, and an artificial lens is slipped into place. The incision is then closed with tiny sutures, and the eye is bandaged for 24 to 48 hours. The patient must get a new eyeglass prescription after the eye has completely recovered.

This procedure may be done through several methods, including extracapsular extraction, which removes the cataract in one piece, or phacoemulsification, in which an ultrasonic probe is used to break up the cataract. The cataract is then aspirated before an artificial lens is implanted.

Glaucoma. One of the most common and severe ocular disorders is a group of diseases known as glaucoma. It is characterized by increased intraocular pressure (IOP), resulting in damage to the optic nerve and blindness if not treated. It rarely occurs in people younger than 40 years of age and usually is seen in people older than 60. The cause is unknown, but there is a hereditary tendency toward the development of the most common forms. Glaucoma is responsible for about 12% of all cases of blindness and strikes about 2% of all persons older than 40 in the United States.

The ciliary body constantly produces aqueous humor, which should circulate freely between the anterior and posterior chambers of the eye and eventually empty into the general circulation. A healthy eye is filled with fluid in an amount carefully regulated to maintain the shape of the eyeball. In chronic open-angle glaucoma, the channels that drain the fluid malfunction, and over time aqueous humor builds up, resulting in increased pressure, which affects the blood supply to the retina and the optic nerve. With acute closed-angle glaucoma, the opening of the drainage system narrows or closes completely, causing a sudden increase in IOP (Figure 34-3).

Patients can have chronic open-angle glaucoma for a considerable length of time before symptoms occur. Early detection through regular ophthalmic examinations that include intraocular pressure measurements is crucial for prevention of permanent vision loss. The frequent need to change eyeglass prescriptions, a loss of peripheral vision, mild headaches, and impaired dark adaptation are some of the signs and symptoms that may be seen.

Acute closed-angle glaucoma has more obvious symptoms; the patient complains of severe pain, headaches, inflammation, photophobia, and seeing halos around light. If untreated, acute glaucoma can cause permanent blindness in a matter of days.

Intraocular pressure is checked using tonometry. The air-puff tonometer records the indentation of the cornea from a puff of pressurized area. This device determines the level of resistance of the eye to an external force without touching the surface of the eye. Gonioscopy can

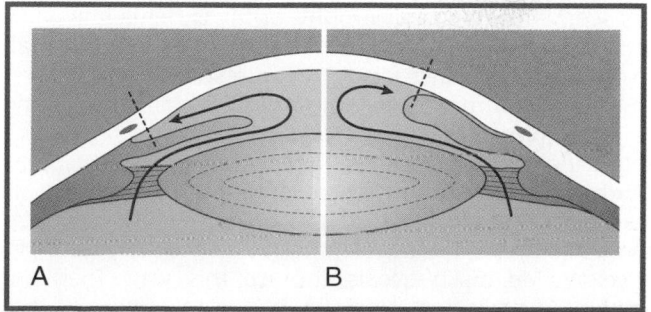

FIGURE 34-3   **A,** Open-angle glaucoma. **B,** Closed-angle glaucoma. (From Damjanov I: *Pathology for the health-related professions*, ed. 2, Philadelphia, 2000, WB Saunders.)

also be used to examine the aqueous fluid drainage system and determine whether the glaucoma is the open- or closed-angle type. An ophthalmoscopic examination can also identify cupping of the optic disc, which indicates atrophy of the optic nerve.

Open-angle glaucoma can be relieved with **miotic** eyedrops or beta-blocker drugs. The combinations of drugs used to treat glaucoma can vary considerably. It is imperative that prescribed eyedrops and oral medications be taken on an uninterrupted basis. Laser surgery may be performed to create an opening or build a new channel for drainage of the aqueous humor. In closed-angle glaucoma, medications to lower IOP are prescribed so that surgery can be performed to create a channel for aqueous fluid to circulate. This is a medical emergency, because the pressure must be relieved within a few hours or permanent vision damage will occur.

Macular Degeneration. The *macula lutea* is the part of the retina that is near the optic nerve and defines the center of the field of vision. Macular degeneration is a progressive deterioration of the macula lutea, which causes loss of central vision so that the patient can only see the edges of the visual field. It is usually painless and develops slowly, affecting sharp vision over time so that reading or other activities that require fine detailed vision become impossible. The condition is age related and caused by changes in the pigment of the retina. There is no known cure for the disease, but recent research indicates that certain vitamins and minerals, including zinc, may be helpful in either preventing the disease or slowing its progression.

Diagnostic Procedures

A complete examination of the eye is technical and requires expensive equipment and the expertise of an ophthalmologist. However, a primary care physician performs some basic examinations and treatments of the eye. The ophthalmoscope is used for examining the interior of the eye. It projects a bright, narrow beam of light through the lens that visualizes the interior parts of the eye and retina. It is helpful in detecting disorders of the eyes as well as certain systemic disorders, such as diabetes mellitus.

The eyelids are examined for edema, which may be the result of nephrosis, heart failure, allergy, or thyroid deficiency. Blepharoptosis, also called ptosis, is a drooping of the upper eyelid that can be caused by a disorder of the third cranial nerve, muscular weakness as seen in muscular dystrophy, or myasthenia gravis.

The pupils of the eyes are normally round and equal. Normal pupils constrict rapidly in response to light and during **accommodation**. This is demonstrated by shining a bright pinpoint light into one eye from the side of the patient's head. The pupil of an illuminated eye constricts, and the pupil of the other eye constricts equally. This test is called *light and accommodation (L&A)*. An older patient's eyes do not accommodate as well as a younger person's do. Each eye is checked this way. Then the patient is asked to look at the physician's finger as it is moved directly toward the patient's nose to check for eye coordination. If the pupils are equal, round, respond normally to light, and adjust and focus on objects at

different distances in a reasonable length of time, the physician will chart the acronym *PERRLA*.

PERRLA	
P	Pupils
E	Equal
R	Round
R	Reactive to
L	Light and
A	Accommodation

Special techniques employed in the ophthalmologist's office include the use of a slitlamp biomicroscope (Figure 34-4). This device is used to view the fine details in the anterior segments of the eye. It may be used to view a foreign body, because it gives a well-illuminated and highly magnified view of the area. The patient with exophthalmia (abnormal protrusion of the eye possibly resulting from an overactive thyroid or from a tumor behind the eyeball) is checked with the exophthalmometer. This instrument is designed to measure the pressure of the central retinal artery. It is helpful in patients with circulatory disease, because it measures the blood pressure in the retinal artery.

Distance Visual Acuity. Distance visual acuity is frequently part of a complete physical examination (Procedure 34-1). It is widely used in schools and industry. It is the best single test available for visual screening. Many cases of myopia, astigmatism, or hyperopia have been detected by this routine test. The most common chart used is the Snellen alphabetical chart (Figure 34-5, *B*). This chart has various letters of the alphabet and is for general use. Patients with limited knowledge of the English alphabet can be tested with the E chart (Figure 34-5, *C*). In addition, there is a chart available that uses pictures as symbols (Figure 34-5, *A*). This chart is used for young children or individuals who do not know the alphabet. The symbol on the top line of the chart can be read by persons with normal vision at 200 feet. In each of the succeeding rows, from the top down, the size of the symbols is reduced so that a person with normal vision

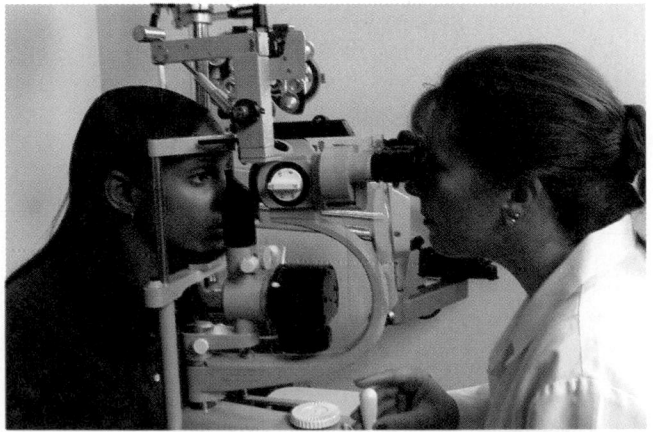

FIGURE 34-4 Slitlamp.

PROCEDURE **34-1**

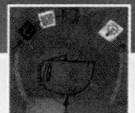

Measuring Distance Visual Acuity Using the Snellen Chart

GOAL: To determine the patient's degree of visual clarity at a measured distance, using the Snellen chart.

EQUIPMENT AND SUPPLIES

- Snellen eye chart
- Eye occluder
- Pen or pencil and paper

PROCEDURAL STEPS

1 Wash your hands.
Purpose: Infection control.

2 Prepare the examination room. Make sure that (a) the room is well lighted, (b) a distance marker is 20 feet from the chart, and (c) the chart is placed at the eye level of the patient.

3 Identify the patient and explain the procedure. Instruct the patient not to squint during the test, because this temporarily improves vision. The patient should not have an opportunity to study the chart before the test is given. If the patient wears corrective lenses, they should be worn during the test.
Purpose: Explanations help gain patient cooperation and alleviate apprehension.

4 Position the patient in a standing or sitting position at the 20 foot marker.

Purpose: Twenty feet is standard testing distance.

5 Position the Snellen chart at eye level to the patient.

6 Instruct the patient to cover the left eye with the occluder and to keep both eyes open throughout the test to prevent squinting (Figure 1).

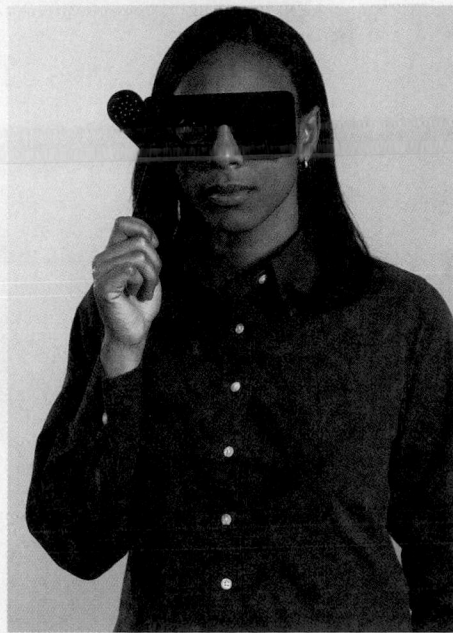

Figure 1

Purpose: The right eye is traditionally tested first.

7 Stand beside the chart and point to each row as the patient orally reads down the chart, starting with the 20/70 row (Figure 2).

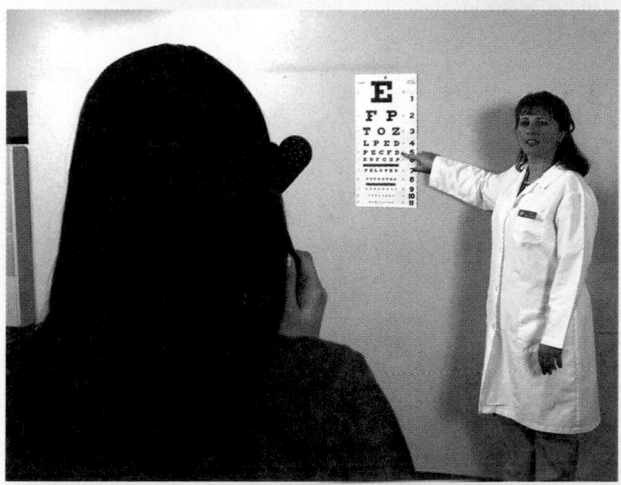

Figure 2

Purpose: Starting with larger letters allows the patient to gain confidence and allows accommodation of vision.

8 Proceed down the rows of the chart until the smallest row the patient can read with a maximum of two errors is reached. If one or two letters are missed, the outcome is recorded with a minus sign and the number of errors. If more than two errors are made, the previous line should be documented.

9 Record any patient reactions in reading the chart.
Purpose: Reactions such as squinting, leaning, tearing, or blinking may indicate that the patient is experiencing difficulty with the test.

10 Repeat the procedure on the left eye.

11 Document the date and time, the procedure, visual acuity results, and any patient reactions on the patient's record. Also record whether corrective lenses were worn.
Purpose: Procedures that are not recorded are considered not done.

See Appendix E for a charting example.

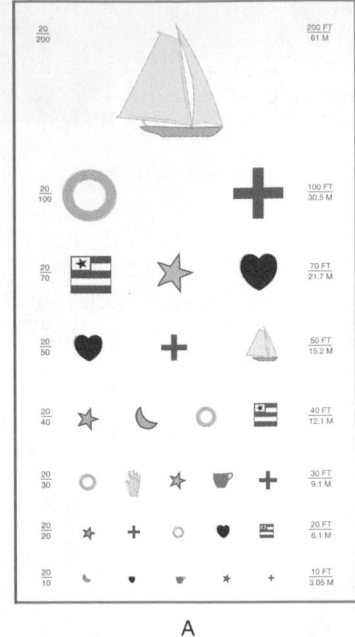

A

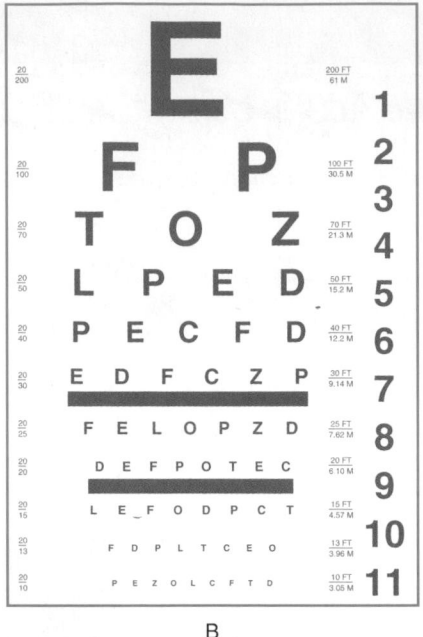

B

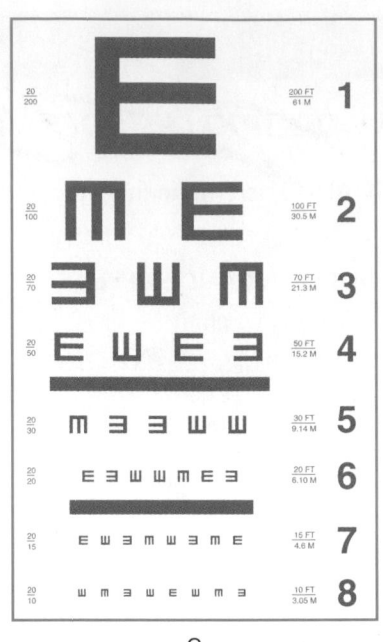

C

FIGURE 34-5 **A** to **C**, Different types of Snellen charts.

can see them at distances of 100, 70, 50, 40, 30, and 20 feet, consecutively.

The patient must not be allowed to study the chart before the test. The room or hall should be long enough so that the 20-foot distance can be marked off accurately. The chart should be hung at eye level and illuminated with maximum light, without glare on the chart. Most adults do not need the standard Snellen chart explained, but if the E chart is used, an explanation must be given as to how the Es are to be read. The patient may point up or down or right or left. If the E chart is going to be used for a child, practice with an index card that has a large E drawn on it before the child is tested. Turn the card in different directions to simulate the position of the "fingers" of the E on the chart, and give the child the opportunity to demonstrate what direction the fingers are pointing by pointing his or her own fingers in the same direction (Figure 34-6).

Because this is a gross screening of distance visual acuity, the eyes are typically tested with corrective lenses, so the patient should not remove glasses or contact lenses unless ordered by the physician. Indicate on the patient's record whether the assessment was done with or without corrective lenses. Record the responses of each eye separately. The response is recorded as a fraction. The numerator (top number) is the distance of the patient from the chart (20 feet), the denominator (bottom number) is the lowest line read satisfactorily by the patient. For example, if the patient reads the 20 line at 20 feet, the fraction 20/20 is recorded for that eye. The last line the patient can read without squinting or straining and with no more than two mistakes is the line recorded in the patient's chart for that eye. The medical assistant should document the outcomes of the test with appropriate abbreviations, using OD (right eye), OS (left eye), and OU (both eyes).

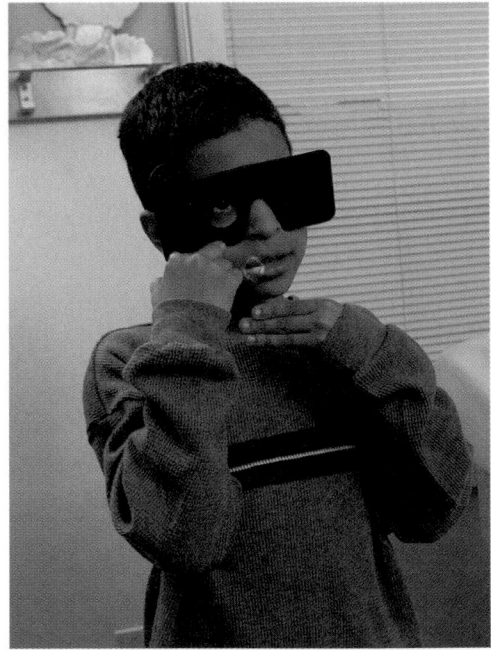

FIGURE 34-6 Visual acuity test with the E chart.

CRITICAL THINKING APPLICATION

Susie Anthony, a 19-year-old patient, is seen today for a general eye examination. The physician orders a routine Snellen test and Kim administers it. Susie wears contacts and with the right eye reads without errors to the 20/25 line but squints and makes three errors at the 20/20 line. With the left eye Susie makes two mistakes at the 20/30 line. How should Kim document this procedure?

60

Nothing can take the place of "the only pair of eyes you will ever have." That is why you are exercising such good judgment in taking care of them as you are now doing.

50

For this reason, you will welcome the suggestion about lenses which are designed and made to give you "greater comfort and better appearance." In man's earliest days he had little use for glasses. He used his eyes chiefly for long distance.

40

He worked by daylight and at tasks with little detail. But now, you use your eyes for much close work—reading, writing, sewing and many other uses which the eyes of primitive man did not know. Now your eyes meet all sorts of lighting conditions, artificial and natural.

30

Many of these conditions produce "overbrightness" or glare. Sometimes it is the direct or reflected glare of sunlight; often it is direct or reflected from artificial light. And very often this glare is uncomfortable—impairs your efficiency. But special lenses, developed by America's leading optical scientists, combat this glare.

25

These lenses give you more comfortable vision and blend harmoniously with your complexion. These lenses are less conspicuous. We are glad to recommend them because they will give you greater comfort and better appearance. Thousands of satisfied wearers testify to their real benefits.

20

You are wise in taking good care of "the only pair of eyes you will ever have." You know how valuable they are, that you can never have another pair. For this reason, you will welcome the suggestion about lenses which are designed and made to give you "greater comfort and better appearance." In man's earliest days he had little use for glasses.

The above letters subtend the visual angle of 5' at the designated distance in inches.

FIGURE 34-7 Near-vision acuity chart.

Near Visual Acuity. Near visual acuity can be tested with the *near-vision acuity chart* (Figure 34-7). This is frequently given to patients to determine presbyopia or hyperopia. If the patient wears corrective lenses, they should be worn during the test. The size of the type on the card varies from newspaper headlines to print similar to that found in telephone books. The test should be given in a well-lit room, with the patient holding the card approximately 14 to 16 inches away. As with the Snellen examination, the near-vision acuity test is given in each eye, starting with the right eye. The eye not being tested should be covered but left open. The patient should be monitored for indications of difficulty, such as squinting or tearing. The patient reads the card, starting at the top, until reaching the smallest print that can be read. The medical assistant should document the number at which the patient stopped reading for each eye, whether corrective lenses were worn, and any symptoms of eye strain exhibited by the patient.

The Ishihara Color Vision Test. Defects in color vision are classified as either congenital or acquired. Congenital defects are caused by an inherited color vision defect and are found most often in males. Acquired defects in color vision occur because of an eye injury or disease. The Ishihara test is a simple, convenient, and accurate procedure that detects total colorblindness as well as the red-green blindness that is prevalent in congenital blindness (Procedure 34-2). The test assesses the perception of primary color as well as shades of colors.

The test booklet contains polychromatic plates made up of colored dots in numerical patterns. The numbers are one color, and the background dots are a different color. Patients with average visual acuity will be able to read the numbers within the dot matrix without difficulty. Patients with color vision defects will not be able to read the number or will see a totally different number. There is also a section of plates that contain colored line trails through a background of dots. These plates are designed to be used with children or adults who are not able to read numbers. In this situation, the patient is asked to take his or her finger and follow the dotted trail through the picture.

The test should be administered in a quiet room that is well illuminated by sunlight and not artificial lighting. If this is not possible, create the best situation possible. If there is a quiet outside patio area, use it or try to set the electric lights to create an artificial sunlight effect. The test uses 14 color plates. The basic test consists of plates 1 through 11. Plates 12 through 14 are used if the patient appears to be having difficulty with the red-green differentiations. The medical assistant records the number of plates that were read correctly. If the results are 10 or greater, the patient is within the average range. If the score is 7 or less, the patient is suspected of having a color deficiency and the ophthalmologist will perform additional assessment tests using more precise color vision testing equipment.

Treatment Procedures

Eye Irrigation. The eye is irrigated to relieve inflammation, remove drainage, dilute chemicals, or wash away foreign bodies. Sterile technique and equipment must be used to avoid contamination (Procedure 34-3). Follow the procedure as prescribed, making sure that the patient is comfortable. Always record the treatment on the patient's chart immediately after completing it. Remember, if it is not recorded, it has not been done.

CRITICAL THINKING APPLICATION

The physician tells Kim to irrigate the left eye of a 22-year-old patient for removal of a foreign body. She is to irrigate it with normal saline solution until clear. How should Kim document this procedure?

PROCEDURE 34-2

Assessing Color Acuity Using the Ishihara Test

GOAL: To correctly assess a patient's color acuity and record the results.

EQUIPMENT AND SUPPLIES

- Appropriate room area with natural light
- Ishihara color plate book
- Pen, pencil, and paper
- Watch with a second hand

PROCEDURAL STEPS

1 Assemble the necessary equipment and prepare the room for testing. The room should be quiet and illuminated with natural light.

Purpose: For testing colors to be seen correctly, natural light is needed.

2 Identify the patient and explain the procedure. Use a practice card during the explanation and be sure that the patient understands that he or she has 3 seconds to identify each plate.

Purpose: An informed patient is a cooperative patient. The first plate is a practice plate and is designed to be read correctly.

3 Hold up the first plate at a right angle to the patient's line of vision and 30 inches from the patient. Be sure both of the patient's eyes are kept open during the test (Figure 1).

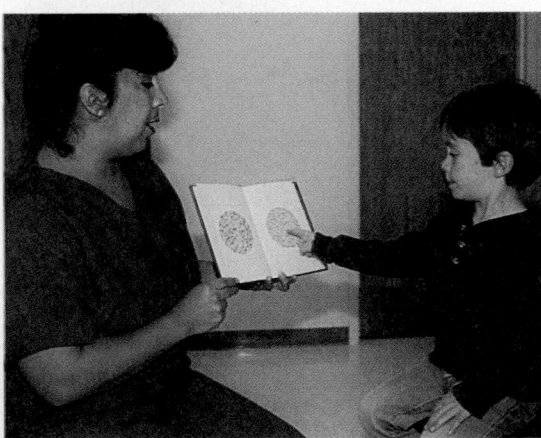

Figure 1

4 Ask the patient to tell you what number is on the plate and record the plate number and the patient's answer (Figure 2).

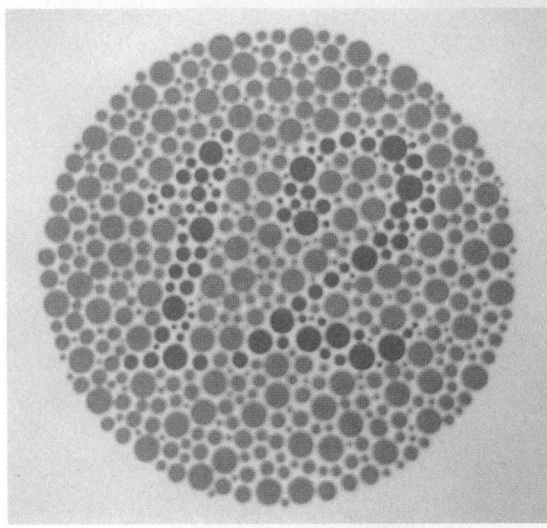

Figure 2

5 Continue this sequence until all 11 plates have been read. If the patient cannot identify the number on the plate, place an X in the record for that plate number. Your record should look like this:

Plate 1 = pass, Plate 2 = pass, Plate 3 = X, Plate 4 = pass, and so on.

6 Include any unusual symptoms in your record, such as eye rubbing, squinting, or excessive blinking.

7 Place the book back into its cardboard sleeve and return the book to its storage space.

Purpose: The Ishihara color plates need to be stored in a closed position away from external light to protect the colors.

8 Record the procedure, including the date and time, the testing results, and any patient symptoms exhibited during the test in the patient's record.

Purpose: Procedures that are not recorded are considered not done.

Foreign bodies in the eye are very irritating and may cause considerable pain. Most foreign bodies are superficial and can be easily removed. Occasionally, foreign particles may be deeply embedded and require eye surgery. When a patient comes into the office and has something in his or her eye, notify the physician immediately.

The first objective of the physician's examination will be inspection. The patient is asked to look to either side and up and down so that the anterior

PROCEDURE 34-3

Irrigating a Patient's Eyes

GOAL: To cleanse the eye (or eyes), as ordered by the physician.

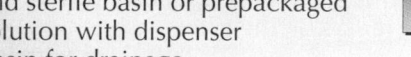

EQUIPMENT AND SUPPLIES

- Prescribed sterile irrigation solution
- Sterile irrigating bulb syringe and sterile basin or prepackaged solution with dispenser
- Basin for drainage
- Sterile gauze squares
- Disposable drape
- Towel
- Nonsterile gloves
- Biohazard waste container

PROCEDURAL STEPS

1 Wash your hands. Put on gloves.
Purpose: Infection control.

2 Check the physician's orders to determine which eye requires irrigation (or whether both eyes require it) and the type of solution to be used.
Purpose: To check the abbreviations: OD (right eye), OS (left eye), OU (both eyes).

3 Assemble the materials needed.

4 Check the expiration date of the solution and read the label three times.
Purpose: To follow the rules for administering medications.

5 Identify the patient, and explain the procedure.
Purpose: Explanations help gain patient cooperation and alleviate apprehension.

6 Assist the patient into a sitting or supine position, making certain that the head is turned toward the side of the affected eye. Place the disposable drape over the patient's neck and shoulder.
Purpose: This position causes the solution to flow away from the unaffected eye so as to reduce the chances for cross-contamination of the healthy eye.

7 Place or have the patient hold a drainage basin next to the affected eye to receive the solution from the eye. Place a polylined drape under the basin to avoid getting the solution on the patient.

8 Moisten a gauze square with solution and cleanse the eyelid and lashes. Start at the inner canthus (near nose) to the outer canthus (farthest from nose) and dispose of the gauze square after each wipe (Figure 1).

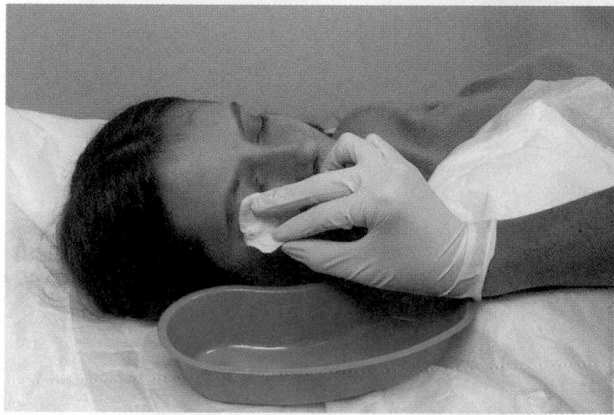

Figure 1

Purpose: Debris on the lids or lashes must be cleansed away before exposing the conjunctiva.

9 If using a bulb syringe, pour the required volume of body-temperature irrigating solution into the basin and withdraw solution into the bulb syringe. If using an irrigating solution in a prepackaged dispenser, remove the lid.
Purpose: Cold solution will cause the patient pain and discomfort.

10 Separate and hold eyelids with the index finger and thumb of one hand. With the other hand, place the syringe or dispenser on the bridge of the nose parallel to the eye.
Purpose: To support and steady the dispenser.

Continued

surface can be inspected. For the physician to fully inspect under the upper lid, the patient must cooperate by looking downward while the physician everts the upper lid using a cotton-tipped applicator. While the lid is maintained in an everted position, any foreign materials may be rinsed away with sterile water or saline solution. If the physician gives the order for you to remove the foreign body, do so through irrigation only. If this technique is unsuccessful, cover both of the patient's eyes with a gauze dressing and notify your supervisor immediately.

 SAFETY ALERT Never attempt to remove a foreign body from the cornea using an

PROCEDURE **34-3—Cont'd**

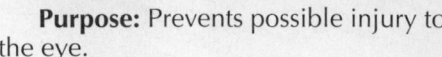
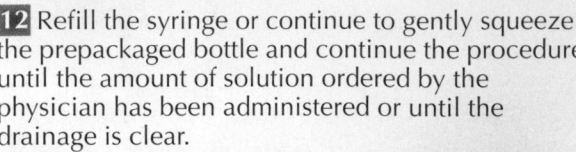

11 Squeeze the bulb or dispenser, directing the solution toward the lower conjunctiva of the inner canthus, allowing the solution to flow steadily and slowly from the inner to outer canthus. Do not touch the eye or eyelids with the applicator (Figure 2).

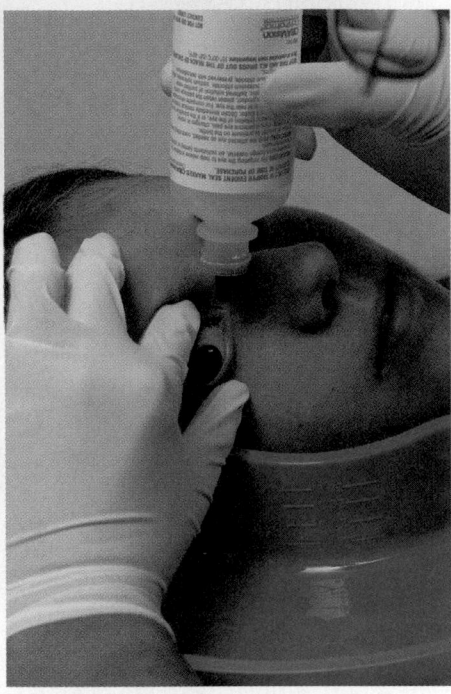

Figure 2

Purpose: Prevents possible injury to the eye.

12 Refill the syringe or continue to gently squeeze the prepackaged bottle and continue the procedure until the amount of solution ordered by the physician has been administered or until the drainage is clear.

13 Dry the eyelid from the inner to outer canthus with sterile gauze. Do not use cotton balls because fibers might remain in the eye.

14 Clean the work area.

15 Remove gloves and wash your hands.
Purpose: Infection control.

16 Document the procedure using appropriate abbreviations; including the date and time; the type and amount of solution used; which eye was irrigated; any significant patient reactions; and the results in the patient's record.
Purpose: Procedures that are not recorded are considered not done.

See Appendix E for a charting example.

applicator, as scratches to the cornea may result, causing scar formation and impairment of vision.

Instillation of Medication. Medication may be instilled into the eye for treatment of an infection, to soothe an eye irritation, to anesthetize the eye, or to dilate the pupils before examination or treatment (Procedure 34-4). Ophthalmic medications come in several forms. Liquid drops are usually in small squeeze bottles with tips that allow one drop at a time to be dispensed, or the bottle may contain a dropper with a small rubber attachment used to dispense the medication by drops. Eye ointments are dispensed in small metal or plastic tubes with an ophthalmic tip that allows you to dispense a small stream of ointment directly into the bottom eyelid.

CRITICAL THINKING APPLICATION

Amy is ordered to administer Humorsol 0.25% one drop to the left eye in a 75-year-old patient recently diagnosed with glaucoma. How should Amy document this procedure?

SAFETY ALERT Whatever the medication, the dispenser should never touch the eye while the prescribed amount of medication is administered.

Aseptic Procedures in Ophthalmology. A major concern in ophthalmologic procedures is the contamination of eye medication applicators. Because of the concern of cross-contamination, the use of stock ophthalmic medications is discouraged. The sterility of all eye medications is critical for good patient care. Newly opened sterile solutions should be used for each patient and either disposed of after instillation or given to the patient for home use. All instruments used for the removal of a foreign body should be sterile.

Examination of the Ear

Otorhinolaryngology is the medical specialty that deals with the ear, nose, and throat. It is frequently referred to as otolaryngology or even as a single specialty of otology or laryngology. Usually, the specialty otorhinolaryngology is referred to simply as ear, nose, and throat (ENT).

Anatomy and Physiology of the Ear

The ears are only a small portion of the actual organ of hearing. Most of this structure lies hidden in the temporal bone. Anatomically, the organ of hearing is divided into three sections: the outer ear, the middle ear, and the inner ear (Figure 34-8).

Outer or External Ear. The outer ear consists of the auricle or pinna, the fleshy part of the ear that you see on the side of the head, and the external auditory canal, the tube that extends from the auricle to the tympanic membrane (eardrum). The auricle collects the sound waves and sends them down the auditory canal.

The skin that lines the auditory canal contains numerous hair follicles, many nerve endings, and ceruminous glands that secrete cerumen (commonly called ear wax), which lubricates the canal. Both the hair and the

---

PROCEDURE 34-4

Instilling Eye Medication

GOAL: To apply medication to the eye(s), as ordered by the physician.

EQUIPMENT AND SUPPLIES

- Sterile medication with sterile eye dropper or ophthalmic ointment
- Disposable drape
- Sterile gauze squares
- Nonsterile gloves

PROCEDURAL STEPS

1 Wash your hands.
Purpose: Infection control.

2 Check the physician's order to determine which eye requires medication (or whether both eyes are to be instilled) and the name and strength of the medication you will be using.
Purpose: To prevent possible medication error.

3 Assemble equipment and supplies.

4 Read the label of the medication three times.
Purpose: To follow the rules for administering medications.

5 Identify the patient, and explain the procedure.
Purpose: Explanations help gain patient cooperation and alleviate apprehension.

6 Put on nonsterile gloves and rinse your gloved hands under warm water to remove all powder from the gloves.
Purpose: Gloves assist you in holding the eye open, but the powder must be removed to prevent eye irritation.

7 Assist the patient into a sitting or supine position. Ask the patient to tilt the head backward and look up.
Purpose: Looking up helps to prevent touching the cornea with the tip of the applicator. It also helps keep the patient from blinking as the medication is instilled. For eyedrops, draw the medication into the dropper. For eye ointment, remove the cap.

8 Pull the lower conjuctival sac downward (Figure 1).

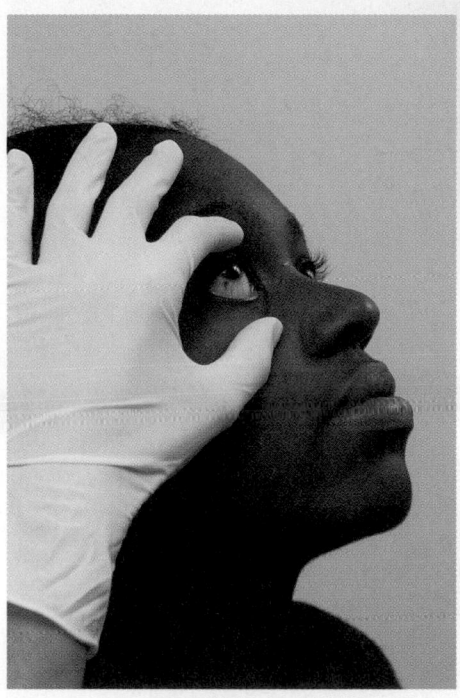

Figure 1

Purpose: Creates a pocket for the medication.

9 Insert the prescribed number of drops or amount of ointment into the eye. For eyedrops, place drops in the center of the lower conjunctival sac, with the tip of the dropper held parallel to the eye and ½ inch above the eye sac. For eye ointment (ung), squeeze a thin ribbon along the lower conjunctival sac from inner to outer canthus, making sure not to touch the eye with the applicator.
Purpose: Placing the medication in the conjunctival sac rather than the eyeball prevents injury to the cornea. Touching the eye with the applicator could injure the eye as well as contaminate the applicator (Figure 2).

Continued

PROCEDURE **34-4—Cont'd**

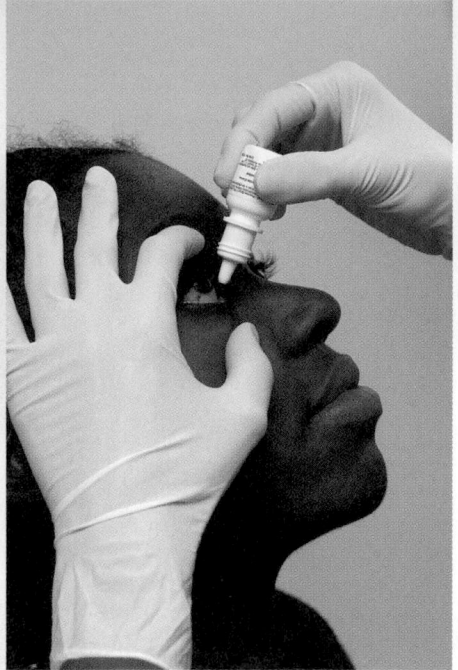

Figure 2

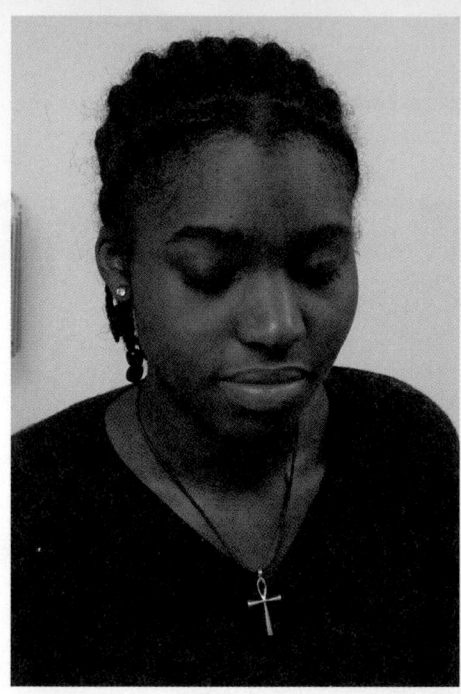

Figure 3

10 Instruct the patient to *gently* close the eye and rotate the eyeball.

Purpose: Gently closing the eye dispels the medication while rotating the eyeball distributes the medication (Figure 3).

11 Dry any excess drainage from inner to outer canthus and explain the medication may temporarily blur vision.

12 Discard the unused medication and clean the procedure area.

13 Remove gloves and wash hands.

Purpose: Infection control.

14 Record the procedure on the patient's chart including the date and time; the name and strength of the medication; the amount of the dose administered; which eye was treated; teaching instructions given if the treatment is to continue at home; and any observations.

Purpose: Procedures that are not recorded are considered not done.

See Appendix E for a charting example.

waxy cerumen help prevent foreign objects from reaching the eardrum. The canal has a slight **S** shape to it and is approximately 2.5 cm or 1 inch long.

Middle Ear. The middle ear, which is sometimes called the *tympanic cavity*, is an air-filled chamber that begins with the tympanic membrane and terminates at the oval window. The middle ear contains the auditory ossicles or bones—the malleus, incus, and stapes. These three tiny bones are linked together through minute ligaments to form a bridge across the space of the tympanic cavity. The malleus is next to the tympanic membrane and the stapes is against the oval window. The eustachian tube opens into the middle ear cavity and

connects to the nasopharynx. It is designed to equalize pressure in the middle ear with that in the external auditory canal. This equalized pressure makes hearing possible. Throat infections may spread to the middle ear through the eustachian tube; this is a very common occurrence in young children.

The tympanic membrane is a thin, disk-shaped tissue that totally seals off the outer ear from the middle ear. Sound waves conducted through the external auditory canal hit this membrane and cause it to vibrate. These vibrations are picked up by the three ossicles and changed from air-conducted sound waves to bone-conducted sound waves. The ossicles transmit the bone-

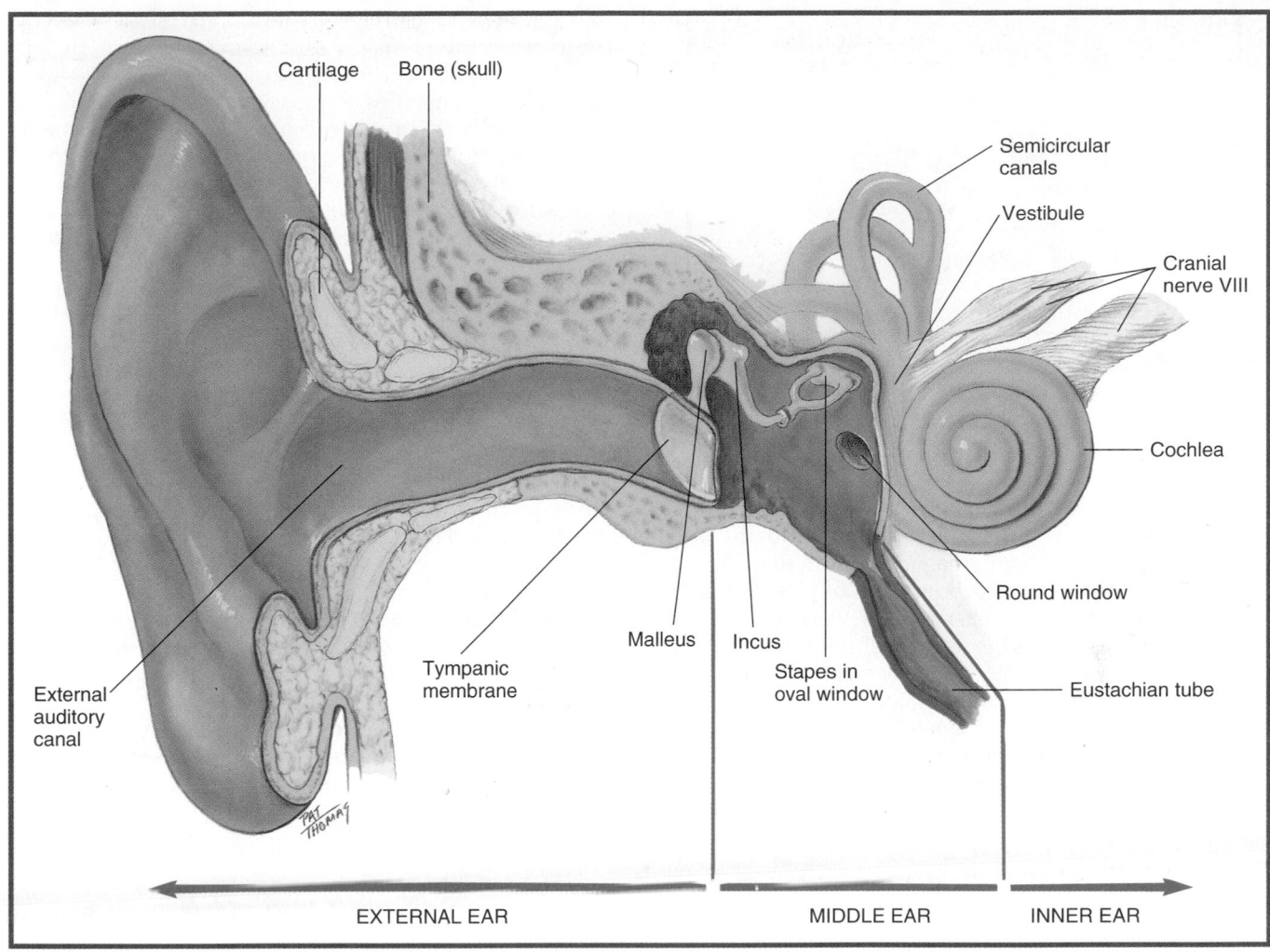

FIGURE 34-8   Anatomy of the ear. (Modified from Jarvis C: *Physical examination and health assessment*, ed. 3, Philadelphia, 2000, WB Saunders.)

conducted sound waves through the middle ear to the oval window, which is the membrane that connects the middle and inner ear. At the oval window the sound waves move into the fluids of the inner ear. This fluid motion excites the receptors, changing the bone-conducted sound into sensory-neural impulses.

Inner Ear. The inner ear is called the *labyrinth* and is divided into the cochlea and semicircular canals, which are joined by the vestibule. The semicircular canals function to maintain equilibrium, and the cochlea is responsible for the sense of hearing.

The organ of Corti, which contains the receptors for sound, is located within the cochlea. These hairlike sensory cells are surrounded by sensory nerve fibers that form the cochlear branch of the eighth cranial nerve. Sound impulses cause the hairs to bend and rub against the nerve fibers, which initiate impulses to travel through the cochlear nerve.

The eighth cranial nerve transmits auditory impulses to the medulla oblongata. Then impulses travel to the thalamus and on to the auditory cortex of the temporal lobe of the brain, where they are interpreted into audible sound and speech patterns.

The semicircular canals are responsible for evaluating the position of the head in relation to the pull of gravity. There are three canals, positioned at right angles to each other, on different planes (Figure 34-9). When the head turns rapidly, these fluid-filled canals must rapidly adjust and send the stimulated change into the central nervous system, which interprets the information and initiates the desired response to maintain balance. When there is repetitive or excessive stimulation to the equilibrium receptors, some people become nauseated and may vomit. This condition is known as *motion sensitivity* or *motion sickness*.

Disorders of the Ear

Hearing Loss. Hearing loss occurs because of two problems: either a conduction problem or a sensorineural impairment. Some individuals experience both conditions.

A conductive hearing loss is caused by a problem that originates in the external or middle ear that prevents the sound vibrations from passing through the external auditory canal, limits the vibrations of the tympanic membrane, or interferes with the passage of bone-conducted

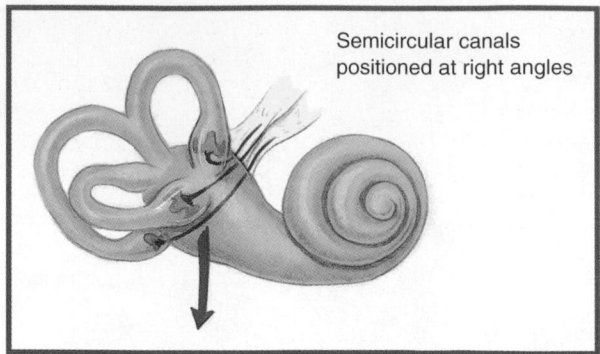

Semicircular canals positioned at right angles

FIGURE 34-9 Semicircular canals. (From Applegate EJ: *The anatomy and physiology learning system*, Philadelphia, 1995, WB Saunders.)

sound in the middle ear. Some of the common causative factors include impacted cerumen; trauma to the tympanic membrane; hemorrhage in the middle ear; **otosclerosis**; and recurrent chronic ear infections. It is the patient with conductive hearing loss who receives the greatest benefit from a hearing aid. If the hearing loss is caused by a malfunction or congenital abnormality of the ossicles, a surgical procedure can be performed to replace the damaged ossicles with manufactured models.

A sensorineural hearing loss results from damage to the organ of Corti or the auditory nerve. Viral infections such as rubella, influenza, and herpes can result in hearing loss as can head trauma or certain **ototoxic** medications. The first sign of drug toxicity is usually *tinnitus*, a ringing in the ears. This sometimes occurs with high doses of aspirin, certain antibiotics (erythromycin and vancomycin), and chemotherapeutic agents. Prolonged exposure to loud noise can also damage the delicate hairs of the organ of Corti, such as a repetitive noise in the workplace or loud music. *Presbycusis*, the hearing loss that affects aging people, results in a reduced number of receptor cells in the organ of Corti and is also classified as a sensorineural loss. Children can be born with a congenital hearing deficit or deafness because of intrauterine infection or trauma (Figure 34-10). If the sensorineural hearing loss cannot be improved by hearing aids, an option is cochlear implants. Cochlear implants are complex devices that use electrical impulses to stimulate the auditory nerve, which then carries the current to the brain to be interpreted as sound. The implants do not create normal hearing but provide increased sound for a person with profound or complete hearing loss.

A mixed hearing loss is a combination of conductive and sensory deafness. This type of loss can result from tumors, toxic levels of certain medications, hereditary factors, and stroke.

Otitis. There are two common types of otitis that are seen in patients in an otologist's practice. The first affects the external ear canal and is called *otitis externa*, or swimmer's ear. Otitis externa may be caused by derma-

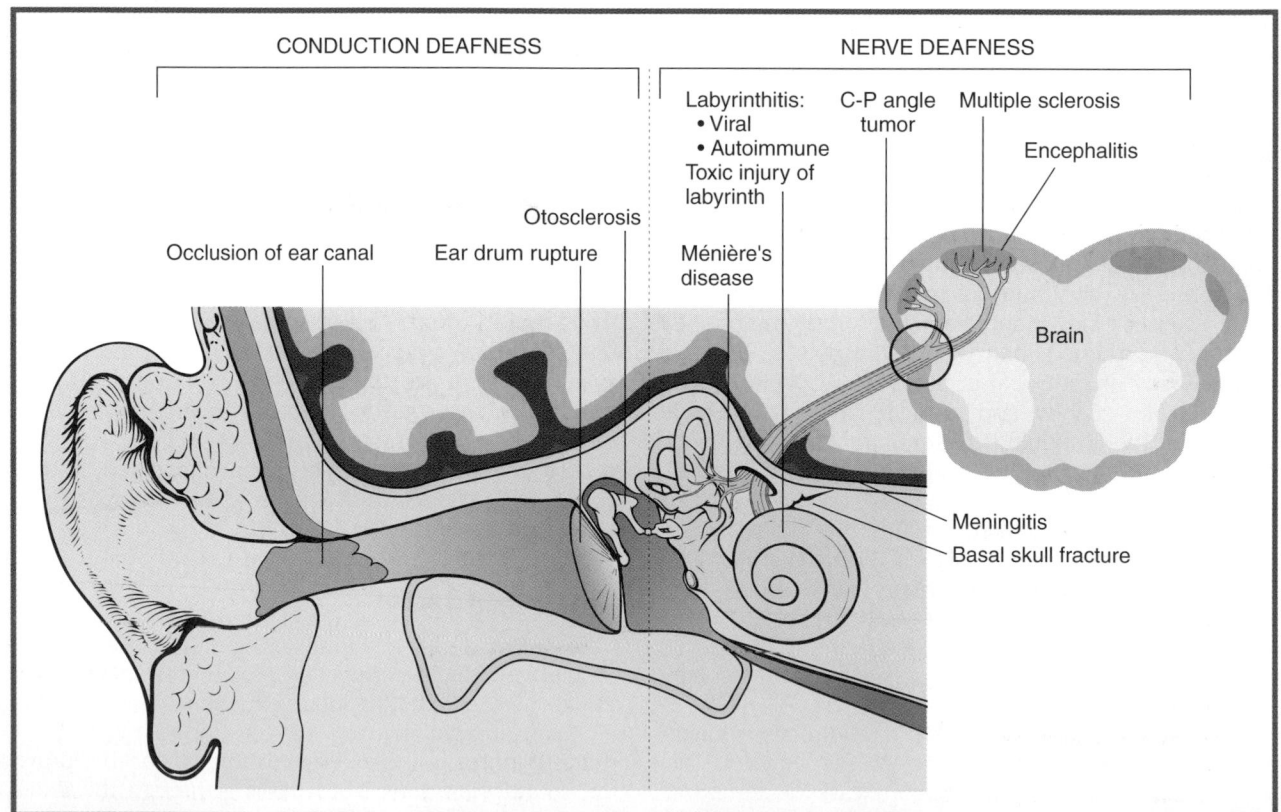

FIGURE 34-10 Causes of deafness. (From Damjanov I: *Pathology for the health-related professions*, ed. 2, Philadelphia, 2000, WB Saunders.)

tological conditions, such as **seborrhea** or **psoriasis**, trauma to the canal, or through the continuous use of earplugs or earphones. Swimmers frequently have otitis externa, because water collects in the ears and mixes with cerumen to form an ideal culture medium for bacteria and fungus. Rubbing can cause additional trauma to the canal and may worsen the condition. Patients with otitis externa complain of severe pain with inflammation and swelling of the external auditory canal, hearing loss, and possibly *purulent* (containing pus) or serous drainage. The inflammation is treated with antibiotic or steroid eardrops and the canal must be kept clean and dry or the condition could become chronic.

Otitis media is an inflammation of the normally air-filled middle ear, resulting in a collection of fluid behind the tympanic membrane. Otitis media can be either serous or suppurative. Serous otitis media occurs because of a build up of clear fluid in the middle ear with patients complaining of a full feeling and some hearing loss. In suppurative otitis media, there is purulent fluid in the middle ear, with fever, pain, and hearing loss. The cause is often associated with an upper respiratory tract infection that has spread through the eustachian tube into the middle ear or as a result of an allergic reaction (Figure 34-11).

Otoscopy reveals the normally pearly gray tympanic membrane is inflamed and bulging. Fluid or pus areas may be visible through the membrane. A *tympanogram* may be done to determine the air pressure of the middle ear and the mobility of the tympanic membrane. If fluid is present in the canal, it can be cultured to determine the causative pathogen. The individual may be given antibiotics, analgesics, and often a decongestant to promote drainage. If this condition becomes chronic, the physician may recommend a myringotomy, which is a surgical incision of the tympanic membrane to drain the fluid, followed by the insertion of a tympanostomy tube to continually drain the middle ear of fluid. This may be necessary to prevent permanent hearing loss because of damage to the ossicles (Figure 34-12).

Impacted Cerumen. Cerumen is normally a soft, yellowish waxy substance created to lubricate the external auditory canal. An excessive secretion of cerumen can gradually cause hearing loss, tinnitus, a feeling of fullness, and otalgia (ear pain). Impacted cerumen that has pushed

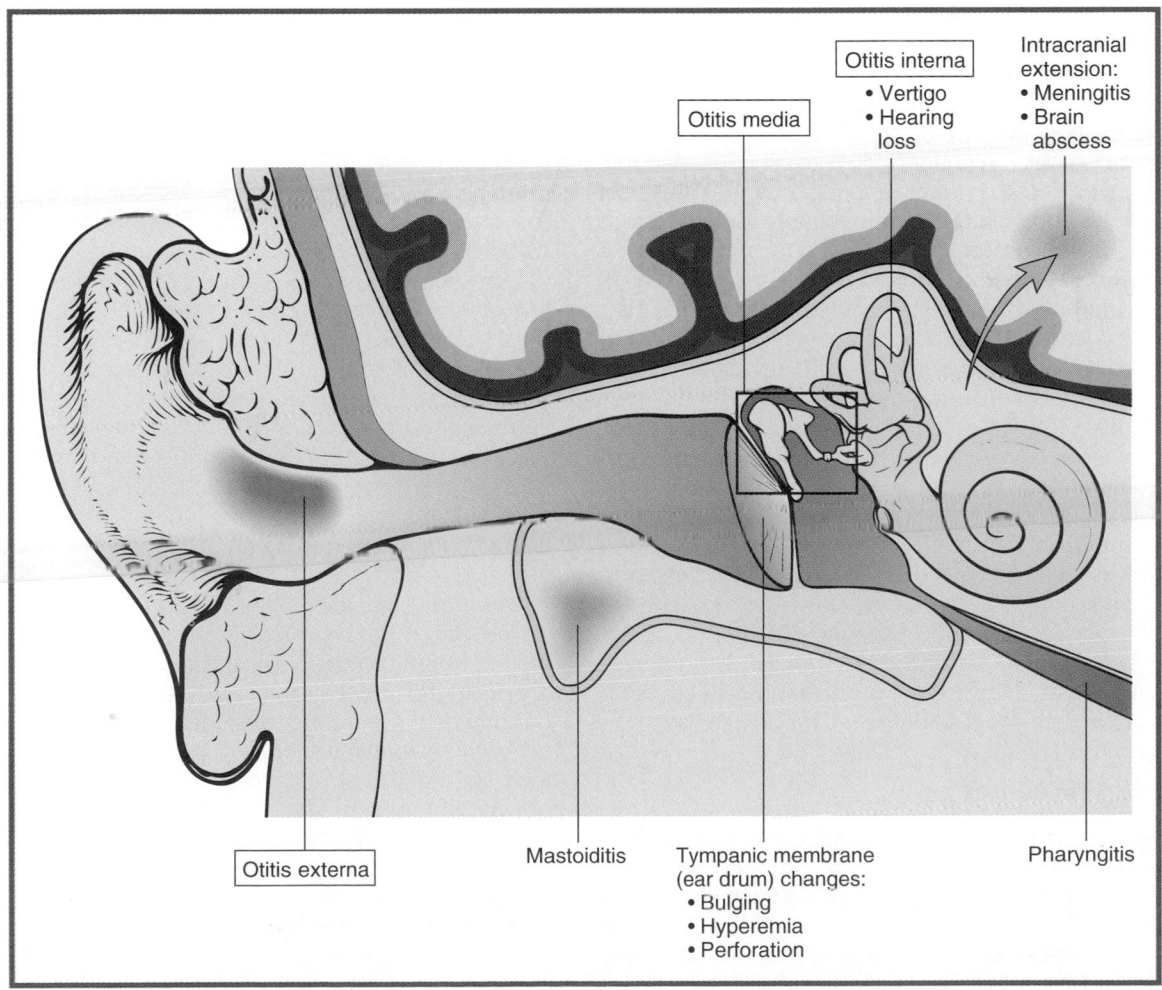

FIGURE 34-11 Inflammations and infections of the ear and surrounding tissues. (From Damjanov I: *Pathology for the health-related professions*, ed. 2, Philadelphia, 2000, WB Saunders.)

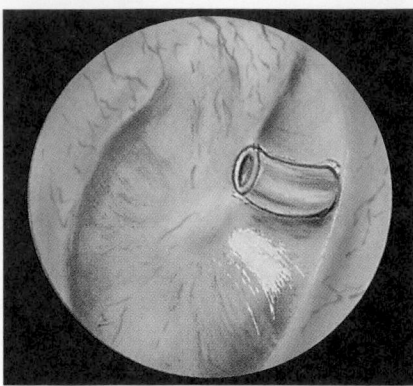

FIGURE 34-12   Insertion of tympanostomy tubes. (From Jarvis C: *Physical examination and health assessment*, ed. 3, Philadelphia, 2000, WB Saunders.)

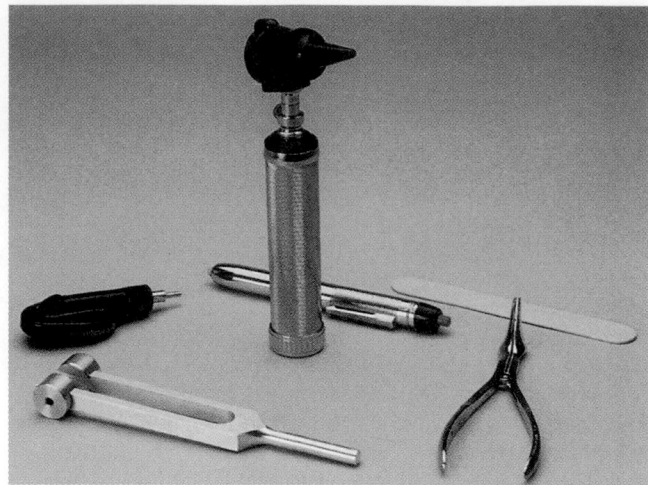

FIGURE 34-13   Otoscopy examination instruments.

tightly up against the eardrum is a frequent cause of conductive hearing loss since the sound vibrations cannot pass through the cerumen to initiate movement of the tympanic membrane. Individuals with psoriasis, abnormally narrow ear canals, or an excessive amount of hair growing within the ear canals are more prone to this condition.

An otoscopic examination quickly reveals this problem. If impacted cerumen is found, it must be removed. This can be done by softening the wax with oily drops, such as carbamide peroxide (Debrox), and then irrigating the ear with warm water until the plug is removed. Because this condition can recur, the patient needs to schedule periodic examinations. If the patient experienced hearing loss because of the impaction, it is immediately remedied with removal of the cerumen.

Ménière's Disease. Although the cause of Ménière's disease is unknown, it results in destruction of the hair cells of the cochlea. It is a chronic, progressive condition that affects the labyrinth and causes recurring attacks of vertigo, tinnitus, a sensation of pressure in the affected ear, and advancing hearing loss. During an acute attack, patients experience nausea, vomiting, and problems with balance. The attacks can last from a few hours to several days, increasing in severity over time. The attacks are treated symptomatically with medications for nausea and vomiting. Patients are placed on salt-restricted diets, and diuretics and antihistamines are prescribed to control edema within the labyrinth. Surgical destruction of the affected labyrinth is an option. Although this relieves symptoms, it may also result in permanent deafness if the cochlea is damaged.

Diagnostic Procedures

An ear examination involves viewing the external auditory canal with an otoscope covered by an ear speculum (Figure 34-13). A normal external auditory canal contains a small amount of cerumen, and the tympanic membrane is pearly gray and concave. In addition to the otoscopic examination, the physician palpates the area around the pinna for abnormalities or sensations. There are a number of tests used to assess hearing acuity, ranging

from simple tuning fork tests to quantitative and qualitative audiometric testing. If a hearing loss is suspected, the next test is usually performed with a tuning fork.

Tuning Fork Testing. Tuning fork tests, as mentioned in Chapter 29, measure hearing by air conduction and bone conduction. In bone conduction the sound vibrates through the cranial bones to the inner ear. There are different-sized tuning forks, each with a different frequency. The most commonly used fork is the *C*, which has a frequency of 1024 hertz (Hz), because this frequency reflects the level of normal speech patterns. To activate the fork, the physician holds it by the stem and strikes the tines softly on the palm of the hand. Striking the tines too forcefully will create a tone that is too loud for diagnostic use. The two testing evaluations that are used to evaluate hearing are the Weber and the Rinne tests. Both of these procedures are commonly used to evaluate conductive and sensory losses.

The *Weber test* is used if the patient states that hearing is better in one ear than the other. The vibrating fork is placed in the center of the top of the head, and the patient is asked in which ear the tone is louder or if the tone is the same in both ears. Because the patient is hearing the tone by bone conduction through the head, the sound should be equal in both ears.

The *Rinne test* is designed to compare air conduction sound with bone conduction sound. In this test the stem of the vibrating fork is placed on the patient's mastoid process, and the patient is advised to raise his or her hand when the sound disappears. The fork is quickly inverted so that the vibrating tines are approximately 1 inch in front of the external ear canal. If the hearing is normal, the patient should still hear a sound. In normal hearing the sound is heard twice as long by air conduction as by bone conduction. The normal response would be that air conduction is greater than bone conduction.

Audiometric Testing. An audiometric test may be done in the otologist's office and performed by medical assistants who have received additional training (Figure 34-14, *A*). Audiometry measures the lowest intensity of sound that an individual can hear. The patient, frequently

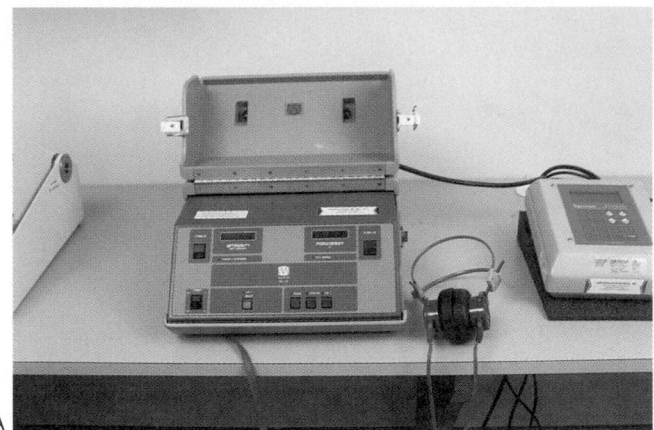

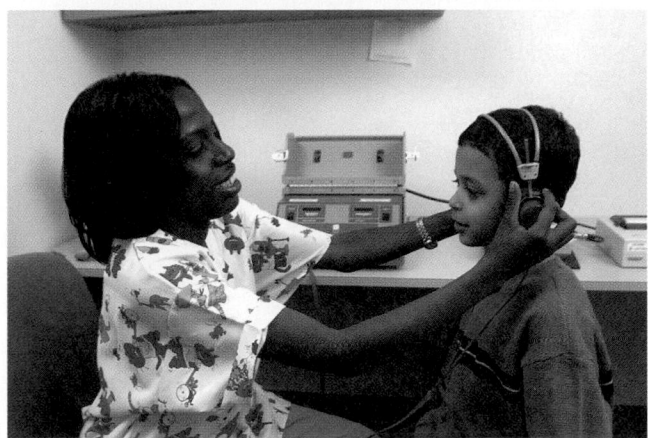

FIGURE 34-14 A, Audiometer. B, Placing headphones.

a child, is assisted in placing headphones over the ears. Each ear is tested by delivering a single frequency at a specific intensity, starting with low frequency tones going up to very high frequencies (Figure 34-14, *B*). The patient is asked to signal when he or she hears the sound. The results are printed on a graph called an *audiogram* (Procedure 34-5).

After the physician completes the screening test procedures, the patient may be given an appointment to see an **audiologist** for audiometric evaluation. The evaluation consists of a battery of tests that assess the level of hearing impairment and provide valuable information as to how the patient may be helped. The first tests are to evaluate speech comprehension and to assess the patient's ability to follow instructions. Once this evaluation is completed, the patient is placed in a sound-proof booth and earphones are placed over the ears. From this point on, the audiologist speaks to the patient and conducts all testing through the earphones. The assessments include testing the frequency, intensity, and audibility of sound. This process takes approximately an hour.

Aseptic Procedures in Otology. Routine examination instruments are sterilized after each use and stored in a clean area. Surgical asepsis must be practiced when changing dressings, placing packs, and performing minor surgery. Dressing forceps must be sterilized after

their use with each patient. Medications, such as eardrops and nose drops, must be handled carefully to avoid contamination.

Treatment Procedures

Ear Irrigation. An ear irrigation is performed to remove excessive or impacted cerumen; to remove a foreign body; or to treat the inflamed ear with an antiseptic solution (Procedure 34-6). When an ear irrigation is ordered by the physician, the medical assistant may perform the procedure if proper training has been completed and the assistant is competent in the technique. Follow the procedure as prescribed, making sure that the patient is comfortable. Always chart the treatment and its results immediately after completion.

CRITICAL THINKING APPLICATION

Kim is ordered to perform a bilateral ear irrigation on a 68-year-old patient with impacted cerumen. She checks the auditory canals before the procedure with an otoscope and sees a large amount of dark brown cerumen in the right ear completely covering the tympanic membrane. The left ear has a moderate amount of golden brown cerumen covering the bottom half of the tympanic membrane. After the procedure both membranes are visible and the patient tolerated the procedure without complaints. How should Kim document the procedure?

Instilling Otic Medications. Medication that is to be instilled into the ear generally is given to soften impacted cerumen, to relieve pain, or is an antibiotic drop needed to fight an infectious pathogen (Procedure 34-7). The patient may be apprehensive and in considerable pain as well as experiencing difficulty hearing, which makes teaching difficult. Wait until after the procedure is completed or on a follow-up visit to inform the patient of the disease process, depending on the condition of the patient.

Examination of the Nose and Throat

If you are working in an ENT specialty office, you will also be assisting in the examination of the nasal cavity and the throat. The nasal cavity is examined to inspect the mucous membrane of the nostrils. The common cold and allergies are the main causes of changes in the mucosa. The physician may use a nasal speculum to visualize the nostrils and examine the nasal sinuses by palpation and transillumination.

The throat is the area that includes the larynx and pharynx; it can be viewed with the aid of a mirror and either a tongue depressor or a gauze square to grasp the tongue. In the nasopharynx, the physician looks for enlarged adenoids (pharyngeal tonsils) and for the orifices of the eustachian tubes. Spraying the throat with a topical anesthetic helps a patient who may have a pronounced gag reflex.

PROCEDURE 34-5

Measuring Hearing Acuity Using an Audiometer

GOAL: To perform audiometric testing of hearing acuity.

EQUIPMENT AND SUPPLIES
- Audiometer with adjustable headphones
- Quiet area

PROCEDURAL STEPS

1 Wash hands, assemble the equipment, and conduct the patient into a quiet area (see Figure 34-14, A).

Purpose: The testing room should be free from distractions and noise to allow the patient to completely concentrate on the hearing evaluation.

2 Explain that the audiometer will measure whether the patient can hear various sound wave frequencies through the headphones. Each ear will be tested separately. When the patient hears a frequency, he or she should raise a hand to signal the medical assistant.

Purpose: Patient education is needed for compliance with the examination.

3 Place the headphones over the patient's ears, making sure they are adjusted for comfort (see Figure 34-14, B).

4 The audiometer tests each ear separately, starting at a low frequency. If the results are not automatically recorded by the machine, the medical assistant documents the patient response to the frequencies on a graph or audiogram. *The medical assistant requires specialized training to conduct this test.*

5 Frequencies are gradually increased to test patient ability to hear. The medical assistant continues to document each response by the patient.

6 The other ear is then tested and the results are documented.

7 Patient results are given to the physician for interpretation.

8 Disinfect the equipment according to the manufacturer's guidelines.

9 Wash hands.

Throat specimens are frequently collected in the physician's office to assist in the diagnosis of strep throat infections. Strep throat is caused by the Group A beta-hemolytic *Streptococcus* bacteria, and, if left untreated, can cause serious complications. Throat cultures are collected by gently swabbing the back of the throat and the surfaces of the tonsils with a sterile swab. The mouth and tongue should be avoided to prevent contamination of the swab with the normal flora of the mouth (Procedure 34-8).

Patient Education

Patients with vision or hearing impairments face serious challenges. Such patients require that the medical assistant use good listening skills, appropriate nonverbal methods for communication, and touch to communicate empathy. Teaching may have to be adapted to meet the special needs of these patients. A person with a vision loss may need large-print forms and handouts, increased levels of lighting, or verbal instructions rather than written ones to reinforce learning. An individual with a hearing deficit may benefit from printed instructions, demonstrations of how to manage treatments, or even sign language interpretation. Family members should be included in the

patient's treatment plan, and referrals to appropriate community or professional resources may be very beneficial to a patient with sensory loss. Each patient must be individually assessed to determine his or her level of needed adaptation.

An important part of home care for patients receiving eye medications is stressing the need for maintaining the sterility of the medication. Patients and/or family members must be taught how to apply the medication and prevent trauma to the eye as well as contamination of the applicator. Patients receiving ear treatments must also understand how to instill the medication.

Legal and Ethical Issues

Diminished sight or hearing may render the patient seriously impaired. To avoid possible accidents and office injuries, always ask a sight- or hearing-impaired patient if he or she requires assistance. When you place the patient in an examination room, offer your arm and tell the patient the approximate distance that you will be walking. If the patient is to have an examination that will involve local anesthesia or eyedrops that dilate the pupil, be sure the patient has recovered and someone is available to take the patient home before allowing him

PROCEDURE 34-6

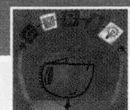

Irrigating a Patient's Ear

GOAL: To remove excessive or impacted cerumen from a patient's ear (or ears).

EQUIPMENT AND SUPPLIES

- Irrigating solution
- Basin for irrigating solution
- Bulb syringe or an approved otic irrigation device
- Gauze squares
- Otoscope
- Drainage basin
- Disposable drape with polylined barrier
- Cotton-tipped applicators
- Disposable gloves

PROCEDURAL STEPS

1 Wash your hands.
Purpose: Infection control.

2 Check the physician's order and assemble the materials needed (Figure 1).

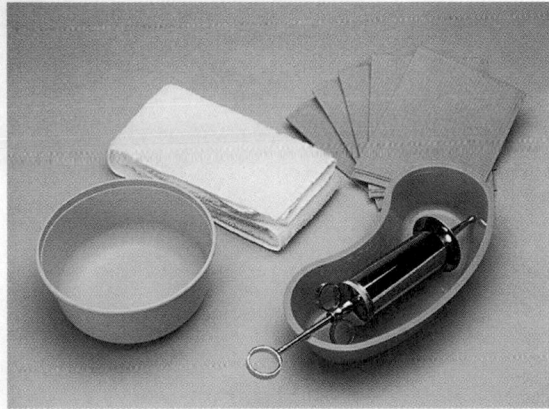

Figure 1

3 Check the label of the solution three times: (a) when you remove it from the shelf, (b) when you pour it, and (c) when you return it to the shelf.
Purpose: Prevent possible medication error.

4 Prepare the solution as ordered. The solution temperature should be at body temperature (98.6° F to 100° F) to help loosen the cerumen.
Purpose: Solutions at 100° F are most comfortable to the patient. Ask the patient if the solution temperature is comfortable.

5 Identify the patient, and explain the procedure.

6 View the affected ear with an otoscope to locate cerumen impaction.

7 Place the patient in a sitting position with the head tilted toward the affected ear. A water-absorbent towel is placed over a polylined barrier on the patient's shoulder, and the collecting basin is placed on the towel flush against the base of the ear. The patient may be asked to assist you by holding the collecting basin in place (Figure 2).

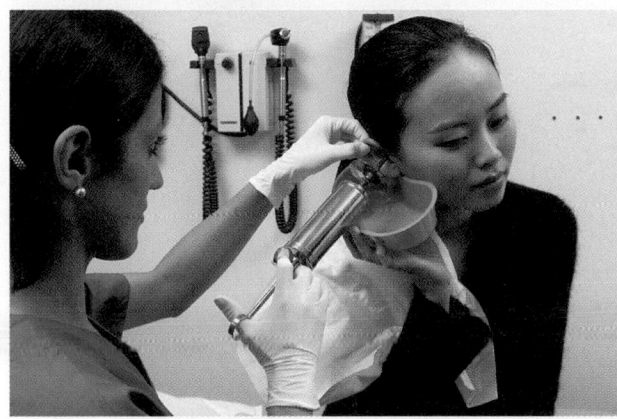

Figure 2

Purpose: This technique will minimize the risk of getting the patient's clothing wet and will aid the water flow into the collecting basin.

8 Apply gloves and wipe any particles from the outside of the ear with gauze squares.
Purpose: This prevents the introduction of foreign materials into the ear canal.

9 Test to be certain that the solution is warm, fill the syringe, and expel air.
Purpose: Trapped air in the syringe will increase the pressure of the irrigation, causing discomfort.

10 Straighten the external ear canal. For adults and children over the age of 3, gently pull the ear up and back; for children younger than 3, pull down and back (Figure 3).

or her to leave the office. Never assume that the patient is capable of leaving alone. If the patient insists on leaving before the designated recovery time, inform the physician and record the time and circumstances sur-

rounding the event in the patient's chart. This information should be signed and witnessed. The physician may want a refusal of care form signed by the patient and placed in the chart.

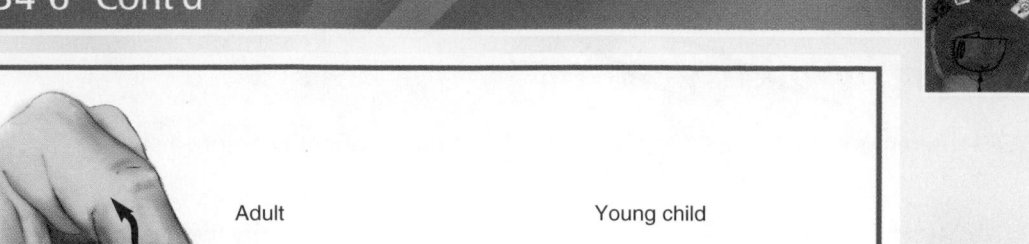

PROCEDURE **34-6—Cont'd**

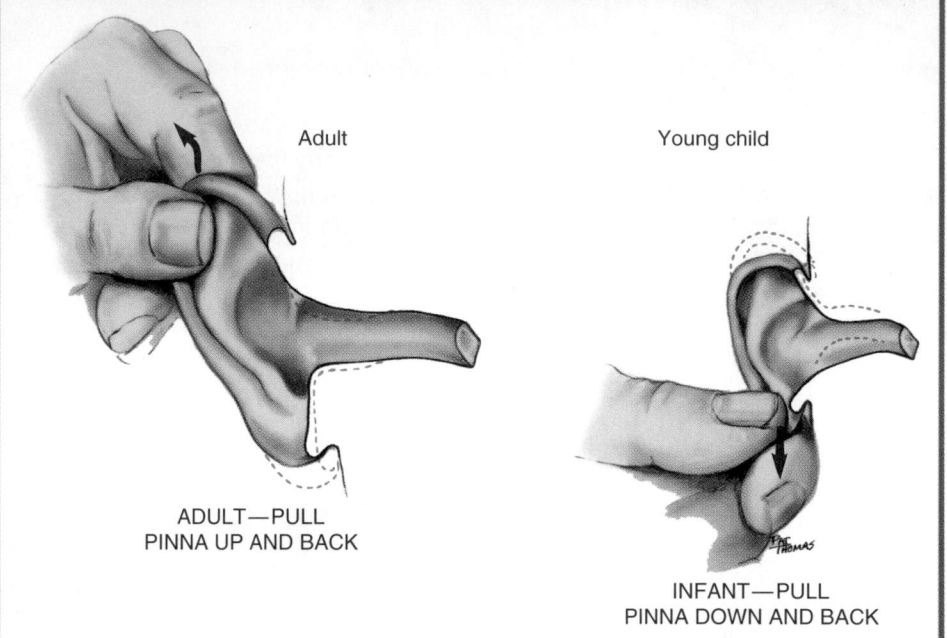

Adult   Young child

ADULT—PULL
PINNA UP AND BACK

INFANT—PULL
PINNA DOWN AND BACK

Figure 3

Purpose: Straightening the canal allows the irrigating fluid to circulate through the canal.

11 Place the tip of the syringe into the meatus of the ear.

12 Gently direct the flow of the solution toward the roof of the canal.

Purpose: This will help to prevent injury to the tympanic membrane and will aid in the removal of the imbedded material.

13 Refill the syringe with warm solution and continue until the material has been removed. Note the particles in the collecting basin to evaluate when the material has been successfully removed.

14 Dry the patient's external ear with gauze squares and the visible ear canal gently with cotton-tipped applicators.

Purpose: Inserting the applicator into the canal may cause serious trauma.

15 Inspect the ear with an otoscope to determine the results.

16 Place a clean, absorbent towel against the freshly irrigated ear and allow the patient to rest quietly while you wait for the physician to return to check the affected ear.

17 Clean the work area, and return all equipment after it has been properly disinfected. Wash your hands.

Purpose: Infection control.

18 Record the procedure, including the date and time; which ear was irrigated, using the appropriate abbreviations—AU (both ears), AD (right ear), AS (left ear); the type and amount of irrigating solution used; the characteristics of the material returned from the irrigation; the visibility of the tympanic membrane after irrigation; and any patient reactions.

Purpose: Procedures that are not recorded are considered not done.

See Appendix E for a charting example.

SUMMARY OF SCENARIO

After observing Kim and asking many questions, Amy is beginning to understand her special responsibilities in the ophthalmology and otorhinolaryngology clinic. She recognizes the need to be familiar with the anatomy and physiology of both the eye and ear as well as to be able to perform specialty-related skills, such as irrigations, medication instillations, and diagnostic procedures. She also realizes she needs to understand the pathological conditions that can occur so she will be able to assist the physician as needed and answer patient questions. Amy has decided to take advantage of educational opportunities at the hospital and through her professional organization so she can continue to learn about this special area of practice.

PROCEDURE 34-7

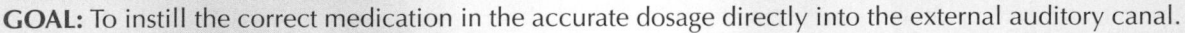

Instilling Medicated Ear Drops

GOAL: To instill the correct medication in the accurate dosage directly into the external auditory canal.

EQUIPMENT AND SUPPLIES

- Prescribed otic drops in dispenser bottle
- Cotton balls
- Disposable gloves

PROCEDURAL STEPS

1 Wash hands and gather the needed equipment and supplies.
Purpose: Infection control and to reduce procedure time.

2 Check the medication label three times: (a) when you remove it from the shelf, (b) when you prepare it, and (c) when you return it to the shelf.
Purpose: To avoid possible medication error.

3 Identify your patient and explain the procedure.

4 Have the patient sit up and tilt head away from the affected ear or lie down on the side with the affected ear upward.
Purpose: Exposes the ear for treatment, gravity helps the medication flow into the canal, and ensures patient comfort.

5 Check the temperature of the medication bottle. If it feels cold, gently roll the bottle back and forth between your hands to warm the drops.
Purpose: Cold medication may increase the pain level or cause symptoms of nausea and vertigo.

6 Hold the dropper firmly in your dominant hand. With the other hand, gently pull the pinna up and back if the patient is an adult or down and back if patient is younger than 3 years old.
Purpose: To straighten the ear canal and make it easier for the medication to reach its designated position.

7 Place the tip of the dropper in the ear canal meatus and instill the medication drops along the side of the canal (Figure 1).

8 Rest the patient on the opposite side of the affected ear and instruct him or her to remain in this position for about 3 minutes.
Purpose: This time will allow the medication to reach the base of the canal and will prevent it from running out of the ear (Figure 2).

9 If instructed by the physician, place a moistened cotton ball into the ear canal.
Purpose: Protects the ear canal and prevents medication from leaking out of the ear.

10 Clean the work area and wash your hands.
Purpose: Infection control.

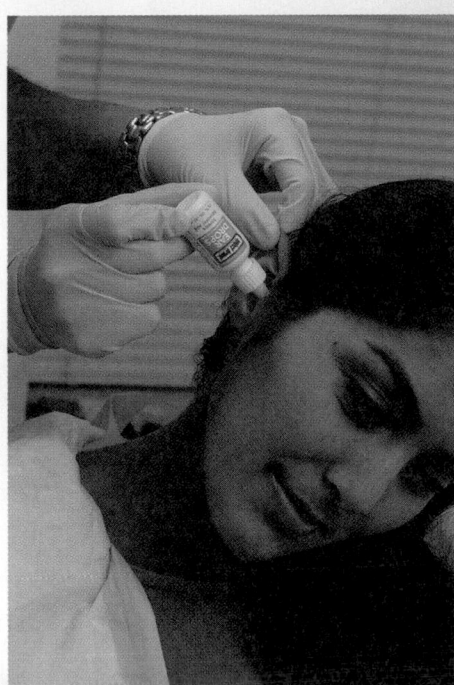

Figure 1

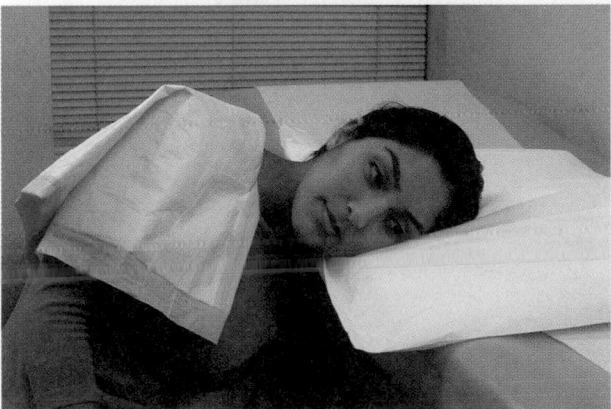

Figure 2

11 Record the procedure using the appropriate abbreviations, including the date and time; the name, dose, and strength of the medication; which ear was treated; and patient reactions on the chart.
Purpose: Procedures that are not recorded are considered not done.

See Appendix E for a charting example.

PROCEDURE **34-8**

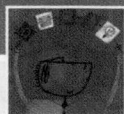

Collecting a Specimen for a Throat Culture

GOAL: To collect a throat culture, using sterile technique, for either immediate testing or transportation to the laboratory.

EQUIPMENT AND SUPPLIES

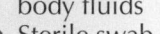

- Nonsterile gloves
- Face protection barrier if the patient is coughing or if there is danger of splattering of body fluids
- Sterile swab
- Sterile tongue depressor
- Transport medium
- Biohazard waste container

PROCEDURAL STEPS

1 Wash and dry your hands.
Purpose: Infection control.

2 Gather the materials needed.

3 Don gloves and face protection if needed.
Purpose: Standard precautions.

4 Position the patient so that the light shines into the mouth.
Purpose: Visualization of the area to be swabbed.

5 Remove the sterile swab from the sterile wrap with your dominant hand, and grasp the sterile tongue depressor with your nondominant hand.
Purpose: Better control of the swabbing process.

6 Instruct the patient to open the mouth and say "ah." Depress the tongue with the depressor (Figure 1).
Purpose: Saying "ah" helps elevate the uvula and reduces the tendency to gag. The tongue is depressed so that you can see the back of the throat.

7 Swab the back of the throat between the tonsillar pillars and especially any reddened, patchy areas of the throat, white pus pockets, purulent areas, and the tonsils.
Purpose: Pathogenic organisms are found in the back of the throat and on the tonsils.

8 Place the swab into the transport medium, label it, and send it to the laboratory. If direct slide testing is requested, return the labeled swab to the laboratory (Figure 2).
Purpose: Transport media prevents the swab from drying. Labeling immediately after collection prevents mixing up specimens.

9 Dispose of contaminated supplies in biohazard waste container.
Purpose: Prevents the spread of infection.

10 Disinfect the work area.

11 Remove gloves; place in a biohazard waste container.

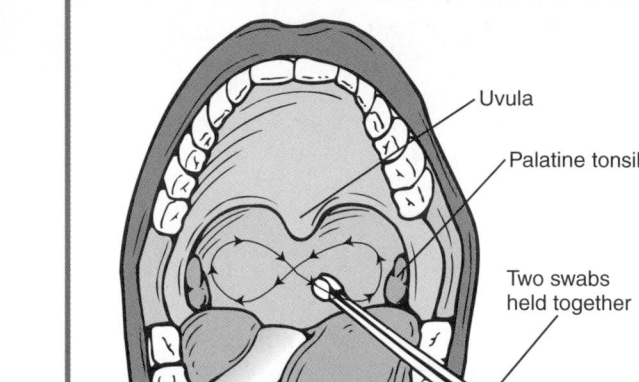

Uvula

Palatine tonsil

Two swabs held together

Tongue blade

Figure 1

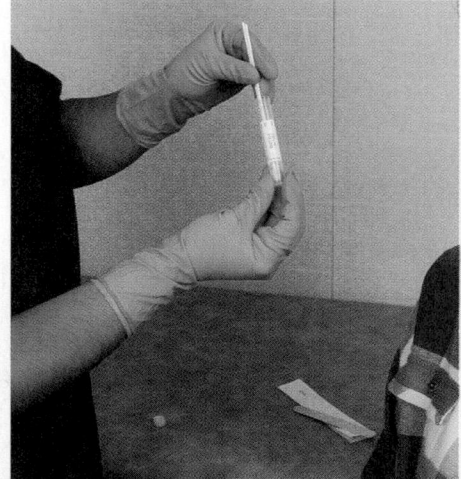

Figure 2

12 Wash your hands.
Purpose: Infection control.

13 Record procedure in the patient's record.
Purpose: Procedures that are not recorded are considered not done.

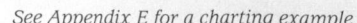

See Appendix E for a charting example.

SUMMARY OF LEARNING OBJECTIVES

- An ophthalmologist is a medical doctor specializing in the diagnosis and treatment of the eye, an optometrist can examine and treat visual defects, and an optician fills prescriptions for corrective lenses.

- The anatomy of the eye begins with the outer covering, the conjunctiva, and the three layers of tissue: the sclera, choroid, and retina. The inner layer is where light rays are converted into nervous energy for interpretation by the brain.

- Vision begins with the passage of light through the cornea, where it is refracted and then passes through the aqueous humor and pupil into the lens. The ciliary muscle adjusts the curvature of the lens to again refract the light rays so they pass into the retina, triggering the photoreceptor cells of the rods and cones. Light energy is then converted into an electrical impulse that is sent through the optic nerve to the brain, where interpretation occurs.

- Refractive errors include hyperopia, myopia, presbyopia, and astigmatism. All are caused by a problem with bending light so it can be accurately focused on the retina. They are usually caused by defects in the shape of the eyeball and can be corrected with glasses, contacts, or surgery.

- Eye disorders can range from problems with eye movement as in strabismus and nystagmus to infections of the eye including hordeolums, chalazions, keratitis, conjunctivitis, and blepharitis. Disorders of the eyeball include corneal abrasions, cataracts, glaucoma, and macular degeneration.

- Diagnostic procedures for the eye begin with a visual examination of the eye using an ophthalmoscope. Next, the eyelids are examined for abnormalities and the pupils are tested for PERRLA. More advanced techniques include the use of a slitlamp to view the fine details of the eye and the exophthalmometer to measure the pressure in the central renal artery. Distance visual acuity is typically assessed with the use of a Snellen chart; near visual acuity is tested with a near-vision acuity chart. A patient can be tested for a color vision defect with the Ishihara test.

- Eye irrigations relieve inflammation, remove drainage, dilute chemicals, or wash away foreign bodies. Sterile technique and equipment must be used to avoid contamination. Medication may be instilled into the eye for treatment of an infection, to soothe an eye irritation, to anesthetize the eye, or to dilate the pupils before examination or treatment.

- The external ear consists of the auricle or pinna, and the external auditory canal, which transmits sound waves to the tympanic membrane. The middle ear is an air-filled cavity that contains the ossicles. The sound vibration passes through the tympanic membrane, causing the ossicles to vibrate. This bone-conducted vibration passes through the oval window into the inner ear. The organ of Corti in the cochlea of the inner ear converts the sound waves into nervous energy that is sent to the brain for interpretation. The semicircular canals in the inner ear maintain equilibrium.

- A conductive hearing loss is caused by a problem that originates in the external or middle ear that prevents the sound vibrations from passing through the external auditory canal, limits the vibrations of the tympanic membrane, or interferes with the passage of bone-conducted sound in the middle ear. A sensorineural hearing loss results from damage to the organ of Corti or the auditory nerve and prevents the sound vibration from becoming nervous stimuli that can be interpreted by the brain as sound.

- There are two common types of otitis that are seen in patients in an otologist's practice. The first affects the external ear canal and is called otitis externa, or swimmer's ear. Otitis media is an inflammation of the normally air-filled middle ear, resulting in a collection of fluid behind the tympanic membrane. Otitis media can be either serous or suppurative. Impacted cerumen that has pushed tightly up against the eardrum is a frequent cause of conductive hearing loss since the sound vibrations cannot pass through the cerumen to initiate movement of the tympanic membrane. Ménière's disease is a chronic, progressive condition that affects the labyrinth and causes recurring attacks of vertigo, tinnitus, a sensation of pressure in the affected ear, and advancing hearing loss.

- The ear examination begins with an otoscopic examination and can include various tuning fork tests and more advanced audiometric testing.

- An ear irrigation is performed to remove excessive or impacted cerumen; to remove a foreign body; or to treat the inflamed ear with an antiseptic solution. Medication that is to be instilled into the ear generally is given to soften impacted cerumen, to relieve pain, or is an antibiotic drop needed to fight an infectious pathogen.

- Examination of the nose and throat begins with examination of the nasal cavity and then visual examination of the throat and the nasopharynx. Throat cultures may be done to determine the presence of a streptococcal infection.

- Patients with vision or hearing impairments face serious challenges and require individualized attention to meet their health education needs. Teaching adaptations may be required to meet the special needs of these patients. Patients with vision losses may need large print forms and handouts, increased levels of lighting, or verbal instructions rather than written ones. Individuals with hearing deficits may benefit from printed instructions, demonstrations on how to manage treatments, or even sign language interpretation. Family members should be included in the patient's treatment plan, and referrals to appropriate community or professional resources may be very beneficial.

CHAPTER 35

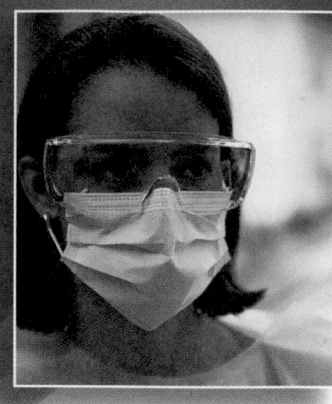

Scenario

Dr. Sam Lee is a dermatologist who employs several medical assistants in his busy private practice. Melissa Bauman, CMA, has worked for Dr. Lee since graduating from a medical assisting program last year. Melissa works as a clinical specialist whose primary responsibilities are to perform telephone screening, prepare patients for procedures, and assist Dr. Lee as needed.

Assisting in Dermatology

Learning Objectives

- Define and spell the terms listed in the vocabulary.
- Explain the major functions of the skin.
- Diagram the anatomical structures of the skin.
- Compare various skin lesions and give examples of each.
- Describe typical integumentary system infections.
- Differentiate between various inflammatory and vascular skin disorders.
- Recognize heat and cold injuries to the skin.
- Compare the characteristics of benign and malignant neoplasms.
- Define grading and staging of malignant tumors.
- Conduct patient education on the warning signs of cancer.
- Describe skin malignancies and their treatment.
- Define the ABCD rule for identifying a malignant melanoma.
- Explain dermatological procedures conducted in the ambulatory care setting.
- Assist with allergy testing procedures.
- Accurately obtain an exudate sample from a wound for laboratory analysis.
- Assist with a skin biopsy.

National Curriculum Competencies

CLINICAL COMPETENCIES

2d. Perform wound collection procedure for microbiological testing

4f. Prepare patients for and assist with procedures, treatments, and minor office surgery

4g. Apply pharmacology principles to prepare and administer oral and parenteral medications

TRANSDISCIPLINARY COMPETENCIES

3b. Instruct individuals according to their needs

3d. Provide instruction for health maintenance and disease prevention

Vocabulary

alopecia Partial or complete lack of hair.

anaplastic Alteration in cells to a more primitive form; cancer-producing cells.

autoimmune Development of an immune response to one's own tissues; the body acts against its own cells to cause localized and systemic reactions.

bilirubin Orange-colored pigment in bile, which when it accumulates leads to jaundice.

cryosurgery Technique of exposing tissue to extreme cold to produce a well-defined area of cell destruction.

debridement Removal of foreign material and dead, damaged tissue from a wound.

ecchymosis Bluish-black skin discoloration produced by hemorrhagic areas.

electrodesiccation Destruction of cells and tissue by means of short high-frequency electrical sparks.

exacerbation An increase in the seriousness of a disease marked by greater intensity in the signs and symptoms.

hyperplasia An increase in the number of cells.

jaundice Yellow discoloration of the skin and mucous membranes due to deposits of bile pigments because of excess bilirubin in the blood.

keratin Very hard, tough protein found in hair, nails, and epidermal tissue.

keratinocytes Any one of the skin cells that synthesizes keratin.

leukoderma Lack of skin pigmentation, especially in patches.

opaque Not translucent or transparent.

palliative Substance that alleviates or eases a painful condition without curing it.

petechiae Small, purplish hemorrhagic spots on the skin.

Raynaud's phenomenon Intermittent attacks of ischemia of the extremities; results in cyanosis, numbness, tingling, and pain.

remission Partial or complete disappearance of the signs and symptoms of a disease.

teratogen Any substance that interferes with normal prenatal development.

The skin, the largest organ in the human body, covers a total area of about 20 square feet in an average-sized adult. Forming the outer boundary of the body, the skin carries out several essential functions: it acts as a barrier to protect vital internal organs against infection and injury, it helps dissipate heat and regulate body temperature, and it synthesizes vitamin D when exposed to ultraviolet light. In addition, the various sensory receptors present throughout the skin enable it to respond to such sensations as heat, cold, pain, and pressure.

The specialty of dermatology deals with the skin and its accessory structures, the hair, nails, and sweat glands, as well as the subcutaneous tissue that lies beneath the skin. A physician specializing in dermatology is called a *dermatologist*.

Anatomy and Physiology

The integumentary system comprises the skin and its accessory organs. Each square inch of the skin contains millions of cells, numerous specialized nerve endings, hair follicles, muscles, sweat glands to cool the body, and sebaceous glands, which release *sebum*, an oily substance that lubricates the skin. These diverse structures and glands are nourished by a permeating, elaborate network of blood vessels. The thickness of human skin varies markedly on different parts of the body, ranging from fairly thin over protected areas, such as the eyelids, to very thick over areas subject to abrasion, such as the palms of the hands and the soles of the feet.

Skin is composed of three layers: the epidermis, which is the thin, uppermost layer; the dermis, which is the thicker layer beneath, often referred to as the true skin, and which makes up about 90% of the skin mass; and the subcutaneous layer, which is composed primarily of fatty or *adipose* tissue (Figure 35-1).

Epidermis

New skin cells called **keratinocytes** are found in the basal cell layer of the epidermis and migrate upward over a period of about 4 weeks. As the cells move toward the surface, they grow flatter and more scaly, eventually losing their nuclei and changing into dead skin cells that contain an inert protein called **keratin**. Keratin, which makes up the outermost layer of the epidermis, forms a protective barrier that helps control water loss from the body. Ultimately, the outermost keratin layer sloughs off as a result of washing and friction. Hair and nails, which are also composed of keratin, are products of the epidermis.

About 95% of the cells in the epidermis are keratinocytes. The other 5% of epidermal cells are pigmented cells, or melanocytes. Melanin is a protein manufactured in the body that gives coloring to the skin and also protects the body from ultraviolet radiation. Skin coloring is determined not by the total number of melanocytes, which is relatively constant for all races, but rather by the rate at which these cells produce melanin. The amount of melanin produced depends on genetics as well as exposure to ultraviolet light. Individuals with albinism, an inherited recessive trait, are unable to produce melanin, so they have white hair and skin and lack pigment in the iris. They have no protection from ultraviolet light, so they must stay out of the sun.

Dermis

The underlying dermis is a thick layer of connective tissue that contains collagen and elastin fibers as well as water and jellylike materials that make the skin compressible. Collagen fibers help to prevent tearing of the skin, and elastin is a flexible fiber that makes the skin resilient. Distributed throughout the dermis are blood vessels, lymph vessels, muscle cells, hair follicles, and sebaceous and sweat glands. There are two types of sweat glands: exocrine glands, which excrete sweat through skin pores to release heat or when a person is stressed, and apocrine glands, which open into hair follicles and

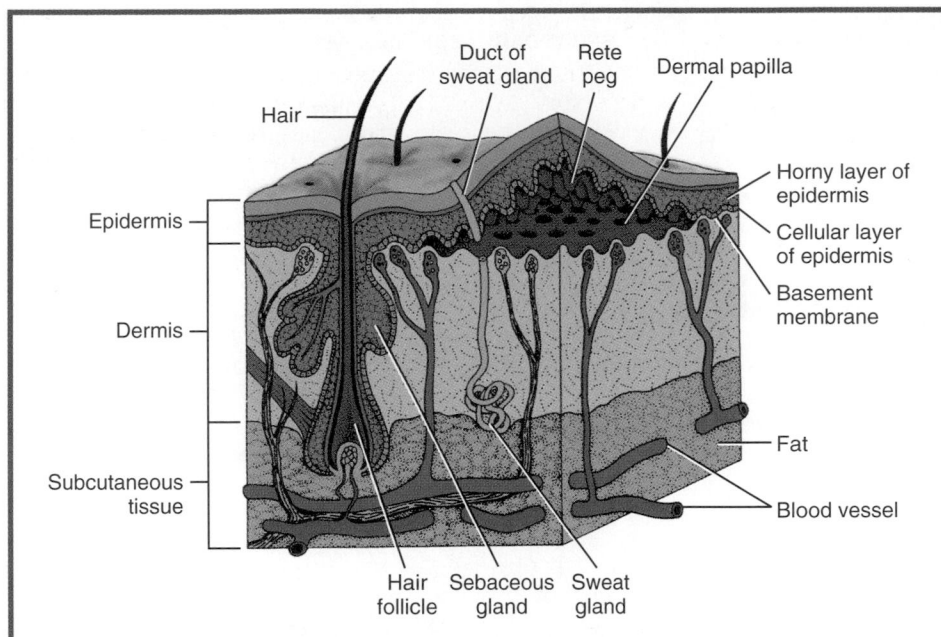

Hair

Duct of
sweat gland

Rete
peg

Dermal papilla

Epidermis

Horny layer of
epidermis

Cellular layer
of epidermis

Basement
membrane

Dermis

Subcutaneous
tissue

Fat

Blood vessel

Hair
follicle

Sebaceous
gland

Sweat
gland

FIGURE 35-1   The three layers of
the skin.

are located in specific areas, including the axilla, scalp, face, and genitalia. Sweat is odorless when excreted, but bacterial action results in odor. A variety of microorganisms called normal or *resident flora* are found on the skin and may increase the risk for integumentary system infections. Healthcare workers are encouraged to perform hand washing before and after each procedure to prevent *transient* microbes from becoming resident flora. Sensory receptors for the nervous system that detect pain, temperature, pressure, or texture are also located in the dermis.

Subcutaneous Layer

The subcutaneous layer consists of fat cells, which provide insulation and serve as a depository for reserve calories. It also contains blood vessels, nerves, and the base of the appendages of the skin. Subcutaneous tissue is unevenly distributed, and as the human body ages, it thins considerably, which can make administering injections or drawing blood on aging patients more difficult.

Diseases and Disorders

Skin is continuously exposed to the environment and may be affected by a wide range of disorders, including infections, inflammation, allergic reactions, and tumors. Many skin problems resolve spontaneously; others can be managed with drug therapy; and still others, such as tumors, large cysts, or moles, may require surgery.

Skin Lesions

Skin lesions may be caused by a systemic problem, such as an allergic reaction or liver disease, or may be a localized response to an infection or allergen. Figure 35-2 describes primary and secondary lesions and gives

examples of each. When communicating with the physician, documenting in the patient chart, or conducting telephone screening, always use correct medical terminology to describe skin lesions, such as "The patient reports widespread maculopapular rash across anterior trunk."

When the medical assistant is gathering details from the patient regarding the characteristics of lesions, some questions that should be considered include:

- What is the color, elevation, and texture of the lesion?
- Is there any pain or *pruritus* (itching)? If pruritus is present, is the area excoriated or inflamed? Is there any drainage, and, if so, what are the characteristics?
- What is the exact location of the lesion, and have there been changes over time?

Primary lesions are those that appear immediately. Macules, papules, plaques, nodules, cysts, wheals, and pustules are all primary lesions. *Secondary lesions* are the result of alterations in a primary lesion. Examples of secondary lesions are scales, crusts, fissures, erosions, ulcerations, and scars. Vesicles formed because of a second intention burn are primary lesions, but if the blisters break and ulcerations form, healing ends in a scar. The ulceration and the scar formation are secondary lesions.

Infections

Bacterial Infections

Impetigo. Impetigo is a common, contagious, superficial infection caused by streptococci or *Staphylococcus aureus*. It usually affects children and initially looks like small vesicles on the face, especially around the nose and mouth, which quickly enlarge and rupture, excreting yellowish exudate. The exudate forms crusty lesions while beneath the crust the area is inflamed and moist (Figure 35-3). Pruritus accompanies the infection, which spreads when the patient scratches. The infection spreads by direct contact with the drainage to other sites or to other

PRIMARY LESIONS

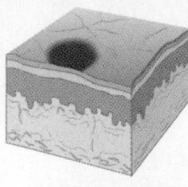

MACULE
Flat area of color change (no elevation or depression)

Example: Freckles

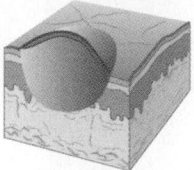

PAPULE
Solid elevation less than 0.5 cm in diameter

Example: Allergic eczema

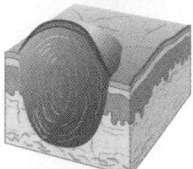

NODULE
Solid elevation 0.5 to 1 cm in diameter. Extends deeper into dermis than papule

Example: Mole

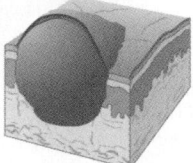

TUMOR
Solid mass—larger than 1 cm

Example: Squamous cell carcinoma

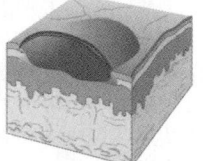

PLAQUE
Flat elevated surface found on skin or mucous membrane

Example: Thrush

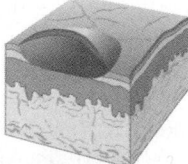

WHEAL
Type of plaque. Result is transient edema in dermis

Example: Intradermal skin test

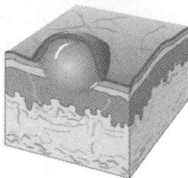

VESICLE
Small blister—fluid within or under epidermis

Example: Herpesvirus infection

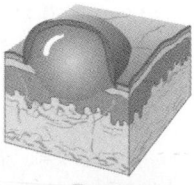

BULLA
Large blister (greater than 0.5 cm)

Example: Burn

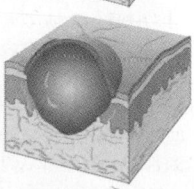

PUSTULE
Vesicle filled with pus

Example: Acne

SECONDARY LESIONS

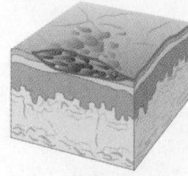

SCALES
Flakes of cornified skin layer

Example: Psoriasis

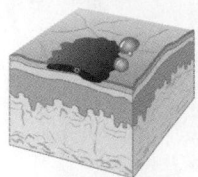

CRUST
Dried exudate on skin

Example: Impetigo

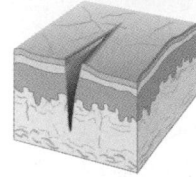

FISSURE
Cracks in skin

Example: Athlete's foot

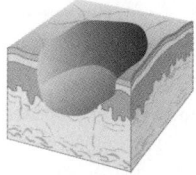

ULCER
Area of destruction of entire epidermis

Example: Decubitus (pressure sore)

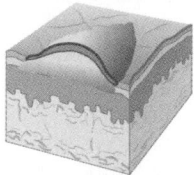

SCAR
Excess collagen production after injury

Example: Surgical healing

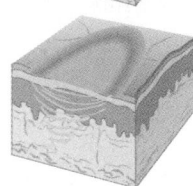

ATROPHY
Loss of some portion of the skin

Example: Paralysis

FIGURE 35-2 Different types of skin lesions.

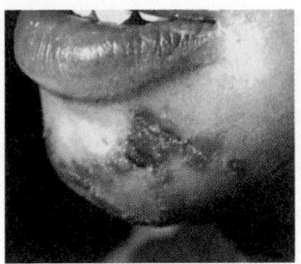

FIGURE 35-3   Impetigo. (From Lookingbill D, Marks J: *Principles of dermatology*, ed. 3, Philadelphia, 2000, WB Saunders.)

children by sharing toys and touching. Consistent hand washing is needed to help break the chain of infection. Treatment consists of properly cleaning the infected areas and applying an antibiotic ointment three or four times a day. If there are multiple lesion locations, oral antibiotic therapy may be necessary.

CRITICAL THINKING APPLICATION

Mrs. Allio calls the office today with concerns about her children being exposed to a child in the neighborhood who was diagnosed with impetigo. She tells Melissa that her 3-year-old woke up this morning with blisters around his mouth. Dr. Lee prescribes polymyxin-bacitracin-neomycin (Neosporin) ointment to be applied three times daily to the affected areas. What should Melissa tell Mrs. Allio about preventing the spread of the infection to her other children?

Acne. *Acne vulgaris* typically begins at puberty and is caused by a number of factors, including inherited predisposition, hormonal fluctuations, exposure to heat and humidity, and the use of oily creams (Figure 35-4). Acne is a disorder of the hair follicle and sebaceous gland unit. Sebum reaches the skin surface through the hair follicles and stimulates the follicle walls, causing a more rapid shedding of the skin cells. This then causes the cells and sebum to stick together and form a plug that promotes the growth of staphylococcal organisms in the follicles. *Comedones* (blackheads), pimples, pustules, or larger abscesses form at the site.

Antiacne medications include the use of topical tretinoin (Retin-A) gel or antibacterial creams, such as benzoyl peroxide. Oral antibiotics, such as tetracycline and erythromycin, at a maintenance dose of 250 mg once or twice daily, can be prescribed to control comedones and pustules. Severe cystic acne can be treated with isotretinoin (Accutane), but it is a strong **teratogen** and should never be prescribed for pregnant women or women not using contraceptives. The use of oral contraceptives may reduce acne outbreaks as well. Dermabrasion can be performed to remove the scars that form from extreme cases of acne vulgaris.

Furuncles and Carbuncles. A *furuncle* or boil is a localized staphylococcal infection that begins as an inflammation of a hair follicle (*folliculitis*) or a skin gland. The affected area is raised, inflamed, and painful

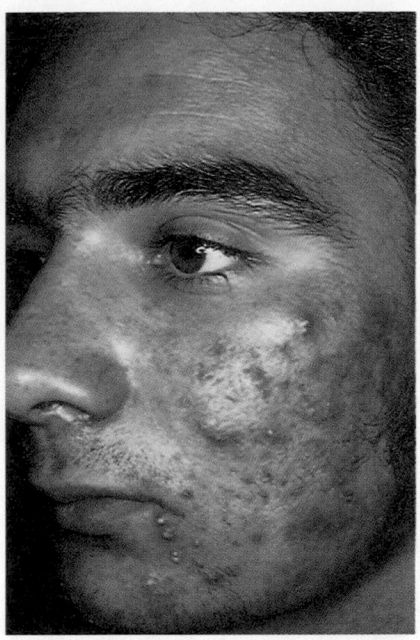

FIGURE 35-4   Acne. (From Hurwitz A: *Clinical pediatric dermatology: a textbook of skin disorders in childhood and adolescence*, ed. 3, Philadelphia, 2000, WB Saunders.)

and may eventually have purulent drainage. A *carbuncle* is a collection of furuncles that have joined to form a large, infected area that may drain through multiple sites or form an abscess. Both infections are treated by oral antibiotics, frequent cleansing of the area, the application of antibiotic ointment, and in some cases, surgical incision and drainage of the purulent material.

Cellulitis. Cellulitis or *erysipelas* is an acute infection of the skin and subcutaneous tissue caused by either streptococcus or staphylococcus that begins from a small cut, secondary to an injury, or at the site of a furuncle or ulcer. The site becomes inflamed, edematous, and painful with red streaks along the lymph vessels that lead from the infection. Oral antibiotic medications are needed to cure the disease, warm compresses are applied locally, and analgesics are given to relieve discomfort. Cellulitis must be treated with caution, because a systemic infection can develop if the lymph glands become involved.

Fungal Infections (Dermatophytoses). Fungal or *mycotic* infections, such as *tinea pedis* (athlete's foot) (Figure 35-5, *A*), *tinea cruris* (jock itch) (Figure 35-5, *B*), and *tinea corporis* (ringworm) (Figure 35-5, *C*), are extremely common. These pathogens tend to live off the dead tissue located in the keratin layer of the epidermis, the hair, or nails and cause almost no inflammation in the underlying skin. The fungus invades the skin where it has been damaged or is consistently moist. All of these lesions are pruritic and are characterized by a distinct border with scaling areas that have a clear center. Secondary bacterial infections may occur with excoriation.

Treatment consists of antifungal topical agents, such as clotrimazole (Lotrimin), ketoconazole (Nizoral), econazole (Spectazole), or nystatin (Mycostatin). Antibiotics

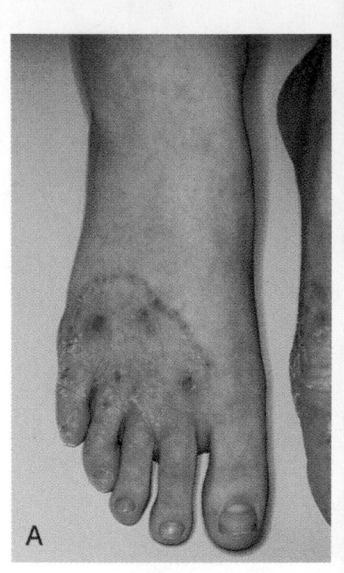

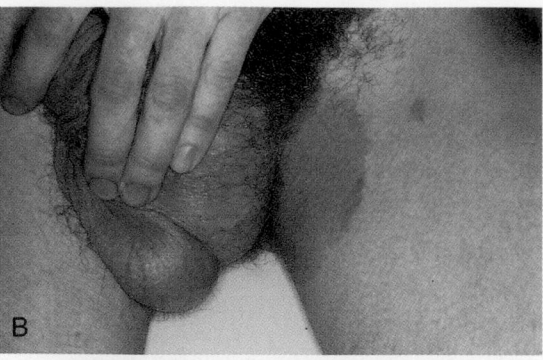

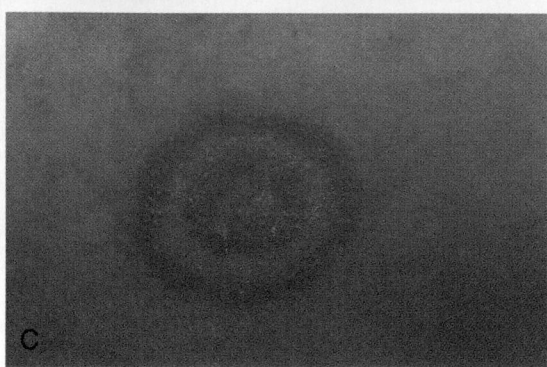

FIGURE 35-5 Fungal infections. **A,** *Tinea pedis.* **B,** *Tinea cruris.* **C,** *Tinea corporis.* (From Callen J, Greer K, Hood A, et al: *Color atlas of dermatology,* ed. 2, Philadelphia, 2000, WB Saunders.)

may be necessary if there is a secondary infection. Because mycotic infections thrive in dark, moist areas, the patient should be advised to keep the site clean and dry and to wear loose clothing if possible. All types of dermatophytosis can become chronic infections if not managed carefully.

Tinea unguium, or *onychomycosis,* is a fungal infection of the toenails and fingernails. Unlike athlete's foot, which occurs on the skin's surface, nail fungus lives in the nail bed and the nail plate. The nail provides the fungus with an extremely well-protected place to live, which is why nail fungus may be especially hard to treat. The primary symptom of nail fungus is in the appearance of the nail. The nail becomes yellow, white, or **opaque**. The texture of the nail also changes and becomes thick and brittle. If the fungus has been present for a long time, the nail can even become twisted or distorted. The most effective way to treat nail fungus is with oral terbinafine hydrochloride (Lamisil), which inhibits the production of the fungal cells.

Viral Infections

Warts. Warts, or *verrucae,* are caused by the human papillomaviruses (HPV) resulting in **hyperplasia** of the epidermis and a raised, cauliflower-like appearance. Verrucae can develop anywhere, but the most common sites are the fingers or the soles of the feet (plantar warts). Genital warts will be addressed in Chapter 38. Most warts resolve themselves over time, but they can be treated with topical chemicals, excised surgically, or removed with cryosurgery.

Herpes Simplex (Cold Sores). Cold sores or fever blisters are caused by the herpes simplex virus type I (HSV-1). The initial infection may be asymptomatic or cause painful ulcers along the gum lines of the mouth or on the lips. After the primary infection, the virus remains

dormant in the trigeminal nerve and can be reactivated by exposure to sun, cold, the presence of another infection such as an upper respiratory infection, or when the patient is under stress. The patient reports a feeling of burning, tingling, or numbness before the eruption of vesicles. The blisters heal in 2 to 3 weeks, but the process may be speeded up by the use of topical antiviral drugs, such as acyclovir (Zovirax) or penciclovir cream (Denavir).

Herpes Zoster (Shingles). *Herpes zoster* is an acute inflammatory disorder that is characterized by highly painful vesicle eruptions on the trunk of the body and occasionally on the face (Figure 35-6). The lesions develop on one side of the body and follow the course of the peripheral nerve, or *dermatome,* that has been infected by the varicella virus, which is the same virus that causes chicken pox. The virus lies dormant in the affected dorsal root ganglia and becomes reactivated in later years as a result of stress or aging.

The onset of the disorder is usually marked by pain along the nerve pathway, and in approximately 3 days lesions appear. The duration of the inflammation ranges from 10 days to 5 weeks. Diagnosis is through the characteristic pattern of painful lesions and may be confirmed by isolating the virus in cell cultures. It can also be detected by the presence of the varicella zoster antibodies in the blood. Treatment focuses on promoting patient comfort with analgesic and antipruritic medications. Corticosteroid medications (Prednisone) and antiviral drugs, including topical or oral acyclovir (Zovirax) and oral famciclovir (Famvir) or valacyclovir (Valtrex), can also be prescribed.

Other Infections

Scabies and Pediculosis. Scabies (itch mite) and pediculosis (lice) are the two most common parasites to infest individuals. Scabies are tiny organisms, barely

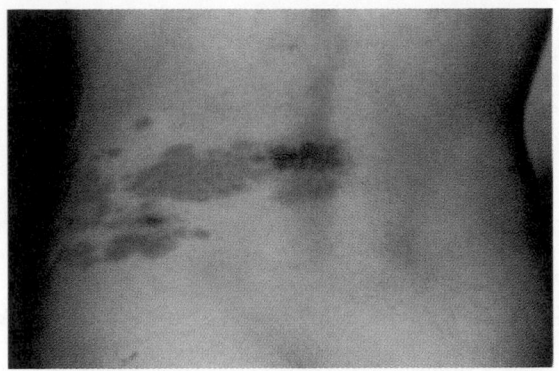

FIGURE 35-6 Herpes zoster (shingles). (From Callen J, Greer K, Hood A, et al: *Color atlas of dermatology*, ed. 2, Philadelphia, 2000, WB Saunders.)

visible with the eye, that burrow into the epidermis (Figure 35-7). Pediculosis consists of three species of lice: the head louse (Figure 35-8, *A*), the body louse, and the pubic louse (Figure 35-8, *B*). Both infestations are highly contagious. Diagnosis of scabies may require scraping the skin at an inflamed area and visualizing the mites under a low-power microscope. Lice can be seen on the hair shafts. Patients describe symptoms of intense itching, possible body rash, and a sensation of something crawling on their skin.

Treatment consists of ridding the body of the parasite, controlling the pruritus, and disinfecting the home environ-

ment to prevent reinfestation. Scabies are treated with a single application of 5% permethrin cream (Elimite) or 1% lindane lotion (Kwell). Medicated shampoo, creams, and/or lotions are used to kill head lice. The treatment must be repeated in 7 to 10 days to destroy the nits (eggs). If a secondary infection has begun, antibiotics may also be prescribed. All family members and other individuals who have had direct personal contact with the infested person must also be treated.

The medical assistant can assist the patient through explanations regarding the washing and/or dry cleaning of all clothing and bedding. Washing must be done in hot water. If clothes worn by the infested person have

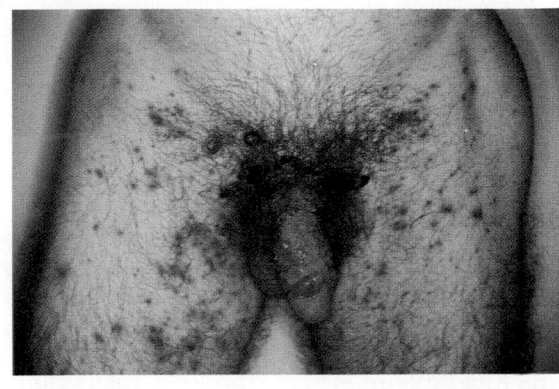

FIGURE 35-7 Scabies rash. (From Callen J, Greer K, Hood A, et al: *Color atlas of dermatology*, ed. 2, Philadelphia, 2000, WB Saunders.)

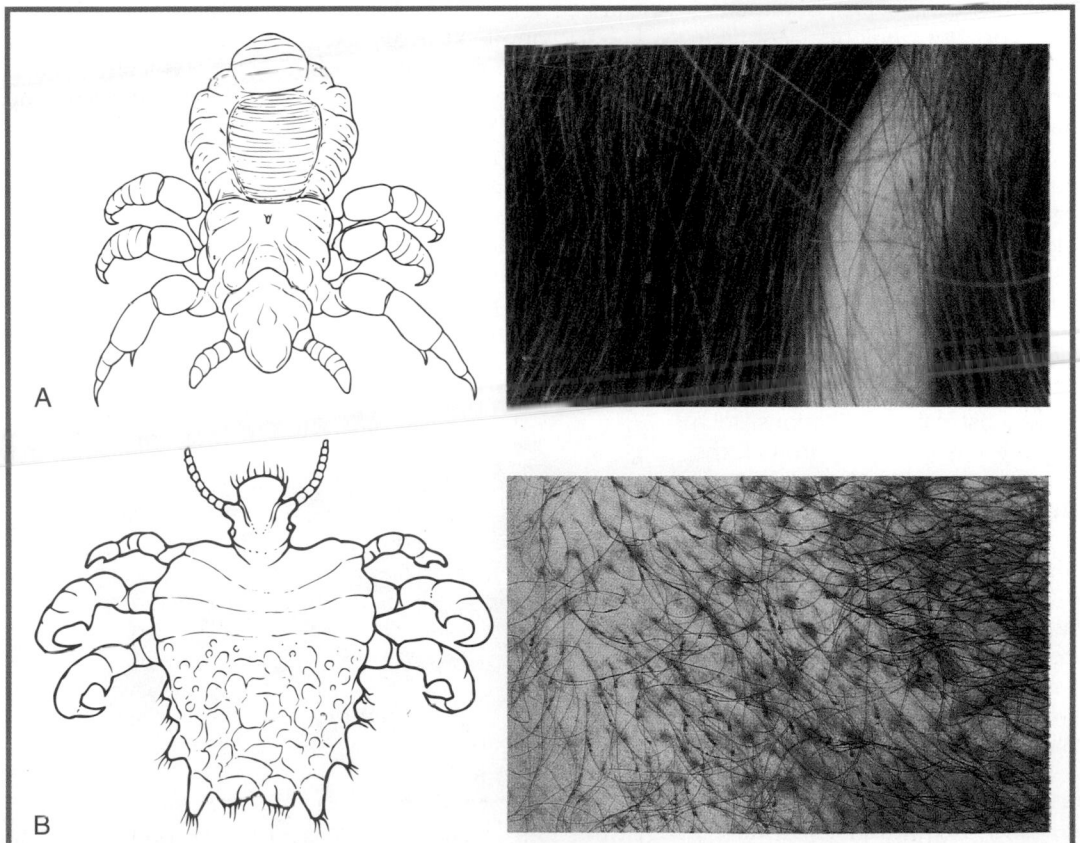

FIGURE 35-8 Pediculosis. **A** *Pediculus humanus capitis* (head louse) and lice in hair. **B**, *Phthirus pubis* (pubic or crab louse) and pubic lice rash. (From Callen J, Greer K, Hood A, et al: *Color atlas of dermatology*, ed. 2, Philadelphia, 2000, WB Saunders.)

been placed back into the closet, all items in the closet must be washed or dry cleaned. Furniture and carpets will need to be washed or vacuumed; and, if possible, both should be sprayed with a surface-disinfecting cleaner.

CRITICAL THINKING APPLICATION

Melissa's young daughter brought home a note today warning of a scabies outbreak in the school. Melissa has a few red marks on her forearms and the areas are quite itchy. Dr. Lee does a skin scraping of one of the areas and views itch mites under the microscope. How should Melissa and her family be treated? Should Melissa remain at work? How should the office and Melissa's home be disinfected to prevent reinfestation?

Inflammatory and Vascular Disorders

Seborrheic Dermatitis. Seborrheic dermatitis is one of the most common, chronic inflammatory conditions of the sebaceous glands. The disorder alters the amount and quality of sebum, resulting in dry or moist greasy-appearing scales and yellowish crusts on the scalp, eyebrows, eyelids, sides of the nose, behind the ears, and the middle of the chest. There are many different forms of the disease, including cradle cap in infants and dandruff. Seborrheic dermatitis of the scalp can be treated with tar- or sulfur-based shampoos; inflammations of the skin are usually treated with topical corticosteroids, such as triamcinolone diacetate (Aristocort), betamethasone valerate (Valisone), or fluocinolone acetonide (Synalar). *Seborrheic keratosis* is characterized by benign, slightly raised, tan to black lesions that occur with aging.

Contact Dermatitis. Contact dermatitis is an acute inflammatory response to a skin irritant or exposure to a substance that causes an allergic reaction. An individual who is allergic to latex gloves or who has been exposed to poison ivy will exhibit the signs and symptoms of contact dermatitis. The patient complains of redness *(erythema)*, edema, pruritus, and vesicles. The patient should be encouraged to wash the affected area immediately after exposure to remove the irritant if possible. Medical treatment includes the application of corticosteroid cream or the use of oral corticosteroid medications, such as prednisone or methylprednisolone (Medrol) if the symptoms are severe.

Eczema (Atopic Dermatitis). Eczema is an idiopathic inflammatory skin disease that tends to occur in patients with a family history of allergies. Its appearance in young children may be caused by food allergies; stress or extremes in temperature can trigger flare-ups in older children. The condition usually improves and may disappear as the child ages. Eczema is characterized by a vesicular rash located on the face, neck, elbows, posterior knees, and behind the ears. It causes pronounced pruritus, which results in excoriation of the affected ?m constant scratching.

?a is diagnosed with a comprehensive family ? examination of the skin. The patient may be asked to investigate possible allergens by making a list of all of the items that might be responsible for the outbreak or undergo allergy testing. The goal of treatment is to reduce the frequency and number of eruptions and relieve the pruritus so the areas do not become excoriated. The primary inflammation is usually treated with topical corticosteroids. Inflamed plaques usually indicate a secondary staphylococcal infection and should be treated with an oral antibiotic.

Psoriasis. Psoriasis is a chronic skin disease that produces discrete pink or red lesions covered with silvery scaling (Figure 35-9). The disease may begin at any age and is noninfectious. Psoriasis was thought to be caused by excessive development of epithelial cells, but recent research confirms that it is an autoimmune response among patients with a family history of the disorder. The affected skin is typically dry, cracked, and encrusted. The lesions may appear on the scalp, chest, buttocks, and extremities.

Psoriasis is diagnosed by observations of the skin, a careful patient history, and/or a skin biopsy. The treatment can only be **palliative**, because there is no cure for the disease. Exposure to ultraviolet light may retard the cell production, and coal tar preparations may be applied to the affected areas. The physician may also order a combination of therapies including methotrexate; a retinoid such as acitretin (Soriatane); the immunosuppressant cyclosporine (Neoral); low-dosage antihistamines; and oatmeal baths to promote patient comfort.

Systemic Lupus Erythematosus. Systemic lupus erythematosus (SLE) is a chronic **autoimmune** inflammatory disease of the connective tissue of the body. The cause is unknown, although women are nine times more likely to develop the disease than men. It can affect any connective tissue in the body but typically causes inflammatory changes in the skin, joints, muscles, and kidneys. SLE usually involves more than one organ, with the patient experiencing periods of **exacerbation** and **remission**. One of the diagnostic characteristics of the disease is a "butterfly" rash that spreads from one cheek and across the nose to the other cheek. Other integumentary system symptoms include erythematous patches and plaques, **alopecia**, and photosensitivity.

The prognosis for SLE depends on organ involvement but is poor for those patients experiencing renal,

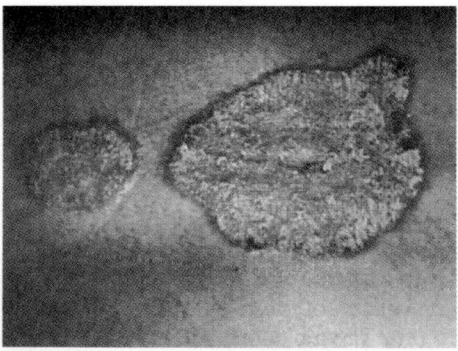

FIGURE 35-9 Psoriasis. (From Callen J, Greer K, Hood A, et al: *Color atlas of dermatology*, ed. 2, Philadelphia, 2000, WB Saunders.)

cardiovascular, or neurological complications. Serious cases are treated with antimalarial drugs (hydroxychloroquine [Plaquenil] or chloroquine hydrochloride [Aralen]) and oral corticosteroids as needed to control the inflammatory reactions.

Scleroderma. Scleroderma is a chronic, progressive, autoimmune disease that affects the blood vessels and connective tissues of the skin, lungs, and internal organs. Integumentary system symptoms include fibrous changes in the skin, which result in *sclerosis* (hardening) of the skin, edema, pallor, pigmentation, and fixation to subcutaneous tissues. These same sclerotic changes can occur in any organ in the body. **Raynaud's phenomenon** may be the first symptom of the disease. The cause of scleroderma is unknown, but it usually occurs in middle-aged women.

There is no cure for the disease and no specific treatment. Physical therapy helps maintain muscle strength, but the prognosis is poor. Patients with scleroderma usually die from cardiac, pulmonary, or renal involvement.

Thermal Injuries

Skin can be damaged and injured by exposure to moderately high or low temperatures over an extended period. It also can be injured in a relatively short time when exposed to very high or low temperatures. The most frequent thermal injuries are burns, which are classified as superficial-thickness (first-degree), partial-thickness (second-degree), or full-thickness (third-degree), depending on the depth of the wound (Figure 35-10).

Superficial (First-Degree) Burn. A superficial-thickness burn shows erythema of the epidermis, blanches with pressure, is painful but without blisters at the site. Sunburn and a steam burn without vesicle formation are examples of superficial burns.

Partial-Thickness (Second-Degree) Burn. A partial-thickness burn destroys the entire epidermal layer and varying depths of the dermis, with blister formation and subcutaneous edema and pain. There is also danger of infection in the blistered area. If the burn is deep enough, there may be some destruction of the hair follicles and the sebaceous glands.

Treatment of Minor Burns. Because burns damage the natural protection of the skin, preventing infection at the site is of primary concern. Medical treatment of superficial- and partial-thickness burns includes gently cleansing the site with a bactericidal solution and **debridement** of broken blisters or dead skin. Blisters that are intact should be left alone. The physician may order the burned area covered with a thin layer of silver sulfadiazine cream and a nonadherent multilayered dressing applied for several days to 1 week. The patient's tetanus immunization status should be reviewed and a tetanus injection administered if needed, and the physician may also order analgesics for pain relief.

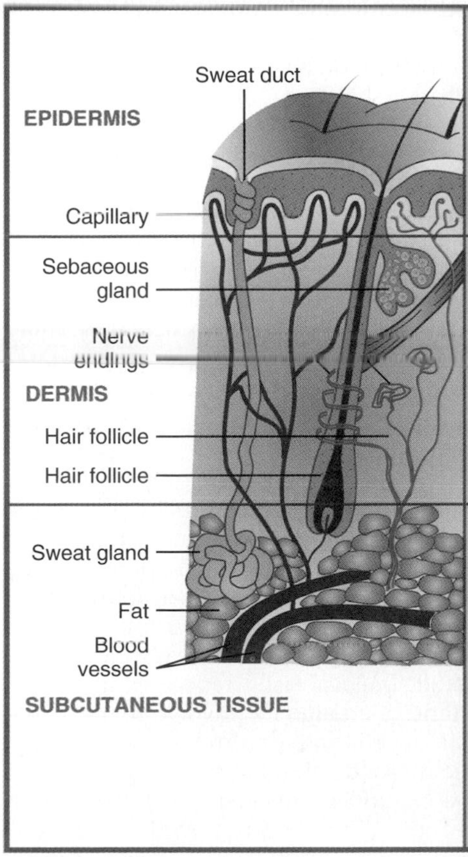

		APPEARANCE	SENSATION	COURSE
EPIDERMIS — Sweat duct, Capillary	SUPERFICIAL BURN	Mild to severe erythema; skin blanches with pressure. Skin dry. Small, thin-walled blisters	Painful. Hyperesthetic. Tingling. Pain eased by cooling	Discomfort lasts about 48 hours. Desquamation in 3–7 days
DERMIS — Sebaceous gland, Nerve endings, Hair follicle, Hair follicle	PARTIAL-THICKNESS BURN	Large thick-walled blisters covering extensive area (vesiculation). Edema; mottled red base; broken epidermis; wet, shiny, weeping surface	Painful. Hyperesthetic. Sensitive to cold air	Superficial partial-thickness burn heals in 10–14 days. Deep partial-thickness burn requires 21–28 days for healing. Healing rate varies with burn depth and presence or absence of infection
SUBCUTANEOUS TISSUE — Sweat gland, Fat, Blood vessels	FULL-THICKNESS BURN	Variable, e.g., deep red, black, white, brown. Dry surface. Edema. Tissue disrupted	Little pain. Anesthetic	Full-thickness dead skin suppurates and liquefies after 2–3 weeks. Spontaneous healing impossible. Requires removal of eschar and skin grafting. Scarring deformities and function loss. Beneath eschar capillary tufts and fibroblasts organize into granulating tissue

FIGURE 35-10 Classification of burns.

PATIENT EDUCATION FOR BURN CARE

- Warning signs of infection include fever, malaise, inflammation, swelling, increased pain, odor, and drainage from the burn area. Any of these should be reported to the physician immediately.
- Review care of the wound, including gentle cleansing with bactericidal solution (such as povidone-iodine solution [Betadine]) and covering the wound with an antibiotic ointment (silver sulfadiazine) so the dressing does not stick to the burn.
- The patient should consume a high-calorie, high-protein diet to maintain weight and promote healing.
- For partial-thickness burns, new skin development takes 6 weeks, with complete healing in 6 to 12 months, depending on the extent of the burn.

CRITICAL THINKING APPLICATION

Thomas Rangoso, a 66-year-old patient, calls the office to report a burn to his right hand and forearm. He fell while passing the stove and burned himself on the hot surface. Mr. Rangoso tells you the area is very red and painful with blisters in the center. He wants to break the blisters and put butter on the burn. Should Mr. Rangoso be seen by Dr. Lee, and what should Melissa tell him about the care of the burn?

Full-Thickness (Third-Degree) Burn. Full-thickness burns destroy all layers of the skin and may involve underlying fat, muscle, nerves, blood supply, and bone. The area appears charred or white, with a firm, leathery skin texture. There is no pain, because the nerve endings are destroyed. Full-thickness burns have the potential of causing major complications, including dehydration, circulatory collapse, respiratory distress, and septic shock. Treatment of major burns includes maintaining the patient's airway, replacing fluids, prevention of infection, and administration of oxygen. Debridement of affected tissue and skin grafts are required for wound healing. Depending on the extent of the burns, the patient may be hospitalized in an intensive care unit or a specialty burn unit.

Burns are also classified according to the percentage of body surface involved, based on the Rule of Nines, as discussed in Chapter 33.

Cold Injuries

Cold injuries are usually less severe than burns, but prolonged exposure to cold can result in infection, gangrene, amputation, and in severe situations, death. Frostbite is caused by exposure to subfreezing temperatures. The damage occurs at the capillary level, which become permanently dilated and unable to regulate local blood flow. The signs and symptoms of superficial frostbite include burning, tingling, numbness, and a white or grayish color of the skin. With deep frostbite the area is hard, mottled, edematous, and blue or gray after thawing with blister formation.

The extent of injury is diagnosed by visual examination and knowing the history of the exposure. Treatment consists of warming the area with immersion in water at 38° to 41° C (100° to 106° F). The affected site should never be rubbed, because that will increase cellular destruction. Vital signs should be monitored and the physician's orders followed explicitly.

Benign and Malignant Neoplasms

A neoplasm is an abnormal growth or tumor that may be either benign or malignant. Table 35-1 outlines the differences between benign and malignant tumors. Invasion and metastasis are the principal criteria used to distinguish between benign and malignant neoplasms. Benign masses are encapsulated, and although they may grow in size, they remain within a confining shell, whereas malignant tumors invade and take over surrounding tissues. Local invasion of surrounding tissue occurs when malignant cells break through the basement membrane that separates epithelial cells from connective tissue. Here the cancerous cells can invade blood and lymph vessels, which can then carry the malignant cells to organs throughout the body. Patients diagnosed with *carcinoma in situ* have a malignant tumor that is confined to the original site of growth without invasion of the basement membrane. Patients with regional spread have evidence of malignant cells in surrounding tissues but no evidence of lymph node involvement. Patients with distant spread, or *metastasis*, show positive lymph node involvement, with possible spread of the tumor into other organs such as the lungs, liver, brain, or bones.

Malignant tumors are also classified according to *grading* and *staging*. After a biopsy of the tumor is obtained, it is sent to the pathologist for microscopic examination. Grading is the histological, or cellular, classification of the tumor that is used in determining the patient's prognosis. The more poorly *differentiated* the cells from the tumor, meaning the less they look like normal cells, the poorer the prognosis. Staging involves using physical examination and diagnostic tests (such as bone or liver scans) to determine the degree of tumor spread. The size and depth of the primary tumor, the level of lymph node involvement, and the presence of metastatic spread determine whether the patient has a carcinoma in situ, a tumor that is localized to the organ of origin, a direct spread beyond the primary organ, lymph node metastasis, or a confirmed secondary tumor growth in a distant metastasis. Grading and staging describe the extent of malignant involvement so the physician can plan appropriate treatment.

There are three methods of obtaining a small piece of tissue for examination under a microscope. In an excision biopsy, the entire lesion may be removed for analysis such as in a wart or mole removal. A punch biopsy involves the removal of a small section from a designated

TABLE 35-1	Differences Between Benign and Malignant Tumors	
Characteristic	**Benign Tumor**	**Malignant Tumor**
Cellular structure and level of differentiation	Same as surrounding tissue	**Anaplastic** changes
Type of growth	Encapsulated mass that expands over time	Infiltrates and metastasizes; can have distant spread through the bloodstream or lymph system to other body tissues and organs
Rate of growth	Usually slow; rarely fatal	May be slow, rapid, or very rapid; almost always fatal if untreated
Destruction of localized tissue	None	Ulceration and necrosis of surrounding tissue common

boosters. These approaches may be used singly or in combination and are usually determined by a specialist in the study and treatment of cancer, the oncologist.

CANCER'S SEVEN WARNING SIGNS

The initial letters of the warning signs spell out the word CAUTION. Any of these warning signs should be reported to the physician immediately. Early detection and self-examination are crucial to cancer survival.

1. **C**hange in bowel or bladder habits
2. **A** sore that does not heal
3. **U**nusual bleeding or discharge
4. **T**hickening or a lump in the breast or elsewhere
5. **I**ndigestion or difficulty in swallowing
6. **O**bvious change in a wart or mole
7. **N**agging cough or hoarseness

---

location within the lesion; usually the center is the optimal site. This can be done with a punch instrument or a large-gauge needle, such as in a breast biopsy. A shave biopsy is done with a scalpel by cutting or shaving off the growth or lesion just above the skin line. This may be used to biopsy a possible squamous cell carcinoma lesion. The medical assistant may help the physician perform these procedures.

ASSISTING WITH A TISSUE BIOPSY

1. Assemble all of the supplies needed for the procedure.
2. Prepare the patient by explaining the procedure.
3. Prepare the site of the biopsy according to office protocol.
4. Assist the physician as needed, using appropriate personal protective equipment according to standard precautions.
5. Label the sample container and prepare it for transport to the testing laboratory. Remember to include the laboratory request forms.
6. Clean the procedure area, properly dispose of all waste materials, and disinfect/sterilize equipment used in the procedure.
7. Wash hands and document the procedure including patient education on biopsy site care.

The ideal treatment of cancer depends on the staging, grading, and type of carcinoma. Possible treatments include surgical removal of the tumor, radiation therapy, chemotherapy, hormone therapy, and immune system

Neoplasms of the Skin

Neoplasms of the skin may be benign or malignant. Examples of benign tumors include birthmarks and moles (*nevi*). A tumor may be benign but have a predisposition to cancer, which means it can go from the benign state to a cancerous one. Whenever a neoplasm is discovered, the physician usually performs a biopsy of the lesion to establish the type of cells involved.

There are three cancerous lesions of the skin: basal cell, squamous cell, and malignant melanoma. Basal cell carcinoma is very slow growing and is the most frequently seen form of skin cancer. The most common sites are areas of the body that are exposed to the sun, such as the face. It appears as a painless, smooth, small, waxy, translucent nodule that may become inflamed and ulcerated. It may be white, brown, or black and have ill-defined borders (Figure 35-11).

Squamous cell carcinoma grows rapidly and is more serious because it has a tendency to metastasize. It appears as a firm, red nodule with visible scales and may ulcerate and form a crust (Figure 35-12).

Malignant melanoma develops from a change in a mole. Sunburns increase the risk of melanoma, and individuals with more moles than average (greater than 100) are also at greater risk. Persons with *congenital nevi* (moles present at birth) are more likely to develop a melanoma than are persons with *dysplastic nevi* (moles that are irregular in shape). Additional risk factors include an inability to tan, light or red hair, fair skin, family history, and the number of childhood sunburns. There are many forms of melanoma, but all are pigmented lesions (usually brown, tan, blue, red, black, or white) that are asymmetrical with irregular borders and are usually larger than 6 mm (Figure 35-13). The staging of the disease is dependent on the depth of the growth. The incidence of malignant melanoma has doubled in the past 10 years and results in more deaths than all

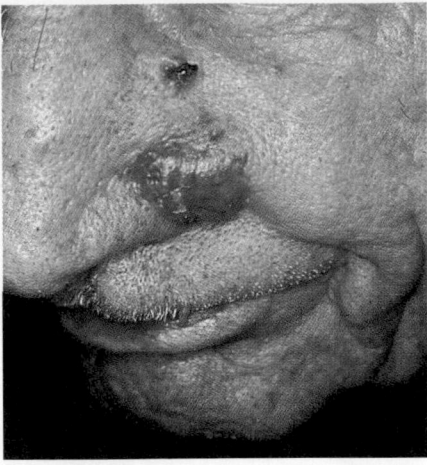

FIGURE 35-11 Basal cell carcinoma. (Modified from Damjanov I: *Pathology for the health-related professions*, ed. 2, Philadelphia, 2000, WB Saunders.)

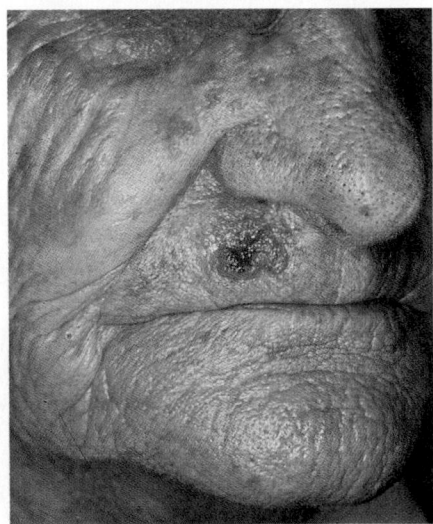

FIGURE 35-12 Squamous cell carinoma. (Modified from Damjanov I: *Pathology for the health-related profession*s, ed. 2, Philadelphia, 2000, WB Saunders.)

other skin diseases. Melanomas often recur or metastasize within 5 years of diagnosis. The patient should be routinely examined for at least 10 years after removal of the melanoma.

EARLY WARNING SIGNS OF MALIGNANT MELANOMA: THE ABCD RULE

If a mole displays any of these characteristics, a dermatologist should examine it immediately.

A	Asymmetry	One half of the mole does not match the other half.
B	Border	Edges of the mole are blurred or irregular.

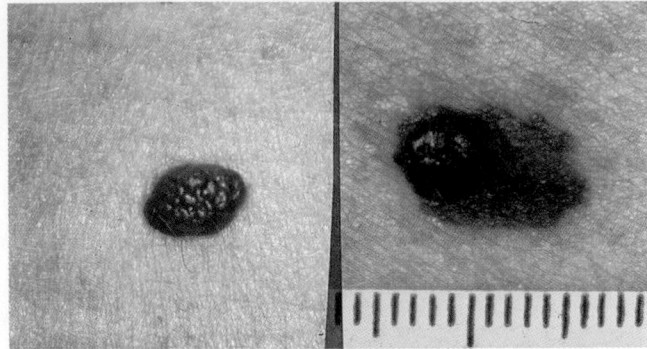

FIGURE 35-13 Pigmented skin lesions. *Left*, Benign pigmented nevus (mole). *Right*, Malignant melanoma. (Courtesy National Cancer Institute, Bethesda, Md.)

C	Color	Color of the mole is not the same throughout, with shades of tan, brown, black, red, white, or blue.
D	Diameter	Mole is larger than 6 mm, about the size of a pencil eraser.

All skin cancers are diagnosed by their appearance, and the diagnosis is confirmed through biopsy. The treatment depends on the type, level of invasion, and location. The physician may choose to surgically remove the tumor or eradicate the tumor with **cryosurgery, electrodesiccation,** or the application of chemotherapeutic agents.

Dermatological Procedures

The integumentary system can reflect both internal and external reactions and disease processes. The skin holds information about the body's circulation, nutritional status, and signs of systemic diseases. Normality of the skin depends on the person's age, sex, and physical and emotional health. It also acts as a mirror reflecting aging changes that proceed in all of the organs of the body. For many people, self-esteem is linked to a youthful appearance. As patients are prepared for a dermatological examination, allow them to express their anxieties. The impairments that most frequently bring a patient to the dermatologist's office are cosmetic disfigurements caused by a skin disease, pain and pruritus, and interference with sensations or movements.

Assisting With the Examination

The dermatologist will examine the visible top layer of skin of the entire body, beginning with the scalp and continuing through to the soles of the feet. This will also include the genital area. The skin assessment is basically accomplished through inspection followed with detailed examination by palpation, diascopy, and special tests.

The *diascope* is a glass plate held against the skin to permit observation of changes produced in the underlying areas by application of pressure. Inspection may include using a magnifying lens and a bright light to closely examine a suspicious lesion or growth. The medical assistant may take photographs of the affected area or chart specific measurements of the lesion to aid in determining future changes.

In the physical examination, concerns about the integumentary system include abnormal coloring, such as cyanosis, pallor, erythema, **leukoderma**, or excessive brown patches. **Jaundice** may indicate an increase in the level of **bilirubin** in the blood. Decreased pigmentation is found in *vitiligo*, which is the acquired loss of melanin and is characterized by white patches. Lesions, ulcers, and bruises may be the result of pathologic conditions. Localized red or purple changes may be the result of vascular neoplasms, birthmarks, or subcutaneous hemorrhages (**petechiae** and **ecchymoses**). Palpation is used to confirm and amplify findings seen by inspection. Inspection and palpation are interrelated in confirming diagnoses. Palpatory findings may include the skin's texture, elasticity, or the presence of edema.

Draping a patient for a skin examination depends on the area to be examined. Remember to expose the area adequately but protect the patient's privacy. Try to make the patient as comfortable as possible and offer support when it is needed.

Allergy Skin Testing. Skin testing to determine patient allergies involves either intradermally injecting or topically applying a small amount of antigen (or groups of antigens) and later examining the test site for a visible reaction.

GUIDELINES FOR SKIN TESTING

1. The patient should stop taking all antihistamines or allergy medication at least 3 days before testing to avoid false-negative results.
2. Recommended sites for allergen injection or application are the anterior forearm and the back.
3. Allergen sites must be specifically labeled and spaced approximately 1½ to 2 inches apart.
4. If the patient exhibits signs of anaphylaxis, notify the physician immediately and prepare emergency supplies. Allergy testing should only be performed when the physician is on-site.
5. Skin testing may cause a mild systemic allergic response resulting in rhinitis, wheezing, and sneezing. The patient should contact the physician if a more severe reaction occurs.

Scratch Test. A scratch test may be performed on any smooth surface of the skin; however, the back is favored in young children because of the large area of skin available. It is also easier to immobilize the child in this position. The skin surface is labeled or numbered in rows 1½ to 2 inches apart. A short scratch is made with a needle or lancet, and a drop of allergen is placed on each scratch or puncture. Fifty or more tests may be done at one time, and a certain pattern is followed so that the site of each allergen can be identified.

A reaction usually occurs within 10 to 30 minutes. If the reaction is positive, a *wheal* (hive) will form at the site of the scratch. The interpretation of the test should always be based on a comparison of this reaction with that of the control, which is a scratch with a plain base fluid, free of any allergy-producing extract.

The interpretation, or reading, of the skin tests is performed by the physician or a trained technician. Reactions are commonly graded from 2 to 4. No precise definition of a reaction can be given, and indeed the intensity may vary among individuals. However, as a general rule, a 2 reaction implies a wheal that is definitely larger than that of the control. A larger wheal is interpreted as a 3, whereas the presence of *pseudopods* (fingerlike extensions around the periphery of the wheal) may be read as a 4. Carefully wipe off the extract to stop the reaction when a strong reaction is occurring. Erythema around the wheal is usually disregarded in the interpretations. Frequently, large or significant reactions are accompanied by local itching. Patients should remain in the office for a minimum of 30 minutes after the completion of the allergy testing procedure in case of a delayed systemic allergic reaction.

Intradermal (Intracutaneous) Test. This test is more accurate than the scratch test. Extracts are injected into the intradermal layer of the skin, with the usual sterile technique, in a dose of 0.1 to 0.2 ml. This method is used for the tuberculin (purified protein derivative [PPD]) test and the Valley Fever coccidioidomycosis test. When using intradermal injections for allergy testing, 10 to 15 allergens may be tested at one time on each arm. The reaction time is identical to that of the scratch test; however, the antigen is more dilute.

Patch Test. This method of testing is of some value in diagnosing dermatitis. In the patch test, the suspected material is placed on the skin (near the original lesion, if possible), covered with a small square of cellophane, and held down with strips of adhesive or transparent tape. Twenty to 30 tests may be done at one time. The reaction is read within 1 to 4 days.

Radioallergosorbent (RAST) Test. This laboratory procedure identifies specific allergens that cause allergic responses such as rashes, hay fever, asthma, or drug reactions. The RAST test is easier to perform than skin testing since it requires a single venipuncture. It is also less painful and less dangerous for the patient and more specific than skin testing. Although skin testing remains the preferred method of diagnosing hypersensitivity, the RAST test may be indicated when the patient cannot stop antihistamine medications, if a skin disorder makes accurate interpretation of skin test results difficult, or if skin tests are negative but the patient's signs and symptoms support further investigation.

CRITICAL THINKING APPLICATION

A new employee in the practice asks Melissa's help in understanding the different methods for testing for allergies. What should Melissa tell her about the various skin tests performed in the office and the venipuncture RAST test?

Treatment of Allergies. For patients with allergies, the physician may prescribe antihistamine medications such as cetirizine hydrochloride (Zyrtec) or fexofenadine hydrochloride (Allegra), or over-the-counter medications for relief of allergy symptoms. Another option is the use of immunotherapy, a series of injections in which minute doses of allergens are administered subcutaneously over time to desensitize the patient's immune system and ultimately develop a resistance to the immune response. This usually requires weekly or bimonthly injections over several years. Some patients are cured, whereas others have only a minor reduction in allergic symptoms. Immunotherapy is a controversial treatment, because it is an expensive, invasive, potentially dangerous treatment with unpredictable results and should be undertaken only in patients with severe allergic symptoms that are not relieved by antihistamine medications.

If a medical assistant is responsible for administering allergy injections, he or she must take great care in preparing the correct dose of each allergen, administering each allergen in a separate site, accurately documenting the procedure and any patient reactions, and observing the patient for a minimum of 20 to 30 minutes after the injections to determine possible systemic allergic responses, such as urticaria, wheezing, or hypotension. If the patient exhibits any localized or systemic reactions, the physician should be notified.

Obtaining a Wound Specimen for Culture. A wound culture specimen is obtained to perform a microscopic analysis of the organisms at the site of a lesion to determine the causative agents of an infection. The physician may order a culture if the wound is inflamed, draining, or the patient has a fever. *Aerobic* cultures are performed to detect organisms that grow in the presence of oxygen and are usually found on the superficial surfaces of the wound. *Anaerobic* cultures check for the presence of organisms that require little or no oxygen and appear in deeper wound sites or areas that have a poor blood supply, such as ulcers or compound fractures (Procedure 35-1). Wound culture results help the physician prescribe the most effective antibiotic for the infection.

Procedures for Appearance Modification

Chemical Peel (Chemexfoliation). Topical agents are used in chemical peels to minimize or remove minor skin features, such as acne scars, hyperpigmentation, and fine wrinkles. Agents used for chemical peels include tretinoin cream 0.05% to 0.1% concentration (Retin-A), alpha hydroxy acid, trichloroacetic acid, or phenol (carbolic acid). During application, care must be taken to prevent the solution from entering the eyes. The use of chemical exfoliating agents may cause the skin to appear inflamed and dry, with crusting and edema. The patient may complain of stinging and burning at the beginning of the treatment regimen. The patient should avoid sun exposure for the length of treatment and use a sunscreen with a minimum sun protective factor (SPF) of 15 when outside, because photophobia (light sensitivity) is a typical side effect of treatment.

Dermabrasion. A *dermabrader* is a hand-held device that mechanically evens the layers of dermal tissue and is effective in the treatment of scars from acne vulgaris. Either topical anesthetics such as ethyl chloride or local injected anesthetics are used for the procedure. Besides the dermabrader, the dermatologist may use a variety of wire brushes, abrasive discs, or other devices to smooth the scar tissue. Standard precautions must be employed, including the use of face and eye guards to avoid aerosol or splatter contamination from the site. The patient should be educated about wound care and signs of infection.

Laser Resurfacing (Photothermolysis). Laser therapy may be used for fine lines and wrinkles, pigmented areas, shallow scars, and tattoo removal. Typically, the patient is instructed to prepare the site 3 to 6 weeks before the procedure with tretinoin (Retin-A), alpha hydroxy solutions, or bleaches. Laser procedures are performed with the patient under local, regional, or general anesthesia. During the procedure it is extremely important that both the patient and all personnel wear the type of eye protection recommended by the laser manufacturer. After the procedure, cool packs are applied to help reduce swelling, and topical antibiotic ointment is used to prevent infection. The treated area will appear inflamed and edematous and can take up to 2 weeks to heal.

Patient Education

There are many opportunities and topics for patient education in the dermatology field. Skin care products are advertised in the newspaper, on billboards, in magazines, and on television. People are willing to try almost anything to keep a youthful appearance. Consult the dermatologist you work for and get approval of skin care procedures that the office can recommend to patients. Sometimes companies that manufacture skin care products will give you samples if you write and tell them that your office recommends a certain product's use to patients. Patients enjoy receiving samples and encouragement to try a new skin care technique.

Another area of patient education involves the potentially dangerous effects of sunlight on the skin. Obtain literature showing how ultraviolet rays cause premature aging and may cause cancerous lesions later in life. You can explain the meaning of sun protective factor in suntanning lotions. Tanning beds should be avoided, especially by persons who have a skin disorder or by individuals taking certain medications, because of the ultraviolet light concentration used in these tanning devices. Providing patients with information about the warning signs of cancer is a vital part of patient education in a dermatology office.

PROCEDURE **35-1**

Collecting a Wound Specimen for Testing and/or Culture

GOAL: To obtain an adequate, noncontaminated sample for culture.

EQUIPMENT AND SUPPLIES

- Sterile culture kit containing tube, swabs, and transport media (for swabbing)
- Sterile culture kit containing syringe and transport media (for aspirating)
- Gauze flats
- Recommended wound cleansing solution
- Clean sterile dressing
- Gloves
- Biohazard container
- Face guard

PROCEDURAL STEPS

1 Wash your hands, gather supplies (Figure 1), and don gloves and face protection.

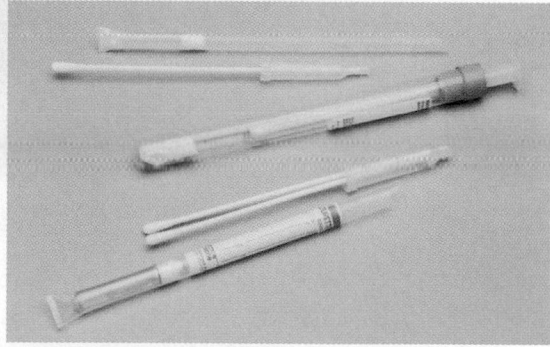

Figure 1

Purpose: Standard precautions.

2 Remove dressing from the wound and dispose of it in a biohazard waste container.
Purpose: Infection control.

3 Observe the wound and make note of the color, odor, and amount of exudate present.
Purpose: Information will be noted for the physician on the patient's record when the procedure is completed.

4 *Swabbing.* Remove the swab from the culture kit, insert the swab into the wound, and saturate it with the exudate. If necessary, use more than one swab, properly labeling each container, to obtain

exudates from the entire wound. If preparing an anaerobic culture, place the specimen in the culture tube as quickly as possible to avoid oxygen exposure and possible destruction of microbes.

5 *Aspirating.* Remove the syringe from the kit, insert the tip into the wound exudate, and draw back the plunger, drawing the exudate up into the syringe.

6 Place the swab into the culture tube and crush the transport media ampule, which is in the transport tube, by squeezing the walls of the transport tube slightly, or place the exudate-filled syringe directly into the transport tube (Figure 2).

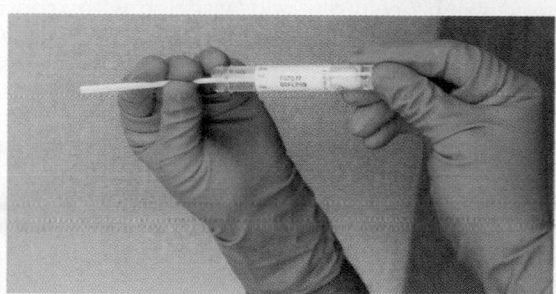

Figure 2

7 Label the culture tube accurately. Include on the laboratory slip the patient's recent antibiotic therapy, the wound site, and the suspected organism.

8 Clean the wound as ordered by the physician and apply a clean sterile dressing to the area. See Chapter 54 for dressing procedure.

9 Clean the area, disposing of all waste materials in biohazard waste container. Remove gloves and wash your hands.
Purpose: Infection control.

10 Place culture tube in the laboratory collection area. Chart the procedure and all wound data on the patient's record.
Purpose: A procedure is considered not done until it is recorded.

If a patient needs help in meal planning because of food allergy, you can help by recommending a nutritional center or a dietetic service, or for other types of allergy you could recommend other possible outside assistance and resource information centers.

Legal and Ethical Issues

When working in a dermatology office, you will hear many patients express concerns regarding a skin disorder. Expressing their concerns, knowing that you are listening, is always helpful, but be careful when offering encouragement about the course and outcome of their treatment. No treatment can restore youth. The improvement achieved may be slow and gradual. Keep encouragement on a positive level. Compliment the patient on small improvements, but let the physician describe the possible course and outcome of the prescribed treatment.

SUMMARY OF SCENARIO

Melissa enjoys her work with Dr. Lee but recognizes the need to keep up with new developments in the field of dermatology. She has learned the importance of giving patients accurate information while conducting telephone screening and always referring questions or concerns to Dr. Lee. Melissa especially enjoys the patient education aspects of working for a dermatologist, including the importance of using sun screens, controlling sun exposure, and informing patients about the warning signs of cancer. Melissa has also learned how to assist Dr. Lee with dermatological procedures, including allergy skin testing, obtaining wound cultures, and assisting with biopsies, chemical peels, dermabrasions, and laser resurfacing.

SUMMARY OF LEARNING OBJECTIVES

■ The skin serves several essential functions: it acts as a barrier to protect vital internal organs against infection and injury, helps dissipate heat and regulate body temperature, and synthesizes vitamin D when exposed to ultraviolet light. In addition, various sensory receptors throughout the skin enable it to respond to heat, cold, pain, and pressure.

■ The skin is made up of three layers: the epidermis, which is the thin uppermost layer; the dermis, which is the thicker layer beneath, often referred to as the true skin and making up about 90% of the skin mass; and the subcutaneous layer, which is composed primarily of fatty or adipose tissue.

■ The diagnosis of skin lesions, as described in Figure 35-2, is based on the color, level of elevation, and texture of the lesion; the presence of pruritus, excoriation, pain, or drainage; and whether the lesion is a primary or secondary growth.

■ Integumentary system infections include bacterial infections, such as impetigo, acne vulgaris, furuncles, carbuncles, and cellulitis; fungal infections, including a variety of tinea growths; viral infections, which cause warts, herpes simplex, and herpes zoster outbreaks; and scabies or pediculosis infestations.

■ Inflammatory and vascular integumentary system disorders include a variety of seborrheic dermatitis inflammations; contact dermatitis; eczema; and autoimmune disorders.

■ The most frequent thermal injuries are burns, which are classified as superficial (first-degree), partial-thickness (second-degree), or full-thickness (third-degree), depending on the depth of the wound. The most important concern in the treatment of burns is the prevention of infection. Cold injuries are usually less severe than burns, but prolonged exposure can result in infection, gangrene, amputation, and in severe situations, death.

■ Benign masses are encapsulated, and although they may grow in size, they remain within a confining membrane while malignant tumors invade and take over surrounding tissues. Local invasion of surrounding tissue occurs when malignant cells break through the basement membrane that separates epithelial cells from connective tissue. Here the cancerous cells can invade blood and lymph vessels, which can then carry the malignant cells to organs throughout the body.

■ Grading and staging describe the extent of malignant involvement so the physician can plan appropriate treatment. Grading is the histological, cellular classification of the tumor. The more poorly differentiated the cells from the tumor, the poorer the prognosis. Staging involves using physical examination and diagnostic tests (such as bone or liver scans) to determine the degree of tumor spread. The size and depth of the primary tumor, the degree of lymph node involvement, and the presence of metastatic spread determine whether the patient has a carcinoma in situ, a tumor that is localized to the organ of origin, a direct spread beyond the primary organ, lymph node metastasis, or a confirmed secondary tumor growth at a distant metastasis.

■ The warning signs of cancer include any change in bowel or bladder habits; a sore that does not heal; unusual bleeding or discharge; a thickening or a lump in the breast or elsewhere; indigestion or difficulty in swallowing; an obvious change in a wart or mole; or a nagging cough or hoarseness. Any of these warning signs should be reported to the physician immediately. Early detection and self-examination are crucial to cancer survival.

■ There are three cancerous lesions of the skin: basal cell, squamous cell, and malignant melanoma. Basal cell carcinoma is very slow growing and is the most frequently seen form of skin cancer. Squamous cell carcinoma grows rapidly and is more serious, because it has a tendency to metastasize. There are many forms of melanoma, but all are pigmented lesions (usually brown, tan, blue, red, black, or white) that are asymmetrical with irregular borders and are usually larger than 6 mm. Treatment depends on the type of lesion, the level of invasion, and location. The physician may surgically remove the tumor or destroy it with cryosurgery, electrodesiccation, or the application of chemotherapeutic agents.

■ The ABCD rule for early detection of a malignant melanoma includes examination of the site for any of the following: asymmetry, irregular border, change in color, and an increase in the diameter. If a mole displays any of these characteristics, a dermatologist should check it immediately.

■ Dermatological procedures include allergy skin testing that can be done with scratch, intradermal, or patch tests; drawing blood for a RAST test; treating allergies with immunotherapy; performing a wound culture; and assisting with appearance modification procedures, including chemical peels, dermabrasion, and laser resurfacing.

KEY INTERNET WEBSITES

- American Academy of Dermatology
- Archives of Dermatology
- The Electronic Textbook of Dermatology
  For active weblinks to each website visit
  http://evolve.elsevier.com/Kinn/

CHAPTER 36

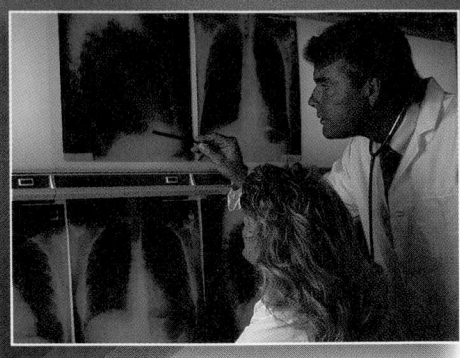

Scenario

Joan Rothman, CMA, was recently hired by United Community Hospital to work for a group of internists. Joan works primarily with Dr. Raj Sahani, a physician who specializes in gastroenterology. Although Joan did very well in school, she has had to learn more advanced information about disorders of the gastro-intestinal tract so she can manage patient questions and understand the diagnostic procedures ordered by Dr. Sahani. Dr. Sahani has asked Joan to research and develop educational packets for common gastrointestinal studies as well as work with other staff members on under-standing procedures related to the gastrointestinal system.

Assisting in Gastroenterology

National Curriculum Competencies

CLINICAL COMPETENCIES

4e. Prepare patients for and assist with routine and specialty examinations

4f. Prepare patients for and assist with procedures, treatments, and minor office surgery

4g. Apply pharmacology principles to prepare and administer oral and parenteral medications

TRANSDISCIPLINARY COMPETENCIES

3b. Instruct individuals according to their needs

3d. Provide instruction for health maintenance and disease prevention

Vocabulary

adhesions Bands of scar tissue that bind together two anatomical surfaces that are normally separate.

anastomosis The surgical joining together of two normally distinct organs.

anorexia Lack or loss of appetite for food.

carcinogens A substance or agent that causes the development of or increases the incidence of cancer.

diaphoresis The profuse excretion of sweat.

emulsification Dispersion of ingested fats into small globules by bile.

endemic Disease or microorganism that is specific to a particular geographic area.

fecalith A hard, impacted mass of feces in the colon.

fissures Narrow slits or clefts in the abdominal wall.

fistulas Abnormal, tubelike passages within the body tissue, usually between two internal organs.

flatus Gas expelled through the anus.

gangrene Death of body tissue as a result of loss of nutritive supply and followed by bacteria invasion and putrefaction.

hematemesis Vomiting of bright red blood, indicating rapid upper gastrointestinal bleeding, associated with esophageal varices or peptic ulcer.

hematocrit Volume percentage of erythrocytes in whole blood.

hemoglobin Protein found in erythrocytes that transports molecular oxygen in the blood.

hepatomegaly Abnormal enlargement of the liver.

ileostomy Surgical formation of an opening of the ileum onto the surface of the abdomen through which fecal material is emptied.

jaundice Yellowness of the skin and mucous membranes caused by deposition of bile pigment; not a disease but a symptom of a number of diseases, especially liver disorders.

ligation Process of tying off something to close it, usually a blood vessel during surgery, with a tie called a ligature.

lithotripsy A procedure for eliminating a stone by crushing or dissolving it in situ through the use of high intensity sound waves.

lymphadenopathy Any disorder of the lymph nodes or lymph vessels.

peristalsis Wavelike movement by which the gastrointestinal tract moves food downward.

polyps Tumors on stems frequently found in the mucosal lining of the colon.

portal hypertension An increased venous pressure in the portal circulation caused by cirrhosis or compression of the hepatic vascular system.

sclerotherapy Injection of sclerosing solutions in the treatment of hemorrhoids, varicose veins, or esophageal varices.

truss Elastic, canvas, or metallic device for retaining a reduced hernia within the abdominal cavity.

Valsalva's maneuver Occurs when one strains to defecate and urinate, uses the arms and upper trunk muscles to move up in bed, or strains during laughing, coughing, or vomiting; causes a trapping of blood in the great veins, preventing it from entering the chest and right atrium and may cause heart attack and death.

Internal medicine is a nonsurgical specialty with several subspecialties. Gastroenterology is one of these subspecialties and covers an extremely wide area known as the gastrointestinal system or the alimentary canal. Gastroenterologists are concerned with the diseases and disorders of the stomach, small intestine, large intestine (colon), appendix, and the accessory organs of the liver, gallbladder, and pancreas. Proctology, a subspecialty of gastroenterology, is concerned with disorders of the rectum and anus. The major purpose of the gastrointestinal system is to prepare, digest, and absorb the necessary nutrients to maintain homeostasis and to excrete the end-products that the body cannot use.

Anatomy and Physiology

The gastrointestinal system is basically a long hollow tube that has the same structural organization from its beginning to its termination (Figure 36-1). It is closely governed by the autonomic nervous system, which gives the entire system its unique ability to move slowly in some locations and to increase the movement in other sections. It is divided into two parts: the upper digestive system includes the mouth, esophagus, and stomach; the lower section consists of the small and large intestines. The gastrointestinal tract is rich in lymphatic tissue, which is very important for the absorption of nutrients from ingested food. Unfortunately, the lymphatic vessels are also the main route for the spread of cancers.

The primary functions of the gastrointestinal organs are threefold; digestion, absorption, and elimination. When food is taken in through the mouth, it is chewed or *masticated* and moistened with saliva. An enzyme released by the salivary glands, salivary amylase, mixes with the food and begins carbohydrate digestion. This mass, now called a *bolus*, is swallowed and the food enters the esophagus. Contractions of the smooth muscles are activated, and the bolus is now moved by **peristalsis**.

At the distal end of the esophagus is the gastroesophageal or cardiac sphincter, which relaxes as the bolus is swallowed so it can pass into the stomach. The muscular walls of the stomach overlap in folds, or rugae, which permit the stomach to expand and hold as much as 1 to $1\frac{1}{2}$ L of food and liquid. The gastric glands located in the stomach mucosa secrete hydrochloric acid, pepsinogen (begins the digestion of protein), and intrinsic factor, which is needed for the absorption of vitamin B_{12}. The gastric contents, now called *chyme*, are slowly emptied through the pyloric sphincter into the small intestine. The small intestine is made up of the duodenum, jejunum, and ileum.

The common bile duct delivers enzymes from the pancreas and bile from the liver to the duodenum, where digestion is completed. The pancreatic enzymes include trypsin for protein metabolism, amylase for digestion of carbohydrates, and lipase for fats. Bile is produced in the liver and stored in the gallbladder and provides the essential function of **emulsification** of fats so they can be absorbed.

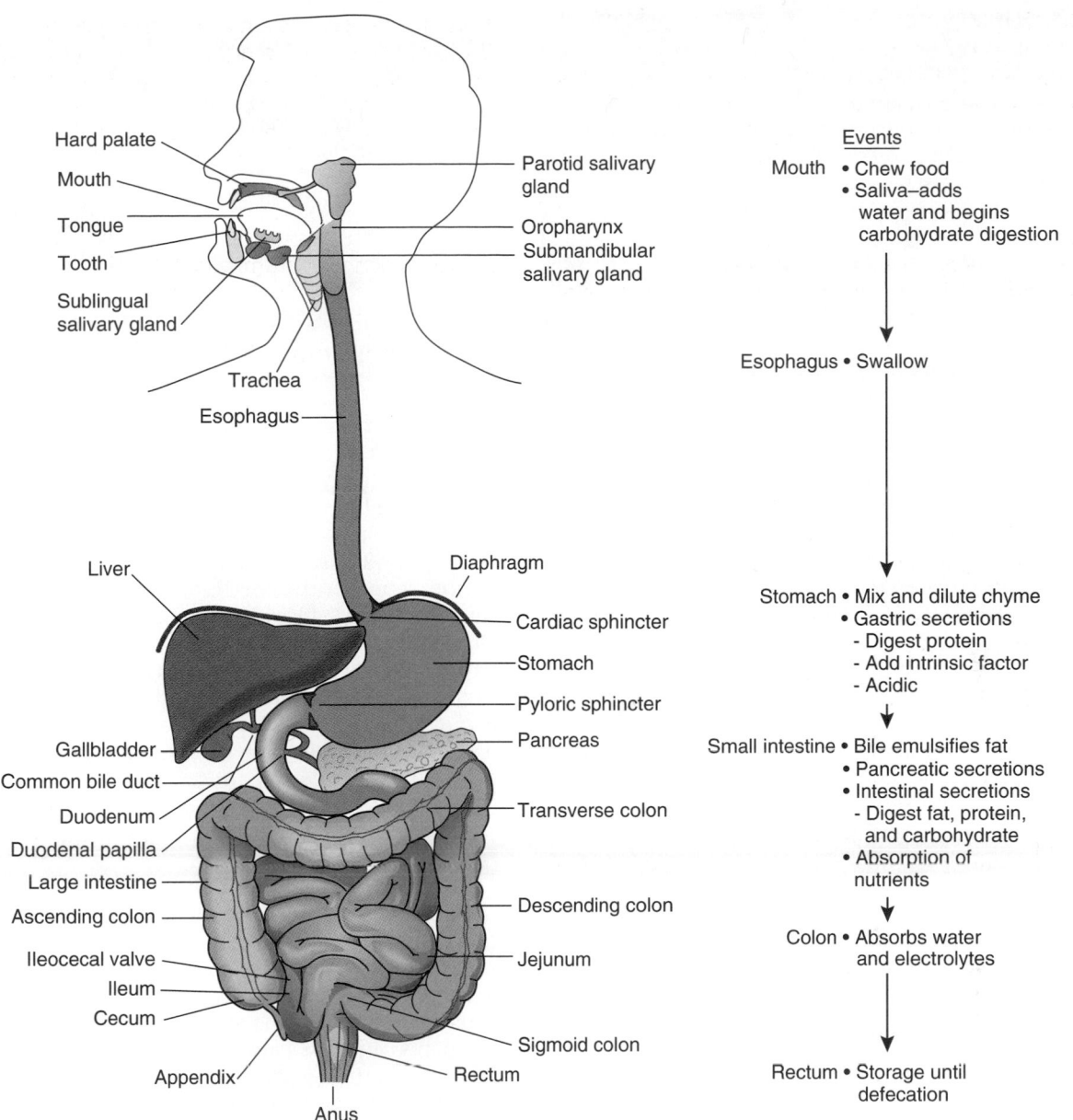

Hard palate
Mouth
Tongue
Tooth
Sublingual salivary gland
Trachea
Esophagus
Liver
Gallbladder
Common bile duct
Duodenum
Duodenal papilla
Large intestine
Ascending colon
Ileocecal valve
Ileum
Cecum
Appendix
Anus

Parotid salivary gland
Oropharynx
Submandibular salivary gland
Diaphragm
Cardiac sphincter
Stomach
Pyloric sphincter
Pancreas
Transverse colon
Descending colon
Jejunum
Sigmoid colon
Rectum

Events

Mouth
• Chew food
• Saliva—adds water and begins carbohydrate digestion

Esophagus • Swallow

Stomach
• Mix and dilute chyme
• Gastric secretions
  - Digest protein
  - Add intrinsic factor
  - Acidic

Small intestine
• Bile emulsifies fat
• Pancreatic secretions
• Intestinal secretions
  - Digest fat, protein, and carbohydrate
• Absorption of nutrients

Colon
• Absorbs water and electrolytes

Rectum
• Storage until defecation

FIGURE 36-1 Anatomy of the digestive system with associated events. (From Gould B: *Pathophysiology for the health professions*, ed 2. Philadelphia, 2002, WB Saunders.)

Once digestion is completed in the duodenum, the second function of the gastrointestinal tract, absorption of nutrients, begins. The small intestine is lined with transverse folds of tissue called *villi*. These overlapping projections greatly increase the surface area available for nutrient absorption. By the time the chyme reaches the terminal end of the small intestine, every nutrient that your body needs at this particular time should have been absorbed. This mass enters the colon or large intestine, which is made up of the cecum (extending from it is the *vermiform* appendix), ascending colon, transverse colon, descending colon, sigmoid colon, rectum, and anus. The colon absorbs large amounts of fluids and electrolytes to prevent dehydration of the body tissues. Once the fluid has been reabsorbed, the remaining solid waste materials, called *feces*, are moved into the sigmoid colon and rectum, and elimination occurs through the anus. This final function is called *defecation*.

CRITICAL THINKING APPLICATION

Dr. Sahani is concerned that some of the staff members do not understand the role of the gastrointestinal system in digestion, absorption, and excretion. He asks Joan to prepare an in-service training on the anatomy and physiology of the gastrointestinal tract. What should Joan include in the workshop?

CHARACTERISTICS OF THE GASTROINTESTINAL SYSTEM

- The abdominal cavity can be divided into 4 quadrants or 9 regions (Figure 36-2).
- The *peritoneum* is a membrane that covers the abdominal wall and organs of the abdominal cavity.
- The *mesentery* is a peritoneal fold that attaches the jejunum and ileum to the posterior abdominal wall.
- The *omentum* is a fold of fatty peritoneal tissue that contains multiple lymph nodes and hangs from the stomach like an apron covering the anterior transverse colon and the small intestine. Inflammation of the omentum results in the formation of scar tissue and **adhesions**.
- The gastrointestinal system digests and absorbs nutrients for all other systems; if it becomes diseased, all other systems are affected.

Diseases of the Gastrointestinal System

Gastrointestinal disorders are probably the most common problem seen in a medical office. Most of the simple problems are managed by a primary care physician. Between 5% and 10% of gastrointestinal problems are referred to a gastroenterologist for diagnosis and treatment. It is assumed that problems that stem from dental disorders are cared for by the dental professions. This chapter concentrates on the gastrointestinal problems most frequently seen, diagnosed, and treated.

Common Signs and Symptoms

A patient with a gastrointestinal problem may complain of multiple discomforts including nausea, vomiting, **anorexia**, diarrhea, constipation, and abdominal pain. It may be difficult for a medical assistant to identify the exact location and quality of the patient's discomfort. When discussing the abdominal pain with the patient, ask the patient to point to or touch the area where the pain is located. This is one way of making sure that the correct quadrant or region is identified and the patient is properly prepared for the physician to examine.

Table 36-1 outlines the typical signs, symptoms, and characteristics that would be seen in patients with gastrointestinal complaints.

CRITICAL THINKING APPLICATION

Two days a week Joan works in the telephone screening area of the practice, where she is responsible for the initial management of all calls from Dr. Sahani's patients. The following problems are typical of a call day from patients. What are some of the questions Joan should ask and subsequently document on each patient's chart?

- The mother of a 7-year-old patient is concerned because her son has been vomiting since yesterday.
- The father of an 18-month-old infant reports that the child has had diarrhea for 2 days.
- A 72-year-old patient is concerned about constipation that is not relieved with laxatives.
- A 22-year-old woman reports acute abdominal pain.

Cancers of the Gastrointestinal Tract

Any organ of the digestive tract can develop cancer. The features of malignant tumors and their treatments were described in Chapter 35. These characteristics, including the abilities to invade surrounding tissues and metastasize through the blood or lymph systems, are true of all cancerous tumors.

Table 36-2 describes some of the common malignant tumors found in the gastrointestinal system. The exact cause of a malignancy may not be known, but exposure to **carcinogens** increases the risk of developing a cancerous tumor. Examples of carcinogens include tobacco and alcohol as well as exposure to chemicals and radiation. Family history and lifestyle factors, such as consuming a diet high in fat and low in fiber, can also increase the risk for certain types of cancer.

Disorders of the Esophagus and Stomach

Hiatal Hernia. A hernia is the abnormal protrusion of part of an organ or tissue through the structures normally containing it. These protrusions can develop in various parts of the body, but most frequently are seen in the abdominal region. Causes of herniation include congenital weakness of the structures, trauma, relaxation of ligaments and skeletal muscles, or increased upward pressure from the abdomen. It is most often found in middle-aged or older individuals. The location of the hernia determines the term by which the protrusion is identified.

In patients with a hiatal hernia, the upper part of the stomach protrudes through the esophageal opening, the hiatal sphincter, of the diaphragm (Figure 36-3). With a sliding hiatal hernia, part of the stomach moves above the diaphragm when supine and slides back down into the abdominal cavity when standing. Part of the fundus of the stomach moves through the weakened hiatus in a paraesophageal hiatal hernia. Food may lodge in the herniated part of the stomach, causing reflux of highly acidic stomach contents into the esophagus, dysphagia, and chronic esophagitis, which may cause fibrosis and stricture. Patients complain of heartburn, frequent belching, and increased discomfort when they cough, bend over, or lie down after eating. *Gastroesophageal reflux disease* (GERD) often accompanies hiatal hernias. Chronic GERD is associated with an increased risk of cancer of the esophagus.

Patients with hiatal hernias are treated medically with omeprazole (Prilosec), esomeprazole (Nexium),

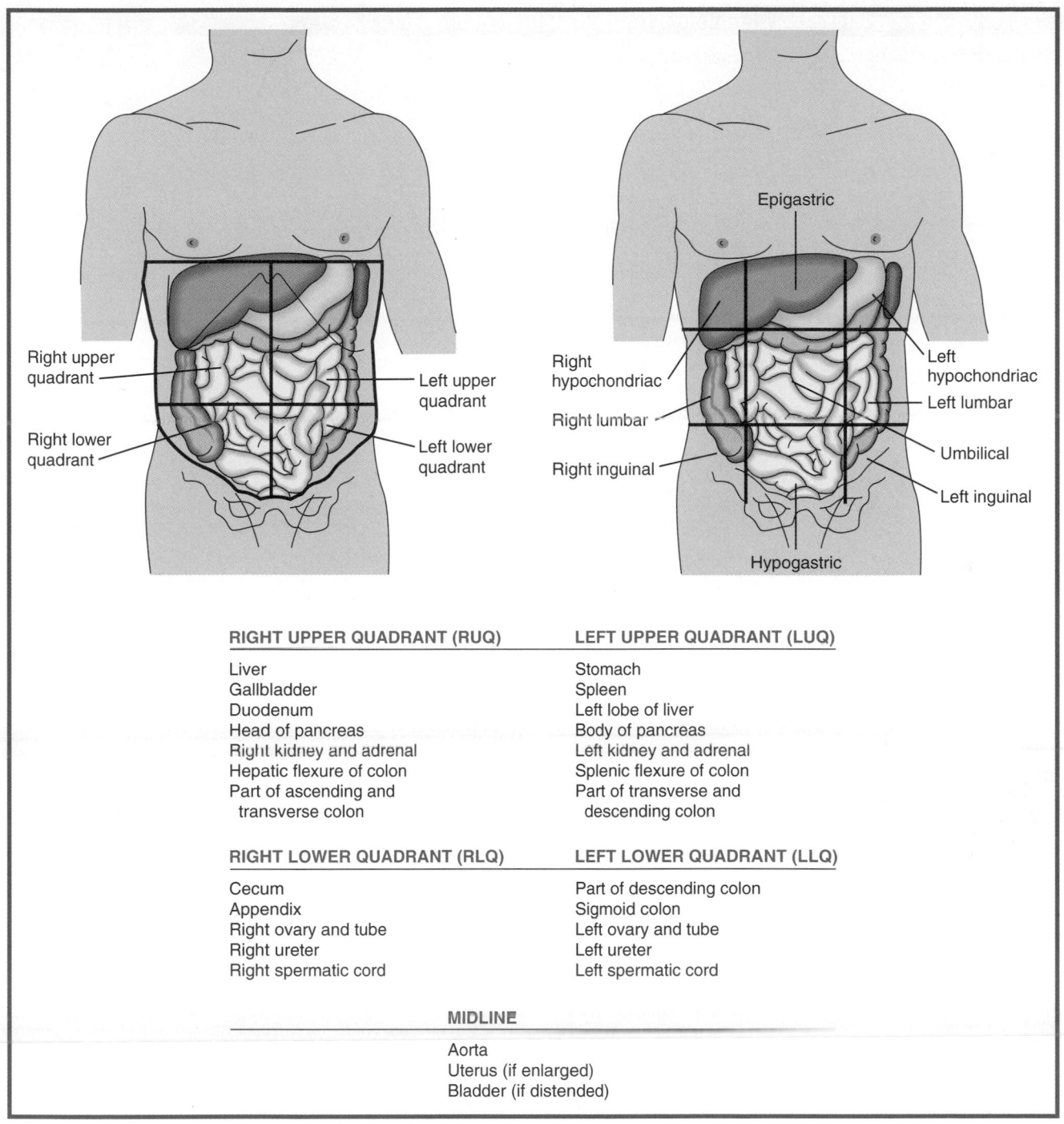

RIGHT UPPER QUADRANT (RUQ)

Liver
Gallbladder
Duodenum
Head of pancreas
Right kidney and adrenal
Hepatic flexure of colon
Part of ascending and
  transverse colon

LEFT UPPER QUADRANT (LUQ)

Stomach
Spleen
Left lobe of liver
Body of pancreas
Left kidney and adrenal
Splenic flexure of colon
Part of transverse and
  descending colon

RIGHT LOWER QUADRANT (RLQ)

Cecum
Appendix
Right ovary and tube
Right ureter
Right spermatic cord

LEFT LOWER QUADRANT (LLQ)

Part of descending colon
Sigmoid colon
Left ovary and tube
Left ureter
Left spermatic cord

MIDLINE

Aorta
Uterus (if enlarged)
Bladder (if distended)

FIGURE 36-2   Abdominal quadrants and regions and the organs located in each.

famotidine (Pepcid), cimetidine (Tagamet), or ranitidine (Zantac). The treatment may also include diet modification including avoidance of caffeine, cigarettes, and alcohol; eating six small meals a day; and weight loss. Surgical repair of a hiatal hernia is complicated and avoided if possible.

Gastric and Duodenal Ulcers. Peptic ulcers occur most frequently in the proximal duodenum (duodenal ulcer) but may also be found in the stomach (gastric ulcer). Both types are characterized by an area of break-down of mucosal membrane that leads to ulceration of the epithelial lining of the duodenum or stomach.

The first signs of a peptic ulcer may be iron-deficiency anemia or a positive stool for occult blood due to the erosion of blood vessels in the organ wall. Patients typically complain of intense pain in the area of the ulcer occurring about 2 hours after the ingestion of food and at night. Gastric ulcers may cause loss of weight, and duodenal lesions often produce nausea and vomiting. Some patients state that eating very small amounts relieves the

TABLE 36-1	Characteristics of Common Gastrointestinal Complaints
Gastrointestinal Complaint	**Characteristics**

Nausea
Vomiting (emesis)
	Patient exhibits pallor, **diaphoresis**, tachycardia
	Caused by:
	    Gastrointestinal irritation
	    Pain or stress
	    Inner ear disturbance
	    Increased intracranial pressure
	
	Important characteristics that should be reported and recorded:
	    Onset, frequency, duration of the problem
	    Yellow or greenish color indicates bile from the duodenum
	    Pyloric stenosis causes vomiting of undigested food
	    Projectile vomiting may indicate increased intracranial pressure
	    Hematemesis causes coffee-grounds vomitus

Diarrhea	Caused by:
	    Infections or inflammation
	    Food allergies
	    Malabsorption syndromes
	
	Important characteristics that should be reported and recorded:
	    Onset, frequency, duration of the problem
	    Dehydration may occur if diarrhea is persistent; occurs more frequently in infants and
	        older adults
	    Presence of blood, mucus, pus
	    Steatorrhea: greasy stools
	    Melena: tarry stools from higher digestive tract bleeding

Constipation	Caused by:
	    Lack of dietary fiber
	    Inadequate intake of fluids
	    Lack of exercise
	    Neurological disorders including spinal cord injuries and multiple sclerosis
	    Side effect of medications (codeine, iron, antacids)
	    Bowel obstructions or tumors
	
	Important characteristics that should be reported and recorded:
	    Onset, frequency, duration of the problem
	    Treatment with over-the-counter medications
	    Diet and fluid intake
	    Presence of watery diarrhea (may indicate fecal impaction)

Abdominal pain	Caused by:
	    Ulcerative diseases
	    Tumors
	    Appendicitis
	    Bowel obstruction
	    Food poisoning
	    Infections or inflammation
	
	Important characteristics that should be reported and recorded:
	    Onset, frequency, duration
	    Exact location (using either quadrants or abdominal regions)
	    Quality of the pain (burning, cramping, sharp, dull, etc.)
	    Degree of pain on a scale of 1 to 10

intensity of the pain. If the ulcerative area is bleeding internally, the patient may have *hematemesis* (blood in the vomitus) or *melena* (coffee-ground and/or tarry black stools). Gastric ulcers are usually found in middle-aged men, whereas duodenal ulcers are seen most frequently in patients who are 45 to 70 years old.

The description of the patient's pain gives the physician a clear suspicion of the disorder. The examination often shows that the patient is guarding the painful area; this is characterized by clutching of the upper abdominal area and keeping the knees drawn up toward the chest. A definitive diagnosis is based on an upper gastrointestinal series (x-ray evaluation) or endoscopy (visualization) of the upper gastrointestinal tract (Figure 36-4). A biopsy of the affected area may be taken during the endoscopy to rule out possible cancer. A sampling of the gastric contents may be collected to establish the level of acidity or presence of blood. A stool test may be ordered to check for the presence of occult blood. Blood tests will also be ordered to establish **hemoglobin** and **hematocrit** levels.

TABLE 36-2	Cancers of the Gastrointestinal Tract	
Tumor	**Characteristics**	**Cause or Contributing Factors**
Oral tumors	White mass in or on mouth that bleeds easily Ulcer or fissure that does not heal Mass is usually not painful	Cancer of the lip—pipe smoking Cancer of the tongue or gums—chewing tobacco
Esophageal cancer	Typically found in the distal esophagus Initial sign is *dysphagia* (difficulty swallowing)	Associated with chronic irritation due to chronic esophagitis, alcohol abuse, or smoking
Gastric cancer	Asymptomatic in early stages Usually not diagnosed until well advanced Prognosis is poor Anorexia, indigestion, weight loss, fatigue Positive occult blood in the stool	Food preservatives, chronic use of nitrates, smoked foods Genetic association Chronic gastritis
Liver cancer	Primary malignant tumors rare; usually a metastasized secondary tumor Initial symptoms mild; anorexia, vomiting, weight loss, fatigue, hepatomegaly, splenomegaly, **portal hypertension** Usually advanced when diagnosed	Primary tumor caused by cirrhosis from hepatitis or chemical exposure
Pancreatic cancer	Weight loss, jaundice Usually advanced when diagnosed Metastasis occurs early; no effective treatment	Cigarette smoking
Colorectal cancer	Usually develops from **polyps** in the colon Metastasis to the liver is common Initial signs depend on location of tumor; changes in character of stool, iron-deficiency anemia, fatigue, weight loss, frank bleeding, or melena	Genetic or familial link Diet high in fat, sugar, red meats, and low in fiber Usually occurs in patients over 55 years of age

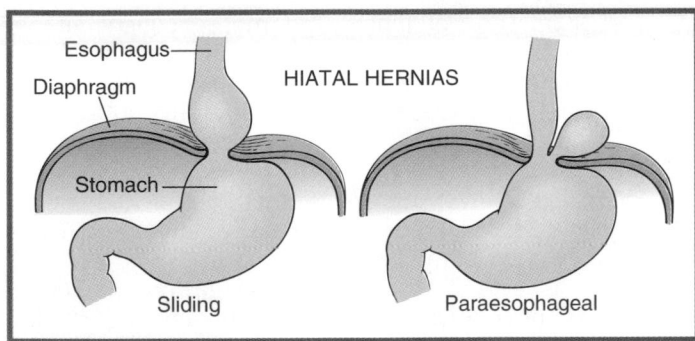

FIGURE 36-3 Hiatal hernias. (From Damjanov I: *Pathology for the health-related professions*, ed. 2, Philadelphia, 2000, WB Saunders.)

Peptic ulcers can appear under a variety of predisposing circumstances, including the use of alcohol, nonsteroidal antiinflammatory drugs (NSAIDs), as well as corticosteroids (Prednisone), severe or chronic stress, cigarette smoking, increased caffeine intake, and genetic predisposition. A major contributor is the presence of the bacterium *Helicobacter pylori (H. pylori)* in the stomach or duodenum of most patients with peptic ulcer disease. The diagnosis can be determined from a culture of gastric mucosa obtained by biopsy at the time of a gastroscopy; however, the *H. pylori* antibodies blood test is easier to obtain and more accurate. The test measures antibody titers and is considered the *gold standard* for detection of the bacteria as well as determining the success of treatment. Although the presence of the bacterium in the gastrointestinal tract does not always cause peptic ulcer disease, destruction of it with a combined treatment of antibiotics (such as clarithromycin [Biaxin] or azithromycin [Zithromax]) and a proton pump inhibitor (omeprazole [Prilosec] or famotidine [Pepcid]) results in rapid healing of the ulceration (Figure 36-5). In severe cases, such as perforation of the gastric wall, surgery may be indicated. Any nonhealing ulcer will be periodically reevaluated through gastroscopy to rule out cancer.

Pyloric Stenosis. *Pyloric stenosis*, which is the narrowing and hardening of the pyloric sphincter at the distal end of the stomach, can be caused by scar tissue from chronic conditions but is typically seen as a congenital defect in infants. The difficulty becomes apparent shortly after birth with projectile vomiting immediately after feeding because of the inability of the stomach to effectively empty. As a result, the baby displays symptoms of failure to thrive, becomes dehydrated, has small and infrequent stools, and is very irritable. Congenital pyloric stenosis typically occurs in first-born males and can be corrected by surgery.

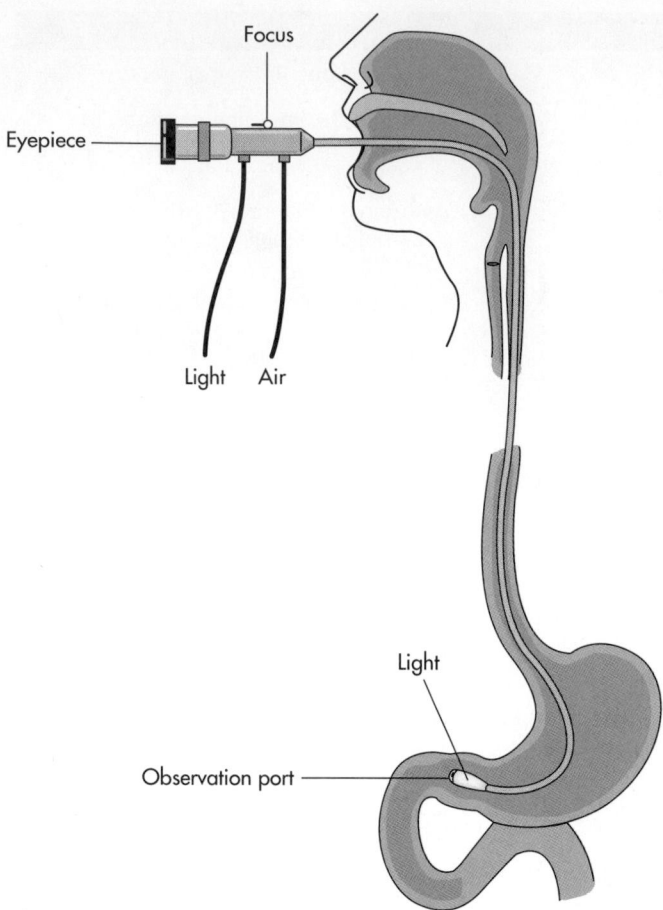

FIGURE 36-4 Fiberoptic endoscopy of the stomach. (From Phipps WJ, Sands JK, Marek JF, eds: *Medical-surgical nursing: concepts and clinical practice*, ed 6. Philadelphia, 1999, WB Saunders.)

Intestinal Disorders

Food Poisoning. Food poisoning is a disorder resulting from the ingestion of food that contains bacterial or toxic material. This includes poisoning from eating mushrooms, foods that contain poisonous insecticides, and foods that have been contaminated with bacteria or have partially decomposed. The disease is usually self-limiting and subsides within 48 hours of onset. Occasionally, it can be much more severe and even life threatening. The more severe cases are usually seen in young children and individuals in a weakened state of health. Food poisoning causes generalized *gastroenteritis*, with sudden and intense symptoms (Table 36-3).

A complete patient history is crucial in determining the diagnosis. Stool and blood cultures may be performed to verify the causative pathogen. If the patient has a remaining portion of the suspected ingested food, this will be sent to the laboratory for analysis. The physician may order an endoscopic examination of the gastrointestinal system in severe cases to determine the extent of the damage or the condition of the mucosal lining of the system.

The patient is stabilized and the symptoms are treated so dehydration is minimized and electrolyte balance is maintained. Antiemetics, such as prochlorperazine (Com-

pazine) and trimethobenzamide (Tigan) rectal suppositories, may be prescribed to control vomiting. Other medications, such as furoxone, loperamide (Imodium), or diphenoxylate/atropine (Lomotil) may be used to control diarrhea. If vomiting and diarrhea cannot be corrected within a reasonable time (determined by age, body size, and health condition), the patient may be hospitalized so that intravenous fluid replacement can be given.

Dumping Syndrome. One of the postsurgical complications of procedures for weight loss, such as gastric clamping with bypass or partial *gastrectomy*, is dumping syndrome. These procedures result in the passage of chyme into the small intestine before it has been completely digested. The result is intestinal distention and increased intestinal motility that can occur both during and immediately after meals. Signs and symptoms include nausea, abdominal cramps, diarrhea, vertigo, tachycardia, and diaphoresis. After surgery, patients should be instructed to eat frequent small meals that are high in protein and low in simple sugars as well as drink fluids between meals rather than with meals. These dietary modifications usually prevent the occurrence of dumping syndrome.

Irritable Bowel Syndrome. Irritable bowel syndrome (IBS) is described as a recurrent functional bowel disorder, because diagnostic studies fail to show an organic cause for the symptoms. The diagnosis of IBS is made if the patient complains of recurrent abdominal discomfort of at least 3 months; abdominal pain that is relieved by defecation; feeling bloated; change in bowel habits with constipation, diarrhea, and mucus discharge; and increased flatulence. The most frequent site of abdominal pain is the left lower quadrant (LLQ). Diagnostic studies, such as a CBC, stool for guaiac, urinalysis, barium enema, and colonoscopy, are performed to rule out other gastrointestinal diseases that have an organic base.

IBS is more common in women. Symptoms usually appear in late adolescence or early adulthood. There appears to be a familial pattern and may account for as much as 50% of the referrals to gastroenterologists because of concern about possible organic disease. IBS is quite common, with an estimated 9% to 20% of the adult population affected. The syndrome is associated with food intolerances, menstruation, and stress levels. Treatment is primarily pharmaceutical with bulk-forming agents (Metamucil); loperamide (Imodium) or diphenoxylate/atropine (Lomotil) for diarrhea episodes; Lactaid if the patient is lactose intolerant; antispasmodic agents (such as dicyclomine [Bentyl]) for cramping and anticholinergic agents (hyoscyamine [Levsin]); and simethicone (Mylicon) for bloating and flatulence. The patient should be encouraged to keep a food diary in an attempt to identify foods that exacerbate the symptoms; to increase fluid and fiber intake; and to avoid spicy, fatty foods as well as caffeine. Routine exercise can also be very helpful in relieving symptoms.

Patients with IBS can become very frustrated and need confirmation that this is a real problem, even though no organic or anatomical changes are apparent. Patients should be encouraged to follow lifestyle recommendations, including actively working to reduce stress. The

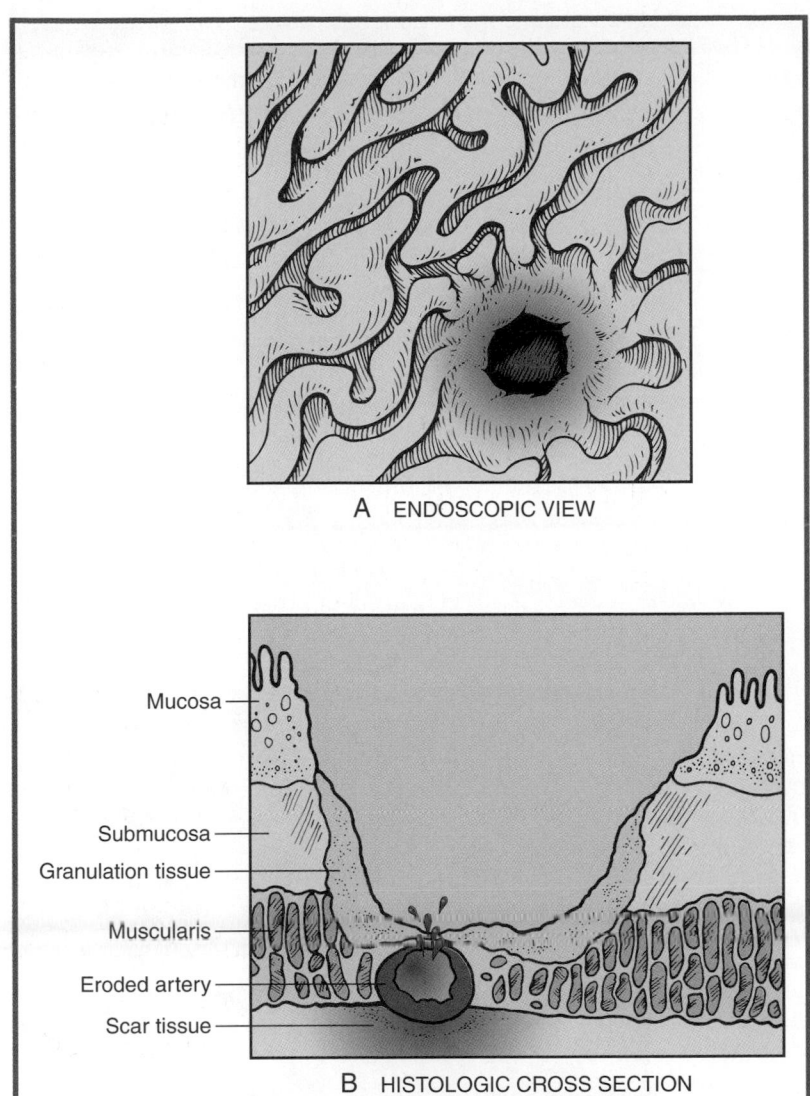

A   ENDOSCOPIC VIEW

FIGURE 36-5   **A** and **B**, Peptic ulcer.

Mucosa

Submucosa

Granulation tissue

Muscularis

Eroded artery

Scar tissue

B   HISTOLOGIC CROSS SECTION

medical assistant plays an important role in providing understanding and support to the patient.

CRITICAL THINKING APPLICATION

Dr. Sahani frequently sees patients with IBS. He asks Joan to prepare a handout for patients describing the disorder, including a description of possible treatments. What should Joan include?

Acute Appendicitis. The vermiform appendix is a narrow pouch about 3½ inches long that extends off of the cecum of the large intestine. It has no known function but can become inflamed and ultimately infected because of obstruction by a **fecalith** or by foreign material. As bacteria multiply, the appendix becomes inflamed and swollen, causing *ischemia* and *necrosis* of the appendix wall. If the infectious material leaks out or bursts from the appendix, a localized infection forms that may become regional if the abdominal peritoneum becomes

involved resulting in peritonitis. Peritonitis is a serious infection that may become life threatening.

Classic signs of appendicitis include right lower quadrant (RLQ) pain; nausea and vomiting; tenderness at McBurney's point, which is located between the umbilicus and the right anterior superior iliac spine; low-grade fever; and *leukocytosis* (increase in the WBC count). The infected appendix is surgically removed (*appendectomy*) and the patient is treated with broad-spectrum antibiotics.

Crohn's Disease. Crohn's disease, also called *regional ileitis* or *regional enteritis*, is an inflammation that may be located anywhere in the alimentary tract but is most common in the small intestine and the ascending colon. The inflammation begins with a localized area of ulcer development that presents as healthy tissue interspersed with areas of affected tissue. Inflammation results in the formation of ulcers that eventually invade deeper into the walls of the intestine, creating scar tissue and partial or complete obstruction at the affected site. If in the small intestine, the damaged wall decreases the ability of the intestine to digest and absorb nutrients and if in the colon, increased motility prevents reabsorption of

TABLE 36-3	Food-Related Gastrointestinal Disorders		
Microorganism	Cause	Incubation Period	Signs and Symptoms
Staphylococcus aureus	Improper hand washing by food handlers; insufficient refrigeration of salads or improper cooking of meats	1-7 hr	Low body temperature; hypotension; acute severe nausea, vomiting, cramps
Escherichia coli	Fecal contamination of food or water; improper cooking of meat or washing of fruits and vegetables	10-12 hr	Vomiting; abdominal cramps; watery diarrhea, may contain blood or mucus
Salmonella	Fecal contamination of food; contaminated work areas; undercooked or raw poultry, eggs, or shellfish	6-72 hr	Acute diarrhea; sometimes vomiting; abdominal cramping and pain; fever
Clostridium botulinum	Bacterial spores in improperly canned or prepared food	12-36 hr	Vomiting or diarrhea possible; neurological complications of vision problems, paralysis, respiratory failure

fluids. Scar tissue from the localized ulceration can ultimately lead to a bowel obstruction or the ulcer may completely invade the intestinal wall resulting in perforation and leakage of intestinal contents into the abdominal cavity. Adhesions may develop from chronic inflammation or fistulas may form between two loops of the intestine or between the intestine and adjacent organs.

Signs and symptoms of Crohn's disease include loose, semiformed stool; melena if the ulcers break through blood vessels; pain or tenderness in the right lower quadrant; anorexia; weight loss; anemia; and fatigue. Most patients cycle through periods of remission and relapse. The cause of the disease is unknown, and there is no cure. Diagnosis is made from a barium enema, and a colonoscopy with biopsy confirms the diagnosis. The goals of treatment are to decrease inflammation, manage symptoms, and provide nutritional support. Sulfasalazine (Azulfidine), which is a both an NSAID and an antibacterial drug, is commonly prescribed. Corticosteroids (such as Prednisone) are used during acute phases. Metronidazole (Flagyl) is an antibiotic prescribed for fistulas, and antidiarrheal agents (Imodium or Lomotil) may also be prescribed. Surgical intervention that involves resection of the diseased bowel, and **anastomosis** may be necessary if an intestinal obstruction occurs or there is fistula or abscess formation. Unfortunately, the disease usually recurs at the site of the anastomosis. The patient may require dietary supplements with a high-protein/high-calorie diet.

Ulcerative Colitis. Ulcerative colitis causes inflammation that usually starts in the rectum and moves proximally through the colon, affecting the lining in a continuous pattern. The disease causes ulcer formation that invades the mucosa and submucosa layers but does not advance through the entire wall of the colon (Figure 36-6). Ulcerative colitis can affect any age group, and although there is a familial tendency, the cause is unknown. The patient presents with complaints of abdominal pain, mucoid stools, and intermittent episodes of

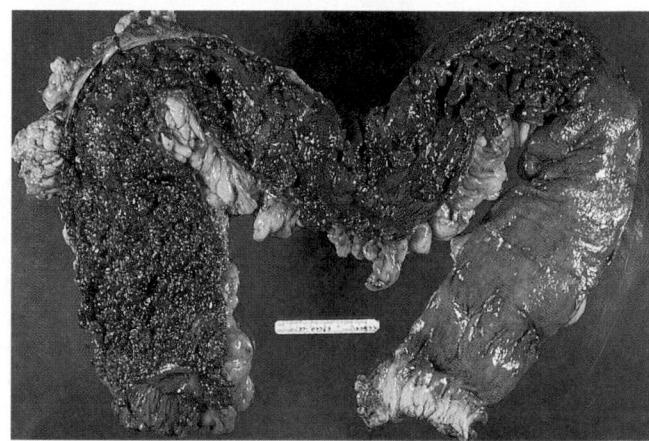

FIGURE 36-6   Ulcerative colitis. (From Damjanov I: *Pathology for the health-related professions*, ed. 2, Philadelphia, 2000, WB Saunders.)

bloody diarrhea. As the disease progresses, the patient may experience as many as 10 to 20 stools per day, with weight loss, fever, and general malaise.

Medical treatment is similar to that for Crohn's disease, but surgical removal of the colon with an **ileostomy** is considered curative for ulcerative colitis. Patients with ulcerative colitis must be screened annually with a colonoscopy since they have an increased risk of colon cancer.

Celiac Disease. Celiac disease is a malabsorption syndrome that is caused by a genetic defect in the intestinal enzyme that metabolizes gluten. Gluten is found in all grains, including any products made from wheat, barley, rye, or oats. If the affected individual eats a product that contains gluten, even a small amount, an antigen-antibody reaction occurs that causes destruction of the villi in the small intestine. The intestine is unable to absorb nutrients; therefore malnutrition occurs. The patient exhibits steatorrhea, abdominal pain, and weight loss. Celiac disease can be treated with strict adherence to a gluten-free diet and using rice with small amounts of corn as replacements for such grains as wheat, rye, barley, and oats.

Diverticular Disease. *Diverticula* are outpouchings or herniations of the muscular lining of the colon, usually the sigmoid colon. Diverticula develop because of chronic constipation and muscular hypertrophy in the colon. *Diverticulosis* is asymptomatic diverticular disease in which multiple diverticula are present in the colon but the patient has no complaints other than mild discomfort, diarrhea, constipation, or flatulence. However, if the herniations become blocked with feces and inflammation develops, *diverticulitis* occurs. Patient signs and symptoms include lower left quadrant (LLQ) cramping, tenderness, or pain; nausea and vomiting; low-grade fever; and leukocytosis. A barium enema or colonoscopy may be done to confirm the presence of diverticula.

Patients with diverticulosis are encouraged to eat a diet that is high in roughage, drink plenty of fluids, and avoid foods with kernels or seeds. The goals are to prevent collection of waste in the herniations and encourage regular, soft bowel movements. If the sites become inflamed, antibiotics are prescribed to treat the infection. Surgery may be necessary if perforation occurs.

Hernias of the Abdomen. Hernias can develop in various parts of the body but most frequently are seen in the abdomen as an organ or part of an organ protrudes through a weakened area in the abdominal muscle wall. The causes of herniation include congenital weakness of the structures, trauma, relaxation of ligaments and skeletal muscles, and increased upward pressure from the abdomen. They are most often found in middle-aged or older persons. The location of the hernia establishes the term by which the protrusion is identified. The types of hernias include umbilical; incisional at the site of a previous surgery; and inguinal hernia, which is a loop of the bowel that protrudes into the inguinal canal of the male (Figure 36-7).

The usual sign of an abdominal hernia is an abnormal lump or bulge that the patient finds while bathing. This bulge is tender, but the pain is mild. The patient may also discover that the bulge can be pushed back into the abdomen, and it will stay that way until there is some type of moving activity, and then it reappears. If there is severe pain, the hernia may be trapped or strangulated if blood flow has been compromised. If immediate medical intervention is not performed, the tissue may die and **gangrene** may set in.

The physician uses palpation to assess an abdominal or inguinal hernia for size and inspect the area with the patient standing and lying down. An inguinal hernia can be detected in a male by having him perform a **Valsalva's maneuver.** The most frequent treatment is surgical repair in the form of a *herniorrhaphy* or hernioplasty. If the person is in poor health, the physician may have the patient fitted with a device called a **truss.**

Hemorrhoids. Hemorrhoids are varicose veins of the anus and rectum and affect about 5% of all adults. There is a familial, hereditary predisposition to the disorder, and it is common in persons with varicose veins of the lower extremities and inguinal hernias. Hemorrhoid formation is related to increased pressure in the rectum often caused by constipation. If the swollen veins are within the rectal wall, they are considered to be internal hemorrhoids; and if they are firm, protruding, and can be felt and/or seen, they are external.

Some patients experience no pain, whereas other patients experience definite rectal pain. Frequently, the patient reports that anal itching and burning discomfort occur immediately after a bowel movement. If the patient must strain to defecate, bleeding and a protrusion of the swollen mass can occur. Often patients will state that it is necessary to bathe the anal area with warm water or even soak in warm water after every bowel movement to relieve the itching and pain.

A proctological examination and inspection of the anal area will reveal external hemorrhoids. Proctoscopy is performed to visualize internal hemorrhoids of the rectum. A hemoglobin level and red blood cell count may be ordered to determine whether there has been any significant blood loss. Hemorrhoids are treated with stool softeners, such as docusate sodium (Colace); a high-fiber diet; and an analgesic ointment applied locally or by suppository to relieve swelling. If these measures do not correct the problem, the next step may be **sclerotherapy** injections, **cryosurgery,** or **ligation.**

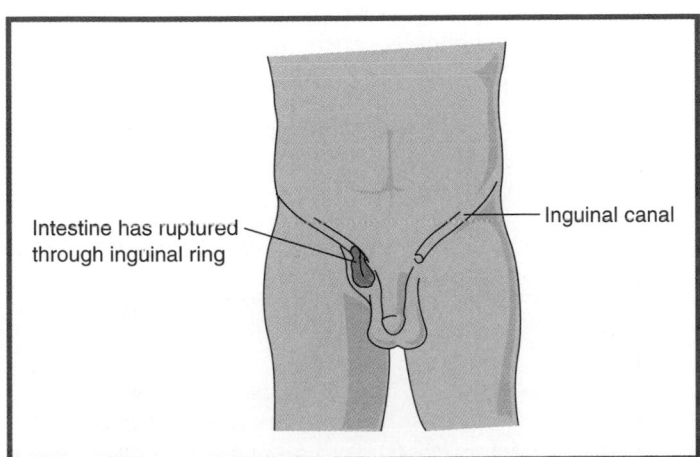

Intestine has ruptured through inguinal ring

Inguinal canal

FIGURE 36-7   Herniated inguinal canal.

Diseases of the Liver and Gallbladder

Hepatitis

The liver is located in the right upper quadrant (RUQ) of the abdomen and its primary functions are to metabolize nutrients and detoxify drugs or other harmful substances. Inflammation of the liver, or hepatitis, may be caused by a localized infection (viral hepatitis), a systemic infection, exposure from chemicals, or a complication of drug metabolism. Mild inflammation temporarily impairs function, but severe inflammation may lead to necrosis and serious complications.

One of the most serious complications of liver inflammation is *cirrhosis*. Cirrhosis is a chronic liver disease in which the lobes of the liver become fibrous and hard and the liver cells degenerate, causing deterioration in liver function. It results in portal hypertension and is an irreversible disease with the only cure a liver transplant. The disease can be a complication of severe viral hepatitis but may also be caused by chronic alcoholism and substance abuse. It is the fourth most common cause of death in men between the ages of 40 and 60. In approximately 30% of cirrhosis cases, the cause cannot be positively established (Figure 36-8).

Viral Hepatitis. Acute viral hepatitis is an infection of the liver that causes an acute inflammatory process of the hepatocytes. There are several forms of this virus, known as hepatitis A, B, C, D, E, and G. Hepatic cells are capable of regeneration; therefore, depending on the degree of liver involvement, the patient may recover completely or develop widespread necrosis, cirrhosis, and liver failure. Chronic inflammation, defined as the presence of the disease for more than 6 months, can occur with hepatitis B, C, and D. This usually results in permanent liver damage and an associated increased risk for liver cancer. Individuals infected with these forms of hepatitis may also become carriers of the disease. Hepatitis carriers are asymptomatic but can transmit the virus to others.

Table 36-4 describes the overall characteristics of the types of hepatitis. Hepatitis A (HAV) is transmitted through contaminated water or shellfish. Some parts of the world are **endemic** for the disease and a vaccine is available. Hepatitis B (HBV) has a relatively long incubation period that makes it more difficult to track the source of the

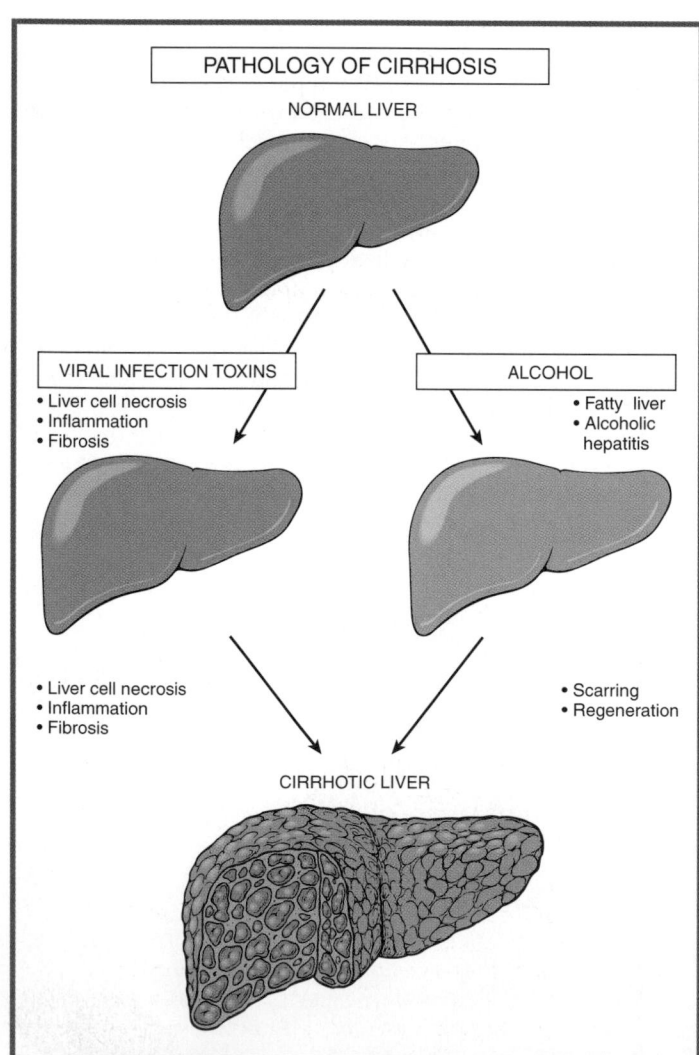

FIGURE 36-8 Pathology of cirrhosis. (From Damjanov I: *Pathology for the health-related professions*, ed. 2, Philadelphia, 2000, WB Saunders.)

TABLE 36-4	Characteristics of Viral Hepatitis Types		
Hepatitis Type	**Mode of Transmission**	**Incubation Period**	**Symptoms**
A (infectious hepatitis)	Fecal-oral	2-6 weeks	Fatigue, weakness, anorexia. Some patients have joint pain, fever, **hepatomegaly**, **lymphadenopathy**, **jaundice**.
B (serum hepatitis)	Blood and body fluids	1-6 months	General malaise, joint swelling, pruritic rash, hepatomegaly, anorexia, nausea, vomiting, dark yellowish-brown urine, jaundice.
C (non-A non-B)	Blood and body fluids; leading cause of posttransfusion hepatitis	2 weeks-6 months	Acute onset of fever, chills, malaise, nausea, vomiting.
D (delta virus)	Blood and body fluids; occurs only in conjunction with hepatitis B	Seen only in patients with hepatitis B	Similar to HBV; increases the severity of HBV disease.
E	Fecal-oral	2-9 weeks	Symptoms similar to hepatitis A; seen in India, Asia, Africa, Central America. Mild form but can cause death in pregnant women.
G	Percutaneous sticks from contaminated needles	Not known	Not defined.

infection. Because the virus is found in all blood and body fluids, it can be transmitted in many ways including needlesticks, human bites from individuals infected with the virus, sexual, and fetal transmission. Immunization of persons who are at increased risk is highly recommended. All healthcare personnel are included in this group, because they are at increased risk of infection through exposure to blood or blood products and body fluids. HBV immunizations are also included as part of pediatric immunizations, which will be discussed in Chapter 39.

As a healthcare professional, a medical assistant cares for sick people on a daily basis who may be carriers of the hepatitis virus. Inhaling droplets released by a cough, holding a patient's hand that was just used to cover the mouth, and discarding a wet baby diaper are all possible ways that exposure can occur. The first line of defense, whether the medical assistant is immunized or not, is employing frequent hand washing and wearing gloves when the possibility of exposure to blood or body fluids exists.

Diagnosis and Treatment. Hepatitis A, B, and C are diagnosed by identifying the virus or the antibodies to the virus in the blood. Another diagnostic test that is very useful is a liver biopsy for tissue examination. Liver function tests are done periodically throughout the course of the disease to determine the degree of liver damage. Patients with hepatitis B, C, and D must be monitored for possible chronic hepatitis and the formation of a carrier state. If patients develop chronic hepatitis or become carriers, *interferon* may be prescribed to control hepatic cell destruction. Otherwise, the treatment for all forms of hepatitis generally consists of bed rest and a high-protein diet.

The best form of treatment for hepatitis B is prevention by being vaccinated against the disease. The vaccine is given in three doses. The first two are given 30 days apart, and the third is given 6 months after the first. As discussed in Chapter 24, OSHA requires healthcare employers to make the vaccine available to employees free of charge. Medical assistant programs encourage students to become vaccinated, because they are also at risk of contracting the disease.

GROUPS AT RISK FOR HEPATITIS A, B, AND C

Hepatitis A: Day care workers and clients, institutionalized residents, individuals traveling to infected areas
Hepatitis B: IV drug users, homosexual men, hemodialysis patients, hemophiliacs, healthcare personnel, those with a history of frequent sexual partners
Hepatitis C: Patients receiving frequent blood transfusions, homosexual men, IV drug users, hospital personnel

CRITICAL THINKING APPLICATION

As a healthcare worker who is constantly exposed to blood and body fluids, Joan is quite concerned about contracting viral hepatitis. What types of hepatitis is she at risk for in Dr. Sahani's office? What can she do to reduce her risk and safeguard herself from contracting these diseases?

Cholelithiasis (Gallstones)

The gallbladder is an accessory organ of the gastrointestinal system that stores the bile excreted by the liver. Cholelithiasis, or gallstones, form in the gallbladder from insoluble cholesterol and bile salt and vary in size and number. The reasons for formation are not always clear, although occurrence is more frequent with a high-calorie, high-cholesterol diet and is associated with obesity (Figure 36-9). It is estimated that 20% of people older than age 65 years develop cholelithiasis, with women three times more at risk than men.

Signs and Symptoms. Most gallstones are asymptomatic and are incidentally discovered during a routine radiograph. Pain usually occurs when the stones move and obstruct the biliary duct. The pain is in the epigastric region and right upper quadrant, often radiating into the right upper back area. Nausea and vomiting may accompany the pain. The pain hits in a wavelike pattern and is called *colicky pain* or *biliary colic*. If the obstruction is not corrected, jaundice may appear.

Diagnosis and Treatment. The physician will base the preliminary diagnosis on the signs and symptoms noted on palpation of the upper right quadrant. To confirm the diagnosis, blood tests may be used to determine signs of infection, obstruction, pancreatitis, or jaundice, and an abdominal sonogram is used to determine the presence of cholelithiasis. A computed tomography (CT) scan may show gallstones and a magnetic resonance (MR) cholangiogram may be ordered to diagnose blocked bile ducts. In addition, a cholescintigraphy (HIDA scan) can be ordered to diagnose biliary tract obstruction. The patient is given an intravenous injection of radioactive material called hydroxy iminodiacetic acid (HIDA) that is taken up by the liver and excreted into the biliary tract. A nuclear scanner then takes pictures of the biliary tract over a 2-hour period.

Treatment is surgical removal of the gallbladder (*cholecystectomy*), which is usually done by laparoscopy. Cholelithiasis may also be fragmented by **lithotripsy** procedures.

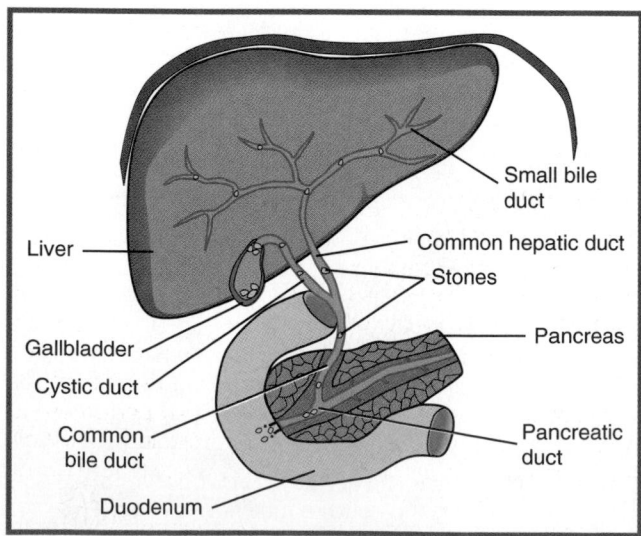

FIGURE 36-9 Gallstones.

Labels: Liver · Small bile duct · Common hepatic duct · Stones · Gallbladder · Cystic duct · Pancreas · Common bile duct · Pancreatic duct · Duodenum

The Medical Assistant's Role in the Gastrointestinal Examination

Emotional factors play an important part in many gastrointestinal problems, often making the separation of functional disorders and organic disorders difficult. Some forms of gastrointestinal disease may demand immediate attention, as in acute appendicitis or acute gastritis with possible hemorrhage. Both may require surgical therapy. Careful questioning is needed to guide the patient to a more precise description of the symptoms. The medical assistant's role as the liaison between the patient and the physician may strongly help the physician in making the diagnosis and getting the patient the treatment needed.

General abdominal discomfort (colic) is common, because abdominal pain is frequently referred pain (Figure 36-10), that is, pain that is felt in the abdomen but is actually being generated from an organ elsewhere. The pain's location may not be directly over the involved organ or over the point of the disorder. The reason for this is that the human brain has no way of determining the felt image for internal organs. However hard to imagine, the pain is referred to a site where the organ was located in fetal development. Even though the organ moves during fetal development, its nerves persist in referring sensations from its primitive or primary location.

The physician may order instillation of rectal suppositories to treat either localized inflammation or constipation or because of a systemic problem, such as vomiting. (Rectal administration of medications is discussed in Chapter 32.) Procedure 36-1 details administration of rectal suppositories.

Assisting With the Examination

When a patient describes and points to the location of the pain being felt, it is important to know the topography of the abdomen and the underlying organs. Record the quadrant or region in which the pain is located so the physician can immediately assess this area when the examination begins. The inspection of the abdomen begins with noting any change in skin color, such as jaundice. *Striae* (silver stretch marks), *petechiae* (small purple hemorrhagic spots), cutaneous *angiomas*, scars, and visible masses may be observed. The contour of the abdomen may be flat, rounded, or bulging in localized areas. A bulging in the right and left lumbar regions (the flanks) may be the result of the presence of free abdominal fluid *(ascites)*.

The physician will use palpation and percussion to evaluate the entire abdominal area. As this is done, the medical assistant should remove the drape from the area to be examined and redrape the patient once the physician has completed the examination segment. In addition, the physician may want notations made of findings as the examination is being done. When the physician wants to examine the anal area, have the patient turn onto his or her left side and assist the patient into the Sims' position. As this is done, be sure the patient remains draped or covered. After the position is achieved, adjust

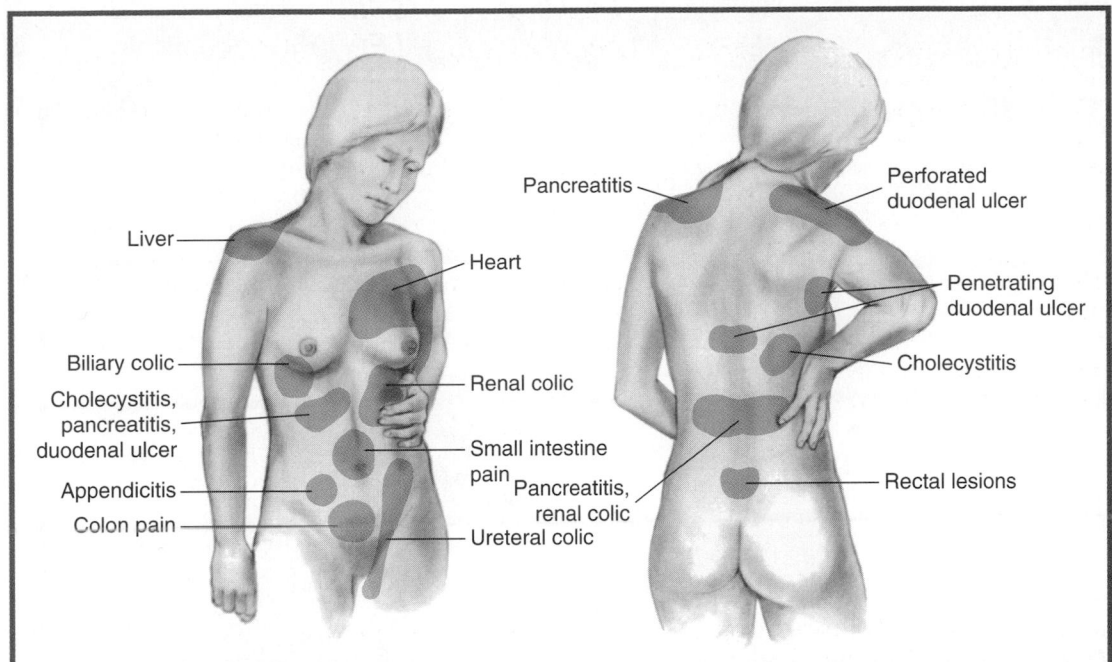

FIGURE 36-10
Common site of referred abdominal pain. (From Jarvis C: *Physical examination and health assessment*, ed. 3, Philadelphia, 2000, WB Saunders.)

the drape so that it can be easily lifted for the final part of the examination.

CRITICAL THINKING APPLICATION

Joan is responsible for initially questioning patients about complaints and clearly documenting this information on the patient chart. What information should Joan include that details each patient's problem and would be helpful in determining the patient's diagnosis?

Diagnostic Procedures

Typical diagnostic procedures for the gastrointestinal system are summarized in Table 36-5. Although the majority of these procedures are not performed in the ambulatory care setting, the medical assistant must still understand the procedure and the recommended patient preparation so adequate patient education can be conducted. If the patient does not adequately prepare for these procedures, the results will be inconclusive and an expensive, time-consuming, uncomfortable test may have to be rescheduled. It is very important that patients completely understand what is required and a handout be given for review at home to confirm verbal instructions given in the office. Physicians may vary in their preference for patient preparation for gastrointestinal diagnostic tests. It is important that the medical assistant refer to the office procedure manual or ask the physician his or her individual preference before conducting patient education.

The unequivocal test for the organs of the entire gastrointestinal system is an endoscopic analysis. The upper gastrointestinal system is examined by passing a soft, flexible tube down the esophagus into the stomach. The colon is examined through an ascending technique, with entrance through the anus. This fiberoptic technology allows the examiner to obtain photographs, filming, and laboratory samples, such as tissue biopsy samples, gastric fluid, pathogens, bile crystals, and cytology samples, during the procedure with only minor discomfort to the patient.

Endoscopic procedures can be used to observe the functioning gallbladder, biliary ducts, and the pancreatic ducts by injecting a dye directly into the vessel ducts of the gallbladder and the pancreas. The examination can then render definitive results regarding patency and function of the organs.

Sigmoidoscopy and Colonoscopy Examinations. Sigmoidoscopy is used to diagnose hemorrhoids, polyps, and diverticular disorders. The sigmoidoscope is a flexible fiberoptic instrument that allows the physician to complete this examination with very little discomfort to the patient. The entire examination can be done with the patient in the Sims' position, which is less traumatic for the patient to maintain than the proctological position. This scope is very thin and bendable so that it can be maneuvered around the curves of the sigmoid colon (Figure 36-11). Because the flexible sigmoidoscope is easier to insert and move, the entire sigmoid colon can be examined (Procedure 36-2). This procedure can be performed in an ambulatory care setting. To examine the entire length of the large intestine, the colonoscope is used. The American Cancer Society recommends that all patients over the age of 50 have a colonoscopy performed for screening of colorectal cancer. This procedure is usually performed in a hospital outpatient area since it requires the use of an IV sedative.

Laboratory Tests. Many of the diagnostic tests for gastrointestinal symptoms are noninvasive. The patient

PROCEDURE 36-1

Inserting a Rectal Suppository

GOAL: To insert the prescribed medication accurately into the rectal mucosa.

EQUIPMENT AND SUPPLIES

- Prescribed suppository medication
- Water-soluble lubricant
- Disposable tissues
- Biohazard waste container
- Disposable gloves

PROCEDURAL STEPS

1 Wash your hands, read the order, and obtain the necessary supplies.

2 Identify the patient and explain the procedure.
   Purpose: Proper identification saves time and avoids possible errors.

3 Ask the patient to remove clothing covering the anal area.

4 Assist the patient into a Sims' position and drape the exposed area (Figure 1).

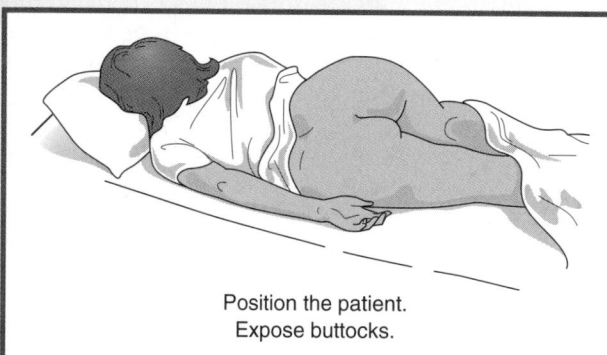

Position the patient.
Expose buttocks.

Figure 1

5 Don gloves.
   Purpose: Infection control.

6 Remove the covering from the suppository and smooth any rough edges on the suppository.
   Purpose: Eliminates any possible trauma to the rectal mucosa.

7 Generously lubricate the suppository with a water-soluble lubricant.
   Purpose: Promotes ease of insertion.

8 With your free hand, gently lift the uppermost buttock (Figure 2).

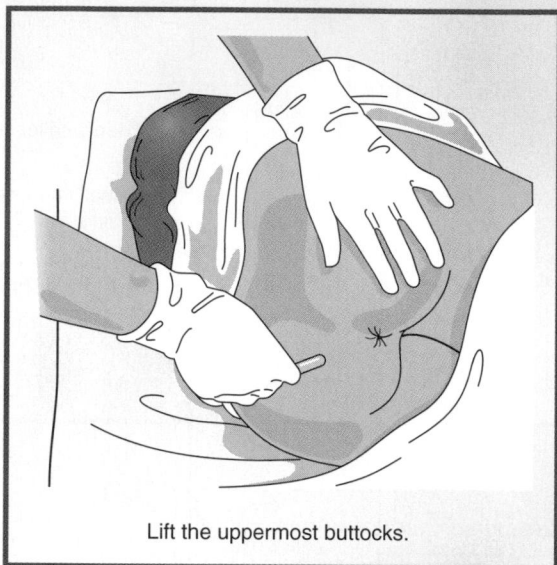

Lift the uppermost buttocks.

Figure 2

9 With your index finger, guide the suppository into the anus, directing it along the rectal wall and away from any fecal masses (Figure 3).

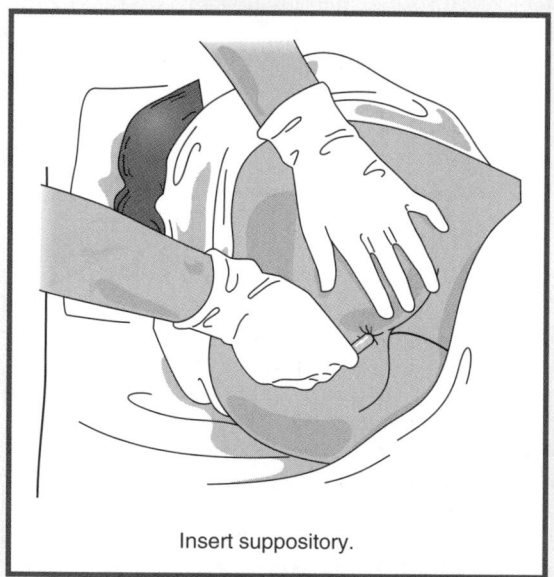

Insert suppository.

Figure 3

PROCEDURE 36-1—Cont'd

10 To prevent immediate expulsion, be sure to insert the suppository beyond the internal sphincter.

11 Use tissue to gently press on the anus for a few minutes to help the patient retain the rectal medication. Then, with the same tissue, wipe any excess lubricant from the rectal area. Dispose of used tissue in a biohazard waste container.

12 Allow the patient to rest for 20 to 30 minutes before he or she gets up and leaves the office.
Purpose: Medication retention.

13 Clean up the area, remove gloves, and wash your hands.
Purpose: Infection control.

14 Record the procedure and any pertinent information on the patient's record.
Purpose: Procedures that are not recorded are considered not done.

TABLE 36-5	Common Diagnostic Procedures for the Gastrointestinal System	
Test	**Description and Purpose**	**Patient Preparation**
Barium swallow	X-ray or fluoroscopic examination of the pharynx and esophagus after swallowing barium sulfate; to diagnose hiatal hernia, esophageal varices, strictures, or tumors.	NPO after midnight; remove all metal objects; do not take medication for GERD.
Upper gastrointestinal and small bowel series	X-ray and fluoroscopic examination of esophagus, stomach, and small intestine after swallowing barium sulfate; to diagnose ulcers, tumors, regional enteritis, and malabsorption syndrome.	Low-fiber diet 2-3 days before, NPO after midnight, no smoking before test. No medications unless approved by physician after midnight. Remove all metal objects. Stool will be chalky and lightly colored 24-72 hr after the test.
Barium enema	X-ray evaluation of large intestine after rectal instillation of barium sulfate; to diagnose colorectal cancer; inflammatory disease of the colon; detect polyps, diverticula, or obstructions.	No dairy products and liquid diet 24 hr before test. Take bowel preparation as supplied by radiology department; enemas until clear. No breakfast; mild laxative or enema after procedure to remove barium. Lightly colored stool for 24-72 hr after test.
Cholescintigraphy (HIDA scan)	Nuclear scan following IV injection of radioactive material. Pictures are taken over a 2-hour period of the biliary tract to determine presence of obstruction from cholelithiasis.	Patient must be NPO 3-4 hours before the test.
Sigmoidoscopy	Endoscopic examination of distal sigmoid colon, rectum, and anal canal. Used to diagnose inflammatory, infectious, and ulcerative bowel disease; tumors; detect hemorrhoids, polyps, fissures, fistulas, abscesses in the rectum and anal canal. Biopsy specimen may be collected.	Clear liquid diet for 48 hr before the test; NPO morning of procedure; bowel preparation with enemas.
Colonoscopy	Endoscopic examination of the large intestine. Detect or monitor inflammatory or ulcerative diseases; locate site of gastrointestinal bleeding; diagnose tumors or strictures.	Clear liquid diet for 48 hr before the test; laxatives; enemas until clear. Large intestine must be completely cleansed. Monitor vital signs before and during procedure.

may be asked to have various radiographs taken of the digestive system which are summarized in Table 36-5. The urine is tested for bilirubin and urinary amylase levels. The stool is tested for occult blood, intestinal ova and parasites, fat excretion, and color.

Occult Blood Screening. Fecal examination is one means of evaluating patients with gastrointestinal bleed-ing, obstruction, parasites, dysentery, colitis, or increased fat excretion. The test for ova and parasites is described in Chapter 52. The American Cancer Society recommends that all patients older than 50 years of age be screened for occult blood. This test, described in Chapter 49, may be performed on younger patients if a familial history indicates a need. Blood is not found in the stool of healthy individuals. If the person is experiencing bleeding of the intestinal wall, the blood is likely to be occult or hidden, which means it cannot be seen with the naked eye.

The physician may collect a random sample during a routine examination, but if it is suspected that the patient has gastrointestinal bleeding, the recommendation is to test three different samples for the presence of occult blood. Patient preparation for this test is a high-fiber diet, with avoidance of red meats, poultry, fish, turnips, and horseradish for 48 to 72 hours before the test as well as throughout the time it takes the patient to collect the ordered fecal samples. The patient is told to stop taking any iron supplements and certain medications, including anticoagulants, steroids, vitamin C, and aspirin products, 48 hours before the test and also during it. If these medications are continued during the testing period, that should be noted on the patient's laboratory slip. Failure to adhere to dietary guidelines or the use of identified medications can cause false-positive test results.

CRITICAL THINKING APPLICATION

Dr. Sahani wants to update patient handouts on the preparations necessary for common gastrointestinal tract diagnostic procedures. He asks Joan to do the initial research and gather pertinent information that should be included. What should Joan include regarding patient preparation for these examinations?

Proctological Examination

Proctology is the branch of internal medicine concerned with the diseases and disorders of the colon, rectum, and anus. The examination of the anal area is done with a 3-inch anoscope or a proctoscope that permits the detection of hemorrhoids, **polyps, fissures, fistulas,** and abscesses. The rectum and the sigmoid colon are examined with a flexible sigmoidoscope, and the descending, transverse, and ascending colon sections (or the entire colon) are examined with a colonoscope.

Many persons are apprehensive about colorectal examinations. To alleviate his or her anxiety, the patient needs to be instructed in exactly what to do before the examination, with reinforcement during the procedure. Let the patient know that some discomfort such as cramping can be experienced. Furthermore, the sensations of expelling **flatus** or of an impending bowel movement may be felt. These sensations are caused by the instrument and the procedure.

Depending on the type and purpose of the colorectal procedure and the physician's preference, the patient may be required to prepare the colon for the examination. Specific patient preparations for common digestive system diagnostic tests are summarized in Table 36-5. A medical assistant must always check the office procedure manual to determine the preferred method of patient preparation for each test since physician orders may vary.

Patient Positioning on a Proctological Table. Positioning for a proctological examination requires an examining table that can be elevated and tilted in the center and lowered at the head and legs. The patient's head and legs are at an angle lower than the buttocks with the patient's body flexed at the hip joint and not at the waist (Figure 36-12). If this flexion is not correct, the patient will experience considerable discomfort, and the bowel will not be displaced forward. A single sheet is draped in and around the anal area. Do not bind the patient's legs together with the drape, because it may be necessary to separate the legs during the examination. This position is often used for a sigmoidoscopic examination, because it straightens the rectosigmoidal area and displaces the lower bowel. It is a convenient position for examining the perineal area, the anus, and hemorrhoids. If the proctologist uses a flexible scope, the patient will be placed in the Sims' position for the procedure.

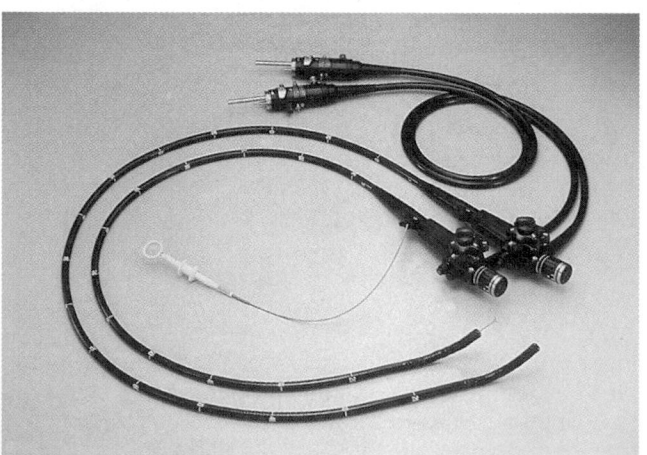

FIGURE 36-11   Flexible colon fiberscopes. (From Phipps WJ, Sands JK, Marek JF, eds: *Medical-surgical nursing: concepts and clinical practice,* ed 6. Philadelphia, 1999, WB Saunders.)

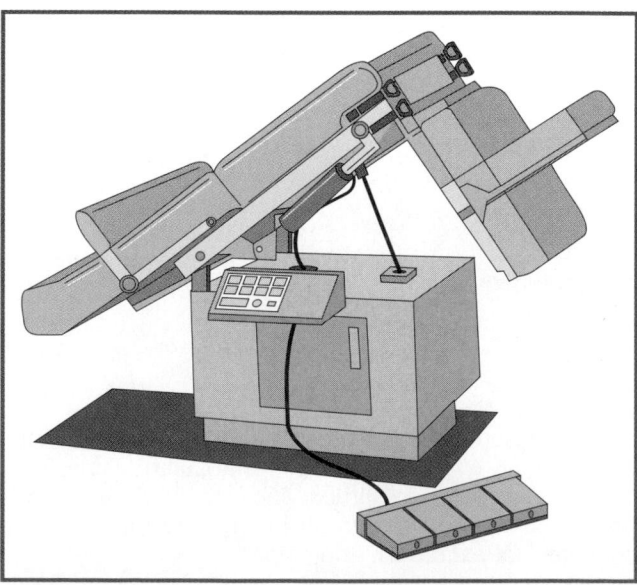

FIGURE 36-12   Proctological examination table.

PROCEDURE 36-2

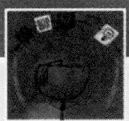

Assisting With a Colon Endoscopic Examination

GOAL: To assist the physician with the examination, to prepare collected specimens as requested, and to promote patient comfort and safety.

EQUIPMENT AND SUPPLIES

- Nonsterile gloves (for medical assistant and physician)
- Appropriate instrument: sigmoidoscope, anoscope, or proctoscope
- Water-soluble lubricant
- Drape and patient gown
- Long cotton-tipped swabs
- Suction source
- Sterile biopsy forceps
- Rectal speculum
- Specimen containers with appropriate preservative added
- Laboratory requisition form
- Tissue wipes
- Biohazard container

PROCEDURAL STEPS

1 Wash your hands and assemble all needed equipment and supplies.
   Purpose: Infection control.

2 Identify the patient and explain the procedure. Be sure the patient completed the proper preparation procedures.

3 Ask the patient to empty his or her bladder.
   Purpose: Aids in patient comfort during the examination.

4 Give the patient an examination gown and instruct him or her to remove all clothing below the waist and put on the gown with the opening to the back. Provide a drape for additional privacy.

5 Obtain and record the patient's vital signs.
   Purpose: Baseline vital signs allow detection of variations that might occur during the examination.

6 Assist the patient onto the table. When the physician is ready, place the patient in the appropriate position for the type of examination ordered.

7 Drape the patient so that only the anus is exposed. A fenestrated drape (drape with a circular opening placed over the anus) may be used in place of the rectangular drape.

8 Don gloves and assist the physician as requested during the examination. This includes the following:

- Lubricating the physician's gloved index finger for the digital examination
- Lubricating the obturator tip of the instrument before insertion
- Plugging in the scope's light source when the physician is ready
- Handing the needed supplies to the physician
- Collecting specimens by holding the container to accept the sample
- Labeling specimens immediately because several specimens may be taken from different areas
- Disposing of contaminated supplies as you are given them by the physician

9 Throughout the examination, observe the patient for any undue reactions. Encourage the patient to breathe slowly through pursed lips to facilitate relaxation.

10 On completion of the examination, cleanse the patient's anal area with tissue wipes. Remove gloves, wash hands, and assist the patient into a resting position; allow the patient time to recover from the procedure. Monitor the patient's blood pressure if indicated.
   Purpose: A drop in blood pressure often occurs after an invasive procedure, and this may cause fainting.

11 Once the patient is stabilized, assist the patient off the table and instruct him or her to get dressed. Show the patient where the sink, towels, and tissues are and provide assistance if needed.

12 Complete all laboratory request forms and specimen-container labels and place specimens in the appropriate location for laboratory pick-up.

13 Apply gloves and clean the work area and all equipment used. The endoscope is first sanitized and then sterilized according to the manufacturer's recommendations. Dispose of gloves in biohazard waste container and wash your hands.
   Purpose: Infection control.

14 Record the procedure and any pertinent information on the patient's record.
   Purpose: Procedures that are not recorded are considered not done.

Patient Education

The gastrointestinal system is responsible for the nourishment of the entire body. When disease interferes with this process, the entire body may become disabled and illness can lead to marked pathological disorders. Listen for a patient's concerns that may indicate a possible problem within this system and its accessory organs. Report these concerns to the physician or note them on the patient's medical record for the physician to read. If the office has information that may assist the patient in dealing with a particular problem, lay out the information for the physician to give to the patient; or with the physician's authorization, talk to the patient and offer suggestions that might help in dealing with a particular concern. Learning to perform and assist with diagnostic procedures can aid the physician in the diagnostic sequence and assist the patient in maintaining a healthy gastrointestinal system, which in turn assists the entire body in homeostasis.

Legal and Ethical Issues

Legally and ethically, the medical assistant's responsibility is to assist the physician and act as the patient's advocate. All information that is discussed between the patient and the physician as well as all testing procedures ordered and done must remain confidential. Confidentiality and trust are very closely linked, and these two issues form the basis for a sound patient-physician relationship. The medical assistant is an important part of that relationship and can strengthen it by practicing ethical professional conduct.

SUMMARY OF SCENARIO

Joan enjoys working with Dr. Sahani and his gastrointestinal patients but is constantly challenged to maintain and update information about diseases and disorders of the system as well as their diagnosis and medical management. Joan must consistently work at applying the correct medical terminology when documenting patient complaints and consider her background in gastrointestinal disorders so she can ask pertinent and detailed questions about patient complaints.

Joan has also had to update her knowledge of patient preparation for diagnostic procedures so patients are adequately prepared for scheduled examinations. She participates in workshops offered by her local professional organization to stay up to date on medications and treatments for gastrointestinal diseases. Joan is looking forward to being actively involved in patient care by continuing to prepare patient education materials and assist Dr. Sahani as needed to provide quality patient care.

SUMMARY OF LEARNING OBJECTIVES

■ The gastrointestinal system is responsible for the preparation, digestion, absorption, and excretion of nutrients and waste materials.

■ The gastrointestinal system begins at the mouth and ends at the anal canal. The digestive process starts in the mouth with mastication and enzyme action; the bolus of food is swallowed and passed from the esophagus into the stomach, where digestion continues with the addition of hydrochloric acid and further enzyme action. Digestion ends in the duodenum, with pancreatic juices and emulsification of fat by bile, which is excreted by the liver and stored in the gallbladder. Absorption of nutrients takes place in the ileum and jejunum with absorption of fluids in the large intestine. Ultimately, waste materials are excreted through the anus.

■ The abdominal cavity can be divided into four sections or quadrants, the right and left upper quadrants and right and left lower quadrants. Another more specific method of dividing the abdominal cavity is with nine regions: the right hypochondriac, epigastric, and left hypochondriac; the right lumbar, umbilical, and left lumbar; and the right inguinal, hypogastric, and left inguinal. The purpose of these anatomical markers is to be able to clearly identify the location of a gastrointestinal problem.

■ Patients with gastrointestinal disorders may complain of nausea with pallor, diaphoresis, and tachycardia; vomiting because of pain, stress, gastrointestinal upset, or an inner ear or intracranial pressure disturbance; diarrhea resulting from an infection, allergy, or malabsorption problem; constipation because of a low-fiber diet or inadequate fluids, as a side effect of medication, or a bowel obstruction or tumor; and abdominal pain that varies in intensity and quality. It is important for the medical assistant to identify the location of the patient's discomfort using either abdominal quadrants or regions and to note the onset, duration, and frequency of all symptoms.

■ Cancers of the gastrointestinal tract can occur in any of the primary or accessory organs of the system. Table 36-2 summarizes the characteristics of gastrointestinal tumors. These can include oral tumors, which present as either a white mass or an ulcer; esophageal, which causes dysphagia; gastric, which causes anorexia and weight loss but is difficult to diagnose in the early stages; liver, which is usually secondary to metastasis from another cancerous site with hepatomegaly and portal hypertension; pancreatic cancer, which is usually advanced when diagnosed; and colorectal cancer, with changes in bowel function and anemia.

■ Esophageal and gastric disorders include hiatal hernias, in which part of the stomach pushes through the hiatal sphincter of the diaphragm causing GERD; peptic ulcers, associated with *H. pylori* infections, which are treated with a combination of antibiotics and proton pump inhibitors; and pyloric stenosis, which is seen most frequently in firstborn male infants, causing projectile vomiting, and must be corrected by surgery. These disorders are usually diagnosed symptomatically and with the use of a barium swallow or upper gastrointestinal series of x-ray films. Medical treatment includes the use of Prilosec, Nexium, Pepcid, Tagamet, or Zantac. Surgery may be indicated for repair of a hiatal hernia or gastric ulcers if perforation occurs.

■ Intestinal disorders include a diverse variety of conditions. Food poisonings cause mild to severe gastroenteritis; symptoms are controlled with antiemetics and antidiarrheal medications. Dumping syndrome, which may occur as a postsurgical complication to weight loss surgery, results in widespread gastrointestinal complaints. IBS is a recurrent functional bowel disorder causing alternating bouts of diarrhea, flatulence, and constipation; it is treated pharmaceutically with bulk-forming agents, antidiarrheals, antispasmodics, and anticholinergics. Acute appendicitis is diagnosed by a positive McBurney's sign and is treated surgically. Regional enteritis, or Crohn's disease, causes localized areas of ulceration in the intestinal tract and is treated medically to decrease inflammation, manage symptoms, and maintain nutritional status. Ulcerative colitis, which causes inflammatory ulcers from the anus and moves proximally through the colon, is treated like Crohn's disease, but surgical removal of the colon is curative. Malabsorption disorders, including celiac disease, result from a genetic defect in the ability to metabolize gluten. Diverticular disease is caused by small herniations of the muscular lining of the colon and is managed with dietary changes and surgery if diverticulitis is advanced. Abdominal musculature can become weakened and hernias can develop that require surgical repair. Hemorrhoids, which are varicose veins of the anus, are treated with stool softeners, high-fiber diets, or surgical repair.

■ Disorders of the liver include hepatitis, either from viral infection or a chemical reaction, such as alcohol abuse or a complication of drug metabolism. Mild inflammation temporarily impairs liver function, but severe inflammation may lead to necrosis and serious complications, including jaundice, cirrhosis, and portal hypertension. The gallbladder stores bile that is excreted by the liver to aid in fat metabolism. If cholelithiasis or cholecystitis develops, the gallbladder may have to be surgically removed to relieve symptoms.

■ Viral hepatitis is an infection of the liver that causes an acute inflammatory process of the hepatocytes. There are several forms of this virus: A, B, C, D, E and G. Hepatic cells are capable of regeneration, so, depending on the degree of liver involvement, the patient may recover completely or develop widespread necrosis, cirrhosis, and liver failure. Chronic inflammation can occur with hepatitis B, C, and D. This usually results in permanent liver damage and an associated increased risk of liver cancer. Table 36-4 describes the overall characteristics of the types of hepatitis. Vaccinations are available for hepatitis A and B.

■ The medical assistant's role in the gastrointestinal examination includes providing patient support and education, gathering and recording specific details about the patient's complaints, instilling rectal medications as ordered, and assisting the physician with the examination and diagnostic procedures performed in the ambulatory care setting.

■ Diagnostic procedures for the gastrointestinal system include laboratory studies, such as liver panels and urinary tests for bilirubin and amylase; and stool tests for occult blood, intestinal parasites, and fat excretion. Radiological and endoscopic tests, detailed in Table 36-5, include barium swallow, upper gastrointestinal series, barium enema, cholescintigraphy, sigmoidoscopy, and colonoscopy.

■ The role of the medical assistant in the proctological examination includes patient support and preparation; positioning and draping the patient for the procedure; monitoring vital signs before and during the procedure; and assisting the physician with the procedure.

KEY INTERNET WEBSITES

- American Gastroenterological Association
- Gastrointestinal site links
- National Institute of Diabetes and Digestive and Kidney Diseases
  For active weblinks to each website visit
  http://evolve.elsevier.com/Kinn/

CHAPTER 37

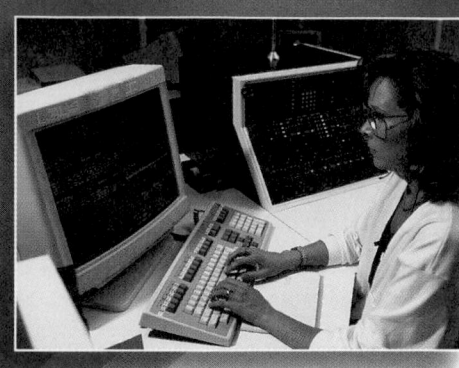

Scenario

Sara Ricci, a CMA with 10 years' experience, works for Dr. Samuel Fineman, a urologist who also manages male reproductive disorders. Dr. Fineman relies on Sara to handle telephone calls from patients, have a clear understanding of the anatomy and physiology of the renal system, and assist him in the clinical area of the practice. Although Sara has worked for Dr. Fineman for almost 2 years, occasionally there are still problems that arise that she is not sure how to manage.

Assisting in Urology and Male Reproduction

Learning Objectives

- Define and spell the terms listed in the vocabulary.
- Describe the organs of the urinary system and their functions.
- Explain the susceptibility of the urinary system to diseases and disorders.
- Identify the primary signs and symptoms of urinary problems.
- Detail common urinary system diagnostic procedures.
- Compare and contrast infections and inflammations of the urinary system.
- Describe urinary tract obstructions and cancers.
- Distinguish between the two methods of treating renal failure.
- Summarize typical pediatric urological disorders.
- Illustrate the organs of male reproduction.
- Determine the cause and effects of prostate disorders.
- Outline common types of genital pathological conditions in men.
- Describe the effects of sexually transmitted diseases in the male patient.
- Summarize the characteristics of HIV infection, diagnostic criteria, and treatment protocols.
- Understand and demonstrate the medical assistant's role in urology.
- Conduct patient education on testicular self-examination.
- Demonstrate with accuracy the catheterization of both a female and a male patient.
- Assist with the urological examination.

National Curriculum Competencies

CLINICAL COMPETENCIES

4e. Prepare patients for and assist with routine and specialty examinations

4f. Prepare patients for and assist with procedures, treatments, and minor office surgery

4g. Apply pharmacology principles to prepare and administer oral and parenteral medications

TRANSDISCIPLINARY COMPETENCIES

3b. Instruct individuals according to their needs

3d. Provide instruction for health maintenance and disease prevention

Vocabulary

albuminuria Abnormal presence of albumin in the urine.

azotemia Retention in the blood of excessive amounts of nitrogenous wastes.

casts Fibrous or protein material molded to the shape of the part in which it has accumulated and thrown off into the urine in kidney disease.

copulation Sexual intercourse.

creatinine Nitrogenous waste from muscle metabolism excreted in urine.

erythropoietin Substance released from the kidney and liver that promotes red blood cell formation.

opportunistic infection Infections caused by a normally nonpathogenic organism in a host whose resistance has been decreased.

urgency Sudden, compelling desire to urinate and the inability to control its release.

Urology is the study of the urinary tract in both male and female patients. The physician who specializes in the diseases and disorders of the urinary system is a urologist. Urologists also specialize in the diseases and disorders of the male reproductive system. There are a wide variety of medical treatments, from radiological to surgical, available to urologists to treat the diseases and disorders of the urinary system.

Anatomy and Physiology of the Urinary System

The urinary tract consists of two kidneys, two ureters, one urinary bladder, and one urethra (Figure 37-1). The main function of the urinary system is to remove waste products from the body. A variety of wastes are produced as by-products of the body's metabolic processes and, if left to accumulate, can become toxic. The urinary system removes salts and nitrogenous waste, which is the product of protein breakdown, in the form of soluble urea from the blood and excrete it through the renal organs. The urinary system also helps to maintain homeostasis by regulating water, electrolytes, and acid-base levels; activating vitamin D, which encourages calcium ion absorption; secreting the hormone **erythropoietin**, which helps control the rate of red blood cell formation; and maintaining blood pressure by the secretion of the enzyme renin.

The kidneys are red-brown, bean-shaped glandular organs. They are located posterior to the peritoneum (retroperitoneal) and against the muscles of the back, roughly between the T12 and L3 vertebrae. The left kidney is located approximately 2 cm higher than the right because of the location of the liver.

The kidneys remove unwanted substances from the blood and form urine for excretion. To perform this crucial function, a great deal of blood circulates through the kidneys—approximately 15% to 30% of the total cardiac output. The blood is delivered to the two kidneys by the renal artery and is distributed through the kidneys by a highway of smaller arteries. The blood is then returned through a pathway of veins, including the renal vein that joins the inferior vena cava through the abdominal cavity.

The outer layer of the kidney, the *cortex*, contains the functional unit of the kidney, the *nephron* unit, where urine is formed as fluid and dissolved substances move between the vascular and tubular structures of the nephron. There are three processes involved in urine formation: filtration, reabsorption, and excretion. The nephron consists of the *glomerulus*, which is a cluster of capillaries extending from the renal artery that are partially surrounded by the *Bowman's capsule*. Fluid and dissolved

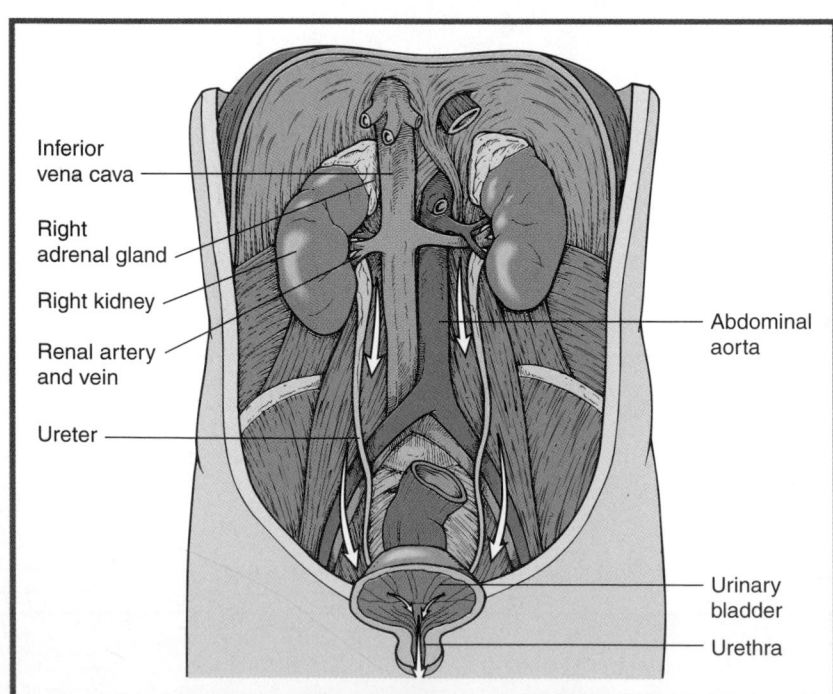

Inferior vena cava

Right adrenal gland

Right kidney

Renal artery and vein

Ureter

Abdominal aorta

Urinary bladder

Urethra

FIGURE 37-1 The urinary system. (From Frazier MS, Drzymkowski JA, Doty SJ: *Essentials of human diseases and conditions, ed. 2,* Philadelphia, 2000, WB Saunders.)

substances move from the glomerulus to the Bowman's capsule and then into the proximal convoluted tubules, where most of the filtrate is reabsorbed by venules and arterioles surrounding the tubules and sent back into the general circulation. Based on the homeostatic needs of the body, the kidneys determine the type and quantity of substances that are reabsorbed. Finally, the remaining substances are passed through the distal convoluted tubules to the collecting tubules and then on to the medulla of the kidney, which contains the distal collection area of the *renal pelvis* called the *calyx* (Figure 37-2).

By the time the waste material reaches the calyx, it is in the form of urine, which is emptied out of the kidneys through bilateral *ureters*. The two ureters are tubular organs about 25 cm long; and with the aid of peristaltic waves generated by the muscle layer, they move the urine from the kidneys to the urinary *bladder*. The urinary bladder is a hollow organ that is lined with smooth muscle that overlaps in rugae formation and easily expands as the bladder is filled. When the bladder is full, sphincters open and urine flows into the *urethra*. The urethra is lined with a mucous membrane and in the male functions as both the urinary canal and as a passageway for cells and secretions from various reproductive organs. In a male, the urethra is about 20 cm long and is divided into three sections: the prostatic urethra (passing through the prostate gland at the base of the bladder), the membranous urethra, and the penile urethra. In a female, the urethra is 3 to 4 cm long. Its proximity to the vagina and anus exposes the renal system to microorganisms that can cause infection. The urethra conveys the urine from the bladder. It passes through the *urinary meatus* and outside the body. The process of urination is known as *voiding* or *micturition*.

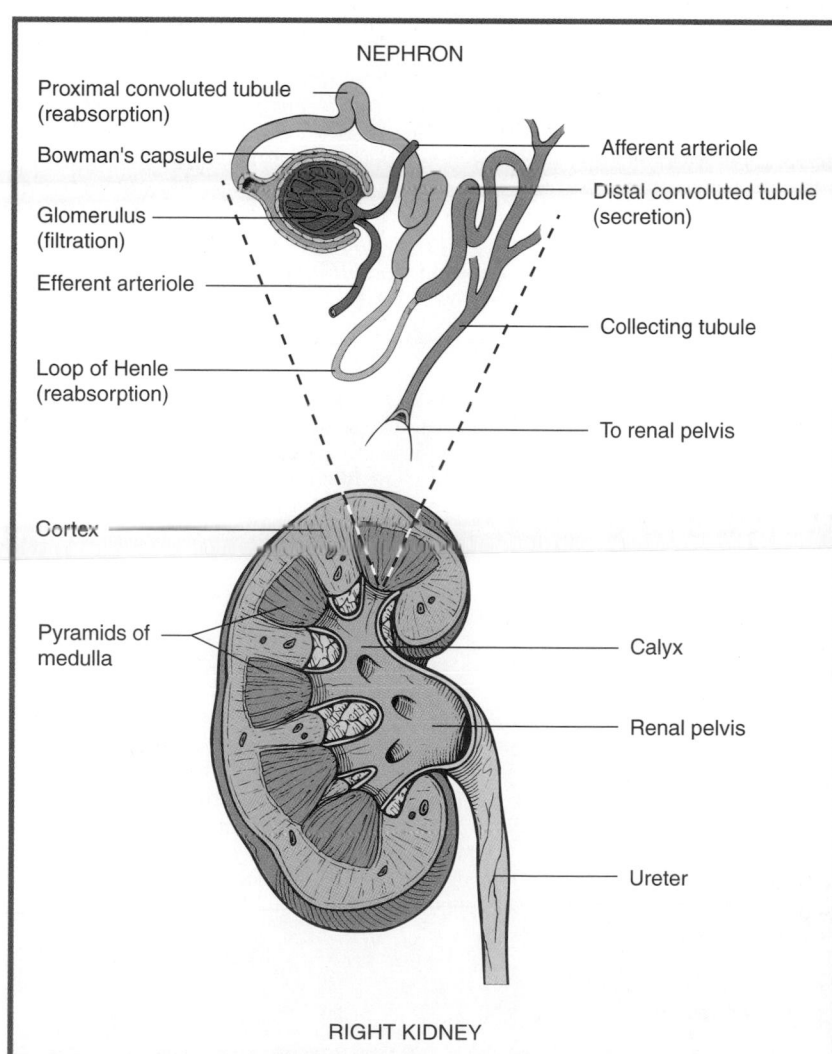

NEPHRON

Proximal convoluted tubule (reabsorption)

Bowman's capsule

Glomerulus (filtration)

Efferent arteriole

Loop of Henle (reabsorption)

Afferent arteriole

Distal convoluted tubule (secretion)

Collecting tubule

To renal pelvis

Cortex

Pyramids of medulla

Calyx

Renal pelvis

Ureter

RIGHT KIDNEY

FIGURE 37-2   The kidney. (From Frazier MS, Drzymkowski JA, Doty SJ. *Essentials of human diseases and conditions, ed. 2,* Philadelphia, 2000, WB Saunders.)

Disorders of the Urinary System

The urinary tract is made up of a continuous mucosal lining that gives organisms entering the urethra a direct pathway through the system. Of the wide range of symptoms that occur in patients with disorders of the renal system, the most common symptoms involve changes in the frequency of urination. Dysuria (difficult or painful urination), **urgency**, retention, and incontinence are all common symptoms. Abnormal functions of any part of the urinary tract can often be determined with urinalysis, blood urea nitrogen (BUN) levels, and with analysis of **creatinine** clearance. Urinalysis is discussed in Chapter 49. Radiological and endoscopic studies are also important in detecting urinary tract diseases. Table 37-1 summarizes common urinary system diagnostic tests.

TABLE 37-1	Common Urinary System Diagnostic Tests	
Test	**Description**	**Patient Preparation**
Kidney-ureter-bladder x-ray (KUB) films	Flat plate films of the abdomen; shows the size, shape, location, malformations of kidneys and bladder; visualizes calculi.	No specific patient preparation; contraindicated in pregnancy.
Renal scanning	Nuclear scans to determine size, shape, and function of the kidney or to diagnose obstruction or hypertension. IV administration of a radioisotope and images taken to see how the isotope is distributed.	Patient should void before the procedure; no sedation or fasting required; drink 2 to 3 glasses of water before scanning; procedure contraindicated in pregnancy.
Cystography and voiding cystourethrogram	X-ray evaluation with contrast dye to study bladder structure or function.	Clear liquids for breakfast; Foley catheter inserted; may take x-ray films while patient is voiding (voiding cystourethrogram); after procedure force fluids to eliminate dye and prevent infection.
Intravenous pyelography (IVP)	IV injected dye with x-ray films taken at intervals to show passage through kidneys, ureters, and into bladder. Diagnose tumors, calculi, obstructions, and congenital renal problems.	Contraindicated in pregnancy and iodine allergies; laxative evening before; liquid diet 8 hours before; adequate fluids before and after; may have enema morning of the study.
Arteriography (angiography)	Injection of dye into the renal artery; computerized fluoroscopy visualizes the blood flow dynamics of the kidneys and serial x-ray films are taken. Used to diagnose stenosis of the renal artery and highly vascular renal cancers.	NPO 2 to 8 hours prior to procedure; administer preprocedure medications as ordered; void before the study; warm flush may be felt when dye is injected; check for allergy to iodine or shellfish.
Renal computed tomography	Can be done with or without contrast dye. Transverse views of the kidney are taken by CT to detect tumors, abscesses, cysts, and hydronephrosis.	If contrast medium is used, fast 4 hours before procedure; scanner may make loud clicking sounds as it rotates around the body; dye may cause flushing, metallic taste, and headache; check for allergy to iodine or shellfish; remove all metal objects.
Renal ultrasonography	High-frequency sound waves are transmitted through the kidneys to detect abnormalities; determine kidney size and diagnose hydronephrosis, polycystic kidneys, and obstructions of the ureters and bladder.	No food or fluid restrictions; noninvasive and painless.
Cystoscopy	Endoscopic view of urethra and bladder for biopsy; measurement of bladder capacity; to find or remove calculi; dilation of urethra and ureters; placement of ureteral stents.	Enemas to clear bowel; force fluids before procedure if local anesthesia is to be used; for general anesthesia, NPO after midnight; preprocedure sedative to reduce bladder spasms; after care: monitor urinary output for 24 hours.
Retrograde pyelography	Dye can be injected into the bladder, ureters, and kidneys through a cystoscope to detect stones and other obstructions. It is also used to replace an IVP for patients with renal failure, with physical blockages, or with allergies to the intravenous dye.	Same as cystoscopy; check for iodine or shellfish allergies.

CRITICAL THINKING APPLICATION

Sara is responsible for scheduling and giving patient preparation instructions for diagnostic radiological and endoscopic procedures. With Dr. Fineman's approval, she has prepared patient handouts that summarize the correct procedures to follow when scheduled for specific urological tests. Today she has a patient that needs to be scheduled for both a cystogram and an intravenous pyelogram (IVP). How should the patient prepare for both of these examinations?

Urinary Incontinence

Urinary incontinence, which is a temporary or chronic loss of urinary control, can be the result of many conditions. Infections of the urinary tract, brain disorders, and tissue damage can all lead to urinary incontinence. This disorder can also be caused by straining or coughing in post-surgical patients and in patients with weak pelvic musculature. When caused in this manner, it is called *stress incontinence.*

Treatment methods for incontinence will depend on the causative factor. Bladder or habit training involves teaching the patient to urinate according to an established schedule rather than when he or she has the urge to void. This is helpful for patients who are incontinent as a result of strokes, Parkinson's disease, Alzheimer's disease, central nervous system lesions, or cystitis. Pelvic muscle exercises (Kegel exercises), in which the patient simulates stopping the flow of urine and holding that contraction for 10 seconds in sets of 20 three times a day, are helpful for patients with stress incontinence as a result of weak musculature.

Intermittent catheterization to empty the bladder for patients with urinary retention is preferable to indwelling catheters, because the use of indwelling catheters often leads to infection. External (condom) catheters can be used for male patients, but they are also associated with an increased incidence of urinary tract infections (UTIs). Chronic incontinence can be treated pharmacologically with anticholinergic preparations including propantheline (Pro-Banthine) or antispasmodic agents, such as oxybutynin chloride (Ditropan).

When all other treatments have failed, surgical intervention in the guise of an artificial bladder sphincter can be implemented. This hydraulically activated mechanism is placed around the urethra, or bladder neck, and is made to open and close by squeezing one of two bulbs implanted under the skin of the scrotum or labia.

Urinary Tract Infections and Inflammations

UTIs occur frequently, because the urinary system has a direct opening to the outside, and urine is an excellent medium for bacterial growth. Most UTIs are ascending, starting with pathogens in the perineal area and infecting the continuous mucosa up through the urethra, bladder, ureters, to the kidneys. Infection and inflammation of the urethra is called *urethritis* and that of the bladder is *cystitis.* The resident flora of the colon, *Escherichia coli,* is the usual causative agent.

Because of the anatomical structure of women—a short urethra and the close relation of the anus—and irritation from the use of tampons, taking bubble baths, and from sexual activity, they are more susceptible to UTIs than men are. Older men with prostatic hypertrophy and resultant urinary retention are also at risk for frequent urinary infections.

Urethritis. Urethritis is an inflammation of the urethra and is more common in men. It results from a gonococcal infection or infection with other pathogenic bacteria or viruses. The symptoms include discharge of pus and an itching sensation at the opening of the urethra. There is a burning sensation during urination, and it can accompany cystitis in women, so sexual partners should be treated as well. Urinalysis may show *hematuria* (blood in the urine) as well as *pyuria* (pus in the urine).

Cystitis. Cystitis, an infection of the urinary bladder, causes inflammation of the bladder wall and urinary urgency. Symptoms vary from very mild to acute discomfort in the lower abdomen, urinary frequency, and painful urination (dysuria). The patient may have systemic infection signs, including fever, general malaise, and leukocytosis. A diagnostic urinalysis shows more than 100,000 bacteria per milliliter of urine, pyuria, and hematuria.

Pyelonephritis. Pyelonephritis, an inflammation of the renal pelvis and kidney, is the most common type of renal disease. It is caused by bacteria that ascend from the lower urinary tract and is associated with conditions such as urinary retention or obstruction that promote urinary stasis and the growth of bacteria. It frequently is preceded by urethritis and cystitis. With pyelonephritis, pus collects in the renal pelvis and abscesses form. Symptoms include fever, chills, nausea, vomiting, and flank (lumbar) pain. The patient reports foul-smelling, dark urine with frequency and urgency.

Diagnostic studies include urinalysis of a clean catch urine sample. It reveals hematuria, pyuria, increased white and red blood cells, **albuminuria, casts,** and the presence of bacteria. Urine cultures are usually done to determine the causative agent.

Treatment of UTIs. Urinary tract infections are treated with antibiotics, such as penicillin, cephalosporin (Keflex), and methoprim-sulfamethoxazole (Bactrim), and forcing fluids to dilute the urine. A follow-up urinalysis should be run to confirm the effectiveness of antibiotic therapy in curing the infection. UTIs tend to recur unless the cause of the infection is removed.

The medical assistant should instruct the patient to finish the entire antibiotic prescription as ordered, the importance of proper hygiene, to completely empty the bladder when the urge to void arises, and for female patients to wipe the bottom from front to back to discourage the spread of *E. coli* in the urethral region. Cranberry juice may be recommended as a prophylactic measure, because it contains substances that discourage *E. coli* growth and helps maintain acidity of urine.

CRITICAL THINKING APPLICATION

Tabitha Allison, a 22-year-old patient of Dr. Fineman's, was diagnosed today with her third UTI in as many months. Patient education on the prevention and treatment of UTIs is needed. What should Sara tell her?

Glomerulonephritis. Acute glomerulonephritis, the degenerative inflammation of the glomeruli, usually develops in children and adolescents about 2 weeks after a streptococcal infection, such as strep throat or scarlet fever. Its symptoms include low-grade fever, anorexia, general malaise, and flank pain. Hypertension and edema may occur because of reduced renal function. A urinalysis shows hematuria and proteinuria. Diuretics such as triamterene/hydrochlorothiazide (Dyazide) or furosemide (Lasix) may be given to control hypertension and reduce edema. Prognosis is usually good; most patients recover spontaneously.

Chronic glomerulonephritis causes progressive, irreversible renal damage that may result in renal failure. At first the patient is asymptomatic, but as the disease progresses and causes more glomerular damage, the patient will develop hypertension, hematuria, proteinuria, *oliguria* (scanty urination), and edema. Chronic glomerulonephritis is caused by an antigen-antibody reaction within the glomerular capsule that ultimately destroys the nephron unit. Treatment is supportive, with an attempt to control symptoms by administering antihypertensives and diuretics. The only cure for the disease is a kidney transplant.

Urinary Tract Obstructions and Cancers

Renal Calculi. Renal calculi, or kidney stones, are created when salts in the urine collect in the kidney or when fluid intake is low, creating a highly concentrated filtrate. They are a common problem and tend to recur if the cause of formation is not treated. Small stones usually do not cause any difficulty until they grow large enough to lodge in the ureters or renal pelvis. An infection can develop from the blockage of urine flow, with resultant stasis. This blockage can also result in *hydronephrosis*, which is a backup of urine causing dilation of the ureters and calyces and increased pressure on the nephron units.

If the stones are located in the kidney or bladder, the patient is often asymptomatic with frequent infections as the only presenting problem. If the stones begin to move or are lodged in the ureters, the patient can experience severe pain in the flank region that radiates into the groin. The pain will persist until the stone is either passed or removed. Small stones can be passed spontaneously, but larger stones require medical intervention.

The physician may perform a cystoscopy to visualize the urethra and bladder and remove any stones found (Figure 37-3). At one time, the only treatment option for calculi in the kidneys or ureters was invasive surgery. Now urologists fragment calculi with either laser lithotripsy or extracorporeal shock-wave lithotripsy (ESWL), which uses vibrations of powerful sound waves to break up the stone. Diagnostic studies are performed to identify the exact location of the calculi. For ESWL, the patient is immersed in water and the intense sound waves are passed through the body at the exact location of the calculi (Figure 37-4). After the procedure, patients complain of flank tenderness and hematuria. Medical treatment includes prevention of recurrence by treating the underlying cause of calculi development. Increasing fluid intake and drinking cranberry juice will help flush the renal system as well as alter the urine pH, which makes conditions less favorable for the formation of calculi.

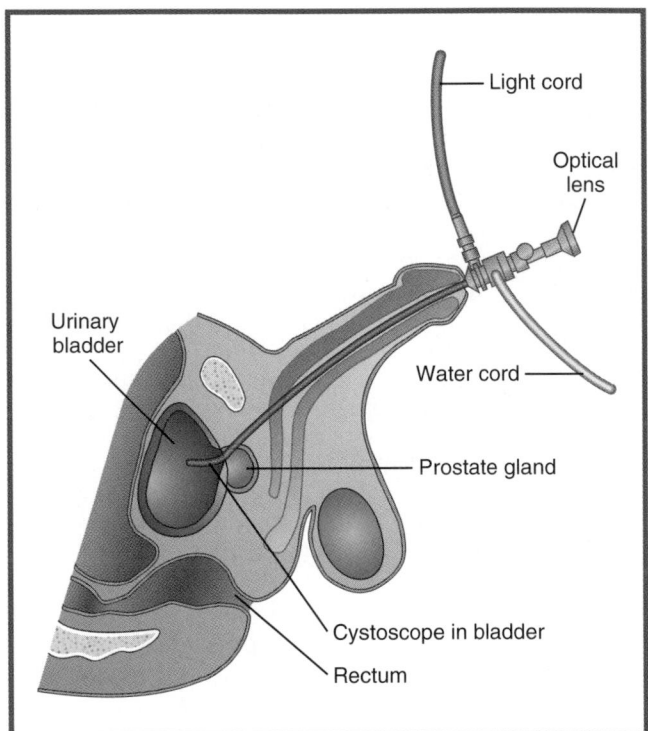

FIGURE 37-3 Cystoscopy.

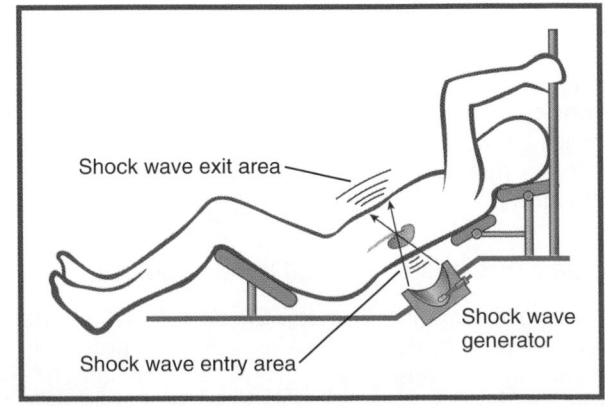

FIGURE 37-4 Extracorporeal shock-wave lithotripsy.

Hydronephrosis. Besides renal calculi, hydronephrosis can also be caused by an enlarged prostate or a tumor. Hydronephrosis can occur bilaterally or unilaterally. The condition is frequently asymptomatic, or patients may complain of mild flank pain as the renal capsule is distended. Urine testing detects hematuria and, if infection develops from stagnant urine, pyuria. It is important to treat hydronephrosis aggressively, because continued pressure from blocked urine flow can cause tissue necrosis and ultimately lead to irreversible kidney damage. Removing the blockage will correct the condition (Figure 37-5).

Polycystic Kidneys. Polycystic kidney is an autosomal dominant genetic disorder that is slowly progressive and irreversible. There are no indications of the disease in children, but as time goes on, normal renal tissue in both kidneys is replaced with multiple grapelike cysts (Figure 37-6). The nephrons and collecting tubules become dilated, fused, and infected. As the cysts enlarge, they compress the surrounding tissue, causing necrosis, uremia, and renal failure. Symptoms do not usually become apparent until the individual reaches adolescence or adulthood. Patients will have a family history of kidney disease or renal failure, flank pain, hematuria, and hypertension. They are also more likely to develop UTIs and

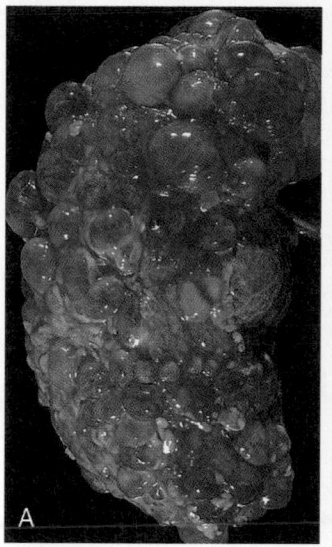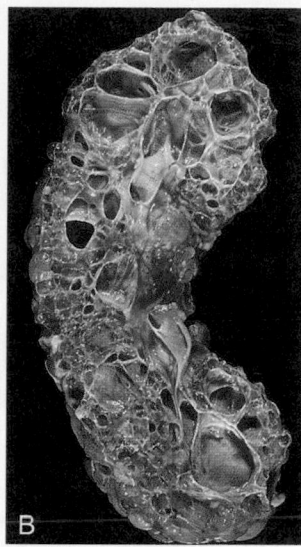

FIGURE 37-6   Polycystic kidney (adult autosomal dominant). **A**, External surface of enlarged kidney, showing cysts. **B**, Bisected, shows large interior cysts. (From Cotran RS, Kumar V, Collins T: *Robbin's pathologic basis of disease,* ed 6. Philadelphia, 1999, WB Saunders.)

renal calculi. Since cyst formation is progressive, these patients will eventually require either renal dialysis or a kidney transplant.

Bladder Cancer. The most common cancer of the urinary tract affects the bladder (Figure 37-7) and is two to three times more common in men than in women. Bladder cancer is characterized by one or more tumors that can reappear. The tumor is invasive and can metastasize through the blood or surrounding pelvic lymph nodes. Testing that can identify recurrence is extremely important. NMP22 is a urine test that identifies recurrence of the disease. This test is twice as sensitive as urine cytology and is painless and inexpensive. It works by identifying the nuclear matrix protein present in the transitional cells of the bladder. Ninety percent of bladder cancers are attributed to these particular cells, called *transitional cells* because of their ability to be cubelike when the bladder is empty and flat when it is full.

The risk for developing this type of cancer increases in persons who smoke, those with recurrent infections, persons who take large amounts of analgesics, and those exposed to aromatic amines and other carcinogenic agents.

Renal Carcinoma. Adenocarcinoma of the kidney is a primary tumor that is initially asymptomatic, so frequently it has metastasized to the lungs, liver, male urogenital system, bone, or brain by the time it is diagnosed. It typically occurs in persons older than 50 years of age and is seen more often in men and smokers. Symptoms of the disease include pain, loss of appetite, anemia, and an increased white blood cell count. Urinalysis will show hematuria. Surgical nephrectomy is the treatment of choice. Although the prognosis for the tumor has improved, the 5-year survival rate is still only about 50%.

Wilms' Tumor. Wilms' tumor, cancer of the kidney in children, is the most common malignancy in children,

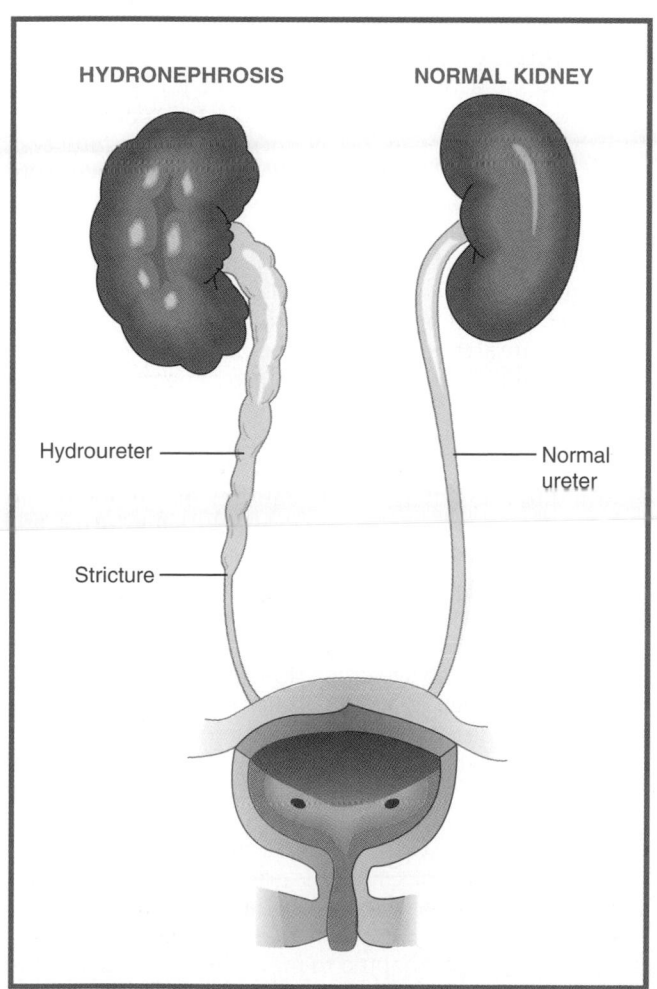

HYDRONEPHROSIS   **NORMAL KIDNEY**

Hydroureter —   — Normal ureter

Stricture —

FIGURE 37-5   Hydronephrosis.

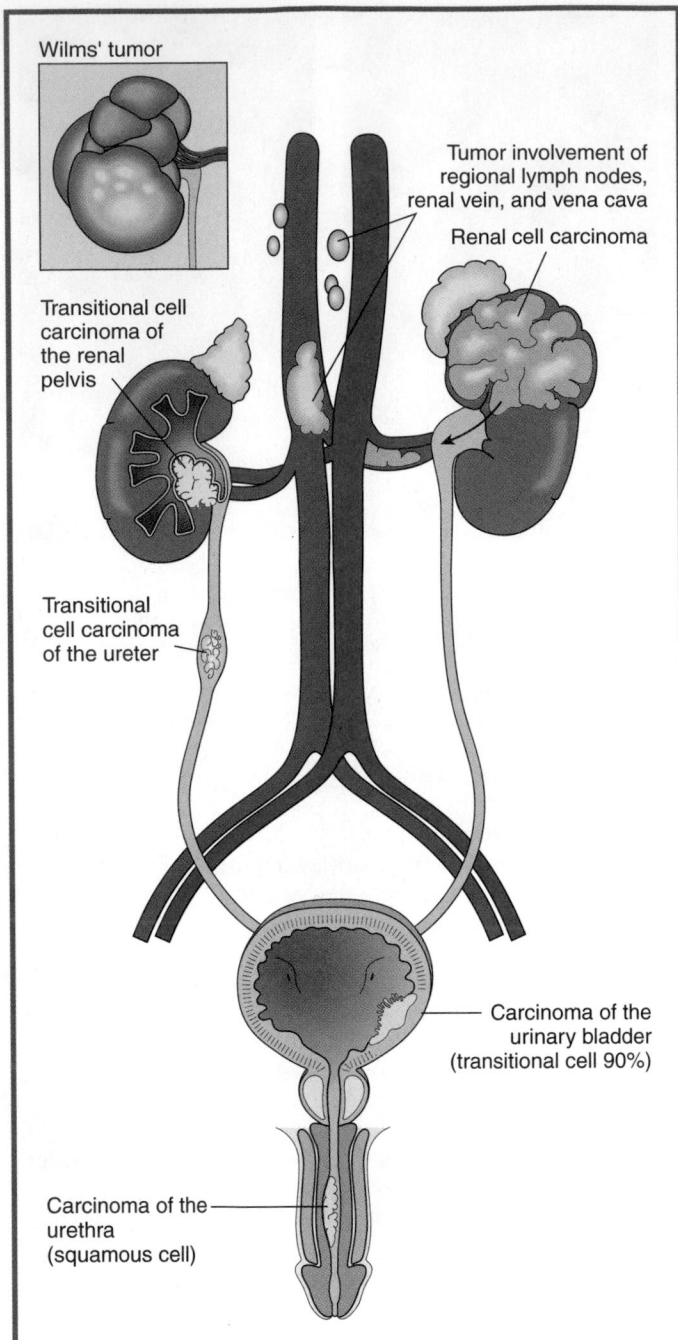

Wilms' tumor

Tumor involvement of regional lymph nodes, renal vein, and vena cava

Renal cell carcinoma

Transitional cell carcinoma of the renal pelvis

Transitional cell carcinoma of the ureter

Carcinoma of the urinary bladder (transitional cell 90%)

Carcinoma of the urethra (squamous cell)

FIGURE 37-7   Neoplasms of the urinary tract. (From Damjanov I: *Pathology for the health-related professions, ed. 2*, Philadelphia, 2000, WB Saunders.)

and is associated with an inherited genetic defect. It usually occurs unilaterally and is diagnosed at about 2 to 5 years of age when caregivers notice an abdominal mass. Combined surgical, radiation, and chemotherapy treatment have improved the prognosis of the disease to a 90% survival rate.

Renal Failure

Acute renal failure has a sudden, severe onset caused by exposure to toxic chemicals, severe or prolonged cir-

culatory or cardiogenic shock that might occur from serious burns or heart disease, or from an acute bilateral kidney infection or inflammation. Blood tests will show elevated BUN and creatinine levels, and the patient will experience acute onset of oliguria. The primary problem must be resolved as quickly as possible to avoid necrosis and permanent kidney failure.

Chronic renal failure is a slowly progressive process that is caused by the gradual destruction of the ability of the kidneys to filter waste materials. This loss of nephron function is asymptomatic at first and results from chronic glomerulonephritis or polycystic kidneys as well as systemic changes from diabetes or hypertension. Once symptoms do appear, the process is irreversible.

Patients with chronic renal failure pass through several stages, starting with an early stage of decreased reserve when there are no apparent clinical signs but serum creatinine levels are consistently higher than average. The middle stage of renal insufficiency is marked by hypertension, an elevation in BUN and creatinine levels, and a low specific gravity of the urine. End-stage renal failure (*uremia*) is marked by oliguria that progresses to *anuria* (no urine output), edema, hypertension, acidosis, and **azotemia**. The end result is that the kidneys can no longer remove waste products from the blood and toxicity develops. To survive, the patient must be placed on dialysis or receive a kidney transplant.

Treatment.   Dialysis, or cleansing of the blood, is used to treat acute renal failure until the problem is reversed or for those patients in end-stage renal disease until a transplant can be performed. There are two forms of dialysis: hemodialysis or peritoneal dialysis (Figure 37-8). The first, hemodialysis, is usually done in an outpatient clinic or hospital. The process uses a machine known as an *artificial kidney* to filter out waste products in the blood and return the cleansed blood to the body. The patient has a cannula or shunt surgically placed in an artery, usually in the arm, that creates an internal fistula. During the procedure the patient's blood passes from the shunt through a tube to the semipermeable membrane of the dialysis machine. The membrane filters waste out of the blood, which then is returned to the patient's vein. Patients on hemodialysis require anticoagulant therapy to prevent the formation of clots during the blood transfer process. Hemodialysis is usually needed three times a week; the procedure takes approximately 3 to 4 hours each time.

Peritoneal dialysis can be done at home, usually at night, or in a dialysis unit. This is a blood-cleansing process by which dialyzing fluid is infused into the patient's abdomen through a catheter that has been implanted into the peritoneal cavity. The catheter has both entry and exit points. A highly concentrated dialyzing fluid enters the peritoneal cavity through the implanted catheter, absorbs waste products, and is then drained from the abdominal cavity by gravity into a container. This process can be controlled either by the aid of a machine or by the patient. It takes longer than hemodialysis but can be adapted to meet the individual needs of the patient and prevents sudden changes in fluid and electrolyte levels in the body.

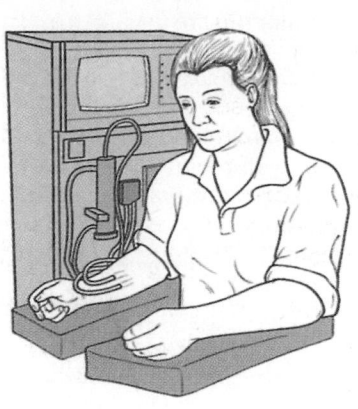
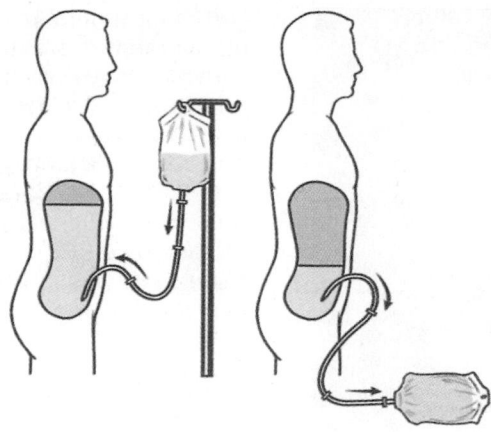

Hemodialysis   Continuous ambulatory peritoneal dialysis

FIGURE 37-8   Dialysis. (From Frazier MS, Drzymkowski JA, Doty SJ: *Essentials of human diseases and conditions, ed. 2,* Philadelphia, 2000, WB Saunders.)

CRITICAL THINKING APPLICATION

Aloysius Gonzales, a 59-year-old patient, is in chronic renal failure. His family is trying to decide whether their father should be brought to the dialysis clinic for hemodialysis or whether they should try to keep him at home and assist with peritoneal dialysis. Sara explains the mechanism of each procedure to the family. What does she include in her description?

Pediatric Urological Disorders

Early detection and treatment of the many urological disorders that occur in children can drastically reduce permanent physical damage to the urinary system.

Enuresis

One of the most common reasons that parents bring a child to a pediatric urologist is enuresis, or bed-wetting. Enuresis is the lack of voluntary control of urination at night or during the day by a child considered to be beyond the age (usually after 5 years old) when control should be acquired. This problem has a familial tendency and is more common in males than females. The urologist first determines whether the problem is physical or psychological. With primary enuresis, bladder control was never established in the child. It may be caused by a physiological problem with bladder control, such as an immature bladder with small capacity, a neurological deficit, diabetes mellitus or insipidus, a urinary tract infection, or may be a psychological problem. Secondary enuresis, when there is a loss of bladder control in a child who has been consistently dry for at least 6 months, can develop because of psychological problems, urinary tract infections, diabetes, or sexual abuse.

A physical and neurological examination and a urinalysis with culture will help determine whether any physical abnormality is present in the urinary system. In most cases, no physical reason is found for the problem. If a psychological problem is suspected, help

from a pediatric mental health professional may be needed. If there are no causative factors, medications that relax the bladder muscles or increase its volume and medications that decrease urine production at night may be useful. Unfortunately, these may have side effects, and parents may decline this treatment. The medical assistant should encourage parents to positively reinforce dryness and avoid punishing or embarrassing the child. An enuresis alarm can be used that is worn at night and is triggered by wetness. The success rate is high (80%), but the device must be used every night until 21 consecutive nights of dryness are achieved.

Urine Reflux Disorder

Another reason for pediatric urology referrals may be urine reflux disorders. Urine reflux is caused by the backward flow of urine in the ureters during voiding. This can be detected early in utero by ultrasonography, or later with a voiding cystourethrogram (VCUG) (Figure 37-9). The test is performed by placing a urinary catheter in the bladder and filling it with a dye or radioactive material that helps visualize the flow of urine. Although a VCUG is an uncomfortable procedure, the benefit of early detection and decreased damage to the kidneys makes the screening worthwhile.

Treatment of reflux is usually determined by grading severity on a 1 to 5 scale, with 5 being the highest. Prophylactic antibiotics are given in low doses daily to avoid damaging kidney infections, which can cause low-grade reflux. However, with higher grade reflux that persists after 4 or 5 years of age or for patients who have breakthrough infections despite the antibiotics, surgical repair of the ureters is necessary. Parents and physicians may also opt for surgery, because the procedure has a high success rate of 95% and poses little risk.

Cryptorchism

A common disorder in young boys involves undescended testes, a condition known as *cryptorchism* (Figure 37-10). Normally, the testes develop in the abdominal cavity of the fetus and then descend into the scrotum

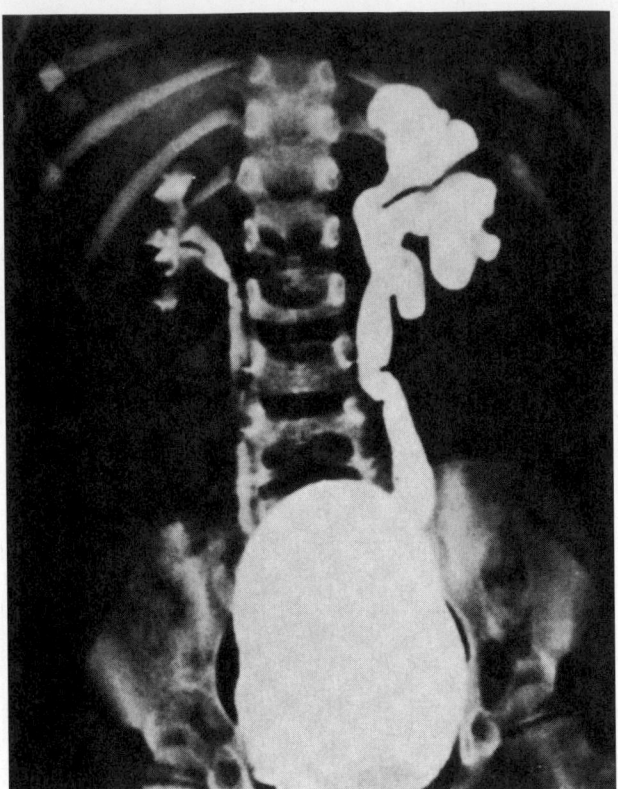

FIGURE 37-9 Voiding cystourethrogram. (From James AE Jr, Squire LF: *Nuclear radiology*, Philadelphia, 1973, WB Saunders.)

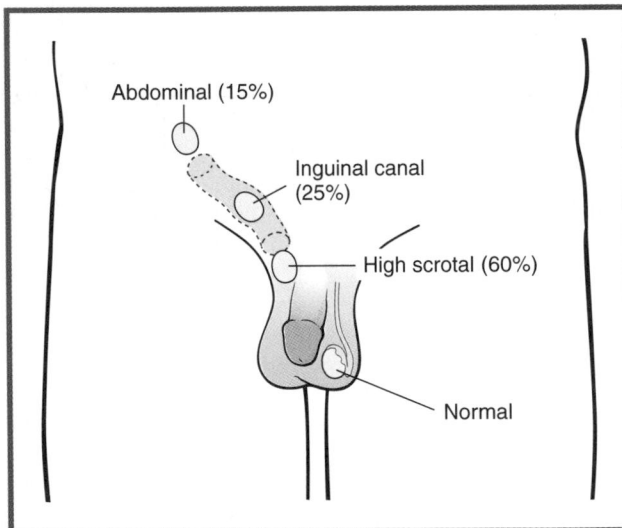

FIGURE 37-10 Cryptorchism. (From Damjanov I: *Pathology for the health-related professions*, ed. 2, Philadelphia, 2000, WB Saunders.)

near the end of the pregnancy. In some instances, however, the path is incomplete or incorrect. Most testes will descend within 3 to 4 months after birth. However, persistent cryptorchism should be treated, because infertility may result because of the effect on sperm of the slightly warmer temperatures in the abdominal cavity, and the increased chance of testicular cancer.

The location of the errant testes will dictate the form of treatment. Testes that are palpable are usually treated with hormones or with an outpatient surgical procedure known as *orchiopexy*, which involves suturing the undescended testicle in the scrotum. If the testicle is impalpable (cannot be felt), laparoscopic surgery is necessary to locate it. This procedure includes inserting the instrument into the abdomen by way of a small incision near the navel. Once found, the testicle is either moved into proper position or is removed. Success rates decrease with testes that are placed higher.

Anatomy and Physiology of the Male Reproductive System

The male reproductive system plays an important role in the continuation of the human species (Figure 37-11). Although not necessary for individual survival, the production, sustenance, and transport of male sex cells are vital to the creation of life.

The primary reproductive organs in the male are a pair of *testes*. Each testis is an oval structure 4 to 5 cm in length and 2.5 to 3 cm in diameter. Each is surrounded by a white, fibrous capsule, and they are contained together in the retractable saclike *scrotum*. The testes consist of lobules that contain the *seminiferous tubule*, which is where *spermatozoa*, the male sex cells, are produced. These cells contain 23 chromosomes, or half of the DNA chain needed to form a complete cell. The sperm cells are tadpole-like structures less than 0.1 mm long that are carried to the *epididymis* for maturation (Figure 37-12).

The epididymis is a long (approximately 6 meters), coiled tube that rests on the top and lateral side of each testis. Peristaltic waves in the epididymis help the sperm move into the *vas deferens*, where the sperm, which is now capable of movement, is stored until ejaculation. Each vas deferens is a muscular, 45-cm tunnel that connects to the epididymis at the base of the structure and passes along the side of the testes. It becomes part of the spermatic cord that passes through the pelvic cavity and ends behind the urinary bladder. Uniting there with the seminal vesicle just outside the prostate gland, it passes through the prostate and into an ejaculatory duct that empties its contents into the urethra.

The *prostate gland* is roughly 4 cm wide and 3 cm thick and surrounds the urethra at the base of the bladder. It secretes a thin fluid with an alkaline pH that neutralizes the acidic sperm-containing fluid and vaginal secretions to provide an optimal pH for fertilization. Secretions from the prostate gland, vas deferens, seminal vesicles, and bulbourethra gland combine with sperm cells to form *semen*. The volume of semen in one ejaculate varies from 2 to 6 ml and averages roughly 100 to 200 million sperm.

Penis

The organ of male **copulation** is the penis. It is a cylindrical organ consisting of an elongated body with a

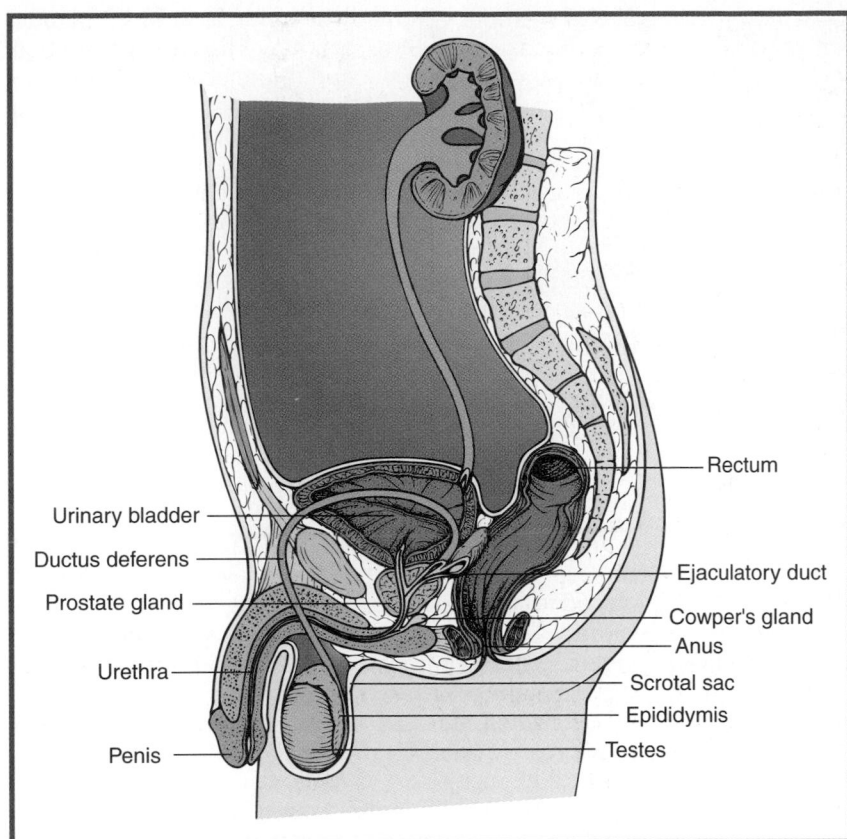

FIGURE 37-11   Male reproductive anatomy. (From Frazier MS, Drzymkowski JA, Doty SJ: *Essentials of human diseases and conditions, ed. 2*, Philadelphia, 2000, WB Saunders.)

Urinary bladder

Ductus deferens

Prostate gland

Urethra

Penis

Rectum

Ejaculatory duct

Cowper's gland

Anus

Scrotal sac

Epididymis

Testes

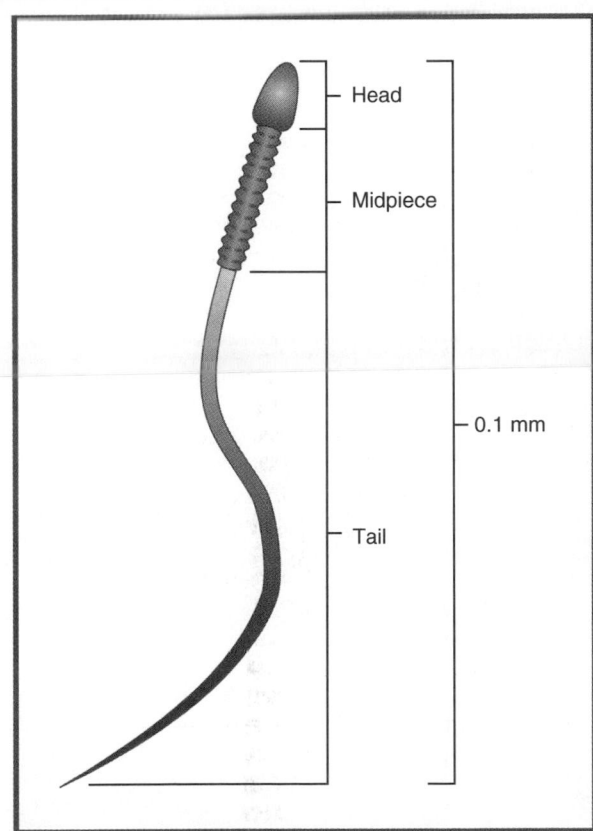

Head

Midpiece

0.1 mm

Tail

FIGURE 37-12   Sperm.

slightly enlarged end, called the *glans penis*. Around the glans penis there is a fold of skin that begins just behind the glans and extends forward to cover it like a sheath. This is called the *prepuce*, or foreskin, and is sometimes removed in a surgical procedure known as *circumcision*. The penis conveys urine and semen through the urethra and outside the body. When transmitting semen to the female tract, the penis must enlarge and stiffen for insertion. This is done when three columns of erectile tissue within the penis become stimulated. The arteries within the penis dilate and the veins compress. This compression of the veins allows a reduction of blood flow away from the penis, causing it to swell. Motor impulses are stimulated by the swelling of the urethra as a result of semen collection, and the contraction of the urethra causes the semen to be ejaculated through the penis.

Hormone Production

Hormone production is also an important aspect of the male reproductive system. As a group, the male sex hormones are called *androgens*. The most influential product of hormone production is testosterone. During pubescence, when the male becomes reproductively functional, the anterior pituitary gland produces gonadotrophic hormones that stimulate the testes to produce testosterone. Testosterone in turn stimulates the testes to enlarge, increases body hair growth, thickens skin and bone, increases muscle growth, and matures sperm cells.

Disorders of the Male Reproductive Tract

There are many diseases and disorders of the male reproductive tract. The most common of these involve enlargement or inflammation of certain organs and malignant tumors. The prostate is the most widely affected organ.

Prostatic Diseases

Prostatitis. The cause of inflammation of the prostate is not always known but usually develops in the presence of infection. Bacterial causes may be either *E. coli* or gonococci in patients with gonorrhea. The common symptoms are dysuria, tenderness of the prostate region, and secretion of pus from the tip of the penis. Treatment is usually with an antibiotic, such as penicillin. Chronic prostatitis may develop from repeated UTIs, urethral obstruction, or retention.

Benign Prostatic Hypertrophy. For men older than 50, the occurrence of enlargement of the prostate is very common. The incidence of benign prostatic hypertrophy increases with age. Swelling of the prostate gland partially blocks the flow of urine, creating a medium for bacterial infection that can lead to cystitis. Benign prostatic hypertrophy is associated with a decrease of testosterone production as men age. The diagnosis is made from patient complaints and a digital rectal examination by which the physician can palpate the enlarged gland (Figure 37-13).

Treatment includes the use of alpha-adrenergic blockers such as doxazosin mesylate (Cardura) or terazosin, which relax the smooth muscles of the prostate and bladder neck. Finasteride (Proscar) may also be prescribed, because it causes a reduction in the prostate, increasing urine flow and providing symptomatic relief. Surgical removal of the prostate gland through the urethra, a *transurethral* resection, may also be performed if pharmaceutical treatment is not effective.

Prostate Cancer. Cancer of the prostate is common in men older than 50 years of age and ranks as the second highest cause of cancer deaths in men, behind lung cancer. The patient may experience many symptoms. Urinary obstruction, increased bouts of urinary infection, and frequent *nocturia* (the need to void at night) are all symptoms of prostate cancer. Prostate cancer spreads rapidly to the bladder and rectum and often metastasizes to the lymph nodes, bones, lungs, and brain. The prognosis is poor unless the tumor is discovered in its early stages of development.

Prostate cancer is diagnosed by a digital rectal examination that identifies a firm or irregular area in the prostate. A blood test, the prostate-specific antigen (PSA) test, is also performed to measure the level of prostatic antigens present, which is compared to standard norms. The levels increase in the presence of prostate cancer. Because of this special finding, the PSA test is believed to be the most reliable test available for mass screening of prostate cancer and for the monitoring of potentially recurrent prostatic carcinomas. The American Cancer Society recommends that the PSA test be used in conjunction with a digital rectal examination annually for all men older than 50 years of age. In addition, PSA screenings should be performed yearly on men over the age of 40 who have a family history of the disease as well as blacks.

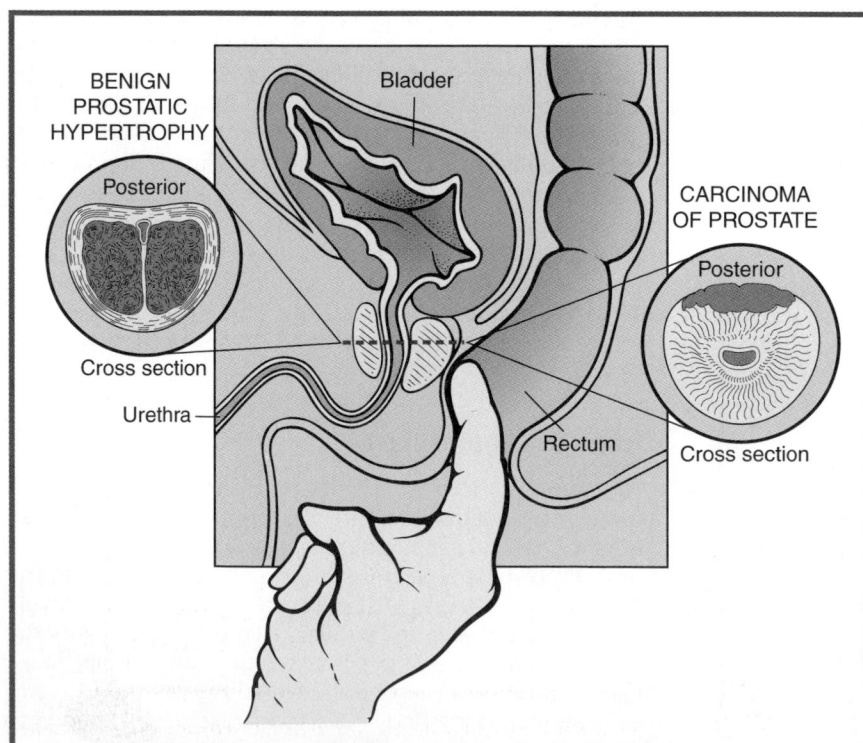

FIGURE 37-13 Benign prostatic hypertrophy and carcinoma of the prostate. (From Damjanov I: *Pathology for the health-related professions, ed. 2*, Philadelphia, 2000, WB Saunders.)

The extent of the prostate cancer will dictate treatment options. Hormone therapy is generally prescribed: estrogen will inhibit the production of testosterone, and testosterone has been proven to increase tumor growth. Surgical options include transurethral resection, in which the prostate gland is removed; orchiectomy, in which the testosterone-producing testicle is removed; radical prostatectomy, in which both the tumor and the testes are removed; or cryosurgical ablation of the prostate. These are debilitating surgical procedures that have side effects, such as impotence and incontinence. An alternative procedure is radioactive seed implantation, a variant of radiation therapy. In this procedure, tiny radioactive seeds are placed directly in the prostate gland through a precisely placed hollow needle. The radiation is quite strong but has a very short range, so that it destroys the tumor and minimizes damage to surrounding tissue. Chemotherapy may be used in advanced cases or in recurrences.

CRITICAL THINKING APPLICATION

Prostate conditions are a common cause for patients seen in Dr. Fineman's practice. Sara decides to review the information on the disorders that affect the prostate gland so she is better able to assist the physician and answer patient questions. What are the important details of prostate disease that Sara should remember?

Pathological Conditions of the Genital Organs

Epididymitis. *Epididymitis* is an inflammation of the tubular epididymis. It is most often attributed to a UTI, prostatitis, or a sexually transmitted disease (STD). Patients experience severe low abdominal and testicular pain as well as swelling and tenderness of the scrotum. If abscesses form and produce scar tissue, sterility can occur if both sides are affected. Antibiotics are the usual treatment. Rest and implementing a diet that avoids irritants such as spicy food and alcohol also encourage healing.

Balanitis. The inflammation of the glans penis and of the mucous membrane beneath it is known as *balanitis*. It occurs most often in uncircumcised patients with narrow foreskins that do not retract easily and in diabetic persons. It has many causes, including allergic reaction to certain chemicals, such as contraceptive foam; buildup of skin secretions, called *smegma*; and urinary tract and yeast infections. Treatment follows causative factors. Antibiotics are used for infections, and cleansing for buildup as well as avoidance of chemicals that cause reactions can help prevent the problem.

Hydrocele. During the descent of the testes, a small canal develops for them to pass through. If the canal does not close after birth, fluid from the peritoneal cavity may pass through and form in the scrotum. This is called a *hydrocele* and must be corrected surgically (Figure 37-14). Acquired hydroceles usually occur after middle age because of a scrotal injury or tumor, or can form in males who sit for extended periods of time, such as aging males in long-term care facilities. It is usually benign but can lead to painful scrotal swelling.

Testicular Cancer. Testicular tumors usually occur in young men and are generally malignant. The primary predisposing factor for development of testicular cancer is cryptorchism, and the tumor has a familial tendency. The patient complains of a hard, painless mass affecting one testicle. Treatment of the tumors is usually a combination of orchiectomy, radiation therapy, and sometimes chemotherapy. Survival rate in stage I is high, almost 95%. Testicular cancer can be detected early with monthly self-examination. Men should be taught to do this 3-minute examination beginning in puberty or at 15 years of age (Procedure 37-1).

The physician may provide pamphlets or a shower card on testicular self-examination (Figure 37-15). There are two ways the medical assistant can approach this teaching intervention. One way is to take the information to the patient, tell him to follow the pictures, and if he has any questions to call for clarification. Will he call? Would you? The second way is to take the pamphlet in and go over the instructions with the patient. Demonstrate the procedure on a model if one is available, or a male medical assistant could observe the patient doing the examination for the first time and provide feedback to ensure the patient knows how to do each step.

Impotence. The inability to achieve and maintain an erection sufficient for intercourse is a condition known as *impotence*. It has many causes, both psychological and physiological. Stress, anxiety, and fear of unsatisfactory performance as well as physical diseases that affect the vascular system, including arteriosclerosis, alcoholism, and diabetes mellitus, can all lead to impotence. Certain medications, such as some hypertensive treatments, have impotency as a side effect. This condition can be treated medically with sildenafil citrate (Viagra).

Infertility. Fertility peaks in men at the age of 25. Infertility may be caused by a problem in the man, a problem in the woman, or a combination of the two. In 10% to 20% of male infertility cases, there is no known cause. For the remaining cases, there can be many

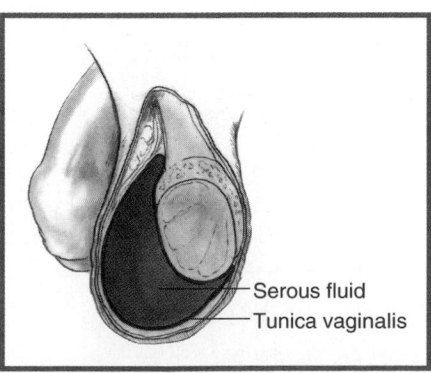

FIGURE 37-14   Hydrocele. (From Javis C: *Physical examination and health assessment, ed 2.* Philadelphia, 1996, WB Saunders.)

PROCEDURE **37-1**

Teaching Testicular Self-Examination

GOAL: To instruct the patient in the steps of testicular self-examination.

EQUIPMENT AND SUPPLIES

- Self-examination pamphlet and shower card
- Demonstration model
- Nonsterile gloves

PROCEDURAL STEPS

1 Wash your hands and collect needed supplies.
Purpose: Infection control.

2 Explain to the patient what you are going to do.
Purpose: Understanding helps with cooperation.

3 Begin by explaining to the patient that testicular cancer may produce no symptoms in the early stages, so it is important to examine the testes once a month for abnormal changes and early detection of the disease. This should begin at puberty or about 15 years of age. It is best to do the examination in the shower or in a warm bath. The total examination takes about 3 minutes.
Purpose: Heat causes the scrotal skin to relax, making the examination easier.

4 Examination of the testes: Start by holding the scrotum in the palms of the hands. Then feel one testicle. Apply a small amount of pressure. Slowly roll it between the fingers and try to find hard, painless lumps (Figure 1).

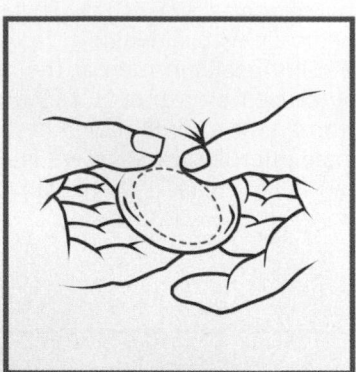

Figure 1

5 Examination of the epididymis: This comma-shaped cord is found behind the testis. Its job is to store and transport sperm. Tender when touched, it is the location of most noncancerous problems. Check for hard spots and lumps (Figure 2).

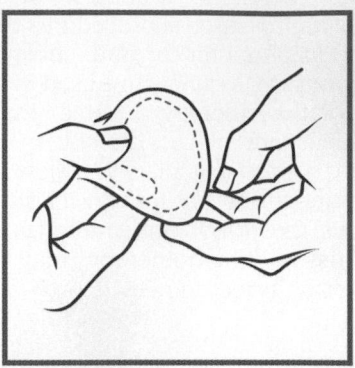

Figure 2

6 Examination of the vas deferens: Continue by examining the sperm-carrying tube that runs up the epididymis. Normally, the vas feels like a firm, movable, smooth tube (Figure 3).

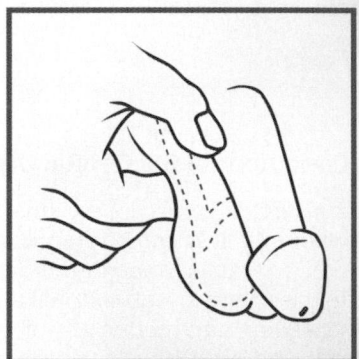

Figure 3

7 Now repeat the entire examination on the other side, beginning with the opposite testis.

8 After completing the examination on the model, ask the patient to do a return-examination using the model. A male assistant can have the patient do a self-testicular examination.

9 Give the pamphlet to the patient, along with the shower card, with instructions to hang it in the shower as a monthly reminder and guide.

10 Record the instructional transaction in the patient's medical record.
Purpose: If it is not recorded, it was not done.

See Appendix E for a charting example.

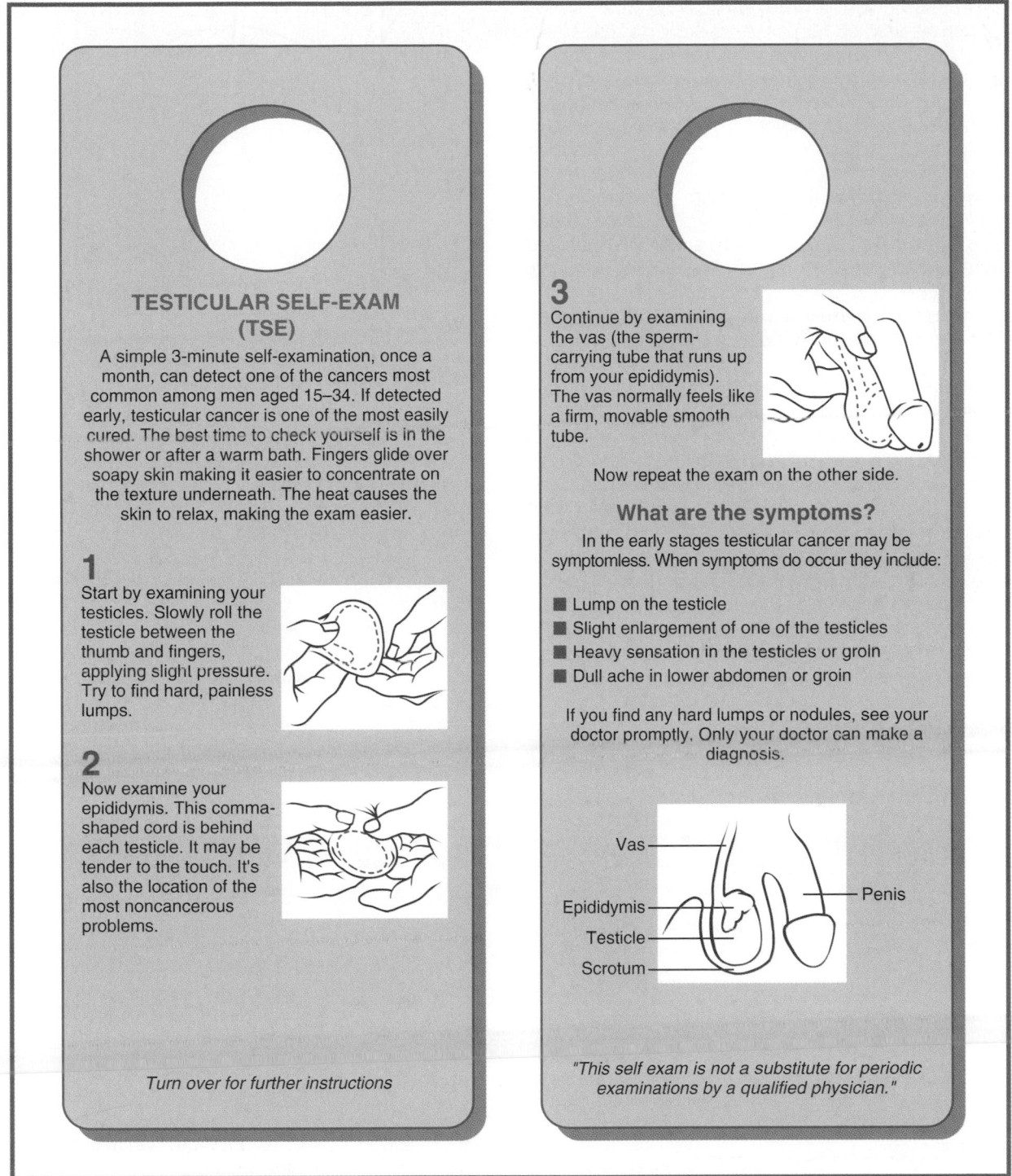

FIGURE 37-15   Self-examination shower card.

causative factors. Cryptorchism, stricture, and varicoceles (dilated spermatic cord veins); low sperm count and motility; obstruction of the vas deferens; and hormonal imbalances are all factors in infertility.

Examination of semen specimens is helpful in making a diagnosis of infertility. These tests determine the presence of sperm, the number of sperm in an ejaculation, and the health and motility of the sperm. The use of

ultrasonography is also helpful for detecting blockages of the vas deferens.

Sexually Transmitted Diseases

Diseases of the male reproductive system can also be acquired during sexual intercourse. No one is immune from these diseases, and it is possible to be infected with more than one at a time. There is no cure for viral STDs, such as HIV or herpes, and bacteria that cause infections are becoming increasingly resistant to antibiotic therapy. STDs are frequently asymptomatic and can cause serious health problems, even death (see Chapter 38 for gynecological pathological conditions). In this chapter we will discuss the signs, symptoms, and treatments for STDs in men (Table 37-2).

Bacterial STDs. Infections with *Gonorrhea* and *Chlamydia* organisms tend to coexist. An affected man develops symptoms associated with acute urethritis and epididymitis. Early detection is done by culturing discharge for the presence of the pathogen. *Chlamydia* is resistant to penicillin; thus, a regimen of antibiotics other than penicillin should be used if the patient has been diagnosed with both conditions.

A syphilitic lesion, called a *chancre*, develops on the male genitalia, usually the penis, within a few days to a few weeks after exposure (Figure 37-16). Syphilis is diagnosed through a complement fixation blood test, the VDRL or RPR. It can be treated successfully with penicillin but can go unnoticed. Without treatment, syphilis advances to a secondary phase indicated by a low-grade fever, headache, sore throat, and a rash that does not itch but that can affect any part of the body. The secondary phase is highly contagious but is still treatable with penicillin. The more advanced stages of the disease can remain undetected or dormant for years. Symptoms that appear years after the primary infection show multisystem involvement.

Viral STDs. Genital herpes causes a blistered, inflamed, painful rash on the penis, scrotum, and urethra. After

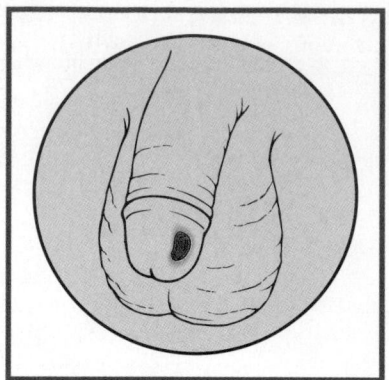

FIGURE 37-16 Syphilitic chancre. (From Frazier MS, Drzymkowski JA, Doty SJ: *Essentials of human diseases and conditions, ed. 2,* Philadelphia, 2000, WB Saunders.)

several days the vesicles rupture, resulting in a painful, ulcerated area. The lesions heal in 3 to 4 weeks, but the herpes virus then migrates to a nerve dermatome. Many factors can reactivate the disease at any time (e.g., stress and upper respiratory infections).

Genital warts are often asymptomatic in men and require preliminary treatment with acetic acid to be visualized. The incubation period for infections from the human papillomavirus (HPV) may be as long as 6 months. HPV infections in women greatly increase the risk of cervical cancer.

Acquired Immunodeficiency Syndrome. The most deadly sexually transmitted disease is acquired immuno-

TABLE 37-2	Sexually Transmitted Diseases in Men	
Disease (Causative organism)	**Signs and Symptoms**	**Treatment**
Chlamydia (*C. trachomatis*)	May be asymptomatic; dysuria; itching and white discharge from penis.	Curable with antibiotic therapy: azithromycin (Zithromax) or doxycycline (Vibramycin).
Genital herpes simplex virus (HSV-2)	Painful genital vesicles and ulcers; erythema and pruritus; tingling or shooting pain 1 to 2 days before outbreak; cycle through episodes. Viral shedding may occur during asymptomatic periods.	No cure, but antiviral therapy during episodes shortens duration of lesions: acyclovir (Zovirax), famciclovir (Famvir), or valacyclovir (Valtrex).
Genital warts (human papillomavirus, HPV)	Most prevalent STD; period of communicability is unknown; genital pinhead lesions may or may not be visible; warts tend to recur.	Goal of treatment is to remove symptomatic warts; cryotherapy for lesions; Podoflox solution or Imiquimod cream to lesions.
Gonorrhea (*N. gonorrhoeae*): bacteria	Dysuria; whitish discharge from penis that may become yellow-green; testicular pain.	Curable with antibiotic therapy: cefixime (Suprax), azithromycin, doxycycline.
Syphilis (*T. pallidum*): spirochete bacteria	Six stages that can affect multiple body systems; 10- to 90-day incubation; initial sign is a painless lesion, or *chancre*, at the exposure site (penis); serous discharge from chancre; lymphadenopathy. If not diagnosed and treated will advance to further stages.	Penicillin G (Wycillin); if patient is allergic to penicillin, doxycycline or tetracycline.
Trichomoniasis (*T. vaginalis*): protozoa	Asymptomatic in men.	Metronidazole.

deficiency syndrome (AIDS), which is caused by the human immunodeficiency virus (HIV). The virus invades T lymphocytes, destroying their ability to fight infection on the cellular level. Approximately 2 to 6 weeks after transmission of the virus, most individuals have flulike symptoms, including fever, *arthralgia* (joint pain), *myalgia* (muscle pain), lymphadenopathy, rash, night sweats, and malaise. After this, it could be 10 years or longer before clinical symptoms of AIDS occur. AIDS is marked by a wide range of **opportunistic infections** that develop because of very low T cell counts. These include *Pneumocystis carinii* pneumonia, candidiasis (yeast infection), Kaposi's sarcoma, dementia, and wasting syndrome. A patient is considered to be HIV positive when antibodies to the virus have been detected in the body, but not to have AIDS until the T cell count is below 200 mm^3 and/or opportunistic infections have been diagnosed.

HIV is transmitted by sexual exposure, intravenous drug use from shared needles, blood and blood products, and from an infected mother to her fetus. The HIV virus is fragile, cannot survive outside the body, and is easily destroyed by chemical disinfectants, such as household bleach. IV drug users who share needles and anyone having unprotected sex of any kind are at increased risk for contracting HIV. Healthcare workers are also at risk from accidental exposure in the workplace and should consistently employ standard precautions to protect themselves and their patients from this deadly disease.

The greatest increase in the incidence of the disease at this time is in young sexually active women. Treatment of infected pregnant women with the protease inhibitor azidothymidine (AZT) decreases the risk of HIV infection in the infant by two thirds. Many physicians recommend that all pregnant women be screened and appropriately treated for the disease to prevent the spread of the infection to newborns.

The most widely used screening test for HIV is the enzyme-linked immunosorbent assay (ELISA) blood test, which detects antibodies to HIV. Unfortunately, it may take up to 12 weeks or more after exposure for the antibody level to be high enough to be detected. Therefore the ELISA test cannot be used to detect the disease in its earliest, most infectious stages. A positive ELISA result is followed by the Western blot test to validate the results. If the ELISA result is negative but there has been reasonable risk that the patient was exposed to the disease, the ELISA should be repeated in 3 to 6 months. Research is currently underway on tests that will detect the presence of HIV infection as early as 2 to 6 weeks after exposure.

A combination of antiviral drugs is used to control the replication of the virus, but there is no cure for the disease. Which medications are selected depends on the clinical manifestations of the disease and the patient's current T cell levels. Research in the treatment of HIV is ongoing, so treatment recommendations are rapidly changing. Therefore, medical assistants working with HIV-positive patients must continually update their knowledge base. Currently, a protease inhibitor is prescribed, such as saquinavir (Invirase, Fortovase), indinavir (Crixivan), or ritonavir (Norvir), and a nucleoside analog,

such as didanosine (Videx), combivir (Retrovir), zalcitabine (Hivid), or stavudine (Zerit) is given with either AZT or 3TC. Pharmaceutical treatment is very expensive, typically more than $1000 per month, and complicated, because the medications must be taken as scheduled two or three times each day. However, current treatment plans have extended the subclinical stage of the disease, so that HIV-positive patients are avoiding opportunistic infections and postponing the development of full-blown AIDS longer than ever before.

The psychosocial needs of a patient diagnosed with HIV are far reaching. Treatment is designed to control the duplication of the virus in the body, but the patient will always be infectious. Prevention of disease transmission includes sexual abstinence, the consistent use of condoms, and precautions with blood spills; these options must be discussed with the patient. Community organizations could serve as a source of counseling and support for HIV-positive patients and their families. All information regarding the HIV status of a patient must be kept in strict confidence, with no documentation on the chart indicating the patient's disease status.

CRITICAL THINKING APPLICATION

The number of patients seen weekly in Dr. Fineman's practice who have sexually transmitted diseases continues to rise. Sara is responsible for telephone screening as well as clinical medical assisting practices. She is constantly being asked questions about the signs and symptoms of STDs and their treatment. What should Sara know about bacterial and viral STDs and their treatment?

The Medical Assistant's Role in Urological and Male Reproductive Examinations

Much of the diagnosis of urinary dysfunction depends on the patient's history, which may include frequency or urgency of urination, dysuria, or incontinence. A major part of the urological examination is urinalysis. The medical assistant must be able to instruct the patient in how to obtain a clean-catch urine specimen (see Chapter 49). It is best to have the patient void during an office visit so that the specimen can be examined immediately. The urologist may need to examine a catheterized specimen, which is collected using sterile technique. A small catheter is introduced into the bladder using sterile technique, and the urine is collected in a sterile container.

Catheterization

Because of the possibility of introducing contagious agents, catheterization is not the ideal method for obtaining a urine sample. Many experts believe that a midstream urine catch is as dependable a specimen as that obtained by an invasive catheterization.

REASONS FOR PERFORMING A CATHETERIZATION

- To relieve urinary retention
- To obtain a sterile urine sample
- To measure the amount of residual urine in the bladder
- To obtain a urine sample when it cannot be obtained by any other method
- To empty the bladder before and/or during surgery or before specific diagnostic procedures

---

Catheters vary in size, type, and construction material. When catheterization is performed to obtain the contents of the bladder, a straight or urethral (usually identified by number) No. 14 French is the most frequently used on female patients, and the coudé, with its slightly curved tip, may be preferred for males. Urologists' offices usually stock sizes 14 to 20 French for adults and sizes 8 to 10 French for children. In addition to the straight and coudé catheters, there is also the Foley or indwelling type, which is designed to remain in the bladder for a period of time. The Foley catheter has a small, inflatable balloon by its tip; when inflated, the balloon allows the catheter to remain in place within the bladder. To remove this type of catheter, the balloon must first be deflated (Figure 37-17). Catheterizations may be performed by the physician or by the medical assistant if he or she is specially trained to do so (Procedures 37-2 and 37-3).

 SAFETY ALERT: This procedure should never be performed by a medical assistant who does not have the necessary training in sterile technique or knowledge of the responsibilities of catheterization.

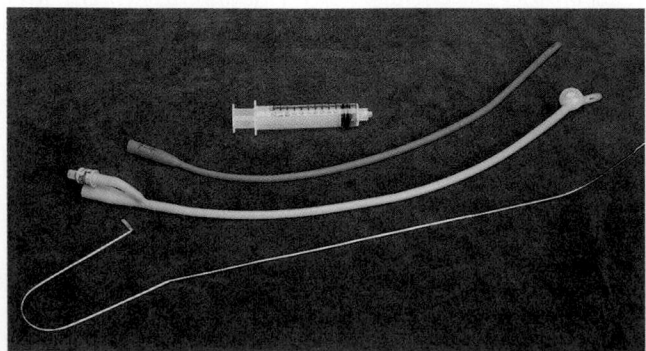

FIGURE 37-17 Types of catheters: straight and Foley with metal catheter guide. A syringe is used to inflate the balloon at the end of the Foley.

Assisting With a Urological Examination

No special instrument set-up is required for a routine urological examination unless a special procedure, such as obtaining a catheterized urine specimen, is to be performed. Most offices use prepackaged disposable units for catheterization and for bladder irrigation.

Both male and female patients disrobe and are given a gown. A woman is placed in the dorsal recumbent position, and a man is seated on the examining table. The physician instructs the patient about what is required. If the patient is a woman and the physician is a man, a female medical assistant must remain in the room with the patient while the patient's genital area is exposed and examined. The primary responsibility during the examination process is to assist the physician with any supplies and equipment needed and to maintain proper draping of the patient.

Assisting With a Male Reproductive Examination

A medical assistant should understand the male reproductive system and provide patient support throughout the examination. The patient should empty his bladder and disrobe before the physician begins the examination. A drape sheet is placed around the patient's waist, covering the lower extremities. A female medical assistant assists only if requested by the physician. The physician inspects the foreskin (if the patient is not circumcised) and the glans penis. The penis and scrotum are palpated for possible masses and tenderness. If the physician uses a transilluminator, the assistant may be asked to darken the room. The patient is also examined for possible inguinal hernias, and a rectal examination of the prostate gland completes the physical assessment.

If the assistant is a man, he may be needed to assist the physician with the examination and aid the patient with draping and positioning. The assistant should watch the patient for signs of discomfort and anxiety; if these signs are noted, he should notify the physician immediately. Answering the patient's questions and reinforcing understanding of the physician's orders are among the assistant's responsibilities.

Vasectomy

A vasectomy is a surgical procedure for sterilizing a male patient (Figure 37-18). It is performed by surgically removing a section of each vas deferens to stop sperm from reaching the prostate and mixing with semen. The sexual characteristics of the patient remain the same, and the ability to have an erection is entirely unchanged.

The procedure can be performed in a physician's office with a local anesthetic agent, such as lidocaine (Xylocaine). The physician makes one or two small incisions with a scalpel to reach and clip the vas deferens bilaterally and then closes the site with sutures. Patients must be aware that sterility is not immediate; some sperm may be present in the ducts. It may take as long as 1 month for the semen to be sperm free. Patients should have two sperm counts 4 to 6 weeks apart to ensure the effectiveness of the procedure.

PROCEDURE **37-2**

Catheterization of a Female Patient

GOAL: To successfully empty the bladder via sterile catheterization.

EQUIPMENT AND SUPPLIES

- Sterile urethral catheterization kit containing:
- Straight catheter
- Sterile drapes
- Sterile lubricant
- Sterile tray
- Two pairs of sterile gloves
- Sterile cotton balls or gauze squares
- Povidone-iodine solution (Betadine)
- Specimen container and laboratory slip
- Waterproof pad
- Gooseneck lamp

PROCEDURAL STEPS

A demonstration model has been used to illustrate this procedure.

1 Wash your hands and collect necessary supplies.
Purpose: Infection control.

2 Explain the procedure to the patient and have the patient remove necessary clothing.
Purpose: Knowledge leads to patient cooperation.

3 Place the patient in the dorsal recumbent position (Figure 1).

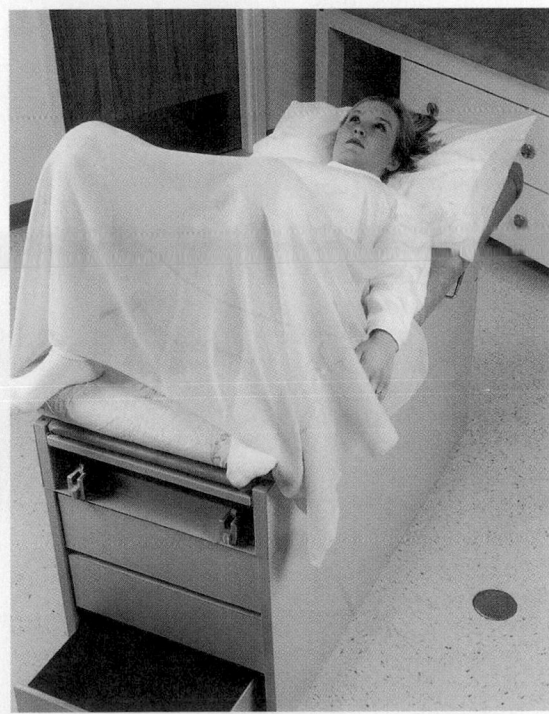

Figure 1

4 Drape the patient's upper body, leaving the genital area exposed.
Purpose: The drape provides a degree of dignity and comfort.

5 Position a gooseneck lamp directed at the genital area.
Purpose: The female urinary meatus may be difficult to identify.

6 Wash your hands and open the catheterization tray on a clean stable surface using sterile techniques; often a Mayo stand is used.

7 Open the sterile underpad drape and hold the underpad so that the undersurface of the two corners encircles your hands. Slide it under the patient while she is lifting her hips off the table. *Be careful not to touch the patient or the table with your hands.* Ask the patient to keep her knees apart.

8 Open the sterile drape and place it over the patient's exposed genital area so that the vulvar area is exposed.

9 Place the insertion kit and any other supplies on the sterile drape between the patient's legs.

10 Put on sterile gloves following sterile procedure (see Chapter 54). Open the sterile povidone-iodine (Betadine) package and pour it over cotton balls or gauze squares in the tray.

11 Open the sterile lubricant package and place it on the sterile field.

12 Open all other items, including the catheter. Stand the specimen container on the tray.

13 With the thumb and index finger of your nondominant hand, separate the patient's labia as widely as possible. *Your nondominant hand must maintain this position throughout the balance of the procedure. Take care that your dominant hand does not touch the patient during the cleansing process.* With your dominant hand, pick up one of the povidone-iodine–soaked gauze squares and wipe from top to bottom on one side of the labia. Discard the used gauze (Figure 2).

Continued

PROCEDURE **37-2—Cont'd**

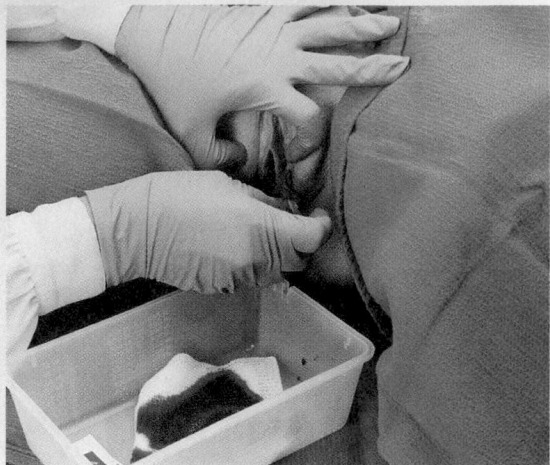

Figure 2

14 Pick up another gauze square and wipe from top to bottom on the other side of the labia. Discard the gauze.

15 Pick up another gauze square and using a circular motion wipe over the urinary meatus from the inside outward. Discard the gauze.

16 With your dominant hand, pick up the catheter about 3 inches from the insertion end and dip the tip into the sterile lubricant. Position the other end of the catheter in the collection compartment of the kit tray.

17 Insert the lubricated tip into the urinary meatus and continue inserting the catheter 2 to 3 inches or until urine begins flowing out the catheter into the kit tray (Figure 3). *Never force the catheter.*

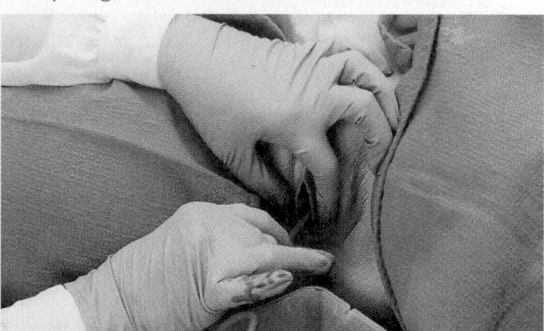

Figure 3

Purpose: Resistance may indicate a problem. Remove the catheter and notify the physician.

18 Let some of the urine flow and then place the specimen container over the end of the catheter and collect the specimen (Figure 4).

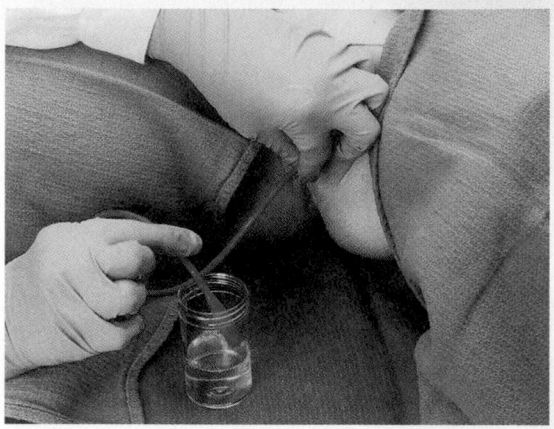

Figure 4

19 When the bladder is completely emptied, and the urine stops flowing, gently remove the catheter. If more than 500 ml of urine drains into the collection tray, clamp the catheter and wait 10 to 15 minutes, then reopen the catheter and allow the bladder to empty.

Purpose: A distended bladder that is emptied too quickly may cause bladder spasm.

20 Secure the lid to the urine specimen.

Purpose: Protects the sterility of the specimen.

21 Remove all supplies, dispose of them according to standard precautions, and wash your hands.

22 Assist the patient off the table and with dressing as needed.

23 Complete the laboratory requisition and record the procedure in the patient's chart, including the number of milliliters of urine removed from the bladder.

Purpose: A procedure is considered not done until it is entered into the patient's record.

See Appendix E for a charting example.

CRITICAL THINKING APPLICATION

Sara routinely sets up for and assists Dr. Fineman with urological and male reproductive examinations. She is also responsible for orienting new employees of the practice and helping them learn the procedures that typically occur in the office. Summarize the role of a medical assistant in helping with these examinations.

Patient Education

Most men under the age of 50 have not seen a physician in years. Medical studies reveal that attitude, not biology, has a lot to do with the difference between men's and women's life spans. Men's misconceptions about their invincibility make them more vulnerable to illnesses and death. The solution to maintaining good health is preventive care, and the first step is establishing a good rapport with a physician of choice. As a general

PROCEDURE **37-3**

Catheterization of a Male Patient

GOAL: To successfully obtain a urinary specimen through catheterization.

EQUIPMENT AND SUPPLIES

- Sterile urethral catheterization kit containing:
- Sterile straight catheter
- Sterile drapes
- Sterile lubricant
- Sterile forceps
- Sterile collection tray
- Two pairs of sterile gloves
- Sterile cotton balls
- Povidone-iodine solution (Betadine)
- Specimen container
- Waterproof pad

PROCEDURAL STEPS

1 Wash your hands and collect the necessary supplies.
Purpose: Infection control.

2 Explain the procedure to the patient and ask him to remove his pants and underwear.
Purpose: Knowledge leads to patient cooperation.

3 Place the patient in the supine position.

4 Wash your hands and open the catheterization kit on a clean surface following sterile technique; often a Mayo stand is used.

5 Hold the sterile underpad so that the undersurface of the two corners encircles your hands. Position it over the patient's thighs under his penis using sterile technique (Figure 1).
Purpose: Provides a sterile field.

6 Put on sterile gloves.

7 Open the fenestrated drape and position it so the opening exposes the penis (Figure 2). Be careful not to touch the patient or the table.

8 Place the sterile kit on the table on top of the sterile drape and open all the supplies as in Procedure 37-2, steps 10 through 12.

9 Grasp the penis below the glans with your nondominant hand. In uncircumcised males, you must pull back the foreskin to see the meatus. You must do this and hold the penis upright with your nondominant hand *only*.

10 Using your dominant hand and forceps, pick up a povidone-iodine (Betadine)–soaked cotton ball and clean around the meatus in circular motions from the center outward. Repeat this a total of three times using a fresh soaked cotton ball each time (Figure 3).

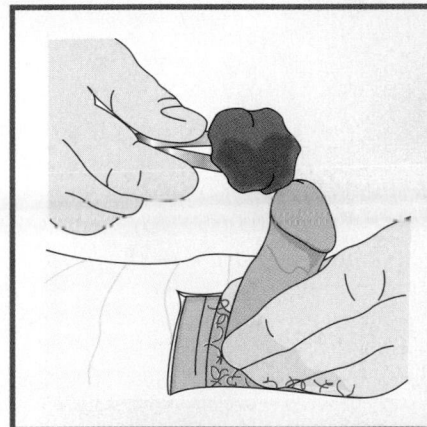

Figure 3

Purpose: Ensures that the urinary meatus is properly cleaned.

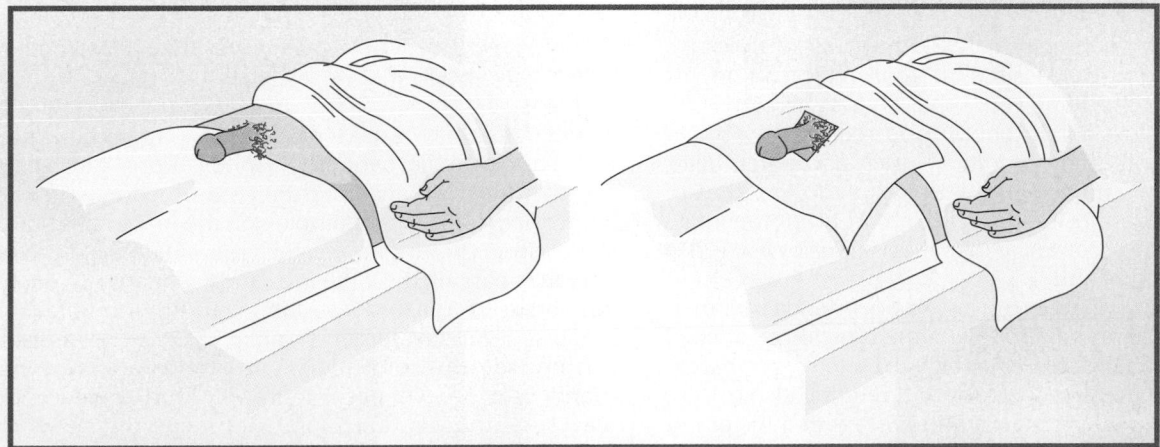

Figure 1 and 2

Continued

PROCEDURE **37-3—Cont'd**

11 With your dominant hand, lubricate the tip of the catheter at least 7 inches. Be sure to put the other end of the catheter into the collection compartment of the kit tray.

12 Hold the shaft of the penis straight and upright with your nondominant hand and apply gentle traction to straighten the urethra. Ask the patient to bear down as if to urinate. Gently insert the lubricated catheter tip into the urinary meatus 6 to 8 inches or until urine begins flowing out of the catheter (Figure 4). *Never force the catheter; if you meet resistance, remove the catheter and notify the physician.*

13 Obtain the specimen (Figure 5) and complete the procedure following steps 19 through 23 of the female catheterization procedure.

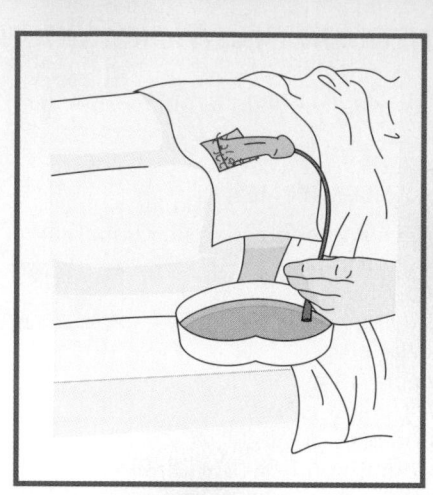

Figure 5

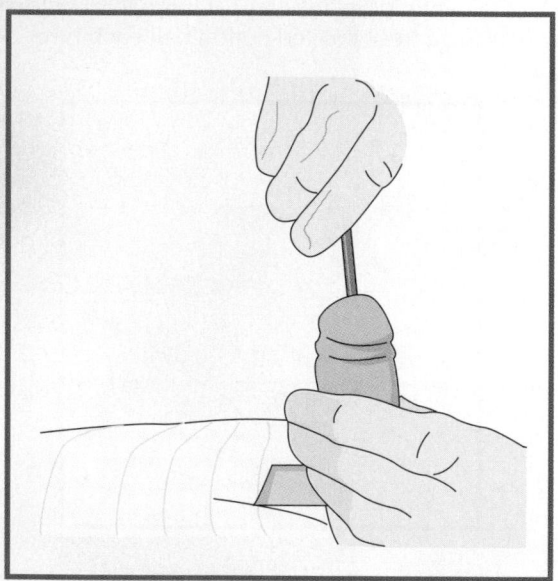

Figure 4

rule, a man in good health should have three checkups in his twenties, from three to four checkups in his thirties, and a checkup every other year in his forties. At the age of 50, a yearly checkup is recommended. In addition to testing for conditions such as cancer, heart disease, stroke, and diabetes, four of the top male health problems, the entire medical team can empower male patients with the knowledge to make responsible decisions regarding good health.

The American Cancer Society recommends that men 50 years of age and older have annual fecal occult stool test and prostate screening (digital rectal examination and PSA blood test), with prostate screening also recommended at age 40 for blacks and men with a history of prostate cancer. In addition, a sigmoidoscopy or complete colonoscopy should be performed initially at the age of

50 and every 3 to 5 years after that to screen for colorectal cancer.

There are many procedures required in a urology setting, and there is a strong need for patient education, especially of male patients. A medical assistant should see this need as an opportunity to become a greater asset to the physician/employer, the patient, and the profession. The urinary system remains a very private, personal part of the patient's body. Patients often feel embarrassed to ask questions about how to obtain the requested urine or semen sample. The medical assistant can provide this information in a sincere, confidential manner to relieve patient anxiety and worry. Using diagrams, models, and handouts helps the patient to understand the disease process and treatment regimen and also encourages patient compliance.

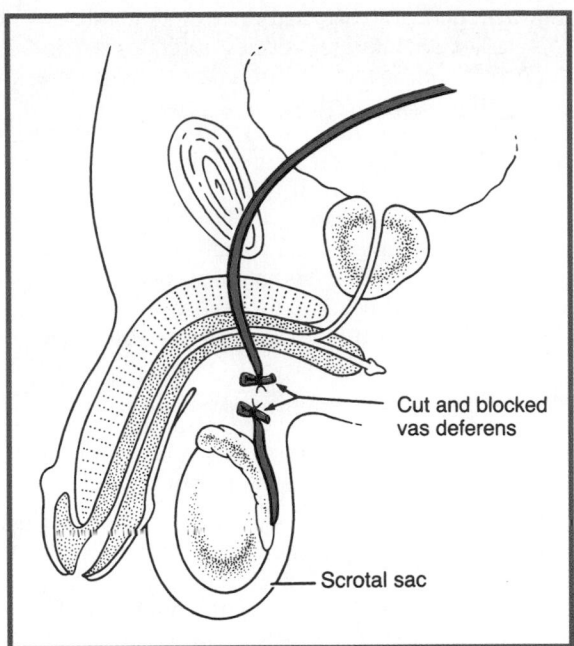

Cut and blocked vas deferens

Scrotal sac

FIGURE 37-18 Vasectomy. (From Chabner DE: *The language of medicine, ed.* 6, Philadelphia, 2001, WB Saunders.)

Legal and Ethical Issues

When working in a urology office, a medical assistant must be very careful to ensure that patients have given informed consent for the procedures to be performed. If the patient refuses a procedure, the assistant needs to have the patient sign the appropriate informed refusal forms; these forms are then included in the medical record. All patient education should be done after the physician has completed the explanation and has given the assistant instructions to do so. Never diagnose, prescribe, or offer comment about a patient's condition. Medical assistants who overstep their professional boundaries may place the physician and themselves in legal jeopardy. Remember that the patient who is legally informed and satisfied with the care received is less likely to find the need to take legal action against the physician and the assistant.

The urology practice manages many sensitive patient issues that require strict adherence to confidentiality guidelines. This is especially true for a patient who has a functional disorder with the reproductive system or is diagnosed with an STD. There are special legal guidelines regarding patients diagnosed with HIV that must be strictly followed to avoid litigation. There should be no evidence of HIV status on the patient's chart, nor should it be mentioned by name in any documentation entries.

SUMMARY OF SCENARIO

Sara enjoys working with Dr. Fineman and the urological patients seen in the practice. She recognizes the need to stay current with information regarding disorders of the system and their treatment. Sara continues to learn on the job and through workshops about the urinary system and current therapies. Her expertise is constantly growing, and she uses this knowledge to help with patient education, manage telephone screening, and assist Dr. Fineman with procedures in the office. She is also working on building a database with local resources, support groups, and Internet sites that could be helpful for patients confronted with urological or male reproductive system problems.

SUMMARY OF LEARNING OBJECTIVES

■ The urinary system is made up of two kidneys located bilaterally in the retroperitoneum, two ureters, the urinary bladder, and the urethra. The main function of the urinary system is to remove waste products from the body. The urinary system also helps to maintain homeostasis by regulating water, electrolytes, and acid-base levels; activating vitamin D, which encourages calcium ion absorption; secreting the hormone erythropoietin, which helps control the rate of red blood cell formation; and maintaining blood pressure by the secretion of the enzyme renin. There are three processes involved in urine formation: filtration, reabsorption, and excretion. The cortex contains the functional unit of the kidney, the nephron unit, through which waste materials are filtered and substances reabsorbed. By the time the waste material reaches the calyx, it is in the form of urine, which is emptied out of the kidneys through bilateral ureters to the urinary bladder. When the bladder is full, sphincters open and urine flows into the urethra.

■ The urinary tract is made up of a continuous mucosal lining, which gives organisms that enter the urethra a direct pathway through the system.

■ A wide range of symptoms occur in patients with disorders of the renal system; the most common involves changes in the frequency of urination. Dysuria (difficult or painful urination), urgency, retention, and incontinence are common symptoms. Abnormal functions of any part of the urinary tract can often be determined with urinalysis, blood urea nitrogen (BUN) levels, and with analysis of creatinine clearance.

■ Diagnostic procedures for the urological system include a kidney-ureter-bladder (KUB) x-ray examination, which involves a flat plate radiograph of the abdomen that shows the size, shape, location, and any malformations of the kidneys and bladder; renal scanning, which is a nuclear scan to determine size, shape, and function of the kidney or to diagnose obstruction or hypertension; cystography or voiding cystography, which is an x-ray examination with contrast dye to study the bladder; an intravenous pyelogram, in which x-ray films are made after a dye is injected to show passage through the urinary system and to diagnose tumors, calculi, or obstructions; a renal arteriogram, in which dye is injected into the renal artery to visualize blood flow through the kidneys; a renal CT, which provides transverse views of the kidneys to detect tumors, abscesses, or hydronephrosis; renal ultrasonography, which can be used to detect functional defects in the kidneys or polycystic disease; cystoscopy, which provides an endoscopic view of the urethra and bladder; and a retrograde pyelogram, which visualizes the bladder, ureters, and kidneys after injection of a dye.

■ Most UTIs are ascending, starting with pathogens in the perineal area and infecting the continuous mucosa up through the urethra, bladder, and ureters, to the kidneys. Infection and inflammation of the urethra is called urethritis and that of the bladder is cystitis. The resident flora of the colon, *Escherichia coli*, is the usual causative agent. Pyelonephritis, an inflammation of the renal pelvis and kidney, is the most common type of renal disease. It is caused by bacteria that ascend from the lower urinary tract and is caused by conditions such as urinary retention or obstruction that promote urinary stasis and the growth of bacteria. Acute glomerulonephritis, the degenerative inflammation of the glomeruli, usually develops in children and adolescents about 2 weeks after a streptococcal infection, such as strep throat or scarlet fever. Chronic glomerulonephritis causes progressive, irreversible renal damage that may result in renal failure and is caused by an antigen-antibody reaction within the glomerular capsule that ultimately destroys the nephron unit.

■ Renal calculi are created when salts in the urine collect in the kidney or when fluid intake is low, creating a highly concentrated filtrate. They are a common problem and tend to recur if the cause of formation is not treated. Small stones usually do not cause any difficulty until they grow large enough to lodge in the ureters or renal pelvis. This blockage can also result in hydronephrosis, which is a backup of urine that causes dilation of the calyces and increased pressure on the nephron units. Polycystic kidney disease is an autosomal dominant genetic disorder that is slowly progressive and irreversible, causing the formation of multiple grape-like cysts in the kidney. As the cysts enlarge, they compress the surrounding tissue, causing necrosis, uremia, and renal failure. Bladder cancer is characterized by one or more tumors that can reappear. The tumor is invasive and can metastasize through the blood or surrounding pelvic lymph nodes. Adenocarcinoma of the kidney is a primary tumor that is initially asymptomatic so it frequently has metastasized before being diagnosed. Wilms' tumor is cancer of the kidney in children resulting from an inherited genetic defect.

■ Acute renal failure has a sudden, severe onset caused by exposure to toxic chemicals, severe or prolonged circulatory or cardiogenic shock that might occur from serious burns or heart disease, or from an acute bilateral kidney infection or inflammation. Chronic renal failure is a slowly progressive process that is caused by the gradual destruction of the ability of the kidneys to filter waste materials. Dialysis is used to treat acute renal failure until the problem is reversed or for those patients in end-stage renal disease until a transplant can be done. There are two forms of dialysis: hemodialysis and peritoneal dialysis. For hemodialysis, a machine known as an artificial kidney is used to filter out waste products in the blood and return the cleansed blood to the body. In peritoneal dialysis, a dialyzing fluid is introduced in the patient's abdomen to absorb waste products, which are drained from the abdominal cavity by gravity into a container. It can be performed by the patient at home.

■ Pediatric urological disorders include enuresis, which is an inability to control urination that may be caused by physical or psychological disorders; urine reflux disorder, which is the backward flow of urine into the ureters when voiding, usually caused by an infection; and cryptorchism, which is the failure of one or both testes to descend into the scrotum and can be corrected with an orchiopexy surgical procedure.

■ The male reproductive system is made up of a pair of testes contained in the scrotum. The testes consist of lobules that contain the seminiferous tubule, where spermatozoa are produced. The sperm cells are tadpolelike structures less than 0.1 mm long that are carried to the epididymis for maturation. The epididymis is a long, coiled tube that rests on the top and lateral side of each testis. Peristaltic waves in the epididymis help the sperm move into the vas deferens, where the sperm is stored until ejaculation. The prostate gland surrounds the urethra at the base of the bladder. It secretes a thin fluid with an alkaline pH that neutralizes the acidic sperm-containing fluid and vaginal secretions to provide an optimum pH for fertilization. The organ of male copulation is the penis, which has a slightly enlarged end called the glans penis. Hormone production is also an important aspect of the male reproductive system. As a group, the male sex hormones are called androgens. The most influential product of hormone production is testosterone, which stimulates the testes to enlarge, increases body hair growth, thickens skin and bone, increases muscle growth, and matures sperm cells.

■ Inflammation of the prostate usually develops in the presence of infection. The common symptoms are dysuria, tenderness of the prostate region, and secretion of pus from the tip of the penis. The swelling of the prostate gland, benign prostatic hypertrophy, partially blocks the flow of urine, creating a medium for bacterial infection that can lead to cystitis. The diagnosis is made from patient complaints and a digital rectal examination by which the physician can palpate the enlarged gland. Treatment includes the use of alpha-adrenergic blockers or surgical removal of the prostate gland through a transurethral resection. Cancer of the prostate is common in men older than 50 years of age and ranks as the second highest cause of male cancer deaths, behind lung cancer. Patients may experience urinary obstruction, increased bouts of urinary infection, and frequent nocturia. Prostate cancer is diagnosed by a digital rectal examination that identifies a firm or irregular area in the prostate and the PSA blood test. The extent of the prostate cancer will dictate treatment options, which include hormone therapy, radiation, chemotherapy, transurethral resection, orchiectomy, or radical prostatectomy.

■ Male genital pathological conditions include epididymitis, usually caused by a UTI, prostatitis, or an STD. Patients experience severe low abdominal and testicular pain as well as swelling and tenderness of the scrotum. The inflammation of the glans penis and of the mucous membrane beneath it is called balanitis. It occurs most often in uncircumcised patients with narrow foreskins that do not retract easily and in diabetic patients. Antibiotics are used for infections, cleansing any buildup of smegma, and avoidance of chemicals that cause reactions can help avoid the problem. Testicular tumors usually occur in young men and are generally malignant. The patient complains of a hard, painless, mass affecting one testicle. Treatment of the tumors is usually a combination of orchiectomy, radiation therapy, and sometimes chemotherapy. Impotence is the inability to achieve and maintain an erection sufficient for intercourse. It has many causes, both psychological and physiological. This condition can be treated medically with sildenafil citrate (Viagra). Male infertility may be caused by cryptorchism, stricture, and varicoceles; low sperm count and motility; obstruction of the vas deferens; and hormonal imbalances. Examination of semen specimens is helpful in making a diagnosis of infertility.

■ There is no cure for viral STDs, such as HIV or herpes, and bacterial causes of infection are becoming increasingly resistant to antibiotic therapy. STDs are frequently asymptomatic and can cause serious health problems, even death. Table 37-2 summarizes the signs and symptoms as well as treatment of STDs in men. Bacterial STDs include gonorrhea and chlamydial infections, which tend to coexist. Symptoms are associated with acute urethritis and epididymitis. Chlamydia is resistant to penicillin; thus, a regimen of antibiotics other than penicillin should be used if the patient has been diagnosed with both conditions. Syphilis begins with a chancre on the male genitalia within a few days to a few weeks after exposure. It is diagnosed with the VDRL or RPR blood test and can be treated successfully with penicillin in the early stages.

Genital herpes is a viral STD that causes a blistered, inflamed, painful rash on the penis, scrotum, and urethra. The lesions heal in 3 to 4 weeks, but the virus can reactivate at any time. Genital warts are often asymptomatic in men and require preliminary treatment with acetic acid to be visualized.

■ The human immunodeficiency virus (HIV) invades T lymphocytes, destroying their ability to fight infection on the cellular level. Approximately 2 to 6 weeks after transmission of the virus, most individuals have flulike symptoms, including fever, arthralgia, myalgia, lymphadenopathy, rash, night sweats, and malaise. After this, it could be as long as 8 years before clinical symptoms of AIDS occur. AIDS is marked by a wide range of opportunistic infections that develop because of very low T cell counts. These include *Pneumocystis carinii* pneumonia, candidiasis, Kaposi's sarcoma, dementia, and wasting syndrome. A patient is considered to be HIV positive when the virus has been detected in the body but not to have full-blown AIDS until the T cell count is below 200 mm^3 and opportunistic infections have been diagnosed. HIV is transmitted by sexual exposure, intravenous drug use from shared needles, blood and blood products, and from an infected mother to the fetus. The HIV virus is fragile, cannot survive outside the body, and is easily destroyed by chemical disinfectants, such as household bleach. The most widely used screening test for HIV is the ELISA blood test, which detects antibodies to HIV. A positive ELISA is followed by the Western blot test to validate the results. A combination of antiviral drugs is used to control the replication of the virus, but there is no cure for the disease. The medications selected depend upon the clinical manifestations of the disease and current T cell levels.

■ The medical assistant's role in a urology practice includes taking a complete patient history, detailing frequency or urgency of urination, dysuria, or incontinence; instructing the patient on how to obtain a clean-catch urine specimen and performing a urinalysis; collecting a catheterized urine specimen; and assisting with a urological or male reproductive examination, which includes providing patient support. Answering the patient's questions and reinforcing understanding of the physician's orders are among the assistant's responsibilities.

KEY INTERNET WEBSITES

- AIDS Clinical Trials Information Service
- AIDS Treatment Information Service
- CDC National AIDS Hotline
- National Association of People With AIDS
- National Kidney Foundation
  For active weblinks to each website visit
  http://evolve.elsevier.com/Kinn/

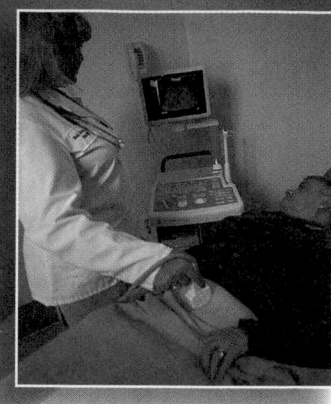

CHAPTER 38

Scenario

Betsy Davis, CMA, was recently hired by the University Women's Hospital to work for Dr. Erin Beck, an obstetrician/gynecologist for a busy family-centered care facility in her community. Betsy has worked for a family practice physician for 3 years, but this is her first position in a specialty practice. Betsy is excited about the opportunity to focus on women's health issues and is especially interested in helping in the obstetrical area of the practice.

Assisting in Obstetrics and Gynecology

Learning Objectives

- Define and spell the terms listed in the vocabulary.
- Identify the major organs of the female reproductive system and explain the primary function of each.
- Trace the ovum through the three phases of menstruation.
- Compare and contrast various contraceptive methods.
- Summarize menstrual disorders and conditions.
- Distinguish between different types of gynecological infections.
- Differentiate between benign and malignant neoplasms of the female reproductive system.
- Compare positional disorders of the pelvic region.
- Summarize the process of pregnancy and parturition.
- Describe the common complications of pregnancy.
- Specify the signs, symptoms, and treatments of menopause.
- Outline the medical assistant's role in the gynecological and reproductive examinations.
- Distinguish between diagnostic tests that may be done to evaluate the female reproductive system.
- Prepare for and assist with the female examination, including a Papanicolaou (Pap) test.
- Teach the patient how to perform a breast self-examination.
- Describe cryosurgery preparation to a patient.
- Determine the estimated day of delivery when given the date of the last menstrual period.
- Assist with the prenatal examination.

National Curriculum Competencies

CLINICAL COMPETENCIES

4e. Prepare patients for and assist with routine and specialty examinations

4f. Prepare patients for and assist with procedures, treatments, and minor office surgery

4g. Apply pharmacology principles to prepare and administer oral and parenteral medications

TRANSDISCIPLINARY COMPETENCIES

3b. Instruct individuals according to their needs

3d. Provide instruction for health maintenance and disease prevention

Vocabulary

adnexal Pertaining to adjacent or accessory parts.

clitoris Small, elongated erectile body situated above the urinary meatus at the superior point of the labia minora.

coitus Sexual union between male and female, also known as intercourse.

colostrum Thin, yellow, milky fluid secreted by the mammary glands a few days before and after delivery.

dilation The opening of the cervix through the process of labor, measured as 0 to 10 cm dilated.

dilatation and curettage The widening of the cervix and scraping of the endometrial wall of the uterus.

effacement The thinning of the cervix during labor measured in percentages from 0 to 100 effaced.

endocervical curettage The scraping of cells from the wall of the uterus.

idiopathic Without an apparent or known cause.

mons pubis Fat pad that covers the symphysis pubis.

multiparous Pertaining to women who have had two or more pregnancies.

myelomeningocele A herniation of a portion of the spinal cord and its meninges that protrudes through a congenital opening in the vertebral column.

neural tube defect Any of a group of congenital anomalies involving the brain and spinal column that are caused by failure of the neural tube to close during embryonic development.

parturition Act or process of giving birth to a child.

stereotactic An x-ray procedure to guide the insertion of a needle into a specific area of the breast.

teratogen Substance that results in severe fetal deformities.

vulva The external female genitalia, which begins at the mons pubis and terminates at the anus.

The branch of medicine that deals with pregnancy, labor, and the postnatal period is known as *obstetrics*, and the branch of medicine that deals with diseases of the genital tract in women is called *gynecology*. Frequently, a physician practices both specialties and is known as an *OB/GYN physician*. Assessment of the female reproductive system is an important part of health care. Often, patients are hesitant and uncomfortable with talking about sexual matters and wait until symptoms are intolerable or disease is advanced before seeking medical care. In addition to the signs and symptoms of disease, the medical assistant must be aware of the patient's emotional state and give support when needed.

Anatomy and Physiology

The Female Reproductive System

The female reproductive system contains both internal and external organs. The internal organs are located within the pelvis and cannot be seen without special instrumentation, such as a vaginal speculum or a laparoscope. The external organs can be seen during the physical examination.

The primary parts of the female reproductive system are the **vulva**, vagina, uterus, fallopian tubes, and ovaries (Figure 38-1). The vulva includes the **clitoris**, the urethral meatus, and the vaginal orifice. These structures are covered by two sets of lips of tissue. The *labia minora* is a thin layer of skin extending from the top of the clitoris to the base of the vaginal opening. The external set is known as the *labia majora*, and these, along with the **mons pubis**, are covered with hair in the adult.

The vagina is the structure that connects the internal and external organs. This tubelike structure is constructed to receive the penis during **coitus**. It is lubricated by a mucous membrane lining, and its walls are made up of overlapping tissue in the form of *rugae* (overlapping tissue) so that the vagina can expand during the birth of an infant. At the distal end of the vagina is the cervix, often called the *neck of the uterus*, which is approximately 1 to 1½ inches long. The *uterus* is an upside-down pear-shaped muscular organ with the sole purpose of housing and nourishing the fetus from implantation shortly after conception until **parturition**. The uterine walls have three layers. The inner layer is the *endometrium*, which is rich in blood and will change in consistency during the menstrual cycle. The middle layer is the *myometrium*. This is the powerful muscular layer that contracts to make the birth of the baby possible. The outer layer is the *perimetrium*, which protects the structure and attaches to ligaments that support and hold the uterus in place (Figure 38-2).

On either side of the **fundus** of the uterus are the fallopian tubes, which are also called the *oviducts*. These tubes extend from the uterus to the ovaries but do not attach to the ovaries. The distal end of the tube opens freely into the abdominopelvic cavity and acts as the passageway for the ovum to the uterus and for the sperm as they search for the ovum. At the distal end of the fallopian tubes are finger-like projections called *fimbriae*. The fimbriae move in a wave-like pattern to draw the released ovum into the tube.

The ovaries are almond-shaped organs that produce and release the egg (ovum) and excrete hormones necessary for the development of secondary sexual characteristics and the maintenance of a pregnancy. The hormones progesterone and estrogen are secreted by the ovaries, and they regulate reproductive function. For pregnancy to occur, the vagina receives the sperm from the male, which move up through the opening in the cervix called the *cervical os*, through the uterus, and into the fallopian tube. As many as 200 to 600 million sperm can be deposited in the vagina, with about 100,000 surviving the acidic content of the vagina to swim toward the egg.

Fertilization occurs when one sperm cell penetrates and fertilizes an egg. Fertilization usually takes place in the distal third of the fallopian tube. The tiny fertilized ovum, now called a zygote, moves by peristalsis and the massaging motion of the cilia that line the fallopian tube into the uterus and implants itself into the uterine wall. After implantation occurs, the placenta forms and will supply the new life with all the nourishment needed for

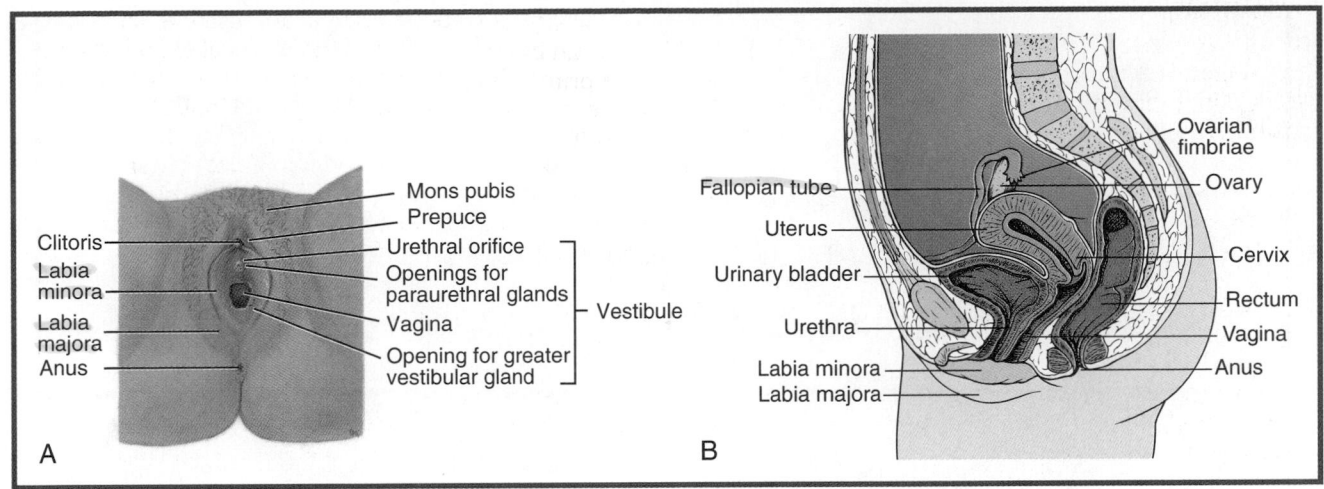

FIGURE 38-1   **A**, Female external genitalia. **B**, Normal female reproductive system. (**A** From Applegate EJ: *The anatomy and physiology learning system*. Philadelphia, 1995, WB Saunders; **B** From Frazier MS, Drymkowski JA: *Essentials of human diseases and conditions*, ed 2. Philadelphia, 2000, WB Saunders.)

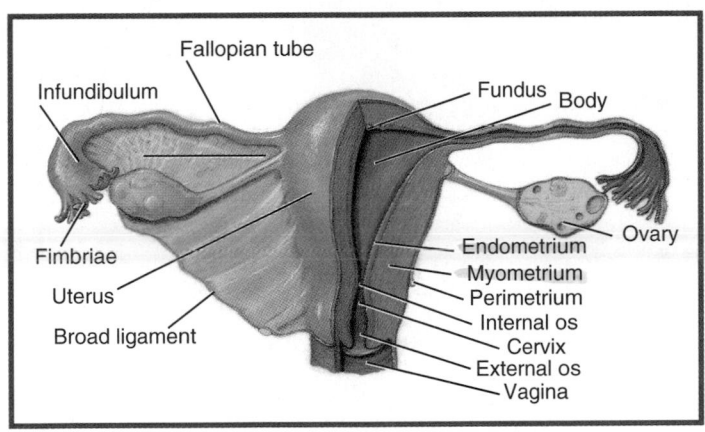

FIGURE 38-2   Uterus and fallopian tubes. (Modified from Applegate EJ: *The anatomy and physiology learning system*, Philadelphia, 1995, WB Saunders.)

its development. Once pregnancy begins, the serum levels of human chorionic gonadotropin (hCG) rise and spill into the female's urine, where it can be detected with a pregnancy test.

Breast Tissue

Mammary tissue develops from increased estrogen secretion, which occurs during puberty. In the center of each breast is a nipple, which is surrounded by a pigmented region called the *areola*. Inside the breast are 15 to 20 lobes with their subunits, lobules of glandular tissue that are separated by connective support tissue and surrounded by adipose tissue. The amount and distribution of the adipose tissue determine the size and shape of the breast (Figure 38-3). Breast tissue also contains mammary glands, which are modified sweat glands that become the organs of milk production as well as a system of ducts for milk collection that open into the nipple. Mammary ducts respond to elevated levels of estrogen and progesterone by increasing in size, resulting in premenstrual fullness and tenderness of the breasts.

Four hormones control the mammary glands. *Estrogen* is responsible for the increase in size, *progesterone* stimulates the development of the duct system, *prolactin* stimulates the production of milk, and *oxytocin* causes the ejection of the milk from the glands.

Menstruation

When a young girl enters puberty, one of the many changes that will occur is *menarche*, or the beginning of the menstrual cycle. This is a normal body process that occurs in every female and is the physiologic way of ridding her body of the thickened uterine wall that occurs during the 28-day cycle known as menstruation. This cycle involves a series of events controlled by the hormones secreted by the pituitary gland and the ovaries. The 28-day cycle is divided into three phases: follicular phase, luteal phase, and menstrual phase.

Follicular Phase (Proliferative Phase). The hypothalamus begins the follicular phase by secreting gonadotropin-releasing hormone (GnRH), which stimulates the anterior pituitary to release follicle-stimulating

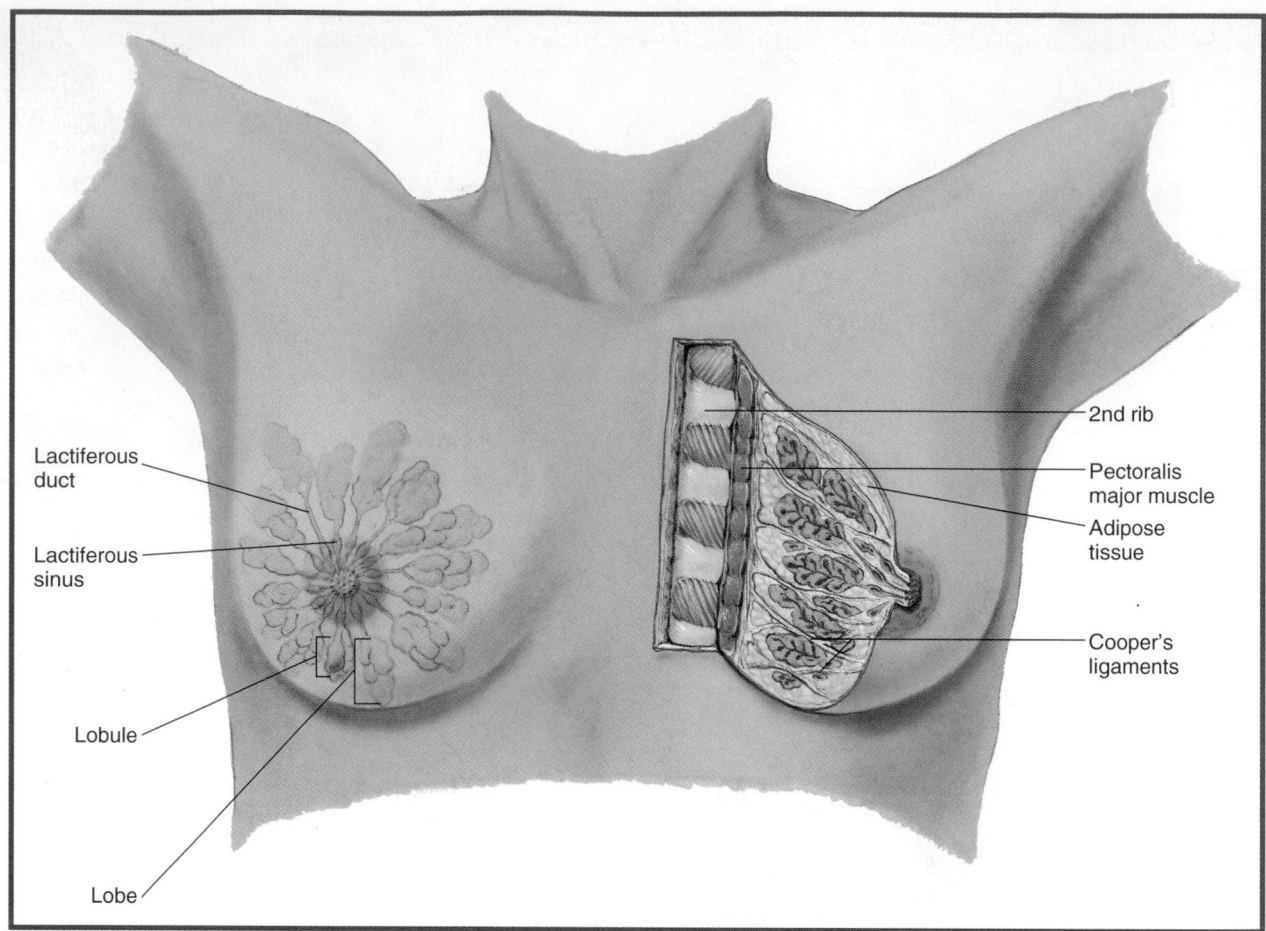

Lactiferous duct

Lactiferous sinus

Lobule

Lobe

2nd rib

Pectoralis major muscle

Adipose tissue

Cooper's ligaments

FIGURE 38-3   Normal female breast. (From Javis C: *Physical examination and health assessment*, ed 3. Philadelphia, 2002, WB Saunders.)

hormone (FSH) and luteinizing hormone (LH). These hormones mature a graafian follicle that contains the ovum. The ovarian follicle secretes estrogen, which stimulates the growth of the endometrium. It takes about 9 days (day 14 of the menstrual cycle) for the graafian follicle to ripen and bulge out from the ovarian wall. This wall becomes thinner as the follicle enlarges until it bursts, allowing the ovum to be liberated into the abdominal cavity. This expulsion of the egg ends the follicular phase. The fallopian fimbriae begin their wave-like motion to fan the ovum into the fallopian tube. The rupture spot on the ovary, now called the *corpus luteum*, begins to secrete progesterone. Ovulation causes an increase in body temperature, and some women experience cramping and tenderness in the lower abdominal area at this time as a result of the graafian follicle rupture.

Luteal Phase (Secretory Phase). Once ovulation is complete, the luteal phase begins (day 15). During this phase, progesterone secreted from the corpus luteum causes extensive growth of the endometrium as it prepares for a possible pregnancy. If conception occurs, the corpus luteum will continue to secrete progesterone until the placenta is well established and can secrete progesterone and hCG to maintain the pregnancy. If conception does not occur, hCG is not secreted and the

corpus luteum will atrophy. Without increased levels of progesterone and hCG, the endometrium breaks down and menstruation begins.

Menstrual Phase. On day 28, menstruation begins. This discharge is made up of necrotic endometrial tissue, mucus, and the blood that was in the endometrial engorgement. As the uterus contracts to shed the excess tissue, a woman may experience cramping pain and irritability. This phase usually lasts about 5 days, and then the follicular phase begins again.

Contraception

A woman's choice of a contraceptive method is based on many factors. To help patients make an informed choice, they should know about the risks, benefits, side effects, costs, failure rates, and convenience of each available method. In addition, although condoms are of only moderate success in preventing pregnancy, they should be used consistently to prevent transmission of sexually transmitted diseases (STDs). The medical assistant may help to conduct patient education on contraceptive methods. Table 38-1 summarizes the characteristics of various contraceptive methods.

TABLE 38-1	Characteristics of Various Contraceptive Methods			
Type	Failure Rate	Characteristics	Contraindications	Side Effects
Condom (barrier method)	2-10%	No prescription or exam needed; easily available; inexpensive		Possible allergic response to latex or spermicide
Diaphragm or cervical cap (barrier method)	2-19%	Must be fitted by clinician; requires instruction on how to insert & remove; spermicide must be used each time; leave in place 6 hr after intercourse (diaphragm)	Latex, rubber, or spermicidal allergy; uterine prolapse; severe cystocele or rectocele	Increased risk for UTI (diaphragm); increased risk abnormal Pap (cap)
Intrauterine device (IUD)	2-6%	Cause endometrial inflammation preventing implantation of a fertilized egg	Cervicitis, vaginitis, endometriosis, pelvic infection, Hx of STD or ectopic pregnancy	Increased risk of PID; spotting in 10-15% of users
Depo-Provera (DMPA)	0.5%	Requires 150 mg IM injection q 3 mo	Intention of becoming pregnant within 1 yr; breast cancer; liver disease	Return of fertility may be delayed 10-18 mo; headache, weight gain, depression possible
Oral contraceptives (OCPs)	1%	Suppress ovulation; atrophy the endometrium	Thrombolytic, liver, or coronary artery disease; breast, liver, reproductive tract cancer; smoker over 35; diabetes; sickle cell disease	Nausea, breakthrough bleeding, breast tenderness, fluid retention; hypertension, elevated lipid levels

UTI, Urinary tract infection; *PID*, pelvic inflammatory disease; *Hx*, history; *STD*, sexually transmitted disease; *IM*, intramuscularly.

FACTORS TO CONSIDER WHEN CHOOSING A CONTRACEPTIVE METHOD

- Is it effective and safe?
- Does it conveniently match your sexual habits?
- Are you at risk for serious side effects?
- Can you afford it?
- Is it reversible?

Barrier Methods

Barrier methods of contraception either kill sperm through the use of a chemical spermicide or prevent their entry into the cervical os. Each method must be used every time intercourse occurs, which means the patient must be motivated to follow through with their use. Barrier methods are relatively inexpensive, and all are reversible.

Patient education for the use of a diaphragm includes the following:

- Examine the diaphragm before each use by holding it up to a bright light to check for holes or cracks.
- Place 1 to 2 tablespoons of spermicidal jelly or cream into the diaphragm dome before insertion.
- *Leave in place for 6 hours after intercourse*; no douching until it is removed.

- Before repeated intercourse, add spermicide to the outside of the diaphragm with an applicator. *Do not* remove the diaphragm until 6 hours after the last intercourse.
- After removal, wash with soap and water, air dry, and inspect for breaks or holes before storing.
- The diaphragm should be refitted if the patient gains or loses more than 10 to 15 pounds; has a miscarriage, gives birth, or undergoes any type of pelvic surgery; or has difficulty voiding or moving bowels with the diaphragm in place.

The cervical cap is a thimble-sized, domed barrier method that fits over the end of the cervix and also is used with spermicidal jelly. It is 92% to 96% effective if used properly. One of the advantages of this barrier method is that the cap can be inserted up to 12 hours before intercourse and can stay in place up to 72 hours without impacting effectiveness or safety.

Hormonal Contraceptives

Depo-Provera (depot medroxyprogesterone acetate) injections are highly effective and undetectable, but the patient must be compliant in returning to the healthcare facility for follow-up and repeat injections every 12 weeks. The initial injection is given during the menstrual cycle or within 5 days postpartum. The injection is given in either a gluteal or deltoid site but should not be massaged after administration. Injections can be given 9 to 13 weeks apart and are safe to use if the patient is breastfeeding.

Almost every patient will experience some menstrual irregularities, but most subside after a series of two injections.

Besides being a highly effective method of birth control, oral contraceptives can be used to treat a wide range of gynecological conditions, including menstrual irregularities, reduction in premenstrual syndrome (PMS) symptoms, treatment of *anovulation*, prevention of ovarian cysts, and may be prescribed to increase bone density. Their effectiveness, however, is based on daily administration. Failure rates are associated with noncompliance and can range from less than 1% in women who are highly compliant to more than 15% in those who do not take the pills as prescribed. Oral contraceptive pills (OCPs) can have serious side effects; so patients should be informed of conditions that require immediate medical attention. These can be remembered with the mnemonic *ACHES*: abdominal pain (new and severe), chest pain (new and severe), headaches (new or more frequent), eye problems (blurred or absence of vision), and severe leg pain. These symptoms may indicate the formation of a blood clot in the abdomen, chest, or leg, or they may be indications of a stroke; blood clot formation and strokes are the most serious complications of taking OCPs.

Permanent Methods

Both male and female patients can undergo surgical procedures that are considered permanent contraceptive methods. In the male, vasectomies were addressed in Chapter 37. For the female, a bilateral tubal ligation can be performed where a portion of both fallopian tubes are excised or ligated. The cost and rate of complications are higher for tubal ligations than for vasectomies. In addition, tubal ligations must be done on an outpatient basis with general anesthesia; so the woman has that additional risk. Both procedures can be reversed, but not always successfully.

CRITICAL THINKING APPLICATION

Dr. Beck's patients often ask questions about birth control methods, including the pros and cons of each. Although Betsy's former employer also prescribed contraceptives, she was not involved in patient education. Dr. Beck expects Betsy to be aware of all birth control options, their characteristics and side effects, and any patient education details that might be requested or appropriate. Betsy has decided to create a reference sheet for herself that includes all these details. What should she include?

Gynecological Diseases and Disorders

Menstrual Disorders and Conditions

Amenorrhea is the absence of menstruation for a minimum of 6 months; with *oligomenorrhea*, the woman has not experienced a period from 35 days to 6 months. The absence of menstruation outside pregnancy could be due to a number of factors, including hormonal imbalances, thyroid disease, ovarian failure, or structural defects in the female sex organs. If a patient has established menstruation that stops, it is usually due to either a hypothalamus or pituitary problem. Suppression of the hypothalamus can occur because of an eating disorder, stress, or extreme exercise resulting in low body-fat content.

Women who do not ovulate and therefore do not go through a monthly shedding of the endometrial wall of the uterus are at greater risk for cancer of the endometrium and the breast. Patients usually are started on oral contraceptives that artificially provide the hormones needed to create a monthly menstrual cycle. These women may experience fertility problems and require further testing and medical intervention to become pregnant.

Abnormal menstrual bleeding is a common cause of OB/GYN visits. *Menorrhagia* is excessive menstrual blood loss, such as a menses lasting longer than 7 days. The physician may ask the patient to count the number of tampons and pads used for several cycles to establish a method of determining an estimate of blood loss. A sign that a woman is losing excessive amounts of blood is iron deficiency anemia. *Metrorrhagia* is spotting or bleeding between menstrual cycles. The physician may prescribe oral contraceptives to atrophy the endometrium and lessen the bleeding. Surgical options for excessive menstrual flow are a **dilatation and curettage (D&C)** or, in extreme cases, a hysterectomy.

Endometriosis. Endometriosis is characterized by the presence of functional endometrial tissue outside the uterus. It is commonly found attached to the ovaries, urinary bladder, fallopian tubes, uterosacral ligaments, intestines, and peritoneum. Many hypotheses have been offered to explain this migration of endometrial tissue, but the most accepted is a retrograde flow during menstruation that causes menstrual fluid and stray endometrial cells to migrate out of the fallopian tubes and implant in the pelvic region. The use of tampons has been suggested as a possible cause. There is also a familial tendency, with ten times greater risk for developing the disorder if the woman has a first-degree relative affected.

The ectopic endometrial tissue responds to routine hormone changes so that it proliferates, degenerates, and bleeds as the endometrium of the uterus does throughout the menstrual cycle. This causes inflammation at the site of the implantation that recurs with each cycle, ultimately leading to adhesions and obstructions of the affected tissue. The primary symptom of endometriosis is *dysmenorrhea* (painful menstruation). More than a third of affected patients also report *dyspareunia* (painful intercourse), and others complain of contact pain in the lower abdomen, pelvis, and back beginning 7 days before menses and lasting 3 days after onset. Other symptoms can include profuse menses, hematuria, rectal bleeding, nausea, vomiting, and abdominal cramps. Infertility is a serious problem for about 70% of the women afflicted with endometriosis.

Conservative treatment through the use of hormones is recommended when the woman wants to have children. Treatment may consist of a laparoscopy to remove the ectopic endometrial tissue. Pharmaceutical treatment includes oral contraceptives used continuously to prevent bleeding or Depo-Provera injections. Lupron (leuprolide acetate) injections may be prescribed intramuscularly every month for 6 months; however, Lupron puts the patient into a state of artificial menopause and can cause menopausal symptoms, including hot flashes, vaginal dryness, and bone density loss. In severe cases, a total hysterectomy may be indicated. There is no cure, but pregnancy, nursing an infant, or natural menopause frequently causes remission (Figure 38-4).

CRITICAL THINKING APPLICATION

Melissa Steiner, a 19-year-old patient of Dr. Beck, was diagnosed with endometriosis when she was 17. She has had two laparotomy procedures and continues to complain of moderate to severe pain before and during menstruation. What can Betsy tell her about the disease to help her understand why she has the pain? Melissa also wants to know about long-term complications, including the impact of the disease on fertility. She asks Betsy to help her understand Dr. Beck's explanation of the disease.

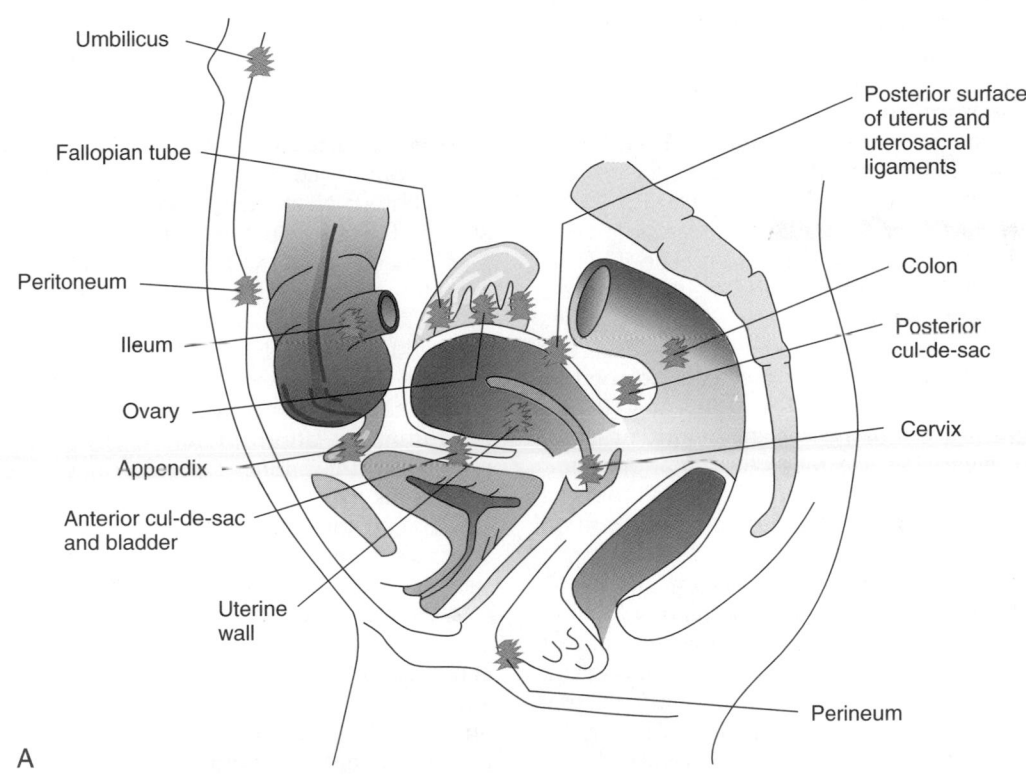

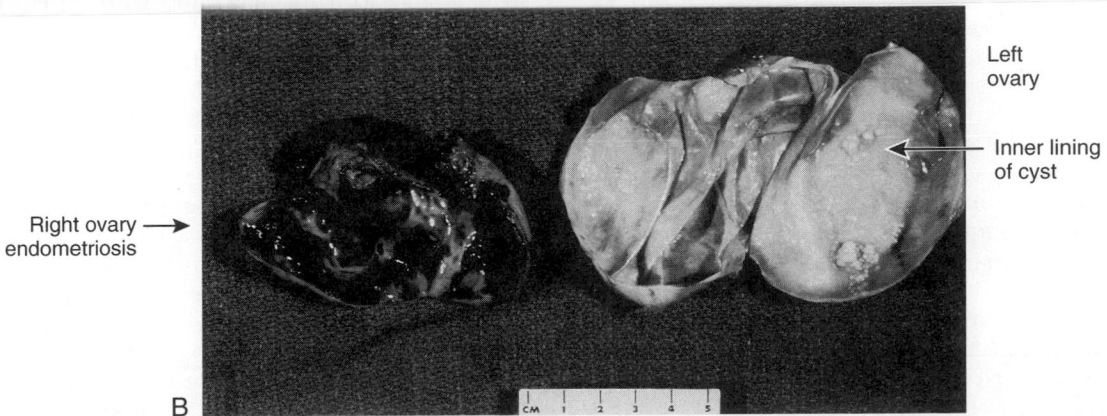

FIGURE 38-4   Endometriosis. **A,** Possible ectopic sites. **B,** Endometriosis involving right ovary (chocolate cyst) and left ovary showing the inner lining of a large cyst with excrescences. (**A** From Gould BE: *Pathophysiology for the health professions,* ed 2. Philadelphia, 2002, WB Saunders. **B** Courtesy RW Shaw, MD, North York General Hospital, Toronto, Ontario, Canada.)

Infections

Candidiasis. *Candida albicans* is the yeast-like fungus responsible for this infection. *Candida* organisms are commonly part of the normal flora of the mouth, skin, intestinal tract, and vagina. Overgrowth of the organism can be caused by antibiotic use, high estrogen levels, oral contraceptives, diabetes mellitus, and immunosuppression disorders, including acquired immunodeficiency syndrome (AIDS). Candidiasis also can be spread through sexual contact. Symptoms include vulvovaginal itching; dry, bright-red vaginal tissue; and odorless, white, "cottage cheese" vaginal discharge. This infection is treated with prescription antifungal medications (Miconazole or Terconazole vaginal suppositories) and over-the-counter medications.

Cervicitis. Cervicitis is an inflammation of the cervix caused by an invading organism. The main symptom is a thick, purulent, whitish discharge with an acrid odor. Dysuria may also be present. Cervicitis can occur after vaginal delivery from an infected cervical laceration. Treatment consists primarily of antibiotics, although cauterization may be indicated when cervical erosion exists.

Pelvic Inflammatory Disease. *Pelvic inflammatory disease* (PID) is any acute or chronic infection of the reproductive system ascending from the vagina (*vaginitis*), cervix (*cervicitis*), uterus (*endometritis*), fallopian tubes (*salpingitis*), and ovaries (*oophoritis*). In these cases, the fallopian tubes may contain pus or may be deformed by chronic attacks of inflammation or adhesions. PID is frequently caused by gonorrhea or chlamydia, or it can develop after pelvic surgery, tubal examinations, and abortion. It accounts for a large percentage of cases of infertility in women, primarily because of the formation of adhesions in the fallopian tubes. The patient may be asymptomatic or complain of purulent vaginal discharge, fever, malaise, dysuria, lower abdominal pain, bleeding, and nausea and vomiting. Cultures are typically done of cervical discharge to determine the pathogenic organism. Treatment should include broad-spectrum antibiotic therapy such as Floxin with Flagyl or Rocephin with Vibramycin. If cultures are positive for an STD, treatment of the partner is necessary for the patient to be cured without reinfection.

Sexually Transmitted Diseases. The list of infectious diseases spread by sexual contact continues to grow. These diseases are considered the most common contagious diseases in the United States. All STDs are transmitted from one person to another through body fluids such as blood, semen, and vaginal secretions during vaginal, anal, or oral sex (Figure 38-5). A summary of STDs was included in Chapter 37.

Table 38-2 summarizes the effect of STDs on women. As mentioned in Chapter 37, the greatest increase in the incidence of human immunodeficiency virus (HIV) at this time is in young, sexually active women. It is possible to pass HIV through the placenta from an infected pregnant woman to her fetus. Treatment of HIV-positive pregnant women with the protease inhibitor azidothymidine (AZT) decreases the risk of HIV infection in the infant by two thirds. Many physicians recommend that all pregnant women be screened and appropriately treated for the disease to prevent the spread of the infection to newborns.

CRITICAL THINKING APPLICATION

A 28-year-old patient was recently diagnosed with an acute gonorrheal/chlamydial infection. She has had human papillomavirus (HPV) since she was 22. Dr. Beck asks Betsy to give her patient education materials, including potential long-term complications of HPV, and to confirm that she understands the signs and symptoms of sexually transmitted diseases in herself and her partner. What should Betsy include in the information?

Benign Tumors

Fibroid Tumors. Uterine fibroid tumors are **idiopathic** benign tumors composed mainly of smooth muscle and some fibrous connective tissue. Fibroids vary in number, size, and location in the uterus and are quite common. Menorrhagia (excessive menstruation) is the primary symptom, although the patient may experience bladder or rectal pressure, pelvic pressure, pain, abdominal distortion, and infertility. Fibroid tumors affect premenopausal women because they consist of estrogen-sensitive cells. Fibroid tumors do not recur and do not undergo malignant transformation; therefore, they have an excellent prognosis. Treatment depends on the severity of the symptoms and the patient's age because fibroid tumors tend to become smaller and calcify after menopause. The masses can be removed surgically, or a hysterectomy may be indicated if bleeding is a serious problem (Figure 38-6).

Ovarian Cysts. Ovarian cysts are sacs of fluid or semisolid material that form on or near the ovaries. They can occur in the follicle or the corpus luteum anytime between puberty and menopause. Most cysts are benign, and those that are small and asymptomatic do not require treatment. Large or multiple cysts may cause discomfort, low back pain, nausea, vomiting, and abnormal uterine bleeding. These can be treated with birth control pills over a period of several months to reduce the size of the cysts. If pharmaceutical therapy is not sufficient, laparoscopy procedures can be done to drain large cysts or remove them. Surgery may be indicated if the cyst ruptures or if *torsion* (twisting and cutting off of the blood supply) of the ovary occurs.

A disorder of the ovaries, *polycystic ovary disease*, is a hormonal problem that causes cysts to develop over enlarged ovaries. Women affected by this disorder have unusually high levels of testosterone, estrogen, and LH and decreased amounts of FSH. This results in anovulation and multiple symptoms, such as amenorrhea, infertility, and *hirsutism* (excessive body hair in a masculine pattern). These women are at greater risk for uterine cancer because the endometrium does not slough off on a monthly basis. Treatment is with oral contraceptive pills to stimulate menses artificially, to lower androgen levels, and to reduce masculine-type symptoms.

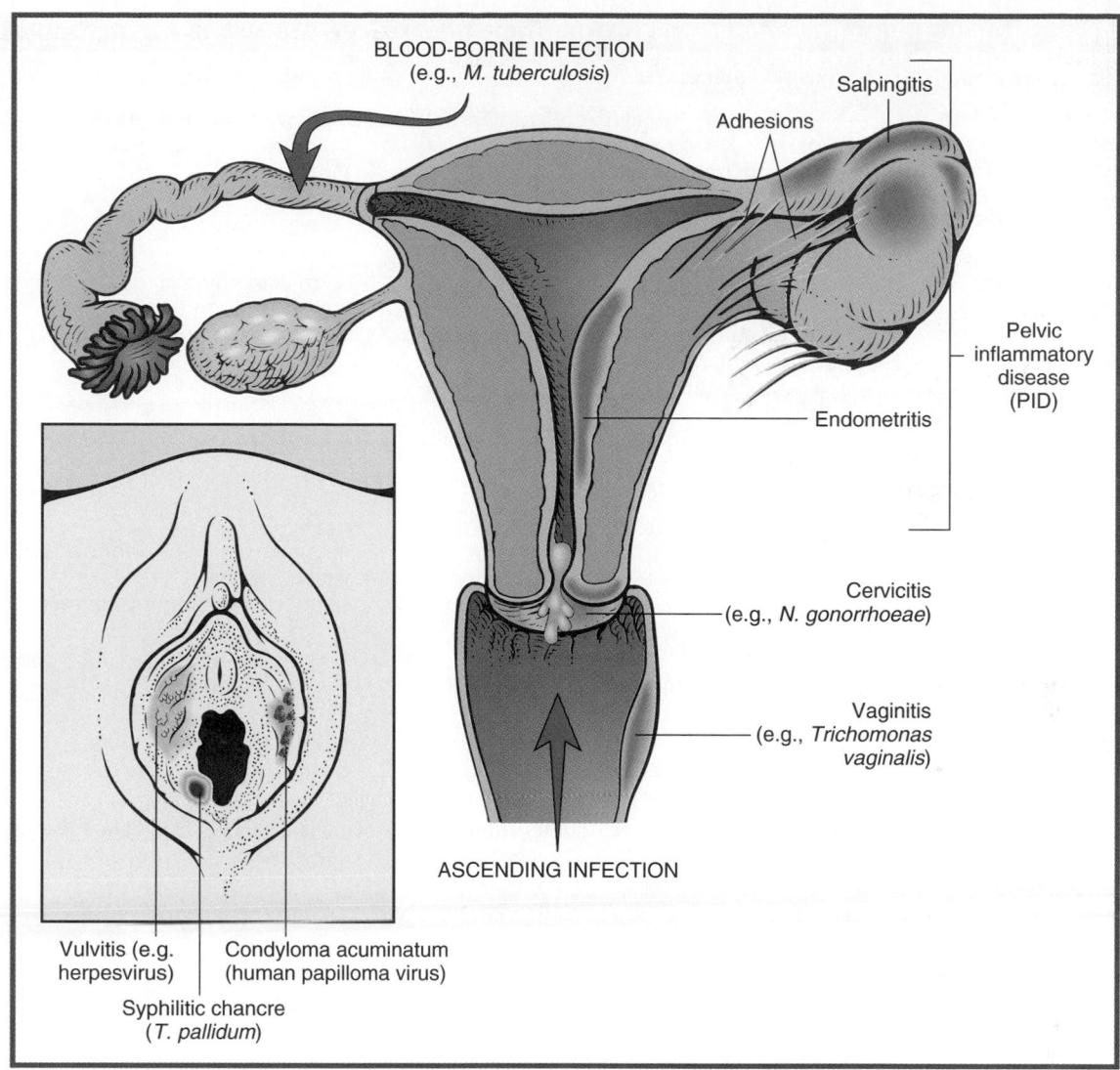

BLOOD-BORNE INFECTION
(e.g., *M. tuberculosis*)

Salpingitis

Adhesions

Pelvic
inflammatory
disease
(PID)

Endometritis

Cervicitis
(e.g., *N. gonorrhoeae*)

Vaginitis
(e.g., *Trichomonas
vaginalis*)

ASCENDING INFECTION

Vulvitis (e.g.
herpesvirus)

Condyloma acuminatum
(human papilloma virus)

Syphilitic chancre
(*T. pallidum*)

FIGURE 38-5   Ascending infections of the female genital organs are usually caused by sexual contact, pregnancy, or instrumentation. Descending infections usually begin in the blood or lymph nodes. (From Damjanov I: *Pathology for the health-related professions*, ed 2. Philadelphia, 2000, WB Saunders.)

Fibrocystic Breast Disease. Fibrocystic breast disease is the presence of multiple palpable nodules in the breasts that are usually associated with pain and tenderness and that fluctuate with the menstrual cycle (Figure 38-7). Over time, the cysts enlarge and the connective tissue of the breast is replaced with fibrous tissue that is dense and firm. The masses may be fibrous tumors that have degenerated or sacs filled with fluid. The cysts feel firm and movable, and the degree of tenderness and size depend on the point in the menstrual cycle, with tenderness peaking just before and during the secretory phase. Several different cellular types of cysts can form, a small percentage of which may be precancerous, especially if the woman has a family history of breast cancer.

Although the risk of breast cancer is only slightly increased with fibrocystic breast disease, the diagnosis of cancerous breast masses becomes more complicated. Because the breasts consistently feel lumpy, breast examinations may not isolate a suspicious mass. In addition, accurate mammography screening is complicated by the dense nature of the cysts, making visualization of a cancerous area more difficult. Because caffeine and high-fat diets aggravate the symptoms of fibrocystic breast disease, diet therapy is often recommended. Patients should be encouraged to perform monthly self-breast examinations and report any changes in the breast immediately.

Malignant Tumors

Most problems encountered with the female reproductive organs are related to abnormal cell growth. Early screening and preventive intervention are essential. Most malignant tumors require surgical removal. Radiation, chemotherapy, and hormone therapy are alternative treatment choices.

Cervical Cancer. The first stage of cervical cancer is asymptomatic, but early diagnosis of cervical cellular changes is possible with a Papanicolaou (Pap) smear. In the invasive stage, the patient will report abnormal vaginal

TABLE 38-2	Sexually Transmitted Diseases (STDs) and Women	
Disease (Causative Organism)	**Signs and Symptoms**	**Treatment**
Chlamydia (*C. trachomatis*)	Dysuria; urinary frequency; abdominal pain; increased or decreased vaginal discharge. May cause endometritis, PID, and urethritis. Transmission to newborn can occur during vaginal delivery; causes neonatal eye infections and pneumonia	Curable with antibiotic therapy; azithromycin (Zithromax), tetracycline, or Vibramycin
Genital herpes simplex virus (HSV-2)	Painful genital vesicles & ulcers; erythema and pruritus; tingling or shooting pain 1-2 d before outbreak; cycle through episodes. Viral shedding may occur during asymptomatic periods. Newborns can be infected by active lesions in vagina at birth. Brain damage, blindness, or death of the newborn may occur. Cesarean section if active lesions at time of birth. Increases risk for cervical cancer	No cure but antiviral therapy during episodes shortens duration of lesions; acyclovir (Zovirax), famciclovir (Famvir), or valacyclovir (Valtrex)
Genital warts (HPV)	Most prevalent STD; period of communicability is unknown; lesions seen more frequently in women; tend to recur; 25% of women with HPV develop invasive cervical cancer. Should be followed with routine (every 3-6 months) Pap smears	Goal of treatment is to remove symptomatic warts; cryotherapy to lesions; Podoflox solution or Imiquimod cream to lesions
Gonorrhea (*N. gonorrhoeae*) bacteria	Dysuria; urinary frequency; abdominal pain; increased or decreased vaginal discharge. May cause endometritis, PID, and urethritis	Curable with antibiotic therapy; Cefixime (Suprax), Azithromycin, Doxycycline
Syphilis (*T. pallidum*) spirochete bacteria	Six stages that can affect multiple body systems; 10- to 90-day incubation; initial sign is a painless lesion, or *chancre*, at the exposure site (vulva or vagina); serous discharge from chancre; lymphadenopathy. If not diagnosed and treated will advance to further stages. Can infect fetus via the placenta, resulting in an infant with congenital syphilis	Penicillin G (Wycillin); if allergic to penicillin, doxycycline or tetracycline
Trichomoniasis (*T. vaginalis*) protozoa	May be asymptomatic. Urinary frequency, urgency, and dysuria; frothy gray vaginal discharge; pruritus	Metronidazole (Flagyl); need to treat partner

PID, Pelvic inflammatory disease; *HPV*, human papillomavirus.

bleeding and persistent discharge as well as bleeding and pain during intercourse. The average age of diagnosis for *carcinoma in situ* (cancerous cells restricted to original site) is currently 35 but continues to drop because of an increasing number of cases occurring in young women. There is a strong link between genital herpes and certain strains of the human papillomavirus and the incidence of cervical cancer. The American Cancer Society recommends that all sexually active women and those over the age of 18 have annual Pap smears (Procedure 38-1). Women with genital herpes and warts may be tested every 3 to 6 months, depending on previous Pap results.

Disposable Pap smear kits are available for ambulatory care use. The physician obtains the smear with a cytobrush that is inserted and rotated in the endocervical canal to obtain endocervical cells for cytology. A cervical spatula then is used to obtain a sample from the vaginal area. The cells are applied to a slide, promptly fixed before drying, and sent to the laboratory for analysis. The medical assistant is responsible for fixing and labeling the slides as well as sending them to the laboratory. In the laboratory, the secretions are examined, and any abnormalities can be identified before symptoms become apparent.

The Pap smear is 95% accurate in detecting cervical carcinoma. It provides grading of neoplastic cervical changes using a cervical intraepithelial neoplasia (CIN) system of II to III, depending on the degree of cellular dysplasia (Figure 38-8). CIN I indicates mild to moderate dysplasia; CIN II, moderate and moderate to severe dysplasia; and CIN III, carcinoma in situ. Patients whose Pap smears indicate dysplasia of any severity should have a colposcopy with biopsy if indicated and possibly an **endocervical curettage** or conization procedure. If adequately diagnosed and treated, carcinoma in situ of the cervix has a 100% survival rate at 5 years.

If the patient is diagnosed with carcinoma of the cervix, it is classified by the following stages:

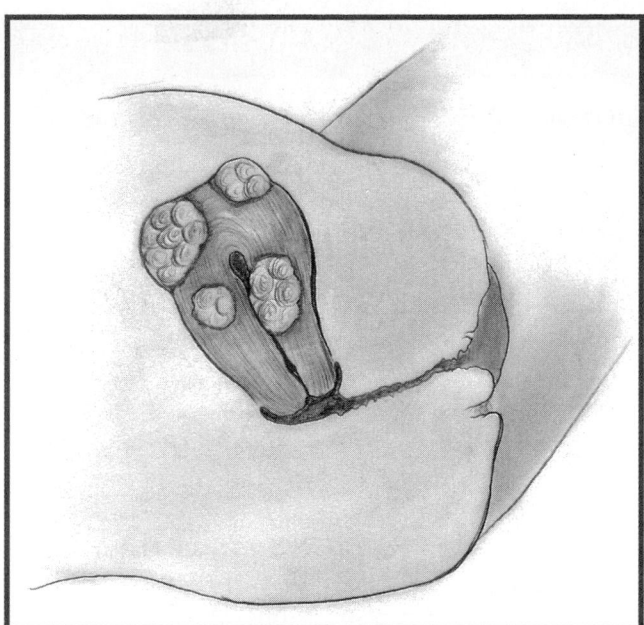

FIGURE 38-6   Uterine fibroid tumors are composed of hormone-sensitive cells. (Redrawn from Jarvis C: *Physical examination and health assessment*, ed 3. Philadelphia, 2002, WB Saunders.)

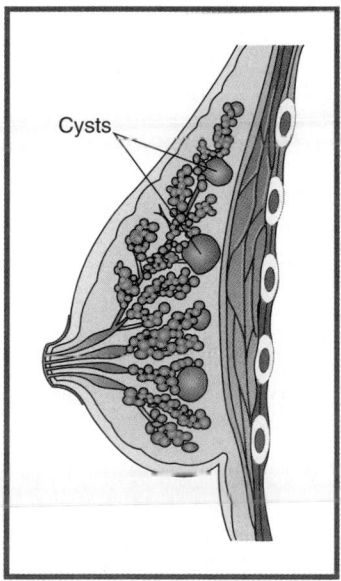

FIGURE 38-7   Fibrocystic breast disease.

- *Stage 0:* Carcinoma in situ
- *Stage I:* Carcinoma of the cervix with no **adnexal** involvement
- *Stage II:* Carcinoma of the cervix with minimal adnexal invasion
- *Stage III:* Carcinoma of the cervix with involvement to the pelvic area
- *Stage IV:* Carcinoma of the cervix with involvement of structures outside the pelvic area

Endometrial Cancer. The inner lining of the uterus, the endometrium, is at increased risk of dysplasia in postmenopausal women who never had children and those who experienced early menarche and late menopause. The disease begins with hyperplasia of the endometrial wall, followed by dysplasia. Early signs are irregular vaginal bleeding and *leukorrhea* (white or yellow) vaginal discharge. Diagnosis usually is made with an endometrial biopsy, and treatment is a complete hysterectomy with radiation and chemotherapy. Because most of these tumors develop after menopause, vaginal bleeding is unusual, which makes it more likely the woman will seek medical attention. Because of this, early diagnosis and treatment lead to a 75% to 80% survival rate.

Ovarian Cancer. Ovarian neoplasms represent the most important pathological disorder of the ovaries. Ovarian cancer is the second most common gynecological cancer but is ranked first in gynecological cancer deaths. In fact, it causes more deaths than all other tumors of the reproductive system. Metastasis has occurred in 75% of the cases before the tumor is diagnosed. Symptoms do not appear until the tumor has enlarged enough to exert pressure on nearby structures, with patients presenting with vague abdominal discomfort, weight loss, and general malaise. Researchers are working to perfect a blood test for the diagnosis of ovarian cancer that would detect the disease in earlier, more treatable stages.

Little is known about how or why ovarian cancer occurs, but pregnancy, breastfeeding, and oral contraceptive use may reduce the risk. Treatment includes a complete hysterectomy (removal of the uterus, fallopian tubes, and ovaries), radiation, and chemotherapy. Ovarian tumors are classified on the basis of their biologic features. About 20% of all ovarian tumors are cancerous, and the recovery rate is linked to the location, stage of the tumor development, and age of the patient.

Breast Cancer. Breast cancer is the second leading cause of cancer deaths in women. According to the American Cancer Society, one in every eight women have a lifetime risk of developing breast cancer and a 1 in 28 risk of dying from the disease. Predisposing factors include family history of breast cancer (especially in mother or sister), early menarche and late menopause, first pregnancy after the age of 30 years or no pregnancy, prolonged use of estrogen replacement therapy, excess alcohol intake, smoking, high-fat diet, and obesity.

Recommendations for screening include a monthly breast self-examination, which the medical assistant should be prepared to teach to all female patients over the age of 20 (Procedure 38-2), and a physical examination by a physician every 3 years to age 40 and yearly after that. A baseline mammogram should be done at age 35, every 2 years from age 40 to 50, and yearly after that. Mammograms should be done more frequently if there are indications of disease.

The indications of concern include a palpable breast mass that is firm and nonmoveable, breast pain, tissue thickening, nipple retraction or dimpling, nipple discharge, and axillary lymphadenopathy. If a breast mass is palpated, a mammogram or ultrasound of the area is ordered and, if indicated, a needle biopsy completed. If a nonpalpable mass is found on a mammogram, a **stereotactic**-guided fine-needle aspiration should be done with possible surgical biopsy as a follow-up.

PROCEDURE **38-1**

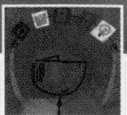

Assisting With Examination of the Female Patient and Pap Smear

GOAL: To assist the physician in examination of a female patient and diagnostic Pap smear.

EQUIPMENT AND SUPPLIES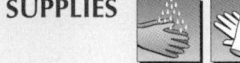

- Patient gown
- Lubricant
- 4 × 4-inch gauze squares
- Laboratory requisition slips
- Drape sheet
- Examination light
- Cervical spatula and cytobrush
- Microscopic slides
- Vaginal speculum
- Uterine sponge forceps
- Disposable examination gloves
- Fixative for Pap smear
- Urine specimen container if needed
- Stool for occult blood test if needed
- Biohazard waste container

PROCEDURAL STEPS

1 Assemble the materials needed, and prepare the room. Prepare the equipment and supplies needed for the Pap smear.

2 Wash your hands. Follow standard precautions.
Purpose: Infection control.

3 Identify the patient, and briefly explain the procedure.
Purpose: Explanations gain patient cooperation and alleviate apprehension.

4 Instruct the patient to empty the bladder and collect a urine specimen if needed.
Purpose: Organ palpations are performed on an empty bladder.

5 Instruct the patient to disrobe completely and to put on a gown. Explain gown opening in the front.

6 Assist the patient into a sitting position at the end of the examination table. Drape the patient and assist the physician with the examination. Provide reassurance to the patient as needed.

7 When the physician is ready to examine the breasts and the abdomen in the supine position, assist the patient into the supine position and drape as needed.
Purpose: To avoid exposing the patient unnecessarily.

8 When the physician is ready to begin the vaginal examination, assist the patient into the lithotomy position. Patient's knees should be relaxed and

rotated outward. Remember always to position the patient underneath the drape.

9 Direct the light source into the perineal area.
Purpose: Facilitates better viewing of the cervix.

10 Don gloves. Warm the stainless steel vaginal speculum in warm water (physician may prefer disposable plastic speculum). Pass the proper instruments to the physician in proper sequence. Physician will need the cytobrush for cervical cells and spatula for vaginal.
Purpose: Teamwork enhances efficiency.

11 Assist the physician with preparation of the slides and labeling (one marked v for vaginal, one marked e for endocervical). Spray fixative immediately about 6 inches from slide. Let dry for 10 minutes.
Purpose: Must fix slides before cells dry; spraying too close could damage smear.

12 Apply the water-soluble lubricant to the physician's fingers.
Purpose: Facilitates the bimanual examination.

13 Physician may do stool for occult blood after rectal examination. Have materials ready.

14 Instruct the patient to breathe deeply through the mouth with hands crossed over the chest.
Purpose: Helps relax muscles.

15 Place the soiled instruments in a basin.
Purpose: Helps produce better aesthetic surroundings.

16 Assist the patient off the table and with dressing if needed.

17 While patient is in the dressing room, clean the room, removing used equipment.

18 Sanitize and sterilize stainless steel equipment. Remove gloves and wash your hands.
Purpose: Infection control.

19 Prepare the Pap smear for transportation to the laboratory. Include patient's LMP date and whether she is on hormone therapy.

20 Record all procedures on the patient's medical record.
Purpose: A procedure is not done until it is entered into the patient's record.

See Appendix E for a charting example.

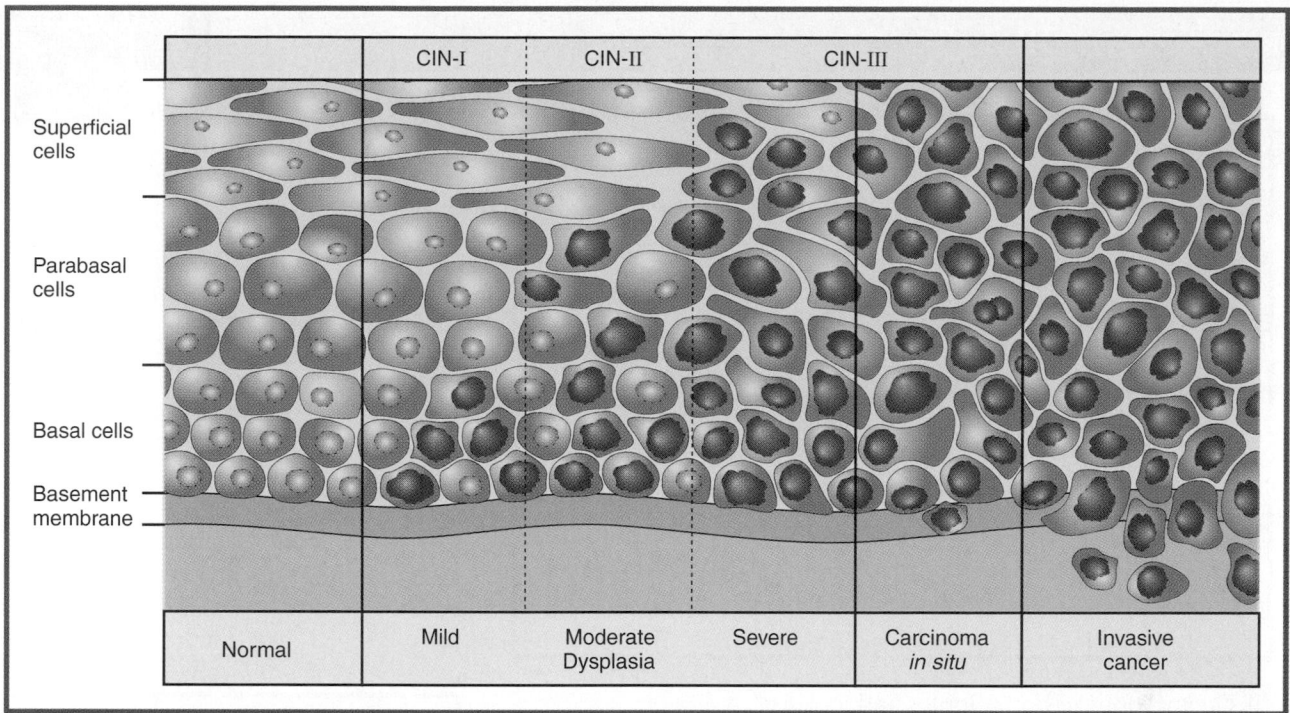

	CIN-I	CIN-II	CIN-III	
Superficial cells				
Parabasal cells				
Basal cells				
Basement membrane				
Normal	Mild	Moderate Dysplasia	Severe	Carcinoma *in situ*	Invasive cancer

FIGURE 38-8 Carcinoma of the cervix. (From Damjanov I: *Pathology for the health-related professions*, ed 2. Philadelphia, 2000, WB Saunders.)

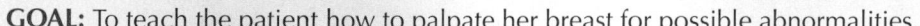

PROCEDURE **38-2**

Teaching the Patient Breast Self-Examination

GOAL: To teach the patient how to palpate her breast for possible abnormalities.

EQUIPMENT AND SUPPLIES

- Instruction pamphlet
- Teaching model (to use to demonstrate the technique before a return demonstration by the patient)

PROCEDURAL STEPS

1 Assemble equipment.

2 Tell patient to examine breast while bathing or showering in warm water. The best time to perform this examination is immediately after the menstrual period is completed because at this time there is minimal breast engorgement. Nonmenstruating women should examine breasts the first of the month.
   Purpose: Fingers will move more smoothly over wet tissue.

3 Have the patient raise one arm. With her fingers flat, she should press gently in small circles, starting at the outermost top edge of the breast and spiraling in toward the nipple. Touch every part of each breast, including the axillary region, gently feeling for a lump or thickening. Use the right hand to examine the left breast and the left hand for the right breast (Figure 1).

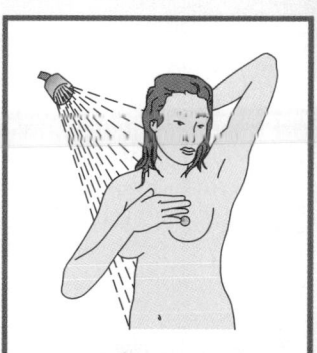

Figure 1

4 After the bath or shower is completed, the patient should continue the examination in front of a mirror with arms at the sides. Then, with the arms raised above the head, look carefully for changes in the size, shape, and contour of each breast. Look for puckering, dimpling, or changes in skin texture (Figure 2).

Continued

PROCEDURE 38-2—Cont'd

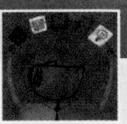

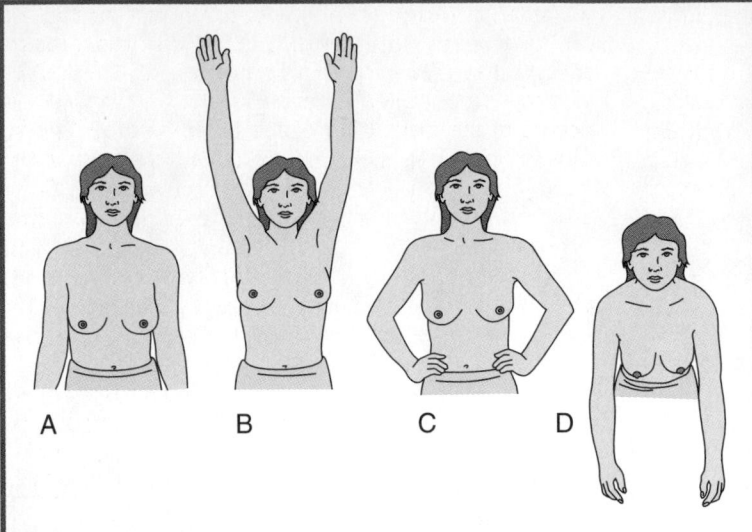

Figure 2

5 Gently squeeze both nipples and look for discharge (Figure 3).

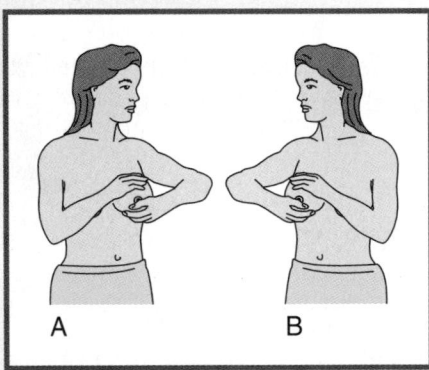

Figure 3

6 Before dressing, lie on a bed. Place a towel or pillow under the right shoulder and the right hand behind the head. Examine the right breast using the left hand. Press gently in small circles, starting at the outermost top edge, including the axillary region, and spiraling in toward the nipple. Repeat with left breast (Figure 4).

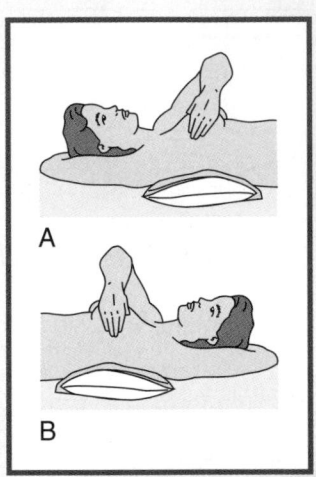

Figure 4

7 The patient should return the demonstration of how to do the breast examination to confirm understanding.

8 Give the patient the instruction pamphlet to use at home. If you have given her the shower card to follow, show her how it will hang inside the shower on a faucet or the shower nozzle and be a quick reference for her.

Treatment of breast cancer is dependent on the type of carcinoma and its staging. These guidelines include:

- *Ductal carcinoma in situ*—simple mastectomy or lumpectomy followed by radiation therapy.
- *Lobular carcinoma in situ*—bilateral simple mastectomy with breast reconstruction.
- *Invasive breast cancer*—lumpectomy with axillary node dissection followed by radiation or a modified radical mastectomy; chemotherapy; tamoxifen 10 to 20 mg daily for 5 years. Larger tumors are treated with systemic chemotherapy to shrink the tumor before surgical removal.

Positional Disorders of the Pelvic Region

The correct anatomical position for the uterus is a slight anterior tip (*anteverted*) and bent over the bladder with the cervix down and back. The uterus may be positioned in various angles because of a congenital anomaly or childbirth. With the aging process and the effect of multiple pregnancies, the muscles and ligaments that support the uterus, bladder, and rectum can stretch or weaken. This weakening of the supportive structures of the pelvic floor can result in multiple structural disorders.

A *cystocele* is a protrusion of the bladder into the anterior wall of the vagina. The bladder becomes angled, and urinary retention is common, along with frequent cystitis. A diagnosis can be made by requesting the patient to bear down as the vaginal opening is examined, allowing the physician to feel the bladder protrusion. A cystocele can result from injury during childbirth, obesity, heavy lifting, chronic coughing, and poor musculature that comes with aging (Figure 38-9).

A *rectocele* is a protrusion of the rectum into the posterior wall of the vagina. Diagnosis can be made by requesting the patient to bear down as the vaginal opening is examined so the physician can palpate the posterior wall. The patient will complain of difficulty with bowel movements and pressure in the pelvic region. Rectoceles are most often seen in postmenopausal women. A rectocele may result from pregnancy, difficult delivery, prolonged labor, obesity, chronic coughing, and lifting heavy objects.

The uterus may also lose supportive structure and drop into the vagina. This structural disorder is called *uterine prolapse*. The prolapse may involve only the descent of the cervix into the vaginal area or may progress to both the uterus and the cervix protruding from the vaginal opening. If severe, all three of these structural abnormalities can be corrected with surgery.

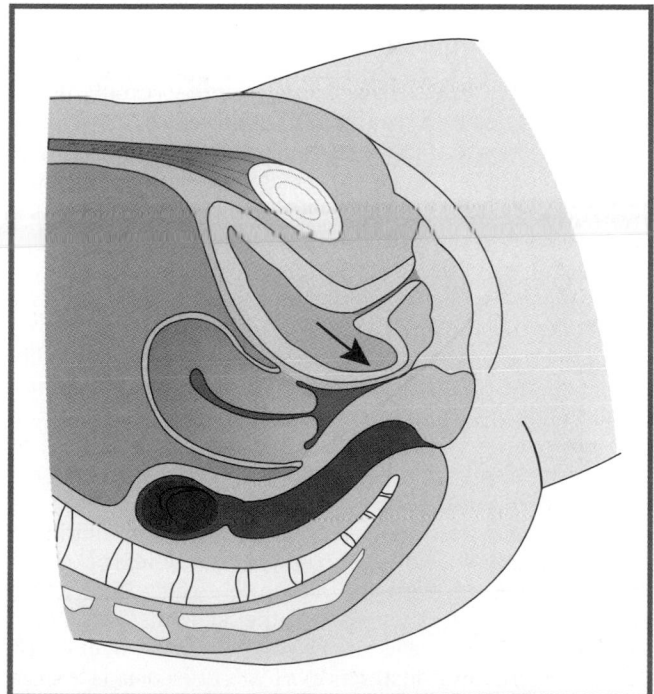

FIGURE 38-9   Cystocele.

Pregnancy

Anatomy and Physiology

When fertilization occurs, the fertilized egg, now called a *zygote*, is formed. The zygote is made up of 23 chromosomes from the ovum and 23 chromosomes from the sperm to form the first complete cell. This cell begins to grow and multiply immediately. Fertilization usually occurs in the distal third of the fallopian tube. The zygote travels down the tube and reaches the uterus in 5 to 6 days, implanting in the uterine endometrium. Enzymes are secreted by the zygote to aid in the implantation process.

After implantation, the placenta forms within the uterine wall. It is derived from maternal endometrium and partly from the *chorion*, the outermost membrane that surrounds the developing zygote. The amnion is the innermost layer of the membranes, and it holds the fetus suspended in an amniotic cavity surrounded by a fluid called the *amniotic fluid*. The amnion and fluid are sometimes known as the "bag of water." In about 25% of pregnancies, the breaking of the amniotic sac signals the onset of labor.

Within 2 weeks of fertilization, the zygote has undergone mitosis and is well established in the uterus. The embryonic period includes the third week of the pregnancy through the end of the first trimester (12 weeks). The *embryonic period* is when all tissues and organs develop. During the second and third trimester periods, the embryo becomes a fetus. This is when cells develop and begin their primary functions, organs mature, and the fetus gains weight and grows in length.

Throughout the pregnancy, maternal and fetal blood never mix. Nutrients and oxygen diffuse from the mother's blood, across the placental membrane, and into the blood vessels of the fetus's umbilical cord. Carbon dioxide and waste materials pass from the umbilical cord, through the placenta, and into the mother's circulatory system for excretion (Figure 38-10).

The placenta also acts as a gland by producing hCG and progesterone to maintain the pregnancy. Low levels of progesterone can lead to spontaneous abortion in pregnant women and menstrual irregularities in nonpregnant women. The average gestation is calculated at 9 calendar months, 10 lunar months, or 266 to 280 days and is divided into first, second, and third trimesters.

First Trimester. The first trimester is the period from the beginning of the last menstrual period through the 14th week. It is a time of multiple physical and psychological changes for the female and is a crucial time for fetal organ development. It is essential that the pregnant woman understand the importance of a nutritious diet and avoidance of potential **teratogens**. The woman may complain of breast tenderness, constipation, headaches, urinary frequency, and nausea and vomiting. Rest, relaxation exercises, plenty of fluids, regular exercise, and small frequent meals will help to relieve these discomforts. It is during this time that the obstetrician obtains a complete health history of the patient, including family, medical, menstrual, and obstetrical histories. The obstetrical history includes the number of times the patient has been pregnant (*gravida*) and the number of times she has given birth to a live infant (*para*).

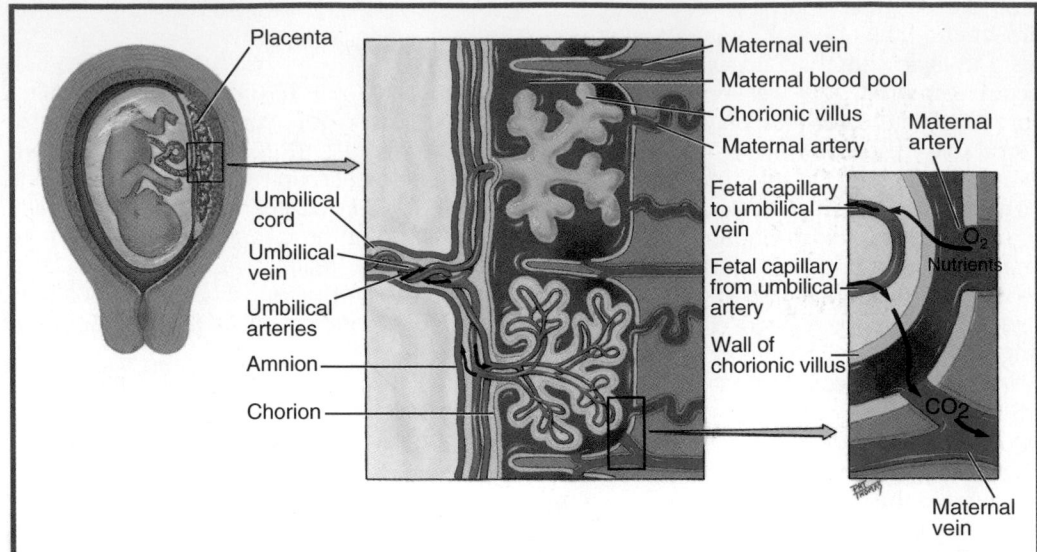

FIGURE 38-10 Structural features of the placenta and exchange of nutrients and wastes between maternal and fetal blood. (From Applegate EJ: *The anatomy and physiology learning system*, Philadelphia, 1995, WB Saunders.)

Second Trimester. The second trimester extends from the 15th through the 28th weeks after the last menstrual period. The uterus has enlarged to above the umbilicus, and the first fetal movements, called *quickening*, are felt by the patient. In addition to the basic health history and physical examination, assessment by abdominal palpation and fetal heart monitoring is conducted. The height of the fundus may be measured in centimeters from the symphysis pubis to the fundus. The mother is evaluated with urine dipsticks to screen for the presence of protein or glucose, and her blood pressure is monitored for signs of hypertension. The mother may complain of backache, dizziness, leukorrhea, and leg cramps from the increasing size of the uterus.

Third Trimester. The third trimester begins at the 28th week and lasts until delivery. This period is marked by rapid fetal growth, with the baby gaining close to one pound per week. The patient continues to be closely monitored. Childbirth preparation classes usually begin during this time. The patient experiences noticeable breast enlargement and may experience occasional discharge from the nipples of the clear sticky fluid **colostrum**. The pregnant woman may complain of uterine cramping (Braxton-Hicks contractions), heartburn, edema, and frequent urination. *Lightening*, the dropping of the fetus into the pelvis, may occur a few weeks before birth, especially in *primigravidas* (women with a first pregnancy).

Parturition

Labor is the physiologic process by which the uterus expels the fetus and the placenta (Figure 38-11). It is divided into three stages:

- *Stage I:* From onset of labor through complete **dilation** and **effacement** of the cervix (see Figure 38-11, *B*). During this time uterine contractions get longer and stronger and closer together until complete dilation and effacement occur and pushing

begins. Stage I is divided into early active (up to 3 cm dilated and 80% to 100% effaced), active (4 to 7 cm dilated and completion of effacement), and transition (8 to 10 cm dilation). The average length of time for primigravidas in Stage I is 9 to 11 hours.
- *Stage II:* From complete dilation and effacement of the cervix through the birth of the fetus (see Figure 38-11, *C*). This is the pushing stage and lasts approximately 1 hour for primigravidas.
- *Stage III:* From the birth of the fetus through the expulsion of the placenta and the amniotic membrane (see Figure 38-11, *D*). Occurs approximately 20 minutes after the birth of the baby.

Pregnancy Complications

Infertility and Abortions. Fertility problems in women can occur for many different reasons, including a history of STDs that have caused scarring or adhesions of the fallopian tubes, failure to ovulate or ovulatory irregularity, congenital anomalies of the reproductive organs, endometriosis, medications that decrease fertility, and increasing age of the woman.

Problems in becoming pregnant can occur at several points in time, the first being abnormal fertilization. Some couples are unable to have a child because of the inability of the sperm and ovum to unite. Ovarian factors are not totally understood; however, it is known that as women age the ova become less viable. If the couple is able to fertilize an egg, another problem that can occur is improper implantation.

An *ectopic* pregnancy refers to a pregnancy that occurs outside the uterus. This can occur in the ovary, fallopian tube, or even the abdominal cavity, but about 90% of the time, it takes place in the fallopian tube. When cells of the forming placenta erode the muscle layer of the tube, bleeding and destruction of the muscular layer can occur, resulting in tubular rupture. Rupture of the fallopian tube containing an ectopic pregnancy is a serious event

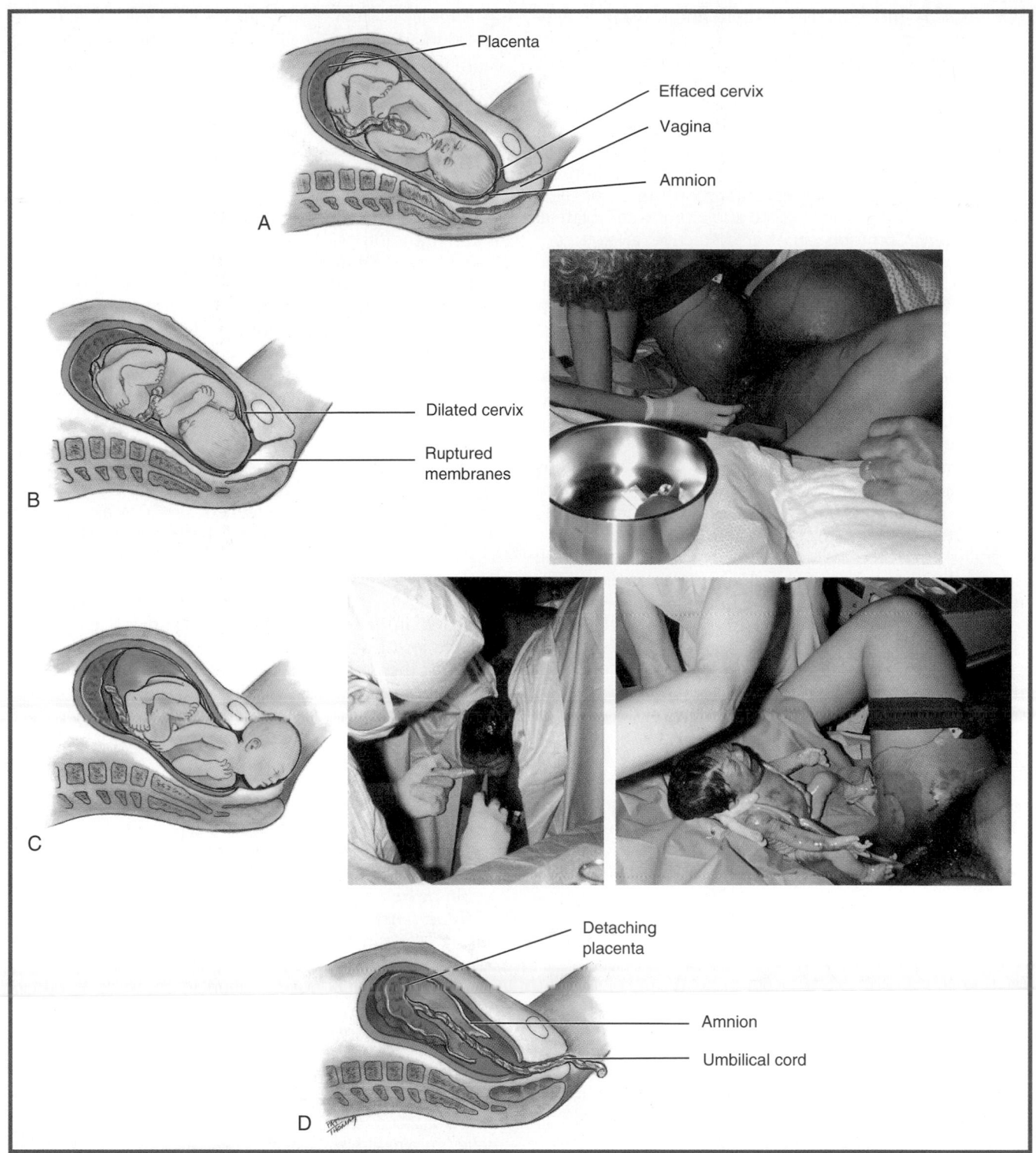

FIGURE 38-11   **A**, Effaced cervix. **B**, Dilation stage. **C**, Expulsion stage. **D**, Placental stage. (From Applegate EJ: *The anatomy and physiology learning system*, Philadelphia, 1995, WB Saunders.)

that requires immediate surgical intervention to prevent fatal hemorrhage.

Once the woman becomes pregnant, there can be problems in carrying the infant to term. An interruption of pregnancy before the term of fetal viability is called an *abortion*. There are several different categories of naturally occurring abortions, including the following:

- *Spontaneous*—abortions that do not have an identifiable cause
- *Complete*—complete expulsion of both fetus and placenta without any medical intervention
- *Incomplete*—expulsion of only parts of the fetus and placenta. A D&C must be done to remove the remaining pieces

- *Missed*—the fetus dies in utero and must be evacuated surgically
- *Threatened*—cervical bleeding but no dilation occurs, and the pregnancy continues uninterrupted

It is estimated that one in three pregnancies will terminate by abortion, and in most cases the causes are not clear. Chromosomal anomalies are frequently detected in an aborted fetus or placenta and may be the primary reason they occur. Spontaneous abortion (miscarriage) is the loss of a pregnancy before the 20th week of fetal development. Common causes are defective development of the embryo, abnormalities of the placenta, endocrine disorders, malnutrition, infection, drug reaction, blood group incompatibilities, severe trauma, and shock. Symptoms include vaginal bleeding of varying degrees of severity and lower abdominal cramping progressing to cervical dilation with rupture of membranes and complete expulsion of the products of conception. Induced abortions are the evacuation of the uterus at the request of the mother.

Placental Abnormalities. Pregnancy complications can occur because of the site of placental implantation. *Placenta previa* is when the placenta implants in the lower uterine segment. If diagnosed early in the pregnancy from routine sonograms, it is possible that the placenta will migrate with uterine wall enlargement. If, however, the previa persists throughout the pregnancy and is implanted on or near the cervix, when the mother goes into labor the dilation and effacement of the cervix can cause the placenta to tear loose (Figure 38-12). It is impossible for complete dilation and effacement to progress without serious oxygen deprivation for the fetus and hemorrhaging in the mother. The signs of placenta previa are painless, bright red vaginal bleeding during or near the last trimester. The diagnosis is confirmed with a sonogram. A cesarean section is done as close to term as possible to prevent complications in both mother and fetus.

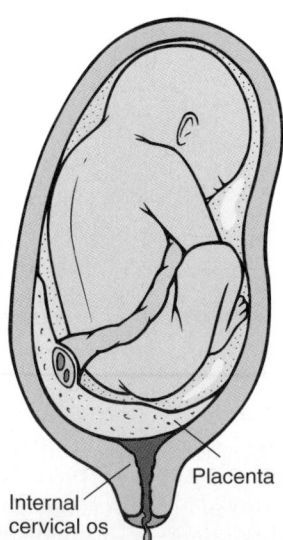

FIGURE 38-12 Placenta previa. (From Frazier MS, Drzymkowski JW: *Essentials of human diseases and conditions*, ed 2. Philadelphia, 2000, WB Saunders.)

Internal cervical os

Placenta

Another placenta problem, *abruptio placentae*, occurs when the placenta detaches from the uterine wall. The pregnant woman reports acute onset of severe abdominal pain with firmness on palpation and hemorrhaging from the vagina. She also exhibits signs of shock, including tachycardia; a thready pulse; hypotension; and clammy, cool skin. The fetus shows signs of distress resulting from lack of oxygen, including decreased fetal heart tones and lack of movement. This is a true obstetrical emergency and requires immediate cesarean delivery to save the infant and mother.

Maternal Disorders

Gestational Diabetes. Any degree of impaired glucose tolerance during pregnancy is diagnosed as gestational diabetes mellitus (GDM). Women at greatest risk are those over age 40; those with a family history of diabetes mellitus; those with a body mass index of more than 25 before pregnancy; smokers; and certain racial groups, including Hispanics, Native Americans, Asian Americans, and blacks.

The most recent recommendations from the American College of Obstetricians and Gynecologists (ACOG) is that all pregnant patients be screened for GDM at 24 to 28 weeks' gestation using a 50-g, 1-hour glucose challenge. The patient is given a concentrated drink equivalent to 50 g of glucose, and blood is drawn 1 hour afterward to measure blood glucose levels. A patient's blood level that is greater than or equal to 130 to 140 mg/dl is considered positive for GDM. Normal glucose levels may be achieved with diet therapy, although some patients require insulin during pregnancy to keep glucose blood levels within normal ranges. The problem with glucose metabolism typically goes away after the birth of the infant, but a small portion of patients may develop Type 2 diabetes later in life.

The medical assistant may perform the blood test as ordered, perform routine urinary dipsticks at each visit, and assist with patient education if GDM is diagnosed. Referral to a dietitian and follow-up with diet counseling would be helpful in diet therapy management.

Hypertension. Most women who develop hypertension during pregnancy usually had a normal blood pressure before becoming pregnant and also during early pregnancy but develop hypertension in the second half of the pregnancy. Gestational hypertension (pregnancy-induced hypertension) can be mild to severe and occurs in about 10% to 15% of pregnancies.

If hypertension is accompanied by proteinuria, the patient is diagnosed as having *preeclampsia*, which occurs in about 2% to 3% of pregnancies. The patient also may have uremia, altered liver function, and a reduced platelet count. If the condition persists, the patient is at risk for severe headaches, vision disturbances, and convulsions either before or during labor. If these symptoms occur, cesarean section is recommended as soon as possible. The mother's blood pressure usually returns to normal quickly after the birth of the infant.

The medical assistant is responsible for monitoring the pregnant woman's vital signs at each visit and performing routine urine dipsticks. Complete and accurate documentation of findings will help alert the physician to possible hypertensive problems.

Menopause

Menopause is the permanent ending of menstruation because of the cessation of ovarian function. It usually occurs between the ages of 42 and 58, but the average age of menopause is 52. Menses may stop suddenly, there may be decreased flow over time, or the time between menses may lengthen until complete cessation occurs. Menopause can be diagnosed only retrospectively. It is only after 12 months of amenorrhea that a woman is said to be in menopause.

Perimenopause begins when hormone-related changes start to appear and lasts until the final menses, for as long as 10 years before menopause. Some women experience few or no symptoms, whereas others have hot flashes, concentration problems, mood swings, irritability, migraines, vaginal dryness, urinary incontinence, dry skin, and sleep disorders. The physician may prescribe low-dose oral contraceptives (Alesse) to balance estrogen and progesterone levels or hormone-replacement therapy (HRT; Premarin or Prempro). He or she may also recommend that the patient consume soy products or take soy supplements for a plant source of estrogen. Vitamin E may help to alleviate hot flashes, and vitamin B_6 helps to create natural serotonin, a neurotransmitter that affects mood. Other factors that help alleviate symptoms are to avoid caffeine and spicy foods to reduce hot flashes, a low-fat diet high in calcium, and regular weight-bearing exercise to help prevent osteoporosis and heart disease.

Medical treatment of menopause focuses on managing uncomfortable symptoms as well as preventing the associated conditions of drops in estrogen, such as osteoporosis and coronary artery disease. Physicians traditionally have treated perimenopause and menopause with long-term HRT for most women; however, recent studies indicate that although HRT *does* protect the menopausal woman from osteoporosis, hip fractures, and colon cancer, at the same time it *increases* the risk of heart attacks, strokes, breast cancer, and blood clots. It is now recommended physicians prescribe HRT to meet individual patient needs rather than as a routine treatment for all menopausal women. The medical assistant should be aware of the physician's recommendations regarding HRT.

CRITICAL THINKING APPLICATION

Rose Conrad, a 69-year-old patient of Dr. Beck, calls because she has read recently the hormone replacement therapy she has been taking for 15 years may be dangerous. Dr. Beck has reviewed her case and agrees that if she is concerned she can stop taking the medication; however, she recommends that Mrs. Conrad try some alternative therapies. What suggestions might Dr. Beck make for nonpharmaceutical treatment of menopause?

The Medical Assistant's Role in Gynecological and Obstetrical Procedures

As the female progresses from menarche through the childbearing years and then through menopause, her medical concerns change and the focal point of the physical examination may change as well. Even though this is true, the overall concentration of the medical office is to keep her physically and mentally healthy. Being able to assist the physician in identifying possible problems before the problem becomes a threat to the patient's health is a major priority in her care. The best way to accomplish this is by listening to the patient. Remember, to the patient, there is no such thing as a routine examination.

Examination Preparation

Examination of the female reproductive system is done to ensure normality of the reproductive organs or to diagnose and treat abnormalities of these organs. Before the physician begins the examination, the medical assistant should obtain a gynecological history, which includes age at menarche, regularity of the menstrual cycle, amount and duration of the menstrual flow, menstrual disturbances, presence of vaginal discharge, and the date of the last menstrual period (LMP). If the patient is to be examined as part of her first prenatal visit, you will need to prepare the patient and the supplies and equipment necessary to obtain pelvic measurements, serologic tests, and laboratory tests (see Procedure 38-1). On follow-up prenatal visits, the medical assistant should collect a urine specimen for urinalysis, weigh the patient, measure the blood pressure, and answer questions about diet and health habits. Any concerns of the patient should be noted and reported to the physician.

The examination room needs to be adequately equipped and the surroundings pleasant. A dressing area with an adjacent toilet should be provided. The dressing area should ensure privacy and should be equipped with tissues and sanitary protection items. Disposable examination gowns also are placed in this room. Supplies should be checked frequently throughout the day.

Assisting With the Examination

This is probably the most emotionally charged medical experience the average female undergoes. Even women with relatively sophisticated attitudes toward their bodies and sexuality may be mortified by the casual, impersonal approach of the medical team during this procedure. Many women fear the physician's findings. Anxieties and fears are best handled through explanations and showing a genuine interest in the patient's concerns.

If the physician is male, the female medical assistant should be present during the examination. The only exception to this rule is when the patient requests that the medical assistant leave the room; if this is done, the request is noted on the patient's medical record. The male medical assistant is usually not in the room during the examination except when it is necessary to assist with a procedure. The physician makes the decision regarding the male assistant's role in the female reproductive system examination. It is the medical assistant's responsibility to support the patient and to assist the physician during the procedure. The procedure should be fully explained to the patient to avoid unnecessary embarrassment and discomfort. During the explanation, the assistant has the opportunity to do some patient teaching.

The patient should be instructed to void, completely disrobe, and put on an examination gown open to the front. The patient should have been advised at the time the appointment was made not to douche or have sexual intercourse for 24 hours before the examination so that vaginal discharges can be evaluated properly and to ensure accurate results of cytologic studies.

Breast Examination. Begin the examination by assisting the patient into a sitting position and by adjusting the gown so that the breast tissue can be easily exposed. The physician will instruct the patient to place her arms above her head, and the assistant should be present to assist the patient if she has difficulty following these instructions. The physician may prefer to examine the breasts with the patient in the supine position. When the patient is instructed to assume a supine position, help the patient and adjust the gown and drape as needed for the physician and for the patient's comfort. A small pillow may be placed under the patient's head for comfort. When the examination is completed, the gown is readjusted to cover the breasts. The physician may choose to discuss breast self-examination with the patient at this time or inform the patient that you will be explaining the technique at the end of the examination (see Procedure 38-2).

Abdominal Examination. After examination of the patient's breasts, cover her breasts and position the drape to allow the physician to palpate the abdomen to confirm normal symmetry and the presence of possible masses. In the case of pregnancy, the level of the fundus is measured to determine fetal growth. For this examination, the patient's arms should be placed at her sides to achieve better relaxation of the abdominal muscles.

Pelvic Examination. The medical assistant should remain in the examination room to provide reassurance to the patient as well as to offer legal protection to the male physician while the patient's vagina and perineal areas are being examined. Furthermore, the lithotomy position is awkward to assume without assistance and may be embarrassing to the patient. Never position the patient in the lithotomy position until the physician is ready to begin the examination. When you assist the patient into the lithotomy position, always keep the patient totally covered.

The medical assistant should stand at the patient's side to be able to observe the patient and also to be able to move quickly if needed by the physician. First, the physician inspects the external genitalia and palpates the perineal body. The patient may be asked to bear down to show any muscular weaknesses that may be the result of lacerations of the perineal body during childbirth. A third-degree laceration may have involved the rectal sphincter and may cause rectal incontinence.

Next, the vaginal speculum, without lubrication, is inserted for examination of the cervix and the vaginal canal and for obtaining the Pap smear. The speculum should be preheated with warm water. Have the patient take some deep breaths to help relax the abdominal muscles. The normal cervix points posteriorly and has smooth, pink squamous epithelium. The abnormalities most frequently seen are ulcerations (erosions), Bartholin cysts, and cervical polyps. Because erosions cannot be palpated, inspection is the only method of knowing their presence. Healed lacerations resulting from childbirth are common in the **multiparous** patient. Pregnancy increases the size of the cervix, and hormone deficiency causes it to atrophy. The vaginal wall is reddish pink and has a corrugated appearance. Vaginal infections change the appearance of the vaginal mucosa. When the Pap specimen is obtained, you may be responsible for applying the fixative to the slide, labeling the slide(s), and preparing the specimen for transport to the cytology laboratory. Be sure to follow the laboratory instructions in the preparation to avoid having to repeat the examination to obtain another specimen.

After the vaginal speculum has been removed, the physician does a bimanual examination; that is, two gloved fingers are lubricated with a water-soluble jelly (lubricant) and inserted into the vaginal canal, and the other hand palpates the abdomen over the pelvic organs and the mons pubis (Figure 38-13). The uterus is examined for shape, size, and consistency. The position of the uterus is noted. The normal uterus is freely movable with limited discomfort. A laterally displaced uterus is usually the result of pelvic adhesions or displacement caused by a pelvic tumor. The fallopian tubes and ovaries are evaluated. The normal tubes and ovaries are difficult to palpate. The physician completes the examination by performing a rectovaginal abdominal examination. A stool for occult blood may be done at this time.

Postexamination Duties

Once the examination is concluded, help the patient into a sitting position and into the dressing room if needed. Using OSHA standard precautions, remove the examination equipment and supplies while the patient is dressing so that when the physician returns to talk to the patient the room is aesthetically neat. Once the patient has left, the room should be cleaned and restocked as necessary and made ready for the next patient.

 SAFETY ALERT: Any instrument that comes in contact with a patient should be disinfected and sterilized before being used for another patient. If the instrument does not penetrate tissue, it can be stored under clean or medically aseptic conditions. Some physicians prefer to use disposable speculum for routine pelvic examinations. Instruments that penetrate the tissue *must be sterilized and stored under sterile conditions.* Examples of such instruments include the

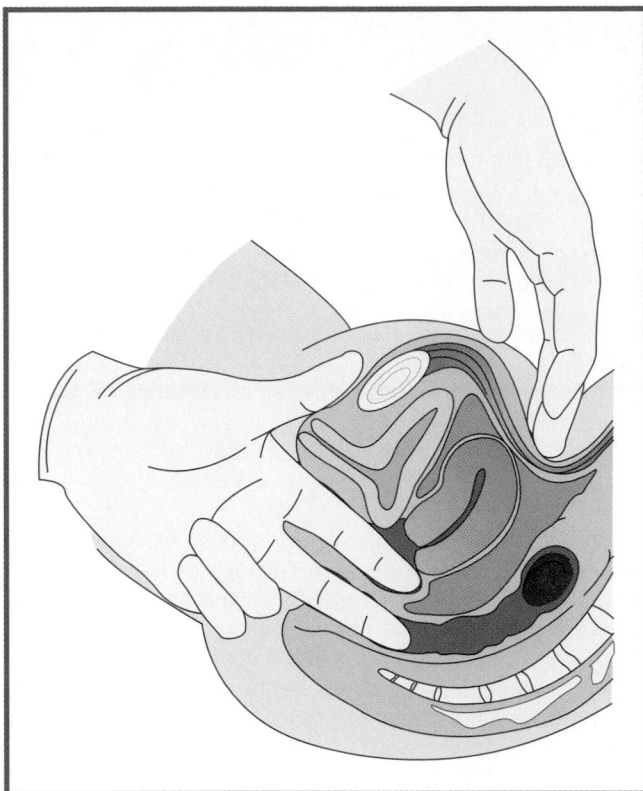

FIGURE 38-13 Bimanual examination.

uterine biopsy punch, uterine tenaculum, and cervical dilators and sounds.

Diagnostic Testing

Sonography

Sonography is a technique that uses high-frequency sound waves to produce images of soft tissues of the body and of accumulations of fluid. It can distinguish between cysts and tumors and is used during pregnancy to determine the number of fetuses, age and sex of the fetus, fetal abnormalities, and position of the placenta. The skin over the area being studied is coated with conductive gel or lotion, and the transducer is pressed lightly against the skin. Once the sound waves reach the underlying body structure, they bounce back to the transducer, which converts the returning sound waves into electrical impulses. The mother must drink three to four glasses of water 1 hour before the procedure and not void so the full bladder can be used as a reference point.

Sonograph technology is divided into two methods. The gray scale image converts sound wave echoes into graphs or dots that form pictures of organs and blood vessels (Figure 38-14). The Doppler method converts the ultrasound into audible sounds that are heard as pulsations and is used in the obstetrician's office to monitor the heartbeat of the fetus. Color-coded Doppler signals, three-dimensional imaging, and contrast medium enhancement of ultrasound image provide more accurate images and data related to organ structure and function.

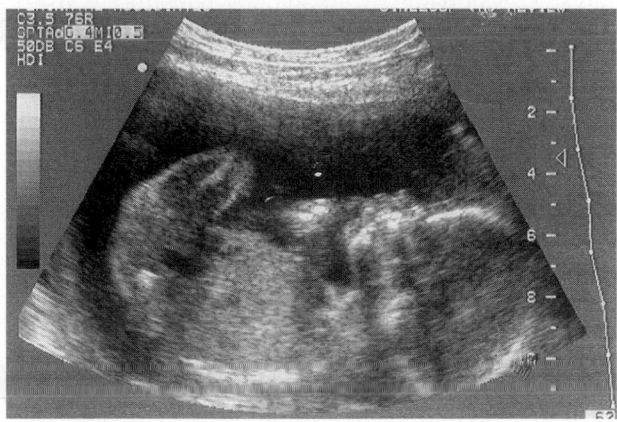

FIGURE 38-14 Sonogram of fetus.

Mammography

Mammography is a specialized x-ray technique that provides images of breast tissue and is performed to identify abnormal masses that would otherwise go undetected under a breast palpation examination (Figure 38-16). Special x-ray equipment is used that compresses the breast firmly during each exposure. Compression is essential to provide the high degree of detail needed to visualize the significant, but often subtle, signs of tumor. This process is not usually painful, but some patients, especially those with fibrocystic breast disease, may find it uncomfortable. If pain persists after the examination, aspirin or ibuprofen is recommended for treatment.

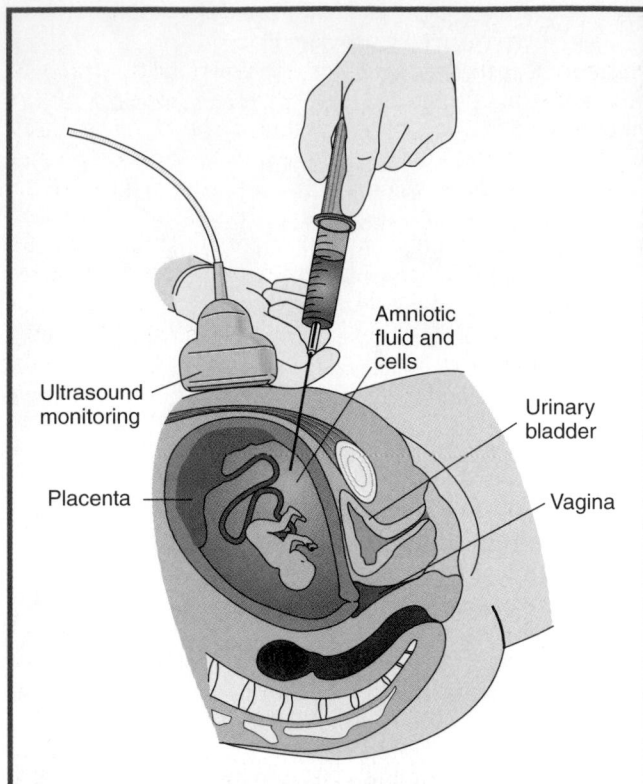

FIGURE 38-15   Amniocentesis.

In preparation for mammography, patients are instructed not to use underarm deodorant and not apply powder or lotions on the breasts or axillary areas. These products may contain ingredients that produce artifacts on mammographic images. This is especially true of antiperspirants that contain aluminum salts. When previous mammograms are available, every effort must be made to obtain them because comparative evaluation is often significant in the radiological diagnosis.

In addition to routine screening examinations and studies for evaluation of known breast lumps, mammographic techniques also may be used to localize needle placement for breast biopsies.

Cancerous tumors of the breast are classified into four stages. Lymph node involvement is classified from a to d; if distant metastasis is present, the tumor is classified as M1.

STAGING OF BREAST CANCER AND AXILLARY LYMPH NODES

Tumor Staging

- Noninvasive mammary carcinomas are classified as stage TIS (tumor in situ)
- Stage I: Tumor less than 2 cm in diameter, either fixed or not fixed to the pectoral muscle
- Stage II: Tumor 2 to 5 cm in diameter, either fixed or not fixed to the pectoral muscle

- Stage III: Tumor larger than 5 cm in diameter, either fixed or not fixed to the pectoral muscle
- Stage IV: Tumor fixed to chest wall or skin

Lymph Node Staging*

a. NO: No regional lymph node involvement
b. N1: Palpable, movable nodes
c. N2: Palpable, fixed nodes
d. N3: Internal mammary lymph node involvement

*Lymph node staging is reported as letters a to d.

Colposcopy

Colposcopy is the visual examination of the vagina and the cervical surfaces through the use of a colposcope. The colposcope is a microscope with a light source and a magnifying lens, making it possible for the physician to locate and evaluate abnormal cells and detect cancer of the cervix in its early stages, examine tissue from which an abnormal Pap smear has been obtained, and monitor areas of the cervix from which malignant lesions have been removed. Colposcopy also can be used to monitor women who are at risk for developing cervical cancer because their mothers were given diethylstilbestrol (DES) during their pregnancy. A cervical biopsy may be performed in conjunction with a colposcopy. One of the major advantages of obtaining a biopsy during a colposcopy is that the instrument visualizes the suspicious area so that the biopsy can be taken from the most atypical area.

The colposcope is not inserted into the vaginal cavity; thus, colposcopy is a relatively safe and painless procedure. Discomfort may occur when the speculum is inserted into the vagina to improve visualization of the tissue. Discomfort and bleeding can occur when tissue is taken for biopsy. Depending on the results of the biopsy, the patient may need a more extensive procedure, a *conization*, which removes a cone-shaped wedge of cervical tissue for either treatment or further analysis.

Cryosurgery

This procedure is often done to treat chronic cervicitis and cervical erosion problems through the use of freezing temperatures. Freezing causes cellular necrosis, and in about 1 month these dead, discarded cells are replaced with healthy cells. The procedure involves placing a probe against the problem area on the cervix and applying liquid nitrogen to the area for about 3 or 4 minutes or until the site is frozen (Procedure 38-3). The patient may experience some pain for about 30 minutes after the procedure and a slight watery discharge for up to a week. If there are any signs of infection, foul discharge, or pain, the patient should call the physician's office. She is advised not to engage in sexual intercourse for 1 month and to expect a heavier than usual menstrual flow for the first period after the procedure.

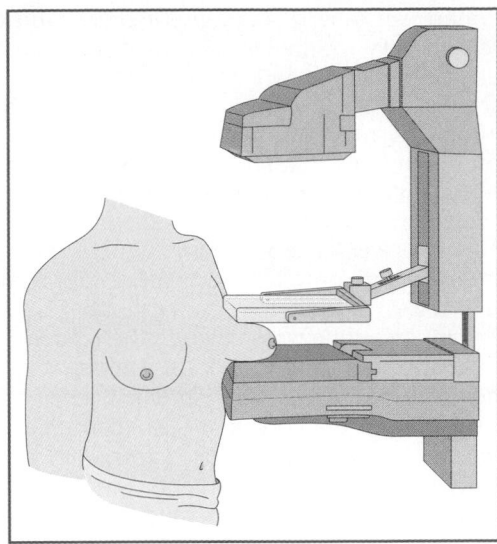

FIGURE 38-16 Proper position of breast for mammogram.

Pregnancy Testing

Pregnancy tests are designed to detect hCG, which is secreted after the ovum is fertilized. It appears in the blood and urine of pregnant women as early as 10 days after conception. Once pregnancy is confirmed, the patient undergoes a complete medical and obstetrical examination, which includes a number of laboratory tests (Table 38-3 and Procedure 38-4). The estimated day of delivery (EDD) is also calculated (Procedure 38-5). The EDD is frequently called her *expected due date*. The EDD can be determined by several methods, including Nägele's rule, the lunar method, or the commercially prepared gestational wheel. Regardless of the method, the EDD is only an educated guess, and most obstetricians rely on sonograms for more reliable data.

Patient Education

The medical assistant can assist the physician by providing information to the patient that promotes sexual health and prevents gynecological and obstetrical disorders throughout the life of the patient.

PROCEDURE **38-3**

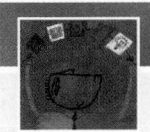

Preparing the Patient for Cryosurgery

GOAL: To prepare the patient and assist the physician in cryosurgery.

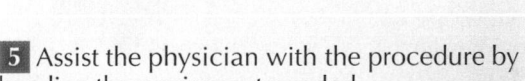

EQUIPMENT AND SUPPLIES

- Cryosurgery machine equipped with liquid nitrogen canister
- Cryoprobe
- Cervical tenaculum
- Cervical ring forceps or disposable cervical swabs
- Vaginal speculum
- 44-inch gauze squares
- Disposable examination gloves
- Gowns and face protection
- Specimen containers
- Biohazard waste container
- Cytology request forms

PROCEDURAL STEPS

1 Assemble equipment.
   Purpose: Expedite procedure.

2 Wash your hands.
   Purpose: Infection control.

3 Obtain the patient's temperature and blood pressure and record them on the patient's record.
   Purpose: To establish an average base range.

4 Drape and assist the patient into the lithotomy position. Don gloves.

5 Assist the physician with the procedure by handing the equipment needed.

6 Encourage the patient to take deep breaths to promote relaxation of the pelvic muscles during the procedure. Observe the patient for any signs of distress.
   Purpose: Patient safety.

7 When the procedure is completed, place the patient in a supine position and allow her to rest while you tidy the room and remove the used supplies. Retake temperature and blood pressure.
   Purpose: Ensure that vital signs and blood pressure return to average range.

8 Help patient sit up and assist her in dressing if needed.
   Purpose: Patient safety.

9 Remove gloves and wash hands.
   Purpose: Infection control.

10 Disinfect and sterilize equipment per manufacturer's directions and return equipment to the proper storage area.

11 Record procedure and final vital sign measurements on the patient's record.
   Purpose: A procedure is not done until it is recorded.

TABLE 38-3	Diagnostic Pregnancy Testing

Complete blood cell count
Blood type and Rh factor
Serologic test for syphilis
Rubella titer
Sickle cell trait or disease (for black patients)
Blood glucose
Papanicolaou smear
Smears for infections (when indicated)
Urinalysis
Pregnancy test

The woman planning a pregnancy or who has just found out she is pregnant may benefit from some simple guidelines for healthy living. These include:

- *Nutrition:* Before pregnancy, emphasize the need for folic acid to prevent **neural tube defects**. The woman can take a supplement or consume dark green, leafy vegetables. Many women have iron deficiency anemia, and eating foods high in iron (red meat or enriched cereal) is helpful. The pregnant woman is meeting the calcium needs of both herself and her fetus and therefore needs about 1000 mg of calcium per day. Most pregnant women should consume about 2500 calories a day. Women of average weight should gain 25 to 35 pounds, but underweight women should gain 28 to 40 pounds for a healthy infant.
- *Alcohol:* Alcohol passes through the placenta to the fetus and can cause serious problems. No one knows how much is safe, so it is a good idea for pregnant women to avoid alcohol completely.
- *Smoking:* Smoking can cause premature birth and low-birth-weight full-term infants. Smoking is linked to an increased risk of otitis media, heart problems, and upper respiratory infections in infants as well as

---

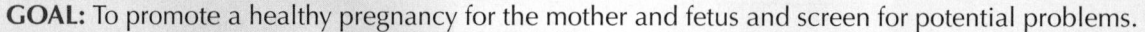

PROCEDURE 38-4

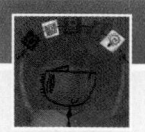

Assisting With the Prenatal Examination

GOAL: To promote a healthy pregnancy for the mother and fetus and screen for potential problems.

EQUIPMENT AND SUPPLIES

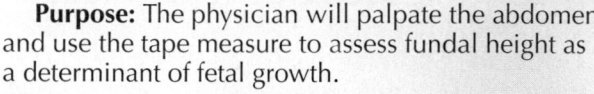

- Scale with height measurement
- Sphygmomanometer
- Stethoscope
- Tape measure
- Doppler fetoscope
- Urine specimen container
- Disposable examination gloves, vaginal speculum, and lubricant if vaginal examination conducted
- Biohazard waste container

PROCEDURAL STEPS

1 Wash your hands, assemble equipment, and identify the patient.

2 Measure and record the patient's weight.
Purpose: The expectant mother's weight reflects maternal nutritional status as well as fetal growth, and an unusual increase in weight may indicate fluid retention.

3 Collect a urine specimen, perform, and record urinalysis results to determine the presence of protein, glucose, or ketones in the urine.
Purpose: Their presence in the urine may indicate disease.

4 Measure and record the mother's blood pressure.

5 Instruct the patient to disrobe from the waist down and put on a gown open to the front so the uterine fundal height can be measured.

Purpose: The physician will palpate the abdomen and use the tape measure to assess fundal height as a determinant of fetal growth.

6 Assist the patient onto the examination table if needed and provide a drape for privacy.

7 Assist the physician as needed throughout the examination.

8 After the examination is completed, assist the patient off the examination table, making sure to observe for signs of dizziness or problems with balance.
Purpose: Lying supine or in a Trendelenburg position places pressure on the aorta, which may result in momentary vertigo when the patient sits or stands.

9 Answer the patient's questions and provide patient education materials needed.
Purpose: Take advantage of "teaching moments" to provide information on diet, health habits, community resources.

10 Discard supplies and disinfect the equipment according to manufacturer's guidelines. Wear disposable examination gloves and follow Occupational Safety and Health Administration (OSHA) guidelines if handling any contaminated items.

11 Wash your hands.

12 Document pertinent information in the patient chart.

PROCEDURE **38-5**

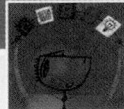

Establishing the EDD Using Nägele's Rule and Lunar Method

GOAL: To establish the patient's due date.

EQUIPMENT AND SUPPLIES

- Calendar for present and following year
- Paper and pencil
- Commercial EDD wheel (optional)

PROCEDURAL STEPS

1 Ask the patient for the date of the onset of the LMP. Be sure that this is the date of the onset and not the date of the termination of the menses.

2 Patient informs you that her LMP was June 7, 2002.

3 Calculate her EDD using Nägele's method.

4 Using Nägele's method: Begin with the date of the first day of her LMP. Count back 3 months and add 1 year plus 7 days.
  Example: LMP = June 7, 2002, May, April, March 7, 2002. Add 1 year and 7 days = March 14, 2003. Thus her EDD is March 14, 2003.

5 Using the same LMP, calculate her EDD using the lunar rule.

6 Using lunar rule:
  Example: LMP = June 7, 2002 + 9 months = March 7, 2003 + 7 days = March 14, 2003.

7 Compare the results for accuracy. Did you obtain the same EDD using both methods?

---

sudden infant death syndrome (SIDS). Pregnant women should not smoke and should not be exposed to secondhand smoke.

- *Medicine:* All chemicals pass through the placenta; so pregnant women should never take any medicine (even over the counter) without the knowledge and approval of the obstetrician. If the medical assistant is managing telephone screening, having a physician-approved list of medications next to the phone will help answer patient concerns.
- *STD Screening:* Should be done before becoming pregnant. Many STDs are asymptomatic in women but treatable. Infants are at risk for serious health problems if exposed to certain STDs in utero or during the birth process.

Pregnant women are usually searching for information about pregnancy and wellness both during and after the birth. Use the waiting room as an education center with videos, books, and pamphlets on health issues and parenting. Maintaining an up-to-date list of community education and support programs would also be helpful. The obstetrical patient who is interested in breastfeeding may need education and support to be successful. The American College of Pediatricians recommends breast milk as the optimal food for newborns. Referral to a breastfeeding support group or lactation consultant will help solve breastfeeding problems and answer maternal questions.

ADVANTAGES OF BREASTFEEDING

For the Infant

- Completely digested by the infant
- Protects against gastrointestinal infection
- Protects against food allergies
- Provides newborn with mother's antibodies to infectious disease
- Associated with higher infant IQ
- Promotes muscular eye and facial development
- Promotes maternal-infant bonding

For the Mother

- Simple, safe, and economical
- Promotes uterine **involution**, which decreases postpartum bleeding
- Decreases the incidence of breast cancer
- Promotes maternal-infant bonding

Legal and Ethical Issues

Many ethical and legal issues arise as a result of missed communication. Listen to what every patient reports, and write down any information that will assist the physician in treating the patient. The issue may appear to be an insignificant problem, but to the patient it may be a major concern. Let the physician be the judge of whether the problem is relevant. As the patient's advocate and the physician's assistant, the medical assistant plays an important role in establishing good communication as a vital link in patient care.

Confidentiality is crucial when dealing with obstetrical and gynecological disorders. Only those health care professionals who are directly involved in the care of the patient should know the purpose of the patient's visit, diagnosis, or treatment. Maintaining patient confidentiality is not only an ethical responsibility, but in the case of HIV status, it is a legal requirement.

The medical assistant may be in the position to recognize and provide assistance to women who are being mistreated. Battered women seldom come forward and tell healthcare workers they are being abused. If the patient reports such problems to the medical assistant or if it is suspected that an abusive situation exists, the medical assistant should not hesitate to report this information to the physician. The American Medical Association (AMA) has developed guidelines to help caregivers recognize victims of abuse. These include:

1. *Know what to look for* including multiple injuries at different sites, especially areas that are normally covered by clothing; the victim may be frightened, anxious, and passive and may have a history of "accidents."
2. *Know what to ask* when collecting a patient history. Even patients who exhibit no signs of abuse should be asked if they have ever been in an abusive relationship; if verbal arguments ever become physical; if their partner acts differently when drinking or using drugs; and if their partner is overprotective and jealous.
3. *Know what to say and do.* A battered woman suffers both physical and emotional abuse. She may begin to believe that she deserves to be mistreated and needs unconditional and nonjudgmental emotional support from the healthcare worker. She needs to be treated with warmth and respect and encouraged to develop a plan of action for when the next violent episode occurs. Suggestions include having immediate access to important documents, keys, money, transportation, the address of a safe house, and phone numbers for the police and local domestic violence hotline if available. The National Domestic Violence Hotline can be reached at 1-800-333-SAFE. It provides 24-hour help for victims seeking local shelters.

SUMMARY OF SCENARIO

After working with obstetrical and gynecological patients, Betsy has learned that a wide range of disorders and conditions can affect a woman's health and pregnancy. She also has learned how to assist with a number of different diagnostic procedures performed in the ambulatory care setting. One of the integral roles of the medical assistant in the OB/GYN practice is reinforcing the physician's patient education efforts. Betsy enjoys this part of the practice but realizes that it involves extensive reading and discussion with Dr. Beck to determine her preferred method of practice.

SUMMARY OF LEARNING OBJECTIVES

- The female reproductive system is made up of the external genitalia, including the vulva, labia majora, and labia minora. The internal organs include the vagina, with rugae formation in the walls so it can expand when the infant is born; the cervix, which must dilate and efface for the vaginal birth of a child; the uterus, whose internal lining is the endometrium and middle lining is the myometrium; the fallopian tubes, which extend from the fundus of the uterus and carry the fertilized egg back to the uterus; and the ovaries, which mature and excrete an ovum.

- The average menstrual cycle lasts 28 days, starting with the follicular phase, during which hormones mature a graafian follicle so that an ovum can be released while at the same time the endometrial wall is thickening. The ovum passes into the fallopian tube, which moves it toward the uterus. The luteal phase then begins, and extensive growth of the endometrium continues; if conception does not occur, the menstrual cycle begins with the breakdown of the endometrium and menstrual flow.

- Barrier contraceptive methods include the use of condoms, diaphragm, or cervical cap. Both the diaphragm and cap use spermicidal agents as well. All barrier methods are relatively inexpensive and reversible but must be used each time there is intercourse. Hormonal contraceptives include Depo-Provera injections every 12 weeks and oral contraceptives, which must be taken daily as prescribed. Hormonal contraceptives have side effects and contraindications, summarized in Table 38-1.

- Menstrual disorders include amenorrhea for a minimum of 6 months and oligomenorrhea, where the woman has not experienced a period for 35 days to 6 months. Abnormal menstrual bleeding includes menorrhagia, which is excessive menstrual blood loss, such as a menses lasting longer than 7 days. Metrorrhagia is spotting or bleeding between menstrual cycles. Endometriosis is characterized by the presence of functional endometrial tissue outside the uterus. The ectopic endometrial tissue responds to routine hormone changes so that it proliferates, degenerates, and bleeds as the endometrium of the uterus does throughout the menstrual cycle. The primary symptoms of endometriosis are dysmenorrhea and frequently dyspareunia.

- Gynecological infections include a yeast infection called candidiasis; cervicitis, which is an inflammation of the cervix from a pathogen; PID, which is any acute or chronic infection of the reproductive system ascending from the vagina (vaginitis), cervix (cervicitis), uterus (endometritis), fallopian tubes (salpingitis), and ovaries (oophoritis); and STDs, summarized in Table 38-2.

- Benign tumors of the reproductive system include uterine fibroids composed mainly of smooth muscle and some fibrous connective tissue. Ovarian cysts are sacs of fluid or semisolid material that form on or near the ovaries. Polycystic ovary disease is a hormonal problem that causes cysts to develop over enlarged ovaries. Women affected by this disorder have hormonal abnormalities that cause anovulation and multiple symptoms. Fibrocystic breast disease is the presence of multiple palpable nodules in the breasts, usually associated with pain and tenderness that fluctuate with the menstrual cycle. Over time, the cysts enlarge and the connective tissue of the breast is replaced with fibrous tissue that is dense and firm. Malignant tumors include cervical, endometrial, and ovarian cancers that vary in their diagnostic features and symptoms. Breast cancer can be of multiple origins, including ductal, lobular, or invasive carcinoma that has invaded surrounding tissue and metastasized. Treatment of all forms of reproductive cancer is dependent on the staging and grading of the tumors.

■ Positional disorders of the pelvic region include a cystocele, which is a protrusion of the bladder into the anterior wall of the vagina. The bladder becomes angled, and urinary retention is common with frequent cystitis. A rectocele can cause a protrusion of the rectum into the posterior wall of the vagina and a uterine prolapse where the cervix has dropped into the vaginal area, or it may progress to both the uterus and the cervix protruding from the vaginal opening. If severe, all three of these structural abnormalities can be corrected with surgery.

■ Pregnancy occurs when the ovum and sperm meet in the fallopian tube and a zygote is formed. The zygote implants in the uterine wall and the placenta begins to form, which provides hormonal support for the pregnancy. The fetus is surrounded by an amniotic sac and floats in amniotic fluid. The fetus's oxygen and nutrient needs are met by maternal blood that passes through the placenta to the umbilical cord; waste materials pass out along the same path. The embryonic period ends at 12 weeks, and by then all tissues and organs have developed. During the remainder of the pregnancy, the organs mature and begin to function, and the fetus grows. Pregnancy is divided into trimesters: the first, second, and third. The first trimester is a crucial time for fetal organ development, the second brings quickening and many physiological changes in the mother, and the third is when organ systems mature and lasts until the birth of the infant. Labor is broken into three stages: dilation and effacement of the cervix; birth; and expulsion of the placenta.

■ The complications of pregnancy begin with fertility problems and the potential loss of the pregnancy from different types of abortions (miscarriages). Placental abnormalities also pose a threat to the well-being of the fetus. These include placenta previa, when the placenta covers the cervical os, and abruptio placentae, when the placenta breaks away from the uterine wall. Both cause maternal hemorrhage, threaten fetal oxygen supply, and require cesarean birth to protect the fetus and mother. Maternal disorders include pregnancy-induced glucose metabolic disorder, GDM, which requires dietary changes and possible insulin therapy during the pregnancy; and hypertension, which may progress to toxemia, a life-threatening rise in blood pressure with edema, uremia, and possible seizure activity.

■ Menopause is the permanent ending of menstruation because of the cessation of ovarian function. Perimenopause begins when hormone-related changes start to appear and lasts until the final menses. Some women experience few or no symptoms, whereas others have hot flashes, concentration problems, mood swings, irritability, migraines, vaginal dryness, urinary incontinence, dry skin, and sleep disorders. The physician may prescribe low-dose oral contraceptives or HRT, soy products or supplements, vitamin E, and vitamin B6; the physician also may recommend avoiding caffeine and spicy foods, maintaining a low-fat diet that is high in calcium, and performing regular weight-bearing exercise.

■ The medical assistant's role in the gynecological and reproductive examinations includes preparing the patient for the examination, equipping the room, making sure supplies are available and properly prepared, assisting with the examination, positioning and draping the patient as needed, assisting with the Pap smear or any other procedures, and providing support and understanding for the patient.

■ Diagnostic tests for the female reproductive system include sonography during pregnancy to determine the number of fetuses, age and sex of the fetus, fetal abnormalities, and position of the placenta; chorionic villi sampling or amniocentesis to perform genetic testing for anomalies or inherited disorders; alpha-fetoprotein (AFP) blood tests to diagnose neural tube defects; mammography, which provides an x-ray image of the breast tissue to identify abnormal masses that would otherwise go undetected under a breast palpation examination; colposcopy procedures that visualize abnormal cervical tissue for evaluation or biopsy; and a variety of tests done during pregnancy.

KEY INTERNET WEBSITES

- Columbia University Health Service
- Mayo Clinic's Women's Health Center
- National Osteoporosis Foundation
- U.S. Public Health Service
  For active weblinks to each website visit
  http://evolve.elsevier.com/Kinn/

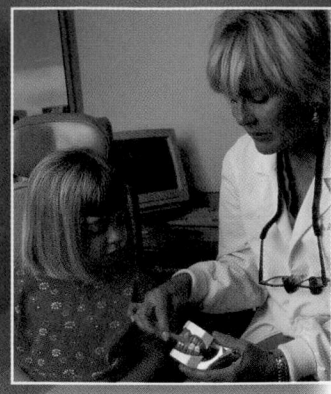

CHAPTER 39

Scenario

Susie Kwong, a CMA with 5 years experience, has been looking for a job and finally decided to accept a position with North Hills Pediatrics, a large, multiphysician practice. Susie's primary responsibility will be to assist in the clinical area, but she will also have to rotate through the telephone triage office as needed. Office policy states that telephone screening employees should manage problems as much as possible, but if patient callbacks are needed, they are to be referred to the physician on-call that day by noon and 5 PM. Although the physicians in the practice have developed specific guidelines for management of patient problems, Susie is anxious about this responsibility, so she requests that she work with the triage staff for several days before she has to start answering incoming calls.

Assisting in Pediatrics

Learning Objectives

- Define and spell the terms listed in the vocabulary.
- Compare childhood growth and development patterns.
- Explain common pediatric gastrointestinal disorders.
- Define intestinal disorders, their signs and symptoms, diagnostic tests, and treatments.
- Classify disorders of the respiratory system in children.
- Distinguish among pediatric infectious diseases.
- Recognize the etiological factors in and signs and symptoms of the two primary pediatric inherited disorders.
- Summarize CDC-recommended immunizations for children.
- Compare and contrast a well-child and a sick-child examination.
- Outline the medical assistant's role in a pediatric examination.
- Specify child safety guidelines for injury prevention and management of suspected child abuse.
- Properly obtain infant head measurements.
- Obtain accurate height and weight measurements and plot growth patterns.
- Accurately obtain pediatric vital signs including vision screening.
- Correctly apply a pediatric urine collection device.

National Curriculum Competencies

CLINICAL COMPETENCIES

4a. Perform telephone and in-person screening
4e. Prepare patients for and assist with routine and specialty examinations
4f. Prepare patients for and assist with procedures, treatments, and minor office surgery
4g. Apply pharmacology principles to prepare and administer oral and parenteral medications
4h. Maintain medication and immunization records

TRANSDISCIPLINARY COMPETENCIES

3b. Instruct individuals according to their needs
3d. Provide instruction for health maintenance and disease prevention

Vocabulary

attenuated Weakened, or changed, virulence of a pathogenic microorganism.

hydrocephaly Enlargement of the cranium caused by abnormal accumulation of cerebrospinal fluid within the cerebral system.

laryngoscopy Visual examination of the voice box area through an endoscope equipped with a light and mirrors for illumination.

microcephaly Small size of the head in relationship to the rest of the body.

rhonchi Continuous dry rattling in the throat or bronchial tube as a result of partial obstruction.

serous Thin, watery, serumlike drainage.

stridor Shrill, harsh respiratory sound heard during inhalation in the presence of a laryngeal obstruction.

suppurative Characterized by formation and/or discharge of pus.

Pediatrics is the medical specialty that deals with the development and care of children and with the treatment of childhood diseases. The age range of pediatric patients is from birth to puberty. Some practices continue to see the child until he or she is 14 to 16 years of age. Occasionally children will continue to see the pediatrician until high school graduation. There are subspecialties within pediatrics, such as surgery, cardiology, and psychiatry.

About 50% of the patients in a pediatric office are there for well-baby or well-child care visits. The roles of the pediatrician and the medical office staff are to supervise and help maintain the health of these patients. Parents must be involved in the care and development of their young children for treatment to be a success. The medical assistant can help by encouraging therapeutic communication among the patient, parents, and medical staff. The trust that a child develops in the care and consideration received in the physician's office forms the basis of good medical care.

Pediatric care actually starts before the child is born, with the promotion of the mother's good general health before conception and during pregnancy. The confidence and enthusiasm of the parents also affect the infant's physical and emotional well-being.

Normal Growth and Development

The terms *growth* and *development* are often used together and refer to the combination of changes that a child goes through as he or she matures. Growth refers to measurable changes such as height and weight; development considers qualitative maturation in motor, mental, and language skills. Pediatric assessment should be individualized for each child according to age, development, condition, and past experiences with healthcare professionals. The pediatrician looks for any signs of growth and development abnormalities by comparing a child's physical, intellectual, and social levels with published national standards. This comparison indicates whether the child is in the appropriate stage of growth and development for his or her chronological age.

Growth Patterns

Physical growth is one of the most visible changes in childhood. The average birth weight is 7 to $7\frac{1}{2}$ pounds, and by 6 months, the baby's birth weight has doubled. Growth slows down slightly, so that at 1 year, birth weight has tripled and length has increased by 50%. By age 2, the child has reached approximately 50% of his or her adult height. Between ages 1 and 2, the child will gain approximately $\frac{1}{2}$ pound per month. Between ages 2 and 3, weight gain will average 3 to 5 pounds and height will increase 2 to $2\frac{1}{2}$ inches. Most children slim down during this period, so that by the time the third birthday arrives, the potbellied toddler has become the characteristic preschooler.

During the preschool period, ages 3 to 6 years, weight increases 3 to 5 pounds a year and height increases at a slower but steady rate of $1\frac{1}{2}$ to $2\frac{1}{2}$ inches per year. By age 4, the child usually doubles his or her birth length. During this time the legs are the fastest growing part, and fatty connective tissue continues to increase slowly until about age 7. This same growth rate continues through the school-age period, 6 to 12 years; and as this period of development ends, the child usually is into a growth spurt that indicates impending puberty.

The growth spurt continues for approximately 2 years, and now the child has reached adolescence, ages 12 to 18 years. During this period, the adolescent gains almost half of his or her adult weight, and the skeleton and organs double in size. These changes are more noticeable in boys than in girls. Weight will increase in girls by 20 to 25 pounds and in boys by 15 to 20 pounds. Girls will grow 5 to 6 inches, and boys will grow 4 to 5 inches. As the growth spurt is completed, the teenager reaches sexual maturity. In the female, sexual maturity is signaled by the onset of the menstrual cycle; and in the male, maturity is determined by the presence of sperm in the semen. Timing of sexual maturity in both sexes varies greatly.

Completion of skeletal growth occurs in girls between 15 and 16 years of age and in boys between ages 17 and 18. Skeletal growth is complete when the growth plates (*epiphyseal plates*) of the long bones of the extremities have completely fused.

Growth charts that can be used to compare the child's individual growth pattern to national standards have been used since 1977, but in 2000 the Centers for Disease Control and Prevention (CDC) revised the charts to reflect cultural and racial diversity (samples are available at http://www.cdc.gov/growthcharts). The CDC charts also take into account both formula-fed and breastfed infants, because breastfed infants may grow differently in the first year of life.

In addition, the CDC growth charts include information on the average body-mass index (BMI) for children 2 to 20 years of age, giving pediatricians another weapon in the fight against childhood obesity. BMI was discussed in Chapter 27 as a way of considering the individual's height and weight. The BMI can be calculated by dividing the child's weight in kilograms by the height in meters squared, or:

$$\text{Weight in kg} \div [\text{Height in meters}]^2$$

Denver II Developmental Screening Test

Each child develops individually and will display differences in attaining developmental plateaus. The Denver II Developmental Screening Test is a standardized tool that is given to children between 1 month and 6 years of age to screen healthy infants for developmental delays, to validate concerns about an infant's development, or to monitor high-risk children for potential problems (Figures 39-1 and 39-2). It should be administered to an infant at 3 to 4 months, again at 10 months, and again to the child at 3 years. Although the test is not difficult to administer, only those trained in the procedure and interpretation of results should administer it. The assessment focuses on five developmental areas:

- *Gross motor skills:* Evaluation of the child's ability to control the body's large muscle groups. EXAMPLES: Standing, kicking, running, and balance
- *Language:* Evaluation of the child's verbal comprehension. EXAMPLES: Word comprehension, following simple commands, use of subjects, and counting
- *Fine motor adaptive skills:* Evaluation of the child's coordination of the fine motor muscles. EXAMPLES: Reaching, grasping, piling blocks, and drawing
- *Personal skills:* Evaluation of child's self-confidence and socialization. EXAMPLES: Playing games, using a fork and spoon, dressing, and brushing teeth
- *Re-screen:* Any child receiving a non-normal finding should be re-screened one to two weeks later to rule out temporary delays such as fatigue or anxiety.

Once the test is completed, the results are analyzed and then determined to be normal, suspect, or untestable. When the results are not normal, the child may be retested with other developmental tests, either by the pediatrician or by a professional pediatric testing agency.

Developmental Patterns

General patterns of child development occur rapidly during the first year of life as the infant progresses from reflex activities, such as grasping fingers and sucking, to learning to manipulate simple objects, such as pulling open drawers or throwing toys out of the crib. In addition to these motor skills, the child also learns verbal patterns, progressing from cooing and crying for attention to speaking first words.

By age 3, the child is showing increased autonomy. Now the child can walk, is toilet trained, sits at the table and eats with the family, can make simple sentences, understands the word "no," and even imitates the parent by using verbal gestures that he or she has seen used. The child's vocabulary consists of up to 900 words.

During the preschool stage, the child becomes increasingly independent and initiates activities. Preschoolers have mastered many gross motor skills and are perfecting their fine motor development. Verbal communication has increased to full simple and even complex sentences but remains quite literal. For example, if you tell a preschool child that you are going to fly to visit Aunt Sue, the child would think you are going to flap your arms and fly. Nonverbal communication skills are also being mastered. The vocabulary now includes more than 2000 words. During this period, children need to develop social skills, such as sharing and taking part in peer-group activities.

The school-age child has perfected fine motor skills and can paint, draw, and play an instrument, enjoys team activities, and expands reading and writing skills. His or her intellectual skills are developing, and social skills are going through refinement as a sense of self-achievement and self-worth is developed. It is during this time that the child learns and tests the rules for socializing outside the immediate family as an independent individual.

The adolescent, or transition, stage is when the individual attempts to establish an adult identity. This usually proceeds through trial and error by experimenting with adult roles and behavior patterns. Traditional values learned in childhood may be questioned, and peer relationships take on new importance. It is during this time that teenagers must develop the emotional maturity and motivation to make beneficial decisions. The family is looked to for encouragement and guidance in making decisions that will help the adolescent develop self-confidence and to become patient and less impulsive and self-centered.

CRITICAL THINKING APPLICATION

Susie receives a call from the mother of a 6-month-old child. The mother has concerns about whether her child is meeting his developmental timetable. What type of information regarding the child's growth and development should Susie gather? If Susie is unable to answer the mother's questions, what should she do?

Diseases and Disorders

The disease process in pediatric patients poses special problems, because children are constantly changing physically and functionally. As a child grows and develops, the immune system matures and, with the aid of routine prophylactic immunizations, the child is fortified with long-term protection against certain infectious diseases.

Gastrointestinal Disorders

Colic. Colic is usually seen in the newborn period or in early infancy. The problem is intermittent. During an attack, the infant draws up the legs, clenches the fists, and has a cry that indicates paroxysms of pain. The abdominal distress of colic usually occurs in the late afternoon and evening. The cause is unknown, but it is thought that overfeeding, swallowing excessive air while eating, and an allergy to cow's milk are all possible causes. Whatever the cause, a colicky infant is

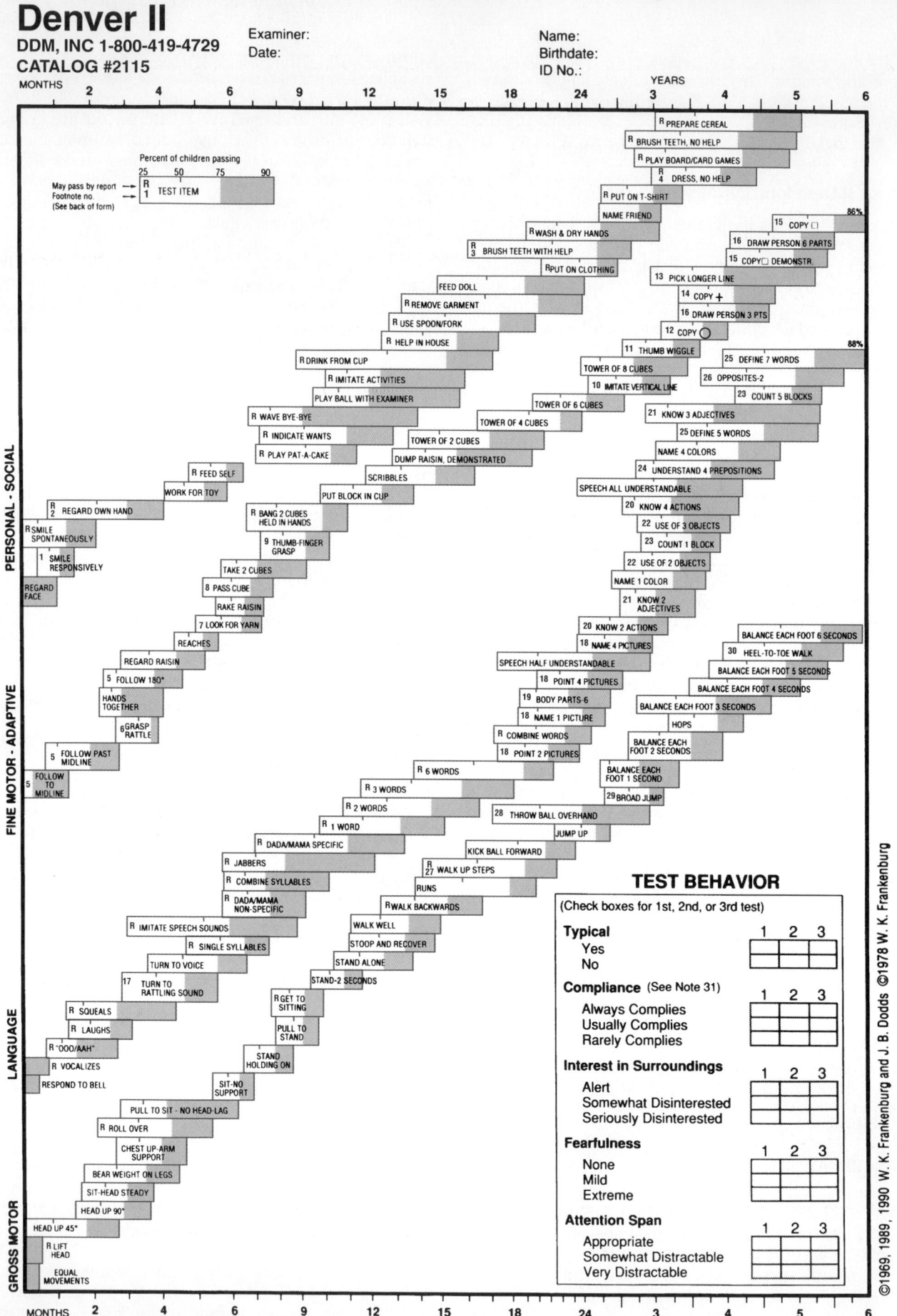

FIGURE 39-1 Denver II Developmental Screening Test (DDST). (©1969, 1989, 1990 W.K. Frankenburg and J.B. Dodds. ©1978 W.K. Frankenburg. Copies can be obtained from Denver Developmental Materials, Inc., (800) 419-4729, www.denverII.com.)

DIRECTIONS FOR ADMINISTRATION

1. Try to get child to smile by smiling, talking or waving. Do not touch him/her.
2. Child must stare at hand several seconds.
3. Parent may help guide toothbrush and put toothpaste on brush.
4. Child does not have to be able to tie shoes or button/zip in the back.
5. Move yarn slowly in an arc from one side to the other, about 8" above child's face.
6. Pass if child grasps rattle when it is touched to the backs or tips of fingers.
7. Pass if child tries to see where yarn went. Yarn should be dropped quickly from sight from tester's hand without arm movement.
8. Child must transfer cube from hand to hand without help of body, mouth, or table.
9. Pass if child picks up raisin with any part of thumb and finger.
10. Line can vary only 30 degrees or less from tester's line. ✓
11. Make a fist with thumb pointing upward and wiggle only the thumb. Pass if child imitates and does not move any fingers other than the thumb.

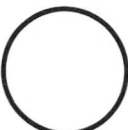   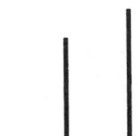   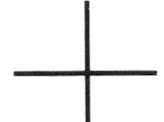   

12. Pass any enclosed form. Fail continuous round motions.	13. Which line is longer? (Not bigger.) Turn paper upside down and repeat. (pass 3 of 3 or 5 of 6)	14. Pass any lines crossing near midpoint.	15. Have child copy first. If failed, demonstrate.

When giving items 12, 14, and 15, do not name the forms. Do not demonstrate 12 and 14.

16. When scoring, each pair (2 arms, 2 legs, etc.) counts as one part.
17. Place one cube in cup and shake gently near child's ear, but out of sight. Repeat for other ear.
18. Point to picture and have child name it. (No credit is given for sounds only.)
    If less than 4 pictures are named correctly, have child point to picture as each is named by tester.

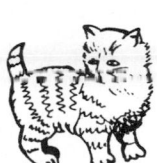   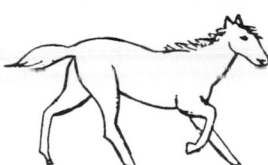   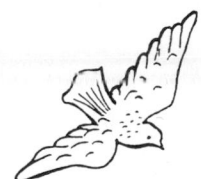   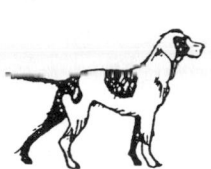   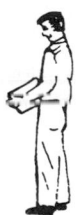

19. Using doll, tell child: Show me the nose, eyes, ears, mouth, hands, feet, tummy, hair. Pass 6 of 8.
20. Using pictures, ask child: Which one flies?... says meow?... talks?... barks?... gallops? Pass 2 of 5, 4 of 5.
21. Ask child: What do you do when you are cold?... tired?... hungry? Pass 2 of 3, 3 of 3.
22. Ask child: What do you do with a cup? What is a chair used for? What is a pencil used for? Action words must be included in answers.
23. Pass if child correctly places <u>and</u> says how many blocks are on paper. (1, 5).
24. Tell child: Put block **on** table; **under** table; **in front of** me, **behind** me. Pass 4 of 4. (Do not help child by pointing, moving head or eyes.)
25. Ask child: What is a ball?... lake?... desk?... house?... banana?... curtain?... fence?... ceiling? Pass if defined in terms of use, shape, what it is made of, or general category (such as banana is fruit, not just yellow). Pass 5 of 8, 7 of 8.
26. Ask child: If a horse is big, a mouse is __? If fire is hot, ice is __? If the sun shines during the day, the moon shines during the __? Pass 2 of 3.
27. Child may use wall or rail only, not person. May not crawl.
28. Child must throw ball overhand 3 feet to within arm's reach of tester.
29. Child must perform standing broad jump over width of test sheet (8 1/2 inches).
30. Tell child to walk forward, ⚭⚭⚭➤ heel within 1 inch of toe. Tester may demonstrate. Child must walk 4 consecutive steps.
31. In the second year, half of normal children are non-compliant.

OBSERVATIONS:

FIGURE 39-2 Instructions for DDST. (©1969, 1989, 1990 W.K. Frankenburg and J.B. Dodds. © 1978 W.K. Frankenburg. Copies can be obtained from Denver Developmental Materials, Inc., (800) 419-4729, www.denverll.com.)

extremely uncomfortable and cries inconsolably throughout the attack.

Treatment consists of determining the cause. Often the child will outgrow the condition before the causative agent can be identified. The usual period for colic is from birth until 4 months of age. In severe cases, the infant may be given a gastric antispasmodic agent and the parent may need counseling and assistance in developing coping techniques.

Diarrhea. Diarrhea can be caused by a variety of microorganisms, including bacteria, viruses, and parasites. However, children can sometimes have diarrhea without having an infection, as when diarrhea is caused by food allergies or as a result of taking medicines such as antibiotics. Diarrhea is diagnosed when the child has two or more watery or apparently abnormal stools within a 24-hour period. The child may not show other signs of illness or may have nausea, vomiting, stomach aches, headache, or fever. If the diarrhea continues for more than 2 days, medical intervention is needed, because prolonged diarrhea, in which fluid loss becomes excessive, can cause dehydration and electrolyte imbalance. Diaper rash and excoriation can produce painful stool elimination.

Treatment consists of observation of the stools both physically and with laboratory analysis for color, consistency, odor, and amount. Infants and small children should be followed up by telephone in 12 hours and then daily until diarrhea has stopped. Parents should be taught indications of dehydration, including lack of tears when crying, lethargy, fewer wet diapers or urination, dry mouth and lips, and weight loss. The physican may recommend the use of oral rehydration therapy such as Pedialyte or sports drinks to help replace electrolytes. A diet of bananas, rice, applesauce, and tea (called the BRAT diet), depending on the child's age and other factors, may be advised. Antibiotics may be prescribed if the causative agent is infectious. The child may require hospitalization to maintain electrolyte and fluid levels if dehydration is severe.

CRITICAL THINKING APPLICATION

Susie receives a call from the grandmother of a 3-year-old child who has had diarrhea since last night. What are some of the questions Susie should ask to determine the seriousness of the problem? Should the child be seen today, even though appointments are already overbooked?

Failure to Thrive

Failure to thrive is a symptom more than a disease but is defined as an infant or young child whose weight is consistently below the third percentile on standardized growth charts. It can be caused by a physiological factor (such as malabsorption disease or cleft palate) or a nonorganic cause that is associated with the parent-child relationship. The physician needs to have an accurately recorded history of the child's birth weight and subsequent length, weight, and head circumference. An accurate family history is important to rule out genetic growth abnormalities or a history of malabsorption problems such as cystic fibrosis or celiac disease. The family must be considered as a whole to effectively treat nonorganic causes, including the use of support groups and parental counseling.

Obesity

It is estimated that more than 30% of school-age children are overweight. Obesity is defined as weighing more than 20% above one's ideal body weight. Children who are more than 40% over their ideal weight should be under a physician-guided weight-loss program. The reasons for childhood obesity vary, including a family history of obesity, inactivity, high-calorie diets, and stress. Rarely, childhood obesity may be caused by metabolic or endocrine disorders. Childhood obesity can lead to serious health problems and self-esteem issues. The pediatrician will recommend a comprehensive diet program that emphasizes healthier eating habits and physical activity. A medical assistant can help by providing educational materials, encouragement for the child and parents, and referral to community education and support programs.

Respiratory Disorders

Common Cold. The common cold, or *infectious rhinitis*, has more than 100 causative pathogens and is highly contagious. It is spread through respiratory droplets from rhinitis, sneezing, or coughing, either from direct contact or from touching contaminated items. The signs include nasal congestion, low-grade fever, and general malaise. Most colds are self-limiting and run their course in about a week. In infants and young children, the primary concern is nasal congestion and loss of appetite. The parent may need to be shown how to use a nasal bulb syringe to suction the nose of an infant (Figure 39-3). Secondary infections in the lower respiratory tract or in the middle ear can occur.

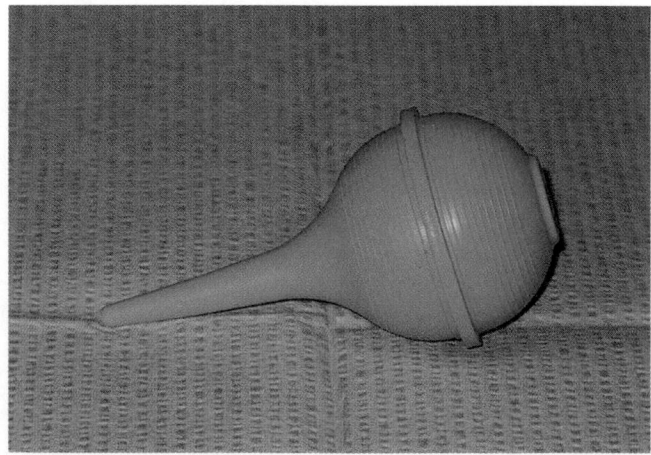

FIGURE 39-3 Nasal bulb syringe.

One of the secondary infections that can occur is *strep throat*, which is caused by group A *Streptococcus* bacteria. It is easily spread when an infected person coughs or sneezes contaminated droplets into the air and another person inhales them. A person can also get infected from touching such secretions and then touching his or her mouth or nose. Symptoms of strep throat infections may include severe sore throat, fever, headache, and swollen glands. If not treated, strep infections can lead to scarlet fever, rheumatic fever, infections of the skin, bloodstream, or ears, and pneumonia. Scarlet fever is characterized by a bright red, rough-textured rash that spreads all over the child's body. Rheumatic fever is a serious disease that can damage the heart valves.

Otitis Media. Infection in the middle ear is usually a side effect of a cold or other upper respiratory tract disorder, but it can also be caused by allergies. Otitis media usually occurs in children under 3 years of age. Symptoms include inflammation of the middle ear, with fluid building up behind the tympanic membrane. The child may cry persistently, tug at the ear, have a fever, be irritable, and be unable to hear well. These symptoms may sometimes be accompanied by diarrhea, nausea, and vomiting.

Otitis media is classified as either **serous** (Figure 39-4) or **suppurative** (Figure 39-5), depending on the composition of the accumulated fluid. The treatment usually consists of analgesics, decongestants, and antibiotics. Some children with chronic ear infections may require an operation—a **myringotomy**—in which a tube is inserted through the tympanic membrane to drain the fluid from the middle ear.

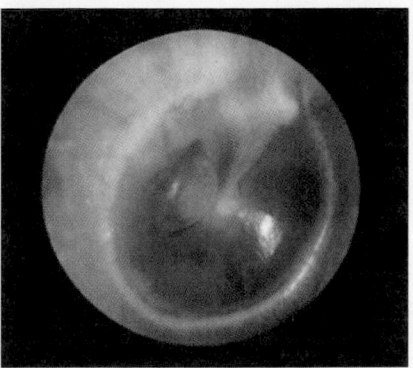

FIGURE 39-4 Serous otitis media. (From Swartz MH: *Textbook of physical diagnosis*, ed 3. Philadelphia, 1997, WB Saunders.)

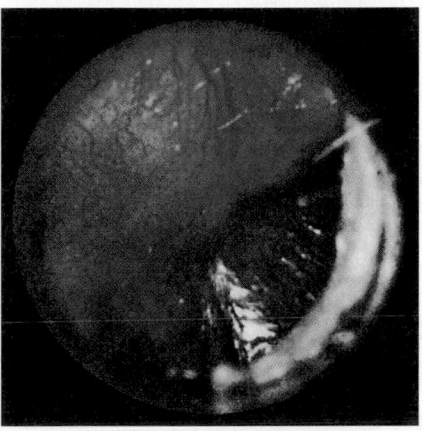

FIGURE 39-5 Suppurative otitis media. (Courtesy Dr. Richard A. Buckingham and Dr. George E. Shambaugh, Jr.)

CRITICAL THINKING APPLICATION

A young mother calls extremely upset about her 4-year-old son. His symptoms started 3 days ago with a cold, but now the child is complaining of a sore throat and an earache. What questions should Susie ask to determine whether the child should be seen today?

Croup. Croup is a viral disorder that affects primarily the larynx with edema and spasm to the vocal cords. This varying degree of obstruction to the cords produces hoarseness, a high-pitched raspy cough, and **stridor** during inhalation. The episodes usually occur at night, and all symptoms may be gone by morning. The infection is usually self-limiting, and the child typically recovers without treatment. Children with allergies may require medical treatment. If the problem becomes chronic or continues for a period of time, it may become necessary to do a **laryngoscopy** or obtain throat cultures to determine the underlying cause.

Bronchiolitis. Bronchiolitis is a viral infection of the small bronchi and bronchioles that usually affects children under 3 years of age. The infection varies in severity and is seen in children with a family history of asthma and children exposed to cigarette smoke. The

child typically has a previous history of rhinitis and cough with acute onset of wheezing and dyspnea. Symptoms occur because of necrosis, inflammation, edema, increased secretions, and bronchospasm in the respiratory pathway. Treatment includes acetaminophen for discomfort and fever as well as a bronchodilator inhaler (albuterol sulfate) for relief of wheezing. Most children fully recover in 2 weeks, but as many as 50% of them will have recurrent wheezing and coughing.

Asthma. Asthma is a chronic breathing disorder and is the most common chronic health problem among children. Asthma is the result of two specific reactions—bronchospasm and inflammation. During an asthma attack, bronchial tubes begin to spasm, thereby decreasing the amount of air that can pass through, while at the same time the inflammatory process causes edema and secretion of mucus. Asthma has a strong hereditary link. Factors that can trigger an attack include:

- Respiratory infections, including infections caused by common cold viruses
- Exposure to cigarette smoke
- Stress
- Strenuous exercise
- Weather conditions, including cold, windy, or rainy days and extreme humidity
- Allergies to animals, dust, pollen, or mold

- Indoor air pollutants, such as paint, cleaning materials, chemicals, or perfumes
- Outdoor air pollutants, such as ozone

Children with asthma have a nonproductive cough accompanied by an expiratory wheeze and shortness of breath. Shallow breathing makes it difficult for the child to speak more than a few words at a time. The child complains of tightness or pressure in the chest, and the physician will hear **rhonchi** on auscultation. An asthma attack can last minutes to days and can develop into a medical emergency. Each child and each attack needs to be evaluated independently.

The therapeutic plan is determined by the severity and frequency of attacks. Children with mild to moderately persistent disease (from symptoms less than twice a week to daily symptoms) should be referred to a specialist. If they experience symptoms 2 or more times per week, they should be on daily antiinflammatory medications either by mouth (zafirlukast [Accolate]) or via inhalers (cromolyn sodium [Intal] or salmeterol xinafoate [Serevent]). "Rescue inhalers" for acute relief of bronchospasm or exercise-induced asthma (albuterol sulfate; Ventolin) should be readily available at all times. Further management of asthma will be covered in Chapter 43.

Influenza. Influenza (flu) is an acute, highly contagious viral infection of the respiratory tract. Its highest incidence is in school-age children, but it is most severe in infants and toddlers. It is transmitted by direct contact with moist secretions. Children tend to have high fevers with influenza and are susceptible to pulmonary complications. There is a broad range in the severity of flu cases, from very mild to life threatening. The virus can destroy the respiratory epithelium, which is one of the body's strong defense mechanisms against bacterial invasion. With the loss of this protective mechanism, bacteria can invade any part of the respiratory tract and cause pneumonia.

There is no medication that cures influenza. Sometimes antibiotics are prescribed to prevent a secondary bacterial infection. The usual treatment consists of bed rest, increased fluids, and a nonaspirin analgesic to reduce fever. Flu vaccines are available but are beneficial only if the individual is vaccinated before the onset of the disease, and these vaccines do not give immunity for all strains of the flu virus. Any child 6 months and older can be vaccinated against influenza. Children in the following groups are at high risk of serious disease with influenza and should be vaccinated:

- Children with chronic lung disease (including asthma) or heart disease
- Children with chronic diseases such as diabetes mellitus or kidney, blood, or suppressed immune system diseases

Infectious Diseases

Conjunctivitis. Pinkeye, also called *conjunctivitis*, was discussed in Chapter 34. It is a common infection in children and is highly contagious, especially in day care centers and schools. It can be caused by a bacterial or viral infection that produces a white or yellowish pus that may cause the eyelids to stick shut in the morning. Health teaching for caregivers of infected children includes the following:

- Use good hand-washing practices and hygiene including proper use and disposal of paper tissues.
- Do not share towels or any other item that comes into contact with the child's face.
- Disinfect any articles that may have been contaminated.
- Children diagnosed with infectious conjunctivitis should be treated with an antibiotic for at least 24 hours before returning to day care or school.

Tonsillitis. Tonsillitis is caused by many infectious agents, but the most frequent is Streptococcus A. The onset is sudden and can become intensely painful in a brief period, with fever and general malaise. The tonsils appear enlarged and inflamed and may be covered with pustules. A throat culture is usually performed to determine the causative organism. The treatment consists of bed rest, liquid to soft diet, analgesic throat spray, and oral antibiotics. The danger is in the secondary problems that can occur, which include rheumatic heart disease and kidney disease.

Fifth Disease. Fifth disease, also called *erythema infectiosum* or "slapped cheek disease," is an infection caused by parvovirus B19. Outbreaks most often occur in winter and spring, but a person may become ill with fifth disease at any time of the year. Symptoms begin with a mild fever and general malaise. After a few days, the cheeks take on a flushed appearance that looks like the face has been slapped. There may also be a lacy rash on the trunk, arms, and legs. Not all infected persons develop a rash.

Most persons who get fifth disease are not very ill and recover without any serious consequences. However, children with sickle cell anemia, chronic anemia, or an impaired immune system may become seriously ill when infected and require medical care. If a pregnant woman becomes infected with parvovirus B19, the fetus may suffer damage, including the possibility of stillbirth. The woman herself may have no symptoms or a mild illness with rash or joint pains.

Fifth disease is spread through direct contact or by breathing in respiratory secretions from an infected person. The patient is most contagious before the onset of the rash. Once the rash appears, the person is no longer contagious.

Varicella (Chickenpox). Chickenpox is caused by a member of the herpesvirus group and is transmitted by direct or indirect droplets from the respiratory tract of an infected person. The incubation period is 14 to 21 days. The child usually runs a slight fever for up to 3 days before the skin eruptions occur and is contagious at this time. The skin lesions continue to erupt for 3 to 4 days and cause intense itching. The infection lasts for about 2 weeks and, in most cases, leaves the child with lifetime immunity. The disease is so contagious in its early stages that an exposed person who is not immune to the virus has a 70% to 80% chance of contracting the disease. A varicella virus vaccine, Varivax, is now available for protection against chickenpox.

Although for most children chickenpox is not a serious disease, newborns or persons with impaired immune systems (e.g., those who are receiving chemotherapy for cancer, have AIDS, or take steroidal medications, such as cortisone or prednisone) may have a severe case or can even die. Chickenpox can be very dangerous for pregnant women, causing stillbirths or birth defects, and can be spread to their babies during childbirth. Occasionally chickenpox can cause serious, life-threatening illnesses, such as *encephalitis* or pneumonia, especially in adults. After infection, the virus migrates to a dermatome and may cause "shingles" or *herpes zoster* (see Chapter 35). An adult with shingles can spread the virus to an adult or child who has not had chickenpox, and the susceptible person can develop the disease.

Meningitis. Meningitis is an inflammation of the membranes that cover the brain and spinal cord. The cause of this inflammation is infection with either bacteria or viruses. Meningitis caused by a bacterial infection (sometimes called spinal meningitis) is one of the most serious types, sometimes leading to permanent brain damage or even death. Bacterial meningitis is most commonly caused by these bacteria: *Neisseria meningitidis* (meningococcal meningitis), *Streptococcus pneumoniae*, or *Haemophilus influenzae* serotype b (*H. influenzae* meningitis). These bacteria are carried in the upper back part of the throat (*nasopharynx*) of an infected person and are spread either through the air (when the person coughs or sneezes) or by direct contact with secretions. However, transmission usually occurs only after very close contact with the infected person.

Symptoms of bacterial meningitis include sudden onset of fever, headache, neck pain or stiffness, vomiting (often without abdominal complaints), and irritability. These symptoms may quickly progress to a decreased level of consciousness (difficulty in being aroused), convulsions, and death. For this reason, if any child displays symptoms of possible meningitis, he or she should receive medical care immediately.

Meningitis caused by *H. influenzae* serotype b (Hib) can be prevented with Hib vaccine, which is given as part of routine childhood immunizations. Some cases of meningococcal meningitis can also be prevented by vaccine. However, this vaccine is not used routinely— usually only during outbreaks or in high-risk children. Many states require reporting of bacterial meningitis cases to the health department, which will probably recommend preventive antibiotics for potentially exposed persons.

Hepatitis B. Hepatitis B virus (HBV) infection can lead to serious and chronic infection of the liver. The virus can be transmitted across the placenta or during the birth process if the mother is infected. HBV can also be transmitted sexually, by blood transfusion, or by direct contact. A child can carry the virus for years and only later develop liver failure or liver cancer as a result. Many states now include immunizations for HBV in the recommended immunization schedule, which is usually begun in the newborn nursery.

Reye's Syndrome. The cause of Reye's syndrome is unknown, but it has been linked to the use of aspirin during a viral illness. It is an acute and sometimes fatal illness characterized by fatty invasion of the inner organs, especially the liver, and swelling of the brain. It is most often seen in children between infancy through puberty (age 16). The syndrome moves through five stages, as shown in Table 39-1.

Prevention is the best treatment, which means children should never be given aspirin. Parents should be advised to use nonsalicylate analgesics and antipyretics, such as ibuprofen and acetaminophen, for fevers or discomfort. Parents should also be warned to read the labels of over-the-counter medication carefully, because cold and flu remedies may contain aspirin.

CRITICAL THINKING APPLICATION

A father of a 10 year-old girl calls this morning concerned about his daughter's symptoms. She has a sore throat, fever, and bright red cheeks. He wants to give her aspirin for the fever. What advice should Susie give the father? What questions should she ask to determine the seriousness of the child's problem?

Inherited Disorders

Cystic Fibrosis. Cystic fibrosis is an autosomal recessive genetic disorder (i.e., both parents are carriers) that causes exocrine glands to produce abnormally thick secretions. The lungs and pancreas are primarily affected, causing a build up of mucus in the lungs and blockage of the pancreatic ducts, which prevents the excretion of pancreatic digestive enzymes and results in malabsorption problems in the child. The child is prone to develop an emphysema-like lung condition as a result of the obstruction of air pathways with mucus. There is also an abnormality in the sweat glands, which produce sweat that is very high in sodium chloride.

Signs and symptoms of cystic fibrosis include a salty taste to the skin, which may be noticed when parents kiss the child, *steatorrhea* (large, greasy, foul-smelling stools), abdominal distention, failure to thrive, chronic cough, and frequent respiratory infections.

The primary diagnostic test is the sweat test, which shows an elevated chlorine level. The treatment of the disease is complicated, requiring a multispecialty approach, because there are so many systems involved. The goals of treatment are to prevent bronchial obstruction through routine chest percussion therapy and the use of bronchodilators and antibiotics for signs of infection. The

TABLE 39-1	Five Stages of Reye's Syndrome
Stage	Signs and Symptoms
1	Restlessness, vomiting, liver malfunction
2	Elevated respiratory rate, hyperactive reflexes, increased liver dysfunction
3	Internal organ tissue changes, coma
4	Loss of brain function, deepening coma
5	Seizures, respiratory arrest, death

child is also given pancreatic enzymes to improve digestion and absorption of nutrients. Cystic fibrosis is a chronic, progressive disease that has no cure, with a life expectancy of 30 to 35 years. Genetic testing can identify carriers, and its presence can be determined through prenatal genetic testing with either chorionic villi sampling or amniocentesis. Cystic fibrosis usually occurs without any warning (parents have no idea they are carriers), so families need support and understanding to cope with the demands of a child with the disease.

Duchenne's Muscular Dystrophy. Muscular dystrophy is an X-linked genetic disease (passed from mothers to sons) that causes progressive muscle degeneration. The disease usually develops before age 5, with muscular weakness, frequent falls, waddling gait, possible swallowing problems, and difficulty climbing stairs. The disorder is diagnosed with a blood test that shows an elevated creatine phosphokinase (CPK) level, electromyography, and a muscle biopsy. As the disease progresses and the necrotic skeletal muscles are replaced with fat and fibrous connective tissue, muscle function is gradually lost. Respiratory insufficiency and infections are common because of involvement of the muscles used for breathing. There is no cure and no specific treatment, except for supportive care. Family counseling is helpful so that family members can learn to cope with the disease. Death usually occurs by age 20 because of respiratory or cardiac complications.

Immunizations

Over the years immunization has helped dramatically reduce potentially lethal childhood infections. Figure 39-6 summarizes immunization recommendations from the American Academy of Pediatrics. This schedule is updated periodically as new vaccines become available and/or research indicates a better method for giving the vaccine. For example, it is now recommended that polio vaccination be given as an injection for better absorption rather than the oral route that was recommended for years.

The CDC recommends immunization against infectious diseases for all children, except those for whom a particular vaccination would pose a risk. Each state develops its own immunization program and methods for enforcement.

Immunizations consist of a vaccine suspension of **attenuated** organisms or their toxins that is administered to stimulate an active immune response, causing the production of antibodies against the specific pathogenic organisms. Booster doses are usually equivalent to one

Recommended childhood immunization schedule*—United States, 2002

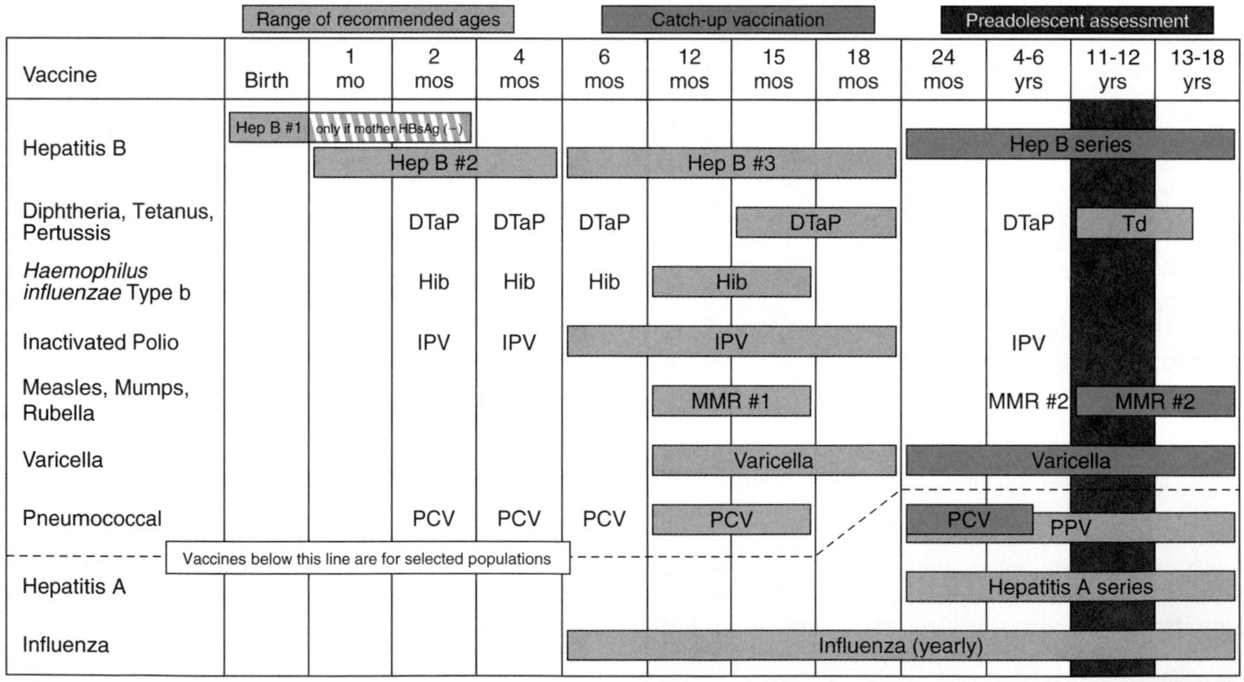

Vaccine	Birth	1 mo	2 mos	4 mos	6 mos	12 mos	15 mos	18 mos	24 mos	4-6 yrs	11-12 yrs	13-18 yrs
Hepatitis B	Hep B #1		only if mother HBsAg (−)							Hep B series		
			Hep B #2			Hep B #3						
Diphtheria, Tetanus, Pertussis			DTaP	DTaP	DTaP		DTaP			DTaP	Td	
Haemophilus influenzae Type b			Hib	Hib	Hib	Hib						
Inactivated Polio			IPV	IPV		IPV				IPV		
Measles, Mumps, Rubella						MMR #1				MMR #2	MMR #2	
Varicella						Varicella				Varicella		
Pneumococcal			PCV	PCV	PCV	PCV				PCV	PPV	
Hepatitis A										Hepatitis A series		
Influenza						Influenza (yearly)						

Range of recommended ages · Catch-up vaccination · Preadolescent assessment

Vaccines below this line are for selected populations

* Indicates the recommended ages for routine administration of currently licensed childhood vaccines, as of December 1, 2001, for children through age 18 years. Any dose not given at the recommended age should be given at any subsequent visit when indicated and feasible. ▇ Indicates age groups that warrant special effort to administer those vaccines not given previously. Additional vaccines may be licensed and recommended during the year. Licensed combination vaccines may be used whenever any components of the combination are indicated and the vaccine's other components are not contraindicated. Providers should consult the manufacturers' package inserts for detailed recommendations.

Additional information about vaccines, vaccine supply, and contraindications for immunization is available at http://www.cdc.gov/nip or at the National Immunization hotline. 800-232-2522 (English), or 800-232-0233 (Spanish). Copies of the schedule can be obtained at http://www.cdc.gov/nip/recs/child-schedule.htm. Approved by the **Advisory Committee on Immunization Practices** (http://www.cdc.gov/nip/acip), the **American Academy of Pediatrics** (http://www.aap.org), and the **American Academy of Family Physicians** (http://www.aafp.org).

FIGURE 39-6 Immunization schedule.

single dose of the initial immunization; for some immunizations, boosters are prescribed at designated intervals to ensure maintenance of immune levels.

Vaccine manufacturers have trade names for each product and have established protocols to ensure potency and stability. All vaccines are tested for safety and effectiveness. In every package of vaccine is an insert that fully describes the vaccine, its use, route of administration, and adverse reactions and symptoms that the parent might observe after immunization that would indicate a potential problem. Untoward responses include high fever, swelling at the site of the injection, urticaria, breathing difficulties, severe headache, and convulsions. Any of these should be reported to the physician immediately. Vaccine storage should follow manufacturer guidelines (e.g., some vaccines must be refrigerated; others must not be exposed to sunlight).

Some vaccines are grown in bird eggs or in a medium made from animal organs, or are weakened with chemicals. Thus a child who is allergic to eggs cannot receive some of the vaccines, such as those for measles/mumps/rubella (MMR) or varicella. It is a medical assistant's responsibility to know potential allergic problems, common symptoms, and adverse reactions to immunizations and to be certain that the parent is informed.

Informed consent must be signed and attached to the child's health record before immunizations are given. Documentation of immunization administration must include the type of vaccine, the manufacturer's lot number, the exact site of administration if an injection is given, and any reported side effects.

Table 39-2 details guidelines for childhood immunizations.

TABLE 39-2	Guidelines for Childhood Immunization		
Vaccine and Disease	**Route of Administration**	**Contraindications (mild illness is not a contraindication)**	**Side Effects**
DtaP Diphtheria, tetanus, pertussis (whooping cough)	IM; Td (tetanus and diphtheria) boosters at 11-12 yr if at least 5 yr since last dose; subsequent booster every 10 yrs	Moderate or severe acute illness; neurological problem; complication such as fever or convulsion after previous dose	Mild fever, anorexia, irritability, drowsiness
HBV Hepatitis B (can use either Energix B or Recombivax HB brands)	IM; may give with all other vaccines but at a separate site; requires three injections	Moderate or severe acute illness; yeast allergy; severe cardiovascular disease	Fever, pain at site, headache, malaise, vomiting
Hib *Haemophilus influenzae* serotype B meningitis	IM; may give with all other vaccines but at a separate site	Not routinely given to children ≥5 years of age; moderate or severe acute illness	Minimal
IPV Inactive poliovirus	SQ or IM; 4 doses; may give with all other vaccines but at a separate site	Moderate or severe acute illness; egg allergy	Uncommon
MMR Measles, mumps, rubella	SQ; may give with all other vaccines but at a separate site	Moderate or severe acute illness; immunocompromised patients (may be given if HIV positive); pregnancy or possible pregnancy in 3 months; egg allergy	Fever
Pneumoccal Pneumococcal pneumonia	IM or SQ; all children 2-23 mo; administer every 6 yr for high-risk patients		
Varicella Varicella (chickenpox)	SQ; may give with all other vaccines but at a separate site; all susceptible children ≥12 mo	Confirmed history of chickenpox; pregnancy or possible pregnancy in 1 mo; moderate or severe acute illness; immunocompromised patients; egg allergy	No salicylates for 6 wk after to prevent possible Reye's syndrome

IM, Intramuscular; *SQ*, subcutaneous.

CRITICAL THINKING APPLICATION

Susie will be administering pediatric immunizations during the well-baby visits that are scheduled today. To prepare for this responsibility, Susie looked up the primary vaccinations, their routes of administration, contraindications, and possible side effects. The first child is here for her 4-month check-up. What immunizations should the child receive and how should they be administered? The baby's father asks if she will get sick from the vaccines. What should Susie tell him?

The Pediatric Patient

A newborn's first physical assessment comes at the time of delivery, when the pediatrician assesses the newborn's ability to thrive outside the uterus. The Apgar score is a system of evaluating the infant's physical condition at 1 and 5 minutes after birth (Table 39-3). Developed by pediatrician Virginia Apgar, the scoring system evaluates the following: Appearance (color); Pulse (heart rate); Grimace (reflex; response to stimuli); Activity (muscle tone); and Respiration (breathing). These parameters are each rated 0, 1, or 2. The maximum total score is 10. Infants with low scores must be given immediate attention.

Well-Child Visits

The frequency of well-child visits varies with the physician and the community. It may follow this pattern: 2 weeks, 4 weeks, 8 weeks, 4 months, 6 months, 12 months, 18 months, 2 years, 5 years, 10 years, and 15 years. These visits focus on maintaining the health of the child through basic system examinations, immunizations, and upgrading of the child's medical history record.

The decision of whether the child is to be seen alone or with the parent depends on the pediatrician and on the age of the child. Often the child will look to the parent for approval before answering or performing a skill; for this reason, the physician may want the child alone. If this is the case, explain to the parent that the physician wants to evaluate the child's independent abilities and that as soon as the testing is completed, the physician will relate the results of the tests.

The medical history is an essential guide to the pediatric examination. With an infant, the physician depends on the caregiver for the history, but as the child gets older, some history may be obtained from the child and clarified or amplified by the parent. Close observation also gives the physician considerable information.

Sick-Child Visits

Sick-child visits occur whenever needed—usually on short notice. For this reason, most pediatric offices keep open appointments in the schedule to accommodate a sick child. The length and frequency of this type of visit depend entirely on the child and the illness. The medical assistant is frequently the first point of contact for a sick child and his or her caregiver. Determining whether the child should be seen immediately or if the problem can wait for an opening in the schedule is crucial to pediatric care. The medical assistant should follow established office policies, but when in doubt about the seriousness of the problem, he or she should ask the office manager or physician for advice. Usually the physician would prefer to see the child rather than delay seeing a patient with a potentially serious condition. Some criteria to consider when conducting telephone screening include:

- If the child is young (less than 2 years old) and the parent reports frequent cycles of crying, lethargy, vomiting longer than 24 hours, diarrhea (more than 6 stools in the last 12 hours), or fever of 101° F (38.5° C) or higher, it is best to see the child right away. He or she cannot verbalize associated pain or problems.

Table 39-4 summarizes some of the action principles for telephone screening of an older child who can communicate his or her symptoms. It is important to focus on the *onset* (When did symptoms first start?), *frequency* (Are symptoms constant, or do they cycle through recurrences?), and *duration* of the problem as well as attempted treatments and their effectiveness. As with any other patient, all telephone communications should be documented to record the reason for the call, the information gathered, and the action taken, including whether the physician was consulted, any orders given, and if and when an appointment was scheduled.

TABLE 39-3	The Apgar Scoring System*		
Clinical Sign	**Assigned Score**		
	0	**1**	**2**
Heart rate	Absent	Under 100	Over 100
Respiratory effort	Absent	Slow and irregular	Good and crying
Muscle tone	Limp	Some flexion of the arms and legs	Active movement
Reflex irritability	No response	Grimace	Coughing and sneezing
Color	Blue and pale	Body pink and extremities blue	Pink all over

*The readings are taken by the pediatrician at 1-minute and 5-minute intervals after birth. At *1 minute*, if the score is 7 or less, some nervous system problems are suspected. If the score is below 4, resuscitation is usually necessary. At *5 minutes*, if the score is at least 8, the child is probably reacting normally.

TABLE 39-4	Action Principles for Telephone Screening
Complaint	**Screening Questions**
Pain	Onset, frequency, duration of pain? On a scale of 1-10, how severe is the pain? Where is the exact location? Was there any accident involved (include details)? Has the pain gotten worse over time? Has the pain interfered with sleep? Is there associated fever, vomiting, diarrhea, or rash?
Gastrointestinal	Onset, duration, frequency of symptoms? Has the child been vomiting longer than 24 hrs without improvement? Is the child receiving clear liquids only? Is the child dehydrated (dry mouth, no urination in 8-10 hrs, listless)? If diarrhea, were there more than 5-6 watery stools in 12 hrs? Does the child have other symptoms (vomiting, fever over 103°F [39.4°C], rapid breathing)?
Respiratory	Onset, duration, frequency of symptoms? Describe the child's breathing. Has the child been diagnosed with a breathing disorder? Is a prescribed treatment being used? Are there any other symptoms (severe headache, stiff neck, fever, cough)? If the child is coughing, what does it sound like? Are there signs of a sore throat or earache?

The Medical Assistant's Role in Pediatric Procedures

The medical assistant is responsible for assisting the pediatrician with examinations; upgrading patient histories; performing ordered screening tests such as vision, hearing, urinalysis, and hemoglobin checks; administering immunizations; measuring and weighing children as needed; and providing patient and caregiver support. A medical assistant must develop a relationship with the pediatric patient that encourages cooperation and compliance with tests and treatment plans. If the child becomes upset, everything that needs to be done during that visit will be done under duress, and the chance for future mistrust will intensify.

Interacting with children requires special techniques, depending on the age of the child. To gain cooperation, a calm, unhurried manner is essential. The tone of voice should be gentle but confident. Using a firm, direct approach about expected behavior is important in gaining the cooperation of older children. Offer reasonable choices when possible, such as, "Would you like your shot in your left or right leg?" *not* "Are you ready for your shot now?" Offering sincere praise for the child during the examination or procedures helps decrease anxiety and builds self-esteem. If the child is having an unusually difficult time, try to discover the reason. If there is a history of a negative healthcare experience, the child may be afraid of what might happen. Each step should be explained in a language the child (and parent) can understand. Children younger than 2 feel better when the parent is holding them or remains very close (Figure 39-7). Preschool children enjoy playing, so making a game out of the situation is helpful (Figure 39-8). Whatever the age of the child, the medical assistant should be sensitive to his or her individual needs and adapt the examination and procedures to meet those needs as much as possible.

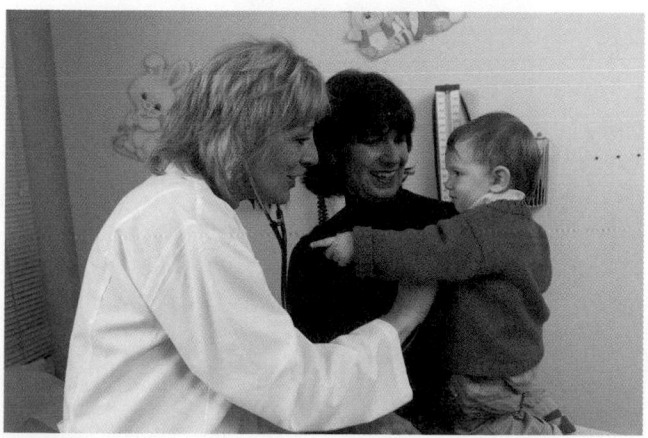

FIGURE 39-7 Sometimes a pediatric patient is more comfortable when held by a parent.

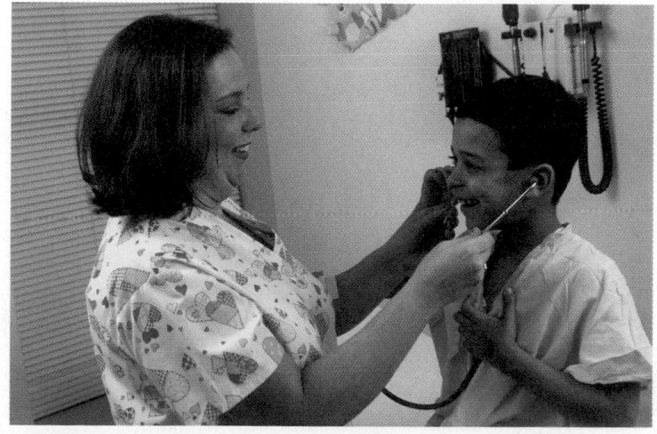

FIGURE 39-8 Making a game out of a procedure.

The sequence of the physician's examination varies and is frequently adapted based on the cooperation of the child. The pediatrician will probably leave procedures and tests that will cause the most objection until the end of the appointment. The physician is constantly evaluating the child's growth and development. A child's alertness and responses tell the physician a considerable amount. In infants and in young children of preschool age, the parent is closely questioned about the child's eating, sleeping, and elimination habits. A school-age child is usually a little more cooperative during an examination and can answer most questions without parental assistance. Adolescent patients should be given the option of not having parents present during an examination. This may permit teenagers to respond more honestly to lifestyle factors as well as protect their privacy.

Measurement

Examination of the child during routine well-child care includes measurement of the circumference of the infant's head to determine normal growth and development (Procedure 39-1). The size of the child's head reflects the growth of the brain. Brain growth is 50% completed by 1 year of age, 75% by age 3, and 90% by age 6. Routine head measurement is recommended in children until 36 months of age and in older children whose head size is not within norms. If the circumference of the head deviates greatly from normal measurements, **hydrocephaly** or **microcephaly** may be suspected. It is important to discover any congenital problem as early as possible so that appropriate treatment measures can be initiated.

The medical assistant should record the child's length or stature, weight, and head circumference on growth charts so the physician can compare the child's measurement statistics with national standards (Procedure 39-2). The growth charts consist of a series of percentile curves that illustrate the distribution of selected body measurements.

The revised CDC 2000 growth charts consist of 16 charts (8 for boys and 8 for girls). These charts represent revisions to the 14 previous charts, as well as the

---

PROCEDURE 39-1

Measuring the Circumference of an Infant's Head

GOAL: To obtain an accurate measurement of the circumference of an infant's head.

EQUIPMENT AND SUPPLIES

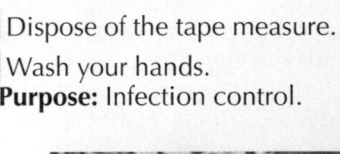

- Flexible disposable tape measure
- Age and sex-specific growth chart
- Patient's chart
- Pen or pencil

PROCEDURAL STEPS

1 Wash your hands.
   Purpose: Infection control.

2 Identify the patient and gain infant cooperation through conversation.
   Purpose: Alleviate anxiety and gain the child's trust.

3 Place the infant in the supine position; an older child may sit on the examination table; alternatively, the infant may be held by the parent.

4 Hold the tape measure with the zero mark against the infant's forehead, slightly above the eyebrows and the top of the ears. Ask the parent for assistance if necessary.

5 Bring the tape measure around the head, just above the ears, until it meets (Figure 1).

6 Read to the nearest 0.01 cm or ¼ inch.

7 Record the measurement on the growth chart and the patient's chart.
   Purpose: A procedure is not done until it is recorded.

8 Dispose of the tape measure.

9 Wash your hands.
   Purpose: Infection control.

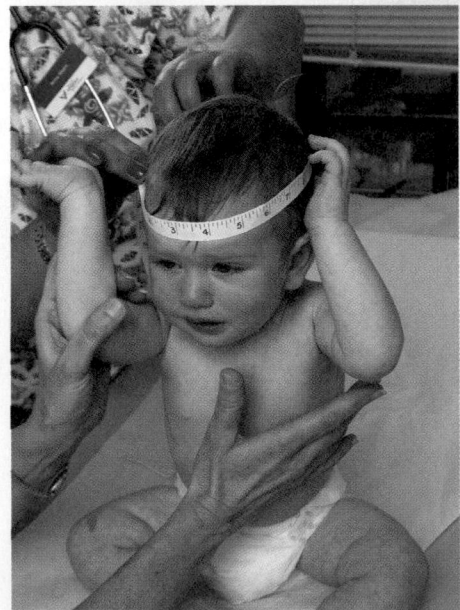

Figure 1

See Appendix E for a charting example.

PROCEDURE **39-2**

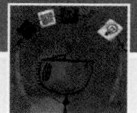

Measuring Infant Length and Weight

GOAL: To accurately measure infant length and weight so growth patterns can be monitored and recorded.

EQUIPMENT AND SUPPLIES

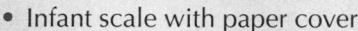
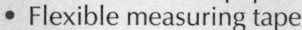

- Infant scale with paper cover
- Flexible measuring tape
- Examination table paper
- Pen
- Infant growth chart
- Biohazard waste container

PROCEDURAL STEPS

Measuring Infant Length

1 Wash your hands, assemble equipment, and explain the procedure to the infant's caregiver.

2 Undress the infant in preparation for measurement of length and weight. You may leave the diaper on until the length measurement is taken, but it must be removed before the infant is weighed.

3 Ask the caregiver to place the infant on his or her back on the examination table, which is covered with paper. If it is a pediatric table with a headboard, ask the caregiver to gently hold the infant's head against the board while you straighten the infant's leg and mark on the paper the location of the heel. If there is no headboard, ask the caregiver to gently hold the infant's head still while you extend the leg for measurement.

4 Measure and record the infant's length with the tape measure.

5 Document the results in either inches or centimeters, depending on office policy, on the infant's growth chart, in the progress notes, and in the caregiver's record if requested. Complete the growth chart graph by connecting the dot from the last visit.

Measuring Infant Weight

1 Wash your hands, assemble equipment, and explain the procedure to the infant's caregiver.

2 Prepare the scale by sliding weights to the left and covering with disposable paper to reduce the risk of pathogen transmission.

3 Completely undress the infant, including the diaper.

4 Place the infant gently onto the center of the scale, keeping your hand directly above the infant's trunk for safety.

5 Slide the weights across the scale until balance is achieved. Attempt to read the infant's weight while he or she is still.

6 Return the weights to the far left of the scale and remove the baby. The caregiver can apply a diaper while you discard the paper covering the scale. If it has become contaminated during the procedure, follow OSHA guidelines for gloves and disposal of contaminated waste. Disinfect the equipment according to the manufacturer's guidelines.

7 Wash your hands.

8 Document the results in either pounds or kilograms, depending on office policy, on the infant's growth chart, in the progress notes, and in the caregiver's record, if requested. Complete the growth chart graph by connecting the dot from the last visit.

See Appendix E for a charting example.

---

introduction of 2 new body-mass index-for-age (BMI-for-age) charts for boys and for girls, ages 2 to 20 years. BMI is the recommended method for determining whether children or adults are overweight or obese. The BMI growth charts can be used beginning at 2 years of age, when height can be measured accurately (Figures 39-9 and 39-10).

Assisting With the Examination

The pediatrician will have a designated set of procedures that the medical assistant will complete before the physician sees the child (Procedure 39-3). Vital signs are measured first (Table 39-5). *Temperature* may be obtained by axillary, oral, or tympanic method. The temperature is most easily obtained using the axillary or the tympanic methods. It is important to remember that the younger the child, the more immature the ability to regulate body heat. Thus the temperature of an infant may fluctuate easily and rapidly. The child's pulse rate is affected in a fashion similar to the adult's and can increase through activity, anxiety, illness, and environmental temperature. If the child is younger than 2, the *pulse* is measured apically by placing the stethoscope on the left side of the chest medial to the nipple. Always count the beats for 1 full minute.

An alternative method of obtaining the pulse of a very young child is to use the brachial artery in the upper arm. After 2 years of age, the child's pulse may be taken at the radial pulse site. Anticipate a higher than adult level pulse rate, because the younger the child, the faster the pulse. The *respiratory rate* is easily obtained in a child, because the chest can be readily observed. Expect the rate to be increased according to the age (the

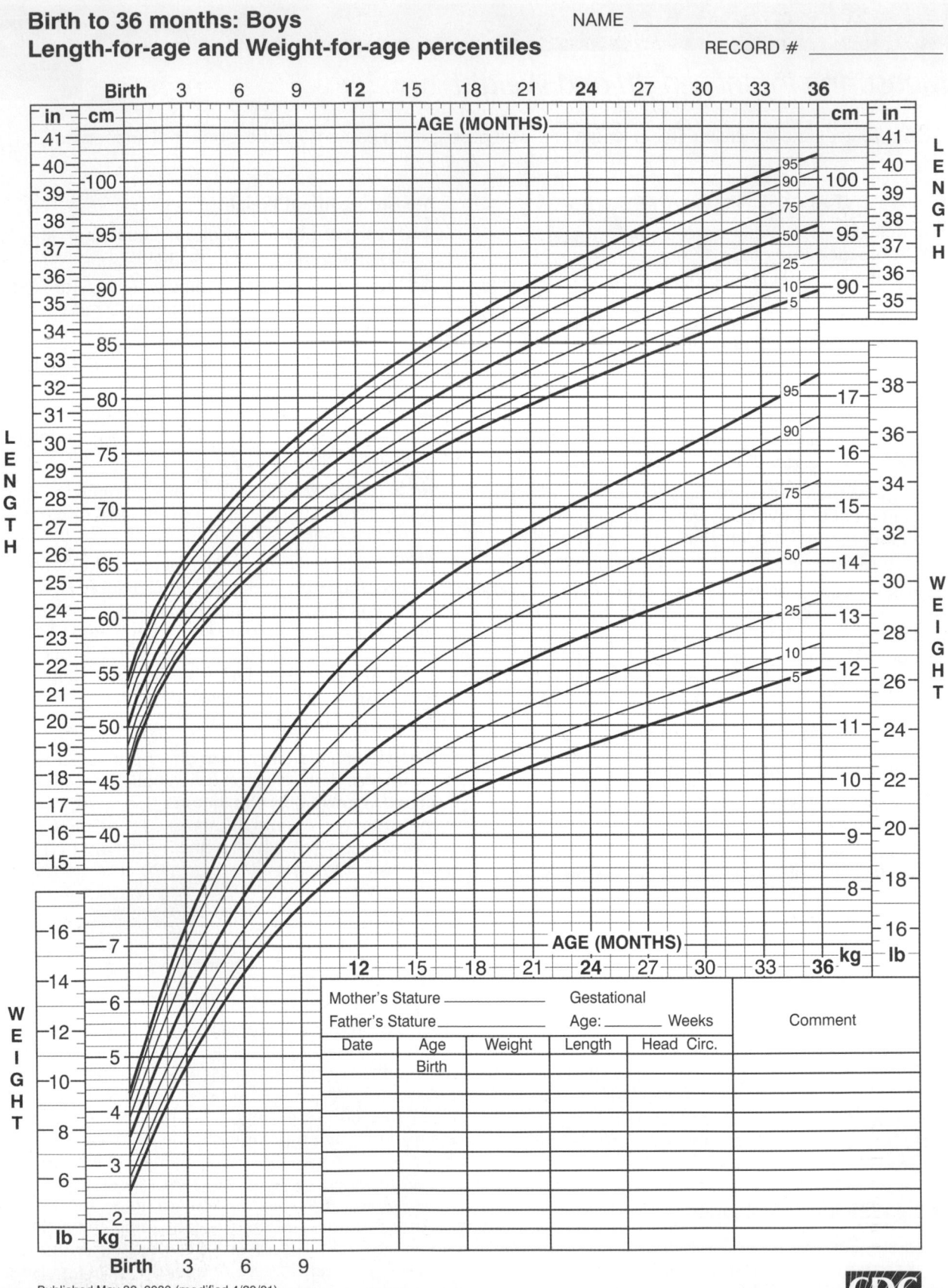

Birth to 36 months: Boys
Length-for-age and Weight-for-age percentiles

NAME _____

RECORD # _____

Published May 30, 2000 (modified 4/20/01).
SOURCE: Developed by the National Center for Health Statistics in collaboration with
the National Center for Chronic Disease Prevention and Health Promotion (2000).
http://www.cdc.gov/growthcharts

FIGURE 39-9   Growth rate graph: males (birth to 36 months).

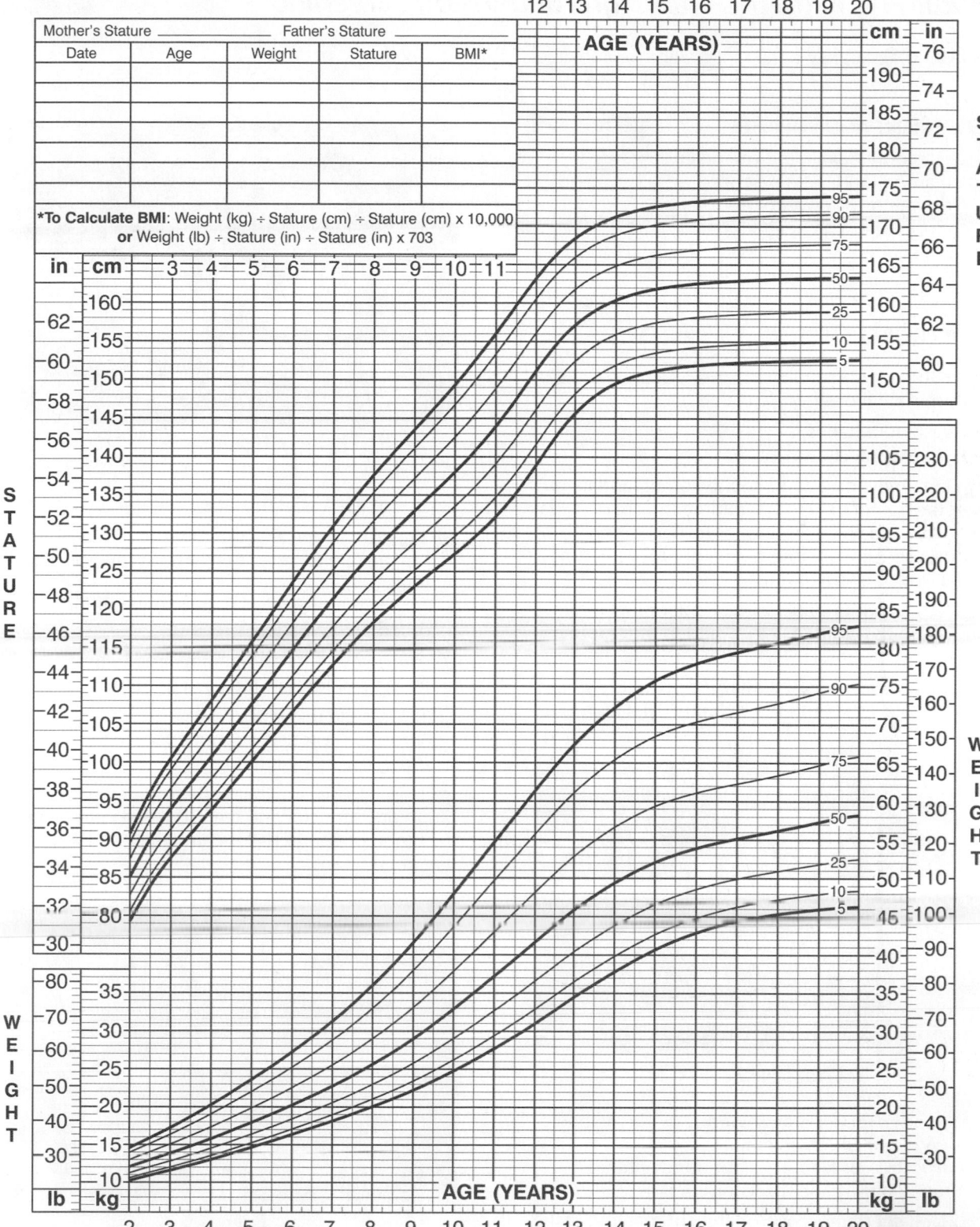

2 to 20 years: Girls
Stature-for-age and Weight-for-age percentiles

NAME _____

RECORD # _____

Mother's Stature _____ Father's Stature _____

Date	Age	Weight	Stature	BMI*

***To Calculate BMI:** Weight (kg) ÷ Stature (cm) ÷ Stature (cm) x 10,000
or Weight (lb) ÷ Stature (in) ÷ Stature (in) x 703*

Published May 30, 2000 (modified 11/21/00).
SOURCE: Developed by the National Center for Health Statistics in collaboration with
the National Center for Chronic Disease Prevention and Health Promotion (2000).
http://www.cdc.gov/growthcharts

CDC
SAFER · HEALTHIER · PEOPLE™

FIGURE 39-10   Growth rate graph: females (2 to 20 years).

PROCEDURE **39-3**

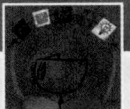

Obtaining Pediatric Vital Signs and Vision Screening

GOAL: To accurately obtain vital signs for and assess vision of a pediatric patient.

EQUIPMENT AND SUPPLIES

- Digital or tympanic thermometer
- Pediatric blood pressure cuff
- Wristwatch with sweep second-hand
- Weight scale with height bar
- Stethoscope
- Snellen E eye chart and oculator
- Pencil and paper

PROCEDURAL STEPS

1 Gather equipment.
Purpose: Efficiency.

2 Wash your hands.
Purpose: Infection control.

3 Explain the procedure to the parent, and if you want the parent to help by holding the child, explain the technique you want him or her to employ.
Purpose: Explanations ahead of time save time and enhance cooperation.

4 Help the child stand in the center of the scale and weigh the child. Ask the child to turn around and obtain the child's height. Record your findings.

5 Obtain tympanic or axillary temperature using the procedure explained in Chapter 28 (Figure 1).

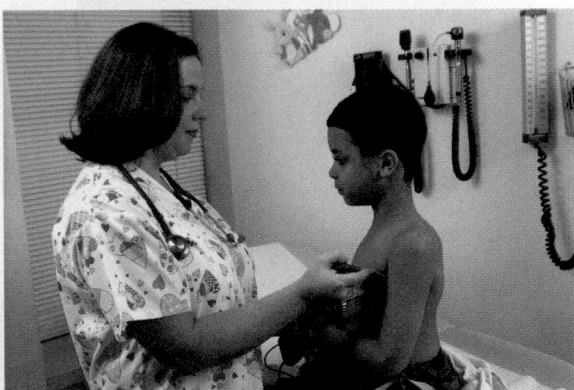

Figure 1

6 Record the temperature. Indicate the method used: A = axillary, T = tympanic.
Purpose: A procedure is not done until it is recorded on the patient's record.

7 Place the stethoscope on the child's chest at the midpoint between the sternum and the left nipple. Listen for the apical beat (Figure 2).

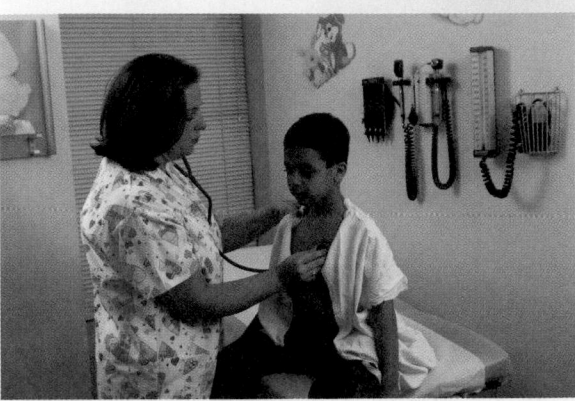

Figure 2

8 Count the apical beat for 1 full minute.

9 Record the apical pulse. Be sure to place an Ap before the rate to indicate that this is an apical pulse reading.
Purpose: A procedure is not done until it is recorded on the patient's record.

10 Place your flat hand on the child's chest and count the respirations for 1 full minute.

11 Record the respiration rate.
Purpose: A procedure is not done until it is recorded on the patient's record.

12 Check to be sure that you have the correct-size blood pressure cuff and then proceed with taking the blood pressure. Follow procedure in Chapter 28 (Figure 3).

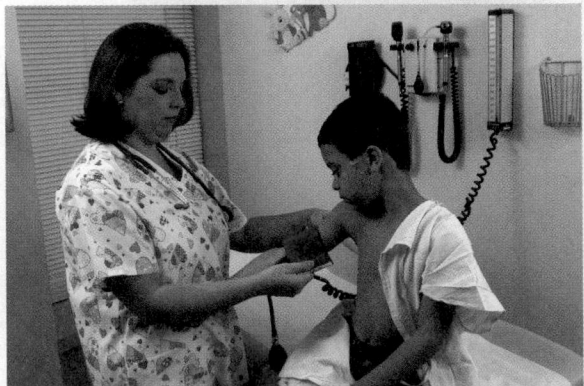

Figure 3

13 Record the blood pressure.

PROCEDURE 39-3—cont'd

Purpose: A procedure is not done until it is recorded on the patient's record.

14 If vision screening is to be done, familiarize the child with the E chart by asking him to make an E point the same way as your E is pointing. Then position the child in front of the pediatric E Snellen chart (Figure 4) and have him match the E sign (using his fingers) with the E on the chart that you are pointing to.

15 Record the vision results:
OD = Right eye; OS = Left eye; OU = Both eyes.
Purpose: A procedure is not done until it is recorded on the patient's record.

16 Compliment the child on his or her performance, and if the parent is present, share the praise with the parent.
Purpose: Builds rapport and encourages self-confidence in the child.

17 Wash your hands.
Purpose: Infection control.

18 Perform appropriate disinfection and return all equipment used to proper storage area.

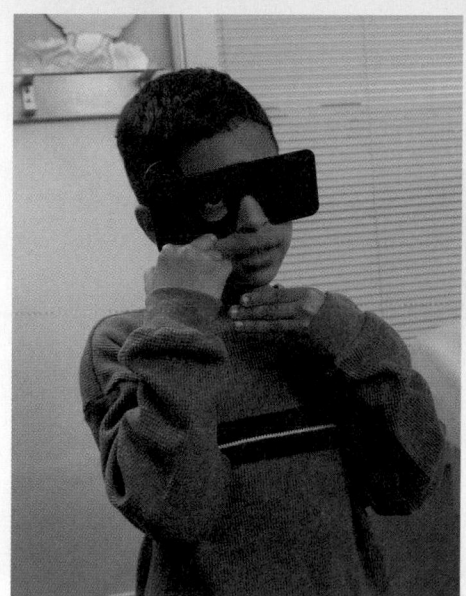

Figure 4

younger the child, the faster the normal respiratory rate) and health of the child. The ratio of four pulse beats to one respiration should remain constant in a healthy child, as in the adult. *Blood pressure* measurements are not included in most pediatric examinations. However, if there is a heart or kidney anomaly, a blood pressure reading may be ordered. The cuff must be the

appropriate width to obtain an accurate reading, and the bell of the stethoscope must be small enough to seal over the site. It is best to use a pediatric stethoscope with a pediatric bell when obtaining an infant's pressure. Blood pressure readings in a young child will be lower than in an adult.

To prevent a small child or infant from rolling the head from side to side during the physician's examination, stand at the head of the table and support the child's head between your hands, making certain not to press on the ears or on the anterior or posterior fontanelles. It is not necessary to drape an infant, but the older child's modesty should be respected. Sincere respect and friendly conversation at the child's level accomplish a great deal. Always be patient with children. Be certain that they understand what is expected. Always involve the parents or caregivers as much as possible.

Obtaining a Urine Sample

The easiest way to obtain a urine sample on a child older than 2 and toilet trained is to give the parent the container and instructions ahead of time. Then when the child appears at the office for the examination, the sample is available to be tested. If the sample is needed while the child is at the office, consult with the parent for the best method to use. If the child is younger than 2 years old, a pediatric urine collection device can be applied to collect the sample (Figure 39-11 and Procedure 39-4). Place this device on the child as soon as the child appears in the office, so that you increase your chances of obtaining the needed sample before the

TABLE 39-5	Reference Ranges for Pediatric Vital Signs

Temperature
Oral: 98.6° F or 37° C
Aural: 100.4° F or 38° C
Axillary: 97.6° F or 36.4° C

Pulse
Newborn: 100-180 beats per minute
3 months-2 years: 80-150 beats per minute
2-10 years: 65-130 beats per minute
Older than 9 years: 60-100 beats per minute

Respirations
Newborn: 30-35 breaths per minute
1-2 years: 25-30 breaths per minute
4-6 years: 23-25 breaths per minute
Older than 7 years: 16-20 breaths per minute

Blood Pressure
Newborn: Systolic < 90; diastolic < 70 mm Hg
1-5 years: Systolic < 100; diastolic < 70 mm Hg
Older than 9 years: Systolic < 120; diastolic < 84 mm Hg
Older than 13 years: Systolic 100 + age; diastolic 30-40 mm Hg less

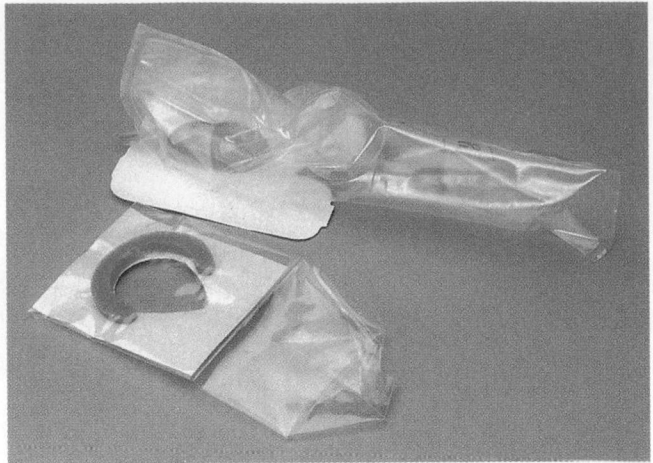

FIGURE 39-11 Urine collection devices.

PROCEDURE 39-4

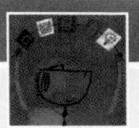

Applying a Urinary Collection Device

GOAL: To properly apply a pediatric urinary collection device.

EQUIPMENT AND SUPPLIES

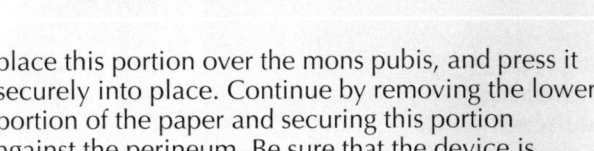

- Pediatric urine collection bag
- Labeled laboratory urinary container
- Laboratory test request form
- Antiseptic wipes
- Biohazard waste container
- Disposable examination gloves

PROCEDURAL STEPS

1 Assemble all needed supplies.
Purpose: Time management.

2 Wash your hands and don gloves.
Purpose: Infection control.

3 Ask the parent to remove the diaper from the child or place the child in a supine position on the examination table and remove the diaper.

4 Cleanse the genitalia with antiseptic wipes.
Male: Cleanse the urinary meatus in a circular motion, starting directly on the meatus, and work in an outward pattern. Repeat with a clean wipe. If the child is not circumcised, retract the foreskin to expose the meatus, and when you have completed cleansing, return the foreskin to its natural position.
Female: Hold the labia open with your nondominant hand and with your dominant hand, cleanse the inner labia, from the clitoris to the vaginal meatus, in a superior to inferior pattern. Discard the first wipe and repeat with a clean wipe.

5 Make sure the area is dry. Unfold the collection device, remove the paper from the upper portion, place this portion over the mons pubis, and press it securely into place. Continue by removing the lower portion of the paper and securing this portion against the perineum. Be sure that the device is attached smoothly and that you have not taped it to part of the infant's thigh.

6 Rediaper the infant, or if the parent is helping, the parent may rediaper the infant at this time. The diaper will help hold the bag in place.

7 Suggest that the parent give the child liquids if allowed and to check the bag for urine at frequent intervals.
Purpose: Increased intake helps increase output.

8 When there is a noticeable amount of urine in the bag, apply gloves, remove the device, cleanse the skin area that was attached to the device, and rediaper the child.

9 Pour the urine carefully into the laboratory urine container and handle the sample in a routine manner.

10 Dispose of all used equipment in a biohazard waste container.

11 Remove gloves, dispose of them in a biohazard container, and wash your hands.

12 Record the procedure in the patient's record.
Purpose: A procedure is not done until it is recorded.

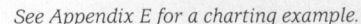

See Appendix E for a charting example.

child leaves. Once the device is in place, the child can be diapered to aid in holding the device properly. Be sure that the adhesive sticks tightly to the child so that the specimen will be in the device and not in the diaper when the child urinates.

In some cases the child may need to be catheterized to obtain the specimen. There are pediatric cath kits available that contain all the supplies needed for this procedure. In getting this kit ready for the pediatrician's use, always remember that this is a sterile procedure. The pediatrician will usually ask the parent to hold the infant's legs apart, and the medical assistant labels and prepares the specimen for the laboratory.

Injury Prevention

Unintentional injuries are the leading cause of death and disability for children in the United States. Injuries cause more childhood deaths than all diseases combined. The primary causes of childhood injuries include motor vehicle accidents, drowning, burns, falls, poisoning, aspiration with airway obstruction, and firearms. Childhood injuries are linked to the child's growth and development level and are therefore often predictable, many times preventable. Young children are totally dependent on caregivers to keep them safe, so constant supervision and a childproof environment are essential for this age group. Older children need to be aware of health hazards and be encouraged to protect themselves from injury, such as using bike helmets, protective padding when skate boarding, seat belts, and so on. The highest incidence of accidental injuries is in children under 9 years of age, but as children grow older, the percentage of deaths from injuries increases. Healthcare workers play a major role in injury prevention. It is the medical assistant's responsibility to make sure that the ambulatory care environment is safe and parents should be educated about potential hazards related to the child's developmental level.

CRITICAL THINKING APPLICATION

The office manager asked Susie if she would check the entire office for potential child safety issues. After inspecting the facility, Susie is concerned about some safety issues, so she decides to create a checklist for future use. What precautions or safety features should she include?

CHILD SAFETY GUIDELINES

- Position healthy full-term infants on their back or side to sleep.
- Stairs should be carpeted and protected with nonaccordion gates.
- Install and maintain smoke detectors on each floor and near sleeping areas.
- Develop and practice a plan of escape in the event of a fire.
- Put a self-latching lock on basement stairs.
- Store dangerous products out of reach (including medicines and vitamins), in cabinets with locks, and in their original containers.
- Keep potentially harmful plants out of reach.
- Post the numbers of the Poison Control Center and the child's physician on all phones.
- Teach children to call 911 as soon as possible.
- Regularly inspect toys for sharp or removable parts.
- Use an approved car seat that is appropriate for the child's age every time the child is in the car and make certain it is properly installed.
- Follow guidelines for placing children in the front seat of motor vehicles.
- Parents should use seat belts *every time* to protect themselves and set a good example.
- All children should wear properly fitting, approved helmets when biking and pads when skate boarding or participating in other impact sports.
- If firearms are in the home, store them unloaded, with the ammunition stored separately, and in a locked container.
- If the child has access to a swimming pool, make certain it is fenced, with self-locking gates.
- All adults and older children should learn cardiopulmonary resuscitation (CPR).

The Adolescent Patient

The adolescent patient may present the greatest challenge to health education and disease management. Adolescence begins with the onset of *puberty*, a time when the child's reproductive system matures and is marked by rapid changes in the endocrine and musculoskeletal systems. The adolescent undergoes rapid growth spurts and the development of secondary sexual characteristics. Health examinations for patients in this age group should include screenings for height and weight; gathering details regarding diet and exercise routines; STD screening and Pap tests if female adolescents are sexually active, especially to screen for human papillomavirus (HPV); review of vaccination history with booster administration as indicated; and assessment of high-risk behaviors such as substance abuse and sexual behavior.

Some of the health problems most frequently seen in adolescent patients include eating disorders (anorexia nervosa and bulimia nervosa), obesity, and injury-related problems. Accidents are the leading cause of death and injury in adolescence and suicide is the third leading cause of death. All healthcare personnel should be on the alert for indicators of suicide including:

- Signs of depression such as headaches, abdominal discomfort, anorexia, fatigue, aggressiveness, drug or alcohol abuse, and sexual promiscuity.
- Verbal statements that hint at the adolescent's intention to commit suicide; talking about dying.
- Actions such as giving away prized objects, withdrawing from social groups, sudden changes in normal behavior patterns, or writing a suicide note.

Child Abuse

The federal Child Abuse Prevention and Treatment Act states that all threats to a child's physical and/or mental welfare must be reported. This means that every teacher, healthcare worker, and social worker—in fact, every citizen—who suspects that a child is being neglected or abused must report this to the proper authority. The agency must record the report, and after three similar reports, the agency must investigate.

When a suspected abuse is reported, the individual must provide his or her name, but this is considered confidential information and will not be given to the child's parent or guardian, nor is it given to the investigating officer. The individual making the report is also protected under the law from any liability for reporting suspicions of child abuse. Figure 39-12 lists some of the signs of abuse the medical assistant should know.

If the medical assistant suspects that a child is a victim of abuse, he or she should consult with the pediatrician immediately, before the patient is seen. In most states, both the medical assistant and the physician can make separate reports to the authorities. However, state laws vary, so the state and local reporting protocols should be outlined in the office procedure manual. Any report made must remain confidential.

Patient Education

In a pediatric practice, the child is usually joined by one or both parents during visits to the physician. Parents need reinforcement, praise, and understanding in dealing with the health and welfare of their child, and they expect to receive such support from the pediatrician and the office staff. Provide parents with information to help them understand their children's behavior and improve their parenting skills. Understanding the normal behavioral characteristics of a particular developmental stage may increase the parents' confidence and reinforce their expectations for their child (Figure 39-13).

The waiting room is an ideal place for parent education. Use the space and resources available to provide up to date information on child health issues as well as local resources for support and assistance. If the pediatrician has pamphlets available, discuss them with the parents. Answer questions when possible or alert the physician so that questions can be answered during the office visit. Every opportunity should be taken to teach parents about sound healthcare. Because so many ambulatory care visits involve infectious disorders, educating children and parents on the following infection control measures may help decrease the spread of disease.

- Children should cover their mouths with a disposable tissue when they cough and blow their noses with disposable tissues.

SIGNS OF ABUSE

Obvious Signals

Previously filed reports of physical or sexual abuse of child
Documented abuse of other family members
Different stories of how an accident happened between parents and child
Stories of incident and injuries found are suspicious
The cause of the injuries are blamed on other family members
Repeated visits to the emergency room for injuries

Findings on Examination

Trauma to the nervous system
Internal abdominal pain
Discolorations/bruising to the buttocks, back and abdomen
Elbow, wrist, and shoulder dislocations

Changes in Behavior

Too eager to please the parent
Overly passive and too compliant
Aggressive and demanding
Parenting the parent—role reversal
Delays in the normal growth and development patterns
Erratic school attendance

Physical Indicators

Poor hygiene
Malnutrition
Obvious dental neglect
Neglected well-baby procedures such as immunizations

FIGURE 39-12 Signs of abuse.

PARENT EDUCATION TOPICS

Normal growth and development
Child safety
Pediatric nutrition needs
Alternative feeding habits
Immunizations
Sexual curiosity
Answering "sex" questions
Toilet training
Adolescent behavior
Adolescent trust vs mistrust
Common health problems

FIGURE 39-13 Parent education topics.

- Only use a tissue once and then immediately throw it away.
- Do not allow children to share toys that they have put in their mouths.
- After a child has discarded a toy that was in the mouth, it should be placed in a bin for dirty toys that is out of reach of others. Wash and disinfect these toys before allowing children to play with them again.
- Make sure all children and adults use good hand-washing practices.

Legal and Ethical Issues

In the United States children are considered to be persons who are growing and developing physically, emotionally, and mentally. Our laws view children as a distinct group, and there are laws and customs dealing with the protection of children's rights. Occasionally in the pediatric office, legal and ethical issues arise, and the entire office staff may be faced with an ethical situation. If this type of situation occurs, the first option is to talk it over with the pediatrician. It may be necessary to have an office staff meeting to identify the conflict, note pertinent laws and facts, consider possible options and the consequences of each, and decide on a course of action. Facing ethical issues confidently may reduce the risk of liability. If the pediatrician's feelings are different from yours, this might be a totally separate dilemma that you will have to deal with. Always remember that as your employer, the physician makes the final decision, and as long as you work in that office, you are required to do things according to that decision.

If something happens that you cannot ethically support, seek the help of the local medical assistant organization. You may find that others have been in similar situations and that they can suggest possible methods to solve the problem.

SUMMARY OF SCENARIO

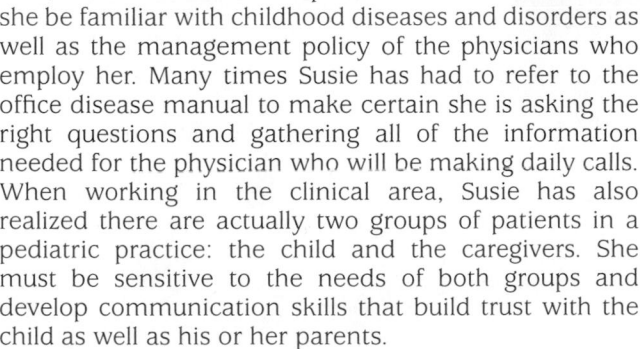

After working with the telephone triage staff, Susie realizes how important it is that she be familiar with childhood diseases and disorders as well as the management policy of the physicians who employ her. Many times Susie has had to refer to the office disease manual to make certain she is asking the right questions and gathering all of the information needed for the physician who will be making daily calls. When working in the clinical area, Susie has also realized there are actually two groups of patients in a pediatric practice: the child and the caregivers. She must be sensitive to the needs of both groups and develop communication skills that build trust with the child as well as his or her parents.

SUMMARY OF LEARNING OBJECTIVES

■ The terms growth and development are often used together and refer to the combination of changes that a child goes through as he or she matures. Growth refers to measurable changes such as height and weight while development considers qualitative maturation in motor, mental, and language skills. By 6 months of age, the child's birth-weight has doubled, at 1 year it has tripled, and length has increased by 50%. By age 2, the child has reached approximately 50% of adult height. This same growth rate continues through the school-age period, 6 to 12 years, which leads into a growth spurt that indicates impending puberty. In adolescence, ages 12 to 18 years, the adolescent gains almost half of his or her adult weight and the skeleton and organs double in size.

■ Child development occurs rapidly during the first year of life and by age 3 the child is showing increased autonomy. During the preschool stage the child becomes increasingly independent, and by school-age the child has perfected fine motor skills and has expanded reading and writing skills. The adolescent, or transition, stage is when the individual attempts to establish an adult identity. This is usually done through trial and error by experimenting with adult roles and behavior patterns.

■ Pediatric gastrointestinal disorders include infant colic; diarrhea that can be caused by a variety of different microorganisms, including bacteria, viruses, and parasites, and is treated medically when it continues for more than 2 days; failure to thrive caused by a physiological factor (such as malabsorption disease or cleft palate) or a nonorganic cause that is associated with the parent-child relationship; and obesity requiring treatment for children who are more than 40% over their ideal weight.

■ Disorders of the respiratory system include the common cold, which may lead to secondary bacterial infections, including strep throat or otitis media because of an accumulation of either serous or suppurative fluid in the middle ear; croup, a viral disorder that affects primarily the larynx with edema and spasm to the vocal cords resulting in a high-pitched raspy cough; bronchiolitis, a viral infection of the small bronchi and bronchioles that has an acute onset of wheezing and dyspnea because of necrosis, inflammation, edema, increased secretions, and bronchospasm in the respiratory pathway; asthma, which causes bronchospasms that decrease the amount of air that can pass through the airways and inflammation of the bronchioles causing edema and secretion of mucus; and influenza, an acute, highly contagious viral infection of the respiratory tract that is transmitted by direct contact with moist secretions and causes high fevers and pulmonary complications.

■ Pediatric infectious diseases include conjunctivitis, caused by a bacterial or viral infection that produces a white or yellowish pus and is highly contagious; tonsillitis, typically caused by beta-hemolytic *Streptococcus* that causes painful, enlarged, and inflamed tonsils with fever and malaise; fifth disease, also called erythema infectiosum, a mild infection caused by parvovirus B19 characterized by a mild fever, general malaise, and flushed cheeks; chickenpox, caused by a member of the herpesvirus group, characterized by a slight fever and skin lesions that last for about 2 weeks and usually leaves the child with lifetime immunity; meningitis, an inflammation of the membranes that cover the brain and spinal cord, caused by bacteria or viruses, with bacterial meningitis more dangerous; hepatitis B virus infection, which can lead to serious and chronic infection of the liver and can be transmitted across the placenta or during the birth process if the mother is infected; and Reye's syndrome, which is linked with the use of aspirin during a viral illness, characterized by fatty invasion of the inner organs, especially the liver, and swelling of the brain.

■ Pediatric inherited disorders include cystic fibrosis, an autosomal recessive genetic disorder that causes exocrine glands to produce abnormally thick secretions and primarily affects the lungs and pancreas, causing buildup of mucus in the lungs and blockage of the pancreatic ducts and resulting in malabsorption problems and an emphysema-like lung condition; and Duchenne's muscular dystrophy, an X-linked genetic disease that causes progressive muscle degeneration and subsequent replacement of muscle fibers with fat and fibrous connective tissue, ultimately causing either cardiac or respiratory failure.

■ CDC recommendations for childhood immunizations are summarized in Table 39-2. It is recommended that all children be vaccinated against diphtheria, tetanus, pertussis, hepatitis B, and the viruses, which can cause some forms of meningitis; polio, measles, mumps, rubella, pneumonia, and chickenpox.

■ Well-child visits are typically scheduled from 2 weeks of age through 15 years of age to focus on maintaining the health of the child with basic system examinations, immunizations, and upgrading of the child's medical history record. Sick-child visits occur whenever needed and usually on short notice. Some criteria to consider when conducting telephone screening include the age of the child and severity of symptoms, including the onset, frequency, and duration of the problem. Table 39-4 summarizes some of the action principles for telephone screening.

■ A medical assistant is responsible for assisting the pediatrician with examinations; upgrading patient histories; performing ordered screening tests such as vision, hearing, urinalysis, and hemoglobin checks; administering immunizations; measuring and weighing children as needed; and providing patient and caregiver support.

■ The medical assistant should be involved in parent education regarding injury prevention in children.

Unintentional injuries are the leading cause of death and disability for children in the United States—injuries cause more childhood deaths than all diseases combined. The primary causes of childhood injuries include motor vehicle accidents, drowning, burns, falls, poisoning, aspiration with airway obstruction, and firearms. Childhood injuries are linked to the child's growth and development level and are therefore often predictable, and many times preventable.

KEY INTERNET WEBSITES

- American Academy of Pediatrics
- Centers for Disease Control and Prevention (CDC)
  - Immunization Information
  - Printable Immunization Sheets
  - 2000 CDC Growth Charts

For active weblinks to each website visit
http://evolve.elsevier.com/Kinn/

Homework. extra Credit

Write Essay on what you learned!

Due week before Final

CHAPTER **40**

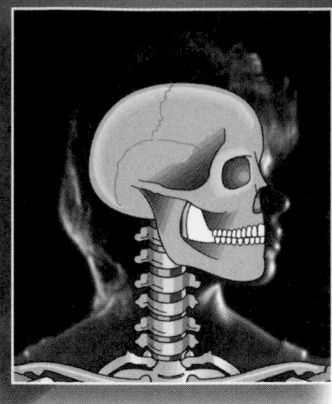

Scenario

Kaiwan Tillman became interested in orthopedics before he even knew what the word meant. When he was in the sixth grade, he broke his right femur when a car hit him while he was riding his bicycle. He spent 2 months in traction in the hospital on an orthopedic floor. His questions about bones, the skeleton, x-ray films, and traction were endless. Fortunately, the staff responded to his youthful enthusiasm by giving him a book about the human skeleton.

In high school his interest grew even more when he worked as an assistant for the football coach. He learned how to wrap ankles, knees, and shoulders and to apply ice to injuries. He was also studying medical assisting along with his regular studies. He was attending the city's only medical arts high school.

On graduation from high school, he had completed the medical assisting curriculum and was fortunate to find a job in a clinic called Sports Medicine Associates. The clinic staff includes three orthopedic surgeons, two physical therapists, and two massage therapists. Kaiwan is most excited to be able to work in this orthopedic clinic, although he was initially somewhat intimidated. Dr. Steve Alexander is the team physician for a local professional baseball team, and part of Kaiwan's responsibilities include assisting Dr. Alexander with treating the team and at the games, both home and away.

Assisting in Orthopedic Medicine

Kim Anthony Aaronson

Learning Objectives

- Define and spell the terms listed in the vocabulary.
- Describe the principal structures of the musculoskeletal system and their functions.
- Differentiate among tendons, bursae, and ligaments.
- List and describe the major disorders of the musculoskeletal system.
- Identify and describe the common types of fractures.
- Explain the common diagnostic procedures used in orthopedics.
- Explain how to use the four most common types of ambulatory devices.
- Describe when and how to use cold applications.
- Describe the effects of heat on the body and why it is an important treatment modality.
- Explain the importance of therapeutic modalities in the treatment of musculoskeletal conditions.
- Compare and contrast active and passive exercise and range of motion.
- Apply cold therapy to an injury.
- Properly use heat application.
- Properly apply therapeutic ultrasound.
- Apply a sling to immobilize an injury.
- Prepare for and assist with a cast application.
- Prepare for and assist with a cast removal.
- Properly fit a patient with crutches and explain the correct mechanics of crutch walking.

National Curriculum Competencies

ADMINISTRATIVE COMPETENCIES

1b. Schedule inpatient and outpatient admission and procedures

CLINICAL COMPETENCIES

1a. Perform hand washing
4c. Obtain and record patient history
4d. Prepare and maintain examination and treatment area
4e. Prepare patient for and assist with routine and specialty examinations
4f. Prepare patients for and assist with procedures, treatments, and minor office surgery

TRANSDISCIPLINARY COMPETENCIES

1a. Respond to and initiate written communication
1b. Recognize and respond to verbal communication
1c. Recognize and respond to nonverbal communication
2a. Identify and respond to issues of confidentiality
2b. Perform within legal and ethical boundaries
2c. Establish and maintain the medical record
2d. Document properly
3b. Instruct individuals according to their needs
3c. Instruct and demonstrate the use and care of patient equipment

Vocabulary

arthritis Inflammation of a joint.

articular Pertaining to a joint.

atrophy Wasting away, decreasing in size.

bursa A fluid-filled, saclike membrane that provides for cushioning and frictionless motion between two tissues.

cartilage Rubbery, smooth, somewhat elastic connective tissue covering the ends of bones.

cervical Neck region containing seven cervical vertebrae.

corticosteroids Antiinflammatory hormones, natural or synthetic.

crepitation Dry, crackling sound or sensation.

diaphysis Midportion of a long bone containing the medullary cavity.

epiphysis End of a long bone.

gait Manner or style of walking.

goniometer Instrument for measuring the degrees of motion in a joint.

inflammation Tissue reaction to trauma or disease that includes redness, heat, swelling, and pain.

kyphotic Relating to normal convex curvature of the thoracic spine region.

ligament A tough connective tissue band that holds joints together by attaching to the bones on either side of a joint.

lordotic Relating to normal concave curvature of the cervical and lumbar spine regions.

lumbar Lower back region containing five lumbar vertebrae.

luxation Dislocation of a bone from its normal anatomical location.

malaise Indefinite feeling of debility or lack of health, often indicative of or accompanying the onset of an illness.

medullary cavity Inner portion of diaphysis containing bone marrow.

NSAIDs Nonsteroidal antiinflammatory drugs.

periosteum The thin, highly innervated, membranous covering of a bone.

prosthesis Artificial replacement for a body part.

reduction The return to correct anatomical position as in reduction of a fracture.

scoliosis Abnormal lateral curvature of the spine.

subluxation Incomplete dislocation of a bone from its normal anatomical location.

synovial fluid Clear fluid found in joint cavities that facilitates smooth movements and nourishes joint structures.

tendon A tough band of connective tissue connecting muscle to bone.

thoracic The region of the back between the cervical and lumbar regions containing 12 thoracic vertebrae.

An *orthopedic physician* diagnoses and treats diseases and disorders of the musculoskeletal system and deals primarily with the bones. *Rheumatologists* are specialists in treating inflammatory joint disorders. *Osteopaths* are doctors of osteopathic medicine (DO) who treat the body from the viewpoint that the body can heal itself when the skeletal system is in proper alignment. *Chiropractors* are doctors of chiropractic (DC) who use manual adjusting procedures to correct subluxations or misalignments of the spine to allow maximal nerve function, thus facilitating the body in maintaining homeostasis and preventing disease.

The musculoskeletal system includes all of the skeletal muscles, bones, joints, and supportive connective tissues (cartilage, tendons, and ligaments). The general functions of the musculoskeletal system include:

- Protection for internal organs
- Support to stand erect
- Movement
- Production of blood cells in the bone marrow
- Mineral storage in the bones

Anatomy and Physiology of the Musculoskeletal System

Muscles

There are more than 600 muscles attached to the human skeleton (Figure 40-1). These muscles account for approximately half of a person's weight and contribute to the body's distinct shape. This chapter is concerned with the skeletal muscles that attach to bones and allow movement. There are two other types of muscles in the body: cardiac (in the heart) and smooth muscle (in organs and blood vessel walls). Both of these are involuntary; a person cannot control their function. Skeletal muscles are voluntary and can be controlled when they contract or relax. Special fibers in skeletal muscles allow them to shorten (contract) and lengthen (relax), causing movement (Table 40-1). These muscles are connected to bone with bands of tough, fibrous connective tissues called **tendons**.

Bones

The human skeleton contains more than 200 bones and makes up about one tenth of a person's weight (Figure 40-2). Bones supply a framework that provides protection for vital organs. In general, the size of a bone is related to how much it moves and how much body weight it must carry. Sometimes the size and shape of a bone are more related to its protective function for the underlying organs.

CRITICAL THINKING APPLICATION

What is the benefit of Kaiwan knowing the names and locations of the major bones of the extremities? How might this knowledge make his job at Sports Medicine Associates more interesting?

Bones are generally categorized by shape, including long, short, flat, rounded, and irregular. A long bone is

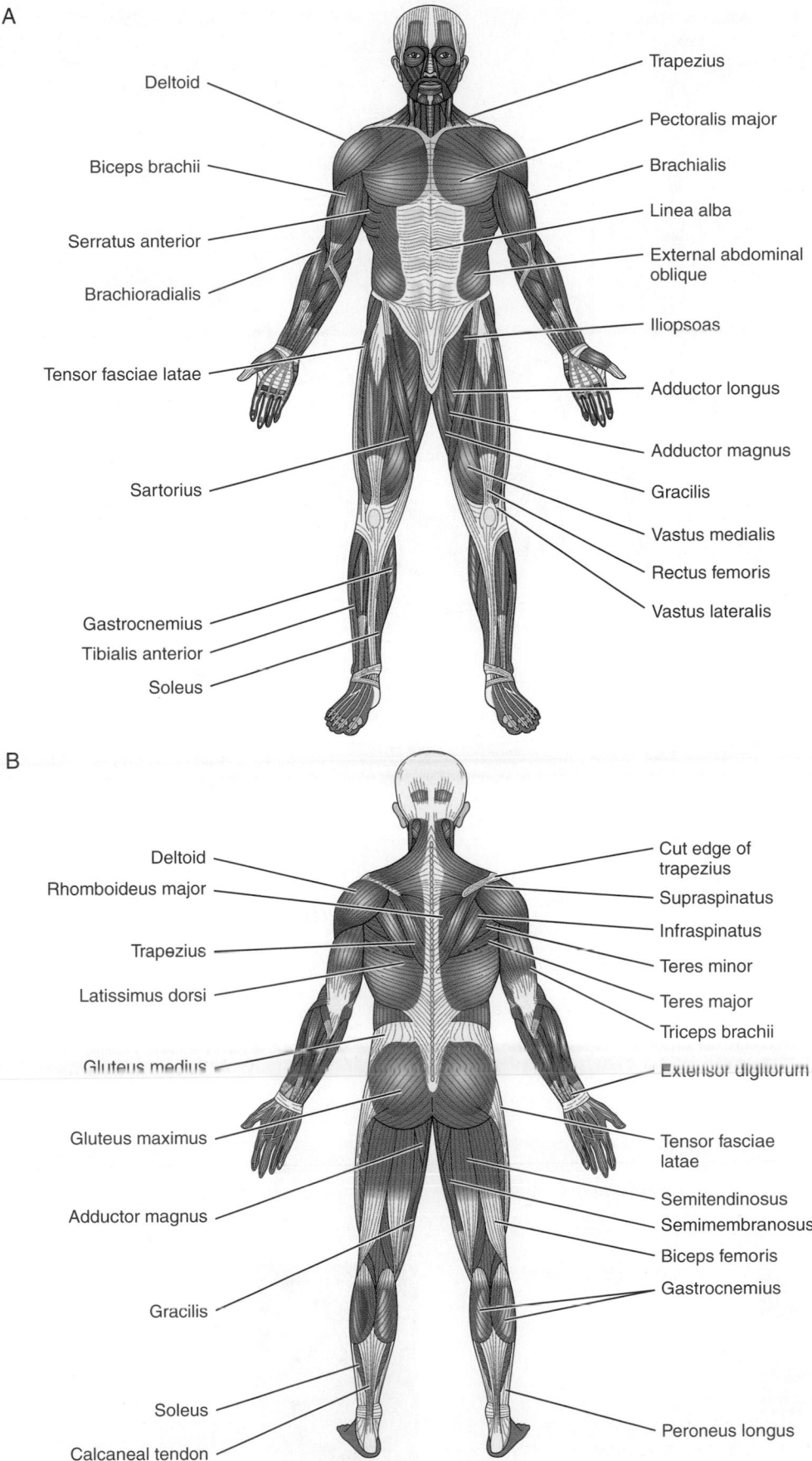

FIGURE 40-1 Muscles of the body. **A**, Anterior view. **B**, Posterior view. (From Chester GA: *Modern medical assisting*, Philadelphia, 1998, WB Saunders, p 275.)

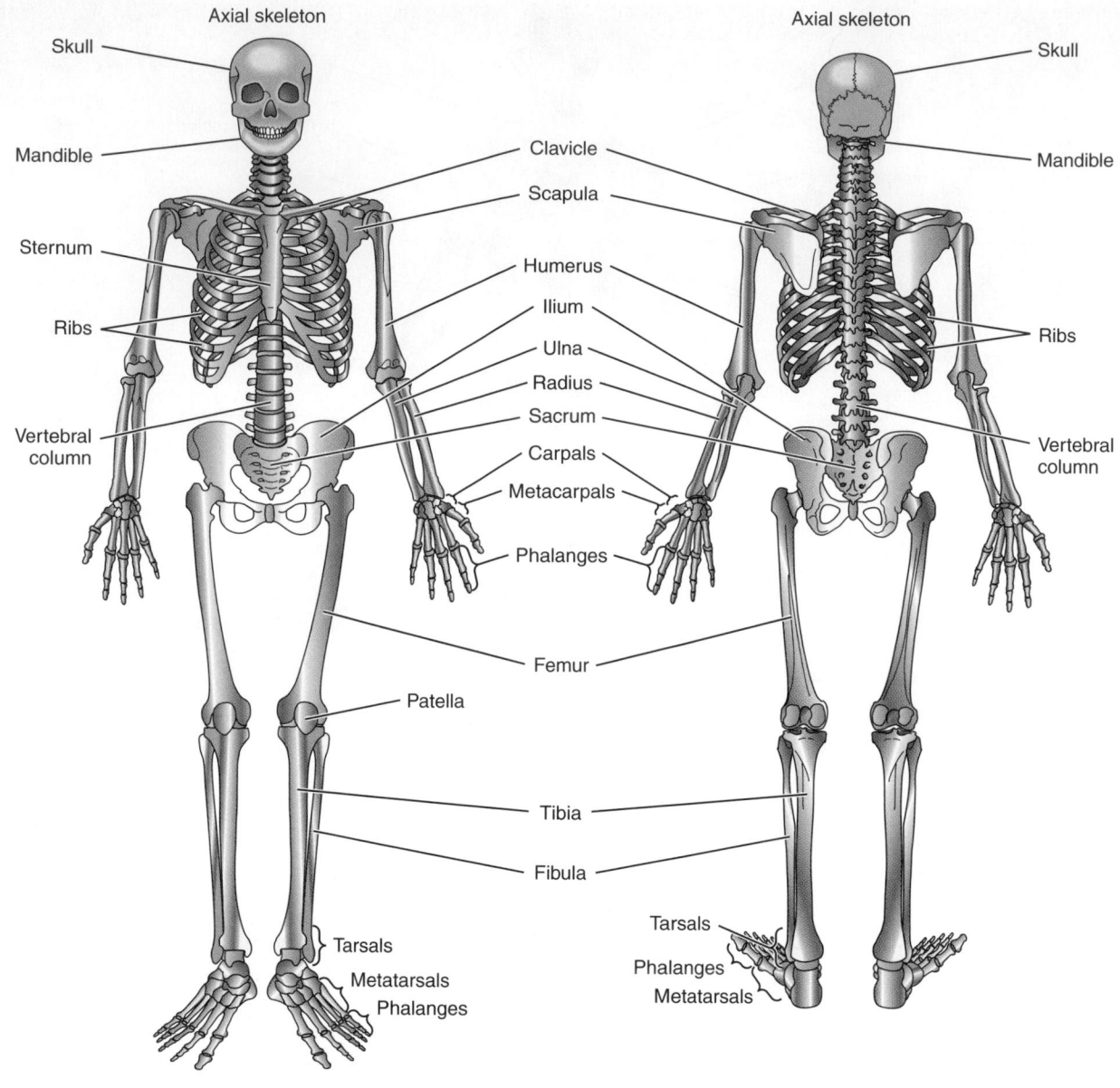

FIGURE 40-2 Axial skeletal bones (listed in outside columns) and appendicular skeletal bones (listed in the middle column). (From Chester GA: *Modern medical assisting*, Philadelphia, 1998, WB Saunders, p 278.)

TABLE 40-1	Types of Body Movement		
Movement	**Definition/Example**	**Movement**	**Definition/Example**
Flexion	Decreases the angle of the joint and brings the two bones closer together.	Circumduction	The circular movement of a limb. It is a combination of abduction, adduction, extension, and flexion.

TABLE 40-1	Types of Body Movement—cont'd		
Movement	**Definition/Example**	**Movement**	**Definition/Example**
Extension	The opposite of flexion; increases the angle or the distance between two bones or parts of the body.	Pronation	Rotation of the forearm that turns the palm of the hand backward or posteriorly.
Hyperextension	Extension greater than 180°; body part is extended beyond its anatomical position.	Supination (see illustration for pronation)	The opposite of pronation. It is the rotation of the forearm that turns the palm of the hand forward or anteriorly.
Abduction	Moving a limb away from the midline or median plane of the body.	Eversion	Turning of the sole of the foot laterally or outward.
Adduction	The opposite of abduction. It moves the limb toward the midline of the body.	Inversion (see illustration for eversion)	The opposite of eversion. It is turning of the sole of the foot medially or inward.
Rotation	The rotation of a bone around its central axis, common in ball and socket joints.	Dorsiflexion	Moving the instep of the foot up and dorsally. It decreases the angle between the foot and the leg.
		Plantar flexion (see illustration for dorsiflexion)	Movement of the ankle joint in which the joint is straightened and the toes are pointed downward.

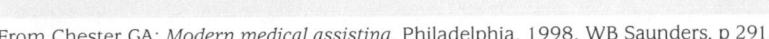

From Chester GA: *Modern medical assisting*, Philadelphia, 1998, WB Saunders, p 291.

made up of a **diaphysis** (shaft) with an expansion at each end called an **epiphysis** (Figure 40-3). The epiphysis is covered with **cartilage** and is attached by ligaments to the epiphysis of another bone, forming a joint. The cartilage decreases the stress of weight-bearing and the friction of movement. The thickness of the cartilage depends largely on the amount of stress placed on a particular joint. The **medullary cavity** is found within the diaphysis and contains bone marrow.

Bone is living, changing tissue that is constantly being remodeled in response to stress or injury. Bone is also a storage location of minerals including calcium and phosphate. Red bone marrow found in the proximal epiphyses of the humerus and femur and in the sternum, ribs, and vertebrae of adults produces blood cells. Bones are covered with a thin membranous tissue called periosteum. The **periosteum** contains many sensory nerves.

Joints

Bones are connected to each other at junctions called *joints*. The two main kinds of joints are *nonsynovial* and *synovial*. In nonsynovial joints, the bones are joined with fibrous cartilage and are immovable, such as the sutures of the skull, or only slightly moveable, such as the vertebrae. Synovial joints are freely moveable because the adjacent ends of two bones are covered with cartilage and are enclosed in a joint cavity that contains a viscous, slippery fluid called **synovial fluid**, which is an excellent lubricant. Synovial joints such as the elbow and knee are basically hinge joints that allow movement in only one plane (Figure 40-4). Other synovial joints, such as the hip and shoulder, allow movement in many planes, thus permitting a wider range of motion than a hinge joint.

JOINT PROSTHESES

Artificial (manmade) joints have been successfully implanted to replace each of the following joints:
- Hip
- Knee
- Ankle
- Shoulder
- Elbow
- Wrist
- Finger

Ligaments, Tendons, and Bursae

Ligaments are powerful, strong, fibrous connective tissue bands that connect bone to bone at the joint and encase the joint capsule. Ligaments allow purposeful joint movement and prevent excessive movement in any particular joint. Ligaments are oblique or parallel to the joint, as in the knee, and surrounding the joint, as in the hip.

A **tendon** is a strong bundle of connective tissue that attaches muscle to bone. Tendons can be flat or round and can pass between muscles, between bones, or through specialized openings between bones.

A **bursa** is a fluid-filled sac that acts as a cushion between bone and tendon, or tendon and ligament. Bursae reduce friction and help muscles and tendons glide smoothly over bone.

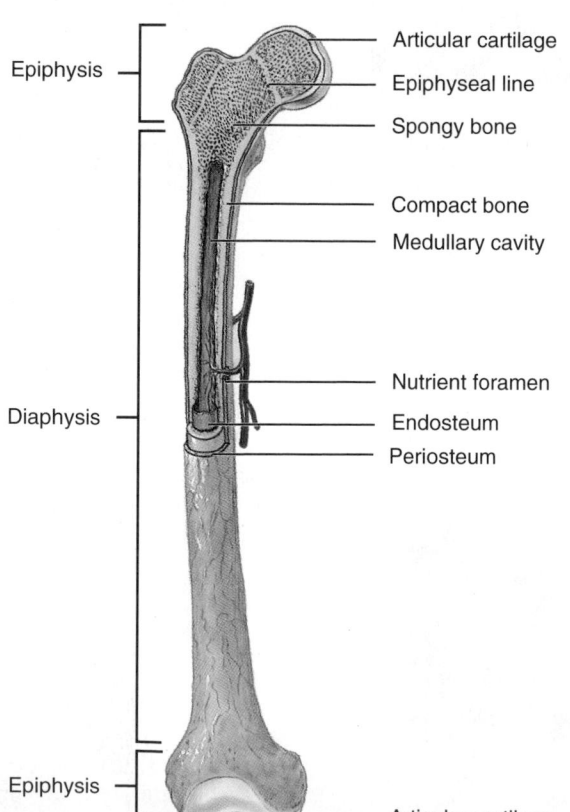

FIGURE 40-3   Long bone features. (From Applegate EJ: *The anatomy and physiology learning system*, ed 2. Philadelphia, 2000, WB Saunders, p 93.)

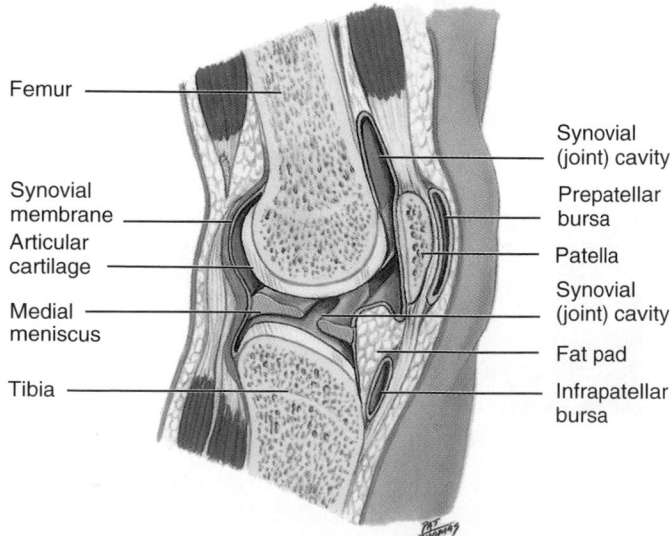

FIGURE 40-4   Sagittal section of the knee joint. (From Applegate EJ: *The anatomy and physiology learning system*, ed 2. Philadelphia, 2000, WB Saunders, p 115.)

Musculoskeletal Diseases and Disorders

Musculoskeletal diseases and conditions can affect any of the muscles, bones, or joints. These problems are common and have a tremendous impact on the normal quality of life. Brittle or deformed bones that are prone to fracture often mark bone disorders such as osteoporosis and osteomalacia. Joint disorders such as osteoarthritis, rheumatoid **arthritis**, and gout can lead to painful, swollen, or inflamed joints. Muscle problems such as sprains and spasms can bring on sudden pain or cause stiffness. Myasthenia gravis, an autoimmune disorder in which there is abnormal transmission of nerve impulses to skeletal muscles, can cause severe muscle weakness (Table 40-2).

Musculoskeletal system trauma quickly leads to **inflammation** in the area of injury. This type of injury is one of the leading causes of time lost from work and for visits to primary care physicians and emergency rooms. As soon as possible after injury, even before being seen by a physician, RICE therapy should be initiated. (RICE stands for *r*est, *i*ce, *c*ompression, and *e*levation.) Thus the injured extremity should not be used, an ice bag should be applied, gentle compression with an elastic bandage should be initiated, and the extremity should be elevated. All of these measures together will decrease swelling, decrease inflammation, and enhance healing. It cannot be stressed enough that the sooner RICE can be implemented, the better.

FROZEN PEA ICE BAG

A bag of frozen peas (or corn) is a most efficient and effective (easily conforming to the shape of a body part) way to immediately ice a musculoskeletal injury. After approximately 20 minutes, put the bag of peas back into the freezer for 30 to 60 minutes to refreeze before applying again.

To maintain musculoskeletal health, it is important to have a significant dietary intake of foods rich in calcium and vitamin D, avoid smoking, and include weight-bearing exercises, such as walking. In addition to these lifestyle measures, medications are sometimes required for conditions that impair normal functioning of this system. The following conditions are seen on a fairly frequent basis in an orthopedic practice.

CRITICAL THINKING APPLICATION

Why is it so important to obtain an accurate history on an injured patient who comes to the office for the first time? What is Kaiwan's responsibility in finding out why a new patient comes for an office visit?

Muscular Disorders

Fibromyalgia. Fibromyalgia is a condition of widespread connective tissue, muscular pain, and often severe fatigue of unknown origin. A patient with fibromyalgia usually complains of diffuse aches and pains all over his or her entire body. It can affect people of all ages and is found more frequently in women than men. Chronic pain and fatigue are the cardinal signs in the absence of any other known cause. The pain is described variously as burning, shooting, throbbing, aching, piercing, or stabbing. Associated conditions can include sleep disorder, irritable bowel syndrome, chronic headaches, temporomandibular joint (TMJ) problems, increased chemical sensitivity, and other musculoskeletal complaints. Although the cause remains unknown, fibromyalgia has been triggered by automobile accidents, bacterial or viral infection, or following the diagnosis of other medical conditions, such as rheumatoid arthritis, lupus, or hypothyroidism. It can be aggravated by changes in weather or temperature, monthly hormonal variations, stress, anxiety, and depression. Diagnosis is made by eliminating any other cause for the symptoms and finding 11 of 18 specific points to be extremely tender to palpation (Figure 40-5). Treatment goals include reducing pain, enhancing sleep, and decreasing anxiety and stress. There is no known cure.

Muscular Dystrophy. Muscular dystrophy is a hereditary disease that affects almost a quarter million Americans. Muscles gradually lose protein and the muscle fibers are gradually replaced with fat so that skeletal muscles ultimately become useless. Duchenne's muscular dystrophy is discussed in Chapter 39, and other forms

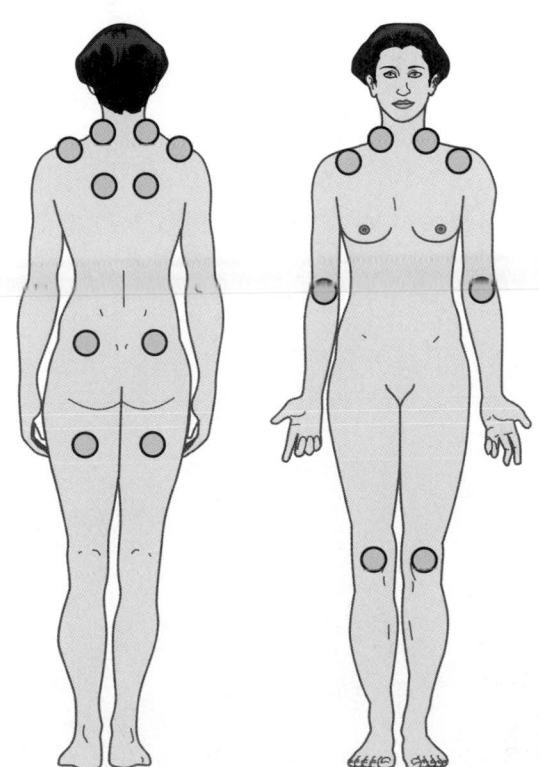

FIGURE 40-5 Fibromyalgia tender points.

TABLE 40-2 Common Musculoskeletal Conditions

Disease	Symptoms/Signs	Diagnostic Procedures	Laboratory Tests	Treatment/Medications
Bursitis and tendonitis	Painful joint with decreased ROM	History, physical examination, x-ray studies to rule out fracture	CBC to rule out infectious arthritis	RICE temporary immobilization, NSAIDs
Carpal tunnel syndrome	Hand and finger pain, numbness, tingling, and difficulty grasping or holding objects, especially in the morning	History, physical examination, compression test	None	Rest, splint, forearm extensor strengthening exercises, surgical decompression in severe cases
Dislocation	Painful joint that looks out of place and has severely decreased ROM	History of trauma, physical examination, x-ray studies	None	Reduce and temporarily immobilize joint
Fibromyalgia	Chronic, severe musculoskeletal pain and generalized weakness	History , physical examination to rule out other causative conditions	As appropriate to rule out other conditions	NSAIDs, rest, decrease stress, muscle relaxer (Flexeril) and tricyclics (Elavil and Thorazine), SSRIs
Fractures	Severe pain, swelling, and decreased ROM	History, physical examination, and x-ray studies	None	Reduction, immobilization, analgesics and NSAIDs
Gout	Painful, inflamed joint, often affects great toe, very sensitive to touch and movement	History, physical examination, microscopic synovial fluid examination for uric acid crystals	Serum uric acid test	Analgesics, NSAIDs
Herniated disk	Depend on location and severity of herniation, back pain, extremity pain or weakness	History, physical examination, CT, myelogram	None	Immobility, physical therapy, traction, muscle relaxants, surgical laminectomy in severe cases
Infectious arthritis	Severely inflamed joint	History, physical examination, microscopic synovial fluid examination for cell count and presence of bacteria	CBC, culture of joint fluid	NSAIDs, corticosteroids, and appropriate antibiotic or antiviral agents
Lupus	Widely disparate presentations of symptoms with no known cause; very difficult to diagnose	Very careful history and physical examination to rule out possible causes of presenting symptoms; frequently this is a diagnosis of exclusion	Diagnostic tests as needed to rule out possible symptom etiologies	Symptomatic relief
Lyme disease	Generalized malaise, fatigue, fever, headaches, myalgias, and polyarthralgias	Careful history and physical examination to look for tick bite location	CBC and perhaps other blood studies	Antibiotics and symptomatic relief

TABLE 40-2 Common Musculoskeletal Conditions—cont'd

Disease	Symptoms/Signs	Diagnostic Procedures	Laboratory Tests	Treatment/Medications
Muscular dystrophy	Increasing difficulty with purposeful movement	History, physical examination, muscle biopsy	None	Supportive treatment including splints or braces, occasionally surgery is indicated
Myasthenia gravis	Profound muscular weakness, frequently starting with facial muscles, can involve any voluntary muscles	History, neurological examination, EMG edrophonium chloride (Tensilon) challenge, neostigmine challenge	Anti-AchR antibody test	Cholinesterase inhibitors, NSAIDs, steroids, immune inhibitors, thymectomy, plasmapheresis
Osteoarthritis	Gradually increasing joint pain and gradually decreasing ROM in affected joint	History, physical examination, x-ray studies and possible CT scan	RA latex test to rule out rheumatoid arthritis, CBC to rule out infectious arthritis	NSAIDs, physical therapy, analgesics, ambulatory support
Osteomalacia	Fractures, muscle weakness and bone pain	History, physical examination, x-ray studies, bone scan	Serum vitamin D, serum calcium, serum alkaline phosphatase, PTH level, occasionally bone biopsy	Vitamin D and calcium supplementation
Osteoporosis	Frequent fractures, exaggerated thoracic kyphosis, decreased height, back pain	History, physical examination, x-ray studies, bone density studies	BMD test, blood calcium level sometimes	Weight-bearing exercise, calcium supplementation, and pharmaceutical treatment with alendronate (Fosamax), etidronate (Didronel), or calcitonin-salmon (Miacalcin)
Rheumatoid arthritis	Severe joint pain and joint deformity	History, physical examination, x-ray studies	RA latex test	NSAIDs, analgesics, joint replacement in severe cases
Scoliosis	Lateral spinal deformity accompanied with back pain	Physical examination, radiographic studies	None	Braces, casts, surgery
Sprain, strain, spasm	Cardinal signs of inflammation, redness, heat, swelling, pain along with decreased ROM	History, physical examination, including active and passive ROM, x-ray studies to rule out fracture	None	RICE and NSAIDs

CBC, Complete blood cell count; *CT,* computed tomography; *EMG,* electromyography; *NSAIDs,* nonsteroidal antiinflammatory drugs; *PTH,* parathyroid hormone; *RA,* rheumatoid arthritis; *RICE,* rest, ice compression, elevation; *ROM,* range of motion; *BMD,* bone mineral density; *SSRI,* serotonin reuptake inhibitor.

can occur in older children and young adults that progress much more slowly. The treatment is activity and exercise that together produce better physical and mental status in the patient. Obesity must be avoided. Splints, braces, and occasionally orthopedic surgery may be needed.

Myasthenia Gravis. Myasthenia gravis is a disease of unknown origin that affects voluntary muscle contraction and can occur in both sexes, all races, and all ages. Frequently the onset involves facial muscle weakness, but this can involve any of the voluntary muscles including the diaphragm. Muscle activity decreases with physical activity and improves with rest. Myasthenia gravis is an autoimmune disorder in which antibodies destroy the receptors (AChR) for the neurotransmitter acetylcholine (ACh) at the neuromuscular junction. When a nerve impulse is received at the muscle, the lack of functioning active receptors does not allow the muscle to get the message adequately. There is no known cure, and the primary treatment involves a medication that inhibits acetylcholinesterase, the enzyme that normally breaks down ACh. This allows ACh to remain at the neuromuscular junction longer than usual so that more of the remaining receptor sites can be activated. Spontaneous improvement and remissions can occur, even with treatment, as part of the normal course of this disease in some patients.

Sprains, Strains, and Spasms. A sprain is a wrenching or twisting of a joint in an abnormal plane of motion or beyond its normal range of motion that results in the tearing of ligaments. There may be concurrent damage to the associated blood vessels, muscles, tendons, and nerves. Probably the most common sprain is the sprained ankle (Figure 40-6), which can result from stepping off a curb or into a small depression and twisting the ankle. Severe sprains are so painful the joint cannot be used. There is a great deal of swelling and reddish to bluish discoloration as a result of ruptured blood vessels in the area.

Diagnosis is made by history and physical examination. Usually x-ray films are obtained to rule out fractures. Treatment includes rest and elevation of the injured joint with no weight bearing to prevent further damage. Elevation of the injured part helps to decrease swelling. Cold application during the first 24 hours helps to reduce pain and swelling. If severe ligamentous injury occurs, immobilization by casting, surgical repair, or both may be required.

CRITICAL THINKING APPLICATION

A patient comes into the clinic hopping on one foot and holding the other in the air. She says she thinks she broke her ankle when she stepped off the curb wrong and fell. What is the first thing Kaiwan should do for this patient? What test will Dr. Alexander most likely order on this patient? Why?

A strain is the overstretching or tearing of a muscle or tendon. This is a much less common injury and it is also generally less severe than a sprain.

Muscle spasm occurs spontaneously and may persist for hours. Muscle spasms and trigger points commonly occur in the neck region, particularly in the trapezius muscle. Trigger points are marble-sized areas of spasm in a muscle. Muscle spasms can be quite painful. Treatment can include massage, direct pressure, ultrasound, stress reduction, stretching exercises, and perhaps muscle relaxants in some cases.

Skeletal Disorders

Fractures. A fracture is a break or crack in a bone that generally is the result of trauma or disease. There are many different types of fractures with each one having its own set of problems (see Table 40-4). The common symptom of all fractures is pain. Other symptoms may include swelling, bleeding, inability to move, misalignment of the bone, and discoloration of the immediate area.

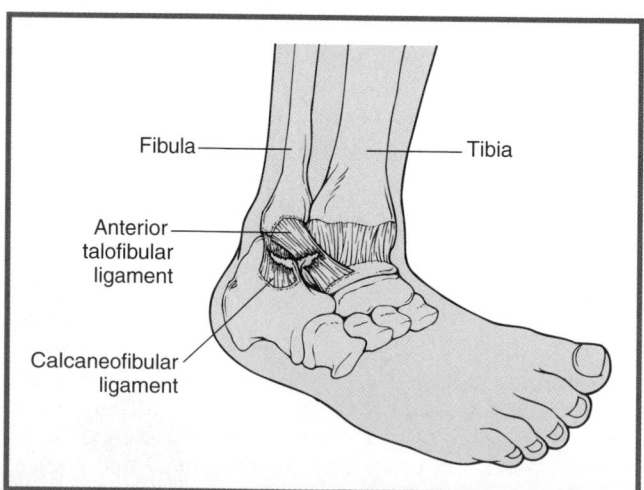

FIGURE 40-6 Ankle sprain. (From Frazier MS, Drzymkowski JW: *Essentials of human diseases and conditions*, ed 2. Philadelphia, 2000, WB Saunders, p 204.)

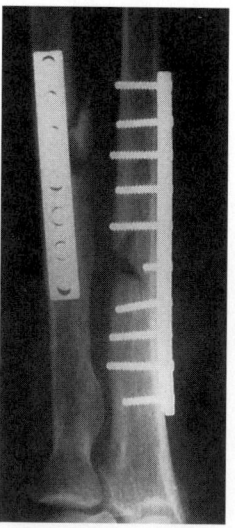

FIGURE 40-7 Orthopedic hardware from open reduction of fractures of the radius and ulna. (From Mettler MA: *Essentials of radiology*, Philadelphia, 1996, WB Saunders.)

When a patient with a suspected fracture comes into the office, you should make him or her as comfortable as possible. First aid includes RICE: Encourage rest by having the patient lie down in a manner that does not put stress on the injured area. Ice should be applied. Control any bleeding with pressure or compression. Do not apply vigorous pressure on a bleeding area if it is over a fracture. Elevate the injured extremity if possible. Be gentle in every aspect of caring for this patient. Do not attempt to straighten the fracture or move it in any way. If the patient must be moved, give support to the joints above and below the suspected fracture before and while moving the patient. The fracture must be confirmed by x-ray examination as soon as possible after arrival. If possible, an x-ray study of the area should be completed before the physician arrives. Table 40-3 identifies the most frequently occurring fractures according to age (Table 40-4 identifies types of fractures and their definitions), which may help in identifying the best course of action before x-rays are taken.

Treatment includes **reduction** and immobilization. Reduction is placing the fractured bone back into its correct anatomical alignment. Reduction of a fracture may be closed or open. Closed reduction is accomplished by manipulating the bone back into its correct position. If this is not possible, or if the fractured bones have pierced the skin, an open reduction will be required, which means reducing the fracture with surgery. During an open reduction, installing metal pins, plates, and screws may facilitate correct bone alignment. These metal implants may be temporary or permanent, depending on the extent of injury (Figure 40-7). After the fracture has been reduced, it must be immobilized by splinting or casting to prevent movement of the fracture site and thus facilitate healing. Immobilization can also be accomplished by taping or wrapping the area, depending on the location and severity of the injury.

Osteomalacia. *Osteomalacia* literally means "softening of the bones." This is a metabolic disease in which there is inadequate calcium, phosphorus, or both available for the building of new bone during growth or remodeling. The skeleton gradually loses calcium and the bones soften and become more flexible. Weight-bearing can gradually change the shape of these softened bones. Symptoms can include decreased endurance, easy fatigability, **malaise**, and generalized bone tenderness and pain. There are two primary causes for this disease. The first is a fat absorption problem in the gastrointestinal tract called *steatorrhea*. The body is unable to adequately absorb dietary fats and they pass through the body in the stool. Vitamin D is normally absorbed with fat so this results in a vitamin D defi-

ciency and poorly absorbed calcium. The second primary cause of osteomalacia is an abnormally increased amount of acid in the body as a result of defective kidney function. The increased acid in the body literally slowly dissolves the skeleton.

Osteomalacia occurring in children is called *rickets*. A much less common cause of osteomalacia can result from dietary vitamin D deficiency and thus inadequate calcium absorption and utilization. This is quite rare, because when exposed to even small amounts of sunlight, the skin makes vitamin D, and nearly all milk sold in the United States is fortified with vitamin D.

Osteoporosis. Osteoporosis is a disease in which calcium in the bone gradually decreases and bones become increasingly fragile until fractures start occurring. Our bones are constantly changing through a process called *remodeling*. This process allows bones to grow and heal. As we age, remodeling naturally breaks down bone quicker than it forms new bone. People over 50 years of age are particularly at risk, and women are four times more likely to develop osteoporosis than men. Osteoporosis is a major public health threat in the United States, affecting more than 40 million individuals. Significant risk is reported in people of all races.

FRACTURES CAUSED BY OSTEOPOROSIS

More than 1.5 million fractures occur yearly from osteoporosis.
- 300,000 fractured hips
- 700,000 fractured vertebrae
- 250,000 wrist fractures
- 300,000 fractures at other sites

The national direct cost for these osteoporotic fractures exceeds $50 million per day.

Osteoporosis is often called the "silent disease," because the progressive loss of bone density occurs without any symptoms. By the time fracture occurs, the disease is quite advanced. Risk factors include being a postmenopausal woman over 50 years of age, of slight build with a family history of osteoporosis, history of amenorrhea, low dietary calcium intake, inactive lifestyle, smoking, and alcohol abuse. Men over 50 years of age with low testosterone levels are also at risk. Osteoporosis occurs in all races, but is slightly more common in whites and Asians.

Diagnosis is made by a specialized form of x-ray evaluation that specifically measures bone mineral density (BMD). This can diagnose osteoporosis before a fracture occurs and thus allow intervention to prevent fractures. Readings are repeated annually to determine the rate of bone loss and to monitor treatment effectiveness. Intervention and treatment include increasing dietary intake of calcium and vitamin D as well as increasing weight-bearing exercise; it can also be treated pharmaceutically with biphosphates (Fosamax and Didronel) and calcitonin-salmon (Miacalcin). Bone density is directly related to the amount of physical stress placed on a bone through weight-bearing exercise. Improvement

TABLE 40-3	Incidence of Fracture Types by Patient Age	
	Under Age 65 (%)	Over Age 65 (%)
Hip	6	54
Arm or leg	62	24
Skull	16	2
Other sites	16	205

TABLE 40-4	Types of Fractures				
Fracture	**Definition**		**Fracture**	**Definition**	
Closed or simple	Broken bone is contained within intact skin		Pathologic	Results from weakening of bone by disease as in osteoporosis or sarcomas	
Open or compound	Skin is broken above the fracture, which is thus open to the external environment, resulting in potential for infection		Nondisplaced	Bone ends remain in alignment	
Longitudinal	Fracture extends along the length of the bone		Displaced	Bone ends are out of alignment	
Transverse	Produced by direct force applied perpendicular to a bone; fracture runs across the bone		Spiral	Have long, sharp, pointed bone ends; produced by twisting or rotary forces; suspicious for child abuse injury	
Oblique	Produced by a twisting force with an upward thrust; fracture ends are short and run at an oblique angle across the bone		Compression	Produced by transmitted forces that drive bones together	
Greenstick	Produced by compression or angulation forces in long bones of children younger than 10; bone is cracked on one side and intact on the other due to softness		Avulsion	Produced by forceful contraction of a muscle against resistance, with a bone fragment tearing at the site of muscle insertion	

TABLE 40-4	Types of Fractures—cont'd				
Fracture	**Definition**		**Fracture**	**Definition**	
Comminuted	Has multiple fragments and is produced by severe direct violence		Depression	Bone fragments of the skull are driven inward	
Impacted	Produced by strong forces that drive bone fragments firmly together				

From Chester GA: *Modern medical assisting*, Philadelphia, 1998, WB Saunders, p 287.

in bone strength and density can easily be measured by the BMD test. The most common BMD test is the pDXA (peripheral dual energy x-ray absorptiometry), which can measure a finger, wrist, or heel. A newer technique using ultrasonography has recently been approved by the FDA; this technique is cheaper and easier to use, making it more readily available for screening purposes.

Spinal Column Disorders

Abnormal Spinal Curvatures. When looking at a patient's back, the spine should be vertically straight. Any abnormal deviation or curvature to the right or left is termed **scoliosis**. Mild scoliosis generally causes no problems and is usually not even noticeable. When scoliosis is severe, it can cause significant back pain and possibly heart or lung problems due to the decreased space in the **thoracic** cavity on one side.

When the spine is viewed from a lateral position, there are four normal curves present (Figure 40-8). The **cervical** region and the **lumbar** region should have curves toward the front of the body; these are called **lordotic** curves. The normal curves in the thoracic region of the spine and the sacrum are toward the back and are called **kyphotic** curves. Loss of cervical lordosis is called *military neck*. Excessive lumbar lordosis is called *swayback*. Excessive upper thoracic kyphosis is called *hunchback* (Figure 40-9).

Diagnosis of these conditions is made by inspection and palpation, and may be confirmed with x-rays. Treatment may include orthopedic devices such as braces, shoe lifts, exercises, and electrical muscle stimulation. In severe cases, rigid casting with or without surgery may be necessary.

Herniated Disk. A herniated disk occurs when the soft nucleus of an intervertebral disk protrudes through a tear or weakened area in the tough outer disk covering (Figure 40-10). This condition occurs most often in

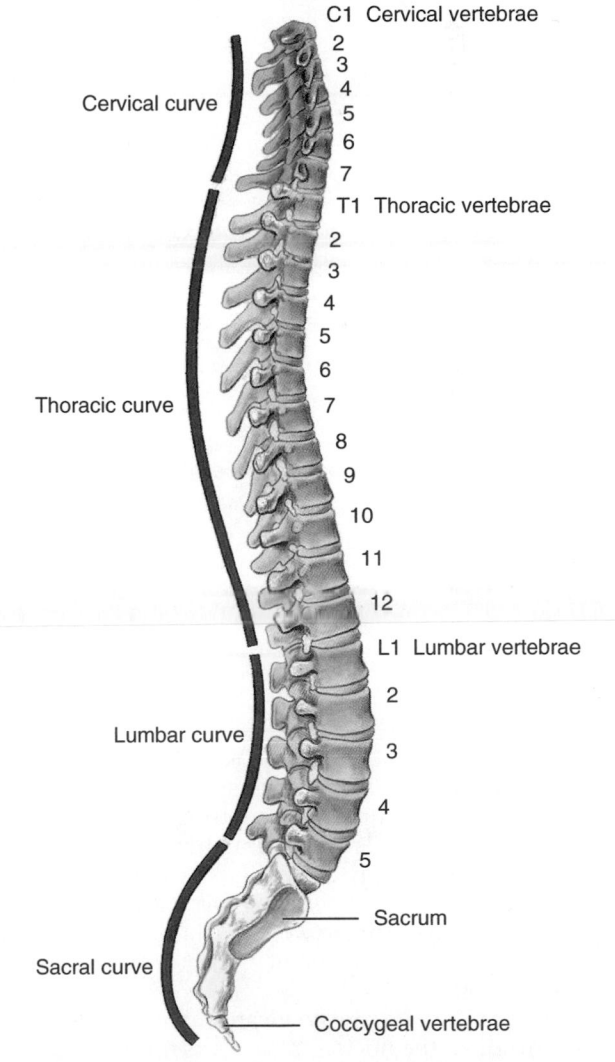

FIGURE 40-8   Normal spine curves. (From Applegate EJ: *The anatomy and physiology learning system*, ed 2. Philadelphia, 2000, WB Saunders, p 103.)

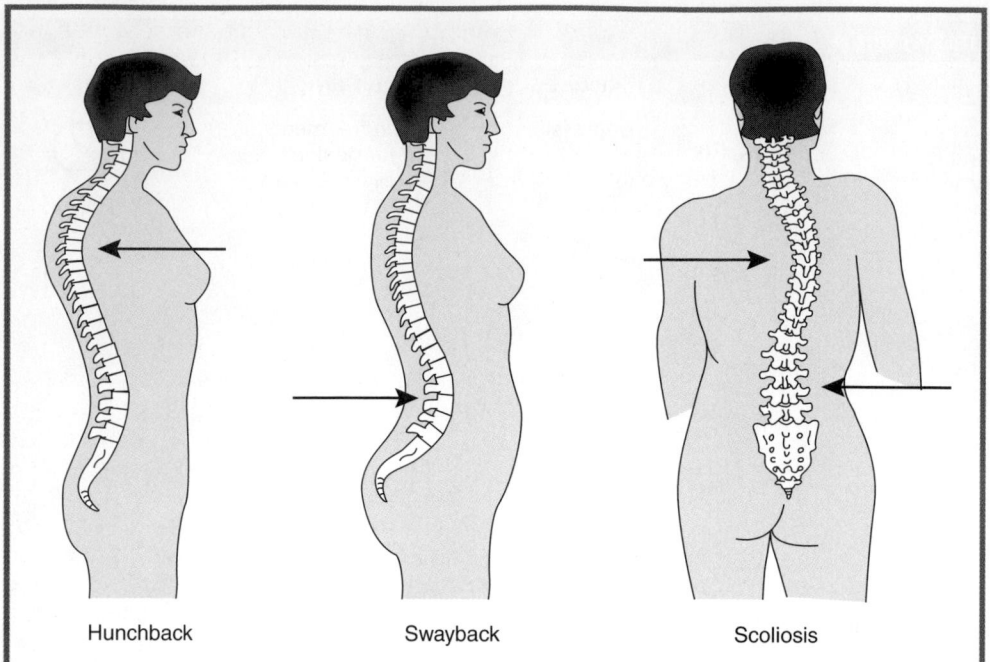

FIGURE 40-9 Spinal curve abnormalities.

Hunchback   Swayback   Scoliosis

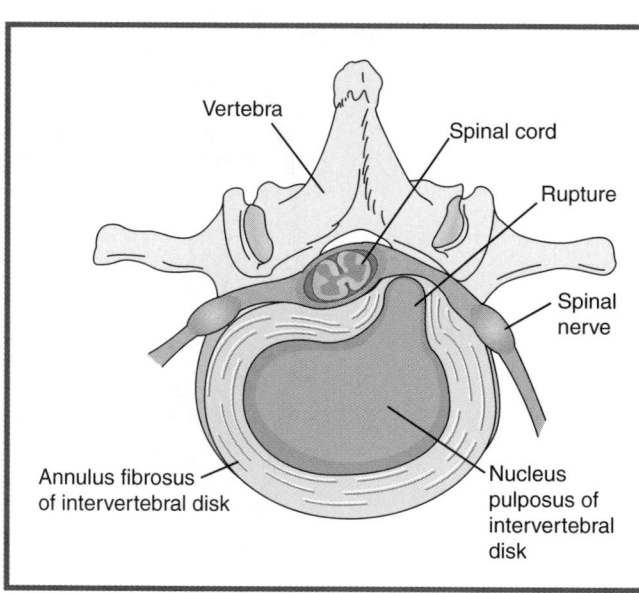

Vertebra

Spinal cord

Rupture

Spinal nerve

Annulus fibrosus of intervertebral disk

Nucleus pulposus of intervertebral disk

FIGURE 40-10 Herniation of vertebral disk.

the lumbar region, frequently in the cervical region, and rarely in the thoracic region of the spine. Disk herniation may be caused by trauma or by putting a sudden strain on the spine while it is in an unnatural position. This frequently occurs when a person lifts a heavy object while bending over instead of squatting and allowing the leg muscles to carry the weight. Herniation may also come on gradually as a result of a progressive deterioration of the disks.

Symptoms depend on the location and the extent of the protrusion of the nucleus beyond its normal location. If the herniation occurs in the lumbar region, it usually results in severe low back pain that can radiate down the leg and cause difficulty walking. If the herniated disk is in the cervical region, there is usually severe neck pain that can radiate down the arms to the fingers.

Diagnosis is made from a careful history, physical examination, and often an MRI. A myelogram may be performed to rule out other spinal conditions. Treatment depends on the severity of the herniation and the symptoms. Conservative treatments can include chiropractic adjustments, physical therapy mobilization of the involved area, and applications of heat or cold. Traction of the affected area is also successfully employed. Muscle relaxants and/or pain relievers may be given. If these measures are ineffective and the patient has recurring pain, numbness, and progressive weakness, surgery may be necessary.

Joint Disorders

Dislocation. Dislocation of a joint is also called a **luxation**, when two bones of a joint are no longer in approximation (Figure 40-11). A **subluxation** is an incomplete dislocation of a joint, meaning that the bones are only slightly out of proper alignment and location. It is possible to have a congenital dislocation, especially of the hip. Common dislocations occur to the finger, thumb, and shoulder and are usually caused by trauma, frequently while a person is playing sports. Symptoms include pain, swelling, loss of motion, and sometimes temporary paralysis. A dislocation requires immediate **reduction** and immobilization to prevent permanent injury to structures adjacent to the joint, such as nerves and major blood vessels. Occasionally surgical reduction and repair may be necessary to stabilize the joint.

CRITICAL THINKING APPLICATION

A patient comes into the office from a sand-lot softball game. After sliding into home plate he was immediately unable to move his right arm and complained of a great deal of pain in his right shoulder. What steps should Kaiwan take to help this patient?

Gout. Gout, which is also sometimes called *gouty arthritis*, is a metabolic disease in which there is an overproduction or improper elimination of uric acid. Needlelike crystals of uric acid appear in the synovial fluid of the affected joint and result in increased sensitivity to touch and severe pain. Gout most often affects the great toe with severe inflammation that even makes walking difficult (Figure 40-12). There are usually periods of remission and exacerbation, but the condition will worsen if it is untreated, resulting in degeneration and deformity of the affected joint.

Treatment includes dietary modification to eliminate purine-containing foods, such as liver, cold cuts, sausage, and alcohol. If a trial of the drug colchicine dramatically relieves the pain, this actually confirms the diagnosis. Precisely how colchicine works to ease the symptoms remains unknown. Other medications that may be beneficial are the uricosuric drugs, because they increase the excretion of uric acid. Drugs that have an inhibitory effect on uric acid production are also used.

Infectious Arthritis. Infectious arthritis usually occurs after some type of systemic or local infection in some other part of the body. It can also occur after a joint has been violated by trauma or surgery. Causes can include bacteria, fungi, and viruses. The joint usually exhibits signs of severe inflammation and shows significantly decreased range of motion (ROM). To determine the diagnosis, the physician may order an x-ray evaluation and bone scan and may draw synovial fluid for microscopic examination and culture. Treatment goals are to decrease inflammation, increase ROM, and treat the causative organism with the appropriate medication.

Lupus. Systemic lupus erythematosus (SLE) is an autoimmune disease of unknown cause. It occurs primarily in women 20 to 50 years of age, although it can occur in both younger and older persons as well. SLE is difficult to diagnose, and the course is entirely unpredictable. The progression and severity vary widely among different patients. The patient develops autoantibodies (antibodies to self) that can attack any tissue or organ in the body, which may result in severe inflammation and tissue changes and destruction. There is no known cure; the therapeutic goal is to have the patient remain as functional and active as possible.

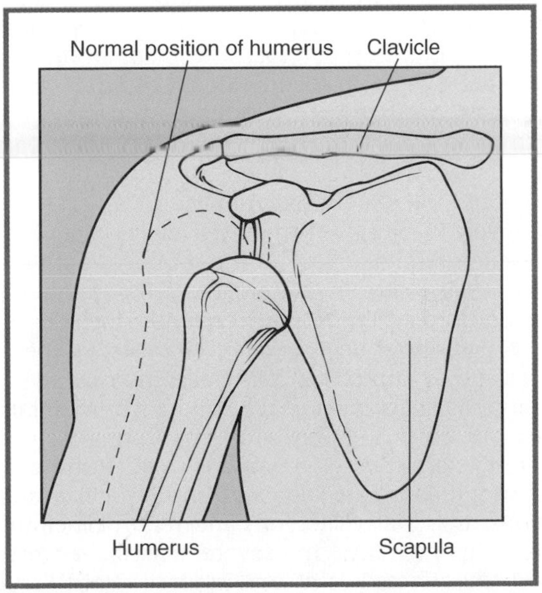

FIGURE 40-11 Luxation or dislocation of the shoulder. (From Frazier MS, Drzymkowski JW: *Essentials of human diseases and conditions*, ed 2. Philadelphia, 2000, WB Saunders, p 205.)

SLE SYMPTOMS

According to the American Rheumatism Association, a patient who has four or more of the following symptoms either chronologically or together is diagnosed as having SLE in the absence of any other known cause:

- Butterfly rash across the face
- Round red macular rash covered with scales
- Photosensitivity
- Painless oral or nasal ulcers
- Noncrosive arthritis affecting two or more peripheral joints
- Pleuritis or pericarditis
- Persistent proteinuria
- Seizures or psychoses
- Hemolytic anemia
- Unidentified immune disorder
- Abnormal antinuclear antibody (ANA) titer

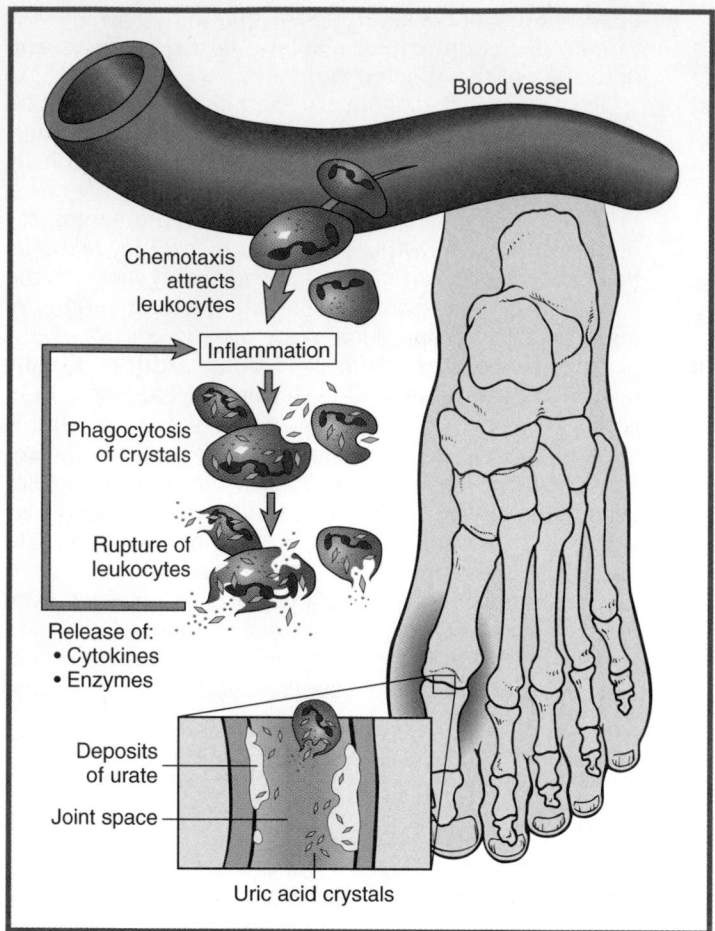

Blood vessel

Chemotaxis attracts leukocytes

Inflammation

Phagocytosis of crystals

Rupture of leukocytes

Release of:
• Cytokines
• Enzymes

Deposits of urate

Joint space

Uric acid crystals

FIGURE 40-12 Gout. Deposits of uric acid crystals in the connective tissue. The inflammation most often affects the joint of the big toe. (From Damjanov I: *Pathology for the health-related professions,* ed 2. Philadelphia, 2000, WB Saunders, p 460.)

Lyme Disease. Lyme disease, which can involve several joints as Lyme arthritis, is an infection caused by the bacteria *Borrelia burgdorferi* and is transmitted to humans by a bite from ticks of the *Ixodes* family. It is named after Lyme, Connecticut, where it is common and was first identified in a cluster of children in 1977. The patient often has complaints of malaise, fatigue, fever, headaches, myalgia, and polyarthalgia. Frequently there is a "bull's-eye lesion" called *erythema migrans* surrounding the area of the tick bite. The severity of Lyme disease varies widely among individuals, from a completely asymptomatic infection to a widely disseminated infection involving the nervous, circulatory, and musculoskeletal systems. The most common late manifestation of the disease is intermittent polyarthalgia. This can become a chronic, debilitating arthritis. Diagnosis is made primarily by taking a careful history, locating the tick bite, and ruling out other causes for the presenting symptoms.

Lyme disease is found in several regions, including coastal areas like northern California, Oregon and Washington, and Wisconsin. It has been spreading rather rapidly across the United States. The most common means of prevention is to avoid being exposed to ticks. Ticks live in woods and overgrown brush. Lyme disease can be treated with antibiotics quite successfully. The effectiveness of treatment depends partly on how quickly the disease is correctly diagnosed.

Osteoarthritis. Osteoarthritis (OA), also called *degenerative joint disease* (DJD), is marked by significant thinning and degeneration of the **articular** cartilage of synovial joints, particularly the knees. Primary OA, which is a part of the normal aging process, can also affect joints of the great toe, lower spine, and distal finger joints. Symptom severity depends on the amount of degeneration that has taken place and ranges from mild to severe. As the articular cartilage disintegrates and wears away, the roughened surface of the bone is exposed and the patient experiences pain and stiffness of the involved joint. Commonly involved joints include the distal interphalangeal (DIP) joints, the first carpometacarpal joint, and weight-bearing joints—hips, knees, and spine. Diagnosis frequently includes x-ray films, which show degenerative changes in the joint surfaces and asymmetrical joint space narrowing.

Treatment goals include relieving pain, maintaining normal motion in the joint, and attempting to prevent crippling deformities. Medications may include analgesics, antiinflammatories, and intraarticular steroid injections. Using a walker or cane may be helpful for maintaining mobility. In severe cases, surgery to remove the affected joint and replace it with a joint **prosthesis** is necessary. All of the following joints can be replaced with prosthetic metal or plastic joints: shoulder, elbow, wrist, finger, hip, knee, and ankle.

CRITICAL THINKING APPLICATION

An 80-year-old male patient with severe arthritis comes into the office complaining of severe joint pain in his knees, hips, and lower back. He cannot possibly get up onto the examination table because of the pain. What should Kaiwan do? Is this patient required to get onto the examination table? Why or why not?

joints may become painful and inflamed. Usually, bouts of arthritis will increase in frequency and severity over time. As this occurs, the joints become damaged and joint swelling and deformity occur. Patients with RA may appear undernourished and chronically ill because of the formation of degenerative lesions occurring in the collagen (connective tissues) in the lungs, heart, blood vessels, and pleura (Figure 40-13). X-ray findings show uniform joint space narrowing, which is different from degenerative changes seen in osteoarthritis.

Rest and exercise seem to be the key elements in treating RA. Therapeutic exercises are designed to prevent and correct deformities, control pain, strengthen weakened muscles, and improve joint function. The most frequently prescribed medications are aspirin (acetylsalicylic acid) and nonsteroidal antiinflammatory drugs (**NSAIDs**), such as indomethacin (Indocin), sulindac (Clinoril), naproxen (Naprosyn), and ibuprofen (Motrin). In severe cases, surgical joint replacement may be necessary.

Rheumatoid Arthritis. Rheumatoid arthritis (RA) can begin at any age but most frequently occurs between the ages of 20 and 40. RA is an autoimmune disease that attacks synovial fluid; its cause is unknown. Early symptoms include malaise, fever, weight loss, and morning stiffness of the affected joints. One or more

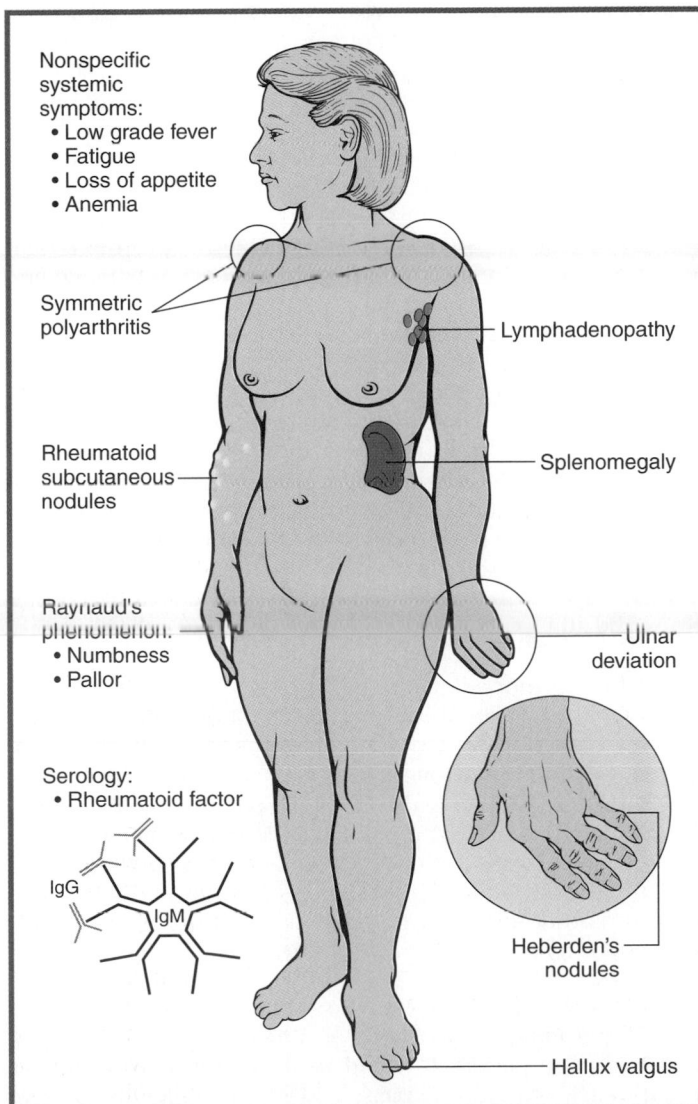

Nonspecific systemic symptoms:
• Low grade fever
• Fatigue
• Loss of appetite
• Anemia

Symmetric polyarthritis

Lymphadenopathy

Rheumatoid subcutaneous nodules

Splenomegaly

Raynaud's phenomenon:
• Numbness
• Pallor

Ulnar deviation

Serology:
• Rheumatoid factor

IgG

IgM

Heberden's nodules

Hallux valgus

FIGURE 40-13 Signs and symptoms of rheumatoid arthritis. (From Damjanov I: *Pathology for the health-related professions*, ed 2. Philadelphia, 2000, WB Saunders, p 458.)

JOINT REPLACEMENT RECORD

In 1999, Mr. Charles N. Wedde of Baroda, Michigan became the Guinness World Record holder for having the most joint prostheses installed. He has had all of the major extremity joints replaced bilaterally, giving him a total of 12 artificial joints. He had the joints replaced because of severe rheumatoid arthritis.

Tendonitis and Bursitis. Tendonitis is one of the most common causes of pain in the shoulder and elbow. Inflammation of tendons may be associated with calcium deposits in the bursae around the joint causing concurrent bursitis. Noting increasing severity of pain when abducting the arm beyond 50 degrees is diagnostic. Treatment includes pain relief and decreasing inflammation so that exercise is possible. This is necessary to prevent permanent shoulder immobility, called *frozen shoulder*. Medications might include analgesics, anti-inflammatories, and injections of long-acting corticosteroids. Cold applications are helpful in relieving pain, whereas heat applications are contraindicated, because they tend to aggravate the calcium tendonitis.

Bursitis is a painful inflammation of a joint bursa that most commonly follows a repetitive movement or prolonged pressure on a joint. The pain is increased with movement of the affected joint. It can also occur from staphylococcus or tuberculosis infections and with some joint diseases including gout and arthritis. Treatment includes not doing the activity that caused the bursitis. The affected area should be protected from excessive pressure and movement. NSAIDs may provide pain relief, and antiinflammatories may be needed in severe cases. Extreme cases may require cortisone injections into the bursa. The best prevention is to limit the underlying causes.

The Medical Assistant's Role in Assisting With Orthopedic Procedures

The role of the medical assistant begins with accurately recording the patient's description of the circumstances surrounding the onset of the problem, what measures were undertaken to alleviate the problem, and what the major concerns presently are. Record the exact location of pain or discomfort, and on a scale of 1 to 10, ask the patient to quantify the intensity of the pain at that time. Also ask and record information about any medications taken, including the names of drugs, dose, frequency, and when they were last taken.

Be sure to offer assistance when escorting the patient to the examination room. Use a wheelchair if necessary. Assist the patient to a comfortable position in the examination room by offering a pillow or folded blanket to support the painful or injured body part. The patient may have limited mobility because of pain, so you may need to provide assistance for disrobing and getting into an examination gown. Be sure the patient is warm enough by offering an additional sheet or blanket. Explain clearly what is happening and what the patient can expect. Notify the physician as soon as the patient is ready for the examination.

Assisting With the Examination

The physician may use inspection, palpation, ROM, and muscle testing to examine the major skeletal muscles and joints. Much of the examination includes comparing the affected side muscles and joints for size, position, and strength with the contralateral side. When the patient is to be in a certain position, it may be helpful to demonstrate the position or movement desired. Watch the patient for the presence of a facial grimace or physical jerk or jump, the "jump sign," during the manipulative and palpatory portion of the examination, as indicators of pain.

As a general rule, the unaffected side is examined first and then the affected side is examined and compared. You may be responsible for making notes during the examination. Keep the patient properly draped and assist the physician by handing the equipment to him or her as needed. Most examinations will require the use of a measuring tape, **goniometer**, blood pressure cuff, stethoscope, and felt-tipped washable marker. Be alert and ready to prevent the patient from falling during the examination. Some of the requested movements and positions may place the injured patient off balance and at increased risk for falling.

Gait analysis is usually done by observing the patient walking in a straight line with or without the patient knowing he or she is being observed. Many gait abnormalities are associated with neurological conditions. Muscular dystrophy or hip dysplasia may produce a waddling gait. When walking, the patient's pelvis on the unaffected side will drop as weight-bearing is shifted to the affected side, producing a very characteristic "hula" motion of both hips.

ROM Evaluation

Often orthopedic injuries severely affect the normal ROM of a joint. Measuring the ROM of specific joints is an objective measure of both the seriousness of an injury and the recovery progress.

When evaluating the ROM of a particular joint, usually both active ROM and passive ROM results are measured and recorded. The joint movement in a single plane is measured with a goniometer. A goniometer has two arms that are fixed together with a hinge joint at one end (Figure 40-14). Each of the arms is lined up with a bone on each side of the joint being tested. The degrees of motion are indicated on a scale on the hinged end of the instrument. To determine the active ROM of a joint, the patient it asked to move the joint as far as possible. To evaluate passive ROM, the patient is asked to relax and the physician moves the joint as far as possible. All ROMs are measured in degrees. During these

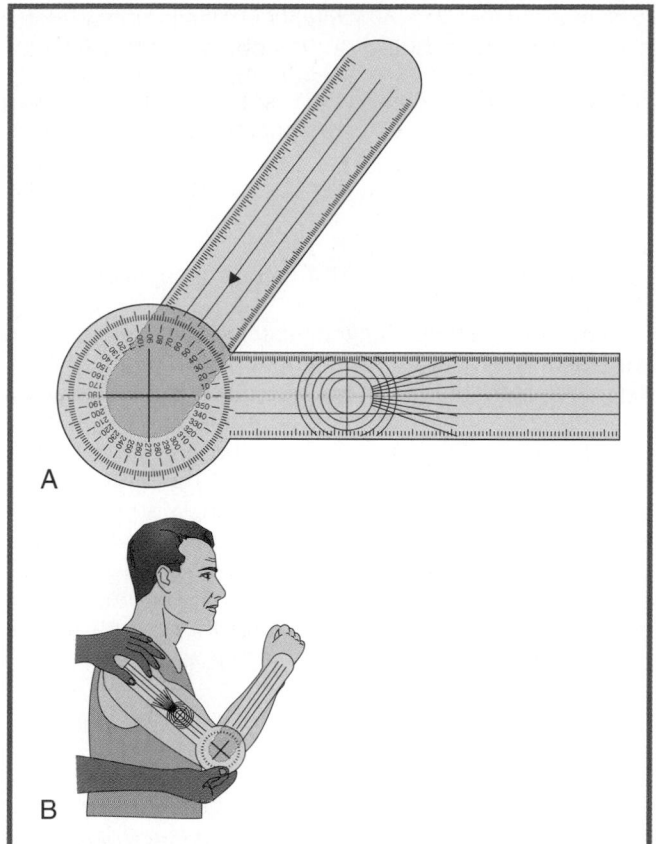

FIGURE 40-14   **A**, Goniometer. **B**, Correct position of goniometer on the arm.

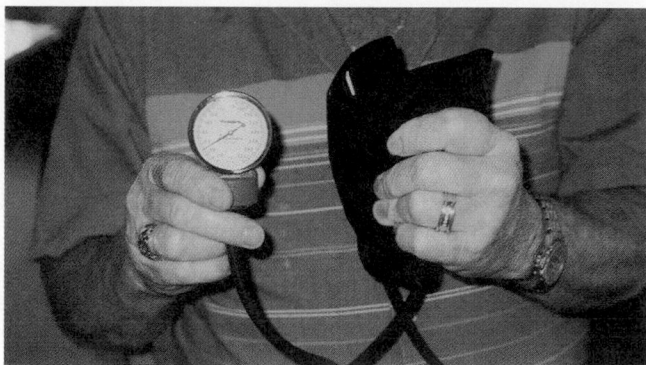

FIGURE 40-15   Assessing strength measurement using a blood pressure cuff.

ASSESSMENT OF STRENGTH USING A BLOOD PRESSURE CUFF

- Roll up an aneroid blood pressure cuff and have the patient hold it on one hand.
- Inflate the cuff to 20 mm Hg pressure.
- Ask the patient to squeeze the cuff as tightly as possible.
- Note the increase in mm Hg pressure on the dial. A normal grip will be above 150.
- Record the hand tested and the results of the test.
- Repeat on the contralateral side.

---

examinations you may be asked to record the degrees of motion for active and/or passive ROM for specific joints as well as noting pain, tenderness, or **crepitation** experienced by the patient during the examination.

CRITICAL THINKING APPLICATION

How can Kaiwan best assist Dr. Alexander in testing upper extremity ROMs on a new patient? What equipment should Kaiwan have ready for the examination? What patient position would best facilitate this examination? Why?

Muscle Strength Evaluation

During the ROM evaluation, the physician will also assess each muscle group for strength. Normal muscle strength allows for complete voluntary ROM in the presence of resistance. This resistance can be gravity, as when rising from sitting to a standing position, or physical, as in pulling, pushing, or lifting an object. Muscle strength is bilaterally equal in normal conditions. The evaluation will be conducted by comparing like muscles in each hemisphere of the body, such as comparing the grip of the right hand with the left hand using a blood pressure cuff (Figure 40-15).

Radiology

Radiology and diagnostic imaging are frequently used to assist in diagnosing orthopedic conditions. Many orthopedic and chiropractic offices have the equipment for taking x-ray films in their office and may employ an x-ray technician. X-ray evaluation is necessary to accurately diagnose fractures, dislocations, and bone and joint diseases. X-ray films can also be used to track the healing of a fracture to determine when it is okay to remove a cast.

A radiograph (x-ray film) is made by projecting x-rays through a body structure, such as an arm or hand, onto a piece of photographic film held in an x-ray cassette (Figure 40-16). Different tissues allow different amounts of x-rays to reach the film. For example, metal stops all x-rays and looks white on the developed film. Bone allows a small amount of x-rays through to the film and appears whitish on the developed film. Air allows for easy transmission of x-rays, so air looks black on the developed radiograph.

At least two views must be taken of any body part that is x-rayed. Most commonly, these are the anteroposterior (AP; taken from front to back) and lateral (taken from the side) views. Additional views may be taken as necessary (Figure 40-17). Specifics about radiology and its use in the medical office are covered in Chapter 47.

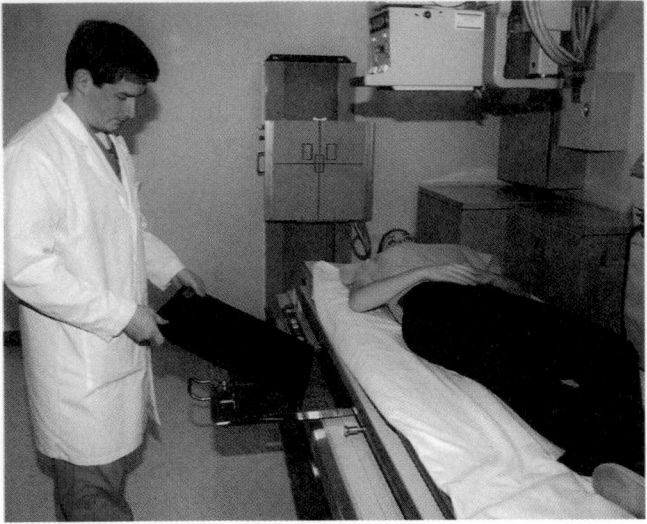

FIGURE 40-16 Proper placement of cassette containing x-ray film.

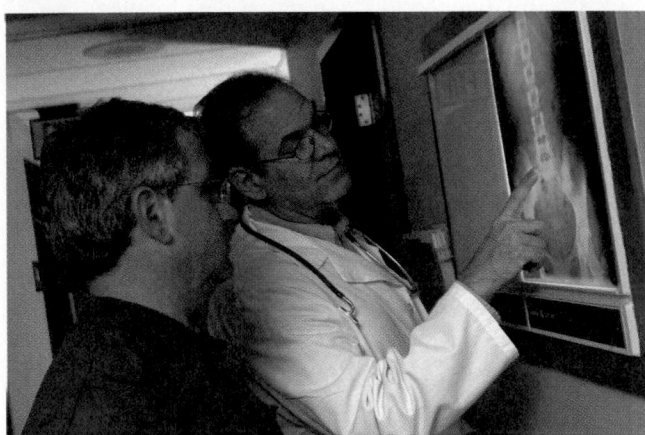

FIGURE 40-17 Reading a lumbar radiograph.

CRITICAL THINKING APPLICATION

A patient who has just been x-rayed stops Kaiwan and wants to see his x-ray films. How should Kaiwan handle this situation? If a patient is in an examination room with her own x-ray film on the view box and she asks Kaiwan to show her where the break is, how should he respond to this request?

Specialized Diagnostic Procedures in Orthopedics

Specialized imaging techniques used in orthopedics include the following:

- Arthrograms: Used to visualize joints
- Myelograms: Used to identify intervertebral disk disorders

- Bone scans: Used to evaluate areas of bone growth, bone density, bone tumors, as well as other bone disease patterns
- Computed tomography (CT) scans: Used to visualize soft tissue such as tumors, masses, lesions, or some spine injuries
- Electromyography and nerve conduction velocity studies: Used to evaluate muscles
- Biopsies of bone and muscle: Used to identify cancerous tumors and other neoplasms and pathogens

When one of these diagnostic tests is necessary, you will need to explain the procedure to the patient. Your explanation should include what will be done, how it is done, where it will take place, and approximately how long it will take. Patients will always be concerned about whether the procedure will hurt. Tell the truth. If the procedure is painful, let the patient know so he or she can prepare for it. Most painful procedures are performed only after the patient has been given a mild sedative. Discuss the procedure in a professional yet empathetic manner. If the patient wishes to talk with the physician about the test, make sure that this happens.

Therapeutic Modalities

Physical agents called modalities are often used in both orthopedic and chiropractic offices to treat orthopedic conditions. These can include the application of cold, heat, baths, diathermy, electric currents, therapeutic ultrasonography, massage, and therapeutic exercises. Cold applications are often used within the first 48 hours after an injury to assist in controlling pain and swelling. Heat application is generally used more than 48 hours after an injury and helps to improve circulation, decrease pain, and maintain muscular and joint function (Table 40-5). Shortwave diathermy creates heat deep in body tissues by the use of radio waves.

General Principles of Cold Application

Cold applications, such as ice packs and cold compresses, act as vasoconstrictors and also cause contraction of the involuntary muscles of the skin ("goose bumps"). These two actions cause a reduced blood supply to the area and cause a numbing effect on the sensory nerve endings. Cold applications can help control bleeding, prevent further swelling and inflammation, and decrease pain. For cold application, disposable, reusable, or home-made ice packs are most commonly used (Figure 40-18 and Procedure 40-1).

Heat Modalities

Heat produces local vasodilation, which causes increased circulation. This accelerates the inflammatory process, promotes local drainage, decreases swelling, relaxes muscles, and repairs tissues and cells. The effects of external heat application depend on the type of heat used, the length of time it is applied, the frequency with which it is applied, the general condition of the patient, and the

TABLE 40-5	Effects of Heat and Cold Application		
Application	**Causes**	**Tissue Response**	**Therapeutic Effect**
Heat	Vasodilation Muscle relaxation Increased metabolism	Increased blood flow More WBCs to area Reduced muscle spasm Local warmth	Increased nutrients to site Faster removal of wastes Phagocytosis Decreased pain Faster tissue repair
Cold	Vasoconstriction Numbness of nerve endings Reduced metabolism Increased blood viscosity	Decreased blood flow Local anesthesia Decreased oxygen need Faster blood clotting	Inhibits swelling Reduced inflammation Decreased pain

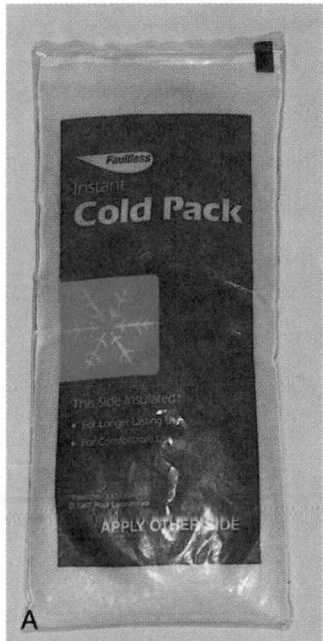 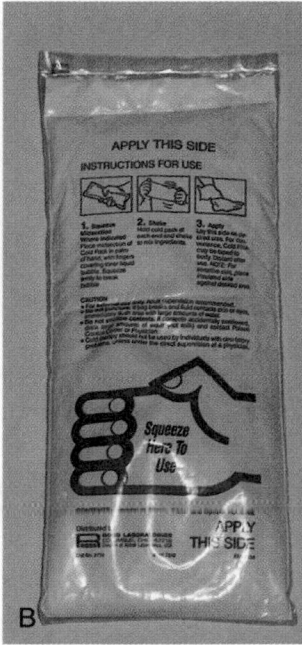

FIGURE 40-18 **A,** Commercial ice pack. **B,** Instructions on the back side.

size of the area needing treatment. Heat application is an excellent therapeutic modality, but it must be used with caution to prevent overheating and burning. Heat application is contraindicated in the following circumstances:

- In the presence of acute inflammatory conditions, particularly during the first 48 hours
- In persons with severe circulatory problems of any kind
- In persons with decreased or abnormal sensation
- During pregnancy or menstruation, because heat can cause uterine contractions
- Over areas containing encapsulated pus
- On blisters from previous burns
- Over scar tissue, because it does not have normal blood supply and easily overheats
- In body areas that contain cancerous tumors
- Over red skin
- Over any metal jewelry and over any area containing metal implants

Body parts may safely be heated to 110° F (44° C) without any tissue damage. Redness appears, because the skin capillaries become congested at the skin's surface. Heat modalities may be either wet or dry and

PROCEDURE 40-1

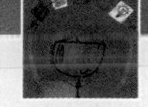

Assisting the Patient With Cold Application

GOAL: To instruct a patient in the correct application of cold to a body area to decrease pain, prevent further swelling, and/or decrease inflammation.

EQUIPMENT AND SUPPLIES
- Ice bag or closeable disposable plastic kitchen food bag
- Small ice cubes or ice chips
- Towel

PROCEDURAL STEPS

1 Wash your hands.

2 Explain the procedure to the patient and answer any questions.

3 Check the bag for possible leaks.

4 Fill the bag with small cubes or chips of ice until it is about two thirds full.
Purpose: Small chips conform more easily to the shape of the body.

5 Push down on the top of the bag to expel excess air and apply the cap.
Purpose: To remove as much air as possible from the bag, because air is a poor conductor of cold.

Continued

PROCEDURE **40-1—cont'd**

6 Dry the outside and cover it with one or two towel layers.

7 Help the patient position the ice bag on the injured area.

8 Advise the patient to leave the ice bag in place for about 20 to 30 minutes or until the area feels numb, whichever is first.

9 Check the skin for color, feeling, and pain.

Purpose: If the area being treated becomes very painful, remains numb, or is pale or cyanotic, the ice bag should be removed and the physician notified.

10 Record the procedure in the patient's chart.
Purpose: A procedure is not considered done until it is recorded.

See Appendix E for a charting example.

can have either superficial or deep effects. Dry heat therapies include heating pads, infrared radiation lamps, ultraviolet radiation, and hot water bottles. More penetrating methods of dry heat application include shortwave diathermy, microwave diathermy, and ultrasound. Moist heat modalities include soaks, whirlpool treatments, hot moist compresses (Figure 40-19), and paraffin baths.

Paraffin Bath. A paraffin bath is especially useful in treating chronic joint inflammation. A mixture of seven parts paraffin and one part mineral oil is melted and heated to approximately 125° F (52° C). The patient's body part, usually a hand, an elbow, or a foot, is dipped into the warm paraffin mixture and removed immediately, leaving a thin coating on the skin. This dipping is repeated numerous times until a thick coating of paraffin remains on the body part (Figure 40-20). The part is then wrapped with plastic and a towel to allow the heat to penetrate into the tissues. The paraffin is kept on for 30 minutes and then is peeled off. The process leaves the skin soft, warm, moisturized, and pliable, with a slight erythema.

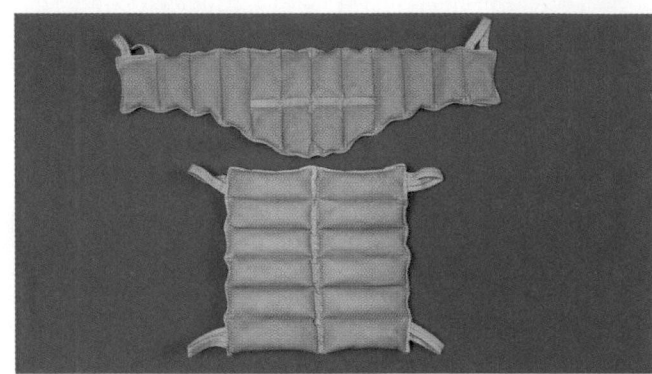

FIGURE 40-19 Commercial hot packs made of canvas that contain a silicone gel.

bottle that is less than half full conforms better to the body surface and is more comfortable (Procedure 40-2).

CRITICAL THINKING APPLICATION

Kaiwan helps a 56-year-old patient with RA to get a paraffin bath treatment for both hands. He did not check the temperature before having the patient put her hands in the bath. When she puts her hands in the bath, she immediately pulls them out and complains that it is too hot. How should Kaiwan handle this situation? What should he say to the patient? What steps should he take to prevent this from occurring with another patient?

PATIENT INSTRUCTIONS FOR APPLYING A HOT COMPRESS AT HOME

1. Moisten a clean hand towel with warm water.
2. Wring it out and fold it to the appropriate size.
3. It should be warm, not hot.
4. Place the folded warm moist compress directly onto the skin.
5. Cover the towel with plastic to keep in the moist heat.
6. Cover the plastic with a dry towel to help maintain the heat.
7. Apply for as long and as often as the physician orders, usually 20-30 min at a time.

Hot Water Bottle. Hot water bottles are often used at home without any concern for correct technique. Patients should be cautioned to keep the water temperature below 125° F (52° C). The hot water bottle can usually be left in place until it becomes cold. If the patient is a child, the temperature should be kept below 115° F (46° C) to prevent burns. Generally, a hot water bottle should not be applied to a child for longer than 15 minutes without a physician's instruction. A hot water

 SAFETY ALERT: Electric heating pads should be left in place no longer than 30 minutes to prevent potential burns.

Therapeutic Ultrasonography

Ultrasound is the energy carried by very high frequency sound waves. Ultrasound works on the same principle

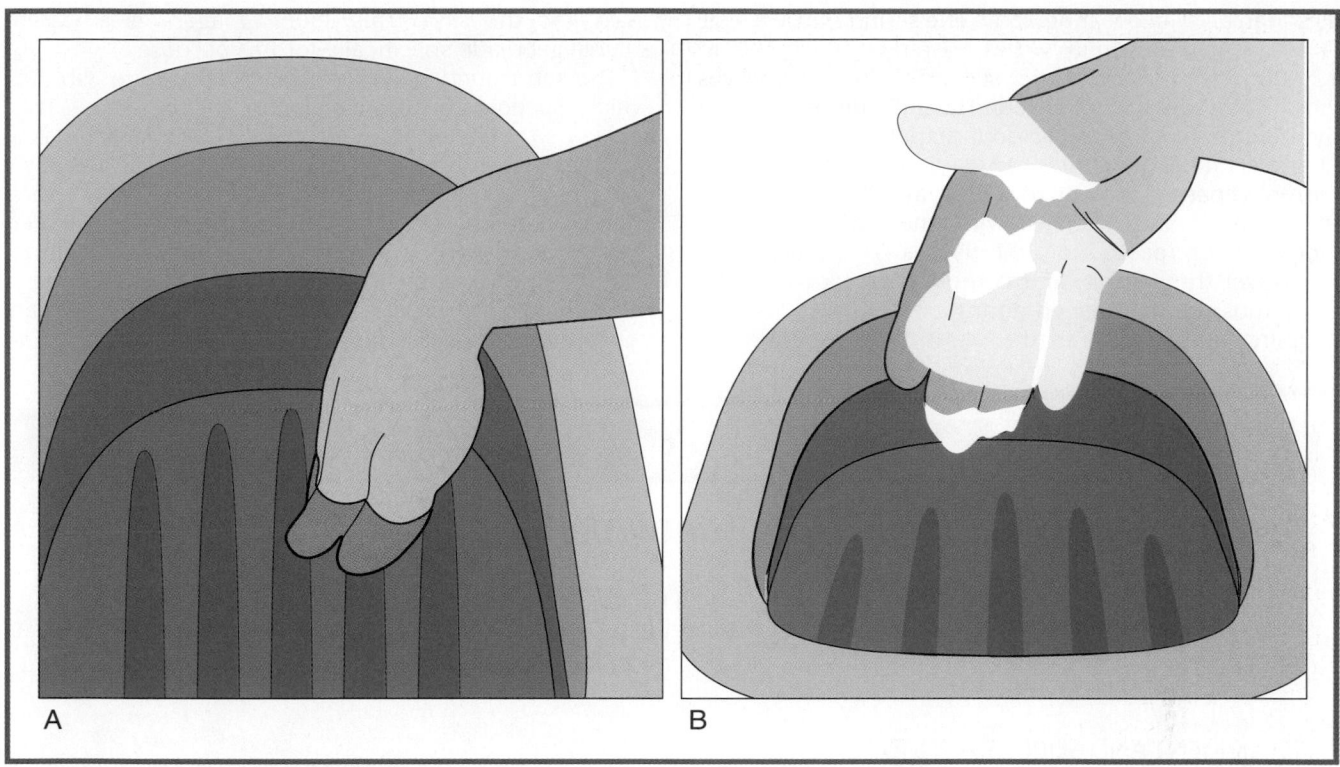

FIGURE 40-20 The paraffin bath is especially helpful for pain relief in patients with arthritis. **A**, The hand is dipped into warm paraffin. **B**, The warm paraffin is left on the hand for about 30 minutes and then is peeled off.

PROCEDURE 40-2

Assisting With Hot Moist Heat Application in the Office

GOAL: To instruct a patient in the correct application of moist heat to a body area to increase circulation, increase metabolism, and relax muscles.

EQUIPMENT AND SUPPLIES

- Commercial hot moist heat packs
- Towel

PROCEDURAL STEPS

1 Wash your hands.

2 Explain the procedure to the patient and answer any questions.

3 Ask the patient to remove all jewelry in the area to be treated.

4 Place one or two towel layers over the area to be treated.

5 Apply the commercial moist heat packs (Figure 1).

6 Cover with the remaining portion of the towel.
Caution: Monitor the patient for complaints of discomfort or signs of potential burns.

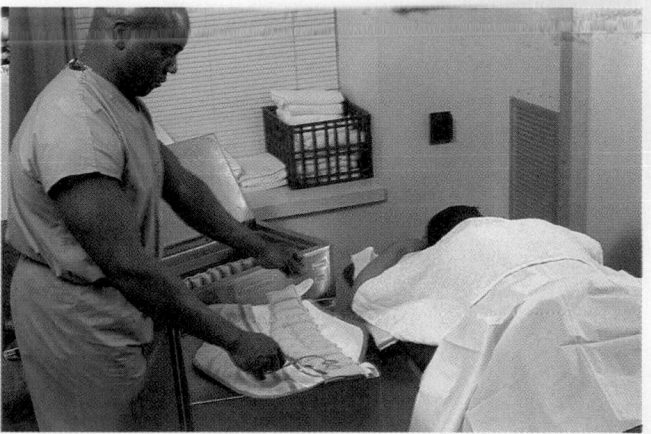

Figure 1

See Appendix E for a charting example.

as sonar, used in oceanography. The sound that we hear is the result of sound waves vibrating from 100 to 12,000 hertz (Hz; cycles per second). Ultrasonic waves vibrate at a rate up to 1 million Hz and cannot be heard by the human ear. The ultrasound applicator contains a quartz crystal that vibrates very rapidly when an electric current is passed through it. The ultrasound applicator is then placed into contact with the body, and the vibrations are passed into the tissues. These waves do not travel through air, and complete contact with the body must be maintained during treatment by using a coupling agent between the ultrasound applicator or

head and the skin. This coupling agent is a water-soluble gel made specifically for this purpose.

The ultrasound waves cause the tissue to vibrate, which speeds up the circulation in the area. This increases the metabolism in the local area, which has a beneficial effect on the body's healing process. Because ultrasound waves travel best through water, they penetrate deeper into body tissues that have a high water content, such as muscles. Because bone has almost no water content, ultrasonography must be used very carefully around bony areas, because the waves can concentrate and cause damage (Procedure 40-3).

PROCEDURE 40-3

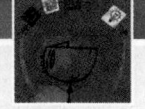

Assisting With Therapeutic Ultrasonography

GOAL: To apply ultra–high frequency sound waves to a patient's deep tissues for therapy. The medical assistant should perform ultrasound therapy only under the supervision of the physician or a physical therapist.

EQUIPMENT AND SUPPLIES

- Ultrasound machine
- Ultrasound gel or lotion (the coupling agent)

PROCEDURAL STEPS

1 Prepare your equipment and wash your hands.

2 Confirm the patient's identity.

3 Explain the procedure and tell the patient to notify you of any discomfort during the procedure immediately during the procedure.
   Purpose: To ensure that the patient does not experience any pain or injury.

4 Ask the patient about the presence of any internal or external metal objects.

5 Position the patient comfortably, with the area to be treated exposed.

6 Apply a warmed ultrasound gel (the coupling agent) liberally over the area to be treated and to the applicator head.
   Purpose: To effectively transmit the sound waves through a water-based medium.

7 Begin the treatment with the intensity control at the lowest setting.

8 Set the timer on the machine to the ordered time.
   Purpose: The timer starts the machine.

9 Slowly increase the intensity control to the ordered amount.

10 Hold the applicator with the head firmly and completely against the patient's skin over the area to be treated (Figure 1).

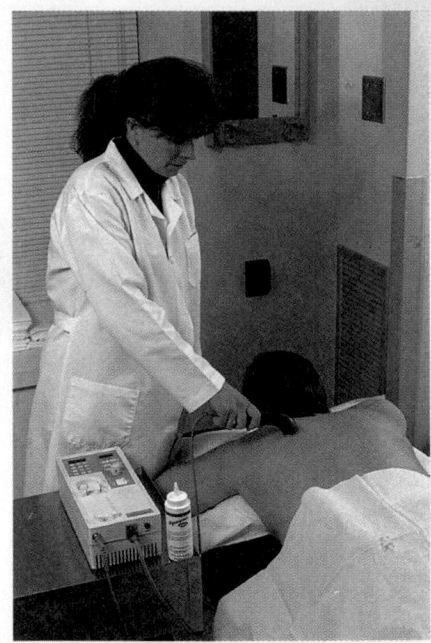

Figure 1

   Purpose: To ensure close contact between the applicator head and the patient's skin.

11 Work the applicator over the area to be treated by moving it continuously in a circular fashion at a speed of 2 inches per second or as directed by the physician.

12 Keep the applicator head in contact with the patient's skin at all times while the machine is on and keep it moving continuously during the treatment time.

PROCEDURE 40-3—cont'd

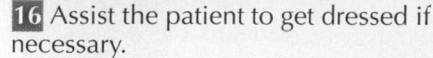

Purpose: Constant motion prevents hot spots from occurring due to the accumulation of excessive ultrasonic waves in one area.

13 When the timer sounds, it shuts off the machine automatically. Then you can safely lift the applicator head away from the patient.

14 Return the intensity control to zero.

15 Remove the ultrasound gel from the patient's skin and from the applicator head with a tissue or paper wipe. Wash your hands.

16 Assist the patient to get dressed if necessary.

17 Record the procedure in the patient's chart, including the date, area treated, intensity setting, duration of treatment, and any unusual occurrences of reactions that may have occurred during treatment. If none occurred, indicate that also.

Purpose: A procedure is not considered done until it is recorded.

See Appendix E for a charting example.

Massage and Exercise

Massage is a form of passive exercise that relieves tension and pain. The systematic, therapeutic stroking or kneading of the body or body part can effectively relieve or significantly reduce both localized and referred pain. You will not usually be asked to apply therapeutic massage to patients, but you should be familiar with the terminology.

THERAPEUTIC MASSAGE TERMINOLOGY

Effleurage: A light, gentle, stroking movement
Friction: Deep stroking that affects the deeper soft tissues, traditionally used for back massage
Petrissage: Kneading or rolling with pressing of the muscles
Tapotement: Rapid, light percussion done with the sides of the hands

---

A growing branch of healthcare employs exercise to aid muscle relaxation, promote healing, and provide relief from tension and pain resulting from stress or a wide variety of physical disorders. Exercise can also be used to restore mobility, coordination, and strength. If the motion in a joint is restricted even for a short time, the joint tissues become dense, hard, and shortened. These changes can begin to occur in as little as 4 days. This can be prevented or decreased by the use of active or passive exercising.

In active exercise the patient initiates and controls movements of a particular part of the body. Special equipment may be used, such as stationary bicycles, treadmills, and/or weight machines. In passive exercise, the therapist moves the body part without the voluntary action of the patient. Both active and passive exercises can be performed to maintain normal ROM or remedy decreased ROM after an injury.

Electric Muscle Stimulation

An electric stimulation unit is a low-voltage machine creating controlled electric current that is applied to the patient through disposable gel electrodes. This low-voltage current is useful for stimulating the motor and sensor nerves that supply muscles. This stimulation provides a passive means of exercising a muscle when a patient cannot activate the muscle voluntarily because of injury. This treatment is used to prevent **atrophy** of a normal muscle.

Another means of using electric stimulation in orthopedics is called a *transcutaneous electric nerve stimulation* (TENS) unit (Figure 40-21). A TENS unit sends a controlled electrical current through electrodes attached to the skin to help control intractable pain. Intractable pain cannot be relieved except through the use of addicting drugs or incapacitating sedation. Patients can use the TENS unit at home.

Walkers

Walkers are usually made of aluminum and can be easily adjusted to fit an individual. Walkers are lightweight, can be folded for storage and traveling, and can be equipped with a front pack to carry items. They can also be fitted with a fold-down seat. The disadvantage of using a walker is it cannot be used on stairs or in small, cramped quarters.

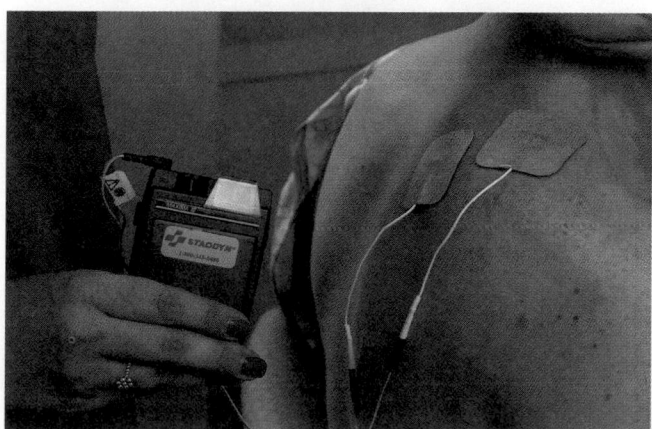

FIGURE 40-21   TENS unit application.

To adjust the height of a walker, have the patient stand by the examination table. The top of the walker should be just below the patient's waist at the same height as the top of the hip bone. When the walker is correctly adjusted to the patient, the patient's elbows will bend about 30 degrees while using the walker (Figure 40-22).

Canes

Canes come in two basic designs (Figure 40-23). The first type is the single-tipped cane, with a curved handgrip. Its use is indicated for individuals who need only minimal assistance with walking. The second type is the legged cane, which has a tripod or quad base. This base provides a greater stability for the patient than a single-tipped cane does. It is heavier and is recommended for patients who need greater support.

To fit the cane properly, have the patient stand up straight and measure the distance from the wrist crease to the floor. If the patient is 70 years of age or older or finds that extra length would feel more comfortable, up to 2 additional inches can be added to the previous measurement. This is the total length of the cane fitted to the patient. The patient's elbow should be bent to approximately 30 degrees when the cane is correctly adjusted to the patient.

Wheelchairs

Wheelchairs provide mobility for patients who cannot walk or who are able to walk only short distances. With a manual wheelchair, the patient uses arm muscles for mobility. Wheelchairs also come with motors that can be controlled by the patient. The patient is referred to an orthopedic appliance store, where the appropriate wheelchair will be fitted to him or her.

 SAFETY ALERT: Always set brakes on the chair before patient is transferred into or out of the chair.

Assisting With Casting

When a cast is used to immobilize a fracture or sprain, you will need to know what type of cast is to be applied (Procedures 40-4 through 40-6). Casting material possibilities include plaster of paris, fiberglass or plastic, synthetic material, or the air cast. Plaster of Paris is the oldest of the casting materials and is formed by briefly soaking rolls of casting material in warm water and then rolling them around the fracture site. It is like a wet bandage and can easily be formed to the extremity, the surface rubbed smooth, and then allowed to dry and harden. This casting material is made of roller gauze that has been impregnated with calcium sulfate, also called plaster of Paris. The fiberglass casting material has impregnated fiber or resin in the roller gauze and is applied in a similar fashion. Fiberglass cast is stronger, weighs less, and is relatively waterproof. If the patient needs to wear a cast only when using the limb, there is a synthetic cast that is a formed boot or sleeve that fits like a sandwich over the fracture and is held in place with

FIGURE 40-22 A properly fitted walker. Note angle of arms and height of walker.

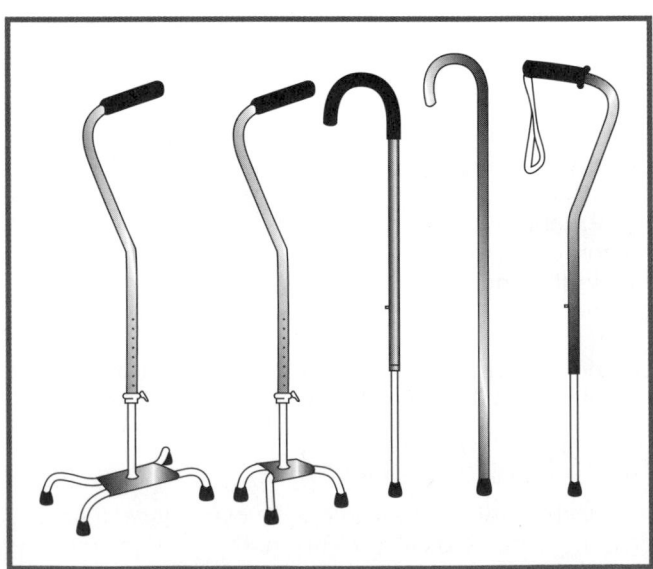

FIGURE 40-23 Types of standard canes.

Velcro tapes. An air cast is a temporary cast that is inflated around the limb to immobilize it. The type of cast to be used will depend on the location and severity of the injury, the age and occupation of the patient, and the physician's preference. After cast application the medical assistant may also have the responsibility of instructing the patient on the use of crutches (Procedure 40-7). This may include proper fitting of crutches and teaching the appropriate technique to avoid further injury to the patient.

CRITICAL THINKING APPLICATION

Kaiwan has just finished helping Dr. Alexander put a cast on the arm of a 6-year-old girl who fell out of her neighbor's tree house and fractured her radius. Her mother wants to take her home immediately when the casting is completed. Should the patient be allowed to leave immediately? Why? What could possibly happen if she left immediately?

Patient Education

Patient education assists you to perform the necessary procedures for your patient and helps to obtain the best possible outcome. An informed patient is better prepared to continue with the intervention at home when this is required. Musculoskeletal conditions, particularly arthritis, are so common that these patients are easy prey for miracle drug promotions. It is important for you to recognize the need for patient education about the condition and to work diligently with the patient and family to encourage participation in effective care programs. When you work with the physician and the physical therapist in helping the patient, you become an important member of the healthcare team. This type of involvement leads to patient satisfaction as well as personal satisfaction and achievement.

PROCEDURE 40-4

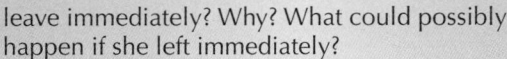

Assisting With Cast Application*

GOAL: To assist the physician in applying a fiberglass cast.

EQUIPMENT AND SUPPLIES

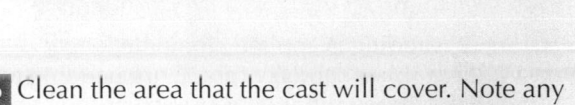

- Rolls of fiberglass casting material
- Stockinette
- Sheet wadding and/or spongy padding
- Tape
- Scissors
- Water
- Basin
- Bandage
- Gloves for physician and medical assistant
- Stand to support foot (lower extremity)

PROCEDURAL STEPS

1 Wash your hands.

2 Identify the patient.

3 Explain the procedure for applying a cast and answer questions before application.

   Purpose: Knowing what to expect will reassure the patient about the procedure. Questions regarding the injury should be directed to the physician.

4 Assemble equipment.

5 Seat the patient comfortably, as directed by the physician. If the cast is being applied to the lower extremity, the toes must be supported by a stand.

   Purpose: The amount of flexion of the ankle can be controlled by supporting the toes so that the patient can more easily maintain the desired position without fatigue.

6 Clean the area that the cast will cover. Note any objective signs and ask about subjective symptoms to chart at the end of the procedure.

   Purpose: The condition of the area under the cast must be noted before the cast is applied. This will be compared with the site when the cast is removed. Clean the area with mild soap solution or as directed. Dry thoroughly.

7 Cut stockinette to fit area cast will cover.

8 Apply stockinette smoothly to area that the cast will cover. Leave 1 or 2 inches of excess stockinette above and below the cast area to finish the cast (Figure 1).

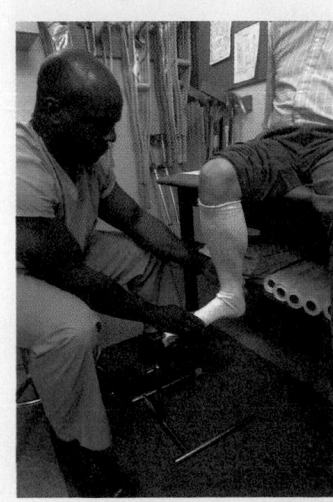

Figure 1

Continued

PROCEDURE 40-4—cont'd

9 Excess stockinette may be cut away where wrinkles form (e.g., at the front of the ankle) (Figure 2).

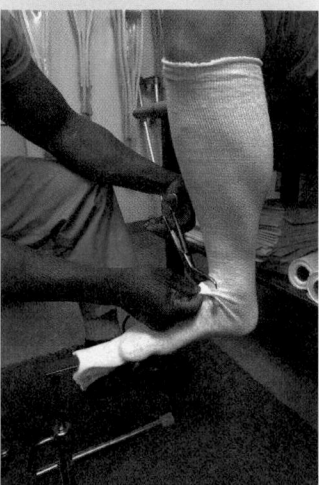

Figure 2

Purpose: Stockinette must lie smooth and cannot be too bulky or wrinkled, as this may cause a pressure wound.

10 Sheet wadding is applied along the length of the cast using a spiral bandage turn. Extra padding may be used over bony prominences such as the bones of the elbow or ankle (Figure 3).

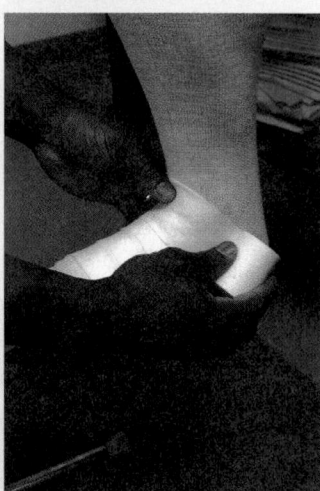

Figure 3

Purpose: Padding the cast helps reduce pressure against bony prominences, which could cause skin breakdown.

11 Don gloves.

12 With lukewarm water in the basin, wet the fiberglass tape as directed by the physician (Figure 4).

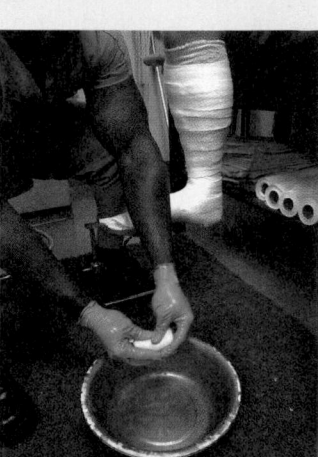

Figure 4

Purpose: Immersing the roll of fiberglass tape in water begins the chemical reaction that will cause the cast to harden. The cast can be shaped while wet and will harden in the shape that is formed.

13 Assist as directed as the physician applies the inner layer of fiberglass tape (shown in the photograph as beige). 1 to 2 inches of stockinette is rolled over the inner layer of the cast to form a smooth edge when the outer layer is applied (Figure 5).

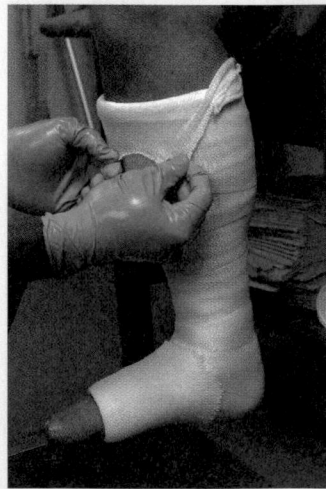

Figure 5

14 Assist as directed by the physician to open and apply an outer layer of fiberglass tape (shown in the photograph as blue) (Figure 6).

PROCEDURE 40-4—cont'd

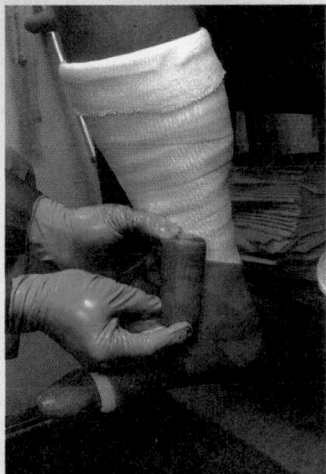

Figure 6

15 Assist to shape the cast as directed. All contours must be smooth (Figure 7).

Purpose: If flat or dented areas develop on the cast, they may cause pressure on the skin below.

16 Discard the water and excess materials. Remove gloves, and wash hands.

17 Reassure the patient, review cast care verbally, and provide written instructions.

18 Document observations and procedure in patient record.

Purpose: A procedure is not considered done until it is recorded in the patient's chart.

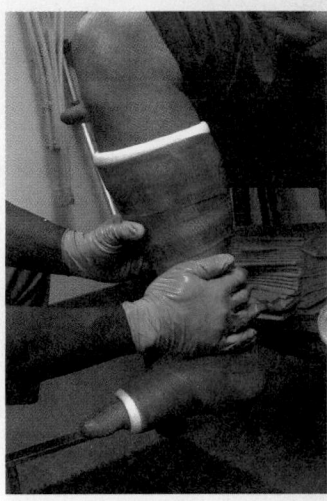

Figure 7

See Appendix E for a charting example.
*Procedure adapted and figures taken from Hunt SA: *Saunders fundamentals of medical assisting*, Philadelphia, 2000, WB Saunders.

PROCEDURE 40-5

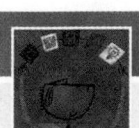

Triangular Arm Sling Application

GOAL: To properly place a casted arm in a triangular sling.

EQUIPMENT AND SUPPLIES

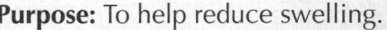

- Triangular-shaped arm sling
- Large safety pins

PROCEDURAL STEPS

1 Be sure that you have a physician's order for a triangular arm sling.

2 Wash your hands and obtain the desired sling.

3 Explain the procedure to the patient.

Purpose: To obtain maximal patient cooperation.

4 Position the patient's injured arm across the chest so that it is parallel to the floor and the patient's waist, with the hand slightly elevated.

Purpose: To help reduce swelling.

5 Carefully slide the triangular sling between the patient's chest and the affected arm.

6 Bring the lower front corner up over the shoulder of the affected side to the neck.

7 Grasp the opposite corner and tie or pin the ends together at the side of the neck.

Purpose: Tying at the side of the neck helps to avoid the headache and muscle discomfort that might be caused by tying at the back of the neck.

8 Fold in the tail and fasten with a safety pin to secure the elbow (Figure 1).

Continued

PROCEDURE 40-5—cont'd

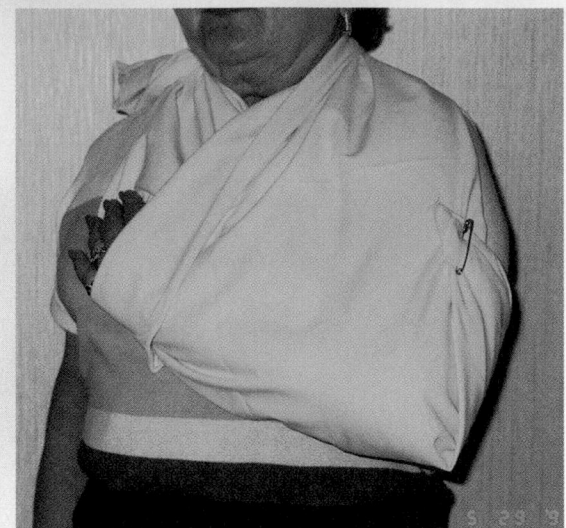

Figure 1

9 Fold the sling edge to form a smooth edge along the wrist.
Purpose: Patient comfort.

10 Record the procedure in the patient's chart.
Purpose: A procedure is not considered done until it is recorded.

Note: If using a commercial sling, follow the manufacturer's instructions for proper application.

PROCEDURE 40-6

Assisting With Cast Removal

GOAL: To remove a cast.

EQUIPMENT AND SUPPLIES

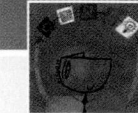

- Cast cutter
- Cast spreader
- Large bandage scissors
- Basin of warm water
- Mild soap
- Towel
- Skin lotion

PROCEDURAL STEPS

1 Explain the procedure to the patient.
Purpose: Allays the patient's fear and anxiety and ensures cooperation.

2 Provide adequate support for the limb throughout the entire procedure.
Purpose: Patient comfort.

3 Make a cut on both the medial side and the lateral side of the long axis of the cast (Figure 1).

4 Pry the two halves apart using the cast spreader (Figure 2).

5 Carefully remove the two parts of the cast.

6 Use the large bandage scissors to cut away the stockinette and padding remaining.

7 Gently wash the area that was covered by the cast with mild soap and warm water.
Purpose: Patient comfort.

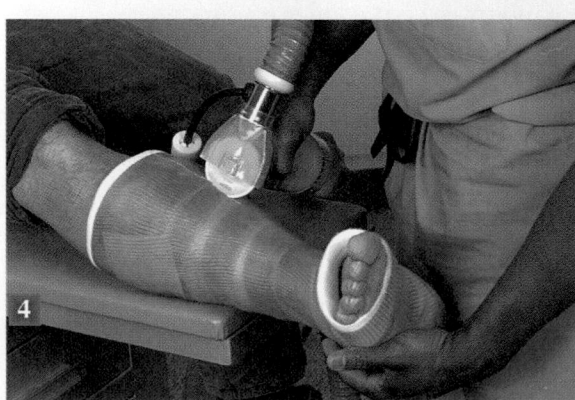

Figure 1

PROCEDURE 40-6—cont'd

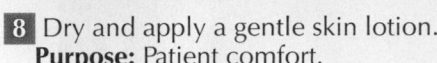
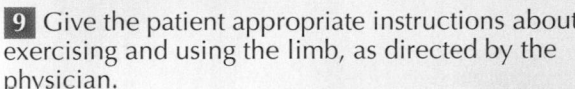

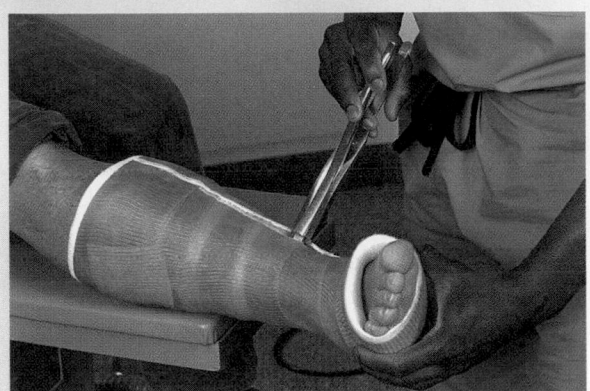

Figure 2

8 Dry and apply a gentle skin lotion.
Purpose: Patient comfort.

9 Give the patient appropriate instructions about exercising and using the limb, as directed by the physician.
Purpose: To enhance continuation of healing, restore lost strength, and prevent injury.

10 Record the procedure in the patient's medical record.
Purpose: A procedure is not considered done until it is recorded.

CRITICAL THINKING APPLICATION

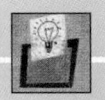

What methods could Kaiwan use to teach a deaf patient how to use crutches?

Legal and Ethical Issues

Working with orthopedic patients may involve triage procedures, assisting with assessments, and performing procedures that directly involve the patient's recovery plan. Many of the procedures in this chapter are not the basic procedures that you will be required to perform when you are first hired as a medical assistant. These techniques all involve additional on-the-job training and practice. Before performing any of the described procedures, you should check with your local and state medical assistant organizations regarding the laws in your state. Whenever you perform the procedures and techniques described in this chapter, you are responsible for them. The following steps are all required before you execute any procedure on a patient:

1. You must have a written order before doing a procedure.
2. You must follow a procedure precisely as it is ordered, without variation.
3. Never advise the patient without permission.
4. Know what instructions the physician gave the patient.

PROCEDURE 40-7

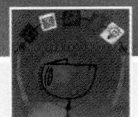

Assisting the Patient With Crutch Walking

GOAL: To properly fit crutches for your patient and teach the patient how to use the crutches properly in three-point walking.

EQUIPMENT AND SUPPLIES
• Crutches

PROCEDURAL STEPS

1 Fit the crutches to the patient so the arm rest is 2 inches below the armpit.

2 Be sure that all wing nuts are tight.

3 Make sure the foam pads at the armpits and around the handgrips are comfortable.

4 Instruct the patient to keep the injured leg as relaxed as possible and slightly bent at the knee.

5 The patient's elbow should be bent from 23 to 30 degrees when holding the handgrip.

6 Place the crutch tips about 6 inches away from and parallel to the toes.

7 Ask the patient to push down on the crutches and lift the body slightly, nearly straightening the arms (Figure 1).

8 Have the patient swing the body forward about 12 inches.

9 Instruct the patient to stand on the good leg, and then move the crutches just ahead of the good foot and repeat.

Continued

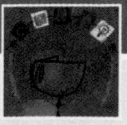

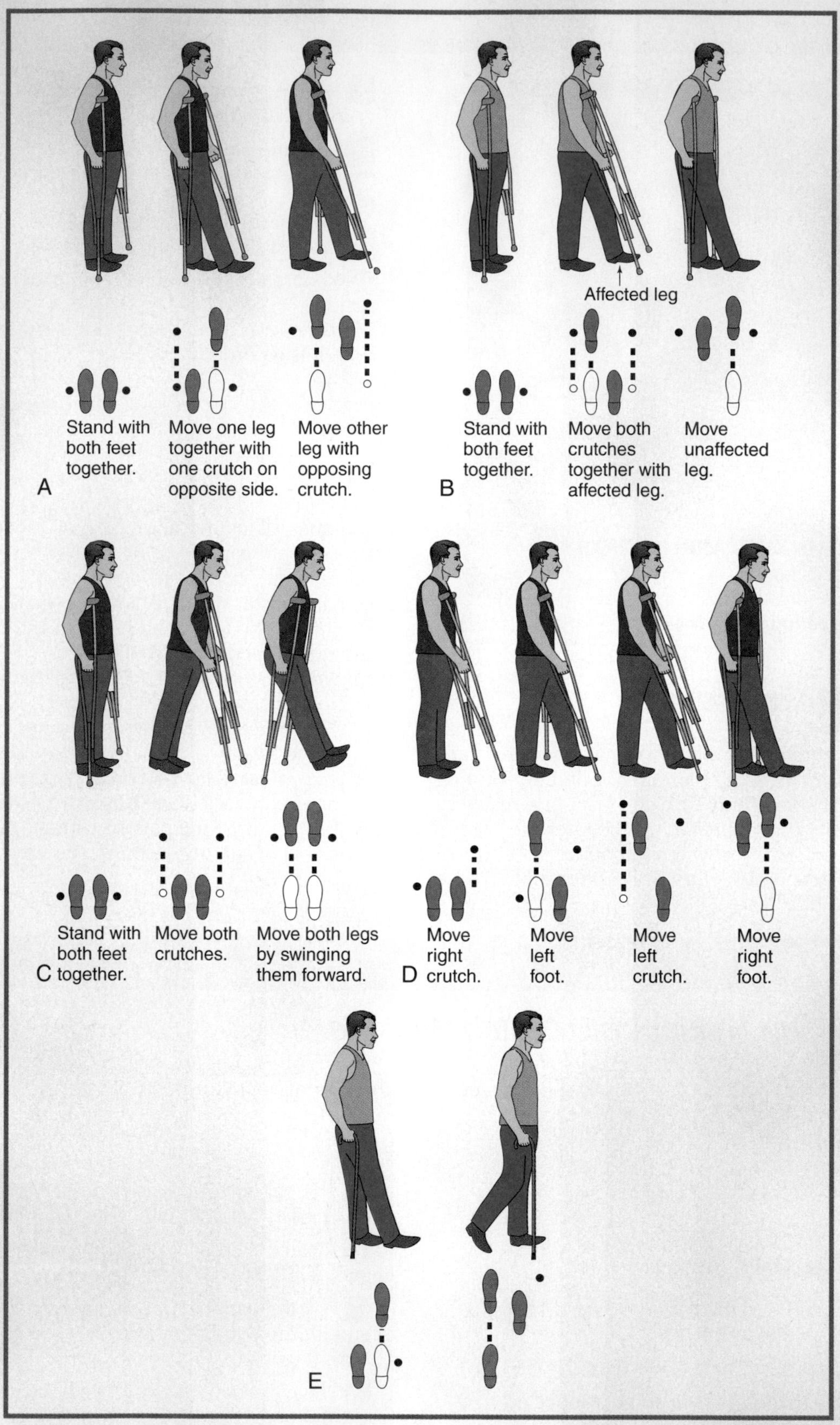

A Stand with both feet together. Move one leg together with one crutch on opposite side. Move other leg with opposing crutch.

B Stand with both feet together. Move both crutches together with affected leg. Move unaffected leg.

Affected leg

C Stand with both feet together. Move both crutches. Move both legs by swinging them forward.

D Move right crutch. Move left foot. Move left crutch. Move right foot.

E

Figure 1

See Appendix E for a charting example.

5. Reinforce the instructions the physician gave the patient.

6. Be sure you are comfortable performing a procedure.

7. If you have any concerns about a procedure, discuss them with the physician or therapist privately before proceeding.

8. Do not perform a procedure if you are uncomfortable; get someone to help you.

Always remember: You are the assistant and this is the physician's patient. The physician is ultimately responsible for every aspect of the patient's care. If you feel uncertain or unsure of any order that the physician has written for a patient, you must get it clarified before you proceed. Always stay within the legal and ethical guidelines of the medical assisting profession in your state.

SUMMARY OF SCENARIO

Kaiwan is becoming more and more comfortable in his position as an orthopedic medical assistant at the Sports Medicine Associates clinic. His enthusiasm is contagious. Patients always comment on his positive, upbeat manner, and the staff all enjoy his youthful energy. Kaiwan shows a great deal of motivation to learn new things and how to better assist the physicians with routine procedures. He always seeks answers to questions that occur with new patients. He has gained a great deal of confidence and now always checks the paraffin bath temperature before starting the treatment with a patient.

One of the most enjoyable aspects of his job continues to be assisting Dr. Alexander with treating the team members and at the games. Kaiwan has attended two sports medicine continuing education seminars with Dr. Alexander. He is now thinking about continuing his education part-time to become a sports trainer while continuing to work at Sports Medicine Associates.

SUMMARY OF LEARNING OBJECTIVES

■ The main structures of the musculoskeletal system include the skeletal muscles, which provide movement; tendons, which connect muscles to bones; bones, which provide support, protection, and mineral storage; and ligaments, which connect bone to bone.

■ Tendons are the tough bands that connect muscles to bones; ligaments provide support by connecting bone to bone and preventing a joint from moving beyond its normal ROM. This is why ligament injury occurs when a joint is forced beyond its normal ROM. Bursae prevent friction between different tissues in the musculoskeletal system.

■ Musculoskeletal system disorders account for more missed days at work and more physicians' office visits than nearly any other medical problem. Musculoskeletal disorders frequently result from trauma, can also be caused by bacteria, fungi, or viruses, or can have an autoimmune cause (see Table 40-2).

■ The common types of fractures are listed in Table 40-4.

■ Common diagnostic procedures routinely performed in the orthopedic office include inspection, palpation, percussion, and x-ray studies. It is necessary to rule out bone fractures in many traumatic injuries, and this can only be done by obtaining x-ray films of the injured area. Other diagnostic tools include CT, MRI, and diagnostic ultrasonography.

■ The most common ambulatory assistive devices are crutches, canes, walkers, and wheelchairs. The most important aspects of using these assistive devices in an orthopedic practice are to fit them properly to the patient and give the patient adequate instruction on how to use the device.

■ Cold should always be used immediately after an injury to help decrease pain and inflammation, to inhibit additional swelling, and to help relieve pain.

■ Heat should be used on injuries after 48 hours to promote circulation and healing, decrease swelling, and cause soft tissue relaxation in the affected area.

■ Therapeutic modalities are critical in the treatment of musculoskeletal conditions because the goals addressed include restoring normal ROM, muscle strength, and function of the injured part as quickly as possible. Other treatment goals include decreasing pain and preserving muscle mass.

■ In active ROM assessment or exercise, the patient provides and controls the movement of the specific body area. In passive ROM assessment or exercise, the therapist provides and controls the movement of a specific body area.

KEY INTERNET WEBSITES

- Arthritis Foundation
- eMedicine: Cast Care
- Skeletal System Photographs
- The Hosford Muscle Tables: Skeletal Muscles of the Human Body
- Virtual Children's Hospital: Musculoskeletal Disease Index
- Virtual Hospital: Skeletal Trauma With X-Ray Images Photographs
  For active weblinks to each website visit http://evolve.elsevier.com/Kinn/

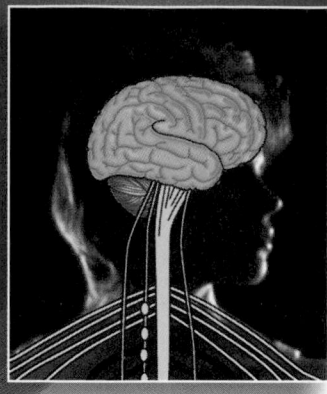

CHAPTER 41

Scenario

Mai Lee is a CMA who has been working in Dr. Kim Song's neurology practice for 2 years. Dr. Song has always been pleased with the pleasantness Mai shows to all patients, even the difficult ones. Mai is conscientious in accurately charting notes on each one of her patients. Dr. Song has just asked Mai to train a new medical assistant in the administrative procedures of the office. He is expanding his clinic hours and wishes to have Mai more involved in assisting him with patients, particularly in the area of patient education. She is excited to have additional responsibilities with Dr. Song's patients, and she is quite happy about the raise in salary that goes along with her new position.

Assisting in Neurology and Mental Health

Kim Anthony Aaronson

Learning Objectives

- Define and spell the terms listed in the vocabulary.
- Correctly label a diagram of main structures of the nervous system.
- Explain the main functions of the central nervous system.
- Explain the main functions of the peripheral nervous system.
- Differentiate between the different layers of the protective covering of the brain.
- Locate, name, and briefly describe the main functions of the three major areas of the brain.
- Recognize the significant symptoms that would suggest a possible neurological condition.
- Identify the most common brain disorders that result from trauma.
- Define the most common work-related neurological condition.
- Name and describe the most commonly used diagnostic procedures to identify neurological disorders.
- Compare the most common mental illnesses.
- Describe three diagnostic tests that might be used during a neurological examination.
- Prepare a patient for a neurological examination or diagnostic procedure.
- Assist with a neurological examination.

National Curriculum Competencies

CLINICAL COMPETENCIES

4a. Perform telephone and in-person screening
4c. Obtain and record patient history
4e. Prepare patients for and assist with routine and specialty examinations
4f. Prepare patients for and assist with procedures, treatments, and minor office surgery

TRANSDISCIPLINARY COMPETENCIES

1b. Recognize and respond to verbal communication
1c. Recognize and respond to nonverbal communication
2a. Identify and respond to issues of confidentiality
2b. Perform within legal and ethical boundaries
3b. Instruct individuals according to their needs

Vocabulary

anomalies Faulty development of the fetus resulting in deformities or deviations from normal.

anoxia Absence of oxygen in the tissues.

ataxia Failure or irregularity of muscle actions and coordination.

atrophy Decrease in the size of a normally developed organ.

aura Peculiar sensation preceding the appearance of more definite disturbance.

benign Not cancerous and not recurring.

collodion Preparation of cellulose nitrate that, when applied to the skin, dries to a strong, thin, protective, transparent film.

coma An unconscious state from which the patient cannot be aroused.

compression The state of being pressed together.

contralateral Pertaining to the opposite side of the body.

cryptogenic Hidden origin.

diplopia Double vision.

embolus Foreign material blocking a blood vessel, frequently a blood clot that has broken away from some other part of the body.

exacerbation Worsening of disease symptoms.

gait How a person walks.

homeostasis Maintaining constant internal environmental conditions compatible with life.

idiopathic Unknown cause.

incontinence Inability to control excretory functions.

ipsilateral Pertaining to the same side of the body.

malignant Cancerous.

occlusion Complete blocking off of an opening.

papilledema Bulging of the optic disc and dilated retinal veins seen by ophthalmoscopic examination of the retina, a sign of increased intracranial pressure.

paresthesia Abnormal sensation of burning, prickling, or stinging.

paroxysmal Pertaining to a sudden recurrent spasm of symptoms.

plaque Abnormal accumulation of a fatty substance.

radiopaque Substance that can easily be visualized on an x-ray.

remission Lessening in the severity of a disease or symptoms.

sheath Covering surrounding the axon of the nerve cell that acts as an electrical insulator to speed the conduction of nerve impulses.

stroke Sudden loss of consciousness or paralysis caused by extreme trauma or injury to an artery in the brain.

syncope Fainting.

thrombus Blood clot.

transection Cross-section: division by cutting across.

The human brain weighs about 3 pounds, requires about the same amount of energy that it takes to light a 20-watt light bulb, stores more than 100 trillion bits of information, and works better than any computer. The matter making up the brain is about 85% water and therefore has a soft texture. Early scientists believed that the brain's function was to cool the blood. Today's scientists have shown us that even though the brain does receive 20% of the body's blood supply, its function is much more complex than cooling blood.

Neurologists specialize in the diagnosis and treatment of medical disorders and conditions of the nervous system. A *neurosurgeon* provides surgical management and treatment for trauma and other conditions requiring surgery. A *psychiatrist* treats neurological conditions that affect behavior.

Anatomy and Physiology

The brain is the "president" or "chief executive officer" (CEO) of the body. It constantly receives information from all parts of the body, including all the organs and systems inside and on the surface. This information is carried to the brain by the peripheral nerves via electrical and chemical impulses. The brain constantly monitors the conditions at all these locations and sends appropriate responses out along nerves to the organs or to the body surface. These responses from the brain can cause some type of reaction in the organs or at the skin. These reactions keep the body running smoothly; this is called maintaining **homeostasis**.

WHEN YOU ACCIDENTALLY TOUCH A HOT IRON

1. Impulses travel to the CNS carrying the information "*hot*."
2. The CNS carries out a hasty analysis and determines there is a heat danger present.
3. The CNS sends a quick and strong message to the finger to move away *now*.
4. You quickly pull your hand away from the hot iron, maintaining homeostasis.

The Central Nervous System

The brain and spinal cord together make up the *central nervous system* (CNS). The *brain* is in the skull in the cranial cavity. The *spinal cord* is a bundle of nervous tissue that extends inferiorly from the brainstem at the base of the brain and exits the skull at the foramen magnum. It descends for about 17 inches within the spinal canal, which courses through the vertebrae of the backbone.

The Brain. The brain accounts for only about 2% of a person's weight, but it requires about 20% of the heart's output of blood. The brain is protected from foreign substances in the blood by a specialized layer of cells in the brain capillaries called the *blood-brain barrier*. The blood-brain barrier closely regulates what substances enter the brain tissue. Oxygen, water, and glucose molecules easily pass into the brain, whereas many chemicals and drugs are prevented from moving into brain tissue. Brain inflammation can increase the ability of many drugs to cross the blood-brain barrier.

The brain is divided into three main areas (Figure 41-1). The *cerebrum* is the largest part of the brain and is where higher learning and most thinking take place. It is divided into right and left sections called *hemispheres*. The right hemisphere usually controls *artistic* functions like drawing, rhythm, and picture memory. The left hemisphere is usually the dominant hemisphere and controls *verbal* functions, such as reading, writing, speaking, and mathematical calculations. The *diencephalon*, located deep in the center of the cerebrum near the superior portion of the brainstem, is made up of the thalamus and the hypothalamus. The *thalamus* is a relay station between different sensory neurons. The hypothalamus is a kind of "vice-president" or "assistant CEO." Its main function is controlling the autonomic nervous system, which is responsible for maintaining homeostasis. Within the cerebrum are four spaces, called *ventricles*, which contain cerebrospinal fluid (CSF). The CSF nourishes, lubricates, and provides some cushioning protection for the brain and the spinal cord.

The *cerebellum* is just inferior to the occipital lobe of the cerebrum and controls balance, equilibrium, posture and muscle coordination. The *brainstem* controls reflexes, and also serves as a sensory relay station for input coming into the brain from the body. The brainstem is probably the most important area of the brain because of its vital role in vision, hearing, respiration, heart rate, blood pressure, and waking and sleeping.

The Spinal Cord. The spinal cord extends from the inferior portion of the brainstem roughly 17 inches inferiorly to approximately the second lumbar vertebra. There are 31 pairs of spinal nerves extending from the spinal cord. At each level, starting just below the first cervical vertebra in the neck, a nerve extends out from the spinal cord *on each side*; thus, a *pair* of spinal nerves originates at each level. At each level, the nerves go to a specific organ or area of the body. The spinal cord carries messages between the spinal nerves and the brain.

Protection. Because both the brain and spinal cord are of critical importance for life, both are well protected. First, they are both encased in some of the thickest bones in the body; then they are surrounded with three membranes called *meninges*; finally, they are cushioned with CSF (Figure 41-2).

The outer layer of the meninges is called the *dura mater* ("tough mother") because it is a tough membrane. The middle layer is the *arachnoid* ("spider") because of its fine spider-web appearance. The innermost layer, which covers the brain and spinal cord, is the *pia mater* ("tender mother"); it is highly vascular and is the thinnest of the three layers.

The CSF is a clear fluid containing some glucose, protein, and chloride (Table 41-1). It is just beneath the arachnoid membrane in the subarachnoid space. Specialized cells in the ventricles produce it constantly. This fluid circulates continuously through the ventricles and around the brain and spinal cord, carrying nutrients and removing wastes.

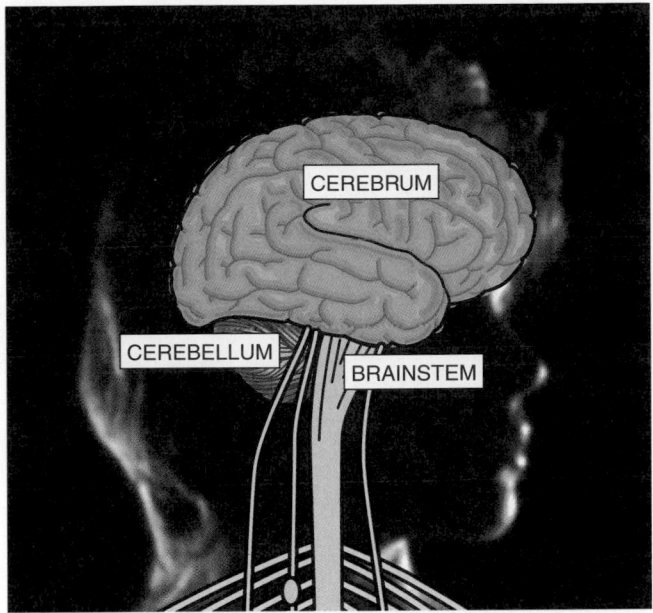

FIGURE 41-1   The brain. (Modified from Chester GA: *Modern medical assisting*, Philadelphia, 1998, WB Saunders, p 345.)

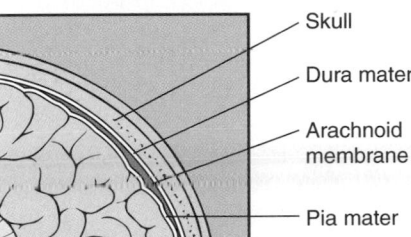

FIGURE 41-2   Protective coverings of the brain. (Modified from Frazier MS, Drzymkowski JW: *Essentials of human diseases and conditions*, ed 2. Philadelphia, 2000, WB Saunders, p 393.)

CRITICAL THINKING APPLICATION

Dr. Song mentions a patient's nervous system function to Mai. The patient hears this conversation and asks Mai, "What is my nervous system?" How should Mai answer this question? What items could she use to help explain the nervous system to the patient?

HYDROCEPHALUS

Hydrocephalus is the abnormal accumulation of CSF within the ventricles of the brain. It is the result of either overproduction of CSF or failure of the CSF to drain properly. If left untreated, hydrocephalus causes gross

HYDROCEPHALUS—cont'd

enlargement of the skull and severe brain tissue damage from the increased intracranial pressure. The only treatment is surgery to place a shunt (tube) from a ventricle in the brain to either the right atrium or the abdominal cavity. This shunt allows the excess CSF to drain away from the brain.

The Peripheral Nervous System

The *peripheral nervous system* (PNS) is made up primarily of nerves that exit the brain or spinal cord. The peripheral nerves exiting the brain directly through the cranium are called *cranial nerves*. The spinal nerves from the spinal cord enter and exit the spinal canal through spaces between each of the vertebrae. Autonomic nerves extend from the CNS at both the brain and spinal cord. Cranial nerves originate from the under side of the brain and relay information to and from the sense organs and muscles of the face and neck (Table 41-2).

Spinal nerves carry information to and from the brain through the spinal cord. *Sensory fibers* in these nerves carry stimuli from the skin and internal organs to the CNS. *Motor fibers* carry messages from the CNS to skeletal muscles, causing them to contract.

Autonomic nerves control homeostasis, or keep the body running smoothly, much like a thermostat controls the temperature in a room. It is an automatic system over which one has no control, and it regulates body functions such as breathing, heart rate, sweating, circulation, and digestion. It also controls the actions of muscles in blood vessel walls, organs, and glands. Just as a thermostat can control both heating and cooling in a room to maintain a comfortable temperature, the autonomic system is made up of two divisions, called the *sympathetic* and *parasympathetic*. The sympathetic system generally causes an increasing effect: it speeds up the heart, increases blood pressure, and widens the airways in the lungs, allowing more oxygen to enter the body quickly. The parasympathetic system generally causes a calming or decreasing effect: slows the heart, narrows the airways, and increases digestive system function (Figure 41-3).

CRITICAL THINKING APPLICATION

A mother brings her 2-year-old son into the office after being referred by her pediatrician. The boy does not seem to have any feeling in his legs. The mother is quite fearful and wants to know whether he has a brain tumor. How should Mai respond to this question?

TABLE 41-1	Typical Cerebrospinal Fluid Laboratory Values				
Condition	Pressure (mm)	Appearance	Cells	Protein (mg/dl)	Glucose (mg/dl)
Normal	50-200	Clear, colorless	0-10 lymphocytes and monocytes	< 45	50-80
Acute bacterial meningitis	200-500	Turbid	100-10,000 granulocytic neutrophils	50-500	Absent or low
Subarachnoid hemorrhage	200-500	Bloody	RBCs	50-1000	50-80

RBC, Red blood cells.

TABLE 41-2	Cranial Nerves and Their Functions	
Number	Name	Function
I	Olfactory	Smell
II	Optic	Vision
III	Oculomotor	Eye movement Pupillary constriction and accommodation
IV	Trochlear	Eye movement
V	Trigeminal	Muscles of chewing General sensations from anterior half of head including entire face and meninges
VI	Abducent	Eye movement
VII	Facial	Muscles of facial expression Tearing, salivation, and taste
VIII	Vestibulocochlear	Hearing and equilibrium
IX	Glossopharyngeal	Swallowing and taste
X	Vagus	Parasympathetic to thorax and abdomen
XI	Spinal accessory	Shoulder and head movements
XII	Hypoglossal	Tongue movements

POLYGRAPH OR LIE DETECTOR TEST

A polygraph (many pictures) actually measures several body parameters that are strongly influenced by the autonomic nervous system. It simultaneously measures and records blood pressure, heart rate, respiratory rate, and the sweatiness of the fingertips. When the person being given the test is stressed, for example, when being deceptive about the answer to a particular question, involuntary changes occur in the above parameters and these show up on the graph. This is an example of your autonomic nervous system at work. When the person is asked a question such as "What day is today?" there is no significant change in any of the measured parameters. Answering this question correctly causes no stress in the individual. Do you think you could beat the polygraph?

The Neuron. The main cell type that makes up nervous tissue, and thus the nervous system, is called the *neuron* (Figure 41-4). The brain contains billions of

individual neurons. Neurons start becoming interconnected during the last 3 months in utero and continue developing into a complex network until about the age of 2 years. Each neuron is made up of the main cell body containing the nucleus and a relatively long extension of the cell called the *axon*, which can be covered with a myelin **sheath**. Many smaller filaments called *dendrites* extend from the neuron body. These dendrites receive the nerve impulse from other neurons and carry it into the cell body. Impulses are carried away from the cell body through the axon to another neuron or to cells in another tissue. The electrical impulse travels down an axon of one neuron and becomes a chemical impulse while moving across the synapse to the dendrite of another neuron. In this second neuron, the impulse again becomes electrical in nature. The impulse is carried across the synapse by chemical neurotransmitters, which bind to specific receptor sites on the dendrites of the next neuron. If the nerve impulse is traveling to a muscle or to any other organ or tissue instead of another neuron, the chemical neurotransmitters bind to special receptors in the target tissue. Messages move throughout the entire nervous system in this manner. Impulses in the neuron are electrical; the impulses become chemical as a specific neurotransmitter is released at each synapse.

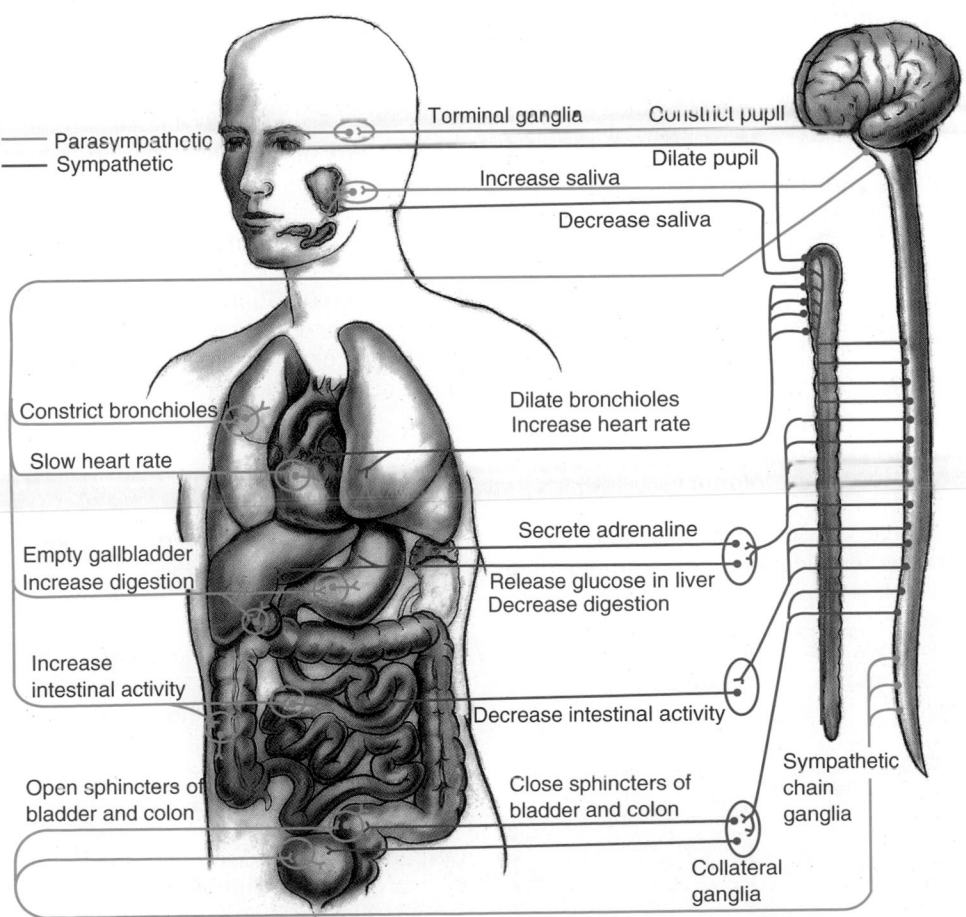

FIGURE 41-3   Structure and function of the autonomic nervous system. (From Applegate E: *The anatomy and physiology learning system*, ed 2. Philadelphia, 2000, WB Saunders, p 176.)

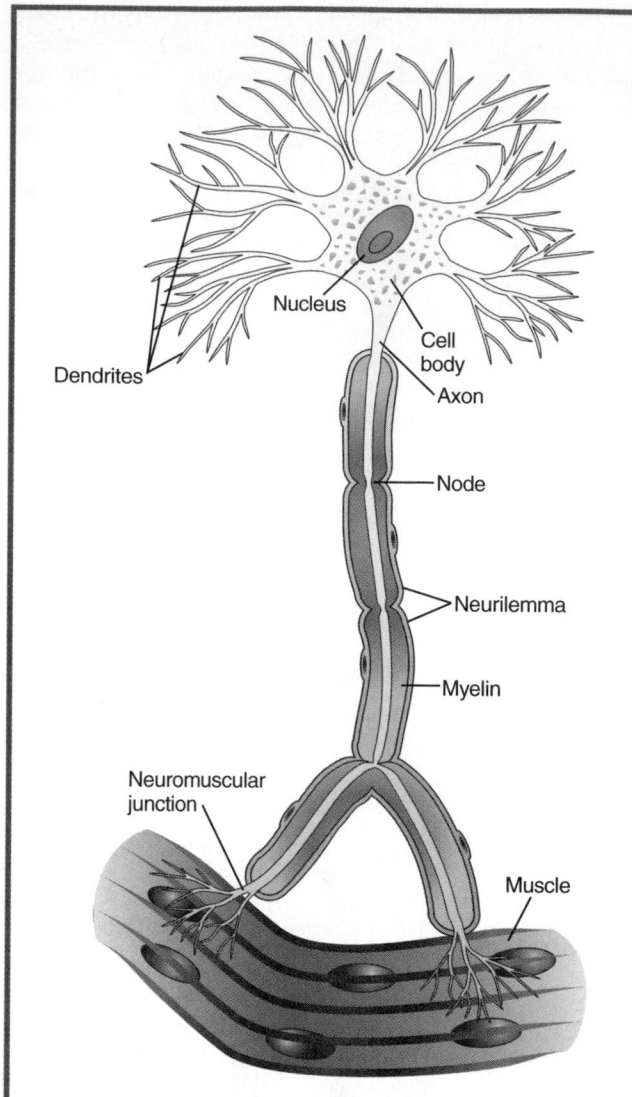

FIGURE 41-4 Neuron.

Diseases and Disorders of the Nervous System

Because the CNS and PNS are so complex, diseases and conditions affecting them can cause an extremely wide range of serious damage. Causes include trauma, infection, congenital **anomalies**, degeneration, tumors, and vascular disorders (Table 41-3).

The medical assistant always should listen carefully when a patient describes his or her symptoms. Many different types of symptoms could indicate a serious neurological condition.

SYMPTOMS THAT SUGGEST POSSIBLE NEUROLOGICAL PROBLEMS

- Recurrent headache
- Periodic memory loss
- Change in sleeping patterns
- Frequently dropping items
- Difficulties with particular speech patterns
- Numbness in a specific body area
- Visual disturbances or abrupt changes in vision
- Loss of consciousness
- Confusion or disorientation as to date, time, and place

Cerebrovascular Disease

Cerebrovascular disease (CVD) continues to be the third leading cause of death and the most frequent cause of crippling disease in the United States. Generally, CVD is related to atherosclerosis of the cerebral arteries and most frequently occurs in older persons. Important genetic factors include hypertension and blood clotting disorders. Atherosclerosis can involve any of the major arteries supplying the brain or any of their branches. The narrowing of these arteries may be gradual from plaque deposits or from the progressive loss of elasticity of the arterial wall. There also may be sudden narrowing, or **occlusion**, when an artery becomes blocked by a **thrombus**.

This disorder usually is diagnosed through cerebral arterial angiography, which is done by injecting a radiopaque dye into the vessel to be visualized and then immediately taking a radiograph. Other confirming tests include magnetic resonance imaging (MRI), computed tomography (CT), and electroencephalography (EEG).

Alzheimer's Disease

Alzheimer's disease, also known as *senile dementia*, is a devastating, chronic, progressive, and degenerative disease of the brain. The patient exhibits slow, increasing loss of recent memory; loss of recognition of people, places, and events; confusion and disorientation; and physical deterioration leading to death. The cause remains unknown, and there is no known cure. Treatment is supportive care only. Alzheimer's disease is addressed in more detail in Chapter 45.

CRITICAL THINKING APPLICATION

Mr. Jackson, a 65-year-old Alzheimer's patient, is coming in for his first visit. He does not respond to verbal commands and is unable to make any intelligible conversation. How can Mai get him into the examination room and into a patient gown while preserving Mr. Jackson's dignity? What are the steps to achieving this goal in this situation?

Cerebrovascular Accident

Cerebrovascular accident (CVA) is the most important clinical manifestation of CVD. CVA is commonly referred to as **stroke** or brain attack, which occurs when a vessel in the brain ruptures or totally occludes as a result of CVD. Cerebral artery ruptures most often are caused by

TABLE 41-3	Common Nervous System Diseases and Conditions			
Disease	**Symptoms/Signs**	**Diagnostic Procedures**	**Laboratory Tests**	**Treatment/ Medications**
Alzheimer's	Short-term memory loss, progressive irreversible confusion and disorientation	History	None	Supportive care Cognex and Aricept Estrogen
Brain tumor	Generally due to increased intracranial pressure; depends on location	History Neurological examination Imaging studies	None	Surgery Radiation Chemotherapy
CVA	Depends on severity; speech difficulties, hemiplegia, confusion, loss of muscle coordination	History Neurological examination CT, MRI	Lumbar puncture	Thrombolytics Antiinflammatories Anticoagulants Hyperbaric oxygen Rehabilitation Supportive care
Encephalitis	Increased intracranial pressure, cerebral edema	History Neurological examination CT, MRI	Lumbar puncture	Antivirals Supportive care
Epilepsy	*Grand mal:* tonic clonic muscle contractions; *petit mal:* momentary absence, stare, amnesia	History Neurological examination CT, MRI, EEG	Blood work	Anticonvulsants
Closed head injury due to trauma	Change in LOC depending on location and severity; headache, increased intracranial pressure	History Neurological examination CT, MRI	Lumbar puncture	Diuretics Decrease intracranial pressure
Meningitis	Headache, nuchal rigidity	History Neurological examination Kernig's, Brudzinski's signs	Lumbar puncture	Antibiotics Anticonvulsants Antiinflammatories
Mental illness	Exhibit emotional, physical, behavioral, or cognitive symptoms that can affect all areas of one's life	History Neurological examination occasionally	Blood work occasionally	Medications Psychotherapy
Migraine	Unilateral throbbing sensation, nausea, vomiting, blurred vision	History Neurological examination	None	Vasodilators Vasoconstrictors
Multiple sclerosis	Problems with vision, sensation, motor function, change in emotions	History Neurological examination MRI	None	Interferon Corticosteroids Antispasmodics Antidepressants
Parkinson's	Resting tremor, shuffling gait, mask-like face	History Neurological examination	None	Anticholinergics Dopamine agonists

CVA, Cerebrovascular accident; *CT,* computed tomography; *MRI,* magnetic resonance imaging; *LOC,* loss of consciousness; *EEG,* electroencephalography.

an occlusion of an atherosclerotic artery or tearing of a weakened section of an artery in the brain. The rupture causes the surrounding brain tissue to become filled with blood, thereby damaging and possibly destroying the affected tissue. An occlusion occurs when an **embolus** or thrombus becomes wedged in an artery and obstructs the flow of blood to an area of the brain (Figure 41-5).

The subsequent symptoms depend on the location of the arterial rupture or occlusion. Some of the most common symptoms include slurred or inaudible speech, sudden confusion, sudden severe headache, difficulty swallowing, dizziness, double vision, loss of consciousness, and paralysis on one side of the body.

Treatment for stroke requires immediate emergency transport to the hospital and most likely admission to the intensive care unit. The most life-threatening problem is brain edema. This swelling is reversed with corticosteroids and diuretics. Thrombolytic drugs and anticoagulants may be given if the cause of the stroke was a blood clot. Hyperbaric oxygen also can be used to increase oxygenation of the brain. An important part of the subsequent recovery will be extensive physical therapy.

STROKE RISK FACTORS

- Hypertension
- Diabetes
- Elevated blood lipids
- Smoking

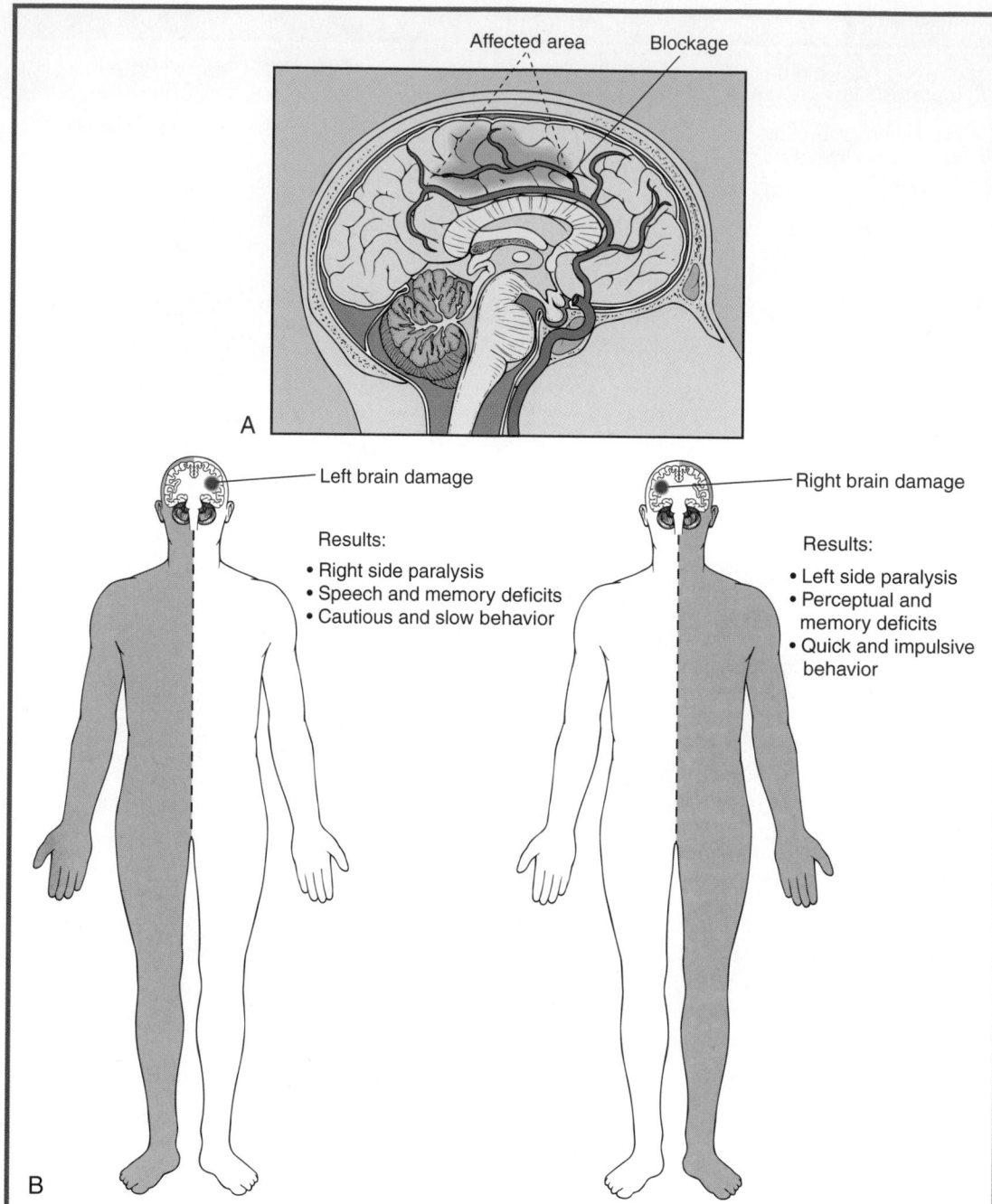

Affected area   Blockage

A

Left brain damage

Results:
• Right side paralysis
• Speech and memory deficits
• Cautious and slow behavior

Right brain damage

Results:
• Left side paralysis
• Perceptual and memory deficits
• Quick and impulsive behavior

FIGURE 41-5
Cerebral artery occlusion and hemiplegia. (Modified from Frazier MS, Drzymkowski JW: *Essentials of human diseases and conditions*, ed 2. Philadelphia, 2000, WB Saunders, p 398.)

B

CRITICAL THINKING APPLICATION

• Mai answers the phone at the clinic to find an anxious female patient on the line who is desperately trying to say something but appears unable to do so. Mai thinks the patient is trying to say something like "help," although it is not clear. Through the caller ID display, she looks up the number in the office computer and learns that it belongs to a 50-year-old patient who came in 2 days earlier for headaches. How should she handle this situation?

• Be sure to think about what she should do, why she should do it, and what might happen if she does nothing.

Transient Ischemic Attacks

Transient ischemic attacks (TIAs), also called *ministrokes*, occur when the blood supply to a particular part of the brain is inadequate for a short period, usually seconds to minutes. They result from the brain tissue becoming ischemic for a short time. These episodes may occur in the days, weeks, or months before a stroke. They can be accompanied by the same symptoms as a stroke, but the symptoms usually dissipate quickly. Patients should be evaluated carefully and treated to prevent possible stroke.

Migraine Headache

Migraine headaches are **paroxysmal** attacks of headaches that can be completely incapacitating and frequently are associated with other symptoms, such as nausea, vomiting, visual disturbances, and throbbing pain in one side of the head. This type of headache occurs differently from one individual to another. Many describe an **aura** before the onset of the headache. This aura often consists of some form of visual disturbance, such as dark lines or spots within the visual field.

Medical science has not yet discovered the underlying cause of migraines, although they do appear to be somewhat hereditary and appear to be triggered by some foods. There is also evidence that a migraine is provoked by constriction of cerebral blood vessels. Diagnosis usually is established from a complete medical history. Additionally, EEG, CT scan, or MRI can be obtained as part of the diagnostic process to rule out other possible causes of the headaches.

Drugs used to treat migraines, such as methysergide maleate, can prevent blood vessel constriction. Other drugs given to abort an acute attack, including sumatriptan succinate, constrict the already dilated blood vessels, which relieves the severe pain. Other treatments include biofeedback techniques and elimination diets.

Epilepsy

Epilepsy is a brain disorder associated with abnormal electrical impulses being generated by some of the neurons in the brain. These errant impulses cause seizures (Figure 41-6). A seizure is characterized by abnormalities in levels of consciousness, sensory disturbances, and impaired motor function. These attacks of altered

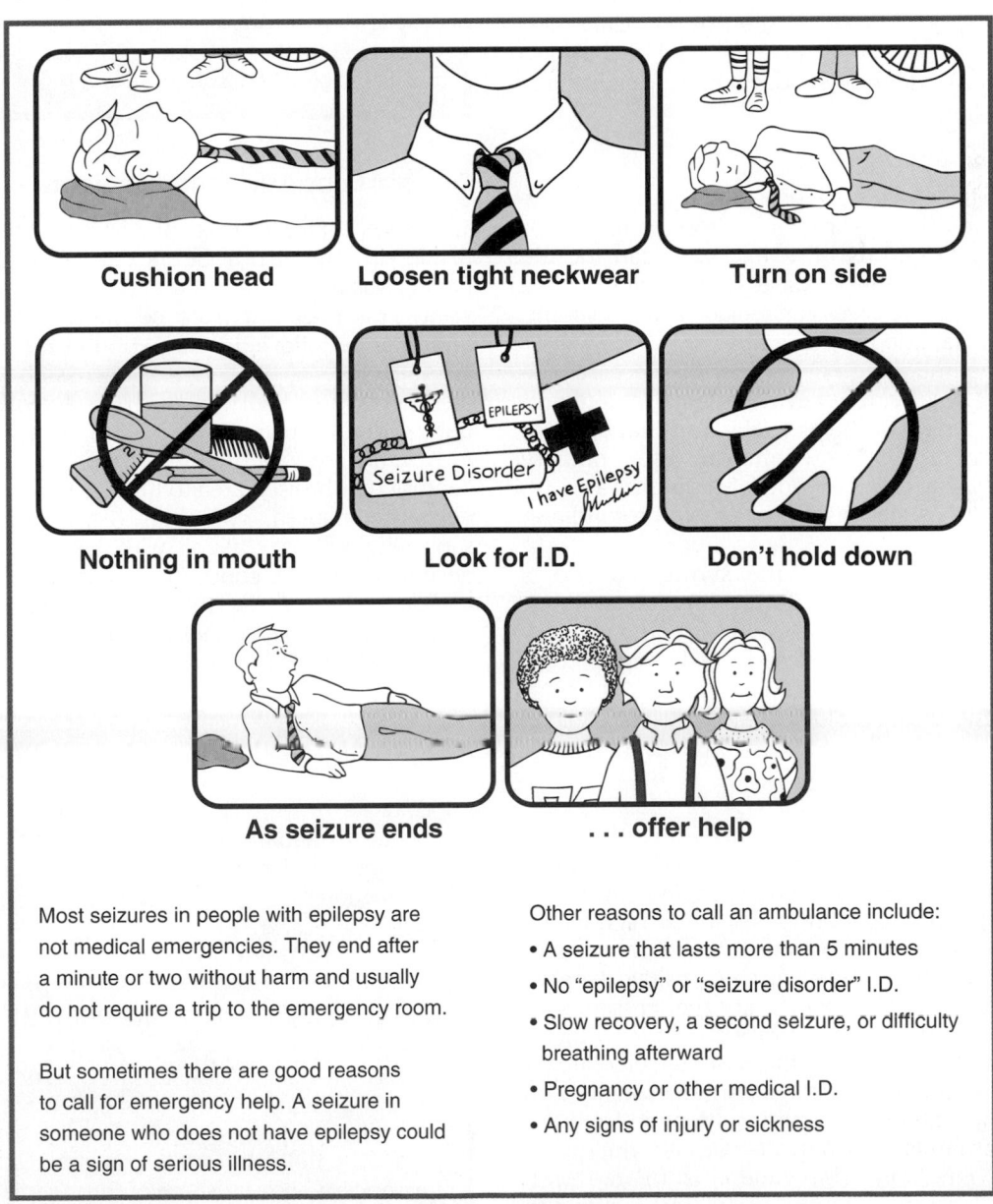

Cushion head

Loosen tight neckwear

Turn on side

Nothing in mouth

Look for I.D.

Don't hold down

As seizure ends

. . . offer help

Most seizures in people with epilepsy are not medical emergencies. They end after a minute or two without harm and usually do not require a trip to the emergency room.

But sometimes there are good reasons to call for emergency help. A seizure in someone who does not have epilepsy could be a sign of serious illness.

Other reasons to call an ambulance include:

- A seizure that lasts more than 5 minutes
- No "epilepsy" or "seizure disorder" I.D.
- Slow recovery, a second seizure, or difficulty breathing afterward
- Pregnancy or other medical I.D.
- Any signs of injury or sickness

FIGURE 41-6   First aid for seizures. (From Epilepsy Foundation of America, Landover, Md.)

cerebral function are the result of uncoordinated and disorganized electrical impulses in the brain. In many cases, the cause is never identified; however, some known causes include high fever, brain tumors, CNS infections, **anoxia**, and traumatic head injury.

The several main types of seizures each may be preceded by a significant aura. When patients experience the aura, they know a seizure is about to occur. The tonic-clonic (grand-mal) seizure causes a sudden loss of consciousness, which results in falling down, and then tonic (stiffening) muscle contractions, followed by clonic (twitching, jerking) muscle contractions of the limbs. Absence (petit-mal) seizures are a less serious form of seizure consisting of momentary clouding of consciousness and loss of contact with reality. Correct diagnosis is dependent on the careful history of the succession of seizures. The EEG is the most commonly used diagnostic test for seizure disorders. Seizures cannot be cured but usually can be controlled effectively by drugs, including phenytoin (Dilantin), phenobarbital, and valproic acid. Most seizures are not medical emergencies in a person with epilepsy but could be a sign of serious illness in someone who does not have epilepsy.

Encephalitis

Most cases of encephalitis are of viral origin and can be transmitted to humans from mosquitoes, animals, or other humans. Symptoms in a mild case can include headaches, muscle aches, malaise, and general flu-like symptoms. More severe cases can include fever, delirium, convulsions, **coma**, and even death.

A quiet, nonstimulating environment is necessary to avoid triggering seizure, to relieve headache, and to promote rest. The patient with cerebral inflammation from encephalitis may suffer from confusion, disorientation, and other behavioral changes. These symptoms are part of the disease and usually disappear when the condition improves.

Patient management treats the symptoms and is aimed at controlling the fever, maintaining electrolytes, and constant monitoring of respiratory and urinary functions. In patients with severe CNS damage, recovery usually is prolonged and physical therapy is necessary to overcome the neurological and musculoskeletal complications.

Meningitis

Meningitis is most commonly an acute bacterial infection of the meninges of the brain and spinal cord. It is characterized by the sudden onset of a high fever, headache, and sometimes vomiting and a severe stiff neck. Brudzinski's and Kernig's signs are positive. Lumbar puncture confirms the diagnosis by the presence of cloudy CSF containing large numbers of white blood cells and bacteria. Culturing the CSF usually allows identification of the causative organism. Meningitis can occur as a complication of an earlier infection from the ears, sinuses, or lungs. It also can occur with no known source of the infection. The patient is treated with analgesics, antibiotics, and appropriate medications to

decrease cerebral edema. Despite treatment, meningitis can be quickly fatal in some patients. Meningitis also occasionally has a viral origin.

BRUDZINSKI'S SIGN AND KERNIG'S SIGN

Brudzinski's Sign

The patient is placed in the supine position. The head is passively flexed toward the chest. If the patient spontaneously flexes the arm, hip, and knee in response to the neck flexion, Brudzinski's sign is present.

Kernig's Sign

With the patient in supine position the physician flexes both one hip and the **ipsilateral** knee to 90 degrees and then attempts to completely straighten the leg by straightening the knee. Kernig's sign is present if pain prevents straightening the leg or the patient involuntarily flexes the **contralateral** knee and hip.

Cerebral Concussion and Contusion

Traumatic injury from a blow to the head frequently results in the victim being "knocked out," and the patient sustains a concussion (Figure 41-7). Loss of consciousness may last from seconds to several minutes and may be followed by a period of disorientation that lasts up to 24 hours. A concussion can cause a disruption in the normal electrical activity in the brain, but the brain usually is not injured permanently.

A more serious injury to the brain can cause a contusion or bruised area to form. Symptoms can include headache, nausea, vomiting, vision disturbances, and sensitivity to light. Talking with the patient may reveal decreased levels of concentration, irritability, or difficulty in recall. Part of the initial assessment may include evaluation of consciousness according to the parameters of the Glasgow Coma Scale (Table 41-4).

CRITICAL THINKING APPLICATION

Dr. Song asks Mai to put together a small brochure explaining the possible dangers of some amusement park rides. What should be included in this brochure?

G-FORCES OF AMUSEMENT PARK RIDES

Emergency room physicians have noticed a steadily increasing number of patients with closed head injuries sustained on amusement park rides. Roller coasters are a great cause for concern because some of them subject

G-FORCES OF AMUSEMENT PARK RIDES —cont'd

riders to G-forces greater than astronauts are subjected to during space shuttle liftoff. "G" refers to gravity. On earth, the G-force is equal to 1. When an astronaut is weightless in space, the G-force is 0. Some rides produce G-forces greater than 3 Gs.

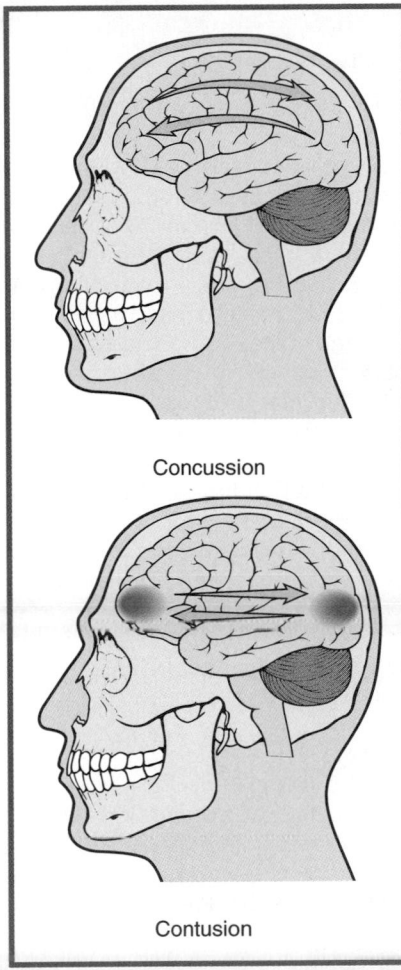

Concussion

Contusion

FIGURE 41-7   Brain concussion and contusion. (Modified from Frazier MS, Drzymkowski JW: *Essentials of human diseases and conditions,* ed 2. Philadelphia, 2000, WB Saunders, p 401.)

Closed Head Injury

When a patient experiences a more severe trauma to the head, significant, serious, life-threatening injury may occur to the intracerebral structures. Subarachnoid hemorrhage may occur when there is a rupture of delicate meningeal blood vessels resulting in blood collecting in the subarachnoid space. This causes rapidly increasing intracranial pressure, which may give rise to sudden, severe headache; nausea and severe projectile vomiting; motor disturbances; visual disturbances; and seizures. In addition to trauma, other predisposing factors that can cause subarachnoid hemorrhage include hypertension, oral contraceptives, family history, and congenital malformations of cranial blood vessels. Treatment includes decreasing the intracranial pressure, sometimes surgically.

Subdural hematoma is the collection of blood in the space between the dura and the brain, usually as a result of a slow bleed from a ruptured blood vessel secondary to trauma. Symptoms of increased intracranial pressure occur slowly as the size of the hematoma increases over days. Signs and symptoms are those associated with increased intracranial pressure and include headache, motor disturbances, nausea and vomiting, seizures, and a decreased level of consciousness. Treatment requires surgery to stop the bleeding and decrease the pressure inside the skull.

CRITICAL THINKING APPLICATION

- Mai is putting together a head injury information sheet for the family of a patient who recently suffered a minor concussion. What symptoms should the family watch for in this situation? How will the family know if they should seek additional medical care?
- Dr. Song said he would approve the leaflet after Mai completed it, but he was called away on an emergency before he saw it. A patient sees it behind the desk and asks to take one. Should Mai let him? Why or why not?

Shaken Baby Syndrome

Shaken baby syndrome is the most common cause of serious head injury in infants. The typical presentation

TABLE 41-4	Glasgow Coma Scale			
Eye Opening				
1—No response	2—To pain	3—To voice	4—Spontaneously	
Best Motor Response (Movement of Arms and Legs)				
1—No response	2—Extension to pain	3—Flexion to pain	4—Localizes to pain	5—Follows commands
Best Verbal Response				
1—No response	2—Incomprehensible sounds	3—Inappropriate words	4—Disoriented and converses	5—Oriented and converses
Scoring				
13 to 15 = Mild head injury		9 to 12 = Moderate head injury		3 to 8 = Severe head injury

is a child of around 6 months who is brought to the clinic or emergency room because of difficulty breathing or marked lethargy. Usually there is little or no external bruising or trauma. Physical findings on examination or autopsy include subdural hematoma and retinal hemorrhages in the back of the eyes. The history given by the caregiver usually indicates that the baby "fell" from the sofa, coffee table, or bed, or was "dropped." On close questioning, the history frequently changes over the first few hours after injury. About one fourth of these infants die of their injuries. The caregiver grasps the child on the chest and violently shakes the infant back and forth. This causes the head to move quickly forward and backward, which causes the injuries.

Spinal Cord Injuries

Spinal cord injuries usually result from severe, accidental trauma to the back or neck. These injuries are most common in the 16- to 30-year-old age group and are associated with automobile and sports accidents. If the cord is completely transected, there will be no nerve impulses traveling between the brain and any of the structures below the injury. The higher the damage to the spinal cord, the more serious the injury becomes. The paralysis resulting from cord **transection** is grouped into one of two categories (Figure 41-8). In *paraplegia*, transection occurs below the midpoint of the spinal cord, and paralysis involves both legs and all other structures below the level of injury. In *quadriplegia*, transection occurs in the upper thoracic or cervical region of the spinal cord, causing paralysis of all four limbs.

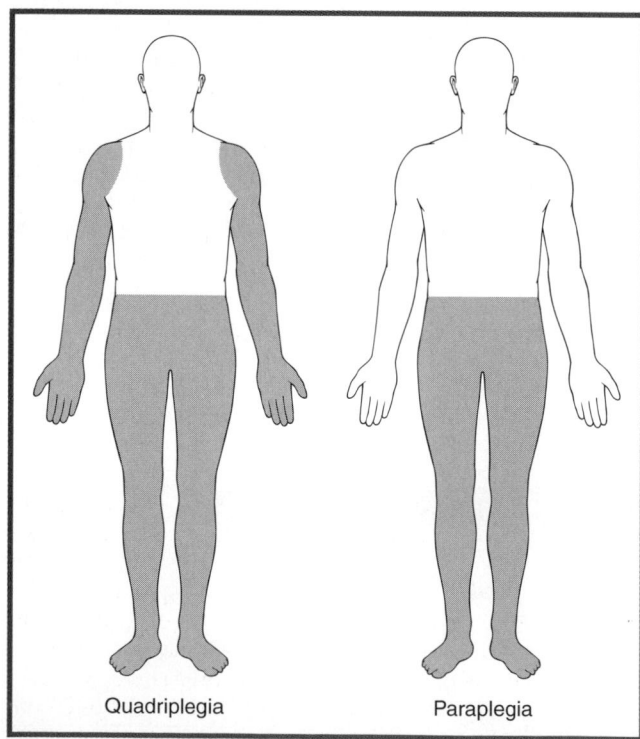

Quadriplegia   Paraplegia

FIGURE 41-8 Types of paralysis: quadriplegia and paraplegia. (Modified from Frazier MS, Drzymkowski JW: *Essentials of human diseases and conditions*, ed 2. Philadelphia, 2000, WB Saunders, p 402.)

Hemiplegia is unrelated to spinal cord injury and occurs when CVA, injury, or tumor occurs on one side of the brain, resulting in paralysis on the opposite side of the body.

No surgery or treatment can successfully restore a transected cord, although this is an area where much research is currently being done. If the spinal cord is injured, but not completely transected, the degree of paralysis will depend on the degree of injury. These patients usually respond well to physical therapy, and their ability to restore motor function is good, although they may always have some functional limitations.

Parkinson's Disease

Parkinson's disease is a progressive, debilitating, crippling disease that affects about one in every 100 adults over the age of 60 years, which means this is a common disease, with more than 60,000 new cases occurring annually in the United States. It affects men more frequently than women. The typical presentation of Parkinson's disease includes muscular rigidity, unilateral pill rolling, tremor movements of the hand, high-pitched monotone voice, and a mask-like facial expression. The patient has a forward-bent posture with the head bowed. Muscular tremors and rigidity increase. The cause is unknown, but some research indicates that it sometimes occurs after a long-time-earlier viral infection. There is a deficiency of the neurotransmitter dopamine in the brain. There is no known cure; giving levodopa (L-dopa), which is turned into dopamine in the brain, is the typical treatment for Parkinson's disease. This is effective only until the dose is increased so high that it causes serious side effects. Sometimes surgical destruction of the most affected area of the brain can produce some relief of symptoms.

Multiple Sclerosis

Nerve fibers made up of bundles of axons in the PNS are covered with myelin sheaths. *Multiple sclerosis* (MS) results from the progressive inflammation and deterioration of these myelin sheaths, leaving the nerve fibers uncovered. This causes a variety of neurological problems, such as visual disturbances, urinary dysfunctions, emotional instability, muscle weakness, and degrees of paralysis. It most commonly begins in women in their early 30s. The cause remains unknown. It is more common in Northern climates and is associated with an autoimmune reaction. It is extremely difficult to diagnose, and diagnosis may be made based on the **exacerbation** and **remission** characteristics of the disease. One of the tests that can assist in diagnosis is lumbar puncture. Increased CSF levels of gamma globulin occur when the disease is present. MRI can show actual plaques on the nerve fibers where the myelin sheath is gone.

There is no cure, and the treatment goals are to alleviate symptoms and delay the progression of the disease. Some patients may live an essentially normal life with only occasional attacks, whereas in other patients the MS progresses, rapidly causing severe incapacitation leading to death soon after the disease onset.

Tumors

Brain tumor is probably one of the most feared medical problems. People often suffer with migraine headaches for years without seeking any medical help because they fear having a brain tumor. Symptoms depend on the type and location of the tumor, but generally the initial symptoms are headaches, vomiting, dizziness, double vision, and changes in muscle strength and coordination. Changes in personality and mental function, seizures, progressive paralysis, loss of speech, and sensory disorders appear as the tumor enlarges.

Conducting radiologic studies such as CT and MRI will confirm the diagnosis. Additional tests may include EEG and lumbar puncture. Ophthalmoscopic examination may reveal **papilledema**. Accurate diagnosis of a brain tumor includes determining its precise location in the brain and determining whether it is **benign** or **malignant**. Approximately half of all brain tumors result from cancer metastasis from other primary cancer sites within the body. Lung cancer, breast cancer, and melanoma frequently spread to the brain by metastasis. Regardless of their origin, as brain tumors grow, they cause serious problems and complications for the patient because of the limited space inside the skull. Treatment of brain tumors can include surgery, chemotherapy, and radiation in any combination.

CRITICAL THINKING APPLICATION

A 34-year-old man has just found out he has a brain tumor, and Dr. Song is going to operate on him next week. Before he leaves the office, he wants to talk to Mai "privately." They go into an examination room and he says to Mai, "Tell me the truth: this is cancer and I'm going to die, right?" How should Mai respond to this frightened patient?

Diseases of the Peripheral Nervous System

Amyotrophic Lateral Sclerosis. *Amyotrophic lateral sclerosis* (ALS), or *Lou Gehrig disease*, is a progressive, destructive neurological disease that results in muscle **atrophy**. It usually begins with small, local, involuntary muscle contractions in the forearms and hands. As ALS progresses, the patient has difficulty with speech, chewing, swallowing, and breathing. Death from failure of the respiratory muscles usually occurs within 6 to 10 years after onset. The cause is unknown, but it most commonly occurs in males over the age of 50.

Bell's Palsy. Bell's palsy affects the seventh cranial nerve of the face. It occurs suddenly and usually subsides spontaneously over several weeks to months. There is muscular weakness and paralysis affecting only one side of the patient's face. The mouth droops on the affected side, and drooling of saliva occurs. The patient cannot close the eye completely on the affected side and may experience taste disturbances. The cause is unknown. Treatment with steroids helps to control edema in the affected area. The eye can be protected with a temporary eye patch.

Peripheral Neuropathy. *Peripheral neuropathy* is not a disease in itself but rather a condition of peripheral nerve dysfunction that can have more than 100 different known causes. It can be **cryptogenic** or **idiopathic**, meaning the underlying cause cannot be identified. The following conditions can cause peripheral neuropathies: diabetes, human immunodeficiency virus (HIV) infection, nutritional deficiencies, and neurological side effects of some medications. Symptoms usually affect the legs and arms and can include muscular weakness and pain or sensory disturbances such as burning, numbness, and tingling.

Symptoms can vary widely from person to person in both number and severity. Patients often experience extreme frustration when trying to explain to the physician the abnormal sensations they are experiencing. Peripheral neuropathies can result from damage or injury to any portion of the neuron. Peripheral neuropathy treatment is most effective when the causative condition is diagnosed and then successfully treated.

Carpal Tunnel Syndrome. *Carpal tunnel syndrome* (CTS) results from **compression** or entrapment of the median nerve as it courses past the carpal bones of the wrist toward the hand. The carpal tunnel contains the median nerve and the flexor tendons of the forearm. Compression of these structures within the carpal tunnel can occur spontaneously but more commonly is the result of repetitive movements. CTS is the most common of the repetitive strain injuries (RSIs). One frequently reported cause is daily use of the computer keyboard for prolonged periods. The symptoms of median nerve compression are pain and **paresthesia** of the radial-palmar region of the hand.

Treatment includes taking breaks from repetitive hand or wrist activities, wearing a wrist support, nonsteroidal antiinflammatory drugs (NSAIDs), ice, and physical therapy. If these treatments do not resolve the problem, surgery may be required to relieve the pressure on the median nerve.

Mental Health

According to the American Psychiatric Association, each year more than 20% of Americans suffer a diagnosable mental condition that adversely affects their work, their relationships with family and friends, and their activities of daily living. Mental health disorders may be caused by any of the following (alone or in combination): changes in brain chemicals, hereditary makeup, psychological disposition, and life experiences. Emotional and physical symptoms can occur for no apparent reason and can remain quite persistent. Emotional symptoms can include panic, apprehension, fear, nightmares, withdrawal, flashbacks, and ritualized repetitive behavior such as constant handwashing. Physical symptoms can include jitteriness, tachycardia, shortness of breath, sleep disturbances, gastrointestinal upset, muscular tension, and cold, clammy hands. Often patients do not associate these symptoms with a mental health disorder and thus do not get appropriate diagnosis and treatment.

Posttraumatic Stress Disorder. *Posttraumatic stress disorder* (PTSD) usually follows a patient's being a part of or witnessing some terrifying, horrendous, or violent physical or emotional event, such as assault, battery, rape, war, natural disasters, acts of terrorism, and serious accidents during which many people are killed or injured. The person who survives the ordeal often has flashbacks; feelings of panic, fear, or guilt; constant replaying of the event in his or her mind; or deep feelings of emotional numbness. Severe depression and inability to function normally in daily activities also may be present. Treatment includes antianxiety and antidepressant medications as well as psychotherapy.

Attention Deficit Disorder. *Attention deficit disorder* (ADD) or *attention deficit hyperactivity disorder* (ADHD) is a condition that frequently includes symptoms such as short attention span, easy distractibility, lack of self-control, extreme displays of impulse, and in some cases hyperactivity. ADD affects between 2% and 6% of the population and affects boys three times more often than girls. Basically, it is present in one student in every classroom in America. It cannot be cured, but treatment with medication and sometimes diet modification can be beneficial.

Depression. *Depression* is a treatable illness characterized by a persistent negative mood that affects the entire physical body as well as the mind. More than 80% of patients treated for depression improve. Depression occurs in one of every five people sometime during their lifetime, and it affects women twice as often as men. It affects people all ages, races, genders, and nationalities; in short, all humans are susceptible. Depression can complicate other illnesses and can lead to suicide when it becomes serious. Frequent causes of depression include stress, medical illness, disappointment, feelings of failure in any area of life, or loss of a job. Although treatment is almost always successful, fewer than half of patients with depression ever seek professional help. Effective treatment can include antidepressants and psychotherapy.

Depression can cause emotional, physical, behavioral, or cognitive (thought) symptoms. The following are the most common symptoms in each of these areas:

- *Emotional:* hopelessness, helplessness, sadness, anger, irritability
- *Physical:* overeating or loss of appetite, sleeping too much or too little, constipation, irregular menses, loss of interest in sex
- *Behavioral:* crying frequently without any particular reason, social withdrawal, decrease in personal hygiene, no motivation
- *Cognitive:* low self-esteem, feeling like a failure, blaming oneself for external problems, continual and overwhelming pessimism, endlessly criticizing oneself

Learning Disabilities. Learning disabilities result from mental confusion affecting a person's ability to link up information in the brain as well as difficulty in interpreting sensory input from the environment. Learning disabilities can adversely affect relationships, school, daily activities, and work. They can cause difficulties in reading, writing, speaking, understanding, coordination, self-control, and attention.

The Medical Assistant's Role in the Neurological Examination

As with other physical examinations, a careful history provides the physician with valuable clues in diagnosing neurological conditions. These may include seizures, **syncope**, **diplopia**, **incontinence**, or any of the subjective symptoms previously mentioned in this chapter. The patient's general health often complicates a neurological diagnosis. The purposes of a neurological examination are to determine whether a nervous system malfunction is present, discover its locations, and identify its type and extent. During the examination, the physician may determine the effect of the symptoms in relationship to the patient's emotional status, intellectual performance, cognitive ability, and general behavior (Procedure 41-1). The patient's grooming and mannerisms are carefully observed. The patient's ability to communicate effectively includes evaluating speech, language, and writing skills. Listen for difficulty in

---

PROCEDURE 41-1

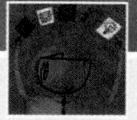

Assisting With the Neurological Examination

GOAL: To assist the physician in obtaining an accurate neurological examination of the patient.

EQUIPMENT AND SUPPLIES
- Otoscope
- Ophthalmoscope
- Percussion hammer
- Disposable pinwheel
- Penlight
- Tuning fork
- Cotton ball
- Tongue depressor
- Small vials of warm and cold liquids prepared according to the physician's instructions
- Small vials of sweet and salty tasting liquids prepared according to the physician's instructions
- Small vials containing substances with distinct odors such as instant coffee, cinnamon, vanilla, etc. prepared according to the physician's instructions

PROCEDURE 41-1—cont'd

PROCEDURAL STEPS

1 Greet the patient and help him or her onto the examination table. Explain the procedure to the patient.
Purpose: To ensure patient cooperation during the examination.

2 During the examination, be prepared to assist the patient in changing positions as necessary, have the necessary examination instruments ready for the physician at the appropriate time during the examination, and record all results from the examination as indicated by the physician.
Purpose: To facilitate a thorough and accurate neurological examination.

3 The neurological examination will generally follow the following order but can be modified according to physician preference:
  a. Mental status examination
  b. Proprioception and cerebellar function
  c. Cranial nerve assessment
  d. Sensory nerve function
  e. Reflexes

4 Complete the documentation of the examination in the patient's medical record.
Purpose: A procedure is not completed until it is accurately documented in the patient's medical record.

---

putting words together, slurred speech, and whether conversation makes sense. If you notice inappropriate changes in the patient, note them on the patient's record for the physician's attention and evaluation.

Physical examination of the neurological system will include evaluation of the cranial nerves. You can assist by helping the patient assume the proper position necessary for each test and by having the instruments the physician will need ready for use. For example, cranial nerve I (the olfactory nerve) is tested by determining the patient's ability to identify familiar odors such as coffee, tobacco, or cloves. Cranial nerve V (the trigeminal nerve) is checked by the patient's ability to differentiate between warm and cold objects held on his or her right and left cheeks.

Peripheral nerve function is evaluated by examining the motor system, including muscular strength, **gait**, and movements. The diameters of the upper arms and the calves of the legs are measured and compared to look for muscle atrophy. Motor functioning can be assessed through the use of the Romberg test, in which the patient will be asked to stand with the feet together, arms horizontal to the body, and eyes closed. The sensory system is examined by noting the patient's ability to perceive superficial sensations, such as a wisp of cotton brushed on the skin, a light pinprick, or hot and cold touching certain areas. Several deep tendon reflexes (DTRs), such as the patellar and Achilles, are tested (Figure 41-9). Stroking the lateral aspect of the sole of the foot with a dull instrument (such as the handle of a reflex hammer or a tongue blade) checks the Babinski reflex. In a positive Babinski test, the great toe dorsiflexes while the other toes fan out. This may indicate a possible stroke or brain lesion. Other diagnostic tests may include skull radiograph, carotid arteriogram, myelogram, EEG, and MRI and CT studies.

Diagnostic Testing

Several diagnostic tests are used to help the physician accurately diagnose conditions and diseases of the neurological system. The most common diagnostic procedures include lumbar puncture, EEG, and various radiographic studies (Table 41-5).

Electroencephalography

Electroencephalography is the recording of changes in electrical impulses in various areas of the brain by

TABLE 41-5	Diagnostic Tests for the Nervous System	
Test	**Procedure and Patient Preparation**	**Results**
Arteriography (angiography)	The patient is usually given a sedative. Then, after injecting a local anesthetic, a catheter is threaded into an artery toward the head. Contrast medium is injected and video fluoroscopic studies are recorded. The patient must remain still during the procedure, which may last up to 1 hr.	Allows visualization of vertebral and carotid arteries, cerebral arterial circulation, leaking vessels, aneurysms, and occluded vessels
CT scan	Patient's head is strapped into a foam block to prevent movement and lies on a moveable table. The table moves into the CT machine that converts an x-ray into a visual image of multiple transverse sections of the brain. Procedure lasts for up to 1 hr and the patient must remain still the entire time.	Visualization of multiple, serial, radiographic sections of a structure differentiating between bone and soft tissues

Continued

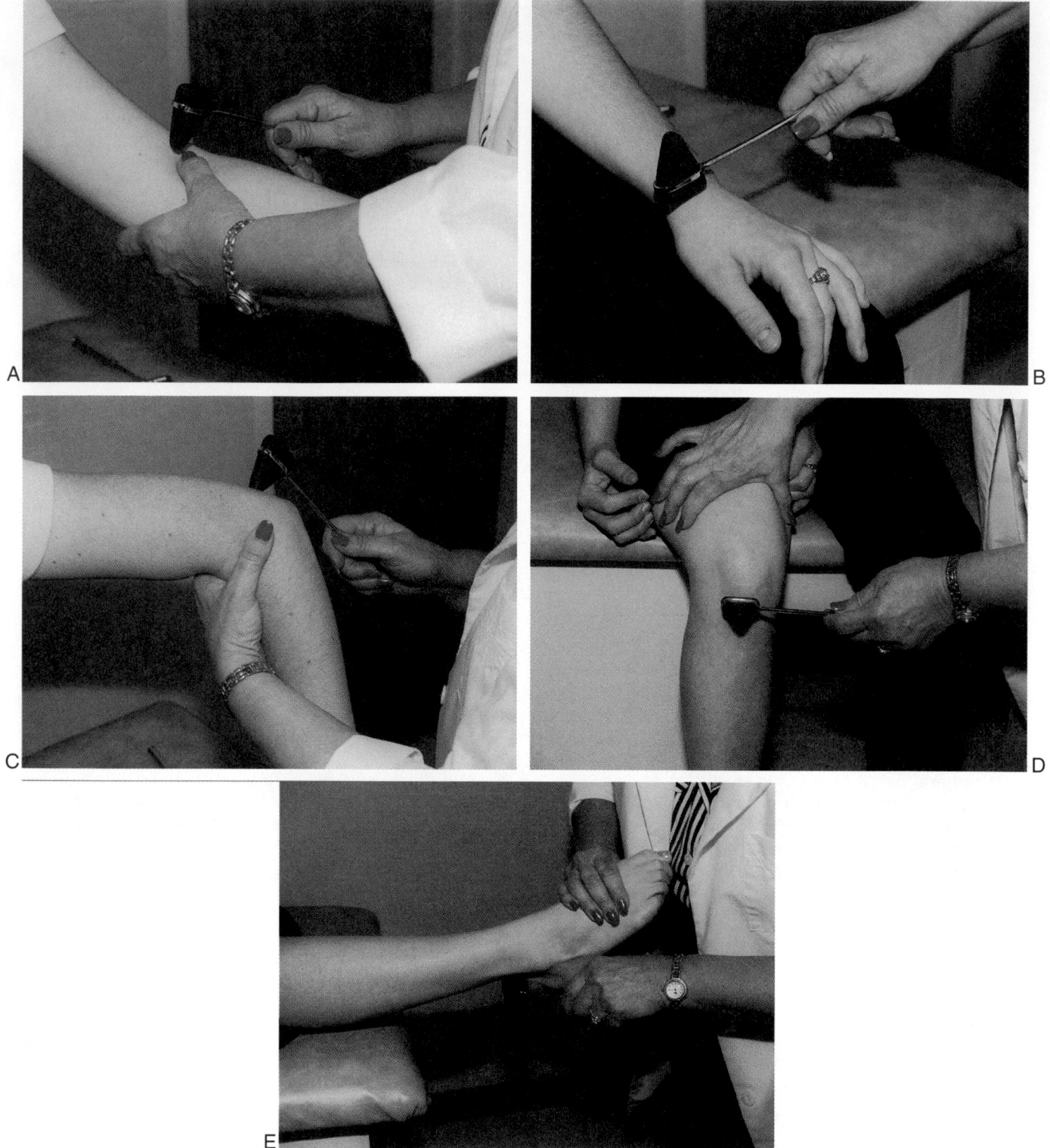

FIGURE 41-9 Testing deep tendon reflexes. **A**, Biceps reflex. Note flexion of elbow. **B**, Brachioradialis reflex. Note flexion and supination of the forearm. **C**, Triceps reflex. Note extension of the arm. **D**, Patellar reflex. Note extension of the leg. **E**, Achilles reflex. Note plantar flexion of the foot.

TABLE 41-5	Diagnostic Tests for the Nervous System—cont'd	
Test	**Procedure and Patient Preparation**	**Results**
EEG	Patient relaxes comfortably on a recliner or bed. Electrodes are attached to the head. The examiner may ask the patient questions, give the patient various forms of visual or auditory stimulation, or have the patient sleep.	Recording of electrical activity of the brain to determine cerebral function, determine origin of seizure activity, diagnose sleep disorders, and determine death
Lumbar puncture	With the patient in a side-lying fetal position, a local anesthetic is injected before a needle is inserted into the subarachnoid space between the third and fourth lumbar vertebrae. The procedure normally takes from 5-20 min and the patient must remain very still during the procedure.	Determine CSF pressure, obtain CSF specimens for testing, reduce intracranial pressure, and for injecting contrast medium for radiographic studies
MRI	Patient's head is strapped into a foam block to prevent movement and lies on a moveable table. The table moves into the MRI machine that converts electromagnetic energy of the body's cells into a visual image. Procedure lasts for up to 1 hr and the patient must remain still the entire time. Patient should not have metal in body.	Like CT, allows visualization of multiple, serial, radiographic sections of a structure; shows images of brain, spinal cord, and surrounding vascular and soft tissue
PET scan	Radioactive isotope is injected into the patient and the brain is scanned to locate areas where the isotope was concentrated. Procedure lasts for up to 2 hr and patient must remain still the entire time.	Radionuclide study can identify areas of increased metabolic activity, vascular abnormalities, and space-occupying lesions
X-ray studies	Patient's head is placed in a specific position in front of the x-ray film; patient must remain still for about 1 min while x-ray is taken.	Bone studies to identify fractures and other bone pathologies

CT, Computed tomography; *EEG*, electroencephalography; *CSF*, cerebrospinal fluid; *MRI*, magnetic resonance imaging; *PET*, positron emission tomography.

means of electrodes placed on the scalp, on the brain surface, or within the brain itself. The electrodes are connected to an amplifier that amplifies the electrical impulses more than a million times. After being amplified, the impulses move an electromagnetic pen that records the electrical activity as brain waves.

The rate, height, and length of the waves vary in different parts of the brain. Every individual has a unique EEG pattern. In a healthy brain, most of the recorded waves are the occipital alpha wave coming from the back of the head. Irregular slow waves are called *delta waves*, which normally are found in deep sleep and in infants and young children. It is abnormal to find a delta wave pattern in an awake adult. Rhythmic slow waves, called *theta waves*, show a decrease in brain activity. Electrical silence (flat-line EEG) indicates no evidence of brain activity and is one of the criteria that determine death. EEG is widely used in studying brain functions and tracing the connections between the parts of the CNS. It is particularly valuable in diagnosing epilepsy, brain tumor, and other brain conditions (Procedure 41-2).

PROCEDURE 41-2

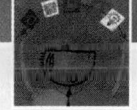

Preparing the Patient for an EEG

GOAL: To prepare a patient properly both physically and psychologically to obtain an accurate and useful EEG recording.

PROCEDURAL STEPS

1 Greet the patient and introduce yourself. Explain to the patient you will go over what is going to happen step by step to ensure the best results.

2 Explain to the patient the purpose of the EEG, how the procedure will be carried out, and what will be expected of the patient during the test.

3 Tell the patient that the electrodes pick up tiny electrical signals from the body and that there is no danger of electrical shock.

4 Explain that the test is painless because the electrodes are attached to the scalp with collodion.

5 If this is a sleep EEG, suggest that the patient stay up later than usual the night before the test so that it will be easier to fall asleep.

Continued

PROCEDURE 41-2—cont'd

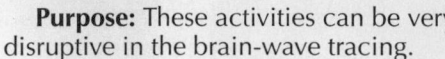
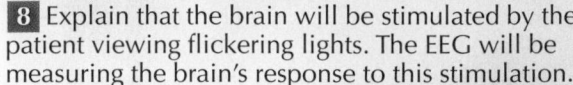

Purpose: Sleep medications are seldom used because they may alter the brain wave pattern.

6 Go over the physical preparation, including the diet to be followed for the 48 hours before the test. This usually includes no stimulants like coffee, chocolate, or sodas, and no meal skipping.

Purpose: Meal skipping may cause hypoglycemia, which alters brain function.

7 Tell the patient that a baseline EEG will be taken at the beginning of the test, and during this time the patient will be asked to avoid all movement, even eye and tongue movement.

Purpose: These activities can be very disruptive in the brain-wave tracing.

8 Explain that the brain will be stimulated by the patient viewing flickering lights. The EEG will be measuring the brain's response to this stimulation.

9 Ask the patient whether he or she has any questions. If so, answer the questions so that the patient understands the procedure clearly.

Purpose: Patients are more likely to be cooperative it they are informed so they will not be unduly apprehensive before and during the test.

10 Document the procedure in the patient record.

Lumbar Puncture

When it is suspected that a patient has a possible infection or inflammation of the CNS, a lumbar puncture (spinal tap) is commonly requested (Figure 41-10). Lumbar puncture is done to collect several milliliters of CSF to be cultured, analyzed for glucose and protein, and examined through the microscope for the presence of bacteria and blood cells. Increased intracranial pressure or an intracranial bleed can also be indicated by lumbar puncture.

Sterile technique always must be used when performing a lumbar puncture. The patient usually is placed on the left side in the fetal position, the lumbar puncture site is injected with a local anesthetic, and then the puncture is performed by inserting a special needle into the sub-arachnoid space. This is done below the inferior end of the spinal cord usually between L-4 and L-5 vertebrae.

After the procedure, the patient must remain flat in bed for about 8 hours. Medical practices usually have a specially equipped room where this procedure is performed. If you are working in such an office, you may be responsible for both assisting with the procedure and monitoring the patient after the procedure until he or she is sent home. You will watch for side effects such as severe headaches, visual disturbances, and pain. You will also have particular office protocols to follow regarding the frequency of vital signs, liquid intake, urine output, and visitors. Lumbar puncture also may be performed in outpatient clinics or surgical centers (Procedure 41-3).

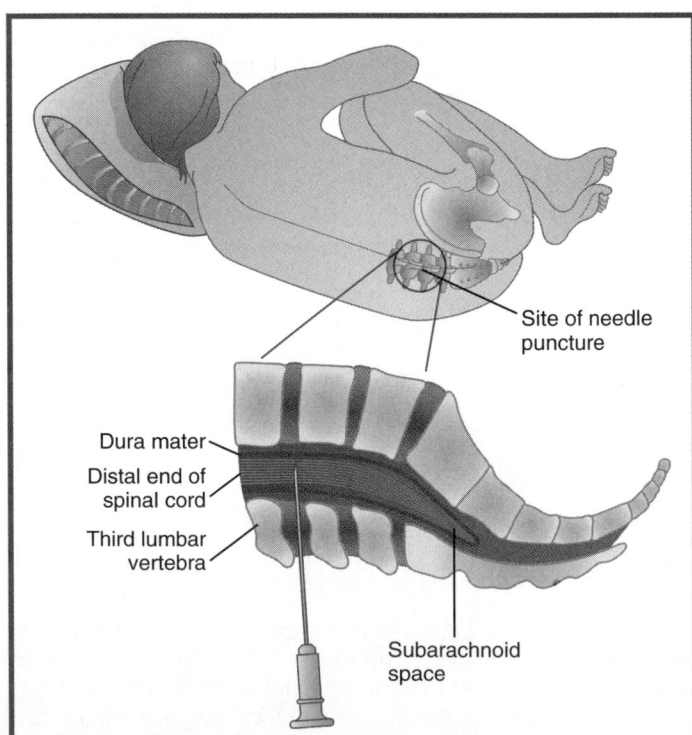

Site of needle puncture

Dura mater

Distal end of spinal cord

Third lumbar vertebra

Subarachnoid space

FIGURE 41-10 Lumbar puncture.

PROCEDURE 41-3

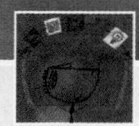

Preparing the Patient for and Assisting With a Lumbar Puncture

GOAL: To prepare a patient properly both physically and mentally for a lumbar puncture to obtain a specimen of CSF for testing.

EQUIPMENT AND SUPPLIES

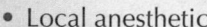

- Local anesthetic
- Sterile, disposable lumbar puncture kit
- Mayo stand
- Sterile gloves
- Permanent marker to label tubes

PROCEDURAL STEPS

1 Greet the patient and introduce yourself. Explain to the patient that you will go over what is going to happen step by step to ensure the best results.

2 Explain to the patient the purpose of the lumbar puncture, how the procedure will be carried out, and what will be expected of the patient during the test.

3 Have the patient void just before the procedure.
Purpose: So the patient can be most comfortable for the duration of the procedure.

4 Give the patient a hospital gown and have him or her put it on with the opening down the back.

5 Place the patient in a left, side-lying fetal position for the lumbar puncture.
Purpose: To give the physician the easiest access to the lumbar region of the spine.

6 Support the patient's head with a pillow as necessary and provide a pillow for between the knees if needed also.
Purpose: Make the patient as comfortable as possible for the procedure.

7 Do a sterile skin preparation of the patient's lumbar region in the usual manner.
Purpose: To prevent bacterial infection at the puncture site.

8 Place the sterile disposable lumbar puncture kit on the mayo stand and open it, establishing a sterile field. Put on sterile gloves and take the fenestrated drape from the kit and drape the lumbar region of

the patient, so that only the L3-4 region of the lower spine is exposed.
Purpose: To isolate the area of the procedure in a sterile field.

9 When the physician is ready to do the lumbar puncture, provide the local anesthetic by holding the vial for the physician or pouring it into the sterile medicine cup on the sterile field of the mayo stand.
Purpose: To expedite the procedure.

10 Reassure the patient and help him or her to hold still during the injection of the local anesthetic and the insertion of the spinal needle.
Purpose: To facilitate accurate insertion of the spinal needle by the physician.

11 Be prepared to hold the top of the manometer steady if requested by the physician.

12 Using the permanent marker, label the specimens #1, #2, and #3 in the order they were collected. This is a critically important step in this procedure.
Purpose: Different tests are done on different tubes. The accuracy of these tests is dependent on which tube they are performed.

13 Complete the laboratory requisition form and prepare the CSF specimens for transport to the laboratory.
Purpose: To ensure that all the necessary tests are ordered correctly.

14 Break down the mayo stand sterile field setup by disposing of sharps, biohazard, and regular waste in the normal manner.

15 Monitor the patient and give liquids as directed by the physician.

16 Document the procedure in the patient's chart.

See Appendix E for a charting example.

CRITICAL THINKING APPLICATION

Dr. Song is going to perform a lumbar puncture on a 10-year-old girl who he suspects has bacterial meningitis. Her mother agrees to the procedure, but while Mai is preparing the girl for the procedure, the mother changes her mind. She is afraid her daughter will become paralyzed by having a needle put into her spine. What should Mai do in this situation?

Computed Tomography

Computed tomography scanning (Figure 41-11) utilizes computer processing to generate an x-ray image showing the various tissue densities in transverse sections (slices) of various body parts as thin as 1 mm in thickness. A liquid contrast medium can be injected into the patient before the procedure to enhance the visible differentiation of the various layers of soft tissue.

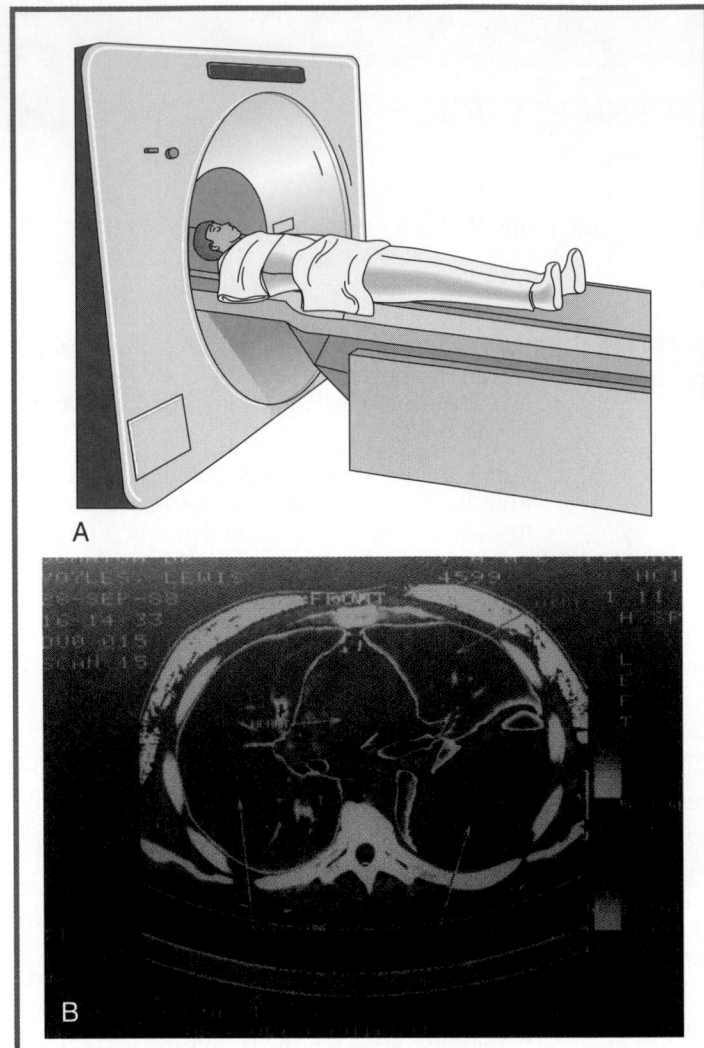

FIGURE 41-11 **A**, Computed tomography (CT) total body scanner. **B**, CT scan.

Magnetic Resonance Imaging

Magnetic resonance imaging can create a hologram to show the precise location of tumor masses, allowing the surgeon to plan a very precise approach through the skull into the brain to remove the tumor (Figure 41-12). Radiologists can make a video from the MRI that peels away the skin, skull, and coverings of the brain to allow the surgeon to view the tumor from all directions with special three-dimensional glasses. This proves helpful for the physician before going into the operating room to remove the real tumor. MRI also can be recorded as serial transverse sections, similar to the CT scan.

Patient Education

The nervous system is the major communication and control system in the human body. It influences and regulates all mental activity, including thought, learning, and memory. It is responsible for homeostasis, or maintaining complete balance in the body. Through its many receptors, the nervous system constantly monitors what is going on inside the body and in the environment outside of the body.

When the nervous system becomes damaged or diseased, signs and symptoms can appear in every other body system. Motor activity can become erratic, or activity level can decrease to the point that the person becomes unable to communicate or function normally. Sometimes these patients seem to be always complaining about something, and no one seems to listen to them.

Your main responsibilities as a medical assistant in neurology will be to observe, listen, and report any changes you observe in patients. Even things that may seem rather slight may give the physician the one clue needed to put a puzzle together to arrive at a correct diagnosis before proceeding to an appropriate treatment. Neurology will not be the specialty in which every medical assistant would like to work because there are few exciting procedures. To enjoy this type of practice, you must have extraordinary communication skills and

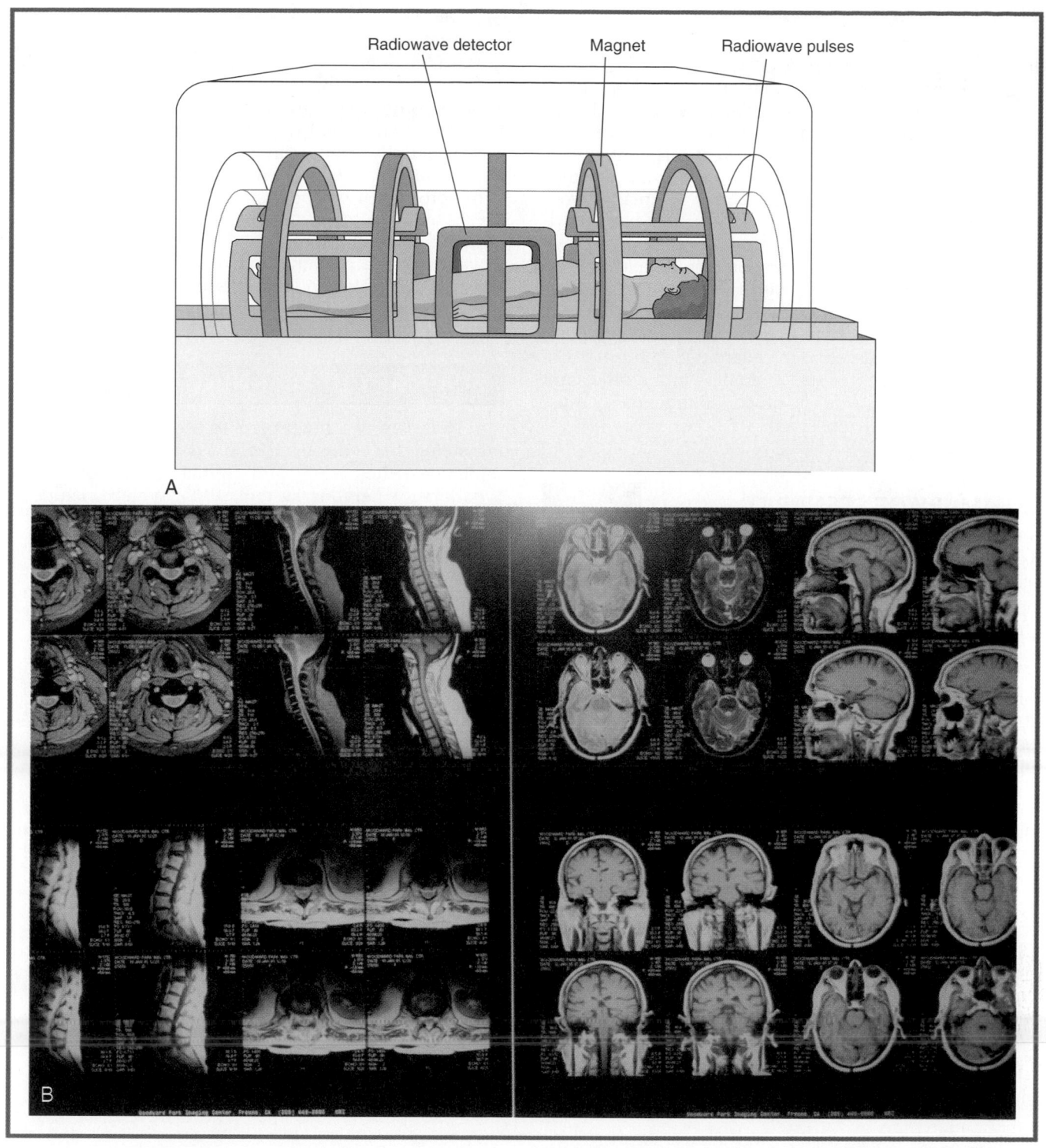

Radiowave detector   Magnet   Radiowave pulses

A

B

FIGURE 41-12   **A**, Magnetic resonance imaging (MRI) unit. **B**, Magnetic resonance images of the skull and spine.

the ability to listen to what patients are telling you. This is important with all patients in neurology, but it is particularly important when a patient calls the office with symptoms. It is mandatory that you grasp the importance and significance of seemingly varied symptoms in the neurological patient. For example, severe headache accompanied by vomiting may be an indication of a serious intracranial problem that needs immediate attention. The medical assistant in a neurology practice must remain alert to these types of situations at all times because neurological emergencies can occur quite rapidly. If you have these skills, assisting in a neurological practice could result in a very rewarding career.

Legal and Ethical Issues

In neurology, you will be faced with many degrees of behavior and personality changes that are all a part of many neurological conditions. Often a patient is not aware of these changes and may appear to feel that there is nothing wrong. You must treat this patient with the same dignity and respect as you would all other patients, despite how the patient may be treating you. Some patients are concerned that loved ones have turned against them and are treating them in an abusive manner. A patient's family may be experiencing severe emotional stress in coping with the patient's behavior. You must remember the medical assistant's code of ethics and the need for total confidentiality. Everything that is said or discussed in the examination room is not to be repeated to other staff members in the office and never discussed outside the office. Confidentiality must absolutely be strictly observed.

SUMMARY OF SCENARIO

Mai has excelled in her new position as clinical assistant and patient educator. She has developed a series of patient information sheets that explain what the nervous system is, what symptoms to watch for after a head injury, the kinds and causes of headaches, what encephalitis is, and what Alzheimer's disease is. Patients like to learn more about these topics, and Mai's information sheets are quite popular with Dr. Song's patients. They often ask for information sheets for other family members and for their friends and neighbors. She also developed a set of information sheets to explain the common neurological diagnostic tests and how best to prepare for them. Mai still talks with each patient to ensure that he or she understands exactly what is going to happen for the test and to ensure that all questions are completely answered.

Mai feels a great deal of personal satisfaction from working with her patients and helping them to get through some trying and anxious times in their lives. The patient she could not understand over the phone was specifically calling Mai for help. Mai called 911 and sent the ambulance to her apartment. The woman was in the process of having a stroke; she was admitted to the hospital. After extensive rehabilitation, she has regained all of her speech and most of her extremity movement. She remains a patient of Dr. Song's and says that she is alive today because of Mai.

SUMMARY OF LEARNING OBJECTIVES

■ There are two main parts to the human nervous system: the central nervous system (CNS), which includes the brain and spinal cord, and the peripheral nervous system (PNS), which includes all of the nerves outside of the CNS.

■ The main function of the nervous system is to control the body and thus maintain homeostasis. It does this by receiving messages in the CNS from the PNS and then sending a response to the appropriate location in the body, again via the PNS.

■ The CNS is well protected, first by bone and then by a series of membranous coverings (meninges) called the dura mater, arachnoid mater, and pia mater.

■ The brain is made up of the cerebrum (all expressions of artistic and verbal processes and thought), the cerebellum (controls balance, equilibrium, posture, and muscle coordination), and the brainstem (vision, hearing, respirations, heart rate, blood pressure, and waking and sleeping).

- Symptoms of possible serious neurological conditions include headache, nausea and vomiting, change in vision, or change in level of consciousness.

- The most common brain disorders resulting from trauma include concussion and contusion. More severe injuries could result in intracranial bleeding.

- The most common work-related neurological condition is an RSI, called CTS.

- Frequently used diagnostic tests in neurology include EEG, lumbar puncture, x-ray, CT scan, and MRI.

- Depression is among the most commonly encountered mental health disorders and has a variety of symptoms that can be overlooked or attributed to some other condition.

- When assisting in neurology, the medical assistant must be particularly careful to recognize signs and symptoms, which frequently are quite subtle but yet can be extremely significant in helping to assess and diagnose the neurological patient accurately.

KEY INTERNET WEBSITES

- National Parkinson Foundation: Explore the autonomic nervous system
- Neuroscience for Kids: Explore the brain and spinal cord (includes explanation and examples of radiography, ultrasonography, computerized tomography, and magnetic resonance)
- Think Quest: Radiology
- University of Adelaide: Head injury (includes some excellent radiographic studies of the head)
- Virtual Hospital: Acute brain injury—a guide for family and friends
- Virtual Hospital: The human brain—dissections of the real brain
  For active weblinks to each website visit
  http://evolve.elsevier.com/Kinn/

CHAPTER 42

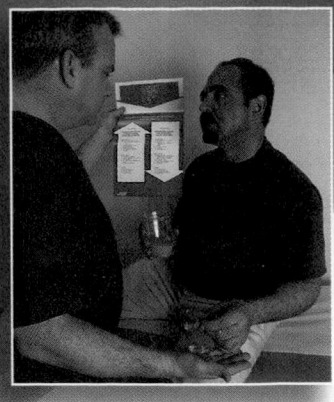

Scenario

Miguel Vasco has been a CMA for 10 years and is concerned about the number of patients diagnosed with type 2 diabetes mellitus. Miguel works in the clinical area for an internal medicine group practice. He assists the physicians in teaching newly diagnosed diabetic patients how to monitor their blood glucose levels and maintain healthy lifestyles.

Assisting in Endocrinology

Carole Stemple Zeglin
Deborah B. Kennedy

Learning Objectives

- Define and spell the terms listed in the vocabulary.
- Anatomically describe the endocrine system.
- Explain the mechanism of hormone action.
- Summarize the characteristics of common endocrine disorders.
- Compare and contrast type 1, type 2, and gestational diabetes mellitus.
- Outline the treatment plan and management of diabetes mellitus.
- Discuss the complications of diabetes mellitus.
- Summarize patient education approaches to diabetes.

National Curriculum Competencies

CLINICAL COMPETENCIES

4e. Prepare patients for and assist with routine and specialty examinations

4f. Prepare patients for and assist with procedures, treatments, and minor office surgery

4g. Apply pharmacology principles to prepare and administer oral and parenteral medications

TRANSDISCIPLINARY COMPETENCIES

1b. Recognize and respond to verbal communication

1c. Recognize and respond to nonverbal communication

3b. Instruct individual patients according to their needs

3d. Provide instruction for health maintenance and disease prevention

Vocabulary

adrenocorticotropic hormone (ACTH) A hormone that stimulates the production and secretion of glucocorticoids; released by the anterior pituitary gland.

follicle-stimulating hormone (FSH) A hormone secreted by the anterior pituitary; stimulates oogenesis and spermatogenesis.

gluconeogenesis The formation of glucose in the liver from proteins and fats.

glycogen The sugar (starch) formed from glucose and stored mainly in the liver.

glycosuria The abnormal presence of glucose in the urine.

growth hormone (GH) Also called somatotropic hormone; stimulates tissue growth and restricts tissue glucose dependence when nutrients are not available.

luteinizing hormone (LH) Hormone produced by the anterior pituitary gland; promotes ovulation.

nocturia Excessive urination during the night.

polydipsia Excessive thirst.

polyphagia Increased appetite.

polyuria Excessive urine production.

prolactin (PRL) Hormone secreted by the anterior pituitary gland; stimulates the development of the mammary gland.

specific gravity Weight of urine compared with an equal volume of water.

thyroid-stimulating hormone (TSH) A hormone secreted by the anterior pituitary gland that stimulates the secretion of hormones produced by the thyroid gland.

Individuals with endocrine system problems are usually seen first by their primary care physician (PCP) and may be referred to either an internist or endocrinologist for specialized care. Patients with certain endocrine disorders, such as diabetes mellitus (DM), may also be seen in clinic settings for follow-up and treatment. The medical assistant may be employed in any of these ambulatory care settings and may be responsible for assisting with diagnostic procedures and specialized examinations as well as patient education. It is important that the medical assistant understand the dynamics behind endocrine system diseases as well as be able to assist patients in understanding how to administer their own medication and prevent long-term complications from their disease.

Anatomy and Physiology of the Endocrine System

Both the nervous system and the endocrine system control the body's physiological responses. The nervous system is electrical in nature and sends immediate messages along a nerve pathway; the endocrine system relies primarily on the bloodstream to carry hormonal messages to a target cell for action. Through hormonal action, the endocrine system regulates all body functions. *Endocrinology* is the study of hormones, their receptor cells, and the results of hormone action.

The word part *endo-* means in or within; the suffix *-crine* means secrete. The endocrine system consists of glands located throughout the body that produce and secrete chemicals known as *hormones*. Hormones function as the body's chemical messengers, transferring information from one group of cells to another. Hormones control growth, mood, system functions, metabolism, sexual maturity, and reproduction. Hormone levels vary and can be affected by outside factors such as illness and stress.

Basic Anatomy

Glands are identified as either exocrine or endocrine. *Exocrine* glands, such as sweat glands and salivary glands, secrete either through a duct or directly onto the surface of the skin or in the mouth. *Endocrine* glands release hormones directly into the bloodstream, where they are transported to target cells for action.

The primary glands of the endocrine system are the hypothalamus, pituitary, thyroid, parathyroids, adrenals, and the reproductive glands, the ovaries, and the testes. Some nonendocrine organs, especially the pancreas, produce and release hormones (Figure 42-1). The hypothalamus, located in the inferior midportion of the brain, is the major connection between the nervous and endocrine systems. The hypothalamus controls the action of the pituitary gland, a pea-sized gland located below the hypothalamus. The pituitary gland is often called the "master gland" because it secretes hormones that regulate multiple endocrine glands.

The pituitary gland is separated into two parts: the anterior and posterior lobes. The anterior pituitary, or *adenohypophysis*, regulates the functions of the thyroid, adrenals, and reproductive glands. It produces **growth hormone (GH), thyroid-stimulating hormone (TSH), adrenocorticotropic hormone (ACTH), prolactin (PRL), follicle-stimulating hormone (FSH), and luteinizing hormone (LH)**. The posterior lobe of the pituitary, or *neurohypophysis*, excretes *oxytocin*, which stimulates the contractions of the smooth muscle of the uterus that occur during labor and the flow of breast milk toward the nipple when an infant breastfeeds. The posterior pituitary also produces antidiuretic hormone (ADH), which helps to control fluid balance by acting on the kidneys (Figure 42-2).

When stimulated by TSH, the thyroid gland produces thyroid hormones, triiodothyronine (T_3) and thyroxine (T_4), that control the body's metabolic rate and that are important factors in bone growth and nervous system development in children. On the dorsal aspect of the thyroid gland are the parathyroids, which release hormones (parathyroid and calcitonin) that regulate the level of calcium in the blood.

On the top of each kidney are the *adrenal glands*, triangular-shaped glands consisting of an outer layer called the *adrenal cortex* and an inner body called the *adrenal medulla*. The adrenal cortex secretes corticosteroid hormones, including cortisol, aldosterone, and adrenal androgens that influence a wide range of bodily functions. The adrenal medulla produces epinephrine, also called *adrenaline*, which stimulates the body's reaction to stress.

The *gonads* produce sex hormones. The male gonads are the *testes*; they secrete *testosterone*, which regulates the development of secondary sexual characteristics, such as voice changes and the growth of facial and pubic hair, and promotes the production of sperm. The female gonads, the *ovaries*, produce eggs or ovum (*oogenesis*) and secrete estrogen and progesterone. The female hormones control the development of breast tissue and other secondary sexual characteristics, regulate menstruation, and play important roles during pregnancy.

The pancreas performs essential endocrine functions by producing insulin and glucagon, which work together to maintain normal blood glucose levels and store glucose for energy.

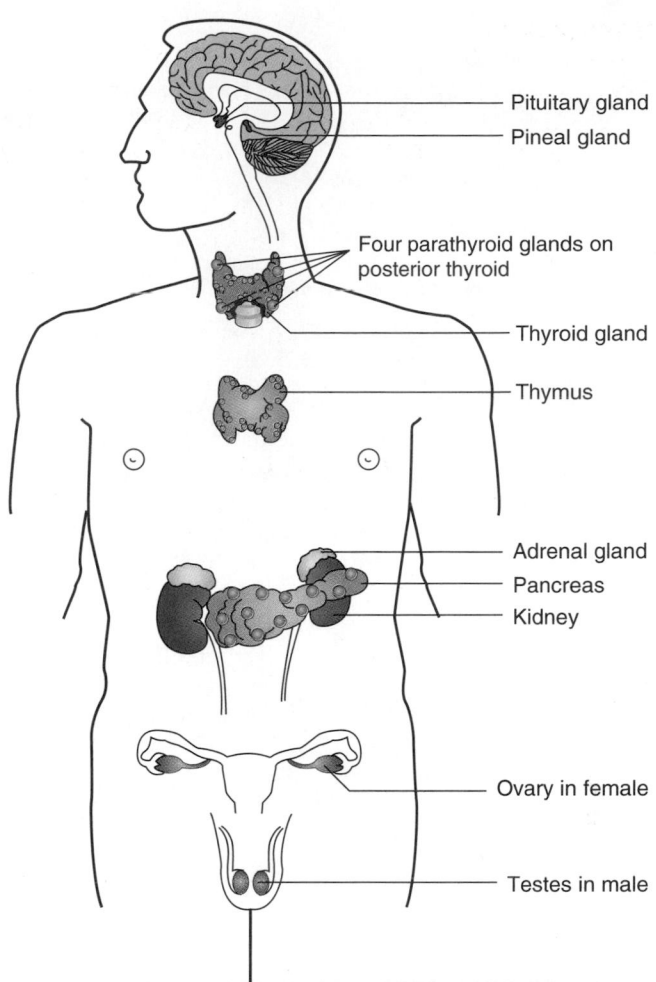

FIGURE 42-1 Location of the endocrine glands (From Gould: *Pathophysiology for the health professions*, ed 2. Philadelphia, 2002, WB Saunders.)

CRITICAL THINKING APPLICATION

Miguel is asked to order patient education supplies for patients with endocrine system disorders. Because he thinks it is important for patients to understand their health problems, he wants to order a brochure that clearly depicts and describes the anatomy of the endocrine system. What glands and organs should be included in the handout?

Mechanism of Hormonal Action

The goal of hormone regulation is to maintain homeostasis. Hormone secretion is regulated by a number of mechanisms, including nervous stimulation, endocrine control (a hormone from one gland, such as the anterior pituitary, stimulates the release of a hormone from another gland), and feedback systems. In the most common feedback system, negative feedback, an endocrine gland is activated by an imbalance and acts to correct the imbalance by stopping the secretion process. For example, if calcium blood levels fall below normal, the parathyroid glands are stimulated to release parathyroid hormone (PTH). PTH acts to increase blood calcium levels. This change in the blood calcium level is detected by the parathyroid gland, which then stops production of PTH. Each hormone that is released into the bloodstream has particular *target cells* for action. The target cells have receptors that attract only specific hormones and permit the hormone to pass through the cell membrane and affect cellular action.

Diseases and Disorders of the Endocrine System

Faulty secretion of any of the hormones, whether too much or too little, can cause health problems for patients. The goal of treatment is either to control the hypersecretion of hormones or to replace hormones that are not being secreted at therapeutic levels.

Posterior Pituitary Gland Disorder

Diabetes Insipidus. When antidiuretic hormone (ADH or *vasopressin*) is not produced or released in sufficient amounts, the patient develops a condition called *diabetes insipidus*. ADH increases the permeability of the renal tubules and collecting tubules in the kidneys, permitting fluid to be reabsorbed and causing the urine to become more concentrated. Without the action of ADH, fluid is not reabsorbed from the renal tubules and is excreted in the urine. A lack of ADH is due to either a tumor in the hypothalamus or posterior pituitary gland or diabetes insipidus may develop because of an inadequate response to ADH in the renal tubules.

The patient presents with **polyuria**, **polydipsia**, **nocturia**, low urine **specific gravity**, and high plasma osmolality (concentration). Diabetes insipidus can cause fatal dehydration if fluid and electrolyte levels cannot be controlled. Replacement therapy with a synthetic vasopressin (desmopressin) nasal spray can be used to treat the disorder.

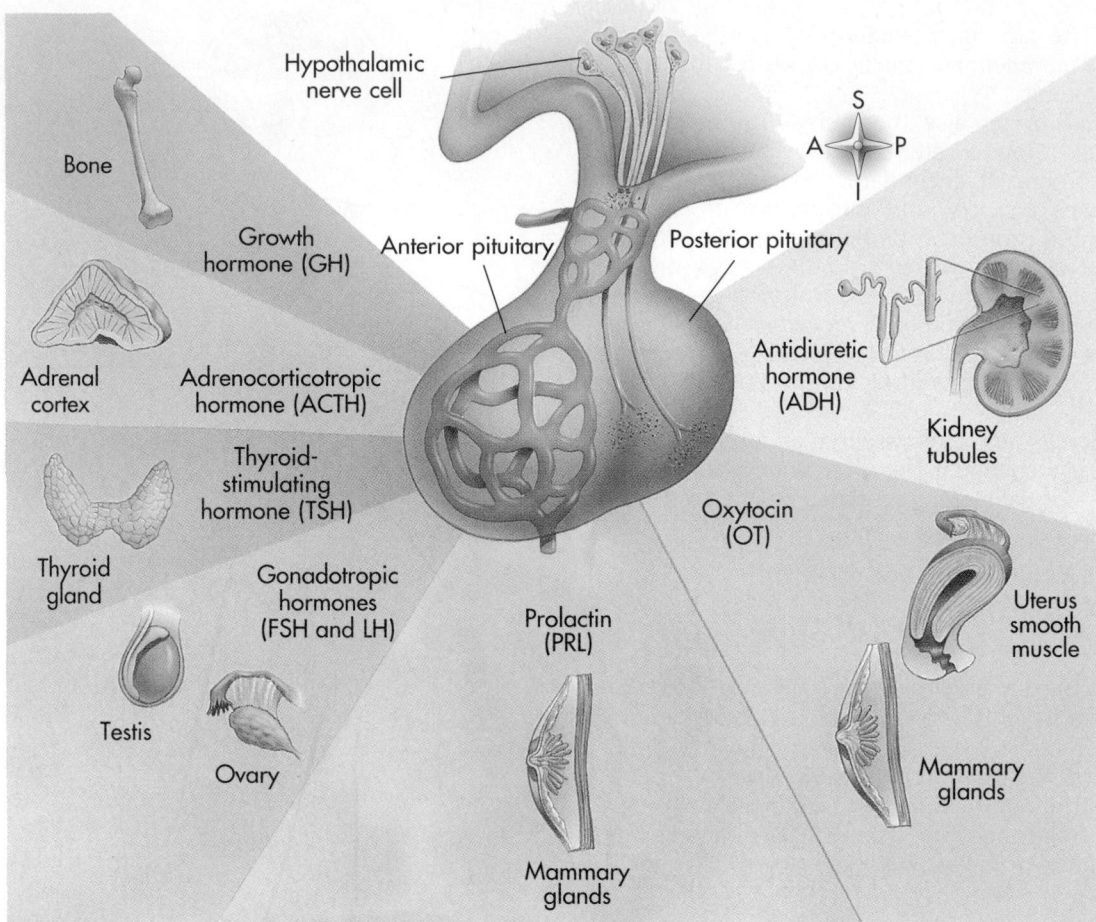

FIGURE 42-2 Pituitary hormones. Principal anterior and posterior pituitary hormones and their target organs. (From Thibodeau GA, Patton KT: *The human body in health and disease*, ed 3. St Louis, 2002, Mosby.)

Diseases of the Anterior Pituitary

Hormones secreted by the anterior pituitary control a number of glandular functions. The effects on the body to altered anterior pituitary gland secretions are dependent on whether the hormones are being produced at an abnormally low level (*hypopituitarism*) or if they are being produced at a very high level (*hyperpituitarism*). If a patient is diagnosed with *panhypopituitarism*, there is a deficiency of all of the hormones produced by the anterior pituitary; thus symptoms will reflect systemic inactivity of all of the glands stimulated by the anterior pituitary hormones.

Growth Hormone Abnormalities. *Hypopituitary dwarfism* occurs when the pituitary gland fails to produce normal amounts of GH. The child's height is impaired, but he or she will have a normal size head and trunk. Hypersecretion of GH causes two different disorders, depending on the developmental age of the patient. Oversecretion of GH in childhood before the epiphyseal plates in the long bones have closed will cause the long bones to grow excessively. Those affected may reach 8 feet or taller. Because GH has a secondary effect on the blood glucose level, these persons may develop DM. Slow-growing, benign adenomas are frequently the cause of gigantism, and treatment consists

of removing the tumor if possible, radiation therapy, or drug therapy.

If there is hypersecretion of GH in adulthood, the disorder is called *acromegaly*. The epiphyseal plates are closed so the long bones cannot grow. Therefore a wide range of manifestations can occur because of the growth of excessive connective tissue and overproduction of bone. Signs and symptoms include an enlarged tongue, overactive sebaceous and sweat glands, coarse skin, and excessive body hair. There is a gradual but noticeable enlargement in the bones of the jaw, face, hands, and feet (Figure 42-3). Advanced acromegaly causes complications such as congestive heart failure, DM, respiratory diseases, or cerebrovascular abnormalities. Treatment of acromegaly requires either surgical removal or irradiation of the pituitary tumor.

CRITICAL THINKING APPLICATION

Many different disorders can occur if there is a problem with the anterior pituitary. Describe two such health problems using your knowledge of target organ action.

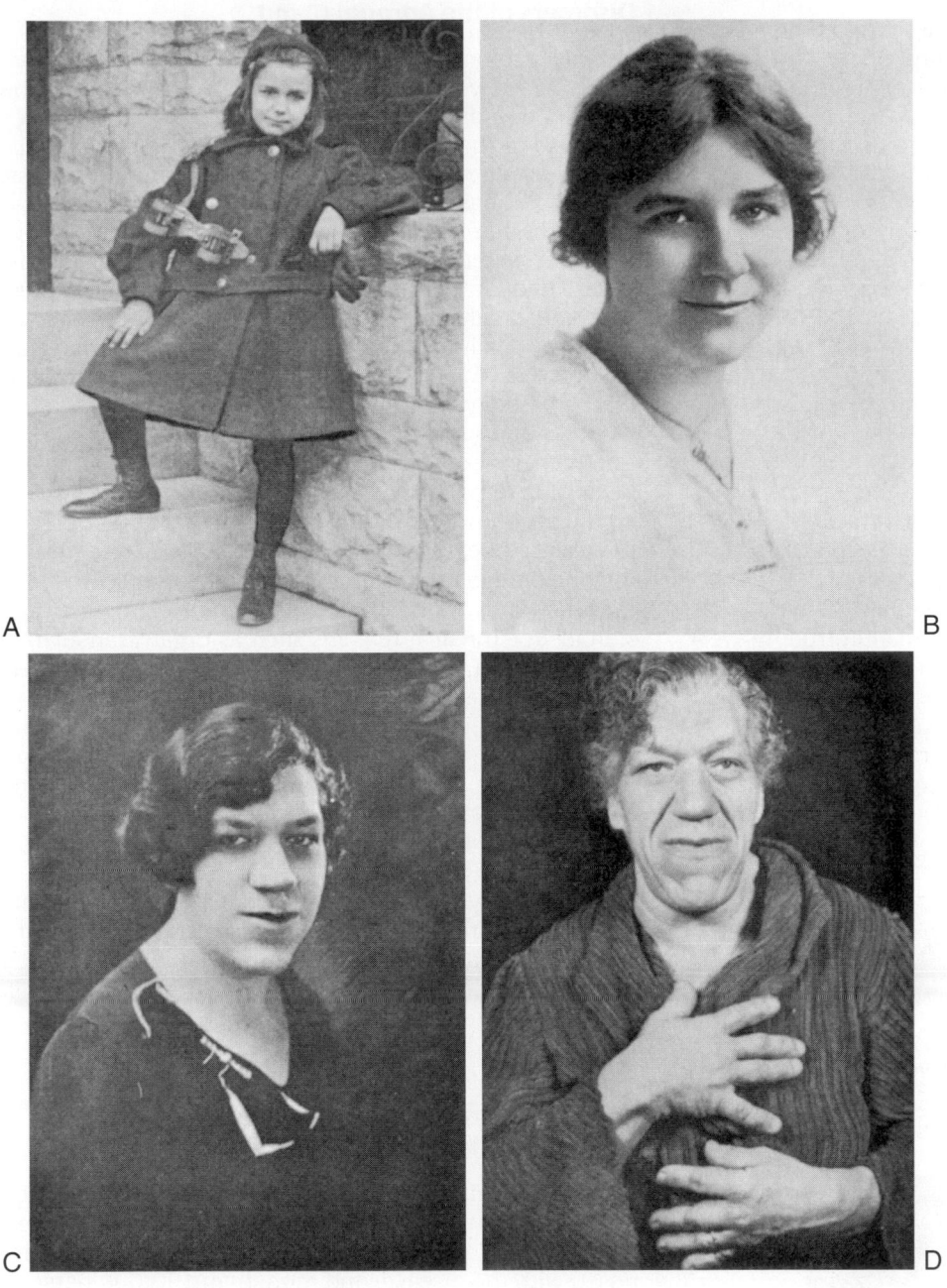

FIGURE 42-3   Progression of acromegaly. **A**, Patient at age 9 years. **B**, Patient at age 16 years, with possible early features of acromegaly. **C**, Patient at age 33, with well-established acromegaly. **D**, At age 52, end-stage acromegaly. (From Clinical Pathological Conference, *Am J Med* 20:133, 1956.)

Disorders of the Thyroid

Hypothyroidism. Deficient secretion of the thyroid hormones may be due to a number of factors. One cause of hypothyroidism is endemic iodine deficiency, a lack of iodine in the diet, resulting in the formation of a simple goiter. A *simple goiter* is any thyroid enlargement that has not been caused by an infection or neoplasm. Endemic goiters occur in certain geographic areas. If more than 10% of the children 6 to 12 years of age in a particular area have goiters, that geographic location is defined as *endemic* for goiters. T_3 and T_4 are produced in the thyroid gland from iodine and are responsible for the regulation of metabolic activities in all body cells. When the thyroid gland is unable to obtain sufficient amounts of iodine from the circulating blood, it enlarges or *hypertrophies*, in an attempt to produce the hormones needed by the body. A decreased amount of thyroid hormones results in a lower metabolic rate, heat loss, and poor mental and physical development. The incidence of iodine deficiency is rare in the United States because of the widespread use of iodized table salt and the distribution of foods from iodine-rich areas. The treatment for a goiter is to reduce its size by prescribing dietary supplements of iodine, thyroid hormone replacement, or surgery.

Improper development of the thyroid in an infant or young child is usually congenital. The absence of adequate levels of thyroid hormones results in a condition known as *cretinism*. Newborns exhibit feeding problems, constipation, sleeping for extreme lengths of time, and a hoarse cry. Symptoms include lethargy, bradycardia, stunted skeletal growth, and varying degrees of mental retardation, depending on the severity and the length of the hypothyroidism.

When severe or chronic hypothyroidism occurs in an adult or older child, the condition is called *myxedema*. The patient exhibits fatigue, weight gain, loss of hair, slower pulse rate, lowered body temperature, muscle cramps, menorrhagia, and thick, dry, puffy skin. Routine tests to diagnose hypothyroidism include radioimmunoassay, a radiologic blood test, for T_3, T_4, and TSH. Adequate doses of thyroxine (Levothroid, Levoxyl, or Synthroid) will restore normal function and appearance. Patients diagnosed with hypothyroidism must take hormone replacement therapy daily for the rest of their lives.

Hyperthyroidism. *Thyrotoxicosis*, a condition in which the serum levels of thyroid hormones are excessively high, can also be caused by a number of factors. Symptoms include weight loss, tachycardia, palpitations, hypertension, agitation, nervousness, depression, tremor, excessive sweating, goiter, and exophthalmia (protruding eyes). *Graves' disease*, an autoimmune disorder that stimulates overactive thyroid hormone production, is the most common cause of thyrotoxicosis (Figure 42-4). The goal of treatment is to control excessive thyroid hormone production through drug therapy (carbimazole, methimazole, and propylthiouracil), radiation to destroy part of the gland, or surgical removal of a section of the gland.

CRITICAL THINKING APPLICATION

One of the internists, Dr. Misha, asks Miguel if he could describe the signs and symptoms a patient with hypothyroidism or hyperthyroidism would exhibit. Summarize his answer.

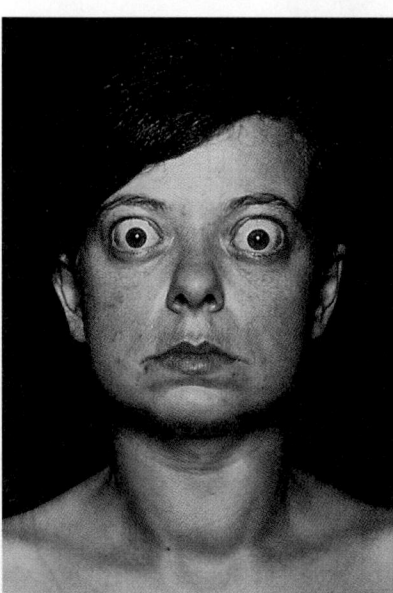

FIGURE 42-4 Exophthalmos in Graves' disease. (From Seidel H, et al: *Mosby's guide to physical examination*, ed 4. St Louis, 1998, Mosby.)

Disorders of the Adrenal Gland

Adrenal insufficiency is called *Addison's* disease. This condition is relatively rare and is caused by an autoimmune reaction that affects the adrenal cortex, which secretes corticosteroid hormones. Symptoms include hypoglycemia, increased pigmentation of the skin, muscle weakness, gastrointestinal disturbances, and fatigue. Cortisol and aldosterone deficiencies lead to retention of potassium and the excretion of water and sodium in the urine. Severe dehydration, low blood volume, low blood pressure, and circulatory shock can occur. Treatment includes long-term daily administration of glucocorticoids, an adequate fluid intake, maintaining a balance of sodium and potassium, and a diet high in complex carbohydrates and protein.

Hypersecretion of the adrenal cortex, causing increased levels of cortisol, is known as *Cushing's syndrome*. Usually a pituitary tumor or tumor of the adrenal cortex causes the release of excessive amounts of ACTH. These tumors may be benign or malignant. Cushing's symptoms also may be seen in persons who are receiving corticosteroids for medical reasons such as organ transplants, severe asthma, or rheumatoid arthritis. Excessive levels of cortisol cause an accumulation of adipose tissue in the trunk, a round or "moon" face, and fat pads in the cervical spine region, causing the formation of a "buffalo hump." The patient also exhibits glucose intolerance because of insulin resistance at the target cell level.

Additional symptoms include hyperpigmentation, muscle wasting, problems with wound healing, hypertension, kidney stones, and osteoporosis. Female patients exhibit menstrual irregularity, and many patients with Cushing's syndrome experience mental disorders such as irritability, depression, or severe psychiatric disorders. Treatment is dependent on the cause of the disorder but includes medication, radiation, and surgery.

Endocrine Dysfunction of the Pancreas: Diabetes Mellitus

Diabetes mellitus is a common hormonal imbalance that has reached epidemic proportions in the United States. About 17 million Americans have been diagnosed with the disease, and more than 190,000 persons die of it each year. DM is characterized by chronic hyperglycemia and problems with carbohydrate metabolism. This problem with glucose management is attributable to lack of insulin production and/or resistance to insulin at the target cell level. The pancreas contains *islets of Langerhans* that produce and secrete the hormones insulin and glucagon. Beta islet cells secrete insulin when the blood glucose level is too high. Insulin is sent through the bloodstream to the target tissue site to conduct glucose into the cell. Glucagon is secreted by the alpha islet cells when blood glucose levels are low, to stimulate the liver to convert glycogen (stored glucose) into circulating glucose.

Without insulin to help transport glucose from the blood into body cells or in the case of cellular resistance to insulin, an individual experiences various symptoms. Some of these symptoms are **glycosuria**, polyuria, polydipsia, **polyphagia**, rapid weight loss, drowsiness,

TABLE 42-1	Insulin Types and Characteristics		
Insulin Type	Onset of Action	Peak Action	Duration
Humalog (Lispro)	10-15 min	30-90 min	4 hr
Regular	30-60 min	2-4 hr	5 to 7 hr
NPH	60-120 min	6-14 hr	24 hr
Lente	60-180 min	6-14 hr	24 hr
Ultralente	6 hr	18-24 hr	36 hr
70:30 (70% NPH, 30% Regular)	70%: 60-120 min	70%: 6-14 hr	70%: 24 hr
	30%: 30-60 min	30%: 2-4 hr	30%: 5 to 7 hr

NPH, Neutral protamine Hagedorn.

fatigue, itching of the skin, visual disturbances, and skin infections. The American Diabetes Association identifies three major types of diabetes: type 1, type 2, and gestational diabetes. If left untreated or managed poorly, DM can have serious, life-threatening consequences such as cardiovascular disease, stroke, hypertension, blindness, kidney disease, nervous system disorders, amputations, pregnancy complications, and diabetic coma (Figure 42-5).

Prediabetes is a condition in which an individual has a higher than normal blood glucose level but not high enough for a diagnosis of type 2 diabetes. It is estimated that another 16 million Americans have prediabetes. Some of the long-term damage to the vascular and cardiac systems may start with prediabetes.

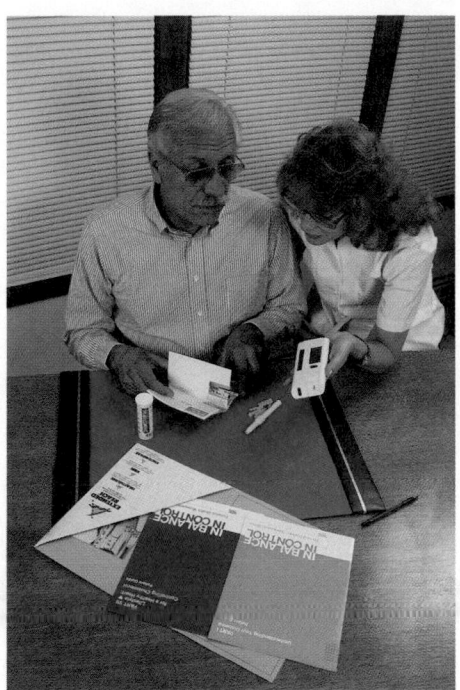

FIGURE 42-5 Educating patients about the risks of diabetes is an important part of the medical assistant's job.

DIAGNOSTIC CRITERIA FOR DIABETES MELLITUS

- Plasma glucose level of >200 mg/dl (norm is 80-120 mg/dl) with the classic symptoms of polyuria, polydipsia, and unexplained weight loss
- Fasting glucose level ≥126 mg/dl (norm is 70-110 mg/dl) on more than one occasion
- During an oral glucose tolerance test (OGTT), a 2-hour glucose level ≥200 mg/dl
- Urinalysis positive for glucose and possibly ketones
- Glycosylated hemoglobin >7% (normal range is 4%-6%)

Type 1 Diabetes. Type 1 diabetes most often develops before the age of 30 and was previously known as either juvenile-onset diabetes or insulin-dependent diabetes. In type 1, the pancreas is unable to produce insulin because of the destruction of the beta islet cells from autoimmune, genetic, or environmental factors. Type 1 diabetes typically has an acute onset and affects 5% to 10% of diabetic cases. Insulin administration is required for the treatment of type 1 diabetes. The goal for insulin therapy is to maintain blood glucose levels as close to normal levels as possible without causing hypoglycemia. Many types and brands of insulin are available, but only genetically engineered human insulin should be used to prevent allergic reactions. At this time, the only method for insulin administration is injection because gastroin-

testinal processes destroy insulin if it is given by mouth; however, multiple studies are in progress with oral, inhaled, and patch forms of the hormone. Subcutaneous administration of insulin was presented in Chapter 32. The medical assistant is usually involved in teaching patients how to administer their insulin accurately. Table 42-1 summarizes the various types of insulin.

ALTERNATIVE INSULIN ADMINISTRATION METHODS

- An insulin pump administers a constant dose of insulin using a small portable pump. The pump is computerized and programmed to deliver a measured dose of insulin by continuous subcutaneous infusion through a catheter. This method more closely resembles the body's normal surge of insulin and is designed to maintain blood glucose levels consistently within normal limits.

ALTERNATIVE INSULIN ADMINISTRATION METHODS—cont'd

• Insulin can be administered through an injector pen that comes in preloaded cartridges for easy use (Figure 42-6). Insulin pens are disposable or refillable and easily portable and so can be used by diabetic patients when they are away from home.

Successful type I diabetic treatment is a complicated combination of insulin injections using various types of insulin in multiple injections (as many as four) throughout the day. The insulin type and dosage are balanced by the patient's typical exercise regimen as well as diet. The patient must monitor blood glucose levels using a glucometer periodically during the day to determine whether they are within the normal range. The physician will typically prescribe glucometer testing in the morning before breakfast, before dinner, and possibly before lunch and bedtime if the patient is having difficulty keeping the levels stabilized. An important responsibility of the medical assistant is to teach the patient how to perform glucometer screening.

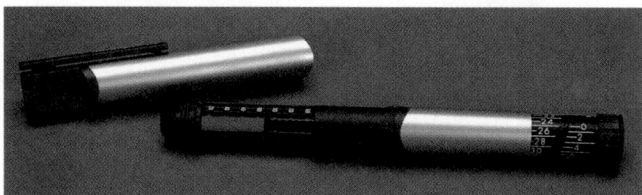

FIGURE 42-6 Nova Pen.

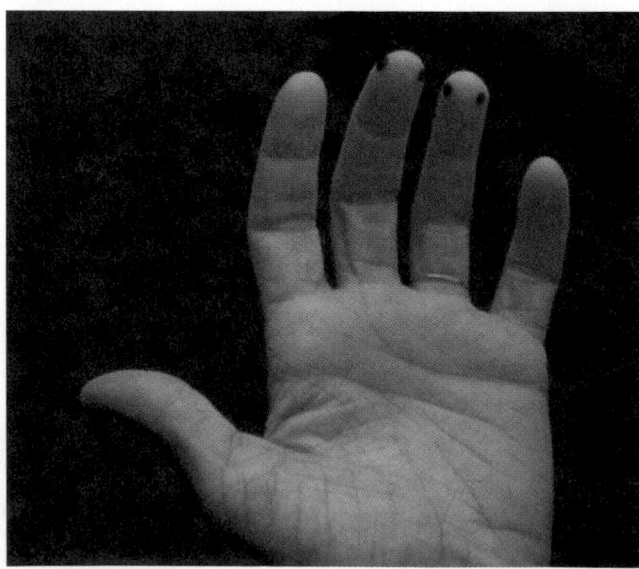

FIGURE 42-7 Capillary puncture sites on fingers.

Most glucometers are palm sized and use very small amounts of capillary blood from a site in the finger (Figure 42-7). Newly developed machines can extract a small amount of capillary blood from the forearm, and noninvasive glucose sensors may be available in the near future. Regardless of the type of glucometer, test results are displayed within seconds, and the results can be stored within most glucometers. The medical assistant should stress that the accuracy of blood glucose results depends on following the instructions for the particular type of glucometer used by the patient. It is important to use the same machine that the patient will use at home when teaching the patient about glucometer screening and to stress keeping a record of glucometer readings to determine long-term serum glucose control.

The patient education intervention should include not only the steps for successfully checking blood glucose levels but also quality control mechanisms as suggested by the manufacturer of the machine (Figure 42-8). Some examples of quality controls include:

• Correctly following the manufacturer's instructions
• Performing instrument maintenance specified by the manufacturer, including correctly cleaning and storage of the instrument
• Checking expiration dates on test strips and solutions and storing these products correctly
• Matching and correctly entering the test strip code into the instrument
• Contacting the physician if test results do not match patient symptoms

---

GLUCOMETER GUIDELINES

---

1. Clean and warm the testing site, usually a fingertip.
2. Obtain a drop of whole blood using a lancet or lancet pen.
3. Follow glucometer directions. The amount and method of blood sample placement vary with manufacturers. Some require a drop of blood to a test strip, whereas others aspirate the specimen using capillary action.
4. Allow the correct amount of time for determination of the glucose level in the specimen. Most glucometers have automatic timers and will display the results on completion.
5. Record the results in a log and, if prescribed by the physician, administer insulin if levels are elevated.
6. Clean and store the instrument according to manufacturer guidelines.

Diabetic patients also need to find the best method for disposal of their syringes and lancets. Local pharmacies or hospitals may offer assistance with disposal of used sharps. If the patient does not have access to a sharps return program, a puncture-resistant container

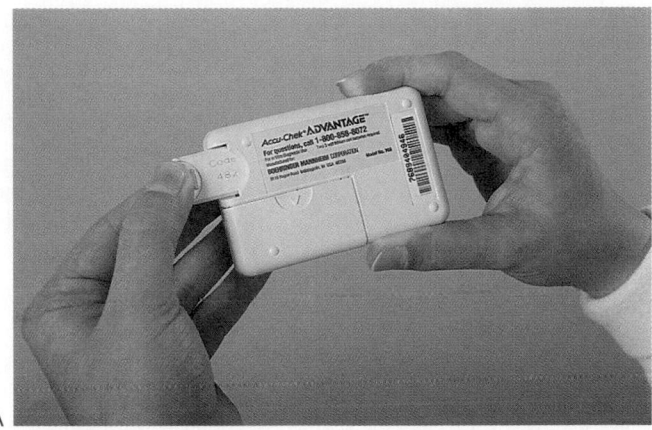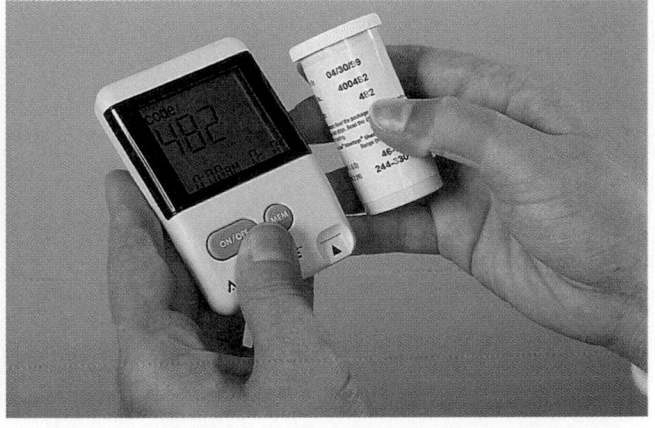

A   B

FIGURE 42-8   Accu-Check Advantage calibration procedure. **A**, The code key is inserted into the monitor. **B**, The code number must match the code number of the vial of reagent strips. (From Bonewit-West K: *Clinical procedures for medical assistants*, ed 5. Philadelphia, 2000, WB Saunders.)

with an opening that can be easily and tightly sealed before disposal is a good choice.

Regardless of the type of diabetes, for treatment to be successful, patients must play an active role in the management of their disease. The medical assistant should consistently encourage patients to be active participants in maintaining blood glucose levels within the normal range and constantly be on alert for possible complications from their disease.

Type 2 Diabetes.   Type 2 DM, once called adult-onset or non–insulin-dependent diabetes, usually develops in adults but may be seen at any age. Factors that increase the risk of developing type 2 DM include a family history, a history of gestational diabetes, impaired glucose tolerance, physical inactivity, and obesity. In this type, the pancreas produces insulin, but not enough, and/or the target cells are resistant to insulin action. Type 2 diabetes is responsible for 90% to 95% of the total cases of diabetes.

Treatment for type 2 diabetes includes weight loss, exercise, dietary restrictions, and oral hypoglycemic medications that act to stimulate insulin production and/or improve tissue response to insulin. Some common oral hypoglycemics are Diabinese, Prandin, Glucophage, Avandia, and Precose. Medications for type 2 diabetes have multiple functions, including stimulation of insulin secretion from pancreatic islet cells in type 2 diabetics with some pancreatic function; decreasing insulin resistance at the cellular level; improving sensitivity to insulin in muscle and adipose tissue; and inhibiting hepatic **gluconeogenesis**.

As with type 1 diabetes, the goal of treatment for type 2 is to maintain blood glucose levels within the normal range. For some patients, exercise, diet, and weight loss are sufficient to control blood glucose levels. Sometimes just the loss of 10 to 20 pounds is enough to bring blood glucose levels under control. Other patients may need medication to maintain normal blood levels; however, levels must be monitored daily with a glucometer to determine the success of treatment. Over time, the type 2 diabetic may require insulin for control of hyperglycemia. Table 42-2 summarizes the characteristics of hyperglycemia and hypoglycemia.

TABLE 42-2	Characteristics of Hyperglycemia and Hypoglycemia			
Disease	**Cause**	**Onset**	**Signs and Symptoms**	**Treatment**
Hyperglycemia: high serum glucose level	Too little insulin Body not able to use insulin properly Too many calories Not enough exercise Illness Stress	Rapid	Polyphagia, polyuria, glycosuria, ketonuria, weight loss, pruritus Possible ketoacidosis with shortness of breath, "fruity" breath, dry mouth, nausea and vomiting, lethargy	Exercise if blood glucose level below 240 mg/dl Decrease caloric intake Physician may alter amount and timing of insulin
Hypoglycemia: Low serum glucose level	Too much insulin Not enough calories Overexercise Type 2 diabetics using insulin-boosting medications	Slow	Shakiness, vertigo, palpitations, diaphoresis, headache, hunger, pallor, fatigue, confusion, irritability, poor judgment, Visual disturbances, seizures, coma	Ingest sugar; glucose tablets recommended Monitor blood levels in 15 to 20 minutes If still low and symptoms persist, take another glucose tablet. *If pass out*, physician can order injected glucagon. CALL FOR EMERGENCY SERVICES

CRITICAL THINKING APPLICATION

Carlos Vespa is a 47-year-old patient who was recently diagnosed with type 2 diabetes mellitus. He is 52 pounds overweight; eats a high-fat, high-carbohydrate diet; and does not exercise. What health issues should Miguel include in his patient teaching intervention? Carlos also tells Miguel he cannot afford the medication prescribed by the physician or the glucometer needed to monitor his blood glucose levels. Is there anything Miguel can do to help Carlos with these issues?

Gestational Diabetes. A pregnant female is diagnosed as having gestational diabetes if she has any two of the following: a fasting blood sugar (FBS) greater than 105 mg/dl; during an oral glucose tolerance test, a 1-hour glucose level greater than 190 mg/dl, a 2-hour glucose level greater than 165 mg/dl, or a 3-hour glucose level greater than 145 mg/dl. Gestational diabetes is considered a risk factor for developing type 2 DM later in life. Some factors that increase the risk of developing gestational diabetes are obesity; maternal age over 40 years; history of delivering infants who weigh more than 10 pounds at birth; a family history of diabetes; previous, unexplained stillbirth; previous birth with congenital anomalies; smokers; and certain ethnic groups, including Hispanics, Native Americans, Asian Americans, and blacks. Some women are asymptomatic, whereas others exhibit classic symptoms of diabetes. Because many pregnant women have gestational diabetes without obvious symptoms, all pregnant women are routinely screened between the 24th and 28th weeks. In obese women, a 30% calorie reduction will reduce hyperglycemia. Some women may require insulin to maintain blood glucose levels within therapeutic range and thereby decrease the possible complications for the fetus. Most women return to normal glucose tolerance postpartum. Because these women are at greater risk for developing type 2 diabetes later in life, patient education should stress weight management, a healthy diet, and regular exercise to maintain normal blood glucose levels.

Complications of Diabetes Mellitus

Acute Complications. There are two acute complications that can occur to diabetic patients, depending on the level of glucose in their bloodstream. If an adult patient's blood glucose level is below 45 to 60 mg/dl, the exhibited symptoms are caused by hypoglycemia. This reaction is related to insulin treatment and may also be called *insulin shock*. Symptoms are those shown with hypoglycemia in Table 42-2. The goal is to prevent such episodes with adequate patient education and reinforcement of individualized medical management of diabetes as well as frequent blood glucose monitoring. The treatment for hypoglycemia is immediate glucose replacement. The recommended form of sugar supplement is glucose tablets because each tablet contains a known amount of glucose. The patient can use other sugar supplements—such as candy, orange juice with sugar, or nondiet soft drinks—but the quantity of glucose in these items is unknown and the patient may actually become hyperglycemic from the ingestion of too much glucose. After the hypoglycemic crisis has ended, if the next meal is more than 1 hour away, the patient should have a mixed protein and carbohydrate snack (peanut butter crackers, cheese crackers) to maintain blood glucose levels until the next meal.

The more serious acute complication is *diabetic ketoacidosis*, or *diabetic coma*. In this case, the diabetic is unable to use glucose for energy because insulin is either absent or insufficient or there is resistance to insulin at the target cell site. Hyperglycemia results with blood glucose levels rising to 300 to 750 mg/dl. Because cells cannot use carbohydrates for energy, the body begins to burn fat. Ketones are waste materials from fat metabolism that build up in the bloodstream and cause it to become more acidic. Although the development of ketoacidosis takes longer than insulin shock, it can become a medical emergency if the patient does not recognize the signs, monitor his or her blood glucose level, and administer insulin as prescribed by the physician.

CRITICAL THINKING APPLICATION

Mr. Vespa returns to the office one week later and tells Dr. Misha he has not been feeling well. Sometimes he feels very shaky, dizzy, and tired; he has been getting headaches and cannot think straight. Dr. Misha orders a glucometer reading, which shows Mr. Vespa's blood glucose level at 65. Dr. Misha's diagnosis is hypoglycemic episodes and asks Miguel to reinforce patient teaching about hypoglycemic and hyperglycemic signs and symptoms as well as treatment. What should Miguel include in the teaching intervention? How can he best reinforce the material so that Mr. Vespa will remember how to manage his disease?

Chronic Complications

MICROVASCULAR DISEASE. Arterial changes at the capillary level can occur within 1 to 2 years of the onset of DM. Hyperglycemic episodes combined with the duration of the disease cause degeneration of tissue arterioles, which results in multiple system disorders, including *diabetic retinopathy*. Diabetes is a leading cause of new blindness in people 20 to 74 years of age and is often a result of 8 to 10 years of diabetes. Ninety percent of patients with type 1 diabetes and 65% of patients with type 2 diabetes will develop retinopathy.

Hyperglycemic episodes damage the blood vessels in the retina; therefore close glucose control helps delay the onset of retinopathy and slows its progression. The disturbances of vision occur from vascular changes in the capillaries of the retina. These complications can lead to retinal detachment and blindness. The diabetic should receive yearly eye screenings and frequent ophthalmologic examinations during routine office visits for early diagnosis of diabetic retinopathy.

Microvascular disease can also cause *diabetic nephropathy*. Kidney disease is present in 10% to 21% of all diabetic persons and is the most common cause of kidney failure in the United States. Diabetic kidney disease is the greatest threat to life in adults with type 1 diabetes. Diabetes damages the small blood vessels in the kidneys and impairs their ability to filter waste from blood. Degenerative changes cause destruction of the glomerular unit and can lead to renal failure. High blood pressure and smoking often are associated with diabetic nephropathy. Because urinary protein is usually the first sign of kidney damage, frequent testing for albuminuria is suggested. Early treatment reduces the progression of kidney disease. Good glucose control can often reverse the early stages of diabetic nephropathy. With disease progression, renal failure may occur, resulting in the need for dialysis and possible kidney transplant.

MACROVASCULAR DISEASE. Macrovascular disease, in the form of atherosclerosis, is a serious health issue for all diabetic patients, especially those with type 2 DM. Persons who have diabetes are two to four times more likely to have atherosclerotic heart disease or strokes. Coronary artery disease (CAD) is the most common cause of death for those with type 2 diabetes. Patients most affected are women at or before middle age. The longer the patient has had diabetes, the greater the risk for CAD. Cerebrovascular accidents (CVA, or strokes) occur twice as frequently in diabetic compared with nondiabetic patients. Hypertension is common in diabetic persons and contributes to the CAD and CVA rates.

Peripheral vascular disease (PVD), a disease process in blood vessels outside the heart, is associated with atherosclerotic changes in small arteries and arterioles and contributes to the incidence of gangrene and amputations in diabetic patients. Patients with type 2 diabetes frequently have signs and symptoms of PVD when first diagnosed. Compromised circulation in the lower extremities causes the formation of ulcers, poor wound healing, and possible progression to gangrene. This progression of PVD may result in amputation of the toes, foot, or leg. Blockage of blood vessels can lead to impotence in diabetic men. About 13% of men with type 1 and 8% of men with type 2 diabetes have impotence from diabetic vascular disease.

DIABETIC NEUROPATHY. Diabetic neuropathy is the most common complication of diabetes, with 60% to 70% of persons with diabetes experiencing some form of diabetic nerve damage. This type of nerve damage is caused by both vascular changes and hyperglycemia. The chief areas that exhibit pathology are the nerves and blood vessels in the eyes, kidneys, legs, and feet. The first signs of diabetic neuropathy are usually numbness, pain, or tingling in the hands, feet, or legs. The loss of sensation in the extremities is important because it affects the patient's ability to be aware of injuries, especially to the feet. Because of peripheral

vascular compromise, foot injuries can develop into ulcers or lesions that can become infected and ultimately lead to gangrene and amputation (Figure 42-9). Even a minor undetected injury, such as a foot blister, can lead to a serious problem for the diabetic patient. Diabetic individuals may also lose temperature sensation and so are more susceptible to heat or cold injuries such as burns and frostbite (Figure 42-10). Diabetic patients should have their feet inspected at every visit to promote early detection and treatment of problems. Healthcare providers should provide verbal

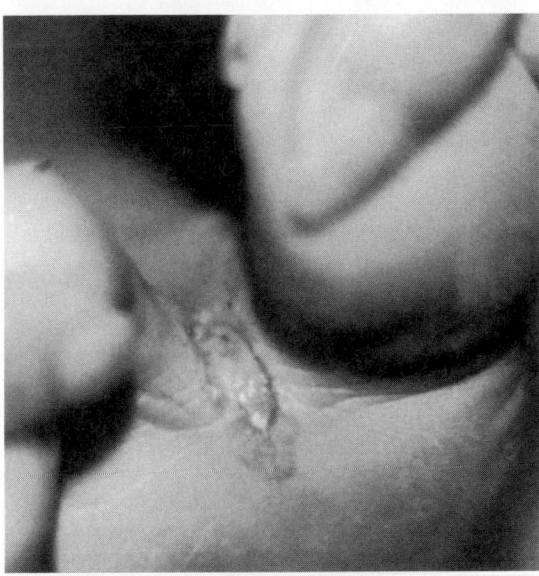

FIGURE 42-9 Ulceration between toes from wearing thong sandals. (From Levin ME: Pathogenesis and general management of foot lesions in the diabetic patient. In Bowker JH, Pfeifer MA, editors: *Levin and O'Neal's the diabetic foot*, ed 6. Mosby, 2001, St Louis.)

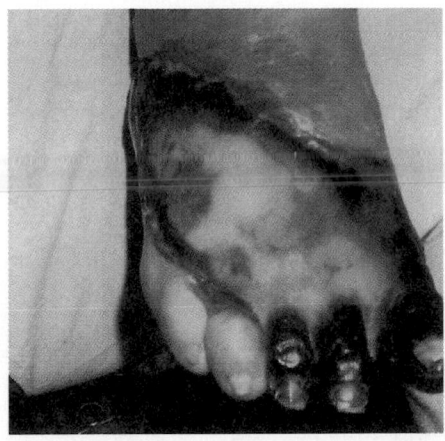

FIGURE 42-10 Diabetic patient with peripheral neuropathy and an insensate foot. Cold packs were applied to the patient's foot for treatment of a sprain. Frostbite developed, and the patient required a transmetatarsal amputation. (From Levin ME: Pathogenesis and general management of foot lesions in the diabetic patient. In Bowker JH, Pfeifer MA, editors: *Levin and O'Neal's the diabetic foot*, ed 6. Mosby, 2001, St Louis.)

and written advice to help prevent or reduce these potentially serious injuries.

DIABETIC FOOT CARE

Diabetic patients need instruction about foot hygiene and foot inspection during *each* visit. Education guidelines should include:

- Wash the feet every day with warm (not hot) water and mild soap.
- Cut nails straight across to avoid ingrown toenails and possible injuries.
- Apply lotion to the feet, especially the heels. If the skin is cracked or red, speak to your doctor.
- Check your feet every day, using a mirror if necessary. Call your doctor at the first sign of redness, swelling, or numbness.
- Speak with your doctor before treatment of corns, calluses, or bunions.
- Do not go barefoot or allow your feet to get too hot or cold.
- Check shoes for foreign objects or rough areas before wearing them.
- Wear comfortable, well-fitting shoes.
- Stop smoking. Smoking causes vasoconstriction, which decreases circulation to the extremities.

INFECTION. All diabetic patients are at increased risk for infection because of a number of different factors. Those with impaired vision and neuropathies have an increased risk of injury because they may not be able to see or feel potentially dangerous items to prevent injury. Once an injury does occur and the integrity of the skin has been compromised, damaged or atherosclerotic blood vessels are unable to deliver the blood needed for healing, and the thickened blood vessel walls impede the release of white blood cells (WBCs) to the area. The WBCs of diabetic patients exhibit reduced phagocytosis, and so their ability to destroy pathogens is limited. In addition, some pathogens multiply rapidly in the glucose-rich environment of diabetic patients. Therefore the best method of controlling infections in diabetic patients is to prevent skin trauma or damage.

CRITICAL THINKING APPLICATION

Mr. Vespa and his wife are scheduled for a long visit today so Dr. Misha can review his treatment plan. Dr. Misha asks Miguel to reinforce the possible complications of diabetes mellitus and criteria for foot care. What should Miguel include in his teaching intervention? How he make sure Mr. and Mrs. Vespa understand the disease, its management, and possible complications?

Diabetic Patient Follow-Up

Experts agree that the best method for prevention of diabetic complications is to maintain blood glucose levels consistently at near-normal ranges. Several laboratory tests can be ordered to monitor patient blood glucose levels. A test that measures the glucose levels in a blood specimen from a fasting individual is an FBS test. Often the test is referred to as an FPG (fasting plasma glucose) and requires a 12-hour fast. The normal range established for fasting plasma glucose is 70 to 110 mg/dl. Even though the physician may order periodic FBS tests, both type 1 and type 2 diabetic patients need to check their blood glucose levels as ordered using home glucometer devices.

A routine test for monitoring long-term diabetes therapy is the glycosylated hemoglobin (HbA_{1C}) test. This test has distinct advantages over routine FBS studies because the FBS reflects glucose levels at a given point in time, whereas the glycosylated hemoglobin test can be drawn every 6 to 8 weeks and reflects serum glucose control over several months. The test measures glucose levels that have been chemically bound to the hemoglobin molecule on the red blood cell (RBC) over a 120-day period (the lifespan of an RBC). The physician can then assess average daily glucose levels over this period. The patient does not need to restrict food or fluid intake for this test and should continue to take prescribed medication before the blood sample is drawn. The patient's total glycosylated hemoglobin level should be as close to a range of 5.5% to 9% as possible. The higher the glycosylated hemoglobin result, the higher the risk that a patient will develop diabetic complications.

Developing a Diabetic Patient Education Plan. Although newly diagnosed persons with diabetes need to be aware of the details and possible complications of their disease, they also need to be informed that a change in diet can be made without disrupting their daily routine. Information regarding diabetes and the need for glucose control must be reinforced at every patient visit. Community resources such as referral to a dietitian for meal planning or a support group may be helpful (Figure 42-11). The medical assistant can research various websites and suggest that these be explored. Other areas that need to be considered are personal and family needs, social activities, typical daily routine, and the individual's medical history.

DIABETIC PATIENT EDUCATION

- Diabetic patients need to understand that physical activity, stress, the presence of disease, medication, and diet all combine to affect blood glucose levels. Having a dietary plan is one step toward self-management.
- The diabetic patient needs to establish a desirable body weight. The medical assistant measures the patient's weight and height

DIABETIC PATIENT EDUCATION—cont'd

and should reinforce the desired weight according to body mass index (BMI) scales and physician recommendations. The medical assistant can supply information about basic nutritional requirements needed either to help the individual maintain his or her ideal body weight or to lose weight.

- The goal of a diet plan is to help maintain a homeostatic blood glucose level. If a healthy blood glucose level is maintained, the patient will avoid complications that can develop with hypoglycemia or hyperglycemia. Basic guidelines considering the person's ethnic influences, age, sex, and physical activity are used to establish a therapeutic meal plan. (Refer to Chapter 27 for meal planning.) Family members should be involved in dietary health teaching and appropriate community resources, such as a registered dietician, should be used to assist with patient understanding and compliance.
- Medical management of diabetes can be quite complicated and overwhelming for many patients. Type 2 diabetics who are prescribed oral hypoglycemics must understand their mechanism of action and accurate dosage. Type 1 and type 2 diabetic patients who require daily insulin must be able to prepare and administer their medication accurately and understand the connection between glucometer readings and insulin dosage. All diabetic patients must be capable of accurate glucometer use and must be aware of the possible complications of their disease.

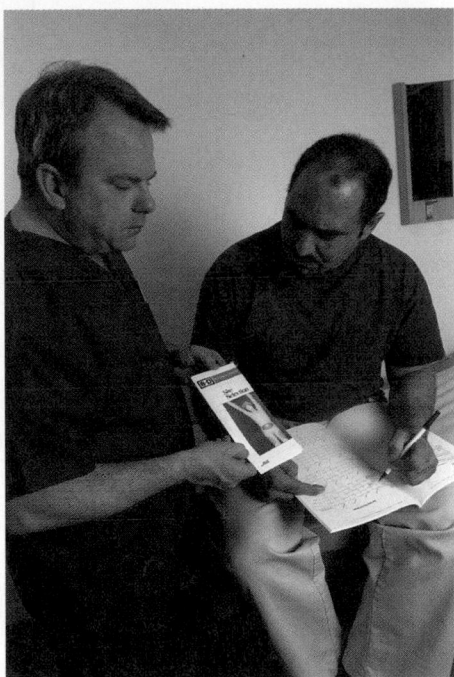

FIGURE 42-11   The medical assistant can use premade education materials to discuss new lifestyle habits with a diabetic patient.

Patient Education

Because patient management of endocrine disorders can be quite complicated, the medical assistant must be certain the patient understands the proper procedures of at-home treatment. By demonstrating a given procedure in the office, the medical assistant can address any inaccurate information or answer any questions the patient may have. Visual materials, such as brochures and procedure cards, are also helpful because they can be taken from the office and used as a reminder. If the patient is taking medication, the medical assistant should review the dosage schedule with the patient, discuss the purpose of the treatment, and clarify any confusion over the physician's instructions. As always, if the medical assistant is uncertain of any procedures or information, he or she should ask the physician for assistance before explaining anything to the patient.

Legal and Ethical Issues

Pathophysiology of the endocrine system can have wide-reaching effects on the functioning of the affected patient. Patient education interventions should be completely documented to have legal proof of the information shared with the patient. Never assume that the patient understands the disease process and treatment recommendations. Suggestions that ensure patient welfare and promote risk management include:

- Advise patients that a medic alert bracelet with his or her diagnosis and medication information is an important safeguard.
- Patients must take medication as prescribed, following directions for dosage, route of administration, and storage and being alert for possible side effects.
- Newly diagnosed diabetic persons should avoid driving until glycemic control is stabilized and should be warned about possible visual impairment from the disease.
- Remember that you are always representing your profession and employer, and respond to each situation accordingly.
- Ask for assistance or further information if you feel unprepared to perform the procedure or to give accurate information.

SUMMARY OF SCENARIO

In his interactions with clients, Miguel has learned to pay attention to both verbal and nonverbal messages. He has used this technique consistently when interacting with Mr. Vespa. Miguel recognizes the complexity of endocrine system disorders and the importance of understanding the anatomy and physiology of the system as well as the most frequently seen endocrine disorders. As a concerned medical assistant, Miguel continues to read professional journals and attend workshops so that he is prepared to answer questions from clients. He is especially interested in diabetes mellitus because there are so many diabetic patients in the internal medicine practice where he works. Miguel never hesitates to ask the attending physicians questions about the disease and its management.

SUMMARY OF LEARNING OBJECTIVES

■ The endocrine system consists of glands located throughout the body that produce and secrete chemicals known as hormones. The primary glands of the endocrine system are the hypothalamus, pituitary, thyroid, parathyroids, adrenals, and the reproductive glands of the ovaries and the testes. Some nonendocrine organs, especially the pancreas, produce and release hormones. Through hormonal action, the endocrine system regulates all body functions.

■ Hormones are chemical transmitters produced by the body and transported to target tissue by the bloodstream. Hormone secretion is regulated by a number of mechanisms, including nervous stimulation, endocrine control, and feedback systems. Each hormone that is released into the bloodstream has particular target cells for action.

■ Hypersecretion or hyposecretion of hormones can cause endocrine disorders. When ADH is not produced or released in sufficient amounts, the patient develops a condition called diabetes insipidus. Gigantism and acromegaly are both diseases of the pituitary gland involving the GH.

When this condition affects children, gigantism is the result; in adults, acromegaly causes excessive growth of the facial area and extremities. Deficient secretion of thyroid hormone may be due to an endemic iodine deficiency resulting in a simple goiter. Improper development of the thyroid in an infant or young child causes cretinism; in an adult or older child, the condition is called myxedema. Adrenal cortex insufficiency is called Addison's disease. Hypersecretion of the adrenal cortex, causing increased levels of cortisol, is known as Cushing's syndrome.

■ Type 1 diabetes usually develops before the age of 30 and is characterized by a complete absence of insulin production. Patients must receive daily injections of insulin to survive. Type 2 diabetes develops gradually because of an insufficient amount of insulin or resistance at the target cell site or both. Gestational diabetes occurs in some pregnancies but typically resolves itself after the infant is born. Affected women may need insulin therapy for glucose metabolism.

■ All diabetic patients must monitor their blood glucose levels on a regular basis to determine the effectiveness of treatment. The treatment of DM is an interaction between exercise, therapeutic diet, weight control, and medication, with emphasis on maintaining serum glucose at a near-normal level. Type 1 diabetic patients require daily injections of a combination of insulins. Type 2 and gestational diabetic patients may be prescribed oral hypoglycemics or insulin if needed.

■ Complications of DM include hypoglycemia; hyperglycemia and diabetic coma; diabetic neuropathy; microvascular diseases, including diabetic retinopathy and nephropathy; macrovascular diseases such as atherosclerosis, CAD, CVA, and PVD; and decreased resistance to infection.

■ Patient education for diabetic patients is an intricate mix of information on the dynamics of the disease; the importance of exercise, diet, and weight control in preventing disease complications and maintaining health; an understanding of the various types of insulin and when and how they should be administered; knowledge about oral medications for type 2 diabetes, their side effects and dosage; home care management including proper use of glucometers and insulin administration; prevention of complications through effective control of blood glucose levels; proper foot care; and monitoring and immediately contacting the physician about infections or disease.

KEY INTERNET WEBSITES

- American Diabetes Association
- Society for Endocrinology
- The Endocrine Society
- The National Library of Medicine
  For active weblinks to each website visit
  http://evolve.elsevier.com/Kinn/

← Diet

CHAPTER 43

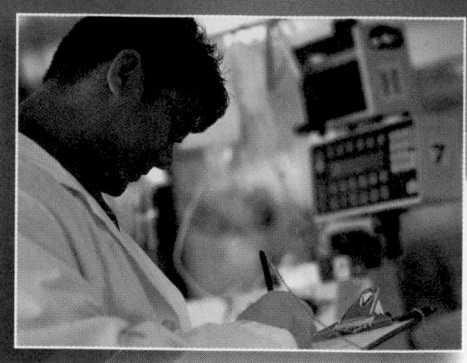

Scenario

Michael McGuire, CMA, works for a primary care physician, Dr. John Samuelson, in the small town in which he grew up. Dr. Samuelson's practice is open to all patients, but there are a large number of individuals with respiratory disease who seek his help in managing their illnesses. Michael has learned in the 6 months since he started to work in the practice how to assist with pulmonary diagnostic tests and how to interact with patients who have respiratory disease.

Assisting in Pulmonary Medicine

Learning Objectives

- Define and spell the terms listed in the vocabulary.
- Describe the organs of the respiratory system and their functions.
- Explain the process of ventilation.
- Employ correct respiratory system terminology in documentation procedures.
- Compare and contrast infections and inflammations of the respiratory system.
- Summarize disorders associated with chronic obstructive pulmonary disease and their treatments.
- Describe cancers associated with the respiratory system.
- Detail common respiratory system diagnostic procedures.
- Demonstrate patient teaching for the use of a peak flow meter and metered-dose inhaler.
- Perform a nebulizer treatment.
- Prepare a patient for pulmonary function testing.
- Obtain an accurate volume capacity spirometric test.
- Correctly employ a pulse oximeter.
- Prepare a patient to collect a sputum sample for culture.

National Curriculum Competencies

CLINICAL COMPETENCIES

4a. Perform telephone and in-person screening

4e. Prepare patients for and assist with routine and specialty examinations

4f. Prepare patients for and assist with procedures, treatments, and minor office surgery

4g. Apply pharmacology principles to prepare and administer oral and parenteral medications

TRANSDISCIPLINARY COMPETENCIES

3b. Instruct individuals according to their needs

3d. Provide instruction for health maintenance and disease prevention

Vocabulary

bronchiectasis Dilation of the bronchi and bronchioles associated with secondary infection or ciliary dysfunction.

chronic bronchitis Recurrent inflammation of the membranes lining the bronchial tubes.

clubbing Abnormal enlargement of the distal phalanges (fingers and toes), associated with cyanotic heart disease or advanced chronic pulmonary disease.

pulmonary consolidation Process of the lungs becoming solidified as they fill with exudates in pneumonia.

tracheostomy Surgical opening through the neck into the trachea for breathing.

virulent Exceedingly pathogenic, noxious, or deadly.

The respiratory system has two primary functions. The first is to exchange oxygen from the atmosphere for carbon dioxide waste. There are two types of respiration: external respiration brings oxygen into the lungs, where carbon dioxide exchange occurs in the blood vessels surrounding the alveoli, and internal respiration is when oxygen is exchanged for carbon dioxide at the cellular level. Cells soon stop functioning and die if they are deprived of oxygen. The second function of the lungs is maintaining the acid-base balance within the body. Failure of this function may result in respiratory acidosis or alkalosis. The respiratory system and the circulatory system work together to supply body cells with oxygen and remove metabolic wastes. The ventilation process is controlled by the respiratory center in the central nervous system and assisted by costal and diaphragm muscles.

PRECONDITIONS FOR NORMAL RESPIRATION

- An open airway leading to the lungs
- Ability of the lungs to expand rhythmically
- Intact alveolar membranes
- Coordination of the intercostal muscles and the diaphragm
- Proper action of the central nervous system's respiratory control center

---

The Respiratory System

The thoracic cage, sometimes called the *rib cage*, is a bony structure that is narrower at the top and wider at the base. It is held in place by the thoracic vertebrae of the spine in the center of the back and the sternum in the center of the anterior aspect of the body. The first seven ribs attach directly to the sternum and are called the *true ribs*. Ribs 8, 9, and 10 fasten one to another, forming the false ribs, and ribs 11 and 12 are the "floating" ribs, or half ribs, because their only attachment is to the thoracic vertebrae. At the base or floor of the rib cage is the diaphragm, a musculotendinous membrane that divides the thoracic cavity and the abdominal cavity (Figure 43-1). The respiratory system is divided into two anatomical regions, the upper and lower tracts.

The Upper Respiratory Tract

The upper respiratory tract, which transports air from the atmosphere to the lungs, includes the nose, pharynx (throat), and larynx (Figure 43-2). As air enters the nasal cavity, it is cleaned by the cilia, warmed by capillary blood vessels, and moistened by mucous membranes. The paranasal sinuses, hollow cavities that are also lined with mucous cells and cilia, open into the nasal cavity. The filtered, warmed, and moistened air moves through the pharynx and past the tonsils, which have an immunity function and help defend the body from potential pathogens. As the air continues toward the lungs, it passes through the larynx. The opening into the larynx is protected by a moveable piece of cartilage, the epiglottis. The larynx, or voice box, is made up of vocal cords, which vibrate when air is exhaled creating the sound of the voice. Once the air passes through the larynx, it enters the lower respiratory tract.

The Lower Respiratory Tract

The lower respiratory tract consists of the trachea, bronchial tubes, and lungs (see Figure 43-2). These structures are also lined with mucous tissue that is covered with cilia. The collection of dust and foreign particles in the cilia initiates the coughing reflex, aiding in expectorating mucus, which may contain possible pathogens. Without these defense mechanisms, pathogens would remain in the lungs, potentially causing disease. Cigarette smoke and other air pollutants slow down or paralyze the cleansing action of the cilia and damage the mucous membrane lining throughout the respiratory tract.

The trachea (windpipe) is a tube that begins at the larynx and extends into the center of the chest, where it divides or *bifurcates* into the right and left bronchi. It is about 5 inches long and is surrounded by C-shaped cartilaginous rings. The open area between the edges of the cartilage allows the esophagus to enlarge when food is swallowed. These rings hold the trachea open regardless of the air pressure changes exerted.

When the trachea bifurcates, it forms the right and left bronchi. It is often said that the bronchial tubes look like a tree hanging in the chest (Figure 43-3). The right bronchus is wider than the left to accommodate the right lung lobes, which are also larger. This means that foreign substances are more frequently seen in the right bronchus. Once the bronchi enter the lungs, they branch into smaller and smaller passageways, much as the vessels do in the circulatory system. This branching continues until it becomes microscopic. These very tiny bronchi are called *bronchioles*. Every tiny bronchiole terminates into microscopic air sacs called *alveoli*. The alveoli are made of thin tissue, only one cell wall thick, which allows the exchange of oxygen and carbon dioxide through the cell wall.

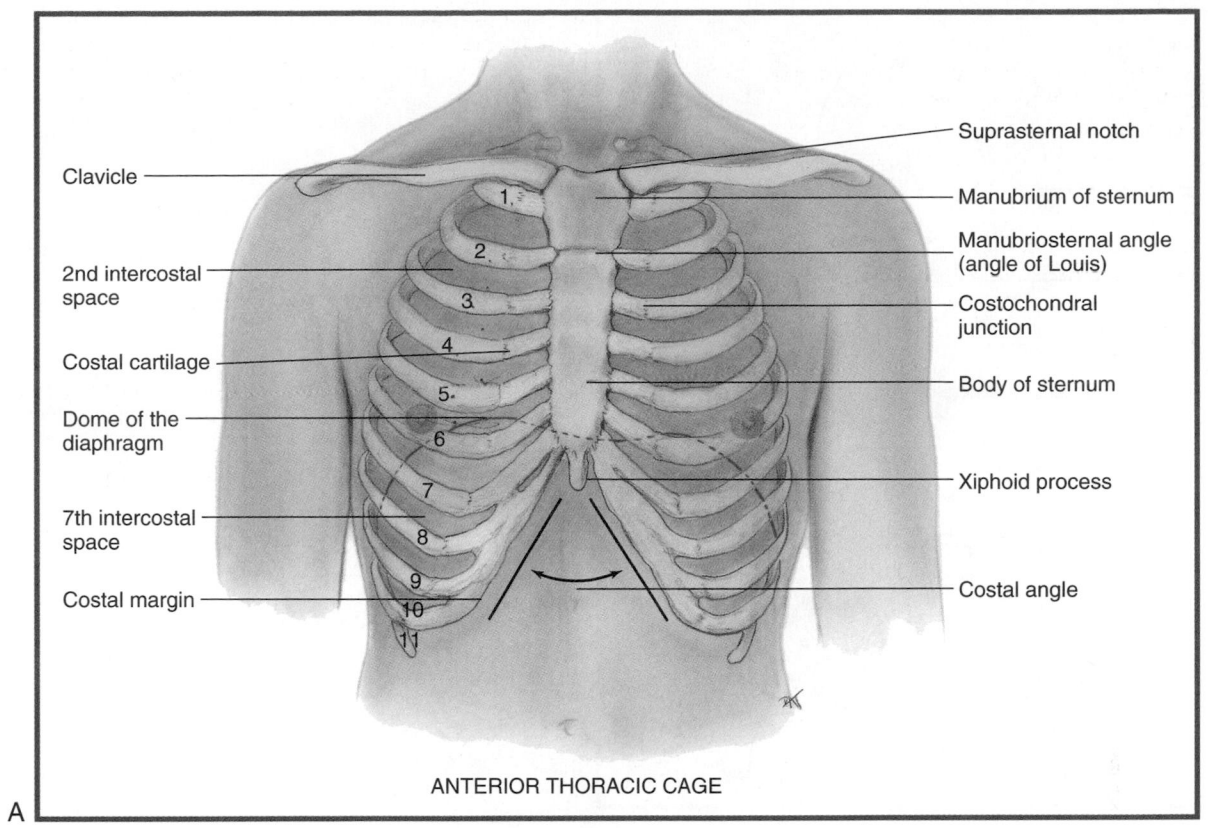

Clavicle

2nd intercostal space

Costal cartilage

Dome of the diaphragm

7th intercostal space

Costal margin

Suprasternal notch

Manubrium of sternum

Manubriosternal angle (angle of Louis)

Costochondral junction

Body of sternum

Xiphoid process

Costal angle

ANTERIOR THORACIC CAGE

A

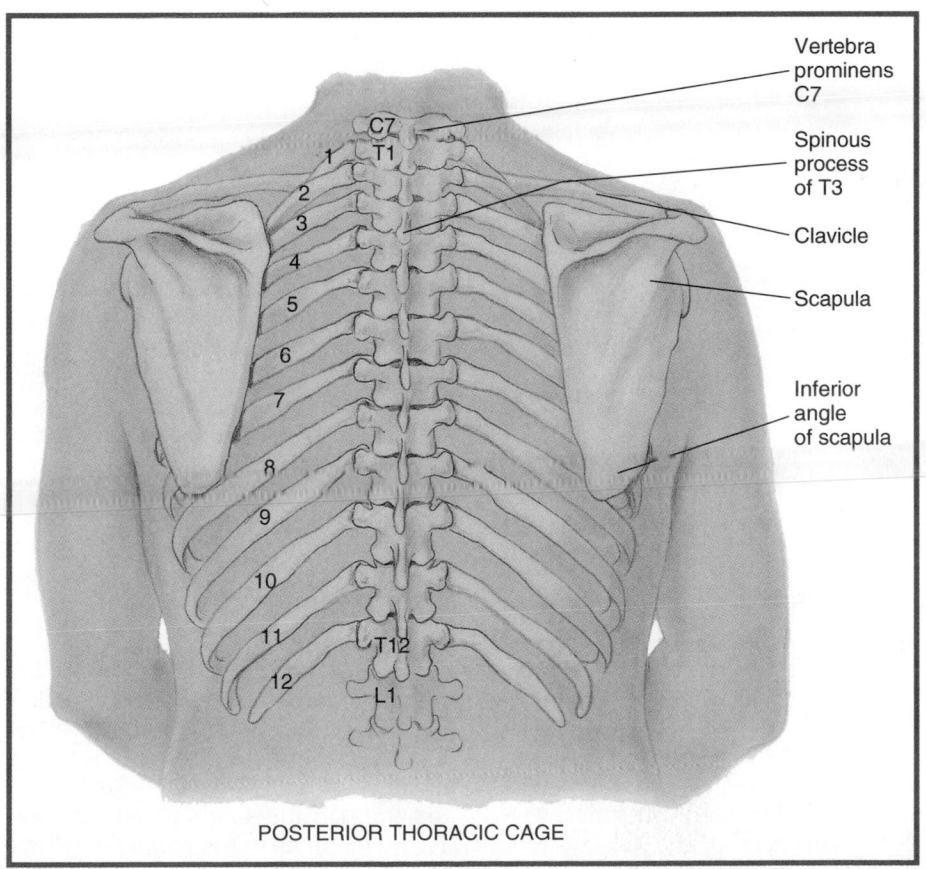

Vertebra prominens C7

Spinous process of T3

Clavicle

Scapula

Inferior angle of scapula

POSTERIOR THORACIC CAGE

B

FIGURE 43-1   **A**, The anterior thoracic cage. **B**, The posterior thoracic cage. (From Jarvis C: *Physical examination and health assessment,* ed. 3, Philadelphia, 2000, WB Saunders.)

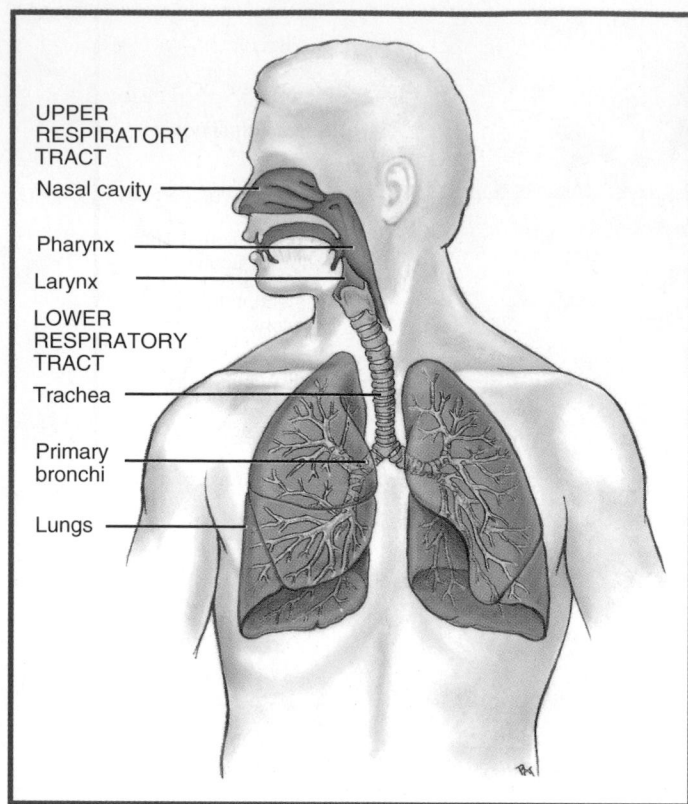

FIGURE 43-2 The upper and lower respiratory tract. (From Applegate EJ: *The anatomy and physiology learning system*, Philadelphia, 1995, WB Saunders.)

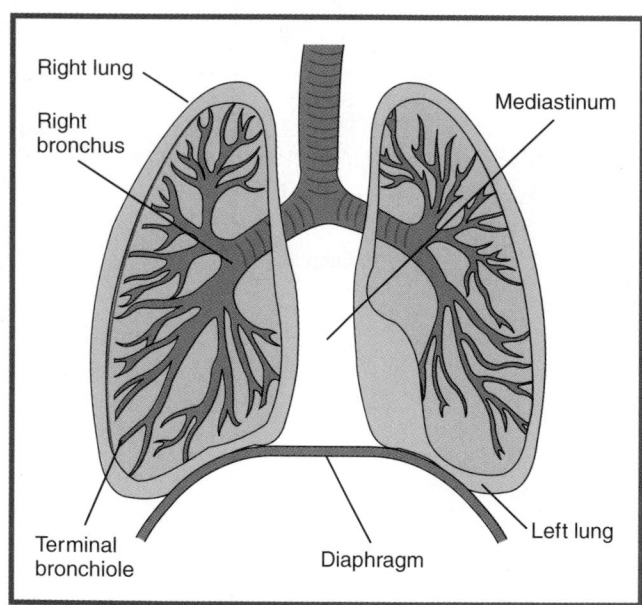

FIGURE 43-3 The bronchial tree.

The bronchial tree and the alveoli are the major structures housed within the right and left lungs. The lungs are soft and spongy because of the air sacs that compose most of their mass. They hang in the right and left sides of the chest, separated by the pericardial sac, which contains the heart. The right lung is divided into three lobes and has a greater volume capacity than the left lung. Each lobe has its own bronchus and blood supply, which makes it possible for one lobe to be removed (*lobectomy*), and the rest of the lung sustain little, if any, damage. The left lung is longer and narrower and has a distinct indentation in the center of it known as the *cardiac notch*, where the left ventricle of the heart is located and an apical pulse is heard. The left lung has only two lobes, an upper and lower (Figure 43-4).

Each lung is encased in a double-layered sac called the *pleural membrane*. The membrane closest to the lung is called the *visceral* pleura, which doubles back to form the *parietal* pleural membrane. Small amounts of pleural fluid fill the space between the two membranes and provide lubrication for the movement of the lungs during inhalation and exhalation.

Ventilation

In the very delicate lung tissue, the bronchioles deposit the oxygenated air into the grapelike structures called the *alveoli*. Surrounding each alveolus is a network of pulmonary capillaries filled with waste air. The oxygenated air moves through the single-celled walls of the alveoli and through the single-celled walls of these capillaries (Figure 43-5). As this is happening, the waste air is forced out of the capillaries, into the alveoli and then into the bronchioles. Air exchange has taken place, the capillaries carry the oxygenated air back to the heart, and the waste

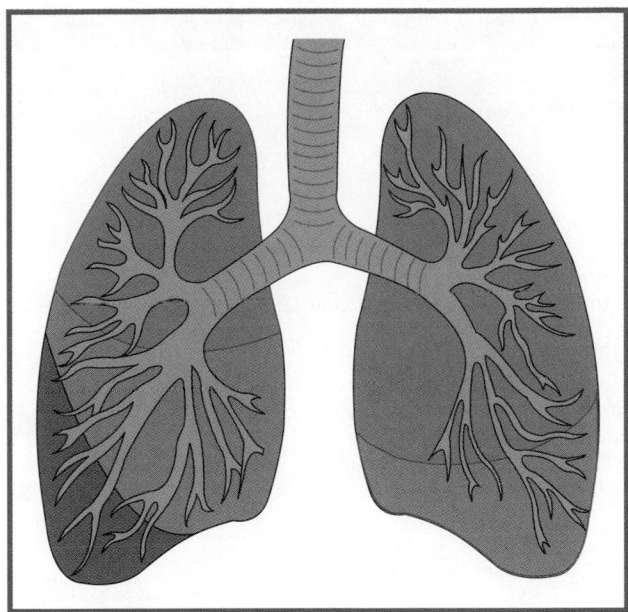

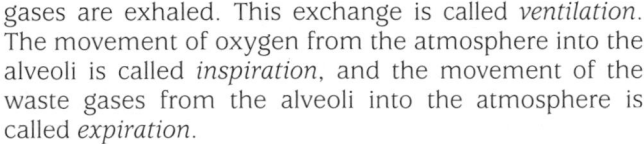

FIGURE 43-4 Lobes of the lungs.

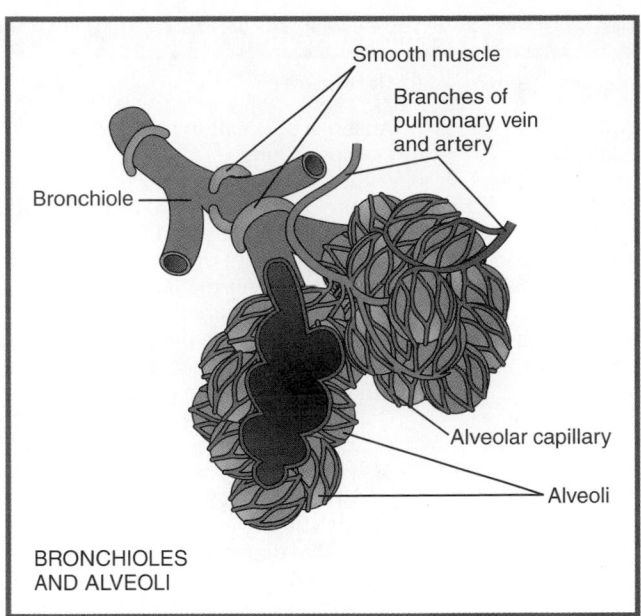

FIGURE 43-5 Alveoli with capillary network.

gases are exhaled. This exchange is called *ventilation*. The movement of oxygen from the atmosphere into the alveoli is called *inspiration*, and the movement of the waste gases from the alveoli into the atmosphere is called *expiration*.

Inspiration

Inspiration begins with a signal from the medulla oblongata in the brainstem. This signal is carried by the phrenic nerve to the major muscle of inspiration, the diaphragm. When the diaphragm receives the signal, it flattens out and pulls downward. At the same moment, the intercostal muscles located between the ribs contract, causing the ribs to move outward and the chest cavity to enlarge. This movement causes the lungs to expand and increase their volume. The more these muscles are contracted, the deeper the inhalation is and the greater the air volume becomes. When an individual is unable to move enough air using the diaphragm and intercostal muscles to meet the body's needs, the individual experiences respiratory distress.

Expiration

The second half of ventilation is expiration. Once inspiration is completed, the diaphragm and intercostal muscles relax, causing the chest to move inward and the lungs to decrease in volume. This movement forces the waste air out of the lungs and back into the atmosphere. This phase of ventilation needs very little energy and takes place with minimal effort by the body. In asthma and/or emphysema, the person has difficulty getting the air out of the lungs, and accessory muscles in the chest are needed to assist the intercostal and diaphragm muscles for complete exhalation.

Respiratory System Defenses

Every part of the respiratory system has a defense mechanism. In the upper respiratory tract, the mucus-covered ciliated surface of the mucous membrane traps particles; through the continuous flow of the mucus back toward the nasopharynx, the particles are swallowed.

The lower respiratory tract is sterile, which is phenomenal considering that each day these airways are exposed to approximately 10,000 L of air containing an endless number of microorganisms and foreign material. It is the ever-changing air flow, inspiration to expiration, that creates a turbulence that makes it very difficult for these invading substances to remain in the bronchi. This, combined with coughing, sneezing, and a functioning immune system, protects the respiratory tract and helps the body maintain homeostasis. Disease occurs when something happens to upset the normal homeostatic chain of events.

Major Diseases of the Respiratory System

Many diseases affect this system; however, the major ones can be divided into infectious diseases, obstructive disorders, and tumors. Respiratory diseases cause common symptoms including sneezing, a productive or nonproductive cough, sore throat or hoarseness, fever, general malaise, altered breath sounds, and changes in breathing patterns. A medical assistant is expected to be familiar with common respiratory terms and use them in documenting patient signs and symptoms. Some common medical terms are listed in Table 43-1.

TABLE 43-1	Respiratory System Terms
Medical Term	**Definition**
Apnea	Absence of breathing
Atelectasis	Collapsed lung
Dyspnea	Difficulty breathing
Empyema	Accumulation of pus in the pleural space
Hemoptysis	Expectoration of blood
Hemothorax	Accumulation of blood and fluid in the pleural cavity
Hypercapnia	Greater than normal amounts of carbon dioxide in the blood
Hyperpnea	Deep, rapid, labored respiration that may occur because of exercise or pain and fever
Hypoxemia	Low level of oxygen in the blood
Orthopnea	Person must sit or stand to breathe comfortably
Pleurisy	Inflammation of the parietal pleura causing dyspnea and stabbing pain; friction rub may be auscultated
Pneumothorax	Collection of air or gas in the pleural space causing the lung to collapse
Pyothorax	Collection of pus in the pleural cavity from infection
Rales	Abnormal sound heard on auscultation produced by passage of air through bronchi that are constricted or contain secretions
Rhinoplasty	Plastic surgery to repair or alter the structure of the nose
Rhinorrhea	Excessive drainage from the nose
Rhonchi	Abnormal sound heard on auscultation caused by thick secretions or spasms
Tachypnea	Abnormally rapid rate of breathing
Thoracotomy	Surgical opening into the thoracic cavity

CRITICAL THINKING APPLICATION

Michael is taking a patient history on a new patient and she reports the following problems: difficulty breathing; sometimes she has to sit up to breathe comfortably; occasionally she coughs up blood and has excessive nasal drainage. Six months ago she experienced very rapid breathing and a blue color to her skin, so she was admitted to the hospital and diagnosed with blood and fluid around her right lung that had become infected and caused her lung to collapse. Based on what Michael knows about respiratory system terminology, how should he document this information?

Infectious Diseases

Respiratory tract infections are in two groups. Diseases of the nose and upper respiratory tract (URIs) are more common than are diseases of the lower respiratory tract (e.g., pneumonia). Respiratory tract infections account for approximately 75% of all clinically diagnosed infections. Only about 5% of these infections involve the lungs. Most lung infections are seen in hospitalized patients, elderly persons, substance abusers, alcoholics, and patients with AIDS. Pneumonia is often the cause of death for debilitated people.

Upper Respiratory Tract Infections

Common Cold. The common cold was discussed in Chapter 39 as an acute inflammatory process affecting the mucous membranes that line the nose, pharynx, larynx, and bronchus. Usually the term *cold* is used when only the membranes of the nose and pharynx are affected; however, the same virus can affect the larynx and the lungs. The viral invasion can be followed by bacterial infections of the pharynx and middle ear. Frequently seen signs of an upper respiratory tract infection (URTI) include nasal congestion and rhinorrhea, sneezing, watery eyes, pharyngitis (sore throat), laryngitis (hoarseness), and coughing. Nasal discharge is usually clear and watery in the early stage but can become greenish yellow as the virus becomes more virulent or when bacteria invade. The patient usually complains of headache, a low-grade fever, chills, and anorexia.

There is at present no cure for the common cold, and the infection usually runs its course in 3 to 5 days. The best way to treat it is by getting plenty of rest and drinking fluids. Taking an over-the-counter cold remedy, cough syrup, and acetaminophen may lessen the discomfort. Echinacea, an herbal remedy, has been found to enhance immunological activity and may be taken to improve the immune system or complement other cold medications. Antibiotics are only prescribed if there is evidence of a secondary bacterial infection.

Sinusitis. The common cold or an allergic reaction can cause one or more of the paranasal sinuses to become inflamed or infected. Inflammation causes edema and the collection of mucus within the cavity, creating a feeling of pressure, either nasal congestion or rhinorrhea, and classic sinus headaches. Treatment is with decongestants, antibiotics, and analgesics.

Allergic Rhinitis (Hay Fever). Although not caused by a pathogenic organism, allergic rhinitis is frequently confused with infectious disease. This disorder affects millions of people every year. It is caused by a reaction of the nasal mucosa to an environmental allergen. The most frequent allergen is plant pollen; this is where the term *hay fever* originated. The sneezing can be controlled with either over-the-counter treatments or prescription antihistamines, such as fexofenadine hydrochloride (Allegra) and cetirizine hydrochloride (Zyrtec), and nasal sprays. The list of possible allergens is extensive. When this condition is seen in the respiratory practice, the patient is usually referred to an allergist for testing and possible immunotherapy.

Patients may have difficulty determining whether symptoms are caused by a cold or an allergy. They are usually suffering from an allergy if the eyes, ears, nose, throat, and roof of the mouth (palate) are itchy; the eyes are red and watery; there is a clear, thin nasal discharge; seasonal symptoms last for weeks or months; and they do not have a fever.

Lower Respiratory Tract Infections

Pneumonia. Pneumonia is both a specific disorder and a general term meaning inflammation of all or part of the lungs (Figure 43-6). Pneumonia may be caused by bacteria, viruses, or other pathogens (Table 43-2). It can also be caused by inhaling irritants or poisonous gas and by aspirating solids or fluids into the lungs. The most frequently seen causative organisms are staphylococci and streptococci.

Pneumonia can occur in any age group but most often affects preschool age children and the elderly (older than 65). Risk factors include smoking, alcoholism, and immunosuppression caused by diseases or treatment. Pneumonia can range from a mild complication to a life-threatening illness and is the fifth leading cause of death in the United States.

The patient usually comes to the office with symptoms of high fever, chills, and general malaise. Signs of the illness include dyspnea, tachypnea, chest pain during inspiration, and a relentless cough with hemoptysis. Auscultation of the chest reveals rales, rhonchi, and other signs of **pulmonary consolidation**. The infection may

TABLE 43-2	Pathogens Causing Pneumonia
Pathogen	Type of Infection
Bacteria	*Streptococcus pneumoniae* *Haemophilus influenzae* *Staphylococcus aureus* Mycobacteria
Virus	Influenza virus
Fungi	*Aspergillus fumigatus* *Candida albicans* *Mycoplasma pneumoniae*
Parasite	*Pneumocystis carinii* (opportunistic infection, seen in immunosuppressed, debilitated, or terminally ill patients)

spread into the pleural cavity, causing empyema and pleurisy.

Diagnosis is confirmed with a chest x-ray evaluation, sputum culture, sensitivity to identify the invading organism and determine appropriate antibiotic therapy, and white blood cell (WBC) count, including a differential count to determine whether the pneumonia is viral or bacterial. If the pneumonia is viral, there will be no increase in the number of white cells; but if it is bacterial, the greater the invasion, the higher the WBC count will be, and the differential count will indicate an elevation in the neutrophil and monocyte levels. Treatment is based on destroying the invading organism. If the organism is bacterial, the treatment of choice is with

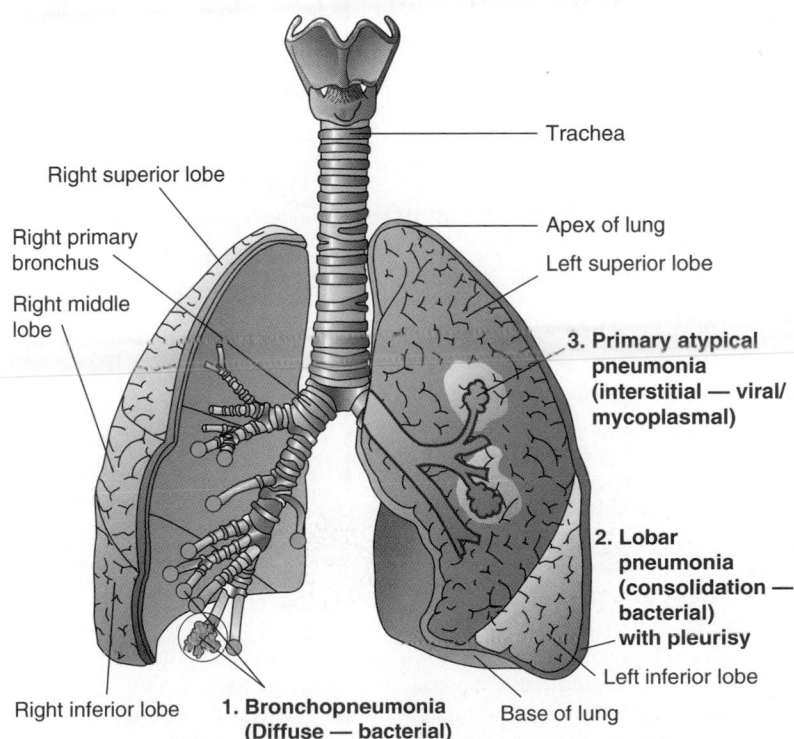

FIGURE 43-6 Types of pneumonia. (From Gould: *Pathophysiology for the health professions,* ed 2. Philadelphia, 2002, WB Saunders.)

antibiotic therapy and lung function therapy until the patient has recovered. If the organism is viral, the patient is given supportive care, such as antipyretics, fluids, and oxygen, until the immune system can control viral spread.

Tuberculosis. For more than 50 years, the incidence of tuberculosis (TB) steadily declined, but since the late 1980s it has shown a serious increase in the United States. This increase is believed to be the result of increased travel and immigration; the number of AIDS patients, who have little resistance to disease; an increase in the number of homeless and malnourished persons; and the overwhelming proliferation of drug-resistant bacteria.

Mycobacterium tuberculosis is the bacterium that causes TB. This organism is covered with a waxy substance that makes it possible for it to survive outside a living host for a long time. It is transmitted by droplets of sputum that are expectorated into the environment by an infected host and inhaled by another person. In the presence of the warm, moist respiratory tract, these organisms can again become active if the individual is susceptible to the disease. TB can also be spread when an infected person coughs or sneezes, releasing airborne infected droplets, which are inhaled and cause an infection if the person is susceptible.

Tuberculosis develops in two stages. The primary infection occurs when the person is first infected with the bacteria and the lungs become inflamed. Cell-mediated immunity takes place, isolating the bacteria and forming a tubercle. At this point, a healthy individual can stop the spread of infection, causing the tubercle to eventually calcify. In this case, the person was exposed to the pathogen but never developed active disease. However, exposed individuals will consistently test positive to tuberculosis skin screening tests and, rather than the PPD (Mantoux test), they should have chest x-ray studies to diagnose active TB. At any time, however, the bacilli in the tubercles can be reactivated, usually because of decreased resistance in the host, and secondary tuberculosis can develop. The patient is now actively infected with the disease, which can spread to the bones, brain, and kidneys (Figure 43-7).

Tuberculosis is diagnosed most frequently in people living in crowded conditions with poor hygiene, who are malnourished, and who have other chronic conditions. It is spreading most rapidly in large cities, in the elderly, nonwhites, alcoholics, and the homeless. Symptoms of the primary infection include an intermittent fever peaking in the afternoon, night sweats, weight loss, and general malaise. As the infection becomes **virulent** within the host, there will be a productive cough with thick, dark, frequently blood-tinged mucus expectorated.

The primary diagnosis of tuberculosis is established through patient signs and symptoms. The infection is suspected with a positive chest x-ray film but confirmed with a sputum culture. Traditional culture methods originally took 4 to 6 weeks to confirm the diagnosis. Because this extended period of time allowed a potentially infectious individual to continue to spread the disease, new culture techniques identify the bacterium as early as 36 to 48 hours. Once the diagnosis is confirmed, the patient

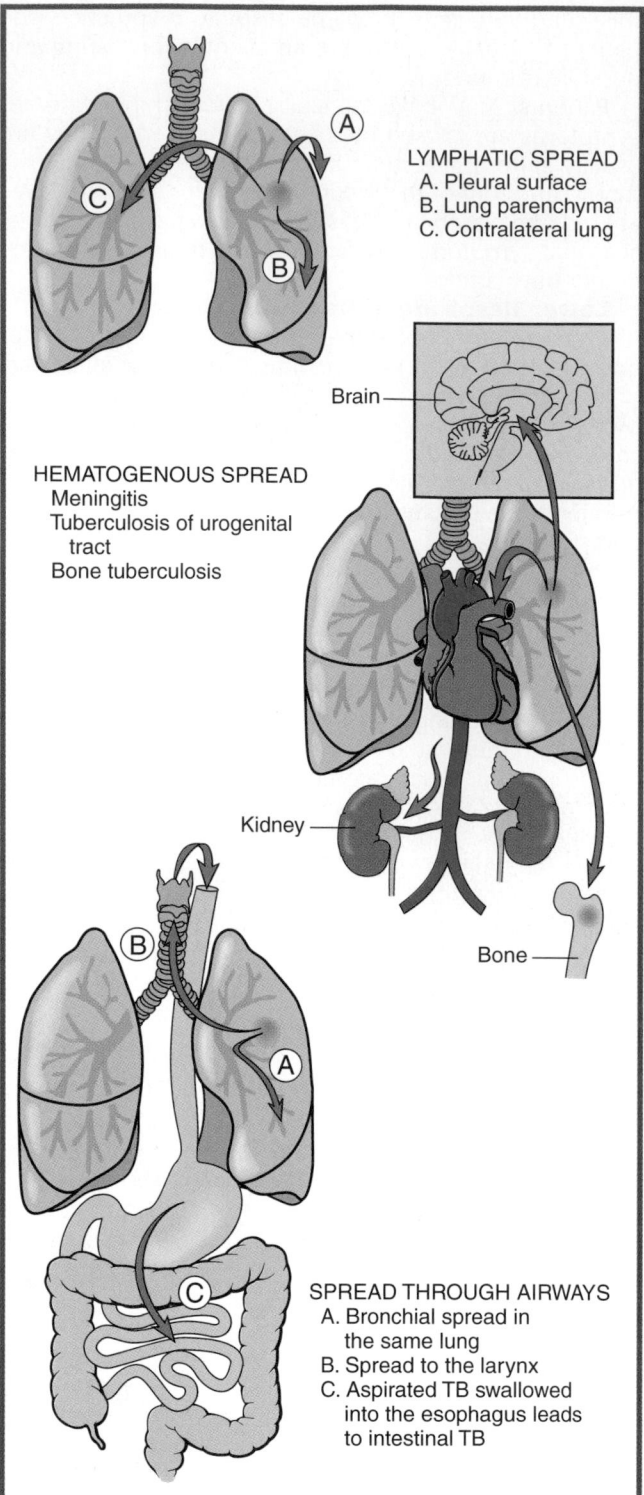

FIGURE 43-7   Spread of tuberculosis. (From Damjanov I: *Pathology for the health-related professions,* ed. 2, Philadelphia, 2000, WB Saunders.)

is prescribed long-term treatment with a combination of drugs to completely eradicate the bacilli. If the patient has tested positive for TB but does not have an active secondary infection, the physician will prescribe isoniazid (INH) 300 mg daily for 6 to 12 months. If the patient has active pulmonary TB, the CDC recommends a four-drug regimen, including INH, rifampin, pyrazinamide, and streptomycin daily for 6 months. The patient is retested, and pharmaceutical treatment is continued for 3 months beyond a negative culture. All tuberculin-negative health-care workers should have a TB skin test annually; workers who are tuberculin positive should have an annual chest x-ray evaluation to screen for the disease.

CRITICAL THINKING APPLICATION

Dr. Samuelson is the primary care physician for a nursing home in the area and is concerned because one of the employees has had a positive result to a Mantoux test. What other tests will Dr. Samuelson order to confirm the diagnosis? If those tests come back positive, how will the patient be treated? What about the other employees and residents of the nursing home?

Chronic Obstructive Pulmonary Disease

Chronic obstructive pulmonary disease (COPD) is a group of diseases with the common characteristic of chronic airway obstruction. Among the diseases included in this group are **chronic bronchitis, bronchiectasis,** and emphysema. Although the mechanism of the obstruction may vary, the patient with COPD is unable to ventilate the lungs freely, resulting in an ineffective exchange of respiratory gases, dyspnea, and productive cough. Over time the patient finds it increasingly difficult to eliminate carbon dioxide from the lungs during expiration.

Asthma. Pediatric asthma was addressed in Chapter 39. Asthma attacks are in response to a number of triggers that cause inflammation and bronchospasm with resultant airflow obstruction. Asthma can develop into a chronic disease characterized by increased activity or sensitivity of the bronchial tubes to external factors, such as environmental irritants, poor air quality, and allergies, or to internal factors, such as stress, exercise, infection, and allergen inhalation. Asthma also has a strong hereditary factor.

Asthma attacks can be mild to severe and can last minutes to days. An asthmatic patient complains of a nonproductive cough, dyspnea, expiratory wheezing, and chest tightness. Because of the difficult breathing, tachycardia, pallor, and diaphoresis may also be present. The patient can only speak a few words at a time and then may need to stop to regulate his or her air intake. When the chest is auscultated, the physician hears diminished breath sounds with wheezes and rhonchi in the lungs. The spasms in the bronchi trap air in the lungs and the inflammatory response creates edema and mucus secretion in the bronchioles. Spirometric evaluation measures the degree of airflow obstruction. Chest x-ray films may also show changes in the lungs from the mucous obstructions. Blood tests include a complete blood cell count with a differential count to determine whether the attack is allergy related.

Asthmatic patients, regardless of their age, should be actively involved in the day-to-day management of their disease. It may be the medical assistant's responsibility to teach the patient how to perform peak flow measurements either daily or at the onset of an attack. Peak flow meters assess the ability of the patient to move air into and out of the lungs. The physician may want the patient to keep a log of daily peak flow results or to use the instrument as an at-home monitoring device when chest tightness and wheezing occur. The meter measures the peak expiratory flow rate, which is the fastest speed at which the patient can blow air out of the lungs after taking in as big a breath as possible. When the patient forcefully exhales, the indicator on the meter rises along the scale and stays at the peak flow value (Figure 43-8).

INSTRUCTING THE PATIENT IN THE USE OF A PEAK FLOW METER

1. Slide the indicator to the bottom of the scale.
2. Hold the meter upright, being careful not to block the opening with the fingers.
3. Have the patient stand up or sit up straight, inhale as deeply as possible, and place his or her mouth firmly around the mouthpiece, forming a tight seal with the lips.
4. Have the patient blow out as hard and as fast as possible, which will slide the indicator up the meter.
5. Take three readings and record the highest value. Slide the indicator to the bottom of the scale before repeating each reading.

If the patient is having an asthma attack, the bronchioles are constricting, becoming edematous, and filling up with mucus, so the patient is unable to exhale strongly enough to raise the indicator to a normal level. If readings are below normal, the physician will prescribe a treatment plan that may include contacting the physician when peak flow levels are below a certain point or starting nebulizer treatments. The physician may recommend an increase in antiinflammatory medication if there is more than a 20% variation in readings from normal. The medication therapy chosen depends on the severity and frequency of acute attacks, but management is necessary to prevent permanent lung damage and emphysema-like changes in the lungs.

The treatment consists of a regimen of medications, including "rescue" inhalers: ipratropium bromide (Atrovent), albuterol (Ventolin), or pirbuterol acetate (MaxAir), which are used to relieve bronchospasms or for exercise-induced asthma (Figure 43-9). Tissue inflammation can be treated with steroid inhalers: flunisolide (Aerobid), triamcinolone acetonide (Azmacort), or fluticasone propionate (Flovent) and/or oral leukotriene-receptor antagonists such as zafirlukast (Accolate) or montelukast sodium (Singulair) taken on a regular basis.

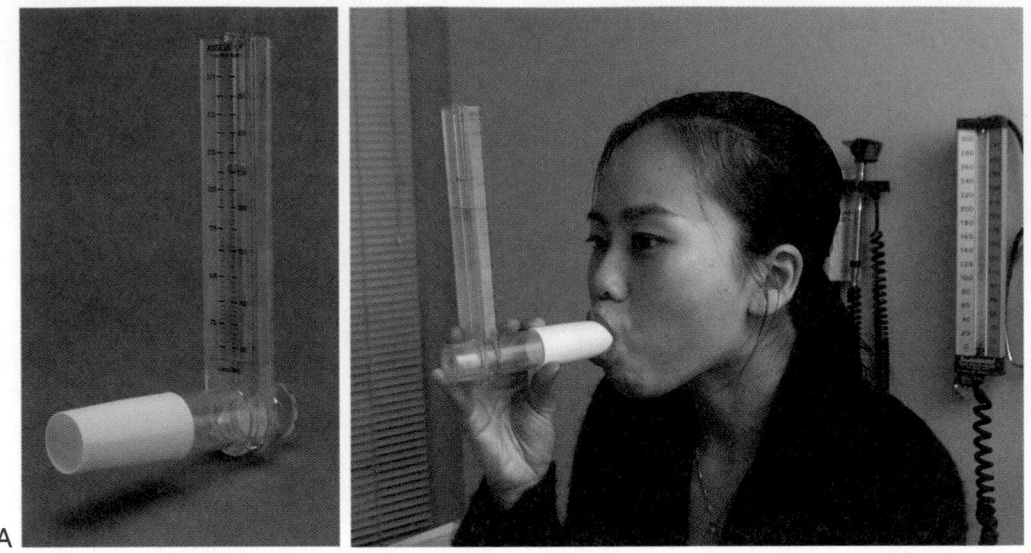

FIGURE 43-8   A, A peak flow meter. **B**, A patient using a peak flow meter.

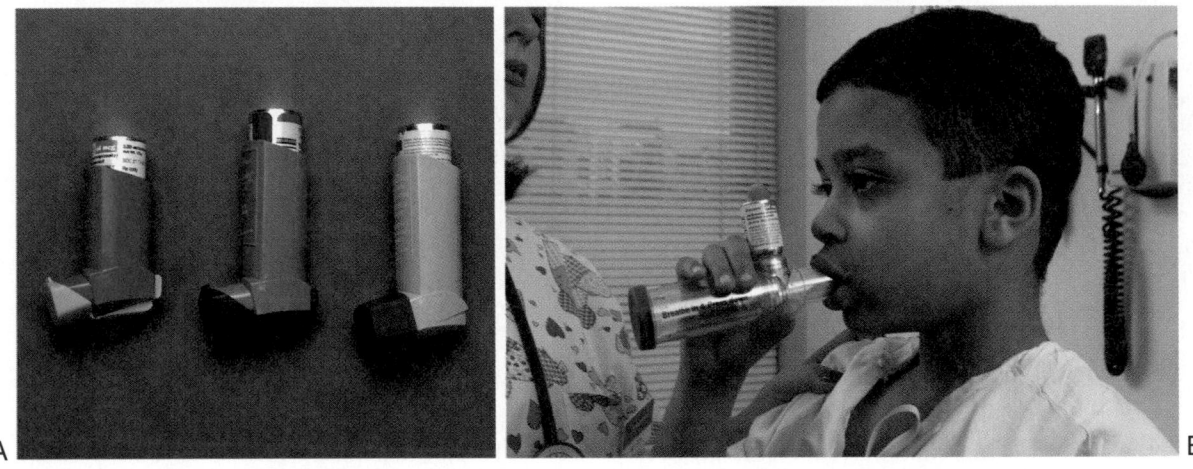

FIGURE 43-9   A, Inhalers. **B**, An inhaler with a spacer.

If an attack is severe, it may require injections of epinephrine, oral corticosteroids (Prednisone), and/or nebulizer treatments with a bronchodilator.

The physician will prescribe particular inhalers with the dosage based on how many "puffs" of a metered-dose inhaler the patient should administer. Metered-dose inhalers (MDIs) consist of a pressurized canister containing medication and a mouthpiece. Most MDIs hold about 200 doses of medication as well as a pressurized gas propellant, which forces the drug out of the canister. When the canister is inverted and depressed a metered dose (premeasured) is delivered through the mouthpiece in aerosol form. Patient teaching is very important to ensure that the patient operates the device correctly so the medication can be administered as ordered. If both a steroid and bronchodilator have been prescribed, the bronchodilator should be taken first, because this will open the airways so the steroid can be better distributed throughout the lungs.

INSTRUCTING THE PATIENT IN THE USE OF METERED-DOSE INHALERS

1. Shake the canister vigorously and place it into the mouthpiece device.
2. The patient should open his or her mouth and hold the inhaler about 1 inch away. (If the patient places the mouthpiece in the mouth, the gas propellant will cause the drug to bounce off the back of the throat, and much of it will be lost around the mouth.)
3. The patient should exhale normally, and while beginning to slowly inhale, he or she should depress the canister, releasing a metered dose of medication.
4. The patient should continue to breathe in until the lungs are full, hold the breath to a

Pneumoconioses. Environmental causes of respiratory diseases include inhaled dusts, fumes, and various kinds of organic or inorganic matter. A majority of these respiratory diseases are occupational: they are the consequence of long-term exposure to unsafe air in the workplace. Although the respiratory system is designed to filter and trap air contaminants, the system becomes overloaded after intense exposure. Therefore particles enter the lungs, and damage increases when the particles are very small and can enter the alveoli, when the individual is exposed to a large quantity of contaminants over a long period, and when there is the added irritation of cigarette smoking.

Some of the occupations that can cause pneumoconiosis include coal mining *(anthracosis)*; insulation manufacture and shipbuilding *(asbestosis)*; and stone-cutting or sandblasting *(silicosis)*. Tissue changes caused by the inhalation of these substances into the lungs are irreversible. Patients develop dyspnea, cough, and emphysema-like changes and have an increased risk factor for cancer of the lung.

Emphysema. Emphysema causes destruction of the alveoli, resulting in overinflation of the remaining alveoli and difficulty with expiration. This is a progressive obstructive disease of the pulmonary system and is irreversible. Cigarette smoking is the primary contributing factor; however, patients who develop emphysema at an early age may have a genetic predisposition to the disease. Other contributors include exposure to pollutants (pneumoconioses) or chronic respiratory disorders (chronic bronchitis or asthma).

The signs and symptoms of emphysema include dyspnea, shortness of breath (SOB), wheezing, production of thick mucus, restlessness, fatigue, anorexia, persistent cough (productive or nonproductive), and peripheral cyanosis with **clubbing**. The patient is typically diagnosed from presenting signs and symptoms and a chest x-ray examination, as well as a pulmonary function test (PFT) that shows increased residual volume and decreased forced expiratory volume.

Patients are encouraged to avoid respiratory irritants and individuals with respiratory infections and to stop smoking. Many of these patients require oxygen therapy and benefit from postural drainage and chest percussion

to expectorate trapped mucus. Nebulizer treatments, which deliver a bronchodilator (Albuterol or Ventolin) by aerosol through either a mouthpiece or mask, may also be prescribed (Figure 43-10).

Patients with emphysema expend a great deal of energy just breathing, so they should consume a high-calorie, high-fluid diet and perform certain exercises, such as pursed-lip breathing, to help them conserve energy. An emphysema patient requires continuous care and support, so getting the family involved in the treatment plan is very helpful. Referral to a pulmonary rehabilitation program or support group is beneficial to both patient and family.

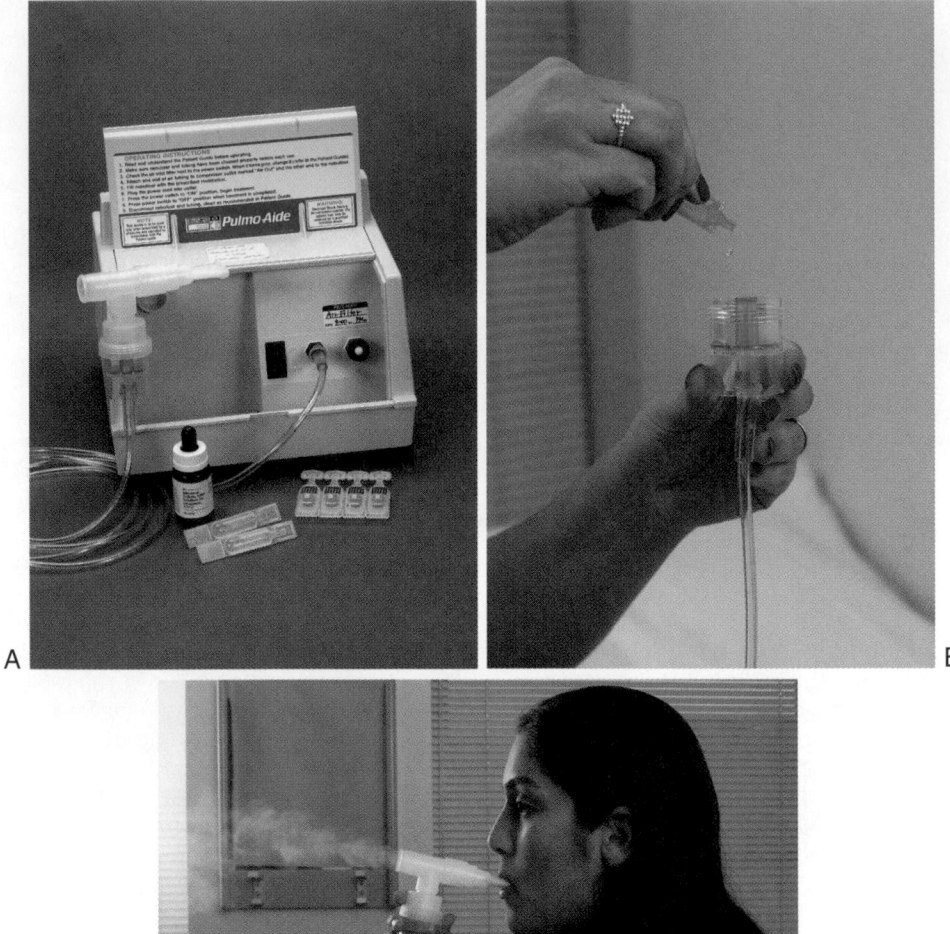

FIGURE 43-10   A, A nebulizer. **B**, Mixing medication and diluent for nebulizer treatment. **C**, Nebulizer treatment.

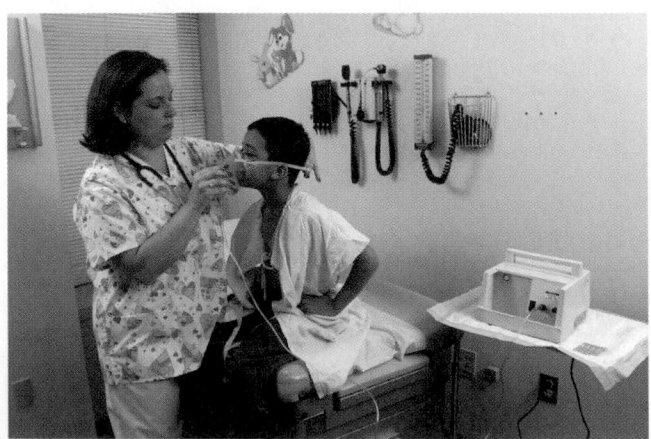

FIGURE 43-11   Nebulizer treatment with mask.

CRITICAL THINKING APPLICATION

Dr. Samuelson has quite a few patients with either asthma or emphysema. Under the direction of Dr. Samuelson, Michael is expected to reinforce patient education and answer patient and/or family questions. Michael decides to make a file on pertinent information and review it with Dr. Samuelson before using it to help coordinate the care of these patients. What information should Michael include in the file? What community resources or groups should be included for patient support?

Tumors

The most prevalent neoplasms of the respiratory system are lung cancer and carcinoma of the larynx.

Lung Cancer. Lung cancer is the leading cause of cancer-related deaths for both men and women in the United States. It is estimated that 80% of lung tumors are linked to cigarette smoking; other risk factors include chronic exposure to second-hand smoke, carcinogens, and genetic predisposition. The risk of developing cancer is higher for patients who started to smoke at a young age and who smoke more than a pack a day for a long period (Figure 43-12).

The lung is a common site for secondary tumors from metastasis as well as primary carcinomas. There are several different cellular types of tumors that can develop in the lungs, but the one seen most frequently is bronchogenic carcinoma, which originates in the epithelial lining of the bronchioles (Figure 43-13). The early symptoms of lung cancer—chronic productive cough, shortness of breath, and chest tightness—are masked by symptoms regularly displayed by habitual smokers. Many times a tumor is discovered accidentally during a routine chest x-ray evaluation or may not be discovered until metastatic symptoms, such as anemia, weight loss, and fatigue, lead to a diagnosis of a primary lung tumor. The patients who do show symptoms usually display local effects of a tumor in the chest such as bronchial obstruction, atelectasis, hemoptysis, chest pain, and pleural membrane involvement. Unless the tumor is diagnosed very early, lung cancer has a poor prognosis. Treatment consists of surgery, radiation therapy, and chemotherapy.

Carcinoma of the Larynx. Carcinoma of the larynx is pathologically linked to smoking and chronic alcohol consumption. Ninety percent of the cases of laryngeal cancer occur in men, with most of those between 60 and 70 years of age. Patients show early signs of hoarseness and loss of voice, *dysphagia* (difficulty swallowing), and occasionally, respiration becomes impaired. Because of these early symptoms, most laryngeal tumors are discovered in their early stages and can be removed with a very good prognosis. Surgical treatment consists of a partial or total laryngectomy. With a total laryngectomy, the voice is permanently lost, and a **tracheostomy** is performed. Patients undergoing such procedures need comprehensive preparation and would benefit from meeting a laryngectomy survivor as well as participating in a support group to deal with postsurgical adjustments.

The Medical Assistant's Role in Pulmonary Procedures

Assisting With the Examination

Preparing a patient for a respiratory examination includes having the patient disrobe to the waist and don a gown with the opening in the front. To assess the status of the

FIGURE 43-12 Classification of lung cancer. (From Damjanov IL: *Pathology for the health-related professions*, ed. 2, Philadelphia, 2000, WB Saunders.)

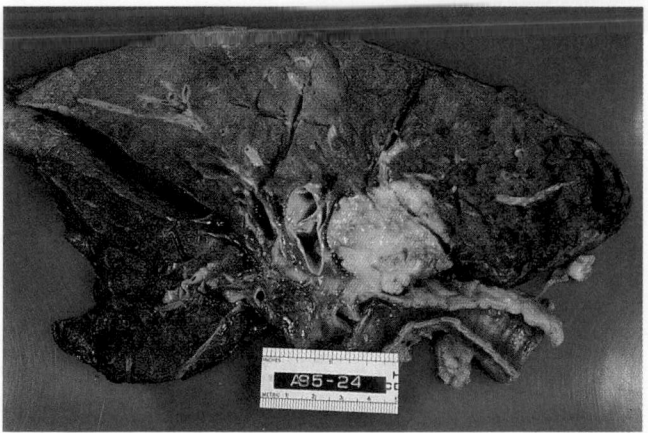

FIGURE 43-13 Lung cancer. (From Damjanov IL: *Pathology for the health-related professions*, ed. 2, Philadelphia, 2000, WB Saunders.)

respiratory system, the physician uses inspection, palpation, percussion, and auscultation on the anterior thorax and then repeats the process on the posterior and lateral thorax. The medical assistant is responsible for assisting the physician throughout the examination, providing the patient privacy and support, and performing diagnostic tests as ordered.

Diagnostic Procedures

Tuberculosis. If the physician orders tuberculosis screening, the medical assistant will administer the Mantoux test (see Chapter 32). The test uses an intradermal injection of purified protein derivative (PPD) from a live tuberculin bacillus culture to test for the presence of tuberculin antibodies. A positive Mantoux reaction indicates the possibility of active or dormant tuberculosis or exposure to the disease. Further testing by sputum culture and chest x-ray examination is required for a definitive diagnosis.

Spirometry Testing. Pulmonary function tests (PFTs) are performed to diagnose a pulmonary abnormality and/or to determine the extent of a pulmonary disease. Lung function measurements are made in the physician office setting with a spirometer (Figure 43-14). Table 43-3 summarizes the aspects of pulmonary function that are measured during a PFT. Successful spirometry requires the application of a consistent technique for preparing the patient, explaining and performing the procedure, and determining the results.

Patient preparation begins when the procedure is scheduled. The patient should be instructed not to smoke and to refrain from using bronchodilators and nebulizers for 6 hours before the test.

The medical assistant may be responsible for conducting this test in the ambulatory care setting (Procedure 43-1). When the patient arrives for testing, the assistant should explain the purpose of the test, determine whether there are any contraindications to performing the test, obtain the patient's vital signs (including height and weight), and explain the maneuver. Spirometry should be described briefly, in simple terms. One statement that works well is, "I am going to have you blow into a machine to see how big your lungs are and how fast the air comes out. It doesn't hurt, but it does require your cooperation and lots of effort."

The next step is to get the patient comfortable and in the proper position. Have the patient loosen any tight clothing, such as a necktie, belt, or bra. There is no significant difference between the sitting and standing positions, but many people become lightheaded and may faint or stumble; thus sitting is a safer position. The patient's legs should be uncrossed, and both feet should be on the floor. The patient's vital signs should be taken and recorded before the procedure.

Explain the maneuver and show the patient the mouthpiece. Explain how the mouthpiece fits into the mouth. Lips should be sealed tightly, and the tongue should not stick out into the mouthpiece. Dentures that fit poorly may be a nuisance and should be removed if you think they will interfere. The chin should be slightly elevated and the neck slightly extended. This position should be maintained throughout the forced expiratory procedure.

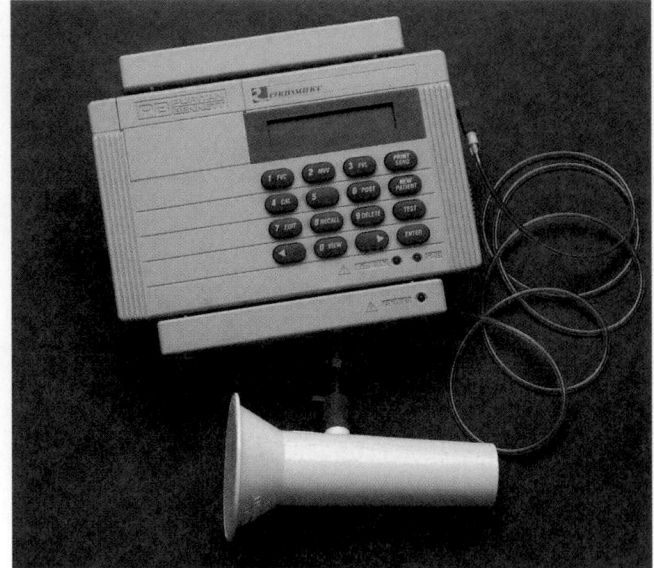

A

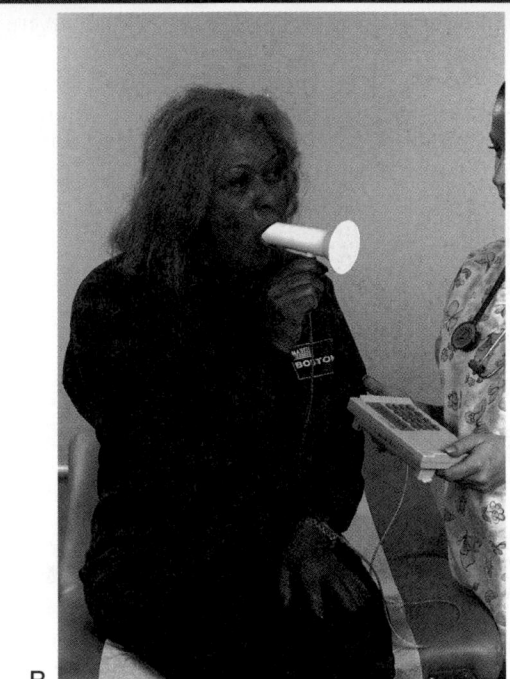

B

FIGURE 43-14 **A,** A spirometer. **B,** Spirometry testing.

Give specific instructions in simple, direct terms. For example: "I want you to take the deepest breath possible, put the mouthpiece in your mouth and seal your lips tightly around it, and then blow into the tube as hard and as fast as you can in one long, complete breath." One analogy that is sometimes helpful to further explain the maneuver is, "It's like blowing out the candles on a birthday cake that don't all go out, so you need to keep blowing the same breath until they do."

Next, demonstrate the maneuver. Many patients will forget some or all of the instructions they just received, so demonstration reinforces exactly what to do. Show the patient proper chin and neck position, how to place the mouthpiece at the right time, and how to blow the air out and continue to blow.

TABLE 43-3	Pulmonary Function Tests	
Lung Function	**Description**	**Patient Instructions**
Tidal volume (TV)	Volume of air inspired and expired during a normal respiration	Patient breathes in and out normally with lips pursed around mouthpiece.
Vital capacity (VC)	Maximum amount of air that can be expired after maximum inspiration	Patient takes deep breath and exhales completely (not forcefully).
Inspiratory capacity (IC)	Maximum amount of air that can be inspired after a normal expiration	Patient breathes in and out normally and then forcibly inhales at the end of the TV.
Expiratory reserve volume (ERV)	Maximum volume of air that can be exhaled after a normal expiration	Patient breathes in and out normally and then exhales forcibly at the end of the TV.
Residual volume (RV)	Volume of air left in lungs after forced expiration	
Functional residual volume (FRV)	Amount of air left in the lungs after a normal expiration	FRV = ERV + RV
Forced vital capacity (FVC)	Amount of air that can be forcefully exhaled from a maximal inhalation	Patient inhales as deeply as possible and then forcibly exhales as much as possible.
Maximal volume ventilation (MVV)	Maximum volume that patient can breathe in and out in 1 minute	Patient breathes in and out as deeply and frequently as possible for 15 seconds (total volume is multiplied by 4).

PROCEDURE 43-1

Performing Volume Capacity Spirometric Testing

GOAL: To perform volume capacity testing.

EQUIPMENT AND SUPPLIES

- Scale with measuring device
- Sphygmomanometer and stethoscope
- Spirometer with recording paper in place
- External spirometric tubing
- Disposable mouthpiece
- Biohazard waste container

PROCEDURAL STEPS

1 Wash your hands and assemble the spirometer.

2 Introduce yourself and confirm the identity of the patient. Determine whether any special preparation was needed by this patient and if it was followed.
   Purpose: If special procedures were *not* followed, the test may have to be rescheduled.

3 Explain the purpose of the test.
   Purpose: To help reassure the patient.

4 Measure and record the patient's vital signs, height, and weight.

5 Explain the actual maneuver.
   Purpose: The patient needs to understand the maneuver so he or she can cooperate fully to obtain best testing results.

6 Be certain the patient is comfortable and in proper sitting or standing position.
   Purpose: Proper positioning is necessary to ensure accurate test results.

7 Loosen any tight clothing, such as a necktie, bra, or belt.

   Purpose: Tight clothing may restrict breathing capacity.

8 Show the patient the proper chin and neck position.

9 Practice the maneuver with the patient and tell the patient, "Inhale."
   Purpose: To relieve apprehension and enhance understanding.

10 Use active, forceful coaching during testing (see Figure 43-14, *B*). Begin by saying, "Blow." Then say, "Blow out hard." Then say, "Keep blowing, keep blowing." Then say, "Don't stop—blow harder."
   Purpose: Coaching improves performance.

11 Give the patient feedback after the maneuver is completed.
   Purpose: Positive feedback and explanations of mistakes in the maneuver will help improve patient compliance.

12 Continue testing until three acceptable maneuvers have been obtained.

13 Place the test results on the patient's chart for physician review. Dismiss the patient only if results are satisfactory.

14 Clean and disinfect the equipment. Discard waste in a biohazard waste container.

15 Wash your hands.
   Purpose: Infection control.

16 Record testing information on the patient's chart.
   Purpose: Procedures that are not recorded are considered not done.

When the demonstration is done, remind the patient of the following points:

- Take as deep a breath as possible.
- Blow air out hard.
- Do not stop blowing until you are told to stop.

Use active and forceful coaching while the patient is performing the maneuver. You may need to raise your voice with some urgency to improve the patient's performance, using such phrases as, "Blow, blow, blow!" "Keep blowing, keep blowing!" and "Don't stop blowing!" After the maneuver, give the patient some feedback on the quality of the test and describe what improvements could be made. Continue to repeat efforts until *three acceptable maneuvers* are obtained. The two best efforts are used to calculate pulmonary function. The physician calculates normal values for each patient based on individual age, height, weight, and sex, which are documented as a percentage. If the patient's best efforts are greater than 80% of pretest calculated values, pulmonary function is considered to be normal. Spirometry tests provide the physician information about the impact of obstruction or pulmonary disease on airflow. If results are less than 60% of the predicted value, the patient may be given bronchodilators and be retested to determine the impact of the inhalant on function.

ACCEPTABLE SPIROMETER TEST

An acceptable spirometer test has five characteristics:

- No coughing
- Good start of test
- No early termination
- No variable flows
- Consistency

Test Results. Place the results of the maneuvers with the patient's chart on the physician's desk when the tests are completed. Many physicians rely on the assistant to include comments pertinent to the testing, such as patient condition during the test and compliance with coaching. If there are any questions regarding the quality of the results, ask the patient to wait while the physician reviews the results. If the patient has delayed taking medication, check with the physician as to when the patient should resume taking it.

CRITICAL THINKING APPLICATION

Michael is in the process of orienting Cinda, a new employee, on how to perform a spirometer test. He has summarized the steps of the procedure on a card next to the machine for easy reference. Cinda knows nothing about the procedure. What would be the best way for Michael to teach her about the test? What information should he include?

Pulse Oximetry. Pulse oximetry is a noninvasive method of evaluating the oxygen saturation of hemoglobin in arterial blood, as well as the pulse rate. It identifies the percentage of hemoglobin that is oxygenated in comparison with the total amount of hemoglobin that is available. Many ambulatory settings have pulse oximeters available to assess a patient's oxygenation status with such disorders as pneumonia, bronchitis, emphysema, or asthma (Figure 43-15, *A*).

To perform the procedure, the medical assistant clips a probe on the patient's earlobe or finger (Figure 43-15, *B* and *C*). A beam of infrared light passes through the tissue and the machine measures the amount of light absorbed by the oxygenated hemoglobin, which is displayed on the digital screen as a percentage. At the same time, the light also measures the patient's pulse rate, which is also shown on the screen. A normal pulse oximeter reading is greater than or equal to 95% (meaning 95% of the total available hemoglobin attachments for oxygen are carrying oxygen). Treatment, such as oxygen or bronchodilator therapies, is usually started when readings are at 90% to 92% or lower.

Obtaining Sputum for Culture. A sputum culture is requested when there are signs and symptoms accompanied by physical evidence of pneumonia, tuberculosis, or other infectious diseases of the lower respiratory tract. The sample is sent to a laboratory equipped to handle bacteriological samples that are potentially infectious. Once the sample arrives at the laboratory, it will be cultured and incubated. The pathogenic organism grown in the culture media will then be identified. If possible, the physician will not start antibiotic therapy until the sputum has been collected. The sample may also be sent to the laboratory for cytological analysis that might suggest a cancerous condition of the lungs or bronchi.

Methods of Collection. In the ambulatory care setting, the primary method for collection of a sputum sample is expectoration (Procedure 43-2), but sputum can be collected by tracheal suctioning and bronchoscopy. If the sample is to be collected by expectoration, most physician practices will have the patient perform the procedure at home with instruction. The medical assistant may be responsible for explaining the procedure to the patient or reinforcing physician instructions. The patient should understand that the best time for sputum specimen collection is in the morning when the patient first wakes up, before eating or drinking. The patient can rinse out his or her mouth with water before collecting the sample to decrease contamination from the oropharynx. The sample is collected from sputum coughed up from the lungs, not from saliva, so the patient should be encouraged to cough deeply and forcefully to collect a satisfactory sample. It may help to have the patient take several deep breaths and then cough. At least 1 teaspoon of sputum should be collected in a sterile specimen cup (the patient needs to know how to handle the specimen cup to maintain sterility), which should be returned to the office or laboratory as soon as possible after the specimen is collected.

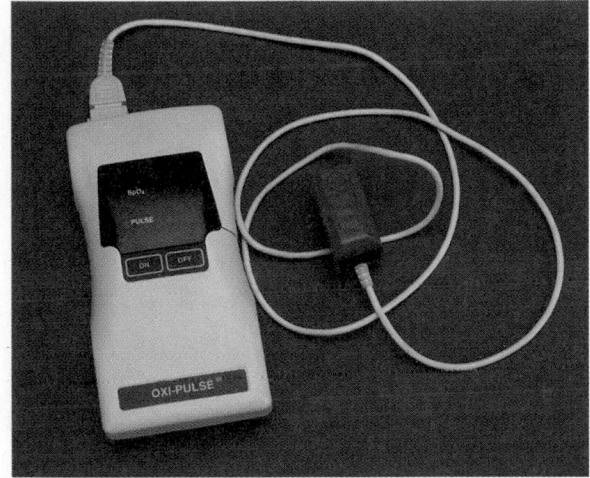

A

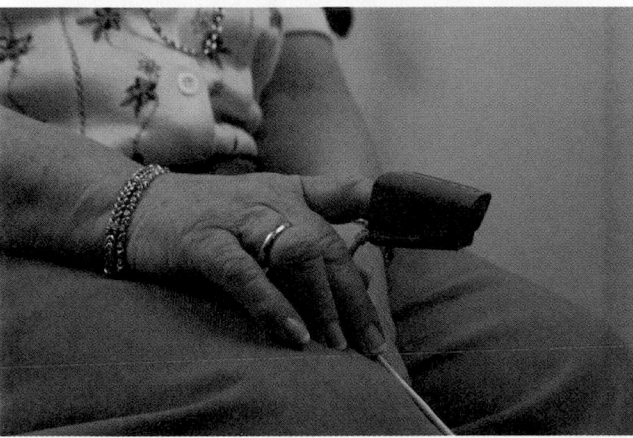

B

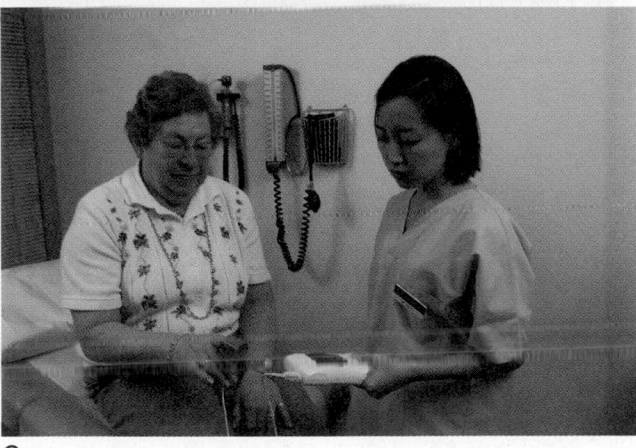

C

FIGURE 43-15 **A**, A pulse oximeter. **B**, A pulse oximetry clip. **C**, A patient with a pulse oximeter.

If the patient is taking antibiotic medications at the time of the specimen collection, this information should be included on the laboratory slip. If the cough does not produce sputum, chest physiotherapy or nebulization (a heated aerosol spray) may be ordered by the physician to induce it. Sputum collection may be required for three consecutive mornings.

Bronchoscopy. Bronchoscopy is typically performed in the outpatient clinic or hospital setting. The medical assistant should be familiar with the procedure, because he or she will probably schedule the test, instruct the patient on preparation, and help answer patient or family questions. Bronchoscopy provides an endoscopic view of the larynx, trachea, and bronchi. The procedure is performed by a pulmonary specialist or a surgeon, usually with a flexible fiberoptic bronchoscope through which the physician can collect biopsy specimens or bronchial washings for cytological evaluation or culture. Laser therapy to treat endotracheal lesions is also possible through the flexible scope.

The patient should remain NPO for 4 to 8 hours before the test to reduce the risk of aspiration. The patient should perform good mouth care before the procedure to reduce the number of bacteria present. Dentures should be removed, and he or she will receive medication before the procedure to aid in relaxation and dry up oral secretions. The patient should be reassured that the procedure does not interfere with breathing.

Before the instrument is inserted, the physician will spray a topical anesthetic (lidocaine) in the mouth and back of the throat to help prevent the gag reflex and reduce any discomfort from passage of the instrument. The tube can be inserted through the nose or mouth, and as it reaches the glottis, more lidocaine is sprayed to control the cough reflex. The physician continues to pass the tube through the bronchi and larger bronchioles, collecting biopsy specimens of any suspicious tissue and obtaining cellular washings if indicated. Because the patient is sedated, it is not an uncomfortable procedure, but there may be hemoptysis for several hours, and the patient may have a sore throat after the procedure. Biopsy and culture reports are usually not available for 2 to 7 days.

Patient Education

It is often said that the greatest fear a person ever has is the fear of the unknown. Often the patient worries and fears the tests that the physician orders. The imagination can create all types of frightening scenarios with even more alarming outcomes. A medical assistant can play a vital role in allaying patient fears by explaining

PROCEDURE 43-2

Obtaining a Sputum Sample for Culture

GOAL: To collect a sputum sample while observing standard precautions.

EQUIPMENT AND SUPPLIES

- Sterile laboratory specimen cup, accurately labeled
- Plastic laboratory specimen bag with laboratory requisition
- Disposable examination gloves
- Face shield with goggles
- Impervious gown
- Biohazard waste container
- Cup of water
- Ginger ale or juice

PROCEDURAL STEPS

1 Assemble the equipment and label the specimen cup.

2 Identify the patient and explain the procedure.
Purpose: An informed patient is more cooperative.

3 Wash your hands and don gloves, face shield, and lab coat.
Purpose: Standard precautions must be followed when collecting potentially infectious materials.

4 Have the patient rinse his or her mouth with water.
Purpose: Any food particles in the mouth will contaminate the specimen.

5 Instruct the patient to take three deep breaths and then cough deeply to bring up secretions from the lower respiratory tract.
Purpose: The organisms for culture must be from the lung fields in the lower respiratory tract.

6 Tell the patient to spit directly into the specimen container and to avoid getting any sputum on the exterior of the container.
Purpose: Sputum on the exterior of the container is considered hazardous.

7 Place the lid on the container securely and then place the container into the plastic specimen bag.
Purpose: Minimize the possibility of spreading the potentially hazardous specimen.

8 Offer the patient a glass of juice or ginger ale.
Purpose: The patient may have a bad taste in his or her mouth after the test, which may cause nausea.

9 If another test is ordered for the next morning, instruct the patient when to come to the office or explain how to complete the procedure at home. Remind him or her to follow the same instructions for preparation.

10 Clean the work area and properly dispose of all supplies.
Purpose: Observe standard precautions.

11 Wash your hands.
Purpose: Infection control.

12 Process the specimen immediately to ensure optimal test results.
Purpose: Microorganisms may propagate or die, creating an elevated or false-negative result.

13 Record the procedure in the patient's record.
Purpose: Procedures that are not recorded are considered not done.

---

diagnostic tests, making certain the patient understands how to prepare for the study and what will be expected of him or her during the procedure. Ensure that the patient receives literature explaining the test ordered to read at his or her leisure before the testing time. Answer all of the patient's questions and consult with the physician regarding concerns or questions before the patient leaves the office.

As medical assistants, we need to be aware of opportunities to give advice and help by answering questions and alerting the physician to possible symptoms that we notice in preparing the patient.

Legal and Ethical Issues

When the respiratory system is mentioned, people generally think of breathing, but this is only one of the activities of the respiratory system. The cells of the body need a continuous supply of oxygen to maintain life. The respiratory system works together with the circulatory system to supply this oxygen and to remove the waste products of metabolism. Too often people take breathing for granted and assume that nothing could possibly happen to their ability to breathe. Sadly, respiratory diseases are the leading cause of death, and that means there are people we know and love who will suffer and die of some of the diseases discussed in this chapter.

If the pulmonary test ordered is an invasive test, such as bronchoscopy, be certain that a written consent form is obtained from the patient and is in the patient's chart. If the patient is to see another specialist, a consent form must be signed to give permission to copy and forward patient information to the consultant. If oxygen therapy is ordered, the physician must write a prescription that specifies the amount of oxygen to be given and the type of device to be used for delivery. The physician may also write an order for a respiratory care practitioner to follow up on the patient at home.

SUMMARY OF SCENARIO

Michael has become very adept at performing respiratory diagnostic procedures and treatments for ambulatory patients. He enjoys interacting with this special group of patients and works at maintaining an up-to-date file on educational and resource assistance in the community. Michael especially enjoys the patient education aspect of caring for persons with respiratory disease. Many of these patients have chronic diseases that will require long-term physician care, and Michael attempts to use those frequent "teaching moments" to reinforce healthy lifestyle habits and confirm patient understanding of treatments.

SUMMARY OF LEARNING OBJECTIVES

- The respiratory system has two primary functions: exchange oxygen from the atmosphere for carbon dioxide waste through external and internal respiration; and maintain the acid-base balance within the body. The respiratory system and the circulatory system work together to supply body cells with oxygen and remove metabolic wastes. The upper respiratory tract transports air from the atmosphere to the lungs and includes the nose, pharynx, and larynx. The lower respiratory tract consists of the trachea, bronchial tubes, and the lungs.

- The bronchioles deposit oxygenated air into the alveoli. Surrounding each alveolus is a network of pulmonary capillaries filled with waste air. The oxygenated air moves through the single-celled walls of the alveoli and through the single-celled walls of these capillaries, and waste is forced out of the capillaries back into the alveoli and then into the bronchioles. This exchange is referred to as ventilation. The movement of oxygen from the atmosphere into the alveoli is called inspiration, and the movement of the waste gases from the alveoli back into the atmosphere is called expiration.

- Table 43-1 lists common respiratory system terms and their definitions. A medical assistant is expected to be familiar with these terms and use them in documenting patient signs and symptoms.

- Upper respiratory tract infections include the common cold, which is caused by a virus and has no cure; sinusitis, which causes edema and the collection of mucus within the cavity, creating a feeling of pressure, either nasal congestion or rhinorrhea, and classic sinus headaches. Lower respiratory tract infections include pneumonia, meaning inflammation of all or part of the lungs that is caused by bacteria, viruses, irritants, or other pathogens; and tuberculosis, caused by the bacterium *Mycobacterium tuberculosis*, which is transmitted by droplets of sputum expectorated by an infected host and inhaled by a susceptible host and which develops into either primary or secondary infections.

- Chronic obstructive pulmonary disease (COPD) is a group of diseases with the common characteristic of chronic airway obstruction. Among the diseases included in this group are chronic bronchitis, bronchiectasis, asthma, pneumoconiosis, and emphysema. Although the mechanism of the obstruction may vary, a patient with COPD is unable to ventilate the lungs freely, resulting in an ineffective exchange of respiratory gases. Treatments include bronchodilator and corticosteroid inhalers, evaluation of peak flow values, and nebulizer treatments.

- The most prevalent neoplasms of the respiratory system are lung cancer and carcinoma of the larynx. Lung cancer is the leading cause of cancer-related deaths for both men and women, and the lung is a common site for secondary tumors from metastasis as well as primary carcinomas. Prognosis is very poor for lung cancer, because early symptoms mimic chronic conditions present in long-term smokers. Carcinoma of the larynx is linked to smoking and chronic alcohol consumption. Owing to early symptoms, most laryngeal tumors are discovered in their early stages and can be removed with a very good prognosis.

- Respiratory system diagnostic procedures include the Mantoux intradermal test for TB; pulmonary function tests, measured with a spirometer, that diagnose a pulmonary abnormality and/or determine the extent of a pulmonary disease; pulse oximetry, a noninvasive method of evaluating the oxygen saturation of hemoglobin in arterial blood as well as the pulse rate; cultures performed on expectorated sputum for identification of infectious pathogens or cytological evaluation; and bronchoscopy, an endoscopic view of the larynx, trachea, and bronchi that uses a flexible fiberoptic instrument through which the physician can collect biopsy specimens or bronchial washings for cytological evaluation or culture.

KEY INTERNET WEBSITES

- American Academy of Allergy, Asthma and Immunology
- American Lung Association
- Cystic Fibrosis Foundation
- National Heart, Lung, and Blood Institute Information Center
- National Institute of Allergy and Infectious Diseases
  For active weblinks to each website visit
  http://evolve.elsevier.com/Kinn/

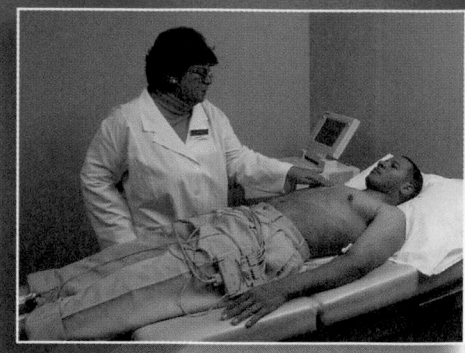

CHAPTER 44

Scenario

Anna Stern, CMA, has been working for more than 3 years as a medical assistant in a variety of physicians' offices. Anna was recently hired to work at City Hospital in the cardiology department. Her job description includes working in the clinical area of the practice as well as assisting attending physicians with patient education and follow-up. Because Anna has never worked for a cardiologist, she is concerned about her knowledge base and competency in cardiac patient care.

Assisting in Cardiology

Learning Objectives

- Define and spell the terms listed in the vocabulary.
- Anatomically and physiologically describe the heart and its significant structures.
- Summarize the risk factors for the development of cardiovascular disease.
- Describe the signs, symptoms, and diagnostic and therapeutic procedures employed with coronary artery disease and myocardial infarction.
- Explain hypertension and its effect on the cardiovascular system.
- Outline the causes and results of congestive heart failure.
- Illustrate the effect of inflammation and valve disorders on cardiac function.
- Anatomically and physiologically describe the circulatory vessels.
- Differentiate between the various types of shock.
- Summarize the characteristics of common vascular disorders.
- Outline typical cardiovascular diagnostic procedures.

National Curriculum Competencies

CLINICAL COMPETENCIES

4a. Perform telephone and in-person screening

4e. Prepare patients for and assist with routine and specialty examinations

4f. Prepare patients for and assist with procedures, treatments, and minor office surgery

4g. Apply pharmacology principles to prepare and administer oral and parenteral medications

TRANSDISCIPLINARY COMPETENCIES

3b. Instruct individuals according to their needs

3d. Provide instruction for health maintenance and disease prevention

Vocabulary

bruit Abnormal sound or murmur heard on auscultation of an organ, vessel, or gland.

intermittent claudications Recurring cramping in the calves caused by poor circulation of blood to the muscles of the lower leg.

Marfan syndrome An inherited condition characterized by elongation of the bones, joint hypermobility, abnormalities of the eyes, and development of aortic aneurysm.

scleroderma Autoimmune disorder that affects the blood vessels and connective tissue, causing fibrous degeneration of the major organs.

In the past, cardiac disease was frequently seen in men but seldom seen in women. That has changed, and today the most frequent cause of illness and death, regardless of gender, is cardiovascular disease. Medical assistants in all specialties often care for patients with heart disorders. Seldom does the cardiologist discover the heart problem. Most patients who see this specialist have already been diagnosed with a suspected heart disorder and were referred to the cardiologist for verification and treatment.

Because of the overwhelming number of people with cardiovascular problems, all medical assistants need to understand this system, be able to recognize early symptoms of potential disorders, perform basic screening tests when ordered by the physician, and assist the physician in the examination of the heart and vessels.

Anatomy of the Heart

The heart is a hollow, muscular organ situated in the thoracic cavity in the mediastinal region, between the right and left pleural spaces. It weighs about 9 ounces and is about the size of a closed fist, with approximately two thirds of it located to the left of the sternum (Figure 44-1). The heart is a muscular pump that provides the force needed to push blood through all the arteries of the body, thus circulating a continuous supply of oxygen and nutrients to the cells and picking up the metabolic waste products from them. Deprived of these vital functions, the cells will die. At the same time, the heart also pushes deoxygenated blood through the pulmonary artery to the lungs for oxygen saturation and then back through the pulmonary veins into the left side of the heart. The average adult heart pumps about 5 L of blood every minute. If the heart loses its pumping action for even a few brief minutes, death or permanent damage can result.

Layers of the Heart

The heart is enclosed in a double-membrane sac called the *pericardium*. The outer layer of the pericardial sac is a tough, protective membrane that connects the heart to the diaphragm; the inner layer, the visceral membrane or *epicardium*, forms the first layer of the heart. Between the two membranes is a small space, the *pericardial cavity*, which contains a few drops of pericardial fluid that permits easy heart movement. The middle layer of the heart is the *myocardium*, the muscle layer that constitutes the largest percentage of the heart wall. Contractions of this muscle layer force the blood from the heart into the vessels. The inner layer of the heart is the *endocardium*, including the heart valves that separate the chambers of the heart and provide a means of blocking the flow of blood from major blood vessels entering and exiting the heart (Figure 44-2).

Heart Chambers and Arteries

The heart is divided into four chambers (Figure 44-3). The *atria*, the top chambers, receive blood, and the *ventricles*, the bottom chambers, pump the blood out. The blood flow through the heart begins in the right atrium, which receives deoxygenated blood from the inferior and superior vena cava. The atria contract, and blood passes through the tricuspid valve into the right ventricle; the ventricles contract, and blood passes from the right ventricle to the lungs via the *pulmonary artery* (the only artery in the body that contains deoxygenated blood). Oxygenation occurs in the lungs, and the now-oxygenated blood returns to the left atria through the *pulmonary veins* (the only veins in the body that carry oxygen-rich blood). The atria contract, and blood passes through the mitral (bicuspid) valve into the left ventricle; the ventricles contract, and oxygen-rich blood is sent out to the body through the *aorta* (the largest artery in the body).

The myocardium requires a continuous supply of oxygen and nutrients, which are delivered through two coronary arteries that branch off the aorta above the aortic valve (Figure 44-4). The right coronary artery nourishes the anterior and posterior myocardium on the right side of the heart, and the left coronary artery does the same on the left side. The left coronary artery quickly divides and forms the left anterior descending artery and the left circumflex artery. Smaller branches of the coronary arteries feed the myocardium and the endocardium. Any interference in blood flow in any of the coronary vessels will alter heart action.

Heart Conduction

A sophisticated electrical conduction system, controlled by the autonomic nervous system and located in the myocardium, stimulates the heart-muscle contractions. These muscle contractions make blood move through the chambers of the heart and the rest of the body. Each electrical impulse passes through the heart muscle in a twisting, spiral motion. These rhythmic waves cause the cardiac cells to beat, which causes the heart to contract.

The cardiac impulse originates in specialized muscle tissue called the *sinoatrial* (SA) node. The SA node rhythmically initiates impulses 70 to 80 times a minute; because it creates the basic rhythm, it is called the *pacemaker* of the heart. It is located in the posterior,

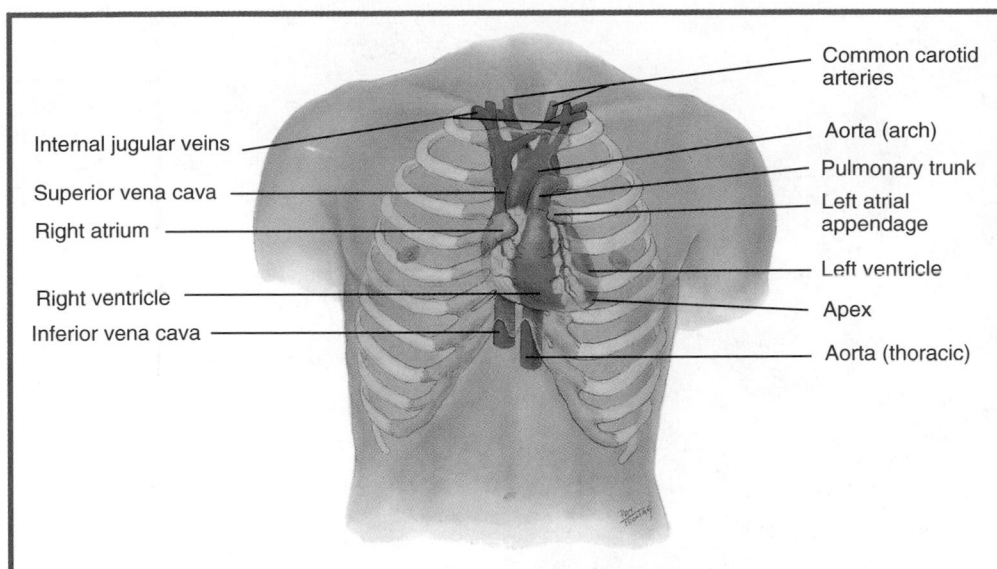

FIGURE 44-1 Location of the heart in the thoracic cavity. (From Applegate EJ: *The anatomy and physiology learning system*, Philadelphia, 1995, WB Saunders.)

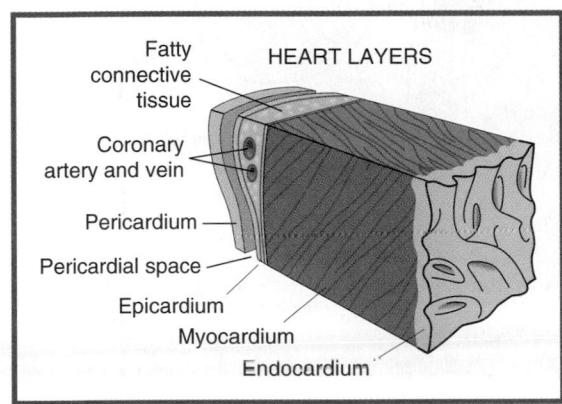

FIGURE 44-2 Layers of the heart. (From Damjanov I: *Pathology for the health-related professions*, ed. 2, Philadelphia, 2000, WB Saunders.)

superior wall of the right atrium, just at the junction of the superior vena cava and the atrium. When it discharges its rhythm pattern into the myocardium, it causes both atria to contract, forcing blood into the ventricles. The wave then passes through a second area of specialized muscle tissue located on the septal wall between the right atrium and right ventricle, called the *atrioventricular* (AV) node. The AV node holds the impulse for a fraction of a second to prevent inappropriately high atrial rates as well as to permit the blood to empty from the atria through the tricuspid and mitral valves. The chordae tendineae, at this moment, close the valves between the atria and the ventricles tightly. Then the AV node releases the charge, sending it down through the bundle of His, located in the septum between the right and left ventricles. This bundle is divided into two main branches, the right bundle located on the right side of the septum and the left bundle located on the left side. From the bundle branches, the transmission of the cardiac wave continues through a mass of cardiac muscle fibers known as the *Purkinje fibers*. The Purkinje

fibers totally encase both ventricles, and the cardiac wave causes the ventricles to contract (Figure 44-5).

Contraction of the atria and the ventricles is also called *depolarization*. After the chambers contract, a period of electric recovery occurs, called *repolarization*, and then the heart returns to resting (*polarization*), which starts the entire cycle again. The normal cardiac cycle consists of atrial contraction, ventricular contraction, and then recovery and heart rest. This cycle maintains the average range of 60 to 100 beats per minute and a normal heart rhythm. It is this electrical force that is traced and evaluated when an electrocardiogram is done. Chapter 46 presents electrocardiograms.

Diseases and Disorders of the Heart

There are many diseases and disorders of the heart and its blood vessels. Disorders that occur when the rhythm of the heart becomes irregular are addressed in Chapter 46. There are multiple risk factors for cardiac disease, including genetic predisposition and familial history; hypertension; diabetes; and elevated blood cholesterol levels. Lifestyle factors, including high-fat, high-caloric diets; obesity; smoking; lack of exercise; and stress, also contribute to premature death by cardiovascular disease. Persons suffering from cardiac disease have similar symptoms, including chest pain, dyspnea on exertion, tachypnea, palpitations (pounding or racing of the heart), cyanosis, edema, fatigue, syncope, and diaphoresis.

Coronary Artery Disease and Myocardial Infarction

Coronary artery disease (CAD) causes about 700,000 deaths in the United States every year. In CAD, the arteries supplying the myocardium become narrowed by atherosclerotic plaques. Platelets stick to the plaque deposits, forming superimposed thrombi, and lipids continue to build up at the site. The process continues, causing

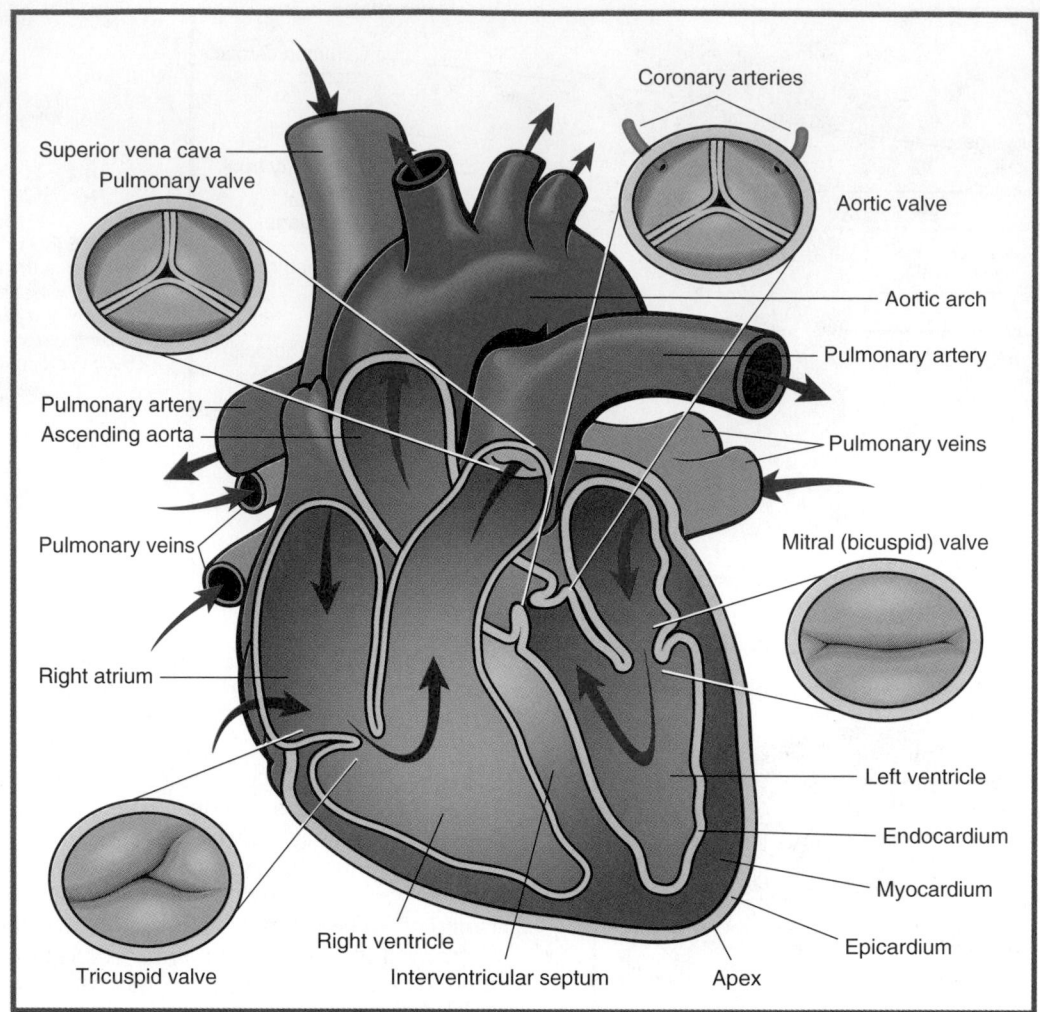

FIGURE 44-3 Chambers of the heart. (From Damjanov I: *Pathology for the health-related professions*, ed. 2, Philadelphia, 2000, WB Saunders.)

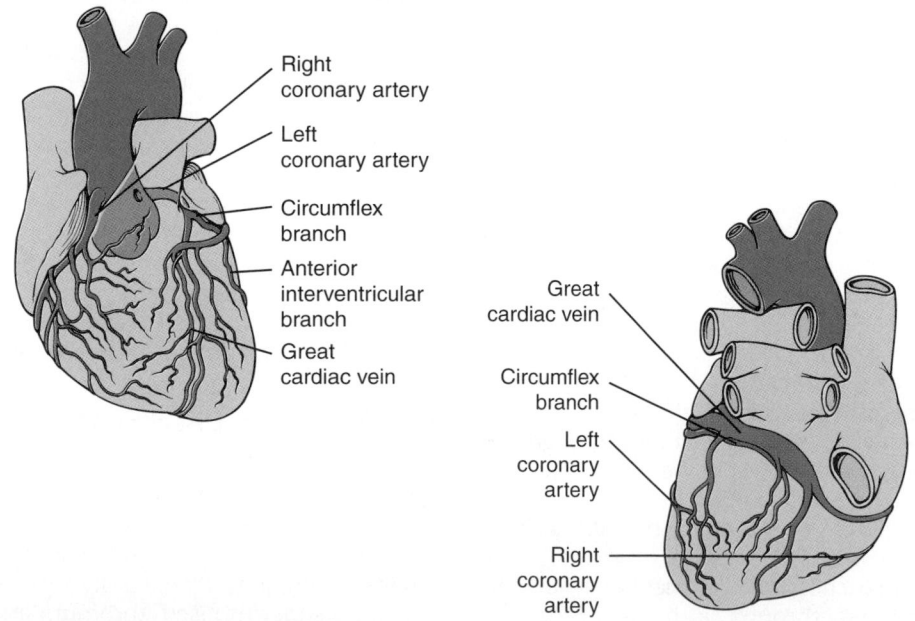

FIGURE 44-4 Coronary arteries. (From Frazier MS, Drzymkowski JW: *Essentials of human diseases and conditions*, ed. 2, Philadelphia, 2000, WB Saunders.)

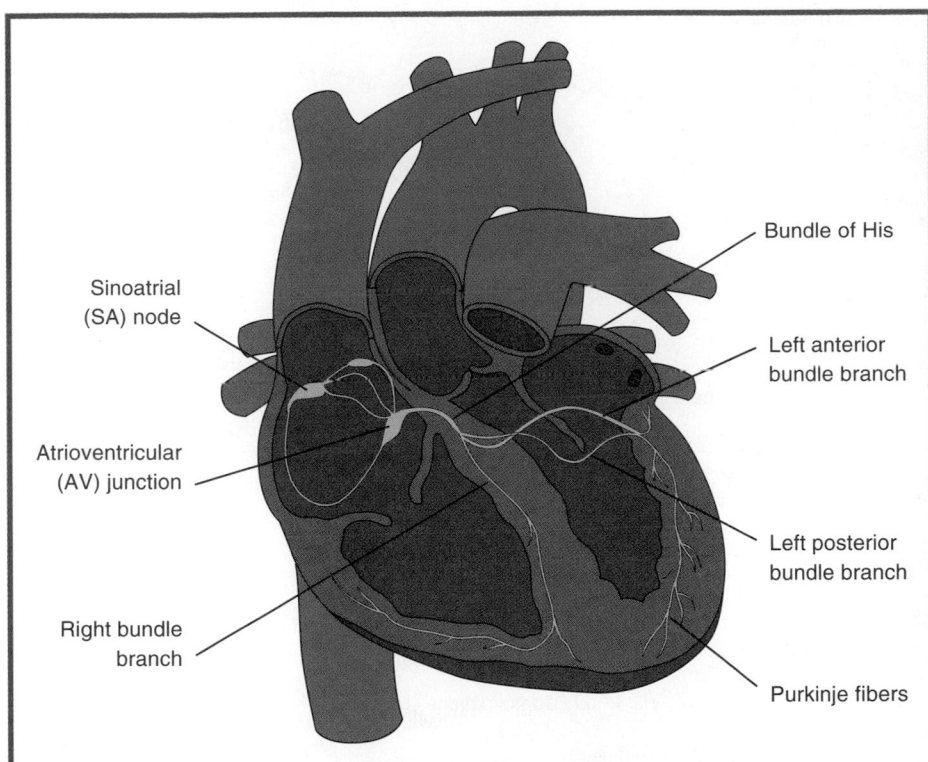

FIGURE 44-5 Cardiac conduction system.

narrowing of the opening (*lumen*) of the arteries and inhibition of the normal flow of blood, thus depriving the heart of an adequate nutritious blood supply (Figure 44-6). The cardinal symptom of myocardial *ischemia* (holding back of blood) is angina pectoris. The features of anginal chest pain are pain behind the sternum that is precipitated by exertion but can be relieved by either rest or sublingual nitroglycerin.

Patients may be asymptomatic until the disease becomes fully developed. The first symptom may be angina, followed by pressure or fullness in the chest, syncope, edema, unexplained coughing spells, and fatigue. A patient reporting any of these symptoms should be seen by the physician immediately. Women may exhibit a different clinical picture than the traditional one expected from men.

The major concern in heart disease is the lack of blood to the myocardium, which occurs when a vessel becomes totally blocked. Ischemia over a prolonged period leads to *necrosis* (death) of a portion of the myocardium, resulting in a myocardial infarction (MI), or heart attack. Symptoms of MI are similar to those of angina, but MI is identified by pain lasting longer than 30 minutes that is unrelieved by rest or nitroglycerin tablets. An MI is life threatening, and intervention must begin within the first hour, or death may occur.

CRITICAL THINKING APPLICATION

A patient who is scheduled for an appointment in 2 days calls the office and reports that she is not feeling well. She complains of a feeling of fullness in the chest, her arms ache, and she is very tired. Although this patient does not have a history of myocardial infarction, what should Anna do?

MYOCARDIAL INFARCTION SYMPTOMS IN WOMEN

- Abdominal or midback pain
- Jaw pain
- Indigestion
- Extreme fatigue
- Aching in both arms

TELEPHONE SCREENING FOR CHEST PAIN

The medical assistant should activate emergency medical services if the patient reports any of the following:
- Current chest pain that is crushing, pressing, or radiating to the arms, upper back, or jaw
- Sweating, difficulty breathing, nausea, indigestion, or dizziness
- A history of coronary artery disease, myocardial infarction, or angina
- A change in the pattern of the angina
- Chest pain that occurs when resting or with minimal exertion

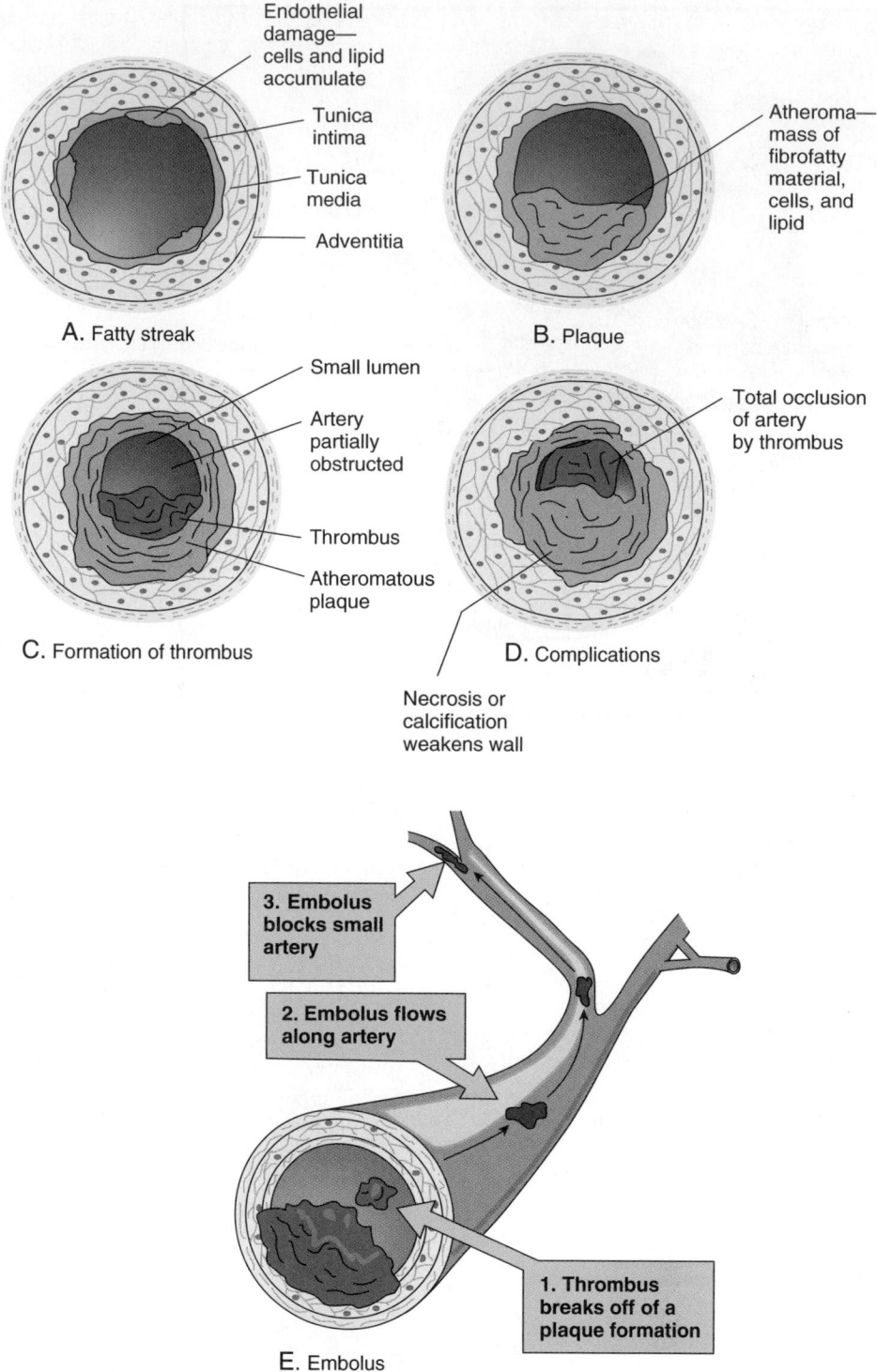

FIGURE 44-6 Development of an atheroma leading to arterial occlusion. (From Gould BA: *Pathophysiology for the health professions*, ed. 3, Philadelphia, 2002, WB Saunders.)

Diagnostic and Therapeutic Procedures. An MI is diagnosed by electrocardiogram (ECG) changes and elevated cardiac enzymes (creatinine phosphokinase [CPK] and lactate dehydrogenase [LDH]) 6 to 12 hours after the episode. These enzymes are released by the necrotic myocardium and may be within normal limits initially but continue to increase for 24 to 49 hours after the MI has occurred. Patients diagnosed with an MI are hospitalized immediately, started on oxygen, and continuously monitored by ECG. Additional diagnostic procedures such as echocardiograms and heart catheterizations are discussed later in this chapter.

Medical treatment includes the use of *thrombolytic* medications, such as streptokinase, to dissolve the coronary artery blockage; however, this treatment must be started within 6 hours of the episode and no longer than 24 hours after initial symptoms to be effective in preventing permanent myocardial damage. This timetable makes it extremely important that patients be identified and treatment started as soon as possible. Additional pharmaceutical treatment includes the use of aspirin and beta-blockers (Tenormin, Lopressor, or Inderal), which decrease the amount of oxygen needed by the myocardium; angiotensin-converting enzyme (ACE) inhibitors (Lotensin, Capoten, or Vasotec) to help prevent left ventricular damage; anticoagulants (warfarin [Coumadin]) for 3 to 6 months to prevent thrombus formation; and anticholesterol agents (Lipitor, Mevacor, or Zocor) to lower blood cholesterol levels and prevent subsequent formation of atherosclerotic plaques.

When blockage or occlusion has taken place in one of the two coronary arteries that supply blood to the myocardium, either percutaneous transluminal coronary angioplasty or coronary artery bypass surgery (CABG) may be indicated. These procedures are discussed later in this chapter. After being discharged from the hospital, patients with CAD that has resulted in an MI face multiple lifestyle changes to prevent the reoccurrence of another episode. Recommendations include no smoking; regular light exercise, such as walking up to an hour three times per week; a diet that is low in salt, fat, and cholesterol; and stress reduction. The medical assistant should be prepared to provide encouragement and reinforce the importance of lifestyle changes to prevent future heart problems. If ordered by the physician, professional referrals to a cardiac rehabilitation program and dietitian also can be helpful.

CRITICAL THINKING APPLICATION

Anna receives a telephone call from a patient who complains of nausea, has difficulty taking a deep breath, and thinks he or she is going to faint. What questions should she ask to determine the seriousness of the problem?

Hypertensive Heart Disease

Chronic elevated blood pressure can result in left ventricular *hypertrophy* (enlargement), angina, MI, or heart failure. Hypertension is also a major cause of stroke and *nephropathy* (kidney disease). Some of the risk factors for developing hypertension include a family history of hypertension or stroke, *hypercholesterolemia* (high blood cholesterol), smoking, high sodium intake, diabetes, excessive alcohol intake, aging, prolonged stress, and race (blacks have a higher incidence than whites).

The two types of hypertension are primary and secondary. *Secondary hypertension* occurs because of a disease process in another body system, such as renal disease or an endocrine disorder. Before secondary hypertension can be properly treated, the underlying disease process must be resolved.

Primary, or *essential*, hypertension is *idiopathic* (unknown cause) and is diagnosed if the patient's blood pressure is consistently above 140/90. The diastolic number is especially important because it reflects the level of peripheral resistance and the resultant workload of the left ventricle. The general rule in diagnosis is that the patient's blood pressure is elevated in two or more measurements taken at least 2 minutes apart with a proper-size cuff. The blood pressure is usually verified in the other arm; if there is a difference, the physician will use the higher value for diagnostic purposes. This process is repeated in a subsequent visit before the patient is diagnosed with essential hypertension. The medical assistant is responsible for accurately measuring and recording the series of blood pressures. Some patients have what is called "white-coat" hypertension, which appears only when they visit the physician. If the patient has a history of this problem, have him or her lie down on the examination table and rest for a few minutes before taking the blood pressure; this may help to get a more accurate reading.

Hypertension has an insidious onset, with the patient showing few, if any, symptoms until permanent damage occurs. Initial symptoms include general malaise and headache, while *epistaxis* (nosebleed), vertigo, nausea, or syncope can occur with prolonged hypertension. Once diagnosed, treatment begins with recommendations to lose weight, decrease the use of salt, control stress, and exercise regularly. If those measures are not successful in lowering the blood pressure, drug therapy is usually started with mild diuretics (hydrochlorothiazide, furosemide [Lasix], or Dyazide) or beta-blockers, calcium channel blockers, and/or ACE inhibitors. If the patient is still not at his or her goal blood pressure level, a second antihypertensive medication may be added. The drug therapy program is designed to fit each patient's needs and response.

The medical assistant can be an interactive part of this therapy by teaching the patient how to take his or her own blood pressure, providing literature that reinforces the necessity of monitoring the blood pressure, and helping the patient to understand that this condition cannot be cured but can be controlled for the rest of his or her life. Continued encouragement and support are needed because compliance with the treatment regimen is difficult for a patient who is not exhibiting any symptoms of disease.

CRITICAL THINKING APPLICATION

Essential hypertension is a common problem for patients seen in the cardiology department where Anna works. What could Anna do to help patients with primary hypertension? What informational materials or community resources would be helpful in gaining patient compliance with treatment?

Congestive Heart Failure

Congestive heart failure (CHF) occurs when the myocardium is unable to pump an adequate amount of blood to meet the needs of the body. Although the problem can have an acute onset, it typically develops over time because of weakness in the left ventricle from chronic hypertension or MI of the ventricular wall, valvular heart disease, or pulmonary complications. Typically, heart failure initially occurs on one side of the heart, followed by the other side. Left-sided heart failure usually results from essential hypertension or left-ventricle disease, whereas right-sided heart failure can develop from lung disease. Right-sided heart failure that occurs because of pulmonary hypertension associated with chronic obstructive pulmonary disease (COPD) is called *cor pulmonale*.

Left-sided heart failure, when the left ventricle cannot completely empty, causes a backup of blood in the lungs, resulting in *pulmonary edema*, a collection of fluid in the lungs. Signs and symptoms include dyspnea, orthopnea, nonproductive cough, rales, and tachycardia. Right-sided heart failure, when the right ventricle cannot maintain complete output, causes a backup of blood in the right atrium, which prevents complete emptying of the vena cava, resulting in systemic edema, especially in the legs and feet. Both types of heart failure cause fatigue, weakness, exercise intolerance, dyspnea, and sensitivity to cold temperatures.

Nonmedication treatment for CHF includes limiting physical activity so that the heart does not have to work so hard, salt restriction, no smoking, stress reduction, and weight control. Patient education for an individual with CHF must stress the importance of monitoring weight gain because a sudden increase in weight may indicate fluid retention. Patients should weigh themselves one to two times per week and report an increase in weight of more than 3 pounds to the physician. Drug therapy begins with diuretics to treat dyspnea and orthopnea and control edema. Other medications may include ACE inhibitors and digitalis (Digoxin) to increase the force of ventricular contractions. Because potassium loss is a common side effect of diuretic and digitalis use, patients may also be prescribed a potassium supplement (KCl). The physician will order routine monitoring of serum electrolytes to determine the need for a potassium supplement so that potential complications can be avoided.

CRITICAL THINKING APPLICATION

Kate Glasgow, a 76-year-old patient with a history of CHF, is in the office today for a checkup. Miss Glasgow does not understand why she needs to stop using salt and does not weigh herself regularly at home. What can Anna do to help this patient understand the importance of her treatment regimen?

Inflammations and Valvular Disorders

Rheumatic Heart Disease. Rheumatic heart disease develops because of an unusual immune reaction that occurs approximately 2 weeks after an untreated beta-hemolytic streptococcal infection. The infection starts as strep throat or an upper respiratory infection but progresses to the creation of antibodies that react with collagen to cause inflammation in the joints, skin, brain, and heart. The inflammation in the heart can involve all layers of heart tissue.

Pericarditis, inflammation of the outer layer of the heart, causes reduced cardiac activity and pericardial *effusion* (collection of blood or fluid in the pericardium).

Myocarditis, inflammation of the muscular lining of the heart, is usually self-limiting but may lead to acute heart failure due to weakening of the myocardial wall. *Endocarditis*, inflammation of the inner lining of the heart and the heart valves, is the most common heart complication. Vegetations form along the outer edges of the valve cusps, causing scarring and stenosis. The mitral valve is affected most frequently, which impacts the ability of the left ventricle to function normally.

Treatment includes the use of antibiotics (penicillin) to eliminate the streptococcal infection completely and antiinflammatory agents for the inflammatory reaction. Follow-up includes the prompt treatment of strep infections and possible antibiotic prophylaxis prescribed before all invasive procedures (such as dental work) to prevent a recurrence of the immune response and additional damage to the heart valves.

Valvular Disorders. Disorders of the valves of the heart may be caused by a congenital defect or an infection such as endocarditis or rheumatic heart disease. Two specific problems can occur with valve disease. The valve can be *stenosed*, or hardened, which restricts the forward flow of blood, or it can be *incompetent*, meaning that it does not close completely, and so blood can leak backward. The most common valve defect is mitral valve prolapse (MVP), an incompetence in the mitral valve, because of a congenital defect or due to vegetation and scarring from endocarditis.

Valve disorders can ultimately lead to ventricular hypertrophy and *cardiomegaly* (enlargement of the heart). Physicians typically prescribe prophylactic amoxicillin, 2 g, 1 hour before an invasive procedure, to prevent further vegetative growth on the valve. Severely damaged valves or serious congenital defects may require surgical replacement of the affected valve.

Blood Vessels

Blood vessels are divided into two systems that begin and end with the heart (Figure 44-7). The *pulmonary system* carries deoxygenated blood from the right ventricle to the lungs and oxygenated blood back to the left atrium. The *systemic system* carries blood from the left ventricle throughout the entire body and back to the right atrium. The vessels are classified according to their structure and function as *arteries*, which carry oxygenated blood away from the heart; *capillaries*, the microscopic vessels that are responsible for the exchange of oxygen and carbon dioxide in the tissue; and *veins*, the vessels that carry deoxygenated blood back to the heart.

Arteries

All arteries, except the pulmonary artery, carry oxygenated blood away from the heart to all the cells of the body. The largest of these vessels is the *aorta*, which starts at the left ventricle and travels through the center of the body into the lower abdomen, where it bifurcates into the right and left femoral arteries with arteries branching off of this system down to the feet. As the aorta passes through the body, arteries branch off from it into

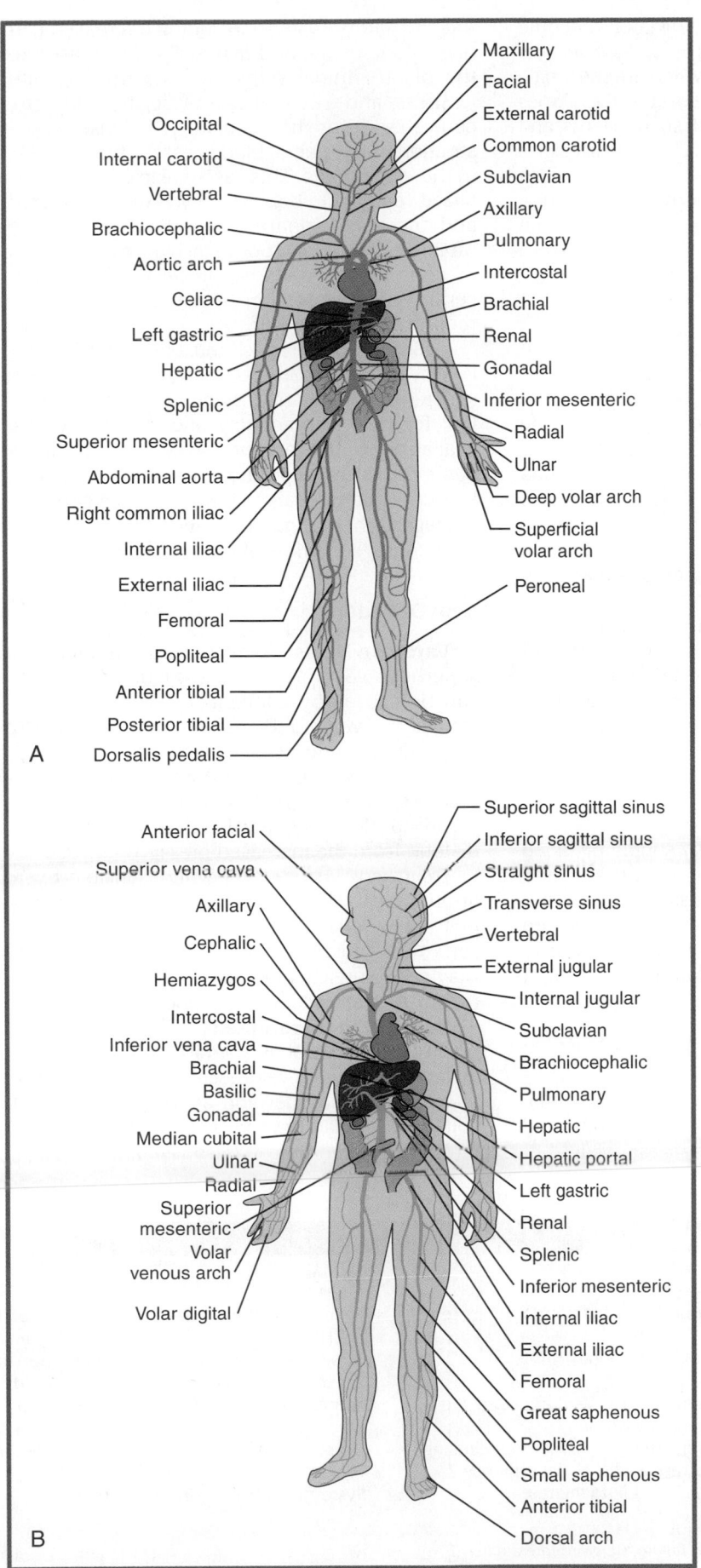

Occipital
Internal carotid
Vertebral
Brachiocephalic
Aortic arch
Celiac
Left gastric
Hepatic
Splenic
Superior mesenteric
Abdominal aorta
Right common iliac
Internal iliac
External iliac
Femoral
Popliteal
Anterior tibial
Posterior tibial
A   Dorsalis pedalis

Maxillary
Facial
External carotid
Common carotid
Subclavian
Axillary
Pulmonary
Intercostal
Brachial
Renal
Gonadal
Inferior mesenteric
Radial
Ulnar
Deep volar arch
Superficial volar arch
Peroneal

Anterior facial
Superior vena cava
Axillary
Cephalic
Hemiazygos
Intercostal
Inferior vena cava
Brachial
Basilic
Gonadal
Median cubital
Ulnar
Radial
Superior mesenteric
Volar venous arch
Volar digital

Superior sagittal sinus
Inferior sagittal sinus
Straight sinus
Transverse sinus
Vertebral
External jugular
Internal jugular
Subclavian
Brachiocephalic
Pulmonary
Hepatic
Hepatic portal
Left gastric
Renal
Splenic
Inferior mesenteric
Internal iliac
External iliac
Femoral
Great saphenous
Popliteal
Small saphenous
Anterior tibial
B   Dorsal arch

FIGURE 44-7   A, Systemic arteries.
B, Systemic veins.

smaller and smaller vessels, which ultimately become microscopic. These vessels are referred to as *arterioles* and terminate into tissue *capillaries*, which are the smallest and most plentiful of the blood vessels. Capillaries are a single epithelial cell thick, and so nutrients and gases can be exchanged on the cellular level. Arterioles deliver *erythrocytes* (red blood cells), which carry oxygen attached to hemoglobin molecules to surrounding tissues. When the blood leaves the capillary bed, the oxygen supply has been depleted, and it now begins the return portion of the blood cycle.

Veins

As the blood leaves the capillary beds, it enters the smallest veins, called *venules*. From this point on, the blood will flow into larger and larger veins until it reaches the largest veins in the body, the *inferior* and *superior venae cavae*. The venae cavae deposit deoxygenated blood into the right atrium, where the blood again begins its trip through the heart, into the pulmonary arteries to the lungs, and then through the pulmonary veins, which will bring the extremely rich oxygenated blood back from the lungs to the left atrium.

The walls of veins are thinner than those of the arteries, and they have valves to prevent the backflow of blood. These venous valves are especially important in the arms and legs because they prevent pooling of blood in the extremities.

Vascular Disorders

The vascular system is constantly busy supplying blood containing oxygen and nutrients to all of our tissues and picking up the metabolic waste from tissue metabolism. For tissues to receive an adequate amount of oxygen and nutrients, the arterial vessels must maintain elasticity and their linings need to remain smooth to prevent occlusion and decreased blood flow.

Shock

There are many different causes for shock (Table 44-1), but they all result in the same signs and symptoms and possible complications. *Shock* is the general collapse of the circulatory system, including decreased cardiac output, hypotension, and *hypoxemia* (decreased oxygen in the blood). Initial signs are extreme thirstiness, restlessness, and irritability. Because the body attempts to compensate for the circulatory collapse with vasoconstriction of peripheral blood vessels, blood can be pooled in the vital organs. This vasoconstriction causes a generalized feeling of cool, clammy skin; pallor; tachycardia; and decreased urinary output. Symptoms progress to a rapid, weak, thready pulse; tachypnea; and altered levels of consciousness. If the process is not reversed, the central nervous system becomes depressed and acute renal failure may occur.

The cause of the shock must be treated for the patient to survive. If the medical assistant identifies a patient in shock, emergency treatment should be started at once. Call for help immediately and if the physician is not available, call 911 for emergency medical care. Place the patient in a supine position, assess vital signs frequently, keep the patient warm, administer oxygen, and elevate the legs (if there is no indication of head or neck trauma) to encourage the flow of blood back to the heart.

Vein Disorders

Varicose Veins. *Varicose* veins are dilated, tortuous, superficial veins in the legs (Figure 44-8). Varicosities can be caused by congenitally defective valves in the saphenous veins and those veins branching off from them. Other contributing factors are pregnancy, obesity, prolonged standing or sitting, and heavy lifting. Whatever the cause, the valves do not completely close, allowing blood to flow backwards, thus causing the vein to distend from the increased pressure.

Treatment includes consistent aerobic exercise and limiting heavy lifting. The legs should be elevated when possible, and support stockings should be worn by persons who must stand for long periods. Varicose veins may need surgical intervention consisting of laser treatments, saline injections, or surgical ligation and stripping.

Deep Vein Thrombosis. *Phlebitis* is an inflammation of the veins that is most commonly seen in the lower legs. When a vein becomes inflamed, a blood clot or *thrombus* may develop at the site. A *thrombus* is a collection of platelets that form a clot and attach to the interior wall of a vessel. *Deep vein thrombosis* (DVT) is a

TABLE 44-1	Types and Causes of Shock	
Type	**Definition**	**Cause**
Cardiogenic	Low cardiac output due to inability of heart to pump	Acute MI, arrhythmias, pulmonary embolism, CHF
Hypovolemic	Excessive loss of blood or body fluids	GI bleeding, internal or external hemorrhage, excessive loss of plasma or body fluids, burns
Neurogenic	Peripheral vascular dilation resulting from neurologic injury or disorder	Spinal cord injury, emotional stress, drug reaction
Anaphylactic	Systemic hypersensitivity to an allergen causing respiratory distress and vascular collapse	Drug, vaccine, shellfish, nuts, insect venom, chemical, allergies
Septic (septicemia)	Systemic vasodilation due to the release of bacterial endotoxins	Systemic infection or bacteremia

MI, Myocardial infarction; *CHF*, congestive heart failure; *GI*, gastrointestinal.

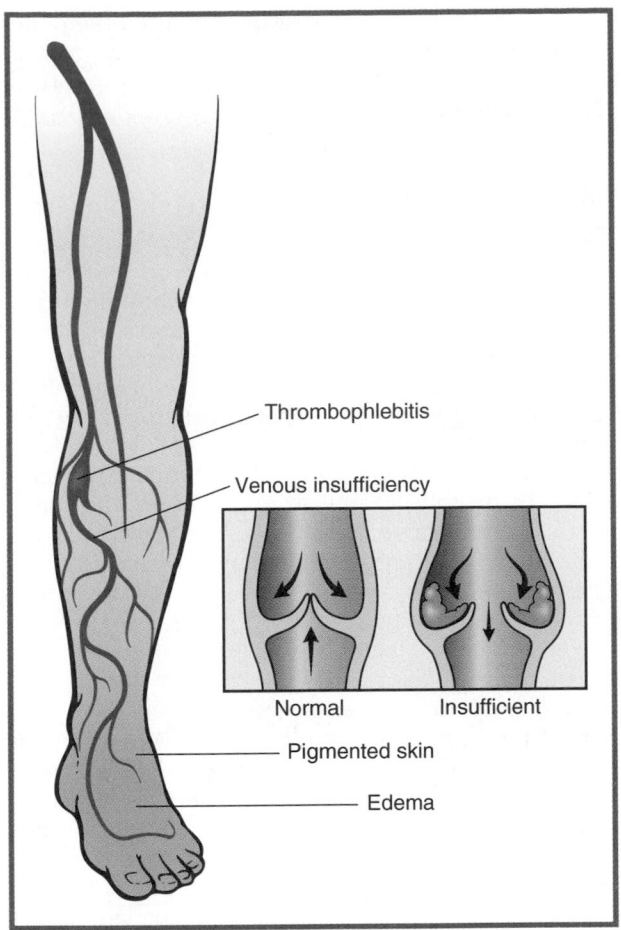

FIGURE 44-8 Varicose veins of the calf. (From Damjanov I: *Pathology for the health-related professions*, ed. 2, Philadelphia, 2000, WB Saunders.)

thrombus with inflammatory changes that has attached to the deep venous system of the lower legs and caused a partial or complete obstruction of the vessel. The most common sites for DVT are the calf veins, but they can also develop in the ileac and femoral veins. Risk factors for the formation of a DVT are recent surgery, immobilization, older age (with increased risk over the age of 50), trauma, obesity, and pregnancy.

In the early stages, about 50% of patients with DVTs are asymptomatic. Some patients complain of calf pain, swelling of the affected leg, warmth, edema, and erythema at the site. If a thrombus becomes dislodged and begins to circulate through the general circulation, it is then called an *embolus*. Pulmonary embolism, the blockage of a pulmonary artery, is the most serious complication of a DVT and may be the first indication that the thrombus was present.

DVTs are typically diagnosed with venous Doppler studies, which use ultrasound to measure the rate of blood flow through the vessel and can accurately detect venous obstruction. Once the diagnosis is confirmed, patients are hospitalized for intravenous anticoagulant therapy (heparin). On discharge, oral anticoagulant treatment (Coumadin) is continued for a minimum of 3 months. Patients will require regular follow-up, including prothrombin time analysis. The medical assistant may

perform venipuncture on these patients and, if so, should follow the guidelines for blood draws on patients taking anticoagulants. In addition, the medical assistant should reinforce the physician's recommendations regarding prevention of future thrombi and precautions regarding anticoagulant use.

CRITICAL THINKING APPLICATION

Alitza Lincoln is a 43-year-old patient who has large varicose veins in both legs and a history of phlebitis. She is a checkout clerk at the local Wal-Mart, and so she stands for extended periods. The physician is concerned about the development of a DVT so instructs Anna on the prevention, signs, and symptoms of a thrombus. Alitza asks Anna what she can do to prevent further problems with the veins in her legs. Anna uses a picture to illustrate the valves in the leg veins and explains preventive measures. What measures should Anna include?

Arterial Disorders

Arteriosclerosis and Atherosclerosis. *Arteriosclerosis* is a general term for the thickening and loss of elasticity of arterial walls that is associated with the aging process. Other conditions that can lead to a hardening of the arterial wall are hypertension, **scleroderma**, and diabetes mellitus. Arteriosclerosis can occur in arteries throughout the body and cause systemic ischemia and necrosis over time.

Atherosclerosis is a form of arteriosclerosis in which there is the formation of an *atheroma*, a buildup of cholesterol, cellular debris, and platelets along the inside vessel wall (Figure 44-9). Cholesterol was discussed in Chapter 27 with recommendations for high-density lipoprotein (HDL) and low-density lipoprotein (LDL) levels. Cholesterol is a nonessential nutrient that can be produced in the liver and forms the base for many of the hormones created in the body. Problems arise from dietary and lifestyle factors that elevate blood cholesterol levels to a dangerous point, causing the formation of atheromas, which ultimately block arteries and cause such disorders as heart attacks and strokes.

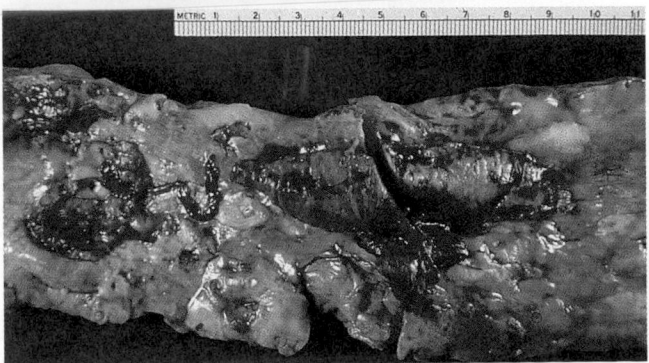

FIGURE 44-9 Atherosclerotic vessel. (From Damjanov I: *Pathology for the health-related professions*, ed. 2, Philadelphia, 2000, WB Saunders.)

Treatment of elevated blood cholesterol levels consists of dietary reductions in saturated fats and foods high in cholesterol and aerobic exercise to elevate HDL levels. Patients are encouraged to stop smoking. Drugs such as lovastatin (Mevacor) and simvastatin (Zocor) may be used to control or reverse plaque buildup. The medical assistant can help in the treatment with encouragement and by educating the patient about risk factors and promoting alterations in lifestyle. Referrals to a dietitian may help patients who are having a difficult time controlling their fat intake.

Aneurysm. An *aneurysm* is a ballooning or dilation of the wall of a vessel caused by weakening of the vessel wall (Figure 44-10). The patient may have an inherited factor for the development of aneurysms, such as in **Marfan syndrome**, but a common cause is the buildup of atherosclerotic plaques, which weaken the vessel wall. Aneurysms usually develop in either the abdominal aorta or the cerebral arteries. In either case, the patient seldom has any signs or symptoms. Occasionally, the patient describes a pounding or pulsating pain in the area of the aneurysm.

An aneurysm can be diagnosed when auscultation of the affected vessel over the area of the aneurysm reveals a **bruit**. Radiologic studies, sonography, and computed tomography all help to confirm the diagnosis. Patients are monitored on a routine basis for changes in the size of the aneurysm. Surgical repair is recommended for all aneurysms 6 cm or larger, but smaller ones can also rupture. If an aneurysm is tender and known to be enlarging rapidly, no matter what the size, surgery is essential. If a rupture occurs, immediate lifesaving intervention must be done.

The medical assistant may aid the physician by observing the patient for signs of pain, mental changes, and changes in pulse and respirations. If any of these signs are observed, the physician must be notified immediately. As with any serious condition, the patient is going to exhibit a high level of anxiety, and the medical assistant's strongest role is to support the patient and the family.

Diagnostic Procedures and Treatments

The cardiovascular examination begins with the medical assistant obtaining the patient's height and weight, temperature, radial and apical pulses, respirations, and blood pressure in both arms. Most cardiologists will also want a complete list of the prescription and over-the-counter medications that the patient is taking, including the strength and frequency of use for each one. A large portion of the physician's examination of the patient focuses on subjective symptoms. The physical examination covers the chest, heart, and vascular systems. General appearance, color of skin, symmetry, clubbing of fingers, jugular vein distention, temperature of extremities, and breathing patterns are a few of the notations that are made by the cardiologist.

Patient support and education are two very strong areas of medical assisting involvement. When patients understand their condition and are encouraged to take an active role in their treatments, they are inclined to comply with the physician's orders in a more precise and orderly fashion. Although cardiovascular diagnostic procedures are not typically done in the ambulatory care setting, the medical assistant should be familiar with the purpose of the tests so patient questions can be answered knowledgeably.

Doppler Studies

Doppler studies can identify occlusions of both veins and arteries from thrombus, emboli, or atherosclerotic plaques. The physician may order arterial Doppler studies for patients with **intermittent claudications**, lack of a pedal pulse, or leg ulcers that refuse to heal. Venous sonography is ordered to assess patients with pronounced varicosities or those with a swollen painful leg to rule out the possibility of a DVT. To perform a Doppler study, a conductive gel is applied to the skin over the test site. The Doppler transducer is moved over the site, directing an ultrasound beam at the vessel being checked (Figure 44-11). The sonographic beam picks up the speed of red blood cells (RBCs) as they travel through the vessel as a "swishing" sound. Variations in RBC velocity indicate either a partial or complete occlusion of the blood vessel. A two-dimensional image of an artery can be produced with a duplex Doppler scan that directly visualizes stenosis or occlusion of the artery. These studies are usually conducted in a vascular laboratory but may be done in a vascular surgeon's office as an initial assessment of the patient or follow-up after bypass grafting. The medical assistant working in this type of practice will require additional training to perform this procedure.

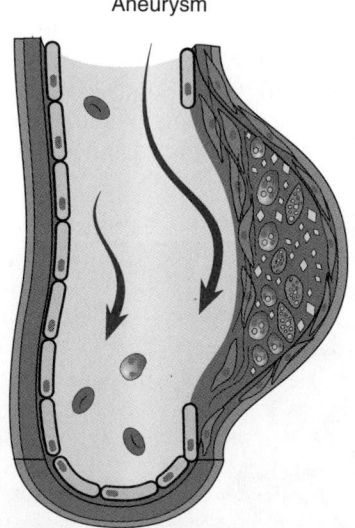

Aneurysm

FIGURE 44-10 An aneurysm because of weakening of the vessel wall. (From Damjanov I: *Pathology for the health-related professions,* ed. 2, Philadelphia, 2002, WB Saunders.)

Angiography

Angiography (arteriography) can be used to visualize any of the arterial pathways in the body (Figure 44-12). A catheter is placed into a major artery, usually the femoral, and advanced to the artery under study. A radiopaque contrast medium is rapidly injected while x-ray films are taken. The study is used to identify abnormal blood vessels, determine blood flow through the vessel, and diagnose arterial anomalies. Angiography can also be used to identify and locate occlusions of the aorta and arteries of the lower extremities. If the radiopaque substance does not pass through the vessel, or only partially passes through, the distal end of the artery will not be visualized or will only be partially visualized on the x-ray films. Arteriosclerotic disease can create a total or partial occlusion; emboli cause total occlusion of the artery. The study can also diagnose the dilation of a vessel from an aneurysm.

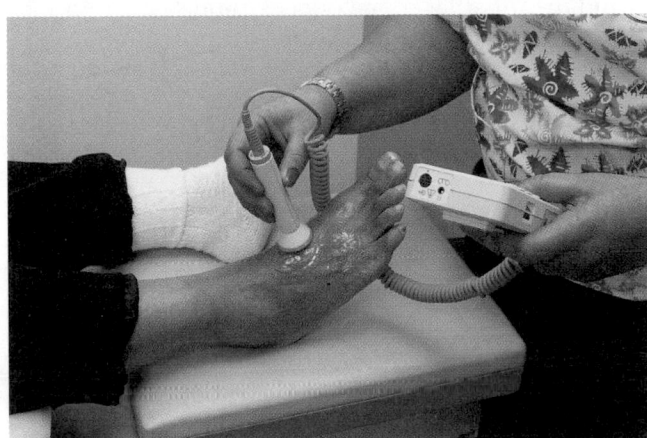

FIGURE 44-11   Doppler study.

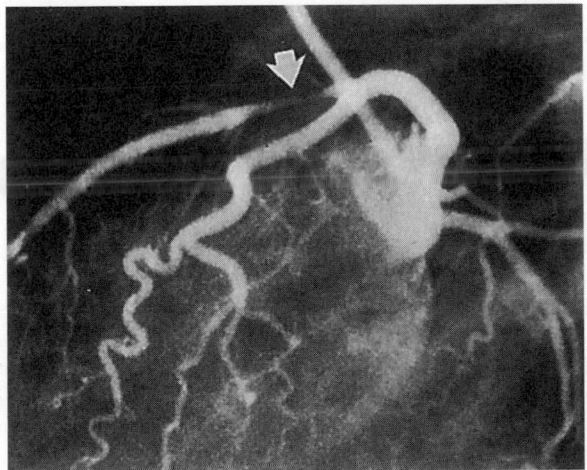

FIGURE 44-12   Coronary angiography shows stenosis *(arrow)* of the left anterior descending coronary artery. (From Braunwald E: *Heart disease: a textbook of cardiovascular medicine,* ed. 4, Philadelphia, 1992, WB Saunders.)

Echocardiography

Echocardiography is a noninvasive sonography procedure that assesses the structure and movement of the various parts of the heart. A high-frequency sound wave from a transducer that is held against the chest wall penetrates the heart. The sound waves bounce off the heart and echo back through the transducer into the machine, where they are converted into a picture that shows the exact size and movement of the parts of the heart that are being measured. Two-dimensional echocardiography can also be done to provide a spatial picture of the anatomical structures of the heart. Echocardiography usually includes color Doppler visualization to show the pattern and velocity of blood flow within the heart and in the great vessels. Backflow of blood, as in a valve that is incompetent, can be identified by changes in color. Echocardiography is used to diagnose pericardial effusion, valvular heart disease, aneurysms, and myocardial wall abnormalities that are seen in CHF or MI.

Cardiac Catheterization and Angioplasty

Cardiac catheterization is used to diagnose or evaluate a variety of heart disorders. Patients who have chronic shortness of breath, vertigo or syncope, chest pain, heart palpitations, arrhythmias, or abnormal stress test or echocardiography results or who have recently experienced an MI are all considered likely candidates for a heart catheterization procedure.

To perform the procedure, a catheter is passed into the heart through a peripheral vein or artery. If the right side of the heart is to be evaluated, the catheter is usually passed through the subclavian, brachial, or femoral vein; the right femoral artery is usually used for left-sided views. As the catheter is passed through the vessels into the heart, pressures are monitored, oxygen levels are measured, and cardiac output is determined. Once the catheter has reached the desired position, contrast medium is injected and fluoroscopy is used to visualize the heart chambers, valves, and coronary arteries. The cardiologist evaluates the condition of these structures, and any deviation from normal is noted.

During the heart catheterization procedure, if atherosclerotic plaques are occluding a coronary artery, percutaneous transluminal coronary *angioplasty* may be performed. When the plaque area is found, a balloon that surrounds the upper portion of the catheter is inflated and the atherosclerotic material is pressed against the vessel walls, relieving the obstruction. Lasers may also be used to dissolve the obstruction, or a coronary arterial *stent*, which is a mesh wire that stretches and molds to the arterial wall, may be inserted and left in place within the vessel to keep the vessel open. If multiple coronary artery occlusions are present, it may be necessary for the patient to have coronary artery bypass surgery. This surgery uses either part of the saphenous vein or an artificial Dacron graft to bypass the occluded, diseased section of the coronary artery. The graft creates a bypass for the blood to flow through to bring nourishment to the ischemic myocardium.

Patient Education

Heart disease and stroke account for more than one third of all deaths. Familial genetics, predisposition, and lifestyle habits such as smoking, lack of exercise, and diet play a significant role in the acquisition of heart disease. Successful management of cardiovascular disease requires major lifestyle revisions for most patients. The medical assistant can help by providing encouragement and support as well as by using community resources to provide assistance for the patient (Figure 44-13).

Places to obtain information include the American Heart Association, workshops and conferences, participation in professional organizations such as the American Association of Medical Assistants (AAMA), and reputable Internet sites.

Because many patients learn best through visual aids, having pictures, brochures, and pamphlets to give them is an effective method for generating learning. Always document education interventions so that on a return visit the information can be clarified or expanded.

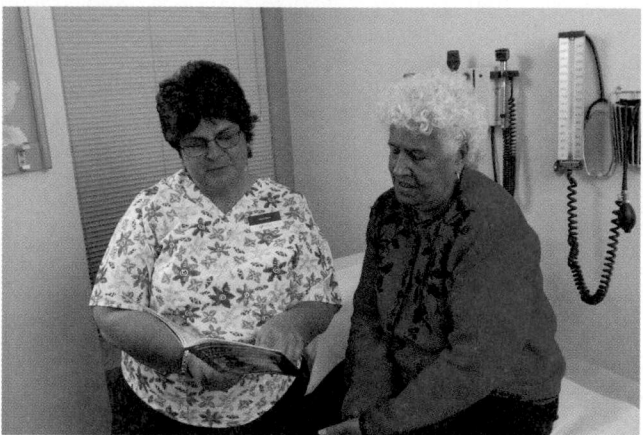

FIGURE 44-13 Patient education.

Legal and Ethical Issues

Diagnostic procedures can have a marked effect on the patient's treatment. When entrusted with performing testing procedures, the medical assistant assumes responsibility for accuracy and performing the tests precisely. This is an important role because the results submitted could strongly influence the therapeutic plan of treatment. Never assume that a test is just routine.

SUMMARY OF SCENARIO

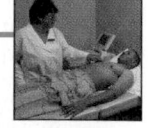

Anna enjoys her new position but recognizes the challenges of interacting with cardiovascular patients. Most patients seen at the clinic must make considerable lifestyle changes to improve health or to prevent further complications from their disease. Anna has found it difficult at times to try to help patients who refuse to quit smoking, do not

exercise regularly, and continue to eat a high-fat diet. She relies on the hospital dietitian for educational support and encourages MI patients to follow the cardiologist's advice and participate actively in the cardiac rehabilitation program offered by the department. She also works hard to stay up to date on cardiovascular medications and treatments because so many of the department's patients have complicated therapeutic plans.

SUMMARY OF LEARNING OBJECTIVES

■ The heart is a muscular organ that pumps blood through all the arteries of the body, thus circulating a continuous supply of oxygen and nutrients to the cells and picking up the metabolic waste products from them. It has three layers of tissue surrounded by a double-membrane sac called the pericardium; the epicardium, or the first layer of the heart; the middle muscular layer of the heart, the myocardium; and the inner layer, the endocardium, which forms the heart valves. The blood flow through the heart begins in the right atrium, which receives deoxygenated blood from the inferior and superior venae cavae. The atria contract, and blood passes through the tricuspid valve into the right ventricle; the ventricles contract and the blood passes from the right ventricle to the lungs via the pulmonary artery. Oxygenation occurs in the lungs, and the blood returns to the left atria through the pulmonary veins; the atria contract, and blood passes through the mitral (bicuspid) valve into the left ventricle; the ventricles contract, and oxygen-rich blood is sent out to the body through the aorta.

■ There are multiple risk factors for cardiac disease, including genetic predisposition and familial history, hypertension, diabetes, elevated blood cholesterol levels, and lifestyle factors, including high-fat, high-calorie diets; obesity; smoking; lack of exercise; and stress.

■ In CAD, the arteries supplying the myocardium become narrowed by atherosclerotic plaque. The process causes narrowing of the lumen of the arteries and inhibition of the normal flow of blood, thus depriving the heart of an adequate nutritious blood supply. The cardinal symptom of myocardial ischemia is angina pectoris, followed by pressure or fullness in the chest, syncope, edema, unexplained coughing spells, and fatigue. Women may exhibit a different clinical picture from the traditional one expected from men. Ischemia over a prolonged period leads to necrosis of a portion of the myocardium, resulting in an MI. Symptoms of MI are similar to those of angina, but MI is identified by pain lasting longer than 30 minutes that is unrelieved by rest or nitroglycerin tablets. An MI is diagnosed by ECG changes and elevated cardiac enzymes 6 to 12 hours after the episode. Medical treatment includes the use of thrombolytic medications to dissolve the coronary artery blockage, aspirin, beta-blockers,

ACE inhibitors, anticoagulants, and anticholesterol agents. When occlusion has taken place in one of the two coronary arteries that supply blood to the myocardium, either percutaneous transluminal coronary angioplasty or CABG surgery may be indicated.

■ The two types of hypertension are primary and secondary. Secondary hypertension occurs because of a disease process in another body system; primary hypertension is idiopathic and is diagnosed when the patient's blood pressure is consistently above 140/90. Chronic elevated blood pressure can result in left ventricular hypertrophy, angina, MI, or heart failure. Hypertension is also a major cause of stroke and nephropathy. Some of the risk factors for developing hypertension include a family history of hypertension or stroke, hypercholesterolemia, smoking, high sodium intake, diabetes, excessive alcohol intake, aging, prolonged stress, and race.

■ Congestive heart failure occurs when the myocardium is unable to pump an adequate amount of blood to meet the needs of the body. It typically develops over time because of weakness in the left ventricle from chronic hypertension or MI of the ventricular wall, valvular heart disease, or pulmonary complications. Typically, heart failure initially occurs on one side of the heart followed by the other side. Left-sided heart failure usually results from essential hypertension or left ventricle disease; right-sided heart failure can develop from lung disease. Left-sided heart failure causes a backup of blood in the lungs, resulting in pulmonary edema. Signs and symptoms include dyspnea, orthopnea, nonproductive cough, rales, and tachycardia. Right-sided heart failure causes a backup of blood in the right atrium, which prevents complete emptying of the vena cava, resulting in systemic edema, especially in the legs and feet. Both types of heart failure cause fatigue, weakness, exercise intolerance, dyspnea, and sensitivity to cold temperatures.

■ Rheumatic heart disease develops because of an unusual immune reaction that occurs approximately 2 weeks after an untreated beta-hemolytic streptococcal infection. The inflammation in the heart can involve all layers of heart tissue. Endocarditis is the most common heart complication. Vegetations form along the outer edges of the valve cusps, causing scarring and stenosis. Disorders of the valves of the heart may be caused by a congenital defect or an infection such as endocarditis or rheumatic heart disease. Two specific problems can occur with valve disease. The valve can be stenosed, which restricts the forward flow of blood, or it can be incompetent so blood can leak backward. The most common valve defect is MVP, an incompetence in the mitral valve, which results from a congenital defect or vegetation and scarring from endocarditis.

■ Blood vessels are divided into two systems that begin and end with the heart. Vessels are classified according to their structure and function as arteries, which carry oxygenated blood away from the heart; capillaries, the microscopic vessels that are responsible for the exchange of oxygen and carbon dioxide in the tissue; and veins, the vessels that carry deoxygenated blood back to the heart.

■ Table 44-1 outlines the various types of shock but all result in the same signs and symptoms and possible complications. Shock is the general collapse of the circulatory system, including decreased cardiac output, hypotension, and hypoxemia. Initial signs are extreme thirstiness, restlessness, and irritability. The body attempts to compensate for the circulatory collapse with vasoconstriction of peripheral blood vessels; as a result, blood can be pooled in the vital organs. This vasoconstriction causes a generalized feeling of cool, clammy skin; pallor; tachycardia; and decreased urinary output. Symptoms progress to a rapid, weak, and thready pulse; tachypnea; and altered levels of consciousness. If the process is not reversed, the central nervous system becomes depressed and acute renal failure may occur.

■ Varicose veins are dilated, tortuous, superficial veins in the legs that develop because the valves do not completely close, allowing blood to flow backwards, thus causing the vein to distend from the increased pressure. Phlebitis is an inflammation of the veins most commonly seen in the lower legs. DVT is a thrombus with inflammatory changes that has attached to the deep venous system of the lower legs and has caused a partial or complete obstruction of the vessel. If a thrombus becomes dislodged and begins to circulate through the general circulation, it is then called an embolus. Arteriosclerosis is a general term for the thickening and loss of elasticity of arterial walls that is associated with the aging process. Arteriosclerosis can occur in arteries throughout the body and cause systemic ischemia and necrosis over time. Atherosclerosis is a form of arteriosclerosis in which there is the formation of an atheroma, a buildup of cholesterol, cellular debris, and platelets along the inside vessel wall. An aneurysm is a ballooning or dilation of the wall of a vessel caused by weakening of the vessel wall.

■ Cardiovascular diagnostic procedures include Doppler studies of the patency of blood vessels; angiography to visualize arterial pathways; echocardiography to assess the structure and movement of the parts of the heart, especially the valves; and cardiac catheterization to visualize the heart chambers, valves, and coronary arteries.

KEY INTERNET WEBSITES

- National Heart, Lung, and Blood Institute
- National Institute of Neurological Disorders and Stroke
- National Stroke Association
  For active weblinks to each website visit
  http://evolve.elsevier.com/Kinn/

CHAPTER 45

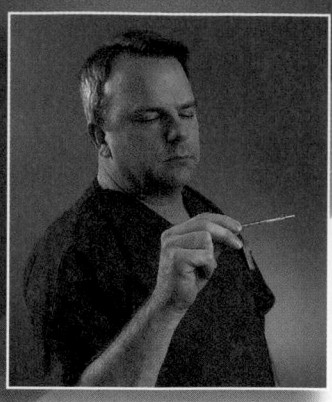

Scenario

Bill Novelli, CMA, works for Dr. Sara Kennedy, a primary care physician in a small town close to where he grew up. Although patients of all ages are seen in the practice, most patients are 65 years of age or older. Bill has learned to recognize the unique communication needs of aging patients and the importance of utilizing family and community resources to maintain optimal health in this special population.

Assisting in Geriatrics

Learning Objectives

- Define and spell the terms listed in the vocabulary.
- Identify the various impacts of an increasing aging population on society.
- Explain the changes caused by aging in each of the body systems.
- Summarize the major diseases and disorders faced by older patients.
- Describe various screening tools for dementia, depression, and malnutrition.
- Explain the effect of aging on sleep.
- Differentiate between independent, assisted, and skilled nursing facilities.
- Summarize the role of the medical assistant in caring for aging patients.
- Determine the principles for effective communication with older adults.
- Identify legal and ethical issues regarding aging patients.
- Role-play the effect of sensorimotor changes of aging.

National Curriculum Competencies

CLINICAL COMPETENCIES

4a. Perform telephone and in-person screening
4e. Prepare patients for and assist with routine and specialty examinations
4f. Prepare patients for and assist with procedures, treatments, and minor office surgery
4g. Apply pharmacology principles to prepare and administer oral and parenteral medications

TRANSDISCIPLINARY COMPETENCIES

3b. Instruct individual patients according to their specific needs
3d. Provide instruction for health maintenance and disease prevention

Vocabulary

collagen Protein that forms the inelastic fibers of tendons, ligaments, and fascia.
costal Pertaining to the ribs.
decubitus ulcer A sore or ulcer over a bony prominence that is due to ischemia from prolonged pressure; a bedsore.
elastin Essential part of elastic connective tissue that, when moist, is flexible and elastic.
lacrimation The secretion or discharge of tears.

According to the U.S. Bureau of the Census, the aging population—those 65 years of age and older—numbered almost 35 million in 2000. This represents 12.4% of the total population of the United States, an increase of 3.7 million since the last census in 1990 compared with an increase of 13.3% for the under-65 population. About one in every eight Americans is older than 65. The "oldest old" (people older than 85) are the most rapidly growing age group, with more than 50,000 persons 100 years of age or older in the 2000 census. It is projected that people older than 65 will represent 16% of the population in 2020 and increase to 20% by 2030. This means that by the middle of the twenty-first century, about 80 million people will be older than 65 years (Figure 45-1). The average life expectancy of an individual who was 65 years of age in 2000 was 17.9 years (19.2 years for women and 16.3 years for men).

As the aging population expands, it will impact all aspects of society. One area in particular will be the greater utilization of health services. To provide better services to the aging consumer, it is necessary to understand the aging process, which includes the physical and sensory changes encountered by older people (Procedure 45-1). This knowledge enables the healthcare professional to recognize the special needs of the aged and to develop therapeutic management and communication skills to effectively care for the older client. Through ongoing research and education about the aging process, many of the old stereotypical beliefs about aging are disappearing.

Aging is a complex physiological, psychological, and social process. Old age is not an illness but a normal life process that people experience in different ways. Lack of exercise, poor nutrition, substance abuse, continual stress, and air pollutants are all factors that cause one to show the effects of aging decades earlier than someone who has practiced healthy living habits.

As people age, they experience changes in their physical appearance and abilities as well as sensory changes in vision, hearing, taste, and smell. These changes do not occur simultaneously or at the same time in everyone; however, sensorimotor changes can have a profound effect on the individual's ability to interact with his or her environment.

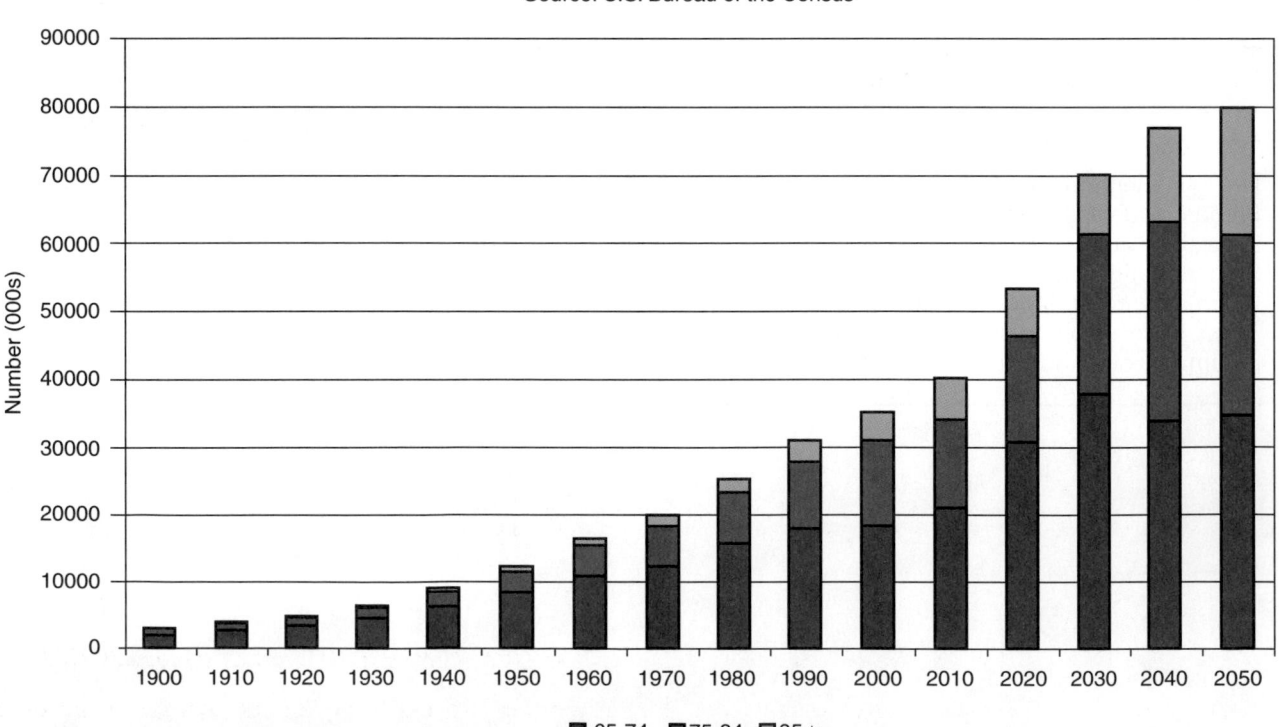

Older Population by Age: 1900-2050
Source: U.S. Bureau of the Census

■ 65-74   ■ 75-84   □ 85+

FIGURE 45-1   Older population by age, 1900-2050. (Source: U.S. Bureau of the Census.)

PROCEDURE **45-1**

Sensorimotor Changes of Aging

GOAL: Role play to better understand the needs of aging persons.

EQUIPMENT AND SUPPLIES

- Yellow glasses, ski goggles, or laboratory goggles
- Pink, white, yellow "pills" (various colors of Tic Tacs work)
- Vaseline
- Cotton balls
- Eye patches
- Tape
- Thick gloves
- Utility glove
- Tongue depressors
- Ace bandages
- Medical forms in small print
- Pennies
- Button shirts
- Walker

PROCEDURAL STEPS

1 Role play vision and hearing loss:
- Put two cotton balls in each ear and eye patch over one eye. Follow your partner's instructions.
- Partner: Stand out of the line of vision (to prevent lip reading) and without gestures, without change in voice volume, tell your partner to cross the room and pick up a book.

2 Role play yellowing of lens:
- Line up "pills" of different pastel colors.
- Partner: Pick out the different colors while wearing the yellow glasses.

3 Role-play difficulty with focusing:

- Put on goggles smeared with Vaseline and follow your partner's directions.
- Partner: Stand at least 3 feet in front of your partner and motion for him or her to come to you (your partner is deaf, so talking will not help).

4 Loss of peripheral vision:
- Put on goggles with black paper taped to sides.
- Partner: Stand to the side out of the field of vision and motion for your patient to follow you.

5 Simulating aphasia and partial paralysis:
- You are unable to use your right arm or leg. Place tape over your mouth. Let your partner know you need to go to the bathroom.
- Partner: Stand at least 3 feet away with your back to your partner and wait for instructions.

6 Problems with dexterity:
- Put thick gloves on your hands and try to sign your name, button a shirt, tie your shoes, and pick up pennies.

7 Problems with mobility:
- Use the walker to cross the room.
- Partner: After your partner starts to use the walker, hand him or her a book to carry.

8 Changes in sensation:
- Put a rubber utility glove on; turn on hot water; test the difference in temperature between the gloved hand and nongloved hand.

9 Summarize and share with the group your impressions of the effect of age-related sensorimotor changes.

MYTHS AND STEREOTYPES ABOUT AGING

- All aging people become senile.
- Disease is normal and unavoidable.
- Older workers are less productive than younger ones.
- Most older people end up in long-term care facilities.
- Most aging people have no interest in, or capacity for, sexual relations.
- Aging people are resistant to change and cannot learn new things.
- Damage to health because of lifestyle factors is irreversible.

CRITICAL THINKING APPLICATION

When Bill first started working with aging patients, he believed many of the stereotypes regarding persons over the age of 65. Since working with Dr. Kennedy, he realizes that many of these myths have no foundation in actual practice. Based on the myths mentioned in the text, what do you think about these beliefs about aging?

Changes in Anatomy and Physiology

The aging process brings about changes in all of the body systems. Table 45-1 summarizes these changes and what can be done to promote healthy aging.

TABLE 45-1	Health Promotion and Body System Changes Associated With Aging	
Body System	**Age-Related Changes**	**Health Promotion**
Cardiovascular	Arteriosclerosis and atherosclerotic plaque buildup reduces blood flow to major organs; hypertension common; CVD no.1 killer of women and men in their 60s	Exercise regularly; control weight; diet rich in fruits, vegetables, & whole grains; monitor cholesterol & blood glucose levels
Central nervous system	Brain shrinks by 10% between 30 & 90; takes longer to learn new material; attention span and language remain same; depression, vascular disease, & drug reactions may be cause	Aerobic exercise to increase blood flow to CNS and maintain mental activities
Endocrine	After 50 women have sharp decline in estrogen and men more gradual decline in testosterone	Possible hormone replacement therapy or natural soy supplements
Gastrointestinal	Decline in gastric juices & enzymes by age 60; decreased peristalsis w/increased constipation; some nutrients not absorbed as well	High-fiber diet to prevent constipation; exercise & folic acid reduce risk of colon cancer
Musculoskeletal	Muscle mass decreases; tendency to gain weight; gradual loss of bone density; deterioration of joint cartilage	Strength training to increase muscle mass; stretching to remain limber; exercise; vitamin D and calcium supplements
Pulmonary	At 55 the lungs become less elastic and the chest wall gradually stiffens, making oxygenation more difficult	Quit smoking and do regular aerobic exercise
Sensory organs	Hearing intact through mid-50s but declines by 25% by 80; oral problems common; skin thins & loses elasticity with age; presbyopia after 40; cataracts common after 60	Avoid exposure to loud noise & use hearing aids; maintain good dental hygiene; avoid sun damage to skin; annual eye examinations & diets rich in dark green leafy vegetables to avoid cataracts & macular degeneration
Urinary	Kidneys become less efficient; bladder muscles weaken; one third of seniors experience incontinence; prostate enlargement common	Pelvic exercises, drugs, or surgery for incontinence; annual PSA monitoring for men
Sexuality	*Men:* Impotence not a symptom of normal aging; men over age 50 may have some altered function. *Women:* Menopause causes vaginal narrowing and dryness, causing painful intercourse	Men should maintain cardiovascular health with exercise, weight control, no smoking. Women use vaginal lubricants or estrogen cream

CNS, Central nervous system; *CVD,* cardiovascular disease; *PSA,* prostate-specific antigen.

Cardiovascular System

Cardiovascular disease is the most frequent cause of illness or disability in the aging population; congestive heart failure (CHF) is the most common reason for hospitalization. Changes in the cardiovascular system are age related, but disease and lifestyle habits such as exercise, diet, and stress control are factors that contribute to these changes. Heart disease is ranked as the leading cause of death among men and women; therefore the proper management of cardiovascular disease can help maintain the health of an aging population as well as reduce mortality rates.

Structural changes occur in the heart due to the aging process. Myocardial cells enlarge, and there are increased deposits of fat and connective tissue, which combine to make the myocardial wall stiffer and increase the amount of time and oxygen needed for the relaxation phase of the cardiac cycle. As a result, cardiac output goes down, making aging persons more susceptible to CHF. In addition, the heart rate of older persons is slower, and during physical exercise there is a decreased ability to maintain maximum heart rate (Table 45-2).

Arteriosclerosis is considered part of the aging process. The vessel walls thicken and become less elastic as a result of the calcification and buildup of connective tissue.

TABLE 45-2	Normal Changes of Cardiac Output
Blood Pumped by Resting Heart (quarts per minute)	**Maximum Heartbeat During Exercise (beats per minute)**
Age 30: 3.6	Age 30: 200
Age 40: 3.4	Age 40: 182
Age 50: 3.2	Age 50: 171
Age 60: 2.9	Age 60: 159
Age 70: 2.6	Age 70: 150

From the American Heart Association.

The ability of the blood vessel to dilate and contract decreases. To maintain an adequate blood supply throughout the body, the heart must work harder to overcome the resistance that is caused by the stiffened vessels. The diastolic pressure remains the same, but the systolic pressure may increase with age. There is also an increased incidence of orthostatic hypotension in older adults. The clinical criterion for alterations in blood pressure from sitting to standing is a drop of more than 20 mm Hg in systolic pressure or a drop of more than 10 mm Hg in diastolic pressure when position is changed. Such a decrease is typically caused by a decrease in the volume of circulating blood and can be an important diagnostic sign for aging patients. The physician may have the medical assistant take orthostatic blood pressures as part of the routine intake protocol on aging patients.

Endocrine System

The most common endocrine system disorder seen in aging patients is type 2 diabetes mellitus. About 10% of the population over the age of 65 are diagnosed with this disease. The average age of patients diagnosed with type 2 diabetes is 60 years. These patients are at increased risk of developing vascular disease, including renal disorders, retinopathy, neuropathy, myocardial ischemia, angina, myocardial infarction, cerebrovascular accidents, and peripheral vascular disease, such as lower-extremity ulcers.

Older patients do not always present with classic diabetic symptoms—polyuria, polydipsia, polyphagia—but may display a variety of problems, including unexplained weight loss, slow wound healing, recurrent bacterial or fungal infections, changes in mental state, cataracts, macular disease, muscle weakness and pain, angina, foot ulcers, and uremia. The range of symptoms is largely attributable to the insidious onset of diabetes in older people, who may have gradually developing hyperglycemia for years before diagnosis.

The treatment protocol for aging patients with diabetes is the same as it would be for other age groups; however, special consideration must be given to the ability of the patient to understand and comply with the therapeutic plan. In addition, because the patient may have other existing health problems that are being treated with medications, the newly diagnosed aging diabetic patient may face a complicated treatment regimen that requires explicit instruction and continual follow-up in the ambulatory care setting. The medical assistant must be aware of any sensory abnormalities, such as decreased vision or fine motor skills, that may interfere with the patient's ability to follow treatment guidelines. Adaptations should be made in the teaching and treatment plans to meet the individual needs of each patient.

Gastrointestinal System

Age-related changes in the gastrointestinal system include a decrease in the production of hydrochloric acid, which affects the digestion of calcium and iron. Secretion of *intrinsic factor*, a protein that allows vitamin B_{12} to be absorbed, also decreases, affecting the function of the nervous system and the formation of red blood cells, and causes excessive fatigue. It is not unusual for aging patients to be seen in the physician's office on a regular basis for vitamin B_{12} injections.

The rate of food passage through the small intestine increases, causing poorer absorption of vitamins and minerals but peristalsis in the colon decreases, making aging patients more susceptible to constipation and diverticular disease. Poor eating habits, reduced fluid intake, and some medications (such as antidepressants, diuretics, antacids containing aluminum or calcium, and antiparkinsonism drugs) also contribute to constipation.

The liver decreases in size after age 70. It is still able to perform vital functions, but the time needed to metabolize drugs and alcohol is increased. All these factors combine to increase the potential of adverse drug reactions in older adults.

Aging persons have an increased incidence of several gastrointestinal system diseases, such as gastroesophageal reflux disease (GERD), peptic ulcers, diverticulosis (related to lack of dietary fiber), cholelithiasis, and colorectal cancer. Dietary counseling and annual screenings should be part of the routine care of aging patients.

Integumentary System

Changes in the appearance and function of the integumentary system are usually due to a combination of ordinary age-related changes and environmental factors, especially the amount of sun exposure over time. Exposure to ultraviolet light from the sun is frequently the cause of wrinkles, age spots, blotches, and leathery-dry, loose skin, all of which are associated with aging. The skin is considered the body's first line of protection against infection and is responsible for preventing the loss of body fluid and regulating body temperature. Changes caused by the ultraviolet light from the sun or from the normal aging process can affect all three layers of the skin: the epidermis, dermis, and subcutaneous tissue.

The cells in the epidermis reproduce more slowly as people age. This slower regeneration causes the skin to appear thinner. The skin becomes more prone to tearing and blistering. There is an increased risk of infections, the healing process takes longer, and older people are more susceptible to bruising. Because the skin can be easily torn, it is important to select an appropriate adhesive when covering a wound or venipuncture site. Vitamin D synthesis, which is a major function of the epidermis, significantly decreases in aged skin, and a decrease in the number of melanocytes increases photosensitivity in aging persons.

The dermis loses 20% of its mass during the aging process, resulting in the paper-thin or transparent skin seen in older adults. The dermis loses much of its vascular supply, making it difficult to regulate temperature and leading to an increased susceptibility to both hypothermia and heat stroke in aging persons. The number of collagen cells in the dermis also decreases with age, causing the skin to sag and wrinkle. Any situation in which an older adult is exposed to extremes of cold or heat should be avoided. Make sure there is a blanket available in the examining room if the air conditioning is on. Inquire about whether the patient is too cold or too hot, and take the necessary steps to make the older patient feel more comfortable.

Atrophy of the subcutaneous layer increases the skin's susceptibility to trauma, and so patients bruise much more easily. Both sweat and sebaceous glands decrease with age, making it difficult for aging persons to tolerate higher temperatures because they perspire less with age. The skin is denied natural lubrication, causing dry skin to be one of the most common complaints among older people. In addition, fat deposits increase in the abdomen of men and in the abdomen and thighs of women as they age.

SUGGESTIONS FOR HELPING THE ELDERLY PREVENT AND TREAT DRY SKIN

- Recommend a home humidifier to obtain artificial humidification.
- Advise elderly patients to bathe less frequently using warm water, not hot water.
- Recommend that patients use a mild soap or cleansing cream such as Aveenobar, Basis, or Dove soap.
- Remind the patient to wear protective clothing in cold weather.
- Suggest establishing a regimen of moisturizers for treatment of dry skin.
- Creams and moisturizers should be applied after getting out of the bathtub or shower to decrease the possibility of falls.

Pain receptors are distributed throughout the skin. Because of age-related changes in the receptors, older persons experience an increased threshold to pain. They may not notice a cut or burn as quickly as a younger person would; thus a burn may become more severe before it is noticed.

Other changes occur in the skin appendages, the nails, and the hair. Hair changes in color, growth, and distribution. Hair grays because of the decreased rate of melanin production and the replacement of pigmented hair with nonpigmented hair. Women lose hair on their trunk and have increased facial hair. Although *alopecia* (male balding) is caused by an inherited trait, aging also causes hair loss. Hair on the eyebrows, nose, and ears becomes coarser and longer in men. Nails of older people take longer to grow and are more brittle. Nails, particularly toenails, thicken as a result of trauma or nutritional causes. Splitting of the nails makes them susceptible to fungal infections.

Seborrheic keratosis, one of the most common benign skin disorders found in the aging population, appears in the form of waxy, greasy papules that vary from a flesh to a dark brown color (Figure 45-2). They are typically found in areas of sun exposure, such as the trunk, back, face, neck, extremities, and scalp. They may be removed for cosmetic purposes but are not dangerous.

CRITICAL THINKING APPLICATION

Mrs. Rose DeLuca is a 71-year-old patient of Dr. Kennedy's who is complaining about the changes that have occurred in her skin in the last several years. Based on what Bill knows about the normal changes that occur in the skin as people age, how can he explain these changes to Mrs. DeLuca, and what suggestions can be made to help with dryness and other typical aging changes?

Musculoskeletal System

As the body ages, changes occur in muscles, bones, and joints, affecting appearance, strength, and mobility. The amount of change depends on diet, exercise, and heredity. Cartilage loss and degeneration, producing osteoarthritis, commonly occur in the weight-bearing joints of older people.

Aging brings a decrease in the strength and speed of muscle contractions in the extremities but only a slight decline in overall muscle endurance. Muscular changes in the aging patient are directly related to the activity level of the individual patient. Research shows that musculoskeletal disease is not an inevitable result of the aging process; however, 40% to 50% of women over the age of 50 years have a serious problem with bone demineralization.

SUGGESTIONS FOR HELPING THE OLDER ADULT WITH MOBILITY, DEXTERITY, AND BALANCE

- Use assistive devices such as adaptive silverware, tub seat or shower chair, electric razor, and reaching devices.
- Assist with gripping devices as needed (wait for the patient to place his or her hand around a cup or help him or her with it before letting go).
- Need more time to complete tasks but prefer to do so independently, so slow down.
- Stroke victims should be supported on the weak side when walking or transferring from chair to examination table.
- Physician may recommend physical therapy for range-of-motion exercises.
- Encourage activity: a lack of activity causes decreased ability to function.

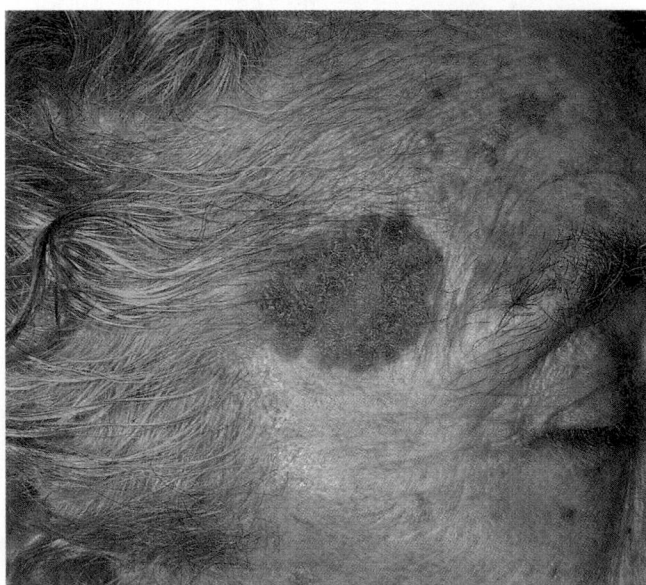

FIGURE 45-2 Seborrheic keratosis. (From Habif TP: *Clinical dermatology: a color guide to diagnosis and therapy*, ed 3. St Louis, 1996, Mosby.)

Osteoporosis. Osteoporosis (see Chapter 40) is the primary cause of hip fractures, which can lead to a loss of independence and complications that ultimately can end in death. The spinal vertebrae also can collapse, producing the stooped posture associated with "dowager's hump." Sometimes bones break because of the sheer weight of the body on them. Often people say they fell and broke a bone when, in reality, the bone fractured, causing them to fall. Multiple factors contribute to the development of osteoporosis, but it is most common in postmenopausal women.

RISK FACTORS FOR THE DEVELOPMENT OF OSTEOPOROSIS

- Female (women have five times greater risk than men)
- Small-boned frame, thin
- Family history of osteoporosis
- Estrogen deficiency before age 45 years from either early menopause or oophorectomy
- Estrogen deficiency resulting from an abnormal absence of menses (eating disorders, excessive aerobic exercise, fibrocystic ovaries)
- Racial background; white and Asian women at highest risk
- Aging
- Extended use of anticonvulsant drugs, prednisone, and excessive thyroid hormone medications
- Sedentary lifestyle, smoking, excessive alcohol intake, lack of calcium and vitamin D when growing up

---

Weight-bearing exercises and calcium and vitamin D supplements are recommended to prevent demineralization of the bones. Medications are available to treat individuals diagnosed with osteoporosis, including calcitonin nasal spray, Fosamax, Actonel, and Evista.

Falls. The risk of injuries from falls increases with age, with falls causing the greatest number of injuries in people over the age of 70 years. Some of the reasons aging persons are at greater risk of falling include sensorimotor changes in vision and mobility, osteoporosis, and stroke. Falls in older patients usually result in fractures because of the presence of osteoporosis in a large percentage of the population. Serious fractures, such as those of the hip, require patients to be immobile for extended periods and open the door to a wide range of debilitating complications such as **decubitus** ulcers, pneumonia, placement in long-term care facilities, and even death. Falls are largely preventable. The medical assistant can play an active role in helping family members as well as patients be aware of the risk factors for falls as well as understand measures that can be taken to prevent falls from occurring.

SUGGESTIONS FOR PREVENTING FALLS

- Perform regular hearing and vision testing so that patients are aware of possible dangers.
- Family and patient should be educated on the side effects of medications, especially those that may make the patient dizzy or sleepy.
- If patient experiences orthostatic hypotension, he or she should rise slowly and stand still for a moment with support before moving.
- Limit the use of alcohol.
- If needed, use assistive devices, a cane or walker, consistently for support.
- Wear low-heeled, rubber-soled shoes with good support.
- Avoid going outside in icy weather.
- Encourage regular weight-bearing exercise for bone strength.
- Hallways, stairs, and bathrooms should be well lit.
- Assess the home for possible danger areas; remove throw rugs; use handrails on steps and grab bars in bathrooms; keep emergency numbers handy.

CRITICAL THINKING APPLICATION

The family of a 73-year-old patient, Mrs. Rita Schaeffer, is concerned about the risk of falls. Mrs. Schaeffer was recently diagnosed with osteoporosis and lives alone. What information should Bill give the family to help them prevent accidents in their mother's home? Her 43-year-old daughter is concerned about developing osteoporosis as well. What preventative methods should the daughter employ to prevent the disease?

Nervous System

Cognitive ability, the ability of a person to think, is influenced by many factors, including a person's general state of health, educational background, and genetic code. The normal process of aging may contribute to a change in the thinking process. The brain begins to get smaller around the age of 50 years and continues to do so as we age because of a loss of fluid within the neurons and the shrinkage of dendrites. Thinning of the dendrites makes it more difficult for messages to be transmitted from one neuron to the next. These factors combine to produce an aging brain that weighs less, is smaller, and has started to pull away from the sheath or cortical mantle. Older neurons process information slower; so the ability to retrieve old information and learn new takes longer. Reaction time also slows and aging persons are distracted easier; however, recent research shows the loss of brain cells is minimal and the older brain is still capable of generating new neurons.

Dementia, the severe loss of intellectual ability, is *not* an inevitable part of aging but rather is the result of an organic disorder. Most men and women remain mentally competent until the end of their lives. Sudden loss of memory, disorientation, and trouble performing the daily tasks of life indicate there is a problem that should be addressed. Many conditions can cause signs and symptoms of dementia, including depression; prescription and over-the-counter drug reactions; alcoholism; malnutrition; thyroid, liver, heart, and vascular disorders; and Parkinson's disease. There are multiple factors that can interfere with mental judgment and motor skills, giving the impression of decreased mental status.

The best way to ensure mental functioning in later life is to remain mentally and physically stimulated. Exercise improves memory and thinking because of its positive effect on vascular health, increasing the amount of oxygen delivered to the aging brain. Other ways to maintain mental function are to be socially active; practice stress-reduction activities; quit smoking; drink alcohol in moderation; use hearing aids and glasses if they are needed to stay in touch with the world; and receive treatment for depression, diabetes, hypertension, and high cholesterol.

RISK FACTORS FOR COGNITIVE DECLINE

- Hypertension, diabetes, heart disease (these decrease blood flow to the brain)
- Environmental exposure to lead
- High stress levels
- Sedentary lifestyle and lack of social interaction
- Low education level
- Smoking and substance abuse

One of the most frequent tests for dementia is the Mini-Mental Status Examination, a 5-minute screening test that was designed to evaluate basic mental function in a number of different areas. The test assesses the patient's ability to recall facts, write, and calculate numbers. It provides the physician with a quick way to determine whether more in-depth testing is needed. Each area of the examination is given a score. These scores show whether the person is functioning within the expected range for his or her age (Figure 45-3).

Alzheimer's Disease. Alzheimer's disease is a progressive deterioration of the brain because of the destruction of neurons, leading to problems with memory, language, thinking, and behavior. Cellular destruction is related to the buildup of amyloid plaques and neurofibrillary tangles within the brain. Patients displaying signs and symptoms of dementia would first be evaluated for organic causes, such as systemic disease or depression. There is no definitive diagnostic test for Alzheimer's disease because it can be confirmed only through examination of the brain on autopsy. If the patient exhibits a gradual onset and progressive difficulty with memory, functional abilities, and behavior and has no evidence of other causes for these disturbances, the physician makes the diagnosis of Alzheimer's disease.

There is a great deal of ongoing research regarding the diagnosis and treatment of Alzheimer's disease. Currently, pharmaceutical treatment includes the use of Cognex and Aricept to delay the advancement of the disease. Estrogen, vitamin E, and ginkgo biloba may also be recommended to delay the onset or slow the decline of affected patients. The goal of treatment is to maintain normal activities as long as possible. Supportive care for family members is absolutely essential because they are the ones faced with caring for a loved one who is suffering progressive memory loss. The medical assistant can be especially helpful in recommending educational workshops, support groups, and stress management skills for caregivers. Multiple resources are available, including online information and support groups that family members may find helpful.

STAGES OF ALZHEIMER'S DISEASE

1. First Stage: Occurs 2 to 4 years leading up to diagnosis; memory loss affects job performance; confusion and disorientation are common; mood or personality changes; difficulty making decisions, paying bills; gets lost easily; withdraws from others; loses things.
2. Second Stage: Two to 10 years after diagnosis; increased memory loss and confusion; shorter attention span; restless; makes constant repetitive statements; exhibits problems with reading, writing, and numbers; may be irritable or suspicious; exhibits motor problems; has difficulty recognizing close friends and family members.
3. Terminal Stage: One to 3 years; does not recognize family; weight loss; unable to care for self; incontinent of bladder and bowel; requires complete care.

CRITICAL THINKING APPLICATION

Maria Angelone is an 86-year-old patient of Dr. Kennedy's who is in the second stage of Alzheimer's disease. Her husband and children are showing signs of stress from the continuous care required by Mrs. Angelone. Her family still does not understand what is happening to her and what to expect in the future. What information can Bill share with them about the disease and what resources could be helpful to the family in dealing with the stress of caring for a loved one with dementia?

Maximum Score	Score	

Patient _____ Examiner _____ Date _____

Orientation

5 ( ) What is the (year) (season) (date) (day) (month)?
5 ( ) Where are we: (state) (county) (town) (hospital) (floor)

Registration

3 ( ) Name three objects: (Apple, Penny, Table) 1 second to say each. Then ask the patient all three after you have said them. Give 1 point for each correct answer. Then repeat them until he or she learns all three. Count trials and record.

Trials _____

Attention and Calculation

5 ( ) Serial 7's. 1 point for each correct. Stop after five answers. Alternatively spell "world" backwards.

Recall

3 ( ) Ask for the three objects repeated above. Give 1 point for each correct.

Language

9 ( ) Name a pencil, and watch (2 points)
Repeat the following "No ifs, ands, or buts." (1 point)
Follow a three-stage command:
   "Take a paper in your right hand, fold it in half, and put it on the floor." (3 points)
Read and obey the following:
   CLOSE YOUR EYES (1 point)
Write a sentence (1 point)
Copy design (overlapping pentagons) (1 point)
Total Score
ASSESS level of consciousness along a continuum _____

Overlapping pentagons

| | Alert | Drowsy | Stupor | Coma |

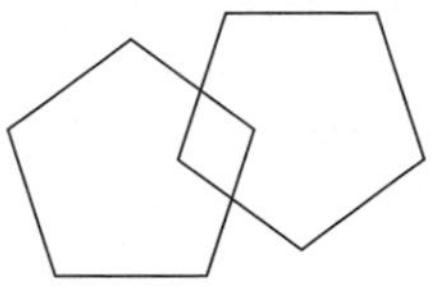

Instructions for Administration of Mini-Mental State Examination

Orientation

(1) Ask for the date. Then ask specifically for parts omitted, e.g., "Can you also tell me what season it is?" One point for each correct.
(2) Ask in turn "Can you tell me the name of this hospital?" (town, country, etc.). One point for each correct.

Registration

Ask the patient if you may test his or her memory. Then say the names of three unrelated objects, clearly and slowly, about 1 second for each. After you have said all three, ask him or her to repeat them. This first repetition determines his or her score (0–3), but keep saying them until he or she can repeat all three, up to six trials. If he or she does not eventually learn all three, recall cannot be meaningfully tested.

Attention and Calculation

Ask the patient to begin with 100 and count backwards by 7. Stop after five subtractions (93, 86, 79, 72, 65). Score the total number of correct answers.
If the patient cannot or will not perform this task, ask him or her to spell the word "world" backwards. The score is the number of letters in correct order, e.g., dlrow = 5, dlorw = 3.

Recall

Ask the patient if he or she can recall the three words you previously asked him or her to remember. Score 0–3.

Language

Naming: Show the patient a wrist watch and ask him or her what it is. Repeat for pencil. Score 0–2.
Repetition: Ask the patient to repeat the sentence after you. Allow only one trial. Score 0 or 1.
Three-stage command: Give the patient a piece of plain blank paper and repeat the command. Score 1 point for each part correctly executed.
Reading: On a blank piece of paper print the sentence "Close your eyes," in letters large enough for the patient to see clearly. Ask him or her to read it and do what it says. Score 1 point only if he or she actually closes his or her eyes.
Writing: Give the patient a blank piece of paper and ask him or her to write a sentence for you. Do not dictate a sentence, it is to be written spontaneously. It must contain a subject and verb and be sensible. Correct grammar and punctuation are not necessary.
Copying: On a clean piece of paper, draw intersecting pentagons, each side about 1 inch, and ask him or her to copy it exactly as it is. All 10 angles must be present, and 2 must intersect to score 1 point. Tremor and rotation are ignored.
Estimate the patient's level of sensorium along a continuum, from alert on the left to coma on the right.

FIGURE 45-3 Mini-Mental Status Examination. (Redrawn from Folstein M, et al: Mini mental state. *J Psych Res* 12:196-198, 1975.)

Pulmonary System

Around the age of 40, there is a decline in the functioning of the respiratory system. The lungs lose their elasticity owing to changes in **elastin** and **collagen**. They become smaller and flabbier. The alveoli (air sacs) enlarge, their walls become thinner, and there is a reduced number of capillaries. As a result, the effective area for gas exchange is reduced. The chest wall may stiffen from osteoporosis of the ribs and vertebrae and calcification of the **costal** cartilage. The respiratory muscles become weaker, making it harder to move air in and out of the lungs. To compensate, older adults rely more on accessory muscles, such as the diaphragm. Weakening of the respiratory muscles and the stiffening of the chest wall make it harder to cough deeply enough to clear mucus from the lungs. Pulmonary function tests reveal a decrease in vital capacity and an increase in residual volume. The incidence of sleep apnea and sleep disorders increases, causing a potential problem with nocturnal hypoxemia. All these factors combine to make the older adult at greater risk for pneumonia and aspiration as well as reactivation of tuberculosis.

Sensory Organs

Vision. By the time a person reaches age 50, structural and functional changes in the eye become noticeable. The eyebrows and eyelashes start to gray. The skin around the eyelids wrinkles, and the loss of orbital fat allows the eye to sink deeper into the orbit. The cornea increases in thickness and has reduced refractive power. There may be the development of a yellow-gray ring (arcus senilis) on the periphery of the cornea. The iris loses pigmentation, and, as a result, most older people appear to have gray eyes.

The lens of the eye continues to grow. As new lens fibers grow, old lens fibers are compressed and pushed to the center, causing the lens to become denser. The lens becomes flatter, thicker, less elastic, and more opaque, progressively yellowing with age. By the age of 70, the lens has tripled in mass. Clouding of the lens causes light rays to scatter, creating glare.

The pupil is designed to adjust to control the amount of light entering the eye. The ciliary muscle that causes the pupil to dilate weakens during the aging processes. As a result, there is a reduction in the size of the pupil, limiting the amount of light available to reach the retina. Tear production normally decreases. Tear glands do not make enough tears, or the tears are of poor quality and do not keep the eyes wet enough. Eye irritation and excessive tearing are a result of decreased **lacrimation**.

During the fourth decade of life, presbyopia develops, which makes it difficult to focus on detailed objects close at hand. This requires the use of corrective lenses to accommodate age-related farsightedness. There is a decrease in the ability to refocus quickly from far to near or near to far. Also, the ability to follow a moving object is decreased. The yellowing of the lens causes it to act like a filter, making it difficult to distinguish certain color intensities. Blues, greens, and violets, which are considered as having short wavelengths, are hard to differentiate, whereas yellows, reds, and oranges are of

longer wavelengths and easier to identify. The loss in the ability to discriminate closely related colors can affect the older person's ability to judge distances or his or her depth perception. This causes an aging person to become more susceptible to falls and accidents. Stairs become a potential hazard because the edges cannot be seen clearly.

Older persons need as much as six times more light to read; however, increasing the level of light does not completely compensate for visual decline since the elderly also experience an increased sensitivity to glare. Glare is probably one of the most painful experiences for the aging eye. Exposed light bulbs, such as those used in chandeliers, and light from highly reflective surfaces such as glass tables and floors can produce excessive glare. The eye has decreased ability to respond to abrupt changes from light to dark or dark to light. Going from a well-lit waiting room into a dim hallway or negotiating the way down dimly lit aisles in a movie theater could be treacherous to an older person.

SUGGESTIONS FOR HELPING THE VISUALLY IMPAIRED OLDER ADULT

- When escorting an older person, whether he or she is visually impaired or not, allow the client to place his or her hand above your elbow. It is easier for the person to follow your movements. This method also provides a source of support and security.
- Use high levels of evenly distributed glare-free light.
- Ask the pharmacist to use large lettering when labeling medicine bottles.
- Use paper that has a nonglare finish and use large print for forms and educational materials.
- Make distinct differences (e.g., size of containers or color coding with bright primary colors) for pills that are similar in size and color.
- Place all objects within the visual field and avoid clutter.
- Give time to adjust to marked changes in light.

Cataracts, Glaucoma, and Macular Degeneration. Eye diseases and disorders that occur frequently in older people are cataracts, glaucoma, and macular degeneration. *Cataracts* are cloudy or opaque areas in the lens that cause blurring of vision; rings or halos around lights and objects; and a blue or yellow tint to the visual field. Surgical lens extraction and implantation with an artificial lens improves vision in 95% of the cases. The procedure is performed in an outpatient facility, either using a small incision to remove the lens or *phacoemulsification* (ultrasonic vibrations), which breaks up the lens and removes it without the need for an incision. Postoperatively, patients must avoid bending or lifting heavy objects for 3 to 4 weeks after the procedure; wearing an eye shield at night and glasses during the day helps to protect the eye until it heals.

Glaucoma is a result of blockage to the outflow of aqueous humor, which causes an increase in intraocular pressure and damage to the optic nerve. If not treated, glaucoma can cause progressive loss of peripheral vision and ultimately lead to blindness, however, it can be treated with medication.

The macula is the part of the eye responsible for sharp vision and color. The damage or breakdown of the macula is called *macular degeneration*, which causes progressive loss of the central field of vision. Macular degeneration is the leading cause of blindness in aging people, and at this time there is no effective treatment or cure. All three of these eye disorders are discussed in more detail in Chapter 34.

Hearing. Hearing loss can produce a profound psychological effect on aging persons, causing depression, social withdrawal, and feelings of isolation. Hearing loss occurs gradually over a long period and may go undetected by the older person and healthcare providers. Lack of attention when being spoken to, inappropriate responses, asking to have statements repeated, and speaking too loudly or too softly are often signs of hearing loss. Changes in auditory ability begin around age 30, and by age 65, 25% of aging people have a hearing impairment, which increases to 65% of those over the age of 80 years. Age-related hearing loss is usually the result of dysfunction or loss of cochlear hairs, resulting in an inability to hear high-frequency sounds and difficulty understanding speech. Hearing impairment is compounded by impacted cerumen, otitis media, otosclerosis, Meniere's disease, long-term exposure to intense noise, and certain ototoxic drugs such as aspirin.

Presbycusis, which is explained in Chapter 34, is associated with normal aging and causes a decreased ability to hear high frequencies and to discriminate sounds. Parts of a conversation may be missed because the sound of the word goes above the 2000-cycle frequency. Often words that sound similar are hard to differentiate. Consonants such as *g*, *f*, *s*, *sh*, *t*, and *z* produce high-pitched sounds that are more difficult to hear and differentiate. Low-frequency pitched sounds, such as the vowels *a*, *e*, *i*, *o*, and *u*, may be more easily heard by people with presbycusis. The inability to hear different frequencies combined with low background noise from groups of people talking, noise from appliances, or busy public places will compromise an older person's ability to hear clearly. Hearing aids, which can be used to amplify speech, also increase background noises, resulting in sensory overload.

Another hearing disorder common among older people is *tinnitus*, a ringing or buzzing in the ear. It can be caused by impacted cerumen, an ear infection, use of antibiotics, or a nerve disorder. Tinnitus can cause difficulty in understanding conversational speech and can make sleeping difficult because of the continuous sensation of ringing in the ears.

There is a direct relationship between hearing loss with its resultant isolation and the development of depression in older adults. Treatable depressions are often overlooked in the elderly population because of coexisting physical illnesses that mask the symptoms of depression. The medical assistant may be able to contribute to information about depression in elderly patients through conversations with the individual and family members. The physician may use, or train the medical assistant to use, the Geriatric Depression Scale short form, which questions the patient about daily activities, interests, and feelings to help diagnose depression in the ambulatory setting (Figure 45-4.)

GERIATRIC DEPRESSION SCALE (SHORT FORM)

Choose the best answer for how you have felt over the past week:

1. Are you basically satisfied with your life? YES / **NO**
2. Have you dropped many of your activities and interests? **YES** / NO
3. Do you feel that your life is empty? **YES** / NO
4. Do you often get bored? **YES** / NO
5. Are you in good spirits most of the time? YES / **NO**
6. Are you afraid that something bad is going to happen to you? **YES** / NO
7. Do you feel happy most of the time? YES / **NO**
8. Do you often feel helpless? **YES** / NO
9. Do you prefer to stay at home, rather than going out and doing new things? **YES** / NO
10. Do you feel you have more problems with memory than most? **YES** / NO
11. Do you think it is wonderful to be alive now? YES / **NO**
12. Do you feel pretty worthless the way you are now? **YES** / NO
13. Do you feel full of energy? YES / **NO**
14. Do you feel that your situation is hopeless? **YES** / NO
15. Do you think that most people are better off than you are? **YES** / NO

Answers in **bold** indicate depression. Although differing sensitivities and specificities have been obtained across studies, for clinical purposes a score >5 points is suggestive of depression and should warrant a follow-up interview. Scores >10 are almost always depression.

FIGURE 45-4   Geriatric depression scale.

SUGGESTIONS FOR HELPING THE HEARING-IMPAIRED OLDER ADULT

- Stand in the line of vision and gently touch the person to get attention.
- Use gestures, pictures, and large, bold print to communicate.

SUGGESTIONS FOR HELPING THE HEARING-IMPAIRED OLDER ADULT—cont'd

- Talk in short sentences into the better ear.
- *Do not* increase the volume of your speech—this also raises the frequency of the voice, which is the hearing most impaired in aging people. Use *expanded* speech—lower the tone of your voice and talk in distinct syllables.
- Avoid background noise. Give instructions in a quiet room with the door closed. If the patient has a hearing aid, make sure it is on.

Taste and Smell. During the aging process, there is a subtle decline in the ability to taste and smell. Deterioration and the atrophy of the taste buds are part of the aging process. The ability to taste salt and sweet flavors is reduced, whereas the ability to detect bitter and sour flavors remains relatively the same. As a result, food tastes bland and unappetizing. Patients on salt-restricted diets and diabetic patients must be cautioned on the use of excessive amounts of salt and sugar. A decrease in the sense of smell accompanies the decrease in taste. This not only affects the individual's enjoyment of food, but it also exposes the person to environmental dangers such as gas leaks, smoke, and other dangerous odors that may go undetected. Checking for gas leaks around stoves and heaters and using smoke alarms reduce some of the danger. Also dating food when it is put in the refrigerator is a good idea.

Nutritional Status. Aging persons, because of the many environmental, social, economic, and physical changes of aging, are at greater risk of poor nutrition, which can adversely affect their health and energy level. It is estimated that 25% of the aging population suffers from malnutrition. Nutrition screening should be part of routine primary care to identify nutritional deficiencies and correct them before disease process occurs or to assist in the treatment of chronic disease. Patients with chronic conditions, such as cardiovascular disease, hypertension, and diabetes, can benefit from nutrition assessments and interventions. Malnourished older patients get more infections; their injuries take longer to heal; surgery on them is riskier; and their hospital stays are longer and more expensive.

The most effective method of assessing a patient's nutritional status is through a comprehensive patient interview that considers all potential barriers to adequate nutrition. The medical assistant can contribute to determining the nutritional status of older patients by considering the following items when conducting patient interviews.

- *Oral health:* Does the patient wear dentures, and do they fit properly? Is there mouth pain? Can the patient swallow without difficulty?
- *Gastrointestinal complaints:* Does the patient have anorexia, nausea, vomiting, diarrhea, or constipation? Is the patient lactose intolerant (increased incidence with age)?

- *Sensorimotor changes:* Is there loss of vision, hearing, or changes in taste and smell? Can the patient feed herself or himself? Does the patient need adaptive utensils?
- *Diet influences:* Can the patient shop for, afford, and prepare food? Are there ethnic or religious influences? Are there any disease-related diet restrictions? What is the alcohol consumption?
- *Social and mental influences:* Is the patient depressed, lonely, isolated? Are support systems available?

CRITICAL THINKING APPLICATION

Multiple changes occur in the senses as people age. Dr. Kennedy asks Bill to develop a handout for patients and family members to help them understand normal, age-related sensorimotor changes as well as adaptations that can be made to improve communication. What information should Bill include?

Urinary System

As the body ages, structural changes in the kidney cause the urinary system to become less efficient. Between the ages of 40 and 80, the kidney loses about 20% of its mass. The number of functional nephron units decreases. There is a reduction in blood flow to the kidney owing to a decrease in cardiovascular efficiency. The reduction of blood flow to the kidney and the decreased number of nephrons cause the kidneys to be less efficient at filtering waste from the blood. This results in a more-diluted, less-concentrated urine. The kidneys require more water to excrete the same amount of waste. Medication takes longer to be removed from the body. Older adults are at an increased risk for toxic levels of medication in the bloodstream because of this reduced filtration rate.

Fibrous connective tissue replaces the smooth muscle and elastic tissue in the bladder. This thickening of the bladder wall decreases the bladder's ability to expand. The bladder's capacity to store fluid comfortably is reduced from 400 to 250 ml. These structural changes in the bladder lead to increased frequency of urination and urinary retention. Older adults are at an increased risk for urinary tract infections because of residual urine. Often sleep is interrupted by the need to void during the night. The sensation of bladder fullness is not recognized as quickly by the older brain. Reduced time between awareness of the need to void and involuntary urination can cause anxiety. Often older adults decrease their fluid intake to prevent possible embarrassment. Unfortunately this causes dehydration and an increased risk of urinary tract infections. Another change is loss of muscle tone in the urethra. Additionally, the pelvic floor muscles in the aging woman relax as a result of decreased estrogen levels or previous pregnancy and childbirth.

Despite these changes, the kidneys have great reserve capacity and are able to continue functioning normally. Urinary incontinence, the involuntary loss of urine, is a significant problem for aging patients but is *not* a normal part of the aging process. Changes in the urinary system make older persons more vulnerable to incontinence, but there are contributing factors such as infection, confusion, difficulty with mobility, and side effects from medications that cause the problem to develop. Incontinence is an emotional as well as a physical problem. To avoid the chance of an embarrassing accident, people with this problem may avoid social occasions or activities they enjoy. Often people are too embarrassed to admit they have this condition or they believe it is just part of aging. Once the condition is diagnosed by the urologist, pelvic floor muscle exercises, medication, or surgery may be recommended.

Reproductive System

Menopause is discussed in Chapter 38. There is a decrease in circulating levels of the female hormones estrogen and progesterone, while androgen levels increase. The results of this decrease are changes in the genital tract. The vagina diminishes in width and length and becomes less elastic. The cervix, uterus, and ovaries decrease in size. Vaginal secretions decrease; therefore, lubrication diminishes and, in some cases, vaginal dryness may be the result. Bacterial or yeast infections may occur because the vaginal secretions are less acidic. Estrogen cream applied to the vaginal tissue may be prescribed by the physician for help with dryness and thinning of the vaginal tissue. The benefits and risks of estrogen replacement therapy should be discussed by the physician with the patient to determine whether it should be used.

Even though sperm production may decline in men older than 50, men remain virile well into old age. Men do experience a change in hormonal levels of testosterone, and these changes can affect the prostate gland, as discussed in Chapter 37. The gland enlarges over time and presses down on the urethra, causing difficulty during urination. Surgery may be required to remove excess portions of the gland. Unfortunately, the operation may cause impotence, which can be treated medically with Viagra (sildenafil citrate).

Men do experience some changes in their sexual functioning. It takes longer for the penis to become erect, longer for an orgasm to occur, and longer to recover. Direct stimulation may be required before an erection occurs, and when it does, it may be less firm when compared with how it was when they were younger.

Some drugs and illnesses can interfere with sexual functioning. Drugs used to control high blood pressure, antihistamines, antidepressants, some stomach acid blockers, diabetes, arthritis, and hardening of the arteries can have an adverse effect on sexual functioning. Often people who have experienced heart surgery or have had heart attacks are concerned about sexual activity. It is important to make patients feel comfortable and not embarrassed to discuss their concerns openly with their physician.

As healthcare providers, it is important to dismiss myths that older patients have lost desire and interest in sexual intercourse. Sex at an older age may become more enjoyable than when the participants were younger. Women are more relaxed because the fear of pregnancy is gone. With their children grown and out of the house, couples have more time and privacy. Older people are more experienced and usually can communicate better with one another. At any age, sexuality may be expressed in other forms such as touching, holding, caressing, and, of course, humor. The ability to laugh and share life experiences with one another plays an important role.

Sleep Disorders

Complaints of sleeping difficulties increase with age. The amount of time spent sleeping may be slightly longer than that of a younger person, but the quality of sleep decreases. Older people are often light sleepers and experience periods of wakefulness in bed. *Rapid eye movement* (REM) sleep is the stage of sleep when people experience dreaming. Non-REM sleep is the period of deepest sleep. The amount of time spent in the deepest stages of sleep decreases with age. Sleep that is disturbed or that leaves the person feeling tired is not part of the aging process and may indicate some underlying emotional or physical problem. Lack of sleep can result in restlessness, disorientation, thick-speech patterns, and mispronounced words. Often these symptoms are mistaken as signs of dementia. Other factors that might influence sleep patterns are medications, caffeine, alcohol, depression, and environmental or physical changes.

Common sleep problems in older adults include dyssomnias, such as periodic limb movement disorder (PLMD), in which the person experiences periodic jerking of the legs during sleep, and sleep apnea, which is common among overweight persons and can occur frequently during the night, causing sleep interruption. Numerous medical conditions can interfere with sleep, including joint and bone pain; Parkinson's disease (because of difficulty changing positions); CHF; chronic obstructive lung disease; diabetes mellitus, which increases nocturia; depression; and certain medications (beta-blockers can cause nightmares, antidepressants increase PLMD, and barbiturates may result in nightmares or hallucinations).

It is important to be aware of the effect of sleep problems because often these can be confused with dementia. Patients who are experiencing difficulty with sleeping should be encouraged to document their sleeping pattern, napping patterns, medications, diet, exercise patterns, and any events that have resulted in a change of lifestyle. They should discuss this problem with their physician. Simple modification of behavioral patterns may resolve the problem. Taking fewer naps, completing exercises several hours before bedtime, changing eating times, decreasing the amount of alcohol and caffeine ingested, drinking a glass of milk before bedtime, or changing medications or the time they are taken are all suggestions that might alter the factors responsible for sleep disturbances.

If behavioral approaches are not effective, medications may be considered for *short-term* use only because they have a high incidence of physical and psychological dependence. The elderly population is especially susceptible to side effects from these drugs, for example, next-day drowsiness and temporary memory loss. Sedatives or hypnotics that may be prescribed include Ambien, Halcion, and Restoril.

Living Arrangements

At any given time, only 5% of the elderly population live in long-term-care facilities. According to information published by the National Institute on Aging, most older people live close to their children and are in frequent contact with them. People prefer to age in place or, in other words, live in their own home environment as long as possible. The reason people are admitted to nursing homes is because they are no longer able to perform activities of daily living, such as bathing, dressing, eating, walking, and maintaining bladder and bowel continence. They also exhibit difficulty with grocery shopping, housekeeping, and money management. Chronic health conditions interfere with the older person's ability to perform these tasks.

Many resources are available that enable seniors to maintain their independence. Outreach programs, such as Meals-on-Wheels, deliver nutritious meals to the homes of older adults. Senior centers serve as a focal point for many activities and a source of information. Transportation services provide rides to doctors' appointments, day care centers, shopping centers, and community events. Home health agencies provide several types of services, which include personal care, shopping, transportation, and meal preparation. Some home health agencies provide a range of activities from patient education to intravenous therapy; medical-social services; physical, speech, and occupational therapies; and nutrition and dietary counseling. Advanced technology allows people to receive services at home that had formerly been provided at a hospital or physician's office only.

Adult day care centers provide socialization, recreation, meals, and, in some centers, physical therapy, occupational therapy, and transportation. These centers provide supervision for older adults who may be taken care of by family members in the evening but need care during the day. They also serve as respite for a caregiver.

Assisted-living facilities can be retirement homes or board and care homes. These facilities are appropriate for older adults who need assistance with some activities of daily living, such as bathing, dressing, and walking. Skilled nursing facilities provide 24-hour medical care and supervision. In addition to medical care, residents receive care that may include physical, occupational, and speech therapy. The objective of treatment is to improve or maintain the person's abilities.

The Medical Assistant's Role in Caring for the Older Patient

Elderly patients in the ambulatory care setting present a specific set of needs that require a certain amount of accommodation by the staff. To reinforce independence, aging patients require more time, but staff members may want to hurry them so the schedule can be maintained. In the best interests of the patient, however, he or she should be treated with respect and given whatever time is needed to prepare for examinations, answer questions, and explain procedures. A system that is sensitive to the needs of older patients will schedule longer periods for appointments; have adequate lighting in the waiting room and forms in large print; have an examination room that is equipped with furniture, magazines, and treatment folders especially designed for older adults; and invite a professional in the management of older patients for in-service training. The primary issue in elder care is effective communication. How you communicate with people is often influenced by what you know or do not know about them. Older people are subject to many changes that affect how they are able to interact with their environment. It is important to recognize these changes as well as our personal perception of older people to break down the barriers that prohibit effective communication.

As people age, they may encounter a reduction in control over their lives owing to physical disabilities, economic constraints, and institutional living. It is important to enable aging people to maintain their dignity and independence. Remember, each patient, regardless of his or her education, socioeconomic status, or age, deserves to be treated with compassion and respect. Ask the patient directly what is wrong rather than discussing the patient with family members. It also is important to listen carefully and to be specific and sincere in responding. When a patient is talking, take time to allow him or her to complete the sentence. Do not finish it for him or her. Give the patient your full attention rather than continuing with other tasks while he or she is speaking. Older people may take a little longer to process information, but they are capable of understanding. Do not hurry through explanations or questions; rather, take time to review a form or give instructions.

SUGGESTIONS FOR EFFECTIVE COMMUNICATIONS WITH AGING PATIENTS

- Address the patient by Mr./Mrs./Miss unless the patient has given permission to use his or her first name.
- All healthcare workers should introduce themselves and their purpose before performing a procedure.
- Face the aging person and softly touch him or her to get attention before beginning to speak.
- Use expanded speech, gestures, demonstrations, or written instructions in block print.
- If the message must be repeated, paraphrase or find other words to say the same thing.

SUGGESTIONS FOR EFFECTIVE COMMUNICATIONS WITH AGING PATIENTS—cont'd

- Observe the patient's nonverbal behaviors as cues to indicate whether he or she understands.
- Provide adequate lighting without glare.
- Allow patients time to process information and take care of themselves unless they ask for assistance.
- Communications should be conducted in a quiet room without distractions.
- Involve family members as needed for continuity of care.
- When leaving a telephone message, remember to speak slowly and clearly and repeat it in the same manner. It is hard to interpret a message, and even more difficult to write it down, if the message was delivered in a hurried manner.
- Use referrals and community resources for support such as:
  - Alzheimer's Association (1-800-272-3900)
  - American Council of the Blind (1-800-424-8666)—provides referrals to state and other organizations that provide services and equipment for the blind
  - American Speech-Language-Hearing Association (1-800-638-8255)—offers information on hearing aids or hearing loss and communication problems in older people and provides a list of certified audiologist and speech pathologists.
  - Arthritis Foundation Information Line (1-800-283-7800)—makes referrals to local chapters and provides information
  - Eldercare Locator (1-800-677-1116)—run by the National Association of Area Agencies on Aging, the help line provides information on contacting local chapters that oversee services to older adults
  - National Institute on Aging Information Center (1-800-222-2225)—provides information on geriatric health issues
  - National Wheels-on-Meals Foundation (1-800-999-6262)
  - Hospice Helpline (1-800-658-8898)—provides information about hospice care and makes referrals to local hospices

Patient Education

The medical assistant must keep the sensorimotor changes that accompany aging and respectful patient communications in mind when conducting patient education with older clients. Remember, the aging process does not affect a person's ability to learn; it just may take longer to process the information and the material may need to be repeated for understanding. Exhibiting sensitivity to the needs of aging learners will ensure successful patient education and improve compliance with prescribed treatment plans. The current aging population is generally respectful toward authority; so if the medical assistant cannot gain patient cooperation, the physician may be able to provide authoritative reinforcement of material.

GUIDELINES FOR EFFECTIVE PATIENT EDUCATION WITH OLDER ADULTS

- May have short-term memory loss, so need to repeat the information using different words.
- Distracted easier, so learning in a group may be difficult.
- Take longer to process information, so teach at a pace that matches patient needs.
- Provide large-print, block-letter handouts for reviewing information at home.
- Involve family members as needed for continuity of care.

CRITICAL THINKING APPLICATION

New staff members in the practice are complaining of having to repeat information to older clients and that they do not pay attention when procedures are being explained. Dr. Kennedy has decided to invite a gerontologist from the local university to present an in-service on healthy aging. She asks Bill to coordinate the in-service and prepare materials requested by the guest speaker. What information regarding caring for the ambulatory aging patient should be included in the workshop?

Legal and Ethical Issues

All patients have the right to know about the medications, treatments, and alternatives available to them. The Patient's Bill of Rights (see Appendix A) informs the patient of his or her rights in a healthcare setting. These rights include the right to privacy about personal and medical information and the right to informed consent, which holds the physician accountable to explain clearly the advantages and risks of any procedures, tests, or treatments. The patient must give permission for medical care and has the right to refuse treatment. The patient has the right to be informed about his or her condition and treatment and the chances of recovery. The patient also has the right to have advance directives explained to him or her.

Consent must be given by the individual undergoing the procedure as long as he or she is judged to be competent, that is, as long as the patient is able to understand the consequences of the procedure. In an emergency situation, or if a court has ruled the patient incompetent, someone else must give consent. This may be a person who was already designated as the durable power of attorney, a close family member (spouse, adult child, parent, sibling), or a court-appointed guardian.

Most states have legal documents available, *advance directives* that provide written instructions specifying the type of medical care a person wishes to receive in the event she or he becomes incapacitated. The document designates a durable power of attorney who is responsible for making medical decisions on a person's behalf if that individual is unable to make his or her own treatment decisions. The document provides a list of specific instructions for the proxy to follow. Various issues may be covered in these documents. Do not resuscitate (DNR) orders allow a patient to refuse attempts to restore heartbeat. The patient may decide to withdraw life-sustaining treatment such as the use of respirators or feeding tubes. A copy of the directive should be kept on file as part of the patient's medical record. It is important to check the laws of the state in which you are practicing about advance directives because these vary among states.

Another legal issue surrounding the care of aging patient is the possibility of elder abuse. Mistreatment of aging persons crosses all social, racial, and economic levels. The abuse may be physical, mental, sexual, material, or financial; neglect or failure to provide adequate care; or self-neglect when aging persons are unable or refuse to care for themselves. The abuse of elders by their caregivers may be difficult to identify. The aging victim feels embarrassed, guilty, or afraid to report the abuse. If abuse is suspected, interviewing the caregiver and questioning the demands of care and self-reported perceptions of stress levels may help the physician detect the problem. Many states now have laws that require reporting suspected elder abuse. Check your state to determine the requirements for healthcare workers.

INDICATIONS OF ELDER ABUSE

- Poor general appearance and poor hygiene.
- Pattern of changing doctors and frequent emergency room visits.
- Skin lesions, signs of dehydration, bruises (signs of new and old bruising together), abrasions, welts, burns, or pressure sores.
- Recurrent injuries due to accidents.
- Signs of malnutrition and weight loss without related illness.
- Any injury that does not fit the given history.

SUMMARY OF SCENARIO

Since working with Dr. Kennedy, Bill has learned to understand the special needs of aging patients. He thought that most older people were chronically sick and would ultimately end up in long-term-care facilities. Now he understands that most older people lead healthy, active lives and that the disorders occurring in later life are usually due to lifestyle factors such as diet and lack of exercise. Bill has also learned how to communicate effectively with older patients and to conduct patient interviews that investigate their physical, mental, emotional, and nutritional health.

SUMMARY OF LEARNING OBJECTIVES

- In the 2000 census, 12.4% of the U.S. population was over the age of 65. About one in every eight Americans is older than 65. The "oldest old" (people older than 85) is the most rapidly growing age group. It is projected that people older than 65 will represent 16% of the population in 2020 and increase to 20% by 2030. The aging population will impact all aspects of society. To provide better services to the aging consumer, it is necessary to understand the aging process, which includes the physical and sensory changes encountered by older people. This knowledge enables the healthcare professional to recognize the special needs of the aged and to develop effective management and communication skills to better service the older client.

- Table 45-1 summarizes the changes in anatomy and physiology that are associated with aging. These changes occur across all body systems. There are normal age-related changes that can be expected and compensated for, but these become more serious problems in the presence of poor health habits and chronic disease. General changes include an increase in arteriosclerosis, an increase in the time needed to learn new material, a sharp decline in estrogen for women and an increased risk of osteoporosis, an increase in malabsorption problems and constipation, a decrease in muscle mass, a tendency to gain weight and deterioration of joint cartilage, decreased elasticity of lung tissue, presbycusis and presbyopia, and enlargement of the prostate and weakening of bladder muscles. All these age-related changes can be managed through regular aerobic exercise and strength training; weight control; a diet rich in fruits, vegetables, and whole grains, and low in fat; avoidance of sun damage to skin; pelvic muscle exercises; and annual physical examinations with health screening.

■ The major health issues for aging people are related to an increase in atherosclerosis and potential cardiovascular disease; hypertension; type 2 diabetes mellitus; a tendency toward hyperthermia and hypothermia; seborrheic keratosis; arthritis; osteoporosis; an increased risk of injury from falls; dementia attributable to metabolic, cardiovascular, or Alzheimer's disease; pneumonia, aspiration, and reactivation of tuberculosis; cataracts, glaucoma, and macular degeneration; depression; malnutrition; urinary tract infections, incontinence, and prostate enlargement; menopausal changes in the vaginal mucosa; sleep disorders such as apnea and PLMD; and the impact of medications on general health.

■ A commonly used screening tool for dementia is the Folstein Mini-Mental Status Examination, a 5-minute screening test that is designed to evaluate basic mental function in the patient's ability to recall facts, write, and calculate numbers. It provides the physician with a quick way to determine whether more in-depth testing is needed. To screen for depression, the physician may use the Geriatric Depression Scale short form that questions the patient about daily activities, interests, and feelings. Nutritional status can be assessed through a comprehensive patient interview that considers all potential barriers to adequate nutrition. The medical assistant can contribute to determining the nutritional status of older patients by considering oral health, gastrointestinal complaints, sensorimotor changes, diet influences, and social and mental influences when conducting patient interviews.

■ Complaints of sleeping difficulties increase with age. The amount of time spent sleeping may be slightly longer than a younger person, but the quality of sleep decreases. The amount of time spent in the deepest stages of sleep decreases with age. Factors that might influence sleep patterns are medications, caffeine, alcohol, depression, and environmental or physical changes. Common sleep problems in older adults include PLMD and sleep apnea.

■ Aging persons prefer to remain within their home environment as long as possible. Adult day care centers can provide supervision for older adults who may be taken care of by family members in the evening but need care during the day. They also serve as respite for a caregiver. Assisted-living facilities are appropriate for older adults who need assistance with some activities of daily living, such as bathing, dressing, and walking. Skilled nursing facilities provide 24-hour medical care and supervision. In addition to medical care, residents receive care including physical, occupational, and speech therapy.

■ The medical assistant's role in caring for the older patient is to develop effective communication skills that are reflective of age-related sensorimotor changes. To reinforce independence, aging patients require more time and so should be scheduled for longer appointments. Adequate lighting in the waiting room with forms in large print; an examination room that is equipped with furniture, magazines, and treatment folders especially designed for the elderly patient; and inviting a professional in the management of the elderly patient for in-service training improve the quality of elder care. Ask the patient directly what is wrong rather than discussing the patient with family members. Give the patient your full attention rather than continuing with multiple tasks while he or she is speaking. Older people may take a little longer to process information but they are capable of understanding. Use referrals and community resources for patient and family support.

■ Effective communication with aging patients includes addressing the patient with an appropriate title; introducing yourself and the purpose of a procedure before touching the patient; establishing eye contact and getting the patient's attention before beginning to speak; using expanded speech, gestures, demonstrations, or written instructions in block print; repeating the message as needed for understanding; observing the patient's nonverbal behaviors as cues to indicate whether he or she understands; allowing time to process information; avoiding distractions; and involving family members as needed.

■ Legal and ethical issues for aging patients include adequate informed consent, the use of advance directives, and staying alert for signs of possible elder abuse.

KEY INTERNET WEBSITES

- Administration on Aging
- Alzheimer's Association
- American Association of Retired Persons
- National Institutes of Health
- National Osteoporosis Foundation
  For active weblinks to each website visit
  http://evolve.elsevier.com/Kinn/

UNIT eight

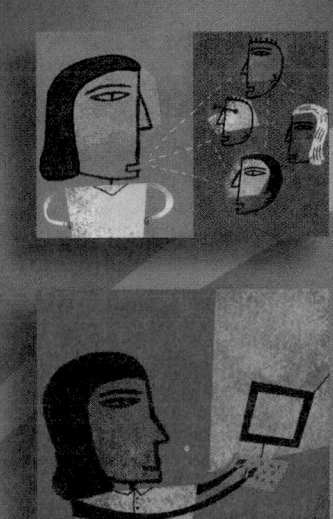

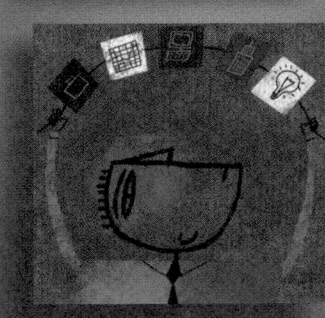

Diagnostic Procedures

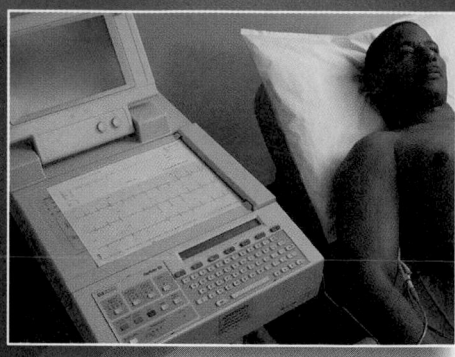

CHAPTER 46

Scenario

Marcus Reyes has been working in the local hospital as a nursing assistant since he was a senior in high school 4 years ago. For the past year he has worked in the coronary care unit. The head cardiologist at the hospital, Dr. Lee, has taken an interest in Marcus by always taking time to answer his questions. Dr. Lee paid for Marcus to go through a medical assisting program at the local community college. Marcus just graduated from the program and is going to work as a medical assistant in Dr. Lee's cardiology practice. Marcus is very enthusiastic but realizes that he has much more to learn on the job to provide the very best patient service possible in Dr. Lee's practice.

Unfortunately, Dr. Lee's previous medical assistant, who was going to train Marcus, had to stop working rather abruptly because of a family emergency out of state and will not be there to train Marcus.

Principles of Electrocardiography

Kim Anthony Aaronson

National Curriculum Competencies

CLINICAL COMPETENCIES

3h. Perform electrocardiograms

Vocabulary

arrhythmia Abnormality or irregularity in the heart rhythm.

atria The two upper chambers of the heart.

atrioventricular (AV) node Part of the cardiac conduction system located between the atria and the ventricles.

bifurcates Divides from one into two branches.

bradycardia Heart rate of less than 60 beats per minute.

bundle of His Specialized muscle fibers that conduct electrical impulses from AV node to ventricular myocardium.

cardiac arrest Condition in which cardiac contractions completely stop.

cardioversion Using electroshock to convert an abnormal cardiac rhythm to a normal one.

defibrillator Machine used to deliver an electroshock to the heart through electrodes placed on the chest wall.

dyspnea Difficulty breathing.

ectopic Originating outside of the normal tissue.

hypertension High blood pressure in which the systolic pressure is above 140 mm Hg or the diastolic pressure is above 90 mm Hg.

infarction Area of tissue that has died from lack of blood supply.

ischemic Characterized by temporary interruption in the blood supply to a tissue or organ.

myocardial Pertaining to the heart muscle.

myocardium Heart muscle.

orthopnea Difficulty breathing when in the supine position.

sinoatrial (SA) node Pacemaker of the heart located in the right atrium.

tachycardia Heart rate over 100 beats per minute.

ventricles The two lower chambers of the heart.

vertigo Dizziness.

Electrocardiography is a painless and safe procedure, the test most frequently used for the diagnosis of heart disease. To perform electrocardiography, electrodes are attached to the patient's skin and connected to wires that go to the *electrocardiograph* machine. The electrocardiograph amplifies the electrical impulses from the beating heart, and a pattern of these impulses is recorded on ECG paper. This record is called the *electrocardiogram* (ECG). The ECG is read and evaluated by the physician and becomes a part of the patient's chart (Figure 46-1).

For the ECG to accurately represent the true cardiac activity of a patient, it must be performed with a high degree of accuracy and skill. A medical assistant must have an understanding of normal cardiac function and the relationship of the ECG markings to normal function. It is the medical assistant's responsibility to ensure that the patient has been prepared mentally and physically and that the equipment is set up properly. When performing the ECG, a medical assistant must be

able to recognize electrical interferences and make appropriate corrections or adjustments. The goal is to obtain the most accurate electrocardiogram possible.

HISTORY OF ELECTROCARDIOGRAPHY

Dutch physiologist Willem Einthoven developed techniques to record the electrical activity of the heart in the late 1800s. He called this recording an *Electro Kardio Gramm;* hence the term *EKG*. Many physicians and other health care providers still call the recording an EKG, although the newer, preferred term is *ECG* for electrocardiogram.

The Electrical Conduction System of the Heart

The Cardiac Cycle

The cardiac cycle includes all of the events occurring in the heart during one single heartbeat. These events include depolarization or contraction of heart muscle, repolarization or recovery of heart muscle, and polarization or relaxation of heart muscle. The cardiac impulse can be recorded by the electrocardiograph, which records both the intensity and the actual time it takes for each event to occur. The ECG measures the electrical conductive impulses of the heart muscle and therefore allows the physician to see any disturbances or disruptions in normal heart activity. Instead of being recorded as an ECG, the cardiac cycle can also appear as a continuously moving pattern on a monitor screen, accompanied by a sound for each beat. On televised programs, you frequently see and hear real ECGs.

The specialized electrical conduction system of the heart (Figure 46-2) initiates each heartbeat. The main part of this system is called the **sinoatrial (SA) node** and is located in the upper back wall of the right atrium. Each cardiac cycle or heartbeat starts with the SA node giving off an electrical impulse that travels throughout the cardiac muscle of the atria, causing them to contract. The SA node controls the rate of heart contraction. This electrical impulse then stimulates the **atrioventricular (AV) node**, which is located in the superior portion of the intraventricular septum. The AV node then sends an electrical impulse through a special group of conduction fibers, the **bundle of His**, to the right and left **ventricles**, causing them to contract. The bundle of His divides into two branches, the *right bundle branch* carrying the electrical impulse to the right ventricle and the *left bundle branch* carrying the electrical impulse to the left ventricle.

Normal sinus rhythm (NSR) refers to a regular heart rate that falls within the average range of 60 to 80 beats/min. Sinus **bradycardia** is a heart rate less than 60 beats/min, whereas a rate of greater than 100 beats/min is called sinus **tachycardia**. In both of these conditions, the rhythm remains even, but the rate is pathological. An irregular cardiac rhythm is called an **arrhythmia**. Conditions that interrupt the conduction pathway, SA node to AV node to bundle of His to right and left bundle branches, can cause arrhythmias.

HEART RATES

- An elephant's heart beats about 20 beats/min.
- A mouse's heart beats about 500 beats/min.

Depolarization and Repolarization

The ECG records a series of waves, or deflections, above or below a baseline on the ECG paper. Each deflection corresponds to a particular part of the cardiac cycle (Table 46-1). The normal ECG cycle consists of waveforms that are labeled the P wave, the Q wave, the R wave, the S wave, and the T wave. The Q, R, and S waves are usually grouped together and called the QRS complex. One entire cardiac cycle can be called the PQRST

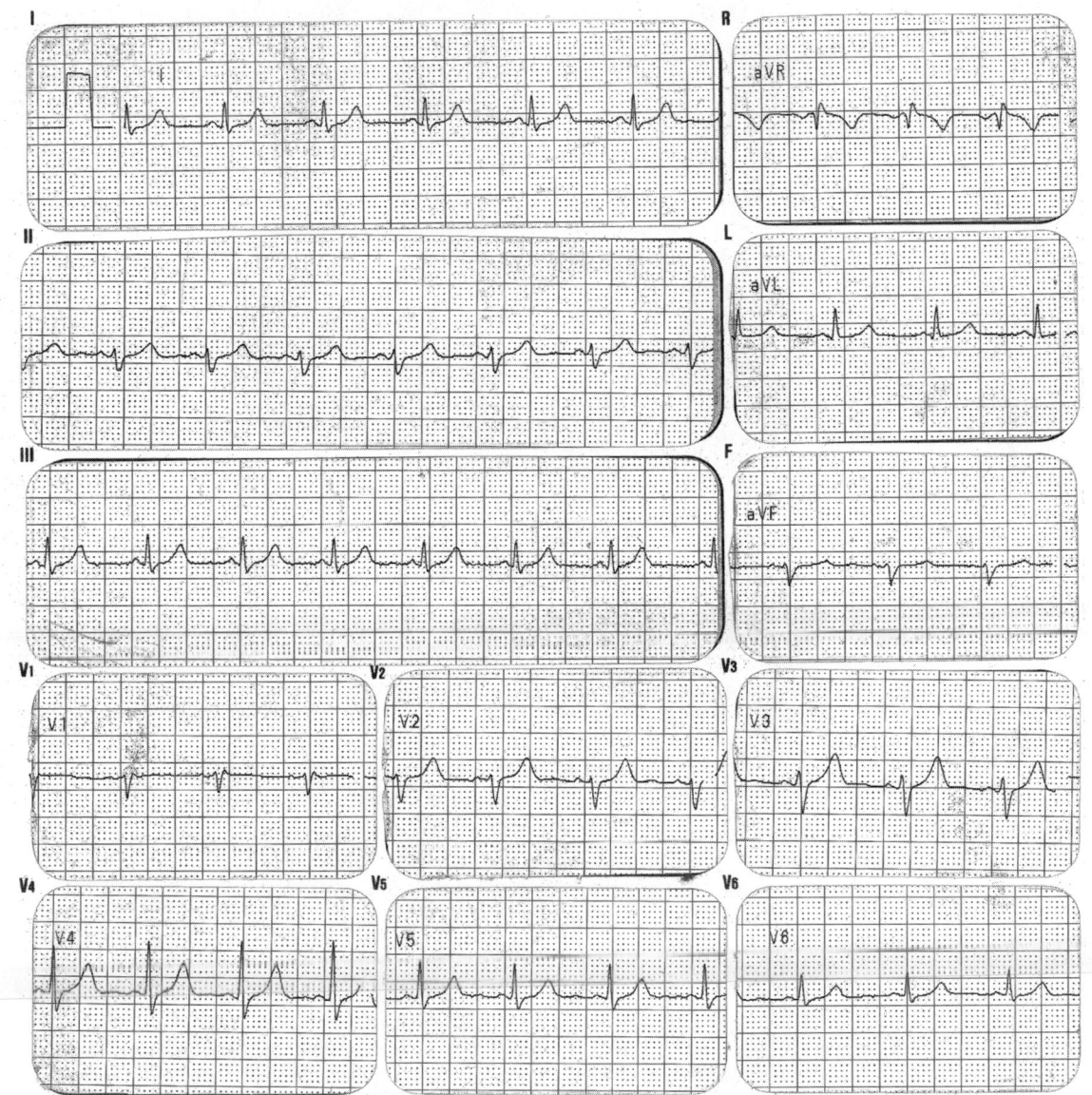

CLIN. DIAG.: *Chest Pain*

ECG DESCRIPTION: *Stat 12 Lead*

INTERPRETATION:

PATIENT: *Jane Doe*

DIG ( ) QUIN. ( ) AGE *29* SEX *F* B.P. *120/80*

ECG REQUEST BY *Dr. Hope U. Arewell*
ATR. RATE *90* VENTR. RATE *90*
INTERVALS: P-R *.12* QRS *.08* QTc
AXIS: *Left Axis Shift*
RHYTHM: *Normal Sinus Rhythm*

INTERPRETED BY: *H. Arewell MD*
DATE:

FIGURE 46-1 A normal ECG. (From Chester GA: *Modern medical assisting,* Philadelphia, 1998, WB Saunders.)

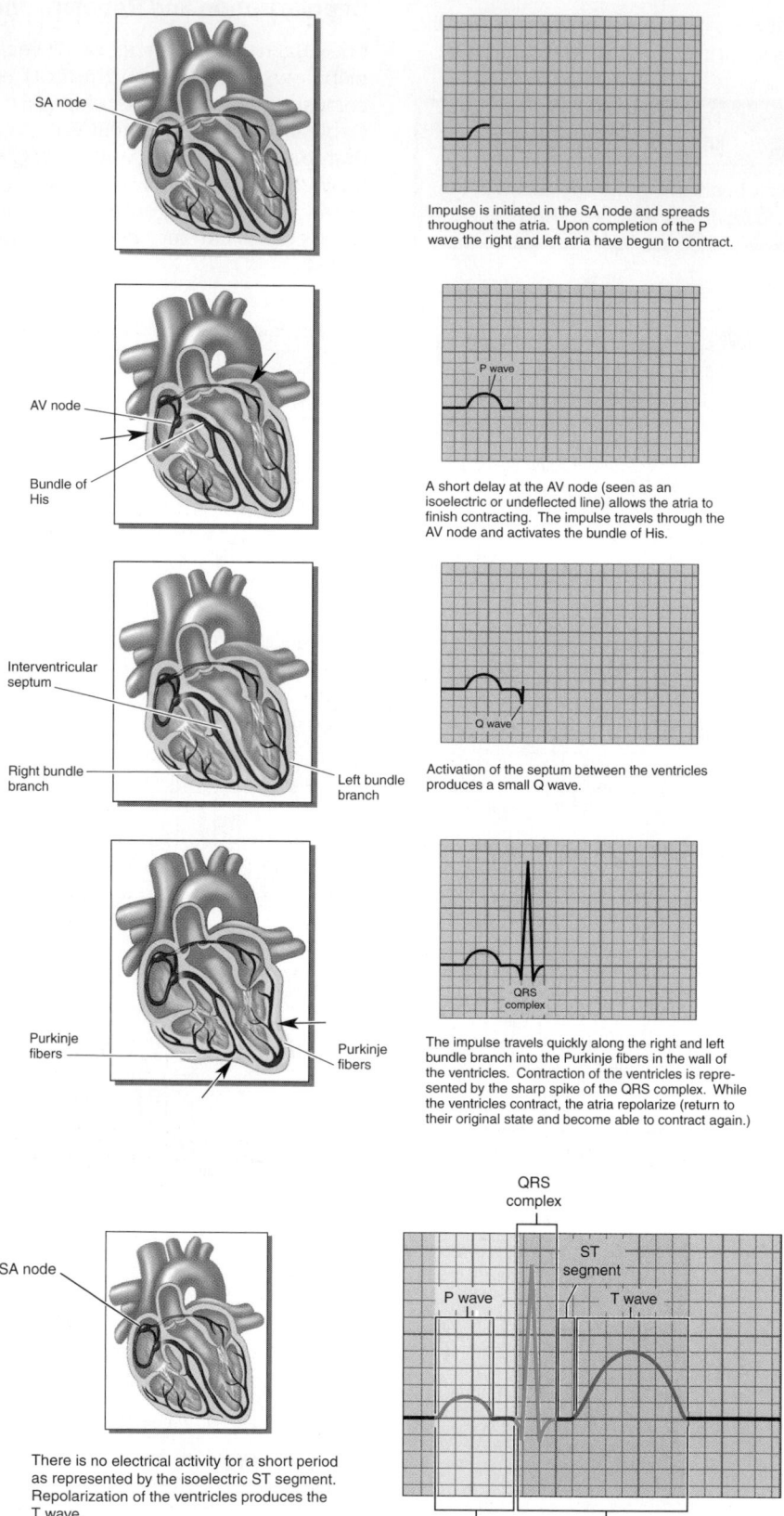

Impulse is initiated in the SA node and spreads throughout the atria. Upon completion of the P wave the right and left atria have begun to contract.

A short delay at the AV node (seen as an isoelectric or undeflected line) allows the atria to finish contracting. The impulse travels through the AV node and activates the bundle of His.

Activation of the septum between the ventricles produces a small Q wave.

The impulse travels quickly along the right and left bundle branch into the Purkinje fibers in the wall of the ventricles. Contraction of the ventricles is represented by the sharp spike of the QRS complex. While the ventricles contract, the atria repolarize (return to their original state and become able to contract again.)

There is no electrical activity for a short period as represented by the isoelectric ST segment. Repolarization of the ventricles produces the T wave.

FIGURE 46-2 Electrical conduction system of the heart. (From Hunt SA: *Saunders fundamentals of medical assisting*, Philadelphia, 2002, WB Saunders.)

complex. In the next section, each part of the ECG will be discussed in more detail.

HOW DID WE GET "PQRST"?

Mr. Einthoven was also responsible for naming the wave in the PQRST fashion. The letters *ABCDE* were already used to describe the unprocessed waves of electrical activity from the heart, so they could not be used. Moving on in the alphabet, *N* and *O* had other distinct usages in mathematics, so the next available letter that began an available sequence was P, which began the second half of the alphabet. Hence he named the processed waves *PQRST*, and the term is used to this very day.

PQRST Complex

The P wave occurs during the contraction of the atria and shows the beginning of cardiac depolarization. The P-R interval is the time from the beginning of atrial contraction to the beginning of ventricular contraction. The QRS complex shows the contraction of both ventricles and also reflects the completion of cardiac depolarization. Repolarization of the atria also occurs during this time, but it cannot be seen on the ECG, because the recording of the much stronger QRS activity overshadows it. The ST segment shows the time between the end of ventricular contraction and the beginning of ventricular recovery. The T wave indicates ventricular recovery or repolarization of the ventricles. After the T wave, there is a time period of complete heart rest, also called *polarization*, which is indicated on the ECG as a straight line. The Q-T interval is the time between the beginning of the QRS complex through the T wave. During this time the ventricles contract and relax. The U wave can occasionally be seen as a small "bump" just after the T wave in patients who have a low serum potassium level or other metabolic disorders.

By measuring the actual configuration and location of each wave in relation to the other waves and to the baseline as well as the intervals between waves and the segments, the physician is able to detect rhythmic disturbances of the heart and to distinguish different types of cardiac disorders.

HEARTBEAT STRENGTH

If you give a tennis ball a quick, vigorous squeeze with your hand, that is about the same amount of force as in a single heartbeat.

The ECG Machine

Most physicians are now using an electrocardiograph (Figure 46-3) that can record three or six leads simultaneously. These are called *three-channel* and *six-channel* ECG machines. In both cases, all limb and chest leads are placed on the patient before the recording starts. When the ECG is started, the machine records all 12 leads automatically and marks each lead with identifying letters instead of the dot-dash coding used on single-strip electrocardiograms. These multichannel ECG tracings take less time to perform, and they can be placed into the patient's chart without mounting. Older ECG machines are single channel and record each of the 12 leads one at a time. These strips must then be cut apart, and each lead's recording is mounted onto the adhesive area of a mounting card.

TABLE 46-1	The Cardiac Cycle	
Stage	**Heart Activity**	**Electric Current**
P wave*	Atrial contraction	Atrial depolarization
PR segment†	Contraction traversing the atrioventricular node	Depolarization traversing the atrioventricular node
QRS complex‡	Ventricular contraction	Ventricular depolarization
ST segment	Time interval between ventricular contraction and the beginning of ventricular recovery	Time interval between ventricular depolarization and ventricular repolarization
T wave	Ventricular contraction subsides	Ventricular repolarization (electric recovery)
U wave (not always present)	Associated with further ventricular relaxation	Associated with further ventricular repolarization
Baseline§	The heart at rest	Polarization
PR interval‖	Time interval between atrial contraction and ventricular contraction	Time interval between atrial depolarization and ventricular depolarization
QT interval	Time interval between the beginning of ventricular contraction and the subsiding of ventricular contraction	Time interval between the beginning of ventricular depolarization and ventricular repolarization (electric recovery)

*Wave: A uniformly advancing deflection (upward or downward) from a baseline on a recording.
†Segment: A portion of an ECG recording between two consecutive waves. Represents the time needed for an electric current to move on.
‡Complex: The portion of the ECG tracing that represents the sum of three waves (contraction of the ventricles).
§Baseline: A neutral line against which waves are valued as they deflect upward (positive) or downward (negative) from the line.
‖Interval: The lapse of time between two different ECG events.

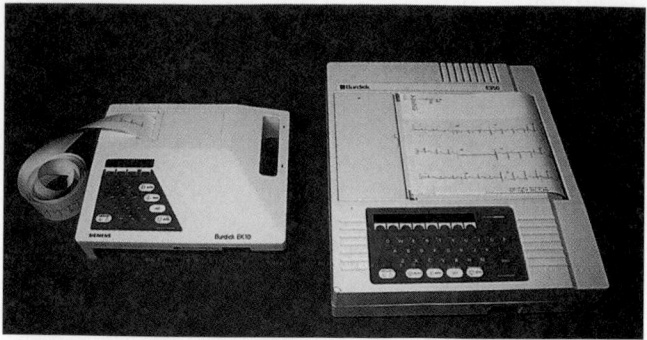

FIGURE 46-3 There are a wide variety of ECG machines, ranging from single to multichannel. (From Chester GA: *Modern medical assisting*, Philadelphia, 1998, WB Saunders.)

CRITICAL THINKING APPLICATION

Marcus has not been taught how to use the kind of single-lead ECG machine in Dr. Lee's office. What steps should he take to learn how to use this machine and feel comfortable and confident using it to obtain ECGs?

Electrocardiograph Paper

Electrocardiograph paper is heat sensitive and pressure sensitive, which means either heat or pressure can cause a mark to appear. The stylus on an ECG machine makes the image on the ECG paper. When the machine is on, the stylus becomes hot and burns a marking on the paper as the paper moves horizontally by the stylus. Because the paper is pressure sensitive, it must be handled carefully to avoid making any additional markings that would blemish the tracing.

ECG paper has horizontal and vertical lines at 1-mm intervals. This is an agreed-on international standard that allows physicians anywhere in the world to interpret a patient's ECG in the same manner. A medical assistant needs to know both the size and the meaning of each square on ECG paper to understand its significance.

Each small square measures 1 mm on each side. Every fifth line, both vertically and horizontally, is darker than the other lines and creates a larger square measuring 5 mm on each side. When running at normal speed, one small 1-mm square passes the stylus every 0.04 second. So one large 5-mm square passes the stylus every 0.2 second. Continuing this logic, in 1 second, five large squares pass the stylus. When examining an ECG, five sequential large squares will show the record of what occurred with the heart during a time span of 1 second. Another way to say this is that normal-speed ECG paper travels past the stylus at a rate of 25 mm per second (Figure 46-4).

The voltage or strength of the heartbeat is also recorded on the paper. One millivolt (mV) of electrical activity moves the stylus upward over 10 mm (two large squares). This is the standard normally used for obtaining an ECG and can be adjusted to match the strength of the electrical activity of the heart. The ECG records both the strength of the electrical activity of the heartbeat in mV and the speed of the heartbeat over time.

Electrodes and Leads

Ten sensors called *electrodes* are placed on the patient's arms (two), legs (two), and chest (six) to pick up the electrical activity of the heart. Ten lead wires from the electrocardiograph, each ending in a small metal clip, are attached to the electrodes. These wires carry the signal of the heart's electrical activity to the electrocardiograph. Most offices use single-use, self-stick, disposable electrodes. Some older ECG machines have only five leads, requiring the single chest lead to be moved to a different chest-wall location to obtain each one of the chest (V) recordings.

The leads to the electrocardiograph carry the cardiac electrical impulses, where they are magnified by an amplifier. These amplified impulses are then converted into mechanical action to be recorded on the ECG paper by a stylus or electrical action to be visualized on a computer monitor.

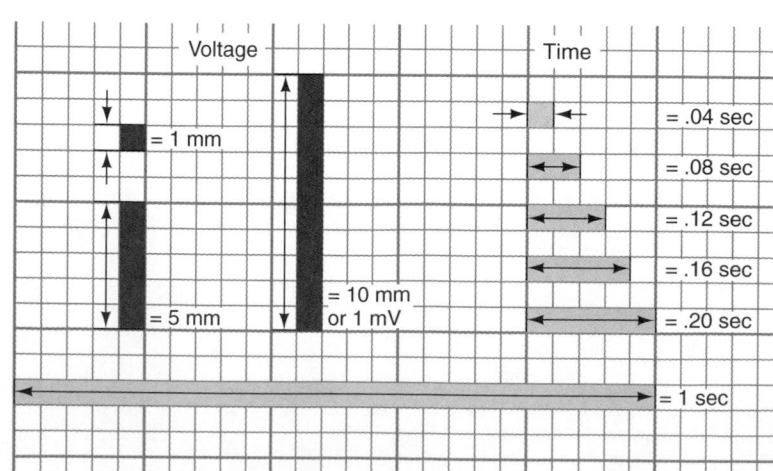

FIGURE 46-4 ECG paper. (From Chester GA: *Modern medical assisting*, Philadelphia, 1998, WB Saunders.)

TABLE 46-2	The Standard Marking Codes	
	Electrodes Connected	Marking Code
Standard of Bipolar Limb Leads		
Lead 1	LA & RA	•
Lead 2	LL & RA	••
Lead 3	Ll & LA	•••
Augmented Unipolar Limb Leads		
aVR	RA & (LA-LL)	—
aVL	LA & (RA-LL)	— —
aVF	LL & (RA-LA)	— — —
Chest or Precordial Leads		
	C & (LA-RA-LL)	V1—•
		V2—••
		V3—•••
		V4—••••
		V5—•••••
		V6—••••••

Courtesy The Burdick Corporation, Milton, WI.

Lead Placement

The standard ECG consists of 12 separate *leads*, or recordings of the electrical activity of the heart, from different angles. Each lead must be *marked* or coded for the physician to know which angle of the heart was recorded. Most machines being used today automatically mark all 12 leads when the *lead selector switch* is turned. However, there may be times when the medical assistant will need to mark each lead manually. A standardized coding system is used to identify each lead. The code consists of a series of dots and dashes. The most common marking system is illustrated in Table 46-2.

Standard Leads. The first three leads recorded are called the *standard* or *bipolar* limb leads, because they

each use two limb electrodes to record the heart's electrical activity (Figure 46-5, *A*). Roman numerals I, II, and III are used to designate these leads.

- Lead I records the electrical activity between the right arm and the left arm.

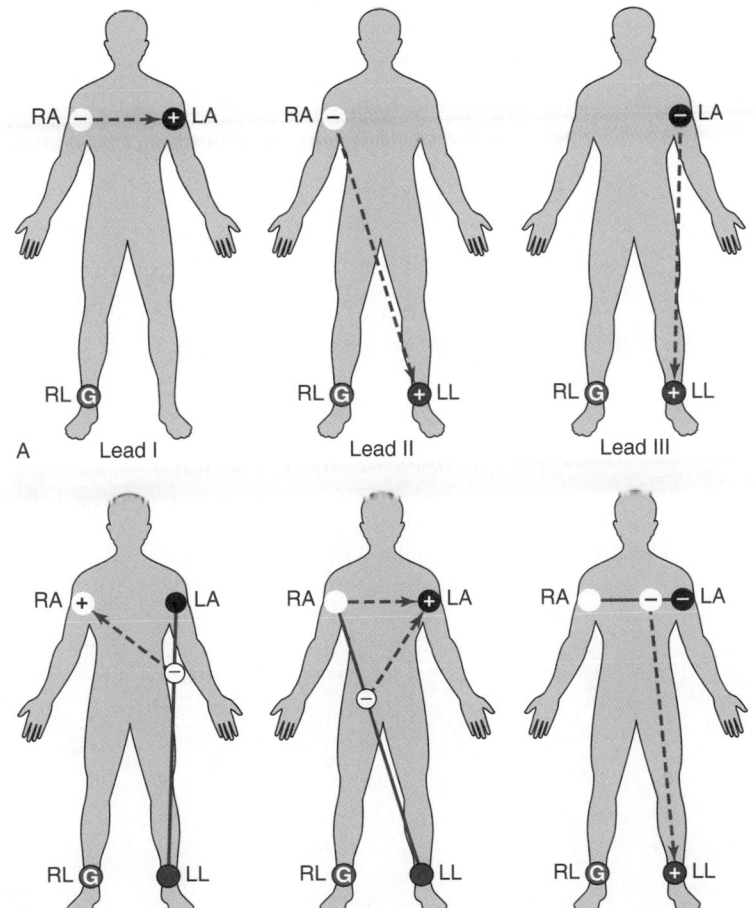

FIGURE 46-5 Standard (A) and augmented (B) limb leads. (From Chester GA: *Modern medical assisting,* Philadelphia, 1998, WB Saunders.)

- Lead II records the electrical activity between the right arm and the left leg.
- Lead III records the electrical activity between the left arm and the left leg.

Augmented Leads. The next three leads are the *augmented* or *combined* leads (Figure 46-5, *B*). These are designated *a*ugmented *V*oltage *R*ight arm (aVR), *a*ugmented *V*oltage *L*eft arm (aVL), and *a*ugmented *V*oltage *F* (aVF) for the left leg. These are all unipolar leads and rely on the right leg for grounding.

- aVR records the activity from midway between the left leg and the left arm to the right arm.
- aVL records the activity from midway between the right arm and the left leg to the left arm.
- aVF records the activity from midway between the right arm and the left arm to the left leg.

Precordial Leads. The *precordial* or *chest* leads are unipolar and are designated V_1, V_2, V_3, V_4, V_5, and V_6. The V means chest, and each of the numbers represents a specific location on the chest. The precordial leads measure the electrical activity between six specific points on the chest wall and a point within the heart (Figure 46-6).

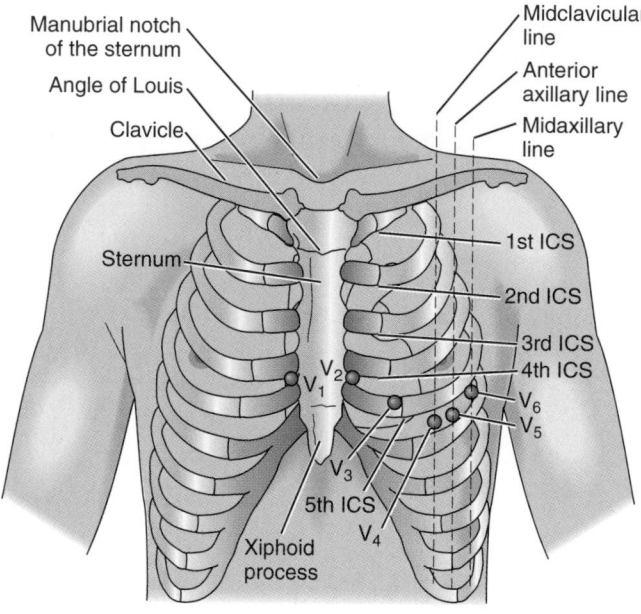

FIGURE 46-6   Chest leads. (From Chester GA: *Modern medical assisting*, Philadelphia, 1998, WB Saunders.)

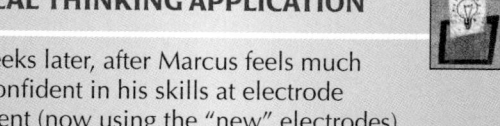
Preparation of the Room and Patient

The room should be in the quietest location in the office and should be as far away as possible from all other electrical equipment, including x-ray machines, diathermy devices, laboratory equipment, centrifuges, fans, refrigerators, and air conditioners. The room should be warm and have adjustable lighting.

The treatment table should be comfortable and wide enough to provide full support for the patient. The table should be wood or have an electrically insulated surface. Position the table so you can work from the side of the patient that is most comfortable for you. Electrocardiographers most often work on the patient's left side, but as long as the electrodes are placed in the proper position, it really makes no difference which side you work from.

Small pillows are helpful for relaxing the patient and providing maximum comfort during the procedure. Offer a pillow for the head and one for under the knees. If a head pillow is used, it should not elevate the patient's shoulders.

The patient should disrobe to the waist and be gowned with the opening down the front; there must be easy access to the patient's extremities. Pantyhose must be removed.

Place the patient in supine position, with arms comfortably at the sides and the legs not touching one another. If the patient has **dyspnea** or **orthopnea**, semi-Fowler's position should be used, or alternatively, the patient can be seated on a wooden chair. Be sure to check with the physician before obtaining an ECG in an alternative position. If a seated position is being used, the patient's feet must rest comfortably on the floor or on a footstool. The legs should not be dangling, nor should there be any pressure on the back of the lower thighs. Note any alternative position on the ECG recording.

The patient should empty the bladder and then rest for at least 10 minutes prior to taking the ECG recording. Check to see if the patient followed all of the instructions in Figure 46-7. Record the patient's vital signs and current medications on the patient's chart.

INSTRUCTIONS FOR PATIENT BEFORE AN ELECTROCARDIOGRAM

Name: _____

Your cardiogram appointment is _____ , _____ at _____ AM
                                         Day   Date   Time   PM

These instructions are simple, but it is important that you follow them. Please call us if you are unable to follow these instructions or keep your appointment so we may make another appointment.

1. There is no discomfort or sensation in having an electrocardiogram. No electricity is put into the patient in any way. Small disposable electrodes are placed on the calf of each leg and on each arm and at different places on the chest. The minute impulse generated by your heart is simply picked up by these electrodes and recorded by the machine.

2. You will be asked to lie down on a comfortable table while the test is being performed by the technician.

3. For your convenience, it is best to wear loose clothing. You will be asked to disrobe to your waist to expose the chest. It will also be necessary to expose your lower legs from the knees down and the upper arms just below the shoulders.

4. The actual test only takes about 5 minutes, but you will be asked to rest for about one-half hour before the test. It is best you do not have a heavy meal for about 2 hours before the test. You should not consume any cold drinks or ice cream or smoke just before the test. It is also advisable to refrain from excessive exercise just before the test. Do not take any medications without the physician's usual instructions and knowledge.

5. During the test, you will be asked to lie absolutely still and relax, because the slightest movement interferes with an accurate tracing. Do not talk.

6. The skin on the legs, arms, and chest must be free from skin ointments, oils, and medications.

7. The technician taking the test is specially trained to perform the test but is unable to tell you the results of the test, because he or she is neither trained nor authorized to make any interpretations of the cardiogram. This is the task of the physician.

FIGURE 46-7   ECG patient instructions.

Explain to the patient the nature and the purpose of the ECG. Chat with the patient while preparing for the procedures. Stress the importance of not moving during the entire procedure and assure the patient that there is no danger of being shocked. Soften the lighting in the room to obtain maximal patient comfort. When you tell the patient to lie still, observe that he or she is breathing normally. Patients will often hold their breath when asked to lie still. Give the patient the opportunity to ask any questions and answer all concerns before beginning the recording.

Applying Leads to the Patient. Disposable, single-use electrodes are placed on the patient's limbs and chest in very specific locations (Figure 46-8). These disposable electrodes are permeated with the necessary electrolyte, as the skin is a poor conductor of electricity. The lead wires from the machine are then connected to the electrodes. Making the proper connections is facilitated by specific lead markings or color-coding on the end of each lead wire (Figure 46-9).

- RA lead is attached to the patient's right arm.
- LA lead is attached to the patient's left arm.
- RL lead is attached to the patient's right leg.
- LL lead is attached to the patient's left leg.
- V_1 lead is attached at the fourth intercostal space at the right sternal border.

- V_2 lead is attached at the fourth intercostal space at the left sternal border.
- V_3 lead is attached halfway between leads V_2 and V_4.
- V_4 lead is attached at the fifth intercostal space at the left midclavicular line.
- V_5 lead is attached on a horizontal line with V_4 at the anterior axillary line.
- V_6 lead is attached on a horizontal line with V_3 at the midaxillary line.

Recording ECG. Warm up the machine according to the manufacturer's instructions. Set the *lead selector control* to STD. Turn the *recorder control* to "on" and then to "run." Using the *position control knob*, center the *stylus* on the baseline. Check the standardization by pressing the *standardization button*; this should cause the stylus to make a 10-mm upward deflection when the sensitivity is set at 1. After the proper standardization is set, turn the *lead selector control* to "automatic." The machine will code each part of the tracing and run the appropriate length of strip. Before removing the leads from the patient, show the recording to the physician for approval. Then remove the leads from the patient, assist him or her into a sitting position, and after the patient rests for several minutes, provide assistance for getting off of the table and dressing if necessary.

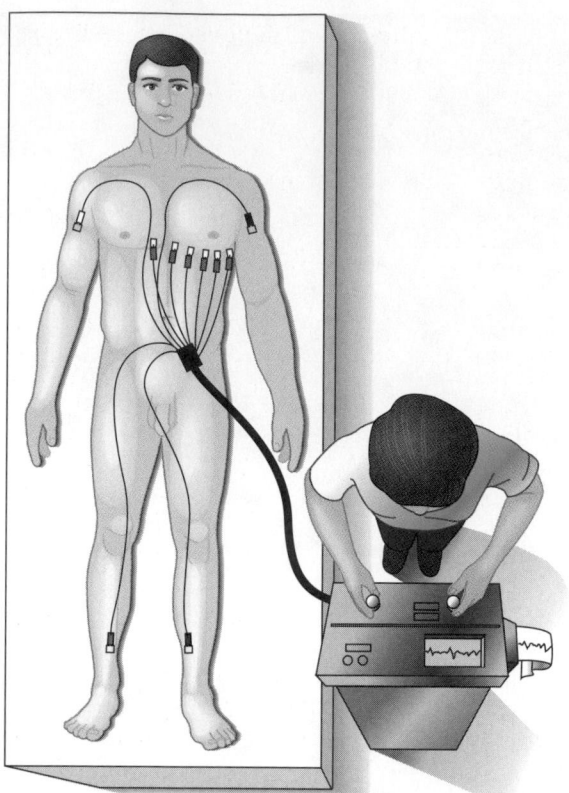

FIGURE 46-8 Lead locations. (From Hunt SA: *Saunders fundamentals of medical assisting*, Philadelphia, 2002, WB Saunders.)

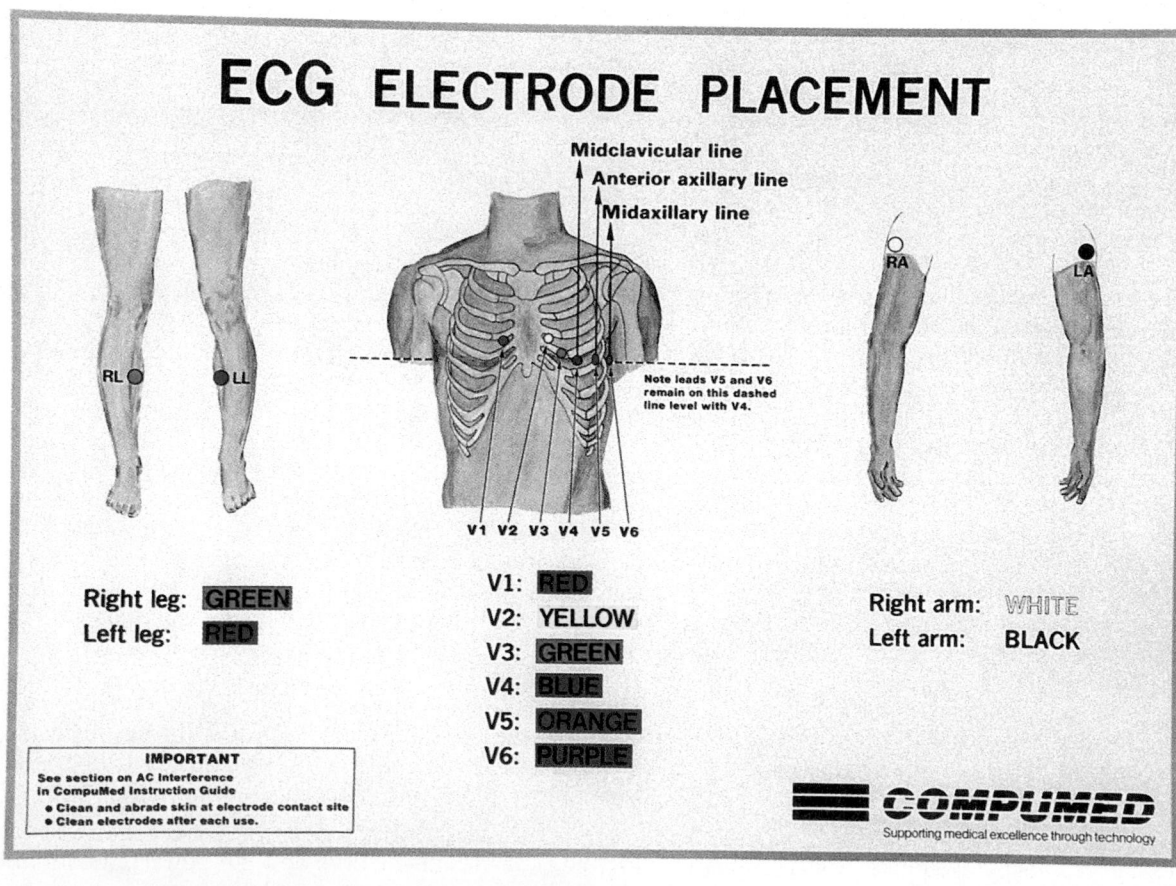

ECG ELECTRODE PLACEMENT

Midclavicular line
Anterior axillary line
Midaxillary line

Note leads V5 and V6 remain on this dashed line level with V4.

RA
LA

RL   LL

V1 V2 V3 V4 V5 V6

Right leg: GREEN	**V1:** RED
Left leg: RED	**V2:** YELLOW
	V3: GREEN
	V4: BLUE
	V5: ORANGE
	V6: PURPLE

Right arm: WHITE
Left arm: BLACK

IMPORTANT
See section on AC Interference in CompuMed Instruction Guide
● Clean and abrade skin at electrode contact site
● Clean electrodes after each use.

COMPUMED
Supporting medical excellence through technology

FIGURE 46-9 Color codes. (Courtesy Compumed, San Diego, Calif.)

Standardization, Sensitivity, and Speed

Standardization has been determined by international agreement so that an ECG can be interpreted in the same way anywhere in the world. This requires the electrocardiograph to be calibrated according to universal measurements. Each time you take a patient's ECG, you must make certain that the machine is correctly standardized.

When a machine is in standard or set at 1 STD, 1 mV of electricity causes the stylus to move vertically 10 mm, or two large squares. When the machine is properly set in this way, it is possible to calculate electrical voltages by measuring the vertical movement of the stylus on the paper. The stylus should deflect exactly 10 mm when the *standardization button* is depressed with a quick pecking motion. The recording of the standardization would be 2 mm wide and rectangular. Each manufacturer's manual explains the exact method of adjustment to obtain a perfect standardization.

At a minimum, standardization must be performed before recording the first lead. Some physicians require a separate standardization in each one of the individual 12 leads.

Most machines have three sensitivity standards that can be selected: $^1/_2$ STD, which deflects the stylus 5 mm or one large square; 1 STD, which deflects the stylus 10 mm or two large squares; and 2 STD, which will deflect the stylus 20 mm or four squares. The appropriate standard is selected in the following manner. If the QRS complex is too tall and is causing the stylus to move off the paper, the STD should be set to $^1/_2$ STD. If the QRS complex is too short, the STD should be set to 2 STD. Figure 46-10 shows what the three sensitivity standards look like when recorded on the ECG paper. Make a particular note when using a standard other than 1 STD.

The usual speed for ECG recording is 25 mm/sec. If the patient's heart rate is very rapid or if certain parts of the complex are too close together, it may be necessary to adjust the paper to run at double speed, or 50 mm/sec. This will extend the recording to twice the normal length. Any change in the speed must be noted on the ECG.

Mounting an ECG Tracing

There are many different types of ECG mounts. Each office selects the mount that is best suited to the type of ECG equipment used in that particular office. It is advisable to select a mount that allows reading of all 12 leads together on one page. The most commonly used mounts are self-adhesive mounting pages that are designed so that an entire test is placed on one side of one page (Figure 46-11). Tracings are usually retained in records for many years, so a mount must last for a long period of time.

Paper clips and staples are never used because they will scratch and mark a tracing. Clear tape should not be used, because it can become sticky or yellow with age. A single photocopy of the ECG can be made without damaging the original. Many offices routinely put a photocopy in the patient's chart, because it is thinner than the mounted ECG.

Regardless of the particular method used, each ECG should be carefully and neatly mounted, with complete information recorded on each one. This must include the following:

- Patient's full name
- Sex
- Age
- Date and time of ECG
- List of all medications and/or supplements the patient takes
- Variations from normal sensitivity and normal speed

Additional notations should be recorded for any variation from the routine such as:

- A very nervous or anxious patient
- Lack of rest before the test
- Smoking immediately before the test
- Failure to follow any pretest instructions

Care must be taken when mounting an ECG. Most tracings are easily scratched or marked, so be careful not to accidentally damage the tracing with watches, rings, fingernails, or clothing buttons. Do not stack other items on top of the open-faced type of mount.

NOTE: If trimming the strip is required for mounting, do not cut off the lead coding (the marking identifying which lead it is) until just before you are ready to mount that particular lead. Double-check each lead code with the mount placement. This is a critical issue with regard to proper ECG interpretation. Some mounts place the precordial leads in horizontal rows, whereas others place them in vertical columns. Take great care not to mount a lead upside down. If you have been requested to show the STD in a lead, be sure to include it where requested. Do not cover the tips of the QRS complexes with the sides of the slotted-type mount. Place the mounted ECG tracing on the physician's desk for evaluation with the patient's medical record and any previous ECG tracings. Physicians nearly always wish to compare the newest ECG with previous ECGs.

Some physicians will wish to see the entire strip before it is mounted and may even choose which sections to mount. If this is the case, be careful to mount the sections indicated by the physician.

CRITICAL THINKING APPLICATION

The office has run out of ECG mounting cards for single-lead ECGs. Marcus has three routine ECGs scheduled for returning patients today. What should he do?

Caring for Equipment

After the ECG recording is satisfactorily completed, remove the tips of the lead wires from the electrodes then remove electrodes from the patient and discard them. The lead wires should be placed carefully on top of the machine to prolong its useful life and to prevent premature wear and tear on the lead wires.

ECG Machine Options

There are many different types of ECG machines, including the older single-channel and the newer 12-channel

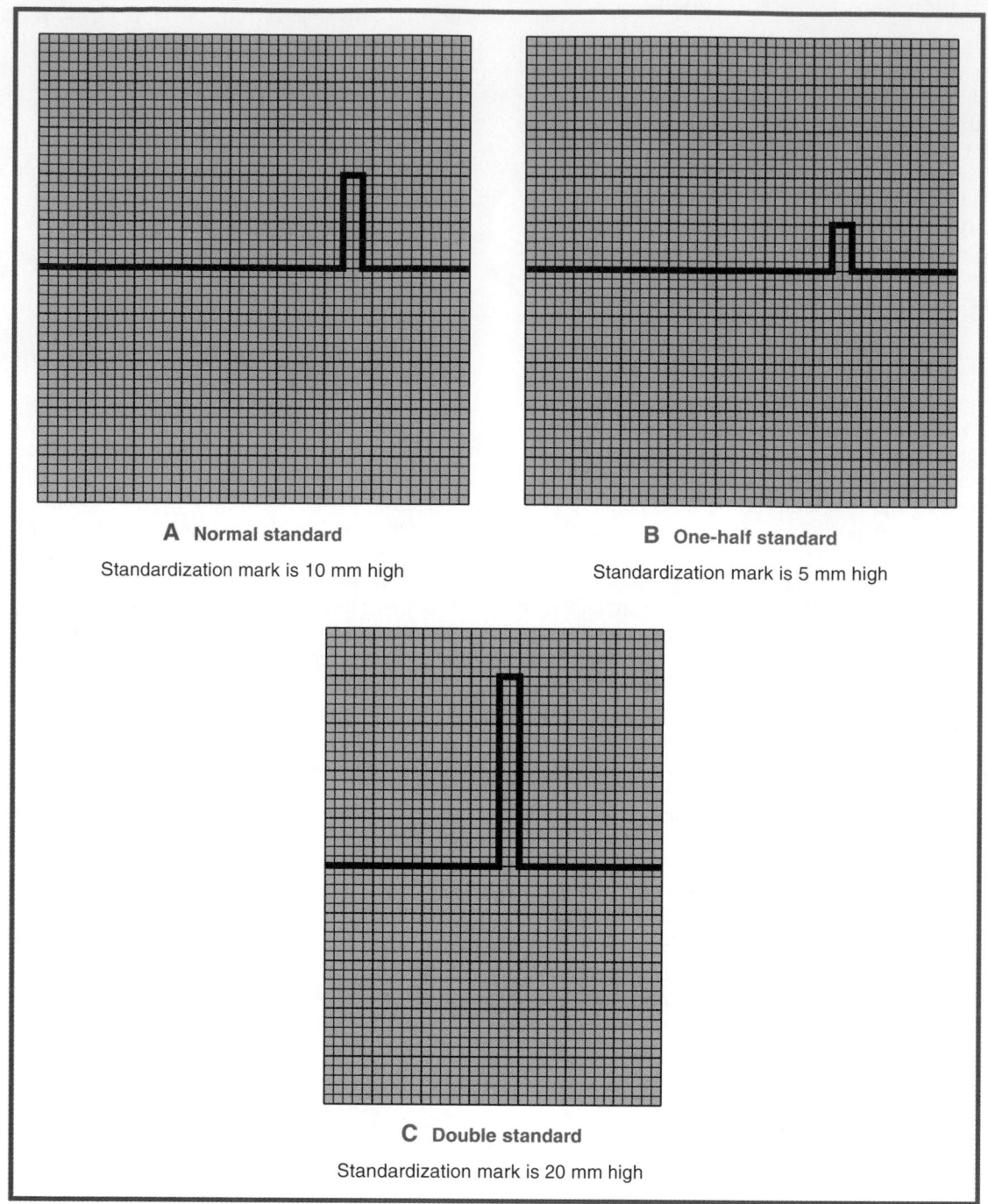

A Normal standard

Standardization mark is 10 mm high

B One-half standard

Standardization mark is 5 mm high

C Double standard

Standardization mark is 20 mm high

FIGURE 46-10 **A** to **C**, Sensitivity standards.

electrocardiographs (Procedure 46-1). Each machine has a slightly different method for attaching the electrodes and lead wires. You must learn the specifics of the equipment you will be using. Read the manufacturer's instruction manual that came with the machine and practice performing an ECG with the equipment before doing one on a patient.

Telephone Transmission. An electrocardiograph with phone transmission capabilities can transmit a recording over a telephone to an ECG data interpretation center. The machine is equipped with a direct ECG fax transmitter. The recording is interpreted by a computer at the data center and verified by a cardi-

ologist. Patient information that may be important to the interpretation such as medications and vital signs is also sent with the ECG data. A printout with the computer-assisted interpretations is returned to the sender by fax or email. This type of reporting allows the physician to begin treatment immediately instead of during a return visit for the interpretation.

Interpretive ECG machines. Interpretive electrocardiographs are equipped with a computer that analyzes the recording as it is being run. With this capability, immediate information on the heart's activity is available and can be valuable for reaching an early diagnosis and initiating immediate treatment. Patient baseline data

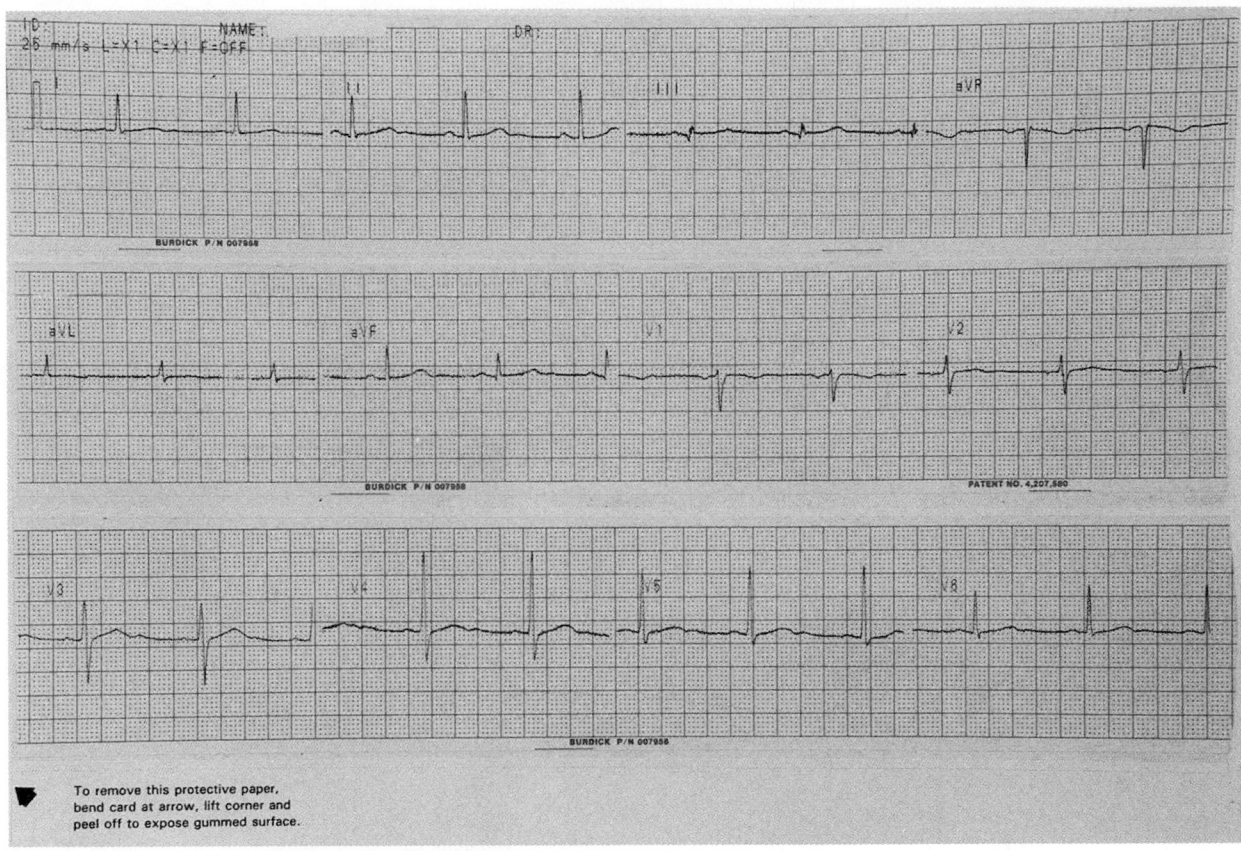

FIGURE 46-11 ECG mount. (Courtesy Burdick Corporation, Melton, Wisc.)

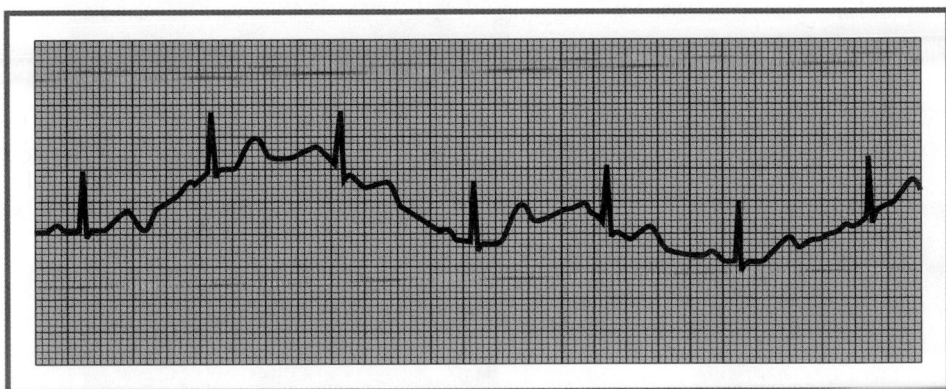

FIGURE 46-12
Wandering baseline.

must be entered into the computer *before* taking the ECG. The computer analysis of the ECG and the reason for each interpretation are then printed on the top of the recording.

Do not allow the patient to read this interpretation. Give the ECG print to the physician immediately. He or she will then decide what to tell the patient.

Artifacts

An artifact is unwanted, erratic movement of the stylus on the paper resulting from outside interference. The electrocardiograph is extremely sensitive to any kind of nearby electrical activity. Electrical artifacts on the tracing make it difficult to accurately interpret the ECG. The medical assistant should have a thorough under-

standing of the causes and remedies of these artifacts. The main types of artifacts include wandering baseline, somatic tremor, alternating current, and baseline interruption.

Wandering Baseline. With the wandering baseline, the stylus gradually shifts away from the center of the paper. This usually results from slight movement of the patient during the tracing or poor electrode attachment (Figure 46-12). This is resolved by reminding the patient to remain as still as possible and can be facilitated by maintaining patient comfort. Metal electrodes can be a major cause of this phenomenon; using disposable, stick-on electrodes should eliminate this cause.

Somatic Tremor. Somatic tremor means muscle movement. Any muscle movement produces a measurable electrical impulse, including skeletal muscle. This

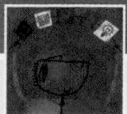

PROCEDURE **46-1**

Obtaining a 12-lead ECG

GOAL: To obtain an accurate, artifact-free recording of the electrical activity of the heart.

EQUIPMENT AND SUPPLIES

- ECG machine with patient lead cable
- 10 disposable, self-adhesive electrodes
- Patient gown and drape
- ECG mounting card if necessary

PROCEDURAL STEPS

1 Wash your hands.
Purpose: Infection control.

2 Explain the procedure to the patient.
Purpose: To alleviate apprehension and gain patient cooperation.

3 Ask the patient to disrobe to the waist and remove socks, stockings, or pantyhose as necessary.
Purpose: Electrodes must be applied to bare skin.

4 Position the patient on the exam table and drape appropriately.
Purpose: To ensure the modesty and comfort of the patient.

5 Turn on the machine to allow the stylus to warm up.
Purpose: To ensure proper machine performance.

6 Label the beginning of the tracing paper with the patient's name, date, time, and current cardiovascular medications, or input information into the machine (Figure 1).

Purpose: To properly identify the ECG recording.

7 At each location you are going to place an electrode, clean the skin with an alcohol wipe (Figure 2).
Purpose: To obtain good electrode adhesion to the skin.

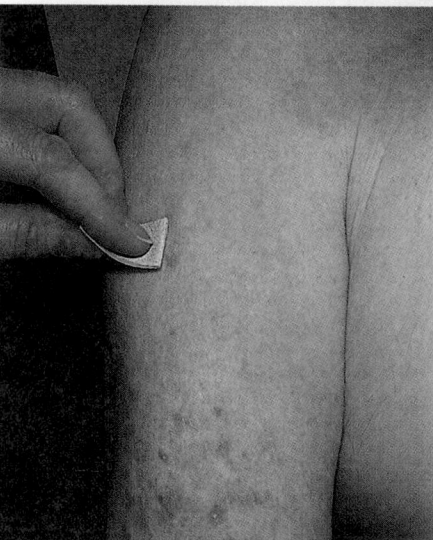

Figure 2

8 Apply the self-adhesive electrodes to clean, dry fleshy areas of the extremities (Figure 3). It may be necessary to shave extremely hairy areas to achieve adequate electrode attachment.

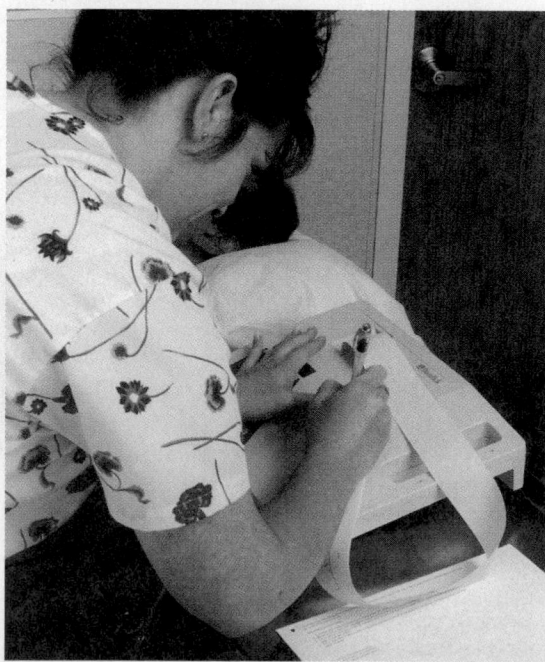

Figure 1

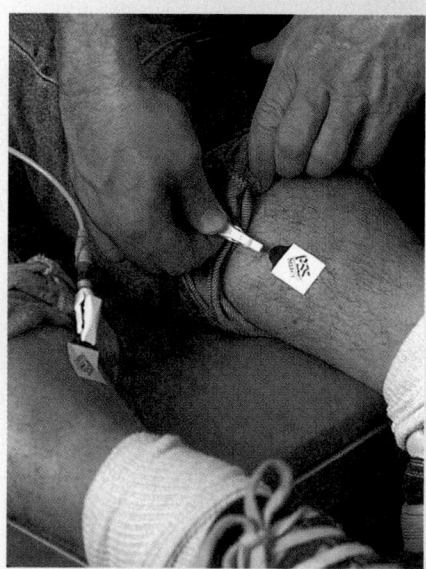

Figure 3

PROCEDURE 46-1—cont'd

9 Apply the self-adhesive electrodes to clean areas on the chest (Figure 4).

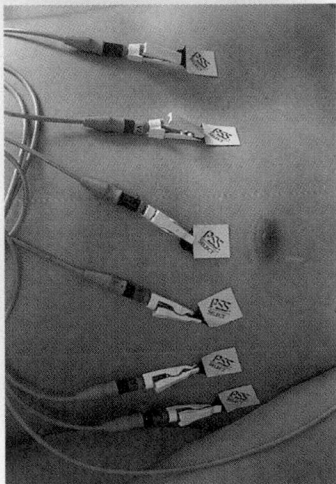

Figure 4

10 Carefully connect the lead wires to the correct electrode with the alligator clips on the end of each lead.

11 Press the AUTO button on the machine and run the ECG tracing. The machine will automatically place the standardization at the beginning, and then the 12 leads will follow in the three-channel matrix.

12 Watch for artifacts during the recording. If artifacts are present, make appropriate corrections, and repeat the recording to get a clean reading.

13 Remove the lead wires from the electrodes, then remove the electrodes from the patient.

14 Assist the patient with getting dressed as needed. Clean and return the ECG machine to its storage area.

15 Mount the ECG or give the unmounted ECG tape to the physician as directed.

16 Wash your hands.

17 Document the procedure in the patient's chart.
Purpose: Procedures are not considered done until they are documented in the patient's medical record.

See Appendix E for a charting example.

additional input causes unwanted stylus movement during the tracing. This shows up on the recording as jagged peaks of irregular height and spacing and a shifting baseline (Figure 46-13). The most common causes include patient discomfort, apprehension, movement, talking, or having a condition that causes uncontrollable body tremors. The patient with uncontrolled tremors needs to be as calm and comfortable as possible to minimize the somatic tremor artifact. The other causes can each be resolved after they have been correctly identified.

AC Interference. Alternating current (AC) interference appears as a series of uniform small spikes on the paper (Figure 46-14). Alternating current that is present in nearby equipment or wiring can leak small amounts of electrical energy into the area in which the ECG is located. The very sensitive electrocardiograph can easily pick up this additional electrical energy signal. This can be minimized by making certain the ECG is plugged into a three-prong, grounded outlet, keeping lead wires uncrossed, unplugging other electrical appliances in the

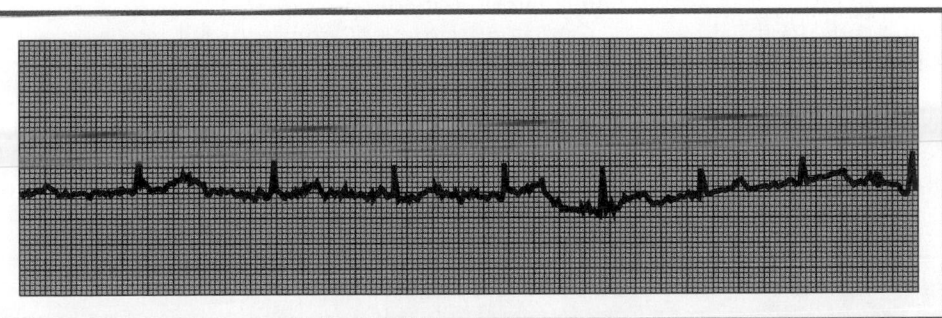

FIGURE 46-13 Somatic tremor.

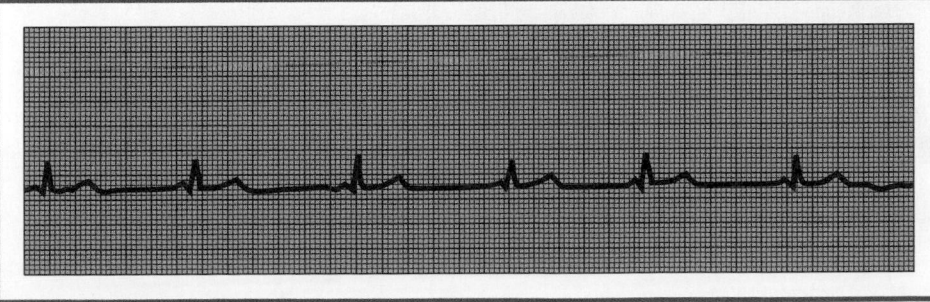

FIGURE 46-14 AC interference.

room, moving the table away from the wall, and perhaps even turning off overhead fluorescent lights. If all of these measures fail, you may need to move to another examination room for the procedure. The last step is to call the manufacturer or your local service representative.

Interrupted Baseline. Baseline interruption occurs when the electric connection has been interrupted. The stylus moves onto the margin of the paper erratically (Figure 46-15). The stylus moves violently up and down across the paper, or it may record a straight line across the top or the bottom of the paper. Noticeable patient movement that dislodges the electrodes causes most baseline interruption. This cause is virtually eliminated by using disposable, stick-on electrodes. Other causes can be a broken wire in the patient cable or cable tips that are attached too loosely to the electrodes.

CRITICAL THINKING APPLICATION

Marcus has just used his last set of disposable, self-adhesive electrodes, and he has two more ECGs scheduled today. What should he do?

Intrepreting a Rhythm Strip

The medical assistant working in the cardiovascular practice needs to be able to recognize rhythm abnormalities that may appear on the tracing. Alerting the physician to the presence of an arrhythmia while the patient is still connected to the machine may give the physician the opportunity to observe the patient while the machine is running or immediately institute some type of therapeutic or prophylactic intervention.

The physician can determine two important heart functions when interpreting the ECG, heart rate and heart rhythm.

Normal Appearances of ECG Complexes

When examining the ECG recording, first look at the characteristics of each of the waves in the recording (Table 46-3). Are the P waves, QRS complexes, and T waves clearly present? Do they have a consistent appearance and do they occur at regular intervals? Are there any odd beats present that do not fit in with the others?

Is the rate normal, fast, or slow? Is the rhythm regular or irregular?

In normal sinus rhythm (NSR) (see Figure 46-1), each beat of the heart is initiated with an impulse from the SA node that then travels, without interruption, along the normal conduction pathway of the heart. In NSR, each beat on the ECG shows a P wave followed by a QRS complex.

Rate

To calculate the heart rate from the ECG recording, count the number of P waves in a 6-second strip (30 large squares) and multiply by 10. In the same manner, you can count the number of P waves in a 3-second strip (15 large squares) and multiply by 20.

Heart rate can also be calculated by counting the number of small squares between two R waves. Then divide that number into 1,500; one minute on an ECG strip passes 1,500 small boxes. When the number of boxes from one cardiac event to the next same event is divided into 1,500 the result is the patient's heart rate. You can practice these by using the ECGs in Figures 46-1 and 46-11.

Typical ECG Rhythm Abnormalities

Common Arrhythmias

Abnormalities in cardiac rhythm are termed arrhythmias. These can result from disturbances anywhere along the electrical conduction pathway in the heart from the SA node through the right and left bundle branches. The best way to determine if an arrhythmia is present is to know what a normal sinus rhythm looks like on an ECG. Study the normal sinus rhythms present in the mounted ECGs in Figures 46-1 and 46-11. NSR or normal sinus rhythm is a heart rate between 60 and 100 beats/min. Any deviations from this should be recognized during the ECG recording and the medical assistant should immediately notify the physician.

Cardiac arrhythmias commonly fall into one of the following broad categories: sinus arrhythmias, atrial arrhythmias, ventricular arrhythmias, and biochemical arrhythmias. The characteristics of several arrhythmias in each of these categories can be compared with NSR in Table 46-4.

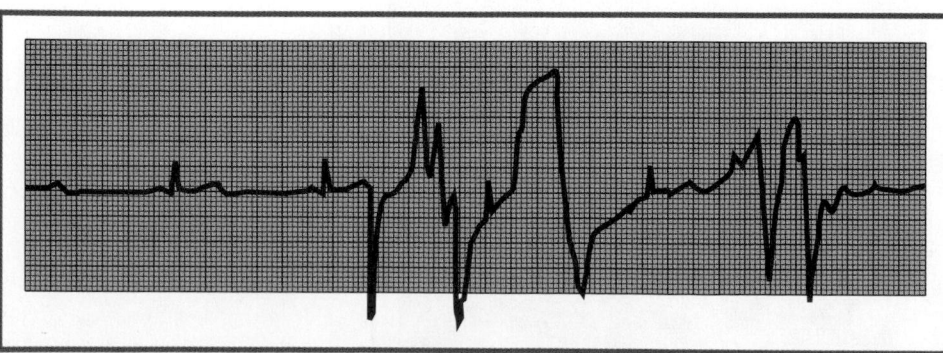

FIGURE 46-15
Interrupted baseline.

TABLE 46-3	Normal Appearances of ECG Complexes	
Wave or Complex	**Duration (in seconds or amplitude)**	**Characteristics to Examine**
P wave	0.06-0.11	Are P waves present? Normal shape (not notched or peaked)? Normal size (< 3 mm)? Do all deflect upward (positive)? Is there one for each QRS? Evenly spaced from QRS?
P-R interval	0.12-0.20	Is it constant?
QRS complex	0.08-0.12 duration R-R interval 0.60-1.00	Do all look the same? Evenly spaced from T waves? Do all point in same direction? Do all QRS complexes appear the same?
ST segment	On baseline (isoelectric line)	Is it on baseline? Could it hide a P wave? Is it constant?
T Wave	5 mm or less in leads I, II, III 10 mm or less in V_1-V_6	Is T wave present? Are all the same? Do all show upward deflection (positive)? Could it hide a P wave?
Q-T interval	Should not be more than half the R-R interval if patient has regular rhythm	Is it constant?
U Wave	Rounded, upright deflection	Is it present?

TABLE 46-4	Types and Causes of Shock		
Name	**Signs and Symptoms**	**Cause**	**ECG Changes**
Sinus Arrhythmias			
Bradycardia	< 60 beats/min	Vagal nerve stimulation; sleep; SA node ischemia; Digitalis toxicity; drugs Can be normal in athletes	Essentially "normal" appearing, but slow
Tachycardia	Nonpathological; heart rate > 100 beats/min pathological	Increased demand for cardiac output; ectopic pacemaker	P wave can be obscured by the ST segment (increasing the ECG speed can reduce this problem)
Atrial Arrhythmias			
PAC	Not pathological if only several per minute	Increased SA node excitability, causing premature beats of atria Can be due to nicotine or caffeine	"Extra" P waves
Flutter	200-350 beats/min	Many ectopic atrial pacemakers, normally unstable and will progress to atrial fibrillation if not corrected	Multiple, sawtooth- appearing P waves before essentially normal-appearing QRS complexes
Ventricular Arrhythmias (see Figure 46-20)			
PVC	Generally none	Ectopic pacemakers originating in ventricles from electrolyte imbalance, hypoxia, acute MI	Widened QRS complex
V-tach	Heart rate > 100 beats/min, always pathological	Damaged tissue around one of the "bundles" causing a difference in conduction speed between the two branches or ectopic pacemaker cells	Rapid rate, irregular pattern that includes "extra" or erratic, irregular, or wide QRS complexes
V-fib*	Shock, unconscious-ness, no pulse	Complete loss of synchronization of conduction system	Erratic deflections on the ECG (can be either coarse or fine) No identifiable ECG waves present
Asystole	< 5 beats/min	Death imminent	Flat line

Continued

TABLE 46-4	Types and Causes of Shock—cont'd		
Name	**Signs and Symptoms**	**Cause**	**ECG Changes**
Biochemical Arrhythmias			
Digitalis toxicity	Abnormal bradycardia, abnormal tachycardia	Digitalis dose is too high	"Swooping" ST segment depression and/or extended P-R intervals
Hypokalemia	Malaise, fatigue, weakness, muscle cramps	Potassium too low, usually from unsupplemented diuresis, from IV fluid administration, or from excessive vomiting	Prominent U waves, T wave and U wave together look like a two-humped camel
Hyperkalemia†	May have none	Potassium too high usually from IV supplementation	Peaked T wave (can be as tall as R wave) and can see widening of all wave forms

*Most life-threatening arrhythmia, frequently precedes asystole if not reversed.
†Life-threatening situation that must be corrected immediately.

Sinus Arrhythmias. Sinus arrhythmias are the result of the SA node firing too slowly or too quickly or from an ectopic source. In sinus bradycardia, the heart rate is less than 60 beats/min. This can be a normal heart rate in well-conditioned athletes, but can be abnormal in other individuals. In sinus tachycardia, the heart rate is more than 100 beats/min. This can be a normal heart rate in a person who is doing aerobic exercise, but can be abnormal in the resting individual.

Atrial Arrhythmias. Premature atrial contraction (PAC) occurs when the atria contract before they should for the next cardiac cycle. This can appear on the ECG as an abnormally shaped P wave or an extra P wave. PACs can be seen in smokers and people who consume large amounts of caffeine. Occasional PACs are not abnormal, but are of medical concern if they regularly occur more than six times per minute. In this situation, the PACs can indicate developing cardiac abnormalities

Atrial flutter occurs when the atria beat at an extremely rapid rate that can be up to 400 beats/min. In atrial flutter the impulses come from many ectopic atrial locations but are blocked at the AV node, which prevents ventricular fibrillation. It is usually reversed with medication to slow the heart or with **cardioversion** (electrical shock).

Ventricular Arrhythmias. PVC or premature ventricular contraction occurs when the ventricles contract before they should for the next cardiac cycle. This can appear on the ECG as an absent P wave, an abnormally shaped T wave, and a widened QRS complex. This is followed by a pause prior to initiation of the next cardiac cycle. PVCs can result from use of tobacco, alcohol, medications containing epinephrine, and occasionally from anxiety. Occasional PVCs are not abnormal, but are of medical concern if they regularly occur more than six times per minute. Pathological PVCs occur in patients with **hypertension**, coronary artery disease, and lung disease.

Ventricular tachycardia (commonly referred to as *V-tach*) causes the ventricles to beat at extremely rapid rates. V-tach can precede V-fib if not reversed with drugs and/or cardioversion. V-tach always reflects a pathological state.

Ventricular fibrillation (commonly referred to as *V-fib*) is the most critical, life-threatening arrhythmia and will result in death quickly if not effectively treated. In V-fib the electrical conduction system of the heart is in total dysfunction. The heart muscle is quivering uncontrollably and is essentially ineffective in pumping any blood during V-fib. Cardioversion with a defibrillator is necessary to restore normal electrical conduction system function.

Asystole is the result of no heartbeat or cardiac cessation and results in a flat line on the ECG (Figure 46-16).

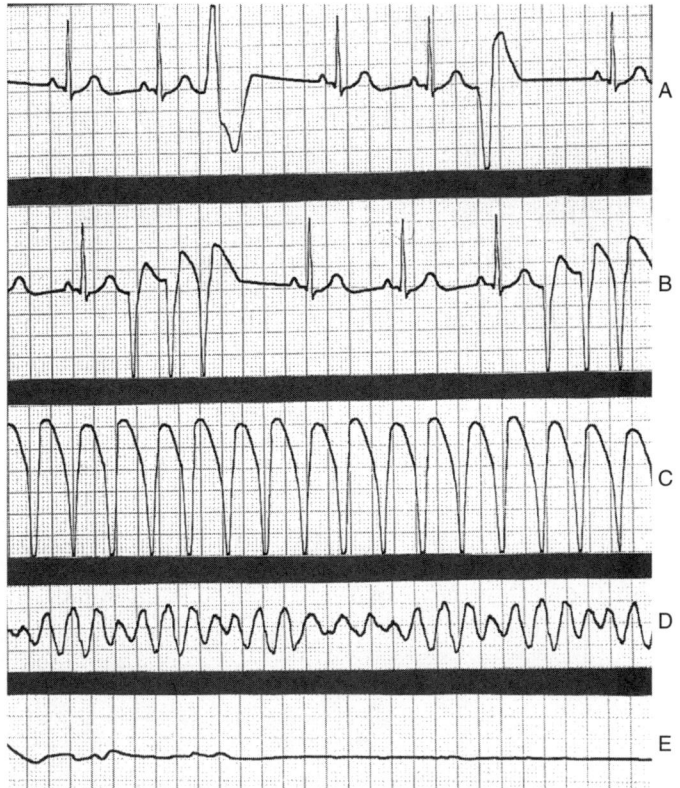

FIGURE 46-16 Ventricular arrhythmias. **A,** PVC. **B,** Three PVCs in a row. **C,** V-tach. **D,** V-fib. **E,** Asystole. (From Chester GA: *Modern medical assisting*, Philadelphia, 1998, WB Saunders.)

Biochemical Arrhythmias. Digitalis, commonly called *Dig* (pronounced *dij*), is a common cardiac drug that is used to slow and strengthen the heartbeat. The heart is quite sensitive to Dig, and too much can prove toxic to the heart and cause ECG changes (Figure 46-17). This condition reverses after reducing the dosage of digoxin or digitoxin (both forms of digitalis).

Potassium is a critical mineral for normal cardiac function. Too much potassium in the blood (hyperkalemia) or too little potassium in the blood (hypokalemia) can both cause life-threatening arrhythmias that must be quickly corrected. Giving intravenous potassium can reverse hypokalemia. Giving a diuretic that does not effectively spare potassium can reverse hyperkalemia.

Pacemaker Rhythms

The implantation of a pacemaker into a patient sometimes corrects cardiac conduction system abnormalities. Electrodes extend from the pacemaker to the cardiac **myocardium**. The pacemaker contains a battery that produces small electrical charges that cause the heart to beat. A pacemaker can be used to stimulate regular contraction of just the atria, just the ventricles, or the entire heart. Pacemakers cause wide variations in the appearance of the ECG, and the firing of the pacemaker or pacing spikes may or may not be visible. Demand pacemakers automatically turn off when the heart beats above a certain rate and turn back on when the rate falls below a certain rate. The surgeon sets these rates before the pacemaker is implanted into the patient.

Automatic Implanted Cardioverter Defibrillator

The automatic implanted cardioverter **defibrillator**, more commonly known as *AICD*, monitors the heart rhythm and delivers a shock to the heart if it detects a dangerous tachycardia. It is a small, battery-operated device that is implanted under the skin in the chest or abdomen. An AICD can be used to reverse V-tach and V-fib, especially after the patient has previously had a **myocardial infarction** (MI), or heart attack. The generator is programmed specifically to treat the patient's particular or potential cardiac arrhythmia.

Heart Attack

Sudden heart attack, or MI, occurs in nearly 1 million Americans each year according to the American Heart Association. Approximately 20% of these patients die before reaching the hospital, and approximately 30% die within 30 days of their heart attack. An MI occurs when a portion of the heart muscle becomes **ischemic** because the blood supply to that area is interrupted.

The heart muscle, **myocardium**, receives its oxygen supply from a network of coronary arteries (Figure 46-18) located on the heart surface. The right coronary artery supplies much of the right side of the heart. The left

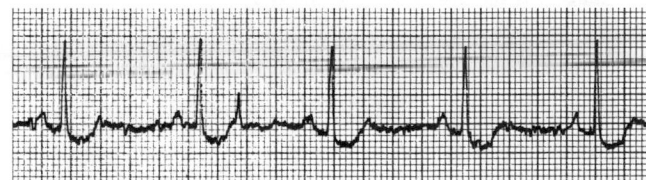

FIGURE 46-17 ECG shows effects of digitalis. Note the "swooping" ST segment. (From Chester GA: *Modern medical assisting,* Philadelphia, 1998, WB Saunders.)

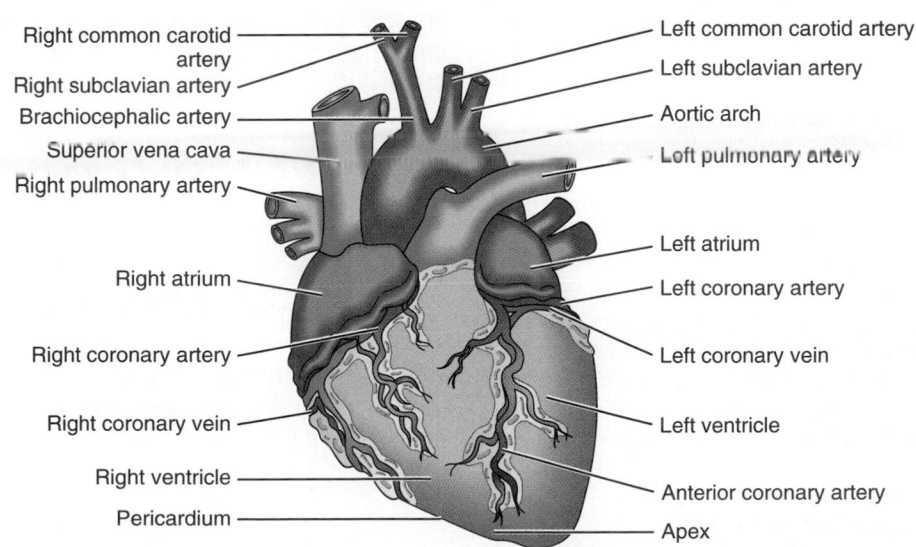

Right common carotid artery
Right subclavian artery
Brachiocephalic artery
Superior vena cava
Right pulmonary artery
Right atrium
Right coronary artery
Right coronary vein
Right ventricle
Pericardium

Left common carotid artery
Left subclavian artery
Aortic arch
Left pulmonary artery
Left atrium
Left coronary artery
Left coronary vein
Left ventricle
Anterior coronary artery
Apex

FIGURE 46-18 Coronary vessels. (From Chester GA: *Modern medical assisting,* Philadelphia, 1998, WB Saunders.)

TABLE 46-5	Phases of MI With ECG Changes	
Phase	When ECG Appear	Specifics Changes Seen on ECG
I. Hyperacute	Occurs in first few hours	ST segment elevation from baseline (this is the earliest indication on ECG); peaked "hyperacute" T waves
II. Fully evolved	After hours or days	Deep T waves; pathological Q waves appear (negative deflection)
III. Resolution	Days to weeks	ST segment returns to normal position; T waves return to normal
IV. Stabilized chronic	Permanent	Pathological Q waves remain

coronary artery **bifurcates** into two main branches: the left circumflex artery, which supplies blood principally to the left lateral and posterior walls of the left ventricle, and the left anterior descending coronary artery, which supplies principally the anterior wall of the left ventricle and the interventricular septum. The left anterior descending coronary artery is sometimes called the *sudden death artery*.

Myocardial infarction frequently causes specific, recognizable changes on the ECG recording. These changes are related to which one of the four phases (Table 46-5) of the MI the patient is in when the ECG is taken. The three most common changes are elevated ST segments, inverted (upside-down) T waves, and abnormal (pathological) Q waves.

The sooner treatment is initiated after the patient's first awareness of a heart attack, the more effective it becomes. Immediate therapy for MI includes administration of nasal oxygen (to increase available oxygen), sublingual nitroglycerin (to dilate coronary arteries), a narcotic analgesic (to eliminate pain), aspirin (to reduce inflammation and decrease clotting time), and possibly a thrombolytic agent to dissolve the clot that is causing the coronary arterial obstruction. Early administration of thrombolytic agents enhances the likelihood of restoring circulation to the myocardium distal to the occluding thrombus (blood clot). After discharge from the hospital, the patient should quit smoking, modify the diet as instructed by a nutritionist, and enter a cardiac rehabilitation program to improve cardiac strength and recovery by exercise.

Complications of acute MI include a sudden episode of atrial fibrillation, V-fib, or bradycardia that may necessitate implantation of a pacemaker.

Related Cardiac Diagnostic Tests

Stress Test

Cardiac stress testing is conducted to observe and record the patient's cardiovascular response to measured exercise challenges (Figure 46-19). Stress testing is performed to accomplish the following:
- To diagnose cardiac disease that cannot be detected by the standard, resting ECG
- To determine an individual's energy performance capacity
- To prescribe a specially designed exercise plan

The stress test is performed while the patient is

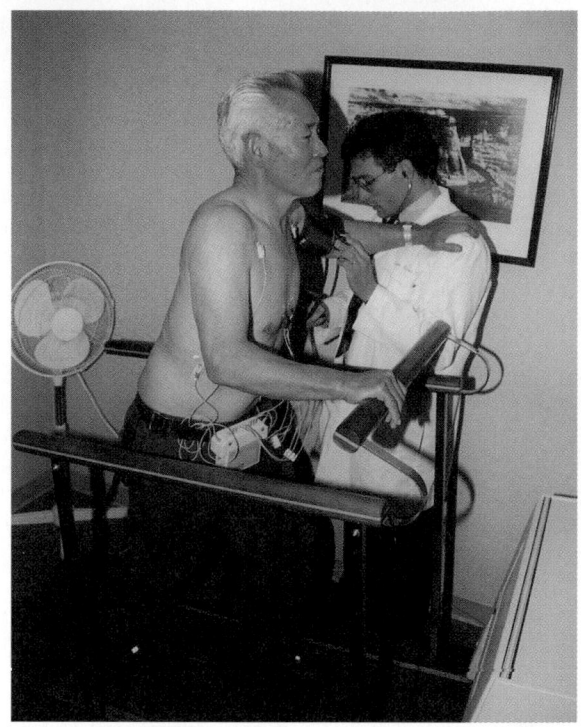

FIGURE 46-19   Cardiac stress test.

exercising on either a bicycle or a treadmill, under careful supervision. The patient must be given the appropriate information explaining the purpose, preparation, and procedure for the test (Figure 46-20).

CRITICAL THINKING APPLICATION

Mr. Sonderford actually had an MI when he was previously at Dr. Lee's office. He has now completed cardiac rehabilitation and is at the office for a checkup. Dr. Lee wants him to be scheduled for a stress test. Mr. Sonderford has never had one before. He confides to Marcus that he is afraid if he takes the test, he will die from another heart attack. How should Marcus handle this situation?

Stress testing can cause **cardiac arrest**. The medical assistant must be able to recognize symptoms of dyspnea, **vertigo**, extreme fatigue, severe arrhythmia, and other abnormal ECG readings that may develop during the

Cardiac Stress Test

Cardiac stress testing (also known as an exercise tolerance test or treadmill test) is a means of observing, evaluating, and recording your heart's response during a measured exercise test. This test determines your capacity to adapt to physical stress.

There are various reasons that your physician may suggest this test for you:

1. To aid in determining the presence of suspected coronary heart disease.
2. To aid in the selection of therapy.
   a. For angina pectoris (tightness or pain in the chest).
   b. Following a myocardial infarction (heart attack).
   c. Following coronary bypass surgery (open heart surgery).
3. To determine your physical work capacity.
4. To authorize participation in a physical exercise program.

Preparation for the Test

1. Avoid eating a heavy meal within 2 hours of your appointment.
2. Take your medications as you usually do, unless your doctor advises you not to take them.
3. Wear a shirt or blouse that buttons down the front with slacks, a skirt, jogging pants, or shorts.
4. Do not wear one-piece undergarments, jumpsuits, or dresses.
5. Tennis shoes are ideal if you have them. Otherwise, wear comfortable flat or low-heeled shoes. Do not wear clogs, sling-backs, crepe soles, boots, or high heels, as they make walking on the treadmill more difficult.

The Procedure

When you arrive in the Cardiology Department, areas of your chest may be shaved (men only) to allow the electrodes to adhere tightly to your chest. A blood pressure cuff will be wrapped around your arm, and an electrocardiogram (ECG) is taken while you are at rest. The technician will then demonstrate how to walk on the treadmill and will answer any questions you may have.

You will then perform a graded exercise test on a motor-driven treadmill. You will begin walking very gradually at a rate you can easily accomplish.

Progressively throughout the test, the speed and grade of the treadmill will be increased, and you will be walking at a faster pace up a slight incline. At no time will you be asked to jog or run, nor will you be asked to exercise beyond your capabilities.

At all times during the test, trained personnel are in the room with you, monitoring your heart rate and blood pressure and observing you for signs of fatigue or discomfort. We do not wish to exercise you to a level that is medically unsafe or physically distressing.

An ECG is taken again when you finish walking. Your cardiologist will immediately interpret the results of the test and explain his or her findings to you. If necessary, medications or treatment will be discussed. A letter with the results of the stress test will be sent to your referring physician.

The entire procedure will take 1 to 1 1/2 hours. If you have any questions regarding the cardiac stress test or any problems with your appointment, please contact us.

FIGURE 46-20   Patient information for a cardiac stress test.

stress test or immediately following the test during the rest period.

All members of a cardiac stress testing team must be prepared to terminate testing immediately if the patient is unable to continue or when abnormalities appear on the monitor. Therefore cardiac stress testing team members need to be certified in CPR and emergency intervention. The physician must always be present in the office during this procedure. In addition to the routine monitoring equipment, oxygen, defibrillator, suction, endotracheal intubation tray, artificial breathing bag, and emergency cardiac medications must be available in case of cardiac crisis.

Holter Monitor

A Holter monitor is a portable system for recording the cardiac activity of a patient over a 24-hour period or longer (Figure 46-21 and Procedure 46-2). It is a small, lightweight device that can be worn while the patient carries out his or her usual daily activities. The Holter can be programmed to record cardiac information continuously or periodically, when activated by the patient when symptoms occur, or during periods of stress.

The patient must keep a journal of all stressful events and activities (as well as of specific details regarding activities when any cardiorelated symptoms occur) during the entire time the Holter is worn. This includes the time, duration, and specific activity, including rush hour traffic, bowel movements, intercourse, climbing

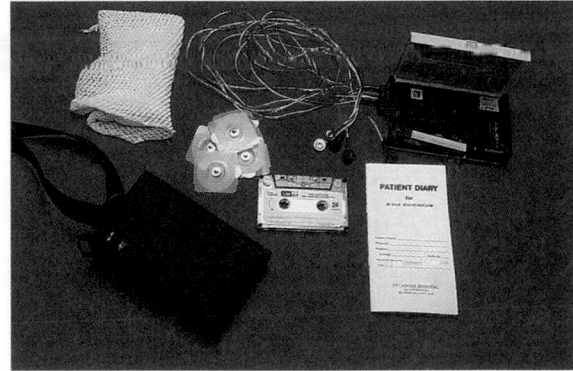

FIGURE 46-21   Holter monitor. (From Chester GA: *Modern medical assisting*, Philadelphia, 1998, WB Saunders.)

stairs, and periods of anger or emotional distress. Some monitors can even record the patient's voice describing a symptom or event so that it can later be correlated with the ECG recording in the same time frame.

Many cardiologists routinely use Holter monitors in their practices. A medical assistant is often responsible for instructing the patient in applying and removing the monitor. The patient must have a full understanding of what is required during monitoring, particularly how to use the event marker in case a significant symptom is experienced. When this marker is used, the patient must also know how to record the event in a written diary. The patient may only take sponge baths during

PROCEDURE 46-2

Applying a Holter Monitor

GOAL: To establish possible correlation between coronary disorders and daily activity.

EQUIPMENT AND SUPPLIES

- Holter monitor and blank magnetic recording tape
- Disposable electrodes
- Razor
- Tape
- Activity diary
- Carrying case with belt or shoulder strap
- Alcohol swabs
- Cloth tape (nonallergenic)

PROCEDURAL STEPS

1 Wash your hands.
Purpose: Infection control.

2 Assemble equipment needed.

3 Install a new battery or fully charged rechargeable battery into the monitor (Figure 1).

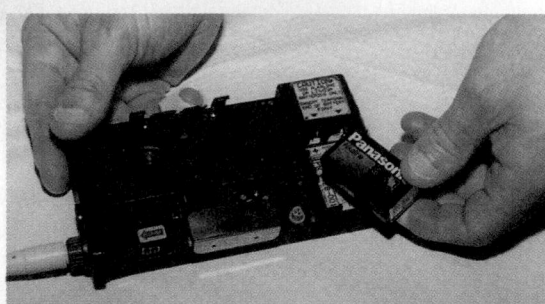

Figure 1

Purpose: A new or fully charged battery ensures accurate monitor function for a 24-hour period.

4 Greet the patient and explain the procedure.
Purpose: An informed patient helps ensure testing accuracy.

5 Ask the patient to disrobe to the waist and sit at the end of the examination table or to lie down.
Purpose: This places the patient at the best working level for the medical assistant.

6 Clean each electrode application site with the alcohol swab and allow the sites to air dry.
Purpose: To remove all surface skin oil to ensure maximal electrode adherence. Clean before shaving to prevent irritation and patient discomfort.

7 If the patient has a hairy chest, dry shave the area at each of the electrode sites.
Purpose: Skin must be hairless to provide maximal electrode adherence.

8 Fold a gauze pad over your index finger and briskly rub the sites (Figure 2).

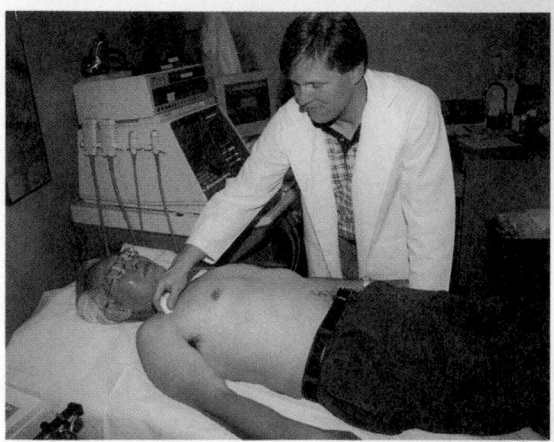

Figure 2

Purpose: Will help electrodes to stick more tightly to the skin.

9 Apply the electrodes to the appropriate sites, making sure to use enough pressure so that they adhere completely to the skin (Figure 3). Rub the edges of each electrode a second time to make certain that the electrode will stay in place.

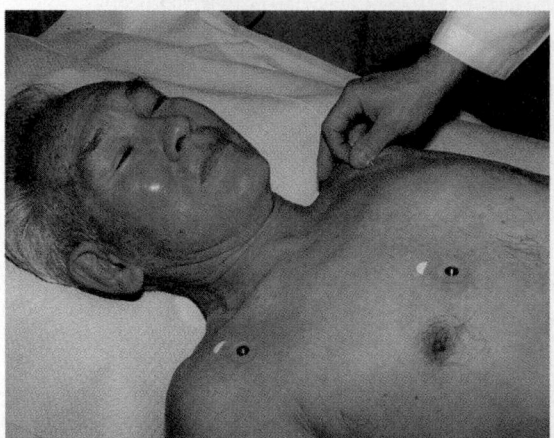

Figure 3

Purpose: Secure attachment of the electrodes is absolutely necessary to produce an accurate tracing.

10 Attach the lead wires to the electrodes and connect the end terminal to the patient cable.

11 Place a strip of cloth tape over each electrode.
Purpose: Aids in securing electrode placement if

PROCEDURE 46-2—cont'd

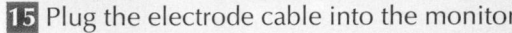

there would be any pulling of the wires during the testing period.

12 Attach the test cable to the monitor and plug it into the electrocardiograph. Run a baseline test tracing.

Purpose: To ensure proper connections of the electrodes and running of the monitor.

13 Help the patient get dressed without disturbing the connected electrodes. Be certain that the cable extends through the buttoned front or out the bottom of the shirt or blouse (Figure 4).

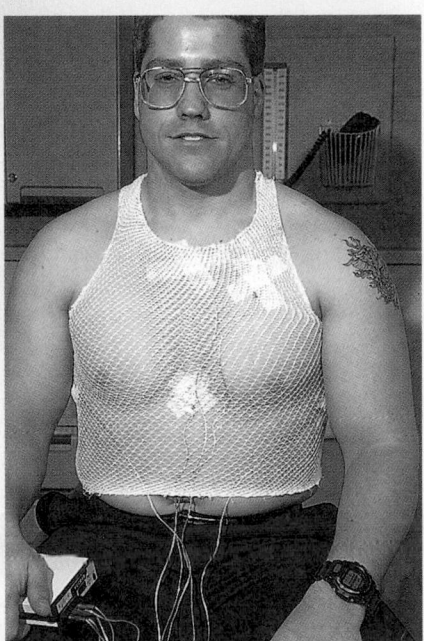

Figure 4

14 Place the monitor in the carrying case, and attach it to the patient's belt or place it over the shoulder (Figure 5). Be sure the wires are not being pulled or bent in half.

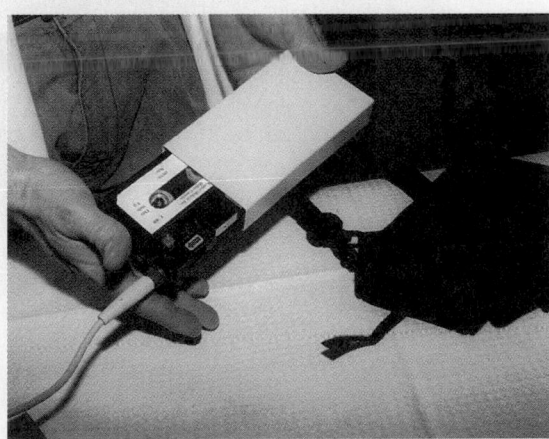

Figure 5

Purpose: Taut or badly bent wires may loosen or malfunction.

15 Plug the electrode cable into the monitor.

16 Record the patient's name, date of birth, and starting date and time of the patient's activity diary.

Purpose: To establish the starting time of the test and cardiac activity.

17 Give the patient the activity diary and advise him or her to begin by writing in his or her present activity (Figure 6).

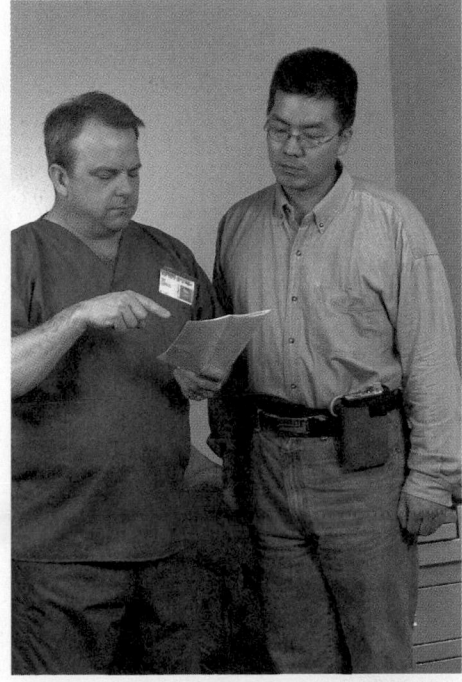

Figure 6

Purpose: Diary must correlate patient's activity with cardiac activity.

18 Give patient appointment for return in 24 hours.

19 Wash your hands.
Purpose: Infection control.

20 Record the procedure in patient's chart.
Purpose: A procedure is not considered done until it is recorded in the patient's medical record.

See Appendix E for a charting example.

the test. The number of electrodes and leads varies with the number of channels on the particular monitor. Electrode placement is determined by the physician or manufacturer guidelines and should be followed precisely. The skin may need to be shaved so that electrodes can be firmly attached. The wires are attached to the electrodes and to the Holter. It is worn on a belt or in a pouch slung over the shoulder or worn around the waist.

At the end of the monitoring period, the patient returns to the office; the monitor is disconnected and the electrodes are removed. The tape and diary covering the testing period are placed into a Holter scanner or computer and the results are analyzed. Any portion of the tape can be printed for further study.

CRITICAL THINKING APPLICATION

Mrs. Jamison was fitted with a Holter monitor at the office yesterday at 4 PM. When Marcus arrived at the office at 8 AM this morning, he found she had left a message with the answering service to call her as soon as possible. When he returned her call, she told him she took a shower last night, and she noticed when she got up to go to the bathroom that the "light is not on" on the monitor. How should Marcus handle this situation?

Heart Scan

One of the newest noninvasive methods of assessing possible cardiac risk is a specialized CT called an *EBT heart scan* (also called an *ultrafast CT*, or electron beam tomography). The heart scan takes less than 5 minutes and does not require any needles or injections. It is a screening tool that allows physicians to visualize the amount of plaque that is present in the coronary arteries by showing the presence of calcium deposits. Calcium makes up approximately 20% of arterial plaque deposits. The EBT heart scan is read, and the physician assigns the patient a calcium score that can be a predictor of future cardiac problems.

Patient Education

Heart disease and stroke account for more than one third of all deaths. Genetic predisposition and detrimental lifestyle habits, such as smoking, lack of exercise, high-fat diets, and obesity, play a significant role in the development of heart disease. There is a constant need for communication skills in your relationship with the patient and with the physician. Talk to the patient about factors that could be changed or modified and give him or her encouragement for any attempt at complying with these suggestions.

Before you can successfully counsel a patient in changing a habit, you will need to obtain background knowledge in possible techniques to use. Places to obtain this information include the American Heart Association, the public library, and the Internet.

Patients like visual aids in learning, and having pictures, brochures, and pamphlets to give to them is an effective method to initiate both patient learning and patient questions. Make a note in the chart of what educational items you give the patient on each visit. On a subsequent visit, ask about the helpfulness of the information, whether the patient tried any modifications, and what the results were. Ask for any suggestions that might help another patient in a similar situation. You may be surprised to learn that patients are inclined to try something new if it has more than one purpose. If they feel that they are helping you prepare a plan for modification and you need their input, they may be willing to try new approaches.

Legal and Ethical Issues

Electrocardiography is a valuable diagnostic tool that continues to be one of the most common procedures used in the diagnosis of cardiac diseases and conditions. The cardiologist compares and measures the patient's heart activity with known values by analyzing the ECG tracing. Comparing an ECG tracing with previous tracings can identify changes in the condition of the heart.

The physician must be able to accurately interpret the ECG tracing and establish its value in correctly diagnosing the patient's condition; therefore the medical assistant has the ethical obligation to complete the task as accurately and carefully as possible. Diagnostic procedures have a profound effect on a patient's subsequent treatment. When you are entrusted with performing testing procedures, you assume full responsibility for the accuracy and precision of each test you perform. This is a critical role in the medical assisting profession. The results you submit will strongly influence each patient's therapeutic treatment plan. No test is ever just routine.

SUMMARY OF SCENARIO

Marcus has now worked at Dr. Lee's office for almost 8 months. He has become quite confident in his ability to quickly and accurately perform the ECG test. He also has learned a great deal about how to effectively communicate with patients regarding their fears and concerns about the various cardiac diagnostic tests. He never forgets to tell a patient the importance of not taking a shower during the 24-hour Holter monitoring period. In 2 months, he and Dr. Lee are going to attend a national meeting of cardiologists in Chicago. There will be 2 days of continuing education classes for medical assistants who work in cardiology. Marcus is very excited to be able to continue learning and to sharpen his skills as a cardiology medical assistant.

He put a chart on the wall of the ECG room showing the correct placement of the chest leads. He referred to it for his first month at Dr. Lee's office. Now he never needs to look at it, because he can confidently place all six of the chest leads on any patient. He says he could literally place them accurately with his eyes closed!

SUMMARY OF LEARNING OBJECTIVES

- The heart beats in response to an electrical signal that originates in the SA node in the right atrium, spreads over the atria, and causes atrial contraction. This impulse continues to the AV node, through the bundle of His, through the right and left bundle branches, and through the Purkinje fibers, eventually causing ventricular contraction.

- The horizontal lines on the ECG paper permit the determination of the intensity of the electrical activity or the relative strength of the heartbeat. The stronger the beat, the greater the vertical deflection on the paper. The vertical lines represent time: the large squares each represent 0.2 seconds; five of them equal one second.

- Taking an ECG requires knowledge of where to accurately place the electrodes and how to accurately connect the leads to obtain the most accurate recording possible. The medical assistant also needs to be able to recognize and correct the most common types of artifacts on the ECG recording.

- Patient preparation for an ECG or a stress test includes explaining why and how the procedure is to be done. When patients understand the test, their fears are allayed, and they are much less likely to be anxious during the testing procedure.

- A P wave results from the contraction or depolarization of the atria. A QRS complex results from the contraction or depolarization of the ventricles. A T wave occurs when the ventricles relax or repolarize, getting ready for the next contraction.

- A 12-lead ECG consists of three limb leads (I, II, and III), three augmented leads (aVR, aVL, and aVF), and six precordial or chest leads (V_1, V_2, V_3, V_4, V_5, and V_6). These leads record the electrical activity from different directions, giving the physician a picture of the function of different areas of the heart.

KEY INTERNET WEBSITES

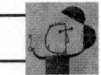

- Automatic Implantable Cardioverter Defibrillator—Patient Information
- ECG Site
- Electrocardiology and Cardiac Arrhythmias (with rhythm strips of each one)
- Most Common Cardiac Arrhythmias
  For active weblinks to each website visit
  http://evolve.elsevier.com/Kinn/

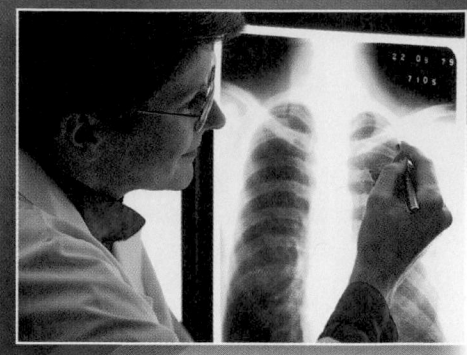

CHAPTER 47

Scenario

Sara Elwood, CMA, is employed by Metro Urgicenter, an urgent care clinic in an urban setting. Metro is staffed around the clock and sees patients with urgent problems that are not immediately life threatening. Facilities at the center include an x-ray department where films of the spine and the extremities are taken to evaluate injuries for possible fractures and chest films are ordered to aid in the diagnosis of patients with respiratory complaints. The center's staff physicians read the x-ray films as they are taken. Afterward, the films are sent to a local hospital for formal interpretation by a physician who is a specialist in medical imaging, a **radiologist**. Sara often assists David Swain, the **radiographer**, by preparing patients for x-ray examinations and processing the films. Sometimes it is her responsibility to send these examinations to the hospital for interpretation and to file them when they are returned. When patients are sent to other facilities for special imaging studies, it is Sara's duty to make the arrangements and provide preliminary explanations of the procedures to the patients.

Assisting With Diagnostic Imaging

Ruth Ann Ehrlich

Learning Objectives

- Define and spell the terms listed in the vocabulary.
- Compare and contrast radiography and fluoroscopy and give examples of appropriate applications of each.
- List and describe three imaging modalities that do not involve x-rays.
- Given examples of diagnostic images, identify the modality used to create them.
- Explain to patients in a general way what they should expect when scheduled for a diagnostic imaging procedure involving x-rays, oral contrast media, intravenous contrast media, computed tomography (CT), magnetic resonance imaging (MRI), diagnostic sonography, or nuclear medicine.
- Explain the procedure and the rationale involved in patient preparation for the following examinations: chest radiography, upper gastrointestinal (GI) series, lower GI series, intravenous urogram, and CT examination of the abdomen with an oral contrast medium.
- Correctly identify the principal components of an x-ray machine.
- List the three body planes and use these terms correctly when discussing radiographic positions and radiographic projections.
- Describe, identify, or demonstrate the following radiographic projections: anteroposterior (AP), posteroanterior (PA), lateral, oblique, and axial.
- Describe the cassette/film image receptor system and explain its function in radiography.
- List precautions to be taken when unloading and loading cassettes.
- Explain the importance of film identification.
- Correctly identify and process a radiograph and reload the cassette.
- Describe the health risks associated with low doses of x-ray exposure like those that are used in radiography.
- List steps to ensure that patients receive the least possible exposure during x-ray procedures.
- Reassure patients who are fearful of radiation exposure from an x-ray examination.
- Describe precautions to ensure the safety of equipment operators and staff during x-ray procedures.
- Describe the risks associated with x-ray exposure during pregnancy and suggest steps to avoid inadvertent exposure to an embryo or fetus.
- Explain the legal responsibilities associated with ownership, retention, and transfer of diagnostic images.
- Explain the legal implications associated with ordering imaging procedures, performing x-ray procedures, and interpreting diagnostic images.

National Curriculum Competencies

CLINICAL COMPETENCIES

4e. Prepare the patient for and assist with routine and specialty examinations.

Vocabulary

angiocardiography Radiography of the heart and great vessels using an iodine contrast medium.

angiography Radiography of blood vessels using an iodine contrast medium.

angioplasty Interventional technique using a catheter to open or widen a blood vessel to improve circulation.

anteroposterior (AP) Frontal projection in which the patient is supine or facing the x-ray tube.

aortogram Radiography of the aorta using an iodine contrast medium.

arteriography Radiography of arteries using an iodine contrast medium.

arthrogram Fluoroscopic examination of the soft tissue components of joints with direct injection of a contrast medium into the joint capsule.

axial projection Radiograph taken with a longitudinal angulation of the x-ray beam; sometimes referred to as a semiaxial projection.

bucky Moving grid device that prevents scatter radiation from fogging the film.

cathartic A laxative preparation.

computed tomography (CT) Computerized x-ray imaging modality providing axial and three-dimensional scans.

contrast media Radiopaque substances used to enhance visualization of soft tissues in imaging studies.

coronal plane Plane that divides the body into anterior and posterior parts.

coulombs per kilogram (C/kg) International unit of radiation exposure.

dosimeter Badge for monitoring radiation exposure to personnel.

embolization Interventional technique using a catheter to block off a blood vessel to prevent hemorrhage.

fluoroscopy Direct observation of the x-ray image in motion.

frontal projection Radiographic view in which the coronal plane of the body or body part is parallel to the film plane; AP or PA.

gantry Doughnut-shaped portion of a scanner that surrounds the patient and functions, at least in part, to gather imaging data.

Gray (Gy) International unit of radiation dose.

intravenous urogram (IVU) Radiographic examination of the urinary tract using intravenous injection of an iodine contrast medium.

latent image Invisible changes in exposed film that will become an image when the film is processed.

lateral projection Radiographic view in which the sagittal plane of the body or body part is parallel to the film.

limited radiography Limited-scope radiography practice, usually in an outpatient setting, that does not require the same credentials needed for professional radiologic technology; also called practical radiography.

lower gastrointestinal (GI) series Fluoroscopic examination of the colon, usually employing rectal administration of barium sulfate as a contrast medium; also called a barium enema.

magnetic resonance imaging (MRI) Imaging modality that uses a magnetic field and radiofrequency pulses to create computer images of both bones and soft tissues in multiple planes.

myelography Fluoroscopic examination of the spinal canal with spinal injection of an iodine contrast medium.

NPO Nothing by mouth, from the Latin *nil per os*.

nuclear medicine Imaging modality that uses radioactive materials injected or ingested into the body to provide information about the function of organs and tissues.

oblique projection Radiographic view in which the body or part is rotated so that the projection is neither frontal nor lateral.

phosphors Fluorescent crystals that give off light when exposed to x-rays.

posteroanterior (PA) Frontal projection in which the patient is prone or facing the x-ray film or image receptor.

rad Conventional unit of radiation dose.

radiograph An x-ray image.

radiographer Person qualified to perform radiographic examinations.

radiography Making diagnostic images using x-rays.

radiologist Physician specialist in medical imaging or therapeutic applications of radiation.

radiolucent Describing a substance that is easily penetrated by x-rays; these substances appear dark on radiographs.

radiopaque Describing a substance that is not easily penetrated by x-rays; these substances appear light on radiographs.

rem Convention unit of radiation dose equivalent.

Roentgen (R) Conventional unit of radiation exposure.

sagittal plane Plane that divides the body into right and left parts.

Sievert (Sv) International unit of radiation dose equivalent.

sonography Imaging modality that uses sound waves to produce images of soft tissues; also called diagnostic ultrasound.

tracer Radioactive substance administered to patient for nuclear medicine imaging procedure.

transducer Part of the sonography machine that is in contact with the patient; the transducer sends high-frequency sound waves and receives the sound echoes that return from the patient's body.

transverse plane Plane that divides the body into superior and inferior parts.

upper gastrointestinal (GI) series Fluoroscopic examination of the esophagus, stomach, and duodenum using oral administration of barium sulfate as a contrast medium.

For more than 100 years, physicians have been using x-ray images to examine the internal structures of the body. The fascinating field of medical imaging now includes a wide variety of diagnostic imaging methods. This chapter provides an overview of imaging modalities and introduces you to radiography. Emphasis is placed on x-ray examinations because these are the procedures most commonly performed in the medical assistant's practice setting.

IMAGING MODALITIES IN RADIOLOGY

- **Angiography:** Imaging of blood vessels with the injection of special compounds called *contrast media*
- **Computed tomography (CT):** A computerized x-ray system that provides axial images (transverse "slices") of all parts of the body
- **Fluoroscopy:** Real-time viewing of x-ray images in motion
- **Magnetic resonance imaging (MRI):** A computerized imaging system that uses a powerful magnetic field and pulses of radio waves to produce images of all parts of the body
- **Mammography:** X-ray imaging of the breast using a special x-ray machine
- **Nuclear medicine:** The injection or ingestion of radioactive materials and the recording of their uptake in the body using a gamma camera
- **Positron emission tomography (PET):** A highly sophisticated computerized form of nuclear medicine imaging
- **Single photon emission computed tomography (SPECT):** A highly sophisticated computerized form of nuclear medicine imaging similar to positron emission tomography (PET)
- **Sonography:** Imaging of soft tissue structures using sound echoes; diagnostic ultrasound

Diagnostic Imaging Modalities

Radiography and Fluoroscopy

Radiography. **Radiography** refers to the making of x-ray images called **radiographs**. X-rays are produced in a vacuum tube when electrons traveling at high speed strike certain materials, such as tungsten. When the x-rays are emitted from the tube, they diverge into space, forming the cone-shaped x-ray beam. The cross section of the x-ray beam at the point of use is called the radiation field (Figure 47-1). The patient or part to be x-rayed is placed in the radiation field, between the x-ray tube and the image receptor or film.

X-rays can penetrate most substances to some degree, but some substances such as metals and bones are more difficult to penetrate and are said to be **radiopaque**. Air, gases, and soft tissues such as fat, skin, and lungs are much easier to penetrate than bone and are said to be **radiolucent**. During the exposure, x-rays from the tube pass through the patient. Some of the x-rays are absorbed by the patient and others are not, resulting in a pattern of varying intensity in the x-ray beam that exits on the opposite side of the patient and exposes the film. The film then has a pattern of exposure, a **latent image**, and must be processed to develop the latent image into one that is visible. On the finished radiograph, radiopaque objects appear light and radiolucent objects appear dark or black (Figure 47-2).

Routine plain films are simple radiographs taken of specific body structures such as the chest or the bones of the extremities or spine. These are the examinations most often performed in physicians' offices and most likely to be performed by medical assistants who are qualified to practice radiography.

Fluoroscopy. **Fluoroscopy** is a technique using special equipment that permits the radiologist to view x-ray images in motion. Fluoroscopy also permits the physician to survey an area quickly, without the delay involved in taking and processing films. Most fluoroscopic units

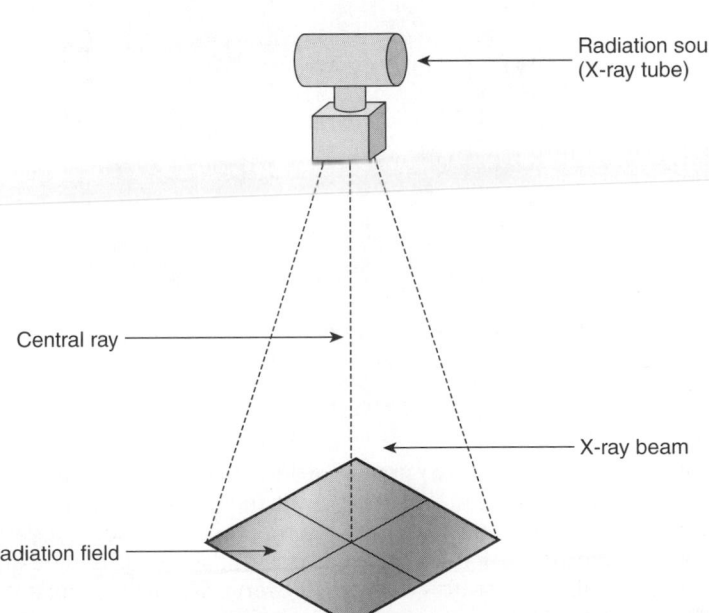

Radiation source (X-ray tube)

Central ray

X-ray beam

Radiation field

FIGURE 47-1 The primary x-ray beam leaves the x-ray tube and diverges into space. The center of the beam is called the *central ray*, and the cross-section of the beam at the point of use is called the *radiation field*. (From Hunkele MM: *Radiography essentials for limited practice*, Philadelphia, 2001, WB Saunders.)

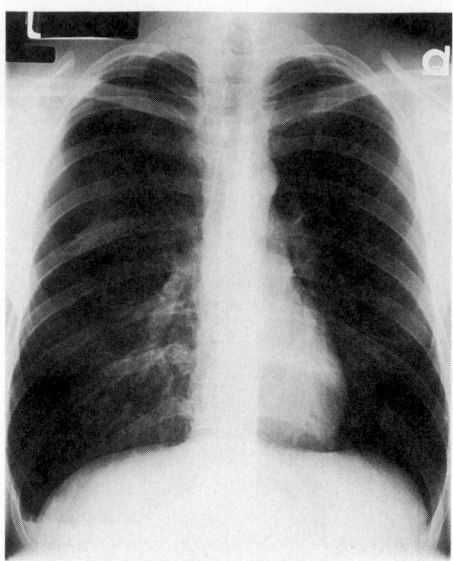

FIGURE 47-2 A chest radiograph demonstrates dark, radiolucent lungs with a light, radiopaque shadow of the spine and heart in the center. (From Hunkele MM: *Radiography essentials for limited practice*, Philadelphia, 2001, WB Saunders.)

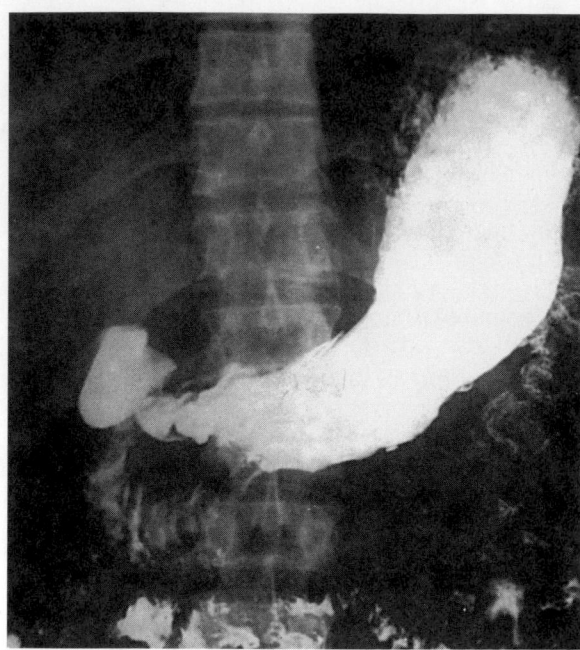

FIGURE 47-3 Radiographic image of the stomach, part of an upper GI series using oral administration of barium sulfate to provide contrast. (From Ballinger PW, Frank ED: *Merrill's atlas of radiographic positions and radiologic procedures*, ed 9, vol 2. St Louis, 1999, Mosby.)

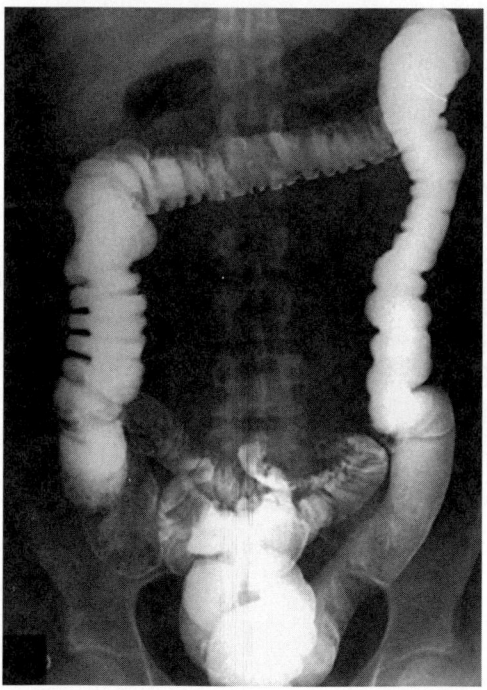

FIGURE 47-4 Lower gastrointestinal (GI) series. Radiograph of the colon filled with barium sulfate administered by way of a barium enema. (From Ballinger PW, Frank ED: *Merrill's atlas of radiographic positions and radiologic procedures*, ed 9, vol 2. St Louis, 1999, Mosby.)

are properly called radiographic/fluoroscopic (R/F) units because they can be used for both radiography and fluoroscopy. This is convenient because most fluoroscopic examinations also have a radiographic component. "Spot films" are taken during fluoroscopy to record the image as seen on the fluoroscope, and sometimes the entire fluoroscopic examination is recorded digitally, on videotape, or on cine (movie) film. After the fluoroscopic portion of the study is completed, larger radiographs are usually taken for comprehensive visualization of the entire anatomical region.

X-Ray Studies Using Contrast Media. Whereas the lungs and the bony structures of the body produce clear x-ray images on plain film radiographs, internal organs such as the stomach and the kidneys are difficult to visualize because they absorb radiation to the same degree as the tissues that surround them. To enhance visualization of these structures, special agents called **contrast media** can be used to fill hollow organs and demonstrate their inner contours. Although gases such as air and carbon dioxide are sometimes used as contrast media, it is far more common to use radiopaque substances such as barium sulfate or iodine compounds. The agent and the technique vary with the structures to be visualized.

Among the most common fluoroscopic examinations are studies of the upper and lower gastrointestinal tract using barium sulfate as a contrast medium. Both require careful patient instruction and advance preparation for a successful study. An **upper gastrointestinal (GI) series** (Figure 47-3) uses oral administration of a barium sulfate suspension to diagnose ulcers, tumors, and other abnormalities of the esophagus, stomach, and duodenum.

A **lower GI series** (Figure 47-4) involves a barium enema to fill the colon and demonstrate its inner surfaces. This procedure is especially useful in diagnosis of polyps, tumors, diverticulosis, and diverticulitis. For

this examination, the inner lining of the large intestine must be clean and free of all fecal matter. The preparation may be complex, taking place over several days. Commercial bowel preparation kits are usually made available by the radiology department to ensure a complete preparation.

Water-soluble iodine compounds are used as contrast media for a wide variety of applications. When injected intravenously, the contrast agent circulates in the blood and is excreted by the kidneys, causing the urine to become radiopaque. Radiography of the kidneys, ureters, and bladder after intravenous (IV) contrast injection is called an **intravenous urogram (IVU)** and is useful in identifying kidney stones, tumors, and other abnormalities of the urinary tract. Preparation for an IVU involves fasting and bowel cleansing, although the preparation is usually less rigorous than for a lower GI series.

Iodine contrast agents can also be injected into joint capsules to produce **arthrograms**, images of the soft tissue components of joints, especially the knee and the shoulder. **Myelography** involves injection of iodine compounds into the spinal canal to demonstrate spinal pathology such as tumors and herniated intervertebral disks. Table 47-1 lists some common radiographic examinations using contrast media, together with the route of contrast administration and the structures that are demonstrated.

Cardiovascular and Interventional Radiography

The highly specialized radiographic procedures that demonstrate blood vessels are collectively known as **angiography**. A cerebral angiogram, for example, demonstrates the vessels of the brain (Figure 47-5); renal angiograms demonstrate the arteries and veins of the kidneys. An **angiocardiogram** is a contrast study that visualizes the interior of the heart chambers and the great vessels that enter and exit the heart, and an **aortogram**, as the name implies, is a procedure that demonstrates the aorta. Selective angiocardiography can be used to demonstrate the coronary arteries. **Arteriograms** are studies of specific arteries and **venograms** are studies of veins.

For all these examinations, iodine compounds are injected for radiographic contrast and a rapid series of

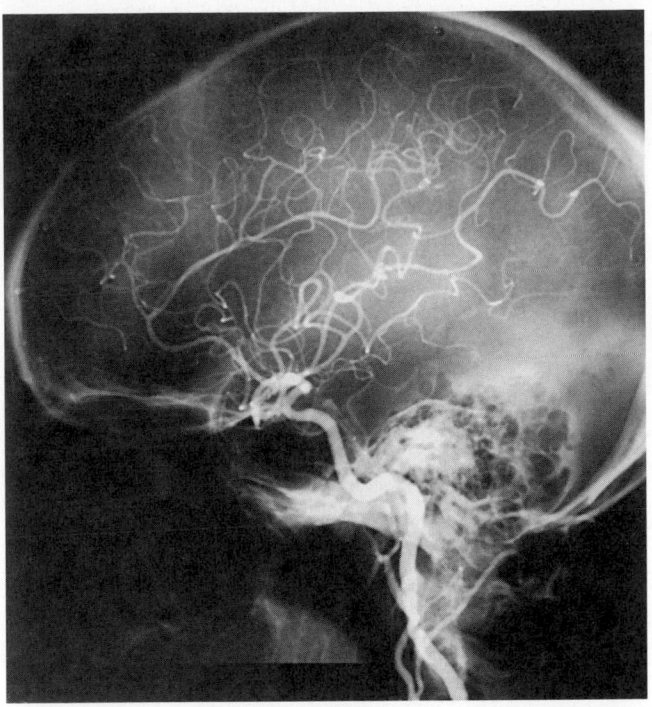

FIGURE 47-5   Cerebral angiogram shows the circulation of the brain enhanced by iodine contrast medium. (From Ballinger PW, Frank ED: *Merrill's atlas of radiographic positions and radiologic procedures*, ed 9, vol 3. St Louis, 1999, Mosby.)

films is taken using highly specialized equipment. Direct injection may be used for some angiographic studies, such as those of the extremities, but the preferred injection method for angiocardiography, aortography, and most arteriography is to use a special catheter. Catheters are placed precisely in the blood vessel of interest using a method called the *Seldinger technique*. A large artery, usually the femoral or brachial, is entered with a large-bore needle and a guidewire is threaded through the needle and into the artery under fluoroscopic control. The needle is then removed, the guidewire

TABLE 47-1	Radiographic Procedures Using Contrast Media		
Examination	**Contrast Medium**	**Route of Administration**	**Structures Visualized**
Angiocardiography	Iodine compounds	Intraarterial injection via femoral or brachial catheter	Heart and large vessels
Angiography	Iodine compounds	Intraarterial or intravenous injection	Blood vessels
Arteriography	Iodine compounds	Intraarterial injection via catheter	Arteries
Arthrography	Iodine compounds	Direct injection into joint capsule	Joints, especially knee, shoulder, and ankle
Barium swallow	Barium sulfate suspension	Oral	Esophagus
Hysterosalpingography	Iodine compounds	Direct injection via cannula	Uterus and fallopian tubes
Intravenous urography	Iodine compounds	Intravenous injection	Kidneys, ureters, and urinary bladder
Lower GI series (barium enema)	Barium sulfate suspension, sometimes also with air	Rectal catheter	Colon
Lymphangiography	Iodine compounds	Direct injection to lymphatic vessels in the feet	Lymphatic vessels and lymph nodes
Myelography	Iodine compounds	Intrathecal injection (spinal tap)	Spinal canal
Upper GI Series	Barium sulfate suspension	Oral	Esophagus, stomach, and duodenum

is left in the vessel, and the catheter is threaded over the wire. The wire is then removed, and the catheter remains in the artery for the duration of the examination. Further manipulation of the catheter may be needed to ensure correct placement in the vessel before injection. For selective catheterization of smaller vessels, the catheter tip is maneuvered into the root of the vessel of interest, such as the coronary, celiac, renal, or carotid artery.

A timed sequence of images is obtained during and after injection of the contrast medium, usually with the aid of an automatic power injector that is electronically coordinated with a programmable film changer and automated exposure control. Digital receptors are replacing the use of film and film changers in some imaging centers, and for some studies such as angiocardiograms, digital fluoroscopy equipment may be used to record the images.

Because these procedures are expensive and involve a relatively high degree of risk, angiography has been replaced somewhat by technological advances in other imaging modalities discussed in this chapter, particularly Doppler ultrasound, nuclear medicine, magnetic resonance angiography (MRA), and computed tomography angiography (CTA).

Despite these advances, angiography continues to be used extensively because it provides the best anatomical demonstration of structures within the circulatory system and also offers the opportunity for immediate therapeutic interventions to treat vascular problems when they are identified. Specialized catheter techniques are used for vessel repair, called **angioplasty**, to widen or open arteries that are narrowed or occluded. **Embolization** refers to therapeutic intervention techniques that decrease or stop blood flow to treat hemorrhage and tumors and to reduce blood loss during surgery.

Computed Tomography

Computed tomography (CT) is the same imaging modality formerly called computerized axial tomography (CAT) scanning. CT uses a special x-ray scanner to produce axial images, slice-like sections in the transverse plane that may be "reconstructed" by the computer to display the anatomical structures in other planes as well. Image characteristics such as brightness and contrast can be manipulated on the computer, and images can be viewed in a variety of formats called "windows" that are designed to enhance visualization of specific tissues (Figure 47-6). Most CT examinations are noninvasive and are not uncomfortable for the patient. The equipment may cause apprehension, however, and careful explanations are necessary for patient cooperation and a satisfactory study.

The CT scanner (Figure 47-7) consists of a movable table with remote control, a circular **gantry** structure that supports the x-ray tube and detectors, an operator console with a monitor, and the supporting computer system. The CT unit also includes both hardware and software to archive and manage data and produce hard copies of the images. During a scan, the x-ray tube rotates around the patient to collect the data. In conventional CT units, the tube makes a complete rotation to gather data for each slice. The table then moves and the

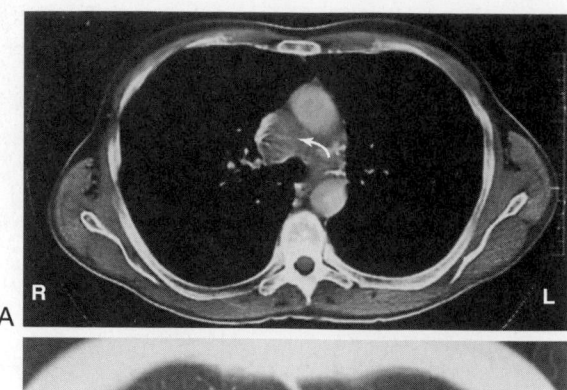
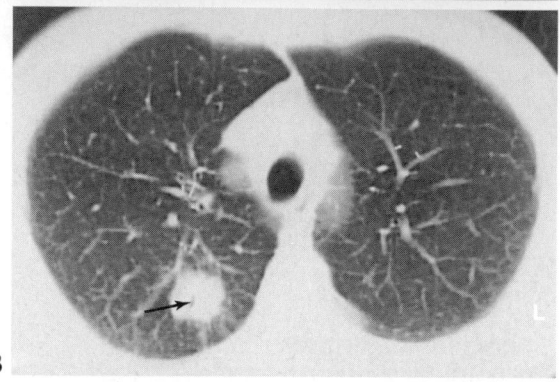

FIGURE 47-6 Two computed tomography windows demonstrate structures of the chest from the same image. **A**, Mediastinal structures are demonstrated in the center of the field, but the lungs are not well seen. **B**, "Lung window" demonstrates the blood vessels of the lungs and a lung tumor *(arrow)*. (Seeram E: *Computed tomography,* ed 2. Philadelphia, 2001, WB Saunders.)

tube rotates again to obtain the next slice. A newer generation of scanner, designated as spiral or helical, scans a spiral path around the patient and can collect data on a larger volume of tissue. These scanners can reconstruct volume information to render three-dimensional images.

The versatility of CT is illustrated by its wide range of applications, including studies of the brain, spine, abdomen, pelvis, chest, neck, and paranasal sinuses. CT is a valuable tool for emergency use, especially in the detection of intracerebral or intraabdominal hemorrhage. It is also used for orthopedic examinations of the extremities and for contrast-enhanced vascular studies known as CTA. CT is useful in localizing both lesions and needle position during needle-aspiration biopsy, a nonsurgical method of obtaining cells for laboratory examination, and is often used with myelography to expand the range of information available.

Although many CT examinations do not require contrast media, the use of contrast agents vastly increases the scope of CT imaging. Studies of the abdomen usually employ oral contrast to help differentiate the GI tract from the surrounding tissues. A special barium compound or an oral iodine preparation is ingested by the patient over a specified period before the study. The amount of contrast and the time period vary depending on whether the examination includes only the upper abdomen or the entire abdomen and pelvis. For these studies, the patient is instructed to fast and to come early to drink the contrast preparation. Some departments have the patient take the contrast home

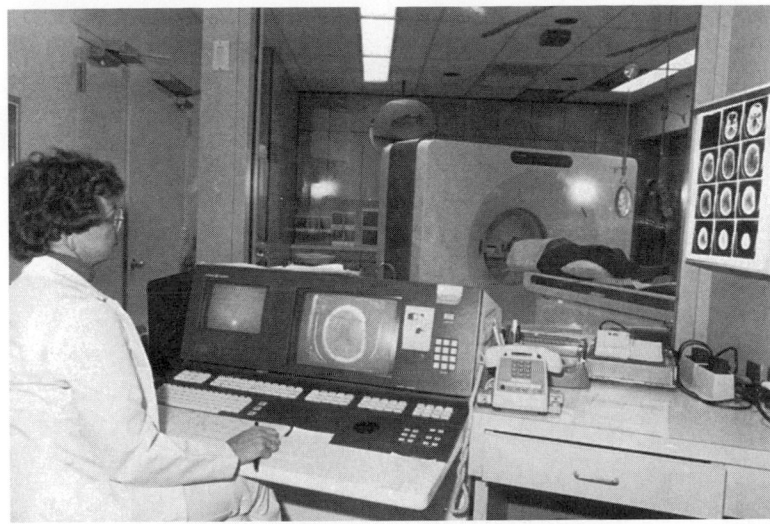

FIGURE 47-7   Computed tomography (CT) technologist monitors the patient while performing a CT scan of the brain. (From Ehrlich RA, McCloskey ED, Daly JA: *Patient care in radiography*, ed 5. St Louis, 1999, Mosby.)

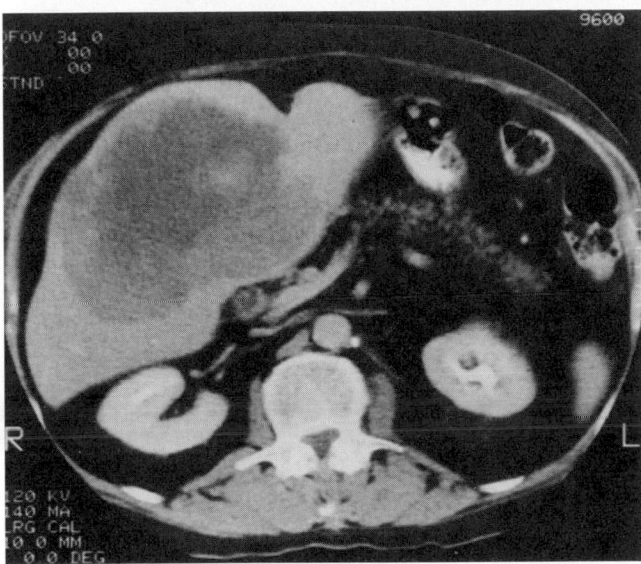

FIGURE 47-8   Axial computed tomography "slice" of the abdomen demonstrates contrast-enhanced liver, kidney, and intestinal structures. (From Ehrlich RA, McCloskey ED, Daly JA: *Patient care in radiography*, ed 5. St Louis, 1999, Mosby.)

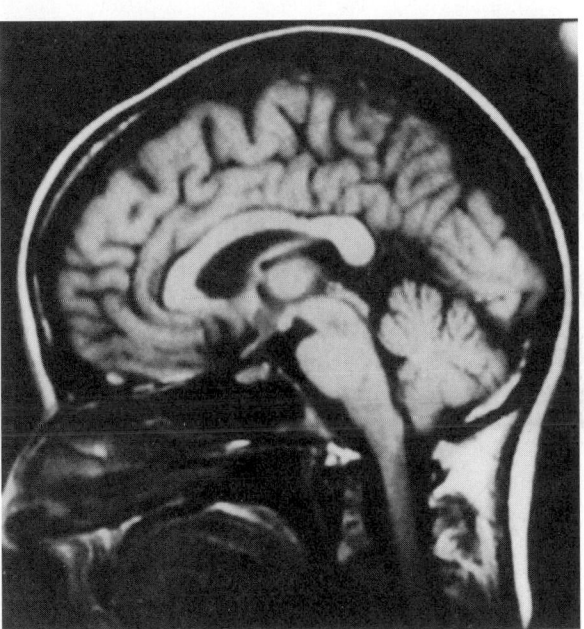

FIGURE 47-9   Midsagittal magnetic resonance image of the brain. (From Ehrlich RA, McCloskey ED, Daly JA: *Patient care in radiography*, ed 5. St Louis, 1999, Mosby.)

with instructions to drink it before reporting for the appointment.

Intravenous injection of an iodine contrast medium may also be employed to increase the contrast level of the patient's tissues. This is advantageous for studies of the chest, abdomen, and soft tissues of the neck because it highlights blood vessels and enhances visualization of vascular organs such as the liver and spleen. The contrast defines the internal structures of the kidneys, ureters, and bladder as it is excreted in the urine (Figure 47-8). In selected cases, IV contrast agents are employed in CT scans of the head to demonstrate brain lesions.

Magnetic Resonance Imaging

Magnetic resonance imaging (MRI) is a noninvasive diagnostic modality that does not use ionizing radiation. A powerful magnetic field and radiofrequency pulses are combined to produce a radio signal in the body that can be detected and processed electronically to provide images on a computer monitor. The images can be managed in a computer database and can also be stored on magnetic tape and photographed with a special camera to produce film copies.

The MRI gantry houses the magnet and the main radiofrequency coil. Conventional gantries are tubular, 5 to 8 feet long, and surround most of the patient's body during the scanning process. An open configuration in gantry design provides better accommodation for large or claustrophobic patients, but it does not always provide image quality equal to that produced by conventional units.

MRI provides excellent imaging of the soft tissues of the nervous system (Figure 47-9) and is useful in the diagnosis of many types of pathology, including brain and spinal cord tumors and diseases such as multiple sclerosis. MRI is also used for diagnosis of herniated intervertebral disks and to obtain images of the soft tissue components of joints, particularly the knee, shoulder, and temporomandibular joint. A more recent advance in MRI is magnetic resonance angiogram (MRA), which uses magnetic resonance technology to study the cardiovascular system. MRA aids in the diagnosis and treatment of heart disorders, stroke, and blood vessel diseases.

Typical scan time for a series of slicelike images ranges from 1 to 10 minutes, and several series demonstrating different body planes and using a variety of radiofrequency pulse sequences may be included in an examination. It is critically important that the patient remain still during a scan series and that the initial position be maintained throughout the study.

Although contrast media are not required for most MRI studies, special paramagnetic agents are sometimes injected intravenously. These agents provide contrast enhancement of certain lesions, particularly brain and spinal cord tumors, and aid in differentiating disk material from scar tissue in postoperative spinal examinations. Contrast injections are also used in MRA studies.

The unique MRI environment requires special safety precautions. Conditions affecting patient safety involve both the powerful magnetic field within the gantry and the thermal effects of radiofrequency pulses on certain materials that could overheat and possibly burn the patient. The principal means of ensuring patient safety during an MRI is careful patient screening before the procedure. Although extensive patient interviews are conducted in the magnetic resonance department, preliminary screening of patients should be conducted by the medical assistant before the appointment is made. The magnetic field or the rapid radiofrequency pulses may be hazardous for patients with artificial heart valves, aneurysm clips, neurostimulators, middle ear prostheses, or intrauterine devices. Cardiac pacemakers are a particular hazard, and *patients with pacemakers cannot have MRI examinations*. Fatalities have resulted from overheating of these implanted devices when patients with pacemakers were scanned. Other conditions that merit assessment before entering the magnetic field include hemolytic anemia, orthopedic pins and screws, and metal fragments or shrapnel in the soft tissues. Most orthopedic hardware is safe in the magnet, although it may compromise image quality in the surrounding area.

Metalworkers who might have steel slivers in their tissues must have a screening x-ray or CT head examination to detect fragments that could damage their eyes or brain because the pull of the magnetic field is so strong that it could cause the fragments to move. Although the energies involved in MRI have not been demonstrated to cause complications with pregnancy, the current philosophy is to avoid examination of pregnant patients except in urgent cases, especially during the first trimester.

Patients should be assured that everything possible will be done to provide assistance in dealing with both physical and emotional discomfort. Few people are completely comfortable for any length of time in a tightly enclosed space. Even patients with no history of claustrophobia may feel anxious when entering a conventional tubular MRI gantry. Occasionally, this anxiety is so severe that it creates panic, preventing the patient from continuing the examination.

Patients may be reassured to know what to expect in advance. They will lie on the MRI table, which will move into the gantry. Plenty of air is available, and no physical discomfort will occur other than the need to lie still. The machine will make a loud "knocking" noise during the scanning process. Earplugs or earphones with recorded music may be offered. Patients can communicate with the technologist through an intercom, and the technologist will be watching them and listening to them from an adjacent area at all times during the procedure. Because no radiation danger exists, a friend or family member may be allowed to accompany the patient. Severely claustrophobic patients may be scheduled at a facility with an open-gantry MRI or may be given an antianxiety medication. Analgesic medications may be administered to patients whose pain makes it impossible to lie still for the duration of the study.

Sonography

Diagnostic medical sonography is a noninvasive procedure that is considered to be very safe for the patient. Sonography was introduced in Chapter 38 because it is used extensively for fetal imaging. This imaging modality, often referred to as *diagnostic ultrasound*, uses high-frequency sound waves to produce echoes within the body. As the echoes return to the sending point, or **transducer**, their strength and timing are interpreted by a computer to produce a map or graphic image of the echo distribution.

The transducer is moved over the surface of the body and the image is viewed in real time on the computer monitor. Special transducer probes can be inserted into body cavities such as the rectum and the vagina to obtain more detailed examinations of the prostate gland and the uterus. Any interface between substances or tissues of varying density produces an ultrasound echo, making sonography an effective technique to visualize the shape, size, and condition of organs such as the heart, spleen, gallbladder, or pancreas (Figure 47-10). Because sonography permits differentiation of fluid from adipose tissue, the presence of an abscess, cyst, or tumor can be demonstrated.

Recent advances in ultrasound technology include computer integration of data to produce three-dimensional images. Special contrast agents containing microscopic bubbles are available for use in cardiac imaging but have not been approved by the U.S. Food and Drug Administration (FDA) for other applications. These agents transmit echoes from within tissues that would otherwise lack image detail.

Doppler ultrasound methodology allows recording of flow phenomena in color and permits demonstration of both arteries and veins. Doppler ultrasound is used extensively to detect vascular disease, such as atherosclerosis in the carotid arteries and venous thrombosis of the lower extremities.

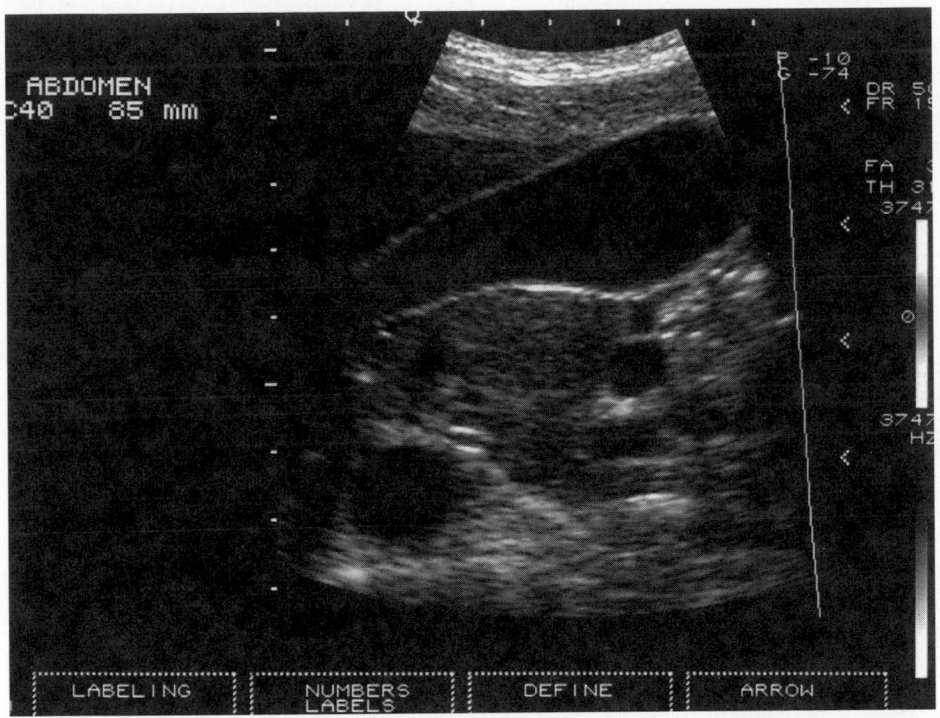

FIGURE 47-10   Abdominal sonogram. (From Ballinger PW, Frank ED: *Merrill's atlas of radiographic positions and radiologic procedures*, ed 9, vol 3. St Louis, 1999, Mosby.)

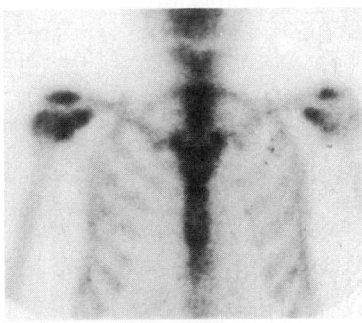

FIGURE 47-11   Bone scan showing increased tracer uptake in right shoulder region due to inflammation.

Nuclear Medicine

Nuclear medicine images are created by scanning the patient after special radioactive materials called **tracers** have been swallowed or injected intravenously. Tracers are similar to substances that are commonly used by the body, and so they enter into the same chemical reactions and are metabolized in a similar way. They are taken up in the target organ or tissue over a period of time that may vary from half an hour to several days. The tracer can then be detected and its location recorded by a special nuclear medicine scanner called a *gamma camera*.

Nuclear medicine scans do not provide clear images of anatomic structures. They are used to obtain information about the *function* of organs and tissues. Abnormal tissues are demonstrated on the image because the tracer is metabolized at a different rate, at a different location, or to a greater or lesser extent than in normal tissue.

Figure 47-11 is an example of a nuclear medicine bone scan. The tracer is absorbed by the bones and appears in greater or lesser amounts depending on the level of metabolic activity within the bone. In this scan, the region of the right shoulder shows a high level of radioactivity that indicates an inflammatory process.

Structures that can be demonstrated by nuclear medicine techniques include the thyroid gland, liver, lungs, brain, skeletal system, kidneys, heart, and blood vessels. One form of tracer flows in the blood, allowing visualization of blood vessels to detect clots and other abnormalities. Thallium stress studies of the heart are nuclear medicine examinations that are particularly useful in the evaluation of cardiac conditions. Table 47-2 lists some common nuclear medicine procedures and their purposes.

The radioisotopes used in nuclear medicine decay within a short time, from a few hours to a few days, and are eliminated in urine or feces. They have a very low level of radioactivity and produce less exposure to the patient than most x-ray examinations. Positron emission tomography (PET) and single photon emission computed tomography (SPECT) are highly specialized nuclear medicine techniques that use different types of tracers and scanners than conventional nuclear medicine, but the basic principle is the same. Radioactive substances from within the body are detected and mapped by specialized equipment to obtain information about the

TABLE 47-2	Some Common Nuclear Medicine Procedures
Procedure	**Purpose**
Bone scan	Helps to detect fractures, tumors, and inflammation; used to determine bone growth
Brain scan	Often used together with other imaging methods to detect tumors and vascular problems
Liver scan	Useful in diagnosing cirrhosis and hepatitis and in detecting tumors and liver abscesses
Lung scan	Often done to detect emboli, blood clots that have traveled through the bloodstream to the lungs
Thallium stress test	Evaluates cardiac condition and response to stress
Thyroid scan	The rate of uptake is an indicator of thyroid function and is also useful in detection of tumors

function of organs, tissues, or systems. These newer modalities acquire digital images that can be reconstructed by the computer to render images in multiple planes and dimensions.

Scheduling and Sequencing Diagnostic Imaging Procedures

One of the most important communications between medical assistants and imaging departments involves the scheduling of multiple diagnostic procedures that may all be ordered at one time by the physician. Consultation is often needed to decide how many procedures can be done in one day and to sequence them in such a way that they will not interfere with each other. For example, an upper GI series usually results in barium sulfate scattered throughout the intestinal tract for several days. Even tiny amounts of residual barium cause complications in radiographic examinations of the urinary tract and biliary system, where tiny opacifications are diagnostically significant. Residual barium in the digestive tract also causes unacceptable artifacts on abdominal CT scans. For this reason, barium studies are scheduled last in any series of procedures.

Some imaging departments will schedule a series of several examinations in one day for patients who are able to tolerate this approach. Radiologists prefer various scheduling practices. For example, some departments schedule gallbladder and upper and lower GI studies on the same day. Others may insist on 2 or 3 days for the completion of the same examinations. You should become familiar with the practice in the institution where you usually schedule patients.

Scheduling several examinations on the same day may be less stressful, resulting in a single bowel preparation, a single period of fasting, and a single trip to the imaging center. There is a limit, however, to the extent of examination a debilitated patient can tolerate. After one study the patient may need to rest.

When fiberoptic studies, such as gastroscopy or sigmoidoscopy, are ordered in conjunction with radiographic examinations requiring barium as a contrast medium, fiberoptic studies are usually done first. This avoids the possibility of the barium interfering with visual assessment during the fiberoptic examination. Patients undergoing gastroscopy should be NPO for 12 hours preceding the examination. They usually receive sedation and a muscle relaxant before the physician inserts the gastroscope. When an upper GI series is to follow, it should be delayed to allow sufficient time for the patient to become responsive and alert before the upper GI series because oral administration of barium to a sedated patient increases the risk that the patient may choke on the barium.

Another study to be considered when sequencing diagnostic procedures is any thyroid assessment test that involves iodine uptake. Because the administration of contrast media containing iodine causes inaccurate results in such tests for at least 3 weeks, thyroid assessment tests (T3 or T4) or nuclear medicine thyroid scans must be performed before any iodinated contrast medium

is administered. The following is a guide to sequencing multiple diagnostic studies for patients undergoing a comprehensive workup.

GUIDE TO SEQUENCING ORDER FOR DIAGNOSTIC STUDIES

- All radiographic examinations not requiring contrast media and any laboratory studies or nuclear medicine procedures involving iodine uptake
- Radiographic examinations of the urinary tract
- Radiographic examinations of the biliary system
- Lower gastrointestinal (GI) series (barium enema)
- Upper GI series

NOTE: *Computed tomography (CT) studies requiring intravenous contrast may be done any time after blood has been drawn for iodine uptake studies. CT studies of the abdomen or pelvis should precede examinations involving barium.*

An additional consideration in patient scheduling involves deciding which patients will need early morning appointments and which can be scheduled later in the day. Imaging departments always begin the daily routine with patients who must fast in preparation for examination so that they will not have to go without food for too long. When scheduling, request early priority for pediatric and geriatric patients because they have the most difficulty being NPO for long periods and extended fasting may actually interfere with their recovery. Diabetic patients who must postpone their insulin until their morning meal may also need priority in scheduling. Diabetic outpatients should be reminded to postpone their morning insulin until the examination is complete, even if they have been scheduled for an early appointment. If an emergency should cause a delay, the patient who has had insulin may suffer a reaction.

CRITICAL THINKING APPLICATION

Mrs. Pellegrini, a 62-year-old diabetic patient, calls Metro Urgicenter at 8:30 AM to confirm her 10:00 AM appointment for an outpatient imaging procedure that requires fasting. On speaking with her, Sara discovers Mrs. Pellegrini has already taken her morning insulin. What should Sara tell Mrs. Pellegrini and David, the radiographer? Should Mrs. Pellegrini keep her appointment or be rescheduled? Why or why not?

Plain Film Radiography

Basic Principles of Exposure

Prime Factors. The radiographer must take a number of factors into consideration in determining the proper technique and exposure factors for an x-ray examination. The four principal exposure factors are called the *prime factors of exposure* and include:

- Milliamperage (mA)—the electrical control setting that determines how rapidly the radiation is produced.
- Exposure time (seconds)—the duration of the exposure
- Kilovoltage (kVp)—the electrical control setting that determines the penetrating power of the x-ray beam
- Source-to-image distance (SID)—the distance between the x-ray tube and the film or other image receptor

The total quantity of radiation in an exposure is indicated by the milliampere-seconds (mAs), the value determined by multiplying the mA times the exposure time.

Technique Charts. A technique chart located near the control console provides the radiographer with a listing of recommended mAs and kVp settings, as well as the SID, for each of the various body parts for different sizes of patients. Some control consoles have "anatomical programming." These computerized units are preprogrammed with the required exposure settings for the selected body part and size.

Radiographic Equipment

The X-ray Tube and Housing. The x-ray tube is the source of the radiation. It is located inside a protective housing (Figure 47-12). The housing incorporates shielding that absorbs any radiation that is not a part of the useful x-ray beam. The housing protects and insulates the x-ray tube itself while providing a base for attachments that allow the radiographer to manipulate the x-ray tube and to control the size and shape of the x-ray beam.

The principal attachment to the tube housing is the *collimator*, a box-like device mounted beneath the opening of the housing. Collimators allow the radiographer to vary the size of the radiation field and to indicate with a light beam the size, location, and center of the field. There is usually a centering light that helps align the cassette tray as well (Figure 47-13).

X-ray Tube Support. The tube housing may be attached to a ceiling mount or a tube stand. Both types of mountings provide support and mobility for the tube. The ceiling mount (Figure 47-14) moves on a system of tracks to allow positioning of the tube at locations throughout the room. This type of tube mount facilitates

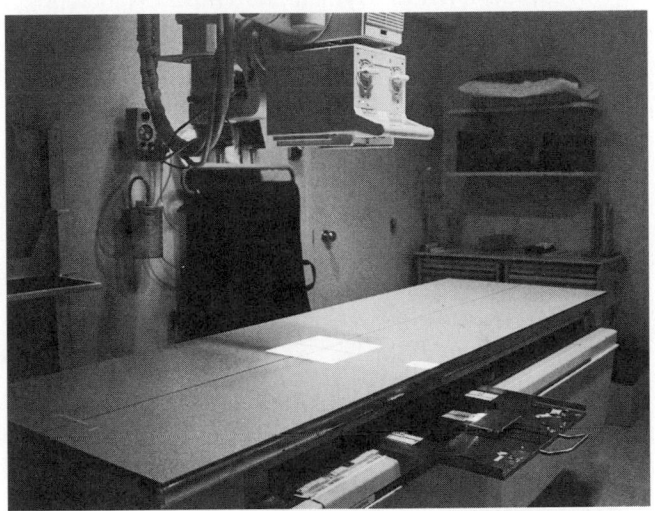

FIGURE 47-13   Collimator light beam demonstrates the radiation field and aids in aligning the cassette tray. (From Hunkele MM: *Radiography essentials for limited practice*, Philadelphia, 2001, WB Saunders.)

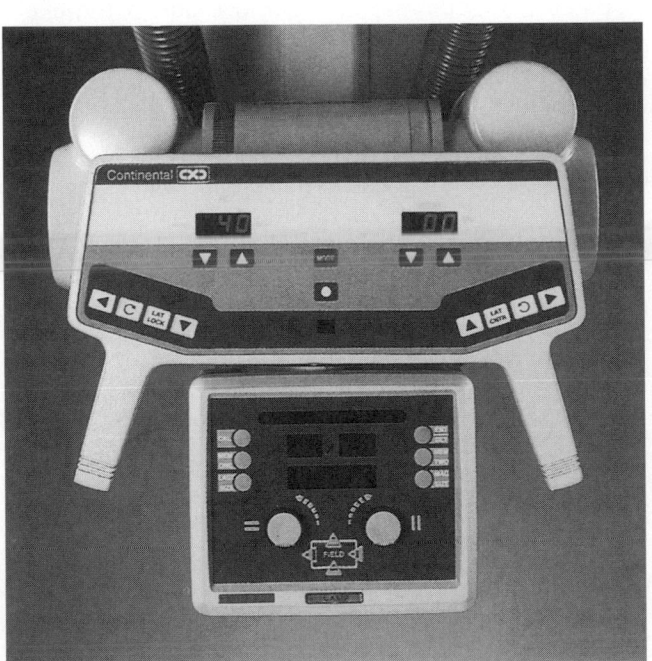

FIGURE 47-12   X-ray tube housing and collimator. (From Hunkele MM: *Radiography essentials for limited practice*, Philadelphia, 2001, WB Saunders.)

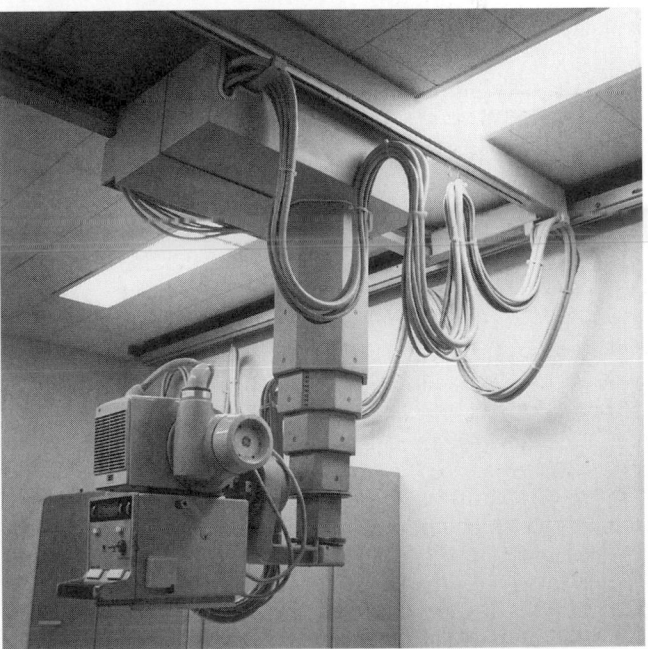

FIGURE 47-14   Ceiling-mount tube support. (From Hunkele MM: *Radiography essentials for limited practice*, Philadelphia, 2001, WB Saunders.)

positioning the tube over a stretcher or placement in various locations. A tube stand (Figure 47-15) is a vertical support with a horizontal arm that suspends the tube over the radiographic table. The tube stand rolls along a track that is secured to the floor (and sometimes also the ceiling), allowing horizontal motion. Outpatient x-ray departments are more likely to have a tube stand.

A system of electric locks holds the tube in position. The control system for all, or most, of these locks is an attachment on the front of the tube housing. To move the tube in any direction, the locking device must be released. Moving the tube without first releasing the lock may damage the lock, making it impossible to secure the tube in position. *Do not attempt to move the tube without first releasing the appropriate lock.* Typical tube motions include:

- Longitudinal—along the long axis of the table
- Transverse—across the table, at right angles to longitudinal
- Vertical—up and down, increasing or decreasing the distance between the tube and the table
- Roll (tilt, angle)—permits angulation of the tube along the longitudinal axis and also allows the tube to be aimed at the wall, rather than the table
- Rotation—allows the entire tube support to turn on its axis, changing the direction in which the tube arm is extended

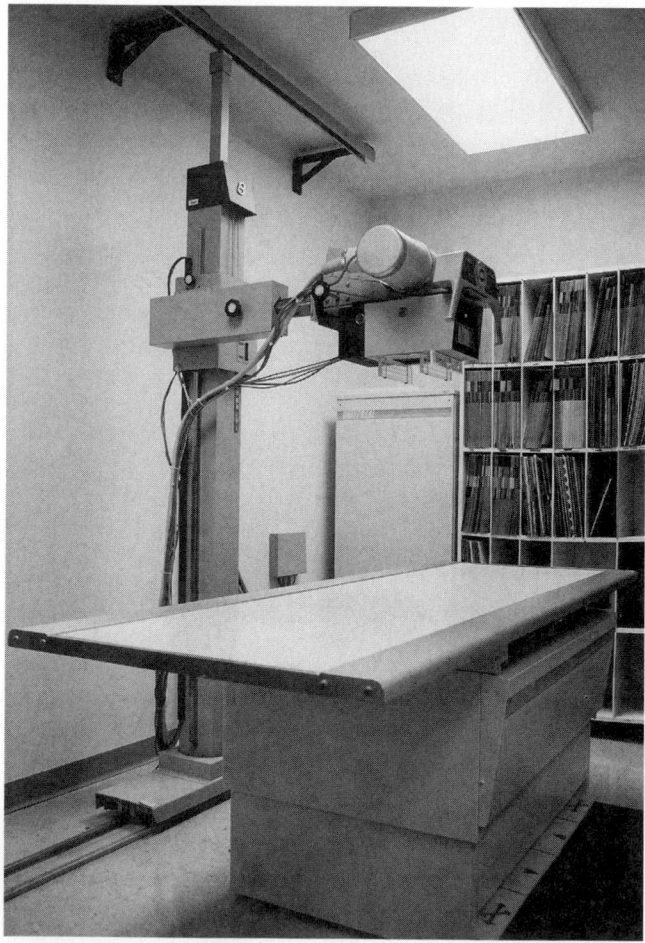

FIGURE 47-15 Tube stand. (From Hunkele MM: *Radiography essentials for limited practice*, Philadelphia, 2001, WB Saunders.)

Radiographic Table. The radiographic table is a specialized unit that is more than just a support for the patient. Some tables are adjustable in height for easy patient access, and some are designed to tilt into upright and Trendelenburg positions. A floating tabletop is a feature that assists in aligning the patient to the tube and film.

SCATTER RADIATION

- Radiation that is scattered or created as a result of the interaction of the primary x-ray beam with the patient or other matter in its path.
- Scatter radiation travels in all directions from the scattering medium and is very difficult to control. Generally, it has less energy than the primary beam.

Grids and Buckys. Beneath the table surface is a moving grid device called a **bucky** (Figure 47-16). The bucky device incorporates the cassette tray that holds the film. The entire unit can be moved along the length of the table and locked into position where desired. The grid is situated between the tabletop and the film. It is a plate made of tissue-thin lead strips, mounted on edge to protect the film from being fogged by scatter radiation that emanates mainly from the patient. Because the strips must be carefully aligned to the path of the primary x-ray beam, precise alignment of the x-ray tube is essential. The bucky device moves the grid during the exposure so that it is not visible on the radiograph. When the table has a floating tabletop, the bucky mechanism and film tray do not move with the tabletop.

Stationary grids that do not move during the exposure are used for the same purpose. A grid may also be incorporated into the front of a special cassette called a grid cassette, which is useful for mobile radiography and other special applications. Grids or buckys are generally used only for body parts that measure more than 10 to 12 cm in thickness. (The average adult's neck or knee measures 12 cm.) When a grid is not needed, the cassette is placed on the tabletop.

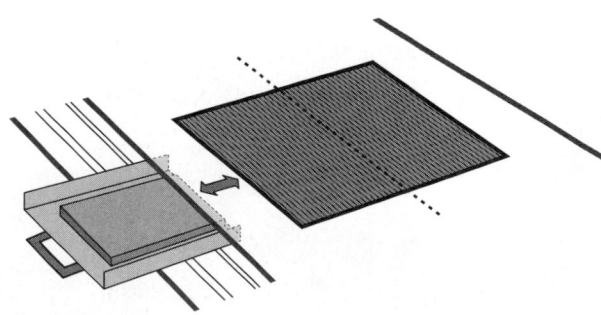

FIGURE 47-16 A bucky grid is under the surface of the x-ray table. (From Hunkele MM: *Radiography essentials for limited practice*, Philadelphia, 2001, WB Saunders.)

SAFETY PRECAUTIONS WHEN MOVING X-RAY EQUIPMENT

- Be sure that footboard and shoulder guard are secure before tilting a table with a patient.
- Check that no equipment is under the table before tilting it.
- Release locks before attempting to move the x-ray tube.
- Move the x-ray tube out of the way before assisting a patient to or from the table to avoid injuring the patient.
- Be sure that equipment is in a safe position before shutting off power to the locks.

Upright Cassette Holder. The upright cassette holder, as its name implies, is a device to hold the film in the upright position for radiography. It is usually placed against a wall, and its height is adjustable. It may incorporate a bucky or stationary grid. When a grid is included, the unit may be referred to as a *grid cabinet* or *upright bucky*. When the patient is to be sitting or standing at the upright cassette holder for radiography, the tube is angled to face the wall and cassette holder. The distance from the tube to the film may be adjusted to 40 inches or to 72 inches, depending on the requirements of the procedure.

Control Console. The control console, located in the control booth, is the access point for the radiographer to determine the exposure factors and to initiate the exposure (Figure 47-17). Radiographic control consoles have buttons, switches, dials, or digital readouts for some or all of the following functions:

- Off/On—controls the power to the control panel
- mA—allows the operator to set the milliamperage (mA), the rate at which the x-rays are produced
- kVp—controls the kilovoltage (kVp) determining the penetrating power of the x-ray beam
- Timer—controls the duration of the exposure
- mAs—some units have an mAs control instead of mA and time settings.
- Bucky—activates the motor control of the bucky device so that the grid will move during the exposure
- Automatic exposure controls—special settings available on certain units that allow termination of exposure when a certain quantity of radiation has reached the film
- Meters or digital readouts to indicate the status of the settings
- Prep (ready or rotor) switch—prepares the tube for exposure and must be continuously activated until exposure is complete
- Exposure switch—initiates the exposure and must be continuously activated until the exposure is complete
- Accessories—other controls may also be present, depending on the equipment and its specific features

Image Receptor Systems

Cassettes and Intensifying Screens. The cassette (Figure 47-18) serves as the film holder during the radiographic procedure. It provides a light-tight, rigid structure to protect the film and also houses the intensifying screens. Most cassettes contain two intensifying screens, one front and one back, and the film is sandwiched between them. Intensifying screens are plates

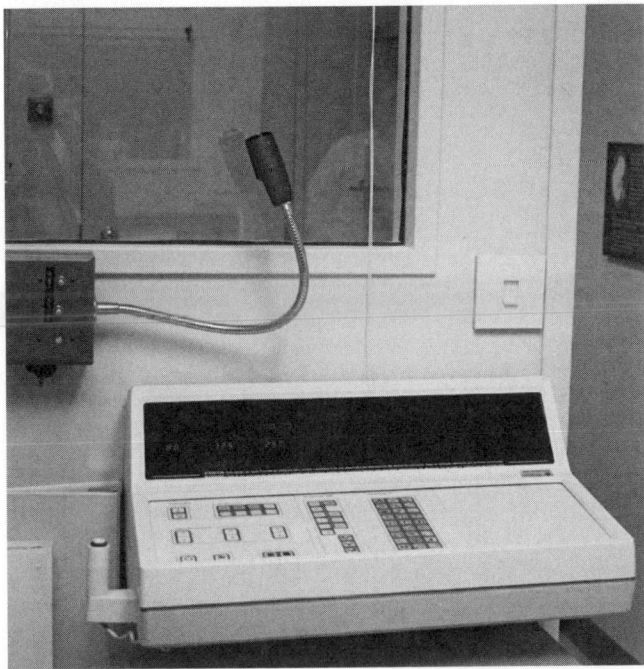

FIGURE 47-17   X-ray control console. (From Hunkele MM: *Radiography essentials for limited practice*, Philadelphia, 2001, WB Saunders.)

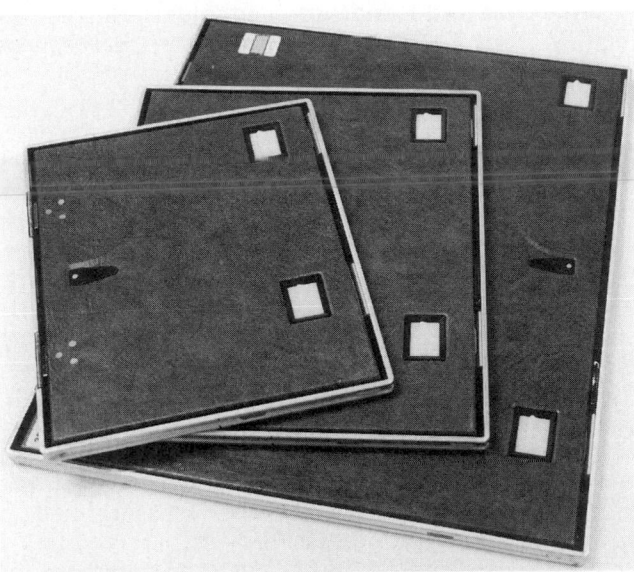

FIGURE 47-18   X-ray cassettes. (From Hunkele MM: *Radiography essentials for limited practice*, Philadelphia, 2001, WB Saunders.)

coated with **phosphors** (fluorescent crystals) that give off light when exposed to x-rays. Their purpose is to reduce the amount of exposure required. Without intensifying screens, as much as 50 to 100 times more exposure would be needed. Intensifying screens greatly reduce patient dose.

Each cassette has a small area where there is no intensifying screen and where exposure is blocked from the film by lead foil. This area is reserved for the photographic imprint of the patient identification. Its location is indicated on the front of the cassette by the position of the identifying label.

Intensifying screens are quite expensive and are easily damaged. Damaged areas, dirt, or stains on the screens prevent light from exposing the film and result in artifacts on the image. For these reasons, it is important to avoid touching the screens and to keep the film processing area free of dust and dirt.

Film. Radiographic film is manufactured with a particular sensitivity to the light emitted by intensifying screens. Green sensitive film is used with screens that emit green light, and blue sensitive film is matched with blue-emitting screens. Film for routine radiography has emulsion coated on both sides of the base so that the film responds to the light from both intensifying screens. This double-emulsion system decreases the exposure required by half. Because both sides of the film are identical, there is no "right" or "wrong" side to a sheet of double-emulsion film.

Film and cassettes come in standard sizes. You will work more effectively in the clinical area when you have learned to recognize them at a glance. The most common sizes are:

- 8 × 10 inches (20 × 25 cm)
- 9 × 9 inches (23 × 23 cm)
- 10 × 12 inches (24 × 30 cm)
- 11 × 14 inches (28 × 35 cm)
- 7 × 17 inches (18 × 43 cm)
- 14 × 14 inches (35 × 35 cm)
- 14 × 17 inches (36 × 43 cm)

Film Care and Handling. Film must be stored correctly to avoid fog, a generalized exposure that reduces image quality. A good storage area is clean, cool, and dry, protected from radiation and processing chemical fumes. Film boxes should stand on edge with the expiration date visible. This date is checked to ensure that older film is used before its expiration date.

To avoid artifacts from improper film handling, be sure your hands are clean and dry, and touch only the corner of the film when removing it from the cassette. Avoid bending and crimping or scraping the film by allowing it to hang vertically when holding it with only one hand (Figure 47-19). To place it horizontally, use both hands and hold by opposite corners.

Film Processing. A comprehensive darkroom orientation is needed before you try to develop patient films. It is especially important to know how to turn on the processor properly and to know when it has warmed up sufficiently for correct processing.

The exposed cassette is taken to the darkroom for processing under safelight conditions. Safelights provide a red or orange light that is quite dim but provides just

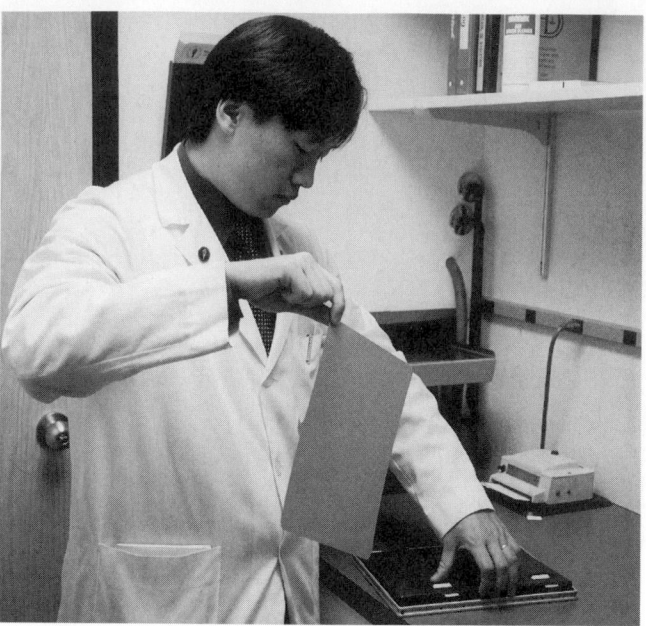

FIGURE 47-19 When holding film with one hand, let it hang vertically. (From Hunkele MM: *Radiography essentials for limited practice*, Philadelphia, 2001, WB Saunders.)

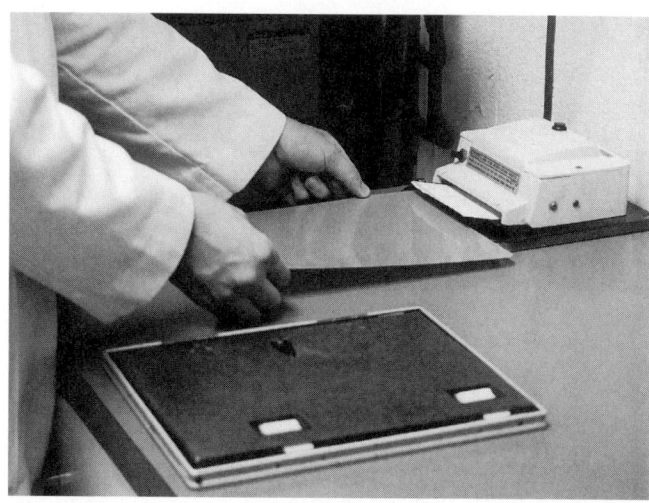

FIGURE 47-20 Film is inserted into printer to stamp it with identification from the printer card. (From Hunkele MM: *Radiography essentials for limited practice*, Philadelphia, 2001, WB Saunders.)

enough illumination for you to see where things are located. Make sure the darkroom door is locked so that no one will open it while you are processing the film.

Film identification is essential for knowing the identity of the patient represented in the image and the date and location of the examination. Serious errors in diagnosis and treatment might occur if films are not correctly identified. The identification information is typed on a card that is inserted into the photographic printer in the darkroom. The printer is used to stamp the information on the film after it is removed from the cassette and before it is processed (Figure 47-20).

The film is then fed into the automatic processor. The cassette is reloaded with one (and only one) sheet of fresh film (Figure 47-21) from the film bin, a storage unit located under the counter. A tone or a red light on the processor will indicate when it is safe to feed another film or to turn on the lights.

The reloaded cassette should be immediately returned to the proper place so that it is ready for use. Correct locations for cassettes are essential because it is not possible to determine by looking at the cassette whether the film is exposed. Only by following the established routines can you be confident that a cassette is unexposed and ready for use.

Daylight Processing. Some departments have a "daylight" system to process film without a darkroom. These systems include a special film processor and a daylight film identification camera, and they use special cassettes. Films can be identified while still in the cassette, and then the entire cassette is fed into the processor. The processor removes and processes the film and reloads the cassette.

Computed and Digital Radiography. Computed radiography (CR) is a radiographic imaging system that does not use film. An image receptor, similar to an intensifying screen, is exposed in a special cassette using conventional x-ray equipment. The radiographer inserts the exposed cassette into a special processor and selects the type of examination from a menu so that the image will be processed correctly. A small beam from a high-intensity laser in the processor converts the latent image to a visible image that is converted into an electronic signal and stored in a computer. The image can then be displayed on a high-resolution monitor. Hard copies can be produced using a laser film printer.

Digital radiography is another type of filmless imaging system. Special radiographic tables and upright cabinets contain digital receptors that react to the pattern of the radiation from the patient and transmit a digital signal directly to the computer system. No cassettes and no processing are involved. Although digital radiography has for some time been used for special applications such as fluoroscopy and angiography, technical limitations and cost factors have prevented widespread adoption of digital systems for general radiography.

Once stored in the computer system, digital images from either CR or digital radiography are organized and cataloged and can be accessed on screen from multiple locations connected to the system network. These digital images can be manipulated electronically to enhance visibility. Conventional radiographs can be added to the system by scanning them with a laser device called a film digitizer.

The computer hardware and software technology used to manage digital images in hospitals and large health care systems is called a picture archiving and communication system (PACS). These systems provide image storage, connect images with patient database information, facilitate laser printing of images, and display both images and information at workstations throughout the network as needed. PACS may include transmission equipment for teleradiology, allowing images to be viewed in remote locations such as a physician's home and receiving images from remote locations such as outlying clinics. PACS technology can transmit images directly over telephone lines and via the Internet.

Radiation Safety

Radiation Units

Two systems are used to measure radiation and radiation dose: the conventional (British) system and the international *(Système International [SI])* units established in 1981. The conventional system is still the most commonly used in the United States. Table 47-3 lists the units used in both systems. The reason for the measurement determines which unit is most appropriate.

The **roentgen (R)** is the conventional unit of radiation exposure. It represents a measurement of radiation intensity and is determined by the interaction of the x-ray beam with air. For example, an x-ray machine might produce 0.01 R during the exposure for a chest radiograph. The corresponding SI unit is **coulombs per kilogram (C/kg)**, specifying the electrical charge in coulombs produced by the exposure of 1 kg of dry air.

The roentgen is not a useful dose unit because dose varies with the depth of measurement and the quantity of radiation energy absorbed in the tissue that is exposed. To measure both therapeutic radiation doses and specific tissue doses received in diagnostic applications, the

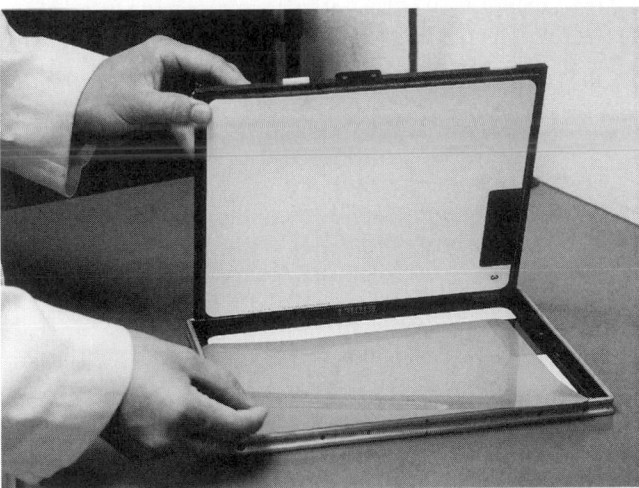

FIGURE 47-21   Reload cassette promptly with a fresh film. Make certain the film is properly situated and secure both latches. (From Hunkele MM: *Radiography essentials for limited practice,* Philadelphia, 2001, WB Saunders.)

TABLE 47-3	Radiation Units	
	Conventional Units	**SI Units**
Units of exposure	Roentgen (R)	Coulombs per kilogram (C/kg)
Units of dose	rad (radiation absorbed dose)	Gray (Gy) 1 Gy = 100 rad
Dose equivalent units	rem (roentgen equivalent in man)	Sievert (Sv) 1 Sv = 100 rem

conventional unit is the **rad**, which stands for *radiation absorbed dose*. It is usually qualified by the specific body part to which it applies. For example, a radiation oncologist may prescribe a treatment involving 150 rad to the pelvis. During the 0.01 R chest exposure, the patient may have received a dose of 0.004 rad *to the thyroid*. Examples of patient dose received in typical radiographic examinations are provided in Table 47-4. The SI unit for dose measurement is the **Gray (Gy)**.

The biological effect of radiation exposure varies according to the type of radiation involved and its energy; equal doses of various types of radiation will not necessarily result in equal biological effects. To measure occupational dose or other exposure that may involve more than one type of radiation, the dose equivalent unit used is the **rem**, which stands for *roentgen equivalent in man*. Dose equivalents are usually assumed to represent whole body dose or dose to unspecified tissues. The report sent by the laboratory that processes the personnel dosimeters will report occupational dose in rem. The SI unit for dose equivalent is the **Sievert (Sv)**.

Because the radiation quantities involved in diagnostic radiology are so small, units may be used that represent $1/1000$ of the common units: milliroentgen (mR), millirad (mrad), and millirem (mrem). It may be confusing to determine which units should be used in a given situation. This is made more difficult by the tendency of many radiographers to use the traditional roentgen, rad, and rem units interchangeably. This practice does not cause serious inaccuracy when speaking only of diagnostic x-rays because exposure to 1 roentgen of x-ray energy will result in approximately 1 rad of absorbed dose, which is equal to a dose equivalent of 1 rem.

Effects of Low-Dose Radiation Exposure

Cellular Response to Exposure. Most cellular effects of radiation exposure are extremely short lived because chemical alterations within the cells are quickly repaired. Even if a cell dies, cell death is an insignificant injury unless the number of cells involved is massive. Some cells may sustain damage that requires several days for the body to repair. The body produces special enzymes that function to repair the DNA protein molecules. Sometimes a cell may be damaged in such a way that its DNA "programming" is changed and the cell no longer behaves normally. This type of injury may eventually result in the runaway production of new, abnormal cells, causing a tumor or malignant blood disease.

The relative sensitivity of different types of cells is summarized in the laws of Bergonie and Tribondeau, which state that cell sensitivity to radiation exposure depends on four characteristics of the cell:

1. *Age:* Younger cells are more sensitive than older ones.
2. *Differentiation:* Simple cells are more sensitive than highly complex ones.
3. *Metabolic rate:* Cells that use energy rapidly are more sensitive than those that have a slower metabolism.
4. *Mitotic rate:* Cells that divide and multiply rapidly are more sensitive than those that replicate slowly.

TABLE 47-4	Typical Doses for Radiographic Examinations		
Examination	Entrance Skin Exposure (mrad)	Mean Marrow Dose (mrad)	Gonad Dose (mrad)
Skull	200	10	< 1
Chest	10	2	< 1
Cervical spine	150	10	< 1
Lumbar spine	300	60	225
Abdomen	400	30	125
Pelvis	150	20	150
Extremity	50	2	< 1

According to these laws, blood cells and blood-producing cells are very sensitive. Cells that are in contact with the environment are quite simple, have relatively short lives, and are quite sensitive. These include the cells of the skin and the mucosal lining of the mouth, nose, and gastrointestinal tract. Some glandular tissue is also particularly sensitive, especially that of the thyroid gland and the female breast. The tissues of embryos, fetuses, infants, children, and adolescents tend to be more sensitive than those of adults because of their age and their higher metabolic and mitotic rates. Nerve cells, which have a long life and are quite complex, are much less vulnerable to radiation injury. Cortical bone cells are also relatively insensitive.

Somatic Effects. Radiation effects may be classified as somatic or genetic. *Somatic* effects are those that occur to the body of the person who is irradiated. Whereas the effects of relatively high doses of radiation are immediate and predictable, the effects of the very low doses associated with radiography are considered long-term effects. They are not easily identified as radiation effects because they occur from 3 to 30 years after exposure and because these same effects also occur in the absence of radiation exposure. Only extensive research with large populations and computer analysis can demonstrate the role of radiation in causing these effects. In other words, radiation causes increased *risk* of these effects, but the effects cannot be predicted with respect to any one individual. Although the individual risk is extremely small, increasing exposure to the entire population poses public health risks that require the attention and concern of everyone involved in applying ionizing radiation to human beings.

The documented latent effects of low doses of ionizing radiation include the following:

- *Cataractogenesis:* The formation of cataracts, clouding of the lens of the eye. This effect concerns radiologists and radiographers who work extensively in fluoroscopy and those who perform other work that involves repeated exposure to the eyes.
- *Carcinogenesis:* Increased risk of malignant disease, particularly cancer of the skin, thyroid, and breast, and *leukemia*, a malignant blood disease associated with radiation exposure.
- *Life-span shortening:* A study of the life span of radiologists who died before 1945 showed that they had shorter life spans than physicians who

did not use radiation in their practices. This group included radiologists who had used radiation since the early days of x-ray science. More recent studies show that occupational exposure no longer has a measurable effect on the life span of radiologists. Nevertheless, because radiation exposure has been linked to life-span shortening, it is a public health concern and another reason to practice a high level of radiation safety.

Radiation and Pregnancy. Radiation exposure poses risks to the developing embryo or fetus. Research has demonstrated that excessive radiation during pregnancy may result in spontaneous abortion, congenital defects in the child, growth retardation, increased risk of cancer and leukemia in childhood, and an increase in significant genetic abnormalities in the children of parents who were exposed in utero. Studies of women exposed to radiation as a result of diagnostic and therapeutic procedures confirm that radiation in excess of 5 rad to the uterus is cause for some level of concern. This is more exposure than is received with most x-ray examinations, but these levels may be encountered with direct exposure to the pelvis, especially with CT examinations or fluoroscopic studies.

Genetic Effects. Genetic effects in the form of changes or mutations to the hereditary material of the reproductive cells may be caused when the ovaries or testes are exposed to radiation. In the female, all the ova cells that the individual will ever produce are present in an immature state at birth. Because no new egg cells are produced as the individual ages, the effect of radiation exposure to the ovaries is cumulative. The genetic effects of radiation to the testes also have a longer-term effect than may at first be presumed because damage to the stem cells that produce the sperm may result in continued production of sperm with the genetic mutation. Most genetic mutations are considered negative or less well suited to survival of the individual than nonmutated cells. Even when these changes are recessive (not apparent in the offspring), they may be passed on to future generations. Public health officials and governments are very concerned about preserving the integrity of the population's gene pool by minimizing harmful, defect-causing radiation, so radiation regulations include rules to minimize radiation dose to reproductive organs.

Radiation Protection

Clearly, exposure to x-rays creates some risk for both patients and radiographers; therefore it is essential for those who apply radiation to human beings to be knowledgeable about radiation safety and to use this knowledge to avoid all unnecessary radiation exposure to patients, to co-workers, and to themselves.

Personnel Safety. In diagnostic x-ray departments, a radiation hazard exists from possible exposure to radiation from the primary x-ray beam or from scatter radiation caused by interaction between the primary beam and the patient or other material in its path. Scatter radiation is present throughout the x-ray room during an exposure. X-rays travel at the speed of light.

They do not linger in the room after the exposure, and they are not capable of making the objects in the room radioactive. The only time a radiation hazard exists is during the x-ray exposure itself.

Because radiographers are considered to be "occupationally exposed individuals," they are prohibited from activities that would result in direct exposure to the primary x-ray beam. This means that they are not allowed to hold patients or cassettes during x-ray exposures and must stand clear of the path of the primary x-ray beam during fluoroscopic and mobile radiographic examinations. Whenever possible, patients should be immobilized without the need for someone to hold them. When infants or children must be held, a parent is usually the appropriate person to perform this duty.

Medical assistants may or may not be considered occupationally exposed persons, depending on their work assignments and the frequency with which they are involved with radiation use. Medical assistants who are not occupationally exposed may occasionally assist with procedures by holding patients or cassettes. When this is the case, the medical assistant should wear a lead apron and should avoid direct exposure from the primary x-ray beam, if possible (Figure 47-22). If the hands will be in the primary beam, lead gloves should also be worn.

Personnel are not exposed to any significant amount of radiation when standing well behind the protective lead barrier of the control booth. X-rays travel in straight lines and do not turn corners. Scatter radiation is not powerful enough to generate additional radiation of concern when it interacts with matter, so it is not necessary for the control booth to be sealed.

Occupational exposure increases when assisting with fluoroscopic procedures or using mobile x-ray equipment. The three principal methods used to protect personnel from unnecessary radiation exposure are time, distance, and shielding.

Because the amount of exposure received is directly proportional to the time spent in a radiation area, dose is decreased when this time is minimized. For example,

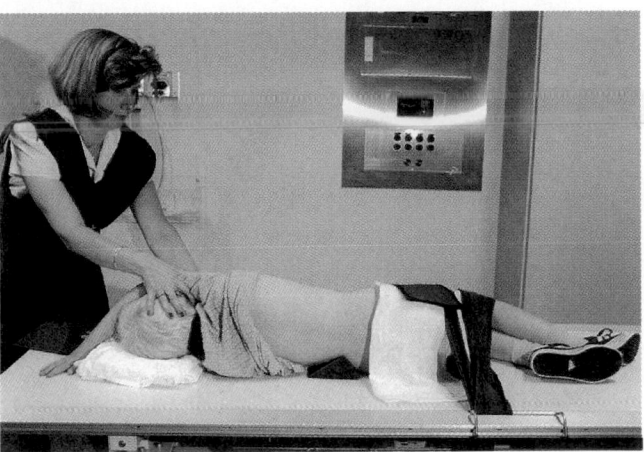

FIGURE 47-22   When holding child for radiographic procedure, wear a lead apron and stay as far from the primary x-ray beam as possible. (From Ballinger PW, Frank ED: *Merrill's atlas of radiographic positions and radiologic procedures*, ed 9, vol 3. St Louis, 1999, Mosby.)

you might shorten the time of exposure by stepping into the control booth during fluoroscopic procedures when not required to be near the patient.

The second method involves using distance. Increasing the distance between yourself and a radiation source decreases your exposure in proportion to the square of the distance, so small increases in distance have a relatively large effect. Mobile x-ray units have long cords on the exposure switches, enabling the radiographer to get as far from the radiation source as possible while making an exposure.

The third method is shielding and is by far the most common method of personnel protection used in outpatient radiography settings. The lead wall of the control booth provides a radiation safety barrier and is the principal defense for personnel. Other types of shielding include lead aprons, gloves, goggles, and thyroid shields. These types of shielding are worn during fluoroscopic procedures and mobile radiographic examinations.

A pre-exposure "safety check" is the method used to be certain that personnel are not accidentally exposed. This safety check ensures that only the required persons are in the x-ray room (usually this means only the patient), that everyone in the control booth is safely behind the lead barrier, and that the x-ray room door is closed. It is also wise to make sure that no cassettes have been left lying about because scatter radiation fog will damage the film. Only the cassette that is in immediate use should be in the x-ray room. X-ray room doors are usually left open or ajar except during exposures. A closed door indicates that it is not safe to enter.

PRE-EXPOSURE "SAFETY CHECK"

Before making an exposure, be *certain* that:
- The x-ray room door is closed
- No nonessential persons are in the x-ray room
- All persons in the control booth are completely behind the lead barrier
- No cassettes are in the room except the one in use

Personnel Monitoring. Devices for monitoring radiation exposure to personnel are called **dosimeters**. They should be worn in the region of the collar and should be outside the lead apron when a lead apron is worn.

Three basic types of dosimeters are commonly used in radiography: film badges, thermoluminescent dosimeters (TLDs), and optically stimulated luminescence dosimeters (OSLs). A film badge consists of one or two pieces of dental film, paper-wrapped and enclosed in a badge-like holder that incorporates several filters. The disadvantage of this type of dosimeter is that the dental film is subject to fog when exposed to heat or fumes, and this exposure could result in a false reading. TLD badges contain one or more lithium fluoride crystals that absorb radiation energy and then emit the energy in the form of light when heated. They are more

durable than film badges and respond only to ionizing radiation exposure. OSL refers to the most recently developed monitoring dosimeter (Figure 47-23), which uses aluminum oxide as the radiation detector. This device provides greater stability and precision plus the ability to reanalyze and confirm results.

Radiation monitor badge service laboratories provide badges, processing service, and reports and keep permanent records of the radiation exposure of each person monitored. Service may be arranged on a weekly, monthly, or quarterly basis. Personnel who receive relatively high doses of occupational exposure change their badges most frequently. Occupationally exposed personnel who are always or nearly always in a control booth during exposures are usually best monitored with quarterly service. Monthly service is a better choice for those who work in fluoroscopy or use mobile x-ray equipment.

Service companies provide an extra badge in every batch that is marked "CONTROL." This badge's purpose is to measure any radiation exposure to the entire batch while in transit. Any amount of exposure measured from the control badge will be subtracted from the amounts measured from the other badges in the batch. The control badge should be kept in a safe place, away from any possibility of x-ray exposure. *It should never be used to measure occupational dose or for any other purpose.*

Exposure reports are sent to the subscriber for each batch, and an annual summary of personnel exposure is also provided. Personnel should be advised of the radiation exposure reported from their badges and should be provided with copies of the annual reports for their own records. Personnel exposed to radiation should not leave their employment without a complete record of their radiation exposure history. Employers are required to provide this information.

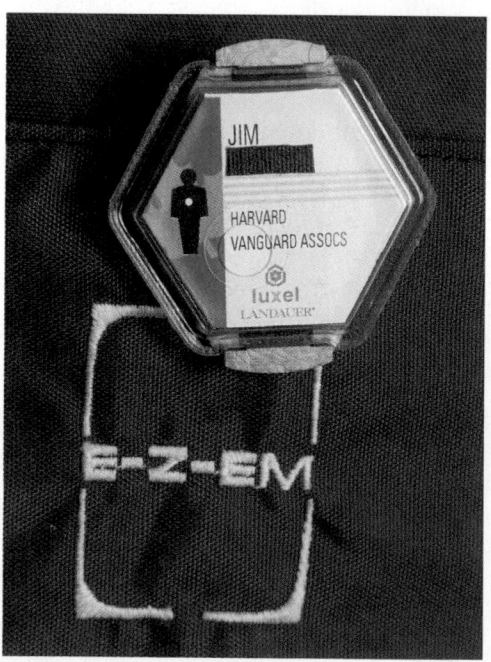

FIGURE 47-23 Optically stimulated luminescence (OSL) dosimeter.

Effective Dose Equivalent Limits. The ALARA principle is the guiding philosophy associated with all radiation use that involves exposure to humans, both patients and workers. It states that all radiation exposure to humans should be limited to levels that are *As Low As Reasonably Achievable.*

The effective dose equivalent (EDE) limiting system is used to calculate the upper limit of occupational exposure that is permitted. For occupationally exposed personnel, the EDE limit is 5 rem (50 mSv) per year. This applies to workers over the age of 18 who are not pregnant and is assumed to be a whole body dose. These limits apply to occupational exposure only and not to exposure that workers may receive as a result of imaging or tests related to their own healthcare.

The established EDE limits ensure that the safety of radiation workers is comparable to that of workers in other safe occupations. The allowable exposure is considered to be so low as to pose an insignificant risk. The occupational exposure received by radiographers is usually well below the established limit.

Occupational Precautions During Pregnancy. Radiation control agencies address the issue of radiation exposure to pregnant radiation workers. The EDE limit of whole-body radiation for the pregnant worker is 0.5 rem over the 9-month course of the pregnancy. When a worker declares that she is pregnant by submitting a written document to her employer, the employer is responsible for providing fetal radiation monitoring and for ensuring that the occupational dose does not exceed the EDE limit for pregnant workers. Here again, the ALARA principle is important. Every effort should be made to minimize exposure, keeping the dose as far below the limit as possible.

For a pregnant radiographer, the safest work assignment would be one in which a permanent lead barrier (control booth) always shields the worker during exposures. Pregnant radiographers, or those of childbearing age who may be pregnant, should pay particular attention to personal safety measures when assisting with fluoroscopy or using mobile x-ray equipment.

Patient Protection

This topic is addressed thoroughly in educational programs for radiographers. The following methods are employed to minimize radiation dose to patients:

- Avoid errors. Double-check requisitions and patient identification so that the right patient gets the right examination.
- Establish good routine procedures and follow them strictly so that careless errors do not necessitate repeat exposures.
- Collimate. Use the smallest radiation field that will encompass the area of clinical interest. In no case should the size of the radiation field be greater than the size of the film.
- Use the highest kVp that is consistent with acceptable film quality. This permits using the least possible mAs to obtain an acceptable exposure.
- Use at least 40 inches SID. This practice limits patient exposure from tube housing leakage and collimator scatter.
- Use the fastest films and screens consistent with the necessary film quality.
- Provide shielding for gonads, eyes, breasts, and thyroid, as appropriate.

Gonad Shielding. Lead shields that prevent unnecessary radiation to the reproductive organs are required when the patient is of reproductive age or younger, whenever the gonads are within the primary radiation field, and when the shield will not interfere with the examination. This applies to most patients under the age of 55 years. A shield device consisting of at least a 0.5 mm lead or equivalent is placed between the x-ray tube and the patient. Shields attached to the collimator (shadow shields) may be positioned by viewing their shadows within the collimator light field. Shields placed on or near the patient's body are referred to as contact shields and are somewhat more effective than shadow shields. Both types meet the legal requirements for gonad shielding. The female shield is placed with its lower margin at the level of the pubic symphysis (Figure 47-24). The male shield is positioned with its upper margin about 1 inch

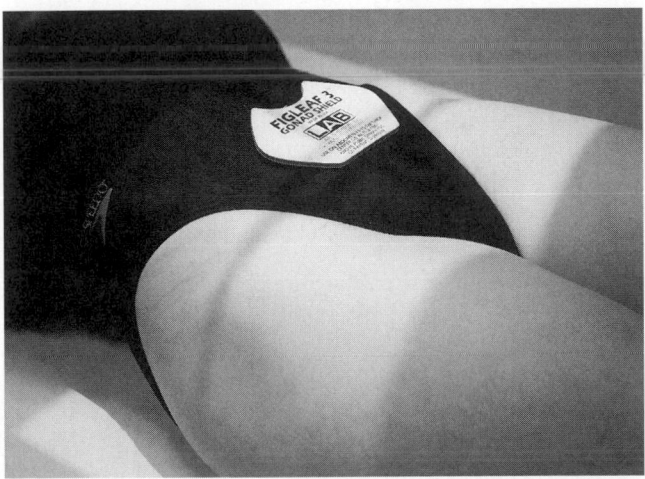
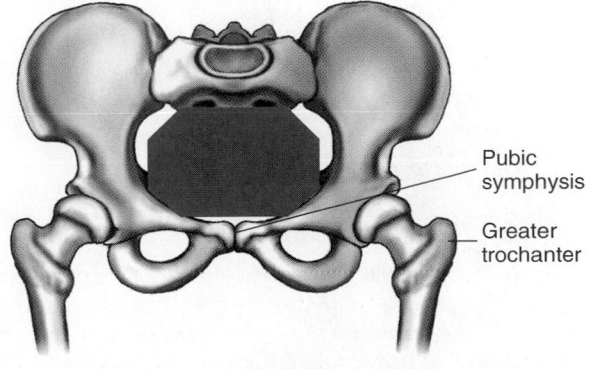

Pubic symphysis

Greater trochanter

FIGURE 47-24   When precise gonad shielding is required for females, place the lower margin of the shield on the upper margin of the pubic symphysis. (From Hunkele MM: *Radiography essentials for limited practice,* Philadelphia, 2001, WB Saunders.)

below the pubic symphysis (Figure 47-25). It is helpful to note that the pubic symphysis is at about the same level as the greater trochanter of the femur, avoiding the necessity of palpating the pubic symphysis for proper shield placement.

Pregnant or Potentially Pregnant Patients. The greatest risks for spontaneous abortion, fetal death, and significant birth defects exist when significant levels of exposure occur during the first trimester of pregnancy. The embryo is most vulnerable to radiation insult while tissues are in the process of differentiation. Unfortunately, this creates the greatest hazard at a time when a woman may not yet be aware she is pregnant.

The public is generally aware that x-rays should be avoided during pregnancy, and this may lead to irrational fears on the part of pregnant women or their families. The chance is extremely remote that a routine x-ray examination of the chest or an extremity would harm the developing child. On the other hand, examinations requiring direct radiation to the pelvis, especially relatively high-dose fluoroscopy studies or CT scans of the abdomen or lumbar spine, may be cause for concern.

Radiation control regulations require that female patients of childbearing age be advised of potential radiation hazards before x-ray examination. This requirement is usually met by posting signs in the radiology department advising women to tell the radiographer before the examination if they may be pregnant. These signs should be written in all languages commonly used in the community.

The patient's physician is in the best position to be aware of an early pregnancy. The patient's history may indicate the possibility of pregnancy, and specific questions to rule out pregnancy should be a part of any medical history that precedes the ordering of pelvic x-ray examinations. If pregnancy is a possibility, an early pregnancy test, easily and quickly performed in the physician's office, may clarify the situation. If the patient is pregnant and the proposed x-ray examination involves direct pelvic radiation, the physician must weigh the potential risks and benefits of the examination and discuss them with the patient before proceeding with

the study. In the case of minor or chronic complaints, it is common to delay the examination until after the child is born. In practice, however, the possibility of pregnancy may not even be considered. This is especially true with accident or injury, where the office visit is brief and the history is limited to the injury complaint. For this reason, it is essential to consider the possibility of pregnancy in any female of childbearing age and to ask specific questions to determine that the physician has addressed the issue of pregnancy before proceeding with the x-ray examination.

CRITICAL THINKING APPLICATION

Ingrid White is gowned and ready for a lumbar spine x-ray examination and Sara asks Ingrid whether there is any possibility that she might be pregnant. Ingrid confides that she and her husband have been trying to conceive for several months, and she is not sure whether she is currently pregnant. What should Sara do?

If an x-ray examination of a pregnant patient must be done, modifications in procedure can help to minimize the dose to the embryo or fetus. If the part to be examined is not the abdomen or pelvis, this area can be shielded with a lead apron. If the abdomen or pelvis is to be evaluated, the number of views or the size of the radiation field may be minimized, resulting in less radiation exposure than that required for a routine procedure. The decision to do a limited study and the determination of the exact limitations to be imposed are prerogatives of the physician.

Radiographic Positioning

Radiographic positioning requires an understanding of commonly used terms. Terms that indicate the surfaces,

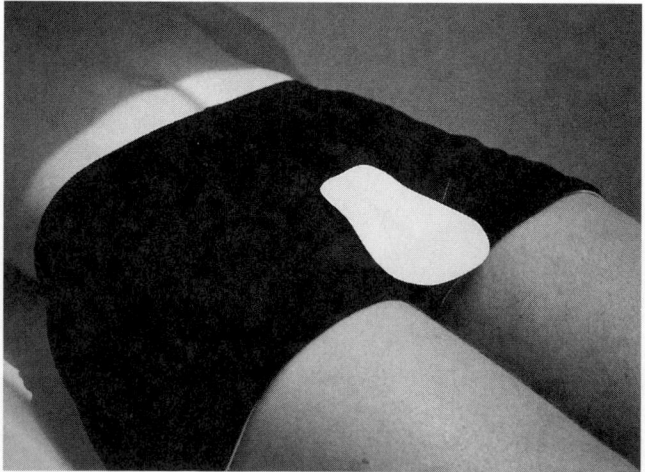
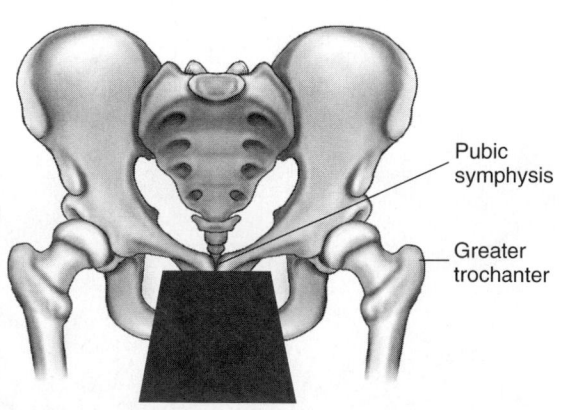

Pubic symphysis

Greater trochanter

FIGURE 47-25 When precise gonad shielding is required for males, place the upper margin of the shield one inch below the pubic symphysis. (From Hunkele MM: *Radiography essentials for limited practice*, Philadelphia, 2001, WB Saunders.)

directions, and planes of various body locations are based on *anatomical position*.

In anatomical position, the subject is standing, facing the observer, with the palms of the hands forward (Figure 47-26). The terms in the list that follows are used to accurately describe locations on and within the body:

- *Anterior:* Forward or front portion of the body or body part
- *Cephalic, cephalad:* Pertaining to the head; toward the head
- *Caudal, caudad:* Away from the head; the opposite of cephalad
- *Distal:* Away from the source or point of origin. For example, the wrist is *distal* to the elbow, being farther from the point of origin of the arm, which is the shoulder.
- *External:* To the outside, at or near the surface of the body or a body part
- *Inferior:* Below, farther from the head
- *Internal:* Deep, near the center of the body or a part; the opposite of external
- *Lateral:* Referring to the side, away from the center to the left or right
- *Medial or mesial:* Toward the center of the body or of a body part; the opposite of lateral
- *Palmar:* Referring to the palm (anterior surface) of the hand
- *Plantar:* Referring to the sole of the foot
- *Posterior:* Backward or back portion of the body or body part; the opposite of anterior
- *Proximal:* Toward the source or point of origin; the opposite of distal
- *Superior:* Above, toward the head; the opposite of inferior

Procedures for radiographic positioning are described using body planes (Figure 47-27). The **sagittal plane** divides the body into right and left parts; the *midsagittal* or *median sagittal plane* divides the body into *equal* right and left parts. The **coronal plane** divides the body into anterior and posterior parts. The *midcoronal* or *midfrontal plane* divides the body into relatively equal parts; it passes through the *external auditory meatus* (the opening of the ear), the center of the shoulder, the *greater trochanter* (the bony prominence in the lateral hip area), and the lateral malleolus (the bony prominence on the lateral surface of the ankle). The **transverse plane** divides the body into superior and inferior portions. It may be drawn at any level.

Body Positions

The following terms are used to describe body positions.

- *Prone:* Lying face down
- *Recumbent:* Lying down. The position may be further described by adding the name of the body surface on which the patient is lying:
  - *Dorsal recumbent:* lying on the back, supine
  - *Lateral recumbent:* lying on the side
  - *Ventral recumbent:* lying face down, prone
- *Supine:* lying face up
- *Upright:* standing or seated

Projections

A radiographic projection indicates the relative positions of the body part, film, and x-ray tube for an exposure.

For a **frontal projection**, the coronal plane of the body or body part is parallel to the film plane and the central ray is perpendicular to both. If the patient is supine, or facing the x-ray tube, the projection is said to be **anteroposterior (AP)** (Figure 47-28). If the patient is prone, or facing the film, the projection is said to **posteroanterior (PA)** (Figure 47-29). Note that these terms indicate the direction of the x-ray beam, from front to back, or back to front.

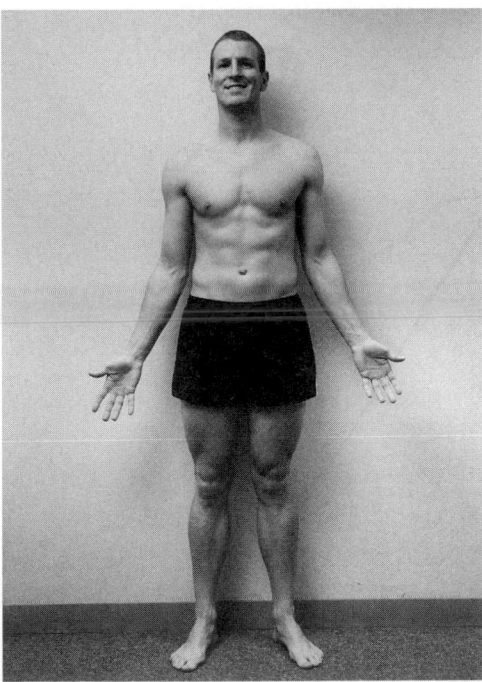

FIGURE 47-26   Anatomical position. (From Hunkele MM: *Radiography essentials for limited practice*, Philadelphia, 2001, WB Saunders.)

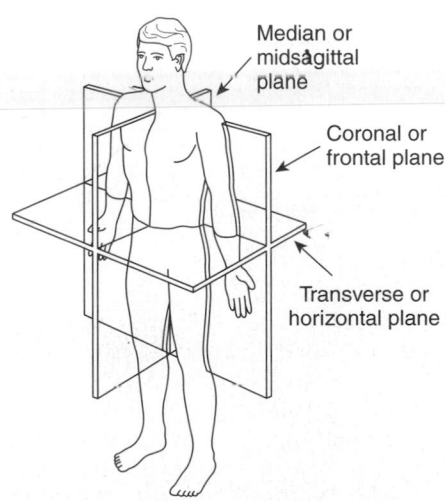

Median or midsagittal plane

Coronal or frontal plane

Transverse or horizontal plane

FIGURE 47-27   Body planes. (From Hunkele MM: *Radiography essentials for limited practice*, Philadelphia, 2001, WB Saunders.)

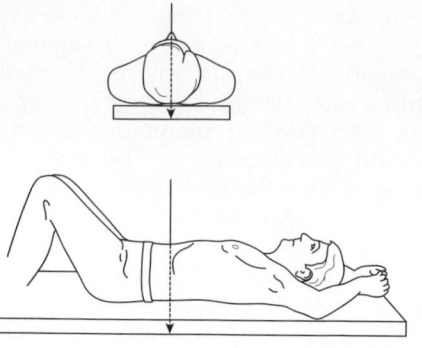

FIGURE 47-28 Anteroposterior (AP) projection. (From Hunkele MM: *Radiography essentials for limited practice*, Philadelphia, 2001, WB Saunders.)

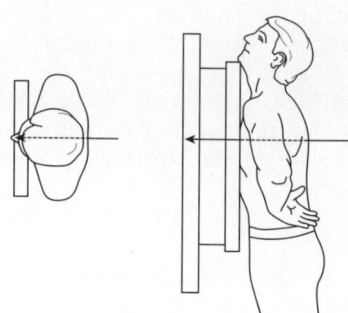

FIGURE 47-29 Posteroanterior (PA) projection. (From Hunkele MM: *Radiography essentials for limited practice*, Philadelphia, 2001, WB Saunders.)

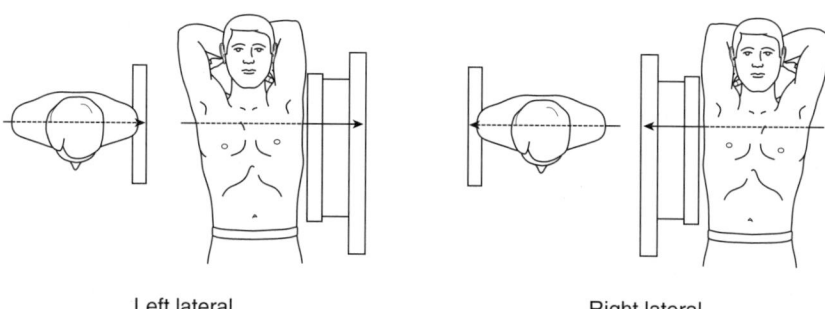

Left lateral   Right lateral

FIGURE 47-30 Lateral projections are named for the side of the body nearest the film. (From Hunkele MM: *Radiography essentials for limited practice*, Philadelphia, 2001, WB Saunders.)

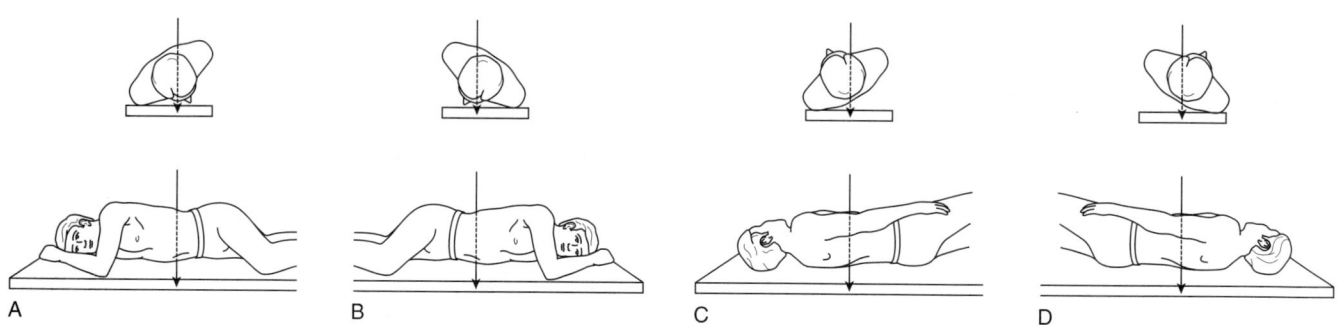

A   B   C   D

FIGURE 47-31 Oblique projections. **A**, Right anterior oblique (RAO). **B**, Left anterior oblique (LAO). **C**, Left posterior oblique (LPO). **D**, Right posterior oblique (RPO). (From Hunkele MM: *Radiography essentials for limited practice*, Philadelphia, 2001, WB Saunders.)

Lateral projections are those in which the sagittal plane of the body or body part is parallel to the film. Lateral projections are always named for the side of the patient that is nearest the film (Figure 47-30).

Oblique projections are those in which the body or part is rotated so that the projection is neither frontal nor lateral. Oblique projections, also, are named for the part of the body that is nearest the film. For example, in a right anterior oblique (RAO) projection, the patient's right, anterior aspect is closest to the film. Figure 47-31 illustrates all four oblique projections: RAO, right posterior oblique (RPO), left anterior oblique (LAO), and left posterior oblique (LPO).

Axial projections, sometimes referred to as semiaxial projections, are radiographs taken with a longitudinal angulation of the x-ray beam. The x-ray beam is angled along the long axis of the body, either cephalad (toward the head) or caudad (away from the head) (Figure 47-32).

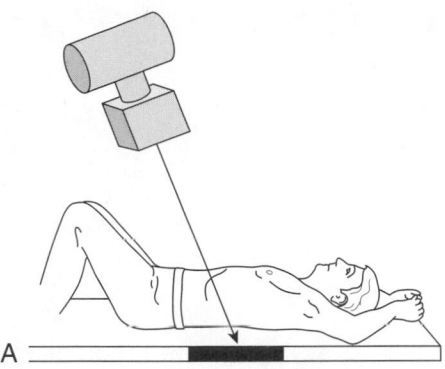
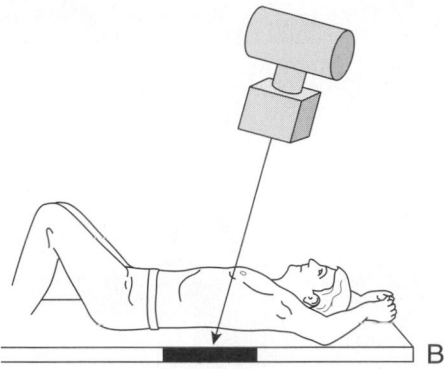

FIGURE 47-32 Axial projections use angulation of the x-ray tube to direct the central ray along the long axis of the body or part. **A**, Cephalad angulation. **B**, Caudad angulation. (From Hunkele MM: *Radiography essentials for limited practice*, Philadelphia, 2001, WB Saunders.)

Basic Radiographic Procedure

Patient Preparation and Explanation

Before a patient is x-rayed, a physician examines the patient and one or more specific x-ray procedures are ordered. The patient should receive an explanation of the procedure and consent to it. This may be handled by the physician or may be delegated to the medical assistant. In most cases, continued acceptance of the procedure is adequate evidence of consent. In some facilities, however, patients may be asked to sign a consent form. If it is your duty to explain the procedure and obtain consent, be certain that you understand the procedure and are prepared to answer patient questions (Procedure 47-1).

PROCEDURE **47-1**

General Procedure for X-Ray Examination

GOAL: To assist with an x-ray examination under the supervision of a physician.

EQUIPMENT AND SUPPLIES

- Physician's order for an x-ray examination
- Patient identification card to imprint radiographs
- X-ray machine
- X-ray cassettes, loaded with film
- Appropriate accessory items for patient comfort and shielding
- X-ray darkroom with automatic processor

PROCEDURAL STEPS

1 Check order and equipment needed. Ascertain whether any special preparations are needed.

2 Introduce yourself, and confirm the identity of the patient. Ascertain whether any necessary preparations were implemented.
   Purpose: If special preparations were not followed, the examination may need to be rescheduled.

3 Explain the procedure to the patient and respond appropriately to any questions or concerns.
   Purpose: Helps to reassure the patient and alleviates fear and anxiety.

4 Place the x-ray cassette correctly (Figure 1).

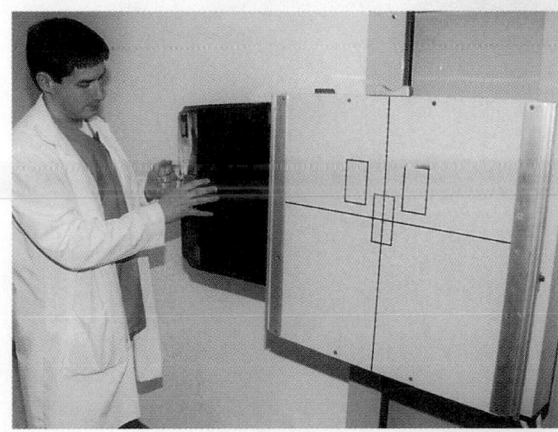

Figure 1

5 Check to make certain that the patient has removed all metal objects from the area to be examined.

Continued

PROCEDURE **47-1—cont'd**

Purpose: Metal objects appear on the film and may obscure important diagnostic information (Figure 2).

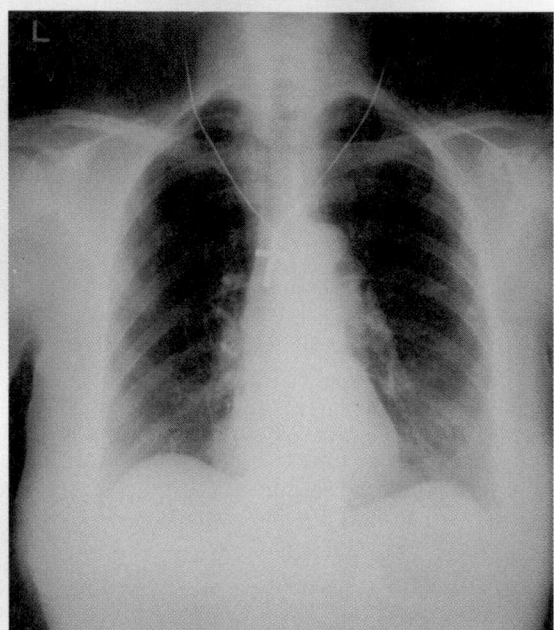

Figure 2

6 Position the patient properly, and immobilize the part, if necessary (Figure 3).

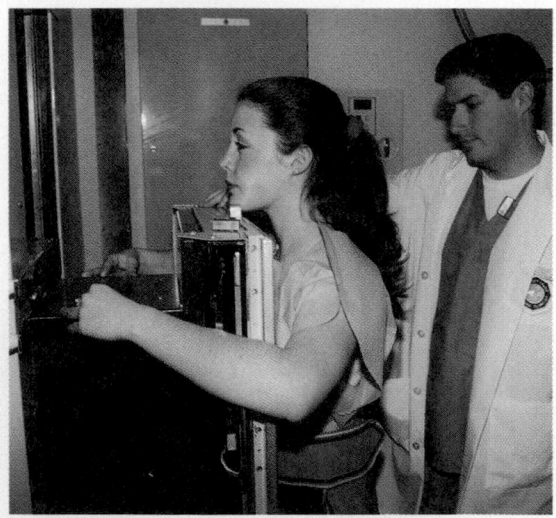

Figure 3

Purpose: Proper positioning and complete stillness are necessary to achieve a clear, readable radiograph.

7 Drape the patient as necessary, and shield the gonads if appropriate (Figure 4).

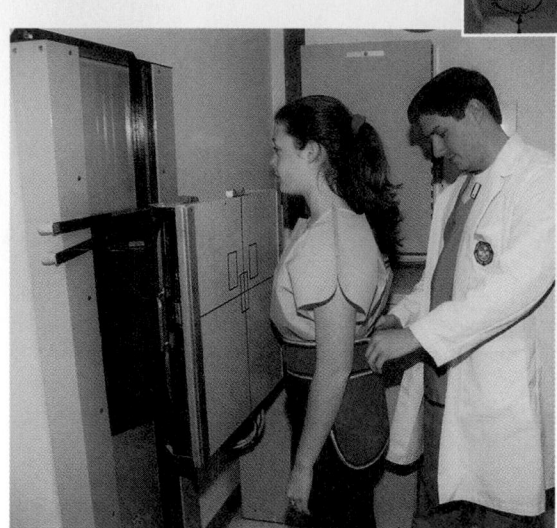

Figure 4

Purpose: Drapes provide warmth and protect patient's modesty; shields are required to minimize potential genetic radiation effects.

8 Align the x-ray tube to the cassette at the proper distance (Figure 5).

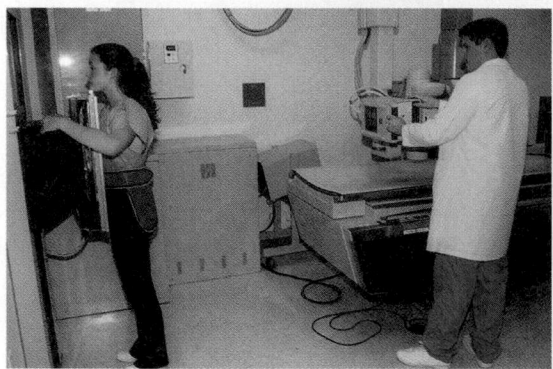

Figure 5

9 Measure the patient's thickness through the path of the central ray and set the control panel for the correct exposure.

Purpose: The measurement is needed to calculate the proper exposure from the technique chart. If the exposure is not correct the image will not be readable.

10 Stand behind a lead shield during the exposure (Figure 6).

Purpose: Lead shields provide protection from scattered radiation.

11 Ask the patient to assume a comfortable position after the examination is completed, and wait until the films are processed.

PROCEDURE 47-1—cont'd

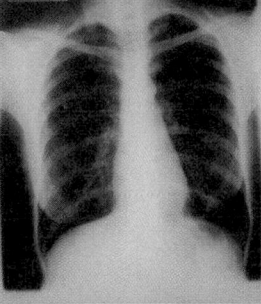

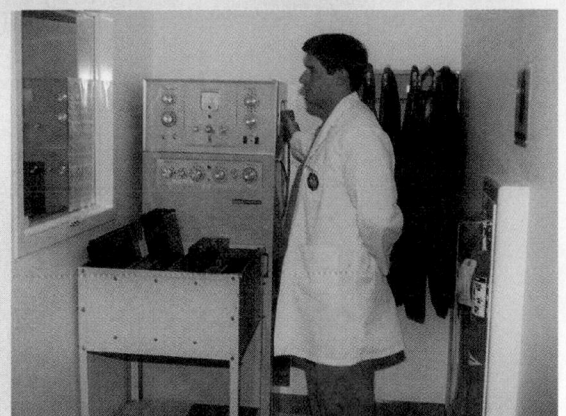

Figure 6

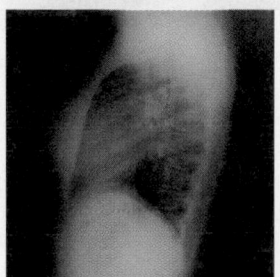

Figure 7

Purpose: In the event that it is necessary to take additional films, the patient will be readily accessible.

12 In the darkroom, remove the film from the cassette, identify the film, and process the film in the automatic processor (Figure 7).

13 Dismiss the patient when all films are satisfactory.

14 Place the finished radiograph(s) in a properly labeled envelope and present it to the physician for interpretation. When it has been read, file it according to the policies of the office.

15 Record the x-ray examination on the patient's chart, along with the final written x-ray findings.

Purpose: A procedure is not complete until it has been recorded.

Patients often express concerns about radiation exposure. You can assure them with confidence that the risks are extremely small and outweigh the health risks of treatment without the information that the examination will provide. It may help to point out that the radiographer is well trained in radiation safety and that the equipment is designed to provide good images with the least possible exposure. You can explain that the amount of radiation involved in the procedure is less than the exposure to natural background radiation that the population receives every year.

Patient preparation for routine radiography involves removing outer clothing from the area to be radiographed and providing a gown if appropriate. Underwear is usually not a problem. No metal objects should be included in the radiation field because these items will appear as artifacts on the images. This includes jewelry, zippers, snaps, underwire bras or other clothing fasteners, and the contents of pockets. Nonmetal objects that are thick or heavy should also be removed. Buttons and the heavy seams in jeans are examples of other clothing items that can cause artifacts on radiographs if they are in the imaging field. Metal items that are not in the radiation field are not a problem, so there is no reason for patients to remove jewelry or clothing that will not be included in the radiographs. When the patient is ready, the next step in the radiographic procedure is to assist the patient into the general position required for the x-ray examination (Figure 47-33). For example, if a hand is to be x-rayed, the patient can be seated at the end of the x-ray table (see Figure 47-33, A). If a chest examination is ordered, the patient will stand at an upright film holder (see Figure 47-33, C). For a spine examination, the patient may need to lie on the table (see Figure 47-33, B).

The radiographer then selects the correct cassette, places a lead marker on it to identify the patient's right or left side, and places the cassette in position for the exposure (Figure 47-34). Next, the patient is positioned precisely and the x-ray tube is aligned to the body part and the film at a specific distance (Figure 47-35). The body part must be measured to determine the proper exposure factors from a technique chart. At this point, lead shields are positioned for radiation protection. The radiographer then goes to the control booth, consults the technique chart, and sets the x-ray control panel to the desired exposure. Final instructions are given to the patient and the exposure is made. If more than one exposure is needed, the film is changed, the patient is repositioned, and the steps are repeated until the examination is complete.

After ensuring that the patient is safe and comfortable, the film is taken to the darkroom for processing. Film processing usually requires less than ten minutes before the film can be evaluated. If the film is satisfactory and no further exposures are needed, the patient is returned to an examination room or dressing room. The radiographer or the medical assistant then readies the x-ray room for the next examination and prepares the films for interpretation.

The films are kept together and given to the physician with the appropriate paperwork. Films are kept in large file envelopes that may contain more than one

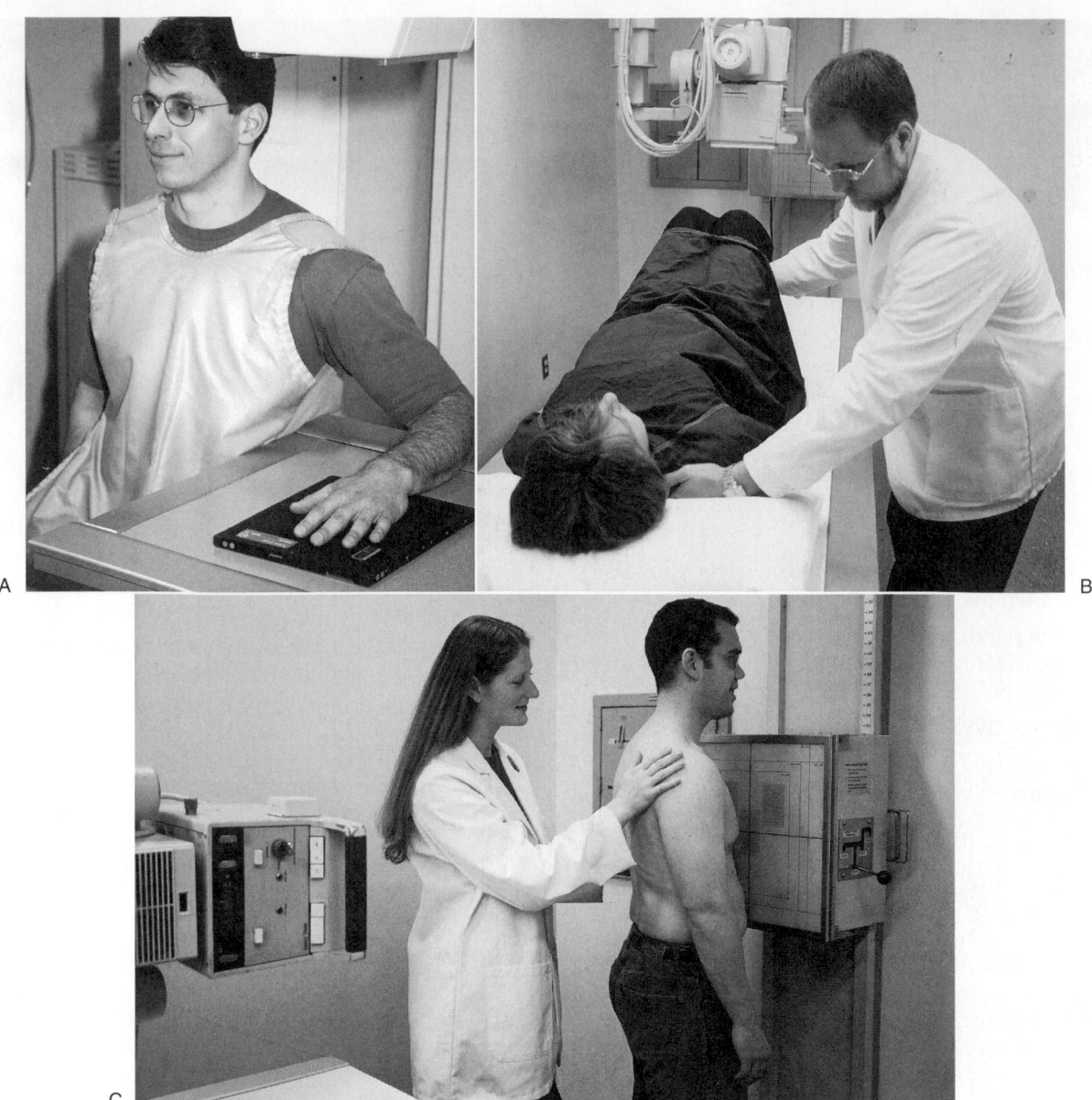

FIGURE 47-33 General positions for radiography. **A**, Patient may be seated at the x-ray table for some upper-extremity examinations. **B**, Radiographer assists patient to lie down for spine radiography. **C**, Radiographer assists patient into position at upright bucky for chest radiographs. (From Hunkele MM: *Radiography essentials for limited practice*, Philadelphia, 2001, WB Saunders.)

examination on the same patient. These envelopes must be accurately identified for proper filing. When images are added to the file, notations are often added to the envelope. After the films have been read, they are promptly filed so that they can be retrieved quickly when needed for future reference. Radiology reports must also be filed. Usually the original is filed in the patient's chart; copies may be filed separately or with the films.

The Role of the Medical Assistant

Depending on your location, you may or may not be legally permitted to take x-rays. Most states require some sort of license or permit to practice radiography. Some, such as New York and New Jersey, grant licenses only to professional radiologic technologists who have completed at least a two-year education program and obtained certification in radiography by the American Registry of Radiologic Technologists (ARRT).

Limited radiography, sometimes called *practical radiography*, is practiced primarily in clinics and physicians' offices. This field developed as nurses, medical assistants, chiropractic assistants, and other health care office personnel were trained to perform basic x-ray procedures in addition to their primary duties. It is called *limited* because the scope of practice is restricted compared to that of registered radiologic technologists. Limited practice does not usually involve the use of

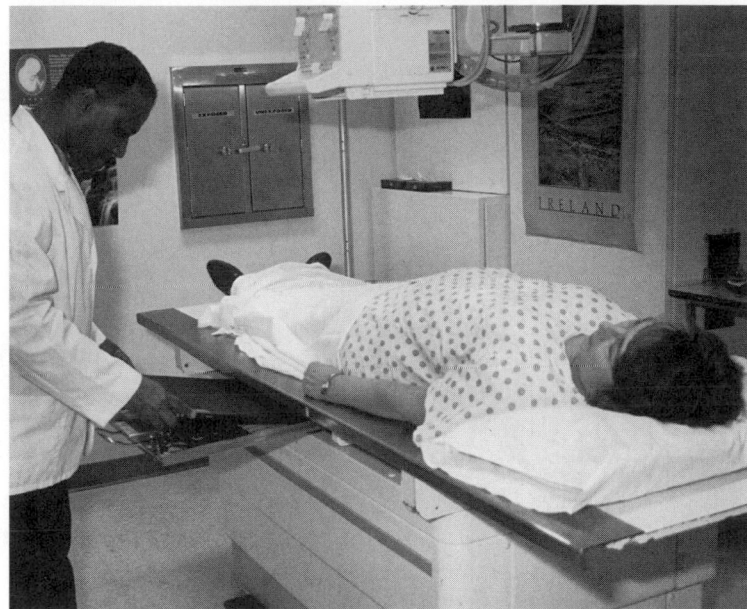

FIGURE 47-34 The cassette must be latched securely in the bucky tray and the tray aligned to the anatomy of interest. (From Ehrlich RA, McCloskey ED, Daly JA: *Patient care in radiography*, ed 5. St Louis, 1999, Mosby.)

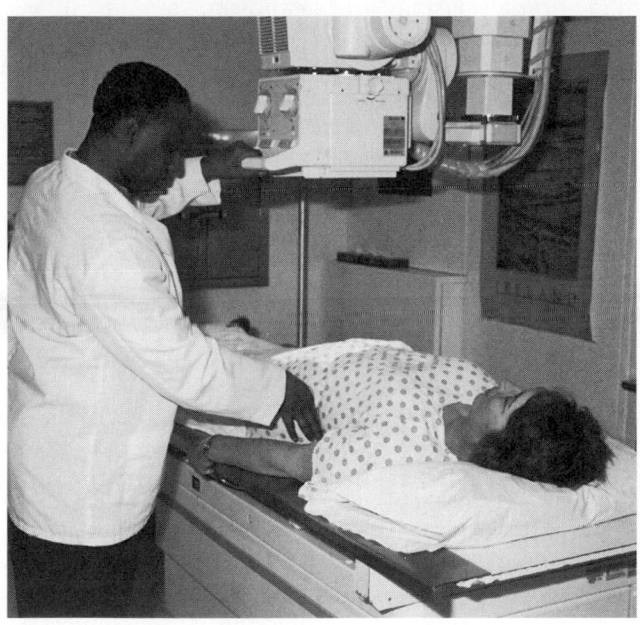

FIGURE 47-35 The x-ray tube must be aligned to the patient and cassette at the proper distance. (From Ehrlich RA, McCloskey ED, Daly JA: *Patient care in radiography*, ed 5. St Louis, 1999, Mosby.)

contrast media, and additional restrictions may be applied depending on the scope of practice permitted in each of the 28 states where limited radiography can be legally practiced.

Even if you are not qualified as a radiographer, it may be helpful to understand the general procedures involved in performing an x-ray examination and to identify those aspects of the process where the medical assistant might be of help to the radiographer. The exact nature of your duties will vary with your qualifications, your place of employment, the size of the staff, and the equipment available.

In summary, the process of radiography involves validation of orders, patient preparation, proper selection of cassettes and film, correct positioning of patient and

equipment, measurement of the part to be examined, protective shielding, correct setting of the exposure controls, and identification and processing of the film. These basic procedures vary considerably depending on the body part to be examined.

Patient Education

When instructing the patient regarding preparation for an examination, it is most helpful to have printed instructions prepared in advance. If more than one alternative is printed on any given paper, be certain to indicate, both orally and in writing, which instructions are to be followed. Review the sheet with the patient slowly, explaining any words or procedures that may not be familiar. Have the patient explain back to you what is to be done. If the patient is too young, too ill, confused, or incapable of understanding and following the instructions, give the instructions (oral and written) to the person who will be responsible for assisting the patient. Be sure to include the telephone numbers of your clinical facility and of the imaging department so that the patient or the patient's family may call if any questions arise after leaving the office.

In preparation for an upper GI series, the patient must fast, avoiding water, smoking, and chewing gum. The NPO order is instituted for a limited period, usually 8 to 12 hours, before the procedure. This ensures that the stomach will be empty at the time of examination so that it will produce an accurate radiographic image of its inner surfaces. Chewing gum and smoking are avoided because they tend to increase gastric secretions.

The preparation for a barium enema involves the use of a bowel cleansing kit. These kits usually contain one or more types of cathartics, a suppository, a low-volume enema, and illustrated instructions in several languages. Research has demonstrated that increased fluid intake enhances the effectiveness of cathartics and aids in minimizing patient discomfort. For this reason, instructions for cathartics are accompanied by a fluid intake schedule that suggests at least 8 ounces of water or clear liquid every 2 hours between noon and midnight on the day preceding the examination. It is helpful to emphasize the importance of fluid intake. The required doses of cathartics have a strong, thorough action that occasionally causes patients to experience painful spasms of the bowel and irritation of the intestinal lining. Persistent diarrhea may last through the night, preventing sleep. Although patients may find this preparation uncomfortable and inconvenient, its effectiveness in cleansing the bowel usually outweighs these considerations. Caution must be exercised in implementing an aggressive preparation for elderly or frail patients who are likely to be adversely affected. A gentler alternative should be available for these debilitated patients. Those with chronic or acute diarrhea may require a lower dosage or less active preparation than is usually given. When decreasing the routine strength or amount of cathartics, several days of a low-residue diet and increased fluid intake become critically important to the success of the preparation. Patients should always be advised of the nature of the action expected from the cathartic when it is given.

CRITICAL THINKING APPLICATION

Dr. Roberts, a physician at Metro Urgicenter, has scheduled Mr. Tillman for a barium enema, and David asks Sara to provide preparation instructions for the procedure to Mr. Tillman. What information should Sara obtain from Mr. Tillman to determine whether the usual bowel preparation is appropriate? If Sara thinks the usual preparation might be too harsh for Mr. Tillman, how should she explain her concern to David and Dr. Roberts? Who should decide whether to implement a variation in protocol—Sara, David, or someone else?

Legal and Ethical Issues

Only licensed practitioners of the healing arts are permitted to order x-ray examinations on humans. The interpretation of diagnostic images is a part of the professional practice of making a diagnosis and is solely the privilege of physicians. Although you may learn to recognize certain conditions represented in diagnostic images, you must never discuss your observations with the patient.

In most states, x-ray machines are required to be licensed, and the personnel who operate this equipment must have a current license or permit. In all states that regulate radiography, the practice is defined as more than simply pushing the exposure button. If you position the x-ray equipment, position the patient, or set the exposure controls, even though you do not make the exposure, you are probably practicing radiography as defined by law. Practicing without a valid license or permit or practicing outside the scope of one's credentials may result in fines, imprisonment, or both. Employers may also be penalized if their employees practice radiography in violation of regulations. *Everyone who practices radiography must be aware of the legal standards that apply to them and take care that their practice conforms to these standards.* This information is available from the agencies listed in Appendix C. Even if you work in one of the nine states that currently have no requirements for practicing radiography, you should be aware that the safe practice of radiography requires additional education and experience beyond that provided in this chapter.

X-ray films and other diagnostic images are the property of the institution or facility where they are taken. Even though the patient may pay for the procedure, this does not mean that the patient owns the films. They are considered a part of the medical record and are subject to the same kinds of requirements with respect to confidentiality, retention, and availability to the patient. Retention periods vary from state to state and are usually 5 to 7 years. Images may be loaned or transferred to other healthcare providers to assist in the patient's care. The patient should sign a release when images or copies of images are to be sent to another healthcare provider, and a record of the date and the name and address of the borrower must be kept when original images are loaned to another facility. This record of the film loan meets the legal requirement to retain the image.

Although it is common practice to have the patient carry the films when referred to another physician, it is preferable to send the films directly to the provider when time permits. When the patient must carry the films, it is a wise idea for the physician to review the films with the patient in advance so that the patient will not misinterpret the images and reach an incorrect conclusion.

CRITICAL THINKING APPLICATION

One of the new medical assistants at Metro Urgicenter, Carla O'Neal, tells Sara she is not qualified to practice radiography in the office's jurisdiction. David has instructed her to position a patient and set up the equipment for an x-ray examination. When Carla stated that she was not yet qualified to practice radiography, David replied, "Don't worry. I'll come by in a few minutes and make the exposure." What should Sara tell Carla, and what should Carla say to David? Should Sara tell someone else at the clinic?

SUMMARY OF SCENARIO

David Swain and the physicians at Metro Urgicenter depend on Sara's assistance to keep the x-ray department running smoothly. Today, for example, she instructed four patients to gown and prepare for routine x-rays. Greg Nolan had PA and lateral views of the chest because of a persistent cough and fever, Margaret and Jeff Barge both needed spine x-rays to rule out possible fractures following a car accident, and Dr. Farnsworth ordered AP and lateral views of Ella Jackson's left hip. Sara processed the films and was proud to see that there were no handling artifacts. This afternoon, Sara made an appointment for Cecile Marsden to have a bone scan at University Imaging Center. She was able to describe the procedure for Cecile so that she would know exactly what to expect. Sara enjoys her work in the x-ray department and is attending evening classes to become certified as a limited radiographer.

SUMMARY OF LEARNING OBJECTIVES

■ Radiography and fluoroscopy are both x-ray imaging procedures with a wide variety of applications. Often both techniques are used for a single study. Radiography produces still images, usually on photographic film, while fluoroscopy enables the radiologist to view the x-ray image directly and to observe motion.

■ Magnetic resonance imaging uses a strong magnetic field and radiofrequency pulses to produce images of all parts of the body, including bone, soft tissue, and blood vessels. Nuclear medicine studies demonstrate the function of organs and tissues by

mapping the radiation given off within the body when radioactive tracers have been ingested or injected into the patient. Sonography is a very safe imaging method that demonstrates soft tissues using high-frequency sound waves.

■ Preparation for chest radiography involves undressing to the waist and donning a gown; for an upper GI series, the patient must fast and avoid water, chewing gum, and smoking for at least 8 hours prior to the examination; preparation for a lower GI series is an extensive bowel-cleansing regimen that may involve a low residue or clear liquid diet, forced fluids, cathartics, a suppository, and a low-volume enema; preparation for an IVU requires some bowel preparation, such as a cathartic on the previous evening and NPO orders for a period before the examination. When a CT examination of the abdomen with an oral contrast medium is scheduled, the patient may be instructed to fast and must arrive at the imaging center from 1 to 2 hours in advance to drink the oral contrast medium.

■ The principal components of the x-ray machine are the tube in its barrel-shaped tube housing. The collimator is mounted on the tube housing. The tube housing with its attachments is mounted on the tube support, which may be suspended from the ceiling or attached to a tube stand that runs in a track on the floor. The radiographic table and an upright cassette holder provide support for the patient and the film, and incorporate a grid device. The control console is where the operator selects the exposure settings and makes the exposure. It is located in the control booth.

■ The three body planes are the sagittal plane that divides the body into right and left parts, the coronal plane that divides the body into anterior and posterior parts, and the transverse plane that divides the body into superior and inferior parts. For a frontal projection (AP or PA), the coronal plane is parallel to the film and the sagittal plane is perpendicular to it. For a lateral projection, the sagittal plane is parallel to the film and the coronal plane is perpendicular to it. Neither the sagittal plane nor the coronal plane is parallel to the film on an oblique projection.

■ For a PA projection, the patient is facing the film with the coronal plane parallel to the film. Lateral projections require the coronal plane to be perpendicular to the film. For an oblique projection, neither the coronal nor the sagittal plane is parallel to the film. For an axial or semiaxial projection, the x-ray beam is angled toward the patient's head or feet along the long axis of the body.

■ The image receptor system for radiography usually consists of a cassette with two intensifying screens that give off light when stimulated by x-ray energy and double emulsion film that lies between the intensifying screens. The film is exposed on both sides, principally by the light emitted from the screens. This system greatly reduces the amount of radiation and exposure time involved in making exposures compared with direct exposure of film by x-rays.

■ Cassettes are unloaded and reloaded in the darkroom under safelight illumination only. Precautions include ensuring that the door is locked; that your hands are clean and dry; and that the film is not creased, bent, or scraped in the process of loading and unloading. Take care that the cassette is reloaded with only one fresh film and latched securely. Keep the loading bench clean to prevent dirt from getting into the cassette.

■ Film identification is essential for knowing the identity of the patient represented in the image and the date and location of the examination. Serious errors in diagnosis and treatment might occur if films are not correctly identified. The identification information is typed on a card that is inserted into a photographic printer in the darkroom. The printer stamps the information on the film after it is removed from the cassette and before it is processed.

■ The health risks associated with radiography are extremely small and consist of a slightly increased likelihood of developing cataracts, cancer, or leukemia. There is also a potential for minimal decrease in life span and for a negative outcome when exposure occurs to the abdominal area during pregnancy. Exposure to the reproductive organs may cause genetic changes that can be passed on to future generations.

■ The following steps are taken to ensure that patients receive the least possible exposure during x-ray procedures: avoid errors that could require repeat exposures, establish good routine procedures and follow them strictly, collimate to the smallest radiation field that will encompass the area of clinical interest, use the highest kVp that is consistent with acceptable film quality, use a tube-to-film distance (SID) of at least 40 inches, use the fastest films and screens consistent with the necessary film quality, and shield the reproductive organs and other sensitive organs (such as the eyes, thyroid, and breasts).

■ The principal safety precaution for x-ray equipment operators and staff is to stay completely behind the lead barrier of the control booth during exposures. Occupationally exposed persons must not hold patients or cassettes during exposures. Any staff required to be in the x-ray room during an exposure should be shielded by a lead apron, should stay as far from radiation sources as possible, and should minimize the time they are in the room.

■ The risks associated with x-ray exposure during pregnancy are very small unless the exposure is in excess of 5 rad to the abdominal area. These risks include the possibility of spontaneous abortion, birth defects, growth retardation, and cancer or leukemia in childhood. Inadvertent exposure during pregnancy is avoided by posting warning signs in the x-ray department and by asking women of childbearing age whether there is any possibility that they may be pregnant.

■ Diagnostic images are the property of the facility in which they are made. They are a part of the legal medical record and must be retained and accessible for a period specified by state law, usually 5 to 7 years. Images may be loaned or transferred to other healthcare providers to assist in the patient's care, in which case the patient should sign a release, the images should be sent directly to the borrowing provider if possible, and a record must be kept of the loan.

■ Only licensed practitioners of the healing arts are permitted to order x-ray examinations and/or to interpret x-ray images.

KEY INTERNET WEBSITES

- Radiological Society of North America
- Radiology.org maintains the list of world radiological associations and publications
  For active weblinks to each website visit
  http://evolve.elsevier.com/Kinn/

CHAPTER 48

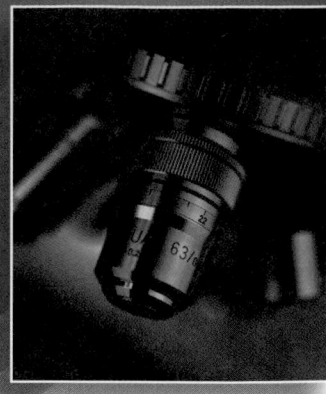

Scenario

Marsha Rollins has been employed for 3 years as a certified medical assistant in a medical practice. The physicians have an active medical laboratory on site and Marsha has become experienced in collecting specimens, performing laboratory tests, and reporting results. Recently she was offered a position in a smaller practice closer to home; she has accepted the position, knowing that her experience will benefit the practice because the physicians would like to expand their on-site medical laboratory testing.

Assisting in the Clinical Laboratory

Robin R. Patterson

Learning Objectives

- Define and spell the terms listed in the vocabulary.
- Discuss the role of the clinical laboratory in patient care and the medical assistant's role in coordinating laboratory tests and results.
- Describe the divisions of the clinical laboratory and give an example of a test performed in that division.
- Compare and contrast the agencies that govern or influence practice in the clinical laboratory.
- List techniques to minimize risks in the clinical laboratory.
- Describe the essential elements of a laboratory requisition.
- Explain the importance of chain of custody.
- Explain the differences and similarities between quality assurance and quality control.
- Convert Greenwich time to military time.
- Name the Fahrenheit temperature and Celsius temperature of three important pieces of laboratory equipment.
- Name the metric units used for measuring liquid volume, distance, and mass.
- Describe the proper use of pipets.
- Explain how dilutions are prepared.
- Name the parts of a microscope.
- Describe the safe use of a centrifuge.
- List quality control measures necessary to ensure sterilization with an autoclave.
- Describe the methods by which materials are prepared for autoclaving.
- Demonstrate the proper use of the microscope.

National Curriculum Competencies

CLINICAL COMPETENCIES

1d. Dispose of biohazardous materials
1e. Practice standard precautions

3a. Use methods of quality control
3g. Screen and follow-up test results

Vocabulary

aliquot A portion of a well-mixed sample removed for testing.

analyte The substance or chemical being analyzed or detected in a specimen.

anticoagulant A chemical added to the blood after collection to prevent clotting.

carcinogenic A substance that is known to cause cancer.

caustic A substance that burns or destroys tissue by chemical action.

cerebrospinal fluid Fluid within the subarachnoid space, the central canal of the spinal cord, and the four ventricles of the brain.

cytology The study of cells using microscopic methods.

diluent A liquid used to dilute a specimen or reagent.

exudates Fluids with high concentration of protein and cellular debris that have escaped from the blood vessels and have been deposited in tissues or on tissue surfaces.

hematoma A sac filled with blood that may be the result of trauma.

hemolyzed A term used to describe a blood sample in which the red blood cells have ruptured.

pipet A cylindrical glass or plastic tube used to deliver fluids.

preservatives Substances added to a specimen to prevent deterioration of cells or chemicals.

referral (reference) laboratory A private or hospital-based laboratory that performs a wide variety of tests, many of them specialized; physicians often send specimens collected in the office to referral laboratories for testing.

resolution The ability of the eye to distinguish two objects that are very close together; the sharpness of an image.

specimen A sample of body fluid, waste product, or tissue that is collected for analysis.

stat A direction that an action is to be taken quickly (from the Latin word *statin*, meaning "at once"); an order found on a laboratory requisition indicating that the test must be done immediately.

teratogenic A substance that is known to cause birth defects.

The Role of the Clinical Laboratory in Patient Care

Laboratory medicine or clinical pathology is the medical discipline that applies clinical laboratory science and technology to the care of patients. The laboratory is the place in which a collected **specimen** is analyzed and evaluated. Tests are performed manually (by hand) or through automation (by using specialized instruments).

Personnel in the Clinical Laboratory

Medical laboratories are located either in hospitals or in nonhospital facilities such as physicians' offices, clinics, public health departments, health maintenance organizations, and private **referral laboratories**. The director of a laboratory facility may be a *pathologist*, a physician specially trained in the nature and cause of disease or a clinical laboratory scientist with a doctorate degree. The laboratory is staffed by various professionally trained personnel, including certified medical technologists (MTs), who have earned a baccalaureate degree, have had additional formal training, and have passed a national certification examination. Other personnel include certified medical laboratory technicians (MLTs) or medical laboratory assistants (MLAs) and certified medical assistants (CMAs). These personnel have completed a specialized training program that is 1 or 2 years in length and have passed a registry examination. One may also find laboratory assistants and phlebotomists, individuals who have received specialized training in the collection and preparation of laboratory specimens.

The agencies granting certifications and titles are described in Table 48-1.

The medical assistant is a multiskilled professional who is trained to perform administrative and clinical procedures, including basic laboratory testing. Laboratory tests are an essential part of a medical diagnosis, an aid to treatment, and, frequently, a control of medication. Only a physician may request laboratory testing for a patient. The medical assistant may be responsible for a number of these testing procedures. To assume this responsibility, the medical assistant must know proper patient preparation, the procedures for each test, and the normal range of results for these tests. The medical assistant must carefully follow all laboratory instructions in obtaining and labeling the specimens and sending them to the laboratory. There must be good communication among the patient, the office staff, and the laboratory personnel. The medical assistant should make the patient feel more at ease with these procedures and thus gain the patient's cooperation.

Clinical Laboratory Testing

Clinical laboratory testing is used in conjunction with a thorough health history and physical examination to provide essential data needed for the diagnosis and management of a patient's condition. The body is considered to be healthy when a state of equilibrium in the internal environment exists. In this state, termed *homeostasis*, the physical and chemical characteristics of body substances (e.g., fluids, secretions, and excretions) will be within a certain acceptable range known as the *normal* or *reference range*. A change in homeostasis results in abnormal test values, outside of the reference range. Abnormal values for a particular test may be seen with more than one pathologic condition. For example, a decrease in hemoglobin levels in red blood cells is seen in iron-deficiency anemia, and it is also noted in hyperthyroidism and cirrhosis of the liver. Thus the physician cannot rely solely on laboratory tests to make a diagnosis but must instead rely on the combination of data obtained from health history, physical examination, and a number of diagnostic and laboratory results.

Tests performed in a clinical laboratory range from simple screening tests to complex *profile* testing. A

TABLE 48-1	Certifying Agencies for Laboratory Personnel	
Certifying Agency	**Title**	**Position**
American Society for Clinical Pathologists	MT(ASCP)	Medical technologist
	MLT-(ASCP)	Medical laboratory technician–certificate
	MLT-AD(ASCP)	Medical laboratory technician–associate's degree
American Medical Technologists	MT(AMT)	Medical technologist
	MLT(AMT)	Medical laboratory technician
Department of Health and Human Services	CLT(HHS)	Clinical laboratory technologist
National Certification Agency for Medical	CLS(NCA)	Certified laboratory scientist
Laboratory Personnel	CLT(NCA)	Certified laboratory technician
International Society for Clinical	RMT(ISCLT)	Registered medical technologist
Laboratory Technology	RLT(ISCLT)	Registered laboratory technician
American Association of Medical Assistants (AAMA)	CMA	Certified medical assistant
Accrediting Bureau of Health Education Schools (ABHES)	RMA	Registered medical assistant
California Certifying Board for Medical Assistants	CCMA-C(CCBMA)	California certified medical assistant–clinical
National Healthcareer Association (NHA)	CCMA	Certified clinical medical assistant
	CPT	Certified phlebotomy technician
	CML	Certified medical laboratory assistant

screening test is one that examines a particular specimen for the presence of a substance that may indicate a disease state. A screening test is not diagnostic for any particular disease but will indicate that the disease state may exist. Screening tests are often done routinely on patients, based on their age, history, or gender. Screening tests are often *qualitative* in that they do not have a numerical value attached to the result; they may simply be reported as positive or negative. The occult blood test for blood in the stool is an example of a screening test. Blood is not normally found in the stool, and its presence may indicate the presence of cancerous lesions. A positive test result indicates that blood is present, but additional testing is required to determine the source of the blood. For example, further testing or examination may reveal that the patient had her menstrual period at the time of collection of the specimen or that she had bleeding hemorrhoids.

A *quantitative* test will have units attached to numerical values. These values often are represented as the amount of **analyte** per given volume of specimen, and it is essential that the results be reported with the units. For example, in a complete blood cell count for a healthy adult, the red blood cells will number 5 million per cubic millimeter ($5.0 \times 10^6/mm^3$), the hemoglobin value will be 15 g per deciliter (15 g/dl), and the hematocrit will be 45%. Generally, the units are printed on the laboratory report, but the medical assistant must always ensure that the values are consistent with the testing being performed.

CRITICAL THINKING APPLICATION

The referral laboratory telephones to report the values on several tests performed on the urine of a client, Cecelia Roberts. Marsha jots down the following: Total protein, 0.12; Blood, moderate; Albumin, 50; Specific gravity, 1.025. What is wrong with the notations she has just made? Are these tests qualitative or quantitative?

The Clinical Laboratory Improvement Amendments

In 1988, Congress passed the Clinical Laboratory Improvement Amendments (CLIA), establishing quality standards for all laboratory testing to ensure the accuracy, reliability, and timeliness of patient test results regardless of where the test was performed. A laboratory is defined as any facility that performs laboratory testing on specimens derived from humans for the purpose of providing information regarding the diagnosis, prevention, and treatment of disease, or impairment of or assessment of health. The CLIA is user-fee funded; therefore all costs of administering the program must be covered by the regulated facilities.

The categorization of commercially marketed in vitro diagnostic tests under CLIA is now the responsibility of the Food and Drug Administration (FDA). The FDA has assumed primary responsibility for performing the CLIA complexity categorization functions, which include the process of assigning commercially marketed in vitro diagnostic test systems to one of three CLIA regulatory categories based on their potential risk to public health: waived tests and moderate- and high-complexity tests.

Waived Tests. Waived tests are:

"laboratory examinations and procedures that have been approved by the Food and Drug Administration for home use or that, as determined by the Secretary, are simple laboratory examinations and procedures that have an insignificant risk of an erroneous result, including those that

(A) employ methodologies that are so simple and accurate to render the likelihood of erroneous results by the user negligible, or

(B) the Secretary has determined pose no unreasonable risk of harm to the patient if performed incorrectly..."

A CLIA database is now available. This database contains the commercially marketed in vitro test systems categorized by the FDA since January 31, 2000 and tests categorized by the Centers for Disease Control and Prevention (CDC) prior to that date. The records can be searched by test system name, specialty/subspecialty, analyte, document number, qualifier, effective date, and complexity.

EXAMPLES OF CLIA-WAIVED TESTS

1. Dipstick or tablet reagent urinalysis (nonautomated) for the following:
   - Bilirubin
   - Glucose
   - Hemoglobin
   - Ketone
   - Leukocytes
   - Nitrite
   - pH
   - Protein
   - Specific gravity
   - Urobilinogen
2. Fecal occult blood
3. Ovulation tests: visual color comparison tests for luteinizing hormone
4. Urine pregnancy tests: visual color comparison tests
5. Erythrocyte sedimentation rate: nonautomated
6. Hemoglobin-copper sulfate: nonautomated
7. Blood glucose by glucose monitoring devices cleared by the FDA specifically for home use
8. Spun microhematocrit
9. Hemoglobin by single analyte instruments with self-contained or component features to perform specimen/reagent interaction, providing direct measurement and readout

Moderate- and High-Complexity Tests. An estimated 10,000 different laboratory tests are performed in the United States every day. Seventy-five percent of them are categorized as moderate-complexity tests by the FDA. Some of these tests are performed in physician's office laboratories (POLs), including hematology and chemistry testing done on an automated analyzer, Gram's staining, and microscopic analysis of urine sediment. High-complexity tests usually are not performed in a POL and include Papanicolaou (Pap) smears, blood typing and cross-matching, and **cytology** testing.

Laboratories that perform moderate- to high-complexity testing must meet CLIA regulations and are subject to unannounced inspections every 2 years. Each laboratory performing these tests must establish a system to maintain the integrity and identification of patient specimens throughout the testing process and ensure the accurate reporting of results. The laboratory also must have established and must follow written quality control and quality assurance procedures and must participate in proficiency testing, a form of external quality control. Three times a year, the laboratory must test samples provided by an approved proficiency testing agency using the same tests that they would use to test a patient's sample. Finally, CLIA regulations specify qualifications and responsibilities for personnel in laboratories, from directors to testing personnel. Personnel requirements are most stringent for high-complexity testing.

Divisions of the Clinical Laboratory

The laboratory is divided into various departments, which may include hematology, chemistry, microbiology, specimen collection and processing, blood bank, coagulation, serology, histology, cytology, toxicology, urinalysis, and special chemistry. The laboratory in the physician's office usually performs procedures in urinalysis, hematology, chemistry, and microbiology.

Urinalysis

Urinalysis includes the physical, chemical, and microscopic examination of urine. In the physical examination, the color, transparency, and specific gravity are noted. Chemical analysis is performed to measure levels of such analytes as glucose, protein, ketones, blood, bilirubin, urobilinogen, nitrites, and pH. Microscopically, the urine is examined for the presence of red, white, and epithelial cells, mucus, casts, crystals, yeasts, parasites, and bacteria. Additional quantitative tests may also be performed in the urinalysis department to confirm routine screening tests.

Hematology

Tests performed in the hematology division may be qualitative or quantitative. Blood cell counts determine the exact number of red blood cells (RBCs or erythrocytes), white blood cells (WBCs or leukocytes), or platelets (thrombocytes) either by manual counting or by automated counting. Qualitative tests determine the characteristics of cells, such as size, shape, and maturity. In addition, the hematology department will perform tests to determine the coagulating ability of blood components.

Chemistry

The clinical chemistry department analyzes blood, **cerebrospinal fluid** (CSF), urine, and joint fluid (synovial fluid). Procedures may include single tests or *profiles*, which include tests for a number of related analytes. Lipid profiles, for example, will include assessments of total cholesterol, triglyceride, and high-density lipoprotein (HDL) cholesterol.

Microbiology

Microbiology involves the study of bacteria, fungi, yeasts, parasites, and viruses. In the microbiology laboratory, microorganisms are grown (cultured) and identified from blood, urine, sputum, CSF, and wound specimens. Susceptibility testing is then performed on these organisms to determine proper antibiotic therapy. Specimens for the microbiology must be collected aseptically in sterile containers.

CRITICAL THINKING APPLICATION

Dr. Watkins has ordered a routine urinalysis with a culture and sensitivity (C&S) test on her patient,

Laboratory Safety

The importance of safety in the laboratory cannot be overemphasized. Most laboratory accidents are preventable by exercising proper techniques and by using common sense. Using safe practices in the laboratory requires a personal commitment and concern for others; an unsafe act may harm an innocent bystander without harming the person who performs the act.

Safety Standards and Governing Agencies

Safety standards for laboratories are initiated, governed, and reviewed by several agencies or committees including the U.S. Department of Labor's Occupational Safety and Health Administration (OSHA); a nonprofit educational organization known as the National Committee for Clinical Laboratory Standards (NCCLS), which provides a forum for development, promotion, and use of national and international standards; the Centers for Disease Control and Prevention (CDC), which is a government agency under the U.S. Department of Health and Human Services; the College of American Pathologists (CAP), a leader in providing laboratory quality improvement programs; and the Environmental Protection Agency (EPA), a government agency whose mission it is to protect human health and to safeguard the natural environment.

Through OSHA, the government has created a system of safeguards and regulations under the Occupational Safety and Health Act of 1970. This system affects nearly every worker in the United States because the regulations apply to all businesses with one or more employees. The regulations are discussed in detail in Chapter 24. Two programs have been mandated by OSHA to ensure the safety of personnel working in clinical laboratories. One covers occupational exposure to chemical hazards; the other covers exposure to bloodborne pathogens. Both of these programs, as they relate to safety in the medical laboratory setting, will be discussed further in this chapter.

Laboratory Hazards

Physical Hazards

Physical hazards in the laboratory can be classified as electrical, fire, and mechanical. Electric shock is a threat when any electrical equipment is in use. It is imperative to keep all electrical equipment in proper repair, and always follow manufacturers' instructions.

Use surge protectors, inspect all cords and plugs frequently, never use extension cords, and avoid overloading circuits. Before servicing, unplug the electrical device and never operate electrical instruments with wet hands. If there is a sink nearby, ensure that electric cords do not come into contact with the water supply. Signs and labels, such as those shown in Figure 48-1, should be placed on specific electrical hazards.

Open flames are rarely used in a laboratory, but the potential for fire still exists. Fires may be ignited by smoking, heating elements, and sparks. Flammable materials should not be stored near any source of ignition. All laboratory personnel should be familiar with the location of fire extinguishers and fire safety blankets. Fire extinguishers should be of the carbon dioxide (CO_2), dry chemical, or halon type—known as the ABC type of extinguisher. The ABC extinguisher can be used on all types of fires. They should be inspected by a licensed inspector on a regular basis and replaced or recharged if used. The medical assistant may be responsible for maintaining records on the care and maintenance of fire extinguishers.

Fire safety blankets should be used to smother flames on burning clothing. However, one should avoid wrapping a victim in a fire blanket, because this may intensify burns. Instead, the flames should be patted out or the victim directed to roll on the blanket.

Emergency phone numbers should be posted on the wall near the telephone, and all personnel should know the location of fire alarms, the fire escape routes, and procedures to follow if exits are blocked. Periodic fire drills should be conducted, and hallways and exits should be kept free of clutter.

Mechanical hazards arise from the use of laboratory equipment. Special care should be exercised when using equipment with moving parts, such as centrifuges, and those that rely on pressure, including autoclaves. Centrifuges, devices that separate liquids from solids, present

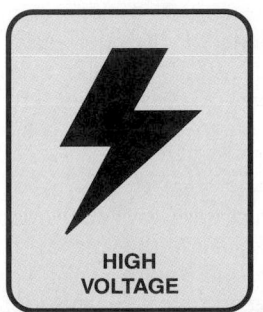
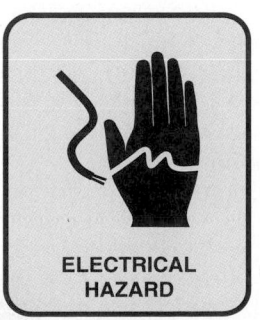

HIGH VOLTAGE　　**ELECTRICAL HAZARD**

FIGURE 48-1　High-voltage and electrical hazard labels. (From Stepp CA, Woods MA: *Laboratory procedures for medical office personnel*, Philadelphia, 1998, WB Saunders.)

a hazard not only from moving parts but also from glassware that might break during centrifugation and from aerosols that might be created if tubes are not capped tightly. Pressurized equipment, such as autoclaves used in sterilization, presents dangers if opened prematurely. Although centrifuges and autoclaves often have built-in safeguards, such as locks that prevent entry until the environment is safe, improper care of the equipment can result in failure of the safety measures.

Chemical Hazards

The clinical laboratory is home to chemicals that are flammable, **caustic**, poisonous, **carcinogenic**, and/or **teratogenic**. Exposure to these dangers can be through inhalation, direct absorption through the skin, ingestion, entry through a mucous membrane, or entry through a break in the skin. OSHA is involved in regulating the standards directed at minimizing occupational exposure to hazardous chemicals in laboratories. The OSHA hazard communication standard (known as the employee "right to know" rule) became law in 1991 and ensures that laboratory workers are fully aware of the hazards associated with their workplace. The law necessitates the development of a comprehensive plan to implement safe practice throughout the laboratory insofar as chemicals are concerned. This *chemical hygiene plan* must outline the specific work practices and procedures that are needed to protect workers from any health hazards that may arise from working with in-stock chemicals. Information and training must be provided to all workers. There must be a *Material Safety Data Sheet* (MSDS) on file for all chemicals in use in the laboratory. OSHA requires the manufacturer of the chemical to make the sheets available, usually as a package insert.

Each MSDS contains the basic information about the specific chemical or product. This includes the trade name, chemical name and synonyms, chemical family, manufacturer's name and address, emergency telephone number, hazardous ingredients, physical data, fire and explosion data, and health hazard and protection information (Figure 48-2).

Following principles of proper handling will reduce your risks of harmful effects. Harmful exposure can be reduced by using proper devices for pipetting; never **pipet** by mouth. If a chemical produces toxic or flammable vapors, work under a fume hood that exhausts air to the outside. In case of accidental exposure to the skin, rinse the affected area under running water for at least 5 minutes. Remove any clothing that is contaminated. If chemicals are splashed in the eyes, flush the eyes with water from an eyewash station for a minimum of 15 minutes. Prompt medical attention must be given to victims of chemical exposure.

Chemicals should be tightly sealed and properly labeled. A hazard identification system was developed by the National Fire Protection Association that provides, at a glance, information on the potential health, flammability, and chemical reactivity hazards of materials. This identification system consists of four small, colored diamond-shaped symbols grouped into a larger diamond shape. The top diamond is red and indicates flammability hazard.

The diamond on the left is blue and indicates hazards to health. The bottom diamond is white and provides special hazard information including radioactivity, special biohazards, and other dangerous situations. Finally, the diamond on the right is yellow and indicates reactivity/stability hazard. The system indicates the severity of the hazard by using numbers imprinted in the diamonds from 0 to 4, with 4 being extremely hazardous to 0 being no hazard (Figure 48-3).

Biological Hazards and Infection Control

Biological hazards, or biohazards, are materials or situations that present a risk or potential risk of infection. Infection with biohazardous material can occur during specimen collection, handling, transporting, or testing the specimen. Potentially infective specimens include blood, body tissue biopsy specimens, urine, **exudates**, and bacterial cultures and smears. Infection can occur through aspiration of a pathogen, accidental inoculation by a needlestick, aerosols created by uncapping specimen tubes, centrifuge accidents, and entry of pathogens through cuts and scratches.

One of the most important OSHA regulations covers exposure to biological hazards. The OSHA-mandated program, Occupational Exposure to Bloodborne Pathogens, must be in place and has been law since 1992 as part of a general *infection control policy*. In addition, the CDC recommends safety precautions regarding handling of all patient specimens. Previously known as *universal precautions*, they are now referred to as *standard precautions* and are published on the organization's web page and in the publication *Morbidity and Mortality Weekly Report*. Chapter 24 covers the specifics of the OSHA-mandated programs.

The recommendations from the CDC include an infection control plan, engineering and work practice controls, personal protective clothing and equipment, sufficient training and education, provision of hepatitis B vaccination, and medical intervention after exposure incidents. The NCCLS also has guidelines for the laboratory worker in regard to protection from bloodborne illness due to contact with patient specimens. The CAP offers a voluntary accreditation program for clinical laboratories that includes biosafety measures. One important precaution that can be taken is labeling of potentially biohazardous material, as described in Chapter 24.

Standard Precautions

Hepatitis B and the human immunodeficiency virus (HIV) are a constant threat to the health and safety of clinical laboratory personnel. Hepatitis B and HIV are both transmitted through exposure to blood and body fluids. Blood and body fluids are the primary substances handled in the laboratory. OSHA mandated the Bloodborne Pathogens (BBP) Standard, which covers all employees who could be "reasonably anticipated as the result of performing their job duties to face contact with blood and other potentially infectious materials." The BBP Standard requires that the laboratory employer have a written exposure control plan.

MATERIAL SAFETY DATA SHEET	MSDS NO. 396
	PAGE 1

SECTION 1   IDENTIFICATION

MANUFACTURER'S NAME: Corelis Corporation
ADDRESS: P.O. Box 93
                      Camden, NJ 08106

EMERGENCY TELEPHONE NUMBER: 1 (800) 733-8690

TELEPHONE NUMBER FOR INFORMATION: 1 (800) 331-0766

ISSUED: 10/99

IDENTITY: 2% Aqueous Glutaraldehyde Solution

PREPARED BY: Regulatory Affairs

PRODUCT CODE: 3345

TRADE NAME: Aldecyde

SYNONYMS: None

CHEMICAL FAMILY: Aldehydes

MOLECULAR FORMULA: $OHCC_3H_6CHO$ (Active)

RTECS #: MA 2450000 (Active)

MOLECULAR WEIGHT: 100

HAZARD RATING – HEALTH: 3 (Serious Hazard)   **FLAMMABILITY:** 0   **REACTIVITY:** 0   **SPECIFIC:** NONE

SECTION 2   HAZARDOUS INGREDIENTS/IDENTITY INFORMATION

COMPONENTS (SPECIFIC CHEMICAL IDENTITY)	CAS #	%	OSHA PEL	ACGIH TLV	OSHA 1910.1200
Glutaraldehyde (active)	111-30-8	2	0.2ppm, C	0.2ppm, C	n/a
Inert buffer salts	n/a		None	None	Nonhazardous
Water	7732-18-5	98	None	None	Nonhazardous

SECTION 3   PHYSICAL/CHEMICAL CHARACTERISTICS

APPEARANCE AND ODOR: 2 components: colorless fluid and liquid salts; turns green when activated. Sharp odor masked with peppermint fragrance.

BOILING POINT: 212°F

SPECIFIC GRAVITY (H_2O=1): 1.003 g/cc

VAPOR PRESSURE (mm Hg): same as water

MELTING POINT: n/a

VAPOR DENSITY (AIR=1): same as water

EVAPORATION RATE (H_2O=1): 0.98

SOLUBILITY IN WATER: complete

pH: 8

FREEZING POINT: same as water

ODOR THRESHOLD: .04 ppm, detectable. (ACGIH)

SECTION 4   FIRE AND EXPLOSION HAZARD DATA

FLASH POINT (METHOD USED): None   **FLAMMABLE LIMITS – LEL:** nd   **UEL:** nd

EXTINGUISHING MEDIA: If water is evaporated, material can burn. Use carbon dioxide or dry chemical for small fires. Use foam (alcohol, polymer or ordinary) or water fog for large fires.

SPECIAL FIRE FIGHTING PROCEDURES: Self-contained breathing apparatus and protective clothing should be available to fireman.

UNUSUAL FIRE AND EXPLOSION HAZARDS: None

TOXIC GASES PRODUCED: None

SECTION 5   REACTIVITY DATA

STABILITY: 212°F

CONDITIONS TO AVOID: None

INCOMPATIBILITY (MATERIALS TO AVOID): None

HAZARDOUS DECOMPOSITION OR BYPRODUCTS: None

HAZARDOUS POLYMERIZATION: Will not occur

FIGURE 48-2   Material safety data sheet (MSDS). (From Bonewit-West K: *Clinical procedures for medical assistants*, Philadelphia, 2000, WB Saunders.)

MATERIAL SAFETY DATA SHEET

MSDS NO. 396
PAGE 2

SECTION 6   HEALTH HAZARD DATA

ROUTE(S) OF ENTRY – INHALATION: yes   SKIN: yes   INGESTION: yes   EYE: yes

SIGNS AND SYMPTOMS OF EXPOSURE:

EYES: Contact with eyes causes damage.

SKIN: Can cause skin sensitization. Avoid skin contact.

INHALATION: Vapors may be irritating and cause headache, chest discomfort, symptoms of bronchitis.

INGESTION: May cause nausea, vomiting and general systemic illness.

EMERGENCY AND FIRST AID PROCEDURE:

EYES: Flush thoroughly with water. Get medical attention.

SKIN: Flush thoroughly with water. If irritation persists, get medical attention.

INHALATION: Remove to fresh air. If symptoms persist, get medical attention.

INGESTION: Do not induce vomiting. Drink copious amount of milk. Get medical attention.

HEALTH HAZARDS (ACUTE AND CHRONIC):
  Acute: As listed above under Signs and Symptoms of Exposure
  Chronic: None known from currently available information.

MEDICAL CONDITIONS GENERALLY AGGRAVATED BY EXPOSURE: None known from currently available information.

LISTED AS CARCINOGEN BY –   NTP: yes   IARC MONOGRAPHS: no   OSHA: no

TOXICITY: ORAL LD50 (Rat)   Toxicity Rating 1: 500-5000 mg/kg.
            OCULAR (Rabbit)   Toxicity Rating 2: Irritating or moderately persisting more than seven days with.
            DERMAL LD50 (Rabbit)   None by dermal route.
            INHALATION LC50 (Rabbit) Irritating but non-toxic at highest concentration achieved (2.89 ppm).

SECTION 7   PRECAUTIONS FOR SAFE HANDLING AND USE

STEPS TO BE TAKE IN CASE MATERIAL IS RELEASED OR SPILLED: For LARGE spills, use ammonium carbonate to "neutralize" glutaraldehyde odor. Collect liquid and discard it. For SMALL spills, wipe with sponge or mop down area with an equal mixture of household ammonia and water. Flush with large quantities of water.

WASTE DISPOSAL METHOD: Triple rinse empty container with water and dispose in an incinerator or landfill approved for pesticide containers. Discard solution with large quantities of water.

EPA HAZARDOUS WASTE NUMBER: n/a

PRECAUTIONS TO BE TAKEN IN HANDLING AND STORING: Use normal storage and handling requirements.

SECTION 8   TRANSPORTATION DATA AND ADDITIONAL INFORMATION

DOMESTIC (D.O.T.): Aldehydes, N.O.S.   INTERNATIONAL (I.M.O.): Aldehydes, N.O.S.

PROPER SHIPPING NAME: Glutaraldehyde   PROPER SHIPPING NAME: Glutaraldehyde

HAZARD CLASS: None   HAZARD CLASS: None

LABELS: None Needed   LABELS: None Needed

REPORTABLE QUANTITY: None   UN/NA: 1989

FIGURE 48-2—cont'd For legend see previous page.

MATERIAL SAFETY DATA SHEET

MSDS NO. 396
PAGE 3

SECTION 9   CONTROL MEASURES

VENTILATION:
ROUTINE: Product should be used in a covered container. Use with standard room ventilation (air conditioning); natural draft.
EMERGENCY: Enhanced ventilation

RESPIRATORY PROTECTION:
ROUTINE: None required
EMERGENCY: Organic vapor cartridge, canister mask

EYE PROTECTION:
ROUTINE: Safety glasses recommended
EMERGENCY: Safety glasses

SKIN PROTECTION:
ROUTINE: Impervious gloves
EMERGENCY: Impervious gloves; Protective clothing; Rubber boots

WORK/HYGIENIC PRACTICES: Avoid contamination of food

SECTION 10   SPECIAL REQUIREMENTS

None

KEY: n/a = Not Applicable
nd = Not Determined
C = Ceiling
PEL = Permissible Exposure Level
RTECS = Registry of Toxic Effects of Chemical Substances
* = Trademark

FIGURE 48-2—cont'd For legend see page 997.

EXPOSURE CONTROL PLAN REQUIREMENTS

- Identification of tasks, procedures, and job classification where possible occupational exposure to blood may occur.
- Establishment of methods that protect employees and comply with OSHA regulations.
- Implementation of a vaccination program for hepatitis B virus.
- Provision of training in the proper use of protective equipment regarding bloodborne pathogens.
- Maintenance of records to show compliance with the BBP Standard.

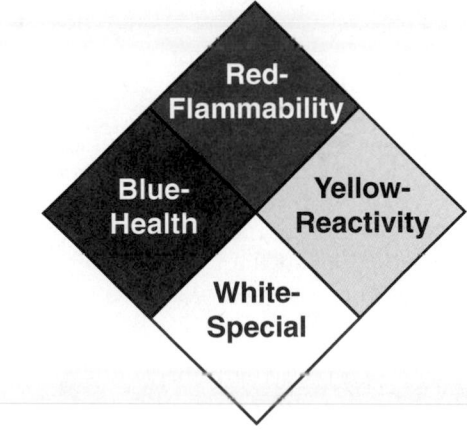

FIGURE 48-3   Identification system of the National Fire Protection Association.

In addition to blood and blood products, the BBP Standard includes "other potentially infectious materials" (OPIM). Urine is the only fluid that is not specifically included in OSHA's BBP Standard. Because blood and blood elements are frequently associated with urine, it must be included and considered as a possible source of exposure.

SAFETY GUIDELINES FOR OTHER POTENTIALLY INFECTIOUS MATERIALS

- Handle and process all specimens as if they contain infectious material.
- Wipe the outside of specimen containers with a germicide.

> **SAFETY GUIDELINES FOR OTHER POTENTIALLY INFECTIOUS MATERIALS—cont'd**
>
> - Dispose of all infectious materials following state and federal guidelines.
> - Clean up spills using a disinfectant (see Chapter 24).
> - Immediately dispose of any chipped or broken glassware in a special disposable container.

Washing the hands is undoubtedly the most effective means of preventing infection. It is the single most effective way of preventing the spread of all infections. Proper hand washing protects you, your patient, and your coworkers because it removes organisms. In the laboratory area it is absolutely required to *wash your hands*:

- When you enter and before leaving this area
- Before and after every patient procedure
- After contact with body fluid even if gloves were worn
- Before and after eating
- Before and after using the rest room

Every laboratory should have a safety manual that covers all safety practices and precautions. The manual should clearly explain procedures to be followed in the event of an accident. A section of the manual should prominently list emergency numbers for ambulance, fire, police, and other security services as well as plans for evacuation. Emergency numbers should also be posted near the telephone, and plans for evacuation must be posted. Second, the manual should give instructions for reporting and documenting accidents, and contain an accident log to record the names and persons involved, the type of accident, and the date it occurred. Copies of this incident report form should be in the manual along with an example of a properly completed form. It is important to note that such a form not only documents the accident but also the steps taken to prevent such an accident from recurring.

Specimen Collection, Processing, and Storage

Laboratory Requisitions and Reports

A patient's medical record should be maintained in an organized manner to promote easy access to the desired information. There are various methods used when filing laboratory reports in a patient's medical record. Many offices compile records in a set order so that the laboratory report sheets follow entry A and precede entry B. Another method is to use standard-sized sheets of a specific color and stagger the reports from the bottom of the sheet upward.

As discussed in Chapter 25, in the source-oriented medical record all like reports are filed in one section. For example, all laboratory reports are together, all surgical reports are together, and all ECG reports are together. The latest test is placed on the top, because it is the most important for the patient's current care and treatment. While in the problem-oriented medical record, all test results are entered and recorded in the objective part of the progress notes, preceded by the number and title of the particular problem.

The medical assistant's responsibility is to make sure that all reports are received for diagnostic tests performed on the patient outside the physician's office. Only after the physician reviews the test results should they be filed into the patient's record.

When the physician requests laboratory testing that must be done outside of the office, a written requisition for the work must be sent to the laboratory with the patient or with the specimen (Figure 48-4). These forms are preprinted, with the most commonly requested test indicated in logical sequence. Patient information must be complete, accurate, and legible.

> **EXAMPLE OF INFORMATION USUALLY REQUIRED WHEN SPECIMENS ARE SENT TO THE LABORATORY**
>
> - Physician's name, account number, address, and phone number
> - Patient's full name, surname first
> - Patient's address
> - Patient's insurance information
> - Patient's age, date of birth, and gender
> - Source of specimen
> - Date and time of collection
> - Specific test (or tests) requested
> - Medications the patient is taking
> - Possible diagnosis
> - Indication of whether test is **stat**

Specimen Collection

The medical assistant is responsible for the collection of many different types of specimens. It is important to recognize that all clinical laboratory results are only as good as the specimen received. The importance of specimen collection cannot be overemphasized. If the test results are to be accurate indicators of the patient's state of health, it is imperative that the concepts of specimen collection be understood and followed exactly. The most common specimens are blood, urine, and swab samples collected from wounds or mucous membranes. Less often, feces, gastric contents, cerebrospinal fluid, tissue samples, semen, and aspirates, such as synovial fluid or amniotic fluid, are submitted for testing. These specimens are analyzed for levels of many chemicals and drugs, types and numbers of cells present, and the presence of microorganisms.

Lab Services

IMPORTANT
Patient instructions and map on back

PHYSICIAN ORDERS

Patient _____ _____ ____ D.O.B. _____ M ☐ Patient
Last Name   First   M.I.   F ☐ SS# __ __ __

Address _____ City _____ Zip _____ Phone # _____

Physician _____
ATTACH COPY OF INSURANCE CARD

Date & Time of Collection: _____
Drawing Facility: _____

Diagnosis/ICD-9 Code _____
(Additional codes on reverse)

☐ ROUTINE   ☐ PHONE RESULTS TO: # _____
☐ ASAP   ☐ FAX RESULTS TO: # _____
☐ STAT   ☐ COPY TO: _____

☐ 789.00 Abdominal Pain   ☐ 414.9 Coronary Artery Disease (CAD)   ☐ 244.9 Hypothyroidism
☐ 285.9 Anemia (NOS)   ☐ 250.0 DM (diabetes mellitus)   ☐ 272.4 Hyperlipidemia
                          ☐ 780.7 Fatigue/Malaise   ☐ 401.9 Hypertension
                          ☐ 272.0 Hypercholesterolemia   ☐ 465.9 URI (upper respiratory infection)

HEMATOLOGY	CHEMISTRY	CHEMISTRY	MICROBIOLOGY
☐ 1021 CBC, Automated Diff (incl. Platelet Ct.)	☐ 5550 Alpha Fetoprotein, Prenatal	☐ 5232 HBsAg	
☐ 1023 Hemoglobin/Hematocrit	☐ 3000 Amylase	☐ 3175 HIV (Consent required)	Source ____
☐ 1020 Hemogram	☐ 3153 B12/Folate	☐ 3581 Iron & Iron Binding Capacity	☐ 7240 Culture, AFB
☐ 1025 Platelet Count	☐ 3156 Beta HCG, Quantitative	☐ 3195 LH	☐ 7200 Culture, Blood x ____
☐ 1150 Pro Time Diagnostic	☐ 3321 Bilirubin, Total	☐ 3590 Magnesium	Draw Interval ____
☐ 1151 Pro Time, Therapeutic	☐ 3324 Bilirubin, Total/Direct	☐ 3527 Phenobarbital	☐ 7280 Culture, Fungus
☐ 1155 PTT	☐ 3009 BUN	☐ 3095 Potassium	Culture, Routine
☐ 1315 Reticulocyte Count	☐ 3159 CEA	☐ 3689 Pregnancy Test, Serum (HCG, qual)	☐ 7005 Culture, Stool
☐ 1310 Sed Rate/Westergren	☐ 3348 Cholesterol	☐ 3853 Pregnancy Test, Urine	☐ 7010 Culture, Throat
	☐ 3030 Creatinine, Serum	☐ 3197 Prolactin	☐ 7000 Culture, Urine
URINE	☐ 3509 Digoxin (recommend 12 hrs. after dose)	☐ 3199 PSA	☐ 7300 Gram Stain
☐ 1059 Urinalysis	☐ 3515 Dilantin	☐ 3339 SGOT/AST	☐ 7355 Occult Blood x ____
☐ 1082 Urinalysis w/Culture if indicated	☐ 3168 Ferritin	☐ 3342 SGPT/ALT	☐ 7365 Ova & Parasites x ____
Urine-24 Hr ____ Spot ____	☐ 3193 FSH	☐ 3093 Sodium/Potassium, Serum	☐ 7400 Smear & Suspension
Ht. ____ Wt. ____	☐ 3066 ▼ Glucose, Fasting	☐ 3510 Tegretol	(includes Gram Stain/Wet Mount)
☐ 3033 Creatinine	☐ 3061 Glucose, 1° Post 50 g Glucola	☐ 3551 Theophylline	☐ 7060 Rapid Strep A Screen (Negs confir by cult)
☐ 3036 Creatinine Clearance (also requires blood)	☐ 3075 ▼ Glucose, 2° Post Glucola	☐ 3333 Uric Acid	☐ 7065 Rapid Strep A Screen only
☐ 3398 Protein	☐ 3060 Glucose, 2° Post Prandial (meal)		☐ 7030 Beta Strep Culture
☐ 3096 Sodium/Potassium	☐ 3049 ▼ Glucose Tolerance Oral GTT		☐ 5207 GC by DNA Probe
☐ Microalbumin 24 Hr ____ Spot ____	☐ 3047 ▼ Glucose Tolerance Gestational GTT		☐ 5130 Chlamydia by DNA Probe
	☐ 3650 Hemoglobin, A1C		☐ 5555 Chlamydia/GC by DNA Probe
SEROLOGY			☐ 7375 Wright Stain, Stool
☐ 8020 ANA (Antinuclear Antibody)			
☐ 8040 Mono Spot			
☐ 3494 Rheumatoid Factor			
☐ 8010 RPR			
☐ 5365 Rubella			

Additional Tests _____

PANELS & PROFILES

☐ ✗ 3309 CHEM 12
Albumin, Alkaline Phosphatase, BUN, Calcium, Cholesterol, Glucose, LDH, Phosphorus, AST, Total Bilirubin, Total Protein, Uric Acid

☐ ▼ 3315 CHEM 20
Chem 12, Electrolyte Panel, Creatinine, Iron, Gamma GT, ALT, Triglycerides

☐ ▼ 3357 CARDIAC RISK PANEL
Cholesterol, HDL, LDL, Risk Factors, VLDL, Triglycerides

☐ ✗ 3048 CRITICAL CARE PANEL
BUN, Chloride, CO2, Glucose, Potassium, Sodium

☐ 3046 ELECTROLYTE PANEL
Chloride, CO2, Potassium, Sodium

☐ ▼ 3399 EXECUTIVE PANEL
Chem 20, Iron, Cardiac Risk Panel, CBC, RPR, Thyroid Cascade

☐ 5242 HEPATITIS PANEL, ACUTE
HAVIgMAb, HBsAg, HBsAb, HBcAb, HCVAb

☐ ▼ 3355 LIPID MONITORING PANEL
Cholesterol, Triglycerides, HDL, LDL, VLDL, ALT, AST

☐ 3312 LIVER PANEL
Alkaline Phosphatase, AST, Total Bilirubin, Gamma GT, Total Protein, Albumin, ALT

☐ ✗ 3083 METABOLIC STATUS PANEL
BUN, Osmolality (calculated), Chloride, CO2, Creatinine, Glucose, Potassium, Sodium, BUN/Creatinine, Ratio, Anion Gap

☐ ✗ 3376 PANEL B
Chem 12, CBC, Electrolyte Panel

☐ ▼ 3382 PANEL D
Chem 20, CBC, Thyroid Cascade

☐ ✗ 3388 PANEL F
Chem 12, CBC, Electrolyte Panel, Thyroid Cascade

☐ ▼ 3391 PANEL G
Chem 20, Cardiac Risk Panel, CBC, Thyroid Cascade

☐ 3393 PANEL H
Chem 20, CBC, Cardiac Risk Panel, Rheumatoid Factor, Thyroid Cascade

☐ ▼ 3397 PANEL J
Chem 20, Cardiac Risk Panel

☐ 5351 PRENATAL PANEL
Antibody Screen ABO/Rh, CBC, Rubella, HBsAg, RPR
☐ 1059 with Urinalysis, Routine
☐ 1082 with Urinalysis w/Culture if indicated

☐ ✗ 3102 RENAL PANEL
Metabolic Status Panel, Calcium, Phosphorus

☐ 3186 THYROID CASCADE
TSH, Reflex Testing

▼ - patient **required** to fast for 12-14 hours

✗ - patient recommended to fast 12-14 hours

LAB USE ONLY

☐ SST		☐ PLASMA	
☐ PURPLE		☐ SERUM	
☐ YELLOW		☐ SWAB	
☐ BLUE		☐ SLIDES	
☐ GREEN		☐ DNA PROBE	
☐ GREY		☐ B. CULT BTLS	
☐ URINE			
☐ BLACK			
☐ OTHER:			

INIT ____

RECV. SPECIMEN: ☐ FROZEN
☐ AMBIENT   ☐ ON ICE

Special Instructions/Pertinent Clinical Information _____

Physician's Signature _____ Date _____
These orders may be FAXed to: 449-5288   7060-500 (7/96)

LAB

FIGURE 48-4 Laboratory requisition form.

Initial identification of the patient is essential, as is collection of the specimen in an appropriate collection container. For example, blood may be collected using a vacuum tube system. These tubes are available in a variety of sizes, with and without **preservatives** and **anticoagulants**. The tubes are color coded so that the color of the stopper denotes which, if any, additive is present (Figure 48-5). Collection in an incorrect tube will result in an unacceptable specimen, and recollection will be necessary. If the specimen is to be tested for the presence of microorganisms, a sterile container must be used. If the patient is to collect the specimen at home, he or she should be provided with the appropriate container and complete instructions for collection.

The medical assistant should always check the laboratory's specimen requirements manual for any unfamiliar tests. The manual lists all specimen collection information. Any unanswered questions should be resolved by calling the laboratory before collecting the specimen. The container must be labeled properly at the time of collection; unlabeled containers should never be accepted for laboratory testing. Labels should include the patient's

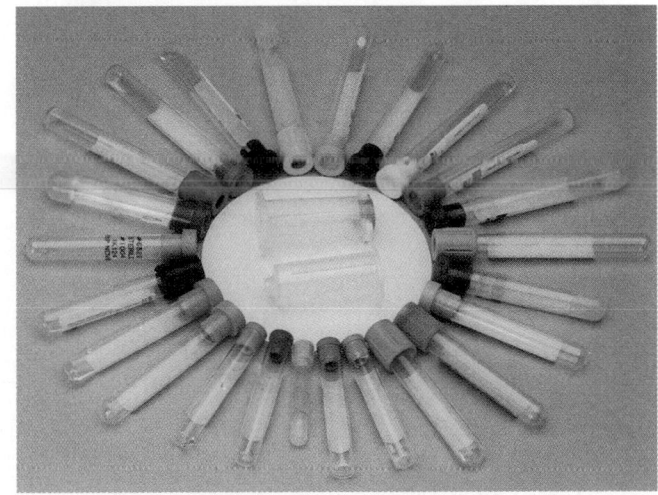

FIGURE 48-5 Vacutainer tubes. Note color-coded tops.

full name and the date; for some specimens the time of collection and the type of specimen should also be included on the label.

If the specimen is to be mailed, it must be carefully packaged to prevent breakage, damage, or contamination by all persons handling it. Containers of liquid specimens may be wrapped in absorbent material and inserted in unbreakable tubes with safe-top lids. The lids are taped shut so that no leakage occurs if the specimen container breaks. Place all specimens in a second container, such as an impervious bag, for transport. The completed requisition goes inside the outermost wrap. Usually, Styrofoam mailers (Figure 48-6) are used because they cushion the sample and also provide insulation. Styrofoam inserts can be shaped to fit around the specimen container. A warning label specifying the etiologic agent or biologic specimen is affixed to the outside of the container. The specimen should be given to the laboratory courier or mailed at a post office immediately so that it is not exposed to temperature extremes. Instructions for properly obtaining, processing, and preparing a specimen for transport are usually supplied to the physician's office laboratory by the testing laboratory. If the instructions are not clear or if you have a question regarding a particular collection, the laboratory will answer your question over the phone.

Avoiding Contamination

A medical assistant must take care to avoid contaminating the specimen as well as himself or herself. Expiration dates on swabs, tubes, transport media, and other collection containers should be checked before these items

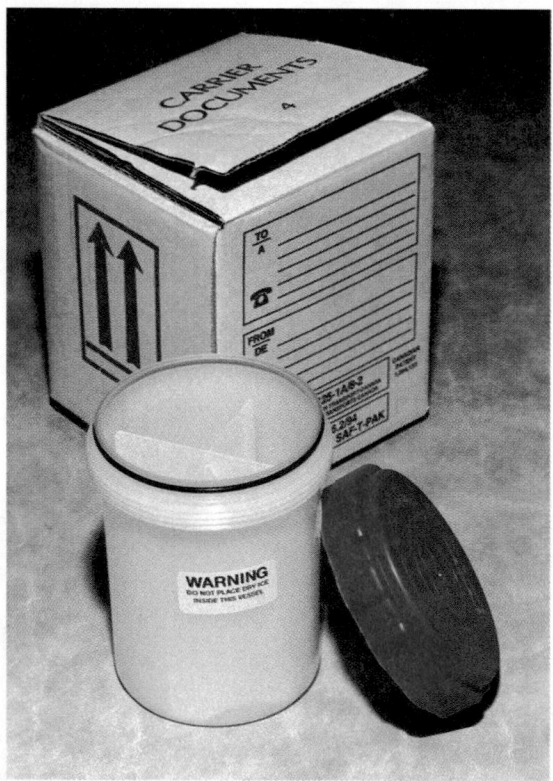

FIGURE 48-6 Specimen mailers.

are used. An improperly handled specimen may become contaminated or may contaminate the surrounding environment. Standard precautions should be followed. All blood and other body fluids from *all* patients should be considered infective.

Sufficient samples should be collected for the tests requested by the physician. Amounts may vary based on the methods used. If a report is returned from the laboratory marked *QNS (quantity not sufficient)*, it indicates a request for an additional specimen. Be certain to clarify any questions concerning the previous specimen by calling the laboratory before collecting a new one.

The specimen collected must be a true representative sample. A swab for a wound culture collected from the surface of the wound generally does not yield the same results as one taken from the depths of the wound. A **hemolyzed** blood specimen, or one taken from an atypical area, such as a **hematoma** or the area above or below an intravenous drip, shows marked differences in many tests. If a large volume of specimen is collected, such as a 24-hour urine or fecal fat specimen, the total volume or weight must be carefully measured and recorded. The specimen must be well mixed before an **aliquot** is removed and submitted for testing.

Proper Handling, Processing, and Storage

The specimen must be handled, processed, and stored according to the instructions to avoid causing any alterations that would affect test results. The medical assistant should determine whether the specimen needs to be kept warm or cool. Specimens such as urine require chilling if testing is not going to be performed immediately. Some cultures or specimens need to be kept at body temperature after collection. Gonorrhea cultures and semen analysis are two such examples, because cooling kills the microorganisms and sperm. When required, serum must be separated from the cells as soon as possible after the specimen has clotted to prevent alterations caused by the metabolism of the cells. Specimens for bilirubin testing must be protected from light. Some specimens need to be frozen to prevent chemical constituents from changing. Laboratory specimen requirements should be consulted to ensure that each specimen is handled and processed properly.

Chain of Custody

When a specimen may be needed as evidence in a court case, certain procedures must be followed for collection and handling of the specimen. Forensic or medicolegal implications require that any results of the testing of a specimen be obtained in such a fashion that they are recognized by a court of law. Specimen processing must be documented meticulously, ensuring that there was no tampering of evidence. *Chain of custody* refers to the stepwise method used to collect, process, and test a specimen. The documentation must be signed by every person who has contact with the specimen, from collection to final reporting of results. Blood alcohol level testing often requires chain of custody handling. Everything needed for collection of the specimen is provided in a kit—even the latex gloves, the vacuum tube, and the needle to collect the blood specimen. Documentation is included and must be signed by all personnel. Medical assistants and phlebotomists have been subpoenaed to testify in court regarding specimens they have collected; therefore it is in your best interest to follow chain-of-custody procedures rigorously.

Quality Assurance and Quality Control

Quality Assurance Guidelines

Quality assurance (QA) is the pledge of health care professionals to work to achieve the highest degree of excellence in the health care given every patient. QA encompasses a comprehensive set of policies and procedures developed to ensure the reliability of laboratory testing. It includes quality control, personnel orientation, laboratory documentation, knowledge of laboratory instrumentation, and enrollment in a proficiency testing program. QA focuses on establishing a series of operating procedures to produce reliable laboratory results for the benefit of the patient, the physician, and the medical assistant who does the laboratory testing.

These policies benefit the physician by reducing the liability for inaccurate reporting of test results. When a physician uses a laboratory test in diagnosing, the results must be compared with *reference values*. Reference values are also useful in assessing the efficacy of a patient's course of treatment. The QA system enables the laboratory to assess, verify, and document the quality of the test results. This documentation is a way of comparing "what is" with "what should be."

Quality Control Guidelines

The objective of *quality control* (QC) in the laboratory is to ensure the *accuracy* of test results while detecting and eliminating error. Physicians' office laboratories play a vital part in QC, because patient treatment is often based on or reinforced by results of laboratory tests. Mandated by law, QC programs monitor all aspects of laboratory activity, from specimen collection through the processing, testing, and reporting steps. Programs check supplies, reagents, machinery, personnel, and actual test performance. Without a QC program, laboratory error is difficult to detect unless the physician would notice test results inconsistent with a patient's history. Undetected laboratory errors may result in harm to the patient.

Specially prepared *quality control samples* are tested daily along with patient samples. The results of testing performed on the quality control samples must be within a pre-established range before the patient results can be reported. The quality control samples, called *controls*, are usually supplied with prepackaged kits intended for use in the small laboratory. The controls should be analyzed at specified intervals. For example, positive and negative controls supplied with pregnancy test kits should be performed with each patient specimen. Urinalysis dipsticks (used for chemical examination of

urine) should be checked daily and each time a new container is opened. Controls for automated chemistry analyses should be performed at specified intervals during the day. Consistent results of controls ensure constant conditions throughout the testing sequence.

Laboratory instrument standardization is important to ensure proper operation and accurate test results. Preventive maintenance prolongs the life of your equipment and reduces breakdowns; it includes daily cleaning as well as adjustment and replacement of parts when necessary. Each instrument should have a log or worksheet to record all changes, including daily maintenance.

GUIDELINES FOR A PREVENTIVE MAINTENANCE PROGRAM

- Follow the manufacturer's instructions for calibration of instruments.
- Read and understand instructions for routine instrument care.
- Perform all preventive maintenance provided by manufacturer's instructions.
- Keep all spare parts available for immediate use.
- Record the name, address, and phone number of a contact person for maintenance or repair.
- Create a maintenance form or use the one provided.

Accurate record keeping is one of the key responsibilities of a medical assistant. A variety of forms are available to assist in recording laboratory information. The primary record is the laboratory master log book in which each procedure performed in the physician's office laboratory is entered with dates clearly shown. Every day that patient tests are performed, QC tests must also be performed. The results of standardization tests and dates when new control vials are begun must be entered, along with the expiration dates of the controls. The records must be retained for a period of years, the exact number determined by state laws and the CLIA '88 mandate. Employee records must be kept confidential and maintained for 30 years.

EXAMPLE OF WHAT TO INCLUDE IN AN EMPLOYEE RECORD

- Employee name and Social Security number
- Hepatitis B virus immunization status
- Copy of *all* results of examinations, medical testing, and follow up necessitated by an exposure incident
- Employer's copy of the examining healthcare professional's opinion in regard to the exposure

CRITICAL THINKING APPLICATION

Marsha is performing a blood urea nitrogen (BUN) test on a sample using an automated BUN analyzer. First she standardizes the instrument and then she runs high, low, and normal controls. Finally she tests the patient's sample and records the value. Explain why she standardized the instrument before she ran the controls, why she ran three controls, and why the patient sample was the last to be tested.

TABLE 48-2	Common Laboratory Temperatures	
	Fahrenheit	**Celsius**
Refrigerator temperature	35°-46°	2°-8°
Freezer temperature	32°	0°
Room temperature	59°-86°	15°-30°
Incubator temperature	98.6°	37°
Body temperature	98.6°	37°
Autoclave temperature	254°	121°

Laboratory Mathematics and Measurement

All laboratory testing, from specimen collection through reporting of results, relies on accurate use of numbers and measurements. Numbers are used, for example, for reporting the time of collection of the sample, the quantity of analyte found in a specimen, the volume of the specimen, dilutions used in sample preparation, and recording quality control results.

Measuring Time

Time of day is often a critical factor in patient care. Medications must be administered, diets must be followed, and specimens must be collected on a particular time schedule. Many clinical laboratories use the 24-hour clock when recording time; this method avoids the confusion that comes with the Greenwich clock that uses the AM (morning) or PM (after noon) designations.

The 24-hour clock system is also known as military time and is expressed with four digits in terms of "hundred hours." Noon is referred to as 1200 (twelve hundred) hours; midnight is 2400 (twenty-four hundred) or 0000 (zero hundred) hours. The military clock is based on a 60-minute hour, just like the Greenwich clock; therefore 5:35 PM is expressed as 1735 (seventeen thirty-five) hours.

Measuring Temperature

Two scales for measuring temperature are currently used; each is divided into units called *degrees*. The Fahrenheit scale is considered to be part of the English system of measurement and is the scale most commonly used in the United States. The Celsius scale, formerly called the *Centigrade scale*, is used in countries that apply the metric system. On the Celsius (C) scale, water freezes at 0° C and boils at 100° C. On the Fahrenheit (F) scale, water freezes at 32° F and boils at 212° F.

Table 48-2 has common laboratory temperatures. The method for converting temperatures from one form of measurement to another is found in Chapter 28.

Units of Measurement

The units of measurement that we commonly use in the United States differ from those used in the clinical laboratory. In everyday life we use the English system of measurement, in which weight is measured in ounces and pounds, length is measured in inches and feet, and volume is measured in cups and quarts. In the laboratory, the metric system and the International System of Units (SI) are used. It is important that the medical assistant memorize and practice these systems so that he or she can communicate professionally.

The metric system is based on a decimal system in which there are basic units and prefixes that indicate a system of division in multiples of ten. The basic units of the metric system are the gram (g) for weight, the meter (m) for length, and the liter (L) for volume. Prefixes are added to each symbol to reduce or enlarge them by units of ten. This information is included in Chapter 31. The most common metric units used in the laboratory are millimeters (mm), centimeters (cm), micrograms (µg), milligrams (mg), grams (g), microliters (µl), milliliters (ml), liters (L), and cubic centimeters (cc). The cubic centimeter and milliliter are used interchangeably in the clinical laboratory.

Quantitative test results are reported using the appropriate units of measurement. Some commonly used designations for reporting analytes are mg, µg, g, dl, and L. Blood glucose, for example, is reported in milligrams per deciliter (mg/dl); hemoglobin levels are reported as grams per deciliter (g/dl).

The International System of Units (Systeme Internationale or SI units) is a system of reporting numbers that are recognized by international organizations such as the World Health Organization (WHO). Many countries have adopted its use; the United States has not completely converted to the SI system.

The SI is an adaptation of the metric system, using a number of the basic units but many are different for reporting results. For example, blood glucose is reported as millimoles per liter (mmol/L), and hemoglobin is reported in grams per liter (g/L). Therefore it is very important to include units of measurement when reporting testing values, double-checking the standard for the laboratory.

Measuring Liquid Volume

Vessels to measure volume in the laboratory can be glass or plastic and may be reusable or disposable. Beakers are wide, straight-sided cylindrical vessels that are used for mixing or reagent preparation. They are not calibrated to hold an exact volume but can be used for estimating volume. Erlenmeyer flasks are used for reagent preparation and have a narrower mouth than a beaker. Like beakers, they are not calibrated.

Test tubes come in many sizes and are often disposable. Test tubes may be sterile and some may be calibrated. Graduated cylinders are used for measuring exact amounts of a liquid. The size of the cylinder should be matched as closely as possible to the volume of liquid being measured for the most accurate reading. In other words, a 50-ml graduated cylinder should not be used to measure 10 ml—a 10-ml cylinder should be used. For the most accurate measurement, a volumetric flask is used. Volumetric glassware, including flasks and pipets, must go through rigorous calibration to ensure the accuracy of the measurement. They are calibrated to single, specific amounts, such as 100 ml or 500 ml, and cannot be used to measure volumes other than those indicated. Figure 48-7 depicts the glassware described.

Pipets (Figure 48-8) are also used extensively in the laboratory. These long glass, cylindrical, calibrated tubes are used to deliver or transfer specified volumes of liquid.

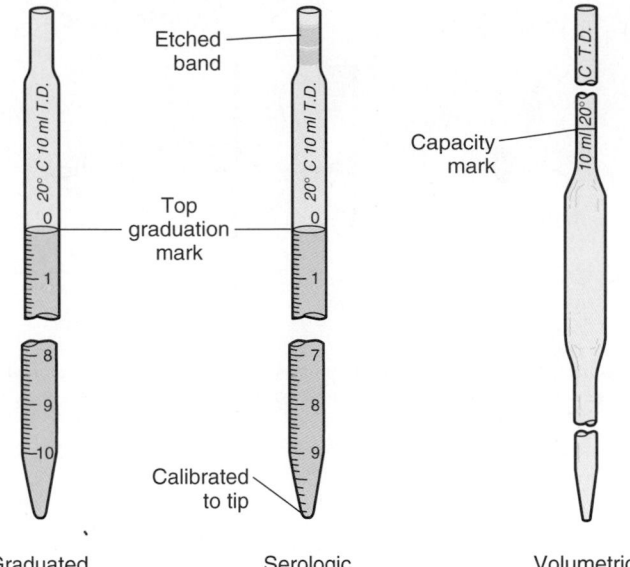

FIGURE 48-8 Types of manual pipets. (Redrawn from Linne JJ, Ringsrud KM: *Clinical laboratory science: the basics and routine techniques*, ed 4, St Louis, 1999, Mosby.)

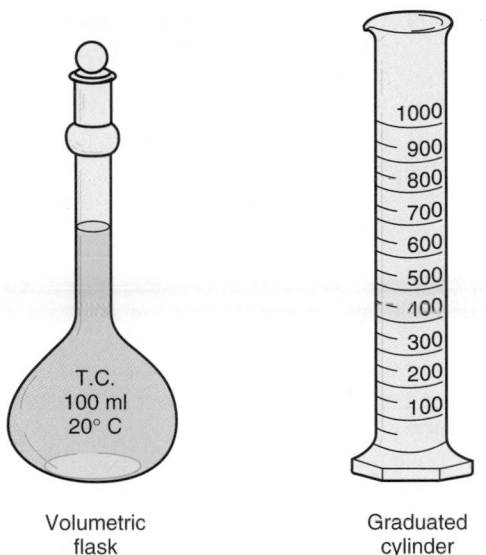

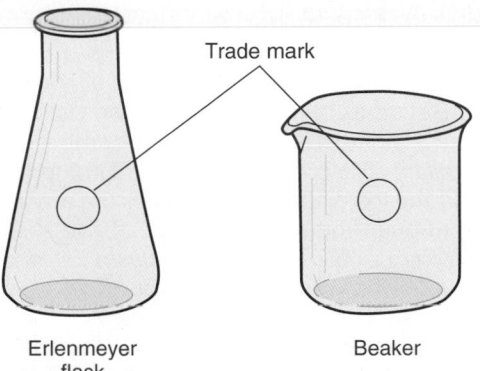

FIGURE 48-7 Laboratory glassware. *T.C.*, To contain. (Redrawn from Linne JJ, Ringsrud KM: *Clinical laboratory science: the basics and routine techniques*, ed 4, St Louis, 1999, Mosby.)

Drawing liquid into the pipet requires a bulb or a vacuum pump–type device; *mouth-pipetting is forbidden*. For most general laboratory procedures, two main types of manual pipets are used: the volumetric pipet, used for transferring, and the graduated pipet, used for measuring. The latter type is classified according to whether it contains or delivers the amount specified. A "to deliver" (TD) pipet will deliver the specified volume by drawing the liquid up to the calibration mark and then allowing it to drain out vertically, unassisted. A small amount of liquid will always remain in the tip of the pipet. A "to contain" (TC) pipet must be emptied completely to deliver the specified amount. When mouth pipetting was routinely being practiced, it was said that these pipets were to be "blown out," meaning that all of the liquid was to be forcibly expelled from the pipet.

A serological pipet is much like the graduated pipet in appearance. The tip opening, however, is large, which permits a fast flow of liquid but less accuracy. The pipet is also calibrated into the tip. Serological pipets are used to prepare dilutions of serum but should not be used in preparation of reagents.

When measuring liquid in a narrow vessel, such as a pipet or a graduated cylinder, you will notice that the liquid has a curvature at the surface. This is called the *meniscus* and should be adjusted so that, at eye level, the bottom of the curve is at the calibration line (Figure 48-9).

Micropipettors (Figure 48-10) are used to deliver very small quantities of liquid—from 1 to 1000 microliters (µl). It is important to follow the manufacturer's instructions for the device, because each may be slightly different. These pipetting devices must be fitted with an appropriate disposable tip. These tips may be sterile, depending on their use. The device is fitted with a piston at the top, which must be depressed before the pipet is filled and when the pipet is drained.

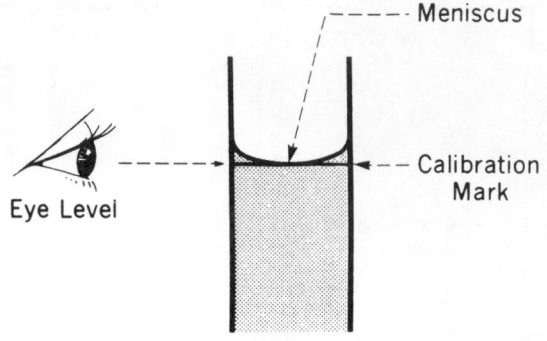

FIGURE 48-9   Reading the meniscus. (From Linne JJ, Ringsrud KM: *Clinical laboratory science: the basics and routine techniques,* ed 4, St Louis, 1999, Mosby.)

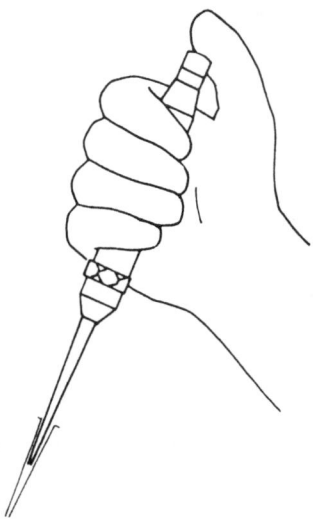

FIGURE 48-10   Piston-type automatic micropipettor. (Modified from Linne JJ, Ringsrud KM: *Clinical laboratory science: the basics and routine techniques,* ed 4, St Louis, 1999, Mosby.)

CRITICAL THINKING APPLICATION

Marsha is preparing a solution and is required to measure a 6-ml volume of saline solution. She has a 10-ml TD pipet. The pipetting device provided by the laboratory uses vacuum to draw up the liquid and forced air to expel it. Marsha knows that she should allow the pipet to drain with the force of gravity, yet she is forced to use a pipetting device. How will she accurately deliver 6 ml?

Preparing Dilutions

When the medical assistant performs laboratory tests, he or she may find it necessary to dilute a body fluid sample with a **diluent,** such as water, saline solution, or a buffer. For example, dilutions must be made when testing for the presence and strength of antibodies in serum, or when a patient's analyte level is grossly elevated and cannot be read by the instrument.

The term *dilution* refers to parts in total volume; it is a statement of relative concentration and represents expressions of concentration, not expressions of volume. For example, a 1:10 dilution can be prepared by measuring 1 ml of sample and diluting it with diluent to 10 ml. This means adding 9 ml of diluent. The same 1:10 dilution can be prepared by mixing 2 ml of sample and 18 ml of diluent or 0.5 ml of sample and 4.5 ml of diluent. Note that the final volume is not the same in each of the above examples, yet each is a 1:10 dilution. Any volume of a dilution can be made as long as the relative amounts of the components remain the same.

Clinical Laboratory Equipment

The Microscope

Every medical laboratory is equipped with a microscope. This indispensable instrument is used to view objects too small to be seen with the naked eye (Figure 48-11). The microscope is used to evaluate stained blood smears, urine sediment, and smears made from body fluids or microbiological cultures. Because the microscope is an expensive and technical instrument, special care must be taken in its operation, care, and storage.

Microscopes have three components: the magnification system, the illumination system, and the framework, which includes all components responsible for positioning the slide and focusing. The *magnification system* of the microscope includes the ocular and the objective lenses. Microscopes are either *monocular* or *binocular.* A monocular microscope has one eyepiece for viewing, and a binocular has two. The *eyepiece,* or *ocular,* is located at the top of the microscope and contains a lens to magnify what is being seen. The usual magnification is 10 times (10×). The *objectives* are attached to the *revolving nosepiece.* Most microscopes have three objectives; each has a different magnifying power. The shortest objective has the lowest power (10×). Low power is used to scan the field of interest and then focus on a particular object. Greater detail is observed with the next longest objective, which is high power (40×). The longest objective, oil immersion (100×), allows for the finest focusing of the object and requires the use of a special oil that is placed directly on the slide.

The *arm* of the microscope connects the objectives and oculars to the *base,* which supports the microscope and contains its light source. The *stage* of the microscope holds the slide to be viewed. Together, the *light source,* the *condenser,* and the *iris diaphragm* compose the *illumination system.* The condenser directs light up through the stage and the iris diaphragm regulates the amount of light passing through the specimen. Just above the base are the focusing knobs. The *coarse adjustment* is used only with low power, and the *fine adjustment* is used with high power and oil immersion lenses.

Microscopes are very precise and expensive instruments that require careful handling. The amount of routine maintenance required depends on the amount of daily use. Dirt is the enemy of the microscope, so it must be kept scrupulously clean at all times. The microscope

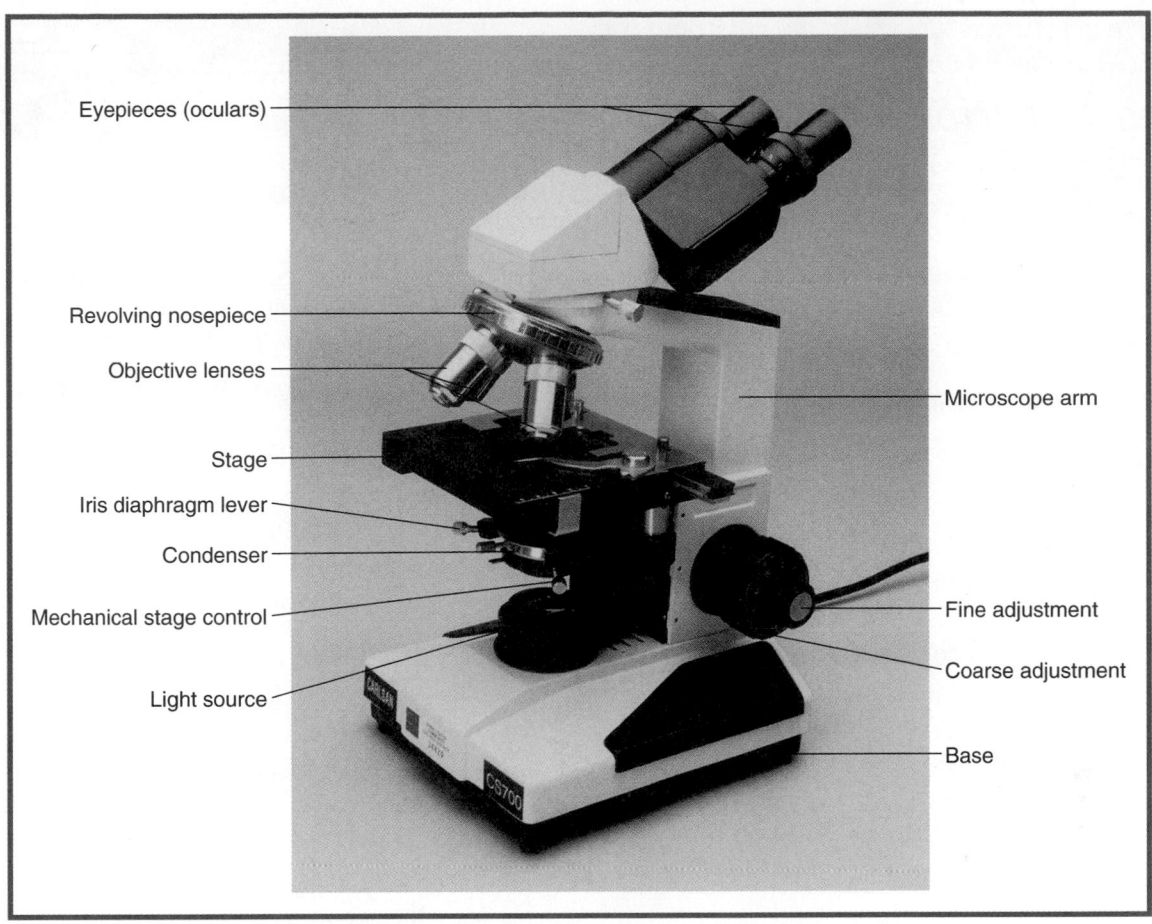

Eyepieces (oculars)

Revolving nosepiece

Objective lenses

Stage

Iris diaphragm lever

Condenser

Mechanical stage control

Light source

Microscope arm

Fine adjustment

Coarse adjustment

Base

FIGURE 48-11   Parts of a microscope. (Courtesy Cynmar Corporation, Carlinville, Illinois.)

should always be stored in a plastic dust cover when not in use. Lenses should be cleaned before and after each use with lens paper and lens cleaner. Any other type of tissue scratches the lenses or leaves lint residue behind. The routine use of solvent cleaners, such as xylene, is not recommended, because these cleaners may loosen lenses. However, xylene can be used to remove oil that has dried on the lenses. Oil, makeup, dust, and eye secretions all can obstruct vision through the lens and cause the possible transmission of infection. The body of the microscope should be dusted with a soft cloth.

The microscope should be placed in a permanent location in the laboratory on a sturdy table in an area where it cannot be bumped. If a microscope must be moved, it should be carried securely, with one hand supporting the base and the other holding the arm. When the microscope is stored, it should be left covered, with the low-power objective in the lowest position. The stage should be centered.

Using a microscope involves focusing and illumination (Procedure 48-1). The image is focused by moving the objective closer to the specimen, and illumination is accomplished by raising or lowering the condenser and by moving the specimen closer or farther away from the objective.

Focusing the microscope is done through movement of the objective or stage, which is controlled by round knobs located on both sides of the microscope. Proper focusing of the microscope begins with the lowest power objective. The coarse adjustment moves the objective very quickly. This knob is used first to bring the specimen into approximate focus. The fine adjustment focus knob then brings the specimen into precise focus. The fine focus moves the objective more slowly to allow the viewer to zero in on the specimen with greater accuracy.

If the microscope is a binocular model, the viewer may find it necessary to adjust the eyepieces to accommodate the distance between the pupils and the individual's point of greatest visual acuity. A gentle push inward or pull outward will adjust the distance between the eyepieces.

The Centrifuge

Centrifugation, which is used when separation of solids from liquids is necessary, involves the application of increased gravitational force achieved by rapid spinning. Centrifugation is used to separate blood cells from serum and solid materials, such as cells and crystals, from urine and is employed in many areas of the clinical laboratory.

Centrifuges (Figure 48-12) are designed for specific uses. They may be bench-top or floor models; some may be refrigerated. Some may have rotors or heads that are interchangeable. A typical clinical centrifuge may have a

PROCEDURE 48-1

Using the Microscope

GOAL: To focus the microscope properly, using a prepared slide, under low power, high power, and oil immersion

EQUIPMENT AND SUPPLIES

- Microscope
- Lens cleaner
- Lens tissue
- Slide containing specimen

PROCEDURAL STEPS

1 Wash your hands.

2 Gather the materials needed.

3 Clean the lenses with lens tissue and lens cleaner.

4 Adjust seating to a comfortable height.

5 Plug the microscope into an electric outlet and turn on the light switch.

6 Place the slide specimen on the stage and secure it.

7 Turn the revolving nosepiece to low power.

8 Carefully raise the stage while observing with the naked eye from the side.

9 Focus the specimen, using the coarse adjustment knob.

10 Switch to fine adjustment and focus the specimen in detail.

11 Adjust the amount of light by closing the iris diaphragm and lowering the condenser.

12 Turn the revolving nosepiece between the high power objective and oil immersion.

13 Place a small drop of oil on the slide.

14 Carefully swing the oil immersion objective into place.

15 Adjust the focus with the fine adjustment knob.

16 Increase the light by opening the iris diaphragm and raising the condenser.

17 Identify the specimen.

18 Return to low power.

19 Lower the stage.

20 Center the stage.

21 Remove the slide.

22 Switch off the light and unplug the microscope.

23 Clean the lenses with lens tissue and remove oil with lens cleaner.

24 Wipe the microscope with a cloth.

25 Cover the microscope.

26 Clean the work area.

27 Wash your hands.

---

rotor that is at a fixed angle, in which the specimen cups are held in a rigid position at a fixed angle; one that has a horizontal head with swinging buckets that swing out horizontally during centrifugation; and a third used for centrifuging capillary tubes for microhematocrit determination (see Chapter 50). Centrifuges may also be equipped with timers to automatically stop centrifugation at a set time.

Directions for the use of a centrifuge are usually given in terms of revolutions per minute (rpm). Spinning generates centrifugal force. General laboratory centrifuges operate at up to 6000 rpm, generating relative centrifugal force up to 7300 times the force of gravity (G). Conventional horizontal centrifuges attain speeds of up to 3000 rpm; angle-head centrifuges can attain higher speeds (up to 7000 rpm).

Centrifuges can be dangerous devices if not used correctly. The most important rule is to ensure that the centrifuge is balanced so that tubes of equal size and containing equal volume are directly across from one another in the rotor holders. Therefore, there will always be an even number of specimens in the centrifuge. If a second specimen of the same volume in the same-sized tube is not available for balance, a tube of water may be used to balance the load. Tubes being centrifuged should also be capped to avoid emission of aerosols. Rubber cups should be placed in the bottom of the carrier cups to avoid breakage of glass tubes.

Centrifuges should never be opened while they are in operation, nor should you attempt to slow a centrifuge with your hands. Most models are equipped with a brake, which should only be used in an emergency, the most common of which is a broken glass tube. In this case, wait until the centrifuge comes to a complete stop and follow the manufacturer's instructions for disinfecting the unit.

Centrifuges should be checked, cleaned, and lubricated regularly to ensure proper operation. A photoelectric device or a strobe tachometer must be used by a certified technician to ensure centrifuge speed to comply with QA guidelines set forth by CAP.

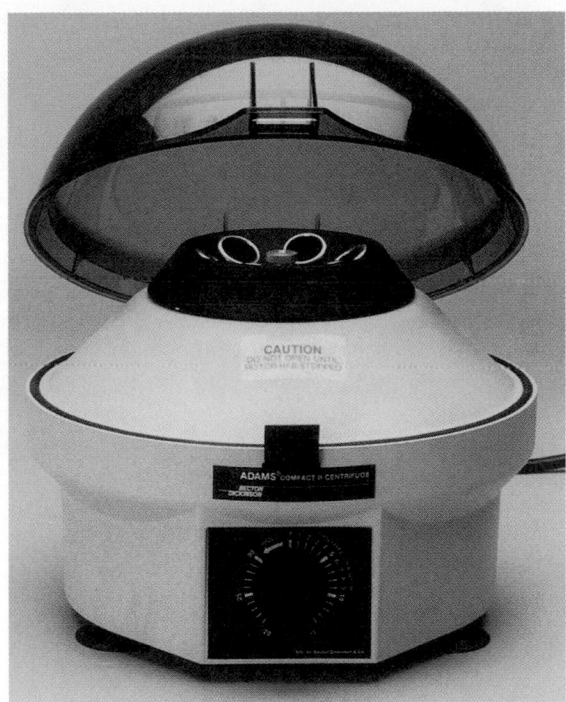

FIGURE 48-12   Centrifuge.

The Incubator

Incubators are cabinets that maintain constant temperatures. Generally used in the microbiology laboratory, they maintain a constant temperature of 35° to 37° C, although other temperatures may be also be appropriate. Some incubator interiors may be enriched with carbon dioxide (CO_2) gas to enhance the growth of pathogenic bacteria; a pressurized tank of CO_2 gas is attached to the cabinet and the concentration is maintained at 10%. Incubators may have warning alarms if the temperature exceeds or falls below a specified range. The temperature should be checked daily and the cabinets should be cleaned regularly with a disinfectant approved by the manufacturer.

The Autoclave

The autoclave is an instrument that uses steam under pressure to sterilize materials that can withstand high temperatures. The principles of operation are explained in Chapter 54.

It is essential that strict QA methods be followed when an autoclave is used. A certified technician should regularly examine the autoclave, and biological and chemical indicators should be checked on a daily basis. Biological indicators include spore preparations that are included in the autoclave load. At the end of the sterilization period, they are incubated and checked for germination. If the spores fail to germinate, the autoclave reached the appropriate temperature. Chemical methods include a special tape that changes color to show the word *autoclaved* when the temperature of the autoclave reaches 121° C.

The autoclave is used in the medical laboratory to sterilize specimens or objects before disposal. For example, throat culture collection devices, contaminated latex gloves, or tubes of blood may require sterilization before disposal. These items are placed in an orange biohazard bag, which is sealed and marked with autoclave tape before autoclaving.

Patient Education

Many testing procedures require that patients be given a specific set of instructions to follow. For example, patients may be required to fast 8 to 12 hours before the collection of blood and urine. They may need to follow a high-carbohydrate diet for several days before a *glucose tolerance test* (GTT). The consumption of some foods and medication must be discontinued. The physician will discuss medication alternatives with the patient. Sometimes it might not be medically advisable to discontinue the medication; this must be noted on the laboratory requisition. The laboratory will then be alerted to the possible drug interferences, and it may be able to use an alternative test method.

Often it is the medical assistant's responsibility to explain to the patient the measures that are to be taken before laboratory testing. Be sure that you have interpreted the physician's orders correctly before explaining the procedure to the patient. Giving the patient written instructions is recommended, with a phone number included on the instruction sheet so that the patient can call if he or she has questions.

Legal and Ethical Issues

If disease did not exist, there would be little need for clinical laboratories. The fact that the human body is susceptible to disease necessitates the existence of laboratory testing. One cannot anticipate or prevent every health and safety risk, but the risks are greatly reduced when everyone who works in the laboratory setting is conscious of safety guidelines.

Use good common sense. Document everything. If you are in doubt about the safety of a procedure, ask your supervisor. If you are aware of a potential safety problem, report it to the person in charge. Your welfare, the welfare of the patient, and the welfare of your co-workers may depend on your commitment to safety.

SUMMARY OF SCENARIO

Marsha's experience in clinical laboratory testing made her a valuable asset to her new employer. A thorough understanding of government rules and regulations, including the CLIA, and the guidelines published by the CDC, the EPA, and OSHA helped Marsha to implement laboratory testing in the clinic, including urinalysis, hemoglobin and hematocrit testing, pregnancy testing, and hemoglobin A1C monitoring. Marsha helped the physicians design a safe, efficient laboratory space with a refrigerator, centrifuge, and biohazard waste station. She developed a rigorous quality assurance program and is now training other medical assistants to perform CLIA-waived testing.

Marsha found it most challenging to determine how to comply with proper medical waste disposal issues. It required her to make several phone calls to state environmental protection agencies, but her diligence was rewarded when the laboratory received certification. Marsha pays close attention to CLIA regulations and receives regular updates of the tests that can be performed in a physician's office laboratory. She is currently determining the feasibility of performing drug screenings for local businesses. Her employers are pleased with her efforts and the patients appreciate the convenience of on-site testing.

SUMMARY OF LEARNING OBJECTIVES

- The clinical laboratory is responsible for analysis of blood and body fluids, providing the physician with test results that become part of the essential data needed to diagnose and manage a patient's condition.

- Most physicians' offices that perform laboratory testing will do so in the areas of urinalysis, hematology, chemistry, and microbiology. Routine urinalysis, complete blood counts, pregnancy testing, and throat cultures are some of the tests that might be performed in a physician's office laboratory.

- Federal agencies that regulate the laboratory include the U.S. Department of Labor, the U.S. Department of Health and Human Services, and the Environmental Protection Agency (EPA). Professional agencies that provide guidelines include the National Committee for Clinical Laboratory Standards and the College of American Pathologists. Although all of the agencies provide recommendations for operation procedures in the clinical laboratory, not all have the power to enforce them. The Department of Labor and the EPA can impose significant fines for failing to follow regulations, but the standard precautions set forth by the CDC are recommended but not enforceable.

- Risks can be minimized in all areas of the laboratory by using common sense and by having a formal safety training program and an up-to-date safety manual.

- The laboratory requisition must have all information needed to identify the patient, the ordering physician, the test ordered, and the specific details regarding the collection (such as time and source) of the specimen.

- Chain of custody is a method used to ensure that a specimen provided by a patient who may be involved in a legal matter is handled in a fashion that will not compromise the test results. All individuals who handle or test the specimen must be identified in writing and provide a signature.

- Quality assurance involves procedures undertaken to ensure that each patient is provided excellent care. Quality control—ensuring that laboratory testing is accurate and reliable—is part of a quality assurance program.

- Greenwich time uses the designations AM and PM, whereas military time uses the 24-hour clock: 3:15 PM is equivalent to 1515 hours.

- Although the Celsius (Centigrade) thermometer is used in the clinical laboratory, in everyday life we commonly use the Fahrenheit system. The incubator is usually set at 37° C (98° F), the autoclave sterilizes at 121° C (254° F), and refrigerator temperature is 2° to 8° C (35° to 46° F).

- Liquid volume is measured in liters, distance is measured in meters, and mass is measured in grams. Prefixes commonly used in the clinical laboratory include *milli* (0.001), *centi* (0.01), *micro* (0.000001), *deci* (0.1), and *kilo* (1000).

- Pipets must be chosen according to the job they are to perform. A pipetting device, such as a bulb or pump, should be attached, and particular attention must be given to the emptying of the pipet. The mouth should never be used in pipetting.

- Dilutions are prepared by mixing volumes of sample, such as blood, body fluids, or reagents, and volumes of diluent, such as water, saline solution, or buffer. The term *dilution* refers to parts in total volume and is an expression of concentration.

- Figure 48-11 provides an illustration of a microscope. The parts of the microscope can be divided into the illumination system (light source, condenser, and iris diaphragm lever), the frame (base, adjustment knobs, arm, stage, stage control), and the magnification system (objective lenses on the revolving nosepiece, oculars).

- Centrifuges are available for different types of centrifugation needs. The proper tube must be used and it must be protected from breakage. Centrifuge loads must be carefully balanced. Specimens must be capped to prevent aerosols. Under no circumstances should centrifuges be opened while they are in operation.

- Autoclaves provide sterilization by exposing materials to steam under pressure. The steam must reach a temperature of 121° C. Specialized tape or spore strips must be used to ensure that the proper temperature has been reached.

KEY INTERNET WEBSITES

- College of American Pathologists
- The Centers for Disease Control and Prevention
- Occupational Safety and Health Administration
- National Committee for Clinical Laboratory Standards
- Environmental Protection Agency
  For active weblinks to each website visit
  http://evolve.elsevier.com/Kinn/

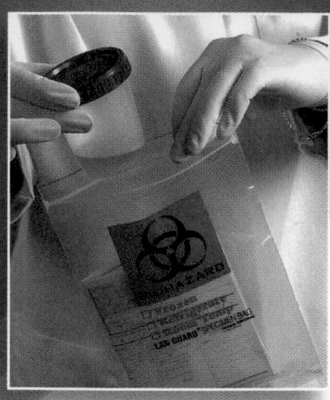

CHAPTER 49

Scenario

As part of her duties as a CMA, Rosa Gonzales performs tests on urine. Urinalysis, she knows, is a very important part of patient care, and a number of tests are performed on urine in the laboratory in Dr. Ronald Hill's busy practice. Dr. Hill most commonly orders routine urinalysis testing, but Rosa also performs some specialized tests.

Assisting in the Analysis of Urine

Robin R. Patterson

National Curriculum Competencies

CLINICAL COMPETENCIES

2e. Instruct patients in the collection of a clean-catch midstream urine specimen

3a. Use methods of quality control
3b. Perform urinalysis
3g. Screen and follow-up test results

Vocabulary

amorphous Lacking a defined shape.

bilirubinuria Presence of bilirubin in the urine.

casts Fibrous or protein materials that are thrown off into the urine in kidney disease.

colony forming units (CFU) Term used when reporting bacteriuria; one CFU represents one bacterium present in the urine sample.

crenate Forming notches or leaflike scalloped edges on an object.

culture and sensitivity (C&S) A procedure performed in the microbiology laboratory in which a specimen is cultured on artificial media to detect bacterial or fungal growth, followed by appropriate screening for antibiotic sensitivity.

enzymatic reaction Chemical reaction controlled by an enzyme.

filtrate Fluid that remains after a liquid is passed through a membranous filter.

glycosuria Presence of glucose in the urine.

ischemia Decreased blood flow to a body part or organ, caused by constriction or plugging of the supplying artery.

mononuclear white blood cell A leukocyte having an unsegmented nucleus; monocytes and lymphocytes in particular.

myoglobinuria Abnormal presence of a hemoglobin-like chemical of muscle tissue in urine that is the result of muscle deterioration.

phenylalanine Essential amino acid found in milk, eggs, and other foods.

polymorphonuclear white blood cell Leukocytes having a segmented nucleus. Also known as PMN (polymorphonuclear neutrophils) or segmented neutrophils.

refractile Causing light to refract, thus creating a sharp boundary or image.

renal thresholds Levels above which a substance cannot be reabsorbed by the renal tubules and is thus excreted in the urine.

supravital Of, relating to, or capable of staining living cells after their removal from a living or recently dead organism.

void To urinate.

A routine *urinalysis* (UA) is one of the more common laboratory examinations used in the diagnosis and treatment of disease. It can be easily and quickly performed, and invasive techniques are generally not needed to collect the specimen. The results of a routine urinalysis can reveal diseases of the bladder or kidneys; systemic metabolic or endocrine disorders, such as diabetes; and diseases of the liver, such as hepatitis or cirrhosis, or obstruction of the bile ducts. Urinalysis is routinely performed on all patients undergoing physical examinations and on those entering the hospital for treatment.

Physiology of Urine Formation

It has been known for centuries that abnormalities in the urine may be indicators of disruption of homeostasis. One of the earliest known tests of the urine was to pour it on the ground and see if it attracted insects. Such attraction indicated "honey urine," which was known to be excreted by persons with skin eruptions. Today urine is still checked for sugar as a means to detect diabetes.

Historically, examination of the urine became a game for quacks and charlatans. Paintings from the Middle Ages show physicians peering into round-bottomed flasks of urine, claiming not only to be able to diagnose disease, but to see into the future by simply looking at the fluid. These charlatans became known as "Pisse Prophets." During the twentieth century, urinalysis became a practical laboratory procedure, and today urine is the most commonly analyzed body fluid in the clinical laboratory.

Urine is analyzed for two reasons. The first is to detect extrinsic conditions—those in which the kidney is functioning normally, but abnormal end-products of metabolism are excreted as a result of an imbalance in homeostasis. The second is to detect intrinsic pathological conditions that involve the kidneys or urinary tract themselves.

The Anatomy of the Urinary Tract

Medical assistants must have a basic knowledge of kidney structure and urine formation to understand the results of a urinalysis. The urinary tract consists of two kidneys, two ureters, one bladder, and one urethra. The functional unit of the kidney is the nephron. There are more than 1 million nephrons per kidney, and each nephron is composed of five distinct areas, each playing a role in urine formation (Figure 49-1). Each nephron consists of a *glomerulus*, which acts in filtering, and a *tubule*, through which the **filtrate** passes. As the filtrate passes through, various changes occur. Certain solutes are reabsorbed, and others are secreted into the kidney for eventual excretion. Nearly all of the water that passes through the glomeruli is reabsorbed.

The glomerulus is composed of a network of capillaries surrounded by a membrane called *Bowman's capsule*. The *afferent arteriole* carries blood from the renal artery into the glomerulus, where it then divides to form a capillary network. Where they reunite, the capillaries form the *efferent arteriole*, through which blood will exit the glomerulus.

The tubular portion of the nephron is composed of the *proximal convoluted tubule*, the *thin-walled segment*, and the *distal convoluted tubule*. The thin-walled descending portion forms a loop known as the *loop of Henle*. Filtrate from several nephrons drains into a collecting tubule, a number of which join to form a *collecting duct*. The collecting ducts join to form the *papillary ducts*, which empty at the tips of the *papillae* into the *calyces*. The filtrate then drains into the renal pelvis and is now called *urine*. Urine passes from the pelvis of the kidney down the ureter and into the bladder, where it remains until it is voided through the urethra.

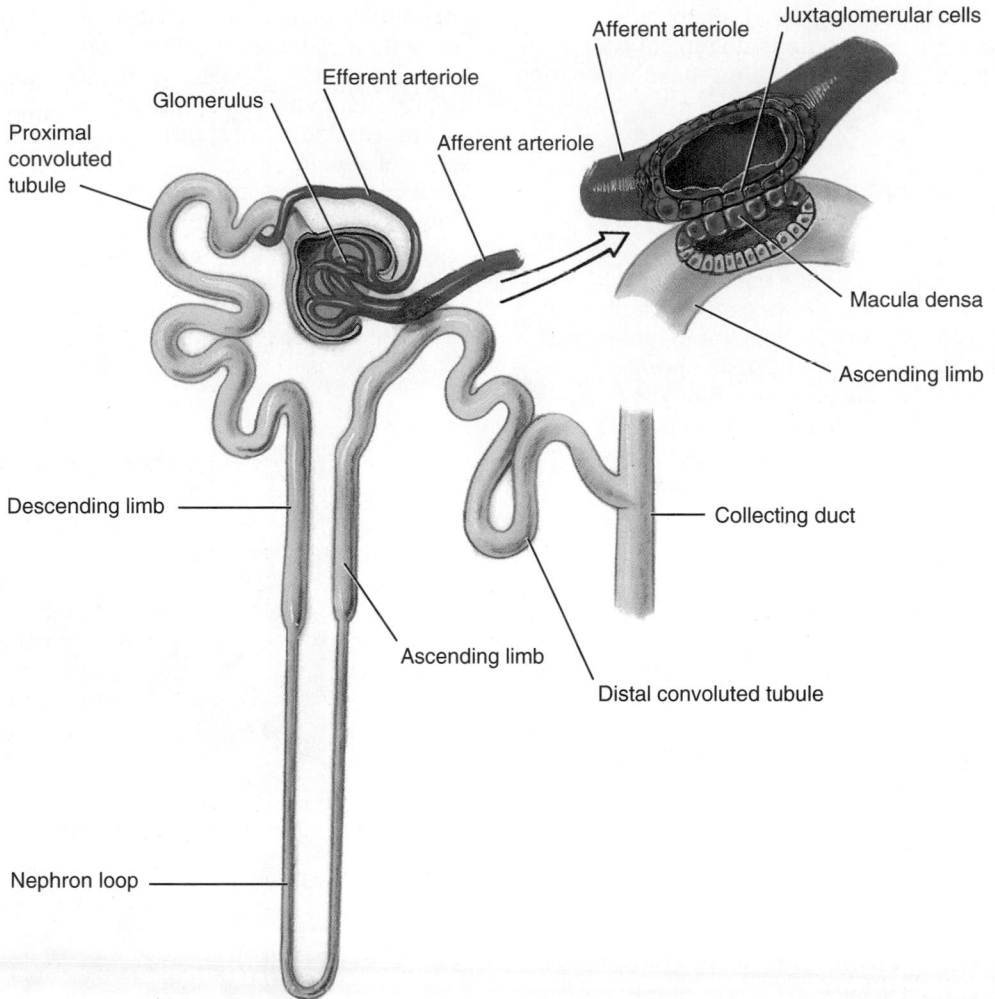

FIGURE 49-1   A nephron. (From Applegate EJ: *The anatomy and physiology learning system*, Philadelphia, 1995, WB Saunders.)

The Formation of Urine

The kidney selectively excretes or retains substances according to body needs and **renal thresholds**. About 1200 ml of blood flow through the kidneys each minute. The blood enters the glomerulus through the afferent arteriole. The capillary walls of the glomerulus are highly permeable to water and the low-molecular-weight solutes of the plasma, and they filter through into Bowman's space and then into the tubules. Many components of the filtrate, including glucose, water, and amino acids, are partially or completely reabsorbed by the capillaries surrounding the proximal tubules. More water is absorbed, and hydrogen and potassium ions are secreted in the distal tubules. Urine is concentrated in the system of collecting tubules and the loop of Henle. The kidneys convert nearly 180,000 ml of filtered plasma per day into a final urine volume of 750 to 2000 ml—approximately 1% of the filtered plasma volume. The largest component of urine is water; the majority of the solutes are urea, chloride, sodium, potassium, phosphate, sulfate, creatinine, and uric acid.

Collecting a Urine Specimen

Containers

The most important requirement for a collection container is that it be scrupulously clean. The physician's office laboratory should provide a container; patients should not use jars from home. Disposable, nonsterile, plastic, or coated paper containers are the most common and are available in many sizes with tight-fitting lids. Special pliable polyethylene bags with adhesive are used for collection of urine from infants and children who are not toilet-trained. For specimens that must be collected over a period of time, large, wide-mouthed plastic containers with screw-cap tops are used. Most routine urinalysis testing, pregnancy testing, and testing for abnormal analytes are performed on urine collected in nonsterile containers.

When urine is to be cultured for bacteria, it is essential that it be collected in a sterile container. Such containers will be recognizable by an intact paper seal over the cap.

It is important to properly label all specimens with name, date, and time of collection and type of collection. Always don gloves before handling filled specimen containers.

Methods of Specimen Collection

Most analyses are performed on freshly voided urine collected in clean containers. This is called a *random specimen*. If the specimen is ordered to be collected when the patient arises in the morning, it is called a *first morning specimen*. These specimens are most concentrated and are best for nitrite and protein determination, bacterial culture, pregnancy testing, and microscopic examination. *Two-hour postprandial urine specimens*, collected 2 hours after a meal, are used in diabetic screening and for home diabetic-testing programs. *Twenty-four-hour urine specimens* are collected over 24 hours to give quantitative chemical analysis, such as hormone levels and creatinine clearance rates (a procedure for evaluating the glomerular filtration rate of the kidneys) (Figure 49-2).

A *second-voided specimen* is usually collected to determine glucose levels; the first void of the morning is discarded, and the second void of the day is collected. A *catheterized specimen* requires the physician or nurse to insert a catheter into the bladder, and a *suprapubic specimen* is collected with a needle inserted directly into the bladder.

The minimum volume for a routine urinalysis is usually 12 ml, but 50 ml is preferred. In any type of collection, it is imperative that the patient receive adequate verbal and/or written instructions. Asking a patient to half-fill the container is acceptable; it is best to have some room at the top of the container because the urine will need to be mixed before analysis. Never haphazardly ask a patient to "fill the cup."

A clean-catch midstream specimen may be ordered when the urine is to be cultured or examined for microorganisms. The clean-catch technique is used to remove microorganisms from the urinary meatus by thoroughly cleansing the area around the meatus and to flush out the distal portion of the urethra. Because the specimen is collected in the medical office by the patient, the medical assistant needs to give complete, understandable instructions to the patient on the method of collection (Procedure 49-1). Failure to do so may

mean that the patient will have to return to the office to allow the collection of another specimen. For culturing, urine should be collected by catheterization or the clean-catch method into a sterile container (Figure 49-3).

Proper handling of specimens is essential. The chemical and cellular components of urine change if they are allowed to stand at room temperature (Table 49-1). These changes can be avoided by refrigerating the specimen if the analysis cannot be performed within 30 minutes after collection. Occasionally, preservatives must be added to prevent the overgrowth of bacteria and resultant loss of glucose; this method is generally used for specimens to be sent to a referral laboratory. Consult

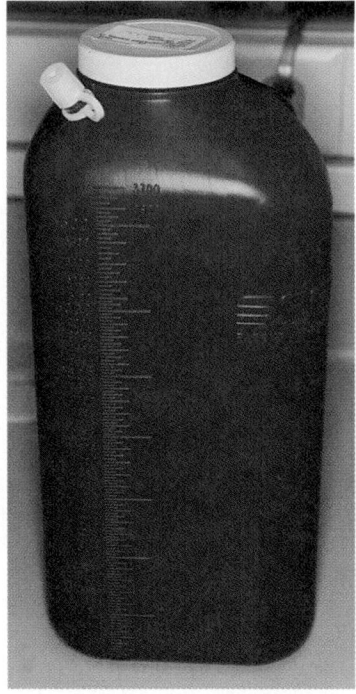

FIGURE 49-2 A 24-hour specimen container.

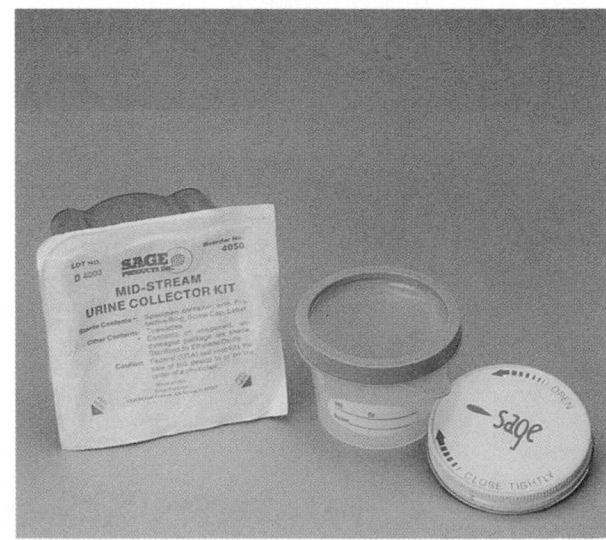

FIGURE 49-3 A sterile container for a midstream specimen.

PROCEDURE **49-1**

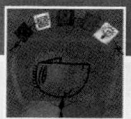

Collecting a Clean-Catch Urine Specimen for Culture or Analysis

GOAL: To collect a contaminant-free urine sample for culture or analysis using midstream clean-catch technique.

EQUIPMENT AND SUPPLIES

- Sterile container with lid and label
- Antiseptic towelettes
- Set of written patient instructions

PROCEDURAL STEPS

1 Label the container and give the patient the supplies (Figure 1).
   Purpose: Labeling the container avoids possible mix-up of specimens.

2 Explain the instructions to adult patients or to the guardians of child patients.
   Purpose: Instructions must be understood if they are to be followed correctly. By talking to the patient, you can determine whether the patient understands or has any questions. (Follow the instructions given in the chapter for obtaining male and female clean-catch samples.)

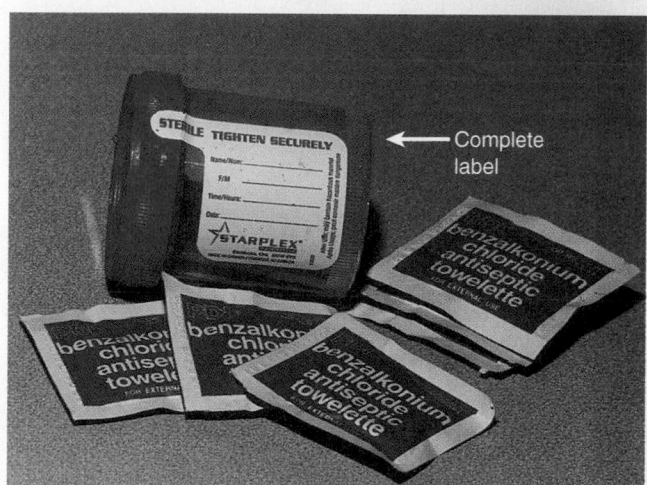

Figure 1

with the referral laboratory manual for the appropriate preservative. Never add a preservative to a specimen that has been collected for culture.

TABLE 49-1	Changes in Urine at Room Temperature
Constituent	**Change**
Clarity	Becomes cloudy as crystals precipitate and bacteria multiply
Color	May change if pH becomes alkaline
pH	Becomes alkaline as bacteria form ammonia from urea
Glucose	Decreases as bacteria metabolize it
Ketones	Decrease
Bilirubin and urobilinogen	Undergo degradation in light
Blood	May hemolyze. False-positives possible due to bacterial peroxidase
Nitrite	May becaome positive as bacteria convert nitrate. Can become negative as bacteria metabolize nitrite.
Casts	Lyse or dissolve in alkaline urine
Cells	Lyse or dissolve in alkaline urine
Bacteria	Multiply twofold every 20 minutes
Yeast	Multiply
Crystals	Precipitate as urine cools. May dissolve if pH changes

CRITICAL THINKING APPLICATION

Dr. Hill has ordered a urinalysis (UA) on the specimen from Mr. Parks, a UA and pregnancy test on the specimen from Mrs. Carpenter, and a UA and **culture and sensitivity (C&S)** on the specimen from Ms. Winfrey. After reviewing the requisitions and entering the patient information into the daily logbook, Rosa notes that Mrs. Carpenter's specimen was collected at 6 AM—3 hours ago. Is this acceptable? Explain your answer. Rosa also notes that the specimen collected in the sterile container from Ms. Winfrey is marked "CCMS." Why is this important?

Instructing Patients in Collecting a Urine Specimen

Most adult patients understand the procedure for collecting a routine (random) urine specimen. However, they do need special instructions for collecting a timed specimen and a midstream clean-catch specimen. The guidelines in the boxes that immediately follow will help you teach patients how to collect urine specimens.

COLLECTING A 24-HOUR SPECIMEN

1. On arising in the morning, **void** into the toilet. Empty your bladder completely. Do not save this urine. Note the exact time, and write it down on the container.
2. Collect all urine voided after this time for exactly 24 hours. Remember that all urine passed at night or during the day in this time period must be saved.
3. Remember to keep the urine cool.
4. At exactly the same time the following morning, urinate completely again. Save this sample. Add it to the collection container. This completes your 24-hour collection.
5. Take all specimens from the 24-hour collection to the medical office, or to the place designated, as soon as possible, maintaining the cool temperature in transit by placing the specimen in a portable cooler or insulated bag.

OBTAINING A CLEAN-CATCH MIDSTREAM SPECIMEN (FEMALE PATIENT)

1. Wash your hands and remove your underclothing.
2. Expose the urinary meatus by spreading apart the labia with one hand (Figure 49-4, *A*).
3. Cleanse each side of the urinary meatus with a front-to-back motion, from the pubis to the anus. Use a separate antiseptic wipe to cleanse each side of the meatus.
4. Cleanse directly across the meatus, front-to-back, using a third cotton ball or antiseptic wipe (see Figure 49-4, *A*).
5. Hold the labia apart throughout this procedure.
6. Void a small amount of urine into the toilet (Figure 49-4, *B*).
7. Move the specimen container into position and void the next portion of urine into it. Remember, this is a sterile container. Do not put your fingers on the inside of the container.
8. Remove the cup and void the last amount of urine into the toilet. (This means that the first part and the last part of the urinary flow have been excluded from the specimen. Only the middle portion of the flow is included.)
9. Wipe in your usual manner, redress, and return the sterile specimen to the place designated by the medical facility.

OBTAINING A CLEAN-CATCH MIDSTREAM SPECIMEN (MALE PATIENT)

1. Wash your hands and expose the penis.
2. Retract the foreskin of the penis (if not circumcised).
3. Cleanse the area around the glans penis (meatus) and the urethral opening by washing each side of the glans with a separate antiseptic wipe (Figure 49-5, *A*).
4. Cleanse directly across the urethral opening using a third cotton ball or antiseptic wipe.
5. Void a small amount of urine into the toilet or urinal (Figure 49-5, *B*).
6. Collect the next portion of the urine in the *sterile* container without touching the inside of the container with hands or penis (Figure 49-5, *C*).
7. Void the last amount of urine into the toilet or urinal.
8. Wipe and redress.
9. Return the specimen to the designated area provided.

GUIDELINES FOR CARING FOR A URINE SPECIMEN OBTAINED AT HOME

1. Do not add anything but your urine into the bottle.
2. Do not pour out any liquid or powdered preservative from the container.
3. If you accidentally spill some of the preservative on yourself, immediately wash with water and call the testing center or designated laboratory.
4. Always keep the collection bottle cool. Refrigerate or keep the bottle in an ice-filled cooler or pail.
5. Keep the cap on the container.
6. You may find it more convenient to urinate into the smaller container provided and then pour the urine into the larger collection bottle.

The Routine Urinalysis

Physical Examination of Urine

The first part of a complete urinalysis is assessment of the physical properties and measurement of selected chemical constituents that are of diagnostic importance (Table 49-2).

Appearance: Color and Turbidity. Normal urine color is a shade of yellow, ranging from pale straw to yellow to amber (Procedure 49-2). Color depends on the concentration of the pigment *urochrome* and the amount of water in the specimen. A dilute specimen should be pale, and a more concentrated specimen should be a darker yellow (Figure 49-6). Variations in color may be caused by diet, medication, and disease. Abnormal colors

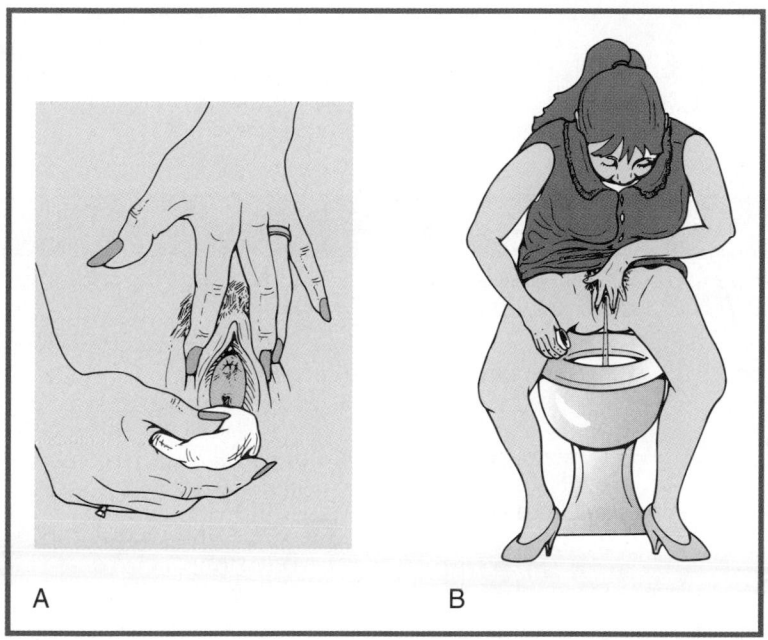

FIGURE 49-4   The procedure for obtaining a clean-catch urine specimen in females. (From Stepp CA, Woods MA: *Laboratory procedures for medical office personnel*, Philadelphia, 1998, WB Saunders.)

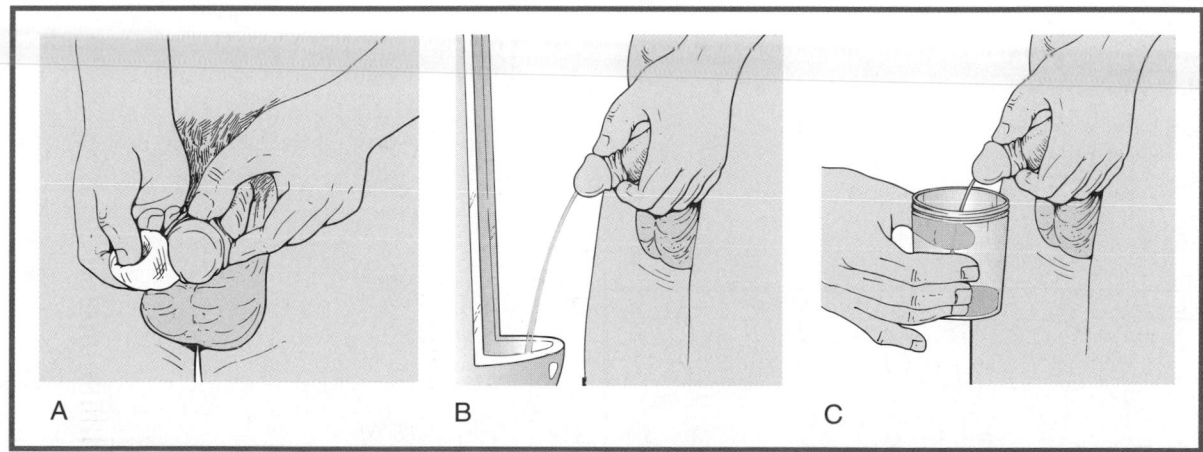

FIGURE 49-5   The procedure for obtaining a clean-catch urine specimen in males. (From Stepp CA, Woods MA: *Laboratory procedures for medical office personnel*, Philadelphia, 1998, WB Saunders.)

TABLE 49-2	Components of the Macroscopic Urinalysis
Physical Property	**Chemical Property Measured by Dipsticks**
Color	Protein
Clarity	Glucose
Specific gravity	Ketones
Amount	Bilirubin
Odor*	Blood: intact red blood cells, hemoglobin, myoglobin
Foam*	Nitrite
	Urobilinogen
	Leukocyte esterase
	Specific gravity†
	pH†

*Not always assessed.
†Physical properties measured on dipsticks.

may be related to pathological or nonpathological factors (Table 49-3).

Both normal and abnormal urine specimens may range in appearance from clear to very cloudy. Cloudiness may be caused by cells, bacteria, yeast, vaginal contaminants, or crystals. Often a urine specimen that was clear when voided will become cloudy as it cools when crystals form and precipitate.

Volume. The amount of urine is rarely measured on a random specimen. With a timed specimen, volume is measured by pouring the entire collection into a large, graduated cylinder. Generally, it is not accurate enough to use the markings on the side of the collection container. Once the volume is measured and recorded, a portion of well-mixed specimen, called an *aliquot*, is removed for testing. The remainder is discarded or stored, depending on the preference of the laboratory.

PROCEDURE 49-2

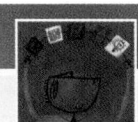

Assessing Urine for Color and Turbidity

GOAL: To assess and record the color and clarity of a urine specimen.

EQUIPMENT AND SUPPLIES

- Urine specimen
- Centrifuge tube

PROCEDURAL STEPS

1 Wash and dry your hands and don gloves.

2 Mix the urine by swirling.
  Purpose: Suspended substances settle when urine stands. If urine is not mixed before assessing appearance, the finding will be incorrect.

3 Label a centrifuge tube if a complete urinalysis is being done.
  Purpose: If a complete urinalysis is being done, a portion of the specimen will be centrifuged for microscopic examination. The centrifuged specimen must be labeled to avoid specimen confusion.

4 Pour the specimen into a standard-size centrifuge tube.

  Purpose: Standard-size containers are a better quality control for assessing color and clarity results.

5 Assess and record the color (Figure 49-6):
  Pale straw
  Yellow
  Dark yellow
  Amber

6 Assess clarity:
  Clear—no cloudiness
  Slightly cloudy—can see light print through tube
  Moderately cloudy—can see only dark print through tube
  Very cloudy—cannot see through tube

7 Clean the work area, remove gloves, and wash your hands.
  Purpose: Infection control.

8 Record the results in the patient's record.
  Purpose: A procedure is considered not done until it is recorded.

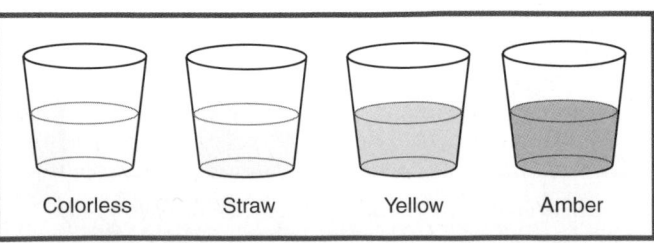

Colorless   Straw   Yellow   Amber

FIGURE 49-6 Colors of normal urine. (From Stepp CA, Woods MA: *Laboratory procedures for medical office personnel*, Philadelphia, 1998, WB Saunders.)

TABLE 49-3	Urine Colors	
Color	**Pathological Cause**	**Nonpathological Cause**
Straw	Diabetes	Diuretics; high fluid intake (coffee, beer)
Amber	Dehydration	Excessive sweating; low fluid intake
Bright yellow		Carotene, vitamins
Red	Blood, porphyrins	Beets, drugs, dyes
Orange-yellow	Bile, hepatitis	Pyridium (phenazopyridine hydrochloride), dyes, drugs
Greenish yellow	Bile, hepatitis	Senna, cascara, rhubarb
Reddish brown	Old blood, methemoglobin	
Brownish black	Methemoglobin, melanin	Levodopa
Salmon pink		Amorphous urates
White (milky)	Fats, pus	Amorphous phosphates
Blue-green	Biliverdin, infection with *Pseudomonas*	Vitamin B, drugs, dyes

The normal volume of urine produced every 24 hours varies according to the age of the individual. Infants and children produce smaller volumes than adults. The normal adult volume is 750 to 2000 ml in 24 hours, with an average of about 1500 ml. Excessive production of urine is called *polyuria*. This is common in diabetes and certain kidney disorders. *Oliguria* is insufficient production of urine and can be caused by dehydration, decreased fluid intake, shock, or renal disease. The absence of urine production, *anuria*, occurs in renal obstruction and renal failure.

Foam. Normally the presence of foam is not recorded, but careful observation of this property can be a significant clue to an abnormality. Foam is the presence of small bubbles that persist for a long time after the specimen has been shaken; they must not be confused with any bubbles that rapidly disperse. White foam can indicate the presence of increased protein (Figure 49-7). Greenish-yellow foam can mean **bilirubinuria**. Caution should be taken in handling such urines, because the color of the foam may mean that the patient has viral hepatitis.

Odor. As with foam, odor is not normally recorded but can be an important clue. Normal urine odor is said to be aromatic. Changes in the odor of urine may be caused by disease, the presence of bacteria, or diet. The odor of the urine of a patient with uncontrolled diabetes is described as fruity because of the presence of *ketones*, which are the products of fat metabolism. An ammonia or putrid smell in the urine can be caused by an infection. The bacteria break down the urea in the urine to form ammonia. Infection usually imparts a putrid odor. Foods such as asparagus and garlic can also produce an abnormal odor in the urine.

Specific Gravity. Specific gravity is the weight of a substance compared with the weight of an equal volume of distilled water. In urinalysis, it is the rough measurement of the concentration, or amount, of substances dissolved in urine. The specific gravity of distilled water is 1.000. Normal specific gravity of urine ranges from 1.005 to 1.030, depending on the patient's fluid intake. Most samples fall between 1.010 and 1.025. Urine specific gravity indicates whether the kidneys are able to concentrate the urine and is one of the first indi-

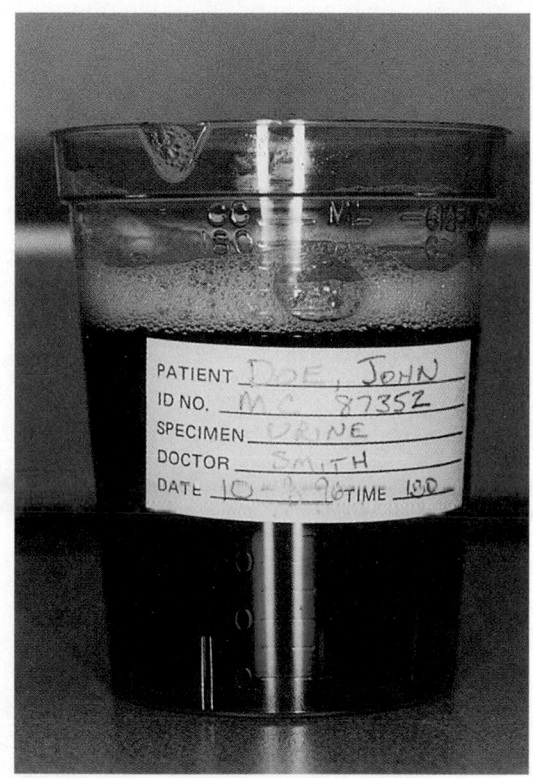

FIGURE 49-7 Dark amber urine with foam indicates possible increased protein and possible hematuria.

cations of kidney disease. The presence of glucose, protein, or an x-ray contrast medium used in diagnostic studies may also increase the specific gravity of urine. To measure the specific gravity of urine, laboratories use reagent strip, urinometer (Procedure 49-3), or refractometer (Procedure 49-4) methods. The reagent strip is the most commonly used method, and it is considered a CLIA waived test. The urinometer method, while accurate, uses a large volume of urine and results in contamination of several pieces of glassware. For these reasons, it is rarely used in specific gravity determination.

PROCEDURE **49-3**

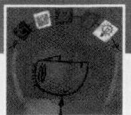

Measuring Specific Gravity Using a Urinometer

GOAL: To calibrate the urinometer to perform a quality control check and to obtain duplicate specific gravity readings.

EQUIPMENT AND SUPPLIES

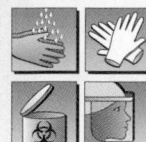

- Urine specimen
- Distilled water
- Urinometer and cylinder

PROCEDURAL STEPS

1 Wash and dry your hands and don nonsterile gloves and eye protection.

2 Fill the glass cylinder two thirds full with distilled water at 20° C (68° F; room temperature).
Purpose: A quantity of 20 to 25 ml is needed to allow the urinometer to float.

3 Read the specific gravity of the distilled water (Figure 1).
Purpose: If the urinometer does not read 1.000, a correction factor or a new urinometer is necessary.

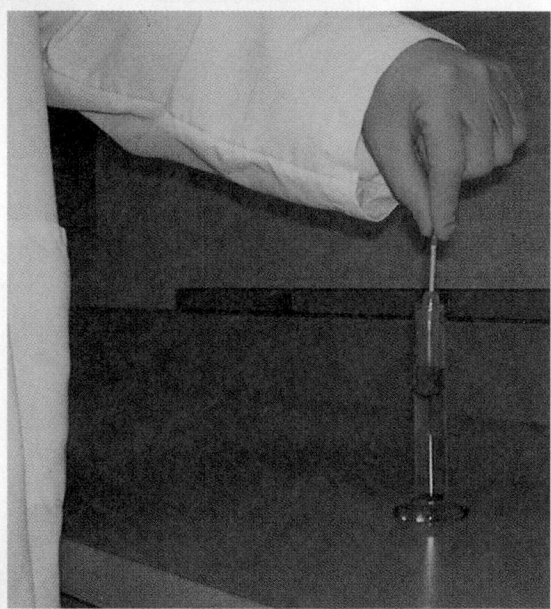

Figure 1

4 Allow the specimen to come to room temperature if it was refrigerated.
Purpose: Specific gravity measured by the urinometer is temperature dependent.

5 Mix the specimen well by swirling.

6 Pour the specimen into the clean glass cylinder to two thirds to three fourths full (Figure 2).
Purpose: A sufficient sample must be present to allow the urinometer to float freely.

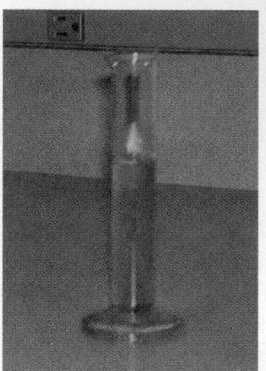

Figure 2

7 Remove any foam using filter paper (Figure 3).

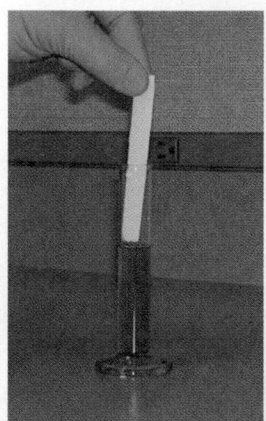

Figure 3

8 With the cylinder on a level surface, gently insert the urinometer in the specimen with a spinning motion (Figure 4).

9 While the urinometer stops rotating in the specimen, read the lower curve of the meniscus, at eye level (Figure 5*).
Purpose: For accurate results, the urinometer must be read at eye level. Adjust your line of vision to the urinometer: do not hold the cylinder in your hand.

10 Clean, disinfect, and dry the equipment, and return it to proper storage.

---

*From Stepp CA, Woods MA: *Laboratory procedures for medical office personnel*, Philadelphia, 1998, WB Saunders.

PROCEDURE 49-3—cont'd

Purpose: Urine salts dried on the equipment cause erroneous readings in later tests.

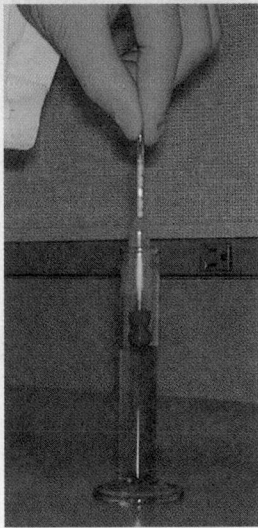

Figure 4

11 Clean the work area. Wash your hands.

12 Record the results on the laboratory form or in the patient's record.

Purpose: A procedure is considered not done until it is recorded.

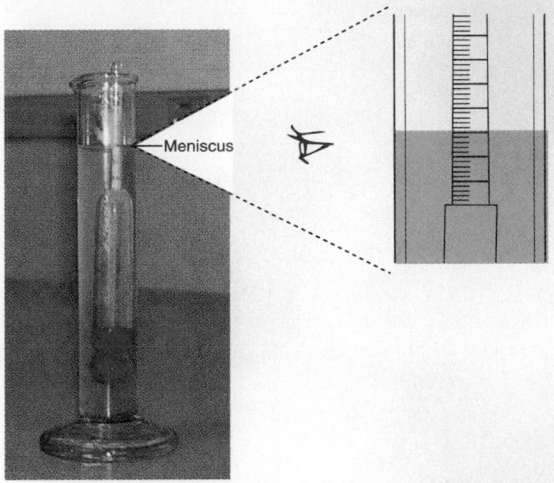

Figure 5

PROCEDURE 49-4

Measuring Urine Specific Gravity With a Refractometer

GOAL: To measure the refractive index of urine using a refractometer. A refractometer is also known as a *total solids* (TS) *meter.*

EQUIPMENT AND SUPPLIES

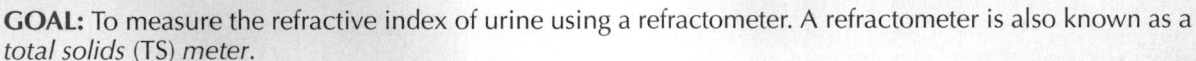

- Urinary refractometer
- Disposable pipet
- Distilled water
- Biohazard waste container

PROCEDURAL STEPS

1 Wash your hands and assemble equipment while the urine specimen reaches room temperature.

Purpose: Measuring specific gravity of cold or warm urine may alter the results.

2 Apply gloves and mix the urine specimen in the collection container.

Purpose: Mixing the urine resuspends solids that have settled during storage.

3 Using a disposable pipet, apply a drop of water to the prism of the refractometer (see Figure 49-9) by lifting the plastic cover. Close the cover and point the device toward a light source such as a window

or lamp. Look into the refractometer and rotate the eyepiece so the scale can be clearly read. The scale reads from 1.000 to 1.035 in increments of 0.001; distilled water should read 1.000.

4 Adjust the refractometer using the small screwdriver provided by the manufacturer if the scale does not read 1.000 (Figure 1*).

Purpose: This step ensures that the refractometer is calibrated properly.

5 Wipe the prism with a soft, lint-free tissue and apply a drop of mixed urine. Close the cover, point the device at a light source, and read the specific gravity on the scale (Figure 2*). Discard the pipet in a biohazard waste container.

Purpose: A soft cloth should be used to prevent scratching the glass prism.

---

*Figures from Stepp CA, Woods MA: *Laboratory procedures for medical office personnel*, Philadelphia, 1998, WB Saunders.

Continued

PROCEDURE 49-4—cont'd

6 Wipe the urine from the prism with a disposable soft, lint-free tissue between samples. When finished, clean with tissue moistened with distilled water. Discard these tissues in a biohazard waste container.

Purpose: Urine must be removed from the prism between samples.

7 Record the results and discard the urine sample.

Purpose: A procedure is not considered finished until it is recorded.

8 Remove and discard gloves and wash your hands.

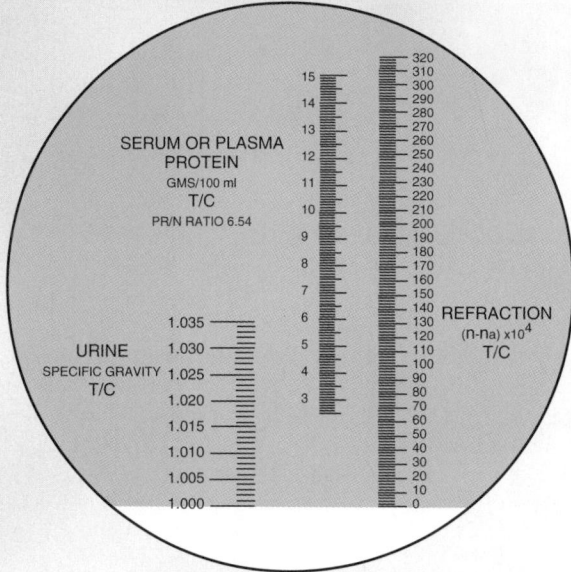

Figure 1

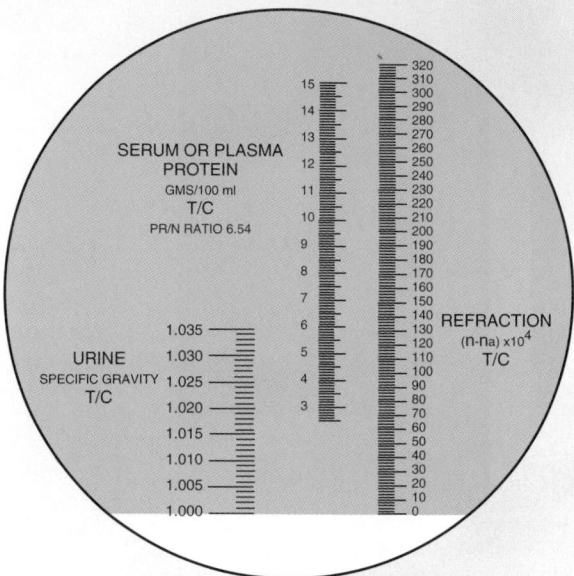

Figure 2

See Appendix E for a charting example.

The *urinometer* is a sealed glass float with a calibrated paper scale in its stem (Figure 49-8). With a slight spinning motion, it is placed into a cylinder containing a urine sample, and the value is read at the meniscus of the urine. It requires a quantity of urine sufficient to freely suspend the float, usually about 20 to 25 ml. If the sample is insufficient to float the urinometer, use a refractometer or record as "QNS" (quantity not sufficient).

A urinometer is fragile, and jarring can cause the paper scale in the stem to shift, resulting in erroneous readings. Occasionally, a damaged urinometer loses its calibration. Thus, the calibration of the urinometer should be checked daily with distilled water. The specific gravity of the distilled water should calibrate at 1.000 at 20° C (68° F; room temperature). For example, if the urinometer reads 1.002 in distilled water, 0.002 must be subtracted from the urine readings. However, it is better to replace the instrument. For each 3° C (37.4° F) that the water temperature measures above 20° C (68° F), 0.001 must be added to the reading. For each 3° C (37.4° F) that the water temperature measures below 20° C (68° F), subtract 0.001 from the reading. Use a laboratory thermometer to determine the water temperature.

A *refractometer* measures the refraction of light through solids in a liquid. The result is called the *refractive index*, which, for our purposes, is the same as specific gravity (Figure 49-9). The refractometer is both

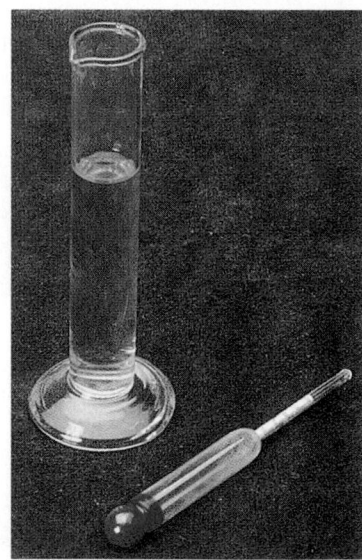

FIGURE 49-8   A urinometer.

faster and easier to use than the urinometer and requires only a drop of urine. One drop of well-mixed urine is placed under the hinged cover of the instrument, and the value is read directly from a scale viewed through an ocular. The refractometer must be

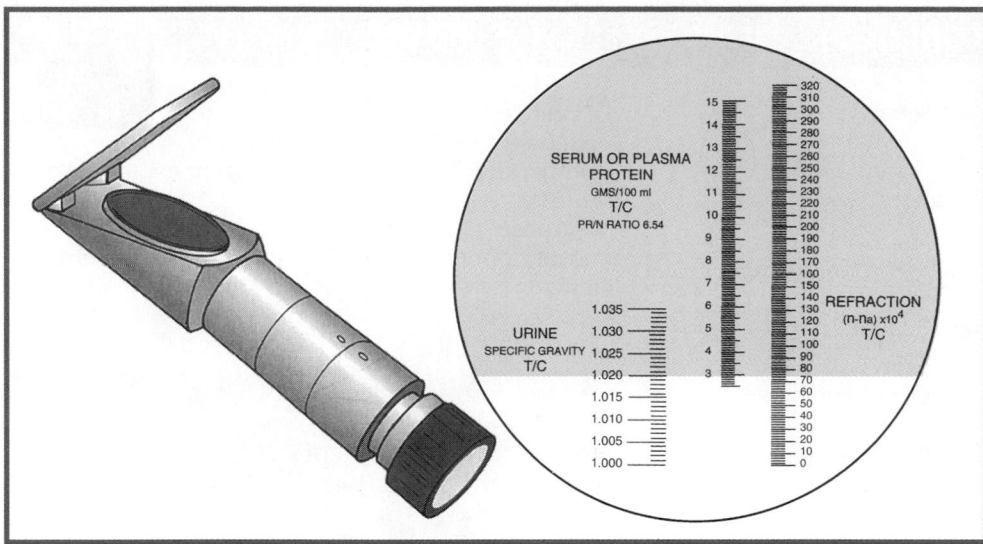

FIGURE 49-9 A refractometer. (From Stepp CA, Woods MA: *Laboratory procedures for medical office personnel*, Philadelphia, 1998, WB Saunders.)

calibrated daily with distilled water, which will read 1.000. Note that the measurement of specific gravity carries no unit of measure after the number.

CRITICAL THINKING APPLICATION

- The requisitions accompanying the urine specimens indicate that all three will require a UA. Rosa performs the physical analysis and notes that Mrs. Carpenter's urine, requiring the pregnancy test, is amber, whereas the other two specimens are pale yellow. Propose possible explanations for Rosa's observations. Should Rosa be concerned about the darker color of Mrs. Carpenter's urine?
- Ms. Winfrey's urine is turbid, whereas Mr. Parks' urine is clear. What might be causing the cloudiness in Ms. Winfrey's urine? Is a cloudy urine cause for concern?

Chemical Examination of Urine

Tests can be performed on urine to detect the presence of certain chemicals, which can provide valuable information to the physician. In certain situations, these chemical test results can be critical to the diagnosis.

Reagent strips (dipsticks) are the most widely employed technique for detecting chemicals in the urine (Procedure 49-5); these strips are available in a variety of types (Figure 49-10). Generally, they are plastic strips to which one or more pads containing chemicals are attached. Tests are available for pH, specific gravity, vitamin C, leukocytes, protein, ketones, glucose, blood, bilirubin, nitrite, urobilinogen, phenylketones, and other chemicals. The presence or absence of these chemicals in the urine provides information on the status of carbohydrate metabolism, liver and kidney function, and the patient's acid-base balance.

Reagent strips are designed to be used once and then discarded. The directions for each strip are located in the package, and these instructions must be followed

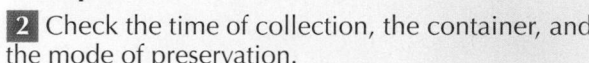

PROCEDURE **49-5**

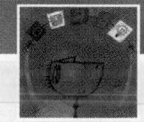

Testing Urine With Chemical Reagent Strips

GOAL: To perform chemical testing on a urine sample.

EQUIPMENT AND SUPPLIES

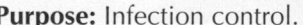

- Urine specimen
- Reagent strips
- Timer

PROCEDURAL STEPS

1 Wash and dry your hands. Don nonsterile gloves and eye protection.

Purpose: Infection control.

2 Check the time of collection, the container, and the mode of preservation.

Purpose: Proper specimen identification and screening of specimens for appropriate collection containers and collection procedures prevent testing of inappropriate specimens.

Continued

PROCEDURE 49-5—cont'd

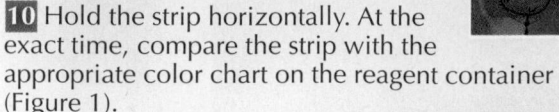

3 If the specimen has been refrigerated, allow it to warm to room temperature.

Purpose: Certain tests are temperature dependent. Testing of cold specimens may cause false-negative results.

4 Check the reagent strip container for expiration date.

Purpose: Do not use expired reagents.

5 Remove the reagent strip from the container. Hold it in your hand or place it on a clean paper towel. Recap the container tightly.

Purpose: Test strips are sensitive to moisture and must be stored in tightly sealed containers. Contamination from chemical residues on countertops can affect results.

6 Compare nonreactive test pads with the negative color blocks on the color chart on the container.

Purpose: Discolored pads have not been properly stored and must not be used for testing.

7 Thoroughly mix the specimen by swirling or inverting.

Purpose: If settling occurs, certain elements may not be detected.

8 Following manufacturer's directions, note the time and simultaneously dip the strip into the urine and remove.

Purpose: Tests are time dependent. Positive tests result in darkening with time.

9 Quickly remove the excess urine from the strip.

Purpose: Excess urine on the strip, or prolonged dipping time, affects test results.

10 Hold the strip horizontally. At the exact time, compare the strip with the appropriate color chart on the reagent container (Figure 1).

Purpose: Holding the strip horizontally prevents runover from one test pad to another and prevents interference from the mixing of chemicals in the test pads.

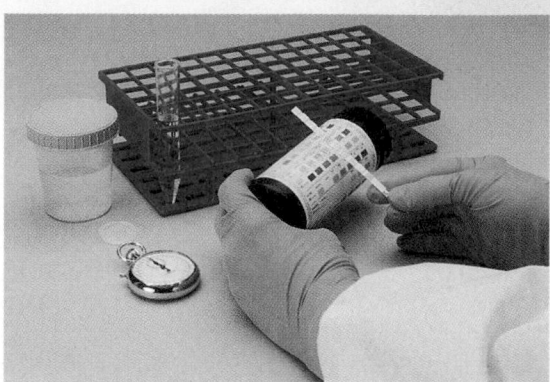

Figure 1

11 Read the concentration.
Purpose: Timing is critical.

12 Clean the work area, remove your gloves, and wash your hands.
Purpose: Infection control.

13 Record the results in the patient's record.
Purpose: A procedure is considered not done until it is recorded.

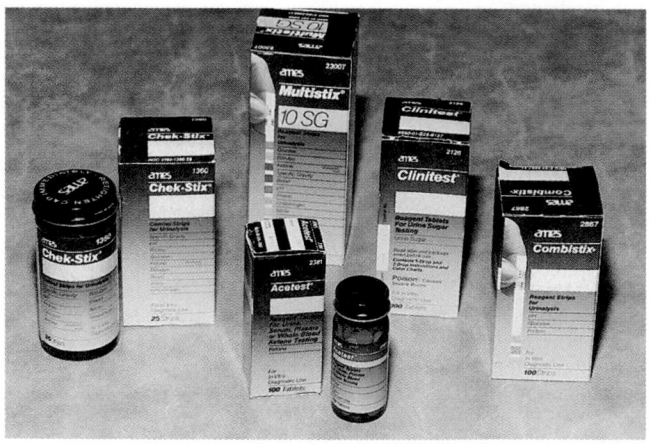

FIGURE 49-10 Examples of reagent strips.

exactly to obtain accurate results. A color-comparison chart is located on the label of the container. In addition to reagent strips, various tablet tests are available.

All strips and tablets must be kept in tightly closed containers in a cool, dry area and should only be removed immediately before testing. Never touch a strip that has been exposed to urine to the color-comparison chart. If both a UA and a C&S are ordered on a specimen, ensure that the urine has been cultured before beginning the UA. Introducing a reagent strip into the urine will contaminate it.

pH. The pH is a measurement of the degree of acidity or alkalinity of the urine. A urine specimen with a pH of 7.0 is neutral (Figure 49-11). Less than 7.0 is acid, and greater than 7.0 is alkaline. Normal, freshly voided urine may have a pH range of 5.5 to 8.0. Urinary pH varies with an individual's metabolic status, diet, drug therapy, and disease. In the case of gross bacteriuria, urine pH is alkaline as a result of bacterial conversion of urea to ammonia. Knowing the pH of the urine will also assist in the identification of crystals if they are found in the urine sediment.

Glucose. Glucose is filtered at the glomerulus, but under normal conditions most of it is reabsorbed by the tubules. The minute quantities normally present in the urine are not detected by reagent strips and tablets. Detectable **glycosuria** occurs whenever the renal tubules cannot reabsorb the filtered glucose load. A positive

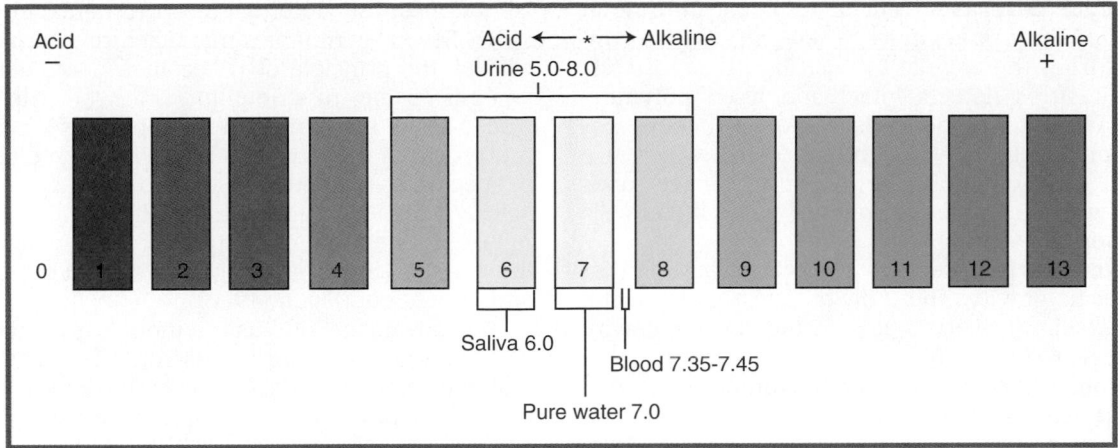

FIGURE 49-11   The pH scale. (From Stepp CA, Woods MA: *Laboratory procedures for medical office personnel,* Philadelphia, 1998, WB Saunders.)

glucose finding is common in urine from diabetic patients and may be the first indication of the disease. The reagent-strip glucose testing method is based on **enzymatic reaction**. It detects only glucose; in other words, it is *specific* for glucose.

Protein.   Protein in the urine in detectable amounts is called *proteinuria* and is one of the first signs of renal disease. We normally excrete a small amount of protein every day; proteinuria may be light to heavy, constant, or sporadic. It may be affected by posture: in orthostatic proteinuria, protein is excreted only when the patient is in an upright position. Generally, first morning specimens from these patients are negative, but protein is found in urine passed throughout the day. Proteinuria is a common finding in pregnancy. It is almost always present after heavy exercise.

Ketones.   Ketone bodies are the end-product of fat metabolism in the body. Acetoacetic acid, acetone, and betahydroxybutyric acid are collectively called *ketone bodies*, or *ketones. Ketonuria* is common in the presence of starvation, low-carbohydrate diets, excessive vomiting, and diabetes mellitus. Because ketones evaporate at room temperature, urine should be tested immediately, or the specimen should be tightly covered and refrigerated if not tested promptly.

Blood.   The presence of blood in the urine may indicate infection or trauma to the urinary tract or bleeding in the kidneys. The blood test pad on the reagent strip reacts with three different blood constituents: intact red blood cells, hemoglobin from red blood cells, and myoglobin, a hemoglobin-like molecule that transports oxygen in muscle tissue.

Hematuria is the presence of intact red blood cells in urine. The color reaction on the reagent strip ranges from yellow through green to dark green when hematuria is present. Hematuria can be caused by irritation of the ureters, bladder, or urethra. It is also a common finding in cystitis and in persons passing kidney stones.

Hemoglobinuria is the presence of hemolyzed red blood cells. True hemoglobinuria is rare. It occurs as a result of intravascular red blood cell destruction and can be caused by transfusion reactions, malaria, drug

reactions, snake bites, and severe burns. **Myoglobinuria** occurs when muscle tissue is damaged or injured, such as in crushing injuries, myocardial infarctions, and contact sports. Muscular dystrophy patients often exhibit myoglobinuria. Hemoglobinuria cannot be distinguished from myoglobinuria by reagent strip testing.

Bilirubin and Urobilinogen.   *Bilirubin* is a product of the breakdown of hemoglobin. Hemoglobin is released from old red blood cells and is gradually converted to bilirubin in the liver and then further to urobilinogen in the intestines. Bilirubin is a bile pigment not normally found in urine. Its presence in urine is one of the first signs of liver disease or other disease in which the liver may be involved, such as infectious mononucleosis.

Bilirubinuria can occur even before jaundice or other symptoms of liver disease are evident. It is the result of liver cell damage or obstruction of the common bile duct by stones or neoplasms (tumors). Excessive bilirubin colors the urine yellow-brown to greenish-orange. Because direct light causes decomposition of bilirubin, urine samples must be protected from light until testing is complete.

Urobilinogen is normally present in urine in small amounts. Increases are seen when there is increased red blood cell destruction and in liver disease. When there is total obstruction of the bile duct, no urobilinogen is formed in the intestines, none is reabsorbed into the circulation, and hence none is present in the urine. Reagent strip methods cannot detect a decrease in urobilinogen.

Nitrite.   Nitrite occurs in urine when bacteria break down nitrate. A positive nitrite test result may indicate the presence of a urinary tract infection (UTI). However, not all bacteria are able to reduce nitrate to nitrite. Negative nitrite tests can also occur when bacteria are insufficient or when the urine has not incubated in the bladder long enough for the reaction to occur. *Escherichia coli*, the organism that causes the majority of UTIs, reduces nitrate to nitrite. False-positive results can occur if a specimen is allowed to sit at room temperature and contaminating bacteria multiply. False-negative results may occur if the bacteria further metabolize the nitrite they have produced.

Leukocyte Esterase. Leukocytes occur in urine in infections of the urinary tract. They can also be contaminants from the vagina. The *leukocyte esterase test* on reagent strips detects intact and lysed **polymorphonuclear white blood cells**. However, it does not detect **mononuclear white blood cells**, which are occasionally present during infections. The test does not react with the small numbers of white blood cells found in normal urine.

Specific Gravity. Reagent strips are available that report specific gravity. The individual test pads on the strip give readings every 0.005 on the specific gravity scale from 1.000 to 1.030, and results are comparable to those from a urinometer or a refractometer.

Phenylketones. *Phenistix* are reagent strips used to detect the presence of phenylketones in the urine. This condition is called *phenylketonuria* (PKU). In this genetically inherited disorder, the body is unable to properly metabolize the nutrient **phenylalanine**.

As high levels of the phenylketones accumulate in the bloodstream, mental retardation occurs. Phenylketonuria is easily treated by limiting dietary intake of phenylalanine in childhood. Because individuals who are properly treated for the disease do not suffer mental retardation, early detection is very important, and the majority of testing is performed on babies.

Limitations to Reagent Strip Testing. The reagent strip is a reliable method for chemical analysis of urine if used properly. The normal urine reference ranges using a reagent strip can be found in Table 49-4. A number of sources of error exist; if the strip is soaked excessively in the specimen, chemicals in the pads may be diluted. If the strip is not held horizontal while being read, colors from one pad may bleed onto another. Finally, certain chemicals, such as ascorbic acid, may affect results of nitrite, glucose, bilirubin, and occult blood tests. Normal levels of vitamin C will not interfere, but if a person consumes large quantities of the vitamin, a special strip can be used to detect interfering levels of vitamin C. If an elevated level is found, the patient should be instructed to discontinue vitamin C intake for 24 hours, then another urine specimen should be collected for testing.

Visual interpretation of color on the reagent strip pads is likely to vary among individuals, and some laboratories use automated instruments to read the strips. Several companies manufacture instruments that employ the principle of reflectance photometry in the analysis of reagent strip color. Once the strip has been placed in the instrument, a microprocessor controls the movement of the strip into the reflectometer. Here light of specific wavelengths is beamed onto the strip. Some light will be absorbed and some light will scatter or be reflected. The amount of light reflected is analyzed by the microprocessor and converted into a digital reading and printed out (Figure 49-12).

The advantage of this method is that timing and color interpretation are consistent. The disadvantage is that the instrument is not able to identify and compensate for urines that are highly pigmented, leading to false positive results. The CMA should be aware of this and manually test urines that are darkly pigmented.

CRITICAL THINKING APPLICATION

Rosa prepares to do the chemical examination of the three urine specimens. Dr. Hill has ordered a UA on the specimen from Mr. Parks, a UA and pregnancy test on the specimen from Mrs. Carpenter, and a UA and C&S on the specimen from Ms. Winfrey. Should she proceed with the chemical analysis of each specimen in exactly the same manner? Explain your answer.

On completing the chemical analysis of the three specimens, Rosa notes several differences among the samples. Mrs. Carpenter's sample has a high specific gravity. Ms. Winfrey's sample reveals an elevated nitrite, a pH of 8, and an elevated leukocyte esterase. Mr. Parks' test results reveal elevated glucose and ketone levels and a specific gravity of 1.035. Based on this information, what are the probable reasons each of these patients visited Dr. Hill today?

TABLE 49-4	Normal Urine Reference Range
	Reference Range
Color	Clear
Character	1.001-1.035
Specific gravity	4.6-8.0
pH	NEG
Protein UA (mg/dl)	NEG
Glucose (mg/dl)	NEG
Ketone (mg/dl)	NEG
Bilirubin (mg/dl)	NEG
Blood/UA (mg/dl)	NEG
Nitrite (mg/dl)	NEG
Urobilinogen (Ehrlich units)	0.1-1.0
White blood cells	NEG

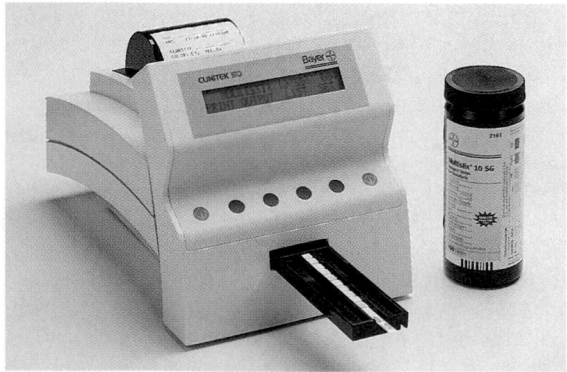

FIGURE 49-12 A Clinitek urine analyzer. (From Bonewit-West K: *Clinical procedures for medical assistants*, ed 5, Philadelphia, 2000, WB Saunders.)

Microscopic Examination of Urine Sediment

The microscopic examination of urine (see Procedure 49-8) consists of categorizing and counting cells, casts, crystals, and miscellaneous constituents of the sediment obtained when a measured portion of urine is centrifuged. The test is not categorized as CLIA-waived, and this would not be performed by a medical assistant without additional training and rigid compliance with CLIA 88 quality assurance protocols for the laboratory, including periodic proficiency testing. The MA, however, should be familiar with preparing the urine for this test and with the possible results. The clear upper portion of the specimen is called the *supernatant*. It is poured off, and a drop of the well-mixed sediment is examined under a microscope. The sediment may be stained with a **supravital** sediment stain to give greater contrast to the formed elements. The most commonly used stain is the Sternheimer-Malbin stain, which consists of crystal violet and safranin. This stain assists in the identification of formed elements by enhancing the detail of internal cellular structure.

Microscopic observation is accomplished most popularly with a brightfield, phase-contrast, or polarizing microscope. With a traditional brightfield microscope, correct light adjustment is essential. The light must be reduced by closing the condenser iris diaphragm to increase the contrast. The condenser should be lowered slightly. Brightfield microscopy is enhanced by the use of stains. Phase contrast microscopy converts variations in refractive index into variations in contrast by fitting a brightfield microscope with a special device known as an *annular ring*, which enhances contrast in living cells and low refractive index components. The polarizing microscope is used most commonly in the urinalysis laboratory to confirm the presence of fat, specifically cholesterol, and for identifying crystals.

Many formed elements will be found in the urine. Some are significant; others are not. Most importantly, the microscopic examination should correlate with the physical and chemical analyses. For example, if the presence of red blood cells is confirmed on the reagent strip, red blood cells should be visible on the microscopic examination, and the urine may appear pink or red-tinged.

Casts. **Casts** are formed when protein accumulates and precipitates in the kidney tubules and is washed into the urine. The protein takes on the size and shape of the tubules; hence the term *casts*. Casts are cylindrical, with flat or rounded ends, and are classified according to the substances observed in them. Certain types of casts are associated with renal pathological conditions; others are physiological and are generally caused by strenuous exercise.

Casts are counted and reported under low-power magnification, but occasionally high-power magnification is needed to identify the type. Because casts tend to migrate to the edges of the coverslip, this area should be examined closely. Casts dissolve in alkaline urine on standing; therefore, examination of a fresh urine specimen is very important.

Hyaline casts are pale, transparent, cylindrical structures that have rounded ends and parallel sides (Figure 49-13). Hyaline casts will be missed entirely if the light

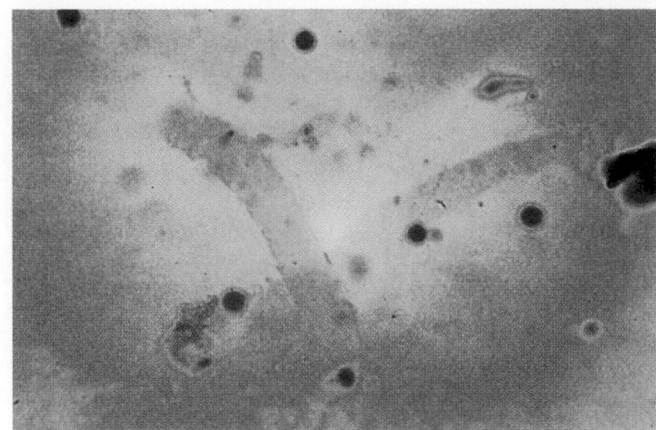

FIGURE 49-13 Hyaline casts. (Sedi-Stain, 400×.) (From Ringsrud KM, Linne JJ: *Urinalysis and body fluids: a color text and atlas*, St. Louis, 1995, Mosby.)

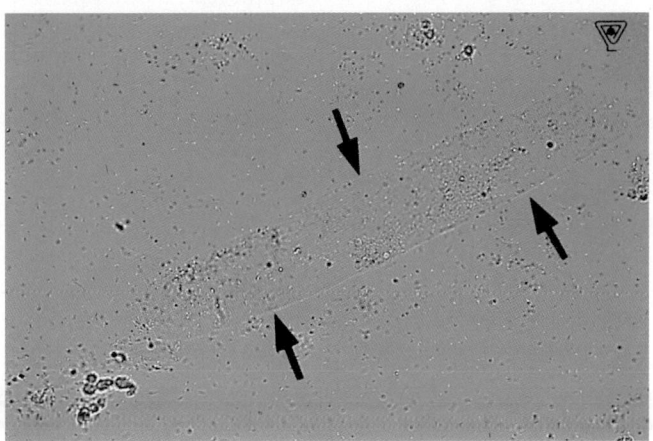

FIGURE 49-14 Hyaline casts. (From Stepp CA, Woods MA: *Laboratory procedures for medical office personnel*, Philadelphia, 1998, WB Saunders.)

is not reduced at the condenser. They are formed when urine flow through individual nephrons is diminished. They can be found in persons with kidney disease but can also be found in urine specimens of normal subjects who have exercised heavily. Occasionally, hyaline casts have granular or cellular inclusions.

White blood cell casts are hyaline casts that contain leukocytes. White blood cells usually have a multilobed nucleus, which differentiates them from renal tubular epithelial cells, which have single, round nuclei. White blood cell casts are seen in pyelonephritis (Figure 49-14).

Finely and coarsely granular casts may be caused by exercise but when present in increased numbers may indicate renal disease. On close examination, granular casts show a hyaline matrix with coarse or fine granular inclusions. The granules are thought to be caused by protein aggregation or degeneration of cellular inclusions (Figure 49-15).

Red blood cell casts always indicate a pathological condition and are highly diagnostic. Red blood cell casts occur in glomerulonephritis. They are hyaline casts with

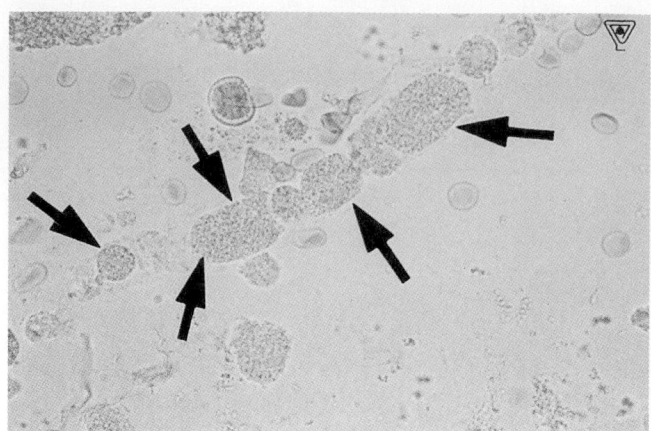

FIGURE 49-15 Granular casts. (From Stepp CA, Woods MA: *Laboratory procedures for medical office personnel*, Philadelphia, 1998, WB Saunders.)

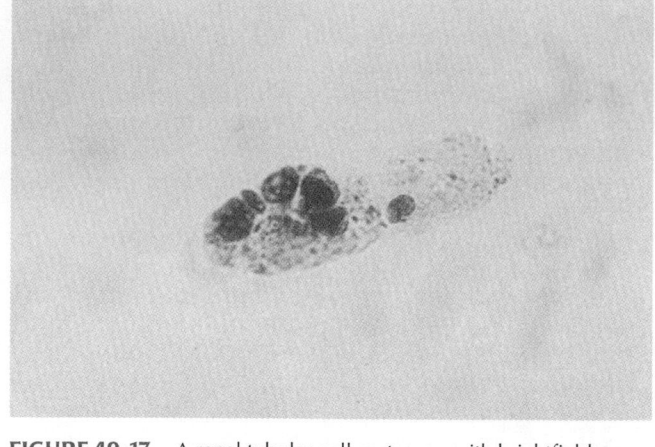

FIGURE 49-17 A renal tubular cell cast, seen with brightfield microscopy. (Sedi-Stain, 400×.) (From Brunzel NA: *Fundamentals of urine and body fluid analysis*, Philadelphia, 1994, WB Saunders.)

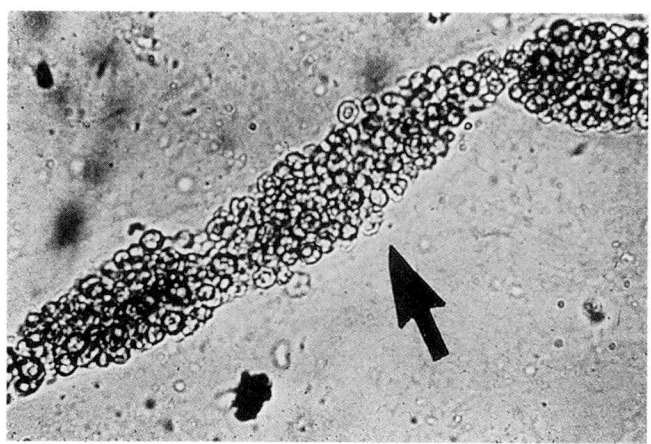

FIGURE 49-16 Red blood cell casts. (From Stepp CA, Woods MA: *Laboratory procedures for medical office personnel*, Philadelphia, 1998, WB Saunders.)

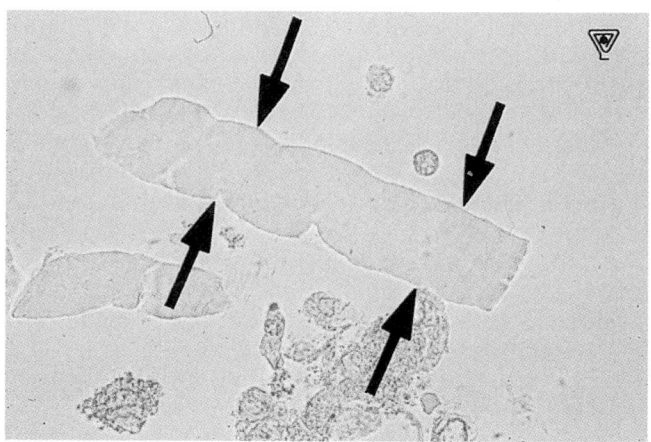

FIGURE 49-18 Waxy casts. (From Stepp CA, Woods MA: *Laboratory procedures for medical office personnel*, Philadelphia, 1998, WB Saunders.)

embedded red cells, and their presence indicates damage to the glomerular membrane. They may appear brown as a result of the color of the red blood cells present (Figure 49-16).

Renal tubular epithelial cell casts contain embedded renal tubular epithelial cells. These casts are easily confused with white blood cell casts, particularly if the cells have started to degenerate. Renal tubular epithelial cell casts are found when there is excessive damage. Causes are shock, renal **ischemia**, heavy-metal poisoning, certain allergic reactions, and nephrotoxic drugs (Figure 49-17).

Waxy casts are rarely seen. They appear as glassy, brittle, smooth, homogeneous structures. They are usually yellowish, have cracks or fissures, and have squared or broken ends. They are considered to be degenerated cellular casts and are found in persons with severe renal disease (Figure 49-18).

Occasionally, more than one type of cell will be found in a single cast. Mixed cellular casts have been reported. Absolute identification of the cell types present may be difficult.

Cells. Cells that are found in urine include epithelial cells, which are derived from the lining of the genitourinary tract. Other cells in urine include red blood cells and white blood cells from the bloodstream. Cells are classified and counted under high-power magnification.

Red blood cells may enter the urinary tract at any point at which there is inflammation or injury. They may be found in normal urine in small numbers, usually less than 1 to 2 per high-power field. Persistent hematuria should be investigated. Red blood cells are pale, round, nongranular, and flat or biconcave (Figure 49-19). They are smaller than white blood cells and have no nucleus. In hypotonic (dilute) urine, they swell and burst. In hypertonic (concentrated) urine, they may **crenate** and wrinkle. When they crenate, they can be mistaken for white blood cells, because the wrinkled surface makes them appear granular. They are often confused with yeast (see Figure 49-26), oil droplets, and droplets of lens cleaner.

White blood cells, also called *leukocytes*, may occasionally be found in normal urine, but increased numbers (usually greater than 5 cells per high-power field) are associated with inflammation or contamination of the

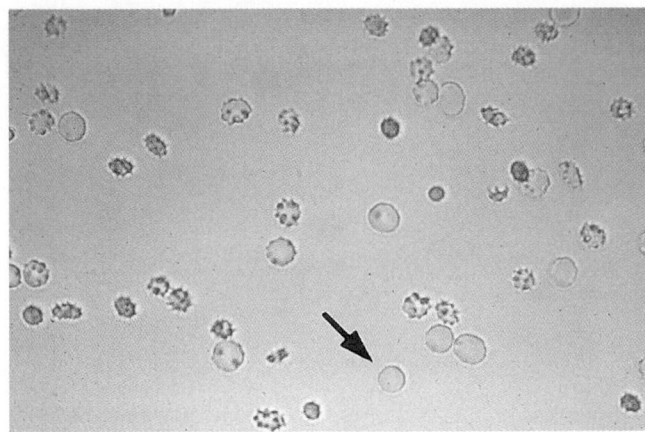

FIGURE 49-19 Red blood cells in urine. (From Stepp CA, Woods MA: *Laboratory procedures for medical office personnel*, Philadelphia, 1998, WB Saunders.)

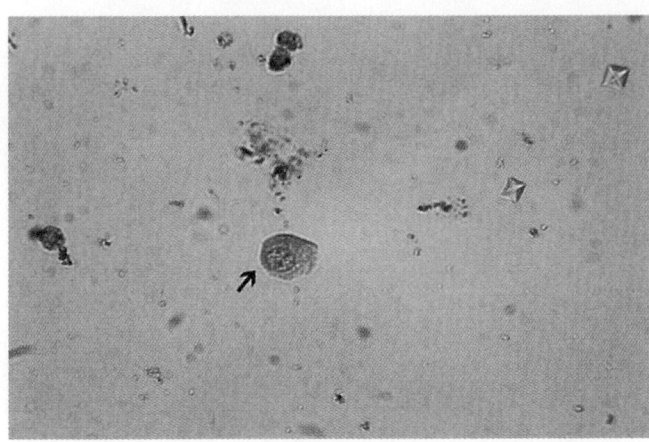

FIGURE 49-21 Renal epithelial cell (*arrow*). (Sedi-Stain, 400×.) (From Ringsrud KM, Linne JJ: *Urinalysis and body fluids: a color text and atlas*, St. Louis, 1995, Mosby.)

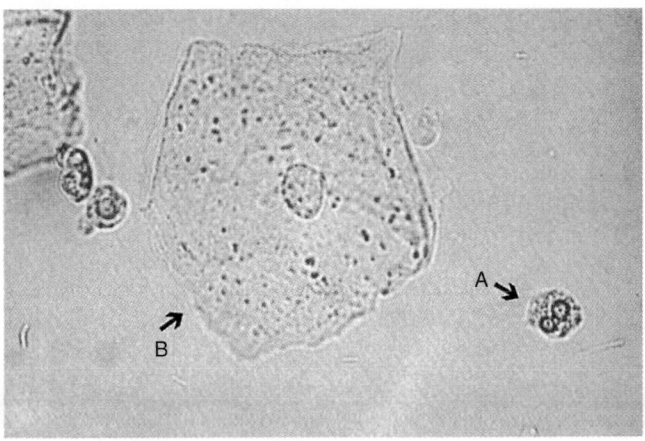

FIGURE 49-20 **A**, A white blood cell. **B**, A squamous epithelial cell. (Unstained, 640×.) (From Ringsrud KM, Linne JJ: *Urinalysis and body fluids: a color text and atlas*, St. Louis, 1995, Mosby.)

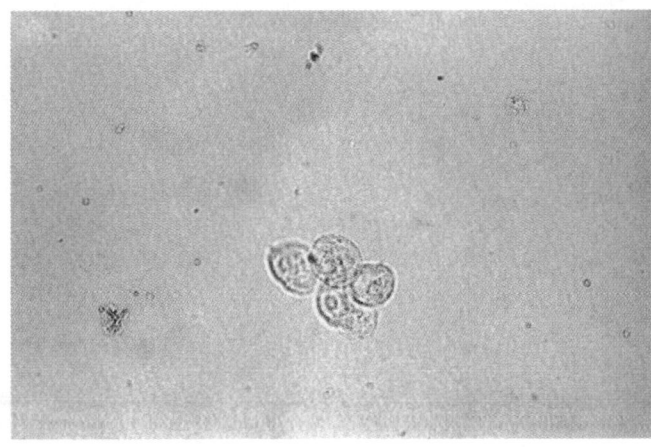

FIGURE 49-22 Cluster of small unstained transitional epithelial cells. (400×.) (From Ringsrud KM, Linne JJ: *Urinalysis and body fluids: a color text and atlas*, St. Louis, 1995, Mosby.)

specimen during collection. White blood cells are larger than red blood cells, have a granular appearance, and usually contain a multilobed nucleus, although nuclear detail may not be evident. Most white blood cells in the urine are neutrophils (Figure 49-20).

Renal tubular or round epithelial cells are somewhat larger than white blood cells, are round to oval, and have a nucleus that is single, large, oval, and sometimes eccentric. A few may be found in normal urine specimens, but their presence in increased numbers indicates tubular damage (Figure 49-21).

Transitional epithelial cells line the urinary tract from the renal pelvis to the upper portion of the urethra. They vary from slightly larger than a round epithelial cell to smaller than a squamous epithelial cell. They are round to oval and may have a tail. Occasionally, two nuclei are seen. When transitional cells are present in large numbers, a pathological condition may exist (Figure 49-22).

Squamous epithelial cells line the lower portion of the genitourinary tract. When present in large numbers in females, they usually indicate vaginal contamination. Squamous epithelial cells are large, flat, irregular cells

and are easily recognized under low-power magnification. They have a single, small, round, centrally located nucleus and often occur in sheets or clumps. Because of their flat nature, the edges of the cells are often rolled or folded (see Figure 49-22).

In identifying epithelial cells, it is helpful to remember the appearance of eggs; round epithelial cells resemble hard-boiled eggs that have been cut in half. Transitional forms resemble poached eggs, and squamous cells resemble fried eggs with large, runny whites.

Crystals. Crystals are common in urine specimens, particularly if they have been allowed to cool. Cooling causes the solid crystals to precipitate out of the urine. The presence of most crystals is not clinically significant, unless they are found in large numbers. With only very rare exceptions, abnormal crystals are seen in acidic urine. Abnormal crystals may be of metabolic origin and are present because of certain disease states or an inherited metabolic condition, or they may be of iatrogenic origin and are present as a result of medication or treatment. Identification of crystals begins with the determination of the pH of the urine, ascertaining

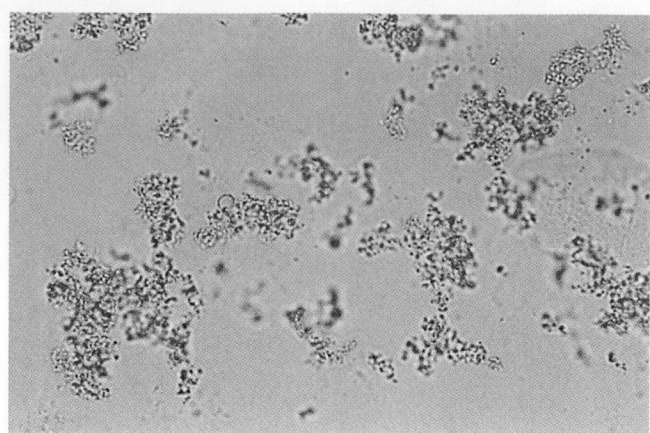

FIGURE 49-23 Amorphous urates. (400×.) (From Ringsrud KM, Linne JJ: *Urinalysis and body fluids: a color text and atlas*, St. Louis, 1995, Mosby.)

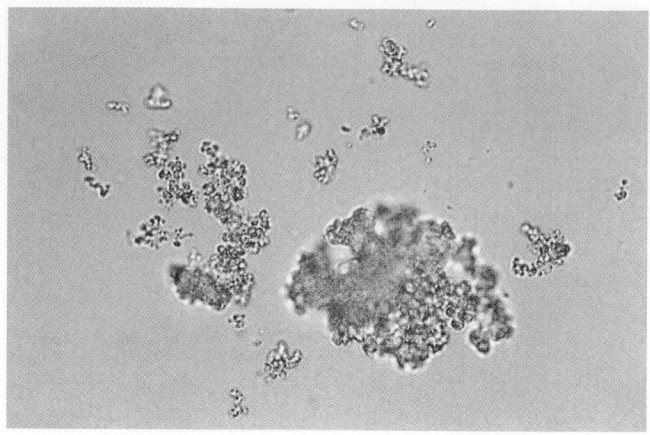

FIGURE 49-24 Amorphous phosphates. (400×.) (From Ringsrud KM, Linne JJ: *Urinalysis and body fluids: a color text and atlas*, St. Louis, 1995, Mosby.)

whether the sample is acidic or alkaline. Next one looks at color, shape, and refractivity. Viewing with a polarized or phase microscope or using a supravital stain can assist in identification. Often a history of medication intake and recent diagnostic testing is helpful.

Identification of crystals is done with the low-power and high-power lenses, and their presence is reported as few, moderate, or many per high-power field. At times crystals can be **amorphous**. Amorphous urates (Figure 49-23) are salts of uric acid and are seen as shapeless granulation in acidic urine. Amorphous phosphates (Figure 49-24) are found in alkaline urine and are seen as fluffy white precipitate. Amorphous crystals are often so profuse they obscure other formed elements in the sediment. It is not always possible to identify crystals without additional chemical testing, which includes solubility testing in acid and base. A sample of crystals found in urine sediment is shown in Table 49-5.

Miscellaneous Findings. *Oval fat bodies* are formed when renal tubular epithelial cells or macrophages absorb fats. The fat droplets contained in the cells vary in size and are quite **refractile**. Oval fat bodies are characteristic of the nephrotic syndrome and are best distinguished by using Sudan III stain, because they are easily confused with other elements (Figure 49-25).

Yeast in urine may indicate vaginal contamination or infection of the urine with yeast (Figure 49-26). It is common in the urine of diabetic patients. Yeasts are easily confused with red blood cells, are usually oval, may show budding, and are more refractile. To differentiate yeast from red blood cells, a drop of sediment is placed on the blood test pad of a reagent strip. Yeast does not react, but red blood cells do. Red blood cells dissolve when a drop of dilute acetic acid (regular white vinegar) is added to the sediment, but the yeast will remain intact.

A few *bacteria* may be found in normal urine specimens. Heavy bacterial concentrations in the absence of white blood cells may indicate that the specimen was allowed to sit at room temperature and the bacteria multiplied. Urine specimens with a putrid odor, numerous white blood cells, and bacteria (Figure 49-27) are

common in urinary tract infections. Bacteria may be bacilli (rod-shaped) or cocci (spherical shaped) and are identified under high-power magnification. They are often motile.

Spermatozoa are often found in the urine specimens of both males and females. In the latter, their presence represents vaginal contamination of the specimen. Sperm usually have pointed, oval heads and long threadlike tails. They may be motile in fresh urine.

The most commonly encountered parasite in urine is *Trichomonas vaginalis* (Figure 49-28). It is usually a vaginal contaminant but may also be found in urine specimens from males. When urine is fresh and warm, the *Trichomonas* may be motile and will be darting about rapidly. *Trichomonas* organisms are pear-shaped protozoa with four flagella. They are larger than round epithelial cells but smaller than squamous cells. *Trichomonas* organisms die when the specimen is cooled.

Mucous threads can be found in most urine specimens. They appear as pale, irregular, threadlike structures with tapered ends. Beginners often confuse hyaline casts with mucous threads. Increased numbers are seen in inflammation and when there has been contamination of the specimen with vaginal secretions (Figure 49-29).

Artifacts and contaminants are often found in urine sediment; training is required to distinguish them and learn to ignore them. As a rule, structures that are apparent when you first view the sediment are unimportant. Starch granules are common artifacts simply because of the extensive use of powdered gloves in the laboratory. The granules are highly **refractile** and dimpled, resembling a pillow with a center button. Fibers are common in the sediment as well and come from clothing, diapers, or digested plant material. Clothing fibers are often long and twisted and are sometimes colored. Diaper fibers can be confused with casts (Figure 49-30). Plant fibers appear in the urine as a result of fecal contamination (Figure 49-31). Hair is distinguishable not only because of the visible rough and fragmented cuticle but also because of the size (Figure 49-32). Finally, air bubbles are common if the coverslip was improperly placed over

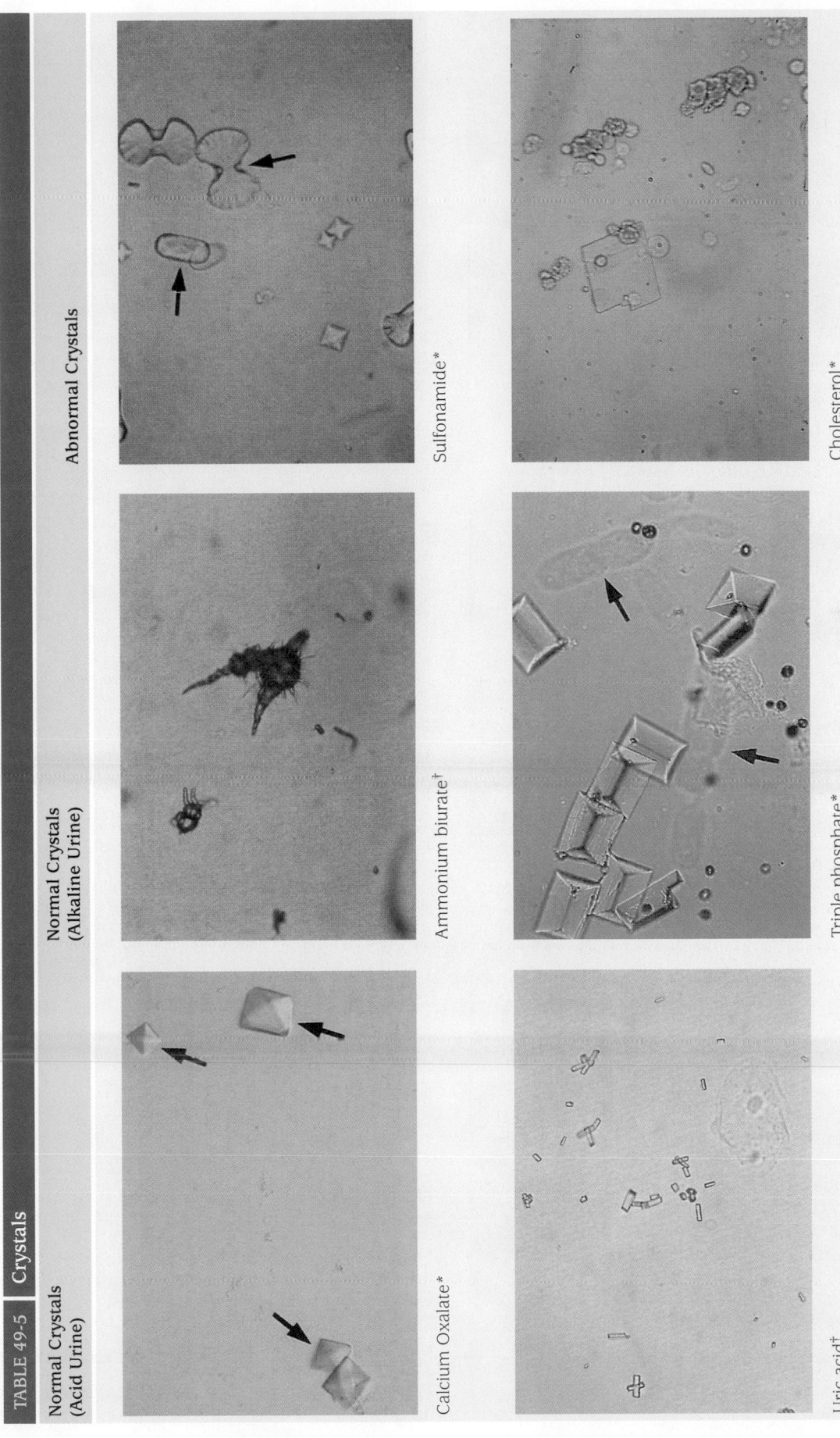

TABLE 49-5 | Crystals

Normal Crystals (Acid Urine)

Normal Crystals (Alkaline Urine)

Abnormal Crystals

Calcium Oxalate*

Uric acid†

Ammonium biurate†

Triple phosphate*

Sulfonamide*

Cholesterol*

*From Stepp CA, Woods MA: *Laboratory procedures for medical office personnel*, Philadelphia, 1998, W.B. Saunders.
†From Ringsrud KM, Linne JJ: *Urinalysis and body fluids: a color text and atlas*, St. Louis, 1995, Mosby.

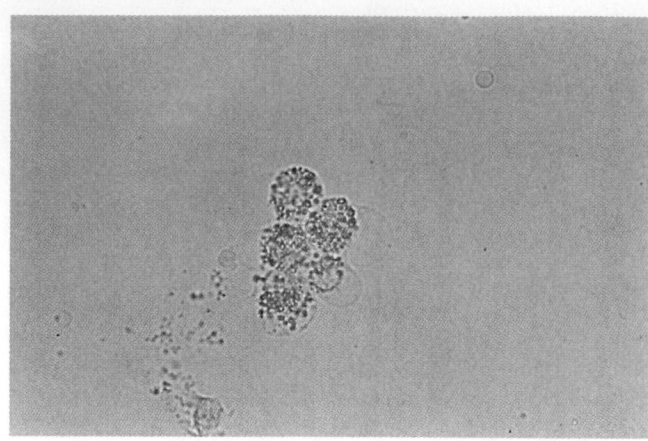

FIGURE 49-25 A small cluster of oval fat bodies. (Unstained, 400×.) (From Ringsrud KM, Linne JJ: *Urinalysis and body fluids: a color text and atlas*, St. Louis, 1995, Mosby.)

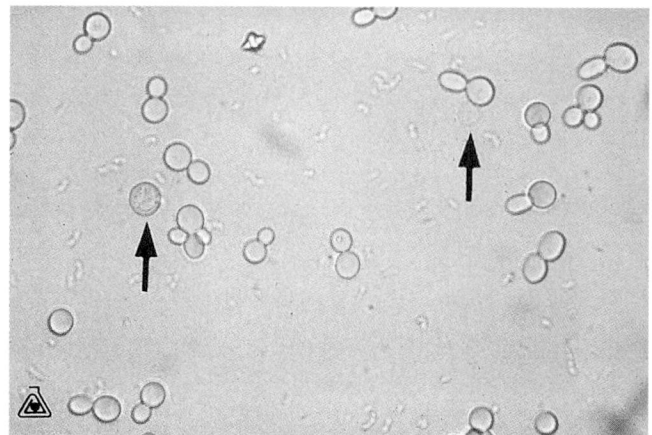

FIGURE 49-26 Yeast in urine. (From Stepp CA, Woods MA: *Laboratory procedures for medical office personnel*, Philadelphia, 1998, WB Saunders.)

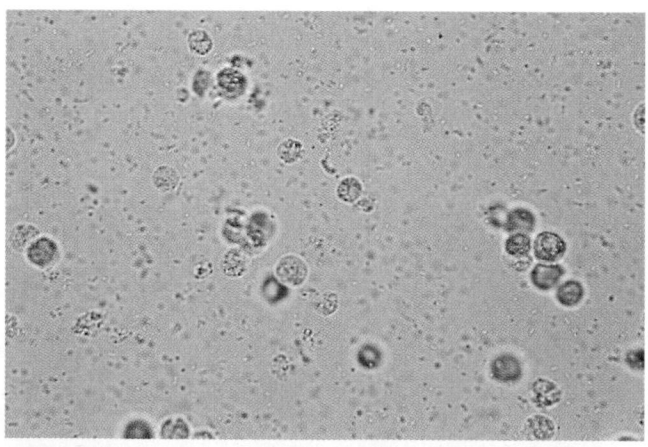

FIGURE 49-27 Many small rod-shaped bacteria appearing like possible cocci and white cells. (Unstained, 400×.) (From Ringsrud KM, Linne JJ: *Urinalysis and body fluids: a color text and atlas*, St. Louis, 1995, Mosby.)

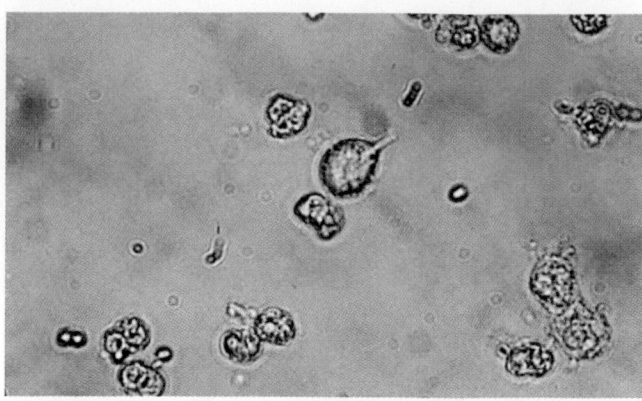

FIGURE 49-28 *Trichomonas* in urine. (From Stepp CA, Woods MA: *Laboratory procedures for medical office personnel*, Philadelphia, 1998, WB Saunders.)

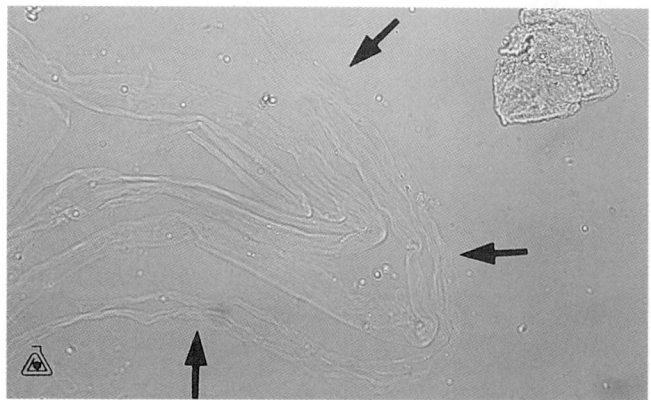

FIGURE 49-29 Mucous threads in urine. (From Stepp CA, Woods MA: *Laboratory procedures for medical office personnel*, Philadelphia, 1998, WB Saunders.)

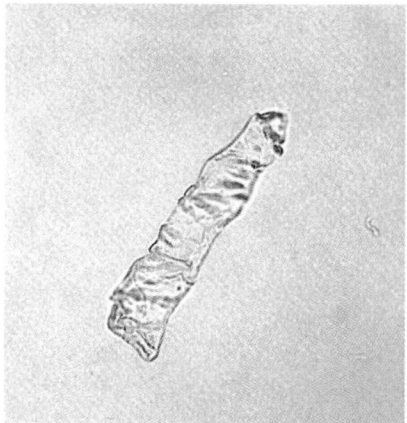

FIGURE 49-30 Diaper fibers. (From Ringsrud KM, Linne JJ: *Urinalysis and body fluids: a color text and atlas*, St. Louis, 1995, Mosby.)

the sediment. Air bubbles are structureless and refractile with a dark outline (Figure 49-33).

Interpretation of the Microscopic Examination

The medical assistant should understand how the findings of a microscopic examination of the sediment

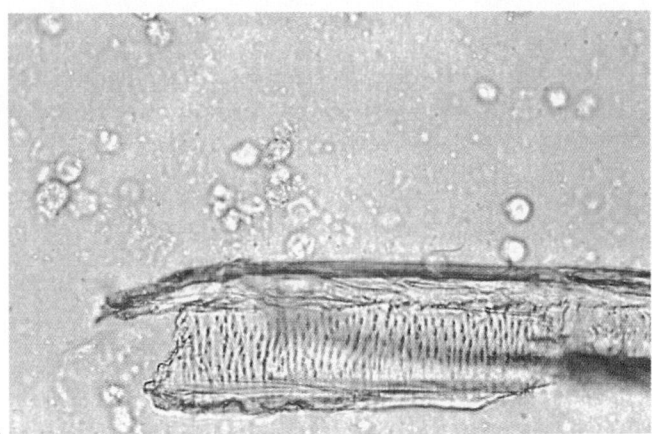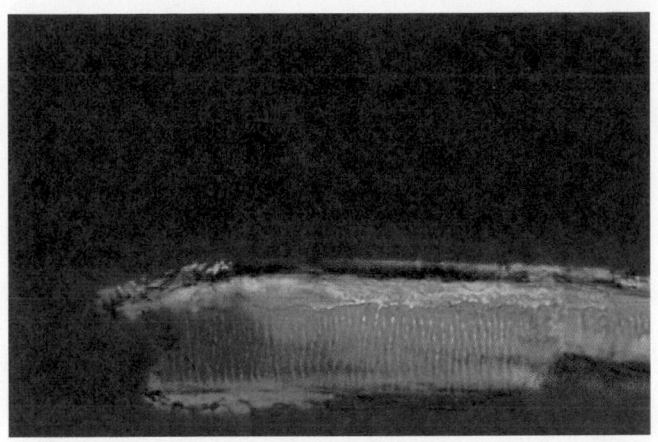

A   B

FIGURE 49-31 Plant fiber, from fecal contamination. Cells and bacteria are also present. (400×.) **A**, Brightfield. **B**, Compensated polarized light showing birefringence. (From Ringsrud KM, Linne JJ: *Urinalysis and body fluids: a color text and atlas*, St. Louis, 1995, Mosby.)

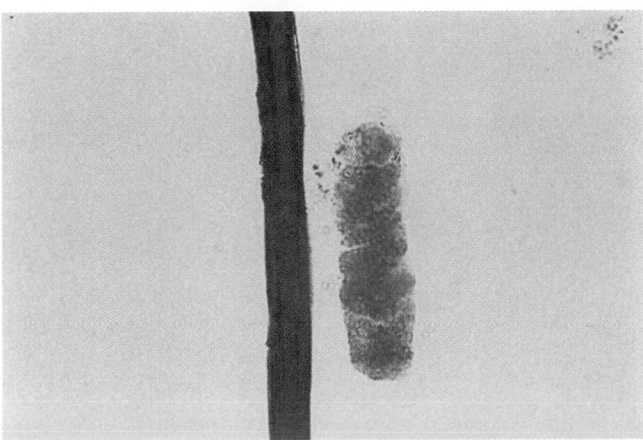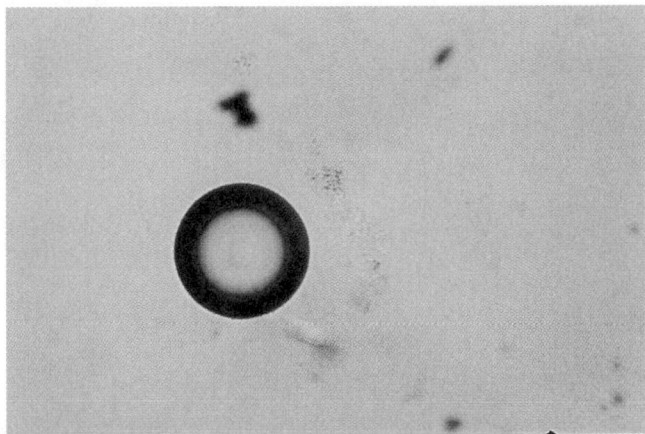

FIGURE 49-32 Fiber, probably hair (*left*); a waxy cast (*right*). (Sedi-Stain, 400×.) (From Ringsrud KM, Linne JJ: *Urinalysis and body fluids: a color text and atlas*, St. Louis, 1995, Mosby.)

FIGURE 49-33 A large air bubble. (400×.) (From Ringsrud KM, Linne JJ: *Urinalysis and body fluids: a color text and atlas*, St. Louis, 1995, Mosby.)

are reported. The sediment is first examined under the low-power objective and low light to locate casts, which generally will be found around the edges of the coverslip. Ten to 15 low-power fields are scanned, and the number of casts is counted and reported. The high-power objective and increased light are then used to identify red and white blood cells, epithelial cells, yeasts, bacteria, and crystals. Ten to 15 high-powered fields should be scanned and the number counted, averaged, and reported. The method of counting varies considerably among laboratories. It is important that all workers in the same laboratory use the same counting and reporting systems. Report the results of the microscopic examination as follows:

1. Separately total the numbers for each element counted, and then average. (Casts, white blood cells, red blood cells, and the three categories of epithelial cells are counted, totaled, and averaged.) Casts, white blood cells, and red blood cells are reported using numerical ranges based on the average:

   0
   0-1
   1-2
   2-5
   5-10
   10-20 and so forth

   Epithelial cells are reported as occasional, few, moderate, or many, according to the following:

   0

0-3	= Occasional
3-6	= Few
6-12	= Moderate
12	= Many

2. Estimate the remaining elements as occasional, few, moderate, or many, according to the following:
   Occasional—not seen in every field
   Few—covers less than a quarter of the field
   Moderate—covers approximately half of the field
   Many—covers the entire field
   Do not report fibers, hair, talc granules, oil droplets, and other artifacts.

   Table 49-6 shows an example of the way in which a microscopic urinalysis would be calculated and reported by a physician or medical technologist.

CRITICAL THINKING APPLICATION

After centrifugation of the three urine specimens, Rosa prepares to view the sediment. She knows she must correlate the findings from the visual and chemical examination she has already performed on these specimens. She reviews the results and notes that Mr. Parks' and Mrs. Carpenter's specimens were clear, but Ms. Winfrey's specimen was turbid. Given the results of the chemical analysis during which Rosa noted an alkaline pH, an elevated nitrite level, and an elevated leukocyte esterase reading, what might the doctor find when examining Ms. Winfrey's specimen?

Additional Testing Performed on Urine

Clinitest. The glucose test on the reagent strip will detect only glucose, which is the most common sugar found in the urine. Sugars other than glucose can appear in the urine as well. Certain metabolic disorders can result in the excretion of sugars such as galactose, fructose, lactose, maltose, or pentoses. *Galactosemia*, a rare pathological condition, is a congenital deficiency in the body's ability to metabolize galactose to glucose; galactosemia results in excretion of galactose in the urine. Seen in infants, it results in failure to thrive, vomiting, and diarrhea. If detected early, galactose can be eliminated from the diet and the child will develop normally. Lactose may be found in the urine of pregnant women or premature infants. Rarely, urine may contain fructose or pentoses (such as xylose or arabinose) as a result of excessive consumption of honey or fruit. Maltose may be excreted in diabetes. Of the many sugars, only the presence of glucose or galactose signifies a pathological condition

The Clinitest (Ames, Inc.), based on the chemical reduction of copper, is commonly used to screen and confirm glycosuria and is used to detect other sugars present in urine (Procedure 49-6). Copper reduction

TABLE 49-6   Calculating a Microscopic Urinalysis

Per Low-Power Field			Per High-Power Field							
Field	Casts	Mucus	WBC	RBC	Squamous Epithelial	Transitional Epithelial	Round Epithelial	Bacteria	Crystals	Other
1	0	Few	16	1	1	0	0	Moderate (rods)	Calcium oxalate —few Uric acid —few	—
2	1 hyaline	Few	32	0	3	0	0	Many	Calcium oxalate —few	Yeast
3	1 coarse granular	Moderate	21	2	3	0	0	Many	Calcium oxalate —few	Yeast
4	1 coarse granular	Few	12	1	5	0	1	Moderate	Uric acid —few	—
5	0	Few	25	0	4	0	0	Many	—	
Total	1 hyaline 2 coarse granular	Few	106	4	16	0	1	Many	Calcium oxalate —few Uric acid —few	Yeast
Average	0.2 hyaline 0.4 coarse granular	Few	21.2	0.8	3.2	0	0.2	Many	Calcium oxalate —few Uric acid —few	Yeast
Report	0-1 hyaline 0-1 coarse granular	Few	20–30	0–1	Few	0	Occasionally	Many (rods)	Calcium oxalate —few Uric acid —few	Yeast

PROCEDURE **49-6**

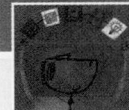

Testing Urine for Glucose With the Clinitest Method

GOAL: To perform confirmatory testing for glucose in the urine using the Clinitest procedure for reducing substances.

EQUIPMENT AND SUPPLIES

- Urine specimen
- Clinitest tablet, tube, and dropper
- Distilled water
- Test tube rack
- Color chart
- Timer

PROCEDURAL STEPS

1 Wash and dry your hands and don nonsterile gloves and eye protection.

2 Holding a Clinitest dropper vertically, add 10 drops of distilled water and then 5 drops of urine to a Clinitest tube.
   Purpose: Holding the dropper vertically prevents altering the size of the drops.

3 Place the prepared tube into the rack (Figure 1).
   Purpose: The tube will become too hot to hold when the tablet is placed into the tube.

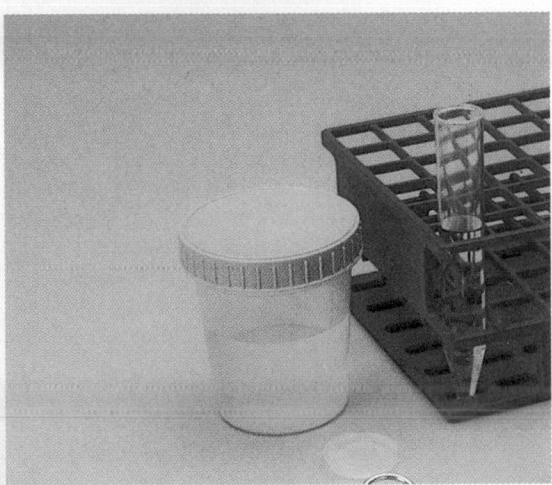

Figure 1

4 With dry hands, remove a Clinitest tablet from the bottle by pouring the tablet into the bottle cap.
   Purpose: Clinitest tablets react with moisture and became caustic. Handling tablets with moist hands could result in hydroxide burns.

5 Tap the tablet into the test tube, and recap the container.

6 Observe the entire reaction to detect the rapid pass-through phenomenon, which means that the glucose level in the urine is very high. (See step 9.)
   Purpose: If pass-through occurs but is not detected, the reading will be falsely low.

7 When boiling ceases, time exactly 15 seconds; then gently shake the tube to mix the entire contents.

8 Immediately compare the color of the specimen with the five-drop color chart, and record your findings (Figure 2).
   Purpose: Color darkens with time. For accurate results, time carefully.

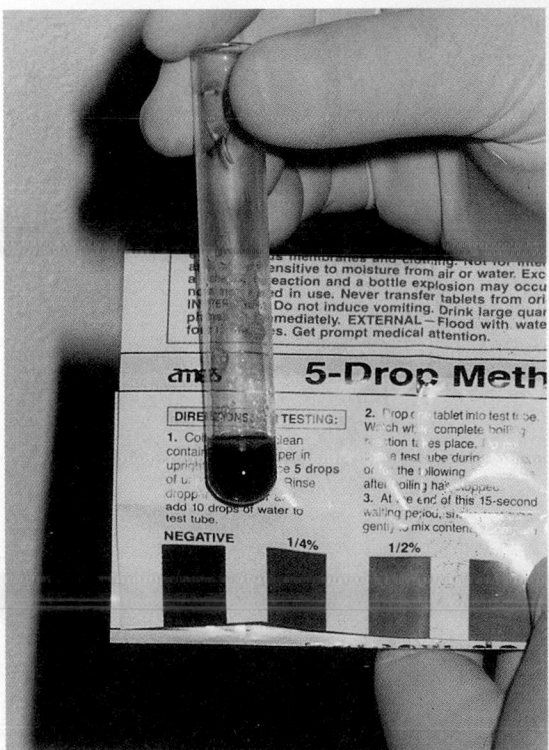

Figure 2

9 If an orange color briefly develops during the reaction, rapid pass-through has occurred, and the test must be repeated using the two-drop color chart.

Continued

PROCEDURE 49-6—cont'd

10 Clean the work area, remove gloves, and wash your hands.

Purpose: Infection control.

11 Record the results:
Negative—clear
Trace—slightly cloudy
1+—can see light print through tube

2+—can see dark print through tube
3+—cannot see through tube
4+—large, fluffy precipitate forms and settles on standing

Purpose: A procedure is considered not done until it is recorded.

---

tests are based on the principle that reducing substances are able to chemically convert cupric sulfate to cuprous oxide, resulting in a color change. A sugar's reducing ability is determined by the presence of a "reducing group" present in all monosaccharides. The Clinitest tablet is dropped directly into a test tube containing diluted urine. A heat-releasing reaction occurs, and after the boiling stops, the color of the tube's contents is compared with a chart provided by the manufacturer.

Acetest. Acetest reagent tablets provide an alternative to strip testing when the urine must be tested for the presence of ketones. Ketonuria results when the body metabolizes stored fat because of inadequate cellular uptake of carbohydrates. This is common in the presence of diabetes, starvation, and excessive vomiting. The Acetest tablet test (Miles, Inc.) is based on the same chemical reaction as the reagent strip test, but its advantage lies in the fact that the tablet can be used with specimens other than urine.

Quality Assurance and Quality Control in Urinalysis. The Clinical Laboratory Improvement Act (CLIA) categorizes the chemical analysis of urine as a *waived test* performed by an instrument or reagent strip. The chemical analysis includes the reagent strip (dipstick) tests for bilirubin, glucose, hemoglobin/blood, ketones, leukocytes, nitrite, pH, protein, specific gravity, and urobilinogen. To perform a microscopic urinalysis procedure, a laboratory must be certified to perform moderate complexity tests. Such a laboratory can also perform waived tests if they meet those qualifications (Procedure 49-7).

To determine the reliability of the reagent strip used in chemical analysis, a commercially available control strip should be employed. One such strip is the Chek-Stix (Bayer Corp.). The plastic control strip has seven pads affixed to it (Figure 49-34). Each of these pads contains synthetic ingredients that mimic human urine when reconstituted in water. After reconstitution, a reagent strip is immersed in the solution and the results are compared with a chart that accompanies the Chek-Stix. Both positive and negative Chek-Stix are available.

Quality control is as important in the microscopic examination as it is in the chemical analysis of urine. To ensure consistency, standardized commercially available systems can be used such as the KOVA System (HYCOR Biomedical) or the UriSystem (Fisher Scientific). These systems may include specially designed graduated

centrifuge tubes with devices or pipets that allow for easy decanting of supernatant and retention of an exact amount of sediment. They also employ specially designed plastic slides with wells or coverslips that accept only a given amount of sediment. Whatever system is used, the NCCLS* recommends the following:

- The urine volume should be 12 ml.
- The specimen should be centrifuged for 5 minutes at a relative centrifugal force of 400 G (i.e., 400 times normal gravity).
- A standardized slide should be used to view the sediment.
- A consistent reporting format should be employed.

Urine Pregnancy Testing. The phrase "the rabbit died" came to be a euphemism for a positive pregnancy test in the late 1920s and early 1930s. About 1927 it was discovered that if you injected the urine of a pregnant woman into a rabbit, there would be hemorrhaging in the ovaries of the rabbit. These bulging masses could not be seen without killing the rabbit to inspect the ovaries, so invariably, every rabbit died, even if the woman was not pregnant. All pregnancy tests detect the presence of human chorionic gonadotropin (hCG), a hormone produced by the placenta and present in urine during pregnancy. After implantation of the fertilized egg in the uterus, the hCG levels in serum double every few days. This rapid rise occurs for approximately 7 weeks and then begins to decline. Within 72 hours of delivery, the hormone disappears.

Today no rabbits are needed to confirm a pregnancy. The most common type of test for pregnancy is the enzyme immunoassay (EIA) test. Many brands are available for laboratory use and are also available over the counter. EIA tests can be so sensitive as to detect the presence of hCG as early as 1 week after implantation or 4 to 5 days before a missed menstrual period. These tests can be performed in as little as 5 minutes, and the results are easy to interpret, usually as easy as reading a color change. For optimal results, the test should be performed on a first-morning voided specimen.

The test is based on reactions that occur between antibodies and antigens. Antibodies are proteins

---

*The acronym NCCLS used to stand for National Committee for Clinical Laboratory Standards, but NCCLS is now a global organization and develops consensus documents for additional audiences beyond the clinical laboratory community. Therefore the organization should be referred to by its acronym, NCCLS.

PROCEDURE **49-7**

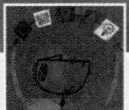

Preparing Urine Specimen for Microscopic Examination

GOAL: To perform a microscopic examination of urine to determine the presence of normal and abnormal elements.

EQUIPMENT AND SUPPLIES

- Urine specimen
- Centrifuge tube
- Centrifuge
- Disposable pipet
- Microscope slide and coverslip
- Microscope
- Permanent marker

PROCEDURAL STEPS

1 Wash and dry your hands. Don nonsterile gloves and face protection.
   Purpose: Infection control.

2 Gently mix the urine specimen.
   Purpose: If the urine is not well mixed, elements that have settled to the bottom of the specimen container will be missed.

3 Pour 10 ml of urine into a labeled centrifuge tube and cap the tube.

4 Place the tube in the centrifuge (Figure 1).

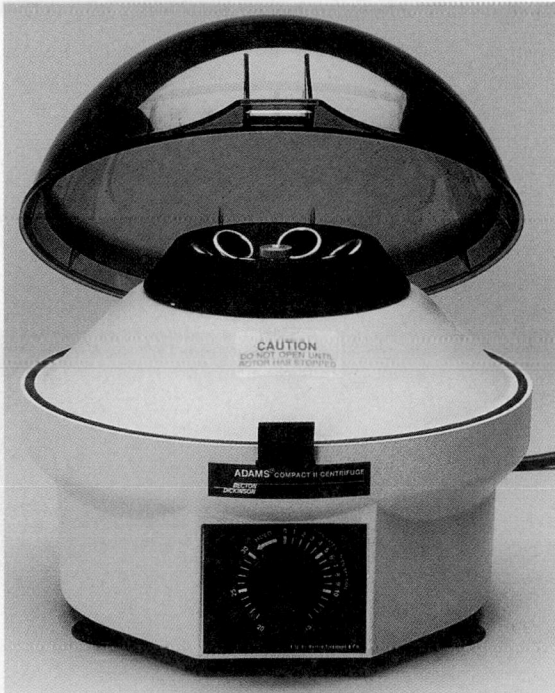

Figure 1

5 Place another tube containing 10 ml of water in the opposite cup.
   Purpose: For proper operation, centrifuges must be carefully balanced. If not properly balanced, damage to the instrument can occur.

6 Secure the lid, and centrifuge for 5 minutes or for the time specified for your instrument.
   Purpose: Timing varies based on the speed and the size of the centrifuge head.

7 Remove the tube from the centrifuge after the instrument has come to a full stop.

8 Pour off the clear supernatant from the top of the specimen by inverting the centrifuge tube over the sink drain (Figure 2*).

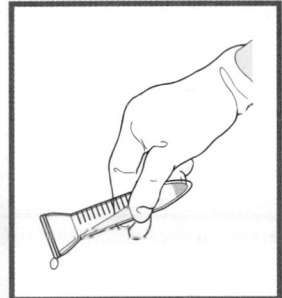

Figure 2

9 Prevent the loss of sediment down the drain.
   Purpose: The sediment is what you will examine under the microscope.

10 Thoroughly mix the sediment by grasping the tube near the top and rapidly flicking it with the fingers of the other hand until all sediment is thoroughly resuspended (Figure 3*).
   Purpose: Elements centrifuge at different rates. Failure to completely mix the entire sediment will cause errors in quantification.

11 Transfer one drop of sediment to a clean, labeled slide (Figure 4*).

12 Place a clean coverslip over the drop, and place the slide on the microscope stage. Remove face protection.

---

*Figures from Stepp CA, Woods MA: *Laboratory procedures for medical office personnel*, Philadelphia, 1998, WB Saunders.

Continued

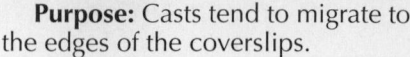

PROCEDURE 49-7—cont'd

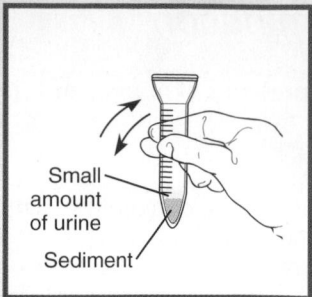

Figure 3

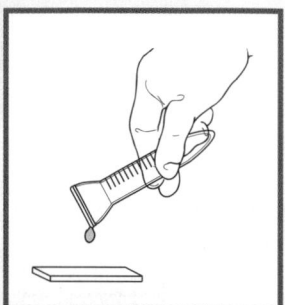

Figure 4

13 Focus under low power, and reduce the light.

Purpose: Mucus and casts are easily missed if reduced light is not used. Constant focusing helps locate them.

14 First, scan the entire coverslip for abnormal findings.

Purpose: Casts tend to migrate to the edges of the coverslips.

15 Examine five low-power fields. Count and classify each type of cast seen, if any, and note mucus if present.

Purpose: Choose five fields so that one is selected from each corner of the coverslip and the last one is chosen from the middle of the coverslip. If you move to an area and there is nothing there, record a zero.

16 Switch to high-power magnification, and adjust the light.

Purpose: As magnification increases, more light is needed.

17 In five high-power fields, count the following elements: red blood cells, white blood cells, and round, transitional, and squamous epithelial cells.

18 In the same five fields, report the following as few, moderate, or many: crystals (identify and report each type seen separately), bacteria (identify as rods or cocci), sperm, yeast, and parasites.

Purpose: These three terms are more easily and universally understood than are exact numbers.

19 Average the five fields, and report the results. Do not remove the slide from the microscope until the physician has verified the results.

20 Clean up the work area, remove face protection and gloves, and wash your hands.

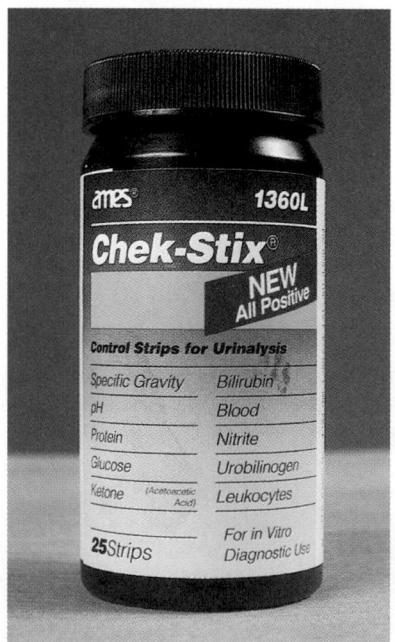

FIGURE 49-34 Chek-Stix control strips. (From Bonewit-West K: *Clinical procedures for medical assistants*, ed 5, Philadelphia, 2000, WB Saunders.)

formed in response to antigens. When in contact with one another, the antibody binds to the antigen if the two are present in sufficient quantity and the antibody is specific for the antigen, like a lock and key. In the EIA test, anti-hCG antibody is bound to a solid membrane in a plastic holder. An absorbent material below the membrane acts as a wick and allows the urine to migrate through the device. If hCG (antigen) is present in the specimen, it attaches to the antibody and is mobilized. As this complex moves over the membrane, it attaches to another antibody and causes a color change on the device. Each testing device has an internal control feature—a line will appear in the Reference/Control region to indicate that the test procedure has been performed correctly. The Wampole PreVue hCG test is one such pregnancy test that can be performed on urine or serum (Procedure 49-8). It is used routinely in many physicians' office laboratories.

Culturing the Urine

Urine cultures are performed to assist in the diagnosis of a UTI and to assess the effectiveness of certain antibiotics in the treatment of the infection. Culturing of

---

PROCEDURE **49-8**

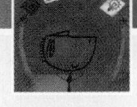

Performing a Pregnancy Test

GOAL: To perform a pregnancy testing of urine using the QuickVue (by Quidel) pregnancy test method.

EQUIPMENT AND SUPPLIES

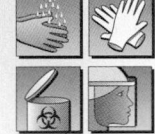

- Urine specimen
- QuickVue test kit

PROCEDURAL STEPS

1 Wash and dry your hands. Put on face protection and nonsterile gloves.

2 Prepare the testing equipment (Figure 1*).

3 Collect the needed specimen.

4 Remove the test cassette from the foil pouch.

5 Add three drops of urine using the dropper that accompanies the kit. Dispose of the dropper in a biohazard bag (Figure 2*).
   Purpose: To ensure accurate test results, specimen amount must be exact.

6 Wait 3 minutes and read the test results.
   Purpose: To ensure accurate test results, timing must be exact.

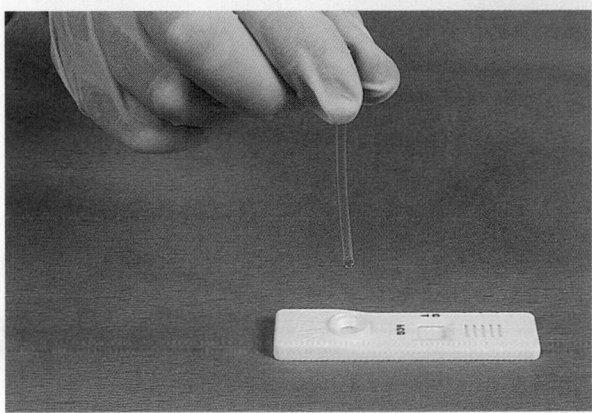

Figure 2

7 Interpret the results (Figure 3*).
   NEGATIVE: A blue control line next to the letter *C* will be present. No line will be present next to the letter *T*.
   POSITIVE: A blue control line next to the letter *C* will appear along with a pink line next to the letter *T*.

   If a blue line does not appear in the *C* area, the test is invalid and the specimen must be retested using another kit. Check the expiration date of the kit before proceeding.

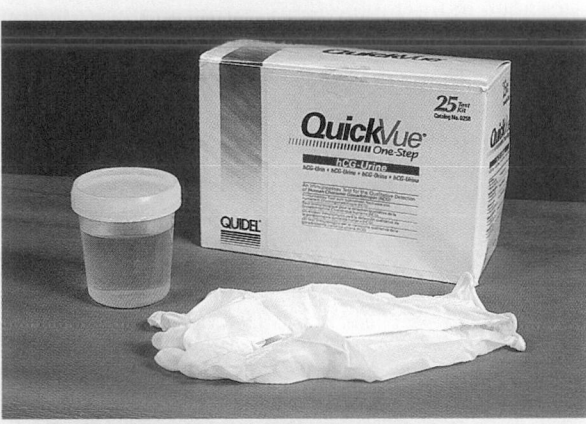

Figure 1

---

*Figures from Bonewit-West K: *Clinical procedures for medical assistants*, ed 5, Philadelphia, 2000, WB Saunders.

Continued

PROCEDURE **49-8—cont'd**

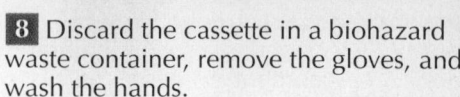

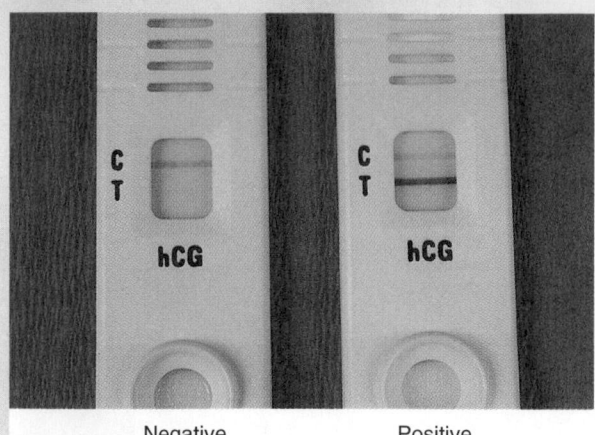

| Negative | Positive |

Figure 3

8 Discard the cassette in a biohazard waste container, remove the gloves, and wash the hands.

Purpose: Infection control.

9 Record the results as either positive or negative.

Purpose: A procedure is not considered finished until it is recorded.

See Appendix E for a charting example.
*Figures from Bonewit-West K: *Clinical procedures for medical assistants*, ed 5, Philadelphia, 2000, WB Saunders.

PROCEDURE **49-9**

Performing a Rapid Urine Culture Test

GOAL: To assess the level of bacteriuria in order to aid in diagnosis of urinary tract infections.

EQUIPMENT AND SUPPLIES

- Clean catch midstream urine specimen
- Uricult test kit
- Incubator
- Biohazard waste container

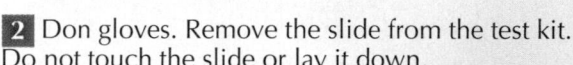

PROCEDURAL STEPS

1 Wash your hands, assemble equipment and specimen. Check the expiration date on the test kit. Label the vial with the patient information (Figure 1*).

Purpose: An expired test kit may yield inaccurate test results.

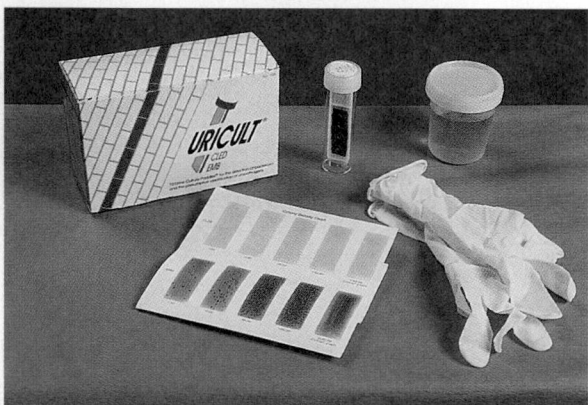

Figure 1

2 Don gloves. Remove the slide from the test kit. Do not touch the slide or lay it down.

Purpose: Touching the slide or laying it down will contaminate the slide.

3 Dip the slide into the urine specimen, tipping the cup carefully if necessary. Alternately, the urine may be poured over the slide, catching it in another container (Figure 2*).

Purpose: The entire slide must be covered with urine for accurate results.

4 Allow excess urine to drain then replace the slide in the protective vial. Screw the cap on loosely.

Purpose: The cap must be loose to allow gas exchange in the tube.

5 Incubate the vial upright in a 35° to 37° C (90° to 98.6° F) incubator for 18 to 24 hours.

Purpose: Incubation for less or more time may produce erroneous results. Disease-causing bacteria will grow best at body temperature, which is 35° to 37° C (90° to 98.6° F).

*Figures from Bonewit-West K: *Clinical procedures for medical assistants*, ed 5, Philadelphia, 2000, WB Saunders.

Continued

PROCEDURE **49-9—cont'd**

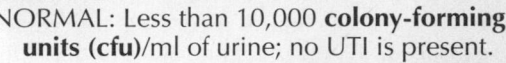

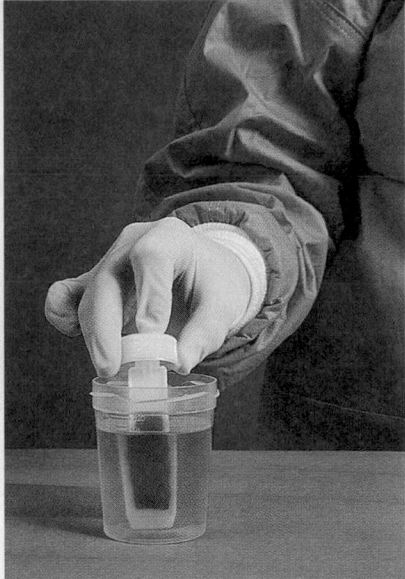

Figure 2

6 After incubation, the test results will be interpreted by a physician or medical technologist by removing the slide from its protective vial and assessing bacterial colony density by comparing the slide with the density chart provided. No actual colony counting is necessary (Figure 3*).

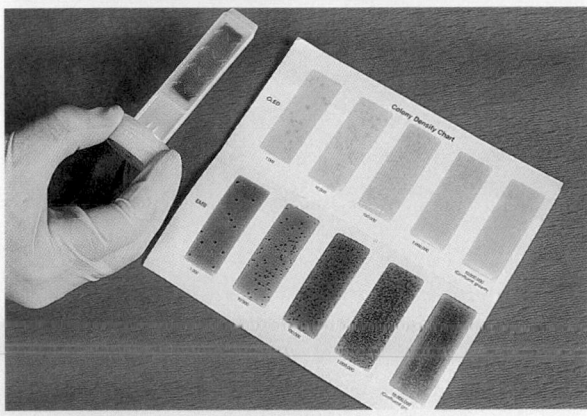

Figure 3

7 The results will be interpreted as follows.

NORMAL: Less than 10,000 **colony-forming units (cfu)**/ml of urine; no UTI is present.

BORDERLINE: 10,000 to 100,000 cfu/ml of urine; a chronic or relapsing infection may be present and the test should be repeated.

POSITIVE: More than 100,000 cfu/ml of urine; a UTI is likely.

8 Return the vial to the protective case and replace the cap.

9 Dispose of the test in a biohazard waste container (Figure 4*).

Purpose: The slide is contaminated. Alternately, the protective case may be filled with a disinfectant. such as 1:10 chlorine bleach before the slide is reinserted.

10 Remove gloves and wash your hands.

Purpose: Infection control.

11 Record the results.

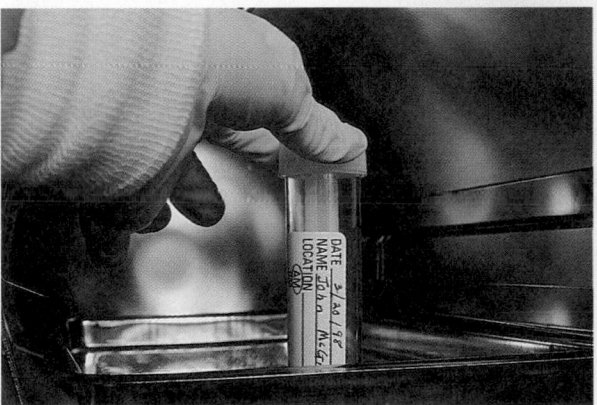

Figure 4

Purpose: A procedure is not considered done until it is recorded.

See Appendix E for a charting example.
*Figures from Bonewit-West K: *Clinical procedures for medical assistants*, ed 5, Philadelphia, 2000, WB Saunders.

specimens using petri dishes and performing an antibiotic sensitivity test is usually handled by a referral laboratory and will be addressed in Chapter 52. Rapid detection systems are also available and are more likely to be used in a physician's office laboratory (Procedure 49-9). Rapid culture kits usually involve a paddle or strip that is coated with a gel-type medium known to support the growth of bacteria. The paddle or strip is removed from its container, dipped in the urine, which has been collected using the clean-catch midstream technique, and then replaced in the container. The device is allowed to incubate, preferably at 37° C (98.6° F) for 18 to 24 hours, after which the density of bacterial growth on the surface is compared to a density chart provided by the manufacturer. Some devices will display color changes that indicate the type of bacterium causing the infection, but interpretation of the results is not to be done by a medical assistant.

Patient Education

Frequently a medical assistant is called on to explain collection techniques to the patient. Patients want to do the procedure correctly but often lack the knowledge of urinary terminology and are embarrassed to or do not know how to ask questions regarding the cleaning of the genital area. When explaining a urinary collection procedure, use pictures and words that the patient will understand. As you explain the procedure in terms that the patient knows, he or she will also feel comfortable in telling you or asking you pertinent details that may have a definite impact on the treatment of the problem. Providing the patient with a clearly written instruction sheet is also helpful. The instruction sheet should be personalized with his or her name, the time to begin collection or testing (if applicable), what supplies should be used, and a phone number to call if questions arise.

Legal and Ethical Issues

Like all other procedures, the test is only as valid as the specimen and the procedure performed on that specimen. You, as the physician's agent, are responsible for that validity when you instruct the patient and when you perform the test.

A medical assistant who is responsible for office laboratory testing must clearly understand the basic concepts of laboratory medicine. To do this, you must stay current with the rapid technological advances in laboratory medicine and assist in establishing a protocol of the tests best suited to your physician/employer.

You have the responsibility for properly collecting specimens and accurately testing them. The office laboratory can provide a real challenge and the opportunity to work with the physician in promoting and improving the health of the patient.

SUMMARY OF SCENARIO

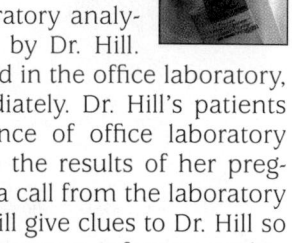

Rosa's capabilities in the laboratory analysis of urine are highly valued by Dr. Hill. Because tests can be performed in the office laboratory, Dr. Hill has the results immediately. Dr. Hill's patients also appreciate the convenience of office laboratory testing. Mrs. Carpenter knows the results of her pregnancy test without waiting for a call from the laboratory and Ms. Winfrey's urinalysis will give clues to Dr. Hill so that he can diagnose a urinary tract infection within minutes. Rosa knows that the laboratory services she provides are an integral part of the excellent patient care provided by Dr. Hill.

SUMMARY OF LEARNING OBJECTIVES

- Routine urinalysis is performed primarily as a screening test to detect metabolic and physiological disorders.

- Urine is formed through a filtration mechanism in the kidney via the nephrons. It is stored in the bladder and voided through the urethra.

- Some urine collections must be timed around meals or fasts. Routine urinalysis requires no special preparation, whereas a clean-catch midstream requires cleansing of the external genitalia. Only urine that will be cultured must be collected in a sterile container.

- The physical examination of the urine involves determination of color, turbidity, and specific gravity. Odor and foam color may be noted.

- The chemical examination of urine involves determination of levels of glucose, pH, protein, ketones, blood, bilirubin, urobilinogen, nitrite, specific gravity, and leukocyte esterase.

- Formed elements in the urine sediment include casts, cells, and crystals. Artifacts may be present, but they are not reported.

- Timed urine specimens are collected to determine the amount of a particular analyte in the urine during a given time frame.

- Proper patient instruction is necessary for an acceptable clean-catch midstream urine. Both men and women are given instructions in cleaning the external genitalia so as to avoid contaminating the urine.

- A complete urinalysis involves physical, chemical, and microscopic assessment. The three must correlate with each other.

- Most testing of urine requires reagent strips or tablets. It is essential that these supplies be stored in dark, cool, moisture-free areas.

- The Clinitest detects reducing sugars, including glucose, in the urine. It is superior to the reagent strip test, because it detects sugars other than glucose.

- Pregnancy testing performed in the physician's office laboratory is based on the same principle as the tests available over the counter. Pregnancy tests detect human chorionic gonadotropin, a hormone produced by the placenta.

KEY INTERNET WEBSITES

- The Internet Pathology Laboratory Urinalysis Tutorial
- MedLine Plus Health Information: The Kidney
- The Microscopic Analysis of Urine
- National Kidney Foundation
- National Institute of Diabetes and Digestive Kidney Diseases
- Urinalysis in Perspective, sponsored by Pfizer and London Health Sciences Center
- The Value of Urinalysis: An Old Method Continues to Prove Its Worth, by Mary Lou Gantzer, PhD
- The Virtual Hospital, University of Iowa Health Care–Urinalysis
  For active weblinks to each website visit
  http://evolve.elsevier.com/Kinn/

CHAPTER 50

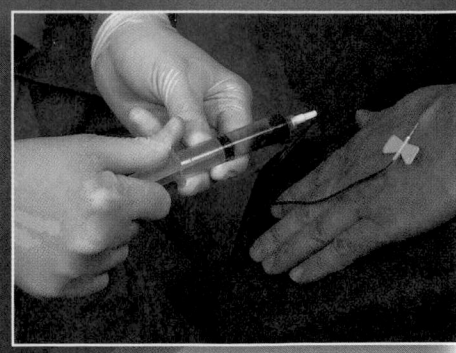

Scenario

Leah Barney, a recent graduate of a CMA program, is a new employee at the Health Alliance Medical Clinic. The class on medical laboratory procedures was Leah's favorite in her medical assisting program at the community college; in this class, she learned phlebotomy. Her instructor said she was a "natural," but she has not had much experience outside the classroom.

Assisting in Phlebotomy

Robin R. Patterson

Learning Objectives

- Define and spell the terms listed in the vocabulary.
- List the equipment needed for venipuncture.
- Explain the purpose of a tourniquet.
- Locate the parts of a venipuncture needle and describe how to handle needles safely.
- Explain why one chooses a syringe for blood collection rather than an evacuated tube.
- Explain why one chooses a winged infusion set (butterfly) rather than an evacuated tube.
- Differentiate whole blood, serum, and plasma and give an example of a test performed with each.
- List at least 10 different stopper colors found on evacuated tubes; identify the additives, and state one use for each.
- State the correct order in which various types of tubes should be collected.
- List, in order, the steps of a routine venipuncture.
- Explain how to apply a tourniquet and three consequences of improper application.
- Describe how to insert a needle properly into the vein and how it should be removed.
- List the veins that may be used for blood collection.
- List situations in which capillary puncture would be preferred over venipuncture.
- Discuss proper dermal puncture sites.
- Describe dermal puncture devices and discuss safety features they may have.
- Describe containers that may be used to collect capillary blood.
- List the steps for capillary puncture.
- Explain why the first drop of blood is wiped away when performing capillary puncture.
- Perform a venipuncture using a syringe.
- Perform a venipuncture using the evacuated tube method.
- Perform a capillary puncture.
- Collect a capillary sample in a microhematocrit tube and in a capillary tube.
- Prepare specimens for transport to the laboratory.

National Curriculum Competencies

CLINICAL COMPETENCIES

1d. Dispose of biohazardous materials
1e. Practice standard precautions

2a. Perform venipuncture
2b. Perform capillary puncture

Vocabulary

antiseptic An agent that inhibits bacterial growth that can be used on human tissue.

bifurcation The point of forking or separating into two branches.

hematocrit The percentage by volume of packed red blood cells in a given sample of blood after centrifugation.

hemoconcentration A situation in which the concentration of blood cells is increased in proportion to the plasma.

hemolysis The destruction or dissolution of red blood cells, with subsequent release of hemoglobin.

plasma The liquid portion of whole blood that contains active clotting agents.

serum The liquid portion of whole blood that remains after the blood has clotted.

stat With no delay; at once.

syncope Fainting.

thixotropic gel A material that appears to be a solid until subjected to a disturbance, such as centrifugation, upon which it becomes a liquid.

*P*hlebotomy, the practice of drawing blood, has its basis in the ancient practice of restoring the four body humors: blood, phlegm, yellow bile, and black bile. The foundation of all medical treatment was to keep these humors in balance by purging, starving, vomiting, or bloodletting. The art of bloodletting was flourishing by the Middle Ages, and both barbers and surgeons performed the art. Barbers advertised with a red (representing blood) and white (representing the tourniquet) striped pole. The pole itself represented the stick the patient squeezed during the procedure. Typically, 16 to 30 ounces (one to four pints) of blood was drained to treat an illness. When the patient became faint, the "treatment" was stopped. Often, bleeding over large areas of the body was accomplished by multiple incisions. George Washington is reported to have died in 1799 after being drained of nine pints of blood within 24 hours to cure a throat infection. In Washington's day, it was believed that one's blood was a carrier of the impurities of disease, and with bleeding new, healthy blood would replace what was lost. By the end of the nineteenth century, bloodletting was declared quackery.

Today, phlebotomy is performed primarily for diagnosis and monitoring of a patient's condition. It involves highly developed procedures and equipment to ensure the comfort and safety of the patient. The high standards necessary for the proper practice of phlebotomy led to the creation of different organizations that develop standards for training. Medical assistants are trained to perform phlebotomy, but their training does not certify or license them as phlebotomists. To be certified or licensed, one must complete course work and training at an accredited institution and then pass a national examination. Continuing education is often required to maintain certification. California and Louisiana are the first states to create state certification requirements.

The most common method of obtaining blood is by venipuncture. In a *venipuncture*, the blood is taken directly from a superficial vein. The vein is punctured with a needle, and the blood is collected in either a syringe or a stoppered tube. The procedure is safe when performed by a trained professional, but it must be performed with care. Much practice is required to become skilled and confident in the technique of venipuncture.

Venipuncture Equipment

Proper collection of blood requires specialized equipment. A complete list of materials used in routine venipuncture is provided in the box shown here. Phlebotomists generally carry the equipment in a portable tray (Figure 50-1). In a physician's office laboratory, there will probably be a permanent location to perform venipuncture. In such cases, you will likely seat patients in a venipuncture chair, which has an adjustable locking armrest to prevent the patient from falling out in the event of fainting.

EQUIPMENT USED IN ROUTINE VENIPUNCTURE

- Double-pointed safety needles
- Evacuated, stoppered tubes
- Needle holder
- Sharps container
- Syringes
- Winged infusion sets (butterfly needles)
- Tourniquet
- Marking pen
- Alcohol swabs
- Gauze pads
- Bandages
- Gloves
- Smelling salts

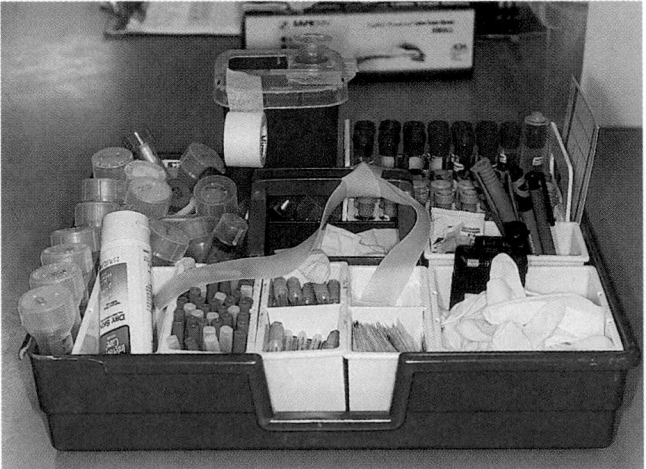

FIGURE 50-1 A fully stocked venipuncture tray. (From Stepp CA, Woods MA: *Laboratory procedures for medical office personnel,* Philadelphia, 1998, WB Saunders, p 122.)

TABLE 50-1		List of Common Stoppers, Additives, and their Laboratory Uses			
Vacutainer Colors*	**Color**	**Hemogard Colors†**	**Additive/Additive Function§**	**Laboratory Use†,§**	**Optimum Volume/ Minimum Volume**
Adult Tubes					
Yellow		Yellow	Sodium polyanetholsulfonate (SPS); prevents blood from clotting and stabilizes bacterial growth	Blood or body fluid cultures	5 ml/NA
Red		Red	None	Serum testing; chemistry studies, blood bank, serology	10 ml/NA
Red/gray (marbled)		Gold	None, but contains silica particles to enhance clot formation	Serum testing	10 ml/NA
Light blue		Light blue	Sodium citrate; removes calcium to prevent blood from clotting	Coagulation testing	4.5 ml/4.5 ml
Green		Green	Heparin (sodium/lithium/ ammonium); inhibits thrombin formation to prevent clotting	Chemistry testing	10 ml/3.5 ml
Green/gray (marbled)		Light green	Lithium heparin and gel for plasma separation	Plasma determinations in chemistry studies	2 ml/2 ml
Yellow/gray (marbled)		Orange	Thrombin	Stat serum demonstrations in chemistry studies	2 ml/2 ml
Lavender		Lavender	Ethylenediaminetetraacetic acid (EDTA); removes calcium to prevent blood from clotting	Hematology testing	7 ml/2 ml
Gray		Gray	Potassium oxalate/sodium fluoride; removes calcium to prevent blood from clotting; fluoride inhibits glycolysis	Chemistry testing, especially glucose/alcohol levels	10 ml/10 ml
Royal blue		Royal blue	Sodium heparin (also sodium EDTA); inhibits thrombin formation to prevent clotting	Chemistry trace elements	7 ml
Pediatric Tubes					
Red		Red			2 ml/NA; 3 ml/NA; 4 ml/NA
Lavender		Lavender			2 ml/0.6 ml; 3 ml/0.9 ml; 4 ml/1 ml
Green		Green			2 ml/2 ml
Light blue		Light blue			2.7 ml/2.7 ml

*Stopper colors are based on Becton-Dickinson Vacutainer tubes.
†Hemogard closures provide a protective plastic cover over the rubber stopper as an additional safety feature.
‡Sterile needles come in a variety of lengths and gauges (bore or opening size). Needles are also made to fit the evacuated tube holder by screwing in or by attaching to the tips of syringes. Most evacuated tube needles have a rubber sleeve to prevent blood from dripping into the holders when tubes are changed; these are called multiple-sample needles. The open end of the needle containing the point has a slanted side (bevel), which must be facing up when the needle is inserted into the vein. Needle positioning is very important in drawing blood. The angle of entry in relation to the skin surface should be 15 degrees. The most common needle size for adult venipuncture is 21 gauge.
§Additives, additive functions, and laboratory uses are the same for both pediatric and adult tubes.
Modified From Rodak BF: *Diagnostic hematology*. Philadelphia, 1995, WB Saunders.

Evacuated Collection Tubes

The evacuated tube (Vacutainer) system is the most common collection system in use. It consists of evacuated tubes of various sizes, with color-coded tops indicating tube contents (Table 50-1). The tube contents include anticoagulants, clot activators, and/or thixotropic gels. The vacuum in each tube is such that a measured amount of blood is drawn into the tube. Tube volumes range from 2 to 15 ml. Be sure to match the needle gauge to the size of the tube; the larger the tube, the greater the vacuum and the more likely blood will hemolyze if a high gauge, small-lumen-sized needle is used.

The size of the tube to be used depends on several factors. Each test performed in the laboratory requires a specific amount of blood. Consult the manual provided by the laboratory to ensure that you are drawing the right amount of blood for the test. Tests can often be combined, reducing the number of tubes that must be drawn. For example, both a complete blood count and an erythrocyte sedimentation rate (discussed in Chapter 51) are performed on a lavender-topped tube. It is not necessary to draw two tubes because the 7-ml volume is sufficient for both tests. When in doubt, call the laboratory. Keep in mind that blood is approximately half cells and half liquid. If a test requires 3 ml of serum, 6 ml of blood must be collected.

Patients often express great concern when several tubes of blood must be drawn. You can allay their fears by explaining that the average adult has a little less than ten pints of blood (5 L). Most adults can relate to donating a unit of blood, which is around a pint (400 to 500 ml). Because the red-topped tube contains 10 ml, you would have to draw 40 to 50 tubes before you have removed a pint.

Tube Additives. All tubes, with the exception of the red-topped tube, contain an additive. *Anticoagulants* are added to prevent blood from clotting. Tubes may be glass or plastic. The additive may be a powder, a liquid visible in the tube, or a liquid sprayed inside the tube by the manufacturer and allowed to dry. The choice of anticoagulant depends on the test to be done.

Ethylenediaminetetraacetic acid (EDTA) found in the lavender-topped tube prevents platelet clumping and preserves the appearance of blood cells for microscopic examination, but it is incompatible with the testing reagents used in coagulation studies. Consult the manual provided by the laboratory before obtaining a specimen from the patient.

Clot activators promote clotting of blood. Silica particles enhance clotting, for example, by providing a surface for platelet activation. Thrombin quickly promotes clotting and is used in tubes drawn for **stat** chemistry testing or in the event a sample is needed from a patient who is taking a prescribed anticoagulant such as heparin.

Anticoagulants prevent blood from clotting, which allows the contents of the tube to be used in two ways. First, the sample can be used as whole blood; second, the sample can be centrifuged and the liquid portion, called **plasma**, can be retrieved. Whole blood is used for tests such as complete blood counts and blood typing, whereas plasma is used for stat chemistry testing and coagulation studies.

If blood is allowed to clot and then centrifuged, the liquid portion is referred to as **serum**. Without a clot activator, blood will clot in 30 to 60 minutes, after which it must be centrifuged. The serum must be quickly separated from the cells because cells may continue to metabolize substances such as glucose or may release metabolites that interfere with testing. **Thixotropic gel** can be found in some tubes, including the SST red-and-gray marbled-topped tube by Becton-Dickinson. This synthetic gel has a density between that of red cells and plasma or serum, and it settles between the two during centrifugation, forming a barrier. This barrier facilitates retrieval of the liquid portion without cellular contamination.

It is important to mix the tube well after collection by inverting it several times (do not shake the tube) and also to avoid a *short draw*, a tube that is not completely filled. Having the proper ratio of blood to additive is crucial. The effects of a short draw are described in Table 50-2. Always be sure to check the tube for an expiration date. Outdated tubes may have diminished vacuum, or the additive may have degraded.

CRITICAL THINKING APPLICATION

- Melissa Machen has been assigned to orient Leah to the clinic and her duties as a CMA. Melissa takes Leah to the laboratory in the clinic. There is a small room with a blood collection chair and a table. What supplies should be on the table to perform venipuncture?
- What else might Leah find in this room?

Order of Collection. In the event that more than one tube must be drawn during a venipuncture, a specified order must be followed so that material from a previous tube is not transferred to the next tube. The National Committee for Clinical Laboratory Standards (NCCLS) developed a set of standards outlining the order of draw for a multitube draw. The same order

TABLE 50-2	Effects of Underfilling
Tube Top Color	**Effect**
Yellow	Decreases possibility of bacterial recovery
Red	Insufficient sample
Red/gray	Poor barrier formation; insufficient sample
Light blue	Coagulation test results are falsely prolonged
Green	False results due to excess heparin
Green/gray	False results due to excess heparin
Lavender	Falsely low blood cell counts and hematocrits; morphologic changes to red blood cells, staining alteration
Yellow/gray	False results
Gray	False results
Royal blue	False results

applies to the filling of tubes when blood is collected in a syringe.

1. Blood culture tubes are collected first because they are sterile.
2. Red-topped tubes are second because they have no additive and thus nothing to transfer to another tube.
3. Light blue-topped tubes are next because other anticoagulants might contaminate the sample collected for coagulation studies.
4. Green-topped tubes are next because heparin is less likely to interfere with EDTA than vice versa.
5. Lavender-topped tubes follow. Because EDTA binds with calcium, this tube is drawn near the end.
6. Red/gray marble-topped tubes are next. They contain clot activator that could interfere with specimens if passed into another tube
7. The gray-topped tube is last because the contents can elevate electrolyte levels or damage cells if passed into another tube.

When collecting only a light blue-topped tube, the NCCLS currently recommends the drawing of a red-topped tube even if the order does not call for it. This is done to prevent any thromboplastin released from the cells during venipuncture from contaminating the blue-topped tube and interfering with coagulation testing. This recommendation is under debate and may change in the future.

A mnemonic that is useful for remembering the order of the draw is: **ST**op; **R**ed **L**ight; **G**reen **L**ight; **R**eady; **G**o (Figure 50-2).

Needles

A critical part of phlebotomy is knowing which needle and which tube or syringe to use in each situation. All needles used in phlebotomy are sterile, disposable, and used only once. Each is housed in a cover, which should be inspected before use to ensure that sterility has not been compromised (e.g., the seal should be intact) and also to ensure that it has no manufacturing defects such as burrs or nicks. Needles have two parts: the *hub* and the *shaft*. Shafts differ in length, ranging from $^3/_4$ to $1^1/_2$ inches. The length of the shaft has no bearing on the venipuncture procedure, but some prefer a longer needle because it is less likely to slip out of the vein, whereas others prefer a shorter needle because it makes patients less uneasy. One end of the shaft is cut at an angle and forms the *bevel*, which creates a very sharp point. The hole in the bevel is called the *lumen*.

Lumen size is important in venipuncture and it is referred to as the *gauge*. Gauge is designated by a numerical value; the higher the number, the smaller the lumen. The blood bank uses a 16-gauge needle to collect pints of blood for transfusions because the lumen is wide, which reduces the chance of **hemolysis**. The smallest gauge needles (23-gauge) are used to collect blood from small or fragile veins, such as those of elderly and very young patients. Routine adult venipuncture requires a 20- to 21-gauge needle. Finally, the hub is the point where the needle attaches to the syringe or the needle holder.

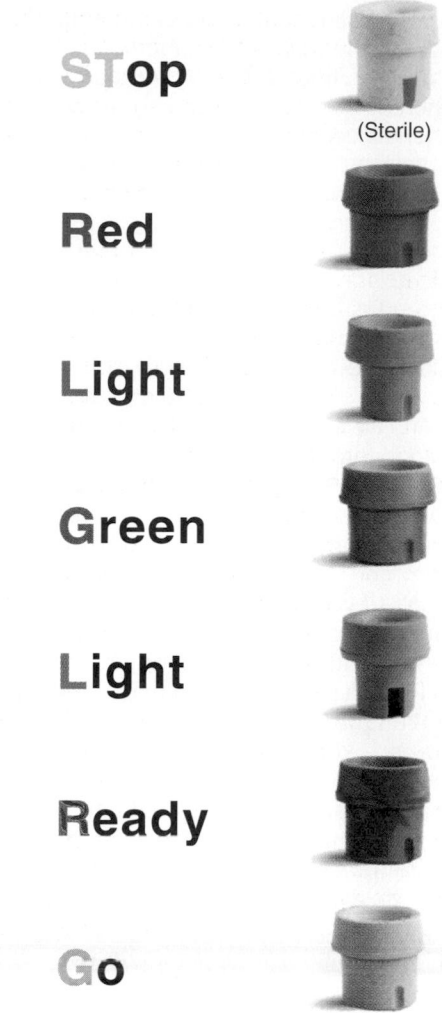

STop
(Sterile)

Red

Light

Green

Light

Ready

Go

FIGURE 50-2 The order of drawing blood. (From Sommer SR, Warekois RS: *Phlebotomy: worktext and procedures manual,* Philadelphia, 2002, WB Saunders, p 147.)

Multisample Needles. Multisample needles are commonly used in routine adult venipuncture. These needles are double pointed (Figure 50-3). One point enters the patient's vein while the other punctures the rubber stopper of the collection tube. Often the point

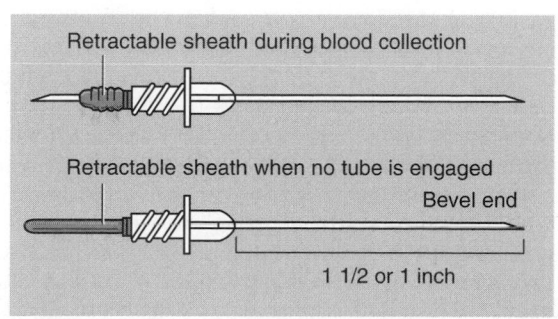

Retractable sheath during blood collection

Retractable sheath when no tube is engaged

Bevel end

1 1/2 or 1 inch

FIGURE 50-3 Multisample needle. (From Sommer SR, Warekois RS: *Phlebotomy: worktext and procedures manual,* Philadelphia, 2002, WB Saunders, p 140.)

that enters the tube is sheathed with a retractable rubber sleeve that allows tubes to be changed without blood leaking into the adapter or tube holder.

Syringes and Syringe Safety Needles. Syringes are used when there is concern that the strong vacuum in a stoppered tube will collapse the vein. The syringe needle fits on the end of the barrel and comes in different gauges as described already. When blood is drawn into a syringe, it must be transferred immediately to another tube because the blood will clot in the syringe barrel. The amount of blood drawn into the barrel depends on how much is to be transferred to stoppered tubes. A special transfer tube adapter is used to transfer the blood to the Vacutainer tube. The adapter connects to the top of the syringe once the needle is capped and removed. The adapter contains an enclosed needle that punctures and delivers the blood into the Vacutainer tube.

Winged Infusion Sets (Butterfly Needles). Butterfly needles (Figure 50-4) are designed for use on small veins such as those in the hand or in pediatric patients. The most common needle size is 23 gauge, and the needle is $1/2$ to $3/4$ inch long with a plastic, flexible butterfly-shaped grip attached to a short length of tubing. One end is fitted into the syringe or the vacuum tube adapter. Often a syringe is used because the vacuum can be controlled more easily. Smaller evacuated tubes, with a less powerful vacuum, are preferable when using a butterfly set.

Needle Adapters. Double-pointed needles must be firmly placed into a needle adapter or tube holder. Usually they are translucent cylinders, and they come in different sizes to accommodate the tube being used. The cylinders often have a ring that indicates how far the tube can be pushed onto the needle without losing the vacuum.

Needle Safety. Healthcare workers who use or may be exposed to needles are at increased risk of needlestick injury. Such injuries can lead to serious or fatal infections with blood-borne pathogens such as hepatitis B virus, hepatitis C virus, or human immunodeficiency virus (HIV). The Centers for Disease Control and Prevention (CDC) estimates that about 1000 accidental needlesticks occur each day in the United States. Several manufacturers have developed safety features that internally self-blunt the needle as it is removed from a patient, and some adapters have special features that permit retraction of the needle after venipuncture to lessen the chance of an accidental needlestick. If at all possible, avoid recapping a needle. Discard the needle in a sharps container immediately after the venipuncture. Some sharps containers have a method for separating the needle from the adapter (Figure 50-5). If you must recap, ensure that the cap is on a flat surface and scoop the cap with the needle using only one hand. Only until the cap is positioned over the needle should you use your other hand to secure the cap over the needle.

According to the CDC, state legislative efforts to improve healthcare worker safety related to needlesticks began in 1998 in California. As of November 2001, 19 other states have enacted some type of legislation related to healthcare worker blood-borne pathogen exposures. These state laws typically require that state

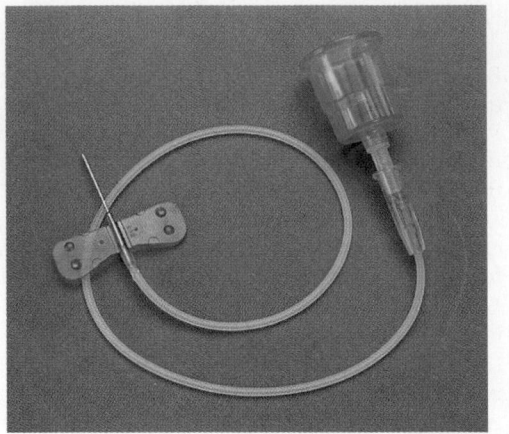

FIGURE 50-4   Winged infusion set attached to an evacuated tube holder with a Luer adapter. (From Sommer SR, Warekois RS: *Phlebotomy: worktext and procedures manual*, Philadelphia, 2002, WB Saunders, p 140.)

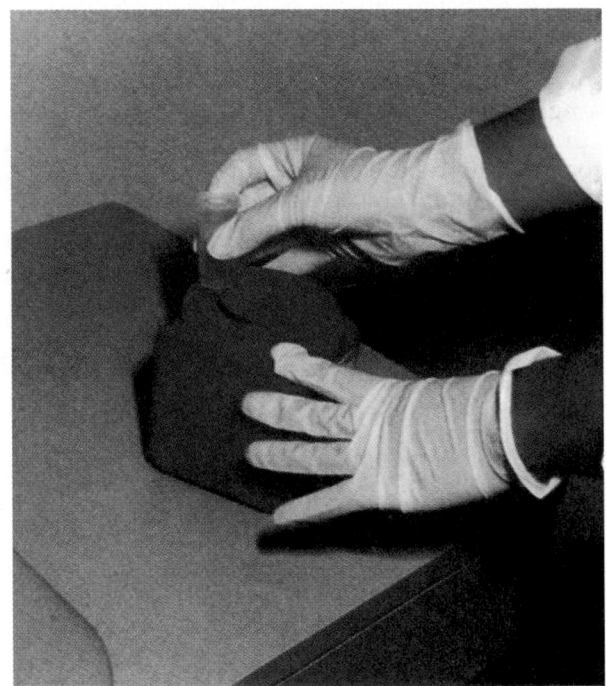

FIGURE 50-5   Needle separation unit.

agencies, such as the department of health or labor, develop a set of administrative regulations to implement the laws. These state laws are aimed at adding additional safeguards for healthcare workers at the state level. This includes adding provisions not in the federal Occupational Safety and Health Administration (OSHA) Bloodborne Pathogen standard or coverage of public employees not regulated by OSHA. Each of these state laws varies in terms of its coverage and scope. Common provisions include requirements for the following:

- Listing of safety devices as engineering controls
- Development of a list of available safety devices by the state for use by employers
- Development of a written exposure plan by employers and periodic review and updates

- Development of protocols for safety device identification and selection by employers and involvement by frontline workers in the process
- Development of a sharps injury log and reporting log information
- Development of methods to increase the use of vaccines and personal protective equipment
- Waivers or exemptions from safety device use under certain circumstances (including patient or worker safety issues, use of alternative effective strategies, market unavailability, and so forth)
- Placement of sharps containers in accessible positions
- Training for workers regarding safety device use

Many of the state laws contain unique requirements, such as surveillance programs, cost-benefit analyses, strict requirements for safety device use, and the use of state-wide advisory boards. Each state law differs as to the time frame for development of its related regulations and the date the laws and regulations become effective.

All healthcare workers should take the following steps to protect themselves and their fellow workers from needlestick injuries:

- Avoid the use of needles where safe and effective alternatives are available.
- Help your employer select and evaluate devices with safety features.
- Use devices with safety features provided by your employer.
- Avoid recapping needles.
- Plan for safe handling and disposal before beginning any procedure using needles.
- Dispose of used needles promptly in appropriate sharps disposal containers.
- Report all needlestick and other sharps-related injuries promptly to ensure that you receive appropriate follow-up care.
- Tell your employer about hazards from needles that you observe in your work environment.
- Participate in blood-borne pathogen training and follow recommended infection prevention practices, including hepatitis B vaccination.

Tourniquets. Before blood can be drawn, a vein must be located. Application of a tourniquet is the most common way to do this and works by preventing venous flow out of the site, causing the veins to bulge.

Various types of tourniquets are shown in Figure 50-6. The tourniquet, usually a thin strip of latex rubber, is tied around the upper arm so that it is tight but not uncomfortable and can be released easily with one hand. Latex tourniquets are inexpensive and easy to disinfect, but some patients are allergic to latex. Other tourniquets with Velcro closures are available and may be more comfortable for the patient, but they have the disadvantage of being difficult to release.

Tourniquets are tied 3 to 4 inches above the elbow immediately before the venipuncture procedure begins. Because it impedes blood flow, leaving a tourniquet on for longer than 2 minutes greatly increases the possibility of **hemoconcentration** and altered test results. Alternately, a blood pressure cuff can be used during a multitube draw and can be released and reinflated as needed to prevent hemoconcentration. Tourniquets are also used when drawing blood from hand and foot veins and are tied on the wrist or ankle, respectively.

Tourniquets can be uncomfortable to patients, especially those with heavy-set or hairy upper arms, if they are not applied correctly. Be sure that the tourniquet is flat against the skin and, if necessary, tie it over the clothing if it is causing the patient discomfort. Tourniquets should be cleaned regularly with soap and hot water and can be easily cleaned between uses with disposable antiseptic towelettes containing benzalkonium chloride.

Antiseptics. To prevent infection, a venipuncture site must be cleansed with an **antiseptic**. The most commonly used is 70% isopropyl alcohol, also known as rubbing alcohol. Prepackaged alcohol "prep pads" are the most commonly used product. The square prep pad is rubbed on the skin in a circular motion, and the alcohol is allowed to dry. Alcohol does not sterilize the skin; it inhibits the reproduction of bacteria that might contaminate the sample. To be most effective, the alcohol should remain on the skin 30 to 60 seconds. Isopropyl alcohol cannot be used when drawing a blood alcohol test. Sterile soap pads, benzalkonium chloride, or povidone-iodine can be used.

If a blood culture is ordered, additional preparation is needed at the venipuncture site to eliminate contaminating bacteria. Povidone-iodine solution (Betadine) is commonly used. For patients allergic to iodine, chlorhexidine gluconate or benzalkonium chloride can

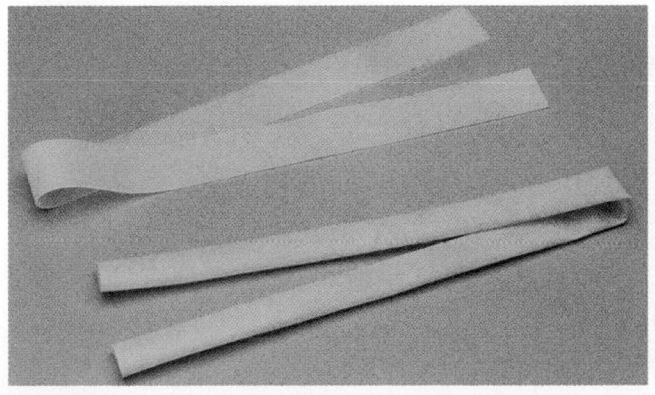
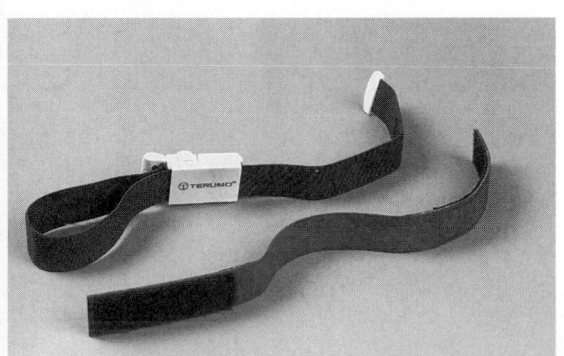

FIGURE 50-6 Examples of tourniquets. (**B** From Flynn JC Jr: *Procedures in phlebotomy.* ed 2, Philadelphia, 1999, WB Saunders, p 80.)

be used. Cleansing the area before a blood culture collection requires more vigorous cleansing than a routine venipuncture.

CRITICAL THINKING APPLICATION

- Melissa calls the first patient into the room. Mrs. Cara Miata is visiting the doctor today to have coagulation studies done. She is a pleasant, talkative woman 88 years of age. Melissa begins to organize her supplies. She examines Mrs. Miata's arms and decides that it would be best to draw from the hand. Why do you think she makes this decision?
- What supplies will she need to draw from the hand? What tubes will she collect?

Routine Venipuncture

Generally, veins in the forearm or the elbow (*antecubital* area) are used for venipuncture (Figure 50-7). The puncture site should be carefully selected after inspecting both arms. Alternative sites may be indicated if the area is cyanotic, scarred, bruised, edematous, or burned. You may use veins on the lower forearm, the back of the hand, or the wrist. Use foot or ankle veins only if the patient has good circulation in the legs and you have received permission from your supervisor or the physician.

Performing a venipuncture involves several important steps with which you must be thoroughly familiar before attempting the procedure. The first step is to select the proper method for venipuncture (syringe or evacuated tube). Next, the patient must be prepared for the procedure. Patient preparation is followed by the actual venipuncture and specimen collection. The final step is care of the puncture site before discharging the patient.

Patient Preparation

All blood collections begin with a requisition, a form from the patient's physician requesting a test. Requisitions may be computer-generated or handwritten and at a minimum must have the following information:
- Patient name
- Date of birth
- Identification number
- Name of physician making the request
- Type of test requested
- Test status (timed, fasting, stat, and so forth)

The venipuncture begins with greeting and identifying the patient. Introduce yourself and explain briefly the purpose and procedure of the venipuncture. If the patient has questions regarding the tests that have been ordered, request politely that they speak to their physician and ask whether they would like to do so before you collect the sample. Obtain verbal consent for performing the procedure simply by asking if you have permission to take some blood from their arm. Always ask the patient if they have experienced problems during routine venipuncture in the past, and take steps to prevent such problems. Your self-confidence in the procedure will be evident to the patient and will help to allay any fears.

Seat the patient in a chair and ask the patient to extend his or her arm. Inspect both arms and ask whether the patient has a preference. Apply the tourniquet, request that the patient make a fist, and palpate for an acceptable vein using your index finger. The vein will bounce lightly. When you have located a vein, remove the tourniquet and assemble the appropriate equipment. Ensure that everything is within easy reach, that the sterile packets are torn open, and that the contents are easily accessible. Wash your hands and apply gloves.

Reapply the tourniquet and quickly relocate the vein. Cleanse the antecubital area with the alcohol, working outward in a circular motion. Do not touch this area after cleansing. Request that the patient clench his or her hand into a fist and then swiftly insert the needle

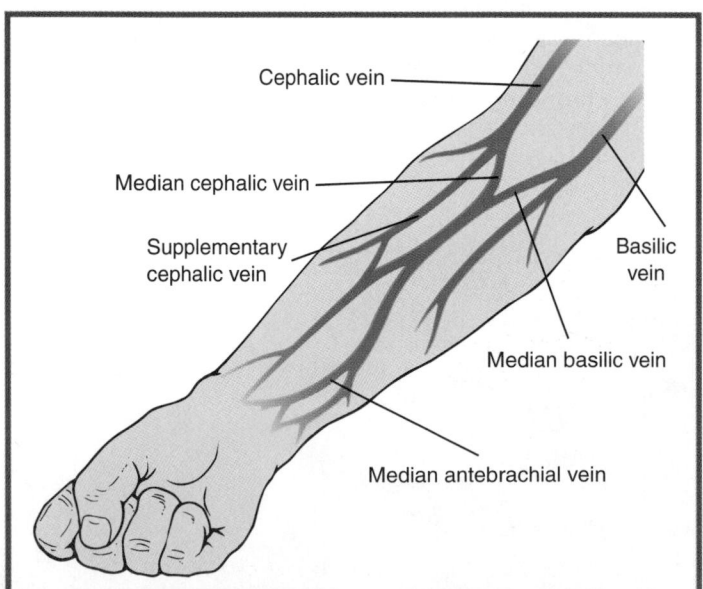

Cephalic vein

Median cephalic vein

Supplementary cephalic vein

Basilic vein

Median basilic vein

Median antebrachial vein

FIGURE 50-7   Veins of the forearm. (From Stepp CA, Woods MA: *Laboratory procedures for medical office personnel*, Philadelphia, 1998, WB Saunders, p 116.)

into the vein at a 15- to 30-degree angle. The bevel should be facing up. Pull back on the syringe plunger or push the evacuated tube onto the double-pointed needle. When blood enters the tube or barrel, request that the patient unclench the fist.

Continue to draw the specimen, checking periodically on the patient's condition. As you near the end of the draw, release the tourniquet. Remove the needle quickly, and then apply the gauze with pressure to the puncture site. Ask the patient to apply direct pressure to the gauze but not to bend the arm. Immediately activate the one-hand safety device to cover the needle and dispose of the entire assembly into a sharps container; then check the puncture site for bleeding or bruising. Apply a bandage and remove the gloves (Figure 50-8), disposing them and the gauze in a biohazard waste container. (Label the tubes and sign or initial the requisition.) Assess the patient's status one last time and then dismiss him or her. Procedures 50-1 to 50-3 outline the proper procedures for collection using a syringe, the evacuated tube method, and a winged infusion set (butterfly needle).

Text continued on p. 1062

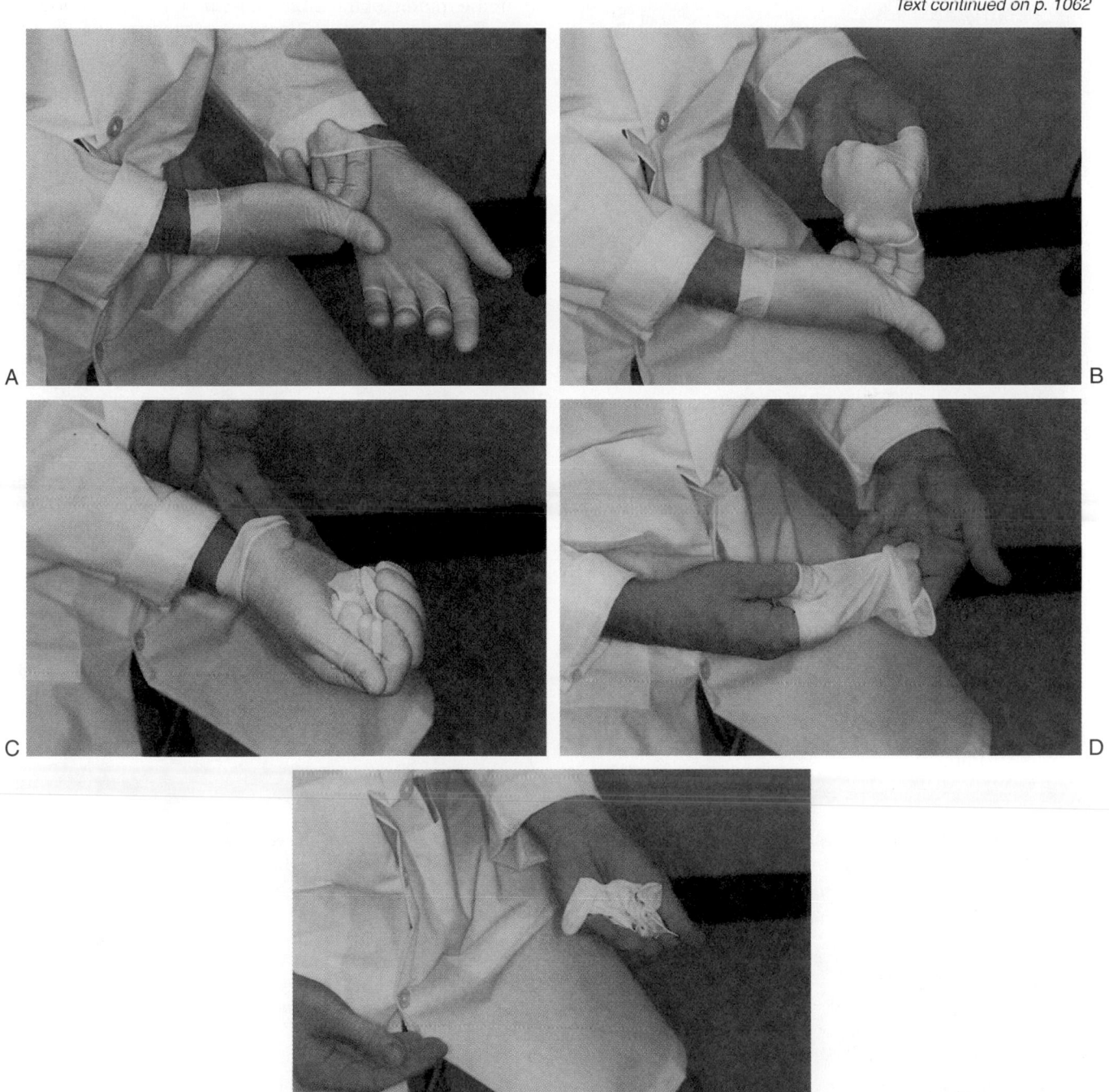

FIGURE 50-8   **A** to **E**, Procedure for removal of gloves. (From Stepp CA, Woods MA: *Laboratory procedures for medical office personnel*, Philadelphia, 1998, WB Saunders, p 125.)

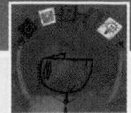

PROCEDURE **50-1**

Collecting a Venous Blood Sample Using the Syringe Method

GOAL: To collect a venous blood specimen.

EQUIPMENT AND SUPPLIES

- Needle, syringe with 21- or 22-gauge needle
- Evacuated tubes appropriate to tests ordered
- 70% isopropyl alcohol
- Sterile gauze pads
- Tourniquet
- Nonallergenic tape
- Permanent marking pen

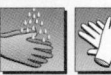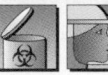

PROCEDURAL STEPS

1 Check the requisition form to determine the tests ordered. Gather the correct tubes and supplies you will need.

Purpose: Allows for proper specimen collection.

2 Wash and dry your hands, and put on face protection and nonsterile gloves.

Purpose: Infection control.

3 Identify the patient and explain the procedure.

Purpose: Ascertain patient identity; explanations help to gain the patient's cooperation.

4 Assist the patient to sit with the arm well supported in a slightly downward position.

Purpose: Veins of the antecubital fossa are more easily located when the elbow is straight.

5 Assemble equipment: Choice of syringe and needle size depends on your inspection of the patient's veins. Attach the needle to the syringe. Keep the cover on the needle.

6 Apply the tourniquet around the patient's arm 3 to 4 inches above the elbow. The tourniquet should never be tied so tightly that it restricts blood flow in the artery (Figure 1*).

Purpose: The tourniquet is used to make the veins more prominent.

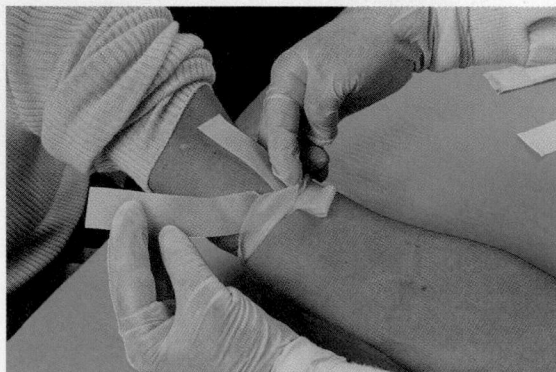

Figure 1

7 Select the venipuncture site by palpating the antecubital space, and use your index finger to trace the path of the vein and to judge its depth. The vein most often used is the median cephalic, which lies in the middle of the elbow (Figure 2*).

Purpose: The index finger is most sensitive for palpating. Do not use the thumb because it has a pulse of its own, which may confuse you.

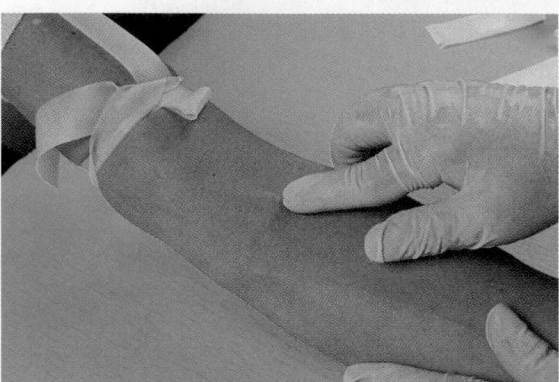

Figure 2

8 Ask the patient to open and close his or her hand several times.

Purpose: Clenching the fist produces engorgement of the vein.

9 Cleanse the site, starting in the center of the area and working outward in a circular pattern (Figure 3*).

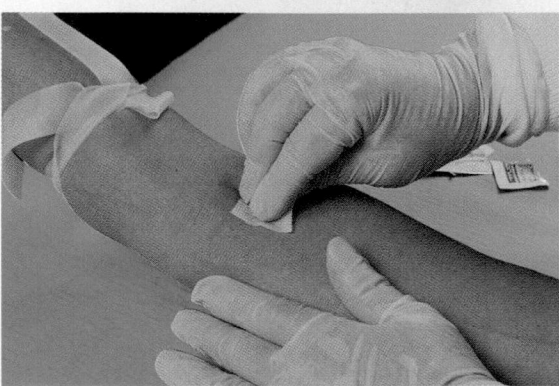

Figure 3

10 Dry the site with a sterile gauze pad.

Purpose: The circular pattern helps avoid recontamination of the area. Puncturing a wet area stings and can cause hemolysis of the sample.

PROCEDURE 50-1—cont'd

11 Remove the needle sheath.

12 Hold the syringe in your dominant hand. Your thumb should be on top and your fingers underneath.

13 Grasp the patient's arm with the nondominant hand while using your thumb and forefinger to draw the skin taut over the site to anchor the vein.

Purpose: Failure to anchor the vein makes puncturing more difficult and painful and may result in a missed vein.

14 Insert the needle through the skin and into the vein with the bevel of the needle up, aligned parallel to the vein, at a 15-degree angle, rapidly, and smoothly (Figure 4*). Request that the patient release his or her fist.

Purpose: The sharpest point of the needle is inserted first.

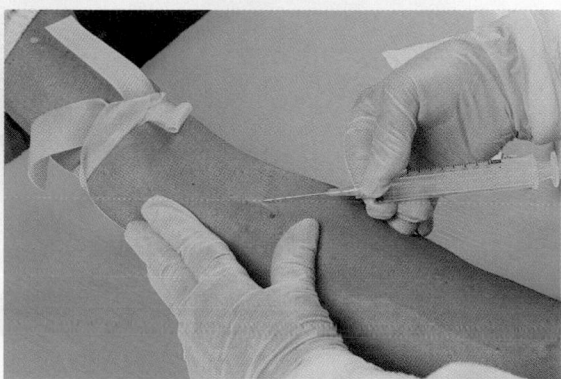

Figure 4

15 Slowly pull back the plunger of the syringe with the nondominant hand. Make sure that you do not move the needle after entering the vein. Allow the syringe or tube to fill to optimum capacity (Figure 5*).

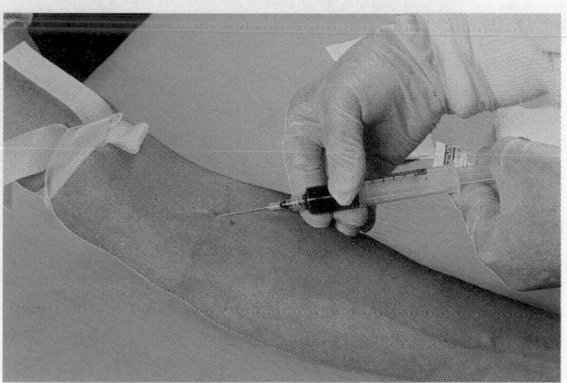

Figure 5

16 Release the tourniquet when venipuncture is complete. It must be released before the needle is removed from the arm (Figure 6*).

Purpose: Removal of the tourniquet releases pressure on the vein and helps prevent blood from getting into adjacent tissues and causing a hematoma.

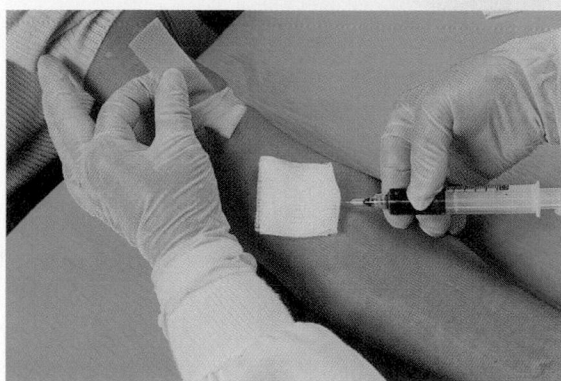

Figure 6

17 Place sterile gauze over the puncture site at the time of needle withdrawal (Figure 7*). Immediately activate the needle safety device and dispose of the entire assembly in the sharps container.

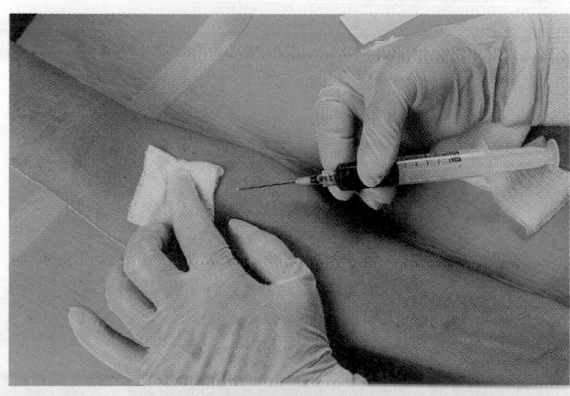

Figure 7

18 Instruct the patient to apply direct pressure on the puncture site with sterile gauze. The patient may elevate the arm.

Purpose: Direct pressure is the best method to stop bleeding. Elevating the arm above the heart also stops bleeding.

Continued

PROCEDURE 50-1—cont'd

19 Transfer the blood to a tube using the syringe Vacutainer adapter. Gently invert tubes to mix anticoagulants and blood. *Label tubes with the patient's name, the date, and the time* (Figure 8).

Purpose: Prevents clotting of blood. Vigorous mixing may cause hemolysis.

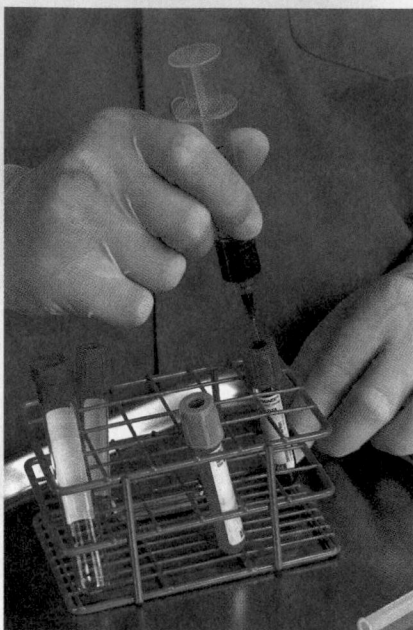

Figure 8

20 Check the puncture site for bleeding.

21 Apply a hypoallergenic bandage (Figure 9*).

22 Dispose of the needle safely. Allow it to drop directly into the disposal unit without touching it with your fingers. Do not recap used needles.

Purpose: Most accidental needlesticks occur when a needle is being recapped. Report any accidents to your supervisor or the physician.

23 Clean the work area, remove gloves and face protection, and wash your hands.

Purpose: Infection control.

24 Complete the laboratory requisition form, and route the specimen to the proper place. Record the procedure in the patient's record.

Purpose: A procedure is considered not done until it is recorded.

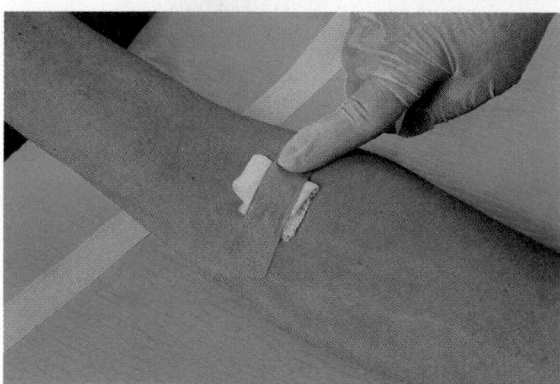

Figure 9

PROCEDURE 50-2

Collecting a Venous Blood Sample Using the Evacuated Tube Method

GOAL: To collect a venous blood specimen.

EQUIPMENT AND SUPPLIES

- Vacutainer needle, adapter, and proper tubes for requested tests
- 70% isopropyl alcohol
- Sterile gauze pads
- Tourniquet
- Nonallergenic tape
- Permanent marking pen

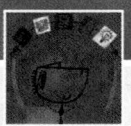

PROCEDURAL STEPS

1 Check the requisition form to determine the tests ordered. Gather the correct tubes and supplies that you will need.

Purpose: Allows for proper specimen collection.

2 Wash and dry your hands, and put on face protection and nonsterile gloves.

PROCEDURE 50-2—cont'd

Purpose: Infection control.

3 Identify the patient and explain the procedure.
Purpose: Ascertains patient identity, and explanations help gain the patient's cooperation.

4 Assist the patient to sit with the arm well supported in a slightly downward position.
Purpose: Veins of the antecubital fossa are more easily located when the elbow is straight.

5 Assemble equipment: Choice of needle size depends on your inspection of the patient's veins. Attach the needle to the Vacutainer holder. Keep the cover on the needle.

6 Apply the tourniquet around the patient's arm 3 to 4 inches above the elbow. The tourniquet should never be tied so tightly that it restricts blood flow in the artery (Figure 1).
Purpose: The tourniquet is used to make the veins more prominent.

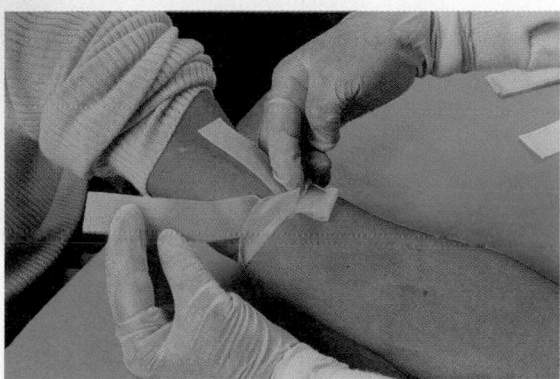

Figure 1

7 Select the venipuncture site by palpating the antecubital space, and use your index finger to trace the path of the vein and to judge its depth. The vein most often used is the median cephalic, which lies in the middle of the elbow (Figure 2).
Purpose: The index finger is most sensitive for palpating. Do not use the thumb, because it has a pulse of its own, which may confuse you.

8 Ask the patient to open and close his or her hand several times.
Purpose: Clenching the fist produces engorgement of the vein.

9 Cleanse the site, starting in the center of the area and working outward in a circular pattern (Figure 3).

10 Dry the site with a sterile gauze pad.
Purpose: The circular pattern helps avoid recontamination of the area. Puncturing a wet area stings and can cause hemolysis of the sample.

11 Remove the needle sheath.

12 Hold the Vacutainer assembly in your dominant hand. Your thumb should be on top and your fingers underneath.

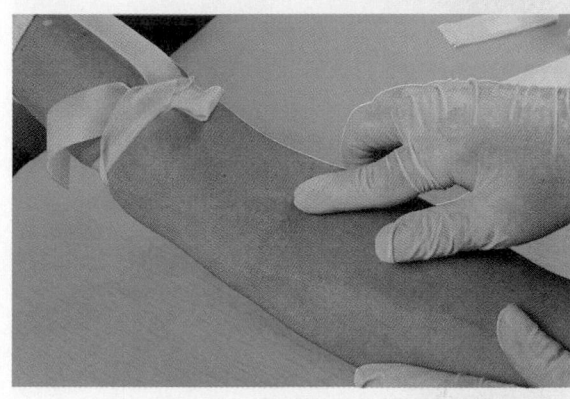

Figure 2

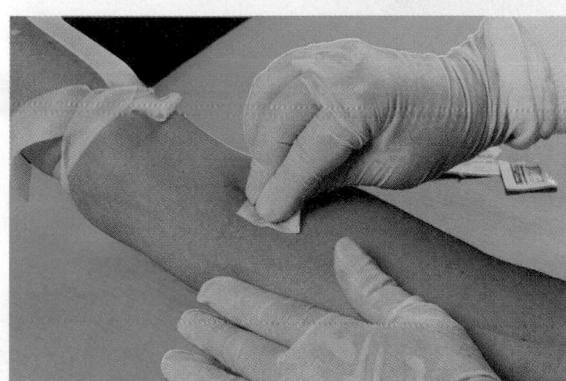

Figure 3

13 Grasp the patient's arm with the nondominant hand while using your thumb and forefinger to draw the skin taut over the site, to anchor the vein.
Purpose: Failure to anchor the vein makes puncturing more difficult and painful and may result in a missed vein.

14 Insert the needle through the skin and into the vein with the bevel of the needle up, aligned parallel to the vein, at a 15-degree angle, rapidly, and smoothly (Figure 4).
Purpose: The sharpest point of the needle is inserted first.

Continued

PROCEDURE 50-2—cont'd

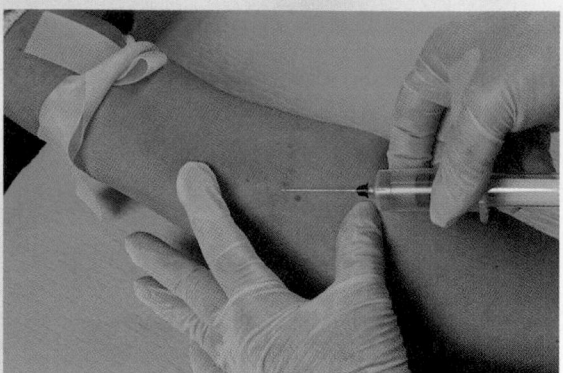

Figure 4

15 Place two fingers on the flanges of the Vacutainer holder and, with the thumb, push the tube onto the needle inside the holder. Make sure that you do not move the needle after entering the vein. Allow the tube to fill to optimum capacity (Figure 5).

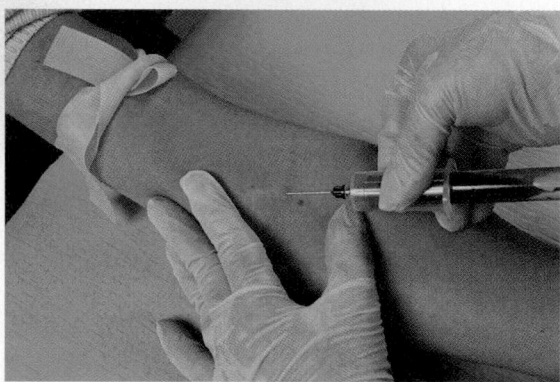

Figure 5

16 Release the tourniquet during the filling of the last tube when venipuncture is complete. *It must be released before the needle is removed from the arm.*

Purpose: Removal of the tourniquet releases pressure on the vein and helps prevent blood from getting into adjacent tissues and causing a hematoma.

17 Remove the last Vacutainer tube from the adapter before removing the needle from the vein (Figure 6).

Purpose: A nontraumatic venipuncture produces the most reliable results. Proper tube filling ensures the correct ratio of blood to additive. Removal of the tube from the holder before removal from the vein prevents any excess blood from dripping from the tip of the needle onto the patient.

18 Place sterile gauze over the puncture site with the nondominant hand at the time of needle withdrawal (Figure 7) and immediately activate the needle safety device. Dispose of the entire unit in a sharps container.

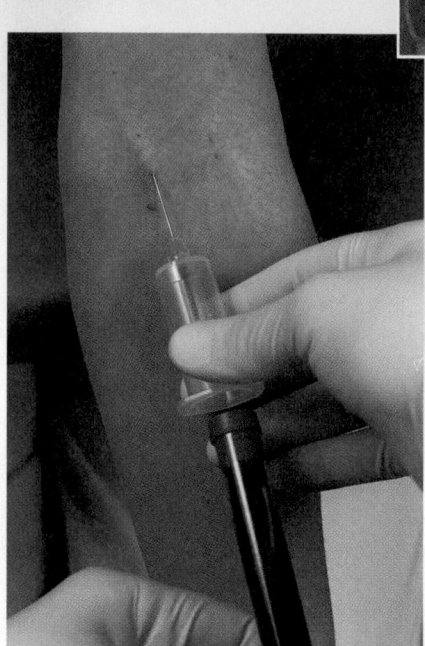

Figure 6

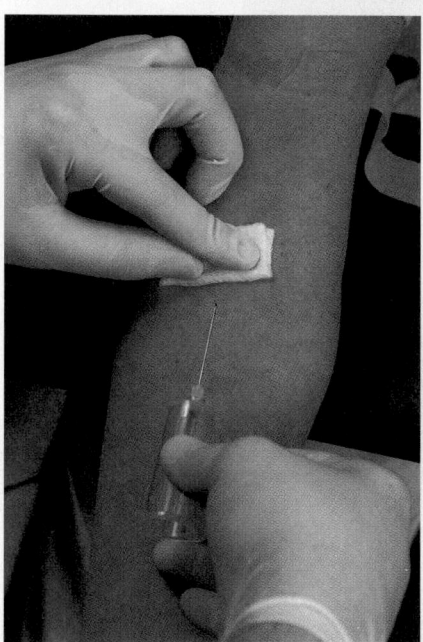

Figure 7

19 Instruct the patient to apply direct pressure on the puncture site with a sterile gauze pad. The patient may elevate the arm.

Purpose: Direct pressure is the best method to stop bleeding. Elevating the arm above the heart also stops bleeding.

PROCEDURE 50-2—cont'd

20 Gently invert tubes to mix anticoagulants and blood. *Label tubes with the patient's name, the date, and the time* (Figure 8).

Purpose: Prevents clotting of blood. Vigorous mixing may cause hemolysis.

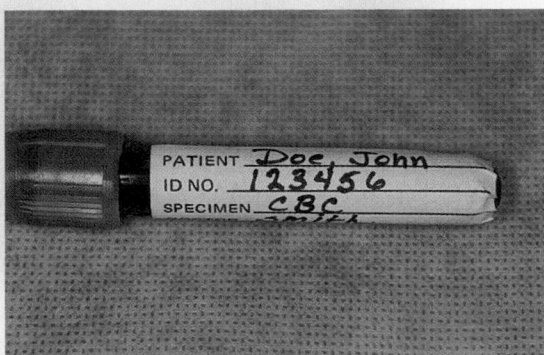

Figure 8

21 Check the puncture site for bleeding.

22 Apply a hypoallergenic bandage (Figure 9).

23 Clean the work area, remove gloves and face protection, and wash your hands.

Purpose: Infection control.

24 Complete the laboratory requisition and route to the proper place. Record the procedure in the patient's record.

Purpose: A procedure is considered not done until it is recorded.

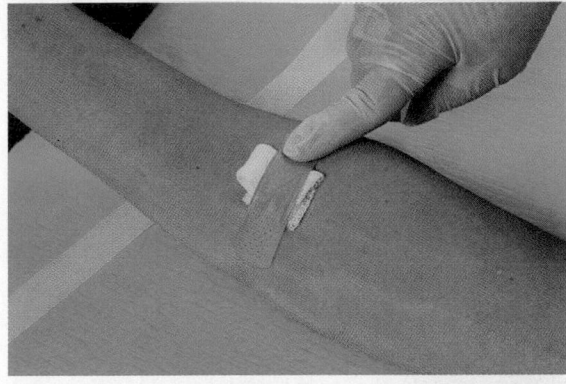

Figure 9

See Appendix E for a charting example.

PROCEDURE 50-3

Performing a Butterfly Draw Using a Hand Vein

GOAL: To obtain the venous sample accurately from a hand vein using the butterfly method.

EQUIPMENT AND SUPPLIES

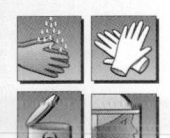
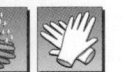
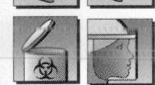

- Tourniquet
- Alcohol pads or other antiseptic preps
- Gauze pads
- Butterfly needle set
- Appropriate pediatric tubes arranged in the order of the draw or
- Luer-Lok syringe
- Sharps disposal container
- Nonallergenic bandage
- Permanent marking pen

PROCEDURAL STEPS

1 Check the requisition and gather the appropriate tubes for the needed tests. Assemble the balance of your supplies.

Purpose: Efficiency in preparation.

2 Wash your hands, and put on face protection and gloves.

Purpose: Infection control.

3 Prepare your patient as for an antecubital draw.

4 Remove the butterfly device from the package and stretch it slightly.

Purpose: To keep the tube from recoiling.

5 Attach the butterfly device to the syringe (Figure 1) or evacuated tube holder (Figure 2).

6 Seat the first tube into the evacuated tube holder.

7 Apply a tourniquet to the patient's wrist, just proximal to the wrist bone.

8 Hold the hand in your nondominant hand with the fingers lower than the wrist.

Continued

PROCEDURE 50-3—cont'd

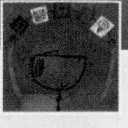

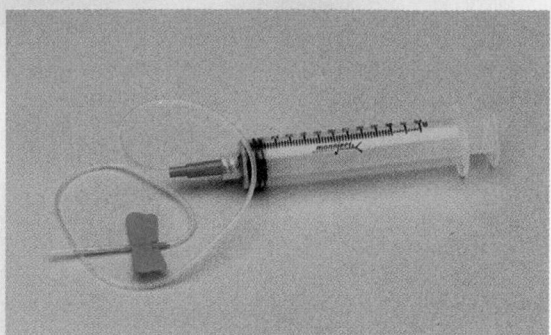

Figure 1

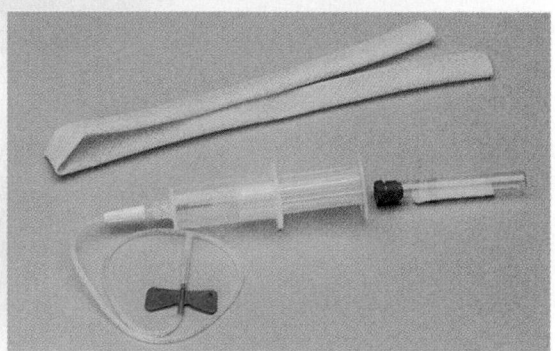

Figure 2

Purpose: This position helps in identifying the veins and draw site.

9 Select a vein and cleanse the site at the **bifurcation**.

10 Using your thumb, pull the patient's skin taut over the knuckles.

11 With the needle at a 10- to 15-degree angle, bevel up, align it with the vein.

12 Insert the needle gently by threading it up the lumen of the vein.

Purpose: So that the needle will not twist out of the vein if you let go of it (Figures 3 and 4).

13 Push the blood collecting tube onto the end of the holder (Figure 5) or draw blood into the syringe

(Figure 6). Note the position of the hands while drawing the blood.

14 Release the tourniquet when the blood appears in the tube.

15 Always keep the tube and the holder in a downward position so that the tube will fill from the bottom up.

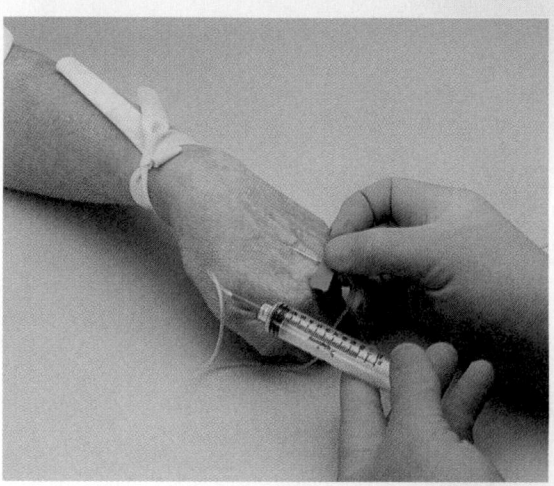

Figure 3

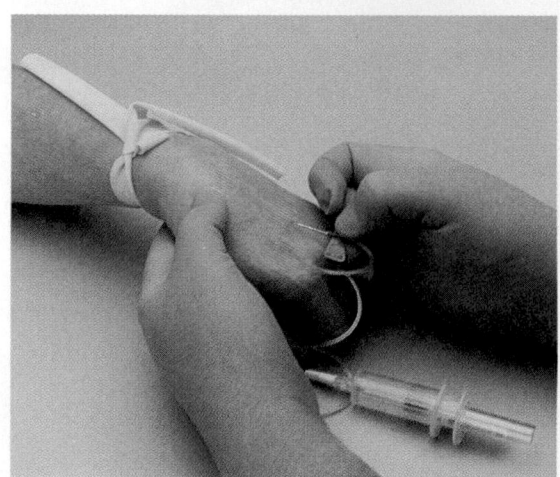

Figure 4

CRITICAL THINKING APPLICATION

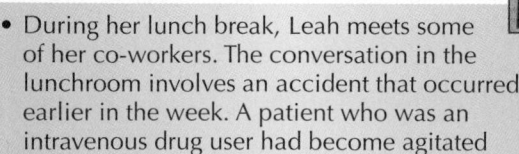

• During her lunch break, Leah meets some of her co-workers. The conversation in the lunchroom involves an accident that occurred earlier in the week. A patient who was an intravenous drug user had become agitated

when their co-worker Louis was administering a tuberculosis Mantoux test. Louis was accidentally stuck with the needle. Describe the actions Louis must take to report and follow up on the incident.

• What measures are available to prevent accidental needlesticks?

PROCEDURE **50-3—cont'd**

16 Place a gauze pad over the puncture site and gently remove the needle.

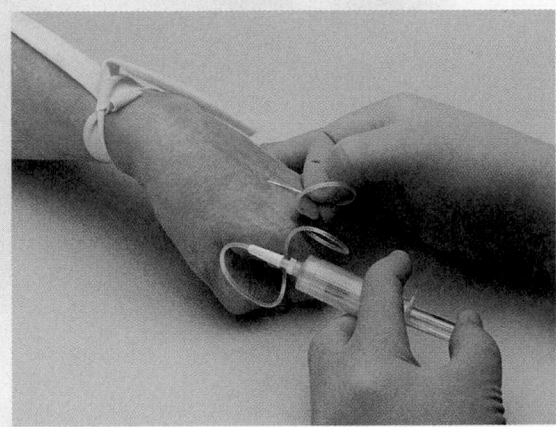

Figure 5

17 Complete the procedure as you would for an antecubital draw (see Procedure 50-2, steps 19 through 25).

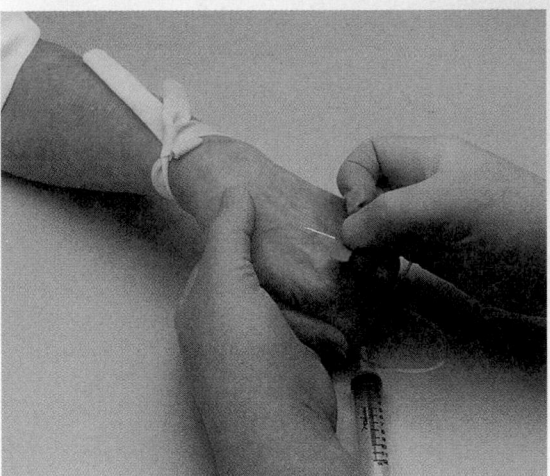

Figure 6

Problems Associated With Venipuncture

Failure to obtain blood can be the result of a number of factors. Determining the cause of the problem may help you to decide whether you will be successful on the second attempt. The first issue before you is to remain calm so that you can think clearly, systematically determining the possible cause of the problem.

A *hematoma* is a large, painful bruised area at the puncture site caused by blood leaking into the tissue, which causes the tissue around the puncture site to swell. The most frequent causes of hematoma formation during the draw are (1) excessive probing to locate the vein, (2) failure to insert the needle far enough into the vein, and (3) the needle going through the vein. A hematoma can form after a draw if you fail to remove the tourniquet before removing the needle or fail to apply adequate pressure on the puncture site or if the elbow is bent while applying pressure. If a hematoma forms, discontinue the procedure stat, apply pressure to the area for a minimum of 3 minutes, and then apply an ice pack to the area. Notify the physician and observe the site to determine whether the bleeding has stopped. An incident report will need to be completed and recorded in the patient's record.

Nerve damage can be a consequence, albeit unlikely, of venipuncture. Preventive measures include avoidance of the basilic vein and blind probing if the vein is missed.

Table 50-3 lists some probable solutions to complications. As a general rule, it is wise to limit yourself to two attempts to obtain blood from any one patient. If you fail on the second attempt, ask the patient whether he or she would prefer having someone else try or whether it would be better to come back at another time. This maneuver lets the patient feel that he or she is in control of the situation. Everyone fails to obtain a needed blood sample at one time or another; so do not feel that you are a failure.

CRITICAL THINKING APPLICATION

During her second week at the clinic, Leah is confident that she can perform phlebotomy on her own. Melissa has been a good mentor, and Leah has done quite a few successful "sticks" without any problems. Today, however, she is just having a bad day. Mr. Godfrey Lawrence has come to the clinic with numerous problems, and Dr. Gupta has ordered several blood tests. Mr. Godfrey is uncooperative when he sees that Leah must draw four tubes of blood. He angrily tells her that she cannot take that much blood out of him—he will have none left. How should Leah deal with this problem?

Specimen Re-collection

Sometimes problems with a sample cannot be determined until the specimen is analyzed in the laboratory. Rejected specimens must be re-collected. The laboratory may reject a specimen for reasons that include the following:

TABLE 50-3	Managing Blood Draw Complications
Possible Complication	**Strategies**
Burned area	Must be avoided, because these areas are prone to infection
Convulsions	Stay calm. *Remove the needle*; then help guide the patient to the floor, protecting him or her from injury. Call for help.
Damaged/scarred veins or infected areas	Look for an alternative site; *do not* draw blood from scarred or infected areas.
Edema	Avoid the area; look for an alternative site.
Hematoma	Adjust the depth of the needle or remove the needle and apply pressure.
Intravenous (IV) therapy/ blood transfusion sites	Blood samples should not be drawn from an arm that is also the site for IV infusion or blood transfusion owing to the dilution factor.
Mastectomy	*Do not* draw blood from the site of the mastectomy, because mastectomy surgery causes lymphostasis, which may produce false results.
Nausea	Place a cold cloth on the patient's forehead, give the patient a basin, in case of vomiting, and instruct him or her to take deep breaths. Alert the physician.
No blood	Manipulate the needle slightly, or remove the Vacutainer and perform the blood draw again using a syringe or butterfly set-up.
Petechiae	Loosen the tourniquet, because this complication usually results from the tourniquet being in place for longer than 2 minutes.
Syncope (fainting)	Position the patient's head between the knees (if in a sitting position). Check and record the patient's pulse, blood pressure, and respiration rate, and continue to observe the patient. *Never leave the patient unattended.*

Modified from Stepp CA, Woods MA: *Laboratory procedures for medical office personnel.* Philadelphia, 1998, WB Saunders.

- Unlabeled or mislabeled specimen
- Quantity not sufficient
- Defective tube
- Incorrect tube used for test ordered
- Hemolysis
- Clotted blood in an anticoagulated specimen
- Improper handling

CRITICAL THINKING APPLICATION

- Leah next must draw a sample from Ms. Danielle Rollins. Ms. Rollins indicates that she has a history of bruising after venipuncture, and sure enough a hematoma begins to rise shortly after Leah inserts the needle. She then notices that Ms. Rollins has become pale and is perspiring. What should Leah do first?
- What other steps should Leah take? Can she still obtain the sample?

Capillary Puncture

Capillaries are small blood vessels that connect small arterioles to small venules. The capillary, or dermal, puncture is an efficient means of collecting a blood specimen when only a small amount of blood is required or when a patient's condition makes venipuncture difficult. Because the requisition will not indicate that the collection is to be made in this manner, you must be familiar with the advantages, limitations, and appropriate uses of this technique. Capillary puncture is warranted in the following:

- Older patients
- Pediatric patients (especially under the age of 2 years)

- Patients who require frequent glucose monitoring
- Patients with burns or scars in venipuncture sites
- Obese patients
- Patients receiving intravenous therapy
- Patients who have had a mastectomy
- Patients at risk for venous thrombosis
- Patients who are severely dehydrated
- Tests that require a small volume of blood
- When venous blood and capillary blood are not identical

Capillaries are bridges between arteries and veins, and thus capillary blood is a mixture of the two. Small amounts of tissue fluid are also present in capillary blood, especially in the first drop. Analyte levels are usually the same in capillary and venous blood with a few exceptions. Hemoglobin and glucose values will be higher in capillary blood; potassium, calcium, and total protein will be higher in venous blood.

Equipment

Skin Puncture Devices. The simplest device for performing dermal puncture is the lancet, a thin, flat piece of steel with a sharp tip. Some devices control the depth of the puncture, and automatic devices deliver a quick puncture to a predetermined depth. Note that the automatic devices for home glucose monitoring make a cut that is too small to collect multiple tests (Figure 50-9). Many devices have safety features, including retractable blades and locks that prevent the device from being reused. Skin puncture devices should always be discarded in a sharps container.

Collection Containers. Depending on the test to be performed, different types of collection devices and containers are available (Figure 50-10). *Microcollection* or *microtainer tubes* hold up to 750 μl of blood and are available with a variety of anticoagulants and additives.

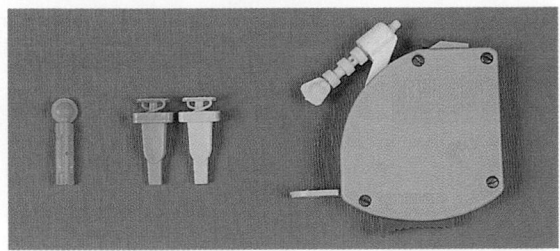

FIGURE 50-9 Skin puncture devices include simple lancets and automated devices that control the depth and width of the incision. (From Bonewit-West K: *Clinical procedures for medical assistants*, ed 5, Philadelphia, 2000, WB Saunders, p 605.)

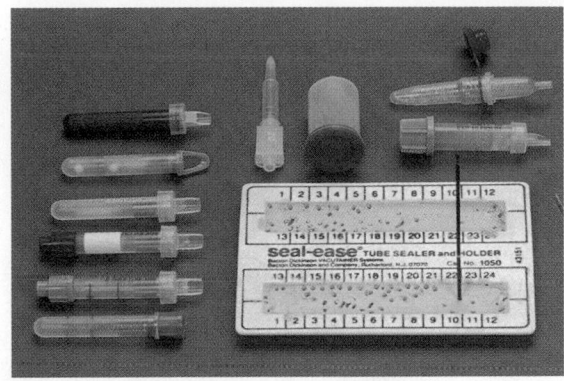

FIGURE 50-10 Microsample containers: microtainer tubes, capillary tube in sealing clay, and Unopette System.

The tops are color coded in the same fashion as evacuated tubes. Blood is collected dropwise into these tubes through a funnel-like device. Capillary tubes are another way to collect blood from a dermal puncture. These are glass or plastic tubes that draw blood by capillary action, that is, the blood fills into these narrow tubes without the need for suction. If the capillary tube is coated with the anticoagulant heparin, a red band will be seen at the top. A common, heparin-coated capillary tube is the *microhematocrit tube* used for determining the percentage of packed red blood cells in the microhematocrit test.

The Unopette system (Becton Dickinson, Franklin Lakes, NJ) is a micropipet and dilution system used for performing manual blood counts. The system includes a reservoir with diluting fluid and a calibrated micropipet. The method for filling a Unopette device is described in Chapter 51.

Manufacturers also provide various collection devices designed to obtain small quantities of blood for "point of care" testing for such analytes as glucose and cholesterol. The blood is either pulled into the collecting device by capillary action after puncture or it is dropped onto a reagent strip which is inserted into the instrument to be analyzed.

Finally, blood from a capillary puncture can be deposited onto filter paper supplied with a test kit. Tests performed on neonates for certain metabolic disorders, such as phenylketonuria (PKU), require that blood is deposited into circles on biologically inactive filter paper (Figure 50-11).

FIGURE 50-11 **A,** An example of filter paper used in neonatal screening. (From Sommer SR, Warekois RS: *Phlebotomy: worktext and procedures manual*, Philadelphia, 2002, WB Saunders, p 221. **A** Modified from Bonewit-West K: *Clinical procedures for medical assistants*. ed 5, Philadelphia, 2000, WB Saunders, p 434.)

Continued

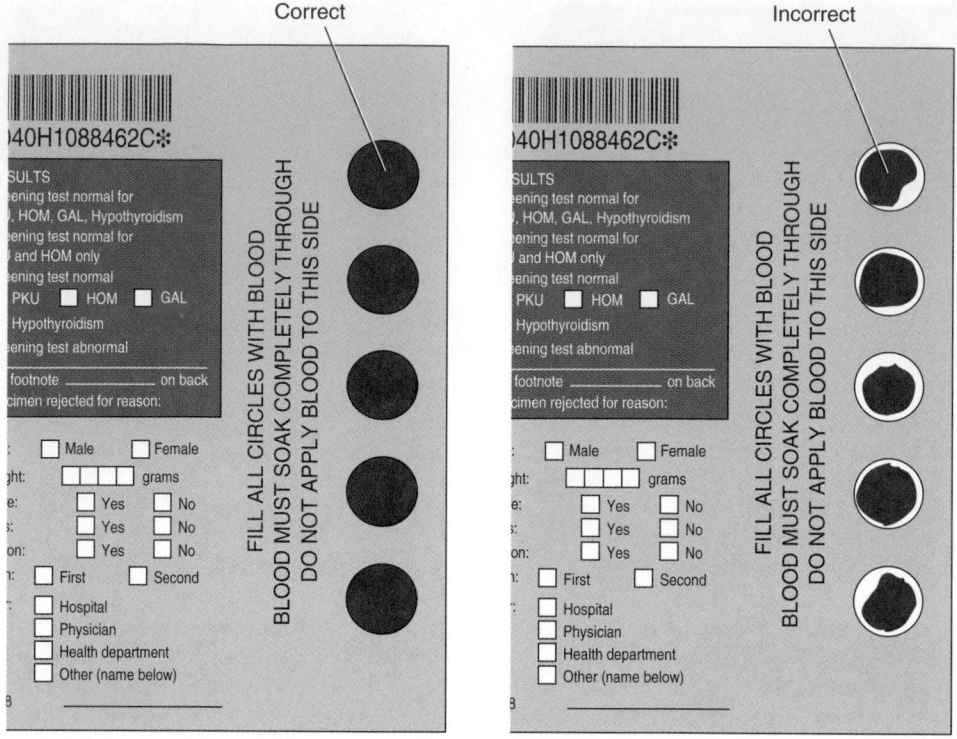

FIGURE 50-11, cont'd **B**, Correct and incorrect ways to fill in the circles. (From Sommer SR, Warekois RS: *Phlebotomy: worktext and procedures manual*, Philadelphia, 2002, WB Saunders, p 221.)

Routine Capillary Puncture

Site Selection. In adults and children, the usual puncture site is the ring finger, but capillary blood can be obtained from the middle finger or heel (Figure 50-12). The thumb is usually too callused, and the index finger has extra nerve endings that make the puncture more painful. The fifth finger has too little tissue for a successful puncture. The puncture is made at the tip and slightly to the side of the finger. Be sure to puncture a fleshy area closer to the center of the finger to prevent damage to underlying bone. Avoid areas that are callused, scarred, burned, infected, cyanotic, or edematous.

For children younger than 1 year, dermal puncture is performed on the medial and lateral surfaces of the plantar (bottom) of the heel. Areas other than these are unsafe and may cause bone or nerve damage to an

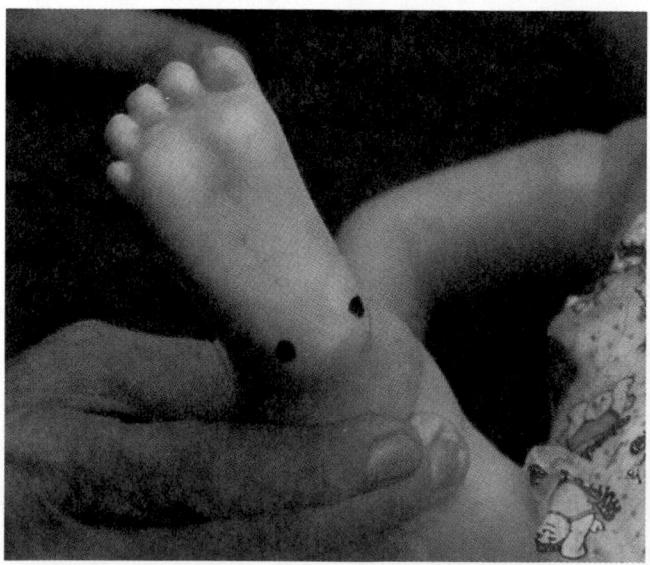
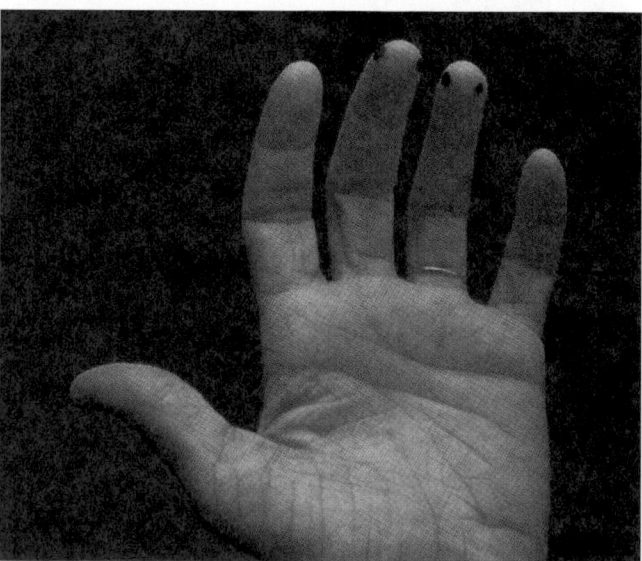

FIGURE 50-12 **A** and **B**, Capillary puncture sites on heel and fingers.

infant. It is advisable to warm the heel before collection. Never place bandages on the heel or anywhere on infants under the age of 2 years. They may peel off and become a choking hazard.

Patient Preparation. Preparation for a capillary puncture is similar to that for venipuncture. Cleanse the finger well with an alcohol prep pad. If the patient's hands are excessively soiled, request that he or she wash the hands before the procedure. If the patient's hands are cold, warm them in warm water, drying thoroughly, or ask him or her to rub or shake them vigorously.

Generally, you must work very efficiently when performing a capillary puncture because blood flow stops quickly. Be sure to have your supplies organized and within easy reach. After puncturing the dermis, it is important to wipe away the first drop of blood. This drop contains tissue fluid that could interfere with test results. Grasp the finger firmly, but do not squeeze or "milk" it. After the devices are filled, ask the patient to apply pressure to the gauze you have placed over the puncture site. Be prepared for blood to contaminate your gloves or surfaces by having spare gloves, extra gauze pads, and disinfectant nearby.

Specimen Handling. Capillary collection devices are often too small to apply a label. The most efficient way to transport capillary tubes is to remove the stopper from a red-topped tube, insert the capillary tubes, sealed-end down, replace the stopper, and label the tube. Microtainer tubes have plastic plugs that fit over the top. They may be placed in either a labeled tube or a labeled zipper-lock bag for transport. Always decontaminate collection devices before delivering them to the laboratory if blood was deposited on the surface during collection. The procedure for routine capillary collection is outlined in Procedure 50-4.

PROCEDURE **50-4**

Collecting a Capillary Blood Sample

GOAL: To collect a capillary blood specimen suitable for testing, using fingertip puncture technique.

EQUIPMENT AND SUPPLIES

- Sterile disposable manual lancet or Autolet with Autolet platforms
- 70% alcohol
- Sterile gauze pads
- Nonallergenic tape
- Supplies for requested test (e.g., Unopettes or capillary tubes)
- Sealing clay or caps for capillary tubes
- Permanent marking pen

PROCEDURAL STEPS

1 Read requisition and gather all of the needed supplies.
  Purpose: Efficiency.

2 Wash and dry your hands. Put on face protection and nonsterile gloves.

3 Explain the procedure to your patient.
  Purpose: Explanations help to gain the patient's cooperation.

4 Assemble the needed materials based on the physician's requisition.
  Purpose: Once the skin has been punctured, the collection must proceed as rapidly as possible so the blood does not clot before the entire specimen has been collected.

5 Select a puncture site (side of middle finger of nondominant hand, outer edge of ear lobe, medial or lateral curved surface of the heel, or the great toe for an infant).
  Purpose: The nondominant hand may have fewer calluses. The side of the finger is less sensitive, and the skin is usually not as thick.

6 Milk, or gently rub, the finger along the sides.
  Purpose: This promotes circulation. If the finger is very cold, you may immerse it in warm water or moisten it with warm towels.

7 Clean the site with alcohol, and dry it with sterile gauze (Figure 1).
  Purpose: Puncturing wet skin is painful and can hemolyze the specimen.

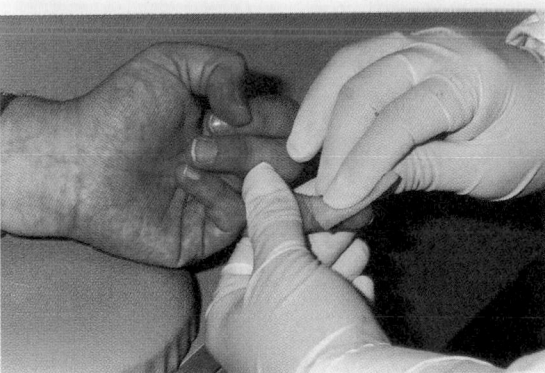

Figure 1

Continued

PROCEDURE 50-4—cont'd

8 Grasp the patient's finger on the sides near the puncture site with your nondominant forefinger and thumb.

Purpose: Firmly holding the site allows control of the puncture.

9 Hold the lancet at a right angle to the patient's finger, and make a rapid, deep puncture on the patient's fingertip (Figure 2).

Purpose: Lancets are designed to puncture at a depth of 3 to 4 mm, which is sufficient to obtain the required drops of blood.

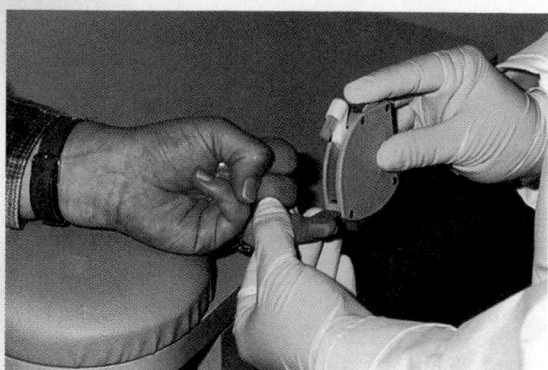

Figure 2

10 Wipe away the first drop of blood (Figure 3).

Purpose: The first drop of blood contains tissue fluid.

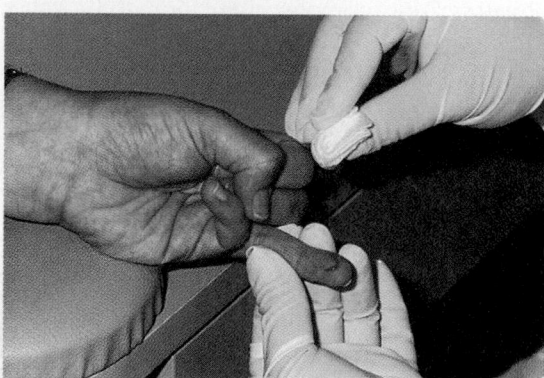

Figure 3

11 Apply gentle pressure to cause the blood to flow freely.

Purpose: Squeezing liberates tissue that dilutes the blood and causes inaccurate results.

12 Collect blood samples.
a. Express a large drop of blood, fill capillary tubes (Figure 4, *A*), and seal the end of the tube in clay (Figure 4, *B*).
b. Wipe the finger with a clean sterile gauze pad, and fill a Unopette (Figure 5).

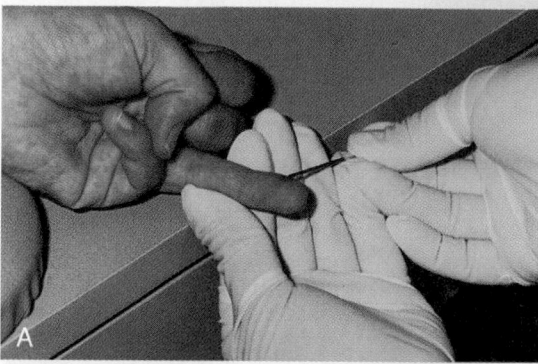

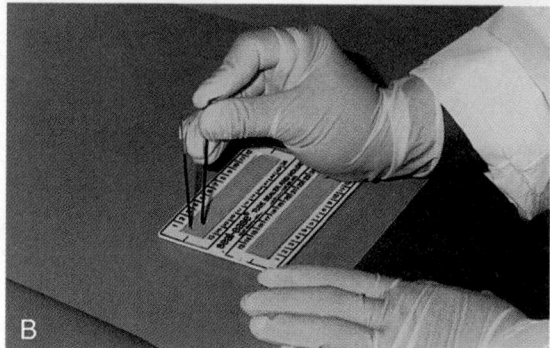

Figure 4

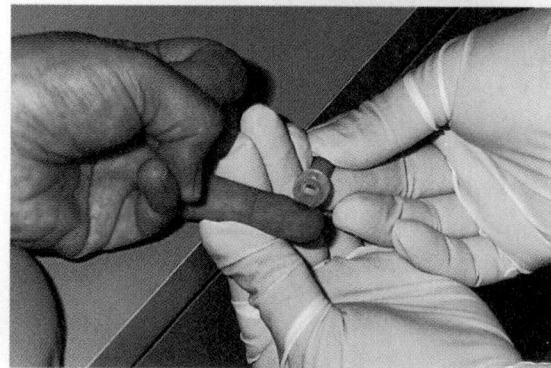

Figure 5

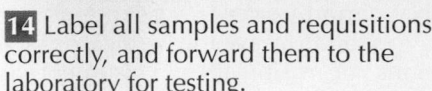

PROCEDURE 50-4—cont'd

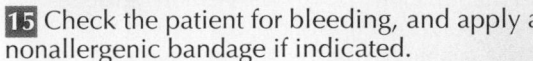

13 Apply pressure to the site with clean sterile gauze (Figure 6).

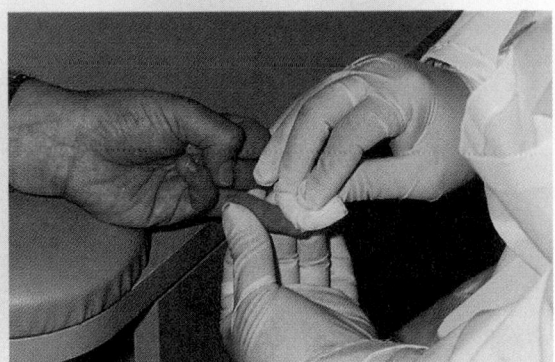

Figure 6

14 Label all samples and requisitions correctly, and forward them to the laboratory for testing.

15 Check the patient for bleeding, and apply a nonallergenic bandage if indicated.

16 Dismiss the patient.

17 Dispose of used materials in proper containers.

18 Clean the work area. Remove face protection and gloves. Wash your hands.
   Purpose: Infection control.

19 Record the procedure in the patient's record.
   Purpose: A procedure is considered not done until it is recorded.

Patient Education

When working as a phlebotomist, the medical assistant must maintain a professional attitude and still be sympathetic to the fears and apprehensions of the patient. By establishing an environment that encourages the patient to relax, the amount of pain and discomfort experienced by the patient during the procedure are kept to a minimum.

If the patient has a positive attitude, you need to provide little explanation about the procedure. Often, the patient can help you by telling from which site the last blood sample was successfully drawn. It is wise to follow the patient's suggestion in choosing the site for the removal of a blood specimen. When a patient is allowed to become an active participant in the procedure, he or she remains more relaxed, talkative, and confident in your expertise as a phlebotomist.

This atmosphere can change dramatically when the patient has had an unpleasant experience and associates pain and discomfort with venipuncture. Such a patient usually is ill at ease, nervous, and apprehensive. When confronted with this scenario, you need to make every effort to perform the procedure quickly, efficiently, and effectively. Once the blood has been drawn and the patient has relaxed, you then will have an opportunity to help the patient develop a positive attitude.

If your patient has a history of **syncope** when blood is drawn, or if you suspect that this patient may faint during the procedure, have the patient lie down. Assemble your equipment and alert the physician before beginning the procedure. This type of professional care may help the patient get through the procedure without a traumatic effect.

Always remember to identify your patient and explain what you are going to do. Answer any questions the patient may have, and perform a skilled venipuncture before anxiety is allowed to set in.

CRITICAL THINKING APPLICATION

- As much as Leah likes children, performing capillary puncture on little fingers is not one of her favorite things to do. Mrs. Spix brings her son Garrett in for a hemoglobin and hematocrit test. Garrett is 5 years old. How can Leah make both Garrett and his mother feel at ease about this procedure?
- What supplies will she need? Explain how she will perform the capillary puncture.

Legal and Ethical Issues

Venipuncture and microcapillary blood collection are invasive procedures in which a sterile needle or a lancet is inserted through the skin. Because the skin is penetrated, drawing blood becomes a surgical procedure and is subject to the laws and regulations of surgery. When performing venipuncture, the rules and regulations must be enforced with no deviations from them.

Be sure to follow the procedures as written and also become familiar with the regulations and standards established by local and state agencies as well as the Clinical Laboratory Improvement Amendment and OSHA regulations. Deviations leave the medical assistant open to accusations of malpractice. Document any situations that arise in which observation of the standard of care comes into question.

On rare occasions, patients who have scarred veins from intravenous drug use may request that they be allowed to draw their own blood. You should never permit this and should always take precautions that your supplies are protected.

Chain of Custody

Blood samples may be collected as evidence in legal proceedings. Blood may be drawn for drug and alcohol testing, DNA analysis, or parentage testing. These samples must be handled with special procedures to prevent tampering, misidentification, or interference with the test results.

Chain of custody is a legal term that refers to the ability to guarantee the identity and integrity of the specimen from collection to reporting of the test results. It is a process used to maintain and document the chronological history of a specimen. (Documents should include name or initials of the individual collecting the specimen, each person or entity subsequently having custody of it, the date the specimen was collected or transferred, employer or agency, specimen number, patient's or employee's name, and a brief description of the specimen.)

Collection kits are available and will contain everything needed for the venipuncture, including the tube, the needle, the chain of custody forms and seals, the antiseptic, and even the tourniquet. Familiarize yourself with these kits before you are required to use them. You may be required to testify at a legal proceeding if you are involved in the collection or testing of a sample involved in a legal proceeding.

SUMMARY OF SCENARIO

Leah has learned that phlebotomy is truly an art. Although she was nervous at first, she has become quite proficient with this new skill. She discovered that her nervousness was "contagious" and that if she remained calm and organized, her patient was more likely to feel at ease with the procedure. She has learned that it is necessary to talk with the patients prior to drawing the blood, not only to allay their fears, but also to get clues regarding past problems or the best site for the draw. She has learned that it is her responsibility to explain what tests are being ordered and how much blood she will draw, but that it is not her responsibility to explain why the tests are being done. Effective communication, she has learned, is the most important aspect of phlebotomy.

SUMMARY OF LEARNING OBJECTIVES

- Venipuncture requires the following equipment: a double-pointed needle, evacuated collection tubes, and an adapter, or a syringe fitted with a needle, a tourniquet, an alcohol prep pad, gauze or cotton, a sterile bandage, latex gloves, biohazard disposal container.

- The tourniquet is used to prevent venous flow out of the site, causing the veins to bulge. This makes veins easier to locate and puncture.

- The venipuncture needle has a shaft with one end cut at an angle *(bevel)*. The other end attaches to the syringe or to an adapter and is called the hub. The opening in the tip is called the *lumen* and is measured in gauge numbers. Needles should be disposed of in a sharps container, and the medical assistant should avoid recapping a needle.

- Syringes are more commonly used for blood collection from elderly patients, whose veins tend to be more fragile; from children, whose veins tend to be small; and from obese patients, whose veins tend to be deep. Using a syringe allows a more controlled draw.

- A winged infusion set (butterfly) is used on blood draws from the hand and from children. The needle has a small lumen and is more easily inserted into small veins.

- Whole blood will coagulate unless mixed with an anticoagulant. Many anticoagulants are available; the anticoagulant must be matched with the test so as not to interfere with results. When clotted blood is centrifuged, the cells and liquid separate and the liquid portion is referred to as *serum*. When anticoagulated blood is centrifuged, the liquid that remains is referred to as *plasma*.

- Evacuated tubes should be collected in a specific order to prevent carryover of tube additives.

- A routine venipuncture begins with greeting and identifying the patient. The medical assistant then assembles the equipment, locates the vein, draws the blood, removes and properly disposes of the needle, tends to the puncture site, labels the tubes, and delivers them to the laboratory. The medical assistant observes standard precautions during the procedure.

- Tourniquets are snugly tied around the upper arm (or wrist for a hand draw) in a fashion that permits easy release. Leaving the tourniquet on for a prolonged period results in hemoconcentration.

- Needles are inserted into the vein at a 15- to 30-degree angle. This angle may have to be increased for obese patients. Do not probe excessively if you are unsuccessful because probing can lead to a hematoma or nerve damage. Before the needle is removed, the tourniquet should be released.

Immediately after removal, pressure should be applied to the puncture site with gauze.

■ The median cephalic vein is the vein of choice for phlebotomy, but blood can be drawn from the cephalic vein and the median basilic vein. Avoid the basilic vein if possible.

■ Capillary puncture is preferred over venipuncture for certain tests, such as hematocrit or hemoglobin analysis, and it is also routinely performed on children under the age of 2 years.

■ The middle two fingers (the lateral sides of each) are generally used for capillary puncture; in infants, the heel is the site of choice. The center of the heel must be avoided.

■ Dermal puncture devices are made of sharp sterile metal. Some are designed to make a cut of a specified depth, and all should have internal safety devices that retract the blade after use.

■ Capillary blood can be collected in microtainer devices, capillary pipets, or on filter paper test cards.

■ Capillary puncture is performed much like venipuncture. No tourniquet is used, however. The first drop of blood is routinely wiped away after the puncture because it is contaminated with tissue fluid.

KEY INTERNET WEBSITES

- Center for Phlebotomy Education
- National Institute for Occupational Safety and Health
- OSHA Publications Office
- Phlebotomy West: International Phlebotomy Newsletter
  For active weblinks to each website visit
  http://evolve.elsevier.com/Kinn/

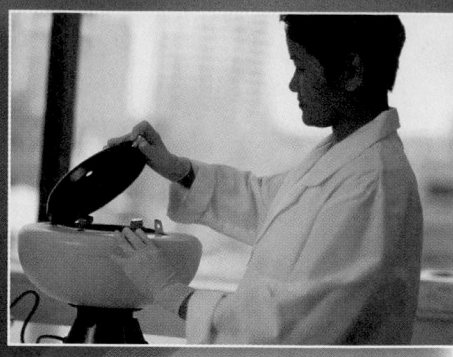

CHAPTER 51

Scenario

Dana Cummings is a certified medical assistant who works as a phlebotomist in the Westhills Family Practice Center. She is preparing to collect blood from Mr. Corrigan, who has had a renal transplant as a result of complications from type 1 diabetes; he is here today for a routine examination. Dr. Fischbach suspects that Mr. Corrigan is anemic and orders an anemia panel in addition to the usual blood work, which consists of a renal panel, hemoglobin A1C level, complete blood count (CBC), and protime.

Assisting in the Analysis of Blood

Robin R. Patterson

Learning Objectives

- Define and spell the terms listed in the vocabulary.
- Name three main functions of blood.
- Describe the role of the hematology laboratory in patient care.
- Describe the appearance and function of the erythrocyte.
- Describe the appearance and function of the granular and the agranular leukocyte.
- Differentiate between T cells and B cells.
- Describe the appearance and function of the thrombocyte.
- Explain the process of clot formation.
- Identify the anticoagulant of choice for hematology testing.
- Explain the purpose of a microhematocrit.
- Explain the role of hemoglobin in the body.
- Identify the tests included in a CBC.
- Explain the use of the hemocytometer.
- Describe the difference between a manual white blood cell count (WBC) and a manual red blood cell count (RBC).
- Describe the difference between a manual blood cell count and an automated blood cell count.
- Calculate RBC indices.
- Explain the reasoning behind performing a differential.
- Describe the appearance of the five different types of leukocytes seen in a normal differential.
- Describe the appearance of the normal erythrocyte.
- Cite the reasons for performing an erythrocyte sedimentation rate test.
- Describe the tests performed to assess coagulation.
- Describe the three means for assessing antigen or antibody presence in a patient's serum that are used in clinical immunology (serology).
- Identify the signs and symptoms of infectious mononucleosis.
- Explain the principle of the heterophile antibody test for infectious mononucleosis.
- Differentiate between the ABO blood groupings and the Rh blood grouping.
- Explain the reasons for testing blood glucose, blood cholesterol, and hemoglobin A1C.
- List five typical chemistry panels, the reason for performing each panel, and the individual tests performed in those panels.
- Explain the reasons for toxicology testing in the clinical laboratory.
- Accurately perform a microhematocrit.

Continued

Learning Objectives—cont'd

- Determine the level of hemoglobin present in a given blood sample.
- Fill a Unopette capillary pipette and transfer to a Unopette reservoir, correctly completing each step in proper order.
- Fill a hemacytometer chamber and correctly complete each step of the procedure in the proper sequence.
- Using a filled hemacytometer, count and calculate a manual WBC or RBC.
- Prepare and stain a blood smear using Wright's stain, completing each step in proper sequence.
- Observe a differential smear and identify various blood cells from a prepared slide.
- Determine a sedimentation rate.
- Secure a capillary blood sample and determine the ABO and Rh grouping of the sample.
- Perform a glucose test using a U.S. Food and Drug Administration (FDA)-approved glucose monitor.
- Perform a cholesterol test using an FDA-approved cholesterol monitor.
- Perform a test for infectious mononucleosis.

National Curriculum Competencies

CLINICAL COMPETENCIES

3c. Perform hematology testing
3d. Perform chemistry testing

3e. Perform immunology testing
3g. Screen and follow-up test results

Vocabulary

anemia A condition marked by deficiency of RBCs.

artifact A structure or feature not normally present but visible as a result of an external agent or action, such as one seen in a microscopic specimen after fixation, or in an image produced by radiology or electro-cardiography.

centrifuge An apparatus consisting essentially of a compartment spun about a central axis to separate contained materials of different specific gravities or to separate colloidal particles suspended in a liquid.

enzyme Any of several complex proteins that are produced by cells and act as catalysts in specific bio-chemical reactions.

hormone A substance produced by one tissue and conveyed by the bloodstream to another to effect physiological activity, such as growth or metabolism.

in vitro Pertaining to a biological reaction that occurs in an artificial environment, such as in a test tube.

metabolite A substance produced by metabolism.

polycythemia vera A condition marked by an abnormally large number of RBCs in the circulatory system.

sensitivity The ability of a test to detect minute amounts of analyte.

serial dilution A process in which a sample, such as serum, is diluted repeatedly for analysis. Most commonly, twofold or tenfold dilutions are prepared.

specificity The ability of a particular antibody to combine with one antigen instead of another.

toxemia An abnormal condition of pregnancy characterized by hypertension, edema, and protein in the urine.

type and cross match Tests performed to assess the compatibility of blood to be transfused.

urea The major nitrogenous end product of protein metabolism and the chief nitrogenous component of the urine.

urease An enzyme that catalyzes the hydrolysis of urea to form ammonium carbonate.

The average body holds 10 to 12 pints of blood. The heart circulates the blood through the circulatory system more than a thousand times every day. More than 70,000 miles of passageways, most of which are narrower than a human hair, carry blood throughout the body. The blood is contained in a closed system of vessels, of which the largest is the aorta and the smallest are the capillaries. The capillaries are only one cell layer thick, and these thin, permeable walls allow certain substances to move back and forth between the blood vessels and the surrounding tissue. The blood contains more than 25 trillion cells, and every second the body replaces eight million old RBCs with eight million new RBCs.

Besides supplying body cells with their needed nutrients and oxygen, the blood also carries away carbon dioxide and **urea**, which are the waste products of normal cell activity. If the blood did not carry away the carbon dioxide and urea, these wastes would accumulate and cause cell damage and possibly **toxemia**. Carbon dioxide is carried in the blood to the lungs, where it is exhaled as part of normal breathing. The blood carries urea to the kidneys where, along with other body wastes, it is excreted in the urine. The blood also distributes **enzymes**, **hormones**, and other chemicals that the body needs for control and regulation of body activities. In addition, the blood functions to maintain the body at a uniform temperature, to keep other body fluids in a state of pH balance, and to carry the hormones from the secreting gland to the tissues where they are needed.

Blood is the second most common body fluid analyzed in the clinical laboratory. Blood testing is done routinely in the hematology, immunology (serology), immunohematology (blood banking), and chemistry sections of the laboratory. The degree of testing on blood you will perform as a medical assistant will depend on the level of service of the physician's office and the Clinical Laboratories Improvement Act (CLIA) regulations. As a medical assistant, you will not perform all of the procedures described in this chapter. Some have been replaced with automated procedures and others are considered highly complex by the CLIA 88 standards and thus are not to be performed by a medical assistant. Nevertheless, these procedures are explained in this text because they provide critical background information necessary to understand the analysis of blood, from the collection of the specimen, to testing, and to the recording of the results.

Hematology

The hematology section of a laboratory deals with the *counting* of RBCs, WBCs, and platelets; *differentiating* WBCs on stained blood smears; *measuring* the percentage of RBCs in blood (hematocrit); and determining the oxygen-carrying capacity of the blood (hemoglobin).

The *complete blood cell count (CBC)* is the most frequent laboratory procedure ordered on blood. It gives a fairly complete look at the components of blood and can provide a wealth of information concerning a patient's condition. The CBC routinely includes the tests shown in the box that follows.

COMPLETE BLOOD CELL COUNT PROCEDURE

- Red blood cell count
- White blood cell count
- Hemoglobin determination
- Hematocrit determination
- Differential white blood cell count
- Estimation of platelet numbers
- Red cell indices

Whole blood is composed of formed elements suspended in a clear yellow liquid portion called plasma. Plasma makes up about 55% of blood by volume. The remaining 45% consists of formed cellular elements, which are the erythrocytes (RBCs), leukocytes (WBCs), and thrombocytes (platelets). These cellular elements all have special functions.

Erythrocytes

Red blood cells, or erythrocytes, are formed in the red bone marrow of the ribs, sternum, pelvis, and skull, and in the ends of long bones in the adult. The immature form of the RBC has a nucleus that disintegrates as the cell matures. Loss of the nucleus results in the familiar shape of the RBC: the biconcave disk, thicker at the rim than in the middle. Erythrocytes transport oxygen from the lungs to the body cells and carry carbon dioxide away from cells, back to the lungs to be exhaled. The main constituent is the red pigment hemoglobin, which is composed of iron and protein. Hemoglobin actually carries oxygen and some carbon dioxide throughout the body.

The life span of an erythrocyte is about 120 days. As the cell nears the end of its life, it becomes more fragile and eventually ruptures and breaks. The iron is reused for new RBC formation, and the protein is converted into a bile pigment.

Leukocytes

Leukocytes, or white blood cells (WBCs), contain a nucleus and are larger than erythrocytes. The prime function of the leukocyte is to protect the body against infection and disease. The five types of leukocytes are classified into granular and agranular groups. The granular leukocytes are called *polymorphonuclear* leukocytes and include the neutrophils, eosinophils, and basophils. They are characterized by their heavily granulated cytoplasm and segmented nuclei. The *agranular* leukocytes are the lymphocytes and monocytes, both of which have clear cytoplasm and a solid nucleus.

Granular leukocytes are phagocytic and engulf invading bacteria and viruses. Unlike erythrocytes, leukocytes function in the tissues. During inflammation, the blood carries the WBCs through dilated vessels to the site of injury. Capillary walls become more permeable, and granular cells squeeze through by ameboid motion. Once at the site of infection or injury, the cells engulf the invading microorganism. Pus contains dead leukocytes, bacteria, and tissue cells.

Agranular leukocytes are responsible for the production of antibodies. Agranular leukocytes include the lymphocytes, which are classified into T cells and B cells based on their functional characteristics.

T cells. T cells make up about 65% to 80% of circulating lymphocytes and have a life span of months to years. This is important in conferring long-lasting immunity to microbial infections. T cells are responsible for immune responses to intracellular parasites, viruses, fungi, and bacteria. Delayed hypersensitivity reactions, such as the response to poison ivy, are mediated by T-cell defenses, as is organ transplant rejection. There are several types of T cells based on function:

- *Cytotoxic or killer T cells*—kill foreign, virus infected, and tumor cells. They produce proteins called *perforans* that induce cell death by punching holes in the cell membrane.
- *Helper T cells*—most numerous type of T cell. They stimulate the activity of other T cells.
- *Suppressor T cells*—inhibit the activity of other T cells.
- *Memory T cells*—respond quickly to the presentation of the same antigen at a later date. They have a long life span.
- *Natural killer cells*—kill cells infected with viruses and tumor cells without prior sensitization.

B cells. B cells are formed in bone marrow and then migrate to other lymph organs, where they multiply and reside. When stimulated, B cells differentiate into plasma cells that produce specific antibodies against an antigen. Antibodies circulate in the plasma or are present in secretions. Some antibodies cause cells to clump and precipitate, whereas others activate the complement system. The *complement system* is a series of reactions between plasma proteins that amplifies the immunologic response to foreign molecules. Activation of the complement system leads to the lysis of microorganisms or their phagocytosis by neutrophils.

Antibodies are protein molecules that attach to antigens. Very small antigens, such as toxin and viruses, can be directly neutralized by antibodies; larger antigens, such as bacteria, require the help of agranular leukocytes. Destroying these pathogens requires three steps:

1. *Antigen processing:* When a macrophage phagocytizes bacteria, proteins (antigens) from the bacteria are broken down into smaller molecules that are then "displayed" on the macrophage surface attached to special molecules called MHC II (major histocompatibility complex class II). Bacterial peptides are similarly processed and displayed on MHC II molecules on the surface of B lymphocytes.
2. *Lymphocyte stimulation:* When a T lymphocyte "sees" the same peptide on the macrophage and on the B cell, the T cell stimulates the B cell to turn on antibody production.
3. *Antibody production:* The stimulated B cell undergoes repeated cell divisions, enlargement, and differentiation to form a clone of antibody secreting plasma cells. Hence, through specific antigen recognition of the invader, clonal expansion, and B-cell differentiation you acquire an effective number of plasma cells, all secreting the same needed antibody. That antibody then binds to the bacteria, making them easier to ingest by white cells. Antibody combined with a plasma component called *complement* may also kill the bacteria directly.

Thrombocytes

Thrombocytes are not true cells but rather cytoplasmic fragments of a large cell in the bone marrow, the megakaryocyte. They are the smallest formed elements of the blood. The typical shape is discoid, but when they are activated, they become globular and form finger-like cytoplasmic extensions called *pseudopodia*.

Clot Formation. In minor injuries, thrombocytes tend to collect and form plugs in blood vessel openings. To control bleeding from vessels larger than capillaries, a clot must form at the point of injury. The coagulation of the blood is also initiated by blood platelets. The platelets produce a substance that combines with calcium ions in the blood to form *thromboplastin*, which in turn converts the protein *prothrombin* into thrombin in a complex series of reactions. *Thrombin*, an enzyme, converts *fibrinogen*, a protein substance, into *fibrin*, an insoluble protein that forms an intricate network of minute threadlike structures called *fibrils*, and causes the blood plasma to gel. The blood cells and plasma are enmeshed in the network of fibrils to form a *clot*.

Blood clotting can be initiated by the *extrinsic mechanism*, in which substances from damaged tissues are mixed with the blood, or by the *intrinsic mechanism*, in which the blood itself is traumatized. More than 30 substances in blood have been found to affect clotting; whether or not blood will coagulate depends on a balance between those substances that promote coagulation (procoagulants) and those that inhibit it (anticoagulants). The coagulation of blood within blood vessels in the absence of injury can cause serious illness or death, especially when a clot forms in the coronary arteries (thrombosis) or cerebral arteries (stroke).

Hemophilia, a bleeding disorder, occurs when a person has a mutation in one of the clotting factor genes. It is a hereditary, sex-linked disorder that affects males of all races and ethnic groups. The mutated gene is on the X chromosome provided by the mother. About 1 in 4000 males is born with the disorder; it is rare, but possible, for a female to be a hemophiliac. People with hemophilia inject themselves with purified clotting factor to prevent bleeding episodes. Internal bleeding, particularly in the joints, is a problem despite treatment and leads to painful arthritis.

Plasma

Plasma is a highly complex liquid that is the carrier for the formed elements and other substances such as proteins, carbohydrates, fats, hormones, enzymes, mineral salts, gases, and waste products. Plasma is composed of about 90% water, 9% protein, and 1% various other chemical substances. When plasma proteins and other components are used up during the clotting process, the remaining liquid is called *serum*.

Collection of Blood Specimens

For most hematology tests, an adequate blood sample can be obtained from capillaries by finger puncture. If a larger sample is required, blood can be obtained from a vein by venipuncture. To perform a complete blood cell count, venous blood is collected in a tube containing an *anticoagulant* that prevents clotting. Ethylenediamine tetraacetic acid (EDTA) is the anticoagulant of choice for hematology testing. It is important that blood is not hemolyzed during collection for hematology testing.

CRITICAL THINKING APPLICATION

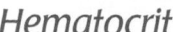

- Dana will collect the specimen for Mr. Corrigan's complete blood cell count (CBC). What tests are included in the CBC? Can any of these tests be performed by capillary puncture? Explain.
- Which vacuum tube will Dana use to collect the CBC?

Hematocrit

The hematocrit is a measurement of the percentage of packed red blood cells in a volume of blood. The test is based on the principle of separating the cellular elements from plasma and is aided by centrifugation (Procedure 51-1). Two or three drops of blood are collected in two capillary tubes and are placed in a specially designed microhematocrit **centrifuge** (Figure 51-1).

After centrifugation, RBCs will be at the bottom of the tube, WBCs and platelets in the center, and plasma on top (Figure 51-2). From this separation, the micro-

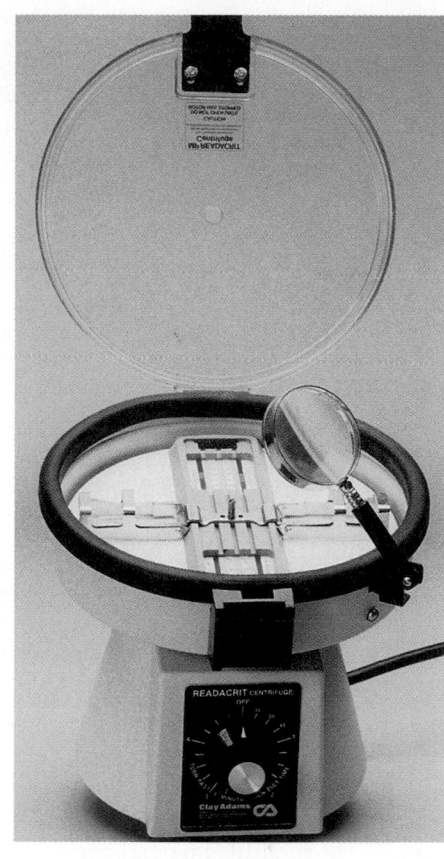

FIGURE 51-1   Centrifuge with capillary tube placement indications.

hematocrit is determined by comparing the concentration of RBCs with the total volume of the whole blood sample. The percentage is read by placing the tubes on a special microhematocrit reader. Some microhematocrit centrifuges have a built-in reading scale that reads

PROCEDURE 51-1

Performing a Microhematocrit

GOAL: To perform a microhematocrit accurately.

EQUIPMENT AND SUPPLIES

- EDTA anticoagulant blood
- Capillary tubes
- Sealing clay
- Centrifuge

PROCEDURAL STEPS

1 Wash and dry your hands. Put on face protection and nonsterile gloves.
  Purpose: Infection control.

2 Assemble the materials needed.

3 Fill two plain (blue-tipped) capillary tubes three-fourths full with well-mixed EDTA anticoagulant blood.
  Purpose: Duplicates should always be done as a means of quality control.

4 Plug the dry end of each tube with a sealing clay.
  Purpose: Sealing the wet end may result in loss of the plug and the sample during centrifugation.

5 Place the tubes opposite each other in the centrifuge, with sealed ends securely against the gasket. Note the tube arrangement in Figure 51-1.

Continued

PROCEDURE 51-1—cont'd

Purpose: The centrifuge must always be balanced to avoid damage. If the clay ends of the capillary tubes are not outermost against the gasket, the sample will spin out of the tubes.

6 Note the numbers on the centrifuge slots and record them.

Purpose: The sample must be identified throughout the entire procedure.

7 Secure the locking top, fasten the lid down, and lock.

Purpose: If the locking top is not firmly in place during the spinning cycle, the tubes will come out of their slots and break. The lid is always locked during centrifugation for safety purposes, that is, to avoid aerosols or broken glass from being ejected.

8 Set the timer, and adjust the speed as needed.

Purpose: The prescribed time is between 3 and 5 minutes. Check the manufacturer's instructions for time and speed.

9 Allow the centrifuge to come to a complete stop. Unlock the lids.

10 Remove the tubes immediately.

Purpose: Tubes left in the centrifuge will show altered results, as the RBC layer spreads horizontally.

11 Determine the microhematocrit values using one of the following methods:

a. Centrifuge with built-in reader using calibrated capillary tubes.
   1) Position the tubes as directed by manufacturer's instructions.
   2) Read both tubes.
   3) The average of the two results is reported.
   4) The two values should not vary by more than 2%.
b. Centrifuge without built-in reader.
   1) Carefully remove the tubes from the centrifuge.
   2) Place a tube on the microhematocrit reader.
   3) Align the clay–RBC junction with the zero line on the reader. Align the plasma meniscus with

the 100% line. The value is read at the junction of the red cell layer and the buffy coat (Figure 1*).
4) Read both tubes.
5) The average of the two results is reported.
6) The two values should not vary by more than 2%.

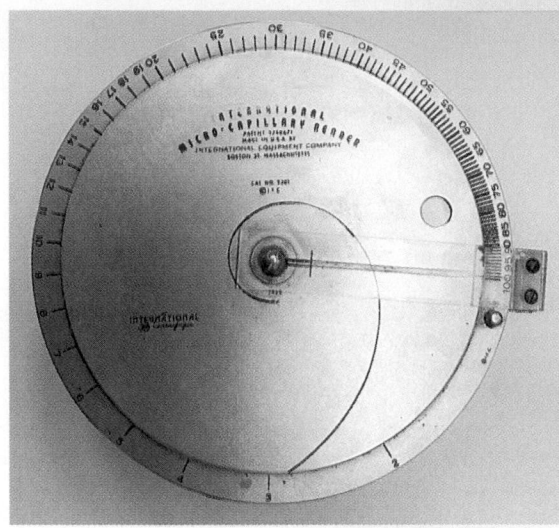

Figure 1

12 Dispose of the capillary tubes in a biohazard container.

13 Clean the work area, and properly dispose of all biohazard materials. Remove gloves and face protection, and wash your hands.

14 Record the results in the patient's medical record.

Purpose: A procedure is not considered done until it is charted.

See Appendix E for a charting example.
*Figure from Stepp CA, Woods MA: *Laboratory procedures for medical office personnel*. Philadelphia, 1998, WB Saunders.

calibrated capillary tubes. Microhematocrits should be performed in duplicate and the average of the two results reported.

The normal values vary with the gender and age of the patient (Table 51-1). The values range from a low of 36% in women to a high of 52% in men. Low microhematocrit readings can indicate **anemia** or the presence of bleeding in a patient; high readings may be caused by dehydration or a condition such as **polycythemia vera**. Values can be influenced by physiologic or pathologic factors, as well as by collection techniques.

The *microhematocrit* is a commonly performed test requested by physicians separately or as part of the CBC. Because it is a simple procedure requiring only a

TABLE 51-1	Hematocrit Reference Values	
Age/Gender		**Hct Value (%)**
Neonate		44-64
Infant		
1 mo of age		35-49
6 mo of age		30-40
Child, 1-10 yr of age		35-41
Adult		
Men		42-52
Women		36-45

Hct, Hematocrit.
From Stepp CA, Woods MA: *Laboratory procedures for medical office personnel*. Philadelphia, 1998, WB Saunders.

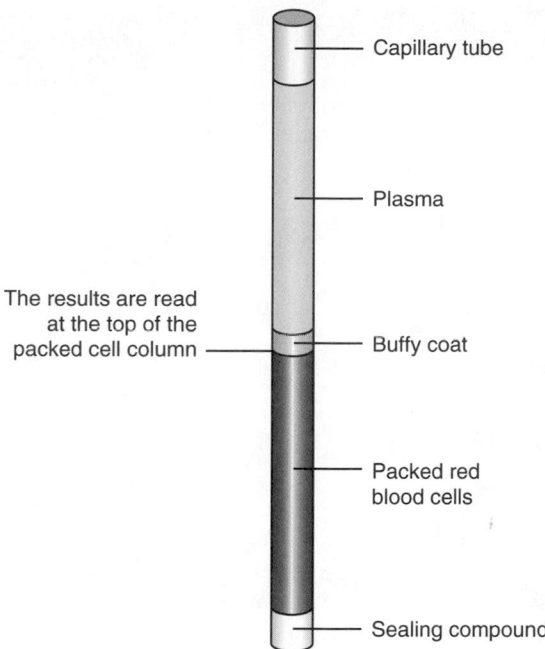

FIGURE 51-2   Hematocrit test results. Cellular elements are separated from plasma by centrifuging an anticoagulated blood specimen, and the results are read at the top of the packed cell column. (From Bonewit-West K: *Clinical procedures for medical assistants*, ed 5. Philadelphia, 2000, WB Saunders, p 623.)

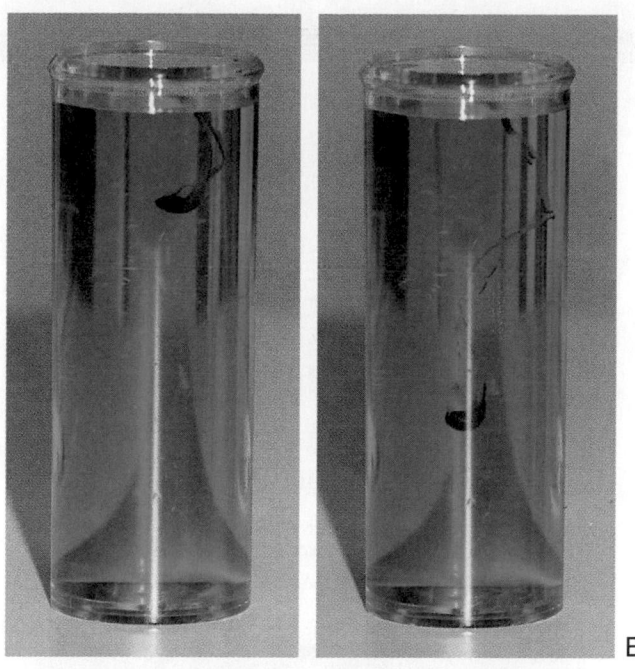

FIGURE 51-3   Copper sulfate specific gravity method for determining hemoglobin values. **A**, A drop of the patient's blood is placed in copper sulfate. The rate and distance it drops determine the level of hemoglobin present. **B**, The level indicates that this patient's hemoglobin is within reference range. (From Stepp CA, Woods MA: *Laboratory procedures for medical office personnel*, Philadelphia, 1998, WB Saunders, p 160.)

small amount of blood, it is an ideal screening test and is often part of a routine physical examination.

Hemoglobin

The hemoglobin determination is a rough measure of the oxygen-carrying capacity of blood. Determining hemoglobin concentration can be performed as part of the CBC or as an individual test. Many methods of determining hemoglobin concentration have been used over the years. The earliest measures simply involved comparing the color of a drop of blood to a chart. Blood that is dark red has more hemoglobin than pale red blood.

The copper sulfate method is another manual method for hemoglobin determination that is often used to screen blood donors. It is based on the principle of specific gravity; when a drop of blood from a patient with normal hemoglobin values is dropped into a copper sulfate solution, it falls rapidly to the bottom (Figure 51-3). If the drop falls slowly or not at all, hemoglobin levels are below reference range.

A *hemoglobinometer* is a device that determines hemoglobin amount either by direct colorimetry or by conversion to another compound (Procedure 51-2). One widely used hemoglobin measurement method is for *cyanmethemoglobin*. A sample of whole blood is diluted

PROCEDURE 51-2

Performing a Hemoglobin Test

GOAL: To determine accurately the level of hemoglobin present in a blood sample using the hemoglobinometer method.

EQUIPMENT AND SUPPLIES

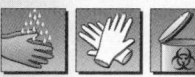

- Hemoglobinometer
- Reagent applicators
- Autolet or blood lancet
- Alcohol preps
- Gauze squares

PROCEDURAL STEPS

1 Wash and dry hands.
   Purpose: Infection control.

2 Collect and assemble all equipment and supplies needed.

Continued

PROCEDURE **51-2—cont'd**

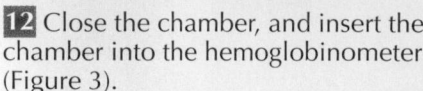

3 Explain the procedure to the patient.

4 Put on gloves.

5 Prepare the clipped chamber by slightly offsetting the cover slide to expose the chamber slide surface.

6 Examine the fingers and choose the site to be used to obtain the blood sample.
Purpose: The site to be used must be free of trauma, calluses, and scarring.

7 Clean the site with alcohol or other recommended antiseptic preparation.

8 Perform a capillary puncture and obtain the blood sample.

9 Wipe away the first drop of blood (Figure 1).
Purpose: This drop may contain tissue fluid.

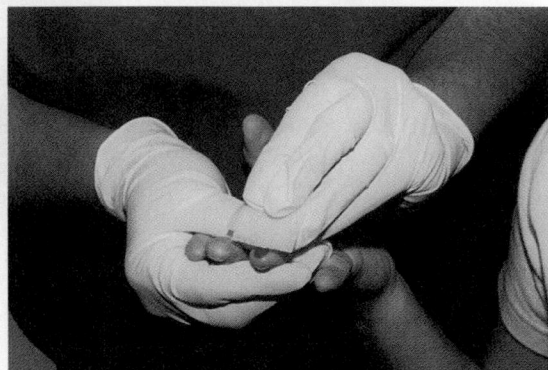

Figure 1

10 Place one large drop of blood on the chamber slide. Do not touch the slide with the finger (Figure 2).
Purpose: Contact of the slide with the skin may alter your results.

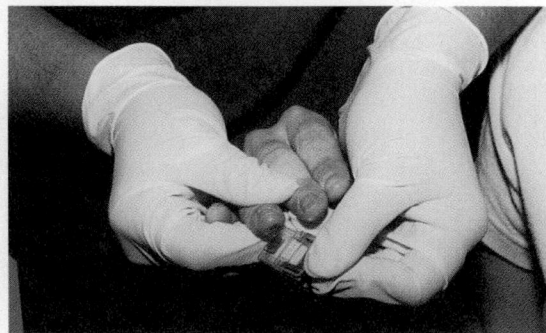

Figure 2

11 Agitate the blood with a reagent stick until the blood appears shiny or transparent. This takes about 45 seconds.
Purpose: To ensure action of anticoagulation.

12 Close the chamber, and insert the chamber into the hemoglobinometer (Figure 3).

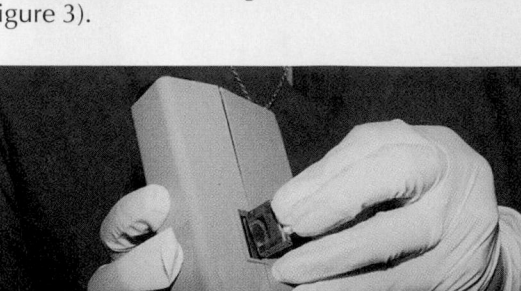

Figure 3

13 Hold the device horizontally at eye level, and turn on the light at the base of the unit with the left hand (Figure 4).

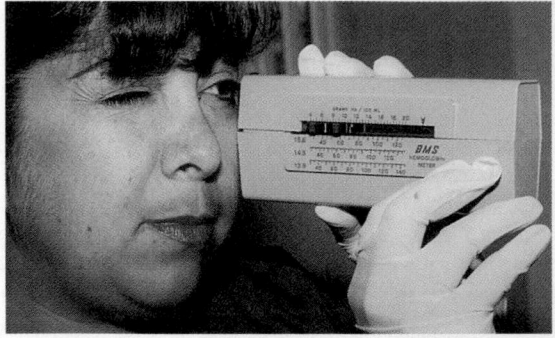

Figure 4

14 Visualize the split green field through the viewer, and with the right hand move the slide adjustment until there is no visible difference between the two hemispheres in the viewer.

15 Read the scale on the right side of the instrument. Your reading will be in grams of hemoglobin per 100 ml of blood.

16 Dispose of the biohazard waste in correct containers, and properly clean the hemoglobinometer chamber and work area. Return equipment to proper storage location.

17 Remove gloves and wash hands.
Purpose: Infection control.

18 Record the test results in the patient's medical record.
Purpose: A procedure is considered not done until it is recorded.

See Appendix E for a charting example.

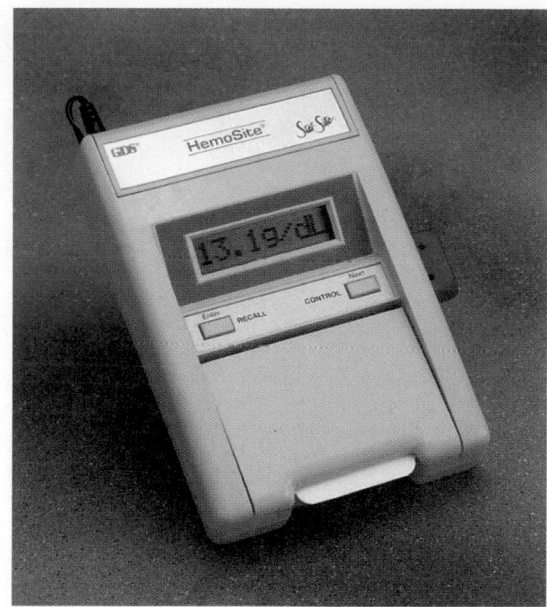

FIGURE 51-4 Hand-held instruments such as the Stat-Site system can analyze hemoglobin quickly and accurately. (Courtesy GDS Technology, Inc, Elkhart, IN.)

TABLE 51-2	Hemoglobin (Hgb) Reference Values
Age/Gender	Hgb Level (g/dl)
Neonate	17-23
Infant (2 mo of age)	9-14
Adult female	12-16
Adult male	15-18

From Stepp CA, Woods MA: *Laboratory procedures for medical office personnel*. Philadelphia, 1998, WB Saunders.

Red Blood Cell Count

The RBC count is a commonly performed procedure and is part of the CBC (Table 51-3). It approximates the number of circulating RBCs. The function of RBCs is to transport oxygen to tissues. The condition where the oxygen-carrying capacity of blood is below normal is called *anemia*. The RBC count is often decreased in anemia. Increases are found in people with dehydration, polycythemia vera, or severe burns and in people who live at high altitudes, as an adaptation to the lower oxygen content of the air.

Normal RBC values range from four million to six million cells/mm³. RBCs are usually higher in males than in females.

in *Drabkin reagent*, which breaks down (lyses) red cells, releasing the hemoglobin into the solution. The chemicals in the reagent react with the released hemoglobin to form the pigment cyanmethemoglobin, which can be measured by using a hemoglobinometer. Other CLIA-approved methods include the STAT-Site M Hgb, a completely portable, battery-operated, hemoglobin analyzer that fits in the palm of the hand (Figure 51-4). Because of the accuracy and noninterpretive nature of newer instruments, the method illustrated on the previous page is quickly being replaced.

Normal hemoglobin values vary throughout life. Values are normally quite high at birth, decline during childhood, and then increase through the teens until adult levels are reached (Table 51-2). Values range from a low of 12.5 g/dl in women to a high of 17.5 g/dl in men. The various factors that affect the hemoglobin level include age, gender, diet, altitude, and disease.

Hemoglobin and hematocrit are often performed together and are referred to as an "H&H." A quick mental calculation should always be done before reporting out H&H results; hemoglobin value × 3 ± 3 should equal the hematocrit value. For example, if the hemoglobin is 15 g/dl, the hematocrit should be between 42% and 48%.

White Blood Cell Count

The WBC count gives an approximation of the total number of leukocytes in circulating blood. The count is performed to aid the physician in determining whether an infection is present or to aid in the diagnosis of leukemia. It may also be used to follow the course of a disease and to determine if the patient is responding to treatment.

The normal WBC varies with age. It is higher in newborns and decreases throughout life. The average adult range is between 4500 and 12,000 cells/mm³. Many factors affect the WBC count. Elevation in WBCs is called *leukocytosis*.

Physiologic increases in the WBC are seen in pregnancy, stress, anesthesia, exercise, exposure to temperature extremes, and after treatment with corticosteroids. Pathologic causes of leukocytosis include many bacterial infections, leukemia, appendicitis, and pneumonia. A decrease in the WBC is called *leukopenia*. This condition may be caused by viral infections or by exposure to radiation, certain chemicals, and drugs.

Methods of Counting Red and White Blood Cells

Manual Counts. Both the RBC and the WBC counts approximate the number of these circulating cells in the blood. These cellular elements are very concentrated; therefore, blood must be diluted for these cells to be counted microscopically. Blood-diluting pipettes and diluting fluids are used for this purpose. Counts are then performed using the diluted blood, a counting chamber called a *hemacytometer*, a hemacytometer coverslip, and a

---

CRITICAL THINKING APPLICATION

Mr. Corrigan's hematocrit value is 37%. What does Dana calculate as the hemoglobin value? Does this test confirm the doctor's suspicions of anemia?

TABLE 51-3	Reference Ranges for a Complete Blood Count				
				Adults	
Test	Neonates	Infants (6 mo)	Children	Men	Women
RBCs	4.8-7.1 million/ mm³	3.8-5.5 million/ mm³	4.5-4.8 million/ mm³	4.5-6.0 million/ mm³	4.0-5.5 million/ mm³
Hematocrit (Hct)	44-64%	30-40%	35-41%	42-52%	36-45%
Hemoglobin (Hgb)	17-21 g/dl	10-15 g/dl	11-16 g/dl	15-18 g/dl	12-16 g/dl
RBC Indices					
MCV	96-108 mm			82-98 mm	
MCH	32-34 pg			26-34 pg	
MCHC	31-33 g/dL			31-37 g/dl	
WBCs	9000-30,000/mm³	6000-16,000/m³	5000-13,000/mm³	4000-11,000/mm³	
Differential WBC count					
Neutrophils	≥ 45% by 1 wk of age	32%	60% for children 2 yr of age and older	50-65%	
Bands	—	—	—	0-7%	
Eosinophils	—	—	0-3%	1-3%	
Basophils	—	—	1-3%	0-1%	
Monocytes	—	—	4-9%	3-9%	
Lymphocytes	≥ 41% by 1 wk of age	61%	59% for children 2 yr of age or older	25-40%	
Platelets	140,000-300,000/ mm³	200,000-473,000/ mm³	150,000-450,000/ mm³	150,000-400,000/mm³	

RBC, Red blood cell; *MCV,* mean corpuscular volume; *MCH,* mean corpuscular hemoglobin; *MCHC,* mean corpuscular hemoglobin concentration; *WBC,* white blood cell.
From Stepp CA, Woods MA: *Laboratory procedures for medical office personnel.* Philadelphia, 1998, WB Saunders.

microscope. It should be noted that a medical assistant would not perform a manual blood count, and manual tests have been replaced by automated methods.

Unopettes. Unopettes are prefilled reservoirs containing a premeasured diluting-fluid unit (Procedure 51-3). This unit comes equipped with a capillary pipette and pipette shield. Unopettes are available for counting erythrocytes, leukocytes, and platelets (Figure 51-5).

Package inserts contain detailed instructions that, when correctly followed, result in a more accurate dilution than with blood-diluting pipettes. Procedure 51-3 describes this moderately complex test.

Hemacytometer. The hemacytometer is used to count the cellular elements of blood. It is a heavy glass slide that, when viewed from the top, has two raised platforms surrounded by depressions on three sides.

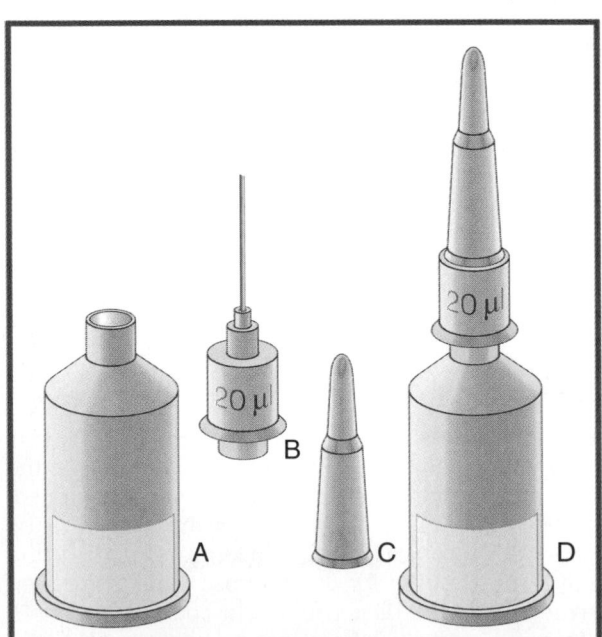

FIGURE 51-5 Components of a disposable blood-diluting unit, such as the Unopette system. **A**, A prefilled reservoir, containing premeasured diluting fluid, is sealed with a diaphragm. **B**, A capillary pipette with overflow chamber and capacity marking. **C**, A pipette shield. **D**, Assembled unit. (From Stepp CA, Woods MA: *Laboratory procedures for medical office personnel,* Philadelphia, 1998, WB Saunders, p 141.)

PROCEDURE 51-3

Filling a Unopette

GOAL: To fill a Unopette pipette with blood properly and to transfer the sample to a Unopette reservoir.

EQUIPMENT AND SUPPLIES

- Unopette unit: capillary pipette, pipette shield, reservoir
- EDTA anticoagulant blood
- Gauze squares
- Test tube rack

PROCEDURAL STEPS

1 Wash and dry your hands, and put on face protection and nonsterile gloves.
Purpose: Infection control.

2 Remove a Unopette reservoir from the storage container, and recap the container tightly.
Purpose: The container is humidified. Loss of the humid conditions will allow evaporation, and the remaining Unopettes will give inaccurate results.

3 Use the pipette shield to puncture the diaphragm of the Unopette reservoir. The hole must be large enough to allow the pipette to enter freely.
Purpose: If the hole is too small, loss of a portion of the sample can occur when the pipette is inserted into the reservoir (Figure 1*).

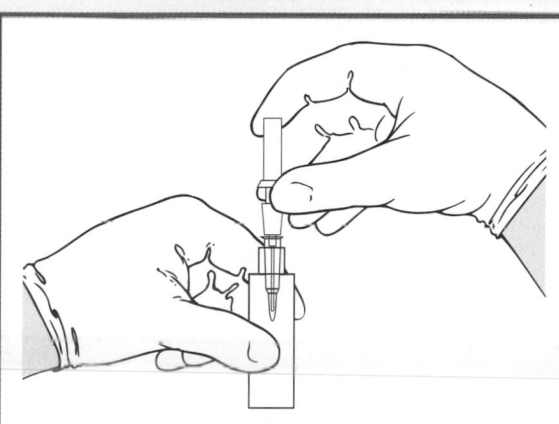

Figure 1

4 Remove the pipette shield.

5 Hold the pipette nearly horizontal.

6 Place the tip of the pipette into a well-mixed tube of blood, and allow the pipette to fill by capillary action until blood reaches the end of the pipette. It will stop by itself (Figure 2).

7 Place a finger over the hole in the end of the pipette to prevent loss of any sample, and carefully wipe the outside of the pipette with gauze to remove all traces of blood (Figure 3).
Purpose: Blood on the outside of the pipette will enter the reservoir and give inaccurate results.

8 Squeeze the reservoir with one hand.

9 While holding your index finger over the hole in the top of the pipette, insert the pipette into the reservoir and seat it firmly in place with a twisting motion.
Purpose: Squeezing the reservoir before inserting the pipette is necessary. It creates a vacuum, which will draw the sample into the reservoir:

10 Release the pressure on the reservoir, and remove your finger from the top of the pipette. The sample will be drawn into the reservoir.

11 Gently squeeze and release the reservoir several times to rinse all blood from the pipette into the reservoir. Liquid should rise to the overflow chamber but should not be forced out of the top of the pipette.

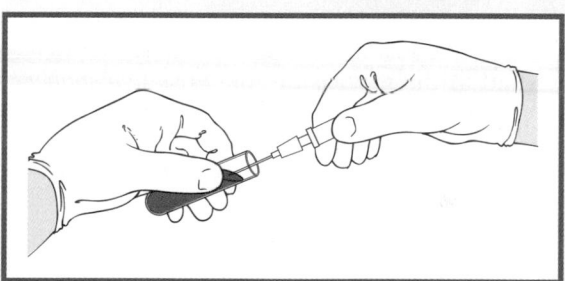

Figure 2

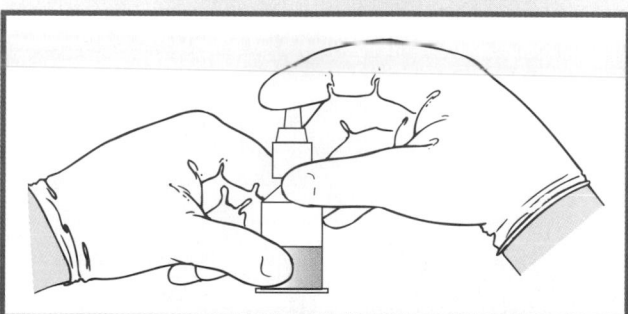

Figure 3

---

*Figure from Stepp CA, Woods MA: *Laboratory procedures for medical office personnel*. Philadelphia, 1998, WB Saunders.

Continued

PROCEDURE 51-3—cont'd

Purpose: The capillary pipette is calibrated to contain an amount of blood. It must be rinsed several times with the diluting fluid to ensure that all the sample has been delivered into the reservoir.

12 Mix the contents of the Unopette gently by inversion or by rolling between the palms of your hands (Figure 4).

13 Identify the Unopette.

Purpose: The sample must be identifiable at all times during the testing procedure.

14 Allow the Unopette to sit for the specified amount of time as stated in the directions.

15 Place the shield on the top of the prepared Unopette to prevent evaporation.

16 Clean the work area by properly disposing of all biohazard materials. Remove the face protection and gloves and wash your hands.

Purpose: Infection control.

17 Record the test results in the patient's medical record.

Purpose: A procedure is considered not done until it is recorded.

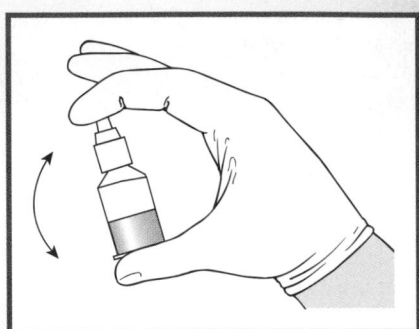

Figure 4

Each raised surface contains a ruled counting area that is marked off by lines etched in the glass. The depressions surrounding these platforms are called *moats*. The raised areas and depressions form an H shape. A special hemacytometer coverslip of uniform thickness is used. The coverslip is positioned on the hemacytometer so that it covers the ruled areas, confines the fluid in the chamber, and regulates the depth of the fluid. The depth of the fluid in the most commonly used *Neubauer-type* hemacytometer is 0.1 mm with the coverslip in place (Figure 51-6).

Each ruled area of the counting chamber consists of a large 3-mm² square. This area, in turn, is divided into nine equal squares, each of which is 1 mm². The WBC

counting area consists of the four large corner squares labeled "W" (Figure 51-7).

The center squares are used to count the RBCs. Each center square is subdivided into 25 smaller squares. Only the four corner and center squares within the large center square are used to count RBCs (see Figure 51-7).

After the coverslip has been positioned, the hemacytometer is filled, or *charged* (Procedure 51-4). This is accomplished by touching the tip of the diluting pipette or Unopette to the point where the coverslip and the raised platform meet (Figure 51-8). The fluid will flow by capillary action into one side of the hemacytometer. The opposite side is also filled.

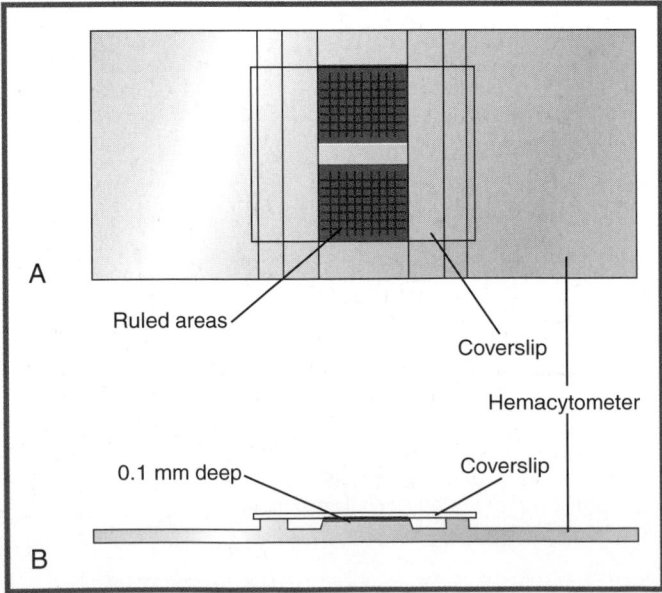

A
Ruled areas
Coverslip
Hemacytometer
0.1 mm deep
Coverslip
B

FIGURE 51-6 Hemacytometer: top (**A**) and side (**B**) views. The blood sample should fill the shaded areas when the chamber is properly filled.

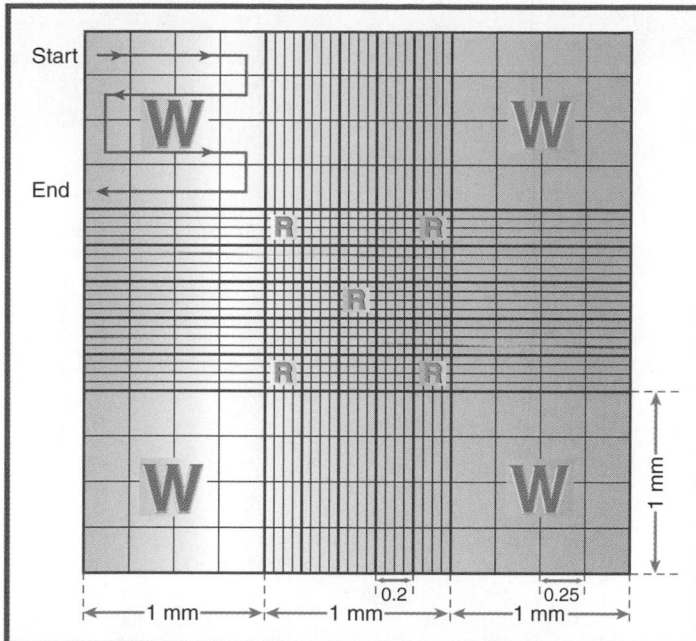

FIGURE 51-7 Arrangement of counting squares. (From Stepp CA, Woods MA: *Laboratory procedures for medical office personnel*, Philadelphia, 1998, WB Saunders, p 141.)

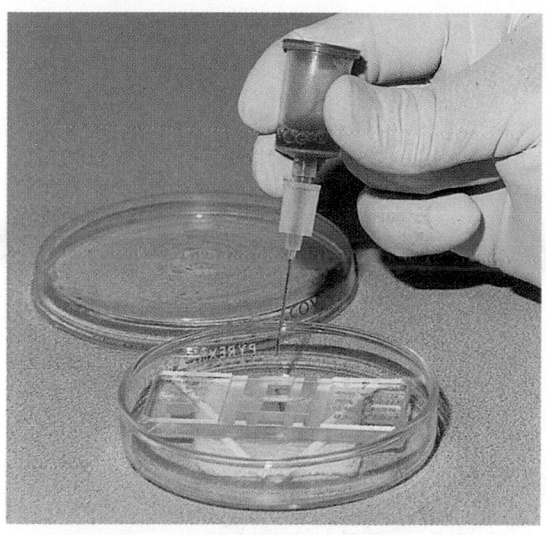

FIGURE 51-8 Charging a counting chamber using a Unopette system. (From Stepp CA, Woods MA: *Laboratory procedures for medical office personnel*, Philadelphia, 1998, WB Saunders, p 142.)

PROCEDURE 51-4

Charging (Filling) a Hemacytometer

GOAL: To fill the hemacytometer for a manual cell count.

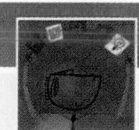

EQUIPMENT AND SUPPLIES

- Neubauer ruled hemacytometer
- Hemacytometer coverslip
- Lint-free tissue
- 70% alcohol
- Blood-diluting pipette or Unopette

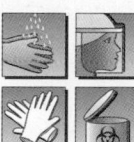

Continued

PROCEDURE 51-4—cont'd

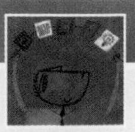

PROCEDURAL STEPS

1 Wash and dry your hands. Put on face protection and nonsterile gloves.
Purpose: Infection control.

2 Clean the hemacytometer and coverslip with 70% alcohol and lint-free tissue, and thoroughly dry.
Purpose: Dirt, fingerprints, grease, or lint interferes with filling and counting.

3 Align the coverslip on the chamber.

4 Convert to dropper assembly by withdrawing the pipette from the reservoir and reseating it securely in reverse position (Figure 1*).

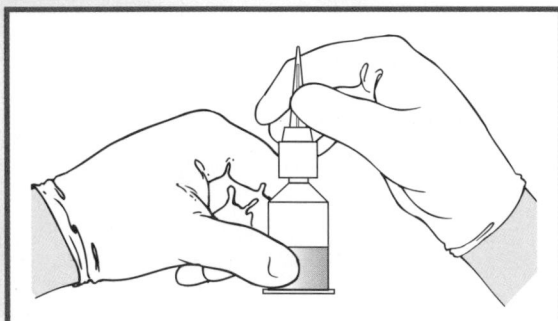

Figure 1

5 To clean the capillary bore, invert the reservoir and gently squeeze the sides, expelling two drops from the well-mixed pipette or Unopette.
Purpose: Diluent in the calibrated stem contains no cells and must be discarded before filling the chamber of the hemacytometer.

6 Touch the tip of the pipette to the edge of the coverslip in the loading area of the chamber (Figure 2).

7 Controlling the flow with the finger on the pipette or by gentle squeezing of the Unopette, fill the chamber in one smooth motion.
Purpose: Chamber fills by capillary action. If the

pipette is not touching the edge of the coverslip, the chamber will not fill properly.

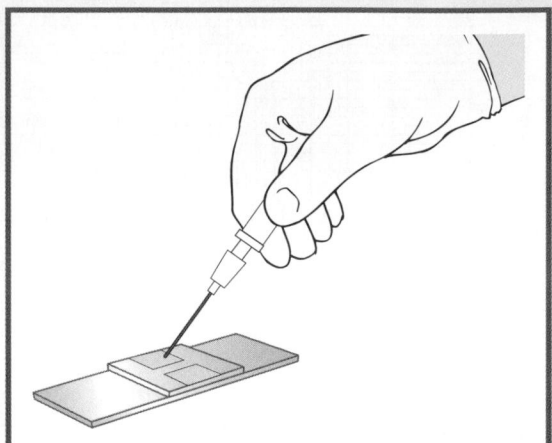

Figure 2

8 Stop filling when the ruled area is full, and do not overfill.

9 Fill both sides of the hemacytometer.

10 Allow the chamber to sit undisturbed for 1 or 2 minutes so that the cells settle, but do not allow the sample to dry.
Purpose: Once the cells have settled in the chamber, the counting procedure is easier. Drying contracts the sample and elevates the count.

11 Clean the work area by properly disposing of all biohazard materials.
Purpose: Infection control.

12 Record the testing results in the patient's record.
Purpose: A procedure is not considered done until it is recorded.

---

*Figure from Stepp CA, Woods MA: *Laboratory procedures for medical office personnel.* Philadelphia, 1998, WB Saunders.

Counting. The hemacytometer is placed on the microscope. WBCs are observed under the ×10 objective, and RBCs are counted under the ×40 objective. A counting pattern of left to right and right to left is used to ensure that cells are counted only once. Counts should begin in the upper left corner square. All cells within the squares are counted. Only cells touching top and left boundary lines are counted (Figure 51-9).

Calculations. Calculations for an RBC are determined by counting both sides of the hemacytometer and obtaining an average. This number is then multiplied by 10,000. For WBCs, the average of the two sides is multiplied by 50.

Automation. Blood cell counts may be performed manually in the physician's office or by an automated counter. Current availability of many different types of instruments has made it possible for the physician's office to become fully automated. Modern instruments range from relatively simple, inexpensive counters to the very complex and expensive instruments. The automated cell counter provides accurate results and does not require a medical technologist to operate it.

Most automated cell counters operate by first diluting the cells in a fluid that conducts an electrical current. Then these diluted cells pass through a special narrow

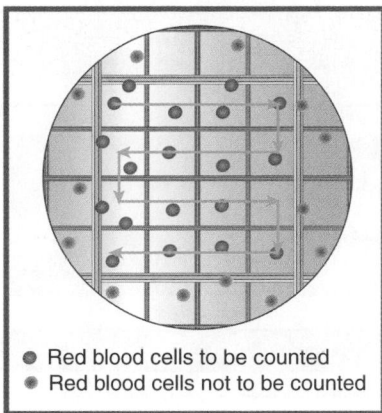

● Red blood cells to be counted
● Red blood cells not to be counted

FIGURE 51-9 Neubauer counting chamber. (From Stepp CA, Woods MA: *Laboratory procedures for medical office personnel,* Philadelphia, 1998, WB Saunders, p 142.)

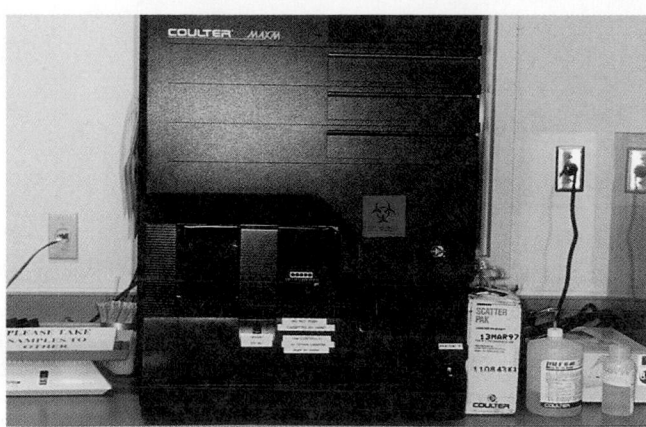

FIGURE 51-10 Automated cell counter. (Courtesy Coulter Corp, Los Angeles, Calif.)

opening in the machine. The passing cells interrupt the flow of current, and each interruption is counted. Some instruments use a laser beam instead of an electric current (Figure 51-10).

Automation improves the accuracy of cell counting and results in greater efficiency. In addition, automation reduces the frequency of handling the individual blood specimen and decreases the risk of exposure to blood-borne pathogens, such as the hepatitis B virus or the human immunodeficiency virus (HIV). It is essential that strict standardization procedures and quality control methods are followed when using automated instruments to perform blood cell counts.

Red Cell Indices

A standard CBC is performed on an automated laboratory instrument that quantitates the amount of hemoglobin as well as the size, shape, and number of RBCs. A variety of calculations are performed to produce indices that provide information about RBC disorders. The standard indices are as follows.

- *Mean Corpuscular Volume (MCV).* MCV is measured directly; the unit is a femtoliter. MCV measures the size of red blood cells and is the most important index for classification of anemias into *macrocytic* with higher than normal MCV and *microcytic* with low MCV.
- *Mean Corpuscular Hemoglobin (MCH) = Hemoglobin ÷ RBC count.* MCH is calculated to give the average mass of hemoglobin in an individual RBC; the unit is a picogram.
- *Mean Corpuscular Hemoglobin Concentration (MCHC) = Hemoglobin ÷ Hematocrit.* MCHC is calculated to provide a measure of the concentration of hemoglobin in the cells.
- *Red Cell Distribution Width (RDW) = standard deviation of MCV.* RDW is calculated to provide a measure of the anisocytosis, or variation in size of the RBCs.

Differential Cell Count

Preparation of Blood Smears

A blood smear enables you to view the cellular components of blood in as natural a state as possible. The morphology of leukocytes, erythrocytes, and platelets can be studied. Their size, shape, and maturity can be evaluated. Examining a blood smear is part of a CBC.

A blood smear is prepared by spreading a drop of blood on a clean glass slide. The slides must be free of dust and grease. The best specimen for a blood smear is capillary blood that has no anticoagulant added. EDTA-anticoagulated blood can be used, provided the smear is made within 2 hours of collection.

There are three kinds of blood smears including the coverglass smear, the spun smear, and the wedge smear. The coverglass smear is often used for bone marrow aspirations and involves placing a drop of blood between two coverslips and pulling them quickly apart. The spun smear uses a centrifuge to distribute the blood on a slide and often has the advantage of being a closed system in that the blood tube is punctured by the instrument and does not have to be handled by the technician. The wedge smear involves placing a small drop of blood one-half inch from the right end of a glass slide. The end of a second glass spreader slide is placed in front of the drop of blood at an angle of 30 to 35 degrees. The spreader slide is brought back into the drop until the blood spreads along the edge of the spreader slide. This is done with a quick but smooth gliding motion. The spreader slide is then pushed to the left with a quick, steady motion, spreading the blood across the slide.

A good smear should cover one-half to three-fourths of the slide. It should show a gradual transition from a thick to a thin end with a feathered edge. It should have a smooth appearance with no ridges, holes, lines, streaks, or clumps (Figure 51-11). The cells should be distributed evenly on microscopic examination.

After the smear has been made, it should be allowed to dry. The slide should be propped up to dry with the thick end down. Do not blow on the slide to dry it. This

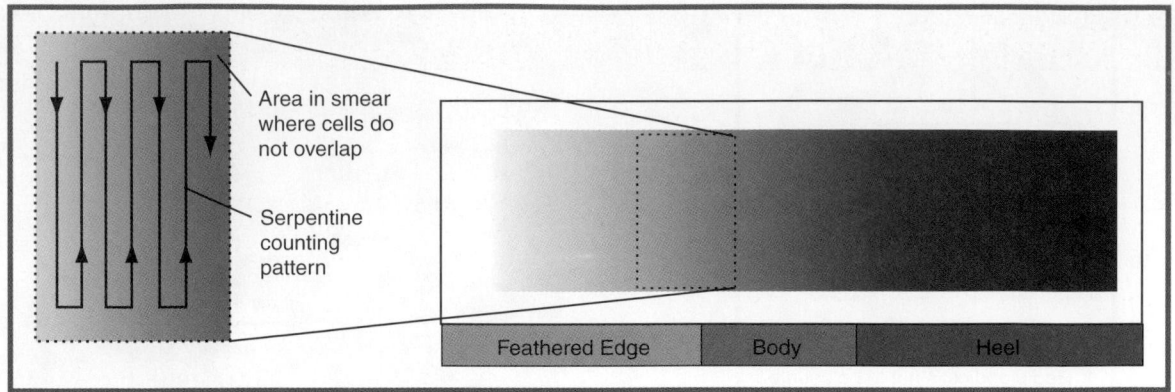

FIGURE 51-11   Serpentine (winding) pattern used to count cells. (From Stepp CA, Woods MA: *Laboratory procedures for medical office personnel*, Philadelphia, 1998, WB Saunders, p 142.)

can cause **artifacts** in the RBCs from the moisture in your breath.

Once dry, the slide is labeled in the thick portion of the smear by writing the patient's name in the dried blood film. If slides with frosted ends are used, the label can be written on the frosted end with pencil or marker.

After labeling, the slide is fixed in *methanol*, a fixative that preserves and prevents changes or deterioration of the cellular components. Many of the quick stains available on the market contain the fixative in the stain.

Staining of Blood Smears

Stains commonly used for examination of blood cells are called *polychromatic* because they contain dyes that will stain various cell components different colors. These stains usually contain *methylene blue*, a blue stain, and eosin, a red-orange stain. These stains are attracted to different parts of the cell. Thus the cells and their structures are more easily visualized and differentiated. The most commonly used differential blood stain is *Wright's stain* (Procedure 51-5).

Wright's stain is applied to the slide for 1 to 3 minutes. A buffer is added on top of the stain, and it is mixed by gentle blowing until a green metallic sheen appears. This usually takes 2 to 4 minutes. The slide is then gently rinsed and allowed to air dry. A properly stained smear should appear pinkish to the naked eye.

PROCEDURE 51-5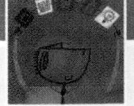

Preparing a Smear Stained With Wright's Stain

GOAL: To prepare and stain a slide that meets the criteria for the performance of a differential examination.

EQUIPMENT AND SUPPLIES

- Clean glass slides
- Transfer pipette or capillary tube
- Wright's stain materials
- EDTA anticoagulant blood specimen

PROCEDURAL STEPS

1 Wash and dry your hands. Put on face protection and nonsterile gloves.
   Purpose: Infection control.

2 Assemble the materials needed.

3 Mix the blood specimen.

4 Dispense a small drop of blood onto a slide, about ½ to ¾ inch from the right end. Use a transfer pipette or capillary tube (Figure 1*).

5 Hold one side of this slide with your nondominant hand.

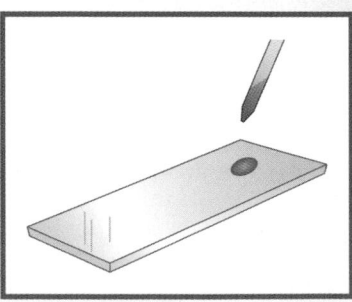

Figure 1

---

*Figure from Stepp CA, Woods MA: *Laboratory procedures for medical office personnel*, Philadelphia, 1998, WB Saunders.

PROCEDURE 51-5—cont'd

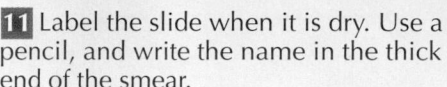

6 Place the spreader slide in front of the drop of blood at an angle of 30 to 35 degrees. Use your dominant hand (Figure 2).

Purpose: An angle of 30 to 35 degrees makes a smear with a good feathered edge.

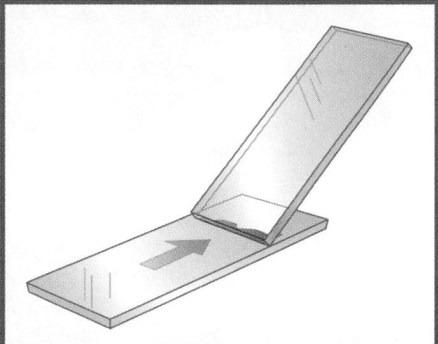

Figure 2

7 Pull back the spreader slide into the drop of blood, and allow the blood to spread to the edges of the slide (Figure 3).

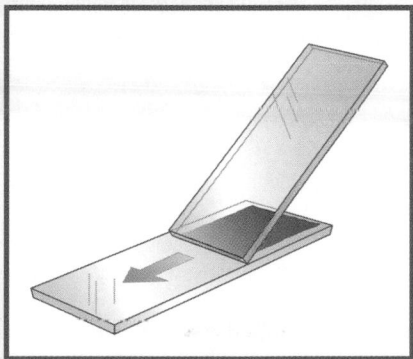

Figure 3

8 Push the spreader slide forward with a quick smooth motion, maintaining the same angle throughout (Figure 4).

Purpose: If the motion is not smooth, ridges will occur in the smear.

9 Rapidly but gently wave the slide to accelerate the drying process.

10 Stand the slide with the thick end down, and allow the slide to complete drying (Figure 5).

Purpose: If the thick end is up, the undried portion of the blood may run down into the dry thin area and ruin the smear.

11 Label the slide when it is dry. Use a pencil, and write the name in the thick end of the smear.

Purpose: Pencil will scratch the name into the smear and will not wash off in the staining process.

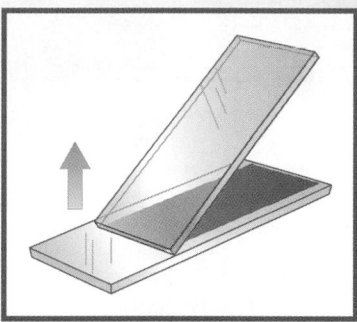

Figure 4

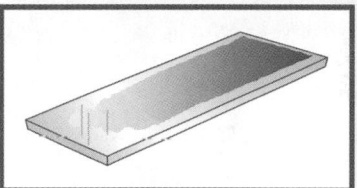

Figure 5

12 Stain according to method used.

Two-step method:
a. Place the smear on a staining rack, with the blood side up.
b. Flood the smear with Wright's stain.
c. Wait for 1 to 3 minutes.
d. Add an equal amount of buffer, drop by drop, on top of the Wright stain.
e. Blow gently, and mix the two solutions until a green metallic sheen appears. This should appear within 2 to 4 minutes.
f. Rinse thoroughly with distilled water.
g. Drain water from the slide.
h. Wipe the back of the smear with gauze.
i. Stand the smear to dry.

Quick stain:
a. Place the smear into solutions according to the manufacturer's instructions (Figure 6, *A* to *D*).
b. Proceed with steps *f* through *i* just listed.

13 Clean the work area. Properly dispose of all biohazard materials. Remove face protection and gloves. Wash your hands.

Continued

PROCEDURE 51-5—cont'd

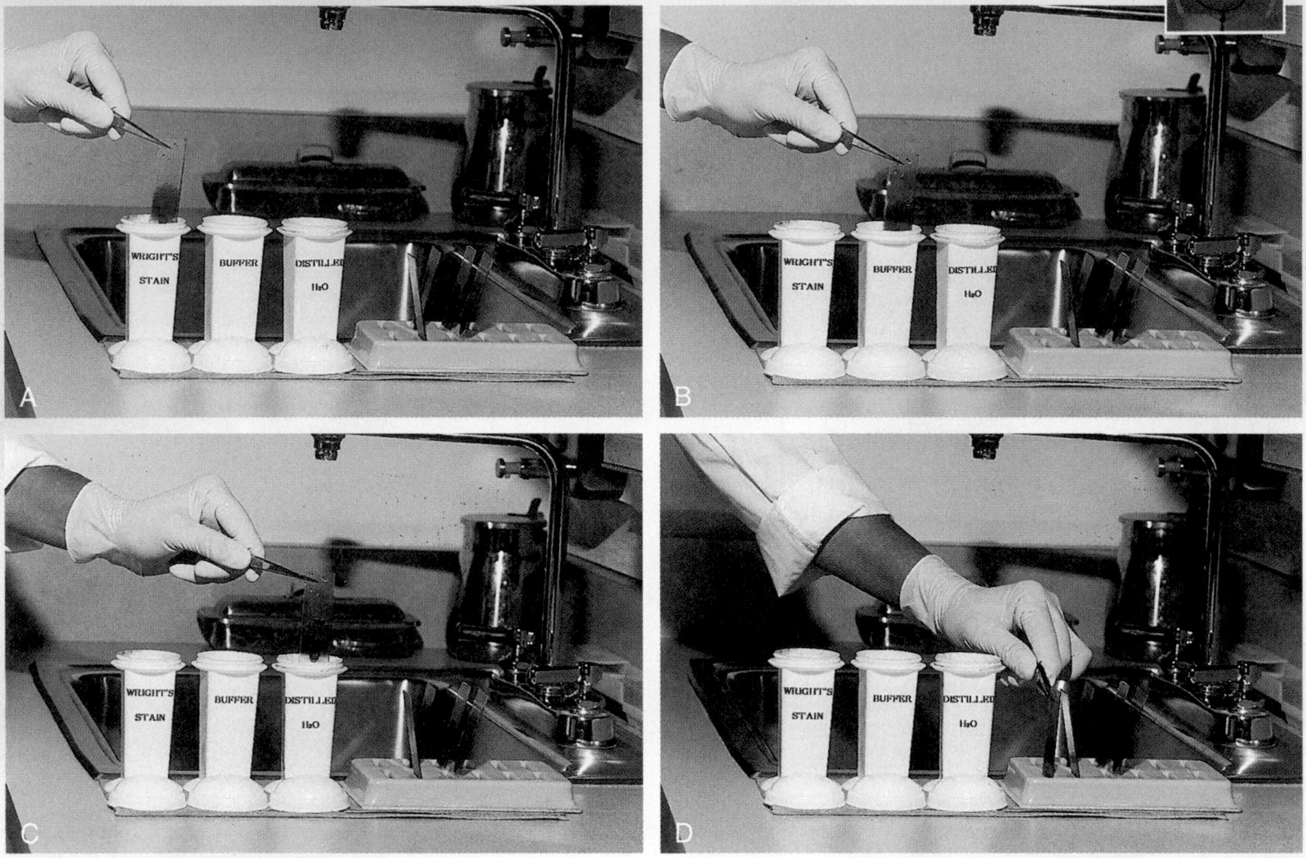

Figure 6

Identification of Normal Blood Cells

Much useful information can be gathered from microscopic identification and evaluation of blood cells in a stained smear. A great deal more information can be acquired from observation of these blood cells than from actual cell counts.

The features of blood cells that you will observe and evaluate are cell size, nuclear appearance, and cytoplasmic characteristics. The results of observing these three features will allow for cell identification, although much practice is required to be able to recognize and classify all the blood cells that may be seen in various disease states. A medical assistant will not perform the differential analysis, but you should be aware of the appearance of formed elements of the blood and the terminology used to describe them.

Cells are examined under the oil-immersion objective. The light should be bright to facilitate the visualization of colors and small structures. The slide is examined near the feathered end of the smear, where cells are barely touching each other and are easiest to identify.

Red blood cells are the most numerous of the cellular elements. They are biconcave disks that have no nuclei. The red cells should appear pinkish tan as a result of the staining of the hemoglobin within the cells (Figure 51-12).

Thrombocytes, or *platelets*, are the smallest of the cellular elements. They may be round or oval. No nucleus is present because the platelet is just a fragment of cytoplasm from a large bone marrow cell. They stain blue.

Leukocytes are the largest of the normal circulating blood cells (Table 51-4). Each of the five types has a

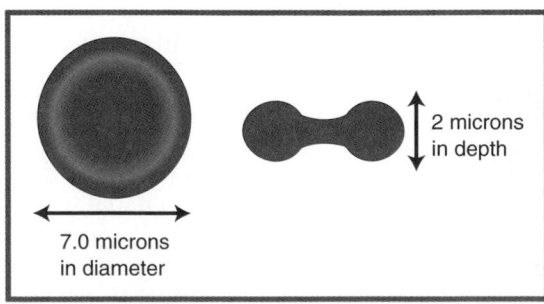

FIGURE 51-12 Red blood cell morphology. (From Stepp CA, Woods MA: *Laboratory procedures for medical office personnel*, Philadelphia, 1998, WB Saunders, p 151.)

TABLE 51-4	Characteristics of Leukocytes					
	Granulocytes				*Agranulocytes*	
	Neutrophil Segmented (mature)	Neutrophil Band (immature)	Eosinophil	Basophil	Lymphocyte	Monocyte
Cell size	10-15 µm	10-15 µm	10-15 µm	10-15 µm	6-15 µm	12-20 µm
Nucleus shape	2-5 lobes connected by thread-like filaments	Band or U-shaped	Bilobed or band	Slightly segmented, granular, or band	Round or oval	Round, indented, or superimposed lobes
Nucleus structure	Coarse	Coarse	Coarse	Obscured by granules	Smudged, lumpy, or clumped	Brainlike convolutions or folded
Cytoplasm amount	Abundant	Abundant	Abundant	Abundant	Scant	Abundant
Cytoplasm color	Colorless to light pink	Colorless to light pink	Colorless to light pink	Colorless to light pink	Sky blue to dark blue	Dull gray to blue-gray
Cytoplasm inclusions	Many tiny tan, pink, or red-purple granules	Many tiny tan, pink with increased red-purple granules	Large rounder oval red to red-orange granules	Large, coarse blue-black granules	None to few round red-purple granules	Ground glass appearance, fine red-purple granules, rare blue granules

From Stepp CA, Woods MA: *Laboratory procedures for medical office personnel*. Philadelphia, 1998, WB Saunders.

characteristic appearance. The granulocytes include neutrophils, eosinophils, and basophils. *Granulocytes* contain distinctive granules in their cytoplasm and may have segmented nuclei. The *agranulocytes* include lymphocytes and monocytes. They have few, if any, granules and non-segmented nuclei. The nuclei of the leukocytes should appear purple, and their cytoplasm may vary from pink to blue or blue-gray. *Neutrophils* are known by a variety of names, including *polymorphonuclear neutrophils (PMNs)*, *segmented neutrophils*, *polys*, and *segs* (Figure 51-13). They are the most numerous WBCs in circulation in adults. They are produced in bone marrow, are released into circulation, and eventually enter tissue to fight off invading microorganisms by engulfing them (phagocytosis). Many types of bacterial infections stimulate increased production of neutrophils.

The *segmented neutrophil* nucleus is segmented into two to five lobes that are connected by a strand. The nucleus stains a dark purple. The cytoplasm is pale pink and contains fine pink or lilac granules.

An immature form of a neutrophil is called a *band or stab*. Instead of having a segmented nucleus where the lobes are separated by a thin filament, the band has an unsegmented nucleus shaped like a horseshoe or a banana. The staining is the same as in the segmented neutrophil. An increase in bands is termed a *shift to the left* and is seen in infections such as bacterial meningitis, pneumonia, appendicitis, strep throat, abscesses, and in chronic granulocytic leukemia.

The nucleus of an *eosinophil* is divided into two or three lobes that stain purple. The cytoplasm stains pink and contains large round or oval red-orange granules. Eosinophils are phagocytic and are associated closely with allergies such as hay fever and with asthma as well as with certain parasitic infestations such as tapeworm and amoebic dysentery.

The nucleus of a *basophil* is segmented and stains light purple. The large, dark blue-black granules contain histamine, heparin, and other compounds that are a part of the allergic response. Basophils are associated with the immediate immune response to external antigens, such as that which occurs in asthma, hay fever, and anaphylaxis.

Lymphocytes are the second most numerous type of WBC in adults. In children, they are usually the most

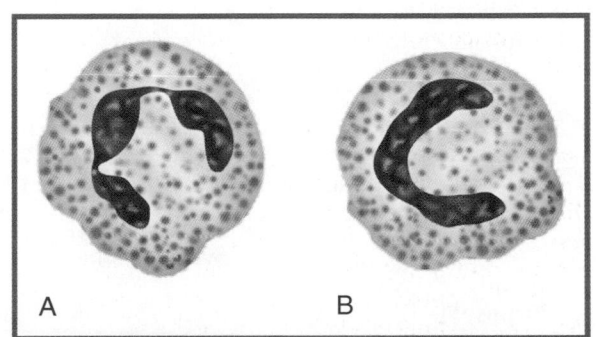

FIGURE 51-13 Neutrophilic cells. **A**, Segmented. **B**, Band. (From Stepp CA, Woods MA: *Laboratory procedures for medical office personnel*, Philadelphia, 1998, WB Saunders, p 151.)

numerous. Their purple-staining nucleus is usually large, oval or round, and smooth. The cytoplasm stains blue. *Lymphs*, as they are commonly called, are responsible for the recognition of foreign antigens and the production of circulating antibodies for immunity to disease. Increased numbers of lymphocytes are found in most viral diseases; in some bacterial infections such as syphilis and tuberculosis; in leukemias; and in young children who are actively making antibodies. In many viral infections, stimulated or reactive lymphocytes, called *atypical lymphs*, are found. These are common in infectious mononucleosis.

Monocytes are the largest type of WBC in circulation. The nucleus may be oval, indented, or horseshoe shaped. The cytoplasm stains a dull gray-blue and may contain *vacuoles*, which appear as clear spaces in the cytoplasm filled with fluid or air. Monocytes are called *macrophages* when they enter tissues and ingest bacteria and debris of cellular breakdown. They are increased in certain viral infections, such as hepatitis and mumps; rickettsial infections, such as Rocky Mountain spotted fever; and bacterial infections, such as tuberculosis and typhoid fever.

Differential Examination

A specific area of a stained smear must be examined when doing the differential count. This area must be

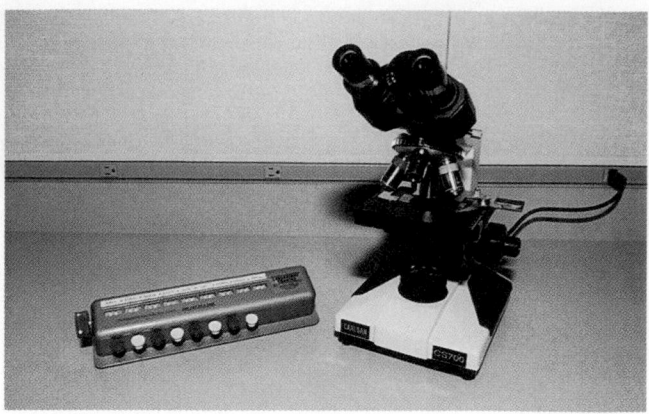

FIGURE 51-14 Microscope with differential cell counter. (Courtesy Cynmar Corporation, Carlinville, Ill.)

where red blood cells are touching but are not clumped when viewed microscopically. After you have located an appropriate area under low power, focus under oil immersion. The differential examination consists of counting and classifying 100 consecutive WBCs while moving in a specific winding pattern through the smear. This pattern must be followed to avoid counting the same cells twice. A tally is kept of the cells observed on a *differential cell counter* (Figure 51-14).

PROCEDURE **51-6**

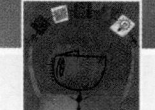

Performing a Differential Examination of a Smear Stained With Wright's Stain

GOAL: To perform a differential cell count, evaluate RBC morphology, and estimate the number of platelets.

EQUIPMENT AND SUPPLIES

- Microscope
- Immersion oil
- Lens tissue
- Lens cleaner

PROCEDURAL STEPS

1 Wash and dry your hands.
Purpose: Infection control.

2 Assemble the materials needed.

3 Clean the microscope with lens tissue and lens cleaner.
Purpose: Dirty optical surfaces interfere with viewing.

4 Place the slide on the stage, with the smear facing up.
Purpose: If the slide is face down, you will not be able to focus under oil immersion.

5 Locate an area of the smear where the RBCs

barely touch each other or slightly overlap, using the low-power objective.
Purpose: If the slide is too thick, the cells will be crowded, small, and difficult to evaluate. If the slide is too thin, the cells will be very far apart and will show the effects of excessive flattening.

6 Focus under oil immersion with the fine-adjustment knob and increased light.

7 Count 100 consecutive WBCs in a winding pattern, identifying each cell encountered (Figure 1*).

8 Record each white cell on the differential cell counter by depressing the appropriate key for each cell.
Purpose: The differential examination must proceed systematically, to avoid missing cells or counting any cell twice.

---

*Figure from Stepp CA, Woods MA: *Laboratory procedures for medical office personnel.* Philadelphia, 1998, WB Saunders.

PROCEDURE 51-6—cont'd

9 Evaluate the RBCs observed in 10 fields. Record any variations in:

    Size—microcytosis, macrocytosis, anisocytosis

    Shape—poikilocytosis, ovalocytosis, target cells, sickle cells, and so forth.

    Content—normochromic or hypochromic

    Purpose: The RBC evaluation gives the physician important information about the RBC population and is an important tool in the assessment of anemias and RBC diseases.

10 Count the platelets in 10 fields, obtain an average, and multiply that average by 15,000 to give an estimate of the platelet count. The normal platelet count is 150,000 to 400,000/mm^3. Report the count as normal, decreased, or increased.

    Purpose: Platelet numbers can be a clue to bleeding disorders.

11 Clean the microscope with lens tissue and lens cleaner.

12 Clean the work area and properly dispose of all materials. Wash your hands.

    Purpose: Infection control.

13 Record the testing results in the patient's record.

    Purpose: A procedure is considered not done until it is recorded.

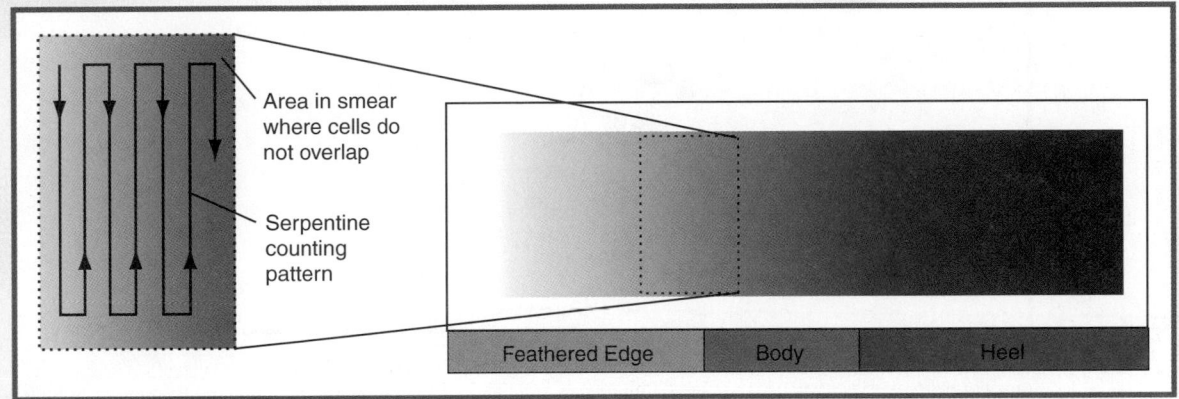

Area in smear where cells do not overlap

Serpentine counting pattern

Feathered Edge | Body | Heel

Figure 1

Normal values for a differential vary with age. Many disease states alter the ratios of the different types of leukocytes. While a medical assistant would not perform a differential examination, Procedure 51-6 is given so that you will understand the process.

Red Blood Cell Morphology

After determining the differential cell count, the RBCs are observed and evaluated. Normally, stained RBCs are the same size and shape and are well filled with hemoglobin. Any variations from the normal state are reported (Figure 51-15).

    Size. Normal-sized RBCs are known as *normocytic*. If the cells are larger than normal, they are *macrocytic*; if smaller, they are *microcytic*. The condition in which different sizes of RBCs are present is called *anisocytosis*.

    Shape. Normal RBCs are round or slightly oval. Cells may be shaped like sickles, targets, crescents, or burrs. *Poikilocytosis* is a significant variation in the shape of red blood cells.

    Content. An RBC with a normal amount of hemoglobin is called *normochromic*. Pale-staining cells are *hypochromic* and have less hemoglobin than normal. Any inclusions in red cells should be reported.

Platelet Observation

On a stained smear, the morphology of platelets is observed for any abnormalities. They are small and irregularly shaped and may vary considerably in size. The average number of platelets seen in 10 to 15 fields is reported. The normal platelet count is 150,000 to 400,000/mm^3. An increase in platelets is called *thrombocytosis*, and a decrease is called *thrombocytopenia*.

Erythrocyte Sedimentation Rate

The erythrocyte sedimentation rate (ESR) is a laboratory test that measures the rate at which erythrocytes gradually separate from plasma and settle to the bottom of a specially calibrated tube in an hour. The test is not specific for a particular disease but is used as a general indication of inflammation. Increases are found in such conditions as acute and chronic infections, rheumatoid arthritis, tuberculosis, hepatitis, cancer, multiple myeloma, rheumatic fever, and lupus erythematosus.

    Normal values vary slightly with age and gender (Table 51-5). Only increased ESR rates are significant.

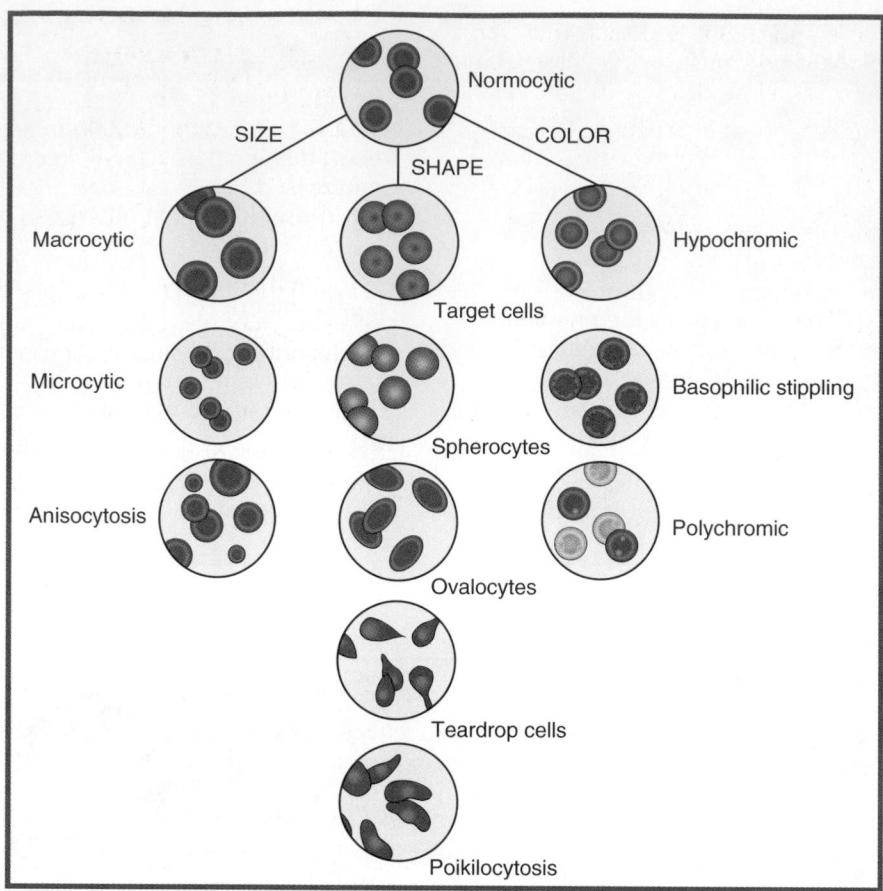

FIGURE 51-15 Abnormal erythrocytes. (Modified from Stepp CA, Woods MA: *Laboratory procedures for medical office personnel*, Philadelphia, 1998, WB Saunders, p 156.)

TABLE 51-5	ESR Reference Values	
	Wintrobe Method (mm/hr)	**Westergren Method (mm/hr)**
Men	0-10	≤ 50 yr of age: 0-15 > 50 yr of age: 0-20
Women	1-20	≤ 50 yr of age: 0-20 > 50 yr of age: 0-30

From Stepp CA, Woods MA: *Laboratory procedures for medical office personnel*. Philadelphia, 1998, WB Saunders.

Several methods of measuring ESR are used, including *Wintrobe* (Figure 51-16), *Westergren* (Procedure 51-7), and *Landau-Adams*. All these methods are based on the same principle and differ only in the amounts of blood needed and the tube size and calibration used.

The International Committee for Standardization in Hematology has selected Westergren's method as the recommended method. A straight glass tube 30 cm in length and 2.55 mm (+/−0.15 mm) in diameter with a bore uniform to 0.05 mm throughout is used. Blood is obtained by clean venipuncture in an EDTA tube and diluted accurately with 1 volume of 109 mmol/L trisodium citrate to 4 volumes of blood. The test should be performed within 2 hours of collection, or within 6 hours if stored at 4° C. The diluted blood sample is drawn to the 200 mm mark in the tube by means of mechanical device or aspiration bulb. The tube is placed vertically in a vibration-and-draft-free environment, not exposed to direct sunlight. After 1 hour, the height of clear plasma above the upper limit of the column of sedimentating cells, measured in mm, is the ESR.

Variations on the standard method have been developed using plastic and disposable glass tubes and capillary tubes for infants. One such method is the SEDIPLAST (Polymedco, Redmond, WA). This closed system incorporates a pierceable stopper that, when pierced by a pipette, ensures a leak-proof seal. An automatic self-zeroing cap and reservoir accurately brings the blood level to the zero-mark and protects from overfilling. A prefilled vial of sodium citrate diluent is provided for dilution of blood prior to testing (see Procedure 51-7).

Quickmode systems have also been developed. Strek Laboratories (LaVista, NE) manufactures the ESR-10, a nonautomated, CLIA-waived test using ESR-vacuum tubes. The tubes automatically draw the correct amount of sample and then are placed in the rack for 30 minutes. Although not CLIA-waived, Strek Laboratories also manufactures analyzers that force readings, allowing results in as little as 10 minutes.

Many factors can affect the ESR. The tube must be totally filled with blood and must not contain air bubbles. The tube must be allowed to sit in a vertical position undisturbed for a full hour. Minor degrees of tilting may increase the sedimentation rate; careful timing is important. Jarring or vibrations from nearby machinery will falsely increase the ESR. *Testing must be performed within 2 hours after blood has been collected.*

Coagulation Testing

Coagulation testing is usually performed in the hematology laboratory. The medical assistant may be asked to perform a test to determine prothrombin time using a hand-held, CLIA-waived instrument that uses whole blood or citrated plasma. The protime (or prothrombin time) is a method of measuring how well the blood clots. Generally, a protime is considered to be prolonged if it is more than 1.2 times the control time. Patients who have problems with delayed blood clotting are given a number of tests to determine the cause of the problem. The prothrombin test specifically evaluates the presence of factors VIIa, V, and X, prothrombin, and fibrinogen. *Prothrombin* is a protein in the liquid part of blood (plasma) that is converted to thrombin as part of

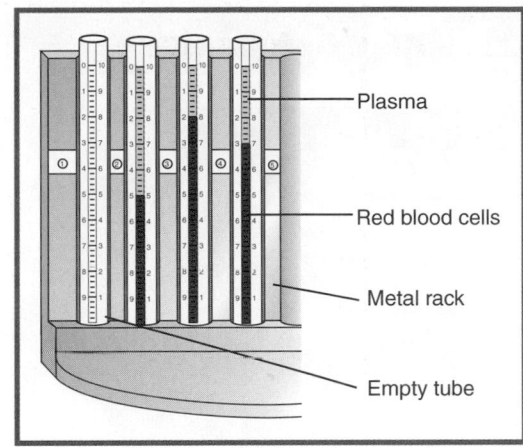

FIGURE 51-16 Wintrobe sedimentation rate system. (From Stepp CA, Woods MA: *Laboratory procedures for medical office personnel*, Philadelphia, 1998, WB Saunders, p 167.)

the clotting process. *Fibrinogen* is a type of blood protein called a *globulin*; it is converted to fibrin during the clotting process. A drop in concentration of any of these factors will cause the blood to take longer to clot.

The protime test is used in combination with the partial thromboplastin time (PTT) test to screen for

---

PROCEDURE 51-7

Performing an Erythrocyte Sedimentation Rate Using a Modified-Westergren Method

GOAL: To fill a Westergren tube properly and to observe and record the findings of an erythrocyte sedimentation rate (ESR) using the Westergren method.

EQUIPMENT AND SUPPLIES

- EDTA anticoagulated blood specimen
- Sediplast ESR system
- Sediplast rack
- Timer

PROCEDURAL STEPS

1 Wash and dry your hands. Put on face protection and nonsterile gloves.
 Purpose: Infection control.

2 Assemble the materials needed.

3 Check the leveling bubble of the Sediplast rack.
 Purpose: The rack must be horizontal to ensure that the tube is vertical.

4 Mix the blood well.
 Purpose: Cells settle when the specimen stands, and blood must always be well-mixed before sampling.

5 Remove the stopper on the blood sample and on the prefilled Sediplast vial. Fill the vial to the indicated line, replace the stopper on the prefilled vial, and invert several times to mix. Recap the blood collection tube.
 Purpose: This dilutes the blood in accordance with the Westergren procedure.

6 Insert the Sediplast pipette through the pierceable stopper on the vial and push down until the pipette touches the bottom of the vial. The pipette will automatically draw the blood up to the zero mark.

7 Insert the pipette and the vial into the rack, ensuring that it is vertical.
 Purpose: A pipette that is not vertical will produce erroneous results (Figure 1*).

8 Allow the tube to stand undisturbed for 60 minutes.
 Purpose: Jarring will increase the sedimentation rate.

Continued

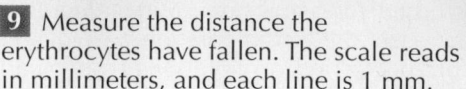

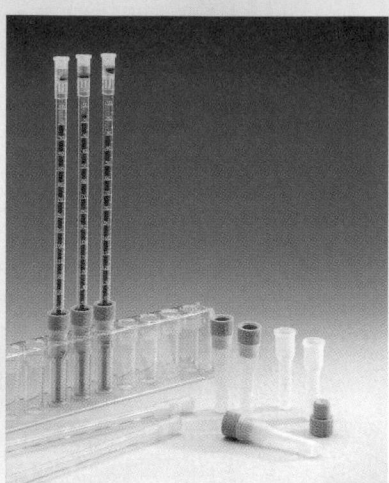

Figure 1

9 Measure the distance the erythrocytes have fallen. The scale reads in millimeters, and each line is 1 mm.

10 Clean the work area, and properly dispose of all biohazard materials. Remove face protection and gloves and wash your hands. Dispose of the pipette in a biohazard container.

11 Record the findings in the patient's medical record.

Remember: The ESR is reported in millimeters per hour.

Purpose: A procedure is considered not done until it is recorded.

*Figure courtesy Polymedco, Inc.

hemophilia and other hereditary clotting disorders. The protime test is also used to monitor the condition of patients who are taking warfarin (Coumadin). Warfarin is a drug that is given to prevent clots in the deep veins of the legs and to treat pulmonary embolism. It interferes with blood clotting by lowering the liver's production of certain clotting factors.

Immunology (Serology)

Serologic testing provides information about past or present infections with bacteria or viruses and also is done to detect certain types of cancers. Testing done in the immunology laboratory is designed to visualize the reaction between antigen and antibody. Antibodies are formed when the body encounters a foreign agent. In the *acute phase* of a disease, antibody level is high; during the *convalescent stage*, antibody level decreases. Once an antigen has been recognized by the immune system and antibodies have been made, the level of antibody to that particular antigen remains at a low but detectable level indefinitely. The amount of antibody at any given time can be measured with serological testing and is referred to as the *titer*. Generally, a titer is performed by preparing **serial dilutions** of serum or plasma; if the 1:100 dilution of a sample is the last dilution to show a reaction between antigen and antibody, for example, the titer is reported as 100.

The reaction between antigen and antibody can be visualized **in vitro** through several means, most commonly agglutination, precipitation, and enzyme-linked immunoassay (or immunosorbent assay). In agglutination and precipitation reactions, latex beads or RBCs from an animal such as a rabbit are needed for visualization. The antigen or antibody is chemically bound to the

bead or cell by the manufacturer. When the corresponding antibody or antigen molecule comes into contact with the bead or cell, they link together and clump (agglutinate). If this reaction occurs in a test tube, the clumps precipitate to the bottom of the tube. If the reaction occurs on a glass or paper surface, such as a slide, the clumps are visible to the naked eye. Antigen and antibody must be present in roughly equal proportions for clumping to occur because the linking is much like lattice-work. If there is markedly more antigen than antibody, or vice versa, the lattice cannot form properly. This represents a false negative reaction and is termed the *prozone reaction*.

Enzyme immunoassays are replacing many of the precipitation and agglutination tests in the serology laboratory because of their enhanced **specificity** and **sensitivity**. There are two general approaches to diagnosing diseases by immunoassays: testing for specific or antigen-specific antibodies. Enzyme-linked immunosorbent assays (ELISA), also known as enzyme immunoassays (EIA), are tests designed to detect antigens or antibodies by producing an enzyme-triggered color change. Solid-phase immunoassay involves the immobilization (attachment) of antigens or antibodies on solid surfaces such as beads, wells in plastic dishes, or plastic cartridges. Generally, when an antigen-antibody reaction occurs, a color change is visible. With some tests, the more intense the color, the higher the concentration of the substance being measured. The commercially available pregnancy tests found in most stores use solid-phase technology in which a plastic cartridge is dipped in urine and a color change is observed if the woman is pregnant.

Most serologic testing done in the physician's office is done with individual testing kits. When performing a serologic test, the first step is to review the package insert provided by the manufacturer. This review will provide valuable information about the test, the principle on which the test is based, the reagents and equipment required, proper specimen collection techniques, preparation requirements, test procedures, and any precautions or warnings that pertain to the procedure. In addition, the inserts provide information regarding quality control, interpretation of results, limitations of the procedure performance characteristics, and references.

The CLIA-waived tests that can be performed by a medical assistant include bladder tumor–associated antigen (BTA), *Helicobacter pylori* antibodies, and infectious mononucleosis antibodies. Most of these test kits involve solid-phase immunoassay.

Bladder Tumor Antigen Testing

The BTA test is a rapid, single-step immunoassay. The disposable test device contains two monoclonal antibodies that detect the presence of an antigen shed by the bladder cells. To use the BTA test, five drops of urine are placed into the sample well of the test device and positive or negative results are provided in 5 minutes. Bladder cancer is one of the most common forms of cancer in the United States. About 53,000 Americans are diagnosed with bladder cancer each year, and approximately 500,000 people are routinely monitored for the disease. The cancer is most common among people over the age of 50, smokers, and workers exposed to chemicals in the rubber, leather tanning, metal, and dye industries.

Testing for *Helicobacter pylori*

Helicobacter pylori is a spiral-shaped bacterium that is found in the gastric mucus layer or adherent to the epithelial lining of the stomach. *H. pylori* causes more than 90% of duodenal ulcers and more than 80% of gastric ulcers. Several methods may be used to diagnose *H. pylori* infection. Serological tests that measure specific *H. pylori* IgG antibodies can determine whether a person has been infected. The biopsy **urease** test is a colorimetric test based on the ability of *H. pylori* to produce urease; it provides rapid testing at the time of biopsy.

Infectious Mononucleosis Testing

Infectious mononucleosis testing can also be performed by the medical assistant (Procedure 51-8). Infectious mononucleosis, also called "mono" or the "kissing disease," is an acute infectious disease caused by the Epstein-Barr virus (EBV). EBV is a member of the herpes virus family and is one of the most common human viruses. Although it is related to the herpes virus, it has nothing to do with cold sores or genital herpes. The virus occurs worldwide; it is especially common in teenagers and occasionally in adults, but it is found most frequently in people between the ages of 10 and 25. Most people have been infected with EBV sometime during their lives. In the United States, as many as 95% of adults between 35 and 40 years of age have been infected.

In children, the infection may pass unrecognized or with a trivial illness lasting only a few days, with sore

PROCEDURE 51-8

Mono-Test for Infectious Mononucleosis

GOAL: To perform and interpret a slide test for infectious mononucleosis.

EQUIPMENT AND SUPPLIES
- Mono-Test kit
- Blood specimen (serum or plasma)

PROCEDURAL STEPS

1 Wash and dry your hands. Glove and put on face protection.
   Purpose: Infection control.

2 Remove the test kit from the refrigerator, and allow the reagents to warm to room temperature. Check the expiration date of the kit.
   Purpose: Outdated or cold reagents do not react as expected.

3 Fill a disposable capillary tube to the calibration mark with serum or plasma (see Chapter 50 for collection of blood). Using the rubber bulb included

in the kit, deposit the specimen in the first circle of the clean glass slide also provided in the kit (Figure 1).

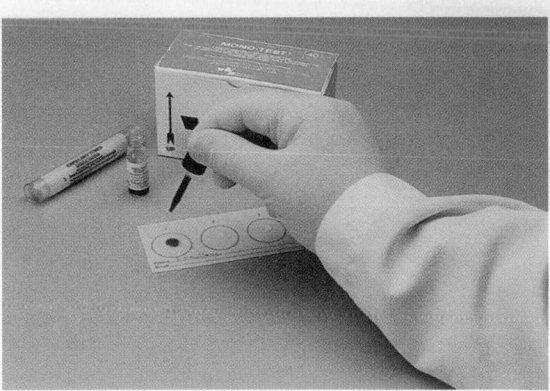

Figure 1

Continued

Purpose: The capillary tube measures the exact amount of sample for accurate testing.

4 Place one drop of negative control in the second circle and one drop of positive control in the third circle (Figure 2).

Purpose: Known controls ensure that reagents are functioning properly.

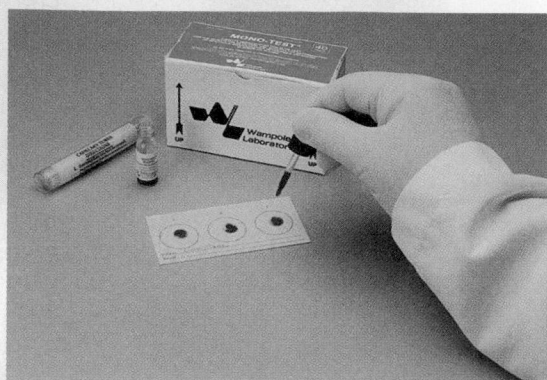

Figure 2

5 Thoroughly mix the Mono-Test reagent by rolling the bottle gently between the palms of the hands. Squeeze the enclosed dropper to mix all the contents of the bottle.

Purpose: Reagent RBCs settle on standing and must be mixed before use.

6 Hold the dropper in a vertical position, and add one drop of Mono-Test reagent to each area of the slide. Do not touch the dropper to the slide.

Purpose: Holding a dropper vertically ensures delivery of the same size drop. If the dropper touches other materials, it becomes contaminated, and results will be inaccurate.

7 Using separate stirrers, quickly and thoroughly mix each area, spreading each area out to 1 inch in diameter.

Purpose: Failure to use a clean stirrer for each area would invalidate the test because of cross-contamination.

8 Rock the slide gently for exactly 2 minutes; observe immediately for agglutination. A dark background is best for viewing.

Purpose: Timing is always important.

9 Interpret the test results, and record them. Agglutination is positive, and no agglutination is negative.

10 Clean the work area. Remove gloves, and wash your hands.

11 Record the test results in the patient's medical record.

Purpose: A procedure is not considered done until it is properly recorded.

---

throat, fever, swollen tonsils and lymph nodes in the neck, which can be indistinguishable from other mild illnesses of childhood. In young people, some of the most common complications include the abrupt onset of fatigue, headaches, aching muscles, faint rash, fever, very swollen tonsils, enlarged lymph glands, and loss of appetite often associated with nausea. There may be a short or prolonged period (days or weeks) after the initial illness when the fatigue continues and the patient may feel dispirited and depressed. Occasionally, complications occur, including the development of a swollen spleen or liver. Heart problems or any involvement of the central nervous system occurs rarely, and infectious mononucleosis is almost never fatal.

Testing for mononucleosis involves a CBC and serologic tests. A CBC will reveal an increased number of lymphocytes that appear atypical on the differential examination. The infected lymphocytes undergo a cellular transformation, causing them to take on the appearance similar to a monocyte (hence the name *mononucleosis*). Most patients exposed to EBV develop a nonspecific antibody response to the virus and produce *heterophile antibodies*. The antibodies react with surface antigens of horse erythrocytes, causing agglutination (clumping) that is visible on the test slide. Solid-phase immunoassay tests are also available for the detection of heterophile antibodies. These tests are similar to the pregnancy test discussed in Chapter 38. Serum, instead of urine, is used.

Immunohematology

The major reason for performing immunohematologic tests is to prevent problems caused by incompatibility of blood types. Compatibility testing (cross matching) is performed to prevent transfusion reactions in patients who are receiving blood transfusions and to identify potential Rh-incompatibility problems in expectant mothers. Rh incompatibility between an expectant mother and the unborn child may result in hemolytic disease of the newborn.

Blood Grouping

There are two major blood antigen systems: the ABO (or Landsteiner) system and the Rh system. In the ABO system, there are four major blood groups: A, B, O, and

AB. A person is either Rh positive or Rh negative. Certain blood types are more common in certain countries. In China, more than 99% of the population has Rh-positive blood. In the United States, about 85% of the population is Rh positive. Blood type is inherited, like eye color. Different kinds of animals have different kinds of blood. Dogs have four blood types; cats have 11; cows have about 800. Among the white population:

- One person in 3 is O positive
- One person in 15 is O negative
- One person in 3 is A positive
- One person in 16 is A negative
- One person in 12 is B positive
- One person in 67 is B negative
- One person in 29 is AB positive
- One person in 167 is AB negative

Determination of ABO Blood Group

The determination of ABO blood groups is a simple test that can easily be performed (Procedure 51-9), but because of the implications of performing the test incorrectly, blood typing is not CLIA-waived. The test detects the presence of A or B antigens on red blood cells based on the presence or absence of agglutination with a known antiserum

When the antigen on a patient's RBCs corresponds to the test antibody, agglutination occurs. If the corresponding antigen is not present on the cells, no agglutination will occur.

In addition to the blood antigens found on RBCs, antibodies are found in plasma. These antibodies appear shortly after birth, and the body never produces an antibody that can combine with its own blood antigen.

PROCEDURE 51-9

Determining ABO Group Using a Slide Test

GOAL: To determine accurately a patient's ABO group using the slide test technique.

EQUIPMENT AND SUPPLIES

- Glass slide with frosted ends
- Anti-A and anti-B serum (Figure 1*)
- Applicator sticks
- Lancet and automatic finger puncture device
- Alcohol preps
- Sterile gauze squares
- Laboratory marking pen or pencil

PROCEDURAL STEPS

1 Reread the physician's orders, and assemble all of the supplies and equipment needed to complete the testing procedure.

2 Wash your hands, and put on face protection and gloves.
   Purpose: Infection control.

3 Explain the procedure to the patient.

4 Label the slides in the frosted area with the patient's name.
   Purpose: To ensure proper identification of testing results.

5 Place one drop of anti-A serum on slide 1, one drop of anti-B serum on slide 2, and one drop of anti-A and anti-B on slide 3.

6 Select the puncture site and perform a finger puncture procedure.

7 Wipe away the first drop of blood.
   Purpose: The first drop of blood may contain tissue fluid.

8 Place one large drop of blood on each of the three prepared slides.

9 Cover the puncture site with a sterile gauze square and instruct the patient to apply gentle pressure to the site.

10 Mix the antiserum and blood thoroughly, using a clean applicator stick for each slide. The mixture should be spread over an area measuring approximately 20 × 40 mm.

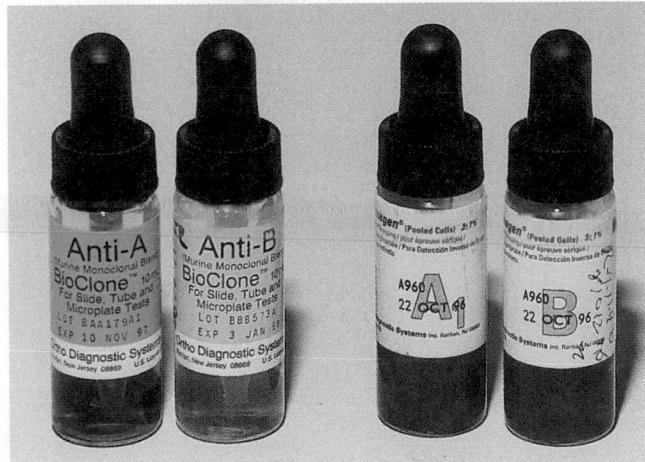

Figure 1

---

*Figure from Stepp CA, Woods MA: *Laboratory procedures for medical office personnel.* Philadelphia, 1998, WB Saunders.

Continued

PROCEDURE 51-9—cont'd

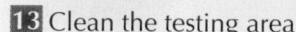

11 Read and interpret the results of the reaction for all slides (Figure 2).

12 Discard all biohazard testing waste in the appropriate container.
   Purpose: Infection control.

13 Clean the testing area.

14 Record the testing results in the patient's medical record.
   Purpose: A procedure is not considered done until it is recorded.

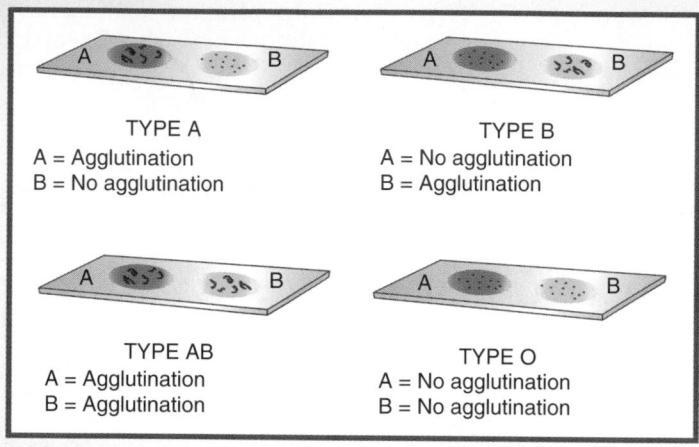

TYPE A
A = Agglutination
B = No agglutination

TYPE B
A = No agglutination
B = Agglutination

TYPE AB
A = Agglutination
B = Agglutination

TYPE O
A = No agglutination
B = No agglutination

Figure 2

The blood group antibodies require that blood transfusions are specific; type A blood should ideally receive type A blood in a transfusion. In emergencies, there may not be time for the laboratory to perform a **type and cross match**, thus, type O negative blood is administered. Type O negative is referred to as the *universal donor* because there are no circulating antibodies to the ABO antigen, nor are there Rh antigens that might sensitize an Rh-negative recipient. Table 51-6 illustrates the compatibility among blood types for transfusion.

TABLE 51-6	Blood Compatibility	
Recipient Blood*		**Compatible with**
RBC Antigen	**Plasma Antibodies**	**Donor Types†**
Type O (no antigens)	Anti-A and anti-B	O
Type A (type A antigen)	Anti-B	O and A
Type B (type B antigen)	Anti-A	O and B
Type AB (type AB antigen)	None	O, A, B, and AB

RBC, Red blood cell.
*Patients with type AB blood are considered to be universal recipients.
†Patients with type O blood are considered to be universal donors.
From Stepp CA, Woods MA: *Laboratory procedures for medical office personnel*. Philadelphia, 1998, WB Saunders.

EXAMPLES OF BLOOD AGGLUTINATION

- Type A blood will agglutinate in the presence of anti-A antiserum but will not agglutinate in the presence of anti-B antiserum.
- Type B blood will agglutinate in the presence of anti-B antiserum but not in the presence of anti-A antiserum.
- Type O blood will not agglutinate in the presence of anti-A antiserum or anti-B antiserum.
- Type AB blood will agglutinate in the presence of both anti-A antiserum and anti-B antiserum.

Determination of Rh Factor

The determination of Rh type is also a simple (although not CLIA-waived) test that can be performed with a minimum amount of equipment (Procedure 51-10). This test detects the presence of D antigens on the surface of RBCs based on the presence or absence of agglutination with anti-D antiserum. When the D antigen is present, agglutination occurs when the anti-D antiserum is reacted with RBCs. If the D antigen is not present, no agglutination will occur. Rh-positive blood will agglutinate in the presence of anti-D antiserum but not in the presence of the Rh control. Rh-negative blood will not agglutinate in the presence of anti-D antiserum, nor will it agglutinate in the presence of the Rh control. There are no naturally occurring antibodies to the Rh

PROCEDURE 51-10

Determining Rh Factor Using the Slide Method

GOAL: To determine accurately the presence or absence of anti-D agglutinations.

EQUIPMENT AND SUPPLIES

- Two glass slides with frosted ends
- Anti-D serum (Figure 1*)
- Applicator sticks
- Lancet and automatic finger puncture device
- Alcohol preps
- Sterile gauze squares
- Laboratory marker or pencil

PROCEDURAL STEPS

1 Check the physician's order, and assemble all the equipment and supplies needed to complete the testing procedure.

2 Wash your hands, and put on face protection and gloves.
   Purpose: Infection control.

3 Label one slide "D" and one slide "C."
   Purpose: To differentiate between the anti-D slide and the control slide.

4 Place one drop of anti-D serum on the D slide.

5 Place one drop of the appropriate control reagent on the C slide.

6 Perform a capillary puncture to secure a blood specimen.

7 To each slide, add two drops of the patient's blood.

8 Thoroughly mix the blood with the anti-D serum, using a clean applicator stick for each slide, and spread the reaction mixture over an area measuring approximately 20 × 40 mm on each slide.

9 Place the slide on an Rh-viewbox.
   Purpose: The viewbox provides warmth, which promotes agglutination, and also provides extra illumination for viewing.

10 Read the results immediately (Figure 2).
   Purpose: Drying of the reaction mixture must not be confused with agglutination.

11 Discard all disposable equipment in the proper biohazardous waste containers.

12 Clean area. Remove gloves and wash your hands.
   Purpose: Infection control.

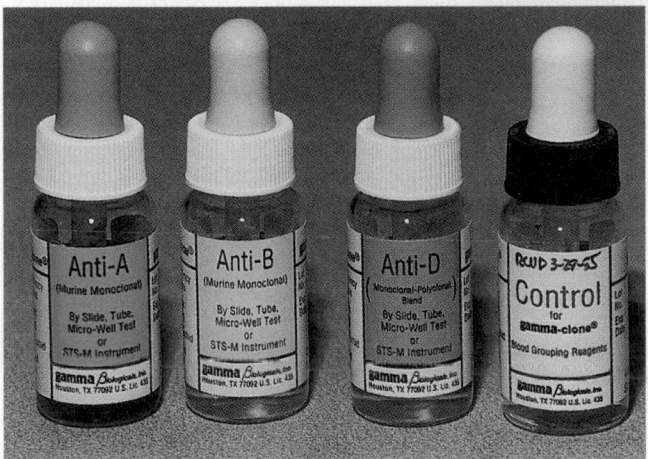

Figure 1

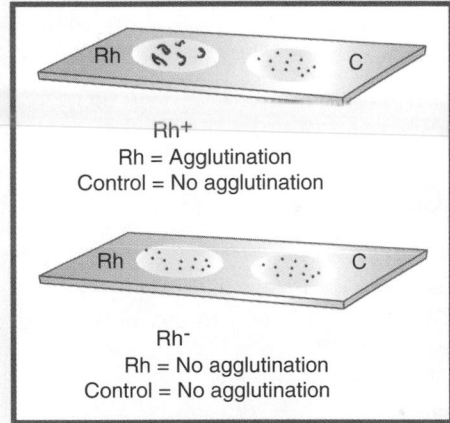

Rh+
Rh = Agglutination
Control = No agglutination

Rh⁻
Rh = No agglutination
Control = No agglutination

Figure 2

*Figure from Stepp CA, Woods MA: *Laboratory procedures for medical office personnel.* Philadelphia, 1998, WB Saunders.

factor. One will develop these antibodies only in the event of exposure to the antigen. This is possible if an incompatible transfusion is administered or if an Rh-negative mother is exposed to the Rh-positive blood of her infant during pregnancy, a miscarriage, abortion, or delivery. When this occurs, a mother may develop antibodies against the D antigen. This usually does not cause a problem during the first pregnancy.

In the event of a subsequent pregnancy with an Rh-positive fetus, the woman's immune system will begin to produce more antibodies because she had been sensitized by the first pregnancy. These antibodies cross the placenta and destroy the RBCs of the fetus, which can lead to anemia, heart failure, or brain damage in the infant and may even cause death. These events are collectively called *hemolytic disease of the newborn* (HDN). The disease is sometimes also called *hydrops* or *blue baby syndrome*.

Until 1968, there was no preventative measure that could be taken. Exchange transfusion, in which all of the infant's blood is replaced, was the only option. Today, however, this can be prevented by the administration of Rh immune globulin products.

Rho(D) immune globulin is a protein solution containing large amounts of Rho(D) antibodies. It is given to the Rh-negative mother by injection after a miscarriage or abortion or after the delivery of an Rh-positive baby. In most cases, it is now also given during pregnancy. The immune globulin prevents the infant's Rh-positive cells from stimulating the mother's immune system, thus preventing HDN.

The source of Rho(D) immune globulin is plasma from women who have had children affected by HDN or from Rh-negative males who are voluntarily injected with Rh-positive RBCs.

CRITICAL THINKING APPLICATION

Before Mr. Corrigan's kidney transplant, he had a type and crossmatch and was determined to be type O Positive. Explain how the test was performed and what the technician observed with the anti-A, anti-B, and anti-D antisera.

Clinical Chemistry

Increasingly, clinical chemistry testing is performed in the physician's office laboratory. Several clinical chemistry tests are CLIA-waived and can be performed by the medical assistant.

Blood Glucose

Glucose is used as a fuel by many cells within the body; under normal circumstances, it is the only substance used by the brain. Maintenance of blood glucose levels within a normal range is vitally important to homeostasis of the human body. Understanding the importance of glucose helps in understanding the reason why glucose is the most frequently tested analyte.

Elevated blood glucose levels are most often associated with diabetes mellitus but may also indicate pancreatitis, endocrine disorders, or chronic renal failure. Diabetes mellitus is a disorder of carbohydrate metabolism that results in elevated blood and urine glucose levels secondary to the inability of the pancreas to produce sufficient insulin.

To check a patient for possible diabetes mellitus, the physician may request a blood glucose tolerance test. For this test, the fasting patient receives an adequate carbohydrate meal of 100 g of glucose by mouth. This is usually given to the patient as a drink that is similar to a sweet fruit punch. The amount may be adjusted according to the patient's weight. If the glucose level does not exceed 100 g/dl at onset of the testing period or 180 g/dl 1 hour after ingestion of the glucose drink, the patient is believed to have a normal glucose level. If the blood glucose level exceeds 200 g/dl, glucose will escape into the urine because the renal tubules are no longer able to absorb the excessive amount present in the glomerulus.

The medical assistant can perform glucose testing using a glucose-monitoring device cleared by the FDA for home use (Procedure 51-11). Blood glucose is routinely monitored by patients with both type 1 (insulin-dependent) and type 2 (non–insulin-dependent) diabetes. Glucose levels may also be monitored by women experiencing gestational diabetes, a condition seen during pregnancy in which the effect of insulin is partially blocked by a variety of other hormones made in the placenta.

Cholesterol

Cholesterol is a fat-like substance (lipid) that is present in cell membranes. It is also needed to form bile acids and steroid hormones. Cholesterol travels in the blood in distinct particles containing both lipid and proteins. These particles are called *lipoproteins*. The cholesterol level in the blood is determined partly by inheritance and partly by acquired factors such as diet, calorie balance, and level of physical activity.

Patients are often confused by cholesterol testing. The confusion is due partly to the way some people use the term *cholesterol*, which is often a catch-all term for both the cholesterol you eat and the cholesterol that is maintained in the body. A high level of low-density lipoprotein, or LDL cholesterol, reflects an increased risk of heart disease, which is why LDL cholesterol is often called "bad" cholesterol. Lower levels of LDL cholesterol reflect a lower risk of heart disease. When too much LDL cholesterol circulates in the blood, it can slowly build up in the walls of arteries that feed the heart and brain. Together with other substances, it can form *plaque*, a thick, hard deposit that can clog those arteries. This condition is known as *atherosclerosis*. If a clot (thrombus) forms where a plaque is, the blood flow can be blocked to part of the heart muscle, causing a heart attack. If a clot blocks blood flow to part of the brain, a stroke results.

PROCEDURE **51-11**

Performing a Blood Glucose Accu-Chek Test

GOAL: To perform accurately a blood test for possible diabetes mellitus.

EQUIPMENT AND SUPPLIES

- Accu-Chek glucose monitor or similar glucose monitoring device
- Accu-Chek glucose testing strip
- Lancet and autoloading finger-puncturing device
- Alcohol preps
- Gauze squares

PROCEDURAL STEPS

1 Reread the physician's order, and collect the necessary equipment and supplies needed to complete the testing procedure.

2 Wash your hands and put on gloves.
   Purpose: Infection control.

3 Ask the patient to wash his or her hands in warm soapy water and then to rinse them in warm water and dry them completely.
   Purpose: Warming the fingers may increase blood peripheral blood flow.

4 Check the patient's index and ring fingers and select the site for puncture.
   Purpose: Site of puncture must be free of trauma.

5 Turn on the Accu-Chek monitor by pressing the ON button (Figure 1*).

6 Make sure the code number on the LED display matches the code number on the container of testing strips.
   Purpose: If code numbers do not match, the device must be reprogrammed with the new code for the test results to be valid.

7 Remove a testing strip from the vial, and immediately replace the vial cover.
   Purpose: Vial must be closed to protect unused strips from possible contamination.

8 Check the strip for discoloration by comparing the color of the round window on the back of the testing strip with the designated "unused" color chart provided on the test strip vial label.
   Purpose: This will establish the validity of the testing procedure.
   Do not touch the yellow test pad or round window on the back of the strip when handling the strip.

9 When the test strip symbol begins flashing in the lower right-hand corner of the display screen, insert the test strip into the designated testing slot until it locks into place. When the test strip is inserted correctly, the arrows on the test strip will be facing up and pointing toward the monitor (Figure 2).

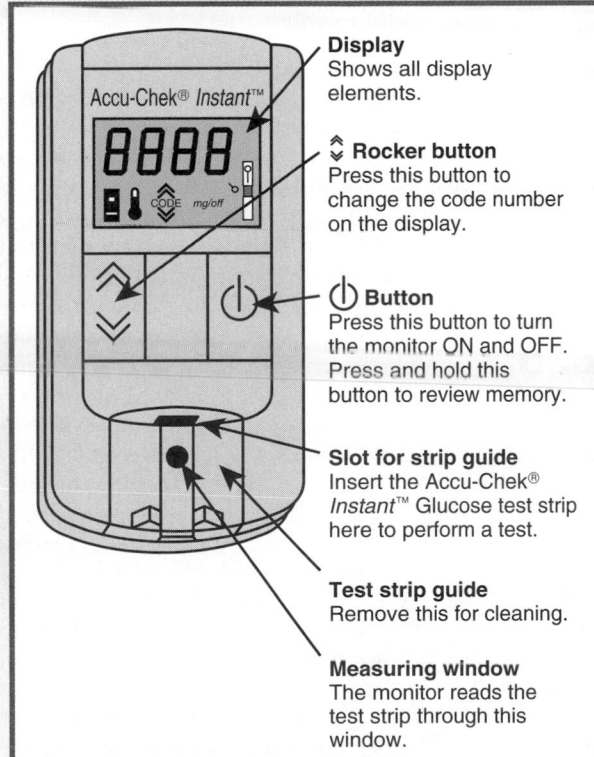

Display
Shows all display elements.

Rocker button
Press this button to change the code number on the display.

Button
Press this button to turn the monitor ON and OFF. Press and hold this button to review memory.

Slot for strip guide
Insert the Accu-Chek® Instant™ Glucose test strip here to perform a test.

Test strip guide
Remove this for cleaning.

Measuring window
The monitor reads the test strip through this window.

Figure 1

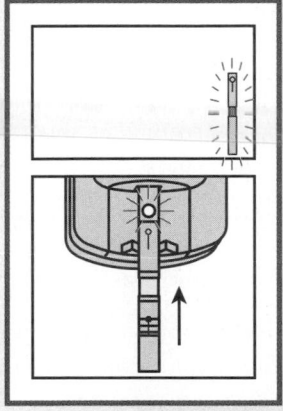

Figure 2

*Figure from Stepp CA, Woods MA: *Laboratory procedures for medical office personnel.* Philadelphia, 1998, WB Saunders.

Continued

PROCEDURE 51-11—cont'd

10 Cleanse the selected site on the patient's fingertip with the alcohol wipe and allow the finger to air dry.

11 Perform the finger puncture, and wipe away the first drop of blood.

Purpose: There may be tissue fluid present in the first drop of blood.

12 Apply a large hanging drop of blood to the center of the yellow testing pad (Figure 3).

a. *Do not touch the pad with the patient's finger.*

b. *Do not apply a second drop of blood.*

c. *Do not smear the blood with your finger.*

d. *Be certain the yellow test pad is saturated with blood.*

13 Give the patient a gauze square to hold securely over the puncture site.

14 The monitor will automatically begin the measurement process as soon as it senses the drop of blood.

15 Read the test result when it is displayed in the display window in milligrams per deciliter.

16 Turn off the monitor by pressing the "O" button.

17 Discard all biohazard waste into the proper waste containers.

Purpose: Infection control.

18 Clean the work area, remove gloves, and wash your hands.

19 Record the testing results in the patient's medical record.

Purpose: A procedure is considered not done until it is recorded.

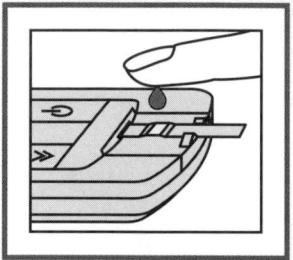

Figure 3

See Appendix E for a charting example.

About one third to one fourth of blood cholesterol is carried by high-density lipoprotein (HDL). HDL cholesterol is known as the "good" cholesterol because a high level of HDL cholesterol seems to protect against heart attack. Medical experts think that HDL tends to carry cholesterol away from the arteries and back to the liver, where it is passed from the body. Some experts believe that excess cholesterol is removed from atherosclerotic plaque by HDL, thus slowing the buildup; however, low HDL cholesterol levels (i.e., lower than 35 mg/dl) may result in a greater risk for heart disease.

It is recommended that adults over the age of 20 have a cholesterol test at least once every 5 years. Total cholesterol, the combination of HDL and LDL, is typically measured (Procedure 51-12); however, the physician may order an HDL determination separately. Both tests are considered screening tests, and elevated results always require additional testing before a diagnosis can be made. In general, total cholesterol levels under 200 mg/dl are considered normal. Results over 240 mg/dl are considered elevated and, based on confirmed testing, place a person in the high-risk category of coronary heart disease. An HDL cholesterol level of 35 mg/dl is considered acceptable. Values below 35 mg/dl place one in a high-risk category.

The total cholesterol and HDL cholesterol are not significantly affected by food consumption; so fasting is not necessary before testing. The physician, however, may request fasting in preparation. If the total cholesterol is elevated, the physician is likely to order a lipid profile, a series of tests that measures total cholesterol, triglycerides, and HDL and LDL cholesterol levels. Triglyceride levels are affected by food consumption, and the patient must be instructed to fast before the test.

Hemoglobin A1C

During the last two decades, diabetes researchers have developed several new laboratory tests that help in the evaluation of blood glucose levels. These tests measure *glycohemoglobin, fructosamine,* and *glycosylated protein*. These tests are not substitutes for monitoring blood glucose levels. Instead, they give different information about the diabetic's health and add a new dimension to the evaluation of diabetes.

The glycohemoglobin test was developed in the late 1970s. Other names that have been used to describe the same test are glycosylated hemoglobin and hemoglobin A1c. This test gives information about the average blood sugar level during the past 2 or 3 months. In the blood, glucose binds irreversibly to hemoglobin molecules within RBCs. The amount of glucose that is bound to hemoglobin is directly tied to the concentration of glucose in the blood.

Because RBCs have a life span of approximately 90 days, measuring the amount of glucose bound to hemoglobin can provide an assessment of average blood sugar control during the 60 to 90 days preceding the test. This is the purpose of the glycohemoglobin tests, most commonly the hemoglobin A1c (HbA1c) measurement. Because the test results give feedback on the previous 2 to 3 months, getting an HbA1c test done every 3 months will provide data on the average blood glucose level. If the glycohemoglobin value is higher

PROCEDURE **51-12**

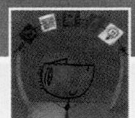

Determining Cholesterol Level Using a ProAct Testing Device

GOAL: To perform and report accurately a ProAct test for cholesterol level.

EQUIPMENT AND SUPPLIES

- ProAct testing device
- Lithium heparin capillary tube and capillary pipette
- Lancets and lancet device
- Sterile gauze
- Alcohol preps
- Biohazard waste container
- Biohazard sharps container

PROCEDURAL STEPS

1 Reread the physician's order, and assemble all the supplies and equipment needed to complete the test.

2 Wash your hands and put on gloves.
Purpose: Infection control.

3 Explain the procedure to the patient.

4 Load the lancet device with a sterile lancet.

5 Examine the patient's index and ring fingers and pick a puncture site.
Purpose: Puncture site must be free of trauma.

6 Cleanse the chosen puncture site with alcohol and allow the site to air-dry.

7 Puncture the site and wipe away the first drop of blood with a sterile gauze square.
Purpose: The first drop of blood may contain tissue fluid.

8 Hold the capillary tube horizontally by the colored end of the tube, and allow the tube to fill. Do not allow air bubbles to enter the tube; if this occurs, discard the capillary tube, and continue drawing the sample with a new tube.
Purpose: Air bubbles may cause erroneous test results.

9 Give the patient a clean gauze square, and ask the patient to apply pressure to the puncture site.

10 Remove a cholesterol testing strip from the container and close the container immediately (Figure 1*).
Purpose: Closing the container will avoid possible exposure of the unused strips.

11 Remove the foil protecting the test area of the strip, and place the strip on a dry, hard, flat surface (Figure 2).

12 Attach the capillary tube filled with blood to the pipette.

13 Squeeze the plunger of the pipette completely to allow a drop of blood to form at the end of the capillary tube.

14 Allow the drop of blood to fall onto the center of the red mesh application zone. Make sure that the tip of the capillary tube does not touch the test strip and that all blood is dispensed (Figure 3).
Purpose: Strip must be saturated with blood to obtain best testing results.

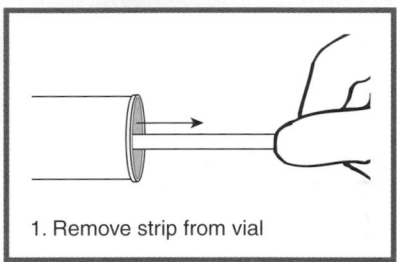

1. Remove strip from vial

Figure 1

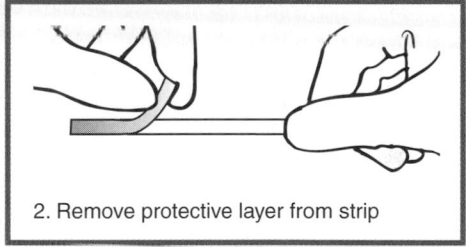

2. Remove protective layer from strip

Figure 2

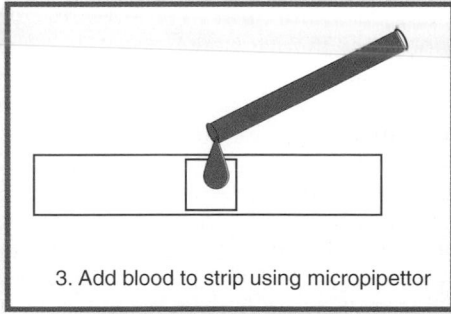

3. Add blood to strip using micropipettor

Figure 3

---

*Figure from Stepp CA, Woods MA: *Laboratory procedures for medical office personnel.* Philadelphia, 1998, WB Saunders.

Continued

PROCEDURE 51-12—cont'd

15 Allow the sample to soak into the red mesh for 3 to 15 seconds.

16 Insert the cholesterol strip into the test port. The ProAct device will count down approximately 160 seconds (Figure 4).

17 Remove the capillary tube from the pipette and discard it in a biohazard container.
Purpose: Infection control.

18 When the measurement time is completed, REMOVE STRIP will appear in the LED display window. Remove the used test strip and the test result will appear on the display (Figure 5).

19 Examine the test area of the used testing strip for

uneven color development before discarding it into the biohazard waste container.
Purpose: If the color appears mottled, the test may not be valid and it is advisable that you repeat the entire testing process.

20 Discard all biohazard testing waste in appropriate containers, clean the testing area, remove gloves, and wash your hands.
Purpose: Infection control.

21 Record the test results in the patient's medical record.
Purpose: A procedure is not considered done until it is recorded.

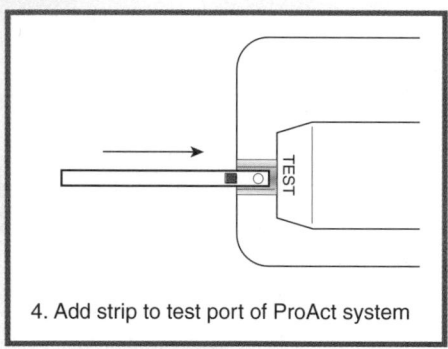

4. Add strip to test port of ProAct system

Figure 4

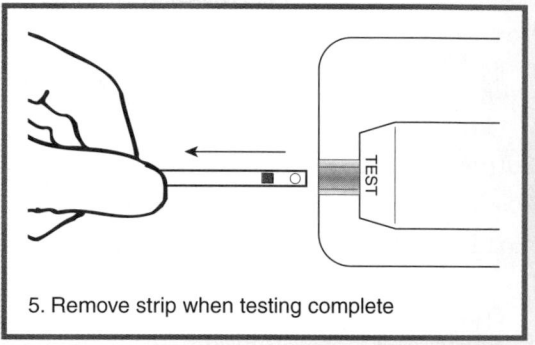

5. Remove strip when testing complete

Figure 5

than the normal range, we know that the average blood sugar has been elevated during the past 2 months.

There are several methods of performing an HbA1c measurement, and the medical assistant can perform HbA1c testing using several CLIA-waived devices. The DCA 2000, made by Bayer Diagnostics, provides HbA1c values in 6 minutes from one drop of capillary blood obtained via a finger stick. Patients can also perform HbA1c testing at home using FDA-approved instrumentation including the A1cNow by Metrika (Sunnyvale, CA) and the A1c At Home by FlexSite Diagnostics (Palm City, FL).

The fructosamine test was developed more recently. *Fructosamine* is a term that refers to the linking of blood sugar onto protein molecules in the bloodstream. Fructosamine levels change more rapidly than glycohemoglobin does. The fructosamine value depends on your average blood sugar level during the past 3 weeks. Therefore it might be able to detect changes in diabetic control earlier than the glycohemoglobin. The fructosamine test could be viewed as complementary to the glycohemoglobin because the two tests are different reflections of diabetes control: glycohemoglobin looks back about 8 weeks, and the fructosamine test looks back about 3 weeks.

Other tests similar to the fructosamine test have been proposed; the glycosylated protein test is an example of

another test that was suggested. Unfortunately, these newer tests are less reliable than originally hoped, and it seems unlikely that either the fructosamine test or the glycosylated protein test will ever become as widely used for monitoring diabetes as the glycohemoglobin level test.

CRITICAL THINKING APPLICATION

Mr. Corrigan routinely monitors his blood sugar. Why is Dr. Fischbach also interested in his hemoglobin A1c levels? What complications of diabetes led to Mr. Corrigan's need for a transplant?

Chemistry Panels

Automated blood chemistry analyzers are often used to perform blood chemistry testing. It is not uncommon for several analytes to be detected at once. A physician may order a chemistry panel, such as a renal or liver panel, that will determine the levels of several related analytes (Figure 51-17). Analytes commonly detected in the chemistry laboratory are listed in Table 51-7. Generally, serum is needed for these tests. Typical panels are shown in Table 51-8.

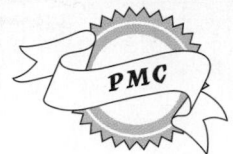

PHYSICIAN'S MEDICAL CENTER
77332 E. CAPITAL DRIVE
ANYTOWN, USA 11123

Ronald J. Haldor M. D.
Kaye M. Jones M. D.
Nicholas C. Stepp M. D.

PATIENT – PLEASE NOTE

If this box is checked, don't eat or drink anything, except water, for 14 hours before going to the lab.

PATIENT NAME _____
LAST _____ FIRST _____ M.I.

ADDRESS _____ DOB _____

CITY _____ STATE _____ ZIP _____ SEX: M F

TELEPHONE # _____ SOCIAL SECURITY # ___ - ___ - ___

ORDERING PHYSICIAN _____ DATE _____

BILLING: ☐ HMO ☐ MEDICARE ☐ MEDI-CAL ☐ OTHER # _____
(Please attach copy of eligibilty card.)
GUARANTOR (If other than patient) _____

☐ PHONE RESULTS TO _____

☐ SEND ADDITIONAL COPIES OF REPORT TO _____

Patient Diagnosis _____

☐ 906 ARTERIAL BLOOD GASES
  ROOM AIR _____
  RESP. ASSIST _____
☐ 105 BLOOD CELL PROFILE (Hgb + Hct)
☐ 862 BILIRUBIN (NEONATAL)
☐ 868 BILIRUBIN (TOTAL & DIRECT)
☐ 100 CBC (Complete Blood Count & Diff)
☐ 3000 ELECTROLYTES
☐   (NA, K, CO2, Cl)
☐   FANA
☐   GLUCOSE
☐ 915 GLUCOSE, PRE-NATAL DIABETIC SCR.
  (1 Hour Post-Glucola)
☐   GLUCOSE TOLERANCE TEST
  # OF HOURS _____ DOSE _____
☐ 3398 HEPATITIS PANEL
  (B-Surf Ag/Ab, B-Core Ab, A-Ab)
☐ 988 LIPID PROFILE
  (Chol, Trig, HDL, LDL, Cardiac Risk)
☐ 3380 LIVER PANEL
  (Alk Phos, Bili, TP, Alb, GGT, SGOT (AST)
  SGPT (ALT), & Consult)
☐ 3006 METABOLIC 7
  (Na, K, CO2, Cl, Glu, Mg)

☐ 3035 PANEL 17
  (Panel 13 + Na + K + Cl + CO2)
☐ 3020 METABOLIC 10
  (Na, K, CO2, Cl, Glu, BUN, Creat)
☐ 3015 METABOLIC 11
  (Met 10 & Phos)
☐ 3160 OBSTETRICAL PANEL 1
  (CBC, UA, ABO/Rh, Antibody Screen,
  Rubella, RPR)
☐ 3172 OBSTETRICAL PANEL 3
  (CBC, ABO/Rh, Antibody Screen,
  Rubella, RPR)
☐ 3445 OBSTETRICAL PANEL 7
  (ABO/Rh, Antibody Screen, Rubella,
  RPR)
☐ 3447 OBSTETRICAL PANEL 7A
  (ABO/Rh, Antibody Screen, Rubella,
  RPR, Hepatitis B Surt Ag)
☐ 3025 PANEL 13
  (Glu, BUN, Creat, Uric Acid, Ca, Tp,
  Alb, Bili, Chol, Alk, Phos, SGOT (AST),
  LDH, Phos)
☐ 3030 PANEL 15
  (Panel 13 + Na + K)

☐ 3010 METABOLIC 8
  (Na, K, CO2, Cl, Glu, BUN)
☐ 3040 PANEL 20 - SMAC
  (Panel 17 + SGPT (ALT) + GGT +
  Osmolality)
☐ 3043 S-1 Panel (Panel 20 + Triglyceride)
☐ 500 PROTHROMBIN TIME (PT)
☐ 505 Partial Thromboplastin Time (PPT)
☐ 7500 RPR
☐ 7515 RUBELLA
☐ 2030 THYROID SCREEN
  (T4, T3, Uptake, Adj T4)
☐ 704 URINALYSIS

BACTERIOLOGY

SPECIMEN SOURCE **(REQUIRED)**
_____
COLLECTION DATE _____
☐ _____ ROUTINE CULTURE
☐ 8919 AFB CULTURE
☐ 8921 FUNGAL CULTURE

ADDITIONAL LABORATORY TESTS:

2804 (4/93)

LABORATORY OUTPATIENT REQUEST

OFFICE USE ONLY

Telephone Order per _____

Order Received by _____

FIGURE 51-17 Panel request form. (From Stepp CA, Woods MA: *Laboratory procedures for medical office personnel*, Philadelphia, 1998, WB Saunders, p 186.)

CRITICAL THINKING APPLICATION

What tests are routinely done as part of the renal panel? What information will these tests give Dr. Fischbach regarding the status of Mr. Corrigan's kidney?

Toxicology

Toxicology is the study of poisonous substances and their effects on the body. The toxicology laboratory will perform testing on body fluids and tissues to monitor therapeutic drugs such as digoxin (a cardiac medication) and theophylline (an asthma medication) or to

detect poisonings by herbicides, metals, animal toxins, and poisonous gases (such as carbon monoxide).

Laboratory testing for illegal drugs or alcohol is also done. It is most commonly done as an employment, insurance, or government requirement. Although serum (blood) testing is a more accurate test for determining current impairment or time of ingestion, urine is the specimen of choice for most routine screening.

Urine Drug Screening. For routine screening, a random specimen is usually collected. Often, there are safeguards to ensure that a specimen is fresh and truly from the patient. In some cases, a strict chain of custody is required (see Chapter 49). The substance being tested for, or its **metabolite**, often remains in urine much longer than the impairment or intoxication lasts. This is one reason that urine screening is favored

TABLE 51-7	Blood Chemistry Tests			
Test	**Abbreviation**	**Normal Values**	**Description**	**Purpose**
Alanine amino-transferase	ALT (SGPT)	< 45 U/L	Enzyme found predomi-nately in liver but also in kidney	To detect liver disease
Albumin		3.5-5.0 g/dl	Protein	To assess water
Alkaline phosphatase	ALP	20-70 U/L	Enzyme found in several tissues	To detect liver and bone disease
Aspartate amino-transferase	AST (SGOT)	< 40 U/L	Enzyme found in several tissues	To detect tissue damage
Blood urea nitrogen	BUN	7-18 mg/dl; 2.5-6.4 mmol/L	Metabolic products of protein catabolism	To detect renal disease
Calcium	CA	8.4-10.2 mg/dl; 2.1-2.6 mmol/L	Mineral	To assess parathyroid function and calcium metabolism
Chloride	Cl	98-106 mmol/L	Electrolyte	To determine acid-base and water balance
Cholesterol	CH, Chol	Total: < 200 mg/dl; < 5.18 mmol/L LDL: < 130 mg/dl; < 3.37 mmol/L HDL: > 35 mg/dl; > 0.91 mmol/L	Lipid	Screening for atherosclerosis related to heart disease
Creatine phosphokinase	CPK	Specific to testing method used	Enzyme found in several tissues	To assess the source of muscle damage (myocardial infarct)
Creatinine	creat	0.2-0.8 mg/dl	Metabolic product of protein catabolism	Screening for renal function
Ferritin		20-50 ng/ml	Iron-carrying protein	To detect the amount of iron stored in the body
Gamma glutamyl-transferase	GGT	0-45 U/L	Enzyme found mainly in liver cells	To detect liver disease
Globulin	glob, Ig	Varies according to type	Protein	To detect abnormalities in protein synthesis and removal
Glucose fasting blood sugar	FBS	70-100 mg/dl; 3.9-6.1 mmol/L	Carbohydrate	To detect disorders of glucose metabolism (diabetes)
Glucose tolerance test	GTT	Varies with time	Carbohydrate	To detect disorders of glucose metabolism (diabetes)
Iron	Fe	35-140 µg/dl	Mineral	To assist in diagnosis of anemia
Lactate dehydrogenase	LDH	< 240 U/L	Enzyme found in several tissues	To assist in the confirmation of myocardial or pulmonary infarct
pH	pH	7.35-7.45		To assess acid
Phosphorus	P	3.0-4.5 mg/dl; 0.97-1.45 mmol/L	Mineral	To assist in the proper evaluation of calcium levels and to detect disorders of the endocrine system

TABLE 51-7	Blood Chemistry Tests—cont'd			
Test	**Abbreviation**	**Normal Values**	**Description**	**Purpose**
Potassium	K	3.5-5.1 mmol/L	Mineral	To assist in diagnosis of acid-base and water balance
Sodium	Na	135-146 mmol/L	Mineral	To assist in diagnosis of acid-base and water balance
Total bilirubin	TB	0.2-1.0 mg/dl; 3.4-17.1 mmol/L	Metabolic product of hemoglobin catabolism	To evaluate liver function and to aid in diagnosis of anemia
Total iron binding capacity	TIBC	245-400 µg/dl		A measure of the potential to transport iron
Total protein	TP	6.0-8.0 g/dl; 60-80 g/L		To assess the state of hydration; to screen for diseases that alter protein balance
Troponin I and T		< 0.4	A cardiac specific protein only found in heart muscle damage	To aid in diagnosis of myocardial infarct
Thyroid stimulating hormone (thyrotropin)	TSH	5-6 milliU/L	Hormone produced by the pituitary	To assess thyroid and pituitary gland function
Thyroxine	T_4	5-12 µg/dl; 64-155 mmol/L	Hormone produced by the thyroid gland	To assess thyroid function
Triglycerides	Trig	30-190 mg/dl; 0.34-2.15 mmol/L		Screening for atherosclerosis related to heart disease
Triiodothyronine	T_3	27-47%	Hormone produced by the thyroid gland	To assess thyroid function
Uric acid	UA	*Male:* 3.4-7.0 mg/dl; 202-416 µmol/L *Female:* 2.4-6.0 mg/dl; 143-357 µmol/L	Metabolic product of protein catabolism	To evaluate renal failure, gout, and leukemia

over serum or blood screening. Some common drug screening tests along with their "maximum detection times" are listed in Table 51-9.

As a medical assistant, you may be responsible for the collection of specimens for toxicology tests. CLIA-waived tests include a saliva alcohol test manufactured by STC Technologies (Bethlehem, PA), which uses a Dacron swab saturated with saliva to detect ethanol. The test is used primarily for workplace testing, most publicly for federally mandated testing of transportation workers but also in private company "drug-free workplace" programs.

The QuickScreen At Home Drug Test is the first rapid drug test kit cleared by the FDA for home use and is also CLIA waived. It is manufactured by Pharmatech (San Diego, CA) and detects amphetamines, methamphetamines, marijuana, cocaine, and opiates. The kit includes a rapid drug-screening device, a wide-mouth collection container, easy-to-read instructions, a handbook with frequently asked questions, and all the materials needed to ship the sample to the laboratory if the screening device indicates the presence of drugs in the sample.

The rapid drug-screening device resembles a credit card in size and shape. It is dipped into a urine sample. The results are read in 10 minutes. "Negative" results indicate that none of the targeted drugs was detected in the urine sample; "inconclusive" results indicate that the device reacted with something in the urine and confirmation testing is required.

TABLE 51-8	Typical Chemistry Panels
Panel	**Component**
Liver	Alkaline phosphatase (ALP) Gamma glutamyltransferase (GGT) Aspartate aminotransferase (AST) Alanine aminotransferase (ALT) Lactate dehydrogenase (LDH)
Anemia	Iron Total iron binding capacity Ferritin Transferrin
Thyroid	Thyroid-stimulating hormone (TSH) Thyroxine (T_4) Triiodothyronine (T_3)
Cardiac	Creatinine phosphokinase (CPK) Troponin I Troponin T
Electrolyte	Sodium Potassium Chloride
Renal	Creatinine Blood urea nitrogen Uric acid Glucose

TABLE 51-9	Commonly Abused Drugs and Body Retention Times
Drug Maximum	**Detection Time**
Alcohol	2-10 hr
Amphetamine	24-48 hr
Barbiturates	
Phenobarbital	2-6 wk (phenobarbital)
Secobarbital	24 hr (secobarbital)
Benzodiazepines (valium class drugs)	3 days to 6 wk (depends on usage)
Cocaine/cocaine metabolites	1 hr to 4 days
Opiates/heroin/morphine	1-2 days
Methadone	2-3 days
Methaqualone	8 days
Phencyclidine (PCP)	1-8 days
Propoxyphene metabolites	6-48 hr
Tetrahydrocannabinol metabolites (THC)	2 days to 11 wk

CRITICAL THINKING APPLICATION

Dr. Fischbach's suspicions of anemia were confirmed. Explain what Dana most likely observed when performing the complete blood cell count (CBC), the differential, and the anemia panel.

Patient Education

Depending on the type of medical office you work in, you may never have the occasion to assist with the procedures discussed in this chapter; however, you will likely be present when patients are advised that these tests are necessary, and so you may be placed in a position to answer a patient's questions about these procedures. By fully understanding the methods used and the testing processes, you will be able to help the patient gain an understanding of the procedures and to offer reassurance. It is important to remember that through knowledge comes acceptance and understanding.

Legal and Ethical Issues

In 1991, many states adopted the Blood Safety Act, which requires physicians to provide patients with information concerning blood transfusion options. This information is given before surgery and before any medical procedure in which there is a possibility that blood transfusion may be necessary. Physicians are also required to note on each patient's medical record that a written summary was given to the patient. As the physician's agent, you share this responsibility. If this is needed for a particular patient, it is the responsibility of every member of the health care team to ensure that this information is supplied to the patient, noted on the chart, and initialed. The written summary has been formally prepared, and copies of it can be requested from the state department of health services.

Be sure to follow the procedures established by your employer and the regulations of your state. If a blood sample drawn is for drug level studies, serology evaluations, or human immunodeficiency virus determinations, the procedure must be performed exactly as the law dictates. Courts of law require absolute adherence to procedures and complete and exact documentation of the chain of events for collecting, handling, and analyzing specimens. Skin preparation for a blood alcohol level test must be done with povidone-iodine (Betadine) rather than alcohol because using alcohol could falsely elevate the blood alcohol level. Many states have statutes that specify exactly how, when, and under what circumstances this testing can be done. You can find out about the regulations for your state by requesting a copy of the legislation from the state hospital association, the state police headquarters, or a state congressman.

SUMMARY OF SCENARIO

Dana knows the important role laboratory analysis of blood plays in patient care. She remains vigilant in both the proper collection of blood specimens and in the reporting and charting of the results. Her job as a medical assistant, she knows, is not without danger. She is exposed to biological and chemical hazards every day but she is confident that the knowledge she gained in school and also in obtaining continuing medical education credit will help her to make safe decisions.

SUMMARY OF LEARNING OBJECTIVES

- Blood supplies cells with needed nutrients, delivers oxygen to tissues via hemoglobin, and removes waste.

- In the hematology laboratory, blood cells are enumerated, WBCs are differentiated, and the oxygen-carrying capacity of blood is determined.

- Red blood cells are also known as erythrocytes because of their red color, which comes from hemoglobin. The biconcave disks lack a nucleus and are responsible for transporting oxygen and carbon dioxide to and from tissues.

- White blood cells are also known as leukocytes. Agranular leukocytes lack granules in the cytoplasm and granular leukocytes have granules. All leukocytes function in fighting infection.

- T lymphocytes are important in immunity and play roles in killing foreign, virus-infected, and tumor cells; assist in antibody production; and keep the immune system in check.

- B cells are responsible for antibody production.

- The thrombocyte, also known as a platelet, is a fragment of a larger cell found in the bone marrow called a megakaryocyte. Thrombocytes play an important role in clot formation, both physically and chemically.

- Clot formation begins with the aggregation of thrombocytes, which release a substance that initiates the clotting cascade, resulting in a network of minute threads that trap plasma and blood cells.

- The anticoagulant required for most hematology testing is ethylenediamine tetraacetic acid (EDTA). The lavender-topped vacuum tube used in phlebotomy contains this anticoagulant.

- The microhematocrit (or hematocrit) test is performed to assess the volume of erythrocytes in relationship to total blood volume by centrifuging a small amount of whole blood in a capillary tube. Whole blood normally consists of slightly less than 50% RBCs. Hematocrit is reported as a percentage and is roughly three times that of hemoglobin.

- Hemoglobin is the RBC protein responsible for oxygen transport from the lungs to the tissues. It gives the blood its red color.

- The complete blood count, or CBC, involves an erythrocyte count, a leukocyte count, a thrombocyte count, a hemoglobin and hematocrit determination, a differential examination of leukocytes, and calculation of red cell indices.

- Enumeration of blood cells and thrombocytes can be done manually using a device called a hemocytometer. Diluted blood samples are placed under the coverslip of the device, observed with a microscope, and counted.

- A manual WBC count uses a diluting device called a Unopette. The diluting fluid contains acetic acid that lyses red cells, making the white cells easier to count. Automated counts are performed with a device that detects cells with either a laser beam or an electrical impulse.

- A manual RBC count uses a diluting device called a Unopette. Automated counts are performed with a device that detects cells with either a laser beam or an electrical impulse.

- Red blood cell indices are calculated using values obtained from the CBC, namely the RBC count, hemoglobin, and hematocrit. They assist the physician in diagnosing blood disorders such as anemia.

- A differential WBC count is performed to assess the numbers and types of WBCs in the blood. A thin smear of whole blood is stained typically with Wright's stain and examined microscopically. In addition, the red cells and platelets are examined for distribution and abnormalities.

- Typical leukocytes seen in the differential examination include the segmented neutrophil, which has a segmented blue nucleus and lavender granules in the cytoplasm; the eosinophil, which appears similar to the neutrophil but has orange granules; the basophil, which appears similar to the neutrophil but has blue-black granules; the lymphocyte, which is a smaller cell with a light blue cytoplasm and large dark blue nucleus; and the monocyte, the largest cell, which has a cerebriform blue nucleus and a light blue cytoplasm that appears to have bubble-like inclusions.

- A normal erythrocyte is circular, evenly stained red-purple, and appears to have a hole or depression in the center.

- An ESR test is performed to assess inflammation and is often used to monitor rheumatoid arthritis. This test measures the rate at which RBCs fall in a calibrated tube in a 60-minute period.

- A prothombin time (protime) and partial thromboplastin time are the most commonly performed tests to assess coagulation capacity. The protime is also routinely performed to assess a patient's response to anticlotting drugs such as warfarin (Coumadin).

- Either antigens or antibodies can be detected in blood serum. This testing, done in the immunology (serology) laboratory, may involve agglutination, precipitation, or enzyme immunoassay.

- Infectious mononucleosis is caused by the Epstein-Barr virus and usually afflicts young adults. Signs and symptoms include fatigue, sore throat, lymphadenopathy, an increased lymphocyte count, and a decreased total WBC count.

- The test for infectious mononucleosis detects heterophile antibodies, which are nonspecific antibodies produced by the immune system when a person is infected with the Epstein-Barr virus. In the physician's office laboratory, infectious mononucleosis is detected either with an agglutination test or with a solid-phase immunoassay.

- Both the ABO blood group and the Rh group result from antigens on the surfaces of RBCs, and both are crucial when it comes to transfusion. There are four different ABO types (A, AB, B, and O) but only two Rh types (positive and negative). Corresponding antibodies are present in the blood for the ABO type (anti-A antibody is found in type B and type O blood, for example), corresponding antibodies are not normally found in the Rh system.

- Blood glucose is monitored routinely in both type 1 and type 2 diabetes and also in women who are experiencing gestational diabetes during pregnancy.

- Cholesterol testing generally refers to assessing levels of HDL cholesterol and LDL cholesterol; it is done to assist in determining one's susceptibility to coronary artery disease.

- Hemoglobin A1C levels are tested to determine average blood glucose level during a 2- to 3-month period before the test is done and assists in management of diabetes.

■ Often clinical chemistry tests are performed in groups called panels. Certain tests that provide information on a disease or syndrome are grouped together. A liver panel, for example, will detect abnormalities in a number of different liver enzymes.

■ Toxicology testing is done to assess levels of drugs or toxins in the body. The drugs can be either therapeutic or illegal. Some employers require workplace drug and alcohol testing on a routine basis.

■ It is essential that strict patient confidentiality be upheld when performing any laboratory testing.

KEY INTERNET WEBSITES

- American Association for Clinical Chemistry
- American Association of Blood Banks
- American Diabetes Association
- American Society of Hematology
- The National Institute of Diabetes & Digestive & Kidney Diseases
  For active weblinks to each website visit
  http://evolve.elsevier.com/Kinn/

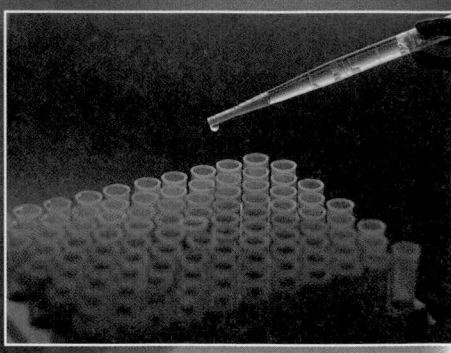

CHAPTER 52

Scenario

Anna McIntyre is a CMA working in a busy family clinic and is responsible for collection and preparation of specimens for transport to a referral laboratory. Anna also receives results over the telephone and transcribes them onto the patients' charts. While most microbiology testing ordered by the physicians in the clinic is sent to a referral laboratory, some tests are performed at the clinic.

Assisting in Microbiology

Robin R. Patterson

Learning Objectives

- Define and spell the terms listed in the vocabulary.
- Cite the protocols for specimen collection.
- Identify the elements needed for microbial growth.
- Describe the bacterial structures used in identification.
- Compare bacteria with viruses.
- Compare bacteria with fungi, parasites, and protozoa.
- Describe the unusual characteristics of chlamydia, rickettsia, and mycoplasma.
- Draw various bacterial morphologies.
- Describe the equipment needed in a microbiology laboratory.
- Describe the different growth media used for culturing.
- List the steps of the Gram's stain.
- Compare rapid culture with standard culture growth methods.
- Describe the method used for antimicrobial susceptibility testing.
- Discuss legal and ethical issues in laboratory testing.
- Prepare direct smears and indirect smears from culture.
- Examine stained smears for the presence of microorganisms.
- Identify bacterial morphologies and Gram reactions through microscopic viewing.
- Inoculate media for culture.
- Perform a rapid strep test.
- Perform a urine culture.
- Secure a collection for pinworms.

National Curriculum Competencies

CLINICAL COMPETENCIES

3a. Use methods of quality control
3f. Perform microbiology testing
3g. Screen and follow-up test results

Vocabulary

antimicrobial agent A drug that is used to treat infection.

asepsis The process of removing pathogenic microorganisms or protecting against infection by such organisms.

broad-spectrum antimicrobial agent A drug used to treat a broad range of infections.

cyst A small capsule-like sac that encloses certain organisms in their dormant or larval stage.

eukaryote A single-celled or multicellular organism whose cells contain a distinct membrane-bound nucleus.

fastidious Requiring specialized media or growth factors to grow.

in vitro Refers to conditions outside of a living body.

macromolecules The molecules needed for metabolism: carbohydrates, lipids, proteins, and nucleic acids.

molecule A group of like or different atoms held together by chemical forces.

microorganism An organism of microscopic or submicroscopic size.

nanometer One billionth (10^{-9}) of a meter.

nosocomial Pertaining to or originating in the hospital, said of an infection not present or incubating before admittance to the hospital.

organelle A differentiated structure within a cell, such as a mitochondrion, vacuole, or chloroplast, that performs a specific function.

pathogen An agent that causes disease, especially a living microorganism, such as a bacterium or fungus.

prokaryote A unicellular organism having cells that lack a membrane-bound nucleus.

pure culture A bacterial or fungal culture that contains a single organism.

specimen A sample, as of tissue, blood, or urine, used for analysis and diagnosis.

tissue culture The technique or process of keeping tissue alive and growing in a culture medium.

transport medium A medium used to keep an organism alive during transport to the laboratory.

viable Capable of living, developing, or germinating under favorable conditions.

wet mount A slide preparation in which a drop of liquid specimen or the like is covered with a coverslip and observed with a microscope.

Microorganisms get a lot of publicity. Bioterrorism became a reality in the United States in the fall of 2001 when *Bacillus anthracis* spores sent through the mail caused anthrax, killing three people. Products line our grocery store shelves declaring their ability to keep us germ free. The evening news reports on the latest outbreaks of "flesh-eating strep," contaminated water supplies, and antibiotic-resistant microbes. No wonder most people have the impression that all microorganisms are harmful. In reality, however, fewer than 1% of known microorganisms are **pathogens**. In fact, without microorganisms, we could not survive.

Microorganisms are responsible for decomposition of waste and natural recycling. Our *normal microbiota*, those organisms present on and in our bodies, ensure that our food is digested; that our blood clots properly as a result of vitamin K production by those inhabiting our intestines; and that pathogens are prohibited from invading our skin, mucous membranes, and gastrointestinal and genitourinary tracts. When the normal microbiota are disrupted because of antibiotic use or hormonal changes, for example, certain organisms that are present normally in low numbers will overgrow, causing a *superinfection*. Vulvovaginal candidiasis, a yeast infection of the vaginal tract, is common in women who are taking **broad-spectrum antimicrobial agents**.

As a medical assistant, you will need to understand the role of microorganisms in both health and disease. The main objective of microbiologic procedures is to identify the organisms responsible for illness so that the physician can properly treat the patient. In addition, responsibilities include preventing **nosocomial** infections and assisting with infection control in the physician's office laboratory and in the society the physician office laboratory (POL) serves. Microbiologic procedures may be performed in the POL or in the microbiology department of a medical referral laboratory.

Chapter 24 discussed the chain of infection and how it can be broken using infection control procedures such as proper handwashing techniques, the use of antiseptics and disinfectants, and sterilization methods. This chapter covers cultivation of microorganisms; detection of infecting organisms by microscopy; detection of specific products of infecting organisms using chemical, immunologic, or molecular techniques; and detection of antibodies produced by the patient in response to an infecting organism (*serodiagnosis*).

Specimen Collection and Transport

Specimen collection and handling are among the most critical considerations in patient care because any results the laboratory generates are directly dependent on the quality of the specimen and its condition on arrival in the laboratory. Specimens for microbiology testing must be collected in such a way as to prevent the introduction of any contaminating microorganisms. This means not only using special sterile collection and transport devices and taking steps to prevent environmental contamination but also making efforts to eliminate or limit normal microbiota from the patient. Such steps include use of antiseptics on the skin before blood or cerebrospinal fluid collection, instructing a patient in the collection of a urine sample using the clean-catch midstream (CCMS) technique (see Chapter 49), or a process as simple as avoiding the mouth and tongue when collecting a throat culture swab.

When collecting specimens for microbiological analysis, the medical assistant should always ask herself or himself two questions: "In what ways can I prevent extraneous microorganisms from contaminating this sample?" and "What can I do to prevent myself from becoming infected while I collect this sample?" Answers to the first question include cleansing the area to be sampled with an antiseptic, opening sterile containers only when necessary, and never touching a sterile swab or collection device to a nonsterile surface. Answers to the second question include wearing a disposable surgical mask while collecting a throat or sputum culture, wearing gloves when receiving a urine specimen from a patient who has just voided, and working with collected specimens in an approved biological hood or cabinet (discussed in Chapter 46).

Ideally, specimens should be collected during the acute phase of an illness and before antibiotics are prescribed. Many types of samples can be collected. Physicians and physician assistants may collect tissue samples or body fluids by needle aspiration. Sterile swabs can be used to collect samples from wounds, the genital tract, and the upper respiratory tract, for example. Serum or whole blood can be used in indirect detection of infection organisms. Urine and feces can be collected in containers by patients at home. The commonality among all specimens collected for microbiology testing is clear instructions for collection. The referral laboratory is responsible for providing a manual of written instructions to the POL, and the POL is responsible for providing clear instructions (preferably written) to the patient, especially if the patient will be collecting the sample in privacy or at home.

Transport of specimens is also crucial. Many different types of transport devices exist, and close attention must be given to their proper use. Microorganisms are living organisms and must be provided with conditions that permit their survival but do not permit their multiplication. If microorganisms are allowed to multiply after their collection, the culture results would not reflect the true disease state. Specialized **transport media**, such as modified Stuart's medium or Amie's medium, are often used in the swabbing devices used for specimen collection (Figure 52-1). These collection devices are typically made of a plastic tube that encases a sterile Dacron swab and a sealed vial of transport medium. After the specimen is obtained on the swab, it is placed in the plastic tube and the transport medium is released, usually by crushing the internal vial. It is essential that the manufacturer's directions be followed to avoid drying of the swab and specimen.

Ideally, a specimen should be transported to the laboratory and cultured immediately after collection. In most situations, however, this is not possible, and the transport device must be handled by a courier en route to a referral laboratory or held in the POL until it can be cultured. For specimens that will be transported by a courier, ensure that the specimens are safely packaged in leak-proof containers marked with warning labels (Figure 52-2). Proper temperature and time of storage are crucial. Most pathogenic organisms prefer temperatures around 37° C and will remain **viable** for up to 72 hours if held at room temperature or refrigerator temperature (4° C). Some organisms, however, will die if exposed to cold temperatures. Cultures for gonorrhea and strep throat should never be refrigerated if they cannot be plated immediately. Always refer to the referral laboratory's procedure manual for directions regarding length and temperature of storage before plating. Likewise, microorganisms have oxygen requirements; some, called *aerobes*, require oxygen to stay alive; others, called *anaerobes*, will die if exposed to oxygen. Collection devices are available for both aerobic and anaerobic collection. Table 52-1 lists the collection, transport, and storage of specimens commonly collected or handled by medical assistants. Figure 52-3 shows some commonly used collection devices.

CRITICAL THINKING APPLICATION

Aaron Mitchell, age 9, was brought in to the clinic this morning at 9:00 AM with scabbing sores on his upper lip. Dr. Chowdry suspects impetigo and orders a wound culture. How will Anna collect this culture? What device might she use? How should she store this specimen until the courier, who does not come until 3:00 PM, arrives? Anna knows that impetigo is highly contagious. How can she protect herself from becoming infected?

While preparing to collect the specimen from Aaron, Anna receives a telephone call from BioStatLab, the referral laboratory the clinic uses. The results from Ms. Tina Walker's urine culture and from Mr. Robert Livore's abscess culture are complete.

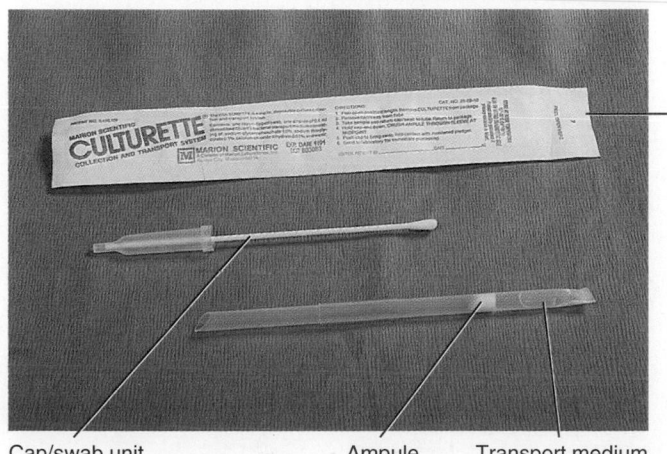

Peel-apart envelope

Cap/swab unit   Ampule   Transport medium

FIGURE 52-1 Culturette collection and transport system. (From Bonewit-West K: *Clinical procedures for medical assistants*, ed 5. Philadelphia, 2000, WB Saunders.)

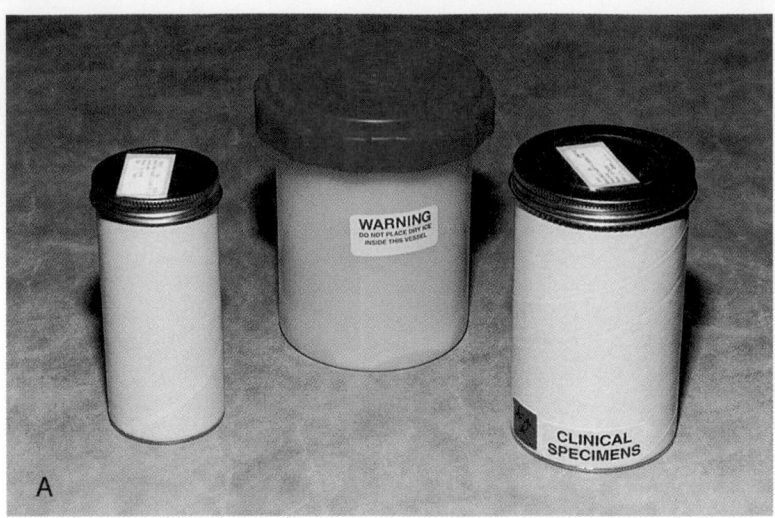
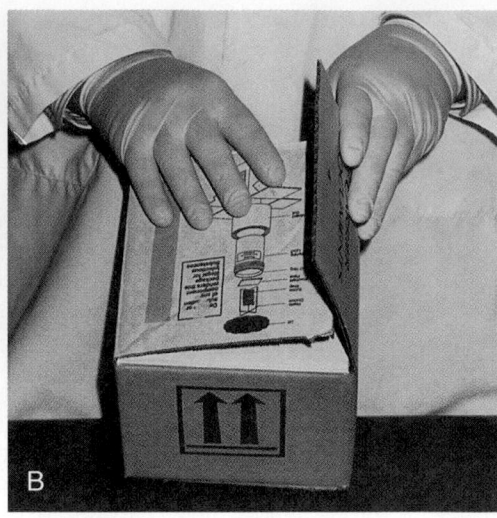

FIGURE 52-2 **A**, Appropriate containers for transport. **B**, Appropriate packaging for transport.

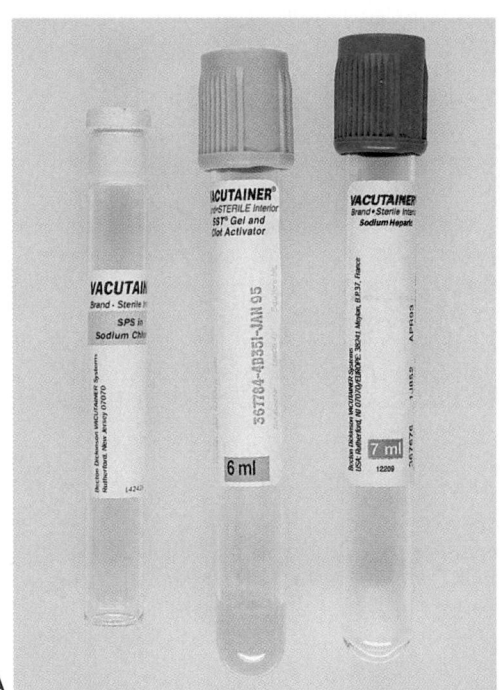
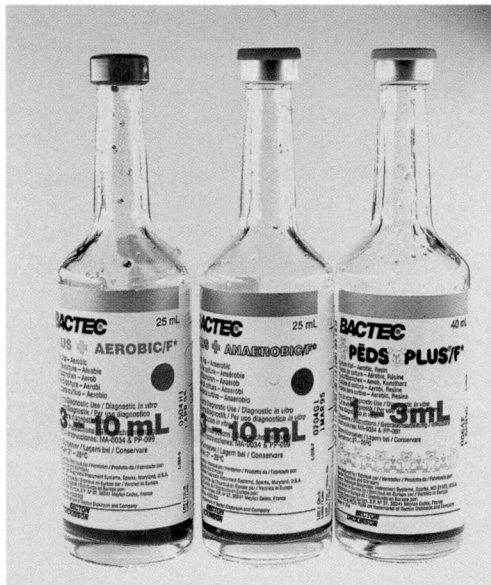
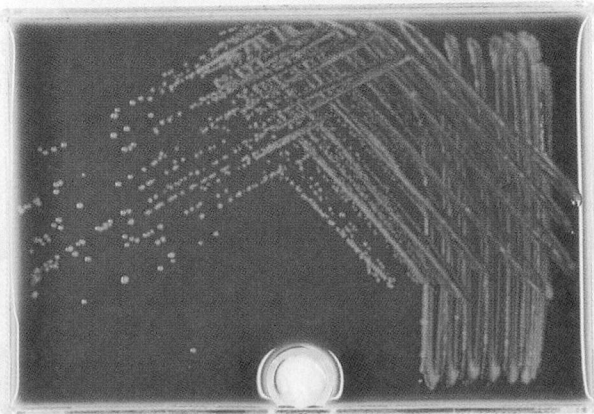

FIGURE 52-3 **A**, Blood collection Vacutainer tubes. **B**, BACTEC blood culture bottles. **C**, JEMBEC plate. (From De la Maza, Pezzlo, Baron: *Color atlas of diagnostic microbiology*. St Louis, 1997, Mosby, **A** and **B** From Becton, Dickinson and Company, Franklin Lakes, NJ; **C** From BBL Microbiology Systems, a division of Becton, Dickinson and Company, Franklin Lakes, NJ.)

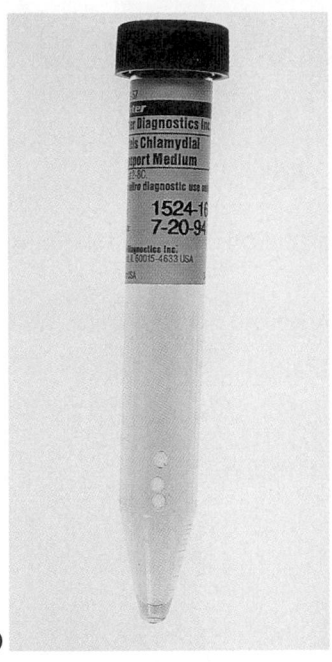

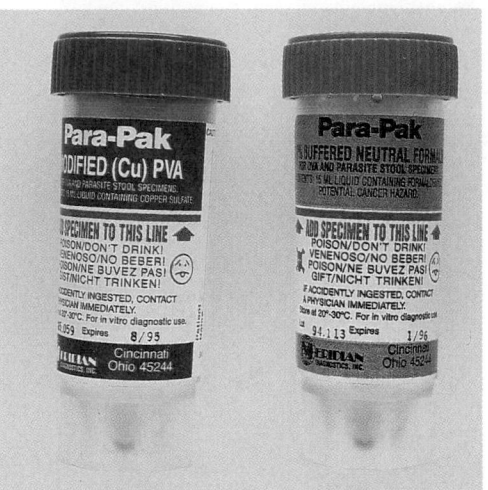

FIGURE 52-3, cont'd **D**, Viral-chlamydial transport medium. **E**, Para-Pak Parasitology Collection Kit. (From De la Maza, Pezzlo, Baron: *Color atlas of diagnostic microbiology*. St Louis, 1997, Mosby; **D** From Baxter Diagnostics, a division of Baxter Healthcare, Deerfield, Ill; **E** From Meridian Bioscience, Inc., Cincinnati, OH.)

TABLE 52-1	Collection, Transport, and Processing of Specimens Commonly Submitted to the Physician's Office Laboratory			
Specimen	**Container**	**Patient Preparation**	**Special Instructions**	**Storage Prior to Processing**
Blood	Blood culture media set or Vacutainer brand blood culture tube with SPS	Disinfect venipuncture site with alcohol swab and Betadine	Draw blood during febrile episodes; draw two sets from right and left arms	Deliver to lab within 2 hours; incubate at 37°C upon receipt in the lab
Body fluids (peritoneal, synovial, pleural, etc.)	Sterile, screw-cap container or anaerobic transporter	Disinfect aspiration site with alcohol swab and Betadine	Needle aspirations are preferable to swab collections	Transport immediately and plate specimen immediately upon receipt in the lab
Eye	Aerobic transport swab		Moisten swab with Amie's or Stuart's medium before collection	May be stored up to 24 hours at room temperature
Stool	Clean, leak-proof container		Transport to lab within 24 hours if storing at 4°C	Plate within 72 hours if storing at 4°C
Rectal swab	Swab placed directly in enteric transport medium		Insert swab approximately 2.5 cm past anal sphincter	Store at 4°C, transport within 24 hours to lab and plate within 72 hours
Gonorrhea culture	JEMBEC transport system or transport device with Stuart's or Amie's medium	Wipe away exudate prior to culture, obtain culture with swab	Do not refrigerate	Transport to lab within 2 hours
Chlamydia culture	Specialized Chlamydia transport media containing antibiotics	Urogenital swabs preferred. Necessary to obtain epithelial cells, not exudate	Transport immediately on ice to lab	Store up to 24 hours at 4°C; inoculate cultures within 15 minutes of collection if swab is not on ice
Skin scraping (fungal culture)	Clean, screw-top tube	Wipe skin with alcohol prep pad	Scrape skin at leading edge of lesion	Can be held indefinitely at room temperature but best to process within 72 hours of collection

Continued

TABLE 52-1	Collection, Transport, and Processing of Specimens Commonly Submitted to the Physician's Office Laboratory—cont'd			
Specimen	Container	Patient Preparation	Special Instructions	Storage Prior to Processing
Sputum	Sterile, screw-cap container	Patient should rinse or gargle with mouth-wash prior to collection	Have patient collect from deep cough; do not collect saliva	Store at 4°C, plate within 24 hours
Throat	Transport swab	Moisten swab with Stuart's or Amie's transport medium	Swab pharynx and tonsils, not mouth, tongue, or teeth	Transport and plate within 24 hours; room temperature storage
Ova & parasite	O&P transport device (with formalin and PVA)	Three specimens collected every other day at a minimum for outpatients	Wait 7-10 days if patient has been taking Pepto-Bismol, Kaopectate, or Milk of Magnesia	Store at room temperature and deliver to lab within 24 hours
Urine	Sterile, screw-cap container	Instruct patient on clean catch mid-stream collection	Hold at 4°C and deliver to lab within 24 hours	Hold at 4°C and plate within 24 hours
Superficial wound	Aerobic transport swab	Wipe area with sterile saline or alcohol prep pad before collection	Moisten swab with Amie's or Stuart's medium before collection	Transport and plate within 24 hours; room temperature storage
Deep wound or abscess	Anaerobic transport device	Wipe area with sterile saline or alcohol prep pad before collection	Aspirate material, excise tissue, or insert swab deep into wound	Transport and plate within 24 hours; room temperature storage

Modified from *Bailey & Scott's diagnostic microbiology*, ed 11, St. Louis, 2002, Mosby.

Classification of Microorganisms

Once the specimen reaches the microbiology laboratory, it will be analyzed for the presence of infectious microorganisms or their components. Although the medical assistant will not be responsible for identifying microorganisms, a working knowledge of the terminology used in classification of microorganisms is essential.

Most cultures handled by the medical assistant have been taken to diagnose bacterial infections. Bacteria are one type of microorganism; other microorganisms include fungi and protozoa. Parasitic worms are studied in the microbiology laboratory but are not considered microorganisms. Viruses, discussed in Chapter 24, are not considered by many microbiologists to be microorganisms simply because they are not, by definition, alive. Viruses consist of a core of either RNA or DNA covered by a protein shell. Alone, they neither metabolize nor reproduce; however, once inside a host cell, viruses use the host cell's **organelles** and **macromolecules** to multiply. Because of this absolute need for a host cell for replication, viruses are called *obligate intracellular parasites*, and they cannot be cultured on artificial media like that used to culture bacteria.

Culturing of viruses must be done in fertilized eggs or in **tissue culture** and will be done by referral or hospital laboratories. Often, instead of culturing a specimen for a virus, antigenic products of the virus or antibodies made by a patient to a virus are detected. For example, in the diagnosis of hepatitis B virus infection, the serum is tested for the presence of hepatitis B surface antigen (HBsAg), a protein found in the shell of the virus. Tables 24-1 and 52-2 list common diseases caused by viruses.

Naming of Microorganisms

Scientists have used the binomial system of nomenclature developed by Swedish botanist Carl von Linne to name all living organisms: animals, plants, fungi, protozoa, and bacteria. This binomial system assigns two names; the first name is the genus, and the second is the species. Both names are either italicized or underlined when written. The genus begins with a capital letter, the species with a lower-case letter. Often, the name reveals some characteristic about the organism. *Neisseria gonorrhoeae*, for example, is a bacterium that was studied extensively by Albert Neisser, and it causes the sexually transmitted disease gonorrhea. When reporting culture results, it is essential that both the genus and species names be recorded. Different species may cause different symptoms or require different antibiotic treatment. For example, *N. gonorrhoeae* causes disease, whereas *N. sicca* colonizes the mouth and does not, under normal conditions, cause disease.

CRITICAL THINKING APPLICATION

Anna listens carefully to the technician from the referral laboratory regarding Mr. Livore's abscess culture and jots down "Staphylococcus" on the reporting form. She pauses when the technician stops and asks what species of staph. Why is this important? What species would be considered normal microbiota, and what species is considered pathogenic?

TABLE 52-2	Common Viral Diseases				
Disease	**Virus**	**Transmission**	**Symptoms**	**Tests**	**Preventions**
Smallpox	Variola major	Direct contact; fomites	Vesicles on entire body, including soles and palms		Eradicated (vaccine is still available)
Infectious mononucleosis	Epstein-Barr virus	Direct and airborne	Sore throat, fever, malaise, lymph gland involve-ment; hepatitis, enlarged spleen	Serology testing for heterophile antibodies; CBC	Avoid direct contact with known cases
Influenza	Myxovirus —Influenza A and B	Droplet and fomites	Fever, body aches, cough		Immunization for the old, young, and debilitated
Warts (verucca)	Human papillomavirus	Direct and indirect contact	Circumscribed outgrowths on skin; most common on hands and feet		
Rabies	Rhabdovirus	Contact with saliva of infected animal (dog, cat, skunk, fox, bat are usual)	Fever, uncontrol-lable excite-ment, spasms of the throat, profuse salivation	Animal's brain tissue examined for Negri bodies	Vaccine available; vaccinate pets
Mumps	Paramyxovirus —mumpsvirus	Direct contact	Pain, swelling of salivary glands; fever	Acute and convalescent titers	MMR vaccine
Measles	Paramyxovirus —measlesvirus	Direct contact; droplets	Fever, nasal discharge, red eyes; Koplik's spots, rash	Serologic	MMR vaccine
Rubella (German measles)		Direct contact; droplets; congenital	Rash, swollen lymph glands; causes severe birth defects	Serologic	MMR vaccine
Common cold	Rhinovirus and many other	Direct; droplets, fomites	Headache, fever, runny nose, congestion		Good hygiene (hand washing)
Polio	Poliovirus	Direct contact; carriers Enter via mouth	Fever, headache, stiff neck and back, paralysis of muscles		Trivalent oral polio vaccine (TOPV)
Molluscum contagiosum warts	Molluscipox virus	Direct contact with infected individual	Small pink or white domes found in clusters	Microscopic evaluation	Avoid contact with infected individual; have existing warts removed

MMR, Measles, mumps, rubella.
Courtesy Kathleen Moody.

CRITICAL THINKING APPLICATION—cont'd

The technician also reports Ms. Walker's test results, indicating that the organism causing her urinary tract infection was identified as *Escherichia coli.* What shape is *E. coli*? How could *E. coli* have infected the urinary tract?

Typical Pathogenic Bacteria

Bacteria are single-celled **prokaryote** organisms that reproduce by binary fission, a process that involves duplication of the chromosome and subsequent fission (splitting in half) of the cell. This process of asexual reproduction results in tremendous numbers of bacteria from a single cell and explains why bacterial infections can quickly overwhelm a person's immune system and cause an infection. Some bacteria reproduce in as little as 14 minutes, whereas others take days to divide. A single *Escherichia coli* cell, which has a reproduction time of about 30 minutes, will theoretically produce 351,843,724,088,831 offspring in a 24-hour period if it has the opportunity to enter the urinary bladder.

Bacteria are often classified by their shape, staining characteristics, and the environmental conditions in which they thrive. Both shape and staining characteristics are direct results of the cell wall composition. Three types of cell wall structures exist among pathogenic bacteria: gram positive, gram negative, and acid fast. These designations are based on reactions in specialized stains used to visualize the bacteria under the microscope. The bacterial cell wall is composed of peptidoglycan (PG), a **molecule** composed of carbohydrate and protein. The gram-positive cell has a thick layer of PG with no lipid layer surrounding it, the gram-negative cell has a thin layer of PG with a lipid layer surrounding it, and the acid-fast cell has a thin layer of PG surrounded by a thick layer of wax-like lipids. Acid-fast bacteria will not stain well in the Gram's stain, and gram-positive and -negative bacteria alike stain negative in the acid-fast stain. After staining in the Gram's stain, gram-positive bacteria stain purple and gram-negative stain pink. After staining in the acid-fast stain, acid-fast-positive bacteria (AFB) stain pink and acid-fast-negative bacteria stain blue.

Bacterial Shapes. Pathogenic bacteria assume three different morphological shapes. Spherical bacteria are termed *cocci* (singular, coccus), rod-shaped bacteria are termed *bacilli* (singular, bacillus), and spiral-shaped bacteria are termed *spirilla* (singular, *spirillum*). Tightly coiled spirilla are called *spirochetes*. Certain arrangements are also seen in different genera and species. When the bacteria are in chains, the prefix *strepto-* is used. When found in pairs, the prefix *diplo-* is used, and when they are found in clusters, the prefix *staphylo-* is used. Cocci in packets of 4 are called *tetrads* and in packets of 8 or 16 are called *sarcinae* (Figure 52-4).

Bacterial Oxygen Requirements. Bacteria are also classified according to oxygen requirements. Those that require oxygen to live are called *aerobes*; those that will die in the presence of oxygen are called *anaerobes*. Some bacteria are flexible concerning oxygen requirements and, although they are anaerobes, can survive in the presence of oxygen. These organisms are termed *facultative anaerobes*. *Mycobacterium tuberculosis*, an AFB, thrives in white blood cells in the lungs, causing tuberculosis. It is an aerobe. On the other hand, *Bacteroides fragilis* is the predominant bacterium found in the intestines. This gram-negative bacillus is an anaerobe. *E. coli*, also an inhabitant of the intestines and the most common cause of urinary tract infections, is a facultative anaerobe.

Bacterial Physical Structures. Bacteria can be classified according to physical structures. Some bacteria have thin, long structures called *flagella* that aid in propulsion. *Proteus vulgaris* is a gram-negative bacillus with many flagella surrounding the cell. It is capable of propelling itself through a stream of urine as it enters the bladder and is the primary cause of nosocomial

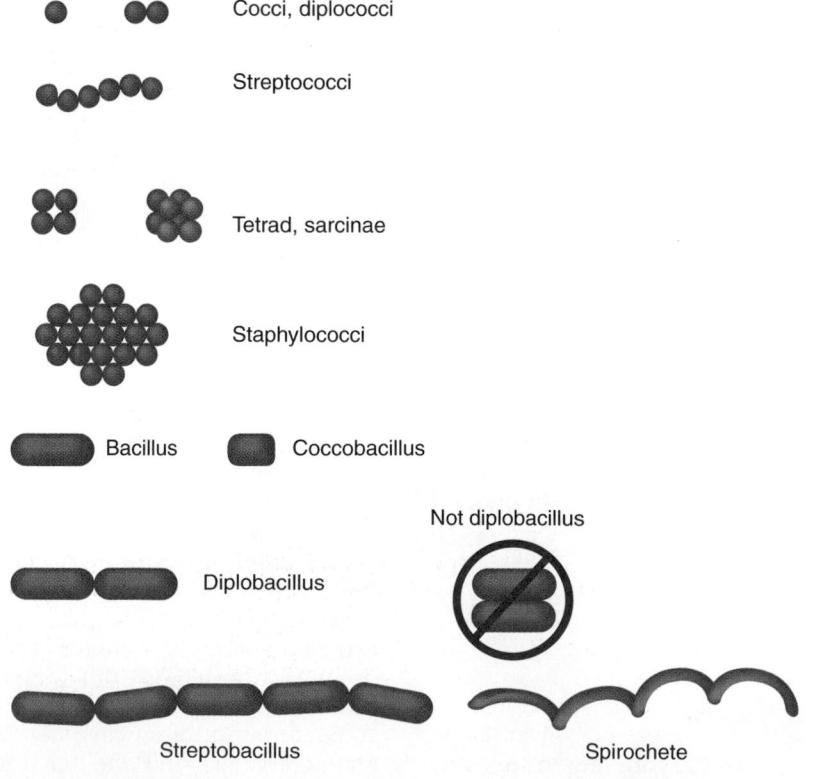

FIGURE 52-4 Typical morphological arrangements of bacteria.

urinary tract infections. Second, some bacteria may have thick gelatinous coats surrounding the cell wall called *capsules. Streptococcus pneumoniae* is nonpathogenic if it is not producing a capsule, but it is the most common cause of pneumonia in older adults when it is encapsulated. The Pneumovax vaccine, which is given to older patients to prevent pneumonia, is composed of highly purified capsular polysaccharides from 23 strains of *S. pneumoniae*. Last, certain bacteria are able to form intracellular structures called endospores that allow the cell to remain viable when environmental conditions are not favorable. *Bacillus anthracis*, mentioned in the chapter's opening paragraph, produces such spores. *Clostridium tetani* is also a spore-former. If spores of *C. tetani* enter a wound and germinate, they cause the disease known as *tetanus*. Tables 52-3 to 52-5 list some important infectious diseases caused by typical pathogenic bacteria.

Unusual Pathogenic Bacteria: *Chlamydia*, *Mycoplasma*, and *Rickettsia*

In the small scale used to measure microorganisms, viruses range between 10 and 100 **nanometers (nm)**. Typical pathogenic bacteria measure between 1000 and 5000 nm. There are tiny, unusual bacteria that fall between the size range of viruses and typical pathogenic bacteria in the genera *Chlamydia*, *Mycoplasma*, and *Rickettsia*. Classification of these organisms has posed a challenge to microbiologists.

The rickettsia are tiny gram-negative bacteria that are transmitted by blood-sucking arthropods. They cannot multiply outside of a host cell, and once inside the host cell, they are able to perform only some of the life-sustaining metabolic reactions on their own. Chlamydia are also tiny bacteria that require host cells for growth and once were considered viruses. Chlamydia, unlike rickettsia, are not transmitted by arthropod vectors.

Mycoplasma are unusual in that they have no PG cell wall, but they are not obligate parasites like rickettsia and chlamydia organisms. Rickettsia and chlamydia will not grow on artificial media in the laboratory, and **tissue culture** or serological testing is required for their identification. Mycoplasma can be cultivated from a patient specimen in the laboratory (Table 52-6).

Fungi

Mycology is the study of fungi and the diseases they cause. Fungi (singular, fungus) are **eukaryotes**, are larger than bacteria, and include the unicellular yeasts and the multicellular molds. Fungi are present in the soil, air, and water, but only a few species cause disease. They are transmitted by direct contact with infected persons, by prolonged exposure to a moist environment, or by inhalation of contaminated dust or soil. Fungal infections may be superficial, affecting only the skin, hair, or nails. Some fungi, however, can penetrate the tissues of the internal body structures and produce serious diseases of the mucous membranes, heart, lungs, and other organs. Fungal infections are resistant to antibiotics used in the treatment of bacterial infections

and must be treated with drugs active against the unusual cell walls of this organism.

A superficial fungal infection is often referred to as a *tinea* (Latin for "ringworm"). Tinea pedis, for example, is athlete's foot; tinea barbae is a fungal infection of the facial hair follicles. The term *ringworm* arose because the infected area is often circular and appears wrinkled in the center as a result of the healing process. Diagnosis of fungal infections can be tedious and is usually based on culturing or microscopic observation of skin scrapings, hair samples, or samples of sputum or mucous membranes. Usually, the samples are treated with potassium hydroxide before microscopic observation to digest away nonfungal material (Table 52-7).

CRITICAL THINKING APPLICATION

Anna notes that it has been 2 weeks since Mr. Livore's culture was sent to the referral laboratory. When the technician tells her that in addition to *Staphylococcus epidermidis*, the culture was positive for the fungus *Sporothrix schenckii*, she understands why it has taken so long. Explain why Anna knows this.

The technician does not provide a list of antimicrobic agents that would be acceptable to treat the infection like she usually does, but Anna is not concerned. Why not? Why would the physician not treat the *S. epidermidis* in Mr. Livore's abscess?

Parasites

Parasitology includes the study of all parasitic organisms that live on or in the human body. In parasitic relationships, the host is harmed as the parasite thrives. Parasites are transmitted by ingestion during the infective stage, direct penetration of the skin by infective **larvae**, and inoculation by an arthropod vector. It is not possible to identify a parasite accurately on the basis of a single test or specimen. Most parasites are identified in urine, sputum, tissue fluids, or tissue biopsy samples (Table 52-8).

Helminths. Helminths are eukaryote parasites called *worms*. Helminths live on or within another living organism and nourish themselves at the expense of the host organism. They can live in animals or humans and are usually transmitted through the soil, by infected clothing or fingernails, or through contact with infected persons or contaminated food or water. Helminths go through the same life cycle as other worms. The adult worm lays eggs (*ova*). The ova develop into larvae. Larvae grow into adult worms, which lay eggs, and the cycle begins again. Diagnosis is usually based on microscopic examination of feces for ova and parasites and on the patient's signs and symptoms (Figure 52-5).

Protozoa. *Protozoa* (singular, protozoon) are single-celled parasitic eukaryotes ranging in size from microscopic to macroscopic (visible to the naked eye). They are present in moist environments and in bodies of water such as lakes and ponds. Protozoa are transmitted

TABLE 52-3 | **Common Diseases Caused by Bacilli**

Disease	Organism	Description	Transmission	Symptoms	Tests/Specimens	Prevention and Immunization
Tuberculosis	*Mycobacterium tuberculosis*	Acid-fast branching bacilli	Inhalation	Pulmonary: cough, hemoptysis, sweats, weight loss. May affect other systems	Sputum for culture; x-ray; skin tests	BCG vaccine (not routinely given in the U.S.)
Urinary tract infections	*Escherichia coli, Proteus sp., Klebsiella sp., Pseudomonas aeruginosa*	Gram-negative bacilli; many flagellated	Ascends urethra; catheterization	Cystitis: frequency, burning bloody urine. Pyelonephritis: flank pain, fever	Clean-catch urine for culture and analysis	Good personal hygiene; always wipe from front to back
Legionnaires' disease	*Legionella pneumophila*	Gram-negative bacillus (stains poorly with usual methods)	Grows freely in water (air conditioning systems)	Pneumonia-like symptoms	Sputum; blood	Isolation
Tetanus (lockjaw)	*Clostridium tetani*	Gram-positive spore-forming bacilli, anaerobic	Open wounds, fractures, punctures	Toxin affects motor nerves; muscle spasms, convulsions, rigidity	Blood	DPT in childhood; T or Td every 10 years
Gas gangrene	*Clostridium perfringens*	Gram-positive spore-forming bacilli, anaerobic	Wounds	Gas and watery exudate in infected wound	Swab, aspirate of wound for culture	Proper wound care
Botulism	*Clostridium botulinum*	Gram-positive spore-forming bacilli, anaerobic	Improperly cooked canned foods	Neurotoxin affects speech, swallowing, vision; paralysis of respiratory muscles, death	Contaminated food; blood	Botulinus antitoxin; boil canned goods 20 minutes before tasting or eating
Diphtheria respiratory secretions	*Corynebacterium diphtheriae*	Gram-positive bacilli, club-shaped		Sore throat, fever, headache, gray membrane in throat	Swabs; Gram's stain, culture; Schick test for immunity	DPT in childhood
Whooping cough	*Bordetella pertussis*	Gram-negative bacilli	Respiratory secretions	Upper respiratory tract symptoms; high-pitched crowing whoop	Swabs for culture	DPT in childhood
Plague	*Yersinia pestis*	Gram-negative bacilli	Via flea bite from infected rodents	Fever and chills, delirium, enlarged, painful lymph nodes	Sputum for culture; blood	Vaccine available; rodent control

BCG vaccine, Bacille Calmette-Guérin vaccine; *DPT,* diphtheria-pertussis-tetanus (vaccine); *T,* tetanus (toxoid); *Td,* tetanus and diphtheria (toxoids).
Courtesy Kathleen Moody.

TABLE 52-4	Common Diseases Caused by Cocci					
Disease	Organism	Description	Transmission	Symptoms	Specimens	Tests	Prevention
Pneumonia	*Streptococcus pneumoniae*	Gram-positive encapsulated cocci in pairs	Direct contact, droplets	Productive cough, fever, chest pain	Sputum; bronchoscopy secretions	Culture, Gram's stain	Vaccine
Strep throat	*Streptococcus pyogenes* (group A strep)	Gram-positive cocci in chains	Direct contact, droplets, fomites	Severe sore throat, fever, malaise	Direct swab	Rapid strep test, throat culture	None
Wound infection, abscesses, boils	*Staphylococcus aureus*	Gram-positive cocci in clusters	Direct contact, fomites, carriers; poor hand washing	Area red, warm, swollen; pus; pain; ulceration or sinus formation	Deep swab; aspirate of drainage	Culture and sensitivity (aerobic and anaerobic)	None
Staphylococcal food poisoning	*Staphylococcus aureus*	Gram-positive cocci in clusters	Poor hygiene and improper refrigeration of foods	Vomiting, abdominal cramps, diarrhea	Suspected food, stool	Culture of food (organism will not be found in stool)	Refrigerate food to prevent toxin production
Toxic shock	*Staphylococcus aureus*	Gram-positive cocci in clusters	Use of absorbent packing materials (e.g., tampons, nasal packs)	Fever, headache, nausea, vomiting, delirium, low blood pressure	Swab, blood	Culture and serology	Change tampon, packing material often
Gonorrhea	*Neisseria gonorrhoeae*	Gram-negative cocci in pairs; intracellular in WBC	Sexually transmitted	*Females:* pelvic pain, discharge; may be asymptomatic *Males:* urethral drip, pain on urination	Swab of cervix, urethra; rectal and pharyngeal swabs in homosexuals	Gram's stain; culture	Avoid unprotected sex
Meningococcal meningitis	*Neisseria meningitidis*	Gram-negative diplococci	Respiratory tract secretions	High fever, headache, projectile vomiting, delirium, neck and back rigidity, convulsions, petechial rash	Nasopharyngeal swabs, cerebrospinal fluid, blood	Gram's stain; culture; cell counts and chemistries	Vaccine; prophylactic antibiotics

WBC, White blood cells.
Courtesy Kathleen Moody.

TABLE 52-5	Common Diseases Caused by Spirilla					
Disease	Organism	Description	Transmission	Symptoms	Tests/ Specimens	Prevention and Immunization
Syphilis	*Treponema pallidum*	Spirochete	Sexually; congenitally	*Primary:* painless sore (chancre) *Secondary:* generalized rash involving palms and soles of feet *Congenital:* birth defects	Blood for serologic tests: VDRL, RPR, FTA-ABS	Avoid unprotected sex
Lyme disease	*Borrelia burgdorferi*	Spirochete	Tick bite	Fever, joint pain, red bullseye rash	Swab for culture	Avoiding tick-infested areas
Pyloric ulcers	*Helicobacter pylori*	Gram-negative, spiral-shaped	Unknown; possibly food and water	Burning pain in stomach, especially between meals	Stomach biopsy for staining and culture; stool for EIA testing	None known
Food poisoning (most common cause in US)	*Campylobacter jejuni*	Paired gram-negative curved rods forming a seagull shape	Contaminated food, water, and milk	Bloody or watery diarrhea	Stool for darkfield microscopy	Sanitary food preparation and control of water and milk supplies

VDRL, Venereal Disease Research Laboratory; *RPR*, rapid plasma reagin (test); *FTA-ABS*, fluorescent treponemal antibody absorption (test); *EIA*, Enzyme immunoassays.
Courtesy Kathleen Moody.

TABLE 52-6	Diseases Caused by *Rickettsia*, *Chlamydia*, and *Mycoplasma*			
Disease	Organism	Transmission	Symptoms	Tests/Specimens
Rocky Mountain spotted fever	*Rickettsia rickettsii*	Tick bite	Headache, chills, fever, characteristic rash on extremities and trunk	Blood for serologic tests; skin biopsy for direct fluorescent microscopy
Typhus	*Rickettsia prowazekii*	Tick bite	Fever, rash, confusion	Blood for serology
Atypical (walking) pneumonia	*Mycoplasma pneumoniae*	Respiratory secretions	Fever, cough, chest pain	Blood, sputum
Nongonococcal urethritis and vaginitis	*Chlamydia trachomatis*	Sexual	May be asymptomatic	Swabs for culture and serologic testing
Inclusion conjunctivitis, pneumonia		Congenital	Severe conjunctivitis in newborns Afebrile pneumonia in newborns	

Courtesy Kathleen Moody.

through contaminated feces, food, or drink. Some pathogenic protozoa inhabit the bloodstream, whereas others inhabit the intestines and genital tract. Diagnosis is usually based on the patient's signs and symptoms and on microscopic examination of stool and blood (see Table 52-8).

Stool specimens are commonly examined for parasitic protozoa and helminths. The stool specimen is collected and placed into two vials, each with a preservative. Most commonly, 10% formalin and polyvinyl alcohol (PVA) are used. From these preparations, a **wet mount** is made to observe motile organisms, a stained smear is made to provide contrast to the existing debris in the stool, and the specimen is concentrated either by sedimentation or flotation to allow recovery of protozoan **cysts** and helminth eggs. The medical assistant should always consult the procedure manual provided by the referral laboratory when an O&P (ova and parasites stool examination) is ordered to ensure proper collection and transport of the specimen.

TABLE 52-7	Common Diseases Caused by Fungi			
Disease	**Organism**	**Predisposing Conditions and Transmission**	**Symptoms**	**Tests/Specimens**
Thrush (oral yeast) vulvovaginal candidiasis or monilia (vaginal yeast)	*Candida* species (yeast)	Oral: during birth; other: following antibiotic therapy, oral birth control, severe diabetes	White, cheesy growth	Swab for KOH prep, culture
Athlete's foot, jock itch, ringworm (tinea)	*Trichophyton* sp., *Microsporum* sp. & others (skin fungi)	Opportunist; direct contact; clothing; prolonged exposure to moist environment	Hair loss, thickening of skin, nails; itching; red, scaly patches	Skin scraping for KOH prep; skin, hair for culture
Histoplasmosis	*Histoplasma capsulatum*	Inhalation of dust contaminated with bird or bat droppings	Mild, flu-like to systemic	Serologic; culture of biopsy material
Cryptococcosis	*Cryptococcus neoformans*	Contact with poultry droppings	Cough, fever, malaise; can become systemic	Sputum culture
Sporotrichosis	*Sporothrix schenckii*	Farmers, florists, people exposed to soil	Skin lesions that spread along lymphatics; can become systemic	Cerebrospinal fluid culture, India ink direct examination, scrapings; serologic KOH, potassium hydroxide
Pneumocystis pneumonia	*Pneumocystis carinii*	Widely prevalent in animals. Occurs in debilitated persons, immunosuppressed; common in AIDS patients	Pneumonia-like	Biopsy

KOH, Potassium hydroxide.
Courtesy Kathleen Moody.

TABLE 52-8	Common Protozoan and Parasitic Diseases			
Disease	**Organism**	**Transmission**	**Symptoms**	**Tests/Specimens**
Malaria	*Plasmodium* sp. (protozoa)	Bite of the *Anopheles* mosquito	Chills, fever (cyclic)	Blood: examination of stained blood for parasites
Toxoplasmosis	*Toxoplasma gondii* (protozoa)	Fecal contamination (cat litter); congenitally	Febrile illness, rash; congenital: jaundice, enlarged liver and spleen, brain abnormalities	Skin test
Amebic dysentery	*Entamoeba histolytica* (protozoa)	Fecal contamination of food and water	Bloody diarrhea, cramping, fever	Stool for O&P
Giardiasis	*Giardia lamblia* (protozoa)	Common in intestinal tract, opportunist; contaminated surface water	Asymptomatic to severe diarrhea and abdominal discomfort	Stool for O&P; intestinal biopsy; string test
Trichinosis	*Trichinella spiralis* (roundworm)	Ingestion of undercooked pork, bear meat	Nausea, fever, diarrhea, muscle pain and swelling, edema of face	Biopsy; blood tests
Tapeworm	*Taenia* sp.	Undercooked meats (beef and pork)	Abdominal discomfort, diarrhea, weight loss	Stool for O&P
	Diphyllobothrium latum	Undercooked fish; common among Norwegians, Japanese	As above, may become anemic	Stool for O&P
Pinworm	*Enterobius vermicularis* (roundworm)	Fecal-oral	Severe rectal itching, restlessness, insomnia	Scotch tape applied to perianal region for ova
Scabies	Itch mite: *Sarcoptes scabiei*	Direct contact; clothing, bedding	Nocturnal itching; skin burrows	Skin scrapings for parasites
Lice	*Pediculus humanus; Pthirus pubis* (crabs)	Direct contact; clothing, bedding, furniture (can transmit other diseases via bite)	Intense itching; skin lesions	Finding adult lice or eggs (nits) on body or hair

O&P, Ova and parasites.
Courtesy Kathleen Moody.

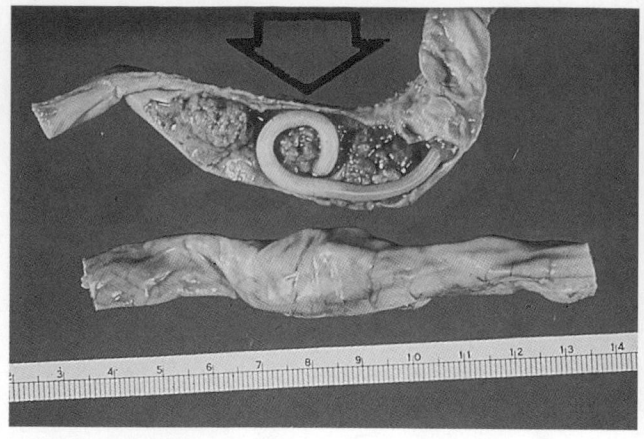
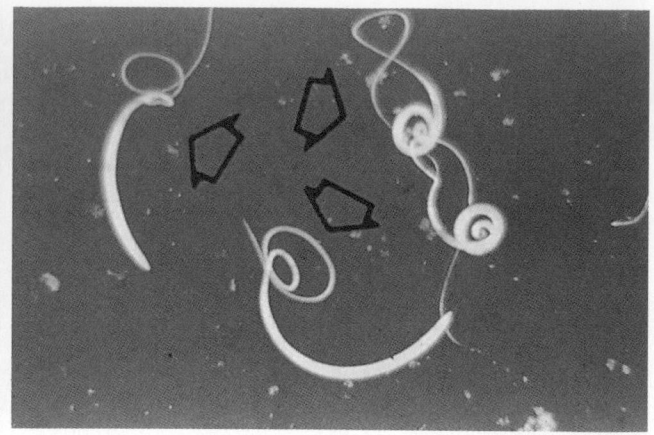

FIGURE 52-5 **A**, Roundworms. **B**, Whipworms. (From Stepp CA, Woods MA: *Laboratory procedures for medical office personnel*. Philadelphia, 1998, WB Saunders.)

The Microbiology Laboratory

The equipment and supplies you will find in a microbiology laboratory vary with the size of the facility. Most laboratories will have a refrigerator, autoclave, safety cabinet, microscope, and incubator (discussed in Chapter 48). In addition, you are likely to find the following equipment and supplies.

Inoculating Equipment

Cultivation and identification of microbes require the use of certain tools. Inoculating loops and needles (Figure 52-6) are needed to transfer samples or microbes to growth media or to slides for staining. Loops and needles may be disposable and presterilized, or they may be made of wire and can be heat-sterilized before and after use. An inoculating loop is shaped like a bubble-wand, and a thin film of liquid will adhere to the loop. The amount of fluid held by the loop can be calibrated; a urine culture requires that a 1-μl sample be applied to the culture media, and special loops are available that deliver this amount. An inoculating needle is thin and pointed and is ideal for sampling single colonies.

Incineration Equipment

Incineration is the fastest way to sterilize reusable equipment such as wire loops and needles and metal forceps that must be sterilized before and after use. Some laboratories will use a Bunsen burner connected to a natural gas supply, but most use an electric incinerator because of the reduced fire hazard (Figure 52-7). An incinerator can also be used to heat fix smears when doing a bacterial stain.

Culture Media

Once a specimen has been properly collected, it must be inoculated onto an appropriate medium (Figure 52-8). Under the proper incubation conditions, the bacteria or fungi in the sample will metabolize and reproduce using the nutrients in the medium and become visible as colonies. Media can be solid, liquid, or semisolid. A liquid

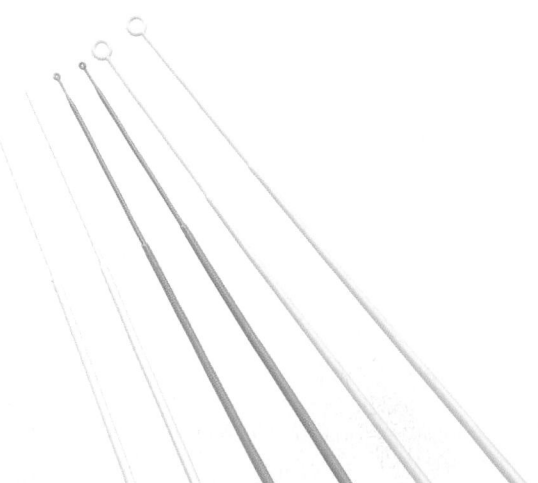

FIGURE 52-6 Inoculating loop and needle. (Courtesy Simport Plastics, Beloeil, Quebec, Canada.)

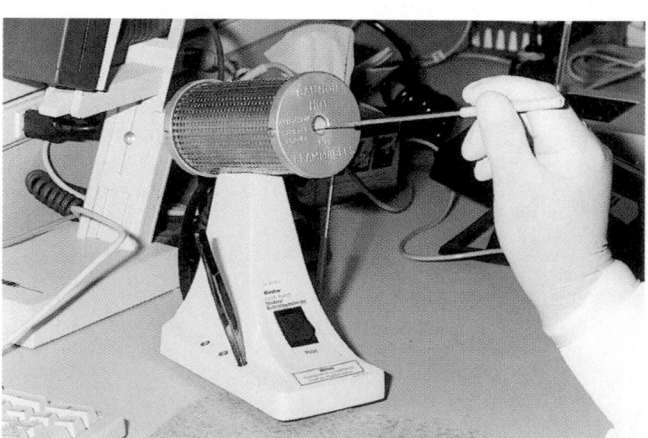

FIGURE 52-7 Loop incinerator. (From Stepp CA, Woods MA: *Laboratory procedures for medical office personnel*. Philadelphia, 1998, WB Saunders.)

medium is called a *broth*. The addition of a powdered extract of seaweed called *agar* to a boiling liquid medium allows it to solidify and remain solid at 37° C. The molten medium can be poured into Petri dishes (a plastic dish with a lid) or into tubes.

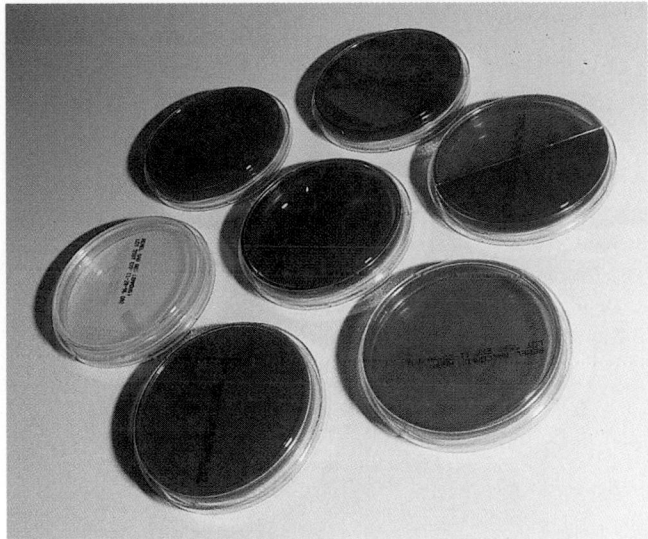

FIGURE 52-8   Media used in cultures. (From Stepp CA, Woods MA: *Laboratory procedures for medical office personnel*. Philadelphia, 1998, WB Saunders.)

> ### THE FOUR DIFFERENT TYPES OF MEDIA
>
> - *All-purpose or nutritive.* All-purpose media is used to support the growth of a wide variety of bacteria but will not support the growth of **fastidious** bacteria.
> - *Selective.* Selective media supports the growth of one type of organism while inhibiting the growth of others through the addition of a salt, dye, antibiotic, or chemical. Phenyl ethanol agar contains alcohol that inhibits the growth of gram-negative bacteria and permits gram-positive bacteria to flourish.
> - *Differential.* Differential media contains chemicals or dyes that alter the appearance of certain bacterial types. Many differential media are also selective. Mannitol Salt Agar contains an increased level (7.5%) of sodium chloride (salt) that selects for staphylococci. It also contains mannitol, a carbohydrate that can be fermented to an acid endproduct by *Staphylococcus aureus*, but not by *S. epidermidis*. The medium contains a pH indicator that turns yellow in the presence of acid. Therefore, if the colony is yellow on the agar medium, it is presumptively *S. aureus*. Differential media are used in biochemical testing.
> - *Enriched.* An enriched medium contains complex organic materials that certain fastidious species must have in order to multiply. Blood agar, needed for the growth of *S. pyogenes*, is made by adding sterile sheep blood to an all-purpose medium. It is widely used in clinical microbiology to cultivate pathogens.

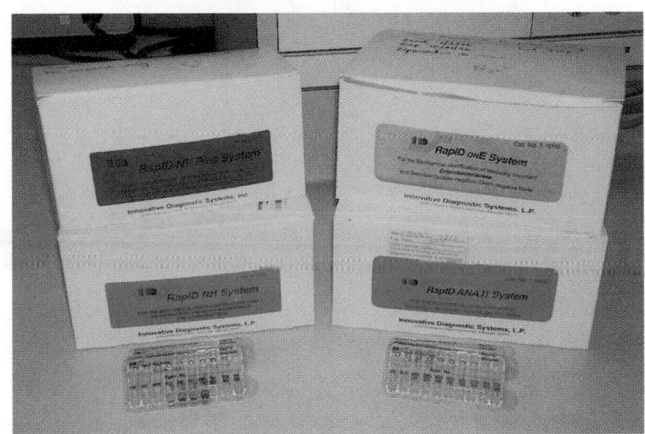

FIGURE 52-9   Rapid biochemical test kits. (From Stepp CA, Woods MA: *Laboratory procedures for medical office personnel*. Philadelphia, 1998, WB Saunders.)

All media should be inspected before use for contamination. New batches of media should be inoculated with control microorganisms to ensure quality. The manufacturer will provide a list of organisms that can be used.

Inoculation of Media

Once the specimen has been collected, it must be "plated" or inoculated onto the appropriate media. If the specimen has been taken on a swab, the swab is rolled onto a portion of the agar medium in a Petri dish, and a sterile inoculating loop is used to spread the sample. If the sample is liquid, such as sputum or urine, a sterile inoculating loop is used to spread the sample.

Several different techniques can be used to spread the sample. The *quadrant streak* is done with a loop to spread the sample thinly over the agar medium in several directions. This effectively separates the bacteria so that they may grow in individual colonies (Figure 52-9). Another technique, used when assessing antibiotic effectiveness or counting colonies, is the *lawn* or *spread streak*. This involves spreading the sample with a swab or loop continuously over the entire plate.

Once the sample is inoculated onto the plate, the plates are incubated in an inverted position so that any condensation that will accumulate on the underside of the lid does not fall down onto the growth. The temperature and conditions of incubation depend on the source of the specimen and the suspected pathogens. Most cultures are incubated in an aerobic atmosphere enriched with 5% carbon dioxide at 37° C. Cultures for fungi are incubated both at room temperature and at 37° C to promote dimorphism, a characteristic of some fungi in which they appear as yeast at 37° C and as a mold at room temperature.

Cultures for anaerobes must be incubated in an atmosphere devoid of oxygen. Special jars called *anaerobe jars* chemically remove oxygen from the environment and are small enough to place in a 37° C incubator (Figure 52-10).

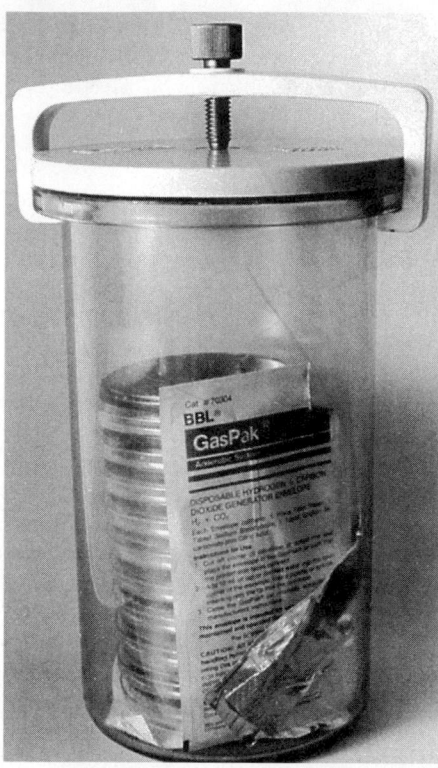

FIGURE 52-10 GasPak anaerobe jar. (Courtesy Becton, Dickinson and Company, Franklin Lakes, NJ.)

Identification of Pathogens in the Microbiology Laboratory

Assessing a Culture

Once the original culture (the *primary culture*) has incubated at the appropriate temperature for 18 to 24 hours, it is examined for evidence of pathogens. Because there are often numerous normal microbiota in addition to the pathogens in samples, it takes a trained eye to spot those organisms that might be causing infection. Suspicious colonies will be subcultured onto the appropriate medium in order to isolate them in **pure culture**. When the organism is in pure culture, staining and additional biochemical testing can be done to identify it at the genus and species level.

Staining

Pathogenic microorganisms are generally colorless, and a microscope is needed to see them. Special *differential stains*, such as the Gram's stain and acid-fast stain, are often used to differentiate bacteria based on biochemical differences. As discussed previously, the Gram's stain differentiates bacteria into two categories according to cell wall thickness, and the acid-fast stain differentiates bacteria into two categories based on the presence or absence of a waxy lipid in the cell wall.

Before a stain can be done, the bacteria must be applied to a labeled slide. A direct smear from a swab can be made or a culture can be stained. Individual colonies growing on the culture medium can be spread into a drop of sterile saline on a glass slide, or material directly from the site of infection can be spread on the slide from the swab used to collect it. The slide is then air-dried and fixed. Either heat or methanol can be used to fix the slide, which results in the material adhering to the slide. Both heat, from either a Bunsen burner or an incinerator, and methanol will cause protein in the sample to denature and stick to the slide, much the same as egg white sticks to a hot frying pan (Procedure 52-1).

PROCEDURE 52-1

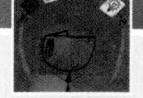

Preparing a Direct Smear or Culture Smear for Staining

GOAL: To prepare a smear for staining from a clinical specimen or from a culture medium.

EQUIPMENT AND SUPPLIES

- Clean glass slides
- Permanent marker
- Incinerator
- Normal saline solution
- Specimen collected on a smear
- 24-hour culture on agar

PROCEDURAL STEPS

Direct Smear

1 Wash and dry your hands. Glove and put on face protection.

2 Label the slide with a permanent marking pen.
   Purpose: Other labels are destroyed in the staining process.

PROCEDURE **52-1—cont'd**

3 Prepare a thin smear by rolling the swab on the slide. Make certain that all areas of the swab touch the slide (Figure 1).

Purpose: Rolling the swab ensures that all parts of the swab come in contact with the slide so that the organisms collected are deposited on the slide. Thin smears are needed for evaluation.

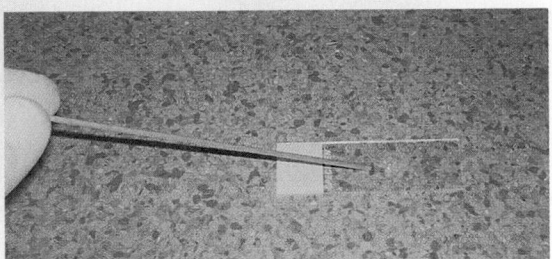

Figure 1

4 Allow the smear to air-dry. Do not wave it or heat-dry it.

Purpose: Waving the slide spreads pathogens. Overheating organisms distorts them.

5 Hold the slide with the smear up. Heat-fix the slide using an incinerator. Check the heating process by touching the slide to the back of the hand (Figure 2). The slide should feel warm, not hot. Check it often by touching the back of the slide to the back of the hand. Cool the slide.

Purpose: Heat-fixing causes materials to adhere to the slide.

Culture Smear

1 Wash and dry your hands. Glove yourself and don face protection.

2 Identify the colonies to be stained by circling them on the back of the plate and numbering them with a permanent marker. Label the slide accordingly.

Purpose: This allows accurate identification of colonies.

3 Apply a small drop of saline solution to the slide, using a loop.

Purpose: Liquid is needed to emulsify the colony. Large drops require a longer drying time.

4 Touch, with a sterile loop, only the top of the colony chosen. Transfer the material picked up to the appropriate area of the slide, and spread it in a circular motion to the size of a dime. Repeat for each colony chosen using a separate slide.

Purpose: Only a small amount of colony is needed for staining.

5 Allow the smear to air-dry.

6 Heat-fix the smear.

7 Properly dispose of all biohazard materials and clean the work area.

8 Remove gloves and wash your hands.

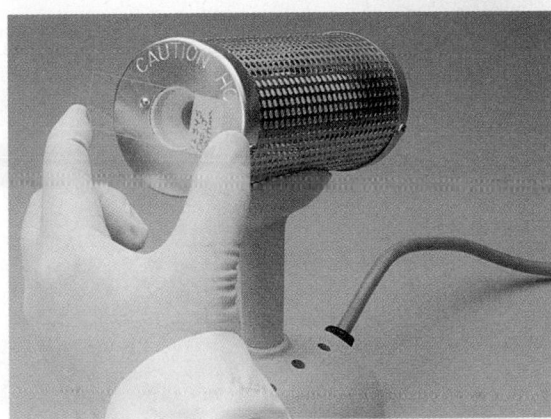

Figure 2

Gram's Stain. The Gram's stain, developed by Dr. Hans Christian Gram more than 100 years ago, is still the most common stain used in the microbiology laboratory. It involves applying a sequence of primary dye, mordant, decolorizer, and counterstain to the slide. The dyes are taken up differently according to the chemical composition of the cell walls (Procedure 52-2). Bacteria react best in the Gram's stain when they are 24 hours old or less. Gram-positive bacteria stain purple, and gram-negative bacteria stain pink or red (Figure 52-11). While not considered a CLIA-waived test, it is useful for the medical assistant to understand the Gram's stain procedure and the microscopic results that are obtained.

Acid-Fast Stain. The acid-fast stain is used in the identification protocol for *Mycobacterium* species. *M. tuberculosis* and *M. avium* complex (MAC) are two important species of mycobacteria. The former causes tuberculosis and can be isolated from sputum samples or tissue samples in infected patients; the latter is a common soil organism that enters through the respiratory tract and disseminates throughout the body. MAC is the third most common cause of death among acquired immunodeficiency syndrome (AIDS) patients. The acid-fast stain involves applying a sequence of primary dye (carbolfuchsin), decolorizer (acid-alcohol), and counterstain (methylene blue). Two procedures can be used, both of which assist in disruption of the waxy cell wall to facilitate staining. In the Ziehl-Neelsen protocol, the primary dye is applied in the presence of heat; in the Kinyoun protocol, the primary dye is mixed with a detergent. Acid-fast-positive bacilli are often referred to as *AFB* (Figure 52-12). associated w/ TB

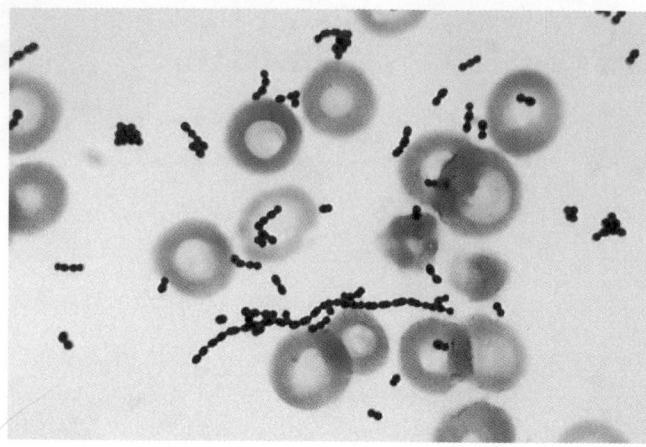 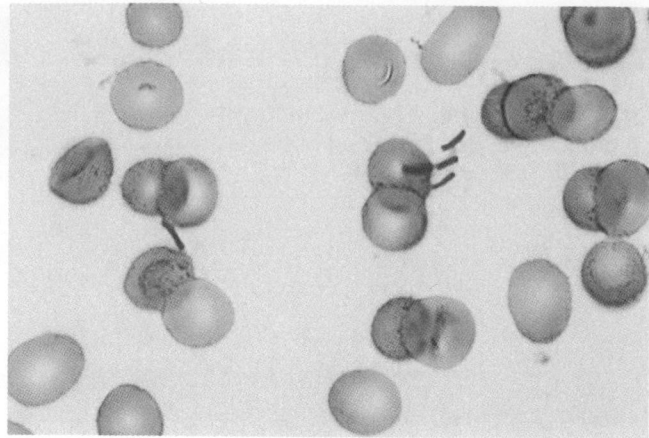

FIGURE 52-11 The Gram's stain. **A,** Red blood cells (RBC) and gram-positive cocci. **B,** RBC with gram-negative bacilli. (From De la Maza, Pezzlo, Baron: *Color atlas of diagnostic microbiology.* St Louis, 1997, Mosby.)

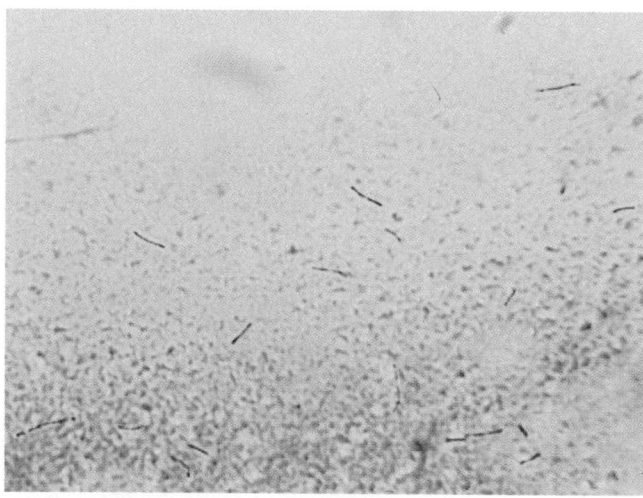

FIGURE 52-12 The acid-fast stain. Pink acid-fast bacilli (AFB) are seen in this smear. (From De la Maza, Pezzlo, Baron: *Color atlas of diagnostic microbiology.* St Louis, 1997, Mosby.)

PROCEDURE 52-2

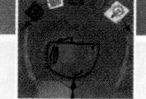

Staining a Smear With Gram's Stain

GOAL: To stain a slide, using the Gram's stain, so that the organisms present are colored appropriately.

EQUIPMENT AND SUPPLIES
- Gram's stain reagents
- Staining rack
- Forceps
- Wash bottle of water
- Prepared smear for staining
- Absorbent paper

PROCEDURAL STEPS

1 Wash and dry your hands.
Purpose: Infection control.

2 Place the slide face up on a level staining rack.

Purpose: If the slide is face down, the organisms will not be stained. If the rack is uneven, the stain will run off the slide surface.

3 Flood the slide with crystal violet. Time for 30 seconds. Figure 1* shows the entire staining process.
Purpose: Crystal violet is the primary stain and colors everything purple.

4 Flood the stain off with a sharp stream of water from the wash bottle. With forceps, tip the slide to remove the water.
Purpose: Using forceps keeps your fingers clean.

PROCEDURE 52-2—cont'd

5 Flood the slide with Gram's iodine (mordant). Time for 30 seconds.

Purpose: Gram's iodine causes the stain to set in the organisms that are gram-positive.

6 Flood the iodine off with water. Grasp the slide with forceps, and hold it nearly vertical.

7 Decolorize by running the decolorizer (alcohol) down the slide until the smear stops, giving off purple stain in all but the thickest portions (about 10 seconds).

Purpose: This is the critical step. The decolorizer removes stain from the organisms that are gram-negative.

8 Rinse the slide with water, and return it to the staining rack.

9 Flood the slide with safranin, and time for 30 seconds.

Purpose: Safranin is the counterstain and stains red everything that has decolorized.

10 Rinse the slide well with water.

11 Wipe off the back of the slide with an alcohol tissue.

Purpose: The back of the slide is cleaned to remove traces of stain, which make examination of the smear difficult.

12 Blot the slide dry between sheets of absorbent paper.

13 Clean the work area. Remove gloves and wash your hands.

14 Record the procedure in the patient's record.

Purpose: A procedure is not considered done until it is properly recorded.

---

*Figure from Stepp CA, Woods MA: *Laboratory procedures for medical office personnel*. Philadelphia, 1998, WB Saunders.

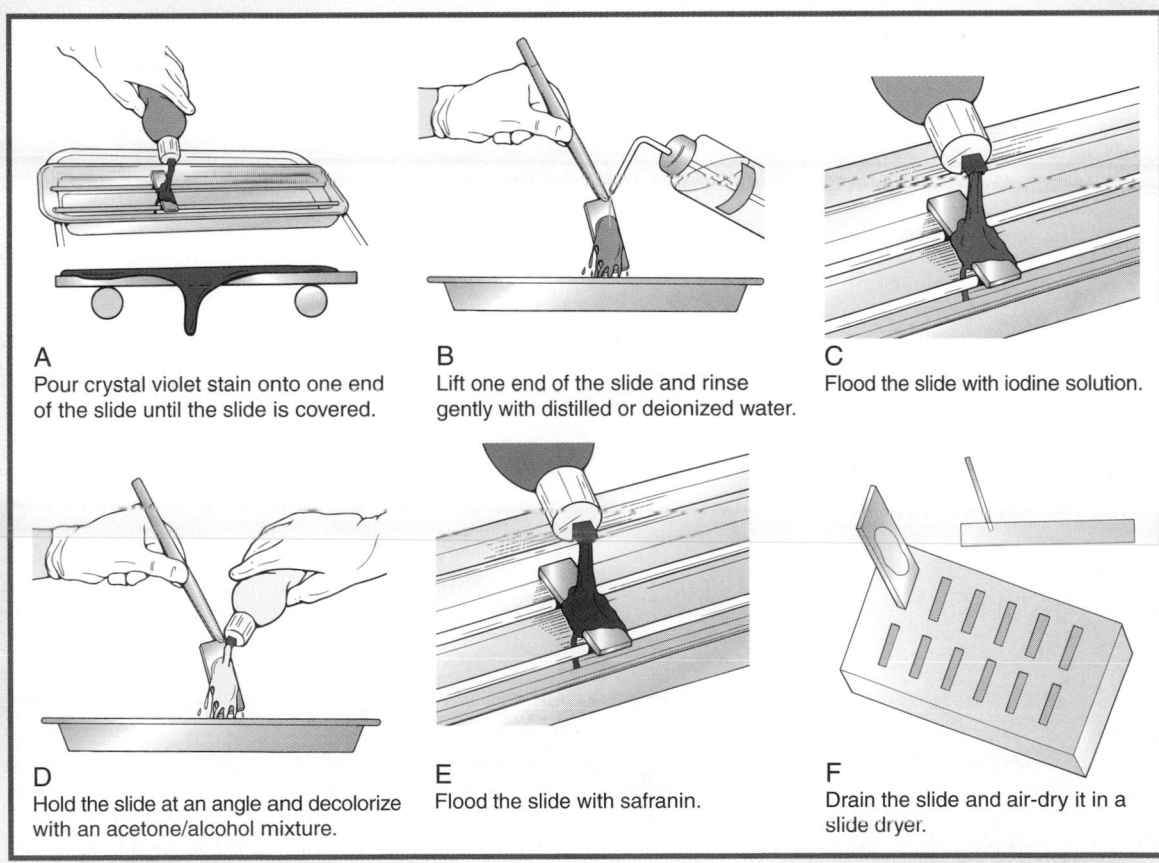

A Pour crystal violet stain onto one end of the slide until the slide is covered.

B Lift one end of the slide and rinse gently with distilled or deionized water.

C Flood the slide with iodine solution.

D Hold the slide at an angle and decolorize with an acetone/alcohol mixture.

E Flood the slide with safranin.

F Drain the slide and air-dry it in a slide dryer.

Figure 1

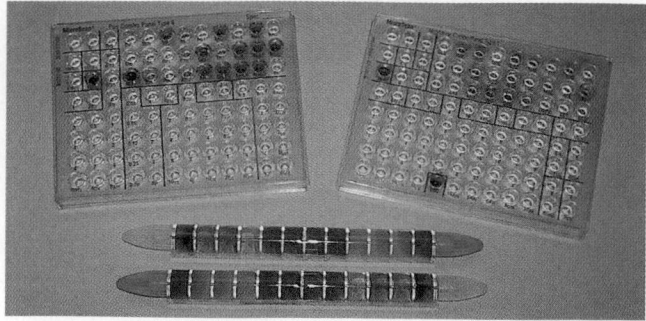

FIGURE 52-13 Enterotube II and Microscan identification tests. (From Stepp CA, Woods MA: *Laboratory procedures for medical office personnel*. Philadelphia, 1998, WB Saunders.)

Biochemical Testing

Once a suspected pathogen is isolated and is in pure culture, biochemical testing must be performed to identify the genus and species. Some of these tests, such as a catalase rapid enzyme test or an oxidase test, take only a few minutes to perform. Others, such as fermentation testing using various carbohydrates, take up to 24 hours to perform. Hundreds of tests are available to identify an organism biochemically, and manufacturers have developed miniaturized multitest systems that speed inoculation and identification (Figure 52-13).

Rapid Identification Methods

Physician's office laboratories with appropriate CLIA certifications are permitted to perform many rapid culture and identification tests. The tests used in a particular laboratory depend on the number of tests performed per month and the amount of refrigerator space available for storage. Dry media tests have a long shelf life, do not require refrigeration, and occupy little incubator space. The rapid culture methods offer presumptive identification of most organisms. Further specialization and sensitivity testing require additional materials, equipment, and procedures. Rapid tests are designed to give the physician a positive indication of the problem so that treatment can be initiated. For a differential or a specific diagnosis, the physician may need additional test results. Some of the rapid tests available determine the presence of *Neisseria* species, *Haemophilus* species, and anaerobes. Clinical Laboratories Improvement Act (CLIA)–waived tests include rapid detection tests for *Helicobacter pylori* and *Streptococcus pyogenes* (group A beta-hemolytic streptococcus).

CRITICAL THINKING APPLICATION

The swab that Anna collected from Aaron at 9:30 AM arrives in the referral laboratory at 4:30 PM. The technician prepares to inoculate the specimen onto the appropriate media. What types of media do you think he would use? What temperature do you think he will use to incubate the specimen? How long will it be before he can call Anna with the results of the culture?

Antimicrobial Susceptibility Testing

Isolating the infectious agent from a patient is only the first step in successful treatment. When a physician wants to determine the appropriate antibiotic through laboratory testing, he or she will order a "culture and sensitivity" test. The "culture" refers to cultivating the organisms, while the "sensitivity" is a test to determine the organism's susceptibility to certain antibiotics. Most bacteria exhibit resistance to **antimicrobial agents**. These patterns of resistance are continuously changing; therefore, they cannot be predicted.

Shifting patterns of resistance require testing of individual bacteria against the appropriate antimicrobial agent.

HOW TO DEFINE THE APPROPRIATE ANTIMICROBIAL AGENT

- Demonstrates the most activity against the infectious agent
- Has the least toxicity to the patient
- Has the least impact on the normal microbiota of the body
- Has the desired pharmacologic characteristics
- Is the most economical

The clinical microbiology laboratory can recommend antimicrobial agents based only on their **in vitro** activity. The final therapeutic outcome is the decision of the physician. The physician bases this decision on numerous factors, including the test results, the physical examination, and the knowledge of the patient. The expertise of a pharmacologist can be helpful in choosing the most effective antimicrobial agent for the patient.

Whenever you are inoculating specimens, **asepsis** must be strictly observed to ensure safety and good results. The organism being tested must also be isolated in pure culture before the test. The test, often referred to as the *Kirby-Bauer Antimicrobial Susceptibility Test*, is performed by inoculating sterile water with the pure culture of bacteria to a specified degree of turbidity. This suspension is then spread with a swab in a lawn on the surface of the appropriate agar medium. Disks, each containing an antimicrobic agent such as penicillin or tetracycline, are placed on the agar with forceps or an automatic dispenser. After incubation, the zone of inhibition (area of no growth) around each disk is measured in millimeters and compared with values provided by the manufacturer of the disks (Figure 52-14). Three determinations are possible: *S*, *R*, or *I*. *S* refers to "susceptible," meaning that the antibiotic is effective against the organism in that particular concentration in vitro; *R* means that the organism is resistant to the

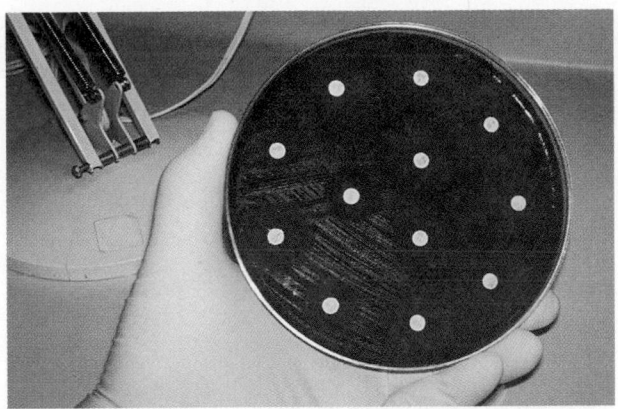

FIGURE 52-14 Antimicrobial susceptibility test. Note the zones of inhibition around 11 of the 12 disks.

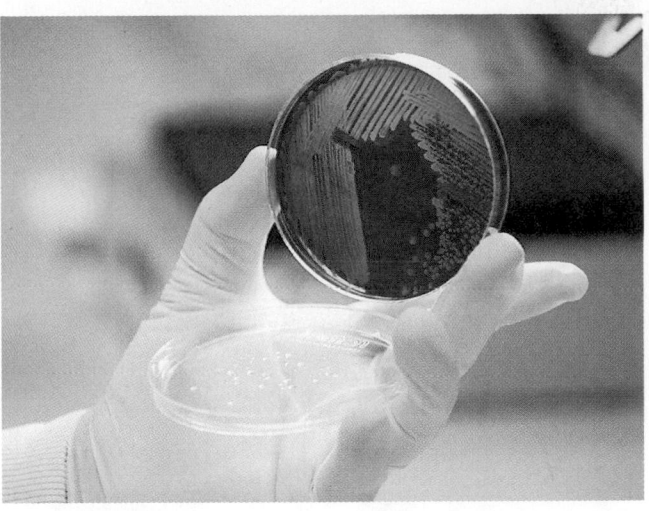

FIGURE 52-15 Beta hemolysis seen as a clear area around the streptococcus colonies. (From Stepp CA, Woods MA: *Laboratory procedures for medical office personnel.* Philadelphia, 1998, WB Saunders.)

antibiotic. The designation *I* refers to intermediate and means that additional testing must be performed to determine the dosage of antimicrobial necessary for therapeutic treatment.

CRITICAL THINKING APPLICATION

Anna has recorded the results of Ms. Walker's urine culture and notes that 10 antimicrobial agents had been tested, but the *Escherichia coli* was susceptible to only five of them. How will Dr. Ling determine which of these five antibiotics would be best for Ms. Walker?

Procedures Performed in the Physician's Office Laboratory

As a certified medical assistant (CMA), you will most likely be involved in patient education and collection of specimens from clients who visit the office. You may also be responsible for performing certain rapid diagnostic tests. Common procedures performed in the POL include the throat culture, the rapid strep test, and the urine culture. Group A beta-hemolytic streptococci (*S. pyogenes*) cause septic sore throat and are capable of producing severe complications if not diagnosed and treated promptly.

Complications include scarlet fever, rheumatic fever, and glomerulonephritis. Swabs from throat cultures are streaked on a sheep blood agar plate, after which a bacitracin differentiation disk is placed on the most heavily streaked first quadrant. This disk contains an antibiotic (bacitracin), which inhibits the growth of *S. pyogenes* and is used for differential diagnosis. Complete clearing of the agar around the colonies indicates beta-hemolysis as a result of a hemolytic toxin produced by the organism, hence the name *beta-hemolytic strep* (Figure 52-15 and Procedure 52-3).

PROCEDURE 52-3

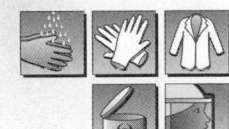

Inoculating a Blood Agar Plate for Culture of Streptococcus pyogenes

GOAL: To inoculate a blood agar plate for the detection of the etiologic agent of strep throat.

EQUIPMENT AND SUPPLIES

- Blood agar plate
- Bacitracin disk or strep A disk
- Incinerator
- Inoculating loop
- Permanent marker
- Swab from patient's throat (see Procedure 34-8)
- Forceps

PROCEDURAL STEPS

1 Wash and dry your hands. Glove and apply face protection.

Continued

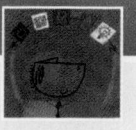

PROCEDURE 52-3—cont'd

Purpose: Infection control.

2 Remove the swab from the container. Grasp the plate by the bottom (media side), and lift the cover, or lift the cover while the plate is on the table.

Purpose: To make handling the plate easier and to prevent contamination of the plate.

3 Roll the swab down the middle of the top half of the plate, then use the swab to streak the same half of the plate. Dispose of the swab properly (Figure 1*).

Purpose: Rolling the swab ensures contact with the surface of the agar.

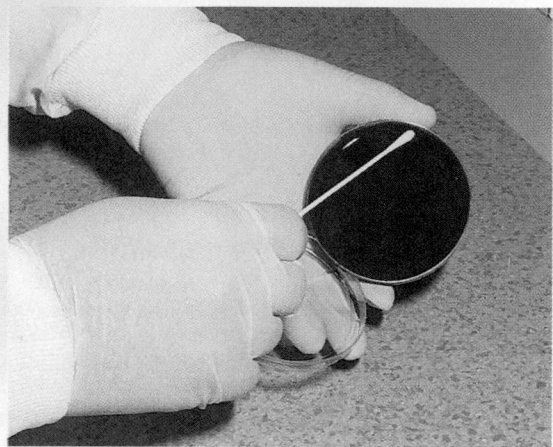

Figure 1

4 Sterilize the loop in the Bacti-cinerator, and allow it to cool (Figure 2).

Purpose: Loops must be sterilized before and after use, to prevent cross-contamination of specimens.

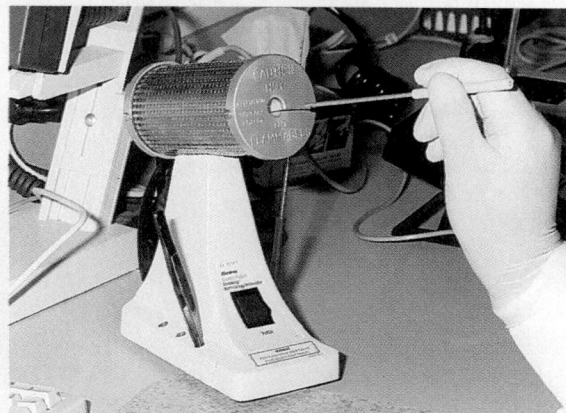

Figure 2

5 Streak for isolation of colonies in the third and fourth quadrants, using the loop. Use the loop to make three slices in the agar in the area of heavy inoculum. Sterilize the loop (Figure 3).

Purpose: Isolated colonies are needed for

observation of colony morphology. The agar is sliced to allow for detection of subsurface hemolysis.

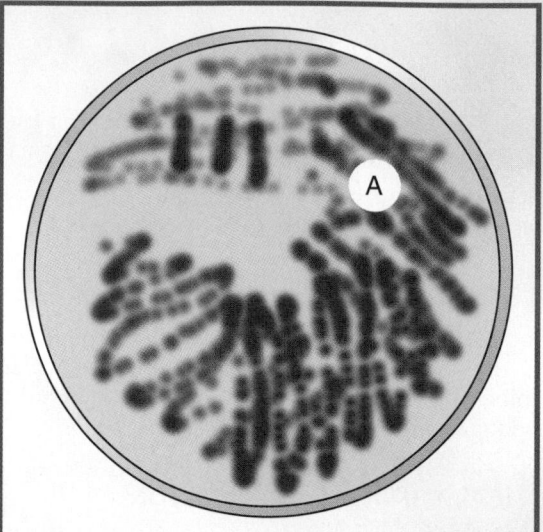

Figure 3

6 Sterilize the forceps and remove one disk from the vial. Place the disk on the agar in the first quadrant. Sterilize the forceps.

Purpose: Group A beta-hemolytic streptococci are presumptively identified by their sensitivity to the disk.

7 Label with permanent marker the agar side of the plate with the patient's name and identification number and the date.

Purpose: Labeling the agar side of dish prevents mixing up specimens.

8 Place the plate in the incubator, with the agar side of the plate on the top.

Purpose: Placing the plate with the agar side up prevents accumulation of moisture on the surface of the agar.

9 Incubate for 24 hours and then examine. Incubate negative cultures for an additional 24 hours.

Purpose: Some hemolysis patterns are not well defined after 24 hours of growth.

10 Clean the work area and properly dispose of all biohazard waste.

11 Remove your gloves and wash your hands.

---

*Figure from Stepp CA, Woods MA: *Laboratory procedures for medical office personnel*. Philadelphia, 1998, WB Saunders.

Rapid strep testing is commonly performed in the POL. The tests can be performed while the patient waits. The patient's throat is swabbed, the swab is placed in an extraction tube, and the extract is tested for the presence of streptococcus antigens (Procedure 52-4). Negative tests should be confirmed with a throat culture; the rapid strep tests are highly specific but not as highly sensitive. This means that if the test is positive, there is a high degree of confidence that *S. pyogenes* is in the sample; if the test is negative, the organism may not have been present in great enough quantity to be detected.

Urine cultures require a procedure that will permit quantitation of the sample. Most laboratories use a variety of differential and selective media along with an all-purpose medium to which one microliter (1/1000 ml) of urine is applied. Each colony that grows on the plate then represents 1000 colony-forming units per milliliter. A system of numerical values has been devised to

---

PROCEDURE 52-4

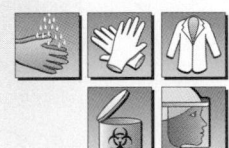

Performing a Rapid Strep Test

GOAL: To perform a rapid strep test to assist in the diagnosis of strep throat.

EQUIPMENT AND SUPPLIES

- Directigen Strep A Test kit
- Timer or wristwatch with sweep second hand
- Throat swab specimen (see Procedure 34-8)

PROCEDURAL STEPS

1 Collect all supplies and equipment needed to perform the test. Bring all reagents and reaction disks to room temperature (minimum of 30 minutes).

2 Wash and dry your hands. Put on gloves and face protection.
Purpose: Infection control.

3 Position all bottles vertically, and dispense reagents slowly as free-falling drops. Avoid reagent contact with your eyes because the reagent is an irritant (Figure 1).

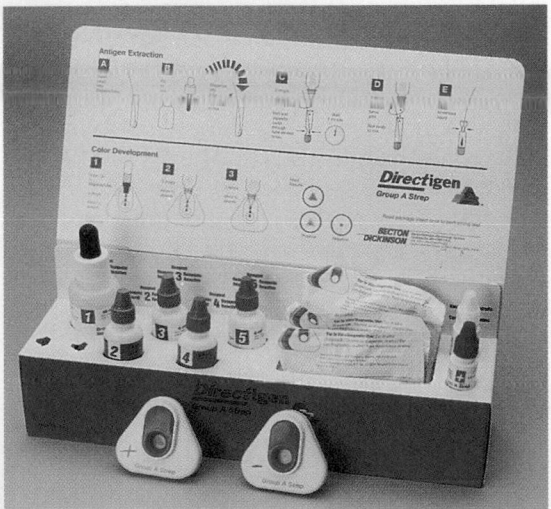

Figure 1

4 Add three drops of reagent 1 to an extraction tube. This solution is pink.

5 Add three drops of reagent 2 to the same tube. The solution should turn yellow.

6 Place the specimen swab in the tube, twirling the swab in the mix.

7 Let stand for exactly 1 minute.

8 Add three drops of reagent 3 to the same tube, again twirling the swab in the tube to mix. This solution should be pink.

9 Express the liquid from the swab by squeezing the tube with the thumb and forefinger and rotating the swab as it is withdrawn. The liquid must be thoroughly removed from the swab. Best results are achieved when the liquid reaches or exceeds the line on the tube.

10 Discard the swab in a biohazard waste container.

11 Remove the reaction disk from the pouch and place it on a dry, flat surface.

12 Pour the entire contents of the tube into the reaction disk.

13 Read the test results when the entire end of assay window turns red (5 to 10 minutes).

14 Properly dispose of all contaminated waste.
Purpose: Items contacting samples are considered potentially infectious.

15 Clean work area, remove gloves, and wash your hands.
Purpose: Infection control.

16 Record the test results in the patient's medical record.
Purpose: A procedure is considered not done until it is properly recorded.

assess the possibility of a urinary tract infection (Procedure 52-5). This is necessary only for specimens that have been collected via the CCMS technique described in Chapter 48. Any microorganisms isolated from a specimen obtained via a urinary catheter are considered pathogenic; specimens other than CCMS or catheter-collected are rejected, and a re-collection is requested.

Numerous self-contained culture systems for urine are available. These systems are ideal for the smaller laboratory that does not want to purchase plate media. Examples of these systems include the Diaslide (Diatech Diagnostics, Boston, MA), Bactercult (Carter-Wallace/Wampole Division, Cranbury, NJ), and Uri-Kit (Culture Kits, Inc, Norwich, NY).

CRITICAL THINKING APPLICATION

The technician from the referral laboratory indicated that Ms. Walker had a urinary tract infection. What numbers will Anna likely write on the laboratory report?

PROCEDURE 52-5

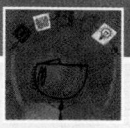

The Urine Culture

GOAL: To inoculate three plates with one microliter of urine in order to quantitate the number of bacteria and aid in the diagnosis of a urinary tract infection.

EQUIPMENT AND SUPPLIES

- Urine specimen, collected CCMS in a sterile container
- Bacti-cinerator
- 1.0 microliter calibrated inoculating loop
- Blood agar plate, MacConkey agar plate, and Columbia nutrient agar plate (or an appropriate selection of all-purpose, differential, and selective media)

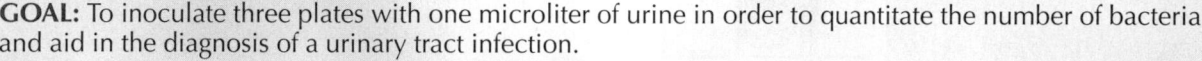

PROCEDURAL STEPS

1 Wash and dry your hands. Glove and apply face protection.
   Purpose: Infection control.

2 With the screw cap lid in place, mix the urine specimen thoroughly by swirling.
   Purpose: Microorganisms settle to the bottom of the specimen when the specimen is allowed to stand.

3 Sterilize the calibrated loop, cool, and dip the tip into the specimen.
   Purpose: The loop must be allowed to cool, or the heat will destroy the microorganisms as the loop comes into contact with the urine specimen, resulting in falsely low colony counts on the culture. Urine on the shaft of the loop will run down the shaft and increase the size of the specimen deposited on the plate, resulting in a falsely elevated colony count on the culture.

4 Deposit the specimen on the plate, as indicated in Figure 1 in Procedure 52-3. Use the loop to streak as shown in Figure 3 in Procedure 52-3.
   Purpose: Careful streaking of the plates is necessary for an accurate count of the organisms present.

5 Inoculate the second and third plates in the same manner.

6 Label the bottom of the plates with the patient's name and identification number and the date.
   Purpose: Labeling the bottom of the plates prevents mixing up of the specimens.

7 Record all information in the patient's medical record.

8 Place the plates in the incubator, with the agar sides of the plates facing up.

9 Incubate for 24 hours, and then count the colonies on the all-purpose medium.

10 The results will be interpreted by a physician or medical technologist as follows:
- >100 colonies = >100,000 colony-forming units (cfu)/ml of urine indicates a urinary tract infection
- 10 to 100 colonies = 10,000 to 100,000 cfu/ml of urine indicates suspicion. The urine may have been allowed to stand at room temperature, which facilitated overgrowth of bacteria; or the patient may have a subclinical infection. Re-collection of the specimen is recommended.
- <10 colonies = 10,000 cfu/ml of urine and indicates normal urethral microbiota
   Purpose: Because the urine was collected by passing through the urethra, some normal bacteria should be present. This system of quantitation accounts for the presence of normal microbiota.

11 Clean the work area, dispose of all biohazard waste, remove gloves, and wash your hands.

Miscellaneous Microbiology Testing

Testing for Pinworms

Enterobius vermicularis, commonly called a pinworm, is a parasite that infests primarily young children. Humans are infected by the ingestion of mature eggs via hand-to-mouth transfers, feces-contaminated fingers, or feces-contaminated foods or liquids or by inhaling eggs in air currents from infected areas. The eggs hatch in the small intestine, with the females migrating out of the anus, usually at night, to deposit the eggs. The eggs adhere to the skin, perianal hairs, sleeping garments, and other clothing items. This results in itching of the anal area, whereby the eggs come in contact with the hands and fingernails of the host.

In children, specimens are best collected late at night or early in the morning before a bowel movement, urination, or bathing. Petroleum jelly–impregnated paraffin swabs or cellulose tape may be used to collect the eggs deposited by the adult worm during the night. Diagnosis is based on laboratory detection of the eggs in fecal smears. If the parent does not feel comfortable about obtaining the needed specimen, instruct the parent to bring the child to the office as soon as he or she awakens in the morning. Advise the parent to not change the child's clothing or change the child's diaper before coming to the office but to bring the child immediately on waking. When the child arrives, have all the needed supplies ready to use and do the procedure immediately (Procedure 52-6).

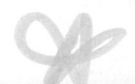

PROCEDURE **52-6**

Performing a Cellulose Tape Collection for Pinworms

GOAL: To obtain a rectal sample using cellulose tape for the purpose of testing for pinworm eggs.

EQUIPMENT AND SUPPLIES

- Glass slide
- Clear cellulose tape
- Wooden tongue depressor
- Toluene
- Microscope
- Gauze or cotton balls

PROCEDURAL STEPS

Ask the patient to assist you with this procedure.

1 Gather and prepare supplies and equipment needed for obtaining the specimen.

2 Place a strip of cellulose tape on a glass slide, starting ½ inch from one end and running toward the same end. Continue around this end lengthwise. Tear off the strip so that it is even with the other end (Figure 1*).

    Note: Do not use Magic transparent tape; use regular clear cellulose tape.

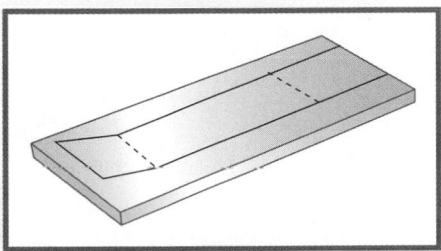

Figure 1

3 Place a strip of paper measuring ½ × 1 inch between the slide and the tape at the end where the tape is torn flush. This will be the specimen labeling area. *As soon as the child arrives, place the child with the attending parent in the prepared examination room.*

4 Wash hands, glove, and apply face protection.
    Purpose: Infection control.

5 Remove the clothing and diaper from the child and lay the child in a prone position, over the parent's lap, with the buttocks in a superior plane.

6 To obtain the perianal sample, first peel back the tape on the slide by gripping the label (Figure 2). With the tape looped (adhesive side outward) over a wooden tongue depressor that is held against the slide and extended about 1 inch beyond it, press the tape firmly against the right and left anal folds (Figure 3).

7 Spread the tape back on the slide, adhesive side down (Figure 4).

8 Smooth the tape using a cotton ball or gauze square (Figure 5).

---

*Figure from Stepp CA, Woods MA: *Laboratory procedures for medical office personnel.* Philadelphia, 1998, WB Saunders.

Continued

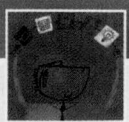

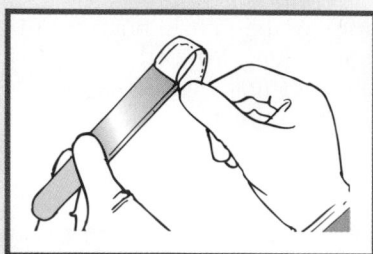

Figure 2

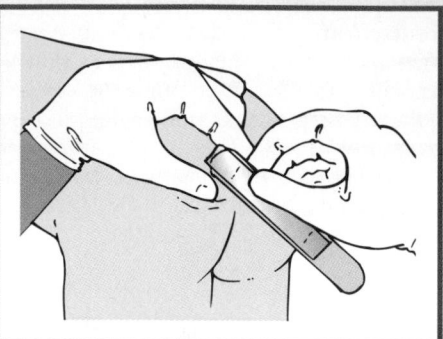

Figure 3

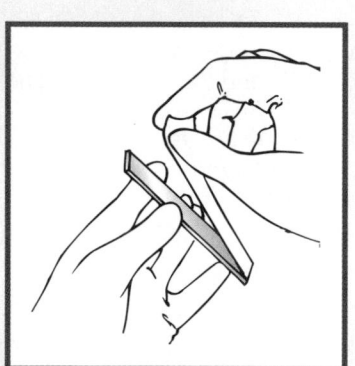

Figure 4

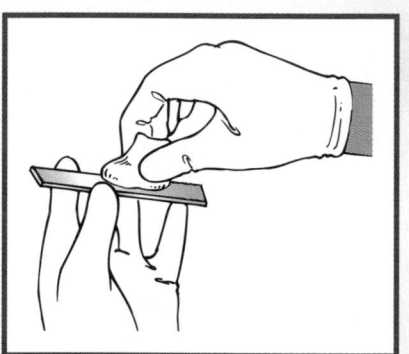

Figure 5

PROCEDURE **52-6—cont'd**

9 Write the patient's name and date on the slide label.

10 Advise the parent that the child can be dressed or assist with dressing the child if needed.

Testing the Sample

11 Lift one side of the tape and apply one drop of toluene before pressing the tape back down on the glass slide.

   Purpose: This will clear the specimen so that any eggs will be visible.

12 Place the prepared slide under the microscope's low-power objective for examination by a physician or medical technologist under low illumination (Figure 6).

13 Dispose of all biohazard waste, clean the work area, remove gloves, and wash your hands.

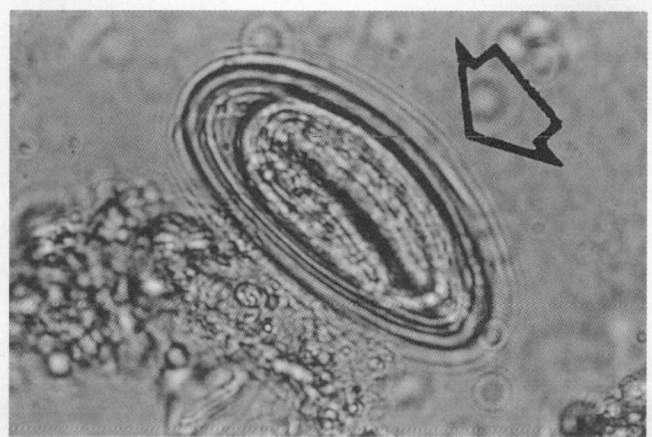

Figure 6

Patient Education

Microorganisms such as bacteria, viruses, fungi, and parasites are responsible for most human diseases. Patient education plays an important role in helping the patient and the patient's family to control the spread of infection. The following is a list of teaching topics that will help you in educating the patient in infection control:

- An explanation of the patient's type of infection—bacterial, viral, fungal, or parasitic
- How infection spreads
- Normal barriers to infection
- Risk factors for infection
- Patient preparation for cultures and serologic, hematologic, and imaging tests, as necessary
- The patient's role in specimen collection
- Handwashing, proper storage and cleaning of personal items, and disposal of contaminated supplies

Explain to the patient that infection does not always occur at the entry site; for example, measles can be transmitted through the respiratory tract or through the conjunctivae by touching an affected patient and then rubbing the eye. Reinforce the need for strict adherence to the prescribed antimicrobial therapy by pointing out the possible complications of noncompliance, such as relapse or systemic involvement. Explain to the patient that inadequate drug therapy (not taking the medication as prescribed) may cause the infection to worsen and spread.

Above all, *always listen to the patient*; be sure that the questions asked are answered. Do not try to answer questions that you are unsure of. Notify the physician of the patient's concerns so that the doctor can include the answers and explanations in the patient's consultation.

CRITICAL THINKING APPLICATION

Aaron's culture was confirmed as *Staphylococcus aureus*. What advice can Anna give to Aaron and his mother concerning contagion of this infection?

Legal and Ethical Issues

Maintaining a laboratory in the office increases the physician's liability. By testing patients' specimens in the office, the physician assumes responsibility for the interpretation and accuracy of the results. As the person in the office who runs the tests and notes the results on the patient's chart, it is your responsibility to maintain optimal accuracy in the testing results. A *quality assurance* (QA) program for POLs may reduce the risks involved and still allow the patient to benefit from the convenience of office testing.

Strict confidentiality is essential. Never release information to anyone other than the patient or legal guardian; however, certain infectious diseases must be reported to the Centers for Disease Control and Prevention (CDC) or local board of health. POLs that have established QA programs, with written policies and procedures that govern their laboratory testing and ensure that these policies are implemented, are in compliance with CLIA regulations. If the office where you are employed does not have laboratory guidelines, suggest developing testing guidelines.

SUMMARY OF SCENARIO

It seems Anna sees something new about harmful bacteria on the television or in the newspaper every day—outbreaks on cruise ships, biowarfare, and smallpox vaccinations have become common topics, yet Anna knows that most bacteria are harmless; we can protect ourselves from infection by using a few simple techniques such as hand washing and keeping the hands away from the face. Anna makes a point of explaining this to the patients she sees at the family clinic and has developed a program on hand washing that she presents to schools and daycare facilities. Prevention, she knows, is the key to controlling infection.

SUMMARY OF LEARNING OBJECTIVES

- Specimens for the microbiology laboratory must be collected in sterile containers. Transport systems are available if the specimen cannot be plated immediately. These systems often contain a transport medium that keeps the organisms alive but does not let them multiply.

- All microbes require nutrients to stay alive. Aerobes will require oxygen; anaerobes will die in the presence of oxygen. Most pathogens prefer an incubation temperature of 37° C.

- Viruses differ from bacteria in that they are not cells. Viruses comprise a core of nucleic acid surrounded by a protein coat. They do not metabolize, and they cannot replicate on their own.

- Bacteria are prokaryotic; fungi, protozoa, and parasites are eukaryotic. Many different species cause disease.

- Identification of bacteria begins with the observation of their morphology. Cocci are spherical-shaped organisms, bacilli are rod-shaped, and spirilla are spiral-shaped.

- Staphylococci are cocci in clusters, streptococci and streptobacilli refer to the organisms arranged in chains, and diplococci and diplobacilli refer to the organisms arranged in pairs.

■ The most important stain in microbiology is the Gram's stain. The four steps involve the addition of the primary stain, crystal violet; the mordant, iodine; the decolorizer, alcohol; and the counterstain, safranin. Gram-positive bacteria stain purple, and gram-negative bacteria stain pink or red.

■ Growth media consists of nutrients selected for certain species. Media can be liquid or can be made solid by the addition of agar. Solid media can be prepared as Petri plates or as tube media.

■ Media can be all purpose and support the growth of many species. It can be selective, permitting only a certain type of microbe to grow. Media can also be differential, allowing differentiation of species based on color changes caused by different biochemical reactions. Enriched media support the growth of fastidious bacteria.

■ Numerous rapid methods have been developed for use in the laboratory. Generally, these tests identify some component of the infectious agent and do not require culture.

■ Antimicrobial susceptibility testing uses disks impregnated with antimicrobial agents dropped onto the surface of an agar plate inoculated with a pathogen. The pathogen will display susceptibility, resistance, or an intermediate reaction to the antimicrobial agent. These determinations are made by measuring the zone of inhibition around each disk and comparing with a chart provided by the manufacturer.

■ The medical assistant must be aware that patient confidentiality is of utmost importance, but certain infections, such as sexually transmitted diseases and tuberculosis, must be reported to the CDC and to the local board of health.

KEY INTERNET WEBSITES

- American Biological Safety Association
- Centers for Disease Control and Prevention (CDC)
- CDC Bioterrorism Response Pages
- Environmental Protection Agency—Microbiology Home Page
- Guidelines for Specimen Collection
- Infection Prevention Online Course
- Material Safety Data Sheets for Infectious Agents
- National Institute of Allergy and Infectious Disease
For active weblinks to each website visit
http://evolve.elsevier.com/Kinn/

extra credit
due 4/20

1 page

UNIT nine

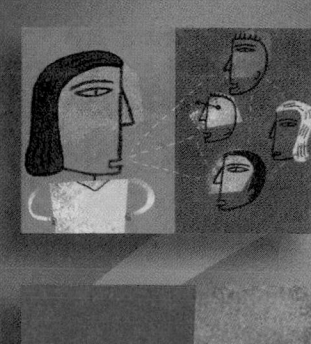
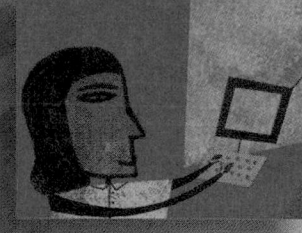
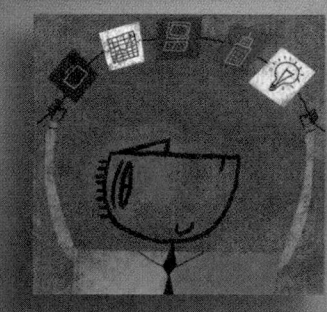

Assisting With Surgeries

CHAPTER 53

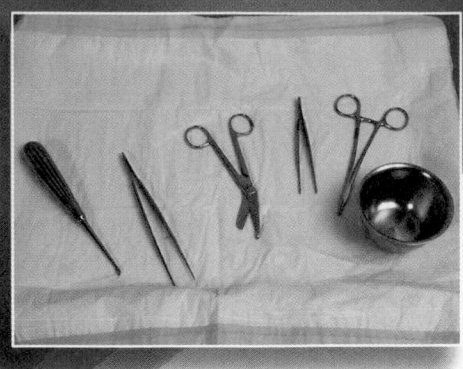

Scenario

Tom Anderson, CMA, works for Dr. Sheila Samanski, a dermatologist who frequently performs minor surgical procedures in the office. Tom assists Dr. Samanski with procedures and is also responsible for maintaining stock supplies in the minor surgery room, including solutions and medications, as well as cleaning, maintaining, and inspecting the surgical instruments. Because no procedures are scheduled for today, Tom is planning to compile an inventory of supplies and equipment and to perform routine maintenance activities.

Surgical Supplies and Instruments

Learning Objectives

- Define and spell the terms listed in the vocabulary.
- Identify the solutions and medications used in minor surgical procedures.
- Outline the general functions of surgical instruments.
- Describe the care of surgical instruments.
- Identify by name the instruments used in minor surgical procedures.
- Identify types of sutures and surgical needles.

National Curriculum Competencies

CLINICAL COMPETENCIES

4f. Prepare patient for and assist with procedures, treatments, and minor office surgery

TRANSDISCIPLINARY COMPETENCIES

4a. Perform an inventory of supplies and equipment
4b. Perform routine maintenance of administrative and clinical equipment

Vocabulary

abscess Localized collection of pus that may be under the skin or deep within the body that causes tissue destruction.

cannula Rigid tube that surrounds a blunt trocar or a sharp, pointed trocar inserted into the body; when withdrawn, fluid may escape from the body through the cannula, depending on where it is inserted.

curettage Act of scraping a body cavity with a surgical instrument, such as a curette.

dilatation Opening or widening the circumference of a body orifice with a dilating instrument.

dissect To cut or separate tissue with a cutting instrument or scissors.

fascia Sheet or band of fibrous tissue located deep in the skin that covers muscles and body organs.

fistula Abnormal, tube-like passage between internal organs or from an internal organ to the body surface.

lumen Open space, such as within a blood vessel, the intestine, the inside of a needle, or an examining instrument.

obturator Metal rod with a smooth, rounded tip that is placed into hollow instruments to decrease injury to body tissues during insertion.

patency Open condition of a body cavity or canal.

polyps Tumors with stems, frequently found on mucous membranes.

stylus Metal probe that is inserted into or passed through a catheter, needle, or tube used for clearing purposes or to facilitate passage into a body orifice.

Office surgery is restricted to the management of minor problems and injuries. The medical assistant is expected to prepare the sterile field and the patient for procedures. Some medical assistants are employed in outpatient surgical facilities and are expected to assist with procedures that were once performed in the hospital. Although these more difficult operations may involve complete gowning and gloving with surgical masks and caps, the two surgical chapters in this text limit discussion and descriptions to the routines necessary to prepare for and assist in minor surgery only. This chapter includes a discussion of surgical supplies and instruments, the care and handling of instruments, and the different types of surgical sutures and needles. It prepares you for Chapter 54, which presents sterilization, preparation of the sterile field, specific minor surgical procedures, and care of the patient.

Minor Surgery Room

When minor surgery is routinely performed, the medical office is designed to include a changing room and a minor surgery room that is separate from the other examining rooms. The larger surgery centers have recovery rooms and family waiting areas. The minor surgery room in the physician office setting should be near a workroom with a sink and an autoclave if the room does not have its own. It should be easy to disinfect and uncluttered to allow easy movement and minimal dust collection. In addition to the operating table, equipment should include a clock with a second sweep, an operating light, sitting stools, and Mayo stands (Figure 53-1). Cabinets with countertops are necessary to serve as a side or back table during the surgery. All surgical supplies are stored in these cabinets. Supplies used in this room should not be used elsewhere, and supplies used elsewhere should not be brought into this room.

Surgical Solutions and Medications

Treatment room supplies include standard solutions and medications that are used in minor surgery and dressing changes. Although the solutions and medications listed here are basic, every practice has preferred items and methods of applying them. The medical assistant uses many of these items; some items are used only by the physician, but the medical assistant is responsible for their care and supply.

Sterile water is kept in two forms. Multiple-dose vials are used as a diluent for medications; larger containers of sterile water are for rinsing instruments that have been in a chemical disinfectant solution.

Sterile physiologic saline solution (0.9%) is also stocked in two sizes. The small multiple-dose vial is used for injection. A larger-size container of sterile saline is used for rinsing and irrigating wounds. These high-quality, commercially prepared products can be purchased from a medical supply company.

The patient's surgical site must be prepared preoperatively with an antiseptic skin cleansing preparation to reduce the number of pathogens. Although isopropyl alcohol and hydrogen peroxide have been used in the past to cleanse wound areas, neither of these provides the antiseptic, bactericidal, and virucidal actions of povidone-iodine (Betadine). Betadine does not cause the allergic problems of the earlier tincture of iodine and is used in several different ways: as a skin preparation for surgery, as a surgical hand scrub for operating room personnel, and as a topical antiseptic ointment. Another antiseptic and antimicrobial cleanser is Hibiclens (chlorhexidine gluconate), which can also be used as a surgical scrub and for patient preoperative skin preparation.

Even minor surgical procedures require the use of anesthetics, which are either injected locally at the site of the procedure or may be sprayed on the skin as a preinjection anesthesia. For patients who find injections of local anesthesia painful or traumatic, the physician may first spray the injection area with a topical anesthetic, such as Fluori-Methane 15%, which is supplied in 3.5-ounce amber glass bottles for either fine or medium spray. Immediately after spraying the site, the physician makes a series of injections around the area with a local anesthetic.

Another topical anesthetic spray is ethyl chloride, a vapo-coolant that controls pain associated with minor

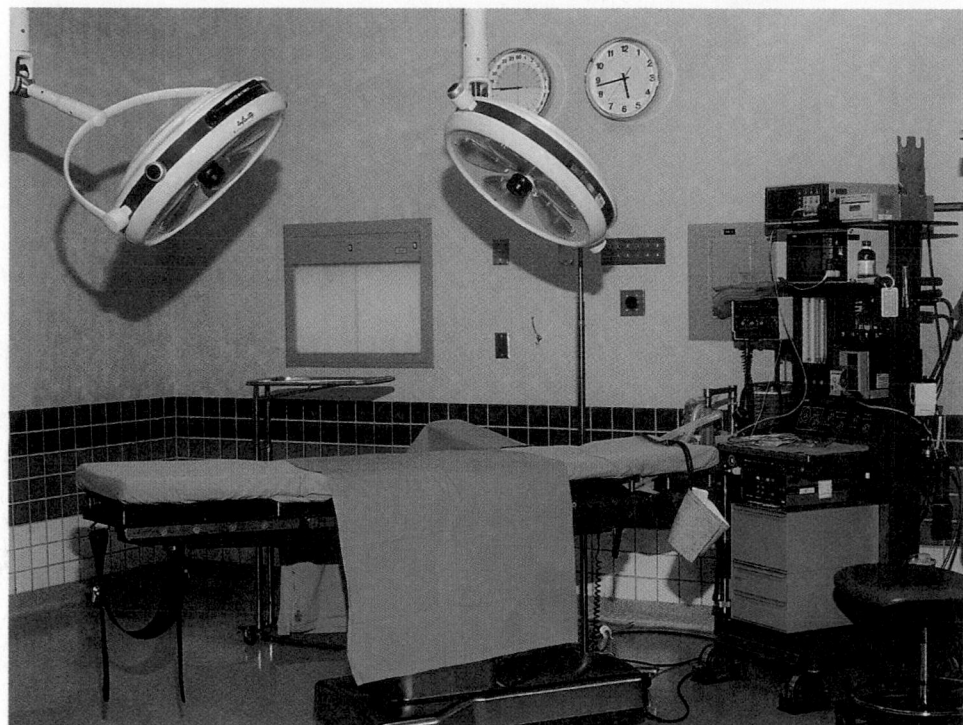

FIGURE 53-1   Operating room and equipment. (Courtesy Fresno Surgery Center, Fresno, CA.)

surgical procedures such as lancing boils or incision and drainage of small **abscesses** by causing localized freezing of the affected area. Because ethyl chloride is highly flammable, it should never be used in the presence of electrical cauterizing equipment and requires the application of petroleum jelly to surrounding areas to protect them from the cooling action of the spray. It has a short duration, and so all equipment must be prepared and the physician ready to perform the procedure before it is applied.

Local anesthetics are injected into the subcutaneous tissue and result in temporary cessation of feeling at the site of injection by blocking the generation and conduction of nerve impulses. There are many different types of local anesthetics, but all share the same suffix of -*caine*. Those that are used most frequently include lidocaine (Xylocaine), Nesacaine, and Sensorcaine. Local anesthetics are purchased in multiple-dose vials of 30 to 50 ml and in varying strengths such as 0.5%, 1%, and 2%. They begin acting relatively quickly, within 5 to 15 minutes; the duration of action depends on the type of anesthetic used, but they usually last from 1 to 3 hours. When highly vascular areas are involved, local anesthetics containing epinephrine may be used. Epinephrine causes vasoconstriction at the site, which keeps the anesthetic in the tissues longer, prolonging its effect. It also minimizes local bleeding. However, epinephrine is not used in areas where decreased circulation may cause problems with healing, such as fingertips or toes.

All tissues removed, or biopsied, from the patient are sent to the pathology laboratory for analysis. A 10% formalin solution is typically used to preserve excised tissue for specimens. Specimen bottles are purchased with preservatives included and should be part of the supplies prepared for a surgical procedure if a biopsy is to be done. The physician will place the specimen in the container, and the medical assistant is responsible for accurately labeling the container with the patient's name, date of collection, and type of specimen.

Sometimes the physician may want to use topical silver nitrate ($AgNO_3$) solution or coated applicator sticks to stop localized bleeding, such as with *epistaxis* (nosebleed) or capillary bleeding at the site of a wound. The applicators must be kept in light-proof brown containers, and the most commonly used strength is 20%. The applicator sticks are convenient for use in the mouth or nose.

ADDITIONAL SURGICAL SUPPLIES

- Wound drains (Penrose drain): rubber drains placed in a wound at the end of a surgical procedure to drain excess fluid
- Sterilized gauze squares or strips saturated with Vaseline (petroleum jelly or petrolatum): used for packing wounds
- Sterilized iodoform gauze strips: $1/4$ to 2 inches wide impregnated with iodoform iodine; used to pack abscesses, acting as a wick to draw out the infection and as a local antibacterial agent (Figure 53-2)
- Surgical sponges: used to absorb blood and protect tissues during surgery
- Syringes and needles: used to inject local anesthetics and irrigate wounds

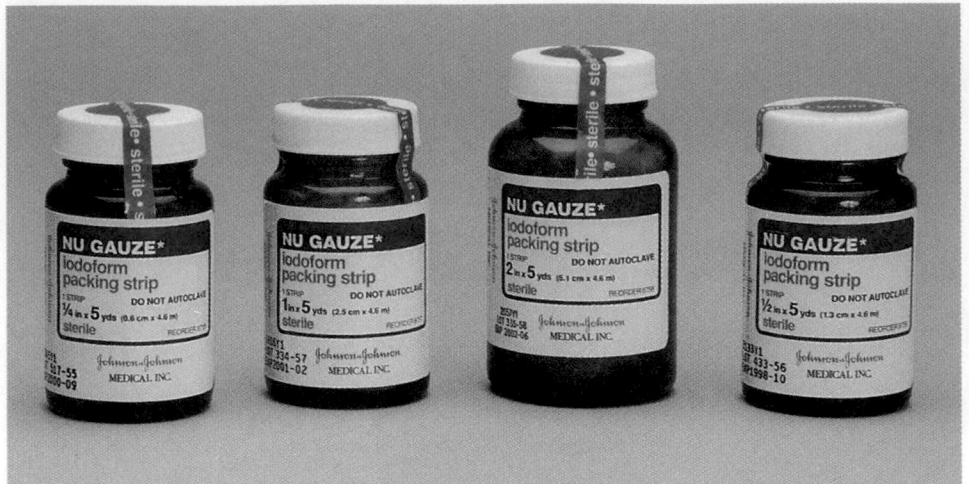

FIGURE 53-2 Iodoform gauze. (Courtesy Johnson & Johnson Medical, Inc., Arlington, TX.)

Surgical Instruments

The medical assistant must know which instruments are used for each procedure and should be able to identify and understand the function of the surgical instruments preferred by the physician. Instruments have clearly identifiable parts and can be visually differentiated from one another (Procedure 53-1). The basic components are the handle, the closing mechanism, and the part that comes into contact with the patient, commonly called the *jaws*. Many instruments can be ordered straight or curved, depending on the operator's preference and the task to be performed.

Instruments have either ring handles (*finger rings*) or spring handles (sometimes called *thumb-handled* or *thumb grasp*). Scissors are an example of a ring-handled instrument; tweezers are spring-handled. Some instruments have a hinge type of mechanism called a *box lock*. A ring-handled forceps is shown in Figure 53-3, *A*; a box-lock mechanism is shown in Figure 53-3, *B*; and a spring-handled thumb forceps is shown in Figure 53-3, *C*.

Ratchets resemble gears and are located just below the ring handles. They are used to lock an instrument into position. Most ratchets can be closed at three or more positions, depending on the thickness of the tissue or materials being grasped. Figure 53-3, *A* and *B* show ratchet-closing mechanisms.

PROCEDURE **53-1**

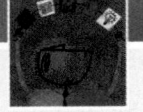

Identifying Surgical Instruments

GOAL: To identify, correctly spell, and determine the use(s) of standard office instruments or those selected by your instructor.

EQUIPMENT AND SUPPLIES

- Curved hemostat
- Straight hemostat
- Dressing (thumb) forceps
- Paper and pencil
- Scalpel and blade
- Dissecting scissors
- Towel clamp
- Vaginal speculum
- Bandage scissors
- Allis tissue forceps

PROCEDURAL STEPS

1 Look for the following parts that determine usage: box-lock, serrations, finger rings, cutting edge, noncutting edge, thumb type, teeth ratchets, and electric attachments.

Purpose: To determine the combination of features and parts for each instrument.

2 Consider the general classification of the instrument: cutting and dissection, grasping and clamping, retracting, or probing and dilating.

PROCEDURE 53-1—cont'd

Purpose: The clue to the name of the instrument may be found by determining the classification.

3 Carefully examine the teeth and serrations.

Purpose: The clue to the name of the instrument may be found by determining its distinctive parts.

4 Look at the length of the instrument to determine the area of the body for which it is used.

Purpose: The clue to the name of the instrument may be found by determining where it can reach.

5 Try to remember whether the instrument was named for a famous physician, university, or clinic.

Purpose: Many instruments are named for the inventor.

6 If the instrument is a pair of scissors, look at the points and determine whether the tips are sharp-sharp, sharp-blunt, or blunt-blunt.

7 Carefully compare the instrument with similar instruments that you know to determine whether it is in the same category or has the same name.

Purpose: The clue to the name of an instrument may be found with the knowledge you already have.

8 Write, with correct spelling, the complete name of each instrument, including its category and use.

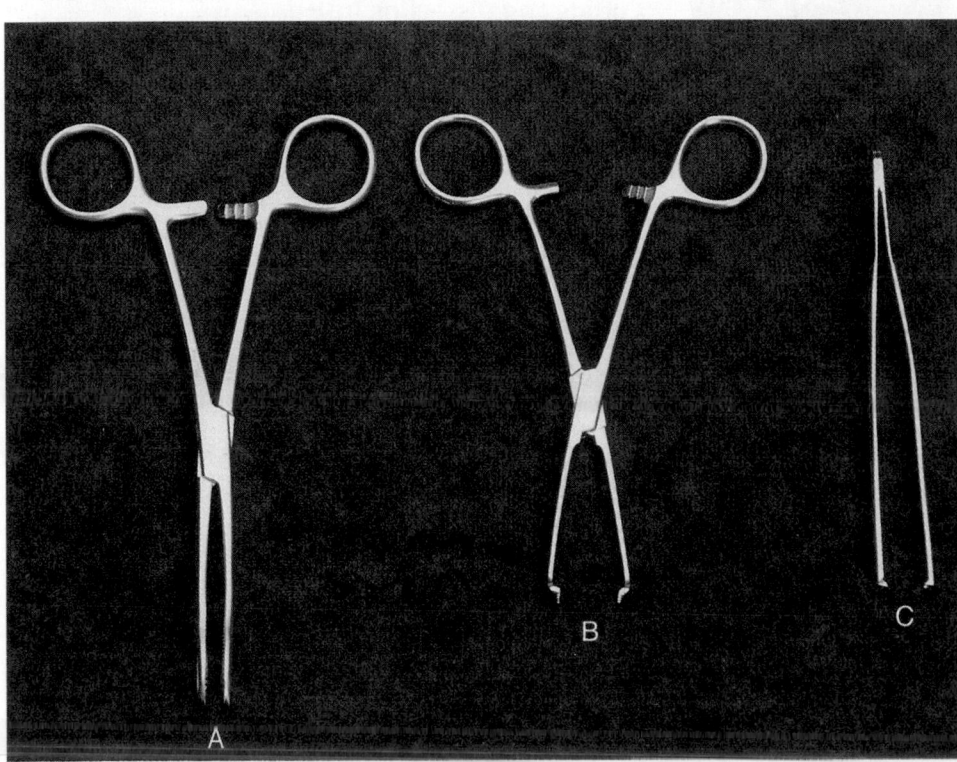

FIGURE 53-3 **A**, Ring-handle forceps. **B**, Box-lock hinge forceps. **C**, Spring-handle thumb forceps.

The inner surfaces of the jaws on some instruments have ridged teeth called *serrations*, and both ring-handled and thumb-type instruments may have them. These serrations may be crisscross, horizontal, or lengthwise (Figure 53-4). Serrations prevent small blood vessels and tissue from slipping out of the jaws of the instrument.

Instrument tips or jaws may be plain tipped or mouse toothed (Figure 53-5, *A*). If the tooth is large, the tip is called *rat toothed* (Figure 53-5, *B*) rather than mouse toothed. Tissue forceps are usually toothed instruments and are identified by the number of intermeshing teeth (e.g., 12, 23, 34). Figure 53-5, *C* shows an Allis tissue forceps. Because this forceps is used to grasp

delicate soft tissues, the teeth are finer, shallower, and more rounded; others are sharper and deeper. Still others have sharp hook-like single or double teeth, such as the tenaculum and vulsellum. Usually, the tenaculum has a single sharp hook on each jaw. The vulsellum has a double hook that resembles the fangs of a snake. Toothed instruments commonly have ratchets for locking into towels or human tissues. Instrument tips may also be either straight or curved, depending on their use.

An instrument is usually named for its use (e.g., splinter forceps, for removing splinters) or after the person(s) who developed it (e.g., Mayo-Hegar needle holder). Many general instruments are identified by the

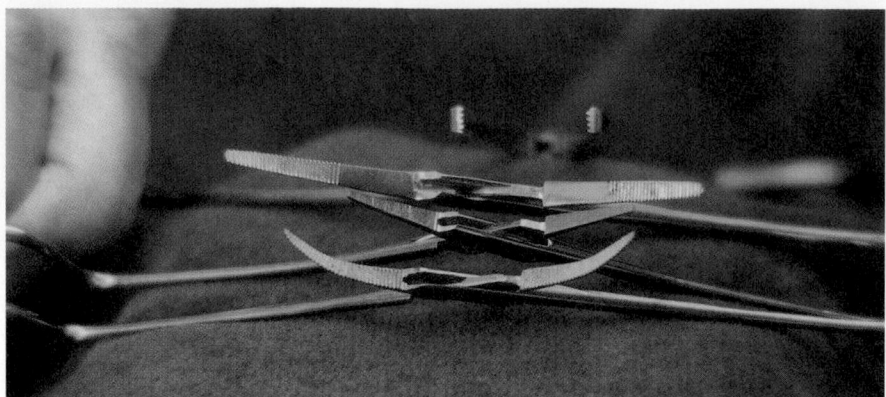

FIGURE 53-4 Instruments with serrations.

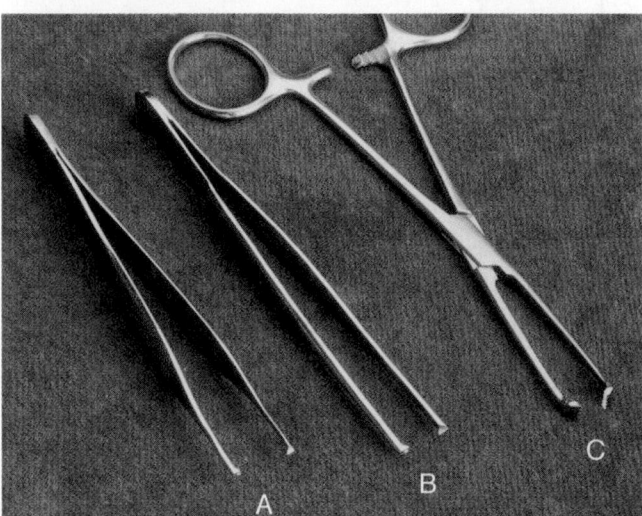

FIGURE 53-5 **A**, Mouse-toothed jaws. **B**, Rat-toothed jaws. **C**, Teeth of Allis tissue forceps.

part of the body where they are used (e.g., rectal speculum and nasal speculum).

There are thousands of surgical instruments with multiple name variations. The same instrument may carry two or three different names, depending on the physician or the part of the country. A physician may ask for a clamp or forceps when a Kelly hemostat is wanted; so it is important to learn the physician's preference in terminology. Learn to recognize the distinctive parts of instruments and the reasons for each part, and you will quickly build a working knowledge of hundreds of instruments.

Classifications of Surgical Instruments

Surgical instruments are generally classified according to their use, and most belong to one of four groups:
- Cutting
- Grasping
- Retracting
- Probing and dilating

Cutting and Dissecting Instruments

These are cutting, incising, scraping, punching, and puncturing instruments. Included are scissors, scalpels, chisels, elevators, curettes, punches, drills, and needles. Instruments with a sharp blade or surface can cut, scrape, or dissect.

Bandage Scissors (Figure 53-6, *A*)

- Probe tip is blunt
- Easily inserted under bandages with relative safety
- Used to remove bandages and dressings

Operating (Surgical) Scissors

Metzenbaum ("Metz") scissors (Figure 53-6, *B*)

- Most frequently used length is 5¼ inches
- Used to cut and **dissect** tissue

Mayo Scissors (Figure 53-6, *C* and *D*)

- Have curved or straight blade tips
- Used to cut and dissect fascia and muscle
- Straight Mayo scissors can be used as suture scissors

Iris Scissors (Figure 53-6, *E* and *F*)

- Usual length is 4 inches
- Have curved or straight blade tips
- Straight tips usually used for suture removal

Littauer Stitch or Suture Scissors

- Blade has beak or hook to slide under sutures
- Used to remove sutures

Scalpel Handle (Figure 53-7, *A* to *C*)

- No. 3 is the standard handle
- No. 3L and No. 7 are used in deeper cavities

Scalpel Blades (Figure 53-7, *D* to *G*)

- No. 15 is commonly used and fits Nos. 3 and 7 handles
- Nos. 10, 11, and 12 are used for specialty incisions and fit Nos. 3 and 7 handles

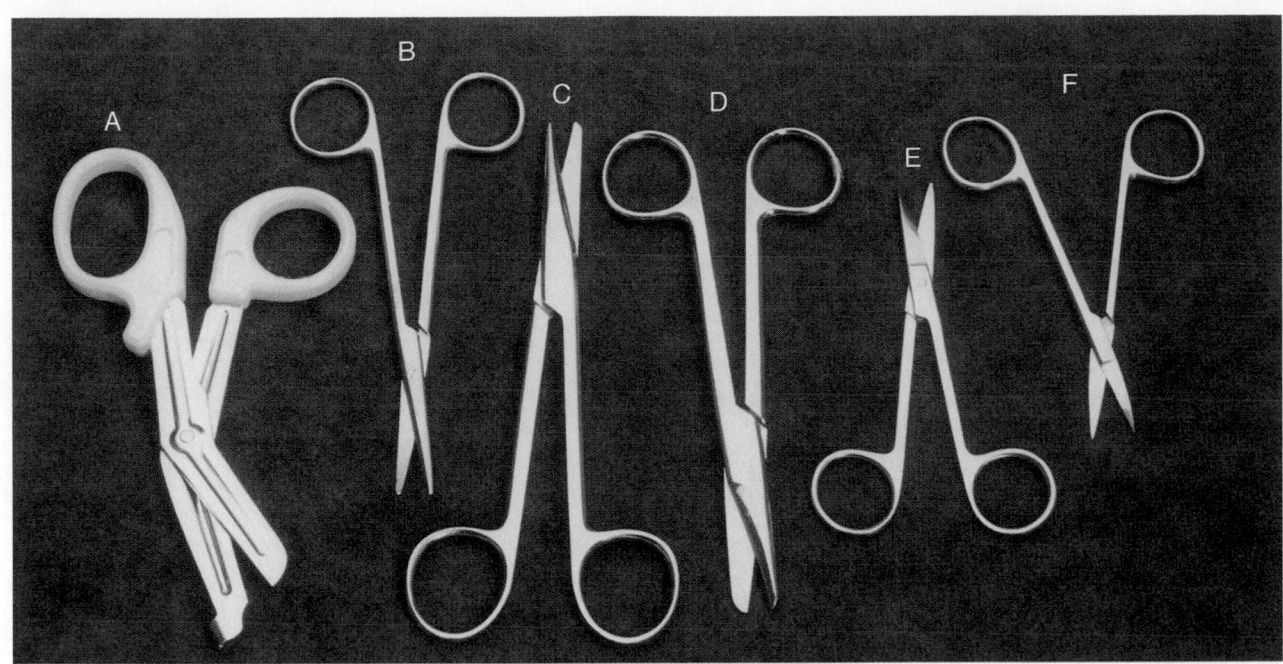

FIGURE 53-6   Operating scissors. **A**, Bandage scissors. **B**, Metzenbaum ("Metz") scissors. **C**, Curved Mayo scissors. **D**, Straight Mayo scissors. **E**, Straight iris scissors. **F**, Curved iris scissors.

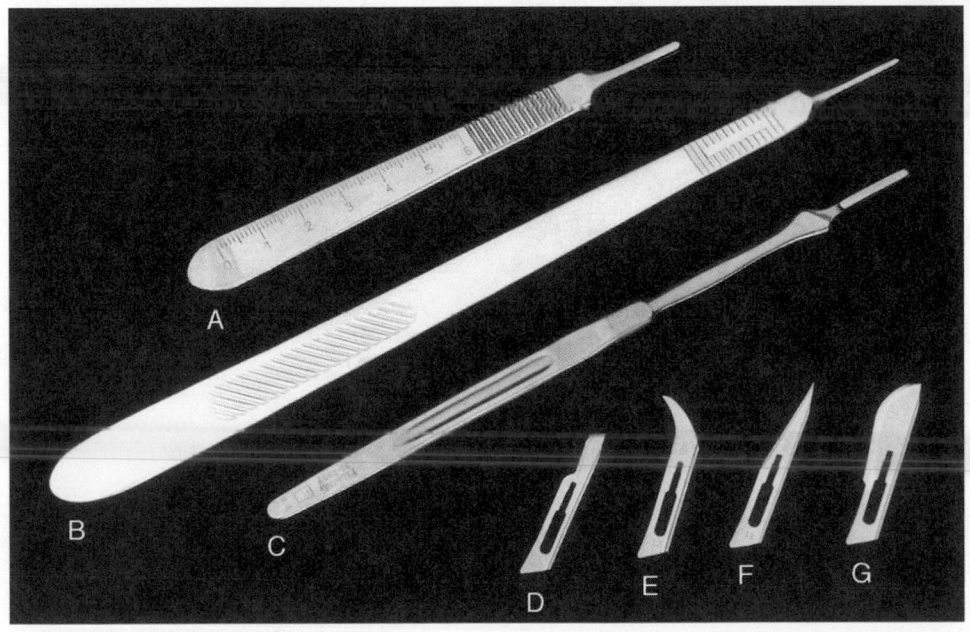

FIGURE 53-7   **A**, No. 3 scalpel blade. **B**, No. 3 long scalpel handle. **C**, No. 7 scalpel handle. **D**, No. 15 blade. **E**, No. 12 blade. **F**, No. 11 blade. **G**, No. 10 blade.

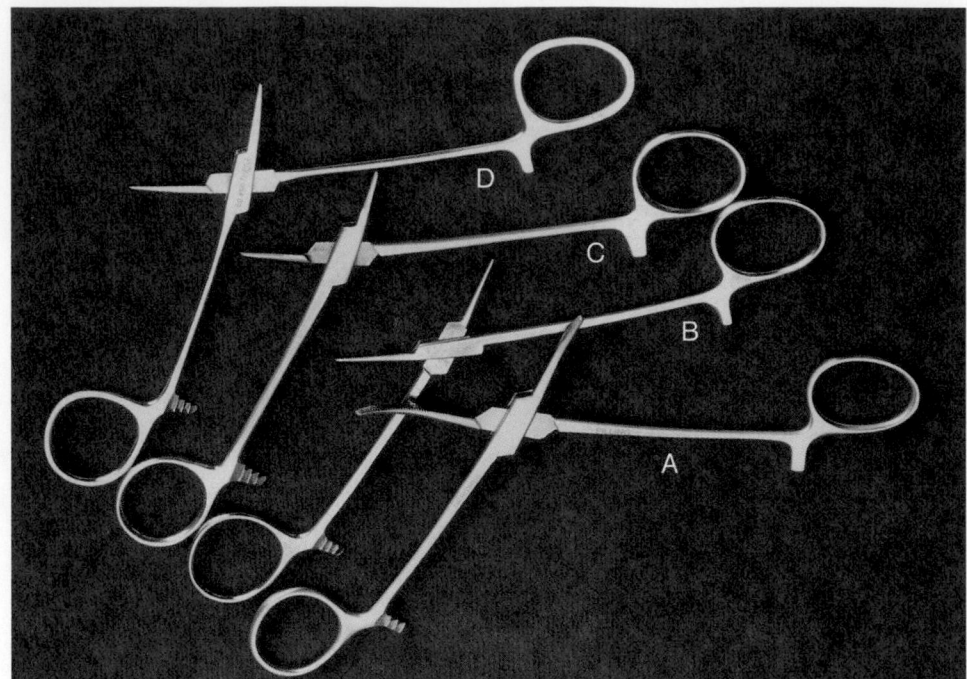

FIGURE 53-8 **A**, Kelly hemostat forceps. **B**, Mosquito hemostat forceps. **C**, Needle holder. **D**, Smooth-tip needle holder.

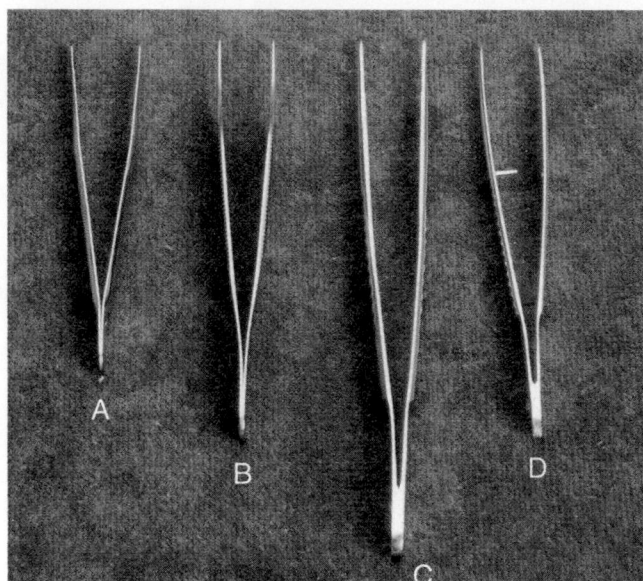

FIGURE 53-9 **A**, Splinter forceps. **B**, Smooth Adson forceps. **C**, Long plain-tip forceps. **D**, Short plain-tip forceps.

Grasping and Clamping Instruments

Clamping instruments are used for many different tasks. Many have a sharp tooth or teeth and are used to retract, hold, and manipulate human **fascia**. The most common clamping instruments are hemostats, which were originally designed to stop bleeding or to clamp severed blood vessels. Some clamping instruments are used to grasp other instruments or sterilized materials. Sometimes hemostats and other clamping instruments are used interchangeably.

Hemostat Forceps (Figure 53-8, *A* and *B*)

- Jaws may be fully or partially serrated, without teeth
- May be curved or straight
- Used to clamp small vessels or hold tissue
- Mosquito forceps (4 inches) are smaller and used for very small vessels
- Crile forceps (5 inches) are medium sized
- Kelly forceps (6 to 7 inches) are larger

Needle Holders (Figure 53-8, *C* and *D*)

- Jaws are shorter and stronger than hemostat jaws
- Jaws may be serrated or may have a groove in the center
- Are 4 to 7 inches in size
- Used to grasp a suture needle firmly

Splinter Forceps (Figure 53-9, *A*)

- Design and construction vary
- Fine tip for foreign object retrieval

Smooth Adson Forceps (Figure 53-9, *B*)

- Same use as the Adson thumb forceps

Plain Thumb (Dressing) Forceps (Figure 53-9, *C*)

- Manufactured in lengths from 4 to 12 inches
- Have varying types of serrated jaws but no teeth
- Used to insert packing into or remove objects from deep cavities

Towel Forceps (Towel Clamp) (Figure 53-10, *A* to *D*)

- May have sharp or atraumatic tips
- Are various lengths from 3 to 6¹/₂ inches
- Used to hold drapes in place during surgery

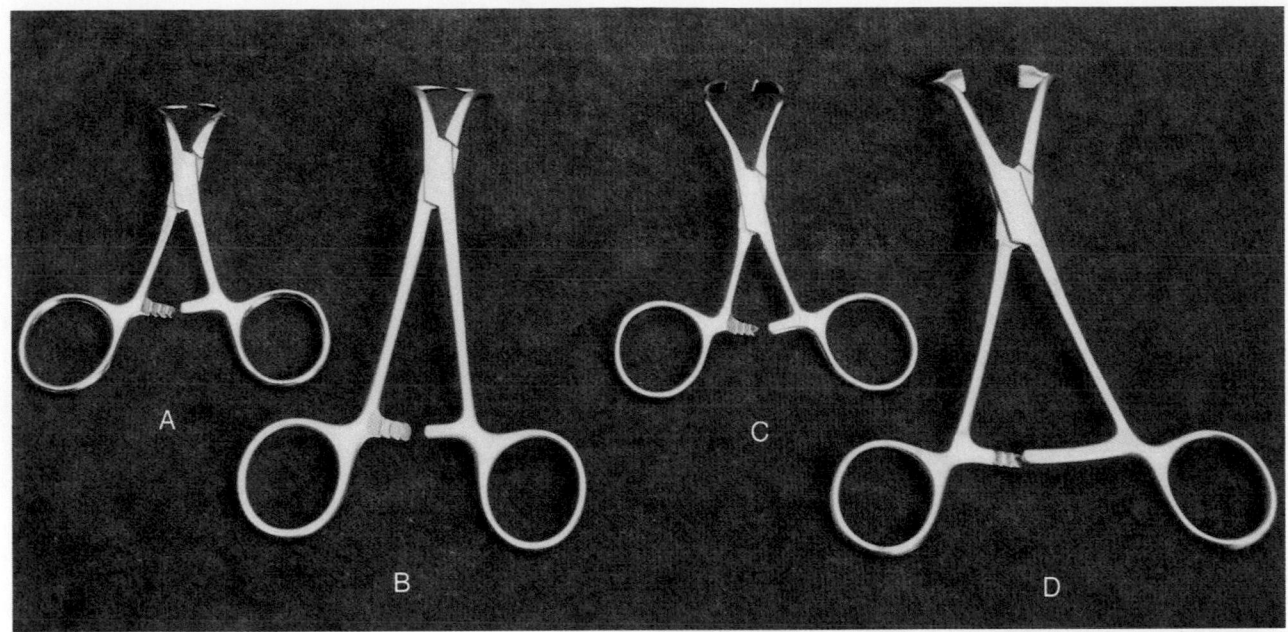

FIGURE 53-10 **A**, Small sharp towel forceps. **B**, Large sharp towel forceps. **C**, Small atraumatic towel forceps. **D**, Large atraumatic towel forceps.

Allis Tissue Forceps (Figure 53-11, *A*)

- Available in different lengths and jaw widths
- Used to grasp tissue, muscle, or skin surrounding a wound

Foerster Sponge Forceps (Figure 53-11, *B*)

- Used to hold gauze squares to sponge the surgical site

Transfer Forceps (Figure 53-11, *C* to *E*)

- Many sizes and lengths are available
- Sterile transfer forceps may be used to arrange items on sterile tray

Adson Thumb Forceps (Figure 53-12, *A* and *B*)

- Usually in 4-inch lengths
- Manufactured with or without teeth
- Used to grasp tissue and in suturing

Bayonet Forceps (Figure 53-12, *C* to *E*)

- Manufactured in different lengths
- Smooth tipped
- Used to insert packing into or remove objects from nose and ear

Plain-Tip Tissue Forceps (Figure 53-12, *F*)

- Manufactured in different lengths
- Atraumatic to tissue
- Used to grasp tissue, muscle, or skin surrounding a wound

Toothed Tissue Forceps (Figure 53-12, *G*)

- Manufactured in 4- to 18-inch lengths
- Pincher grip
- Used to grasp tissue, muscle, or skin surrounding a wound

Retractors

Retracting instruments hold tissue away from the surgical wound (incision). Depending on physician preference, skin hooks and Senn retractors are used to retract during most minor surgical procedures. These instruments are hand-held and are used for skin retraction. Self-retaining retractors, such as the Weitlaner, remain extended by mechanical means.

Army-Navy Retractor (Figure 53-13, *A*)

- Hand-held
- Used to retract small incisions

Four-Prong Rake Retractor (Figure 53-13, *B*)

- Pronged end may be sharp or dull
- Manufactured in different lengths

Senn Retractor and Skin Hook (Figure 53-13, *C* and *D*)

- Used to retract small incisions or to secure a skin edge for suturing
- Flat end is a blunt retractor
- Three-prong end may be sharp or dull

Weitlaner Retractor (Figure 53-13, *E* and *F*)

- Used to retract incisions
- Self-retaining
- Available with sharp or blunt teeth
- Available in different lengths

Crile Malleable (Ribbon) Retractor (Figure 53-13, *G* and *H*)

- Used to hold back margins of large wounds and connective tissue or organs from the surgeon's viewing field.

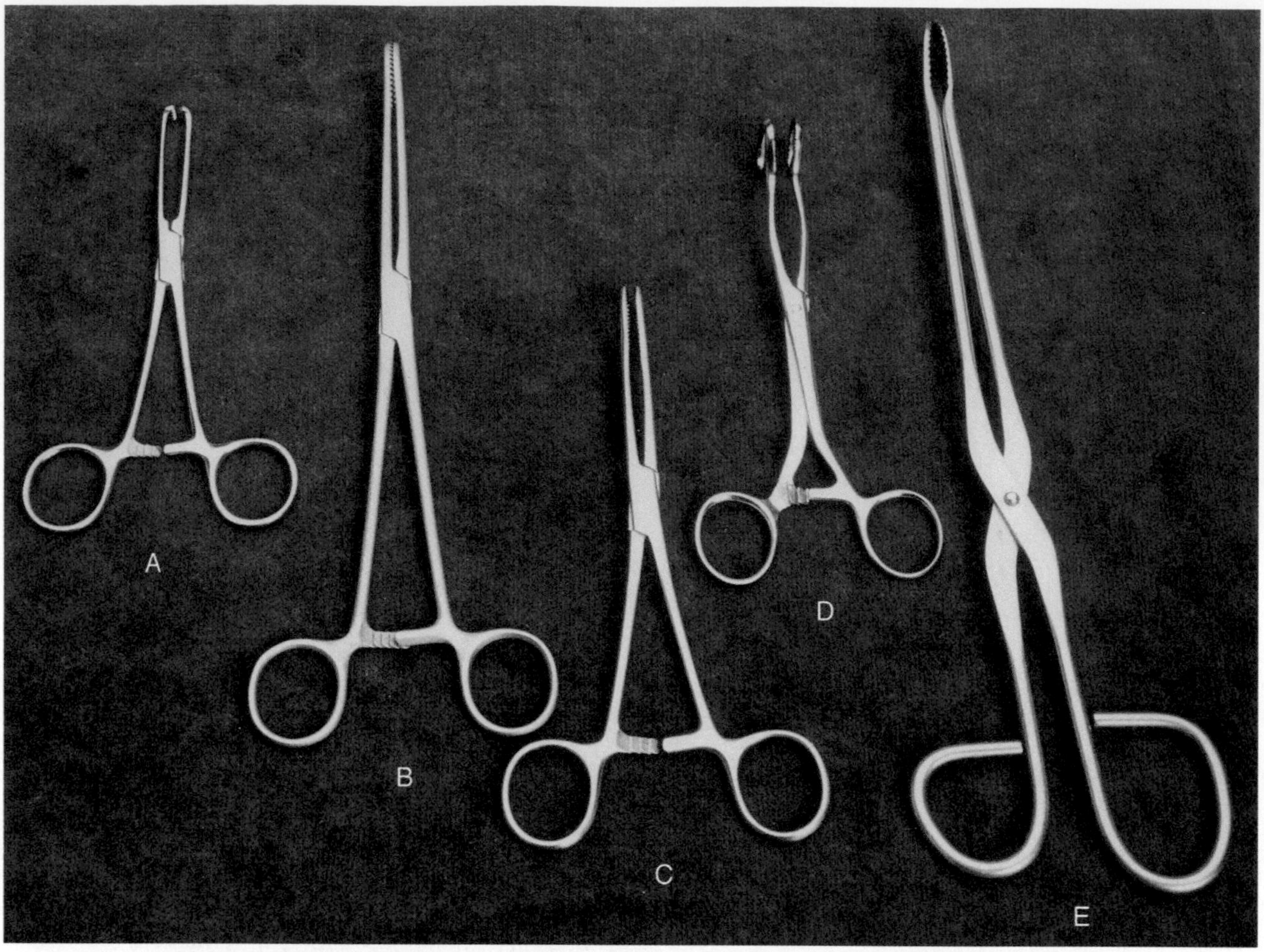

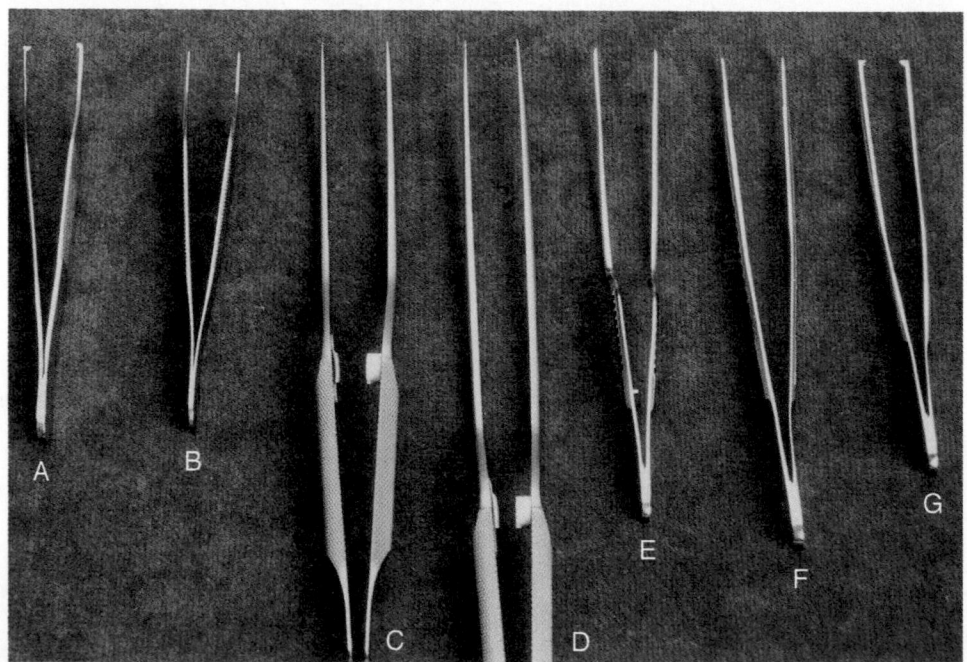

FIGURE 53-11 **A**, Allis forceps. **B**, Foerster sponge forceps. **C**, Straight transfer forceps. **D**, Short transfer forceps. **E**, Long transfer forceps.

FIGURE 53-12 **A**, Toothed Adson forceps. **B**, Smooth Adson forceps. **C**, Medium long bayonet forceps. **D**, Long bayonet forceps. **E**, Short bayonet forceps. **F**, Plain-tip tissue forceps. **G**, Toothed tissue forceps.

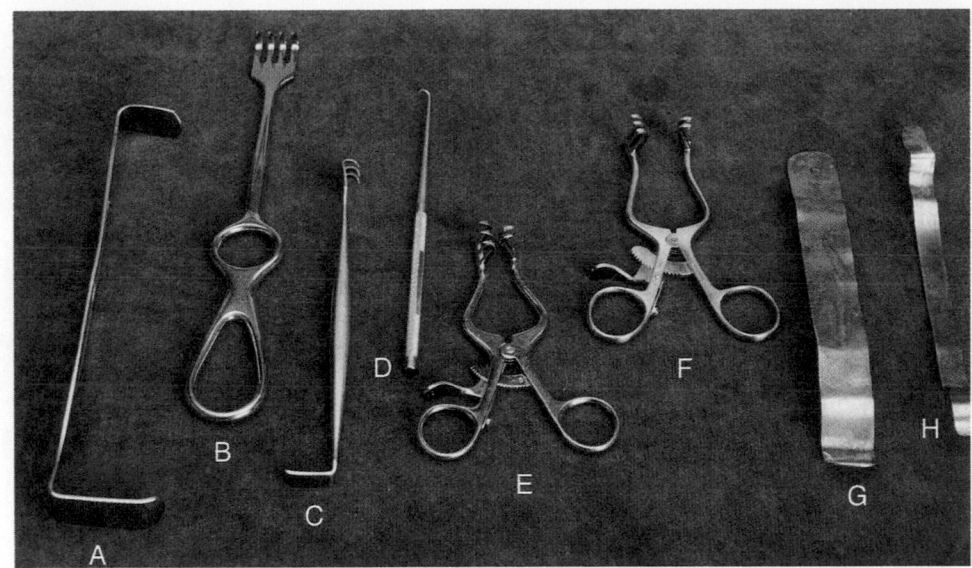

FIGURE 53-13 **A**, Army-Navy retractor. **B**, Four-prong rake retractor. **C**, Senn retractor. **D**, Single skin hook. **E**, Sharp 3/2 Weitlaner retractor. **F**, Dull 3/2 Weilaner retractor. **G**, Wide Crile (ribbon) retractor. **H**, Narrow Crile (ribbon) retractor.

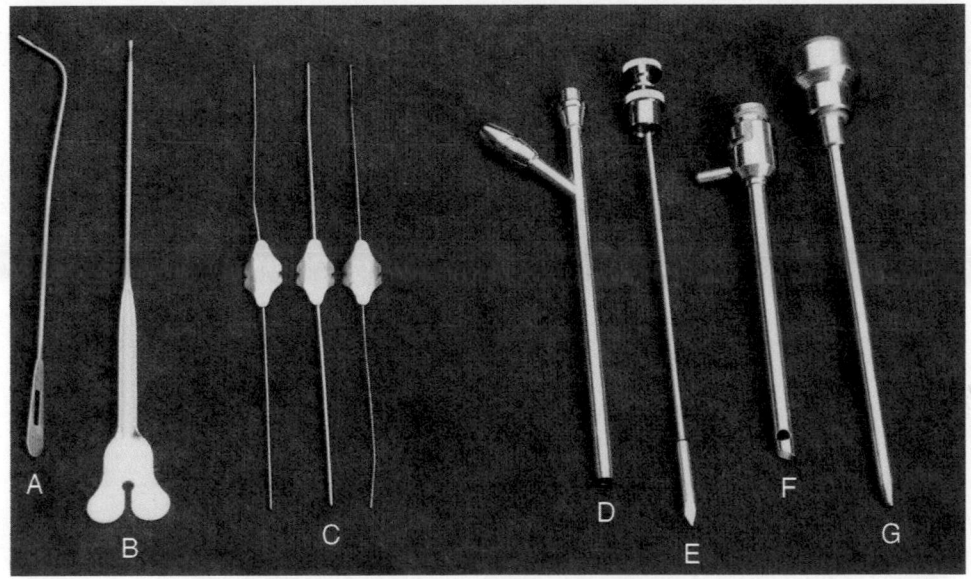

FIGURE 53-14 **A**, Probe. **B**, Grooved director. **C**, Lacrimal duct probes. **D**, Double-ended cannula. **E**, Sharp trocar. **F**, Cannula. **G**, Blunt-tip obturator.

Probes and Dilators

These instruments are used for both surgery and examinations. Probes can be used to search for a foreign body in a wound or to enter a **fistula**. Dilators are used to stretch a cavity or opening for examination or before inserting another instrument to obtain a tissue specimen.

Probes (Figure 53-14, *A* to *C*)

- Length ranges from 4 to 12 inches; available with or without bulbous tip
- May be smooth or have a grooved director
- Used to find foreign bodies embedded in dermal tissue or muscle or to trace a wound tract

Trocars and Obturators (Figure 53-14, *D* to *G*)

- Consist of a sharply pointed **stylus (obturator)** contained in a **cannula** (outer tube)
- Available in various sizes
- Used to withdraw fluids from cavities or for draining and irrigating with a catheter

Specula (Figure 53-15, *A* to *D*)

- Most common dilator used
- Valves are spread apart, dilating the opening
- Used to open or distend a body orifice or cavity

Nasal Specula (see Figure 53-15, *A* and *B*)

- Valves can be spread to facilitate viewing
- An applicator or snare can be introduced through the valves
- Used to spread the nostrils for examination

Specialty Instruments

Although all instruments fall under the same four categories as the surgical instruments just discussed, the remaining instruments are organized into specialty groupings. Presenting the instruments in this manner makes it easy to see how the instruments relate to particular examinations. In addition to recognizing the name and use of each instrument, the medical assistant must organize and set out the instruments needed for each particular examination in what is called a tray setup.

Gynecology

Foerster Sponge Forceps (Figure 53-16, *A*)

- Used in the same way as the dressing forceps
- Tips are round and serrated

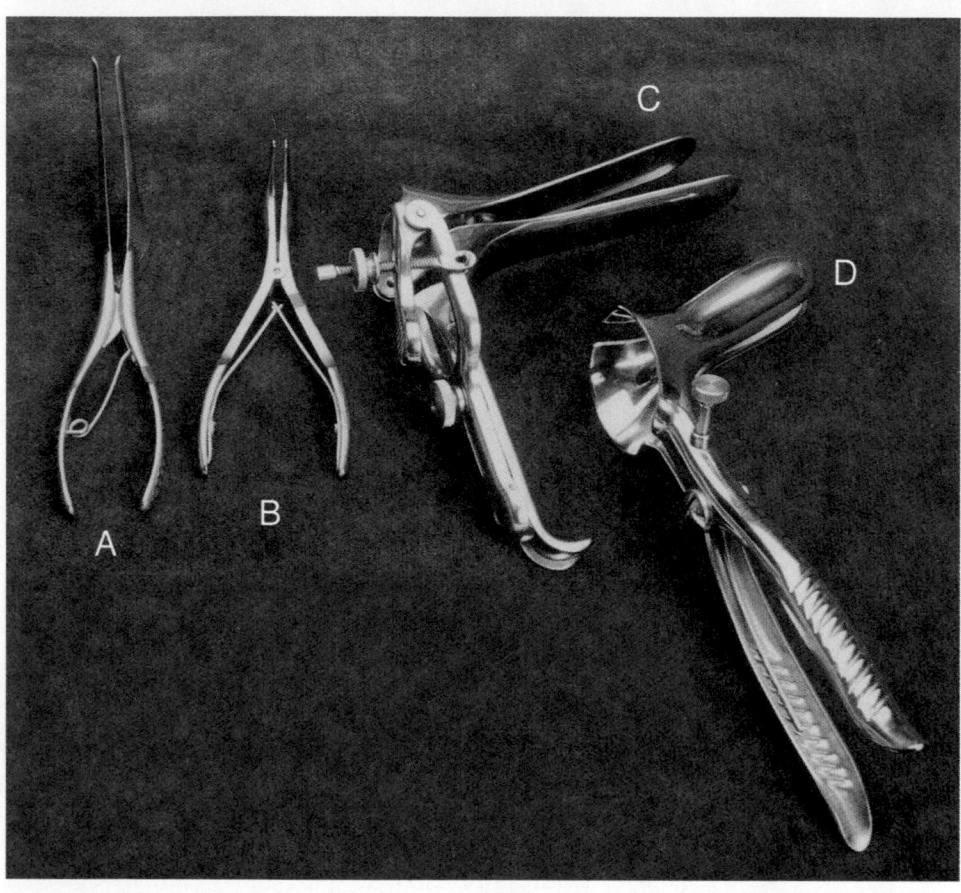

FIGURE 53-15 **A**, Long nasal speculum. **B**, Short nasal speculum. **C**, Graves vaginal speculum. **D**, Anal speculum, self-retaining.

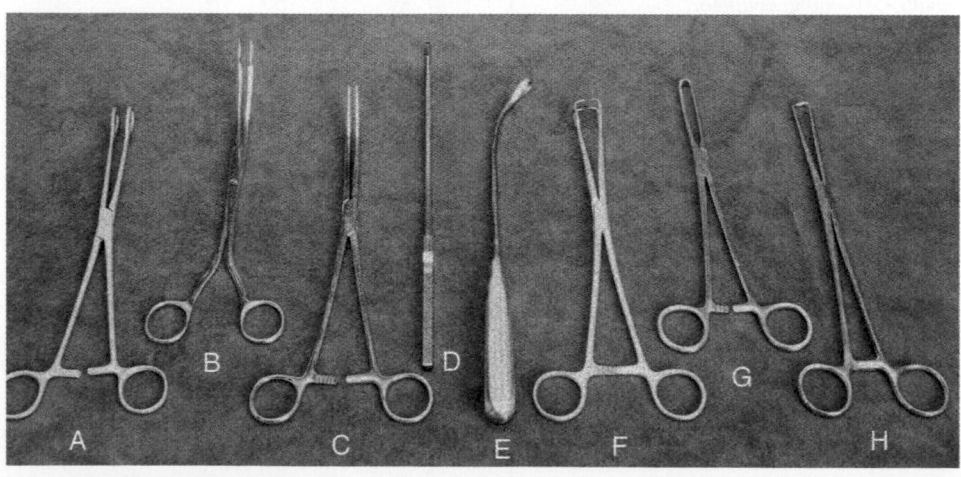

FIGURE 53-16 **A**, Foerster sponge forceps. **B**, Placenta forceps. **C**, Bozeman uterine dressing forceps. **D**, Endocervical curette. **E**, Sime uterine curette. **F**, Schroeder uterine vulsellum forceps. **G**, Long Allis forceps. **H**, Schroeder uterine tenaculum forceps.

Placenta Forceps (Figure 53-16, *B*)

- Used to remove tissue from the uterus

Bozeman Uterine Dressing Forceps (Figure 53-16, *C*)

- Used to swab the area or apply medication
- Designed to hold sponges or dressings
- Capable of reaching the cervix through the vagina

Endocervical Curette (Figure 53-16, *D*)

- Smaller than the uterine curette
- Used the same as the uterine curette

Sims Uterine Curette (Figure 53-16, *E*)

- Used to remove **polyps**, secretions, and bits of placental tissue
- Manufactured in several sizes
- Hollow and spoon shaped, used for scraping

Schroeder Uterine Vulsellum Forceps (Figure 53-16, *F*)

- Used to hold tissue (such as cervix) while obtaining a tissue specimen or to lift the cervix to view the fornix

Long Allis Forceps (Figure 53-16, *G*)

- Same as Allis forceps
- Used in deeper body cavities

Schroeder Uterine Tenaculum Forceps (Figure 53-16, *H*)

- Used in the same way as the vulsellum forceps
- Have very sharp, pointed tips

Hegar Uterine Dilators (Figure 53-17, *A*)

- Used to dilate the cervix for **dilatation** and **curettage**
- Available in sets
- Double or single ended

Sims Uterine Sounds (Figure 53-17, *B*)

- Used to check the **patency** of the cervical os or the urethral meatus

Ophthalmology and Otolaryngology

Krause Nasal Snare (Figure 53-18, *A*)

- Has a wire loop at the tip that can be tightened
- Used to remove polyps from the nares

Metal Tongue Depressor (Figure 53-18, *B*)

- Used to depress the tongue for oral examinations

Hartmann "Alligator" Ear Forceps (Figure 53-18, *C*)

- Has a 3½-inch shaft and is made in a variety of styles
- Action of the jaw similar to that of an alligator's jaw
- Used to remove foreign bodies or polyps

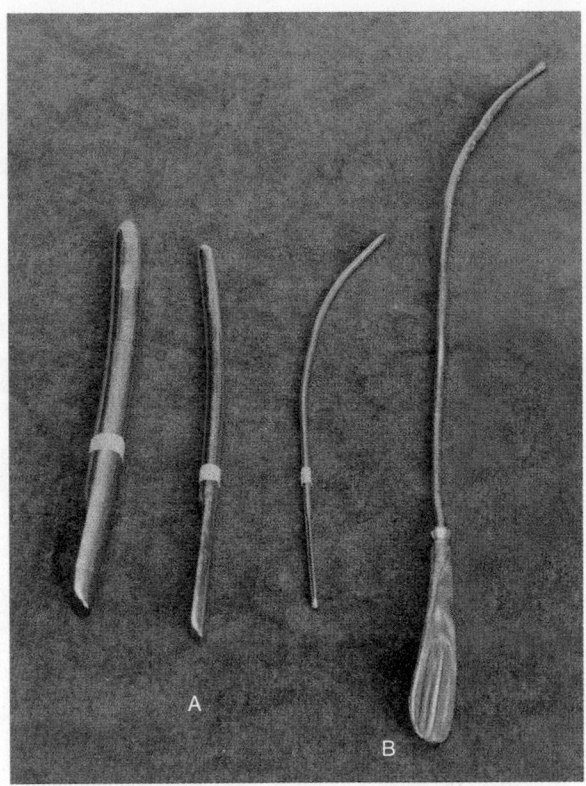

FIGURE 53-17   **A**, Uterine dilators. **B**, Sims uterine sounds.

Laryngeal Mirror (Figure 53-18, *D*)

- Made in various sizes
- May have a nonfogging surface
- Used for examination of the larynx and postnasal area

Ivan Laryngeal Metal Applicator (Figure 53-18, *E*)

- Holds cotton in place with its roughened end. Used to swab or sponge throat or postnasal tissue
- Six to 9 inches long with curved end for use in throat or postnasal areas
- Used to remove foreign bodies imbedded in the pharynx

"Buck" Ear Curette (Figure 53-18, *F*)

- Made with sharp or blunt scraper ends
- Manufactured in various sizes
- Used to remove foreign matter from the ear canals

Sharp Ear Dissector (Figure 53-18, *G*)

- Used to remove debris from the ear canal

Biopsy

Cervical Biopsy Forceps (Figure 53-19, *A*)

- Available with or without teeth
- Used to obtain cervical specimens for diagnostic examination

Rectal Biopsy Punch (Figure 53-19, *B*)

- Manufactured with interchangeable stems

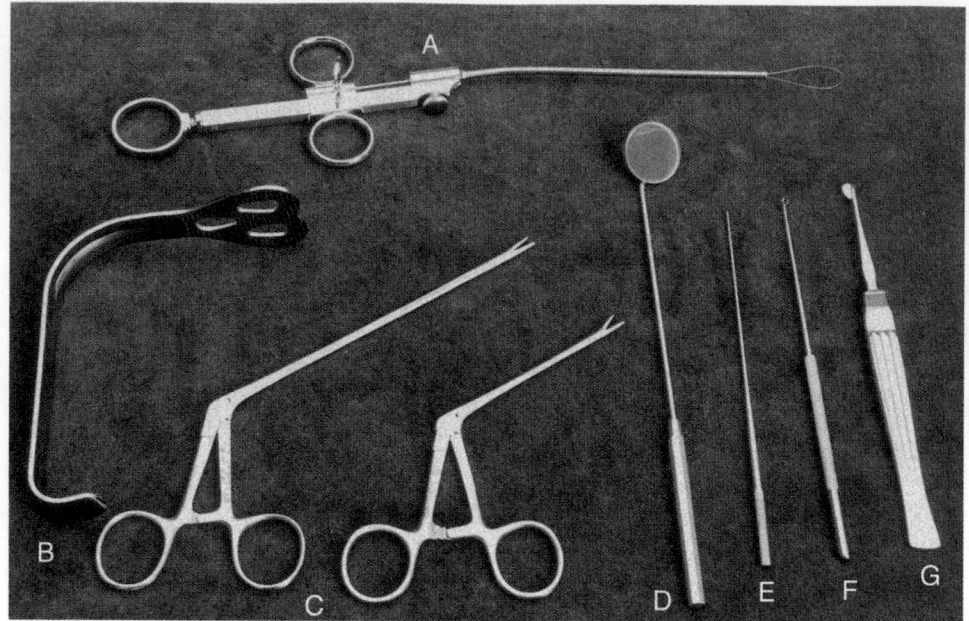

FIGURE 53-18 **A**, Krause nasal snare. **B**, Metal tongue depressor. **C**, Long and short alligator forceps. **D**, Laryngeal mirror. **E**, Ivan metal applicator. **F**, "Buck" ear curette. **G**, Sharp ear dissector.

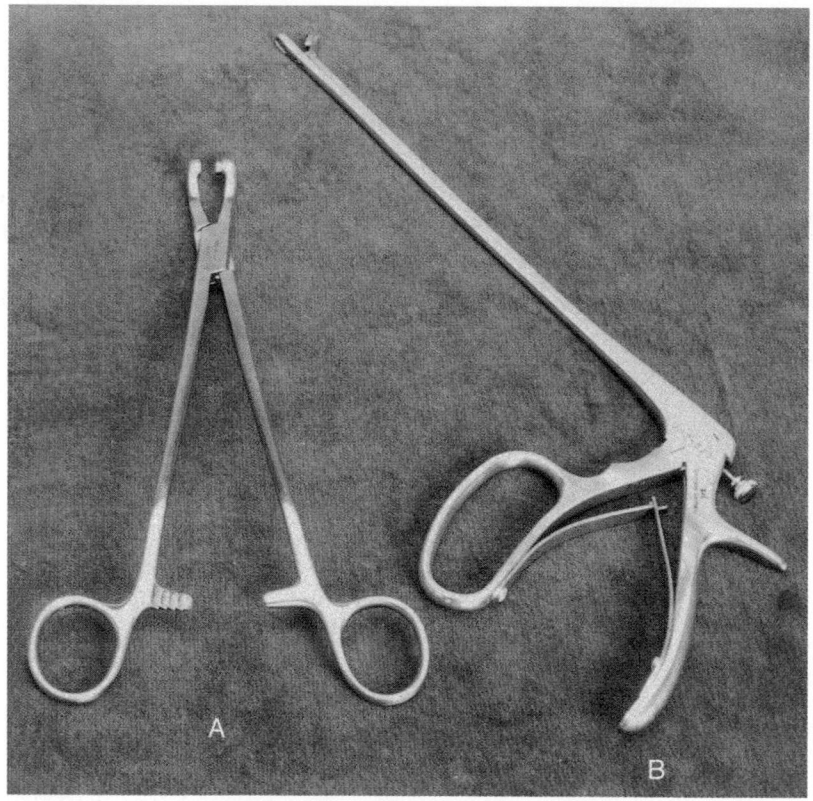

FIGURE 53-19 **A**, Cervical biopsy forceps. **B**, Rectal biopsy punch.

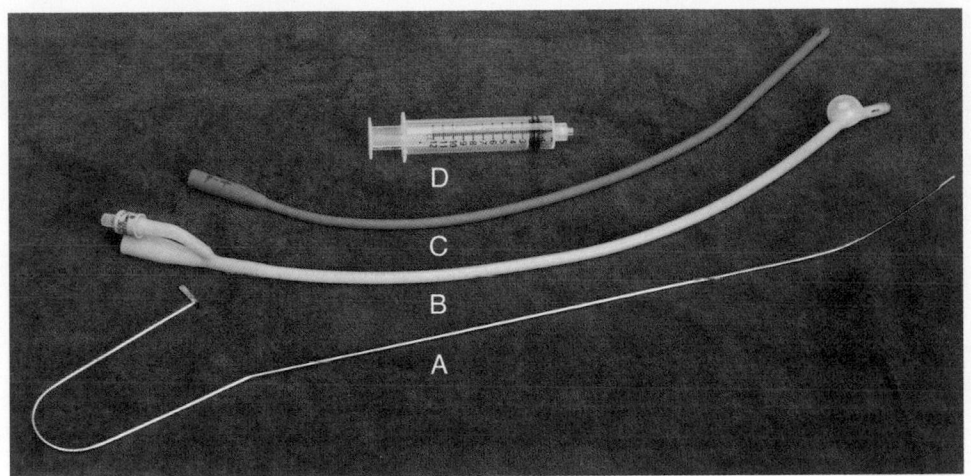

FIGURE 53-20 **A**, Metal catheter guide. **B**, Foley catheter with inflated balloon. **C**, Red Robinson catheter. **D**, 12-ml Luer-Lok syringe.

- Available in different lengths and styles
- Used through a proctoscope or sigmoidoscope

Silverman Biopsy Needle

- Manufactured with a split cannula
- Stylus is removed, and cannula is inserted to retrieve specimen.
- Needle biopsy can eliminate the need for surgical incision

Genitourinary

Catheter Guide (Figure 53-20, *A*)

- Metal guide
- Used with extreme caution
- Used by the physician when it is impossible to insert a catheter by normal means

Foley Catheter With Inflated Balloon
(Figure 53-20, *B*)

- Manufactured in sizes 8 to 32 French with a double rubber lining toward the tip
- After insertion, sterile solution injected into the inner lining (inflating the balloon) to hold it in the bladder
- Used as an indwelling catheter

Red Robinson catheter (Figure 53-20, *C*)

- Soft rubber urethral catheter in sizes 8 to 32 French (each French unit is equal to 1.3 mm)
- The higher the number, the larger the **lumen**
- Inserted temporarily into the bladder for drainage or to obtain a specimen

12-ml Luer-Lok Syringe (Figure 53-20, *D*)

- Used for injecting amounts greater than 5 ml

Colon-Rectal

Sigmoidoscope

- Used to internally view the anus, rectum, and sigmoid colon
- Used with a fiberoptic light source; may use photography or video setup

CRITICAL THINKING APPLICATION

Tom is preparing instrument and supply packs for specific procedures performed by Dr. Samanski. One of the packs he is preparing for the autoclave is for removal of a nasal polyp. Based on your understanding of typical and specialty instruments and supplies, what items should Tom include in the instrument pack?

Care and Handling of Instruments

Because instruments are expensive and the physician's skill is dependent on their quality, the medical assistant must properly care for each instrument to maximize its life and ensure that every part is in safe working order.

Most instruments are made of fine-grade stainless steel. The term *stainless* is usually taken too literally. Although stainless steel does resist rust and keeps a fine edge and tip longer, even the best stainless steel may develop water spots and stains, especially if water with a high mineral content is used. Proper hardness and flexibility are important. Inexpensive instruments that are chrome plated may be too brittle or too soft. In addition, mistreatment of chrome-plated instruments can cause minute breaks in the finish, which may become a source of contamination or may tear the surgeon's gloves.

All instruments should be carefully examined when they are purchased. Scissors should be tested to see whether they shear the full length of the blades completely to the tip. If the scissors cut a piece of cloth cleanly and do not chew at any point, even at the tip, they are functioning correctly. Teeth and serrations should be checked to see whether they intermesh completely and whether the jaws are even on the sides and tip. Each instrument should be felt over its entire surface for any rough areas that may tear or snag the surgeon's gloves or act as a future source of contamination. Box-locks and hinges must work freely but should not be too loose. Thumb- and spring-handled instruments must have the correct tension and meet evenly at the tips. After inspection, instruments should be cleaned and checked again for possible faulty workmanship before sterilization.

Under no circumstances should instruments be bundled together or allowed to become entangled. Avoid mixing stainless steel instruments with others made of different metals. This may cause electrolysis and result in etching. Even mixing stainless steel with chrome-plated instruments is best avoided. If an instrument is accidentally dropped, it may be permanently damaged. If scissors are dropped with the blades partially open, there may be a nick at the point where the blades cross.

After the surgical procedure, contaminated instruments should be placed in a basin of disinfectant solution with heavier instruments on the bottom of the basin and lighter, more delicate instruments placed on top. Always unlock each instrument before immersion in the chemical decontaminate to permit cleansing of the entire surface area. Never allow blood or other coagulable substances to dry on an instrument because they will be difficult to remove. If immediate disinfection is not possible, the instruments should be rinsed well and placed in a cold water solution with a blood solvent and mild detergent. The detergent increases the wetting ability of the water, giving the instrument surfaces better exposure to the solution. It is best to use a detergent that has a neutral pH, with low suds action and easy rinse off. Manufacturer recommendations for the correct dilution and time of immersion of the various disinfectants and blood solvents must be strictly followed for the chemicals to be effective.

When the surgical procedure is completed, the receiving basin for the instruments should be transferred from the surgical area to the cleaning and sterilization room. It is important to remove used instruments from the patient's view as soon as possible. After decontamination is completed, instruments should be thoroughly rinsed and either washed by hand or washed mechanically using an ultrasonic washer.

Some delicate instruments, such as microsurgical and lensed instruments, should be washed by hand with a mild, low-suds, neutral pH detergent solution and a soft brush. The instruments should be cleaned while submerged to avoid airborne spread of microorganisms. Throughout the cleaning process, the medical assistant should wear heavy utility gloves to avoid possible contaminant exposure. Instruments should then be rinsed with distilled water, dried with a lint-free cloth, and inspected for proper function before packing for sterilization.

Mechanical washing, such as with an ultrasonic washer, can be used for most instruments and is an especially good method for cleaning sharp instruments to avoid possible injury.

An ultrasonic cleaning unit uses sound waves while instruments are immersed in a cleaning solution to clean contaminants from instrument surfaces. The unit then rinses and dries the instruments, leaving them ready for the sterilization process. Manufacturer guidelines should be used with rubber and plastic materials.

After disinfection and inspection, the instruments are ready for the sterilization process. This procedure is discussed in Chapter 54.

Commercially prepared disposable packs are available for most minor surgical procedures. They save time and eliminate cleaning and autoclaving reusable stainless steel instruments but may be cost prohibitive for individual practices.

> ### CRITICAL THINKING APPLICATION
>
> Tom is responsible for inspecting and caring for all of the surgical instruments in the minor surgical room as well as cleaning and preparing contaminated instruments for autoclaving. Tom is in the process of writing an addition to the office policies and procedures manual on the management of surgical instruments. Based on what you know about the care and handling of surgical instruments, what should Tom include in the policy?

Drapes, Sutures, and Needles

Disposable surgical drapes are available in several different materials and sizes and typically have an opening (fenestration) for the operative site. The drape is placed over the operative area using sterile technique after the patient's skin preparation has been completed. This procedure is presented in Chapter 54.

Sutures

The word *suture* is used as both a noun and a verb. As a noun, it refers to a surgical stitch or to the material used to close a wound. As a verb, it refers to the act of stitching. Modern surgery and the use of sutures began in 1865, when Lister developed antisepsis and the disinfection of suture materials. Many kinds of materials have been used over the centuries, including precious metals, horse hair, animal tendons, and cotton and linen cord. Most of the improvements in suture materials and techniques have occurred in the past 50 years.

A suture may also be used as a ligature. This is a strand of suture material used to tie off a blood vessel or to strangulate tissue. If a ligature is used to tie off an internal tubular structure, it must last permanently or long enough for the structure itself to disintegrate.

Types. Sutures may be classified as either *absorbable* or *nonabsorbable*. Many different suture materials are available, each having its advantages and disadvantages. The following are commonly used suture materials in minor surgical procedures (Figure 53-21).

Absorbable Suture. The absorbable suture is dissolved by the body's enzymes during the healing process. It is used when deep incisions or lacerations require inner layers of sutures to close the wound. Absorbable suture material is also used in areas where suture removal is difficult, as in oral surgery. An example of an absorbable suture material is surgical catgut, which is obtained from sheep, cattle, or pig intestine. Plain catgut is used in tissues that heal most rapidly, such as mucous membranes and

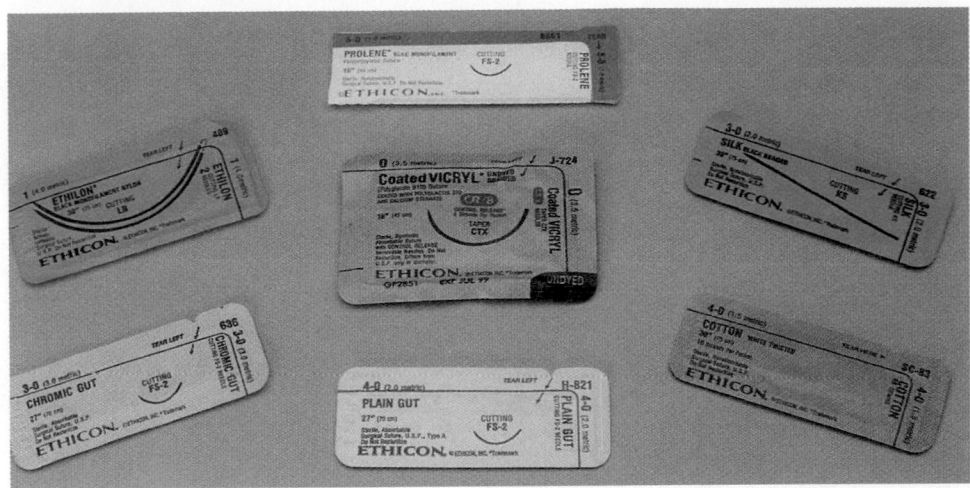

FIGURE 53-21 Suture packets labeled according to size, type, length, and type of needle point and shape.

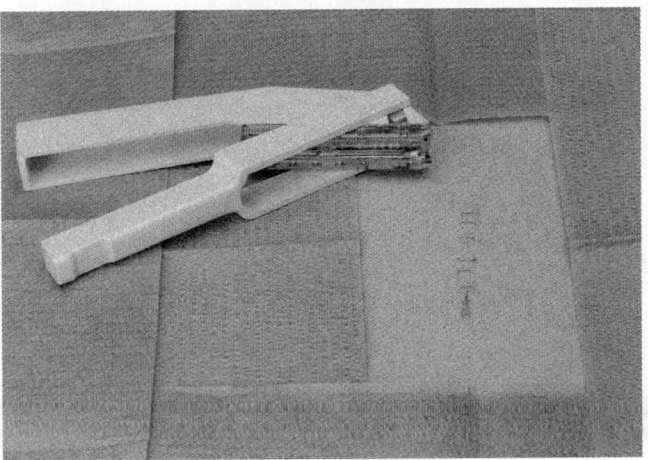

FIGURE 53-22 Disposable skin stapler.

subcutaneous tissues. Chromic catgut is coated with chromic salts, which delays the absorption of the suture material up to 80 days.

Catgut was once the absorbable suture material of choice but has been replaced in recent years by Vicryl, a synthetic absorbable suture made of polyglactin. It may take as long as 11 weeks to be absorbed.

Nonabsorbable Suture. Nonabsorbable suture material is left in the wound site until healing is complete. It is frequently used in minor surgical procedures performed in the medical office because most of the suturing required is superficial and in areas where sutures can be removed after healing has taken place. A common non-absorbable suture material is silk because it is strong and easy to tie. It is treated with a coating to prevent tissue drag and flaking. Polyester fiber suture is one of the strongest nonabsorbable sutures along with surgical steel. These fine filaments are braided and have great tensile strength. Nylon suture is strong and has a high degree of elasticity. It is primarily used for skin closure. Owing to its elasticity and stiffness, many knots must be used because the knots tend to untie if placed incorrectly.

Surgical staples can also be used for skin closure. They are made of stainless steel or titanium and are available in different sizes. They are applied and removed with specific staple instruments (Figure 53-22).

Suture Sizing and Packaging. Suture material comes in a variety of diameters and lengths. The diameter of the suture strand determines its size, with the smaller gauges below 0 (pronounced *aught*) and the larger gauges above 0. For instance, 2-0 is thinner than size 0, which is thinner than size 2. Sutures as thin as size 11-0 and as thick as size 7 are available. The sizes from 2-0 to 6-0 are the most frequently used in the medical office. The length of the suture may vary and strands are precut in 18-, 24-, 54-, and 60-inch lengths (Figure 53-23).

Needles

Surgical needles are chosen according to the area in which they are to be used and the depth and width of the desired suture. They are classified according to shape, which may be straight or curved (Figure 53-24). Most sutures are applied with curved needles because they allow the physician to penetrate the surface and then back up again on the other side. The sharper the curve of the needle, the deeper the surgeon can pass it into the tissue. The point of a needle can be a taper or a cutting edge. A taper is used on delicate tissues. The cutting edge needle is used on the skin. It lacerates the skin as the needle is passed through. This is advanta-geous on tougher tissues, such as connective tissue.

Most needles are manufactured with the thread attached, or *swaged*, to the needle. These atraumatic needles do not have an eyelet and cause the least amount of tissue trauma as they are passed through the tissues. Manufacturers package the suture strands with the suture needle attached in peel-apart sterile dispos-able packages. These may be obtained single, individu-ally packed, or as multipack sutures in a variety of needle types and sizes with a wide range of suture materials and lengths. The most common needle type for minor skin repair is the curved, cutting-edged, swaged needle.

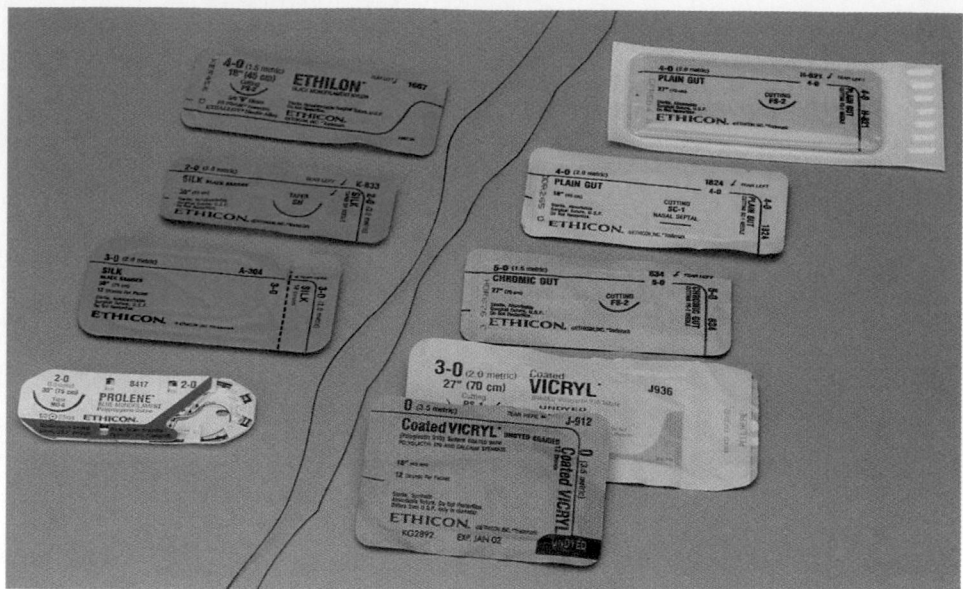

FIGURE 53-23   Suture packets (and opened suture strands) with and without needles.

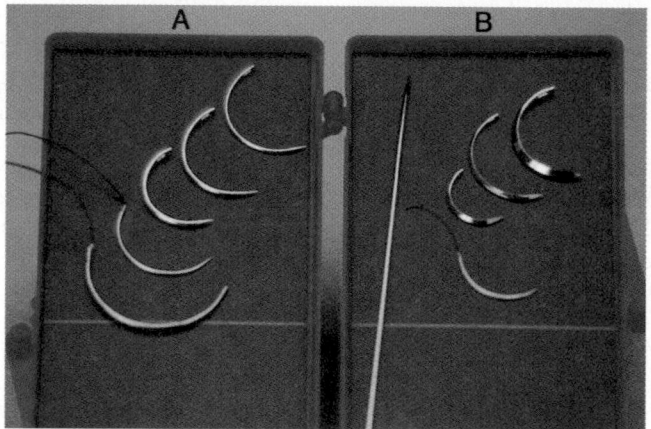

FIGURE 53-24   Surgical needle shapes. **A**, Taper point. **B**, Cutting point.

Patient Education

Patients may have questions concerning the instruments the surgeon is using. The medical assistant can assist the patient by answering his or her questions to help alleviate any fears. Explaining patient preparation for the procedure, how it will be conducted, and what to expect afterward helps make the procedure easier to perform and encourages the patient to follow the physician's advice and orders.

Legal and Ethical Issues

When surgical procedures are done in the medical office, awareness of legal responsibilities is imperative. The medical assistant must know what surgery is planned and whether the patient has been informed regarding the procedure. In the surgical setting, the medical assistant must realize the full extent of his or her role as the "patient's advocate" and the "physician's agent."

The medical assistant should confirm the fact that the physician has explained the surgery to the patient and that the patient fully understands all aspects of the procedure that will be performed. This means that when the patient signs the consent for surgery, he or she is fully informed. Increasing the patient's understanding ensures greater compliance with presurgical preparations, the surgical procedure, and postsurgical care.

SUMMARY OF SCENARIO

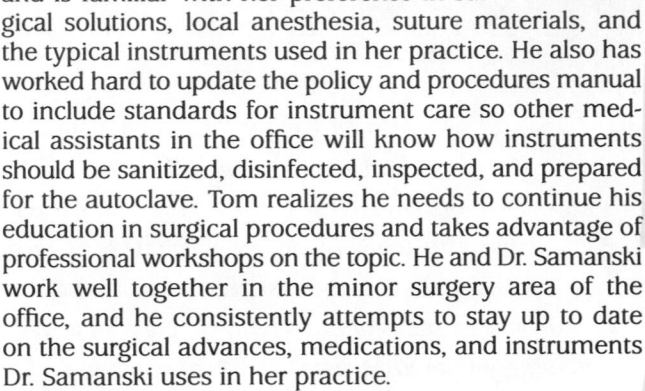

Tom has worked for Dr. Samanski for 2 years and is familiar with her preference in surgical solutions, local anesthesia, suture materials, and the typical instruments used in her practice. He also has worked hard to update the policy and procedures manual to include standards for instrument care so other medical assistants in the office will know how instruments should be sanitized, disinfected, inspected, and prepared for the autoclave. Tom realizes he needs to continue his education in surgical procedures and takes advantage of professional workshops on the topic. He and Dr. Samanski work well together in the minor surgery area of the office, and he consistently attempts to stay up to date on the surgical advances, medications, and instruments Dr. Samanski uses in her practice.

SUMMARY OF LEARNING OBJECTIVES

■ The solutions used in minor surgery include sterile water for mixing with medications or rinsing instruments; sterile saline for injection or wound irrigations; antiseptic skin cleansers such as Betadine or Hibiclens for site preparations; local anesthetics, including ethyl chloride or Fluori-Methane topical applications as well as lidocaine, Nesacaine, or Sensorcaine injectables. These local anesthetics may come packaged with or without epinephrine. The physician may also use topical silver nitrate to control local bleeding.

■ Surgical instruments are classified according to their use as either cutting, grasping, retracting, or probing and dilating tools. The components of the instrument include the type of handle, the closing mechanism, and the jaws. Instrument tips may be either straight or curved.

■ Surgical instruments are expensive and must be cared for properly to maintain function and maximize life. Instruments must be examined when purchased for proper working order and possible faults with mechanisms. Stainless steel instruments should be kept separate from other metal types. Each instrument must be cleaned according to manufacturer guidelines, unlocked, and disinfected immediately after use. Some instruments must be washed by hand in a mild, low-suds neutral pH solution and soft brush. Most instruments can be cleaned with an ultrasonic washer, which is an especially good method for sharp instruments to avoid possible injury.

■ The instruments used in minor surgical procedures are dependent on the type of procedure and physician preference. Many disposable prewrapped surgical packs can be purchased; however, if packs are wrapped and autoclaved in the ambulatory care setting, it is important to be familiar with what is needed for a particular procedure as well as what the operating physician prefers.

■ Suture material is available as absorbable for internal sutures or nonabsorbable for skin closures. Catgut or Vicryl are the two most popular absorbable materials; nonabsorbable sutures can be made out of silk, nylon, or staples. Suture materials range in size, with smaller gauges for finer tissues below 0 (aught) and thicker gauges above 0, and they come in various lengths. Surgical needles are either straight or curved. The sharper the curve, the deeper the surgeon can pass the needle. Most needles are manufactured with the suture material attached. A wide range of suture material is packaged attached to a variety of needle types. The medical assistant must ask the physician for his or her preference.

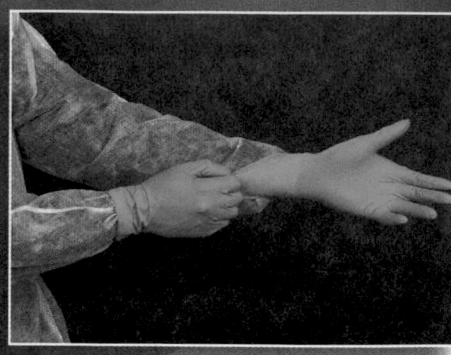

CHAPTER 54

Scenario

Melissa Gelbart has been a surgical medical assistant for Lakeside Surgical Associates for just over 1 month. She was hired to work as an administrative medical assistant at the front desk, but when one of the surgical assistants unexpectedly quit, the supervisor of surgery offered Melissa the position. At least she was familiar with a number of the patients, most of the staff, and the kinds of outpatient surgeries that were performed on a daily basis. Surgical asepsis and assisting with surgery were her favorite topics when she was in medical assisting school. She is very enthusiastic to get into the operating room, but they are starting her out in the supply and sterilization area. The supervisor of surgery wants her to become familiar with all of the surgical trays and instruments used daily at Lakeside Surgical Associates. It will probably be about 4 months until she gets to start working in the surgical suite.

Surgical Asepsis and Assisting With Surgical Procedures

Kim Anthony Aaronson

Learning Objectives

- Define and spell the terms listed in the vocabulary.
- Define the concepts of aseptic technique.
- Explain the differences among sanitization, disinfection, and sterilization.
- Explain the types and uses of sterilization indicators.
- Discuss the legal and ethical concerns regarding surgical asepsis and infection control.
- Conduct patient education in aseptic technique and surgical procedures.
- Demonstrate proper hand-washing technique for surgical asepsis.
- Clean and wrap instruments and equipment for autoclaving.
- Load, run, and unload an autoclave properly.
- Open a sterile pack to create a sterile field.
- Transfer sterile instruments and pour solutions into sterile field.
- Assist with minor surgical procedures.
- Assist with suturing.
- Remove sutures.
- Properly apply dressings and bandages to surgical sites.
- Apply sterile gloves and gown.
- Remove contaminated gloves.
- Perform a surgical skin prep.

National Curriculum Competencies

CLINICAL COMPETENCIES

1a. Perform hand washing
1b. Wrap items for autoclaving
1c. Perform sterilization techniques

1d. Dispose of biohazardous materials
1e. Practice standard precautions
4f. Prepare patients for and assist with procedures, treatments, and minor office surgery

Vocabulary

antiseptic Substance that kills microorganisms.

asepsis Being free from infection or infectious materials.

contamination Becoming unsterile by contact with any nonsterile material.

diseases Pathological processes having a descriptive set of signs and symptoms.

disinfection Destruction of pathogens by physical or chemical means.

edema Swelling between layers of tissue.

infection Invasion of body tissues by microorganisms that then proliferate and damage tissues.

microorganisms Living organisms that can only be seen with a light microscope.

pathogens Disease-causing microorganisms.

permeable Allows a substance to pass or soak through.

spores Thick-walled dormant form of bacteria, very resistant to disinfection measures.

sterilization Complete destruction of all forms of microbial life.

Asepsis means freedom from infection or infectious material. *Medical asepsis* is the destruction of organisms *after they leave the body*. The principles of medical asepsis are implemented to prevent reinfection of a patient and prevent cross-infection to another patient or to ourselves. Isolating potential microorganisms and pathogens by following standard blood and body fluid precautions by disinfecting or sterilizing objects as soon as possible after they are contaminated does this quite effectively. This creates a nonsterile but clean environment.

Surgical asepsis is the complete destruction of organisms *before they enter the body*. This technique is mandatory for any procedure that invades the body's skin or tissues, such as surgery. Everything that comes in contact with the patient should be sterile, including surgical gowns, surgical drapes, surgical instruments, and the gloved hands of the surgeon and surgical assistants. Any time the skin or a mucous membrane is punctured, pierced as in venipunctures or injections, aseptic techniques must be practiced. Urinary catheterizations, injections, and some specimen collections, such as venipuncture and biopsies, are performed using aseptic technique.

Sterile Technique

There is no mystery about surgical aseptic technique. Handling sterile items requires a degree of dexterity and vigilance that can only come with practice. It requires a great deal of concentration and planning of all movements in the area and of all procedural steps. The procedures covered in this chapter are for minor surgery; they are also the same techniques that are used for major surgery. To develop sound knowledge of sterility and sterile technique, use the following memory aid: *Everything sterile is white,* and *everything that is not sterile is black.*

There is no gray! Sterile surfaces must NEVER come into contact with nonsterile surfaces. If this occurs, the sterile surface immediately is considered contaminated or unsterile. Here absolute honesty is important. This is called a "break" in sterility or a "break" in the sterile field. During any procedure, everything must stop at this point and the "break" must be corrected immediately. Any break could lead to serious wound **contamination**, postoperative **infection**, and even death.

This chapter discusses in detail how to establish and maintain a sterile field.

Personnel

Hands and hair are two of the greatest sources of contamination. With practice, you will learn to know what may be touched with your hands and what must be touched only with sterile gloved hands. Hair that falls freely over the shoulders and forward gives off a cloud of bacteria with every movement. It must always be secured back and up, not touching the shoulders. Sterile field rules include:

- Air currents carry bacteria, so body motions over a sterile field and talking should be kept to a minimum.
- Sterile team members should *always* face each other.
- *Always* keep the sterile field in your view. *Never* turn your back on a sterile field or wander away from it.
- Nonsterile persons or items should never cross the sterile field.

Sterile Field

A sterile field is any sterile surface on which sterile items are placed. In the office, a sterile field will most often be set up on a Mayo stand (Figure 54-1). In surgery, a sterile field is created by draping sterile towels (either disposable or from autoclaved packs) over a Mayo stand or table. The surgical site on the patient's skin is prepared (or "prepped," as it is called in healthcare practice) and then draped with sterile towels or drapes so it also becomes a sterile field.

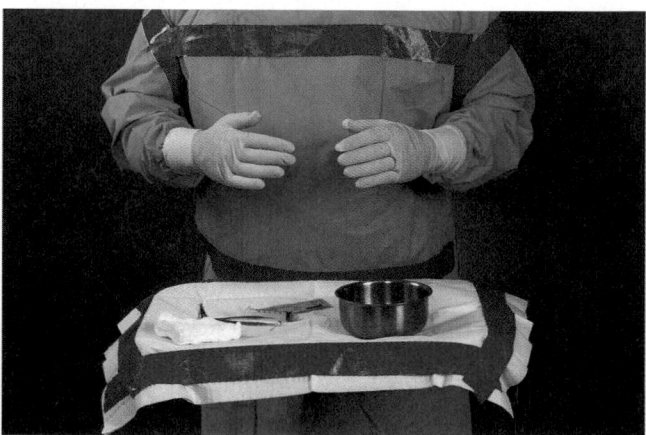

FIGURE 54-1 Sterile field (outlined in red).

Sterilization

Sterilization reduces the likelihood of contamination to patients, physicians, medical assistants, and other surgical staff. To ensure proper sterilization for surgical aseptic procedures, an area should be set aside in each office for just this purpose. The area should be divided into two sections, one *dirty* and one *clean*. The *dirty* section is used for receiving contaminated instruments and other materials at the conclusion of surgical procedures. This area should have a sink as well as receiving basins, proper cleaning agents, brushes, sterilizer wrapping paper or cloth, sterilizer envelopes and tape, sterilizer indicators, and disposable gloves. Designated waste containers are needed for gloves worn when handling contaminated items. The *clean* section should be reserved for receiving the sterile items after they are removed from the sterilizer. Clear, clean plastic bags in which to store sterile packs may be kept in the *clean* area. Both areas should be spotlessly clean and well organized.

CRITICAL THINKING APPLICATION

Melissa has spent the first few days reading the surgical supply and sterilization room procedure manual. Why is this important before she starts working with instruments? What information in this manual would be most important to Melissa as she starts this new position? Why?

All items must be properly sanitized and disinfected before sterilization occurs. Sterilization can be achieved by moist heat in an autoclave, by gas, and by chemicals. Most medical offices use the autoclave method.

Autoclave

Steam under pressure in the autoclave (Figure 54-2) is the best method of sterilization, because it kills all **pathogens** and **spores**. Pressurized steam is fast, convenient, and dependable. The pressure allows for heat higher than the boiling point, and when combined with moisture, these two factors create a very effective mechanism for killing all **microorganisms**. When steam is admitted into the autoclave chamber, it simultaneously heats and wets the object, coagulating the proteins present in all living organisms. When the cycle is complete and the chamber cooled, the steam condenses and explodes the cells of microorganisms, thus destroying them. To be effective, the steam moisture must contact *all* surfaces to be sterilized. Steam under pressure is capable of much faster penetration of fabrics and textiles than dry heat, but its use has definite limitations if the proper techniques are not followed.

The recommended temperature for sterilization in an autoclave is 121° to 123° C (250° to 255° F). Unwrapped items should be sterilized for 20 minutes, small wrapped items for 30 minutes (Table 54-1), and large or tightly wrapped items for 40 minutes.

TABLE 54-1	Sterilization Chart		
Article	**Method**	**Temperature (F)**	**Time**
Gauze, small, loosely packed	Autoclave	250°	30 min
Gauze, large, loosely packed	Autoclave	270°	30 min
Gauze, small, tightly packed	Autoclave	250°	40 min
Gauze, large, tightly packed	Autoclave	270°	40 min
Gauze, tightly packed	Dry heat	320°	3 hr
Gauze, loosely packed	Dry heat	320°	2 hr
Glass syringes in tubes	Autoclave	250°	30 min
Glass syringe in muslin	Dry heat	320°	1 hr
Instruments on tray, muslin under and over	Dry heat	320°	1 hr
Instruments on tray, muslin under and over	Autoclave	250°	15 min
Solutions in flasks with gauze plug	Autoclave	250°	30 min
Glassware unwrapped	Dry heat	320°	1 hr
Glassware wrapped	Autoclave	250°	30 min
Petroleum jelly, 1-oz jar	Dry heat	340°	1 hr
Petroleum jelly, 2-oz jar	Dry heat	320°	2 hr
Petroleum gauze in instrument tray	Dry heat	320°	150 min
Powder, 1-oz jar	Dry heat	320°	2 hr
Powder, small glove packs	Autoclave	250°	15 min

Remember to always place an indicator in areas where there is doubt that the steam will penetrate.
Do not measure by chamber pounds. A thermometer and indicator are the reliable methods of judging a killing temperature.

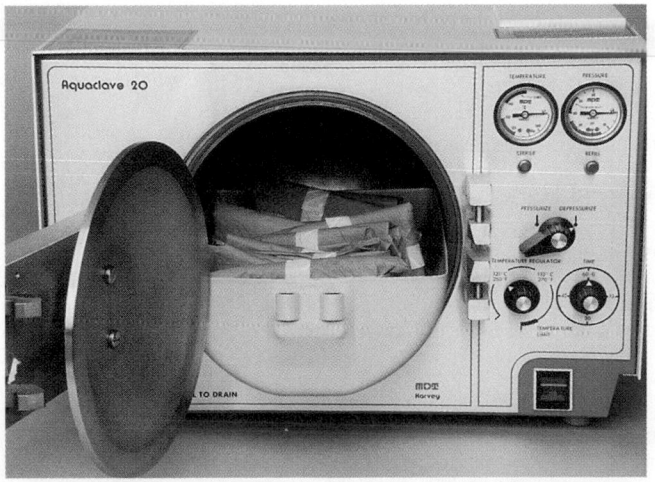

FIGURE 54-2 Steam autoclave. (Courtesy Aquaclave by MDT.)

Incorrect operation of an autoclave may result in superheated steam. If steam is brought to too high a temperature, it is literally dried out, and the advantage of a higher heat is diminished. Wet steam is another cause of incomplete sterilization. Wet steam results from failing to preheat the chamber, which causes excessive condensation in the interior of the chamber. Condensation is necessary, but too much prevents the sterilization process from being properly completed. It can be compared with taking a hot shower in a cold bathroom, which results in heavily steamed mirrors, walls, and towels. If fabric packs become too saturated to dry during the drying cycle, the packs will pick up and absorb bacteria from the air or any surface on which they are placed. Placing cold instruments in a hot chamber also increases condensation. Other causes of wet steam include opening the door too wide at the end of the cycle or allowing a rush of cold air into the chamber. Overfilling the water reservoir may produce this same effect.

The main cause of incomplete sterilization in the autoclave is the presence of residual air. Without the complete elimination of air, an adequately high temperature cannot be reached. Air and steam do not mix. Because air is heavier than steam, it will pool wherever possible. One tenth of 1% (0.1%) residual air trapped around an instrument will prevent complete sterilization. This is especially dangerous in older autoclaves that do not have a chamber thermometer separate from the pressure gauge. Adequate chamber pressure does not guarantee a proper chamber temperature. All release valves and discharge lines must be kept clean and free from dirt and lint (Table 54-2).

Wrapping Materials. Maintenance of sterility depends completely on the wrapper and method of wrapping (Procedure 54-1). The wrapping material must be permeable to steam but impervious to contaminants, such as dust and insects. A double thickness of material should be used.

Acceptable wrapping materials for autoclaving should be made of a substance that allows the steam to penetrate while preventing pathogens from entering during storage and handling. A wrapper should not be used if it is torn or has a hole in it. Clean muslin and disposable autoclave paper are examples of autoclave instrument wraps (Figure 54-3).

Wrapping Instruments. The method used to wrap instruments for autoclave sterilization must allow the pack to be opened without becoming contaminated. To protect the package contents, the following rules are followed:

- Muslin wrappers must be inspected for holes before each use and must be discarded if any holes are found.
- All hinged instruments are wrapped in the open position to allow full steam penetration of the joint.
- Place a gauze sponge around the tips of sharp instruments to prevent them from piercing the wrapping material.

TABLE 54-2	Tips for Improving Autoclaving Techniques	
Problem	**Causes**	**How to Correct**
Damp linens	Clogged chamber drain	Remove strainer; free openings of lint.
	Goods removed from chamber too soon after cycle	Allow goods to remain in sterilizer an additional 15 min with door slightly open.
	Improper loading	Place packs on edge; arrange for least possible resistance to flow of steam and air.
Stained linens	Dirty chamber	Clean chamber with Calgonite solution; never use strong abrasives, such as steel wool; rinse thoroughly after cleaning.
Corroded instruments	Poor cleaning; residual soil	Improve cleaning; do not allow soil to dry on instruments; sanitize first.
	Exposure to hard chemicals (e.g., iodine, salt, and acids)	Do not expose instruments to these chemicals; if exposure occurs, rinse immediately.
	Inferior instruments	Use only top-quality instruments.
Spotted or stained instruments	Mineral deposits on instruments	Wash with soft soap and detergent with good wetting properties.
	Residual detergents from cleaning	Rinse instruments thoroughly.
	Mineral deposits from tap water	Rinse with distilled water.
Instruments that have soft hinges or joints	Corrosion or soil in joint	Clean with warm, weak acid solutions (10% nitric acid solution); rinse thoroughly.
	Jaws and shanks out of alignment	Have instrument realigned by qualified instrument repair professional.
Ebullition, or caps that blow off solutions	Exhausting chamber too rapidly	Use slow exhaust, cool liquids, or turn autoclave off and let cool on its own; that is, let the pressure decrease at its own rate.
Steam leakage	Worn gasket	Replace.
	Door closes improperly	Reopen door and shut carefully; have serviced if unable to close door properly.
Chamber door does not open	Vacuum in chamber (check chamber pressure gauge)	Turn on controls to starting steam pressure; wait until equalized, then vent and open door.

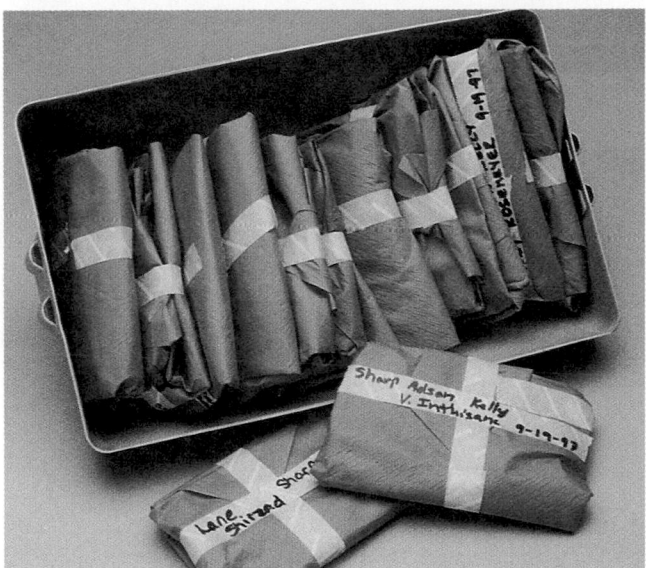

FIGURE 54-3 Autoclave paper wrap. Note chemical lines of indicator tape before autoclaving.

- If a number of instruments are to be placed on a stainless steel tray for wrapping, first place a double-folded towel on the tray and then position the instruments. This helps to protect them.
- When using sterilizing bags, insert the jaws of the instruments first to ensure that the grasping end of the instrument can be reached easily when the bag is opened.
- Indicate on the wrapper what is in the package or label it with a code. This code should correspond to a list of instruments that is stored with the pack after sterilization.

- Label the contents as noted, the sterilization date, and your initials. Use a permanent marker, never a ballpoint pen.

Whether you are wrapping one item or many items together on a tray as a surgical pack, the procedure is the same. Be sure to pick a wrapper that is large enough to adequately cover the items to be sterilized.

CRITICAL THINKING APPLICATION

Melissa has now moved to processing instruments and trays. She notices one of her co-workers never inspects a muslin wrapper before wrapping a pack. What is the significance of Melissa's observation? How should she handle this situation? Why?

Sterilization Indicators. Sterilization is achieved only when steam reaches an optimal temperature for a designated length of time and has penetrated to the center of the articles. To eliminate constant doubt about whether complete sterilization has been achieved, indicators are used. These indicators show, by melting or changing color, that a certain temperature has been reached for a certain period of time.

Autoclave Tape. Autoclave tape, a commonly used sterilization indicator, contains a chemical dye that changes color when exposed to steam (Figure 54-4). The tape is not an absolute indication that the proper sterilization time and temperature have been maintained; it merely indicates that a high temperature has been reached while the article was in the autoclave. Its main function is to verify that the package has been autoclaved.

PROCEDURE **54-1**

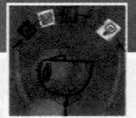

Wrapping Instruments and Supplies for Steam Sterilization in an Autoclave

GOAL: To place dry, checked, sanitized, and disinfected supplies and instruments inside appropriate wrapping materials for sterilization and storage without contamination.

EQUIPMENT AND SUPPLIES

- Dry, checked, sanitized, and disinfected items
- Assorted wrapping materials
- Autoclave tape
- Indicator tape
- A waterproof felt-tipped pen

PROCEDURAL STEPS

1 Collect and assemble already sanitized and disinfected items to be wrapped. Gloves may be worn.

2 Place the wrapper to be used on a clean flat surface.

3 Place the item (or items) diagonally at the approximate center of the wrapping material. Make sure the size of the square is large enough for the items (Figure 1).

Purpose: Each of the four corners must fold over and completely cover the items, with a few extra inches of overlap for folding back a flap.

Continued

PROCEDURE **54-1—cont'd**

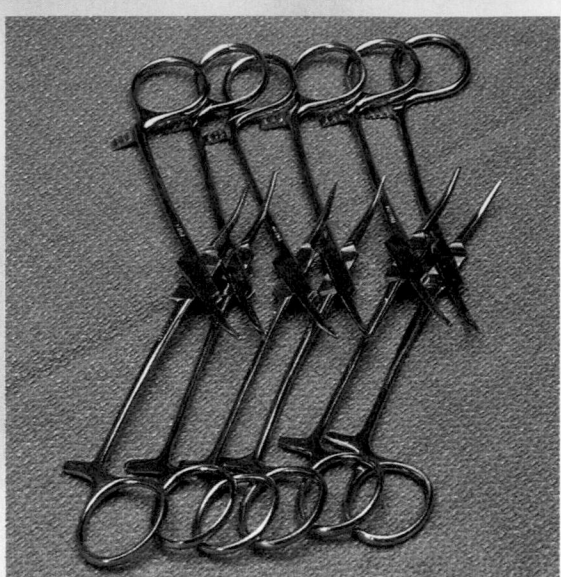

Figure 1

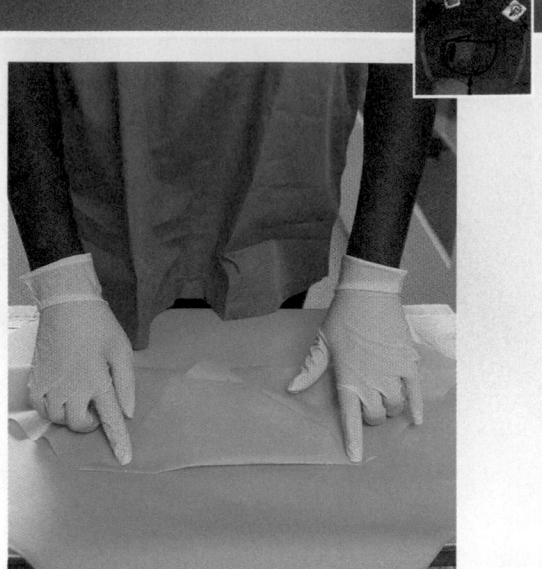

Figure 2

8 Repeat the above step with each corner, making sure to turn back a portion each time. (Figures 3 and 4).

4 With the squares that are cloth fabric, use two pieces if the cloth is single layered, or follow the manufacturer's recommendation when using commercial autoclave wrapping paper.

Purpose: To ensure sterility until the sterile item is needed for use.

5 Open any hinged instruments. If the instrument is sharp, its teeth or tip should be shielded with cotton or gauze.

Purpose: To prevent puncture of the package or the operator.

6 If the package is to contain several items, place a commercial sterilization indicator inside the package at the approximate center.

Purpose: To ensure that the autoclave is reaching effective levels of heat and pressure.

7 Bring up the bottom corner of the wrap, and fold back a portion of it.

Purpose: This folded-back flap is the only part of each wrapper corner that can be touched when opening a sterile package (Figure 2).

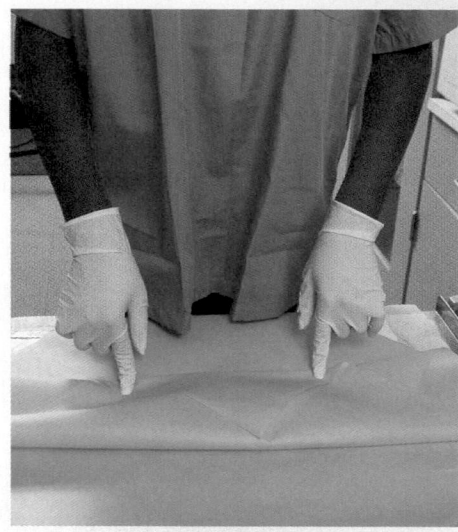

Figure 3

Sterilization Indicator Strips. A strip indicator contains a temperature-sensitive dye that changes color when the proper combination of steam, temperature, and time has been achieved. At least one indicator strip should be placed with each load deep within the packs or in places that seem inaccessible to steam.

Sterilization Indicator Bags. Sterilization indicator bags are very convenient. They are made of disposable paper or thermostable plastic and can be used to sterilize and store a variety of small surgical items. The bag is permeable to steam and provides a barrier against airborne bacteria during storage. An indicator is printed on each bag and appears when the bag has been autoclaved.

Culture Tube Test. An excellent system for testing the effectiveness of your office autoclave is the culture test. It is a bioindicator that consists of a double-walled

PROCEDURE **54-1—cont'd**

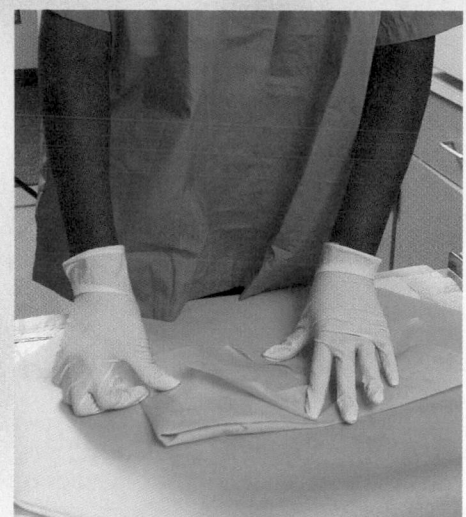

Figure 4

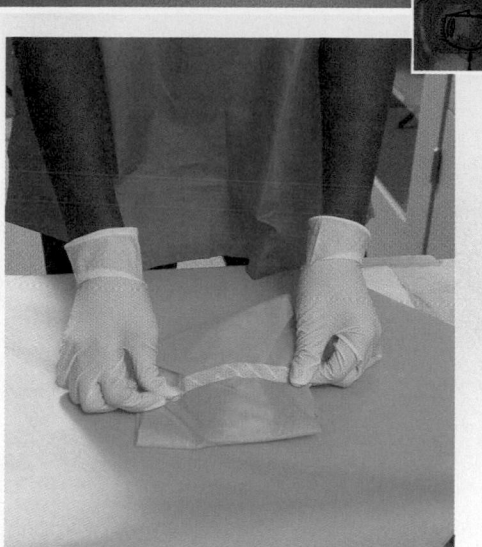

Figure 6

9 Fold the last flap over (Figure 5).

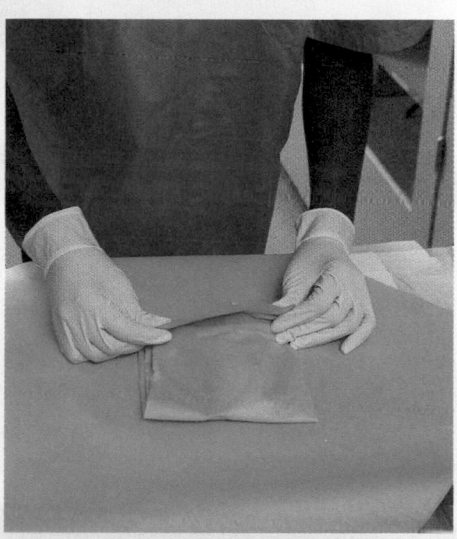

Figure 5

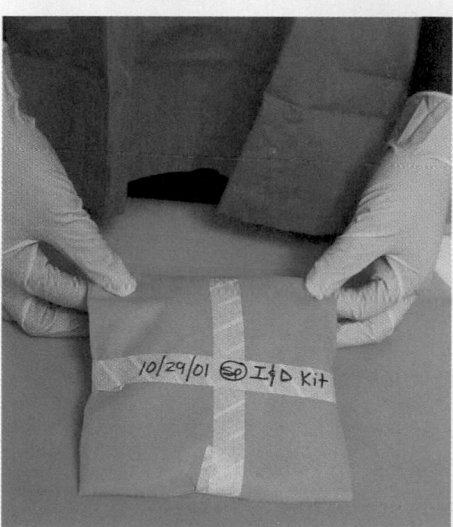

10/29/01 ℠ I&D Kit

Figure 7

10 Secure with autoclave tape (Figure 6).

11 Secure with autoclave tape and label package with the date including year, contents, and your initials (Figure 7).

Purpose: To know what is in the pack at a later date, whether the shelf life has expired (expiration date), and who performed the task. As a general rule, most office-autoclaved packs are considered sterile (usable) for up to 28 days.

tube that, when broken, releases a microorganism into a culture medium. If the sterilization cycle is defective and the microorganisms still live, growth should occur within 24 hours. A culture can be incubated in the office in a water bath or a dry block heating unit set at 37° C (98.6° F).

Quality Assurance Records for Office Sterilization. Every office should have specific protocols to follow for

quality assurance evaluation of the autoclave. This is done at specific intervals that depend on the volume and frequency of autoclave use. A log must be kept of the type of control test done, when it was performed, and the testing results. If the testing results indicate that the sterilization was inadequate, a report must be made and filed. This report will identify the nature of the problem and how and when it was corrected. This

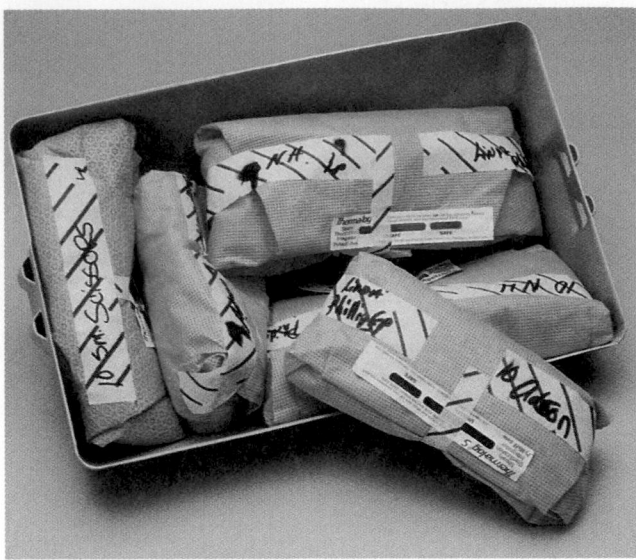

FIGURE 54-4 Wrapped autoclaved instruments with strip indicators on packages.

report will also contain proof of correction by indicating the date and time of a first, subsequent, and successful sterilization run.

Loading the Autoclave. Prepare all packs and arrange the load in a way that will allow maximum circulation of steam and heat (Procedure 54-2). Articles should be resting on their edges (see Figure 54-2). The packs should never be crowded tightly; instead, make several loads. Jars, bottles, and trays must be wrapped and placed on their sides if they are to be used to store sterile items. Covers on jars and containers should be put to one side or left open to allow steam to penetrate. Extreme care must be taken not to contaminate jars when replacing their lids after autoclaving is complete.

Instruments may be autoclaved unwrapped if they are to be used immediately or do not need to be sterile when used later. Perforated trays are used for sterilizing unwrapped instruments. Place a lint-free towel under and over the instruments to facilitate drying and to prevent contamination when removing them from the autoclave.

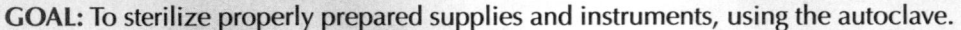

PROCEDURE 54-2

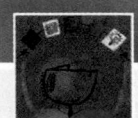

Operating the Autoclave

GOAL: To sterilize properly prepared supplies and instruments, using the autoclave.

EQUIPMENT AND SUPPLIES

- An autoclave
- Wrapped items ready to be sterilized

PROCEDURAL STEPS

1 Check the water level in the reservoir and add distilled water as necessary.

Purpose: Too much or too little water may alter the effectiveness of the equipment. Tap water will leave lime deposits in the chamber.

2 Turn the control to "fill" to allow water to flow into the chamber. The water will flow until you turn the control to its next position. Do not let the water overflow.

3 Load the chamber with wrapped items, then space them for maximum circulation and penetration.

Purpose: Ensure sterilization of all items.

4 Close and seal the door.

Purpose: The door must be closed or the heated water in the chamber will evaporate.

5 Turn the control setting to "on" or "autoclave" to start the cycle.

6 Watch the gauges until the temperature gauge reaches at least 121° C (250° F) and the pressure gauge reaches 15 pounds of pressure.

Purpose: Proper temperature and pressure must be reached before sterilization can begin.

7 Set the timer for the desired time.

8 At the end of the timed cycle, turn the control setting to vent.

Purpose: This releases the steam and pressure. The water at the bottom of the chamber will drain back into the reservoir.

9 Wait for the pressure gauge to reach zero.

10 Open the chamber door a fourth of an inch.

Purpose: To allow steam to escape faster.

11 Leave the autoclave control at vent to continue producing heat.

Purpose: To dry the items faster.

12 Allow complete drying of all articles.

13 Using heat-resistant gloves or pads, remove the items from the chamber and place the sterilized packages on dry, covered shelves or open autoclave door and allow items to cool.

14 Turn the control knob to "off," and keep the door slightly ajar.

Purpose: Allows the inside of the autoclave to dry completely.

Unloading Guidelines. When the sterilization cycle is complete, release the pressure following manufacturer's instructions. Once the pressure gauge reads "0," stand back from the door and, with oven mitts, open the door about $1/4$ inch. Allow the load to dry for at least 15 minutes (this will vary according to the type of autoclave and the size of the load). Capillary attraction is the action that draws moisture through the surface of materials. Packs can act like a sponge, attracting outside moisture and microorganisms. Touching a wet pack allows microorganisms on your hands to penetrate the wrappings, making the contents of the pack unsterile. Dry, wrapped packs may be removed with clean, dry hands, but it is safer to wear oven mitts to reduce the possibility of burns from the hot instruments inside the packs. If possible, allow all packs to cool in the autoclave with the door open. Place the packs on a dry, dust-free surface inside an enclosed cupboard or drawer for storage. Avoid placing the packs on cold surfaces, because hot packs may cause condensation, and moisture will contaminate the contents.

Shelf-Life of Sterilized Packs. Each office will have its own strict guidelines regarding the shelf-life of sterile packs. Generally, double-wrapped muslin and double-wrapped paper packs are considered sterile for up to 28 days from the date of sterilization. Another way to say this is that these types of packs have a 28-day expiration date (or a 28-day shelf-life) from the date of sterilization. Nonpermeable plastic-wrapped packs are considered sterile for up to 6 months from the sterilization date. All sterile packs should be stored on dry, dust-free, covered shelves or in drawers. Fabric wrappers must be inspected for holes and laundered after each use. A damaged pack or a broken seal renders the package unsterile; spills of any fluid onto a package will also contaminate it. When a pack is no longer sterile for any reason, including expiration date, the contents must be reprocessed as if the pack had been used for surgery. The contents must be sanitized, disinfected, wrapped, and sterilized as usual.

CRITICAL THINKING APPLICATION

Melissa discovers a number of packages of paper-wrapped sterile instruments that have no dates on them. The indicator tape shows that they have been autoclaved. What should she do with these packs? Why?

Gas Sterilization

There are a variety of gas sterilizers on the market. Each has its own very specific operating guidelines to ensure operator safety. Because of the long processing times, very specific OSHA requirements for gas ventilation, and the associated hazards of reproductive organ damage and cancer, it is unrealistic to use gas sterilization in the physician's office.

Chemical Sterilization

In the medical office, chemical sterilization is used for instruments that cannot be exposed to the high temperatures of steam sterilization. The sterilizing chemical solution must be mixed exactly according to the instructions on the bottle. The solution must be marked with the date of preparation and expiration. Materials to be sterilized must be submerged in this chemical bath for 8 hours or more. Items are removed with sterile forceps and must be rinsed with sterile water to remove all traces of the chemical before using on a patient. It is then dried with a sterile towel. You must avoid skin contact with the sterilizing solution because it is very caustic.

Scrub, Gloves, and Gown

The instruments are sterile and ready for surgery. Now the attention is drawn to the medical assistant. In a sense, the goal is to make you as sterile as possible so that your microorganisms do not contaminate the sterile field or the operative site of the patient. To ensure surgical asepsis, the following procedures (Procedures 54-3 to 54-7) must be learned and followed precisely as appropriate for the surgery to be performed. Practice these procedures until you can accomplish each one quite automatically.

The Medical Assistant's Role in Asepsis

Medical asepsis *directly* affects the health and well-being of the patient, physician, and office staff. The spread of pathogens in the office can be controlled only through effective sterilization of all reusable equipment.

A medical assistant must develop an inner sense for aseptic procedures. *It is important that these techniques be performed on such a routine basis that they become an unbreakable habit.* Conscientious attention must be given to sterilizing *all* items at *all* times. Frequent checking and rechecking of solutions and procedures helps to ensure that they are effective and are employed without any "breaks" in technique. Using single-use, disposable items is the best method of infection control and is being used more frequently in medical offices. However, when disposable equipment is used, the assistant must be conscious of disposal guidelines and provide the office and the environment with continuous protection.

Surgical Procedures

Common Office Minor Surgical Procedures

Common surgical procedures that are routinely performed in the primary care office include suturing, cyst removal, incision and drainage of an abscess, and biopsy. The medical assistant should be proficient in explaining each of these procedures to the patient, preparing the patient and the room, assisting the physician

Text continues on page 1181.

PROCEDURE 54-3

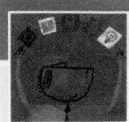

Performing Surgical Hand Scrub

GOAL: To scrub your hands with surgical soap, using friction, running water, and a sterile brush to sanitize your skin before assisting with any procedure that requires surgical asepsis.

EQUIPMENT AND SUPPLIES

- Sink with foot or arm control for running water
- Surgical soap in a dispenser
- Towels
- Nail file or orange stick
- Sterile brush

PROCEDURAL STEPS

1 Remove all jewelry.
  Purpose: Jewelry harbors bacteria and is not permitted in surgical asepsis.

2 Inspect your fingernails for length and your hands for skin breaks.

3 Turn on the faucet and regulate the water to a comfortable temperature.

4 Keep your hands upright and held at or above waist level (Figure 1).
  Purpose: Water running from the nonscrubbed area above the elbow down to the hands can carry bacteria back onto the hands. All areas below the waist are considered contaminated during all surgical procedures.

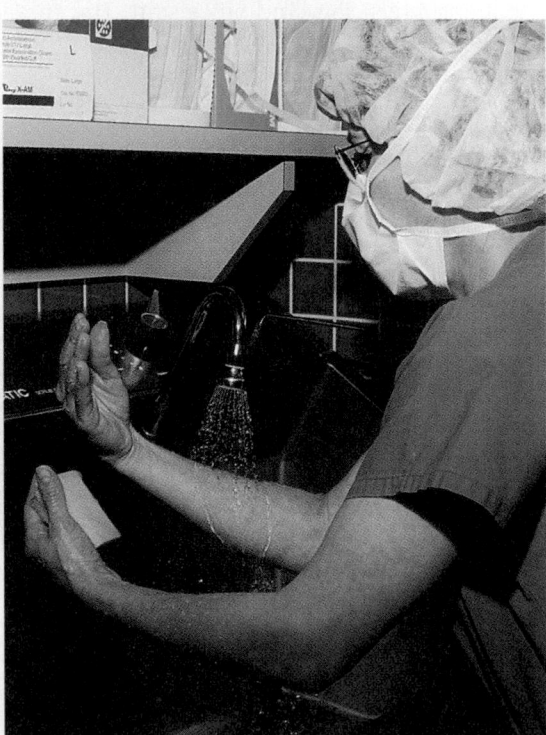

Figure 1

5 Clean your fingernails with a file, discard it, and rinse your hands under the faucet without touching the faucet or the insides of the sink basin (Figure 2).

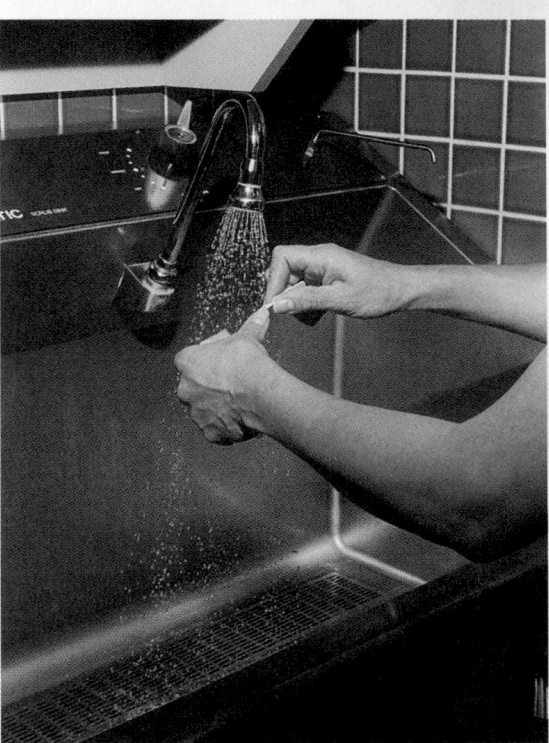

Figure 2

6 Allow water to run over your hands, apply acceptable solution, lather while holding your fingertips upward, and remember to rub between the fingers (Figures 3 and 4). The scrub process should take at least 5 minutes for each hand/arm.
  Purpose: The surfaces of the fingers have four sides.

7 Wash wrists and forearms while holding your hands above waist level (Figures 5 and 6). Rinse arms and forearms without touching the faucet or the insides of the sink basin.
  Purpose: Always keep away from the contaminated faucet and basin.

PROCEDURE 54-3—cont'd

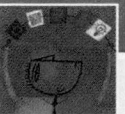

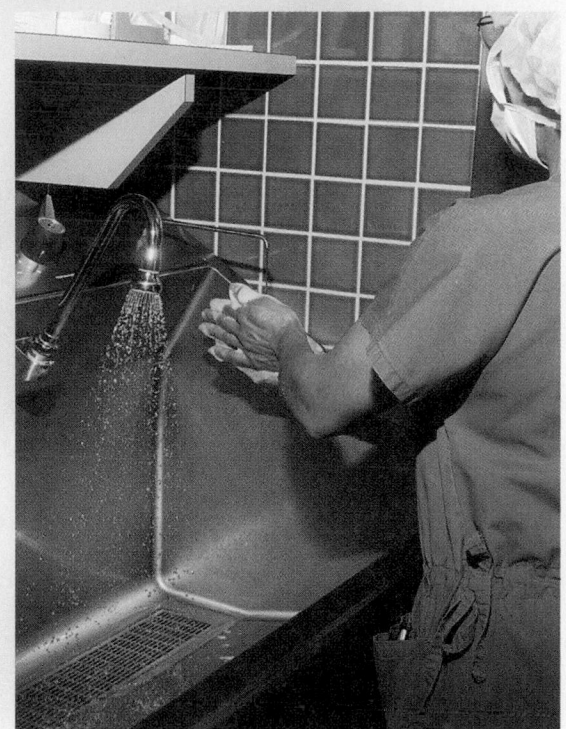

Figure 3

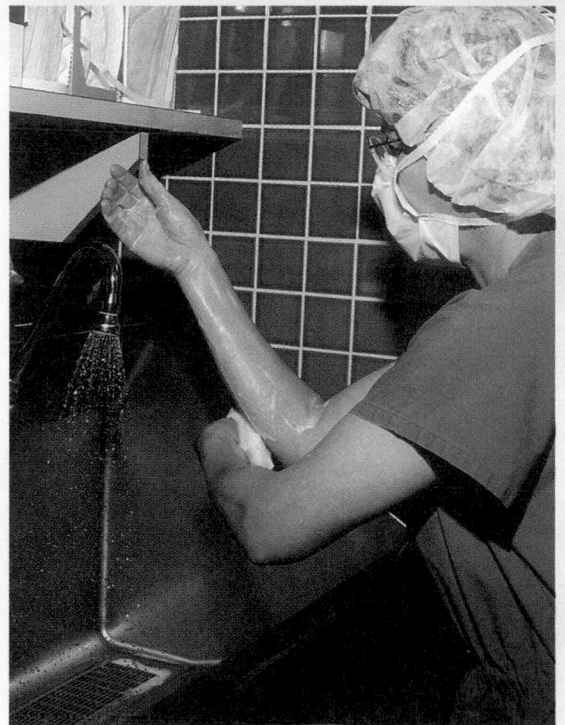

Figure 5

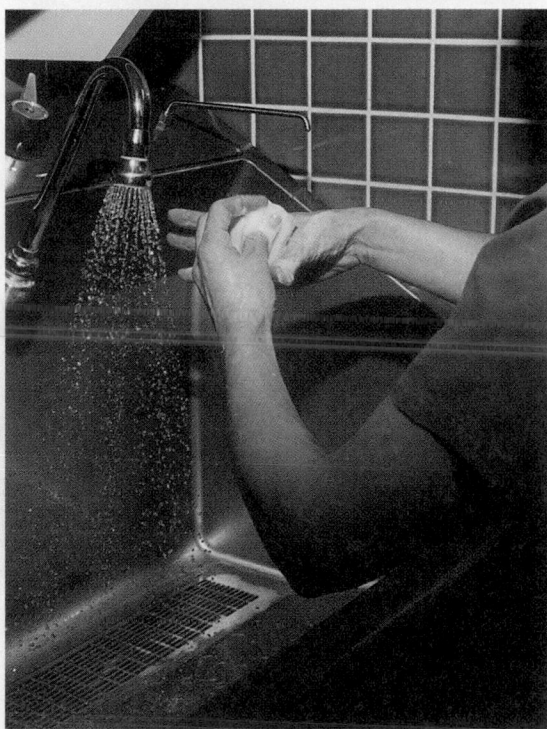

Figure 4

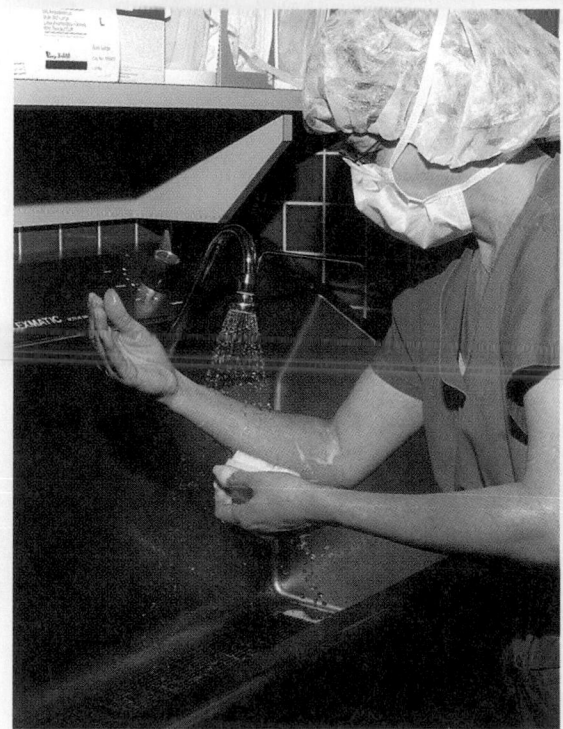

Figure 6

Continued

PROCEDURE 54-3–cont'd

8 Apply more solution and repeat the scrub on the other side, remembering to wash and use friction between each finger with a firm, circular motion (Figures 7 and 8).

9 Scrub all surfaces with a brush, being careful not to abrade your skin. The second washing process should take at least 5 minutes (Figures 9 and 10).

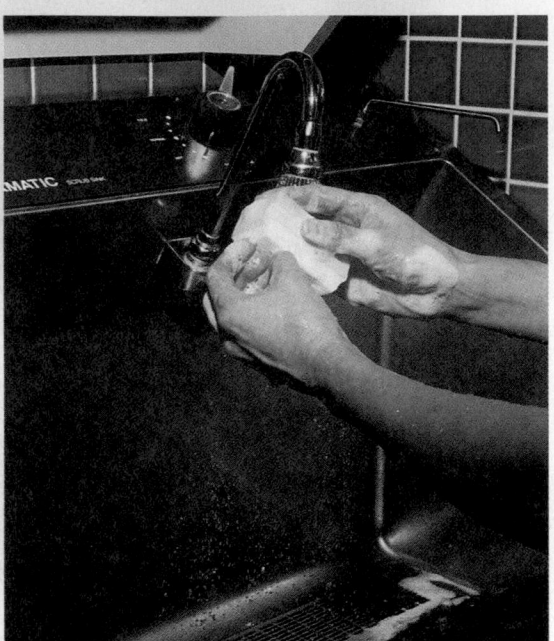

Figure 7

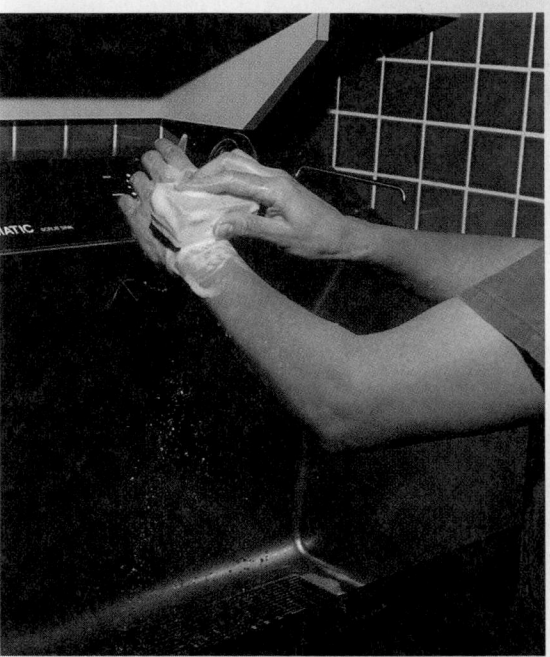

Figure 9

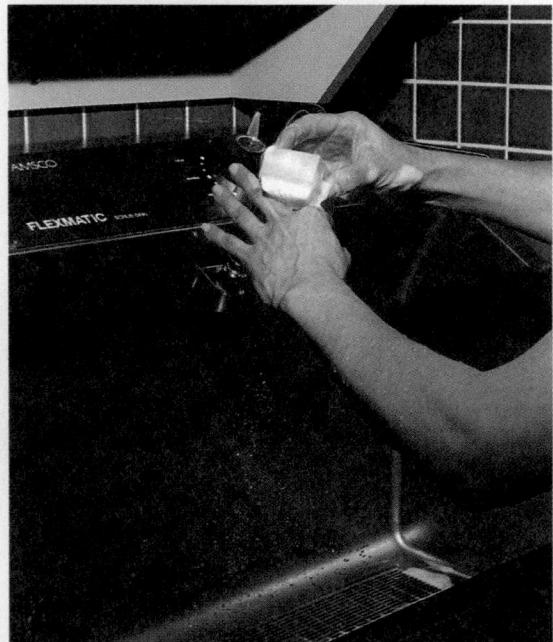

Figure 8

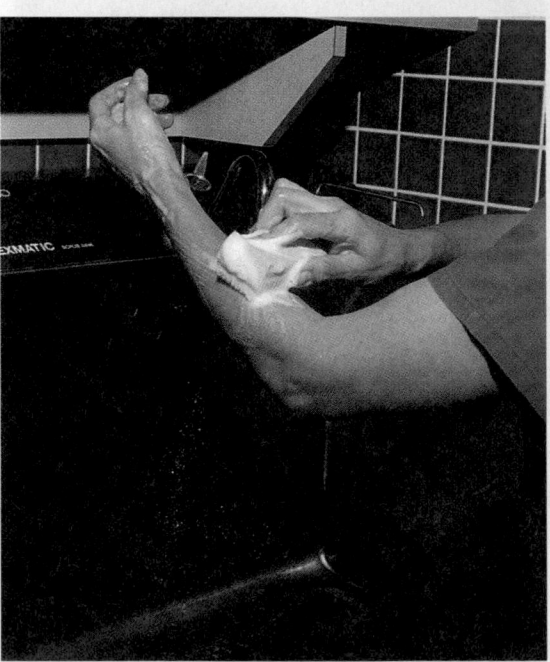

Figure 10

PROCEDURE 54-3—cont'd

10 Rinse thoroughly, keeping your hands up and above waist level. Discard scrub brush (Figures 11 to 13).

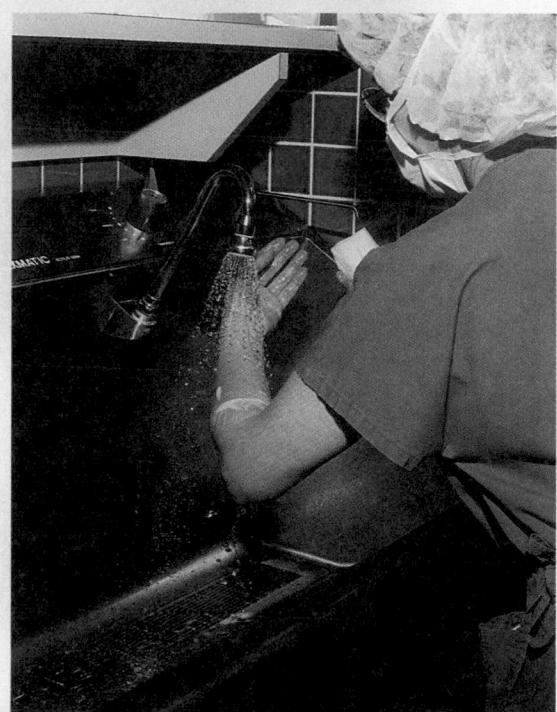

Figure 11

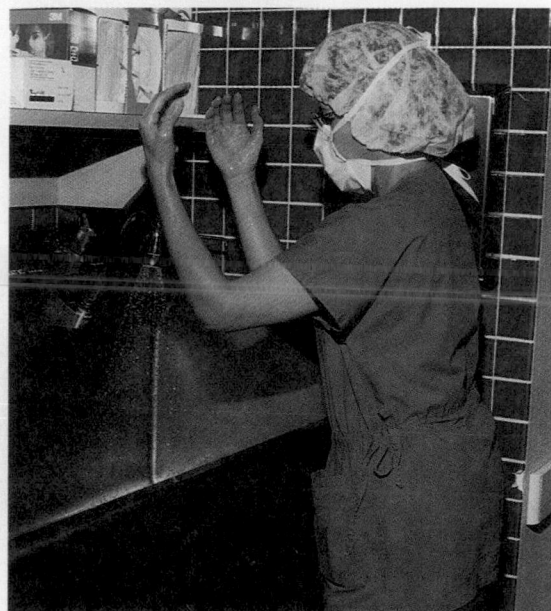

Figure 12

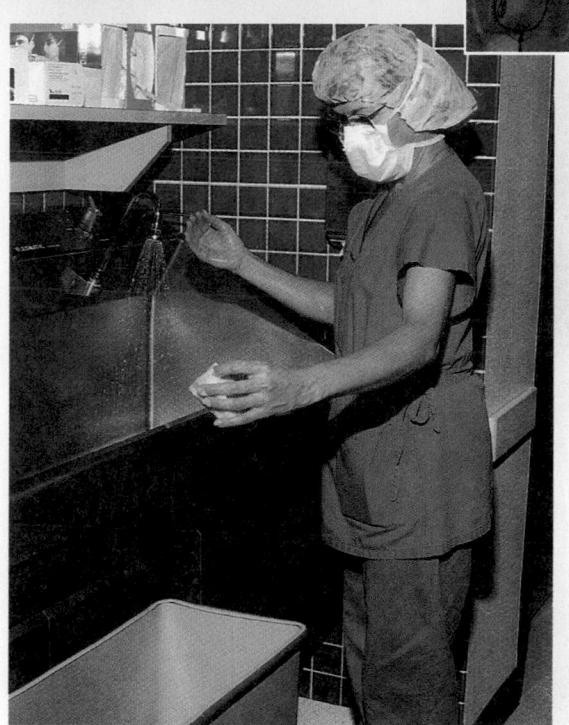

Figure 13

11 Turn off the faucet with the foot or forearm lever, if available.

Purpose: To separate the clean hands from the contaminated faucet handles.

12 Dry your hands with a sterile towel (Figures 14 and 15). Use the opposite end of the towel for the other hand (Figures 16 and 17).

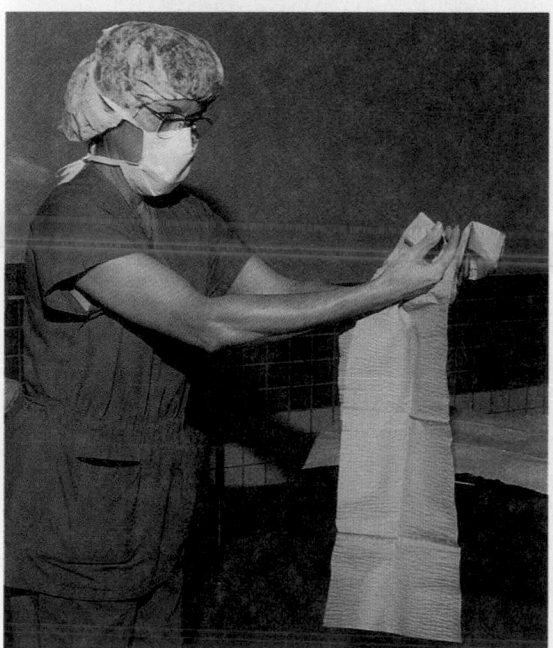

Figure 14

Continued

PROCEDURE **54-3—cont'd**

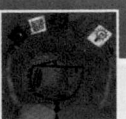

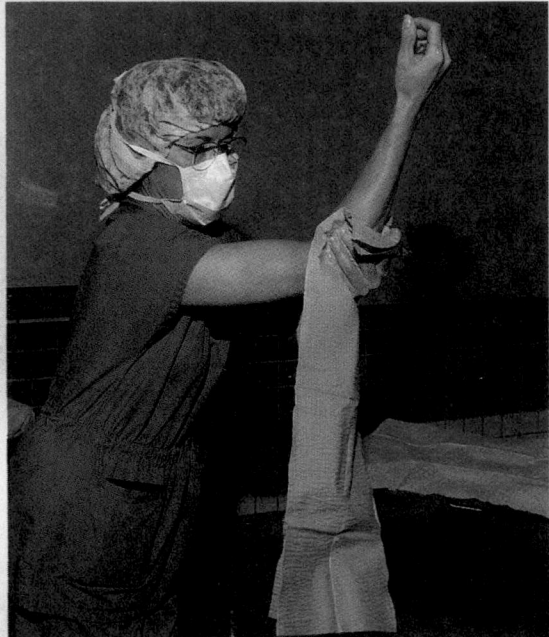

Figure 15

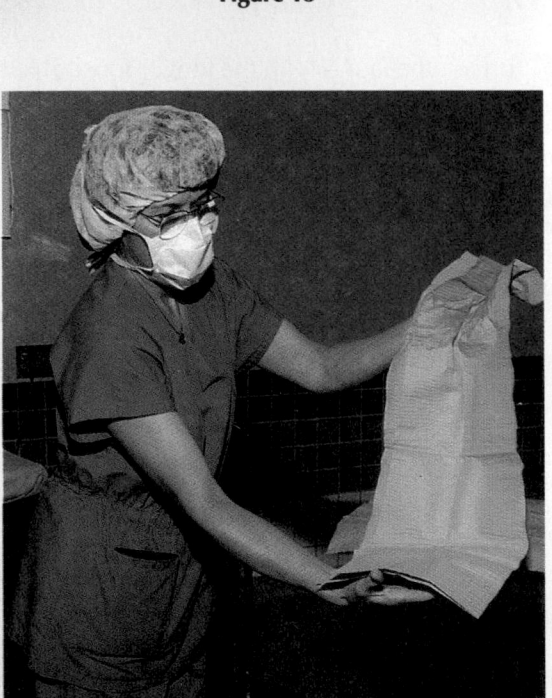

Figure 16

Purpose: To keep your clean hands from touching the part of the towel that comes into contact with your forearms, which are not as clean as your hands. If you are to gown and glove for a procedure, you will be required to use a sterile towel.

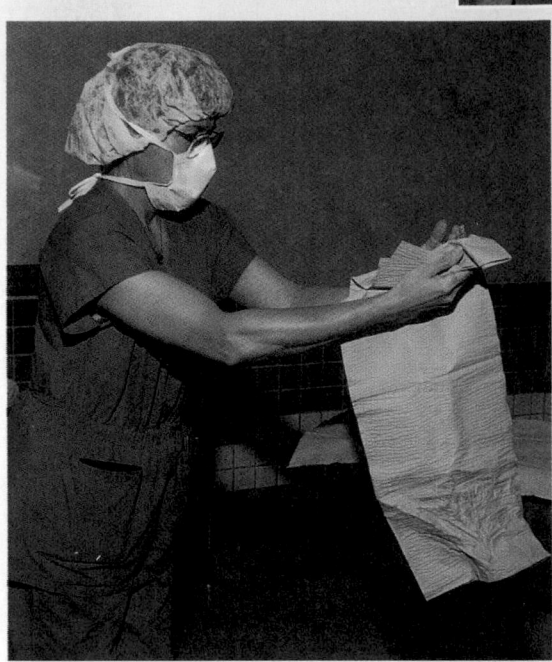

Figure 17

13 Using a patting motion, continue to dry the forearms (Figure 18). Discard the towel and keep your hands up and above waist level (Figures 19 and 20).

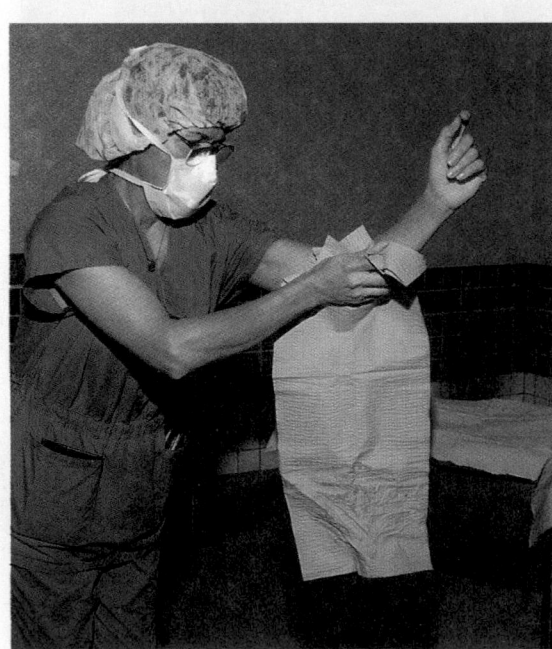

Figure 18

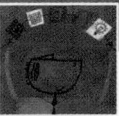

PROCEDURE 54-3—cont'd

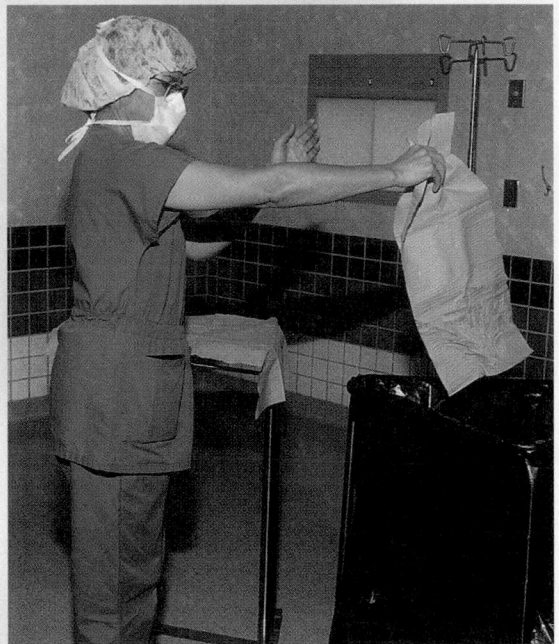

Figure 19

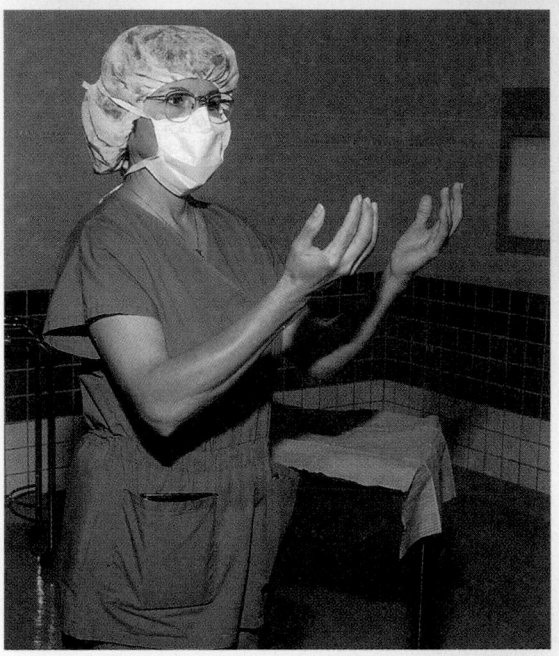

Figure 20

CRITICAL THINKING APPLICATION

After completing a surgical scrub before assisting with a minor surgical procedure, Melissa sneezes. She does not touch her face, but instinctively raises her hands toward her face in the "sneeze range." Can she go ahead with putting on her sterile gloves? Why or why not?

with the surgery, and applying a sterile dressing and bandage after the procedure is completed.

These procedures are all quite similar. Each one requires appropriate skin preparation and draping with a fenestrated drape, also called an *eye sheet*. This is a surgical drape with an approximately 3-inch hole in the center. This opening is placed directly over the surgical site after the site has been suitably prepped. A minor surgery tray is opened and a sterile field is created on a

Text continues on page 1192.

PROCEDURE 54-4

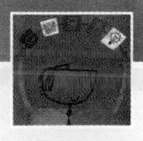

Putting on Sterile Gloves

GOAL: To apply your own sterile gloves before performing sterile procedures.

EQUIPMENT AND SUPPLIES

• Pair of packaged sterile gloves in your size

PROCEDURAL STEPS

1 Open the glove pack. Remember, a 1-inch area around the perimeter of the glove wrapper is considered not sterile.
   Purpose: The open glove pack is a sterile field.

2 Perform the surgical hand scrub.

3 Dry your hands well.
   Purpose: Gloves do not slide easily over moist hands.

4 Glove your dominant hand first.
   Purpose: This will set up your dominant hand to do the more difficult step, which is to apply the second glove.

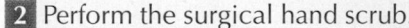

Continued

PROCEDURE 54-4—cont'd

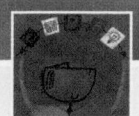

5 With your nondominant hand, pick up the glove for your dominant hand with your thumb and forefinger, grabbing the top of the folded cuff, which is the inside of the glove, being careful not to cross over the other sterile glove (Figure 1).

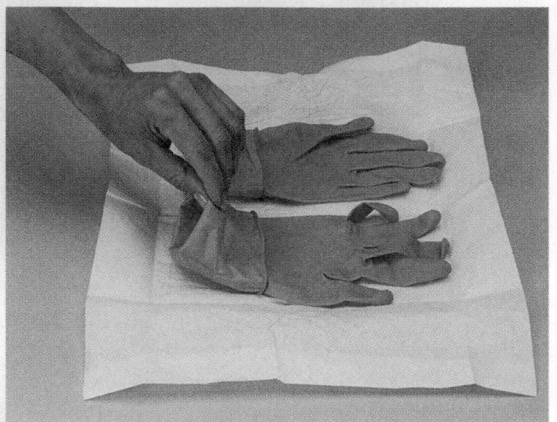

Figure 1

Purpose: The inside of the glove will be next to your skin and is considered not sterile.

6 Lift the glove up and away from the sterile package.
Purpose: Movement over a sterile field must be kept to a minimum.

7 Hold your hands away from you and slide your dominant hand into the glove (Figure 2).

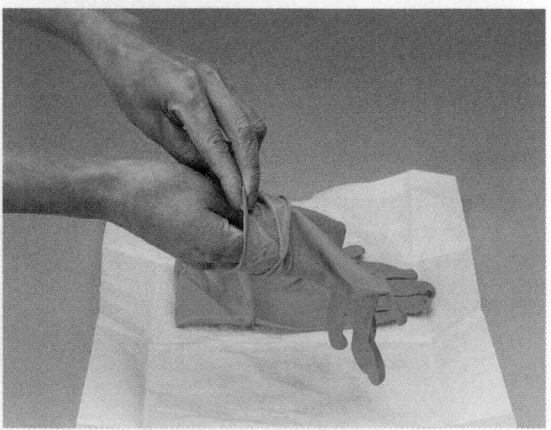

Figure 2

8 Leave the cuff folded (Figure 3).
Purpose: You will unfold the cuff later.

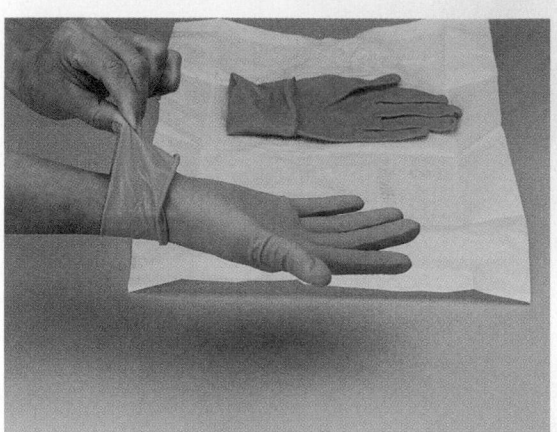

Figure 3

9 With your gloved dominant hand, pick up the second glove by slipping your gloved fingers under the cuff so that your gloved hand only touches the outside of the second glove (Figure 4).
Purpose: Sterile surfaces must always touch sterile surfaces.

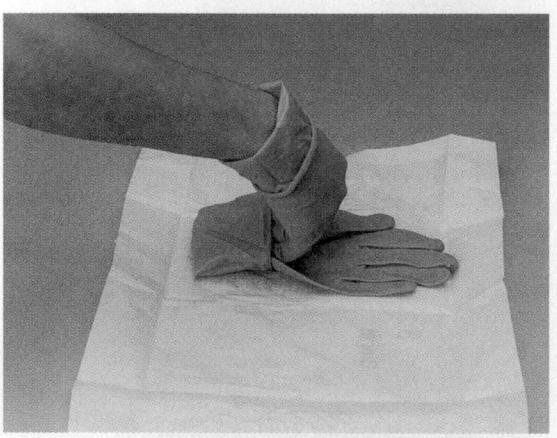

Figure 4

PROCEDURE **54-4**–cont'd

10 Slide your second hand into the glove, without touching the exterior of the glove or any part of your hand (Figures 5 to 7).

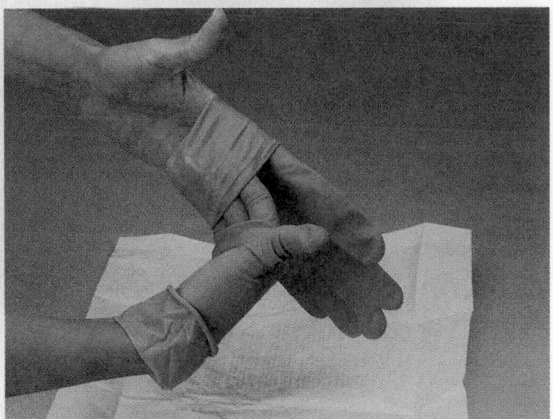

Figure 5

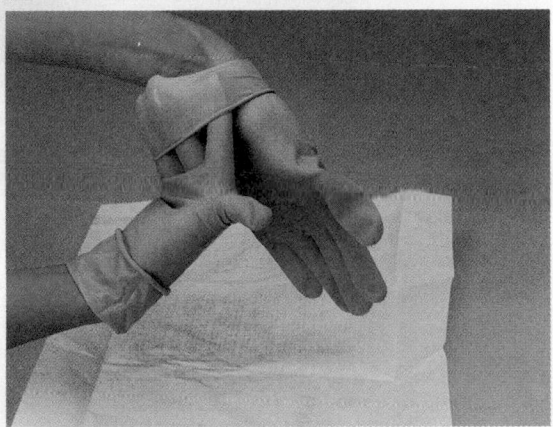

Figure 6

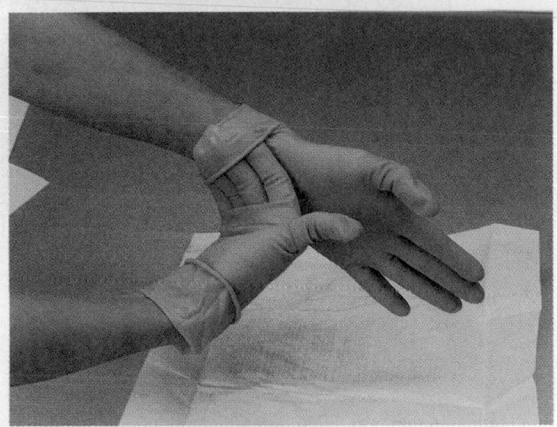

Figure 7

11 Still holding your hands away from you, unroll the cuff by slipping the fingers up and out. Do not touch your bare arm with any part of the sterile glove (Figure 8).

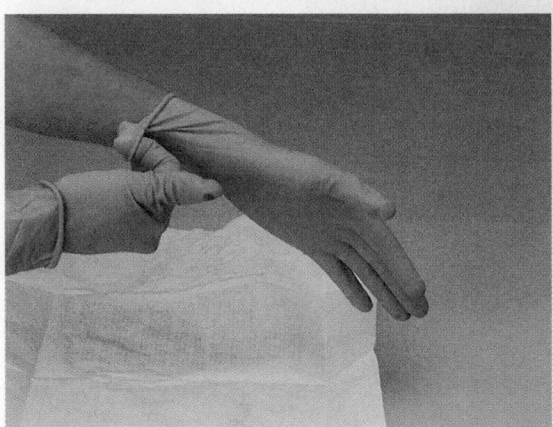

Figure 8

12 Now, slip your gloved fingers up under the first cuff and unroll it, using the same technique (Figures 9 to 11).

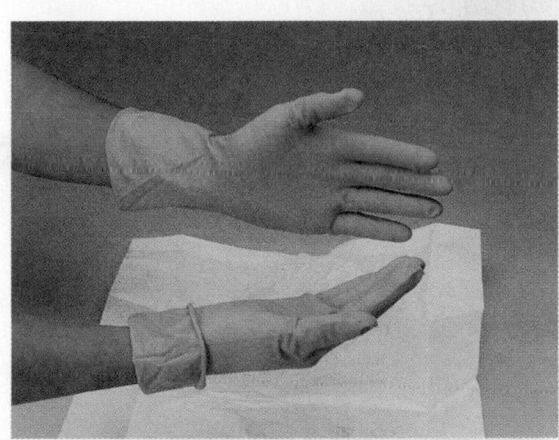

Figure 9

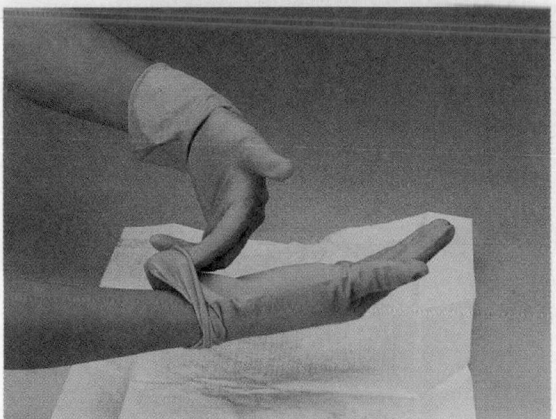

Figure 10

Continued

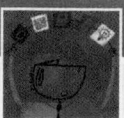

PROCEDURE **54-4—cont'd**

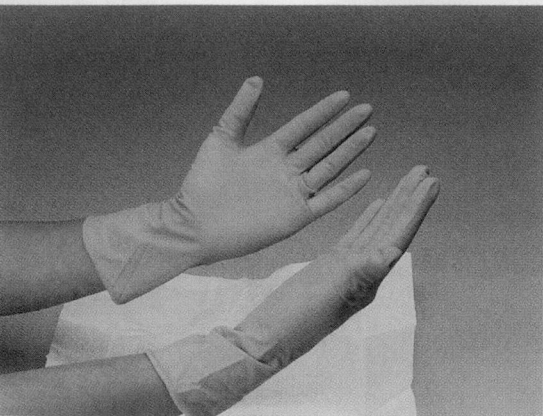

Figure 11

PROCEDURE **54-5**

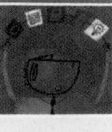

Donning a Sterile Gown

GOAL: To don a sterile gown before assisting with a surgical procedure.

EQUIPMENT AND SUPPLIES

- Sterile gown and gloves (opened on a waist-high counter or Mayo stand, in an opened area to dress)
- NOTE: A mask, goggles, and hair cover are worn.

PROCEDURAL STEPS

1 Scrub, using aseptic technique. Remember to keep your hands up and above waist level (Figure 1).
   Purpose: Protect the patient from your resident bacteria.

2 Grasp the sterile gown by the collar and gently lift it from the sterile gown wrapper (Figures 2 and 3).
   Purpose: The sterile gown will not be contaminated by the edges of the wrapper.

3 Hold the gown away from your body. Allow it to gently unfold, grasping only the inside of the gown (Figures 4 and 5).
   Purpose: Only the inside of the gown touches you; the outside of the gown must remain sterile.

4 Slip your hands into the sleeve openings. Remember to touch only the inside of the gown (Figure 6).
   Purpose: Keep the outside of the gown sterile and away from contaminants.

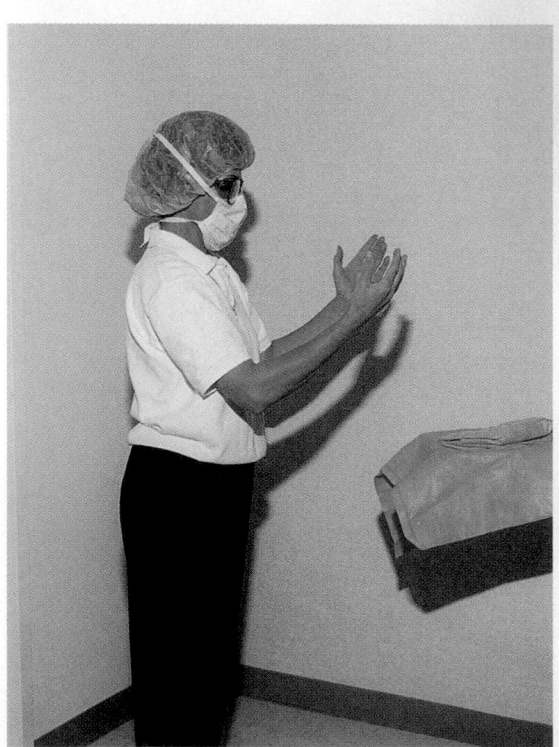

Figure 1

PROCEDURE 54-5—cont'd

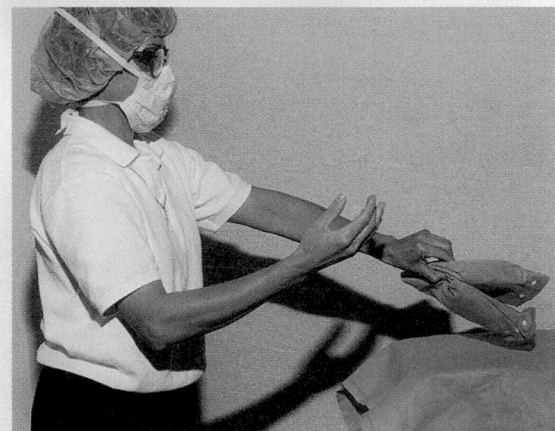

Figure 2

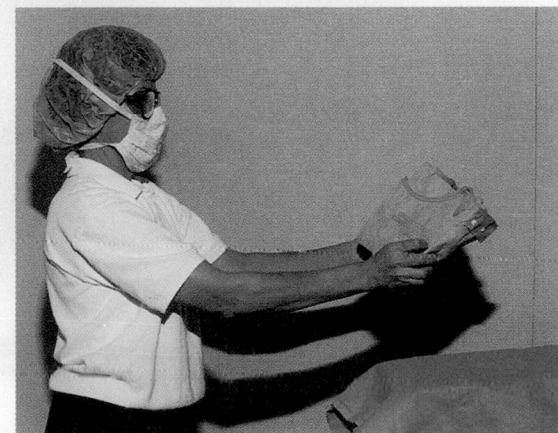

Figure 3

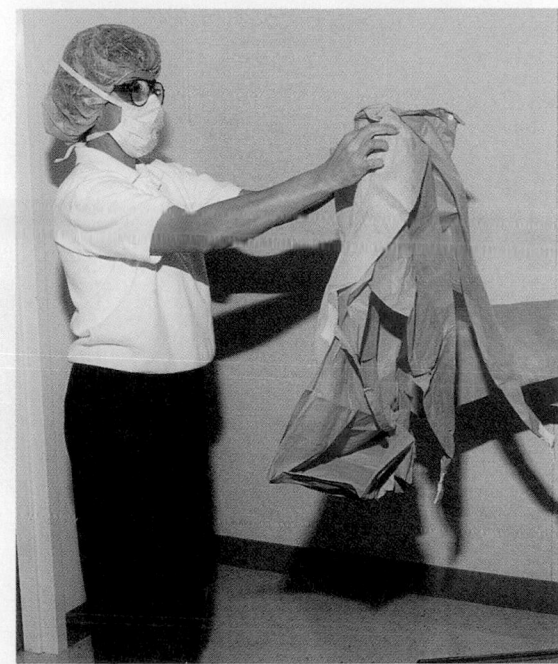

Figure 4

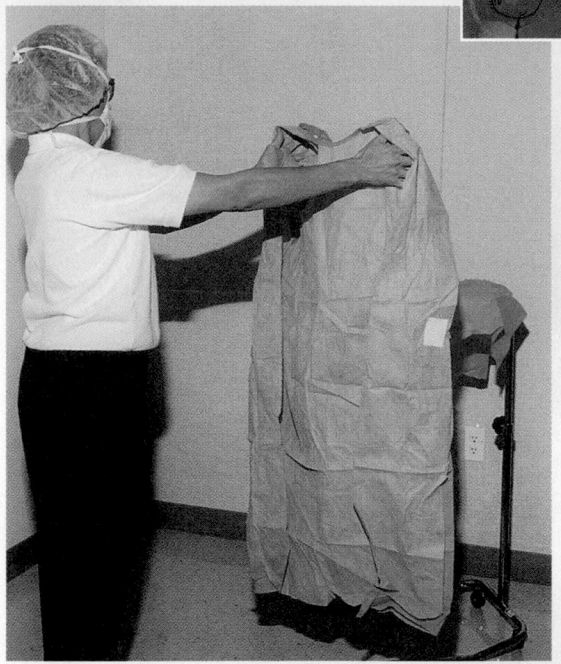

Figure 5

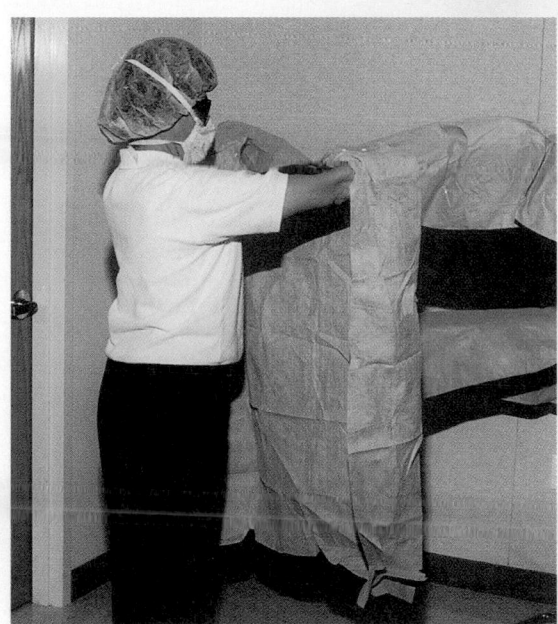

Figure 6

5 The hand and forearms are advanced only to the edge of the gown cuff.

Purpose: The hands are kept covered to avoid contamination of the gown.

6 The circulating assistant touches only the inside of the gown, pulling the gown over the scrub assistant's shoulders (Figure 7).

Continued

PROCEDURE **54-5—cont'd**

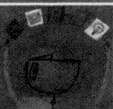

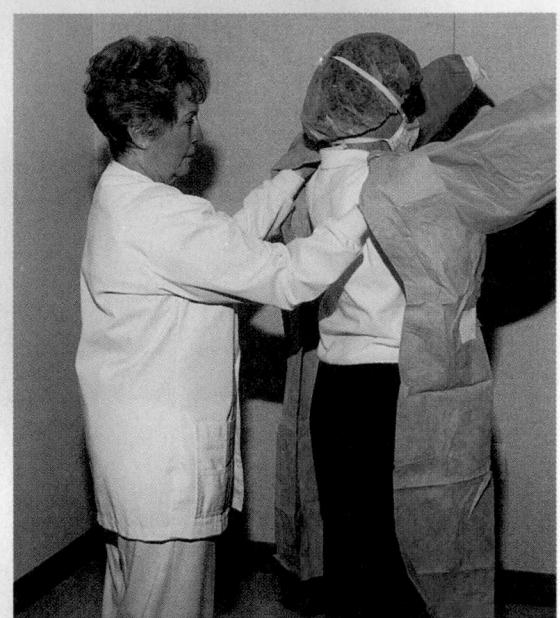

Figure 7

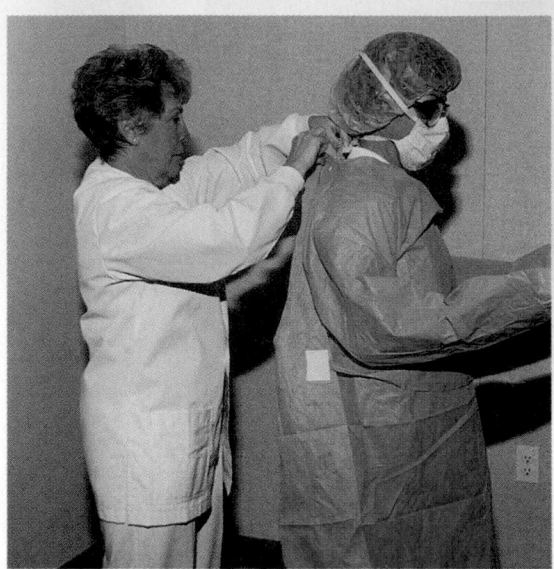

Figure 9

7 The waistline and neck ties are tied (Figures 8 and 9).

Purpose: The gown is fastened to prevent contamination from a flapping gown while applying sterile gloves.

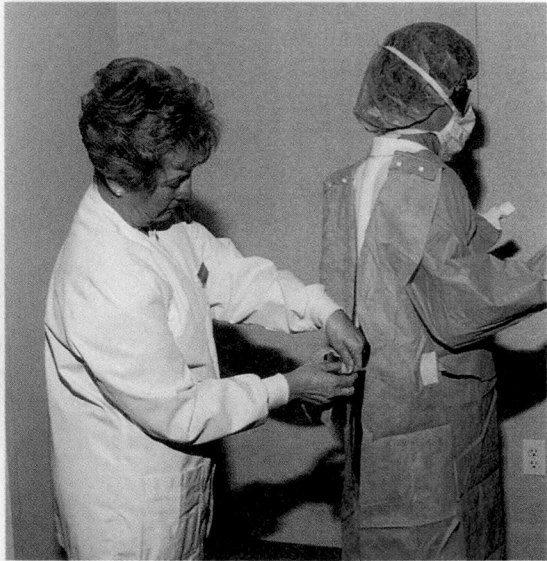

Figure 8

PROCEDURE 54-6

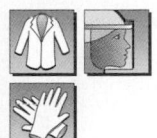

Gloving With a Sterile Gown On

GOAL: To apply sterile gloves while dressed in a sterile gown before assisting with a surgical procedure.

EQUIPMENT AND SUPPLIES

- Sterile gloves, opened on a sterile field
- NOTE: A mask, goggles, hair cover, and a sterile gown are worn. The gloves are applied with the hands covered by the sterile gown to avoid contamination.

PROCEDURAL STEPS

1 Glove your nondominant hand first.
   Purpose: The dominant hand does the most difficult step, which is to apply the first glove.

2 Lift the glove with your major hand, and use your thumb and forefinger to grasp the top of the folded cuff (Figure 1). Remember, your hands are covered with the sterile gown sleeves.
   Purpose: Movement over a sterile field must be kept to a minimum.

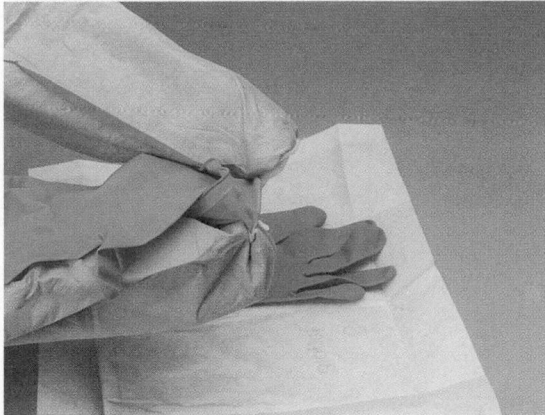

Figure 2

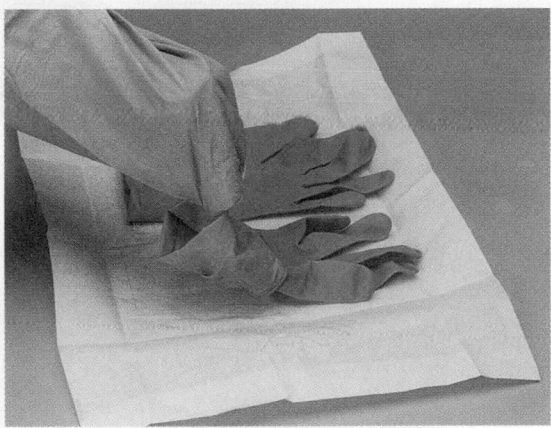

Figure 1

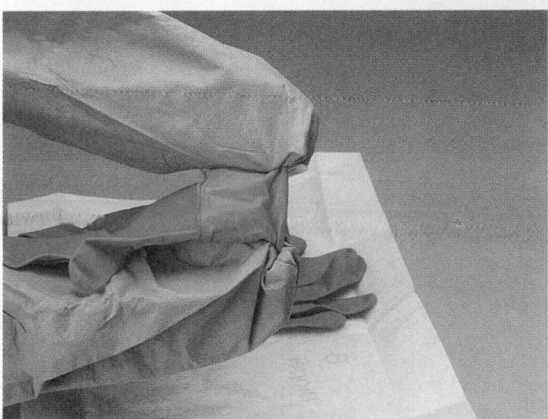

Figure 3

3 Place the glove in the palm of your nondominant hand, with glove fingers pointing to elbows (Figure 2).
   Purpose: Your bare hand will only touch the inside of the glove as it slides into the glove.

4 Grasp the inside of the cuff with your fingers and gently stretch the glove cuff (Figure 3).
   Purpose: Sterile surfaces touch only sterile surfaces.

5 Pull the glove over your hand as you push through the gown cuff (Figures 4 to 6).
   Purpose: Your bare hand touches only the inside of the glove.

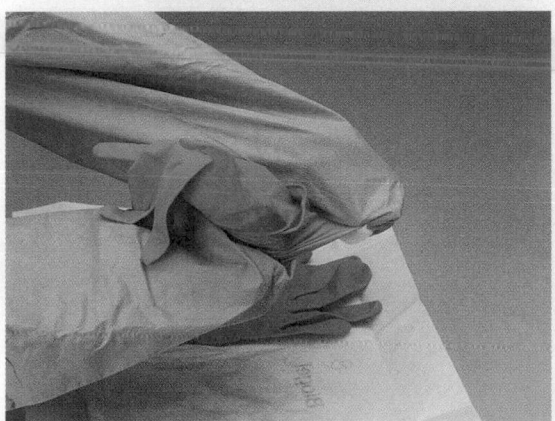

Figure 4

Continued

PROCEDURE **54-6—cont'd**

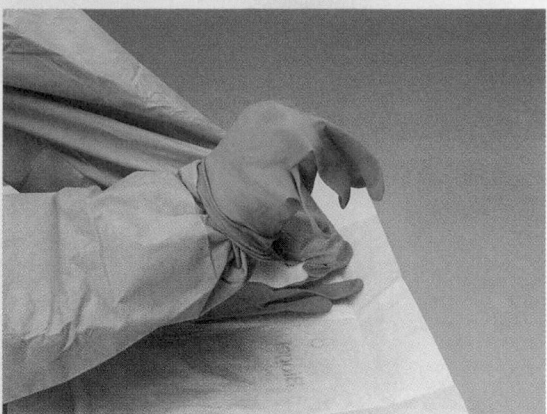

Figure 5

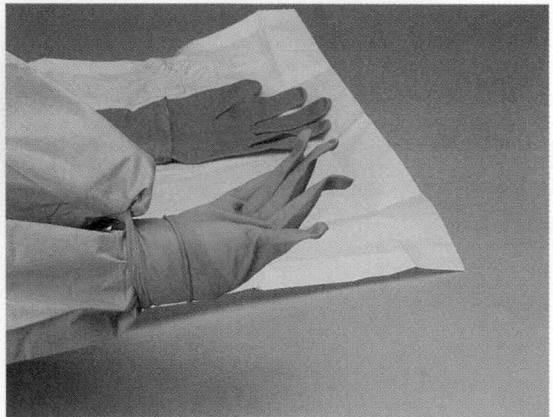

Figure 6

6 Gently slide your fingers in the glove (Figure 7).

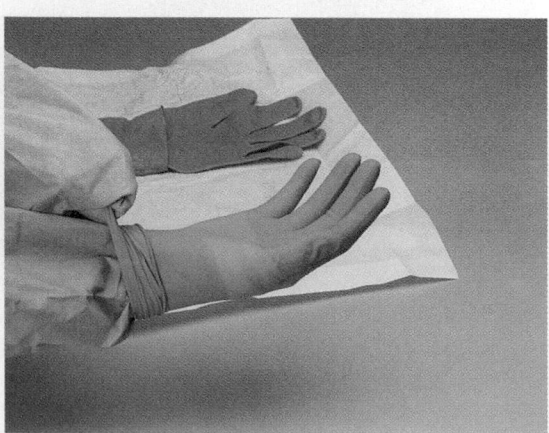

Figure 7

7 With your minor gloved hand, slip your fingers under the cuff of the second glove (Figure 8).

> **Purpose:** Sterile items touch only sterile items.

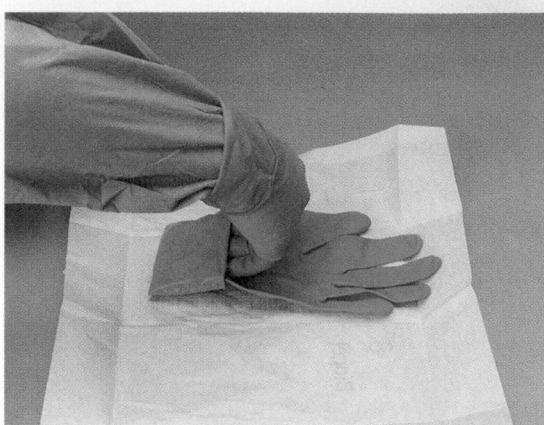

Figure 8

8 Follow steps 3, 4, 5, and 6 for the second glove (Figures 9 to 12).

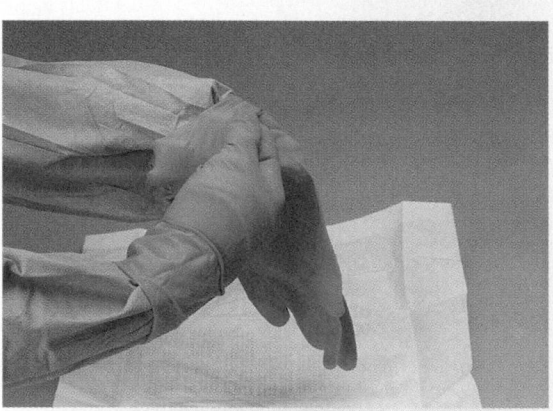

Figure 9

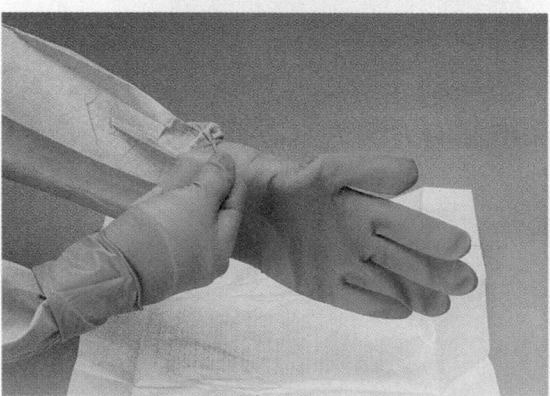

Figure 10

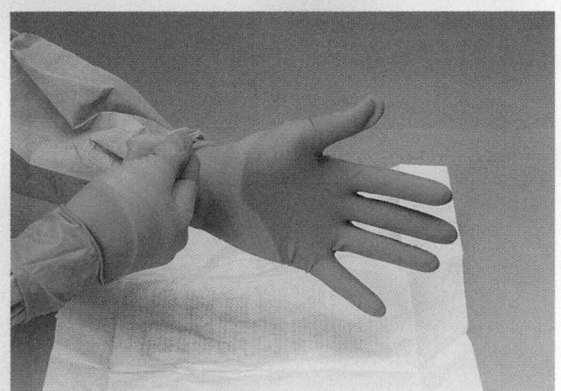

Figure 11

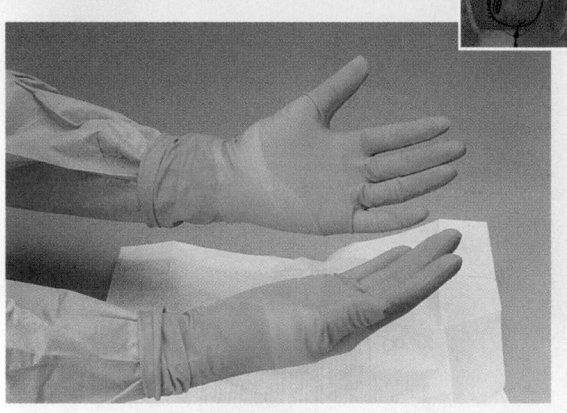

Figure 14

10 The outside sterile gown ties may now be tied with the circulator's assistance (Figures 15 to 18).

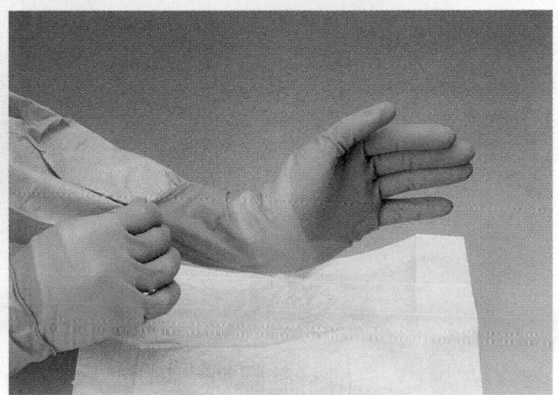

Figure 12

9 The cuffs may now be adjusted (Figures 13 and 14).

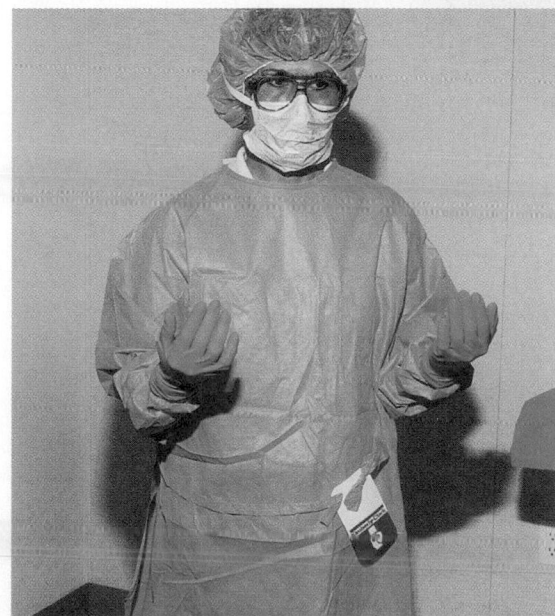

Figure 15

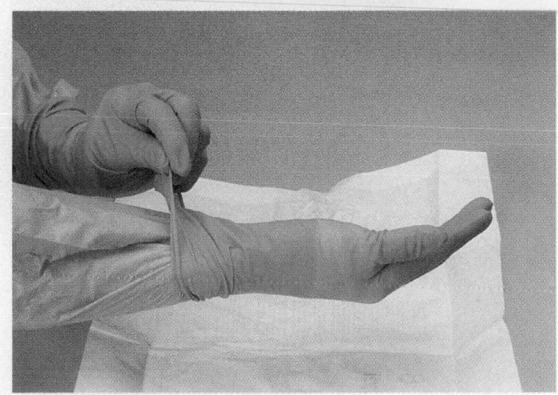

Figure 13

Continued

PROCEDURE **54-6—cont'd**

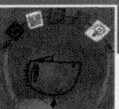

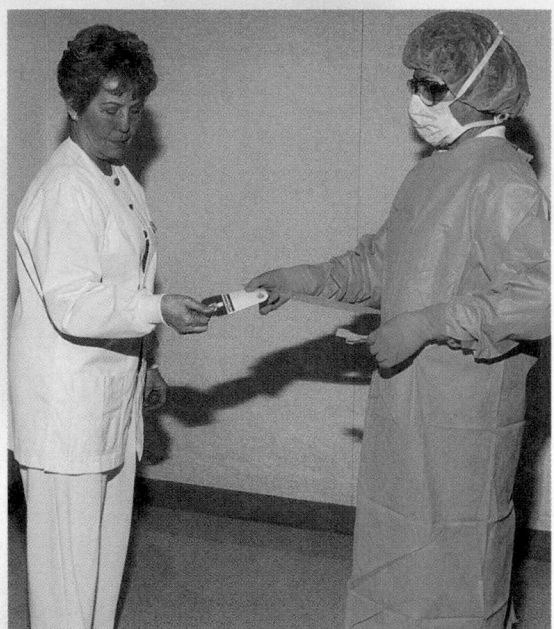

Figure 16

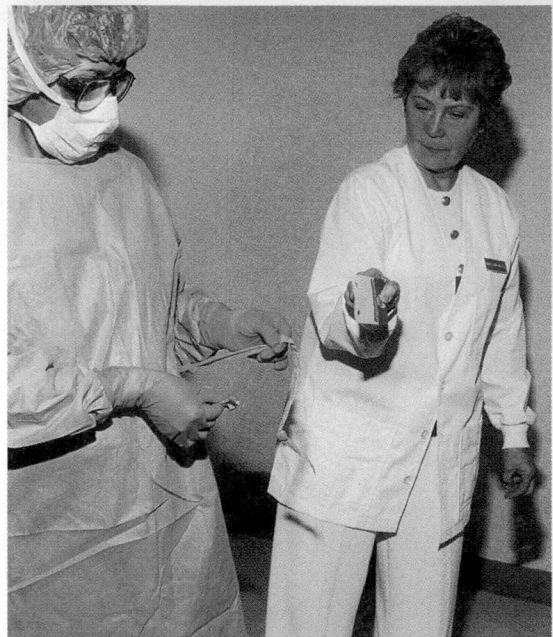

Figure 18

11 The circulator grasps the red part of the tag by the corner (Figures 17 and 18).

Purpose: This will be discarded after the scrub assistant is able to fasten the waist ties. Nonsterile areas do not touch sterile areas.

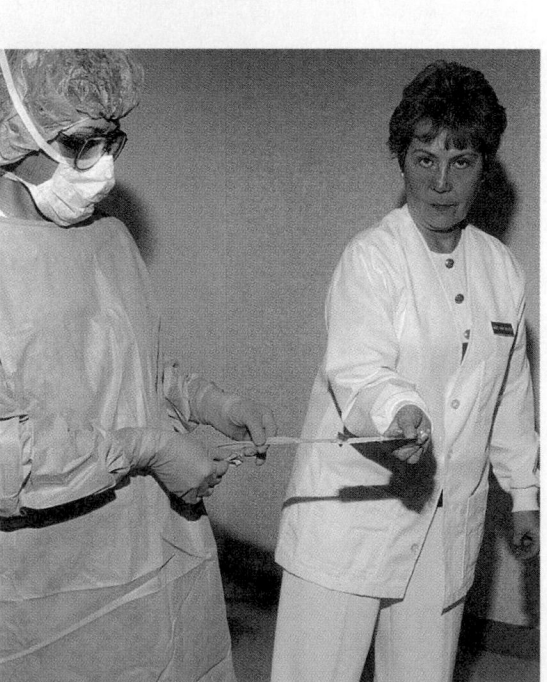

Figure 17

PROCEDURE **54-7**

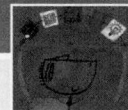

Removing Contaminated Gloves

GOAL: To properly remove and dispose of contaminated gloves following a procedure.

EQUIPMENT AND SUPPLIES

- Contaminated gloved (sterile or nonsterile) hands
- Biohazard or regular disposal container as required

PROCEDURAL STEPS

NOTE: The following procedure is written for someone who is right-handed. If you are left-handed, simply reverse each one of the hand designations for this procedure.

1 Using the left hand, grasp the outside of the cuff of the glove on the right hand. Be careful not to touch the right arm during this step (Figure 1).

   Purpose: You do not want to contaminate your skin with the contaminated glove.

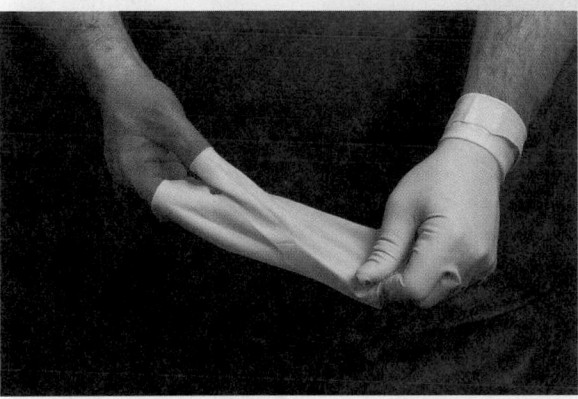

Figure 2

3 Now the contaminated right glove is inside out in the left hand. Using only the left hand, ball this dirty glove in the palm of the hand (Figure 3).

   Purpose: This will keep the right hand glove inside of the right hand glove as the left glove is removed.

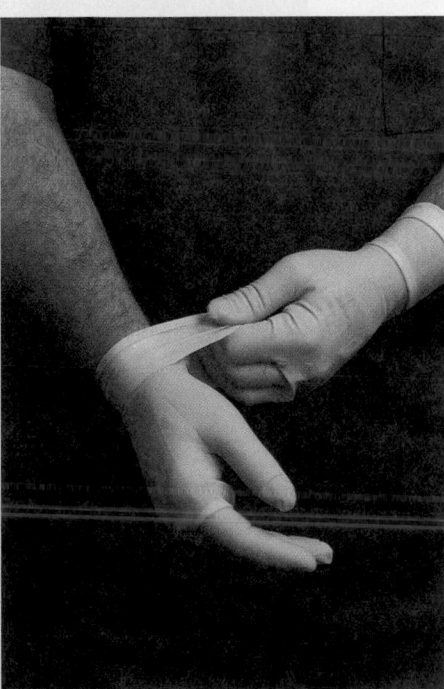

Figure 1

2 Take the glove completely off of the right hand by pulling it away from the fingers and pulling it inside out (Figure 2).

   Purpose: The contaminated surface of your right glove is now on the inside.

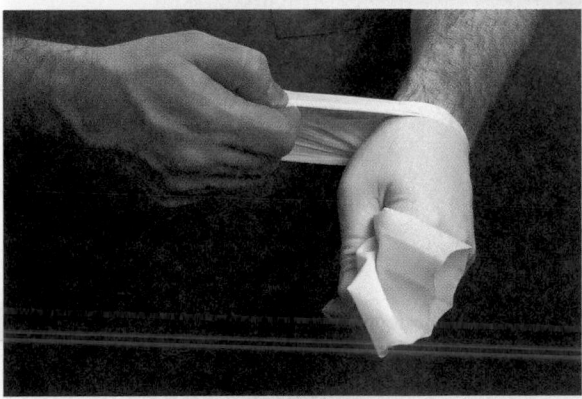

Figure 3

4 Now use the right hand to carefully grasp inside of the cuff of the right glove and pull it off over the hand (and the other glove), turning it inside out as this is done (Figure 4).

   Purpose: The inside of the second glove is the cleanest side, so the inside can now be touched with an ungloved hand.

Continued

PROCEDURE 54-7—cont'd

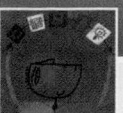

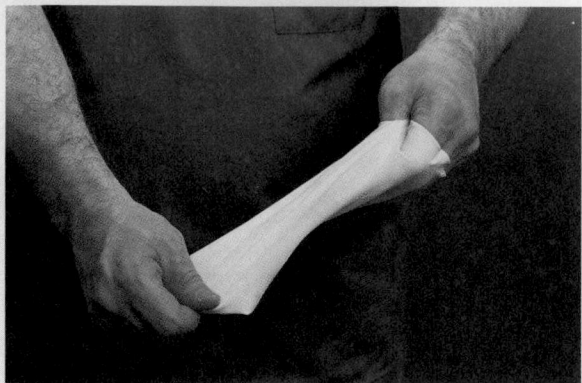

Figure 4

5 Dispose of the gloves in the proper disposal receptacle, or a biohazard bag if they are contaminated with blood or body fluids (Figure 5).
   Purpose: Proper handling of biohazardous waste.

6 Wash your hands.
   Purpose: To remove glove powder residue, and as an extra protection against possibly transferring microorganisms to another patient.

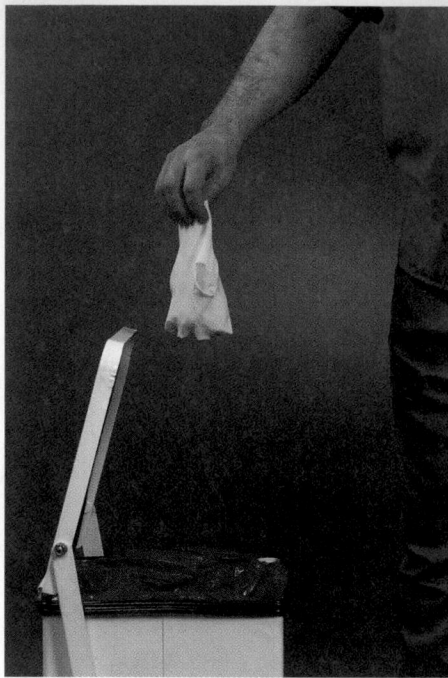

Figure 5

CRITICAL THINKING APPLICATION

After one assists with a minor surgical procedure, can gloves ever just be thrown in the regular trash? Must used gloves always be disposed of in a biohazard container? Why or why not?

Mayo stand. Sutures, knife blade, and any other instruments are added to the field, according to the surgeon's preference. Have a local anesthetic ready, also according to the physician's preference.

After achieving suitable local anesthesia, the physician will open the skin with an incision. If a cyst is being removed, the physician will dissect around it and usually try to "deliver" it from the wound intact. If the procedure is an incision and drainage (I&D), foul matter will start oozing out of the wound immediately after the skin is incised. The wound is drained completely and flushed out with copious amounts of sterile saline solution. Frequently, a drain will be placed in the wound and left for several days. If the procedure is a biopsy, a small amount of tissue will be sliced away and placed in a specimen container with preservative. The specimen container must be carefully labeled with the appropriate patient demographic information, date, and what the tissue specimen is, and then sent to the laboratory, where it will be fixed, stained, and examined microscopically for changes or abnormalities.

Electrosurgery. Electrosurgery is also known as *electrocautery*. An electrosurgical unit (ESU) uses high-frequency current to cut through tissue and coagulate blood vessels. When the electric current comes in contact with tissue and blood cells, they are vaporized, producing carbon and steam. This process seals blood vessels, minimizing cellular oozing and bleeding. Electrosurgery may be used to destroy granulations and small polyps.

Necessary components are the electrosurgical unit's power source, the grounding cable and pad, and the active electrode (a pencil-like instrument with a tip and cord). Tips are disposable and are used according to the type of procedure being performed. The two most commonly used tips are the needle and flat.

The surgeon, holding the pencil-like instrument, touches the tissue with the tip and activates the electric current with a switch on the instrument or a foot pedal. The electric current is then delivered to the tissues, and tissue is vaporized at the site of contact.

IMPORTANT TIPS ABOUT THE GROUNDING PAD

• Carefully inspect the pad, cable, and skin before the procedure.

IMPORTANT TIPS ABOUT THE GROUNDING PAD—cont'd

- Place the pad close to the operative site.
- The pad must be tight against the patient's skin.
- Apply the pad to a fleshy area like the thigh.
- Do not place the pad over a bony area.
- Do not place the pad over body hair.
- Do not place the pad over metal implants or a pacemaker.
- Carefully inspect the pad site on the skin after the procedure.

Laser Surgery. *LASER* or *laser* is an acronym for *L*ight *A*mplification by *S*timulated *E*mission of *R*adiation. These light waves were first used in medicine with the treatment of diseases of the retina. Their application was later expanded to photocoagulation therapy and then to thermal vaporization, coagulation, and ablation of tissue.

Lasers are used in the following types of surgery: ophthalmic, genitourinary, gynecological, orthopedic, neurological, laryngological, otological, rhinological and sinus, vascular, thoracic, gastrointestinal, and plastic and reconstructive. Laser equipment is found in hospitals, surgery centers, and medical offices.

A laser key should be accessible to authorized persons only. A medical assistant must be specially trained to operate a laser before assisting with laser surgery. Laser equipment requires very careful handling, care, and maintenance. Laser light destroys tissue and can harm the patient, the physician, and you if improperly handled. A full laser safety program should be completed before assisting in laser procedures.

MEDICAL ASSISTANT'S FUNCTION DURING LASER SURGERY

- Observe the surgical field through safety goggles for possible contamination, and protect patient's eyes.
- Keep wet sponges ready.
- Remove any flammable item from the CO_2 laser's path.
- Assist with the suctioning of the plume to maintain a clear visual field.
- Have a basin of sterile normal saline solution and a filled irrigating syringe ready.
- Watch each application of the laser beam, anticipating needs for protective supplies, special equipment, or instruments.

Microsurgery. Microsurgery involves the use of an operating microscope in many types of surgical procedures. One of its major uses is in ophthalmological surgery. It is also used on otological, rhinological and sinus, laryngological, neurosurgical, microvascular, gynecological, and genitourinary procedures. A medical assistant must acquire basic knowledge about the operation and care of a microscope.

The basic components include the light source, eyepieces (also called the oculars), lenses, and cord. Accessory pieces include assistant and observer lenses, cameras, video recorders, television monitors, and printers. These are all valuable for both documentation and teaching purposes. Disposable sterile drapes and handle covers are used on the microscope during surgical procedures.

Surgical microscopes are expensive, delicate instruments and require extreme care when handling and cleaning. They may easily be bent or damaged through careless or inattentive handling. All lenses and cords should be carefully inspected before and after each use.

Endoscopic Procedures. A miniature telescope or long tube with an optical system and a light source is used to examine a hollow organ or cavity, such as the urinary bladder, bronchus, larynx, colon (Figure 54-5), stomach, uterus, abdomen, joints like the knee, wrist, and shoulder, as well as other parts of the body. Direct visualization is necessary for diagnostic purposes or to perform surgical procedures. Endoscopes may be rigid (for example laparoscope or hysteroscope), semirigid, or flexible (colonoscopes, bronchoscopes, gastroscopes). All are delicate and expensive, and require extreme care in handling to protect them from damage.

Accessory equipment used with endoscopes includes a fiberoptic light cable, a light source, an irrigator for

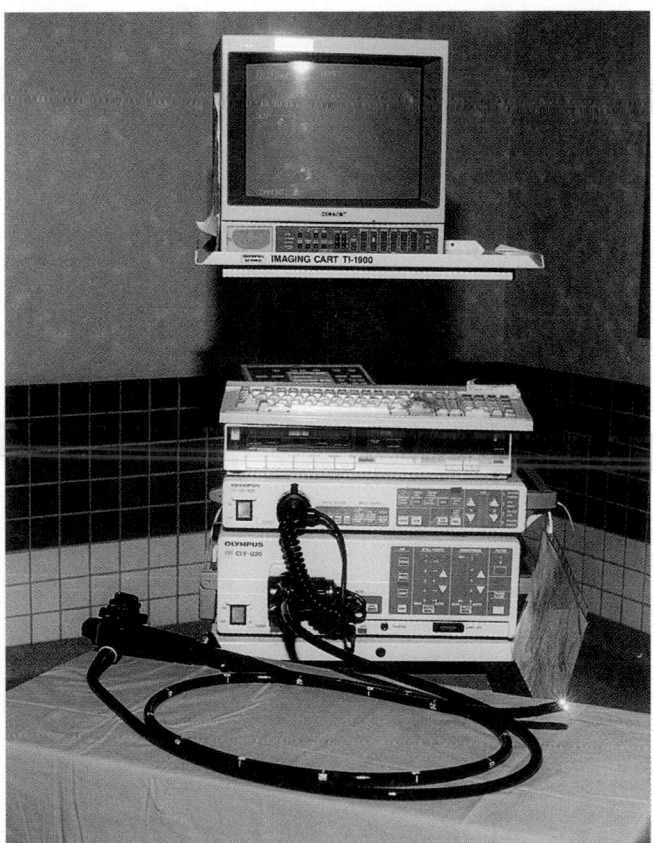

FIGURE 54-5   Flexible colonoscope with monitor and video recorder.

solution installation and suction, a camera, a monitor, a printer, and a video recorder. The fiberoptic light cable consists of hundreds of glass fibers. It is important to protect it from being bent, dropped, kinked, squashed, or smashed. The light source can become very hot and must be kept out of contact with the patient, the physician, the staff, and any flammable material, such as surgical draping. All equipment must be checked before and after use. Always follow manufacturer's recommendations for use, care, and maintenance of equipment.

Cryosurgery. In cryosurgery, a very low temperature probe is used to destroy tissue by freezing it on contact. The probe temperature is usually below –20° C (–4° F). This cold temperature is achieved by circulating liquid nitrogen through the tip of the probe. A local anesthetic is usually administered before cryosurgery. Cryosurgery is used to treat cancers of the skin, prostate, liver, pancreas, and kidney. Using cryosurgery is, in many situations, less invasive than traditional surgery, and therefore generally has fewer associated complications. Cryosurgery is often performed in an office setting or in an outpatient surgery center.

The Medical Assistant's Role in Surgery

Minor surgery is restricted to the management of minor problems and injuries. Most medical assistants are expected to glove and assist with preparation of the sterile field and the patient. The following procedures can be successfully used for assisting with minor surgery in the medical office, clinic, and outpatient surgery center. Individual practices and preferences may modify some of these procedures. You should be flexible and adapt to the preferences of your employer.

Preparation of the Patient

Whether minor surgery is performed because of an unforeseen accident or is a planned, elective procedure, the patient needs psychological care as well as physical care. A patient facing any surgical procedure suffers from fear of pain, fear of disfigurement, and often the fear of cancer being discovered. An injured patient may feel anxious about medical bills or possible loss of employment. Because surgery is a frightening and dehumanizing experience, the medical assistant must take the time, both preoperatively and at the time of surgery, to help the patient through these fears and anxieties. The best method is to help the patient talk about the procedures and voice any concerns.

Questions should be answered directly, but you should answer only those questions that are within your scope of experience and the policies of the office. If you cannot answer a question, assure the patient that you will relay the question to the physician before the procedure, *and then be sure to do so*. What may seem to be a minor or unimportant question to you may be very frightening to the patient. A good technique is to write down the question while you are with the patient and then give it to the physician. The minor-surgery room can look very

frightening to the patient, so unless the patient is sedated, try to make conversation with the patient while you prepare for the physician's arrival.

Physical preparation may involve obtaining blood and urine samples for tests the day before surgery, completing forms and consents, and gathering a current history concerning any recent illnesses or medications and allergies. Before the day of surgery, preoperative instructions may include a shave prep, cleansing enemas, food intake restrictions, special bathing, and administration of a sedative medication.

On the day of surgery, the patient's vital signs are recorded, the patient is assisted in undressing if necessary, and then is asked to empty the bladder. Keep the patient on schedule, but never appear to rush the process.

Preoperative Instructions. When office surgery is planned, certain procedures should be followed before the appointment. These should include:

- Having the necessary consent forms ready to sign.
- Giving the patient all necessary preoperative instructions, such as medications to be used and special skin-cleansing instructions.
- Telling the patient to bring a relative or friend to drive him or her home after the surgery.
- Instructing the patient to leave jewelry and other valuables at home.
- Calling the patient the day before the scheduled surgery to confirm any special instructions.

Informed Consent. The physician must have the patient's written informed consent before beginning any surgical procedure. To sign an informed consent form permitting the physician to legally perform the surgery, the patient must understand what procedure will be performed, why it should be done, the potential risks and benefits of the surgery, alternative treatments (including no treatment), and the possible risks of any alternative treatment. This legal requirement is not simply met by having the patient sign an operative permit; a discussion must occur during which the physician provides the patient or the patient's legal representative with enough information to decide whether to proceed with the proposed surgical treatment. After this discussion, the patient either consents to or refuses the surgery. The patient then signs or refuses to sign the consent form. If the patient signs with an X, the medical assistant should write "patient's mark" beside the X, and in addition, have a family member witness the signature. The discussion must be fully documented in the patient's medical record. A copy of the signed form must also be included in the patient record. Treatment may not exceed the scope of the permit.

NOTE: The patient must not be under the influence of any sedative medication at the time he or she signs the consent form. This condition must *never* be violated.

CRITICAL THINKING APPLICATION

Melissa is preparing a patient for a breast biopsy. The consent form has previously been signed and is in the chart. In chatting with the patient while completing the final set up for the procedure, it

Positioning. Have the patient disrobe sufficiently to completely expose the surgical site. There is much risk of contamination in performing a procedure while either you or the patient is holding back clothing that may slide into the area where the physician is working. Clothing may also act as a tourniquet or may make it difficult to apply a proper dressing or bandage. The patient's clothing may also be stained with the skin-disinfecting solution or may prevent a large area from being properly prepped.

It is equally important to position the patient as comfortably as possible. An uncomfortable position can be held for only a limited time, and the patient will have to move, often in the middle of a procedure, if you have not ensured their comfort from the beginning. If the patient is not comfortable, his or her muscles may stiffen or ache unnecessarily after the surgery. When deciding on the correct patient position, consider where you and the physician will stand or sit, where the instruments will be placed, and where other needed equipment will be. If the patient has an open wound that will need irrigation during the procedure, wear nonsterile gloves to assist the patient into position. If there is active and profuse bleeding, a gown and gloves should be worn. If there is danger of blood and body fluid contamination to your face, wear goggles and a mask.

Skin Preparation. The human skin is a reservoir of bacteria and cannot be sterilized. Resident organisms cannot be completely removed or destroyed. Transit bacteria can also be harmful, so a great deal of care must be given to cleanse the patient's skin of bacteria as much as possible. Cleansing the patient's skin before surgery with surgical soap and an antiseptic is called a *skin prep*. A good skin prep sharply decreases transference of harmful organisms to the incision site. A gloved assistant performs the skin prep (Procedure 54-8). Sometimes the patient may be instructed to repeatedly cleanse the surgical area with bacteriostatic or antiseptic soap several days before the surgery. The medical assistant or physician may need to shave the surgical area before the skin prep. Disposable skin prep trays and razors are commonly used in a physician's office.

PROCEDURE 54-8

Skin Prep for Surgery

GOAL: To prepare the patient's skin for a surgical procedure to reduce the risk of wound contamination.

EQUIPMENT AND SUPPLIES

A disposal skin prep kit or an autoclave skin prep containing the following:
- Gauze sponges
- Cotton-tipped applicators
- Antiseptic soap
- Sterile gloves
- Two small stainless-steel bowls
- Antiseptic
- *Optional:* cotton balls, nail pick, scrub brush
- A waste receptacle

PROCEDURAL STEPS

1 Wash your hands and dry them carefully. Follow standard precautions.
   Purpose: Moisture on your hands contaminates the pack.

2 Instruct the patient on scrub procedure.
   Purpose: To ensure cooperation and keep the patient comfortable.

3 Expose the site. Use a light if necessary.

4 Open your skin prep pack.

5 Add the surgical soap and antiseptic solutions to the two bowls.

6 Arrange the items with sterile gloved hands.
   Purpose: The opened skin prep pack is a sterile field.

7 If needed, place two sterile towels at the edges of the area to be scrubbed.
   Purpose: The area must be scrubbed up to the sterile towels, which will be beyond the opening of the surgical drape when the drape is applied.

8 Start at the incision site and begin washing with the antiseptic soap on a gauze sponge in a circular motion, moving from the center to the edges of the area to be scrubbed (Figure 1).
   Purpose: Circular motion from inside to outside drags contaminants away from the incision site.

9 After one complete wipe, discard the sponge, and begin again with a new sponge soaked in the antiseptic solution.
   Purpose: After one circular sweep, the sponge is now contaminated with skin bacteria and debris.

Continued

PROCEDURE **54-8—cont'd**

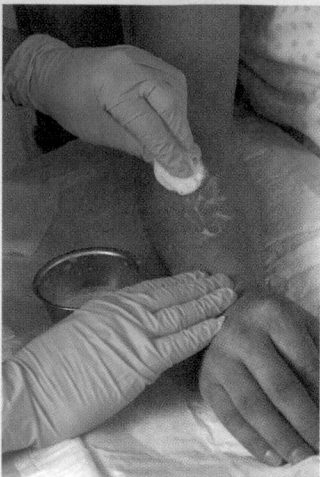

Figure 1

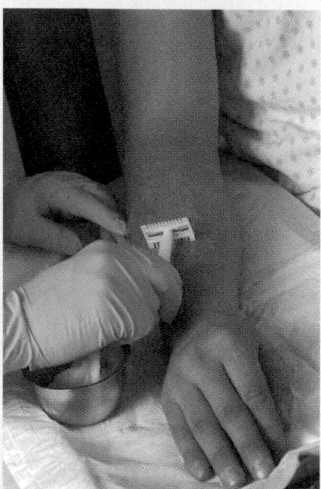

Figure 2

When you return to the incision site for the next circular sweep, you must use sterile material.

10 Repeat the process, using sufficient friction for 5 minutes (or follow office policy for the length of time required for a particular prep).

11 If there is hair growth, the area may need to be shaved. Hold skin taut, and shave in the direction of growth (Figure 2). After shaving, scrub the skin a second time.

    Purpose: Hair should be removed before any invasive procedure, to limit the potential for infection. (Also, care should be taken to avoid injuring the patient for the same reason.)

12 Rinse the area with sterile solution (Figure 3). Check that no solutions are pooling under the patient.

    Purpose: The solution will irritate or burn the skin.

13 Dry the area, using the same circular technique with dry sponges. The area may be dried by blotting with a third sterile towel.

14 Paint on the antiseptic with the cotton-tipped applicators or gauze sponges, using the same circular technique and never returning to an area that has already been painted (Figures 3 to 5).

15 Place sterile drape and/or towel over the area. Patient is now ready for surgery.

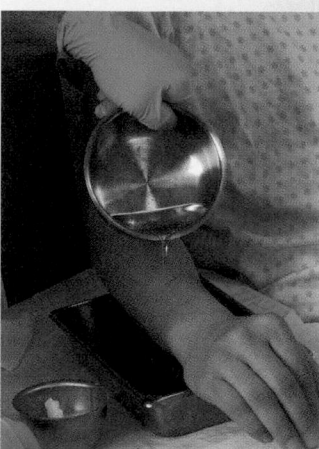

Figure 3

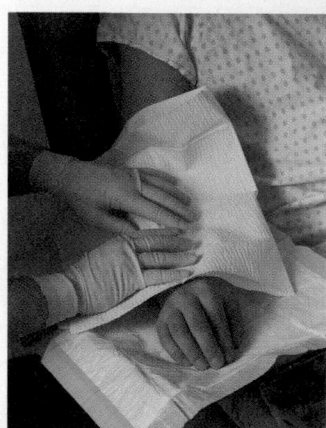

Figure 4

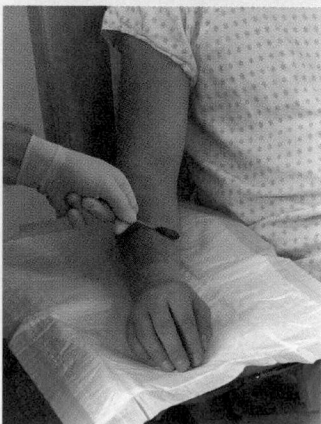

Figure 5

Preparation of the Room

After receiving an assignment to assist in a minor surgical procedure, study the physician's care preferences, review the procedure, and note the materials that are needed. Next, prepare the room and gather the supplies to be used (Table 54-3). Sterile supplies are opened just before the procedure. Opened materials that have been exposed longer than 1 hour, usually because of a delay, are considered unsterile. Supplies should not be placed where they can be knocked over or dropped. Wrapped sterile supplies that fall to the floor must not be used. Once supplies are opened, the sterile field should be covered with a sterile drape, and a team member should stay in the room to monitor them.

Setting Up a Sterile Field. The circulating assistant opens the packs, beginning with the pack that provides the sterile surface for the remaining sterile items, also known as the *sterile field* (Procedure 54-9). The Mayo tray is usually prepared as soon as the scrub assistant is gloved and ready to manage the sterile field. Drapes, towel packs,

additional sponge packs, and other sterile packages are stacked on the side or back table. Items from this table may be added, if needed, during the procedure (Procedures 54-10 and 54-11). A basin or biohazard container for waste is placed nearby for use during the surgery.

Assisting the Physician During Surgery

The physician is ultimately responsible for the patient; however, the medical assistant is responsible for ensuring that everything the assistant and the physician will use in caring for the surgical patient is accounted for, ready for use, and prepared in a safe and sterile manner (Procedure 54-12). A surgical conscience painstakingly ensures the practice of good aseptic technique and demands that breaks in aseptic technique be corrected immediately without regard to delays or embarrassment.

Every team will have preferences regarding the sequence they follow during routine minor surgery. Once a routine is established, it should be followed in

TABLE 54-3	Single Assistant Preparation for Minor Surgery

1. Wash your hands; gather all supplies.
   Sterile side (Mayo tray): Two towel packs, skin prep pack, patient drape pack, instrument pack, miscellaneous pack(s), three glove packs, masks, goggles, aprons, or gowns
   Nonsterile side (side counter): Syringes, suture material, anesthesia solutions, additional sponges, dressings, bandages, transfer forceps, waste basin, waste receptacle, nonsterile gloves, masks, goggles, aprons, or gowns
2. Escort patient into the room.
3. Greet and converse with patient.
4. Position patient on table.
5. Wash your hands.
6. Open first towel pack.
7. Open skin prep pack.
8. Pour soap and antiseptic solutions.
9. Expose the site to be prepped.
10. Scrub with the surgical hand wash.
11. Glove and arrange prep items within sterile field.
12. Place sterile towels at skin scrub boundaries using sterile technique.
13. Prep the patient's skin.
14. Discard skin prep materials.
15. Discard gloves; wash your hands.
16. Open table drape pack on Mayo stand to create sterile field.
17. Open instrument pack (packs), and transfer instruments to sterile field. Add sterile syringe unit.
18. Add sterile items as requested.
19. Physician joins you and converses with the patient.
20. Open the physician's glove pack (the physician now gloves).
21. Open the patient drape pack (the physician now drapes the surgical site).
22. Cleanse and hold up anesthesia vial for the physician to withdraw anesthesia with sterile syringe (the physician will now administer the anesthesia).
23. Repeat surgical hand wash; reglove with a new glove pack.
24. Arrange sterile field instruments and other materials for safety and in sequence; check instrument condition.
25. Unwind suture materials; load the first suture into the needle holder.
26. Place two gauze sponges at the site.
27. Assist with the procedure.*
    For the physician—pass instruments; maintain field; anticipate needs; cut sutures.
    For the patient—retract tissue; sponge blood from wound; apply bandage; and care for specimen.
28. Escort the patient to recovery area and check vital signs as instructed.
29. Record and prepare specimens.
30. Clean the room; clear materials; discard gloves.
31. Chart the procedure on the medical record.
32. Help the patient to prepare to leave the office.
33. Disinfect and sterilize equipment at the first available time.

*By law, the assistant may not clamp tissue, place sutures, or alter body tissues in any way.

PROCEDURE 54-9

Opening a Sterile Pack and Creating a Sterile Field

GOAL: To open a sterile pack that contains a table drape, using correct aseptic technique.

EQUIPMENT AND SUPPLIES

- A sterile pack (autoclaved linen or disposable) that will serve as a sterile table drape or field
- Mayo stand or countertop
- Disinfectant and gauze sponges

PROCEDURAL STEPS

1 Check that the Mayo stand or countertop is dust free and clean. If it is not, clean with 70% alcohol or another disinfectant and towel.

Purpose: Although some areas cannot be sterile, steps must be taken to keep contamination to a minimum.

2 Wash your hands and dry them carefully.

Purpose: Moisture on your hands contaminates the pack.

3 Place the sterile pack on the Mayo stand or countertop and read the label.

Purpose: Most medical offices have a limited supply of autoclaved packs. To open a wrong package could mean not having enough sterile supplies for a different procedure.

4 Check the expiration date (Figure 1). If using an autoclaved pack, check the indicator tape for color change.

Purpose: An expired pack is not considered sterile. Autoclave indicator tape changes color after the sterile processing cycle.

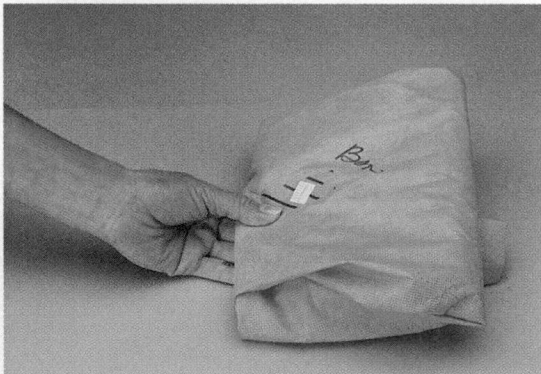

Figure 1

5 Position the package so that the outer envelope flap is face up and at the top as you look at the package.

Purpose: This positions the pack for correct opening, using aseptic technique.

6 Open the first flap away from you (Figure 2).

Purpose: Otherwise, you will be reaching over a sterile field for the other three flaps.

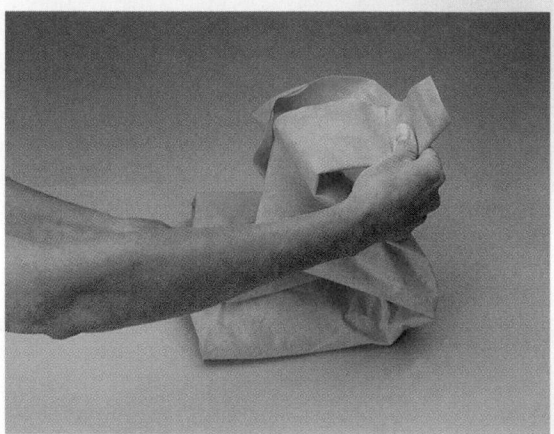

Figure 2

7 Pull away the two side flaps, one at a time. Be careful to lift each flap by reaching under the small folded-back tab and without touching the inner surface of the pack or its contents (Figures 3 and 4).

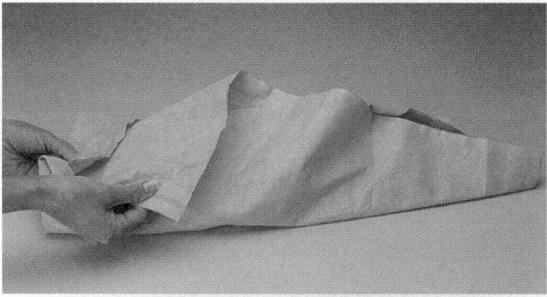

Figure 3

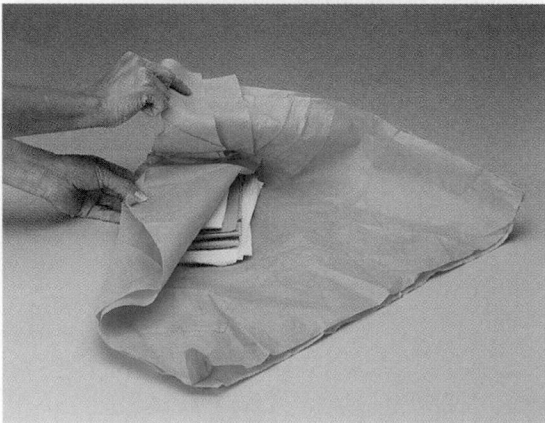

Figure 4

PROCEDURE 54-9—cont'd

8 Pull the last flap toward you by its tab, exposing the towel (Figure 5).

9 You now have a sterile drape as a sterile field to work from and for the distribution of additional sterile supplies and instruments (Figure 6).

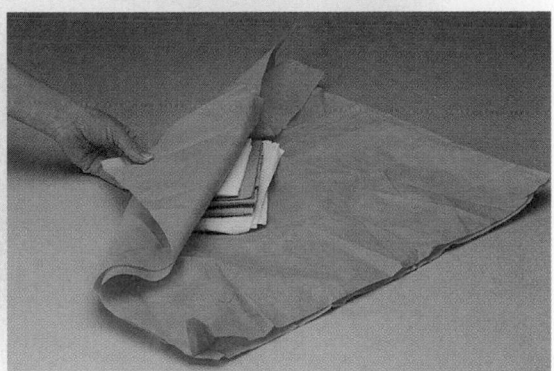

Figure 5

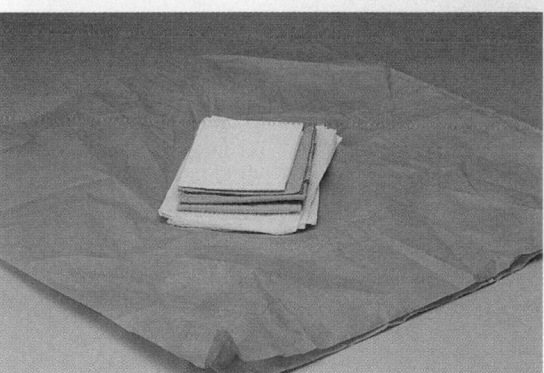

Figure 6

PROCEDURE 54-10

Using Transfer Forceps

GOAL: To move sterile items on a sterile field or transfer sterile items to a gloved team member.

EQUIPMENT AND SUPPLIES

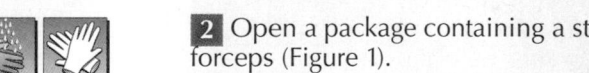

- Sterile item to move or transfer
- Sterile wrapped transfer forceps
- Mayo stand set-up with a sterile field and sterile instruments

PROCEDURAL STEPS

1 Wash your hands and dry them carefully.
  Purpose: Water on your hands makes gloving difficult.

2 Open a package containing a sterile transfer forceps (Figure 1).

3 Using aseptic technique, handle sterile forceps by ring handle only. Always point forceps tips down.
  Purpose: If the tips are turned upward, any solution encountered will run onto the nonsterile area and then back down over the sterile end when the tips are turned down again, thus contaminating the forceps.

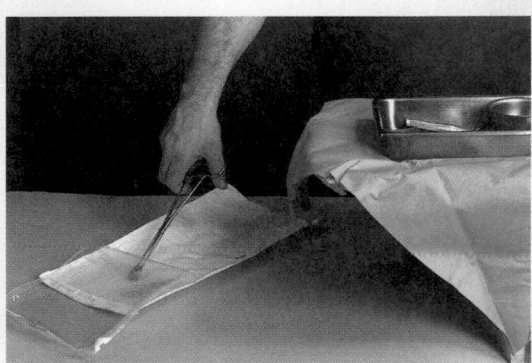

Figure 1

Continued

PROCEDURE 54-10—cont'd

4 Grasp an item on the sterile field with sterile forceps, points down, and move it to its proper position for the procedure, making sure not to cross the sterile field with the hand or contaminated end of the forceps (Figure 2).

5 Or, transfer an instrument from the autoclave to the sterile field.

6 Remove the transfer forceps after one-time use.

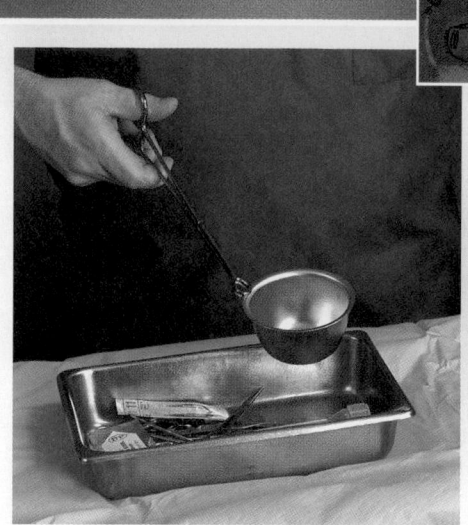

Figure 2

PROCEDURE 54-11

Pouring Solutions onto a Sterile Field(s)

GOAL: As a circulating assistant, pour a sterile solution into a stainless-steel bowl or medicine glass that is sitting at the edge of a sterile field.

EQUIPMENT AND SUPPLIES

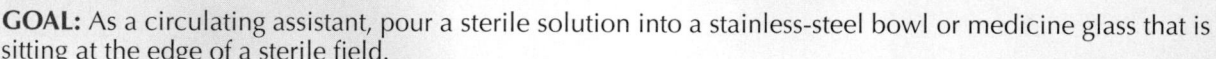

- A bottle of sterile solution
- A sterile bowl or medicine glass
- A sterile field
- A sink or waste receptacle
- NOTE: The sterile bowl should be placed near one edge of the field and the perimeter of the 1-inch barrier.

PROCEDURAL STEPS

1 Wash your hands and dry them carefully.
   Purpose: Moisture on your hands may cause the bottle to slip from your hand.

2 Read the label of the ordered solution.
   Purpose: Always perform the three label checks before administering any solution or medication.

3 Place your hand over the label and lift the bottle. NOTE: If the container has a double cap, set the outer cap on the counter inside up, then proceed.

4 Lift the lid of the bottle straight up, and then slightly to one side, and hold the lid in your nondominant hand facing downward.
   Purpose: Air currents carry contaminants that could settle on the inside of the lid.

5 Pour away from the label (Figure 1).
   Purpose: Spills down the side of the bottle stain or make the label unreadable.

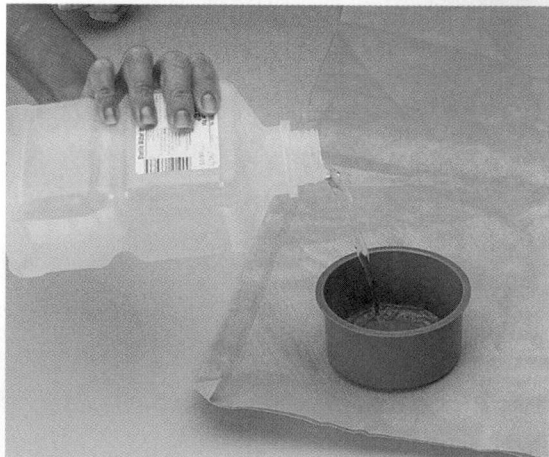

Figure 1

6 If the container does not have a double cap, pour off a small amount of the solution into a waste receptacle.

PROCEDURE **54-11—cont'd**

Purpose: To rinse any contaminants off the bottle lip. NOTE: If the container has a double cap, skip this step and proceed to step 7.

7 Pour away from the label, into the bowl, without allowing any part of the bottle to touch the bowl and without crossing over the sterile field (Figure 2).
Purpose: The bottle exterior is not sterile.

8 Tilt the bottle up to stop the pouring while it is still over the bowl.
Purpose: Solutions spilled on the sterile field may contaminate the field.

9 Remove the bottle from over the sterile field.
Purpose: Motion over a sterile field should be kept to a minimum.

10 Replace the cap (or caps) off to the side, away from the sterile field.

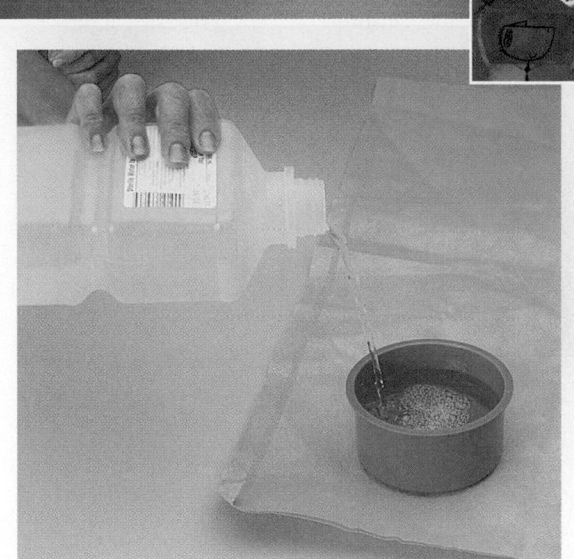

Figure 2

every case. Sample set-ups for various types of minor surgery are provided in Table 54-4.

The scrub assistant sorts and places the scalpels, hemostats, scissors, tissue forceps, and retractors on the sterile field according to their sequence and frequency of use (Figure 54-6). Scalpels and sharp instruments should be conspicuously placed so that they do not accidentally harm a team member. If the scrub assistant has not previously prepped the patient, the circulating assistant now performs the patient skin prep. The circulating assistant opens the drape pack. The physician enters the room after scrubbing and then gloves. The physician drapes the patient with towels or a fenes- trated drape as the scrub assistant hands the drapes, one at a time. In many offices, the scrub assistant alone drapes the site. Once the site is draped, the Mayo stand is positioned below the site and the scrub assistant stands opposite the physician over the patient.

Local Anesthesia. The circulating assistant cleans the vial of local anesthetic medication with an alcohol swab and holds the vial so the physician or scrub assistant can easily read the label. The scrub assistant or physician lifts the syringe from the sterile field, reads the label, and draws the appropriate amount of anesthetic into the syringe without touching the circulating assistant holding the vial. The physician then

TABLE 54-4	Set-ups for Minor Surgeries			
Procedure	Side Counter	Sterile Field	Comments	Postoperative Care
Suture repair	Local anesthetic, dressings and bandages, splints or guards, tape, drape, gloves, sterile normal saline solution	Syringe and needle, hemostats (3), scissors, sponges, suture material and needle, tissue forceps or skin hook, needle holder	If an emergency patient arrives in the office with a pressure dressing over a laceration, do not remove the pressure dressing until the physician is ready to suture. If the patient's pressure cloth *must* be removed, have ample sterile dressings ready to apply immediately. Ask the patient the possible length, depth, and exact location of the laceration. Usually there is limited cleansing of a wound because of the bleeding. If not, let the physician instruct you on the necessary cleansing.	Frequently, clean lacerations in a moderately protected area will not be dressed but left open. The patient will be instructed to keep the area clean and dry. Some lacerations may be closed with adhesive Steri-strips. These are becoming increasingly popular, because they reduce the chance of infection and do not leave suture scars.

Continued

TABLE 54-4	Set-ups for Minor Surgeries—cont'd			
Procedure	**Side Counter**	**Sterile Field**	**Comments**	**Postoperative Care**
Needle biopsy	Specimen container with prepackaged fixative or preserving solution, laboratory form and label, local anesthetic, gloves	Biopsy needle, syringe and needle, sponges	A biopsy is the examination of tissue removed from the living body. Biopsies are usually done to determine whether a growth or swelling is malignant or benign; however, they may be done as a diagnostic aid in other diseases or infections. A needle biopsy may be done by aspiration with a needle and syringe or by a special biopsy needle. The specimen is then sent to a pathologist for either a cytological or histological examination.	Usually there is no special dressing required after a needle biopsy. A Band-Aid is often sufficient.
Cyst removal	Local anesthetic, disinfectant (skin prep), laboratory form, dressing (size depends on site), gloves, drape, specimen container with prepackaged fixative or preserving solution	Kelly hemostats (2 straight and 2 curved), dressing forceps (2), suture and needle, scissors s/s or s/b, dissector (physician's choice), skin hook, syringe and needle, knife handle with blade No. 11 or No. 15, tissue forceps (2), Allis forceps, needle holder, sponges	A sebaceous cyst is a benign retention cyst of a sebaceous gland containing fatty substance of the gland. It is also called a *wen*. It may occur any place on the body, with the exception of the palms of the hands and the soles of the feet. It is more common on the neck and shoulder; and because it is frequently the source of irritation, it is removed. Ordinarily, the cyst is attached only to the skin and moves freely over the underlying tissue. For cosmetic reasons, the physician will make the incision on the natural skin crease lines.	See suture repair above or apply a small dressing depending on size of incision.

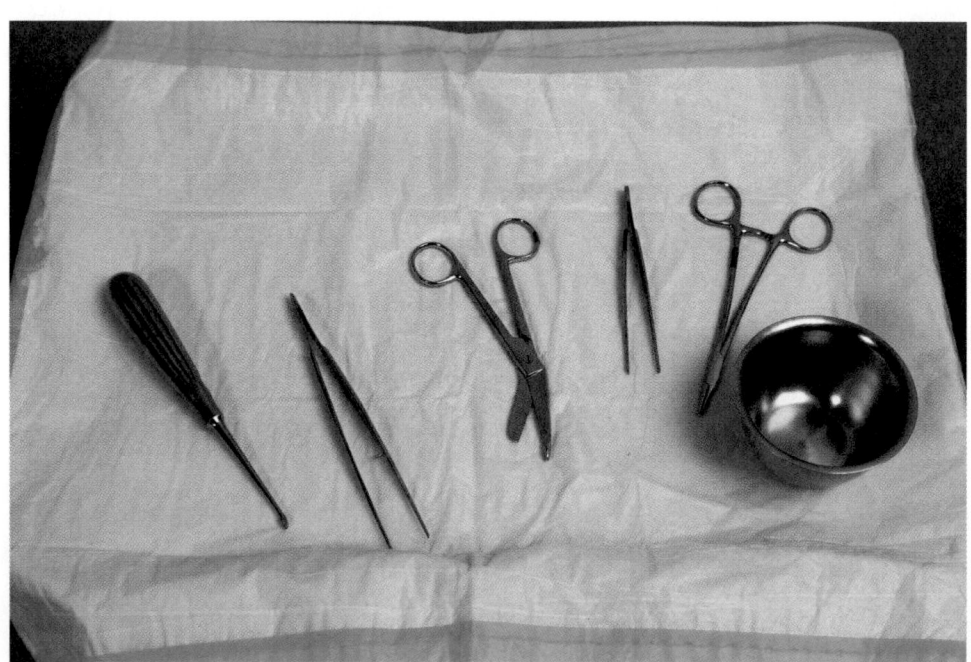

FIGURE 54-6 Mayo stand with surgical set-up on sterile field.

injects the anesthetic at the surgical site. The scrub assistant places a sponge on the patient, next to the surgical site, for sponging blood at the time of the first incision or to sponge an open injury as the first step in the procedure. The local anesthetic medication is administered either directly into the lesion or into the tissues surrounding the site to be incised. After the local anesthetic has taken effect, the physician begins the procedure.

Passing Instruments. During a procedure, the scrub assistant must protect the sterile field from contamination. Notify the physician if there is a break in sterile technique; dispose of soiled sponges into the biohazard waste container, and anticipate the surgeon's need for instruments. The physician may verbally request instruments or may use hand signals (Figure 54-7). As the team works together over time, the physician may not need to give any signals because the assistant will be able to anticipate what instrument is needed next during the procedure.

Instrumentation is logical: if the physician requests a suture, scissors will be needed next to cut the suture strand. In the case of sudden hemorrhage from a bleeding vessel, the physician will need an appropriately sized hemostat. In gaining experience, the assistant watches, listens, and learns to judge what will be needed or performed next. Pass instruments with a firm and purposeful motion so that the physician will not have to

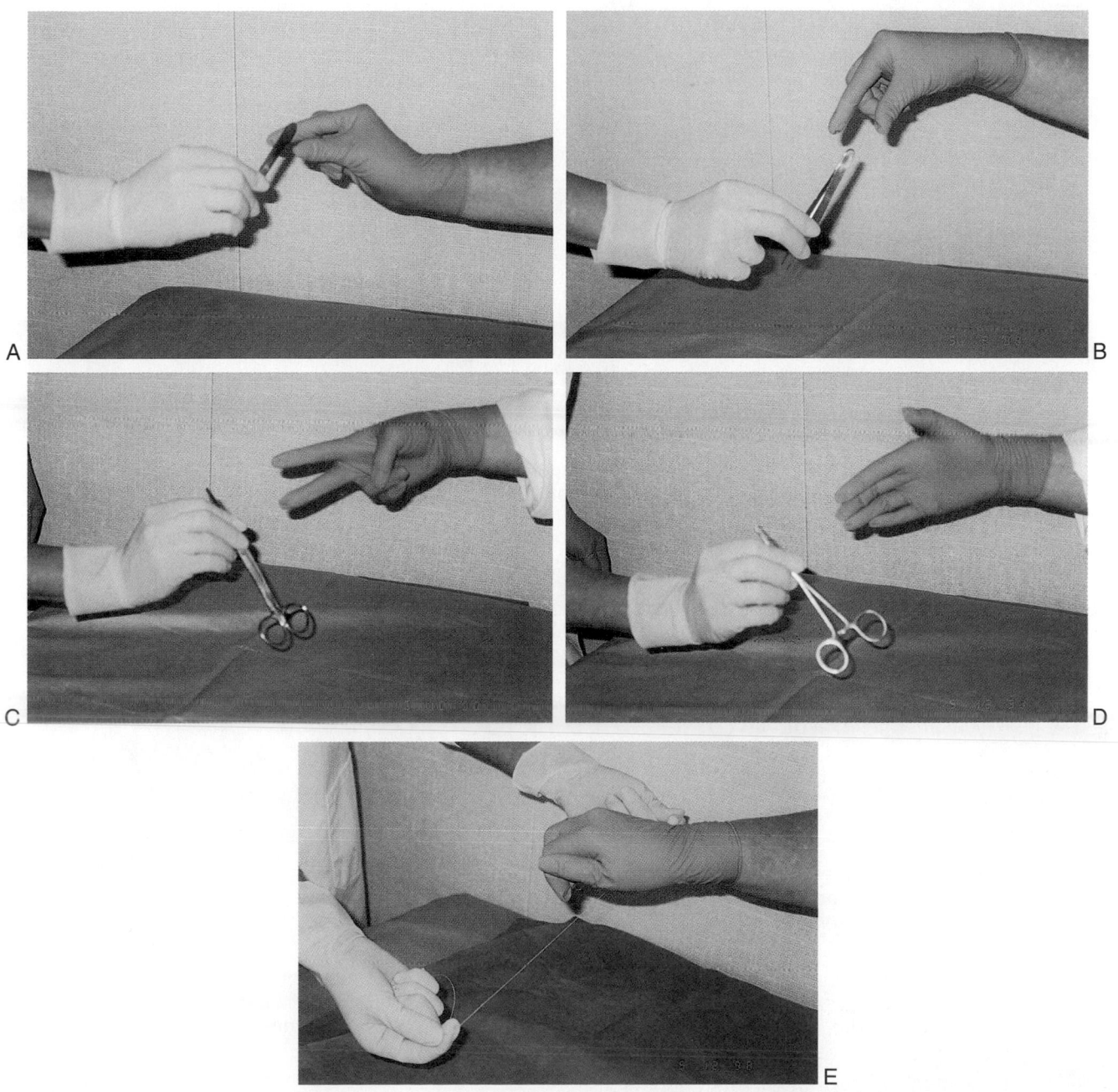

FIGURE 54-7   Passing sterile surgical instruments. **A**, Scalpel. **B**, Forceps. **C**, Scissors. **D**, Clamp. **E**, Free suture pass (free tie).

look up. Wait until you feel the physician grasp the instrument, so it will not drop onto the patient or to the floor. Pass instruments so that you and the physician are protected from injury. Pass the scalpel blade down and present the handle to the surgeon. Hold all instruments by their tips and pass the handle ends into the physician's palm or fingers. Avoid painful slapping of the instrument into the surgeon's hand, as you commonly see on TV and in the movies. Correct passing produces a faint, gentle "snap" as the instrument contacts the surgeon's gloved hand.

CRITICAL THINKING APPLICATION

While passing the scalpel to the surgeon while assisting with an I&D, Melissa feels the blade "slice" through her glove. She quickly and secretly looks at it and notices a "very tiny" nick in her glove. Since this is a "dirty" procedure, she decides to say nothing and continue assisting with the procedure. Is her reasoning sound here? What is the best approach to handling this situation? Why? Evaluate Melissa's reasoning in this situation.

Specimen Collection. If a specimen is collected during a procedure, it is placed in a sterile glass or basin. Do not remove the specimen from the sterile field until the physician gives the order. The surgeon may want to examine the specimen again during the surgery.

Completing the Surgical Procedure. At the conclusion of the procedure, the physician will begin the wound closure (Procedure 54-13). The techniques and methods of tissue closure vary greatly and it would be impossible to describe or illustrate all of them. There are two basic methods of suturing: the continuous running suture, and the interrupted suture, in which each knot is placed and tied one at a time, so that if one breaks, the others keep the wound closure intact (Figure 54-8). For the majority of skin closures in a medical office, the interrupted technique is used.

The scrub assistant mounts the suture and needle in the needle holder and passes it to the physician, handle first. As the physician closes the wound, the scrub assistant assists by cutting the suture and sponging the site. The physician places the first interrupted suture at the midpoint of the incision. Then each side of the first suture is mentally divided in half again, and the next two sutures are placed at each of these midpoints. The rest of the sutures are placed using the same technique until the wound edges are completely approximated.

PROCEDURE **54-12**

Assisting With Minor Surgery

GOAL: To maintain the sterile field and to pass instruments in a prescribed sequence during a surgical procedure that involves the making of a surgical incision and the removal of a growth.

EQUIPMENT AND SUPPLIES

- Open patient drape pack on the side counter
- Mayo stand covered with a sterile drape
- Packaged sterile gloves (two pairs)
- Needle and syringe for anesthesia medication
- Vial of local anesthetic medication
- Sterile drape
- Scalpel handle and No. 15 blade
- Allis tissue forceps
- One skin retractor
- Three hemostats
- Supply of gauze sponges
- Biohazard waste receptacle
- Needle with suture material

PROCEDURAL STEPS

1 Wash your hands. Dry thoroughly.
Purpose: Gloving is difficult with moist hands.

2 Apply sterile gloves, using aseptic technique. Set up the sterile field with instruments and supplies, in the sequence to be used (Figure 1*). Cover the sterile field with a sterile drape.

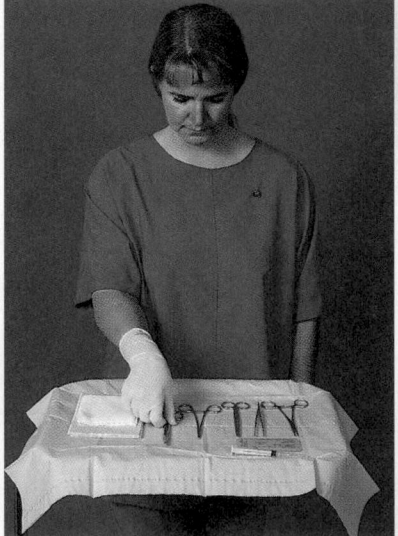

Figure 1

---

*Figure from Bonewit-West K: *Clinical procedures for medical assistants,* ed. 5, Philadelphia, 2000, WB Saunders.

PROCEDURE 54-12—cont'd

3 Apply sterile gloves, using aseptic technique, and prep the patient's skin with surgical soap and antiseptic solution. Instruct the patient of prep procedure.

Purpose: Infection control and to ensure the patient's cooperation.

4 Scrub, using the surgical hand wash procedure. Follow standard precautions.

5 Dry your hands thoroughly.

6 Apply sterile gloves, using aseptic technique.

7 Position the Mayo stand near the patient and the operative site (Figure 2).

Purpose: Motion over a sterile field should be kept to a minimum.

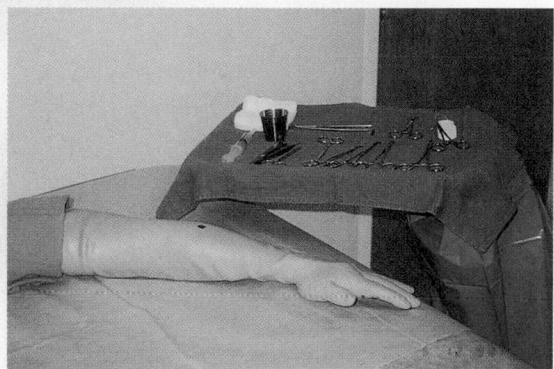

Figure 2

8 Lift the patient drape from the open pack without touching the drape to any of the pack edges.

Purpose: The 1-inch perimeter around the sterile field is considered nonsterile.

9 Grasp the patient drape by holding one edge or corner in each hand (Figure 3).

10 Drape the surgical site without touching any part of the patient or the operating area with your gloved hands (Figure 4).

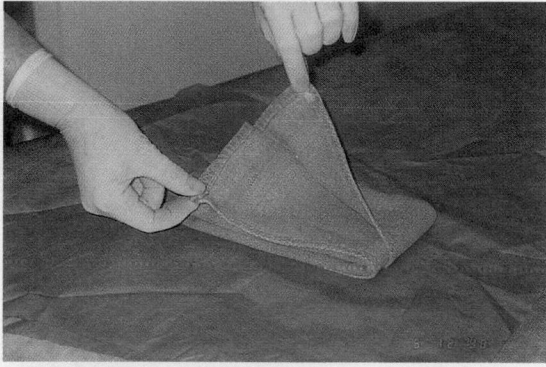

Figure 3

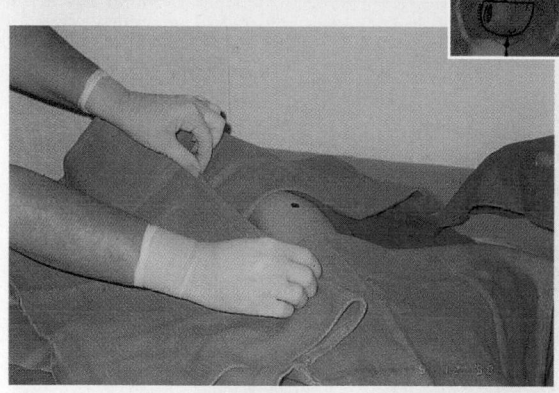

Figure 4

11 After removing gloves, circulating assistant holds local anesthetic so physician can read the label. Physician withdraws the desired amount using sterile technique (Figure 5).

Purpose: The vial of local anesthetic medication cannot be held after both team members are gloved.

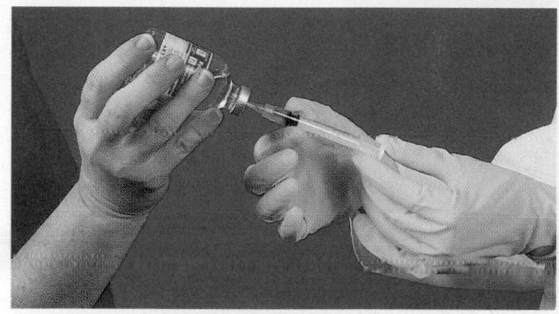

Figure 5

12 The surgeon injects the local anesthesia, and the assistant should apply sterile glove using aseptic technique.

Purpose: Everyone should read the medication label before dispensing or administering a medication.

13 Position yourself across from the surgeon. Arrange the sterile field. Check instrument condition and placement location on Mayo stand (Figure 6).

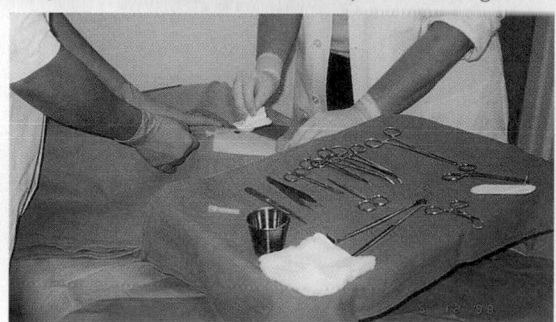

Figure 6

Figure from Bonewit-West K: *Clinical procedures for medical assistants*, ed. 5, Philadelphia, 2000, WB Saunders.

Continued

PROCEDURE 54-12—cont'd

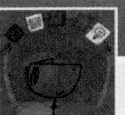

14 Place two sponges on the patient, next to the wound site (Figure 7).

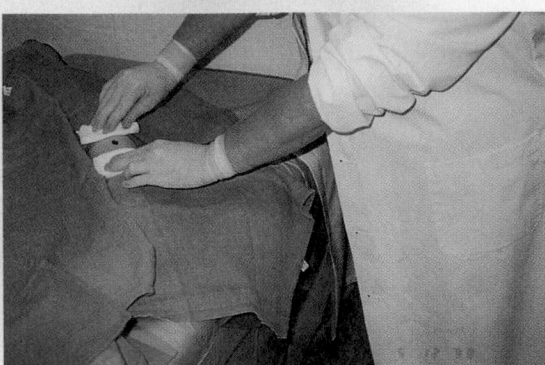

Figure 7

15 Grasp the scalpel blade with a hemostat and mount the scalpel blade onto the scalpel handle. Keep all sharp equipment conspicuously placed on the sterile field (Figure 8).

Purpose: Sharp instruments that are not clearly visible may injure a team member.

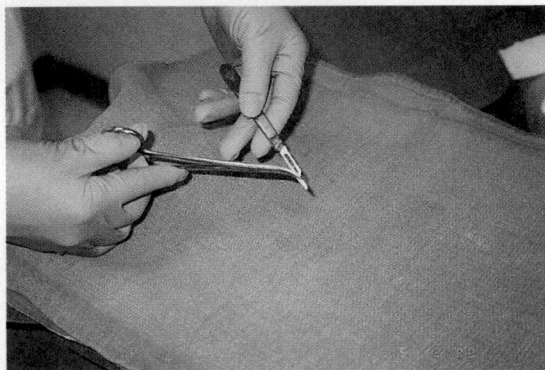

Figure 8

16 Pass the scalpel, blade down and handle first, to the surgeon or the surgeon will reach for it himself or herself. The surgeon will take the scalpel with the thumb and forefinger in the position ready for use (Figure 9).

Purpose: To protect the surgeon and yourself from injury.

17 Grasp an Allis tissue forceps by the tips and pass it to the surgeon to grasp a piece of the tissue to be excised (Figure 10).

18 Pass the handles into the surgeon's open palm with a firm and purposeful motion. A gentle "snap" is heard as it contacts the surgeon's gloved hand.

Purpose: The surgeon will not have to look up to receive the instrument.

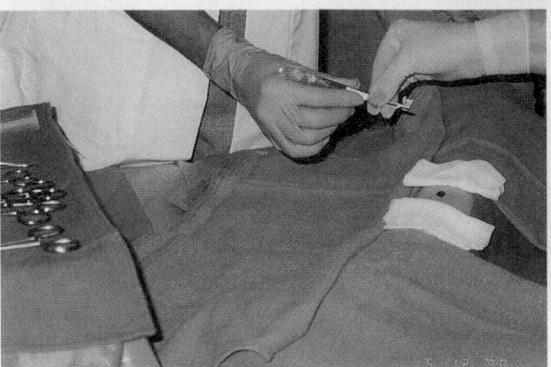

Figure 9

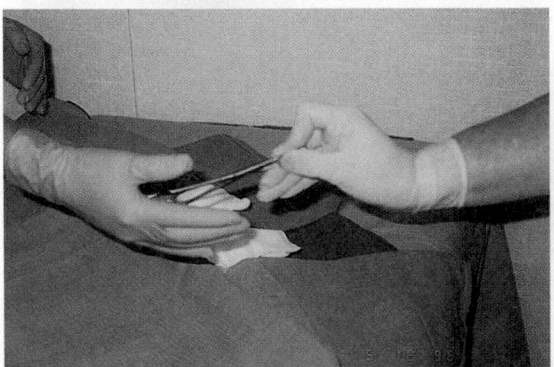

Figure 10

19 Dispose of soiled sponges, using the biohazard waste receptacle.

20 Hold clean sponges in your hand, to pat or sponge the wound, as needed (Figure 11).

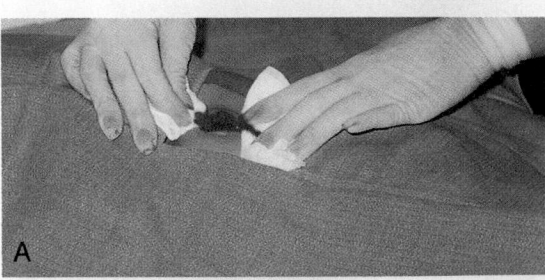

A

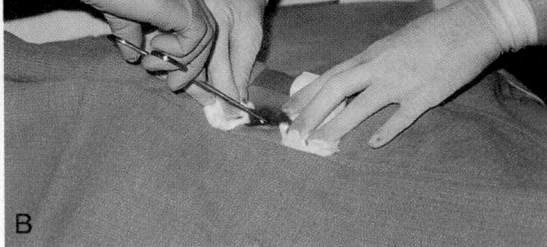

B

Figure 11

PROCEDURE **54-12—cont'd**

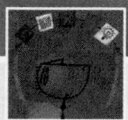

21 Safely position the specimen (if any) where it will not be disturbed on the sterile field (Figure 12).

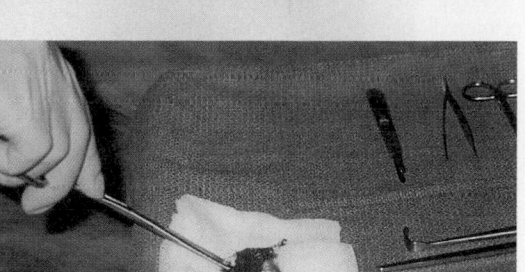

Figure 12

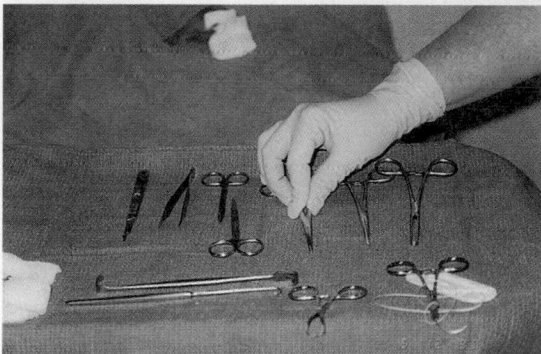

Figure 13

22 If there is a bleeding vessel, or if a hemostat is requested, pass the hemostat in the manner described in steps 17 and 18.

23 Receive instruments, and place them on the sterile field (Figure 13).

24 Continue to sponge blood from the wound site.
   Purpose: A clear sterile field expedites the procedure.

25 Retract the wound edge, as needed, with a skin retractor.

26 Continue to monitor the sterile field and assist the surgeon as needed.

27 Pass the surgeon the needle and suture material to close the wound (Figure 14).

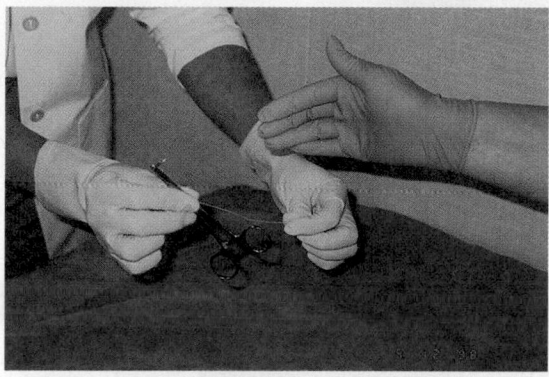

Figure 14

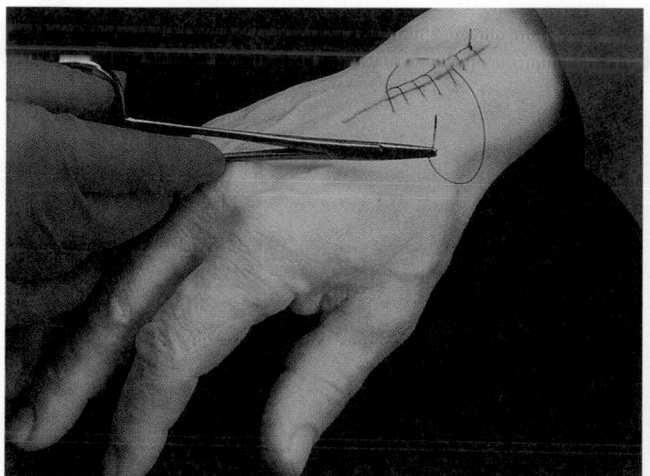

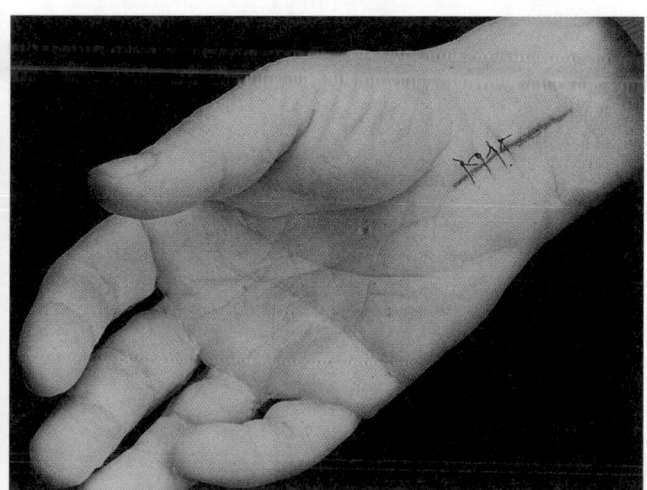

FIGURE 54-8   **A**, Continuous (running) suture placement. **B**, Interrupted suture placement.

After the skin closure, the wound site is cleaned with wet (using normal saline solution) and dry sponges by the surgeon or the scrub assistant. Care must be taken not to disturb the wound edges or sutures. Next, sterile dressings are placed over the incision (Procedure 54-14) and the drapes are removed. Lift the drapes directly off the patient with minimum movement so as not to disturb the dressing or stir up the air currents. The circulating assistant or the surgeon then applies the bandage and tape to the dressing. Do not take away the Mayo stand with instruments until the patient has left the room or the surgeon instructs you. If there is an unexpected contamination of the wound site during the dressing application, more materials will be needed from the sterile field.

PROCEDURE 54-13

Assisting With Suturing

GOAL: To assist the surgeon in wound closure, using sterile technique.

EQUIPMENT AND SUPPLIES

- Sterile field on Mayo stand
- Surgical scissors
- Suture material
- Sterile gloves
- Needle holder
- Gauze sponges

PROCEDURAL STEPS

NOTE: This procedure may be a continuation of Procedure 54-12. If done independently, you must perform the surgical scrub and glove before beginning step 1.

1 Hold the curved needle point in your minor hand, 4 to 5 inches over the sterile field (Figure 1).

Purpose: Always work over a sterile field and take care not to puncture gloves with the sharp needle.

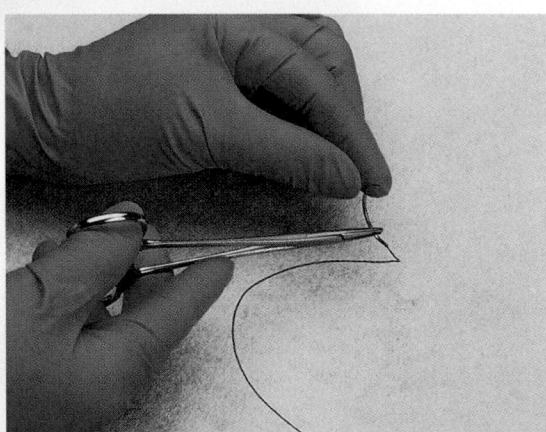

Figure 1

2 With the needle holder, clamp the suture needle at the upper third of its total length (Figure 2).

Purpose: Clamping in the middle weakens and may distort the shape of the needle. Clamping too near the thread may cause the suture to detach from the needle. Clamping at the lower third of the needle damages the needle point.

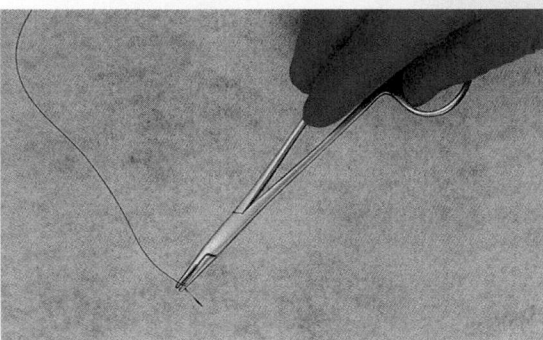

Figure 2

3 With your dominant hand, hold the needle holder halfway down its shaft, at the box-lock, with the suture needle point up.

4 With your nondominant hand, hold the suture strand, and pass the needle holder into the surgeon's hand (Figures 3 and 4).

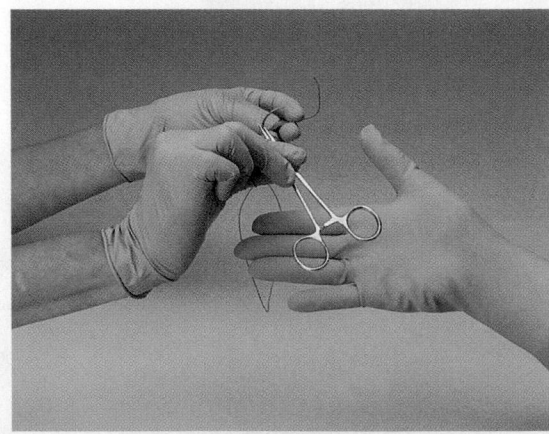

Figure 3

PROCEDURE 54-13—cont'd

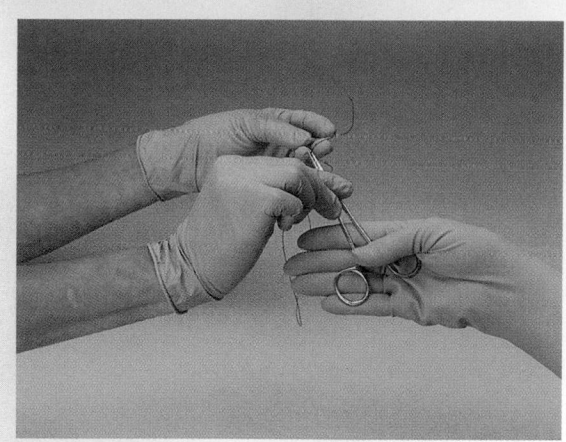

Figure 4

5 Pick up the surgical scissors with your dominant hand and a gauze sponge with your nondominant hand.

6 After the surgeon has placed a closure suture, knots it, and holds the two strands taut, cut both suture strands in one motion. Cut between the knot and the surgeon, at the length requested, about ⅛ inch.

Purpose: Too long a suture may irritate the patient during recovery, and too short a suture may untie during recovery.

7 Gently blot the closure once with the gauze sponge in your nondominant hand.

Purpose: Rubbing or friction may damage the wound edges.

8 If additional strands of suture are needed, repeat the process.

Surgical Room Clean-Up

While the circulating assistant escorts the patient from the room, the scrub assistant clears the sterile field. Standard blood and body fluid precautions must be followed. The scrub assistant should not remove gloves until all contaminated materials are properly removed and handled. Disposable items are placed in appropriate waste cans and sharps containers, and the linen is placed in the linen hamper. The room should be checked for any blood spills or other contamination. Remove the contaminated gloves and wash your hands.

Use clean gloves to decontaminate, sanitize, and disinfect the room, including the table, Mayo stand, side and back tables, any other equipment in the room, and the floor. The used instruments and linens are washed and resterilized for future use. Label any specimens and prepare them for transport to the laboratory. The surgeon and medical assistant both document the procedure in the patient's medical record.

Postoperative Instructions and Care

The patient is given time to rest after the surgery. If a sedative was administered, make certain that the patient is sufficiently recovered to avoid injury after the surgery or during the journey home. If the patient has been given a topical or local anesthetic, explain to the patient that the anesthesia effect will wear off and that there may be discomfort at the operative site. Check with the physician if pain medication has *not* been prescribed. If medication has been prescribed, review the purpose of the medication and directions for its use with the patient and his or her companion. Before the patient leaves the office, a follow-up appointment should be made.

Postoperative care extends for the total recovery period, not just for the time of immediate care before the patient leaves the office. Most medical assistants are responsible for teaching patients to care for themselves at home after surgery. The concentration of a postoperative patient is diminished after the stress of surgery, so all instructions should be given to the patient in writing. They should be simple in style and easily understood by the patient and the caregiver at home. These instructions can be preprinted forms for each type of surgery, or a general form with checked boxes for particular postoperative instructions that apply specifically to the individual patient (Figure 54-9).

Warning Signs. Explain to the patient the importance of calling the office if there are any questions or changes that they are concerned about. If the patient does not call within the next 24 hours, you should call the patient. Many patients tend to "ride it out" or say they did not want to disturb you. Never allow the postoperative patient to leave the office without the physician's knowledge and approval. Tell the patient to call the office immediately if he or she notes redness around the operative site, bleeding from the wound, fever, swelling, or increasing or severe pain. The wound should be kept clean and dry, and the patient should be taught how to change the dressing if needed.

Follow-Up. If the healing process is a long one, or if the wound becomes wet or infected, the patient may return for a dressing change. Notify the physician immediately. Check the patient's medical record and follow the physician's instructions carefully. Follow standard precautions; wear gloves and other protective barriers, as appropriate. Place the patient in a comfortable position, explain what you will be doing, and adequately expose the area to be redressed. Try to obscure the wound site from the patient's view, and do not reveal any unpleasant reactions by either comment or facial expression. If at any time you determine that the wound may be infected, stop and have the physician examine it. Generally, no bandaging material should be reused, including reusable Ace wraps. They

POSTOP INSTRUCTIONS FOR _____

☐ Elevate your arm.
☐ Elevate your leg.
☐ Limit food intake to _____.
☐ Limit activity to _____.
☐ Do not bathe or shower.
☐ Sponge bath only.
☐ Change dressing as instructed
☐ Call the office for fever, redness, pain, swelling, or bleeding.
☐ Take_____ every 4 hours as needed for pain.
☐ Return to school/work in _____days.
☐ Call the office tommorrow before _____p.m.
☐ Your next appointment is on M T W Th F S _____ at _____.

FIGURE 54-9 An example of preprinted postoperative patient instructions.

should absolutely never be reused if there is any evidence of soiling.

Tape applied directly to a patient's skin is not a good dressing immobilizer. If tape is used, always keep it to a minimum. If there is tape holding a dressing in place, always remove it by *pulling toward the wound.* If it is adhering to a hairy area of the body, lift the outer tape edge with one hand and slowly and gently separate the underlying hair and skin from the tape with the thumb of your other hand. Peel the skin from the bandage, not the bandage from the skin. Never rapidly "rip" tape from the body—the patient's skin may be injured. If the tape is not irritating to the patient, it may be advisable to leave the tape in place until total healing has taken place.

After the physician examines the wound, the medical assistant will either apply a new dressing or remove the patient's sutures (Procedure 54-15).

Caring for Wounds. A wound is an interruption in the continuity of body tissues, and can be external, internal, or both.

Types of Wounds. A wound can be intentional (from a surgical incision) or accidental, and may be open or closed (Figure 54-10). An open wound has an outward opening where the skin is broken, causing the underlying tissues to be exposed. A closed or nonpenetrating wound does not have an outward opening, but the underlying tissues are damaged, as in a hematoma, contusion, or bruise. Closed wounds are usually the result of some type of blunt trauma to the body. An aseptic (clean) wound is not infected with pathogens. Septic wounds are infected with pathogens.

Open wounds may be classified according to the appearance of their openings. An incised wound has a clean edge and is made with a cutting instrument. An incised wound may be the result of intentional surgery,

PROCEDURE 54-14

Applying/Changing a Dressing

GOAL: To properly apply a dressing at the completion of a surgical procedure.

EQUIPMENT AND SUPPLIES
• Sterile dressing material or Telfa

PROCEDURAL STEPS

1 Before the sterile drape is removed from the patient, and with sterile gloves in place, the dressing is picked up from the sterile field, placed on the wound, and held.

   Purpose: To prevent introducing microorganisms to the wound area.

2 The drape is then removed while switching hands to hold the dressing in place.

Purpose: To keep the wound as clean as possible.

3 The dressing is secured with paper tape and/or an appropriate bandage.

   Purpose: To keep the wound covered and protected.

4 The procedure is documented in the patient's medical record.

   Purpose: A procedure is not completed until it is recorded.

_____

See Appendix E for a charting example.

PROCEDURE 54-15

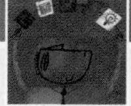

Suture Removal

GOAL: To remove sutures from a healed incision, using sterile technique and without injury to the closed wound.

EQUIPMENT AND SUPPLIES

Suture removal pack containing the following:
- Suture removal scissors
- Gauze sponges
- Thumb dressing forceps
- Steri-Strips or Band-Aids
- Skin antiseptic
- Biohazard waste container
- Sterile gloves

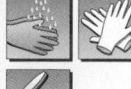

PROCEDURAL STEPS

1 Assemble necessary supplies.

2 Wash and dry your hands. Follow standard precautions.

3 Instruct patient of procedure and to lie or sit still during procedure.
 Purpose: To ensure cooperation during the procedure.

4 Position patient comfortably and support the area.

5 Place dry towels under the patient area.

6 Open the suture removal pack, and apply sterile gloves.

7 Place a gauze sponge next to the wound site.
 Purpose: To place the removed sutures.

8 Grasp the knot of the suture with the dressing forceps, without pulling.

9 Cut the suture at skin level (Figure 1).

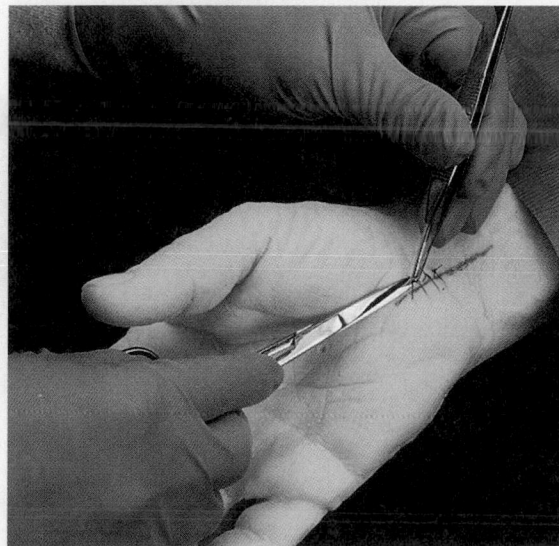

Figure 1

10 Lift, do not pull, the suture toward the incision and out with the dressing forceps (Figure 2).

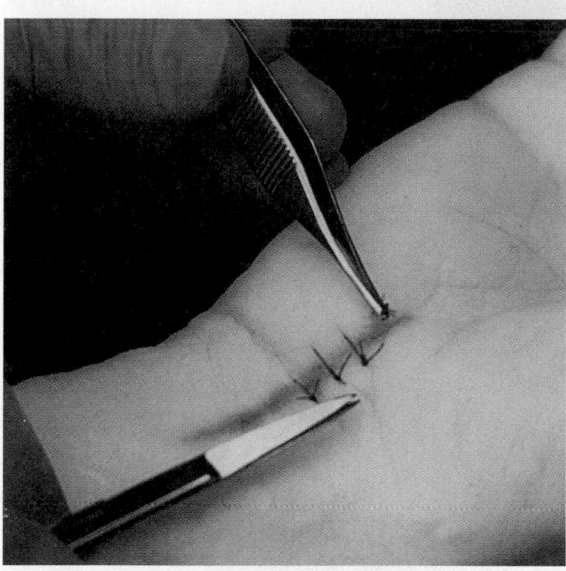

Figure 2

11 Place the suture on the gauze sponge, and check that the entire suture strand has been removed.
 Purpose: Suture fragments left in a wound may cause irritation and/or infection and may prolong the healing process.

12 If there is any bleeding, blot the area with a sterile gauze sponge before continuing.

13 Continue in the same manner until all the other sutures have been removed.

14 Remove the gauze sponge with the sutures on it and dispose of contaminated materials in the biohazard waste container.

15 The surgeon may apply Steri-Strips or a Band-Aid for added support, strength, and protection.

16 The patient is instructed to keep the wound edges clean and dry and not place excessive strain on the area.

17 Document the procedure, wound condition, and patient education on wound care.
 Purpose: A procedure that is not documented was not done.

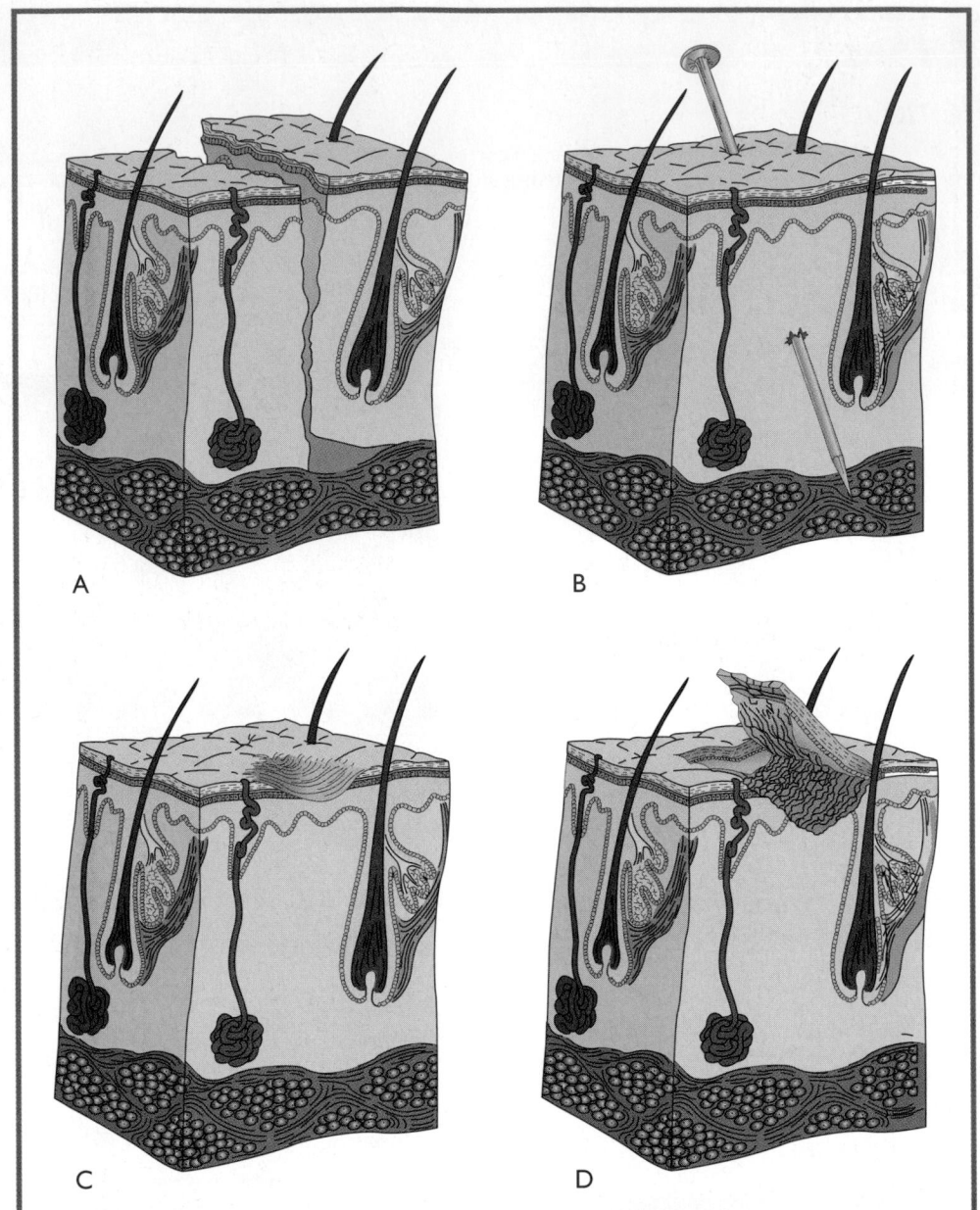

FIGURE 54-10 Types of wounds. **A**, Laceration—jagged, irregular breaking or tearing of tissues, usually caused by blunt trauma. **B**, Puncture—skin is pierced by a pointed object, such as a pin, nail, splinter, or bullet. **C**, Abrasion—superficial wound, scraping of the skin. **D**, Avulsion—tissue forcibly torn or separated, caused by accidents.

an accident, or a knife wound. A lacerated wound has torn or mangled tissues and is made by a dull or blunt instrument. A penetrating or puncture wound is caused by a sharp, slender object, such as a needle or ice pick, and passes through the skin into the underlying tissues. A perforated wound is a penetrating wound that passes through to a body organ or cavity, such as a gunshot wound.

Wound Healing. All wounds go through a healing or repair process that has three phases. The lag phase occurs first when the blood vessels contract to control hemorrhage, and blood platelets form a network in the wound that acts like glue to plug the wound. After a cascade of chemical reactions, fibrin is released into the

wound and clotting begins. The fibrin continues to collect RBCs, and the clot dries into a scab. About 12 hours later, special WBCs arrive to clear away bacteria and dead tissue. Within 1 to 4 days, the fibrin threads contract and pull the edges of the wound together under the scab.

The second phase, proliferation, is the wound healing and new growth period, lasting from 5 to 20 days. It is during this phase that the tissues repair themselves. New cells form and the wound continues to contract and seal. If the wound is a clean surgical incision, complete contraction usually takes place during this phase, and there is little scarring or permanent fibrous tissue (cicatrix) formation.

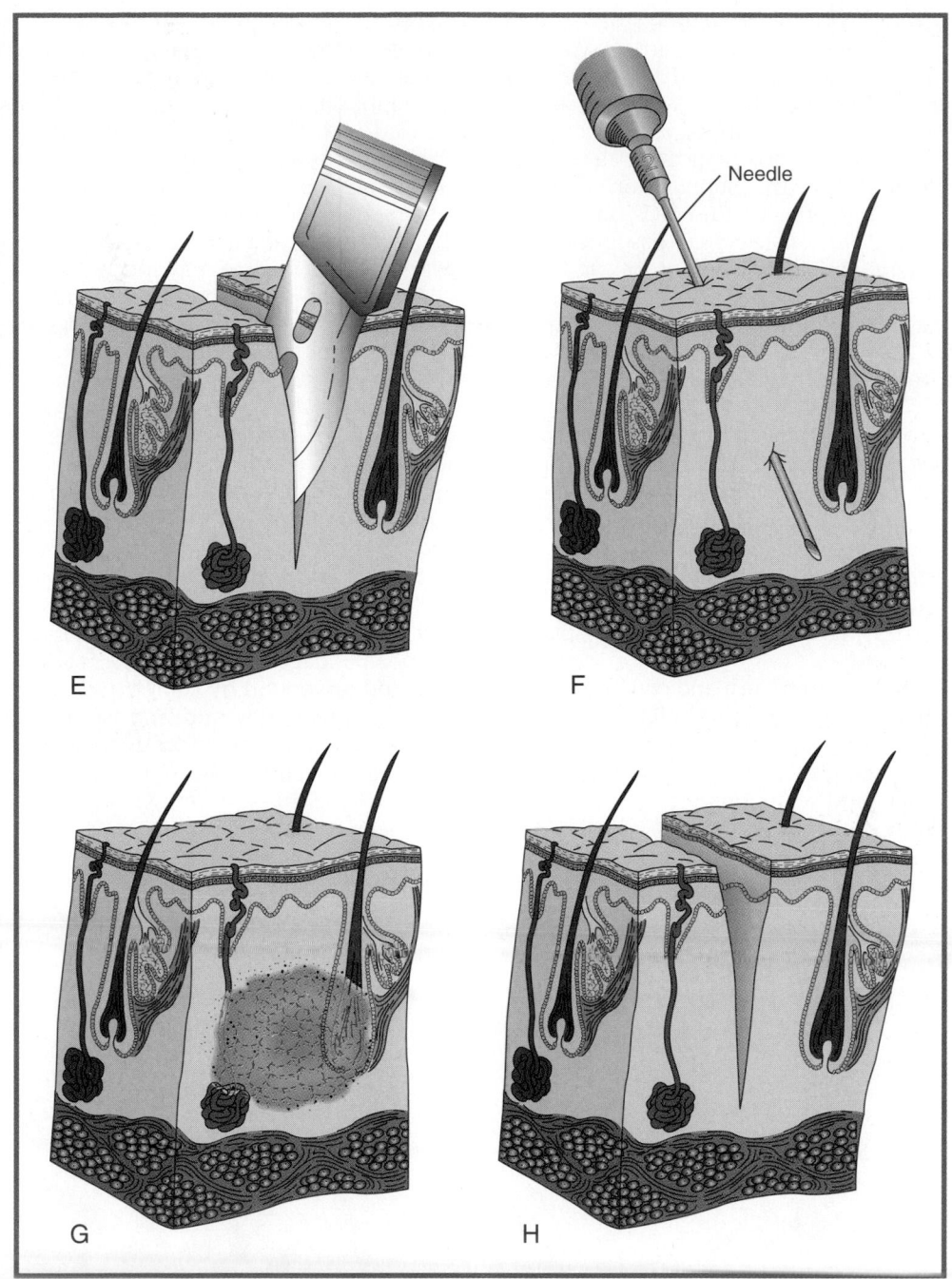

Needle

FIGURE 54-10—cont'd   Types of wounds. **E**, Surgical incision—a neat, clean cut. **F**, Hypodermic puncture —injection under the skin. **G**, Contusion—closed nonpenetrating wound in which blood from broken vessels accumulates in tissues. **H**, Incision—neat, clean cut from sharp objects, such as glass, knives, or metal.

The final or remodeling phase occurs from the twenty-first day onward. Clean, shallow wounds may contract in the first two stages; large or mangled wounds require the time and cellular activity of this third phase to build a bridge of new tissue to close the gap of the wound. The cells produce a fibrous protein substance called collagen (connective tissue) that gives the wounded tissues strength and forms scar tissue. Scar tissue is not true skin; it is usually very strong, but it lacks the elasticity of normal skin tissue. Scar tissue is also devoid of normal blood supply and nerves.

Wounds are classified by the way they repair themselves. The clean, surgical wound that has been sutured closed and heals quickly without much scarring does so by *first intention*. Tissues that are severely damaged, purposely kept open, or fail to close are said to heal by granulation (healing from the bottom of the wound outward), which is called *second intention*.

Several factors influence the healing process. People who are young, in good general health, and have adequate nutrition heal more rapidly. Adequate protection and rest to the injured area also enhance the healing process. Destruction or reinjury during the second phase can delay healing and increase scarring. Wounds are susceptible to infection because the normal skin barrier is broken. If there is debris in a wound as the result of the breakdown of the various cellular components, this dead (necrotic) tissue acts as a culture medium for bacterial growth. Suppuration (pus) is necrotic tissue with bacteria, dead WBCs, and other products of tissue breakdown. Necrotic tissue must be removed. Removal of debris is called *debridement*, which may occur naturally or be performed surgically.

Sometimes the physician may prefer no dressing or bandage on small wounds. This is called *open wound healing*. Some advantages to open wound healing include the following:

- It allows air to freely circulate around the wound.
- The wound is not irritated or rubbed by a dressing.
- The wound stays dry, which inhibits bacterial growth, reducing the chance of infection.
- Sutures stay dry and hold together better.
- Any preexisting infection remains localized and is not spread by the dressing or bandage.

Dressings. A dressing is a sterile covering placed over a wound to:

- Protect the wound from injury and contamination
- Maintain constant pressure to minimize bleeding and swelling
- Hold the wound edges together
- Absorb drainage and secretions
- Hide temporary disfigurement

A dressing usually consists of a strip of lubricated mesh gauze, a nonstick Telfa pad, or a clear dressing placed over a sutured wound (Figure 54-11). Gauze sponges may be placed over nonadhering material, depending on the physician's preference. Body cavities or wounds that need to remain open for a time are dressed with long, thin packing material that is often impregnated with an antiseptic or lubricant. This is sometimes called *packing*. A good dressing must be effective and comfortable and must remain in place. If the dressing covers a hairless area, it may be anchored with tape, but no tape may touch the wound.

Frequently, small, clean lacerations may be closed with special adhesive strips called *Steri-Strips* (Figure 54-12). These strips reduce the chance of infection and do not leave suture scars. Steri-Strips are used on areas of the body that are protected from movement and stress. They are often used on the face. Because they are a suture replacement, only the physician should place them. They are placed on the wound in the same sequence and at the same intervals as interrupted sutures and are left in place until they fall off or the wound heals.

Bandages. Bandages hold dressings in place and also help maintain even pressure, support the affected part, and help protect the wound from injury and contamination. Bandages can be gauze, cloth, or elastic cloth rolls and are bound by clips, tape, or ties. Dressing and bandages frequently appear easy and simple to apply; however, special skill is required to apply a functional dressing (Procedure 54-16). Bandages that are too loose fall off; those that are too tight may compromise circulation and further harm the patient. Patients do not feel that good medical care has been given if bandages are messy or uncomfortable.

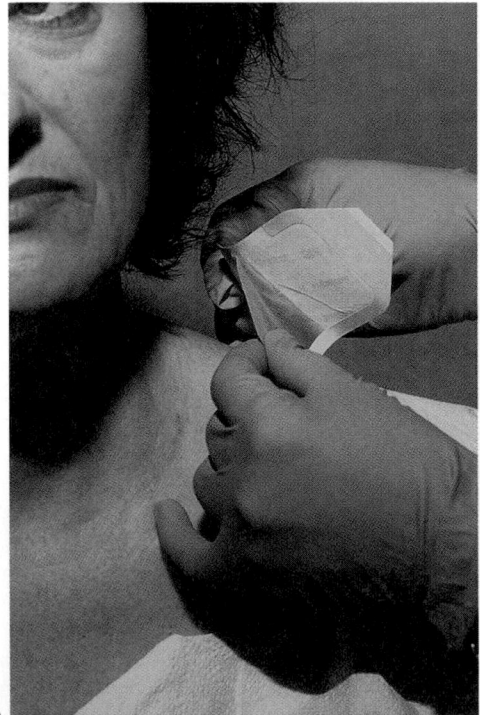 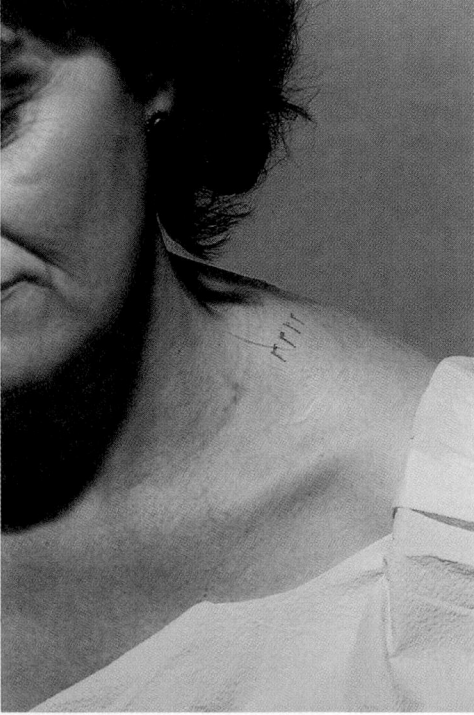

A   B

FIGURE 54-11 **A**, Placing a clear dressing on a sutured wound. **B**, Clear dressing in place over a sutured wound.

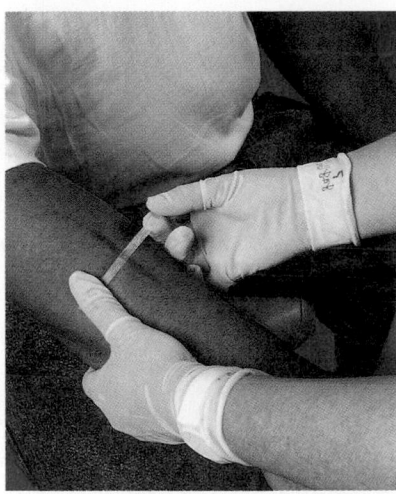

FIGURE 54-12 Steri-Strips on a wound. (From Bonewit-West K: *Clinical procedures for medical assistants,* ed. 5, Philadelphia, 2000, WB Saunders.)

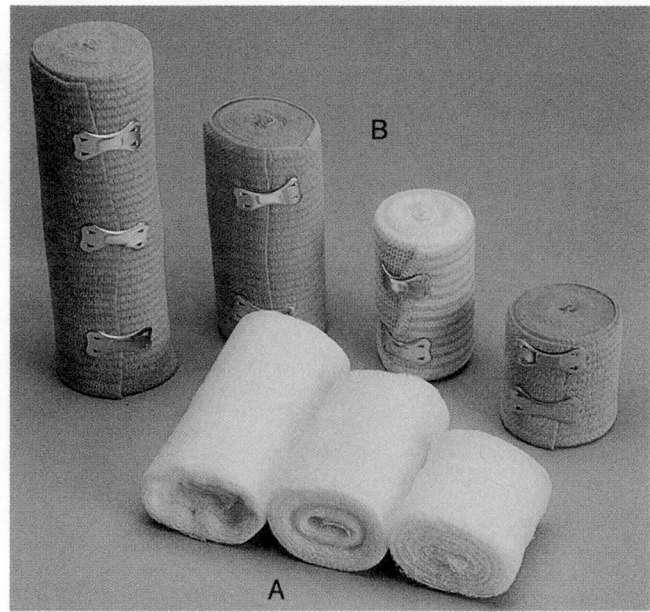

FIGURE 54-13 **A**, Kling bandages. **B**, Roller bandages.

Plain roller gauze is seldom used. It is difficult to handle, because it must be applied with reverse spiral turns if the area is uneven. It has no elasticity and tends to bind. It also tends to slip, because it does not adhere to itself. Wrinkled crepe-type roller bandages (e.g., Kling) are preferred, because they easily conform to various shapes of the body and adhere to themselves (Figure 54-13, *A*). A bandage should always be applied over a dressing.

Plain elastic cloth bandage (e.g., Ace) or elastic roller cloth with adhesive backing makes a flexible and secure cover (Figure 54-13, *B*). When applying an Ace elastic roller bandage as a pressure bandage, especially to the lower limbs, it is essential to keep the bandage consistent in spacing and tension to ensure even pressure. Even, gentle pressure stimulates circulation and healing. Uneven pressure causes constriction points that can create pressure sores, ulcers, or **edema**. Roller bandages are usually applied from the distal to the proximal part of the area. Bandaging can remain even and snug if it is wrapped from a smaller to a larger circumference. Elevate the limb while you are bandaging and work with the roller facing upward, close to the patient's skin. Elastic bandages are excellent for bandaging the hand and wrist (Figure 54-14) and the foot and ankle (Figure 54-15).

Seamless tubular gauze bandage, with or without elastic, is superior material for covering round narrow surfaces such as fingers or toes. It can be used as either a dressing or a bandage. A tubular gauze bandage is applied with a cagelike applicator (Figure 54-16). Work with the U-shaped cutting channel of the applicator toward the patient. Start in the middle of the area to be dressed and anchor the dressing, if there is one, with a small piece of tape. Hold the applicator in the dominant hand, and control the tension flow with your fingers as the applicator is gradually rotated and the material slides off. Tubular dressing may be applied with or without slight pressure. Beyond the tip of the bandaged part, give the applicator a full half-turn, place the applicator again over the part, and repeat the process,

being careful not to create a tourniquet effect when you reverse the applicator. When the desired thickness of the bandage is reached, cut the gauze and anchor the final dressing by tape or by tying at the wrist. This lightweight gauze should never be used as a stockinette under a cast. Patients should be advised to call the physician's office if there is any problem with the dressing.

Patient Education

There are many ways a medical assistant can help the patient. The best time to instruct your patient in aseptic techniques to be used at home is while you are performing an aseptic procedure. For example:

- While washing your hands before a procedure or examination, explain to the patient that hands should be washed before meals; after sneezing, coughing, or nose blowing; after using the bathroom; before and after changing a bandage; and after changing an infant's diaper.
- Explain to the patient how using disposable tissues to cover the nose and mouth when coughing or sneezing decreases the possibility of transmitting illness between household members.
- Discuss proper ways for disposing of used tissues, especially when one member of the household is suspected of having a communicable disease.
- Instruct the patient regarding the differences between sterile and clean dressings and bandages. Show him or her step by step how to change a dressing properly and then how to dispose of the contaminated items.

A medical assistant's duty may include calling the patient the day before surgery to confirm the scheduled surgical procedure and appointment time. Explaining the procedure and what to expect during and after

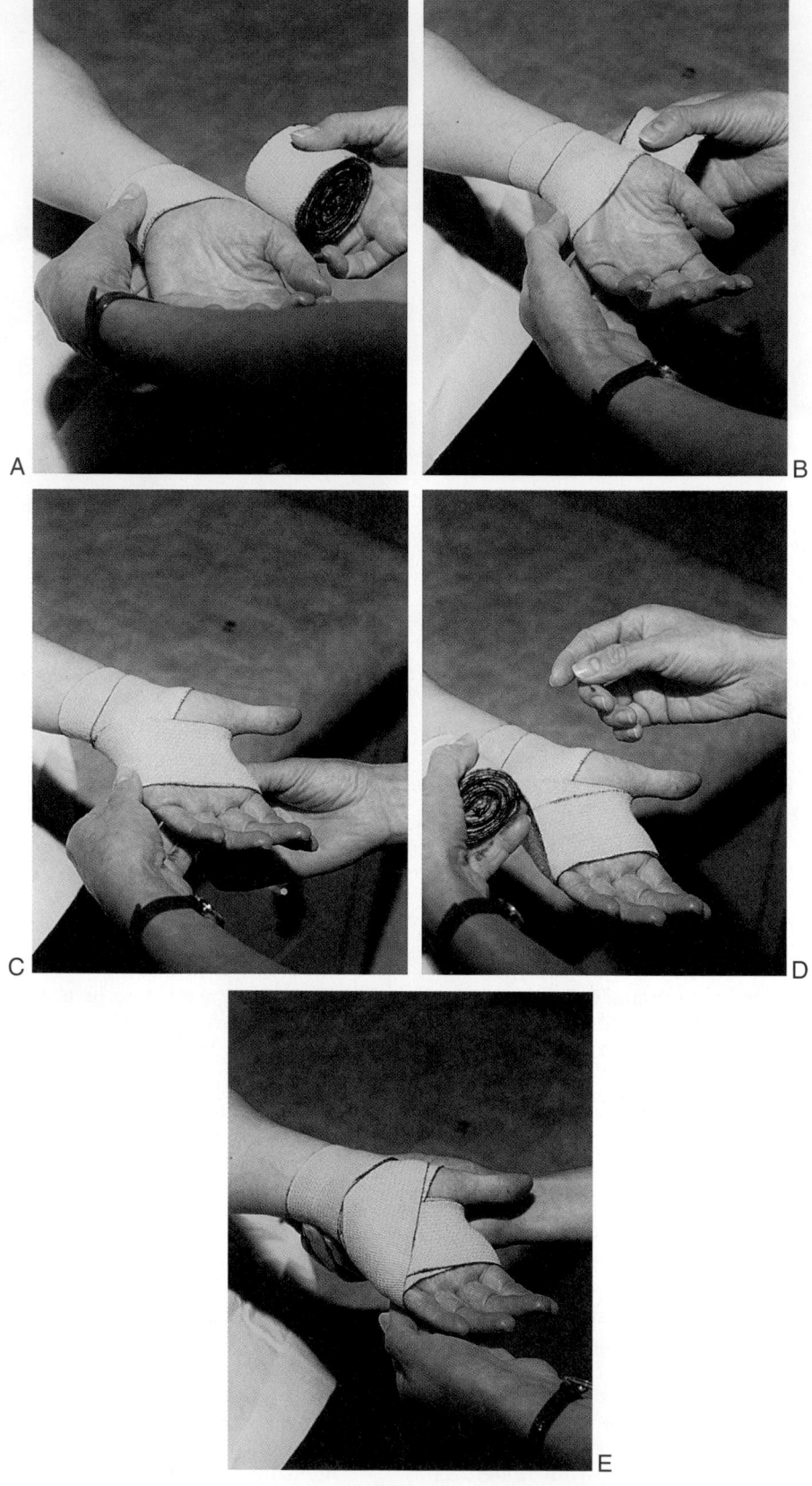

FIGURE 54-14 **A,** Use combination of recurrent and figure-of-eight turns for the hand.
B, Start at wrist. **C,** Applying a roller bandage to the hand. **D,** Roller bandage applied to the
hand. **E,** Maintain consistent tension while applying bandage.

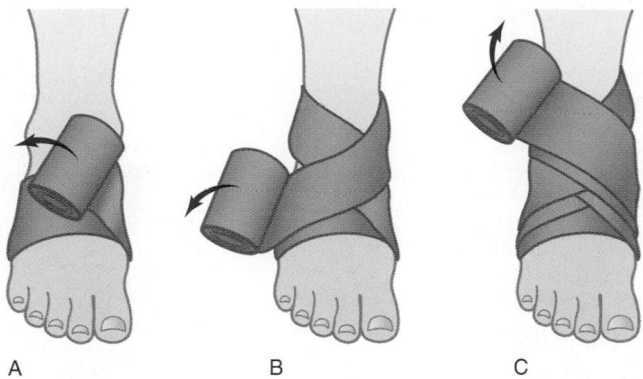

A   B   C

FIGURE 54-15   Use of the figure-of-eight turn for the ankle. (From Leake MJ: *A manual of simple nursing procedures*, Philadelphia, 1971, WB Saunders.)

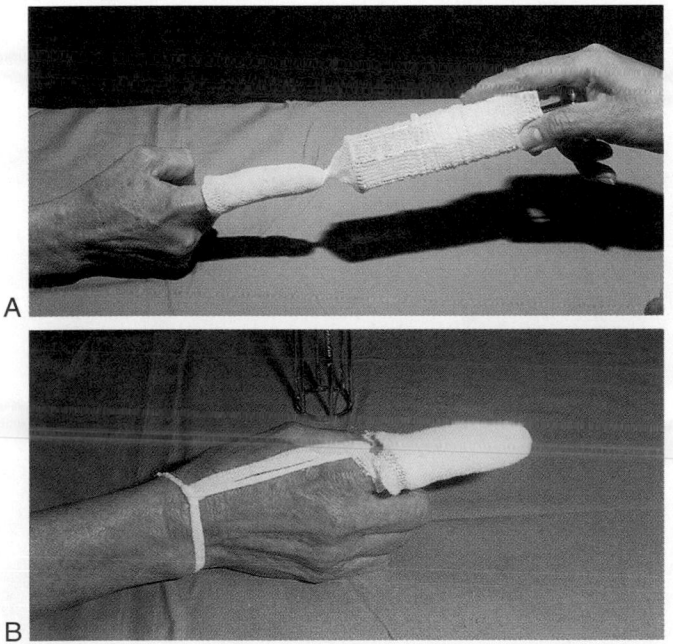

A

B

FIGURE 54-16   **A**, Tube gauze applied with even tension, twisting at fingertip before applying next layer. **B**, Tube gauze bandage applied and secured by tying at the wrist.

PROCEDURE 54-16

Bandaging Using Gauze and Elastic Dressings

GOAL: To apply an elastic bandage to the forearm.

EQUIPMENT AND SUPPLIES

• One 3- or 4-inch elastic bandage.

PROCEDURAL STEPS

1 Choose the proper size bandage for the size of the arm you are bandaging.
   Purpose: To provide proper support for the area.

2 Start at the distal point and hold the roll so the bandage can be rolled away from you (Figure 1).
   Purpose: To easily apply the bandage by unrolling it.

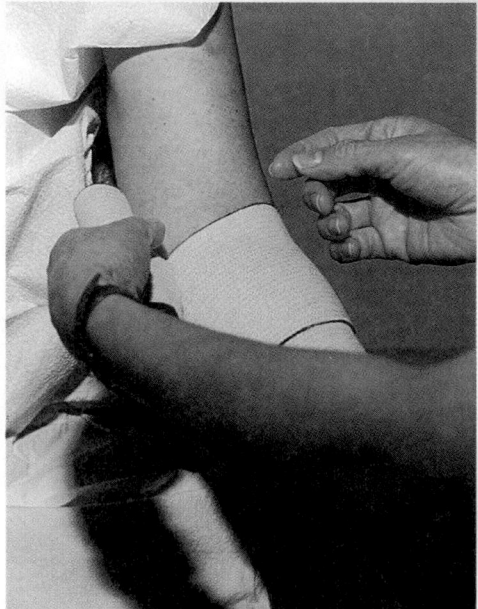

Figure 2

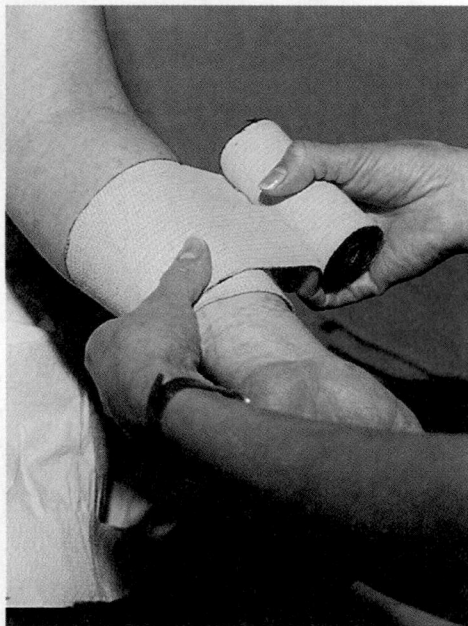

Figure 1

3 Keep the roll close to the patient and keep it facing upward (Figure 2).

4 Maintain even tension and spacing as you continue to apply the bandage up the forearm.
   Purpose: To maintain even, light pressure over the entire area.

5 When crossing a joint, slightly flex the joint (Figure 3).
   Purpose: To facilitate patient comfort and maintain normal circulation.

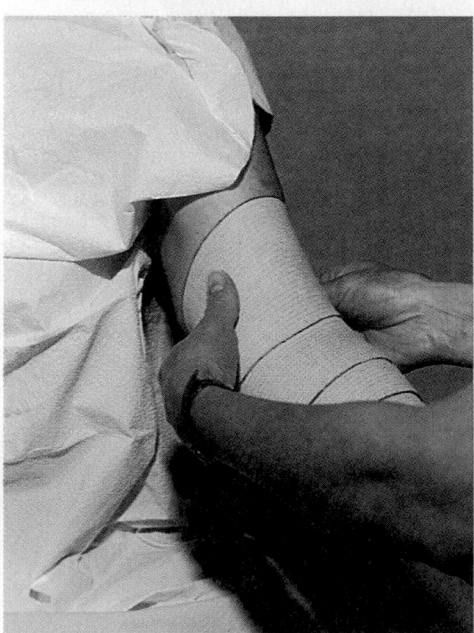

Figure 3

PROCEDURE 54-16—cont'd

6 Fasten the end of the bandage with clips or tape (Figure 4).

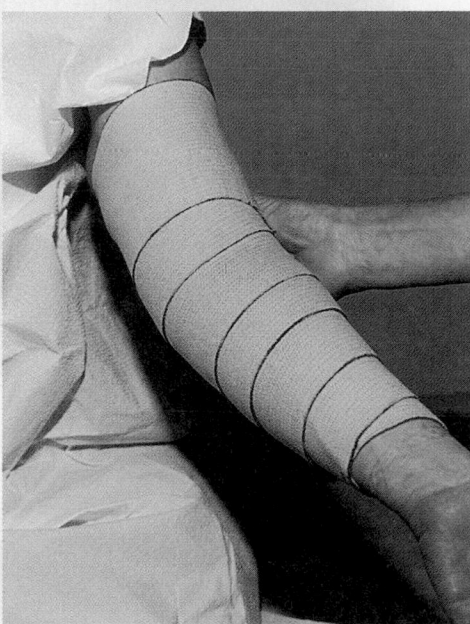

Figure 4

7 Check the nail beds for cyanosis.
   Purpose: To ensure that the bandage is not acting as a tourniquet if applied too tightly.

8 Check the radial pulse.
   Purpose: To ensure that the bandage is not acting as a tourniquet if applied too tightly.

9 Have the patient move his or her fingers.
   Purpose: To check that there is normal nerve function.

10 Document the procedure in the patient's medical record and patient instruction regarding bandage care and replacement.
   Purpose: The procedure is not completed until it is written down, dated, and signed.

See Appendix E for a charting example.

CRITICAL THINKING APPLICATION

Melissa applies a figure-of-eight elastic bandage to the hand and wrist of a patient who came into the office for suturing after cutting her hand while trying to cut frozen meat. She immediately sends the patient home after applying the bandage. She does not complete the chart at that time because the office is quite busy. Discuss all of your concerns regarding this situation. In what ways were office procedures ignored here? What would be a worst-case scenario for the outcome of this situation? How can this be corrected after the fact?

surgery will prepare the patient and help to calm the patient's fears or concerns. Lying still during surgery is important, and eating a light meal the night before should be encouraged. Bathing before coming to the office will help reduce the amount of bacteria on the skin, and wearing comfortable loose clothing is recommended. Sometimes in the course of general conversation, the medical assistant can pick up hints of concern that the patient may have and can direct the conversation into a discussion of these concerns.

Patients should be informed that they may need someone to accompany them home. There will be a bandage applied after surgery, and it must be kept clean and dry. There may be pain, and the physician will probably prescribe pain medication. An appointment will be given for a return visit and examination.

Legal and Ethical Issues

Many minor surgical procedures previously performed in the hospital are now being done in a medical office, surgery center, or clinic. As insurance companies continue to recognize the cost-effectiveness of performing minor surgical procedures in these settings, the role of the medical assistant continues to expand.

Personal discipline is the primary concern in surgical asepsis. Often the assistant is alone when performing a surgical aseptic procedure; if contamination occurs, no one may know except the medical assistant. It is the surgical assistant's responsibility to begin the procedure again with clean supplies if it is *possible* that contamination occurred. One of the medical assistant's main responsibilities is to carry out sanitization, disinfection, and sterilization procedures with precision and with total effectiveness. *There is no room for compromise.*

Patients should have absolute assurance that they are being taken care of in an aseptic atmosphere and under the most stringent aseptic conditions. This assurance is just as important for the protection of the office staff as it is for the patient. Allowing the physician to assume that the correct aseptic techniques have been employed in the preparation of equipment and allowing him or her to use contaminated equipment on a patient can result in claims of malpractice and charges of battery. Absolute, uncompromising honesty on the part of the assistant builds self-respect and contributes to professional achievement and satisfaction.

To have a good understanding of the subject, you must become familiar with the various techniques of sanitization, disinfection, and sterilization. Ignorance or carelessness can be dangerous and is inexcusable before the law.

The medical assistant must know what procedure is to be performed and whether the patient has been informed regarding the procedure. In the surgical setting, the medical assistant must realize the full extent of his or her role as *patient advocate* and *physician agent*.

Confirm that the physician has explained the procedure to the patient and that the patient fully understands all aspects of the procedure that will be performed. This means that when the patient signs the consent for surgery, he or she is fully informed. Legal action can occur when complications arise from failure to complete procedure and consent forms. If the surgery is to be sterilization for birth control, it is essential to follow the stipulated regulations of your state. Law often requires a waiting period.

The surgical procedure is expedited when the patient is given instructions and knows what to expect. When the physical and psychological needs of the patient are met, one can be assured that the patient has sufficient information to be comfortable. Increasing the patient's understanding ensures greater compliance with the presurgical preparations and the surgical procedure, and the patient will be more inclined to follow instructions and advice after surgery.

Finally, the medical assistant must practice perfect aseptic technique. A break in technique may invite infection and possible legal action. It is the medical assistant's duty to protect the patient. A major responsibility for the medical assistant is self-commitment to adhere strictly to aseptic technique and to *immediately correct any break in technique*.

SUMMARY OF SCENARIO

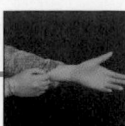

Melissa is finding her surgical medical assisting position at Lakeside Surgical Associates to be rewarding, exciting, and challenging. She enjoys coming to work every day and has learned all aspects of her position much more quickly than most of her peers. Melissa frequently reads the latest information on new developments in minor surgery practice. Her concern for her patient's well-being makes her stand out, and the clinic constantly gets positive comments on her level of professionalism.

Melissa has made several mistakes during her first year as a surgical medical assistant, but she has learned from each situation and has never covered up a mistake. She has communicated with her supervisor and the surgeon whenever she realized later that she did not follow procedure. This allowed errors to be discussed, corrected if possible, and will most likely result in her not making similar mistakes again.

Melissa is a team player who always works to ensure that surgical procedures occur with the most efficiency. She consistently tries to anticipate the surgeon's and patient's needs both before and during surgery. Her cooperative, supportive manner is appreciated by everyone on the surgical team, and she is the most-requested assistant at Lakeside Surgical Associates.

SUMMARY OF LEARNING OBJECTIVES

■ Using proper surgical aseptic technique is the primary means of preventing unnecessary postoperative infections in surgical patients. A "break" in technique at any step of the way can have dire consequences for a patient. Everyone on the surgical team is responsible for preventing and correcting breaks in technique.

■ Indicator devices can be used to prove that a package was indeed in the steam autoclave during a sterilization run. Other indicators can prove that the contents of the package were exposed to a sufficient temperature for a sufficient length of time to achieve sterilization.

■ The legal and ethical concerns with regard to infection control affect everyone on the surgical team to a large degree. It is necessary for all individuals involved in the surgical care of a patient to be aware of all legal and ethical practices that apply for excellent patient care. The most important legal concern for all involved is the area of informed consent, without which surgery cannot be legally performed on a patient without risking the possibility of battery. The consent also clearly limits what procedure can be done.

■ Education of the surgical procedure takes many forms, from information sheets or pamphlets to be given to the patient before surgery, to having conversations with the patient about the procedure, and giving them postoperative information sheets to prevent and minimize complications. The informed patient is more relaxed, cooperative, and much more pleasant to deal with than the uninformed, frightened patient who did not receive adequate explanations from the surgical office staff.

KEY INTERNET WEBSITES

- Introduction to Aseptic Technique
- Steps of Chemical Sterilization
- Surgical Aseptic Technique
- Wound Care Information Network—Phases of Wound Healing
  For active weblinks to each website visit
  http://evolve.elsevier.com/Kinn/

UNIT ten

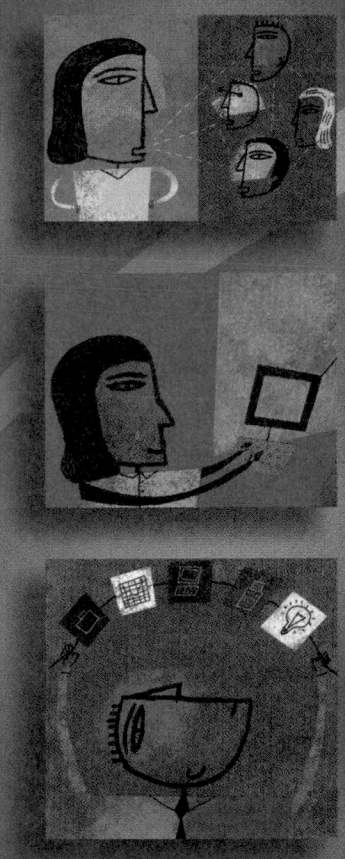

Career
Development

CHAPTER 55

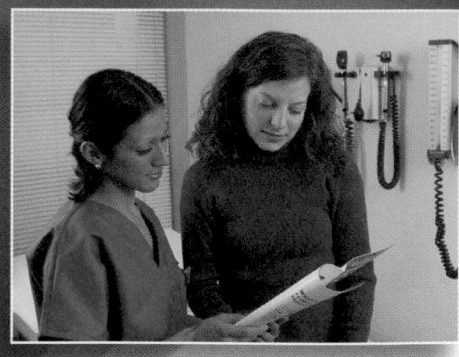

Scenario

Lisa Walker is 1 month away from graduating from her medical assisting program. She has been an excellent student and is looking forward to beginning her career in the medical field. Lisa wants to begin her job search now to minimize the time during which she is not employed after her externship ends.

Lisa has participated in several volunteer activities while she has been attending school. She plans to list these experiences on her resume. She met many office managers and physicians while doing volunteer work, and she will be contacting those people in hopes of obtaining more job leads.

Lisa began saving for interview clothing when she first began school. She is on a strict budget, but she found several outfits appropriate for interviews at second-hand clothing shops and discount stores. Her best-looking suit cost only $20!

Not a person afraid to interview, Lisa looks forward to sharing her skills and experience with potential employers. She looks on each interview as a practice session for the next one, and this helps her to relax more and present a true picture of herself to the office manager. She has a great smile and projects a natural friendliness and positive attitude.

Lisa has given much thought to what she wants from her first job as a medical assistant. She knows that she may not start at a high salary, but she also realizes that there are benefits and perquisites ("perks") when working in a physician's office. She plans to commit to working for 2 years on her first job, gaining experience before looking for the next job at a higher salary.

Lisa is excited about her future as a medical assistant. She is ready to put the training she received to work with actual patients. She plans to perform exceptionally well at her externship site and to go above and beyond her designated duties to impress the staff in that facility, who will become references for her first paid position. Lisa is dedicated to becoming the best medical assistant possible and becoming indispensable to her employer.

Career Development and Life Skills

Vocabulary

appraisals Act of giving an expert judgment of the value or merit of; also, evaluations of work performance.

counteroffer Return offer made by one who has rejected an offer or job.

default Failure to pay financial debts, such as a student loan.

deferment Postponement, especially of a student loan.

genuineness Expressing sincerity and honest feeling.

intolerable Not tolerable or bearable.

mock Simulated; intended for imitation or practice.

networking Exchange of information or services among individuals, groups, or institutions; also, meeting and getting to know individuals in the same or similar career fields and sharing information about available opportunities.

pertinent Having a clear, decisive relevance to the matter at hand.

proofread To read and mark corrections.

ramifications Consequence; outgrowth; something produced by a cause or necessarily following from a set of conditions.

rectify To correct by removing errors.

subtle Ingenious; artful; delicate.

succinct Marked by compact, precise expression without wasted words.

synopsis Condensed statement or outline.

vocation The work in which a person is regularly employed.

Each day that a person exists is a small portion of a whole—in this case, the person's entire lifetime. The events that happen during a day, no matter how small, shape the future. In the same way, the events that happen in the life of a medical assistant play a role in shaping his or her career. Every day, he or she "writes a resume"—through actions that will reveal strengths, highlight skills, and summarize the accomplishments— that builds on the medical assistant's **vocation**. Each duty performed becomes a part of the medical assistant's sum of experience and is important in the overall growth of the individual. Each action taken can have an impact on the future for the medical assistant. If the actions are professional, accurate, and performed to his or her utmost ability, the resume that the medical assistant is writing through these actions will be one that will lead to greater opportunities. If the medical assistant performs poorly, the resume will be one that will not reflect trustworthiness and dependability. The small decisions that are made every day are those that greatly affect the overall impressions that the medical assistant makes in the workplace.

Approximately 85% of persons seeking employment have never had any type of formal training in the job search process. A newly graduated medical assistant should take advantage of job search training for three reasons:

1. The training will decrease the amount of time spent searching for a job.
2. The training will increase the chances of receiving better wages through negotiations.
3. The training will help to eliminate the fears of looking for work and interviewing.

What Does the Employer Want?

Employers have three basic desires when they are interviewing individuals for a job:

1. They want a person who has a neat appearance and looks as if he or she fits the job (Figure 55-1).
2. They want an individual who is dependable and can prove that he or she has been a reliable team member in other job positions.
3. They want a person with the skills to do the job.

From the beginning of the job search process, a medical assistant's attitude is the most critical part of his or her potential success in getting a job (Figure 55-2). A good attitude is not a trait that can be developed overnight. For this reason a medical assistant must have a positive

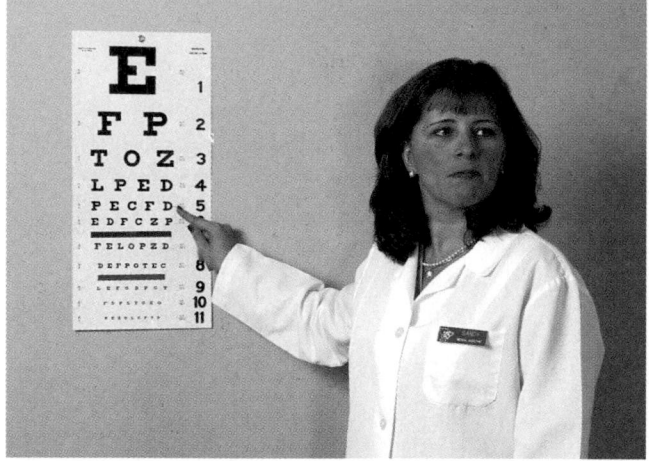

FIGURE 55-1   A professional appearance is mandatory in the medical office.

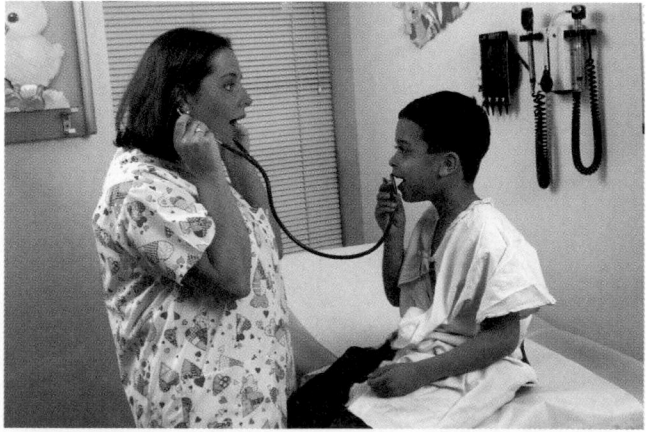

FIGURE 55-2   A great attitude is the best personal asset. Employers in the medical profession want medical assistants who will exhibit a positive attitude with the patients.

outlook in all situations, so the **genuineness** of his or her demeanor will be clear during job interviews.

Assessing Strengths

Before promoting himself or herself as a potential employee, a medical assistant must first determine the strengths that make him or her a valuable team member. There are three types of skill strengths: job skills, self-management skills, and transferable skills.

Job skills are the abilities that the medical assistant needs to perform the job. This includes such skills as venipuncture, filing insurance, answering the telephone, scheduling appointments, giving injections, and other tasks.

Self-management skills relate to the medical assistant's personality and character traits. They include such attributes as honesty, integrity, and enthusiasm.

Transferable skills can be taken from one job to another. For instance, if the medical assistant has the ability to communicate effectively, this skill can be used on every job. Leadership is a transferable skill, as are the ability to follow directions and the ability to manage people.

Developing Career Objectives

Each medical assistant has a reason for entering the healthcare field. This basic desire should influence decisions concerning his or her career choices. Because medical assisting is such a versatile profession, a medical assistant will have numerous options after graduation.

It is wise to take some time to think about what the medical assistant wants from his or her career. While he or she is attending school and subsequently completing an externship, ideas may surface about what specialty to enter.

When developing career objectives, the medical assistant should start by asking several questions:

- Where am I today?
- Where will I be in 5 years?
- Where will I be in 10 years?
- What additional skills do I need to get where I want to go?

Write down the questions and answers and go into specific detail. Set realistic goals and develop a plan as to how and when they will be reached. It is helpful to put a list of goals in a prominent place at home, where they will be seen every day. Some people use the front of the refrigerator, and some post the goals on the mirror in the area where they get dressed every day. Having the written goals in a visible place helps to keep them in mind even on the more difficult days, when the goals seem far from sight.

Knowing Personal Needs

A medical assistant must evaluate all of the needs that he or she requires in a work situation. Most people have a minimum salary that they require, as well as certain benefits. For example, if the medical assistant is a single mother, she may require a moderate salary and insist on health insurance benefits. We also have intrinsic needs, which are those internal desires that are important to us personally.

A helpful activity is to write a **synopsis** of a typical day on an ideal medical assisting job. Imagine the type of office, the job title, the daily duties, and the salary and benefits that would be a part of the ideal job (Figure 55-3). This will help to develop a focus and a goal to work toward as the medical assistant's career develops.

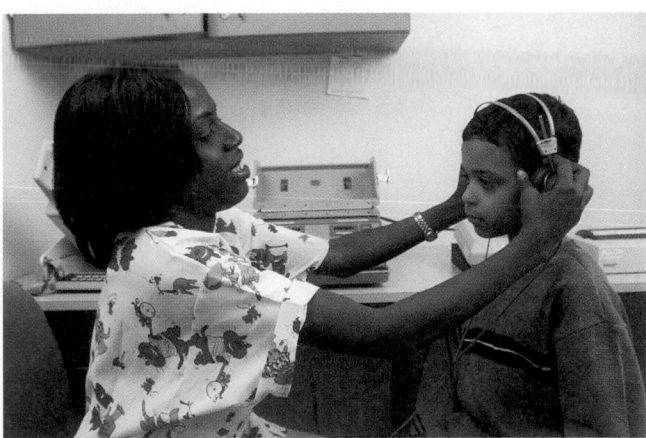

FIGURE 55-3 Enjoyment of the job is paramount. Medical assistants should enjoy their job and give compassionate, friendly care to all patients.

Finding a Job

Many people have misconceptions about the job market that exists today. Graduation from a medical assisting program does not guarantee that the student will obtain employment. Completion of the program will give the medical assistant the job skills needed to work, but a good attitude and positive outlook are essential for success in the job search.

Some job seekers assume that potential employers will not interact with students until they graduate. However, prospecting before graduation is a smart idea, and there are **subtle** ways of introducing oneself to a facility without bluntly asking for employment. Many also think that they must have work experience to be hired, but employers are more interested in attitude and teachability than a long resume full of experience. In fact, many physicians like hiring students fresh from school so that they can teach them how they want procedures done.

The Two Best Job Search Methods

Although there are many ways to find employment, two methods have proved to be the best and most effective. These are networking and direct contact with employers.

Networking is the exchange of information or services among individuals, groups, or institutions. When related to a job search, networking involves meeting and getting to know individuals in the same or similar career fields, and sharing information about available opportunities. A medical assistant should begin to form a network of friends, business associates, co-workers, and acquaintances early in training, and he or she should stay in contact with these people throughout the job search effort (Figure 55-4).

Networking is not limited to job searching, and many organizations are formed to develop networks of individuals or groups that assist each other and refer clients to each other. However, these groups are useful to the person who is looking for employment, and by attending meetings and get-togethers held for networking purposes, the medical assistant may happen into the ideal job he or she has been looking for.

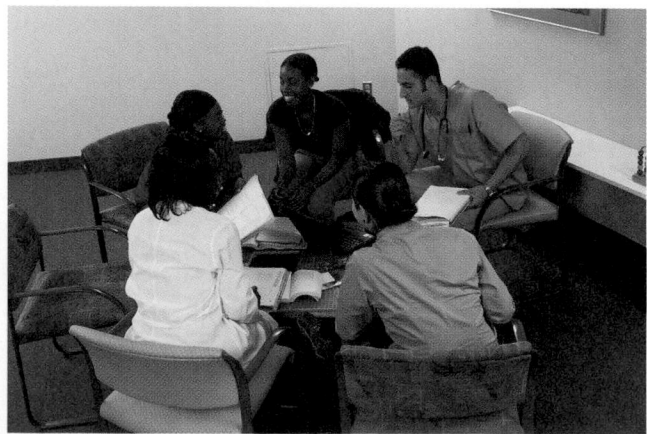

FIGURE 55-4 Stay in touch with classmates. Classmates are excellent networking contacts and may be able to provide job leads.

CRITICAL THINKING APPLICATION

Lisa knows that networking is a great way to secure employment. She is making a list of people with whom she can share her resume or inform that she is now ready to seek employment as a medical assistant. How many people can you think of who are good prospects for networking?

Direct contact with employers is also an effective method of job searching. Medical assistants often know of specific clinics or facilities that they would like to investigate as job possibilities. Compile a list of these places and learn as much about them as possible. If the facility has a website, read it thoroughly. Ask for brochures about the employer. Some have an annual report that lists details about the organization. All of this information will help the medical assistant get a good basic idea of why the facility exists and what it does for the community.

Contact with employers does not necessarily begin only after the student has graduated. Students can begin networking and contacting employers from the very start of their enrollment at school. The student may wish to keep a file on potential employers. Make a list of facilities that are good prospects for employment and then begin researching them. Call to find out who supervises medical assistants in the facility. In a physician's office, this is usually the office manager. Then call the office manager and ask to make an appointment to learn about the facility. Even the busiest people are usually willing to help a student investigate healthcare facilities in the area.

Do not express to the office manager that the objective of the appointment is a job offer. The goal at this point is to learn about the facility, what it offers the community, and what roles the medical assistants in the facility perform. Suggest that the appointment be set at his or her convenience. Then treat the appointment like an actual job interview, dressing appropriately and arriving on time. Have a list of questions about the facility prepared in advance, and do not take too much of the office manager's time. Take notes about what the office manager says about the facility, so that they can be referred to on graduation, during the actual job search.

After the appointment with the office manager, ask for a business card and always send a thank-you note or letter. *Do not fail to remember this critical point!* This helps the office manager to remember the name of the medical assistant and is a pleasant addition to the daily mail. Everyone enjoys being recognized for his or her efforts, and the office manager will appreciate the thank-you note.

Toward the time that he or she is to graduate, the medical assistant may wish to perform an externship at one of the facilities visited early in training. Check with school regulations to determine whether this is possible. Then the office manager can be approached about allowing the student to extern in the office. Be sure to follow school guidelines when investigating these possibilities.

Some schools allow students to secure their own externship sites, but this must be discussed with the externship supervisor at school. Performing an externship at a medical facility is usually the first practical experience the student will have in the medical field and can be used as a reference in building a resume.

After the externship is completed, the medical assistant may wish to send a resume to all of the office managers met through the direct contact efforts made earlier in his or her training. A professional resume with a cover letter that refers to the earlier meeting will prompt the office manager to remember the student. Ask in the cover letter whether any opportunities exist in the facility. Express that the facility and staff were impressive on the first meeting and that it would be an exciting place to begin a career. In the letter, request that if the office manager does not have any positions available at that time, the resume be kept on file or passed along to an acquaintance who is looking for an additional staff member.

Traditional Job Search Methods

The more traditional job search methods may be effective but are usually not as successful as networking and contacting employers directly.

Newspaper Ads. Newspaper ads normally produce a huge number of applicants and resumes for the employer. A resume or application will have to stand out in the crowd to be noticed when it arrives at the facility. Some applicants use clear envelopes, which draw attention to the resume quickly in a stack of mail.

Employment Agencies. Employment agencies usually charge a fee for their services. Even when the employer pays the fee, the medical assistant may be offered a lower wage to compensate for the fee. These agencies can be useful, however. In salary negotiation, the agency will know the salary range the employer is willing to pay. This means that medical assistants can command a salary within that range and not be short-changed by asking for a salary that is much lower than the employer was willing to pay.

CRITICAL THINKING APPLICATION

Lisa keeps an eye on the ads in local newspapers that mention a need for medical assistants. What current ads in local papers are interesting and would prompt sending a resume?

Professional Societies. Joining local chapters of medical assistant organizations helps the student in many ways. Not only will valuable information be exchanged at the meetings, but the medical assistant may also hear of positions that are coming available in various medical facilities. This is a form of networking.

Volunteering. By volunteering in medical offices or facilities, the medical assistant will meet other professionals who may be able to provide job leads. Volunteer activities should be added to the resume, because these valuable experiences can often be used in the physician's office as well. It does not matter that the position was not a paid job; experience counts, whether paid or not.

Mailing Resumes. Mailing a large number of resumes is not a very effective method of job search. Out of 100 resumes sent, one or two potential employers may respond with a request for an interview. It is much more effective to network first, and then follow up with a good cover letter and resume. Resumes can be used when contacting employers directly, and this approach allows the medical assistant to meet at least one employee of the facility when the document is delivered. Be sure to ask for a business card and write down the name of the person to whom the resume was delivered. For impressive facilities, send a note of thanks to the person who accepted the resume, asking to be considered for future positions.

Cold Calling. Cold calling is contacting employers by phone and prospecting for available positions. If the medical assistant asks, "Are you hiring?" at the beginning of the conversation, he or she should expect a negative answer and has just wasted the call. This is all but useless in the job search effort. However, an assistant who calls for information about the clinic and schedules an appointment with the office manager may have more success. Never attempt to get a job over the phone. Even when interested employers call and ask questions, attempt to set up an interview to discuss your qualifications in person.

Performing Well on Externships. Performing well on externships may be one of the best ways to secure a job. If an opening exists, the medical assistant extern is already oriented to the practice and may be the perfect fit for the job. Perform duties assigned on the externship as if they were final examinations at school. Even when the office does not have a position available at that time, there may be one soon, or the office manager or physician may know of an office that has an opening. Do the best job possible, and there may be an employment offer waiting at the conclusion of the externship.

Developing a Resume

A **resume** is a fact sheet that summarizes an applicant's qualifications, education, and experience. A medical assistant must determine what to include in the resume, remembering that he or she is "selling" himself or herself to an employer (Procedure 55-1).

There are many types of resumes. Three of the most common include the chronological resume, the functional resume, and the targeted resume. A chronological resume highlights the medical assistant's abilities in a logical order, such as most recent jobs back to the beginning of the individual's career (Figure 55-5). A functional resume highlights specific skill sets, emphasizing the most important abilities or the most valuable experiences that the medical assistant has performed (Figure 55-6). A targeted resume is perhaps the most effective: it emphasizes the skills that relate specifically to the job for which the medical assistant is applying (Figure 55-7).

PROCEDURE 55-1

Preparing a Resume

GOAL: To write an effective resume for use as a tool in gaining employment.

EQUIPMENT AND SUPPLIES

- Scratch paper
- Pen or pencil
- Former job descriptions, if available
- List of addresses of former employers, schools, and names of supervisors
- Computer or word processor
- Quality stationery and envelopes

PROCEDURAL STEPS

1 Perform a self-evaluation by making notes about your strengths as a medical assistant. Consider job skills, self-management skills, and transferable skills.

Purpose: To determine the strongest aspects of your abilities so that they can be highlighted on the resume.

2 Explore formatting and decide on a professional resume appearance that best highlights your skills and experience. Use the templates available in word processing software or design your own.

Purpose: To construct an attractive document.

3 Place your name, address, and two telephone numbers where you can be contacted at the top of the resume.

Purpose: To make certain that potential employers have a means of contact.

4 Write a job objective that specifies your employment goals.

Purpose: To give the prospective employer an idea of what you are looking for in a medical assisting position.

5 Provide details about your educational experience. List degrees and/or certifications obtained.

6 Provide details about your work experience. Include all contact information and names of supervisors. Do not include salary expectations or reasons for leaving former jobs.

Purpose: No negative information should be put on the resume. Salaries should be discussed—if a certain salary is listed on the resume, it may limit the amount that the facility will offer the medical assistant.

7 Prepare a cover letter and a list of references. Send the references with the resume only when requested.

8 Type the resume carefully and make certain that there are no errors on the document.

Purpose: Resumes submitted with errors are often discarded without consideration.

9 Proofread the resume. Allow another person to read it as well and look for missed errors.

Purpose: To make certain that the resume is error free.

10 Print the resume on quality paper. Review the resume again for errors and to assure that it looks attractive on the printed page.

11 Target each resume to a specific person or position. Do not send generic resumes to each prospective employer.

Purpose: Targeted resumes get better results during the job search.

12 Follow up on all resumes that are distributed with a phone call to arrange an interview.

Purpose: A resume sent without follow-up is usually ineffective.

A medical assistant should target the resume toward the specific job that he or she is applying for. This means that the job requirements should be compared with the skills on the resume, and those skills should be highlighted in the document (Figure 55-8). Of course, to do this effectively, the medical assistant must actually know the job requirements. One can assume that clinical and administrative duties will be similar from place to place, but the ad for the position may provide further information about the scope of duties for the position. A medical assistant should read these carefully and emphasize that those are a part of his or her skill set on the resume.

A good way to approach the resume is to compose it on a computer and save it to the hard drive or a disk.

Then, as each job opportunity presents itself, the resume can be modified to fit the job. For instance, if the resume lists back-office skills first and the job is for an administrative position, the administrative skills should be moved to the top to draw more attention to them. This is easy to accomplish when the resume is on a computer, because the medical assistant can cut and paste where necessary to make changes and save several versions of the resume. Then an original can be printed on quality paper for every job for which he or she applies.

A resume is an important job search tool, but it should never be expected to get the medical assistant a job on its own merit. It is but one of many tools that should be used when looking for employment.

Ruby Dunham
9362 Caesar Creek Road
Mytown, OH 45458
(937) 555-1899

Education

• 1998: A.S. in Medical Assisting, Community College, Mytown, OH

Experience:

1995–present: Medical Transcriptionist, Community Hospital, Mytown, OH

• Transcribe 55 wpm
• Specialist in medical terminology
• Excellent attendance record
• Detail oriented
• Increased personal productivity each quarter

1990–1995: Secretary, State University School of Medicine, Mytown, OH

• Coordinated schedules of four full-time professors
• Maintained office supply and assistant budget
• Created final examination scheduling guidelines for department
• Developed excellent written communication skills
• Familiar with a variety of office machines

1986–1990: Shift Manager, Burger World, Mytown, OH

• Managed 10 employees, including hiring, training, evaluating, and firing
• Developed excellent oral communication skills and team player concept
• Improved inventory supply techniques, reducing losses by 10%
• Maintained cleanliness standards highest in chain
• Developed customer-focused service goals for store

FIGURE 55-5 Chronological resume.

Developing a professional resume takes some time and effort, and it will prove to be a good investment. Give the document some thought and follow generally accepted guidelines for its construction.

CRITICAL THINKING APPLICATION

Lisa has drafted her resume and given a copy to her placement director. She has recommended that Lisa remove the mention of her volunteer experience, because it was not in the medical field. Should Lisa do this? Why or why not?

Critical Resume Errors

The first error that should be avoided on a resume is just that—any error. There should be no errors at all on a resume. Many employers will automatically disqualify a job candidate if an error is found on a resume.

One medical assistant who was having a difficult time finding a job consulted her placement director at school. The director suggested that she come in for a **mock** interview. About halfway through the interview, the placement director realized the problem. The medical

Max Bryan
1234 Rolling View Court
Mytown, OH 45431
(937) 555-3137

OBJECTIVE

• An entry level position in medical assisting, with the opportunity to utilize and refine skills and training

EDUCATION

• 1998: A.S. in Medical Assisting, Community College, Mytown, OH. Dean's list senior year, cumulative GPA 3.5

STRENGTHS

• Possess excellent interpersonal and communication skills
• Demonstrate consistent positive attitude and high energy
• Caring and compassionate
• Responsible, self-motivated, precise in work
• Experienced in customer-focused service

ACCOMPLISHMENTS

• Tutored students in medical assisting and 12-lead EKG courses. Received excellent evaluations and positive results
• Certified Medical Assistant, active member of local AAMA
• Experienced in MS Office programs
• Consistent "excellent" ratings in clinical externships

COMMUNITY ACTIVITIES

• 1995–present: Organized, recruited, and trained 20 others for church hand bell choir, direct weekly practices and monthly performances
• 1996–present: Teach community CPR twice yearly to high school students
• Vice-President Student Government, Community College, Mytown, OH. Recruited members, organized fund-raisers, campaigned successfully for policy changes

EMPLOYMENT

•1996–present: Tutor, Community College, Mytown, OH
• Waiter, Scott's Place, Mytown, OH

FIGURE 55-6 Functional resume.

assistant had worked for 2 years at a local grocery store and had misspelled the name of the store on the resume. Thinking from an employer's point of view, a person who cannot spell the name of a facility where she worked for 2 years, and cashed a paycheck with the name on it as well, might well make critical errors in charting or in other aspects of her duties. Within a week after this error was corrected, the medical assistant found a job.

Never list salary expectations on the resume. If the medical assistant lists a salary of $25,000 on the last job held, the future employer might not offer more than $26,000 to $27,000, realizing that this is a step up from the last salary. However, if they were willing to pay $32,000, the medical assistant has lost an opportunity for much higher wages.

Avoid using "I" or other personal pronouns on the resume. If abbreviations are used on the resume, be sure

Roscoe Patterson
3472 Vienna Woods Lane
Mytown, OH 45449
(937) 555-8874

Job Target:

• A long-term medical assistant position in a busy and varied medical office

Education:

• 1992: BA in Art History, State University, Mytown, OH
• 1998: AS in Medical Assisting, Community College, Mytown, OH

Capabilities:

• Excellent interpersonal skills and caring attitude
• Detail oriented, with strong analytical and problem-solving abilities
• Utilize solid organizational and time-management abilities in coordinating multiple projects
• Self-starter, take initiative to ensure jobs get done properly and efficiently
• Upbeat, personable, and highly energetic
• Ability to communicate in Spanish and American Sign Language

Accomplishments/Achievements:

• Campaigned for and raised consistent 15% annual increase in contributions and grants, allowing expansion of exhibits and needed renovations to art museum
• Maintained museum budget with 100% accountability
• Organized annual "Art Ball" for 100 contributors under budget
• Museum employee of the year 1995
• Certificates in CPR and EKG; Certified Nursing Assistant; will sit for CMA exam this November

Work History:

• 1998–present: Certified Nursing Assistant, Friendly Nursing Home, Mytown, OH
• 1992–1998: Assistant to the Curator, Mytown Museum of Art, Mytown, OH

FIGURE 55-7   Targeted resume.

USEFUL ACTION WORDS

Accelerated	Manage
Actively	Motivated
Adapted	Organized
Administered	Originate
Analyze	Participated
Approve	Perform
Completed	Pinpointed
Conceived conduct	Plan
Control	Proficient
Coordinate	Program
Created	Proposed
Delegate	Proved
Demonstrate	Provide
Develop	Recommended
Direct	Reduced
Effect	Reinforced
Eliminated	Reorganized
Established	Responsibilities
Evaluate	Revamped
Expanded	Review
Expedite	Revise
Founded	Schedule
Generated	Significantly
Improved	Simplify
Increased	Solve
Influence	Strategy
Implemented	Streamline
Interpret	Structure
Launched	Successfully
Lead	Supervise
Lecture	Support
Maintain	Teach

FIGURE 55-8   Use action words when describing skills on the resume.

to spell them out for clarity the first time they are used, if they are not well-known abbreviations. Never include personal information, such as height, weight, age, marital status, number of children, or any other information that is not **pertinent** to the job requirements.

Do not list dates along the left-hand side of the paper. This is distracting and draws attention away from the points that should be emphasized. A resume must be visually appealing and easy to read. The medical assistant should make good use of spacing, margins, indentions, capitalizing, and underlining to ensure an attractive document. **Proofread** the document several times to be sure there are no errors. It is helpful to have someone else proofread it, because many times the writer of a document misses errors when proofing.

Never include a photograph with the resume. Photographs can be a discriminatory factor in the hiring process, and the medical assistant should be wary of any employer who requests a photograph with the resume.

One of the most senseless errors common to resumes is not having the appropriate contact informa-

tion, such as an address and telephone number. Two phone numbers are suggested, such as a cell phone and a home phone, so that there is a better chance of reaching the candidate when it is time to schedule an interview.

The Argument of Length

Professionals disagree about the acceptable length of a resume. One page may be considered the ideal length, but a person with 20 years' experience in the job market will never get all of his or her skills on one page. A medical assistant without previous work experience may easily fit the resume on one page.

Recent trends indicate that a good rule of thumb is to allow one page for every 6 years of experience. If a person has a 20-year career in healthcare, the resume would be approximately three pages long. This is a general guideline, however; the document should be as **succinct** as possible, while clearly communicating the strengths and experiences of the applicant.

The Purpose of a Resume

The purpose of a resume is *not* to get the medical assistant a job, although this is a commonly held belief. The purpose of the cover letter is to get the employer to look at the resume. The purpose of the resume is to get the applicant an interview. The purpose of the interview, of course, is to get the job. Remember this, and use the resume as a tool, along with other strategies for job searching.

The medical assistant should be the person to write the resume, or at the very least, have a hand in its composition. Professional resume services may be helpful, but the person who knows the most about the experience and education gained is the medical assistant.

CRITICAL THINKING APPLICATION

Lisa has been asked by a potential employer to email her resume. She has used an unusual font on her cover letter and the top of the resume. What concerns should Lisa have about emailing the document? How can Lisa make certain that her document arrives in a readable format when sending it electronically?

The Cover Letter

When sending a resume, always include a cover letter (Figure 55-9). This is the introduction to the resume and the person sending the document. A cover letter should always be sent to an individual, not to the facility or "to whom it may concern." A simple phone call will usually reveal the name of the person to whom the resume should be sent. Ask for the name of the office manager, or if this information is not obtained, address it specifically to the physician.

Make the cover letter brief and interesting. Use the same paper stock weight and color as the resume. Be sure to include contact information, such as an address and at least two phone numbers, even if these are on the attached resume. The supervisor may have separated the two documents, so there must be a method of contact on each one. Never start a cover letter with the sentence, "I saw your ad in the newspaper" or a similar phrase. Be creative with the opening line and try to capture the attention of the reader.

A cover letter should be one to three paragraphs long. The final section should include a call to action that will prompt an interview. If the document concludes with a request for a meeting, the medical assistant should state when he or she will call for a time and date.

Job Applications

Many facilities require a job application along with a resume (Figure 55-10). Arrive 15 minutes before the scheduled interview to allow time to fill out an application.

Brutis Walter
2345 Morrow Court
Mytown, OH 45310
(937) 555-7426

May 23, 1998

Andrea Foreman, CMA
Office Manager
Family Health, Inc.
123 Timberleaf Drive
Mytown, OH 45432

Ms. Foreman:

I will be graduating from Community College with an A.S. in Medical Assisting on June 9 and am interested in an entry-level medical assistant position in your office. I will consider part-time or temporary work to gain experience in a diverse office such as yours.

My training includes hands-on experience in pediatrics, cardiology, internal medicine, obstetrics, and geriatrics. My administrative training would allow me to fill in wherever needed in the office. I am highly motivated and have supported myself and paid my own way through college. I understand responsibility and am a true team player. Belinda Mallet, RN, a fellow church member, told me the office will be short-staffed this summer owing to vacations and a maternity leave. I believe I could help your office run smoothly this summer, and beyond.

I look forward to hearing from you. I am available Tuesday and Thursday afternoons and Friday mornings until graduation. I will call you next Tuesday to set up an appointment for an interview.
Thank you for your consideration.

Very truly yours,

Brutis Walter

FIGURE 55-9 Cover letter.

Job applications can be considered a legal document if the person is hired. Therefore they should be neat and filled out correctly and completely. Always read the application before filling it out, so that directions make sense and information is not placed in the wrong area of the form. Carry a planner or address book to the interview so that former employers' and supervisors' names, addresses, and phone numbers are handy. The medical assistant should not be in a position that he or she must ask for a phone book to get an address. Have all of this information ready for the time that it is needed.

Applications often ask for a date that the medical assistant is available for work. Be careful with this question. If the applicant currently has a job, yet writes that he or she is "immediately available," it may indicate that the applicant intends to quit without notice. On the other hand, the current employer may be aware that the person is seeking other employment and may have granted him or her permission to quit immediately once a new job is found.

Be careful on the sections that ask the reason for leaving former positions. Think about the answers that are listed in those spaces, and try to put the information in as positive a light as possible. Ask the advice of the

APPLICATION FOR POSITION / Medical or Dental Office
AN EQUAL OPPORTUNITY EMPLOYER

(In answering questions, use extra blank sheet if necessary)

No employee, applicant, or candidate for promotion, training or other advantage shall be discriminated against (or given preference) because of race, color, religion, sex, age, physical handicap, veteran status, or national origin.

PLEASE READ CAREFULLY AND WRITE OR PRINT ANSWERS TO ALL QUESTIONS. DO NOT TYPE.

Date of Application

A. PERSONAL INFORMATION

Name - Last	First	Middle	Social Security No.	Area Code/Phone No. ( )

Present Address: - Street | (Apt #) | City | State | Zip | How Long At This Address?:

Previous Address: - Street | City | State | Zip | Person to notify in case of Emergency or Accident - Name:

From: | To: | Address: | Telephone:

B. EMPLOYMENT INFORMATION

For What Position Are You Applying?:	☐ Full-Time ☐ Part-Time ☐ Either	Date Available For Employment?:	Wage/Salary Expectations:

List Hrs./Days You Prefer To Work | List Any Hrs./Days You Are Not Available: (Except for times required for religious practices or observances) | Can You Work Overtime, If Necessary? ☐ Yes ☐ No

Are You Employed Now?: ☐ Yes ☐ No | If So, May We Inquire Of Your Present Employer?: ☐ No ☐ Yes, If Yes:
Name Of Employer: | Phone Number: ( )

Have You Ever Been Bonded? ☐ Yes ☐ No | If Required For Position, Are You Bondable? ☐ Yes ☐ No ☐ Uncertain | Have You Applied For A Position With This Office Before? ☐ No ☐ Yes If Yes, When?:

Referred By / Or Where Did You Learn Of This Job?:

Can You, Upon Employment, Submit Verification Of Your Legal Right To Work In The United States?: ☐ Yes ☐ No
Submit Proof That You Meet Legal Age Requirement For Employment? ☐ Yes ☐ No

Language(s) Applicant Speaks or Writes (If Use Of A Language Other Than English Is Relevant To The Job For Which The Applicant Is Applying:

C. EDUCATIONAL HISTORY

Name & Address Of Schools Attended (Include Current)	Dates From	Thru	Highest Grade/Level Completed	Diploma/Degree(s) Obtained/Areas of Study
High School				
College				Degree/Major
Post Graduate				Degree/Major
Other				Course/Diploma/License/ Certificate

Specific Training, Education, Or Experiences Which Will Assist You In The Job For Which You Have Applied.

Future Educational Plans

D. SPECIAL SKILLS

CHECK BELOW THE KINDS OF WORK YOU HAVE DONE:

☐ BLOOD COUNTS	☐ DENTAL ASSISTANT	☐ MEDICAL INSURANCE FORMS	☐ RECEPTIONIST
☐ BOOKKEEPING	☐ DENTAL HYGIENIST	☐ MEDICAL TERMINOLOGY	☐ TELEPHONES
☐ COLLECTIONS	☐ FILING	☐ MEDICAL TRANSCRIPTION	☐ TYPING
☐ COMPOSING LETTERS	☐ INJECTIONS	☐ NURSING	☐ STENOGRAPHY
☐ COMPUTER INPUT	☐ INSTRUMENT STERILIZATION	☐ PHLEBOTOMY (Draw Blood)	☐ URINALYSIS
OFFICE EQUIPMENT USED: ☐ COMPUTER	☐ DICTATING EQUIPMENT	☐ POSTING	☐ X-RAY
		☐ WORD PROCESSOR	☐ OTHER:

Other Kinds Of Tasks Performed Or Skills That May Be Applicable To Position: | Typing Speed | Shorthand Speed

(PLEASE COMPLETE OTHER SIDE)

FIGURE 55-10 Application for employment. (Courtesy Bibbero Systems, Inc., Petaluma, Calif. 94654, (800) 242-2376, www.bibbero.com.)

E. EMPLOYMENT RECORD

LIST MOST RECENT EMPLOYMENT FIRST   May We Contact Your Previous Employer(s) For A Reference? ☐ Yes ☐ No

1) Employer | Work Performed. Be Specific:

Address   Street   City   State   Zip Code

Phone Number (   )

Type of Business | Dates   Mo. Yr.   Mo. Yr.
                   From   To

Your Position | Hourly Rate/Salary
               Starting   Final

Supervisor's Name

Reason For Leaving

2) Employer | Worked Performed. Be Specific:

Address   Street   City   State   Zip Code

Phone Number (   )

Type of Business | Dates   Mo. Yr.   Mo. Yr.
                   From   To

Your Position | Hourly Rate/Salary
               Starting   Final

Supervisor's Name

Reason For Leaving

3) Employer | Worked Performed. Be Specific:

Address   Street   City   State   Zip Code

Phone Number (   )

Type of Business | Dates   Mo. Yr.   Mo. Yr.
                   From   To

Your Position | Hourly Rate/Salary
               Starting   Final

Supervisor's Name

Reason For Leaving

F. REFERENCES — FRIENDS / ACQUAINTANCES NON-RELATED

(1)
Name   Address   Telephone Number   (☐ Work ☐ Home)   Occupation   Years Acquainted

(1)
Name   Address   Telephone Number   (☐ Work ☐ Home)   Occupation   Years Acquainted

Please Feel Free To Add Any Information Which You Feel Will Help Us Consider You For Employment

READ THE FOLLOWING CAREFULLY, THEN SIGN AND DATE THE APPLICATION

"I certify that all answers given by me on this application are true, correct and complete to the best of my knowledge. I acknowledge notice that the information contained in this application is subject to check. I agree that, if hired, my continued employment may be contingent upon the accuracy of that information. If employed, I further agree to comply with Company/Office rules and regulations."

Signature: _____   Date: _____

FIGURE 55-10, cont'd   For legend see previous page.

placement counselor if unsure what to say in these sections.

If there are sections available for listing special skills and qualifications, fill them out fully. Describe CPR and first aid certifications and any professional organizations joined. If references are requested, list the name, title, employer, and a means of contact. Be sure to get permission before using someone as a reference.

One of the most common mistakes on the job application is writing "see resume." This is an indication of laziness and must be avoided. Even if the exact information is found on the resume, the application must still be completed in its entirety. Additionally, most job applications include a disclaimer that states that if a false or incomplete statement is made on the application, the individual can be dismissed from any position for which he or she was hired.

The Job Interview

A medical assistant may interview with the office manager, the physician, or both. It is possible that other staff members may be brought in for a portion of the interview. This is especially true in offices that have a cohesive team of employees.

The interview is usually the most stressful of the job search steps. Some individuals dread job interviews and become extremely nervous at the prospect of interviewing. Others are very comfortable and consider the interview as much for their own purposes as for the employer's.

There are four phases to interviews. These are the preparation, the interview itself, the follow-up, and the negotiation.

Preparation for the Interview

When preparing for an interview, the medical assistant should learn everything possible about the employer. Look on the Internet for information about the facility. Practice answering potential interview questions. Prepare an outfit to wear to interviews. It is wise to drive to the interview site on a day preceding the interview date if the location is unfamiliar to avoid getting lost on the day of the important event. The better prepared the medical assistant is, the more comfortable he or she will be while interviewing.

When preparing on the day of the interview, be conservative with wardrobe choices. Be sure clothing is fresh and wrinkle free and shoes are shined. It is a good idea to carry a planner or other method of taking notes during the interview. This makes a good impression and indicates interest in the job. Always arrive 15 minutes early for the interview. Do not use heavy perfumes or colognes, do not chew gum, and avoid excessive jewelry. Never take anyone along on a job interview, especially children, even if they are older children.

Pay particular attention to other aspects of appearance (Figure 55-11). Be sure that the hair is clean and styled attractively, and that teeth are clean and breath is fresh. Nails are also important and should be clean and

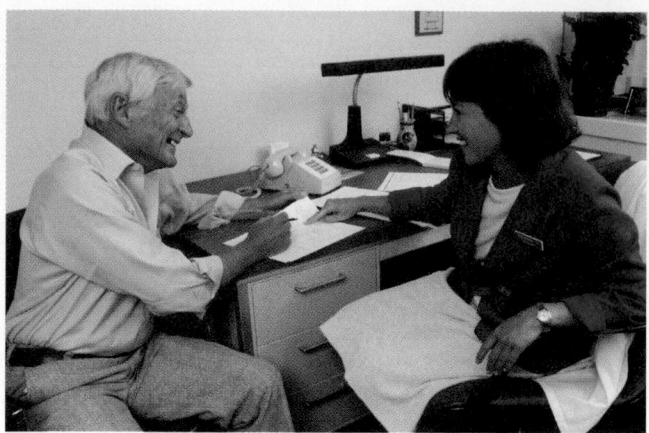

FIGURE 55-11 Present a professional appearance during the job interview and be sure to smile often!

well groomed, because the medical assistant will want to give the interviewer a firm handshake.

The Interview

During the actual interview, maintain good eye contact. Many supervisors refuse to hire people who seem uncomfortable with making strong eye contact. Never take control of the interview. Allow the supervisor to ask questions at his or her own pace. Do not fidget in the chair, and observe the interviewer's body language for clues as to how interested he or she might be. Do not volunteer any negative information, be honest, and do not exaggerate experience or lengths of employment. Never speak negatively about former employers.

Remember that the interview is centered on the medical assistant, so freely discuss the skills and attributes that will be brought to the job. The better prepared the medical assistant is, the smoother the interview will be. Be able to prove the skills claimed, and explain how they meet the needs of the company or facility. Avoid a "know-it-all" attitude, which indicates overconfidence and reluctance in taking direction. Always express an interest in the employer and its projects as opposed to what the employer can do for the employee. Ask intelligent questions at the end of the interview if given the opportunity (Figure 55-12).

Before the interview ends, the medical assistant should ask when a decision will be made, and if it would be acceptable to call to follow up.

CRITICAL THINKING APPLICATION

Lisa is enjoying a good interview when the supervisor, a man, asks her if she is married. When Lisa replies that she is not, he asks if she has a steady boyfriend. What might the supervisor's motive be with this line of questioning? How should Lisa respond? Are these questions inappropriate, or do they serve a purpose?

TOP 100 INTERVIEW QUESTIONS

1. Tell me about yourself.
2. Why do you want to work for this company?
3. Why should I hire you?
4. How do you work under pressure?
5. What type of job or salary do you expect to make in 5 years?
6. How do you handle criticism?
7. What do you think your co-workers think about you?
8. What is your opinion of the company you last worked for?
9. Describe your last supervisor.
10. What is your view of management?
11. What would you like to change about yourself and how would you do it?
12. What is your best asset?
13. What adjectives would you use to describe yourself?
14. What aspects of your life are you most happy with?
15. How would you describe the perfect job?
16. Why did you leave your last job?
17. Why did you choose this type of profession?
18. What salary do you expect?
19. What are your strongest and weakest personal qualities?
20. What motivates you?
21. What have you learned from some of your previous jobs?
22. What personal characteristics are necessary for success in your chosen field?
23. What do you know about this facility and our competitors?
24. What were your major courses of study in school?
25. Do you plan to continue your education?
26. Did school meet your expectations or were you disappointed?
27. How did you pay for your education?
28. Sell this pen to me.
29. To what extent do your grades reflect how much you have learned?
30. Do you feel your education was worthwhile?
31. What were the major responsibilities of your last job?
32. What has been your most rewarding experience at work?
33. What was your single most important accomplishment for the company on your last job?
34. What was the toughest problem you have ever solved and how did you do it?
35. How do you see yourself fitting in with our company?
36. What skills did you learn on your last job that can be used here?
37. What would you do if you were fired in two years?
38. What kinds of additional education do you think you need to meet your career goals?
39. How long do you plan to stay with our company?
40. What immediate contribution could you make if you came to work for us today?
41. Do you feel that you have received good general training?
42. If you were starting school all over again, what courses would you take?
43. How much money do you hope to earn in 5 years? 10 years?
44. Do you think that your extracurricular activities were worth the time spent?
45. Are you interested in making money or do you have other reasons for entering this career field?
46. Do you prefer working with others or by yourself?
47. Can you take instructions or criticism without being upset?
48. Tell me a story.
49. What do you know about the opportunities in the field in which you are trained?
50. How long do you expect to work?
51. Have you ever had any difficulty in getting along with a co-worker, classmate, or instructor?
52. Which of your school years was most difficult?
53. Do you like routine work?
54. Define cooperation.
55. Will you fight to get ahead?
56. Do you have an analytical mind?
57. Are you willing to go where the company sends you?
58. What job in this company would you choose if you could?
59. Do you think that employers should consider grades?
60. What have you done that shows initiative and willingness to work?
61. What benefits did you receive from your last employer?
62. What has been your most important accomplishment during your school years?
63. Have you ever helped to reduce operating costs, and how?
64. Have you ever developed or helped develop any programs, and how did you do this?
65. What do you think determines a person's progress in a company?
66. What would you do if a personal problem interfered with your work?
67. What would you do if you became bored with your job?
68. What would you do if you had a personality clash with a supervisor?
69. How will you be getting to work each day?
70. Do you have reliable transportation?
71. How do you feel about working with someone who is HIV positive?
72. What person has most influenced your life?
73. What is the last book you read?
74. Who do you most admire?
75. Who is your favorite relative?
76. What will previous supervisors say about you?
77. What makes a good supervisor?
78. Why would you be successful in this job?
79. Why have you held so many jobs?
80. Can you explain this gap in your employment history?
81. Have you ever been fired from a position?
82. Do you have adequate child care arrangements that will allow you to be at work when scheduled?
83. What is your philosophy of life?
84. How many other positions are you considering?
85. Why were your grades in school so low?
86. Are you a member of any professional organizations?
87. How old were you when you began to support yourself?
88. Do you participate in continuing education activities or seminars?
89. Have you had the hepatitis B injection series?
90. Where did you perform your externship?
91. How many days of school did you miss?
92. Why did you decide to attend the college/school you attended?
93. What kind of boss do you prefer?
94. How do you usually spend your weekends?
95. Why types of people seem to rub you the wrong way?
96. What planning procedures do you use?
97. What frustrates you about your current job?
98. What is unique about you?
99. What have you done that indicates you are qualified for this job?
100. Do you have any questions?

FIGURE 55-12 Top 100 interview questions.

Follow-Up After the Interview

Follow-up is critical after an interview. Always send a written thank-you letter to the person who conducted the interview. Many employers wait to see who sends a thank-you letter before making the final hiring decision. Limit follow-up calls to no more than once or twice a week. Most employers will give an indication of when the hiring decision will be made. The company should notify all those who interviewed once a decision has been made, unless there were specific protocols set during the interview in this area. For instance, if the office manager said that a decision will be made on Friday, and the final three candidates will be called for a second interview, then the medical assistant knows if a call is not received to continue the job search. Never place all your hopes on one job—continue to prospect until an offer is made.

REASONS PEOPLE DO NOT GET HIRED

Below is a rank order list of reasons that interviewers do not hire job candidates. The list is compiled from the results of a nationwide survey of 153 companies performed by North Central Technical Institute.

1. Poor personal appearance
2. Lack of interest or enthusiasm
3. Overemphasis on money
4. Poor voice, diction, grammar
5. Lack of planning
6. No purpose or goals
7. Condemnation of past employers
8. Poor eye contact
9. Limp, fishy handshake
10. Late to interview
11. Lack of tact
12. Lack of maturity
13. Lack of courtesy
14. Asking no questions
15. Overbearing "know-it-all"
16. Lack of confidence and poise
17. Failure to participate in activities
18. Making excuses, evading unfavorable factors on record
19. Indecisiveness
20. Just shopping around
21. No interest in company
22. Sloppy application blank
23. Wanting a job for a short time
24. Unwillingness to relocate
25. Cynical attitude
26. Low moral standards
27. Laziness
28. Intolerance or strong prejudices
29. No sense of humor
30. Narrow interests
31. Inability to take criticism
32. No appreciation for the value of experience
33. Radical ideas
34. Too aggressive during interview

The Negotiation

The negotiation stage of job acceptance can be as stressful as the actual interviews. A medical assistant should know the lowest salary he or she can afford and then ask for a little more than that figure. Bracket salary requests: instead of asking for $12.00 per hour, ask for a salary in the "mid to high twenties." Let the employer mention a figure first, or a range of salary. Usually the person who mentions a salary range first has the disadvantage. If the medical assistant requests $12.00 per hour and the facility was willing to pay $15.00 per hour, the medical assistant will probably get $12.00.

Never say "no" to a job offer on the spot. Request at least 24 hours to consider the offer. A medical assistant should not let the salary amount be the main factor in the decision to accept a position. Consider whether the position carries any authority, the benefits, the hours, the distance from home, and the potential for advancement before accepting or rejecting a job offer.

You Got the Job!

Once the job offer has been made and accepted, a start date will be determined (Figure 55-13). Before the first day, use the computer to map several ways to get to work. Because the medical assistant may be unsure of traffic flow, leave home extra early the first day so that arrival on time is guaranteed.

Most employees are placed on a 30- to 90-day probationary period, during which employment may be terminated if the employee's performance is not satisfactory. It is also an opportunity for the employer and employee to learn about each other. The medical

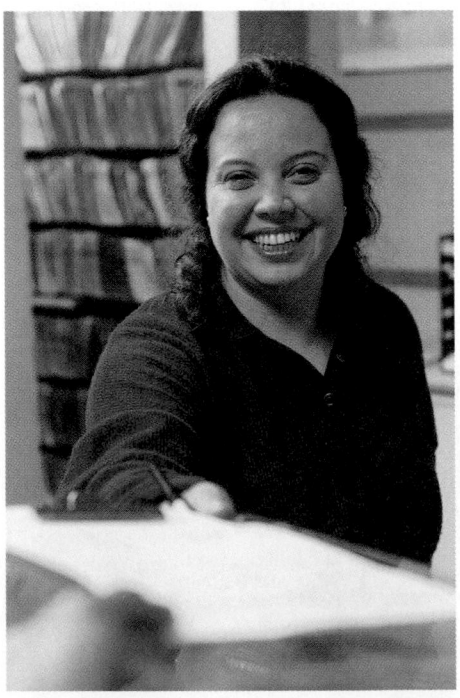

FIGURE 55-13   Congratulations, you're hired! The first job after school is an exciting experience for a medical assistant.

assistant will interact with other co-workers, with patients, and with providers. A new medical assistant should volunteer to help others and efficiently complete the duties assigned. Use the probationary period as a testing ground, carefully observing ways in which the office might run in a smoother manner. However, do not make numerous suggestions for change during this period. Discover why certain methods are used and make an effort to fit in with the rest of the team before suggesting that the routine of the office be changed. Remember, the people at the office may have been employed for substantially longer periods and may resent suggestions from a new staff member. Learn the office's rhythms, procedures, and culture first and demonstrate a team-oriented attitude.

Common Early Mistakes

Some medical assistants make mistakes early on a new job. Never be disruptive to the office by gossiping or complaining. A medical assistant must realize that there may be different ways of performing procedures and that the way he or she was taught in school is probably not the only correct way. Be open to learning new ideas, concepts, and procedures. Although some mistakes are to be expected, be certain that once a mistake is pointed out, it is corrected. Do not make the same mistakes over and over.

Supervisors may or may not work very closely with the medical assistants. Some will be expected to carry out orders on their own. Do not make too much supervision necessary or force the office manager to constantly check the work that is done. Finish all assigned duties in a timely manner and avoid procrastination. When problems arise, communicate them openly with the supervisor and attempt to find a quick resolution. Last, limit absences and tardy days to a minimum and miss work only when absolutely necessary—especially during the probationary period.

How to Be a Good Employee

There are several ways in which a medical assistant can be a better employee. First and foremost, arrive for the scheduled shift on time and do not leave early. Even the best medical assistant cannot benefit an office when he or she does not come to work. Be honest and demonstrate trustworthiness and professionalism. Get along with co-workers in the facility. A medical assistant should be able to resolve simple problems with others easily without involving the supervisor. Reflect a friendly attitude to others, even if they are difficult to get along with.

A medical assistant should constantly be performing assigned duties and not expect frequent breaks in the medical office. Most offices are fast paced, and the supervisor will expect the medical assistant to keep up with the activity. Even when there are slow periods, there is always a counter to clean or filing to do. Be supportive of the leadership in the facility and ask for more responsibility if necessary. Take initiative to perform duties that are cumbersome or repetitive, and get them done quickly.

It is vital to treat the patients with compassion. Remember that they are not always at their best when ill, so be kind and courteous to them and their families. The patients are the reason that the facility exists. Treat them with great respect and care.

CRITICAL THINKING APPLICATION

On Lisa's second day at the externship site, she clearly sees a co-worker taking and using a controlled drug from the storage area. What should Lisa do? What potential problems will this situation prompt? Who should Lisa report this incident to, if anyone?

Dealing With Supervisors

Supervisors appreciate employees who come to them when there are questions but who are able to handle minor decisions on their own. Never hesitate to approach supervisors when there is an issue at hand that needs their attention. Do not allow a situation to go unaddressed and then say, "I didn't want to bother you with that." It is the responsibility of the office manager to deal with difficult issues, and these should be handled immediately when they arise.

A medical assistant should never attempt to cover up a mistake; admitting the error is a much better approach to solving the problem. When talking with the supervisor, do not hesitate to speak or avoid the subject. State the problem clearly and explain what routes are available to **rectify** the situation. Work with the supervisor to resolve issues and accept the advice given with a positive attitude.

Performance Appraisals

Performance **appraisals** are usually done after the initial probationary period and annually after that. The performance appraisal is designed to inform the employee of his or her strengths and weaknesses on the job, according to the supervisor's point of view. Most of these appraisals offer a scale to rate the employee's performance, such as 1 to 5. Do not expect to receive a perfect appraisal, because employees are seldom perfect in all aspects of their jobs. If the supervisor gives perfect scores to an employee, there is no room for growth or improvement. It is the rare employee who completes all duties without any errors. When asked to sit down with your supervisor for a performance appraisal, go into the meeting open to addressing areas that may need improvement. Ask questions and work with the supervisor to improve in the areas that may need more effort or a different approach.

If the employee strongly disagrees with any area of the performance appraisal, discuss this with the supervisor. There may have been misunderstandings as to the duties involved. Clarify this and strive to do better next time.

Asking for a Raise

Most facilities have some type of schedule for pay increases. Some offer a cost of living increase on an annual basis; others use a merit system, offering raises only when earned and deserved based on performance.

There may come a time when the medical assistant feels the need to ask for a raise. Before doing so, do a little self-reflection to determine whether a raise is in order. Has attendance been exemplary? How many times was the medical assistant tardy? Does he or she work well with little supervision? Has he or she performed all the expected duties well and in a timely manner?

Approach the supervisor at a relatively calm part of the day, and ask how a salary raise might be earned in the near future. Do not expect a raise of more than 4% to 5% at any given time. If the supervisor is unable to grant a raise, determine whether the reasons are valid. If they are not, the medical assistant may wish to pursue other employment options. It is always easier to find a job if one already has a job, so do not quit outright unless the work environment is **intolerable**. Begin networking again and discover the options available.

Leaving A Job Professionally

Always offer at least a 2-week notice when resigning from a job. Give the supervisor a written notice of resignation, and take this to him or her in person. Do not just leave it on a desk or place it in the interoffice mail.

It is a dangerous practice to resign from a job just to attempt to get a salary increase. Once the employer doubts the employee's loyalty, the future is usually not bright for the employee at that facility. Resign only after a final decision has been made. If the medical assistant is resigning to take another position, expect the current employer to make a **counteroffer**. However, be wary about accepting counteroffers. What led to looking for a new job in the first place? Has the situation been resolved? Ask these questions before agreeing to stay with the current employer.

Life Skills

To be successful in the job search, the medical assistant must have the basic entry-level skills needed to perform in the workplace. Even more important, however, he or she must develop certain life skills that are essential to excel in any profession. If these skills are not developed and refined, the medical assistant may find fewer opportunities and advancements available, as well as less impressive salaries and benefits.

The most important life skill one can possess is the willingness to change. There are many employees who insist on doing things the same way they have always been done, and they resist any changes in policy or procedure. However, a medical assistant who does not welcome change and work hard at it is a failure waiting to happen.

Personal Growth

Personal growth is a comprehensive term that applies to many aspects of a person's mental, physical, and spiritual health. This growth is a result of goals that are set for self-improvement. Without clear goals, people rarely experience personal growth that is initiated from within. There may be growth that is a result of some outside influence, but a conscious effort toward personal growth is an innate decision.

No matter how great the training or how many opportunities are placed in front of a person, fear and doubt can sabotage efforts to improve the self-image, confidence, and future potential of an individual. Personal growth involves such traits as self-control, self-esteem, problem-solving skills, decision-making skills, and stress management.

STEPS FOR ACHIEVING GOALS

- Decide what you want.
- Write the goal down.
- Set the date of accomplishment.
- Read it three times daily.
- Think of the goal often.
- See yourself accomplishing the goal.
- Develop a plan of action for reaching the goal.
- Do not discuss the plan with others who might be discouraging.
- Be confident.
- Act successful, and you will be!

Self-Control. Self-control is a vital trait in the medical office. Some patients may not be at their best because of their illness, and this may make them less than cordial toward the staff. Remember that this is usually a temporary situation. A medical assistant must exercise self-control and not respond in kind to patients who are disagreeable.

Self-control is important in other areas of the medical office. Never remove drugs from the storage areas without permission, and be careful when dealing with petty cash. A medical assistant must get enough rest during the work week so that he or she can care for the patients in an enthusiastic manner.

Self-Esteem. Everyone has certain strengths and weaknesses. Good self-esteem is the result of knowing what those strengths are and overcoming the weaknesses. It is having a positive outlook about the self and others. A person with good self-esteem is motivated, able to express love, and capable of handling criticism. A person's self-esteem will improve if he or she has developed adaptive skills. Especially in the medical profession, one thing that is guaranteed in the workplace is change. Change can be positive or negative; this depends on the way it is viewed by the individual.

A person is not doomed to live with poor self-esteem forever. With a degree of effort and open-mindedness, an individual can work toward better self-esteem, which can make a tremendous difference in the individual's future potential.

Problem-Solving Skills. For individuals to work together, they must have a degree of trust and be willing to make suggestions for the good of the group. The phrase "two heads are better than one" is still true when it comes to problem solving. Employees usually want to play a part in solving the problems in the workplace, and they appreciate knowing that their opinions make a difference. A medical assistant who can listen to the concerns of others and is willing to give and take will be an excellent problem-solver.

Decision-Making Skills. People who know how to make good decisions are usually successful. Thinking through a decision requires logic, and it is best to take some time to carefully think of all of the "pros and cons." Unfortunately, a medical assistant may not always have time to consider decisions in a leisurely fashion, especially when dealing with emergencies. A good decision-maker is honest when identifying the real problems and attempts to keep personal feelings isolated from the process.

There are several steps toward making a sound decision. The problem must be specifically defined and evaluated so that the individual understands clearly what needs to happen to resolve the situation at hand. Gather as much information as possible and consider all alternatives. It is sometimes helpful to choose an alternative, and then consider all of the **ramifications** of making a decision using that alternative. Then, when the best alternative is determined, the decision should be made and put into action. Care should be taken to avoid making a decision simply because it is easy and comfortable, because more problems could arise later as a result of not addressing the true problem in the beginning.

CRITICAL THINKING APPLICATION

Lisa has been on several interviews and likes the prospect of working for three different physicians. If an offer is made at each office, how can Lisa decide which to accept? What will help Lisa make this decision?

Stress Management. The demands of the medical profession make it a stressful environment at times. Stress is not always bad. In fact, some stress is a positive motivator toward a goal. A stressor is a stimulus that prompts a reaction from the body. Positive stress, or *eustress*, includes exhilarating activities or success, which often leads to higher expectations from the person experiencing the eustress. The opposite is distress, which includes disappointment, failure, or embarrassment. Stress management is a conscious effort toward controlling the stressors and resulting reactions so that the body and mind operate evenly, even when stress is present in an individual's life.

By learning to recognize the signs of stressful overload, a medical assistant can possibly ward off the negative reactions that are so physically and mentally draining to the body. Many people notice a headache or fatigue when overly stressed. Breathing correctly is one way to reduce stress. Often, an accelerated breathing pattern that is quick and shallow is a stress indicator. Breathing from the abdomen at a slower pace, inhaling through the nose, and exhaling through the mouth may help reduce tension. Taking time for relaxing activities and getting plenty of exercise are other methods of stress reduction.

Planning a Budget

A newly graduated medical assistant should formulate a simple budget and attempt to live within that budget. It is helpful to track spending with checkbook ledgers, bill stubs, receipts, and daily records for 3 months before developing a firm budget, so that there is a realistic accounting of where money goes when it leaves the checkbook. Use that information to design a spending plan for monthly income that accounts for monthly, quarterly, and annual expenses, as well as special activities.

Even when making only a small salary, building savings is important. A medical assistant should set aside 5% to 10% of the net income in a savings account. The money in savings should not be touched except in emergencies. It is even better to establish an emergency fund, which would ideally hold 3 months' salary. This way, there is enough cash to pay bills for 3 months in case of a sudden job loss or emergency. No one can do this immediately when beginning a new job, but it can be done over a period of time if one is committed to the effort.

Avoid going into debt whenever possible. If credit cards are used, they should be used conservatively and not for impulse purchases. Instead of using credit, set spending goals and save for a purchase or use lay-away programs. Make more than the minimum payment on credit cards to avoid excessive interest from accruing on the account. Everyone should work toward being debt free as soon as possible.

Limit housing and utilities to no more than 30% of the net income. Other monthly installment debt should total less than 15% of the net income. Many financial institutions figure a debt ratio when they consider loaning money to an individual. If that debt ratio is too high, the bank may not lend money, even to a person with stellar credit.

Student Loans. Student loans are extremely important. Loans are designed to provide the opportunity to obtain a good education. They must be paid back. If an individual allows a student loan to **default**, he or she becomes ineligible for future student loans until the original loan is paid back. There is never a reason for a student loan to default. The medical assistant should contact the company that services the student loan and explain any problems that are keeping him or her from repaying the debt. These companies want to work with students to clear their accounts. Often a deferment is available, which allows the student to postpone the payments for a period of time (Figure 55-14). Deferments may be

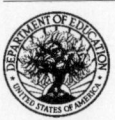

SCH

IN-SCHOOL DEFERMENT REQUEST
Federal Family Education Loan Program

OMB No. 1845-0005
Form Approved
Exp. Date 09/30/2005

WARNING: Any person who knowingly makes a false statement or misrepresentation on this form or on any accompanying documents shall be subject to penalties which may include fines, imprisonment or both, under the U.S. Criminal Code and 20 U.S.C. §1097.

SECTION 1: BORROWER IDENTIFICATION

Please enter or correct the following information.

SSN |___|___|___| – |___|___| – |___|___|___|___|

Name _____

Address _____

City, State, Zip _____

Telephone - Home ( ) _____

Telephone - Other ( ) _____

E-mail Address (optional) _____

SECTION 2: DEFERMENT REQUEST

Before answering any questions, carefully read the entire form, including the instructions and other information in Sections 5 and 6.

■ I meet the qualifications for the deferment checked below and request that my loan holder defer repayment of my loan(s):

❏ While I am enrolled at an eligible school as a **FULL-TIME STUDENT**. (For borrowers with a FFEL Program loan.)

❏ While I am enrolled at an eligible school as a **LESS THAN FULL-TIME BUT AT LEAST HALF-TIME STUDENT**. (For borrowers who, on the date they signed the promissory note, did not have an outstanding balance on a FFEL Program loan made **before July 1, 1987**.)

NOTE: *Your promissory note or other loan documents may state that a borrower with an outstanding balance on a FFEL Program loan made **prior to July 1, 1993**, must receive another loan in order to qualify for a half-time student deferment. This requirement was eliminated by the Higher Education Amendments of 1998. **Effective October 1, 1998**, no FFEL Program borrower who is eligible for a deferment based on enrollment as at least a half-time student is required to receive another loan in order to qualify for this deferment.*

SECTION 3: BORROWER UNDERSTANDINGS AND CERTIFICATIONS

■ **I understand that: (1)** I am not required to make payments of loan principal during my deferment. Interest will not be charged on my subsidized loan(s) during my deferment. However, interest will be charged on my unsubsidized loan(s). **(2)** I have the option of making interest payments on my unsubsidized loan(s) during my deferment. **(3)** I may choose to make interest payments by checking the box below. Interest that I do not pay during the deferment period will be capitalized by my loan holder.

❏ I wish to make interest payments on my unsubsidized loan(s) during my deferment.

(4) My deferment will begin on the date the condition that qualifies me for a deferment began, as certified by the authorized official who completes Section 4 of this form. **(5)** My deferment will end on the earlier of the date that I no longer meet the condition that qualifies me for the deferment, or the ending date of that condition as certified by the authorized official. **(6)** If my deferment does not cover all my past due payments, my loan holder may grant me a forbearance for all payments due before the begin date of my deferment or—if the period for which I am eligible for a deferment has ended—a forbearance for all payments due at the time my deferment request is processed. **(7)** If I am eligible for a post-deferment grace period on loans made before October 1, 1981, my loan holder may grant me a forbearance on my other loans for this period so that I can begin repayment of all my loans at the same time. I understand that my loan holder may capitalize the interest that accrues on my other loans during the six-month period and that this will increase the principal balance of my other loans. **(8)** My loan holder may grant me a forbearance on my loans for up to 60 days, if necessary, for the collection and processing of documentation related to my deferment request. Interest that accrues during the forbearance will not be capitalized.

■ **I certify that: (1)** The information I provided in Sections 1 and 2 above is true and correct. **(2)** I will provide additional documentation to my loan holder, as required, to support my deferment status. **(3)** I will notify my loan holder immediately when the condition(s) that qualified me for the deferment ends. **(4)** I have read, understand, and meet the eligibility criteria of the deferment for which I have applied.

Borrower's Signature _____ **Date** _____

SECTION 4: AUTHORIZED OFFICIAL'S CERTIFICATION

NOTE: *As an alternative to completing this section, the school may attach its own enrollment certification report listing the required information.*

I certify, to the best of my knowledge and belief, that the borrower named above:

(1) is/was enrolled as (check the appropriate box) ❏ a full-time student ❏ at least a half-time student

during the academic period from |___|___| – |___|___| – |___|___|___|___| to |___|___| – |___|___| – |___|___|___|___| and

(2) is reasonably expected to complete his/her program requirements on |___|___| – |___|___| – |___|___|___|___|.

Name of Institution _____ OPE-ID _____

Address _____ City, State, Zip _____

Name/Title of Authorized Official _____ Telephone ( ) _____

Authorized Official's Signature _____ **Date** _____

Page 1 of 2

FIGURE 55-14 In-school deferment form. Do not allow student loans to default. Contact the financial aid office at your educational institution for assistance and answers to questions about student loans.

SECTION 5: INSTRUCTIONS FOR COMPLETING THE FORM

Type or print using dark ink. Report dates as month-day-year (MM-DD-YYYY). For example, 'January 31, 2002' = '01-31-2002'. An authorized school official must either (A) complete Section 4, or (B) attach the school's own enrollment certification report listing the required information. If you need help completing this form, contact your loan holder.

Return the completed form and any required documentation to the address shown in Section 7.

SECTION 6: DEFINITIONS FOR IN-SCHOOL DEFERMENT REQUEST

- The **Federal Family Education Loan (FFEL) Program** includes Federal Stafford Loans (both subsidized and unsubsidized), Federal Supplemental Loans for Students (SLS), Federal PLUS Loans, and Federal Consolidation Loans.

- A **deferment** is a period during which I am entitled to postpone repayment of the principal balance of my loan(s). The federal government pays the interest that accrues during an eligible deferment for all subsidized Federal Stafford Loans and for Federal Consolidation Loans for which the Consolidation Loan application was received by my loan holder **(1)** on or after January 1, 1993, but before August 10, 1993, **(2)** on or after August 10, 1993, if it includes *only* Federal Stafford Loans that were eligible for federal interest subsidy, or **(3)** on or after November 13, 1997, for that portion of the consolidation loan that paid a subsidized FFEL Loan or a subsidized Federal Direct Loan. I am responsible for the interest that accrues during this period on all other FFEL Program loans.

- **Forbearance** means permitting the temporary cessation of payments, allowing an extension of time for making payments, or temporarily accepting smaller payments than previously scheduled. I am responsible for the interest that accrues on my loan(s) during a forbearance. If I do not pay the interest that accrues, the interest may be capitalized.

- The **holder** of my FFEL Program loan(s) may be a lender, guaranty agency, secondary market, or the U.S. Department of Education.

- **Capitalization** is the addition of unpaid interest to the principal balance of my loan. This will increase the principal and the total cost of my loan.

- An **authorized certifying official** for an In-School Deferment is an authorized official of the school where I am/was enrolled as a full-time or at least half-time student.

SECTION 7: WHERE TO SEND THE COMPLETED DEFERMENT REQUEST

RETURN THE COMPLETED DEFERMENT REQUEST AND ANY REQUIRED DOCUMENTATION TO:
(IF NO ADDRESS IS SHOWN, RETURN TO YOUR LOAN HOLDER)

SECTION 8: IMPORTANT NOTICES

Privacy Act Notice

The Privacy Act of 1974 (5 U.S.C. 552a) requires that the following notice be provided to you:

The authority for collecting the requested information from and about you is §428(b)(2)(A) et seq. of the Higher Education Act of 1965, as amended (20 U.S.C. 1078(b)(2)(A) et seq.) and the authority for collecting and using your Social Security Number (SSN) is §484(a)(4) of the HEA (20 U.S.C. 1091(a)(4)). Participating in the Federal Family Education Loan (FFEL) Program and giving us your SSN are voluntary, but you must provide the requested information, including your SSN, to participate.

The principal purposes for collecting the information on this form, including your SSN, are to verify your identity, to determine your eligibility to receive a loan or a benefit on a loan (such as a deferment, forbearance, discharge, or forgiveness) under the FFEL program, to permit the servicing of your loan(s), and, if it becomes necessary, to locate you and to collect on your loan(s) if your loan(s) become delinquent or in default. We also use your SSN as an account identifier and to permit you to access your account information electronically.

The information in your file may be disclosed to third parties as authorized under routine uses in the appropriate systems of records. The routine uses of this information include its disclosure to federal, state, or local agencies, to other federal agencies under computer matching programs, to agencies that we authorize to assist us in administering our loan programs, to private parties such as relatives, present and former employers, business and personal associates, to credit bureau organizations, to educational institutions, and to contractors in order to verify your identity, to determine your eligibility to receive a loan or a benefit on a loan, to permit the servicing or collection of your loan(s), to counsel you in repayment efforts, to enforce the terms of the loan(s), to investigate possible fraud and to verify compliance with federal student financial aid program regulations, to locate you if you become delinquent in your loan payments or if you default, to provide default rate calculations, to provide financial aid history information, to assist program administrators with tracking refunds and cancellations, or to provide a standardized method for educational institutions efficiently to submit student enrollment status.

In the event of litigation, we may send records to the Department of Justice, a court, adjudicative body, council, party, or witness if the disclosure is relevant and necessary to the litigation. If this information, either alone or with other information, indicates a potential violation of law, we may send it to the appropriate authority for action. We may send information to members of Congress if you ask them to help you with federal student aid questions. In circumstances involving employment complaints, grievances, or disciplinary actions, we may disclose relevant records to adjudicate or investigate the issues. If provided for by a collective bargaining agreement, we may disclose records to a labor organization recognized under 5 U.S.C. Chapter 71. Disclosures may also be made to qualified researchers under Privacy Act safeguards.

Paperwork Reduction Notice

According to the Paperwork Reduction Act of 1995, no persons are required to respond to a collection of information unless it displays a currently valid OMB control number. The valid OMB control number for this information collection is 1845-0005. The time required to complete this information collection is estimated to average 0.16 hours (10 minutes) per response, including the time to review instructions, search existing data resources, gather and maintain the data needed, and complete and review the information collection. *If you have any comments concerning the accuracy of the time estimate(s) or suggestions for improving this form, please write to:*

U.S. Department of Education, Washington, DC 20202-4651

If you have any comments or concerns regarding the status of your individual submission of this form, write directly to the address shown in Section 7.

FIGURE 55-14, cont'd   For legend see previous page.

available when the student is unemployed, attending school to continue his or her education, suffering economic hardship, completing a graduate fellowship, completing rehabilitation training, or in other situations. Contact the lender to find out whether a deferment is in order.

TOP TEN WAYS TO AVOID DEFAULT ON A STUDENT LOAN

1. Understand your rights and responsibilities regarding your repayment obligation as well as your repayment options.
2. Borrow for college expenses only. Borrow only the amount you need and only what you can reasonably expect to be able to repay.
3. Keep all records regarding your loan. Make copies of all letters, canceled checks, and any forms you sign.
4. Notify your lender or servicer when you have a change of address, phone number, or name, or if you change schools or your enrollment status.
5. Seek help as early as possible if you have any difficulty maintaining your student loan repayment arrangement.
6. If you have any questions, talk to your lender or student loan guarantor about the particular terms of your loan.
7. Keep credit card debt to a minimum or avoid credit card debt completely.
8. Create and maintain a budget that is within your monthly income.
9. Consider making nominal student loan payments while in school. This will reduce the amount you owe after graduation.
10. Make loan payments on time.

Courtesy Texas Guaranteed Student Loan Corporation, http://www.tgslc.org.

The Guideline Budget

Dealing with personal finances can be a stressor. Developing a realistic budget will assist a medical assistant in planning his or her spending. When careful planning is implemented, more can be accomplished with less money if a commitment has been made to staying on budget and resisting the temptation to spend.

Dangerous Habits. Some individuals practice dangerous habits related to finances. For instance, if this month's bills are arriving and last month's have not been paid, frustration and depression may result. Some people may even avoid opening letters or bills just so they do not have to deal with seeing the balance due. Writing checks on funds that are not in the checking account is not only unwise—it is also illegal. All states

have laws related to insufficient fund checks, and most legislation considers this a form of theft. It is possible to be arrested for writing "hot" checks. People headed for financial disaster also purchase daily items, such as bread and milk, with a credit card. All of these behaviors are signs of financial trouble.

A sample budget outline is shown in Figure 55-15. Take an honest look at each item listed and determine what amount is spent monthly in each category. Compare these amounts with the monthly income and see if the current budget is positive or negative. Remember that the gross salary is the amount earned before taxes and other deductions. The net salary is the take-home pay. Adjustments may be needed to bring the budget into balance.

Closing Comments

The period surrounding graduation will be a celebration, but also a busy time for which much planning is required. Cooperate with the school when securing externship sites and make an effort to obtain a site that will be of the most benefit to the career desired. Do not take an externship just because it is close to home. Think about the skills that will be offered and learn as much as possible. Then perform well, so that the staff and physicians are happy to offer a good reference to potential employers.

Even though this educational experience has ended, remember that there is constantly something new to learn in the medical profession. Join professional societies and participate in as many educational seminars and continuing education classes as possible. Remain in a continual state of learning and be determined to be the best medical assistant you can be.

Patient Education

Some patients assume that the people who assist the physician in the office are all nurses. The medical assistant should always specify that he or she is a medical assistant, especially when making initial introductions. There should never be any representation that the medical assistant is the "office nurse." If a patient uses that term, he or she should be corrected in a friendly manner.

A medical assistant may find it necessary to educate the patient as to the definition of a medical assistant. An occasional rare patient may not have heard of the term. Explain the type of training that was completed, emphasizing that medical assistants are trained specifically for working in a physician's office. If patients have any questions about the medical assistant's qualifications, refer them to the office manager or physician.

Legal and Ethical Issues

Remember to be completely honest when completing a job application and offering information on a resume.

MONTHLY INCOME	AMOUNT
Net Income	
Spouse Net Income	
Child Support	
Other Income	

MONTHLY EXPENSES	AMOUNT
Rent	
Gas	
Electric	
Home/Renters Insurance	
Water/Sewage	
Trash	
Home Telephone	
Cell Telephone	
Pager	
Cable TV/Satellite	
Internet/DSL	
Child Care	
Lawn Care	
Clothing	
Food - Home	
Food - Work or School	
Food – Eating Out	
Laundry/Dry Cleaning	
Medical Expenses	
Dental Expenses	
Life Insurance	
Medical Insurance	
Dental Insurance	
Eyeglasses	
Prescriptions	
Automobile Payment	
Automobile Insurance	
Repairs	
Gas/Oil	
Furniture	
Beauty/Barber Shop	
Pet Expenses	
Student Loan	
Other Loans	
Credit Cards	
Church/Charities	
Birthdays	
Anniversaries	
Christmas	
Vacation Planning	
Entertainment	

FIGURE 55-15 The guideline budget.

Most facilities stipulate that if an individual is not truthful on these documents, his or her employment can be terminated once the deception is discovered. Employers are more interested in honesty and a forthright explanation than in minor problems that affect the job performance.

If a medical assistant has had some brush with the law that requires disclosure on the job application, the best policy is to be honest and deal with the ramifi-

cations of telling the truth. Most businesses can verify whether a potential employee has any type of criminal record. A solid explanation of the facts, admission of a past mistake, and excellent, current references will often prompt an employer to have faith and make a positive decision about extending employment.

SUMMARY OF SCENARIO

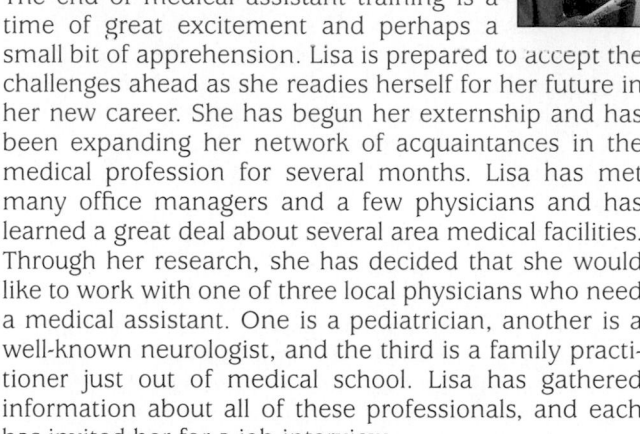

The end of medical assistant training is a time of great excitement and perhaps a small bit of apprehension. Lisa is prepared to accept the challenges ahead as she readies herself for her future in her new career. She has begun her externship and has been expanding her network of acquaintances in the medical profession for several months. Lisa has met many office managers and a few physicians and has learned a great deal about several area medical facilities. Through her research, she has decided that she would like to work with one of three local physicians who need a medical assistant. One is a pediatrician, another is a well-known neurologist, and the third is a family practitioner just out of medical school. Lisa has gathered information about all of these professionals, and each has invited her for a job interview.

Lisa knows that she will need to be at her best, so she takes care of herself and gets plenty of rest. She has a long list of interview questions and has taken the time to write out answers to the questions in preparation for her interviews. She is careful about her grooming every day that she reports to the externship, because she knows that the physician at her site is her first reference in the medical field. In addition, she knows that she may be called for an interview any day that might be scheduled just after her workday ends. Looking professional prepares her for this each day.

Lisa is comfortable during her interviews because she is well prepared. She has identified her strengths and can share them with a potential employer. She is focused on her objectives and knows what the minimum requirements will be for her to accept a position. She has a healthy self-esteem, and her good decision-making skills will help her to determine which position will be right for her. Her enthusiasm and excitement show in her eyes, and she is dedicated to making a difference in the lives of her patients and co-workers.

SUMMARY OF LEARNING OBJECTIVES

■ Because approximately 85% of individuals do not have any formal training in job search skills, taking the time to learn the best methods will place the medical assistant at an advantage. Training decreases the time spent looking for work and increases the benefits and salary offered when using good negotiating skills. The medical assistant will also be more comfortable during interviews and throughout the job search process.

- Employers have three basic expectations of their medical assistant employees. They want an employee with a good appearance, who looks as if he or she fits in the medical profession. A medical assistant should also be dependable and have the skills to do the job for which he or she was hired.

- There are three types of skill strengths that may be used by employees. Job skills are those used to actually perform a job, such as venipunctures or scheduling appointments. Self-management skills are usually a part of the medical assistant's personality; these include honesty and dependability. Transferable skills are those that can be taken from one job to another or used on any job. Examples include the ability to communicate effectively and lead and manage individuals.

- Networking and contacting employers directly are the two best methods of job searching. Networking involves developing a network of individuals that can assist in finding employment. This group may include co-workers, other students, relatives, or friends who provide leads to potential employers. Contacting employers directly includes taking resumes to specific offices or setting appointments to gain knowledge about the facility, then later using that knowledge during the job search. These two methods are more effective than most traditional means of finding a job.

- Any error on a resume should be avoided. Be sure that everything is spelled correctly, but do not rely on the computer's spell-check feature alone. Proofread the document and have someone else proofread it to catch errors that may be overlooked. Salary expectations should never be stated on the resume, and a photograph should not be included. Do not include personal information, such as height and weight.

- Demographic information on other employers should be taken to interviews and kept handy when filling out job applications. A medical assistant should never have to ask for a phone book to look up the address of a former employer. This demonstrates a lack of preparation and planning on the part of the potential employee.

- The four phases of the interview process include the preparation, the actual interview, the follow-up, and the negotiation. The preparation includes all efforts made before the actual interview in obtaining information about the company, deciding on the wardrobe, and making sure nails are groomed and shoes are shined. The interview itself is designed to help the employer and potential employee get to know each other and discover whether they are compatible. The follow-up is perhaps the most critical stage, wherein the medical assistant should send a thank-you letter and continue to stay in touch with the facility until the job is filled. The negotiation includes discussion of the salary and benefits that will be offered to the new employee.

- The probationary period is a time for the new medical assistant to become oriented to the facility. It also allows the employer to assess whether the medical assistant fits with the team and performs the duties of the job in a satisfactory way. During this time, the medical assistant should demonstrate that he or she is a productive team member with an excellent attitude. There should never be idle time; instead, look for ways to assist others when all duties are completed.

- A new employee in the medical office should avoid arriving late or any absences, especially during the probationary period. Never participate in office gossip, and make a good attempt to get along with every employee. A medical assistant should not make excessive supervision necessary and should be open to learning new ways of performing procedures. Fit in with the team, and the job will be more rewarding.

■ No employee is perfect, so performance appraisals rarely have perfect ratings. Even an employee who is doing an excellent job has room for improvement in some area. Without comments that suggest improvement, the employee may not feel that the position offers growth potential. Constructive comments will help a medical assistant to perform better and take on more responsibility.

KEY INTERNET WEBSITES

- All Job Search
- America's Job Bank
- Career Job Search
- Career Journal
- Monster.com—Tough Interview Questions
- National Center for Self-Esteem
  For active weblinks to each website visit
  http://evolve.elsevier.com/Kinn/

APPENDIX A

A Patient's Bill of Rights*

1. The patient has the right to considerate and respectful care.

2. The patient has the right to and is encouraged to obtain from physicians and other direct caregivers relevant, current, and understandable information concerning diagnosis, treatment, and prognosis.

Except in emergencies when the patient lacks decision-making capacity and the need for treatment is urgent, the patient is entitled to the opportunity to discuss and request information related to the specific procedures and/or treatments, the risks involved, the possible length of recuperation, and the medically reasonable alternatives and their accompanying risks and benefits.

Patients have the right to know the identity of physicians, nurses, and others involved in their care, as well as when those involved are students, residents, or other trainees. The patient also has the right to know the immediate and long-term financial implications of treatment choices, insofar as they are known.

3. The patient has the right to make decisions about the plan of care prior to and during the course of treatment and to refuse a recommended treatment or plan of care to the extent permitted by law and hospital policy and to be informed of the medical consequences of this action. In case of such refusal, the patient is entitled to other appropriate care and services that the hospital provides or transfer to another hospital. The hospital should notify patients of any policy that might affect patient choice within the institution.

4. The patient has the right to have an advance directive (such as a living will, health care proxy, or durable power of attorney for health care) concerning treatment or designating a surrogate decision maker with the expectation that the hospital will honor the intent of that directive to the extent permitted by law and hospital policy.

Health care institutions must advise patients of their rights under state law and hospital policy to make informed medical choices, ask if the patient has an advance directive, and include that information in patient records. The patient has the right to timely information about hospital policy that may limit its ability to implement fully a legally valid advance directive.

5. The patient has the right to every consideration of privacy. Case discussion, consultation, examination, and treatment should be conducted so as to protect each patient's privacy.

6. The patient has the right to expect that all communications and records pertaining to his/her care will be treated as confidential by the hospital, except in cases such as suspected abuse and public health hazards when reporting is permitted or required by law. The patient has the right to expect that the hospital will emphasize the confidentiality of this information when it releases it to any other parties entitled to review information in these records.

7. The patient has the right to review the records pertaining to his/her medical care and to have the information explained or interpreted as necessary, except when restricted by law.

8. The patient has the right to expect that, within its capacity and policies, a hospital will make reasonable response to the request of a patient for appropriate and medically indicated care and services. The hospital must provide evaluation, service, and/or referral as indicated by the urgency of the case. When medically appropriate and legally permissible, or when a patient has so requested, a patient may be transferred to another facility. The institution to which the patient is to be transferred must first have accepted the patient for transfer. The patient must also have the benefit of complete information and explanation concerning the

need for, risks, benefits, and alternatives to such a transfer.

9. The patient has the right to ask and to be informed of the existence of business relationships among the hospital, educational institutions, other health care providers, or payers that may influence the patient's treatment and care.

10. The patient has the right to consent to or decline to participate in proposed research studies or human experimentation affecting care and treatment or requiring direct patient involvement, and to have those studies fully explained prior to consent. A patient who declines to participate in research or experimentation is entitled to the most effective care that the hospital can otherwise provide.

11. The patient has the right to expect reasonable continuity of care when appropriate and to be informed by physicians and other caregivers of available and realistic patient care options when hospital care is no longer appropriate.

12. The patient has the right to be informed of hospital policies and practices that relate to patient care, treatment, and responsibilities. The patient has the right to be informed of available resources for resolving disputes, grievances, and conflicts, such as ethics committees, patient representatives, or other mechanisms available in the institution. The patient has the right to be informed of the hospital's charges for services and available payment methods.

A Patient's Bill of Rights © 1992 by the American Hospital Association.
*These rights can be exercised on the patient's behalf by a designated surrogate or proxy decision maker if the patient lacks decision-making capacity, is legally incompetent, or is a minor.

APPENDIX B

Claim Form Comparison Charts

Appendix B lists and compares the CMS-1500 form requirements for each type of payor. The large table covers every box of the CMS-1500 form for common payors. Special considerations for other, less common payors are covered in smaller tables at the end of this appendix.

Claim Form Comparison Chart

Block	Commercial	BC/BS*	Medicare	Medicaid	TRICARE	Workers' Compensation
1	Enter X in "Other" box	Enter X in "Other" box	Enter X in Medicare box	Enter X in Medicaid box	Enter X in CHAMPUS box	Enter X in FECA box
1A	Insurance ID number—omit dashes	BCBS ID number, 2sp, group identification number if provided	Enter Medicare ID number from health insurance card	Enter insured's Medicaid ID number	Enter sponsor's SSN	Enter patient's SSN
2	Enter FULL name of patient (all CAPS no punctuation)	FULL name of patient—for case studies all CAPS no punctuation	Enter patient's name as appears on card (all CAPS no punctuation)	Enter patient's name as it appears on card (all CAPS no punctuation)	Enter FULL name of patient (all CAPS no punctuation)	Enter FULL name of patient (all CAPS no punctuation)
3	Birth date using eight digits MM DD YYYY (use spaces)	Birth date using eight digits MM DD YYYY and X sex block	Birth date using eight digits MM DD YYYY (use spaces)	Birth date using eight digits MM DD YYYY (use spaces)	Enter patient's birth date MM DD YYYY and sex	Enter patient's birth date—MM DD YYYY and sex
4	Enter SAME (if patient and policyholder are same person)	Enter SAME (if patient and policyholder are same person)	Leave blank	Leave blank	Sponsor's name if other than patient, enter SAME if patient is sponsor	Enter employer's name if known
5	Enter patient's mailing address, ZIP, phone number—spaces—no (), -, or punctuation	Enter patient's mailing address, ZIP, phone number—spaces—no (), -, or punctuation	Enter patient's mailing address, ZIP, phone number—spaces—no (), -, or punctuation	Enter patient's mailing address, ZIP, phone number—spaces—no (), -, or punctuation	Enter patient's mailing address, ZIP, phone number—spaces—no (), -, or punctuation	Enter patient's mailing address, ZIP, phone number—spaces—no (), -, or punctuation
6	Enter X in appropriate box—relationship to policyholder	Enter X in appropriate box—relationship to policyholder	Leave blank	Leave blank	Enter X in appropriate box	Enter X in OTHER box
7	If policyholder's address same as in block 5, enter SAME	If policyholder's address same as in block 5, enter SAME	Leave blank	Leave blank	Enter sponsor's duty station/mailing address; if same as patient's—SAME	Enter address and phone number of employer if known
8	Enter X in appropriate box	Enter X in appropriate box	Enter X in appropriate box	Leave blank	Enter X in appropriate box	Enter X in EMPLOYED box
9	Enter NONE (leave 9A-9D blank)	9-9D leave blank	Leave 9-9D blank	Leave 9-9D blank	Enter NONE/9A-9D blank	9-9D leave blank
10A	Enter X in NO box if visit is not related to an on-the-job injury	Enter X in NO box if visit is not related to an on-the-job injury	Enter X in NO box if visit is not related to an on-the-job injury	Enter X in No box	Enter X in YES box	Enter X in YES box
10B	Enter X in appropriate box; yes indicates possible third party liability	Enter X in appropriate box; yes indicates possible third party liability	Enter X in appropriate box; yes indicates possible third party liability	Enter X in No box	If YES selected, sponsor must complete DD 2527	Enter X in appropriate box
10C	Enter X in appropriate box; yes indicates possible third party liability	Enter X in appropriate box; yes indicates possible third party liability	Enter X in appropriate box; yes indicates possible third party liability	Enter X in No box	If YES selected, sponsor must complete DD 2527	Enter X in appropriate box
10D	Leave blank for case study purposes	Leave blank for case study purposes	Leave blank unless eligible for Medicaid	Leave blank	Leave blank	Leave blank
11	Enter group policy name of number if on patient's card	Leave blank	NONE unless change from Medicare secondary to Medicare primary status	Leave blank	Enter NONE	Leave blank

Claim Form Comparison Chart—Cont'd

Block	Commercial	BC/BS*	Medicare	Medicaid	TRICARE	Workers' Compensation
11A	Enter birth date and sex of person, if other than patient (policyholder/subscriber)	Enter birth date and sex of person, if other than patient (policyholder/subscriber)	Leave blank	Leave blank	Leave blank	Leave blank
11B	Enter name of employer, if identified on patient's ID card	Enter name of employer, if identified on patient's ID card	If applicable, enter description of change from Medicare secondary to primary and date effective	Leave blank	Leave blank	Enter name of patient's employer
11C	Enter name of carrier for patient's policy	Enter name of carrier	Leave blank	Leave blank	Leave blank	Enter name of workers' compensation carrier
11D	Enter X in NO box if covered by only one insurance policy	Enter X in NO box if covered by only one insurance policy	Leave blank	Leave blank	Enter X in appropriate box	Leave blank
12	Enter "SIGNATURE ON FILE" if patient has signed an Authorization for Release; assume one has been signed	Enter "SIGNATURE ON FILE" if patient has signed an Authorization for Release; do not enter date	Enter "SIGNATURE ON FILE" if patient has signed an Authorization for Release; case studies — assume one has been signed	Leave blank	Enter "SIGNATURE ON FILE"	Leave blank
13	Enter "SIGNATURE ON FILE"	Leave blank	PAR-SOF/nonPar—leave blank	Leave blank	Leave blank	Leave blank
14	Enter date of first symptom—MM DD YYYY	Enter date of first symptom—MM DD YYYY	Enter date of first symptom—MM DD YYYY	Leave blank	Information appreciated but not required	Enter date symptoms/injury occurred
15	Enter date of prior episode of same illness if documented in patient's record	Leave blank	Leave blank	Leave blank	Information appreciated but not required	Enter date if in patient's documentation
16	Enter dates patient unable to work if documented in patient's record	Leave blank	Leave blank	Leave blank	Information appreciated but not required	Enter dates if available
17	Enter full name and credentials of referring physician	Enter full name and credentials of referring physician	Enter full name, NOT credentials of referring/ordering etc, physician	Enter full name and credentials of referring/ordering physician, etc.	Enter referring provider; if referred from a military facility, enter name of facility	Enter name and title of referring health care provider, if applicable
17A	PAR providers—enter PIN/nonPAR SSN	Enter UPIN of any provider named in block 17	Enter UPIN of physician in block 17	Enter Medicaid number of provider in block 17	Enter referring physician's EIN	Enter SSN (no spaces or hyphens) of block 17
18	Enter admission/discharge dates if inpatient status	Enter admission/discharge dates if inpatient status	Enter admission/discharge dates if inpatient status	Enter admission/discharge dates if inpatient status	Enter admission/discharge dates if inpatient status	Enter admission/discharge dates if inpatient status
19	Local use; for case studies leave blank	For case studies leave blank or X in NO box	Various information	Local use	Leave blank	Leave blank

Claim Form Comparison Chart—Cont'd

Block	Commercial	BC/BS*	Medicare	Medicaid	TRICARE	Workers' Compensation
20	Enter X in NO box if all laboratory tests performed in provider's office—for case studies—NO	Enter X in NO box if all laboratory tests performed in provider's office; for case studies—NO	Enter X in NO box if all laboratory tests performed in provider's office; for case studies—NO	Enter X in appropriate box	Enter X in NO box	Enter X in appropriate box
21	Enter ICD-9 codes—no decimals	Enter ICD-9 codes—no decimals	Enter ICD-9 codes—no decimals	Enter ICD-9 codes—no decimals	Enter ICD-9 codes	Enter ICD-9 codes
22	Leave blank	Leave blank	Leave blank	For case studies leave blank	Leave blank	Leave blank
23	Enter authorization number when required by patient's insurance plan	Enter authorization number when required by patient's insurance plan	Enter authorization number if one assigned	Enter authorization number if one assigned	Enter prior authorization number	Enter preauthorization number
24A	Enter FROM date MMDDYYYY—no spaces TO not filled in if for single procedure entry	Enter FROM and TO date MMDDYYYY—no spaces TO not filled in if for single procedure entry	Enter FROM date MMDDYYYY—no spaces TO not filled in if for single procedure entry	Enter FROM date MMDDYYYY—no spaces TO not filled in if for Medicaid	Enter eight-digit date with no spaces in FROM column, no TO if single procedure entry	Enter eight-digit date with no spaces in FROM column, no TO if single procedure entry
24B	Enter Place of Service code	Enter Place of Service code	Enter Place of Service code	Enter Place of Service code	Use appropriate two-digit code	Use appropriate two-digit code
24C	Enter Type of Service code	Leave blank	Leave blank	Enter Type of Service code	Use appropriate code	Use appropriate code
24D	Enter CPT or HCPCS number	Enter CPT or HCPCS number	Enter CPT or HCPCS number	Enter CPT or HCPCS number	Enter CPT code or HCPCS number	Enter CPT or HCPCS number
24E	Enter reference number (1-4) from block 24D For case studies enter only one number	Enter reference number (1-4) from block 24D For case studies enter only one number	Enter reference number (1-4) from block 24D For case studies enter only one number	Enter reference number (1-4) from block 24D For case studies enter only one number	Enter reference number (1-4) from block 24D For case studies enter only one number	Enter reference number (1-4) from block 24D For case studies enter only one number
24F	Enter fee charged	Enter fee charged	Enter fee charged/nonPAR limiting fee	Enter fee charged	Enter fee for procedure	Enter fee for procedure
24G	Enter number of units/days of service or procedures reported in 24D	Enter number of units/days of service or procedures—use 3 digits: 1 = 001 10 = 010	Enter number of units/days of service or procedures reported in 24D	Enter number of units/days of service or procedures reported in 24D	Enter number of units/days reported in 24D	Enter number of units/days reported in 24D
24H	Leave blank	Leave blank	Leave blank	Enter E, F, B as appropriate	Leave blank	Leave blank
24I	Enter X if documentation indicates a medical emergency existed	Leave blank	Leave blank	Enter X or E if appropriate	Enter X if services provided in emergency department	Enter X if patient given emergency care
24J	Leave blank	Leave blank	Solo—blank/Group-NPI	Leave blank	Leave blank if services performed by 2 providers	Leave blank
24K	Leave blank	Leave blank	Solo—blank/Group-PIN	Leave blank	Leave blank if services performed by 2 providers	Leave blank

Claim Form Comparison Chart—Cont'd

Block	Commercial	BC/BS*	Medicare	Medicaid	TRICARE	Workers' Compensation
25	Enter EIN and X in appropriate box Be sure to enter hyphen	Enter EIN and X in appropriate box Be sure to enter hyphen	Enter EIN and X in appropriate box Be sure to enter hyphen	Enter Tax ID number if available; enter X in appropriate box	Enter billing's entity Tax ID Number	Enter billing's entity Tax ID Number
26	Enter number for patient's account	Enter number for patient's account	Enter number for patient's account	Enter number for patient's account	Enter patient's account number	Enter patient's account number
27	For case studies enter case study number For case studies enter X in NO box	For case studies enter case study number Enter X in YES if PAR; NO if not PAR	For case studies enter case study number Enter YES or NO to accept assignment	For case studies enter case study number Enter X in YES box	Enter X in appropriate box/NO for case study	Leave blank
28	Enter total charges	Enter total charges	Enter total charges	Enter total charges	Enter total charges	Enter total charges
29	Enter amount patient has paid/blank if 0	Leave blank	Enter amount patient has paid/blank if 0	Leave blank	Amount received from other health insurance	Leave blank
30	Enter balance	Leave blank	Leave blank	Leave blank	Enter balance due	Leave blank
31	For case studies enter provider's full name, credentials, and date completed—MMDDYYYY	For case studies enter provider's full name, credentials, and date completed—MMDDYYYY	For case studies enter provider's full name, credentials, and date completed—MMDDYYYY	For case studies enter provider's full name, credentials, and date completed—MMDDYYYY	TRICARE requires provider/supplier personally sign claim	For case studies enter provider's full name, credentials, and date completed—MMDDYYYY
32	Enter data if services performed were not in provider's office or patient's home	Enter data if services performed were not in provider's office or patient's home	Enter data if services performed were not in provider's office or patient's home	Enter data if services performed were not in provider's office or patient's home	Enter information if services performed were not in provider's office or patient's home	Enter information if services performed at a site other than provider's office
33	Enter information	Enter information	Enter information	Enter information and Medicaid number in PIN box	Enter information and TRICARE provider number	Enter information; leave PIN and GRP blank—study

Other Payors

Block	Medicare With Medigap
1–8	Same as for Medicare
9	Enter name of enrollee in Medigap if different from block 2
9a	Enter word Medigap and policy/group number
9b	Enter Medigap enrollee's birth date and sex
9c	Leave blank if Medigap PlanID is known; if PlanID not known, enter abbreviated mail address
9d	Enter Medigap PlanID number; if number not available, enter plan name
13	Enter "SIGNATURE ON FILE"

Block	Medicare-Medicaid Crossover
1a	Enter X in both Medicare and Medicaid boxes
10d	Enter abbv "MCD" followed by ID number
27	NonPAR must accept assignment

Block	Medicare–Secondary Payor
1	Enter X in Medicare and Other boxes
4	Enter primary policyholder's name; if policyholder is patient enter SAME
6	If block 4 is completed, enter relationship
7	Enter address and phone number of policyholder in block 4; if same as block 5, enter SAME
11	Enter policy/group number of primary plan; blocks 4 and 7 must be filled out
11a	Primary policyholder's birth date and sex if patient not policyholder
11b	Employer's name for group plan
11c	Primary plan name or PlanID; primary EOB must be attached to claim
16	Enter dates if patient is employed and unable to work
29	Enter patient payment for service on form EOB from primary; will show payments

Block	TRICARE With Supplemental Policy
9a	Policy or group number of other policy
9b	Enter other insured's date of birth, X in appropriate box for sex
9c	Enter name of employer/school
9d	Enter name of insurance plan or program, name of other insurance coverage

Block	TRICARE As Secondary Payor
11	Insured policy group, FECA number if insurance primary; to TRICARE/enter Medicare if appropriate
11a	If different from block 3 enter information
11b	Enter employer/school if applicable
11c	Enter insurance plan or program
11d	Enter X in appropriate box
29	Enter only payments from other insurances

State Licensing Agencies for Radiology

Arizona
State of Arizona Medical Radiologic Technology Board of Examiners,
4814 South 40th Street,
Phoenix, AZ 85040
Phone: 602-255-4845

California
State of California Radiologic Health Branch,
714 P Street,
Sacramento, CA 95814
Phone: 916-445-6695

Colorado
Colorado State Medical Board, 1560 Broadway, Suite 1300,
Denver, CO 80202-5140,
Phone: 303-894-7714

ITEP Exam Processing Center, PO Box 7871,
Colorado Springs, CO 80933
Phone: 719-392-2452

Connecticut
Department of Public Health,
Bureau of Health Systems Registration,
Capitol Avenue,
MS #12APP,
PO Box 340308,
Hartford, CT 06134
Phone: 860-509-7562 410

Delaware
State of Delaware Office of Radiation Control,
Robbins Building,
PO Box 637,
Dover, DE 19903
Phone: 302-736-4731

Florida
State of Florida HRS Radiation Control
Phone: 850-487-1004
850-487-3451

Hawaii
State of Hawaii Radiologic Technology Board,
Department of Health Noise and Radiation Branch,
591 Ala Moana Boulevard,
Honolulu, HI 96813-2498
Phone: 808-548-4383

Illinois
State of Illinois Division of Radiologic Technologist Certification,
Illinois Department of Nuclear Safety,
1035 Outer Park Drive,
Springfield, IL 62704
Phone: 217-785-9915

Indiana
State of Indiana Radiological Health Section,
PO Box 1964,
Indianapolis, IN 46206-1964
Phone: 317-633-0150

Iowa
State of Iowa Department of Health,
Lucas State Office Building,
Des Moines, IA 50319-0075
Phone: 515-281-3478

Kentucky
State of Kentucky Radiation Control Branch,
275 East Main Street,
Frankfort, KY 40621
Phone: 502-564-3700

Louisiana
Louisiana State Radiologic Technology Board of Examiners,
3108 Cleary Avenue, Suite 207,
Metairie, LA 70002
Phone: 504-838-5231

Maine
State of Maine Radiologic Technology Board of Examiners,
State House Station #35,
Augusta, ME 04333
Phone: 207-582-8723

Maryland
State of Maryland Public Health Engineer,
2500 Broening Highway,
Baltimore, MD 21224
Phone: 301-631-3300

Massachusetts
State of Massachusetts Radiation Control Program,
150 Tremont Street, 11th Floor,
Boston, MA 02111
Phone: 617-727-6214

Minnesota
*Department of Health—Radiation Control Section,
121 E. Seventh Place,
PO Box 64975,
St. Paul, MN 55164
Phone: 612-215-0941

Mississippi
*State Dept of Health Professional Licensure,
PO Box 1700,
Jackson, MS 39215-1700
Phone: 601-987-4153

Montana
State of Montana Department of Commerce,
Board of Radiologic Technologists,
1424 Ninth Avenue,
Helena, MT 59620
Phone: 406-444-4288

Nebraska
State of Nebraska Division of Radiological Health,
301 Centennial Mall South,
Lincoln, NE 68509
Phone: 402-471-2168

New Jersey
State of New Jersey Department of Environmental
    Protection,
Bureau of Radiological Health,
CN 415,
Trenton, NJ 08625-0415
Phone: 609-987-2022

New Mexico
State of New Mexico Radiation Protection Bureau,
PO Box 968,
Santa Fe, NM 87504-0968
Phone: 505-827-2773
505-827-2941

New York
Bureau of Environment Radiation Protection,
New York State Department of Health,
Room 325,
2 University Place,
Albany, NY 12203
Phone: 518-458-6482

Oregon
Health Licensing Boards,
Oregon State Health Division,
PO Box 231,
Portland, OR 97207
Phone: 503-229-5054

Ohio
Ohio Department of Health,
Ms. Margaret Cipkala Wanachick,
Chief, Radiologic Technology Section,
246 N. High Street,
PO Box 118,
Columbus, OH 43266-0118
Phone: 614-752-4319

Pennsylvania
Bureau of Professional and Occupational Affairs,
State Board of Medicine,124 Pine Street,
PO Box 2649,
Harrisburg, PA 17105-2649
Phone: 717-783-4858

Puerto Rico
Puerto Rico Examination Board for Radiology and
    Radiotherapy Technologists,
Physical address:
800 Roberto H. Todd Avenue,
Suite 202,
Santurce, Puerto Rico
Postal address:
Call Box 10200,
San Juan, PR 00908-0200
Phone: 787-725-8161
Present President: Mr. Eduardo Brito, R.T., M.P.H.

Rhode Island
Rhode Island Department of Health,
Division of Professional Registrations,
3 Capitol Hill,
Providence, RI 02908
Phone: 401-277-2827

Tennessee
State of Tennessee Board of Medical Examiners,
283 Plus Park Boulevard,
Nashville, TN 37217
Phone: 615-367-6231

Texas
Texas Department of Health,
Medical Radiologic Technology Program,
1100 West 49th Street,
Austin, TX 78756-3183
Phone: 512-459-2960

Utah
Utah Department of Commerce,
Division of Occupational and Professional Licensing,
Heber M. Wells Building,
160 East 300 South,
Salt Lake City, UT 84145-0805
Phone: 801-530-6403

Vermont
State of Vermont Board of Radiologic Technology,
Division of Licensing and Registration,
Office of the Secretary of State,
Pavilion Office Building,
Montpelier, VT 05609-1101
Phone: 802-828-2886

Virginia
Commonwealth of Virginia,
Department of Health Professions,
    6606 W. Broad Street, 4th Floor,
Richmond, VA 23230
Phone: 804-662-7664

Washington
Washington State Office of Radiation,
Olympic Building S. 220,
217 Pine Street,
Seattle, WA 98101-1549
Phone: 206-464-6840

West Virginia
West Virginia Radiologic Technology Board of
    Examiners,
1715 Flat Top Road,
Cool Ridge, WV 25825
Phone: 304-787-4398

Wyoming
State of Wyoming Board of Radiologic Technologist
    Examiners,
1312 Monroe Avenue,
Cheyenne, WY 82001
Phone: 307-778-7319

For further information contact the Association of Educators in
Radiological Sciences, Inc. (AERS), PO Box 90204, Albuquerque,
New Mexico 87199-0204, Tel. 1-505 823-4740, e-mail
aers@att.net; website http://www.aers.org/
*Indicates that state licensure requirements are pending.

English-Spanish Phrases

Are you having pain? Where?
¿Siente usted dolor? ¿Dónde?

What does the pain feel like?
¿Qué tipo de dolor es?

How long have you had problems with this?
¿Desde cuándo tiene este tipo de problemas?

When did it start?
¿Cuándo comenzó?

Does your child have a temperature?
¿Tiene fiebre su hijo?

Have you given your child any medication?
¿Le ha dado alguna medicina a su hijo?

Are you allergic to any medication?
¿Es usted alérgico a algo?

How did your child get hurt?
¿Cómo se lastimó su hijo?

What is your name?
¿Cómo se llama usted?

How old are you?
¿Qué edad tiene?

Do you take any medication regularly?
¿Toma usted alguna medicación con regularidad?

How many times have you been pregnant?
¿Cuántas veces ha estado embarazada?

How many children were born alive?
¿Cuántos niños sanos ha dado usted a luz?

Who is your closest relative?
¿Quién es su familiar más cercano?

Do you speak English?
¿Habla usted inglés?

Can someone come with you the next time who does speak English?
¿Puede acompañarle alguien que hable inglés la próxima vez?

Can you read English?
¿Sabe usted leer en inglés?

Does someone in your family read English?
¿Alguien de su familiar sabe leer en inglés?

My name is...You are...
Yo soy... Usted es...

Please put the gown on.
Por favor, póngase la bata.

Your blood pressure is...
Su presión arterial es de...

Your blood sugar is...
Su nivel de azúcar en la sangre es de...

The doctor recommends a low fat diet.
El médico recomienda una dieta baja en grasa.

Does this hurt?
¿Le duele esto?

Do you have medical insurance?
¿Tiene usted seguro médico?

Please point to where it hurts.
Por favor, indíqueme dónde le duele.

Where do you work?
¿Dónde trabaja usted?

Have you seen blood in your urine?
¿Ha visto algo de sangre en su orina?

Do you have pain when urinating?
¿Siente algún dolor al orinar?

Please fill out this form.
Por favor, llene este formulario.

Do you have an insurance card?
¿Tiene usted una tarjeta del seguro?

Do you have a telephone? What is the number?
¿Tiene usted teléfono? ¿Cuál es el número?

Please come back to see the doctor on...
Por favor, regrese para ver al médico el...

All days of the week.
Todos los días de la semana.

All months of the year.
Todos los meses del año.

All times.
A todas horas.

All numbers (to 31).
Todos los números (hasta el 31).

The doctor wants you to see another doctor.
El médico quiere que la vea otro médico.

Go to the hospital.
Vaya al hospital.

Call the ambulance now.
Pida una ambulancia ahora mismo.

Take your medication as ordered.
Tómese la medicación tal como se le indicó.

These are the side effects of your medication.
Su medicación tiene algunos efectos secundarios.

Thank you.
Gracias.

You are welcome.
De nada.

Please.
Por favor.

Please come this way.
Venga por aquí, por favor.

Please come with me.
Acompáñeme, por favor.

Please wait here to see the doctor.
Por favor, espere aquí para ver al médico.

You may leave now.
Ya puede marcharse.

We need to get a blood sample.
Necesitamos una muestra de su sangre.

We need to get a urine sample.
Necesitamos una muestra de su orina.

You owe "xxx" today.
Hoy debe abonar "xxx".

Who should we call to pick you up?
¿A quién debemos contactar para que lo recojan?

Please go to the lab at this address.
Por favor, vaya al laboratorio que está en este lugar.

When did you last eat?
¿Cuándo comió por última vez?

Have you had nausea?
¿Ha tenido náuseas?

Have you vomited?
¿Ha vomitado?

Please sign your name here.
Por favor, firme aquí.

Take this medicine (3) times a day.
Tómese esta medicina (3) veces al día.

This paper allows us to file your insurance.
Este papel nos permite presentarle su caso al seguro.

This paper allows the insurance company to pay the doctor.
Este papel es para que el seguro le pague al médico.

The doctor will see you now.
El médico le puede ver ahora.

Good morning.
Buenos días.

Good afternoon.
Buenas tardes.

Here is information (written) about your illness.
Aquí se incluye información (escrita) sobre su enfermedad.

Please follow these directions.
Por favor, siga estas instrucciones.

It is nice to meet you.
Es un placer conocerle.

Thank you for coming.
Gracias por su visita.

Take care of yourself.
¡Cuídese!

Do you drink?
¿Toma usted alcohol?

Do you smoke? How much?
¿Fuma? ¿Cuántos cigarrillos al día?

Have you had this problem before?
¿Ha tenido antes este problema?

Procedure Charting Examples

Procedure 28-1 Obtaining an Oral Temperature Using a Digital Thermometer		
Date	Time	Note
3/27/XX	10:05 AM	T – 97.7°F orally _____ C. Ricci, CMA

Procedure 28-2 Obtaining an Aural Temperature Using the Tympanic Thermometer		
Date	Time	Note
3/30/XX	2:20 PM	T – 101.2°F (T) _____ C. Ricci, CMA

Procedure 28-3 Obtaining an Axillary Temperature		
Date	Time	Note
4/2/XX	9:30 AM	T – 98.2°F (A) _____ C. Ricci, CMA

Procedure 28-4 Obtaining Rectal Temperature		
Date	Time	Note
4/10/XX	3:30 PM	T – 100.4°F (R) _____ C. Ricci, CMA

Procedure 28-5 Obtaining an Apical Pulse		
Date	Time	Note
4/22/XX	4:10 PM	AP – 92 irregular _____ C. Ricci, CMA

Procedure 28-6 Assessing the Patient's Pulse (radial pulse)		
Date	Time	Note
5/6/XX	8:35 AM	P – 72, reg _____ C. Ricci, CMA

Procedure 28-7 Determining Respirations		
Date	Time	Note
5/12/XX	1:15 PM	R – 18 _____ C. Ricci, CMA

Procedure 28-8 Determining a Patient's Blood Pressure		
Date	Time	Note
5/19/XX	3:20 PM	BP – 120/80 Ⓛ arm _____ C. Ricci, CMA

Orthostatic Hypotension Documentation:		
Date	Time	Note
5/19/XX	3:25 PM	BP – 120/80 sitting, BP – 102/68 standing Ⓛ arm _____ C. Ricci, CMA

Procedure 28-9 Measuring a Patient's Height and Weight		
Date	Time	Note
5/26/XX	11:07 AM	Wt – 136¹/2 lb, Ht – 64¹/4 in ———————————————————————— C. Ricci, CMA

Procedure 32-1 Dispensing and Administering Oral Medications		
Date	Time	Note
6/8/XX	9:45 AM	Aldomet tab 250 mg po administered per physician order ————— Dorothy Gaston, CMA

Procedure 32-4 Giving an Intradermal Injection		
Date	Time	Note
6/17/XX	11:00 AM	0.1 ml PPD administered to Ⓛ mid-forearm. Pt given directions to read site in 48 hrs and
		return postcard to office. ——————————————————— Dorothy Gaston, CMA

Procedure 32-5 Administering a Tuberculin Tine Test		
Date	Time	Note
6/22/XX	2:00 PM	Tine test administered to Ⓡ mid-forearm. Pt scheduled to return 6/24/XX to have test read.
		————————————————————————— Dorothy Gaston, CMA
6/24/XX	4:10 PM	Area slightly inflamed, no induration noted at site of Tine test. Test read as negative. ———
		————————————————————————— Dorothy Gaston, CMA

Procedure 32-6 Giving a Subcutaneous Injection		
Date	Time	Note
7/1/XX	12:15 PM	15 U Novolin 70/30 administered SC per order to Ⓡ posterior upper arm. No problems noted.
		————————————————————————— Dorothy Gaston, CMA

Procedure 32-7 Giving an Intramuscular Injection		
Date	Time	Note
7/6/XX	9:30 AM	200,000 U Penicillin G administered IM per physician order to Ⓡ mid-deltoid region.
		Patient observed for 30 min post-injection. No complications noted. ———————
		————————————————————————— Dorothy Gaston, CMA

Procedure 32-9 Giving a Z-Track Intramuscular Injection		
Date	Time	Note
7/13/XX	1:25 PM	1 ml INFeD administered Z-Track IM in Ⓡ dorsogluteal site. Injection site not massaged
		after administration. No evidence of skin discoloration after administration.———————
		————————————————————————— Dorothy Gaston, CMA

Procedure 33-3 Administering Oxygen		
Date	Time	Note
7/24/XX	3:05 PM	R – 28 and labored. Oxygen initiated at 4 L/min via nasal cannula per physician order. Pt
		observed for signs of dyspnea and tachypnea.————————— Cheryl Skurka, CMA

Procedure 33-4	Responding to a Patient With an Obstructed Airway	
Date	Time	Note
7/22/XX	8:35 AM	Pt in waiting room coughing forcefully but clutching throat. After confirming pt choking,
		abdominal thrusts administered until foreign body expelled. Pt breathing without difficulty;
		R – 18. Situation reported to physician.———————————————— Cheryl Skurka, CMA

Procedure 33-5	Caring for a Patient Who Fainted	
Date	Time	Note
7/29/XX	4:18 PM	Pt in waiting room states she feels faint. Pt lowered to floor, clothes loosened, and legs
		elevated. Physician notified. P – 88 and regular, R – 22, BP 112/66. Syncopal episode
		persisted for 90 sec, feeling of vertigo lasted 10 minutes post-syncope. Pt transferred to
		exam room via wheelchair after recovery.———————————— Cheryl Skurka, CMA

Procedure 34-1	Measuring Distance Visual Acuity Using the Snellen Chart	
Date	Time	Note
8/01/XX	2:20 PM	Visual acuity exam completed c̄ Snellen eye chart. OD 20/40; OS 20-30 –1; OU 20/30 c̄
		corrective lenses. No squinting noted. ———————————————— Kim Tau, CMA

Procedure 34-3	Irrigating a Patient's Eyes	
Date	Time	Note
8/06/XX	9:00 AM	OD irrigated with 500 cc normal saline. Sclera clear post-irrigation. No c/o discomfort.———
		———————————————————————————————— Kim Tau, CMA

Procedure 34-4	Instilling Eye Medication	
Date	Time	Note
8/8/XX	1:45 PM	Thin ribbon of Neosporin ophthalmic ung applied in lower conjunctival sac of OS. No pt
		complaints. Pt instructed on homecare application of med including washing hands before
		and after procedure and taking care not to touch eye with applicator. ———————
		———————————————————————————————— Kim Tau, CMA

Procedure 34-6	Irrigating a Patient's Ear	
Date	Time	Note
8/12/XX	10:15 AM	AS irrigated with 500 cc warm saline soln. Large amt of dark brown cerumen expelled. Post-
		irrigation TM visible and pearly gray. No c/o discomfort. ——————— Kim Tau, CMA

Procedure 34-7	Instilling Medicated Ear Drops	
Date	Time	Note
8/12/XX	3:22 PM	ii gtts Auralgan otic soln administered to AD. No c/o discomfort. Pt instructed on home use.
		———————————————————————————————— Kim Tau, CMA

Procedure 34-8   Collecting a Specimen for Throat Culture

Date	Time	Note
8/14/XX	8:35 AM	Throat specimen collected via swab from tonsillar area. Sent to University Laboratories for
		Strep testing. ————————————————————————— Kim Tau, CMA

Procedure 37-1   Teaching Testicular Self-Examination

Date	Time	Note
8/19/XX	11:12 AM	Pt shown and successfully demonstrated testicular self-exam on model. Given pamphlet and
		shower card for home use. ———————————————— Dorothy Gaston, CMA

Procedure 37-2   Catheterization of a Female Patient

Date	Time	Note
8/22/XX	1:22 PM	Pt catheterized for 150 cc dark yellow turbid urine. Sample sent to lab for UA, C&S. ————
		—————————————————————————————— Sara Ricci, CMA

Procedure 38-1   Assisting With Examination of the Female Patient and Pap Smear

Date	Time	Note
8/23/XX	2:00 PM	Pap smear prepared. Slides placed for pick-up by University Laboratory for cytology.————
		—————————————————————————————— Betsy Davis, CMA

Procedure 39-1   Measuring the Circumference of an Infant's Head

Date	Time	Note
8/24/XX	10:15 AM	Head circumference: 43 1/2 cm ————————————— Susie Kwong, CMA

Procedure 39-2   Measuring Infant Length and Weight

Date	Time	Note
8/24/XX	10:20 AM	Wt 17 lb 4 oz Length 27 in —————————————— Susie Kwong, CMA

Procedure 39-4   Applying a Urinary Collection Device

Date	Time	Note
8/24/XX	10:15 AM	Urine specimen collected for culture. Placed for pick-up by North Hills Laboratory.————
		—————————————————————————————— Susie Kwong, CMA

Procedure 40-1   Assisting With Cold Application

Date	Time	Note
8/27/XX	1:45 PM	Ice pack applied to Ⓡ knee for 20 min. No c/o of discomfort. Pt instructed to continue ice
		application q 3 hrs while awake for 24 hrs at 20 min intervals. To call physician if edema
		persists. ———————————————————————— Kaiwan Tillman, CMA

Procedure 40-2	Assisting With Hot Moist Heat Application in the Office	
Date	Time	Note
9/2/XX	8:35 AM	Commercial hot pack applied to lumbar region for 20 min. Pt states muscle cramps relieved.
		Instructed to continue hot packs q 2 hrs for 20 min prn for relief of muscular pain. To return
		to office 9/5/XX for further evaluation. ———————————— Kaiwan Tillman, CMA

Procedure 40-3	Assisting With Therapeutic Ultrasound	
Date	Time	Note
9/6/XX	4:33 PM	Ultrasound treatment applied to Ⓡ lower back @ 3 watts X 6 minutes. No pt discomfort
		during procedure. Pt states pain relief, increased muscle relaxation.———————
		———————————————————— Kaiwan Tillman, CMA

Procedure 40-4	Assisting With Cast Application	
Date	Time	Note
9/7/XX	3:17 PM	Applied short fiberglass cast to Ⓡ leg. Skin under cast is clean and intact. Pt given written
		instructions on cast care. ——————————————— Kaiwan Tillman, CMA

Procedure 40-7	Assisting the Patient With Crutch Walking	
Date	Time	Note
9/8/XX	1:50 PM	Pt instructed in crutch walking using 3-point gait on steps and floor. Pt understands he is to
		be non-weight bearing on Ⓡ leg. Demonstrated techniques without difficulty.———
		———————————————————— Kaiwan Tillman, CMA

Procedure 41-3	Preparing the Patient For and Assisting With a Lumbar Puncture	
Date	Time	Note
9/15/XX	8:32 AM	Lumbar puncture performed by Dr. Song. 30 cc of CSF placed for pick-up by North Hills
		Laboratory. Pt to remain in prone position for at least 8 hours. Pt to be given instructions
		for home care and pain relief upon leaving the office.——————— Mai Lee, CMA

Procedure 46-1	Obtaining a 12-lead ECG	
Date	Time	Note
9/22/XX	12:45 PM	12-lead ECG recorded without incident.———————— Marcus Reyes, CMA

Procedure 46-2	Applying a Holter Monitor	
Date	Time	Note
9/29/XX	3:10 PM	Holter monitor applied per physician order. Pt given instructions to leave leads in place until
		she returns to office tomorrow afternoon. Understands to record cardiac symptoms in diary,
		to use event marker if symptoms occur, and not to shower until monitor removed.
		———————————————————— Marcus Reyes, CMA

Procedure 49-4   Measuring Specific Gravity Using a Refractometer

Date	Time	Note
10/1/XX	9:28 AM	SG: 1.010 ————————————————————————————— Rosa Gonzales, CMA

Procedure 49-9   Performing a Pregnancy Test

Date	Time	Note
10/2/XX	3:47 PM	LMP: 8/16/XX. QuickVue pregnancy test: Positive. ————————— Rosa Gonzales, CMA

Procedure 49-10   Performing a Rapid Urine Culture Test

Date	Time	Note
10/4/XX	1:10 PM	Uricult: Normal (<10,000 cfu/mL) ———————————————— Rosa Gonzales, CMA

Procedure 50-2   Collecting a Venous Blood Sample Using the Evacuated Tube Method

Date	Time	Note
10/5/XX	1:45 PM	Venous blood drawn from Ⓡ arm for CBC with differential and SMA 12. Placed for pick-up by
		Health Alliance Labs. ————————————————————— Leah Barney, CMA

Procedure 51-1   Performing a Microhematocrit

Date	Time	Note
10/7/XX	11:25 AM	Hct: 44. ——————————————————————————— Dana Cummings, CMA

Procedure 51-2   Performing a Hemoglobin Test

Date	Time	Note
10/9/XX	9:25 AM	Hb 15.5 g/dL. ————————————————————————— Dana Cummings, CMA

Procedure 51-11   Performing a Blood Glucose Accu-Check Test

Date	Time	Note
10/11/XX	8:30 AM	Pt last ate on 10/10 @ 12:30 AM. FBS: 92 mg/dl Dana Cummings, CMA

Procedure 54-14   Applying/Changing a Dressing

Date	Time	Note
10/12/XX	2:15 PM	Dressing change completed to wound on Ⓛ mid-forearm. Area slightly inflamed, mod amt of
		serosanguineous drainage noted. Site cleansed and sterile dressing applied. Pt instructed on
		home wound care and to notify physician if drainage changes, inflammation increases, or fever
		occurs. ——————————————————————— Melissa Gelbart, CMA

Procedure 54-16   Bandaging Using Gauze and Elastic Dressings

Date	Time	Note
10/22/XX	9:35 AM	Spiral elastic bandage applied to Ⓡ forearm. Pt denies bandage too tight. Fingers warm to
		touch. ——————————————————————————— Melissa Gelbart, CMA

Glossary

abscess Localized collection of pus that may be under the skin or deep within the body that causes tissue destruction.

academic degree A title conferred by a college, university, or professional school on completion of a program of study.

accommodation Adjustment of the eye for seeing various sizes of objects at different distances.

account A statement of transactions during a fiscal period and the resulting balance.

account balance The amount owed on an account.

accounts payable Debts incurred and not yet paid.

accounts receivable Amounts owed to the physician.

accounts receivable ledger A record of the charges and payments posted on an account.

accounts receivable trial balance A method of determining that the journal and the ledger are in balance.

accreditation The process through which an organization is recognized for adherence to a group of standards that meet or exceed expectations of the accrediting agency.

accrual basis of accounting Method of accounting in which income is recorded when earned, and expenses are recorded when incurred.

act The formal action of a legislative body; a decision or determination of a sovereign state, a legislative council, or a court of justice.

adage A saying, often in metaphorical form, that embodies a common observation.

adhesions Bands of scar tissue that bind together two anatomical surfaces that are normally separate.

adnexal Pertaining to adjacent or accessory parts.

adrenocorticotropic hormone (ACTH) A hormone that stimulates the production and secretion of glucocorticoids; released by the anterior pituitary gland.

advent A coming into being or use.

advocate One who pleads the cause of another; one who defends or maintains a cause or proposal.

affable Being pleasant and at ease in talking to others; characterized by ease and friendliness.

agenda A list or outline of things to be considered or done.

aggression A forceful action or procedure intended to dominate; hostile, injurious, or destructive behavior, especially when caused by frustration.

albuminuria Abnormal presence of albumin in the urine.

aliquot A portion of a well-mixed sample removed for testing.

allegation A statement by a party to a legal action of what the party undertakes to prove, an assertion made without proof.

allied health fields Occupational disciplines in which professionals involved with the delivery of healthcare or related services assist physicians with the diagnosis, treatment, and care of patients in many different specialty areas.

allocating Apportioning for a specific purpose or to particular persons or things.

allopathy A word coined by Samuel Christian Hahnemann to contrast homeopathic medicine with mainstream medicine; medicine supposedly characterized by an effort to counteract the symptoms of a disease by administration of treatments that produce an opposite effect from the symptoms.

allowed charge The maximum amount of money that many third-party payors allow for a specific procedure or service.

alopecia Partial or complete lack of hair.

alphabetical filing Any system that arranges names or topics according to the sequence of the letters in the alphabet.

alphanumeric Systems made up of combinations of letters and numbers.

ambiguous Capable of being understood in two or more possible senses or ways; unclear.

amblyopia Reduction or dimness of vision with no apparent organic cause; often referred to as lazy eye syndrome.

ambulatory Able to walk about and not be bedridden.

amenities Something that contributes to comfort, enjoyment, or convenience.

amenity Something conducive to comfort, convenience, or enjoyment.

amino acids Organic compounds that form the chief constituents of protein and are used by the body to build and repair tissues.

amorphous Lacking a defined shape.

analyte The substance or chemical being analyzed or detected in a specimen.

anaphylaxis Exaggerated hypersensitivity reaction that, in severe cases, leads to vascular collapse, bronchospasm, and shock.

anaplastic Alteration in cells to a more primitive form; cancer-producing cells.

anastomosis The surgical joining together of two normally distinct organs.

ancillary Subordinate; auxiliary.

ancillary diagnostic services Services that support patient diagnoses (e.g., laboratory or radiology services).

ancillary therapeutic services Services that support patient treatment (specialists or surgery).

"and" In the context of ICD-9-CM, the word "and" should be interpreted as "and/or."

anemia A condition marked by deficiency of RBCs.

angiocardiography Radiography of the heart and great vessels using an iodine contrast medium.

angiography Radiography of blood vessels using an iodine contrast medium.

angioplasty Interventional technique using a catheter to open or widen a blood vessel to improve circulation.

animate Full of life; to give spirit and support to expressions.

annotating To furnish with notes, which are usually critical or explanatory.

annotation A note added by way of comment or explanation.

anomalies Faulty development of the fetus resulting in deformities or deviations from normal.

anorexia Lack or loss of appetite for food.

anoxia Absence of oxygen in the tissues.

anteroposterior (AP) Frontal projection in which the patient is supine or facing the x-ray tube.

antibody Immunoglobulin produced by the immune system in response to bacteria, viruses, or other antigenic substances.

anticoagulant A chemical added to the blood after collection to prevent clotting.

antigen Foreign substance that causes the production of a specific antibody.

antimicrobial agent A drug that is used to treat infection.

antiseptic Pertaining to substances that can be used on human tissue that inhibit the growth of micro-organisms, such as alcohol and povidone-iodine solution (Betadine).

aortogram Radiography of the aorta using an iodine contrast medium.

apnea Absence or cessation of breathing.

appeal A legal proceeding by which a case is brought before a higher court for review of the decision of a lower court.

appellate Having the power to review the judgment of another tribunal or body of jurisdiction, such as an appellate court.

applications software Software programs designed to perform specific tasks.

appraisal Act of giving an expert judgment of the value or merit of; also, evaluations of work performance.

arbitration The hearing and determination of a cause in controversy by a person or persons either chosen by the parties involved or appointed under statutory authority.

arbitrator A neutral person chosen to settle differences between two parties in a controversy.

archaic Of, relating to, or characteristic of an earlier or more primitive time.

archived To have filed or collected records or documents.

arrhythmia Abnormality or irregularity in the heart rhythm.

arteriography Radiography of arteries using an iodine contrast medium.

arthritis Inflammation of a joint.

arthrogram Fluoroscopic examination of the soft tissue components of joints with direct injection of a contrast medium into the joint capsule.

articular Pertaining to a joint.

artifact A structure or feature not normally present but visible as a result of an external agent or action, such as one seen in a microscopic specimen after fixation, or in an image produced by radiology or electrocardiography.

artificial intelligence The aspect of computer science that deals with computers taking on the attributes of humans. One such example is expert systems, which are capable of making decisions, such as software that is designed to help a physician diagnose a patient, given a set of symptoms. Game-playing programs and programs that are designed to recognize human speech are other examples.

ASCII codes Acronym for American Standard Code for Information Interchange; a code representing English characters as numbers where each is given a number from 0 to 127.

asepsis Being free from infection or infectious materials; the process of removing pathogenic microorganisms or protecting against infection by such organisms.

assault An intentional, unlawful attempt of bodily injury to another by force.

assent To agree to something, especially after thoughtful consideration.

assets The entire property of a person, association, corporation, or estate applicable or subject to the payment of debts.

assignment of benefits The transfer of the patient's legal right to collect benefits for medical expenses to the provider of those services, authorizing the payment to be sent directly to the provider.

asystole The absence of a heartbeat.

ataxia Failure or irregularity of muscle actions and coordination.

atria The two upper chambers of the heart.

atrioventricular (AV) node Part of the cardiac conduction system located between the atria and the ventricles.

atrophy Wasting away; decrease in the size of a normally developed organ.

attenuated Weakened, or changed, virulence of a pathogenic microorganism.

audiologist An allied health care professional specializing in evaluation of hearing function, detection of hearing impairment, and determination of the anatomical site of impairment.

audit A formal examination of an organization's or individual's accounts or financial situation; a methodical examination and review.

audit trail   The path left by a transaction when it has been completed, often referred to when tracking medical services used by patients or researching claims.

augment   To make greater, more numerous, larger, or more intense.

aura   Peculiar sensation preceding the appearance of more definite disturbance.

authenticated   Proof of; with regard to medical records, it applies to a signature, initials, or computer keystroke by the maker of the record who verifies that the record is correct.

authorization   A term used in managed care for an approved referral.

autoimmune   Disturbance in the immune system in which the body reacts against its own tissue. Examples of autoimmune disorders include multiple sclerosis, rheumatoid arthritis, and systemic lupus erythematosus.

axial projection   Radiograph taken with a longitudinal angulation of the x-ray beam; sometimes referred to as a semiaxial projection.

azotemia   Retention in the blood of excessive amounts of nitrogenous wastes.

backup   Any type of storage of files to prevent their loss in the event of hard disk failure.

bailiff   An officer of some U.S. courts usually serving as a messenger or usher, who keeps order at the request of the judge.

balance sheet   A financial statement for a specific date that shows the total assets, liabilities, and capital of the business.

bank reconciliation   The process of proving that a bank statement and checkbook balance are in agreement.

banners   Advertisements often found on a web page that can be animated to attract the user's attention in hopes that he or she will click on the ad, be redirected to the advertiser's home page, and purchase from the site or gain information from the site.

battery   A willful and unlawful use of force or violence on the person of another; an offensive touching or use of force on a person without his or her consent.

beneficence   The act of doing or producing good, especially performing acts of charity or kindness.

beneficiary   Individual entitled to receive benefits from an insurance policy or program, or a governmental entitlement program offering healthcare benefits. Also called a *participant, subscriber, dependent, enrollee,* or *member.*

benefits   Services or payments provided under a health plan, employee plan, or some other agreement, including programs such as health insurance, pensions, retirement planning, and many other options that may be offered to employees of a company or organization; the amount payable by an insurance company for a monetary loss to an individual insured by that company, under each coverage.

benign   Not cancerous and not recurring.

bevel   Angled tip of a needle.

bifurcates   Divides from one into two branches.

bifurcation   The point of forking or separating into two branches.

bilirubin   Orange-colored pigment in bile, which when it accumulates leads to jaundice.

bilirubinuria   Presence of bilirubin in the urine.

biophysical   Pertaining to the science dealing with the application of physical methods and theories to biologic problems.

birthday rule   Under law, when an individual is covered under two insurance policies, the insurance plan of the policyholder whose birthday comes first in the calendar year (month and day—not year) becomes the primary insurance.

bit   The smallest unit of information inside the computer, represented by either the digit "0" or "1"; eight bits equal one byte.

blatant   Completely obvious, conspicuous, or obtrusive, especially in a crass or offensive manner; brazen.

bond   A durable, formal paper used for documents.

bookkeeping   The recording of business and accounting transactions.

bounding pulse   Pulse that feels full because of increased power of cardiac contractions or as a result of increased blood volume.

bradycardia   A slow heartbeat; a pulse below 60 beats per minute.

bradypnea   Respirations that are regular in rhythm but slower than normal in rate.

broad-spectrum antimicrobial agent   A drug used to treat a broad range of infections.

bronchiectasis   Dilation of the bronchi and bronchioles associated with secondary infection or ciliary dysfunction.

bronchoconstriction   Narrowing of the bronchiole tubes.

bruit   Abnormal sound or murmur heard on auscultation of an organ, vessel, or gland.

bucky   Moving grid device that prevents scatter radiation from fogging the film.

bundle of His   Specialized muscle fibers that conduct electrical impulses from AV node to ventricular myocardium.

bundled codes   Procedures or services that are grouped together and paid as one.

burnout   Exhaustion of physical or emotional strength or motivation, usually as a result of prolonged stress or frustration.

bursa   A fluid-filled, saclike membrane that provides for cushioning and frictionless motion between two tissues.

byte   A unit of data that contains eight binary digits, or bits.

cache   A special high-speed storage that can either be a part of the computer's main memory or can be a separate storage device. One function of a cache is to store websites visited in the computer memory for faster recall the next time the website is requested.

candidiasis   Infection caused by a yeastlike fungus that typically affects the vaginal mucosa and skin.

cannula   Rigid tube that surrounds a blunt trocar or a sharp, pointed trocar inserted into the body; when withdrawn, fluid may escape from the body through the cannula, depending on where it is inserted.

capitation Payment method used by many managed care organizations wherein a fixed amount of money is reimbursed to the provider for patients enrolled during a specific period of time, no matter what services received or number of visits made.

caption A heading, title, or subtitle under which records are filed.

carcinogenic A substance that is known to cause cancer.

carcinogens A substance or agent that causes the development of or increases the incidence of cancer.

cardiac arrest Condition in which cardiac contractions completely stop.

cardiac arrhythmias Irregular heartbeat resulting from a malfunction of the electrical system of the heart.

cardioversion Using electroshock to convert an abnormal cardiac rhythm to a normal one.

carrier As related to insurance, a company that assumes the risk of an insurance policy.

carrier-direct system A system for electronic data submission in which the medical facility has a computer system designed to transmit claims to a specific carrier directly, without first passing through a clearinghouse.

cartilage Rubbery, smooth, somewhat elastic connective tissue covering the ends of bones.

case management The process of assessing and planning patient care, including referral and follow-up to ensure continuity of care and quality management.

cash basis of accounting Method of accounting in which income is recorded when received, and expenses are recorded when paid.

cash flow statement A financial summary for a specific period that shows the beginning balance on hand, the receipts and disbursements during the period, and the balance on hand at the end of the period.

casts Fibrous or protein material molded to the shape of the part in which it has accumulated and thrown off into the urine in kidney disease.

categorically Placed in a specific division of a system of classification.

cathartic A laxative preparation.

caustic A remark or phrase marked by sarcasm; a substance that burns or destroys tissue by chemical action.

CD burner A device that is capable of "writing" data onto a blank compact disk (CD) or copying data from one CD to a blank CD.

centrifuge An apparatus consisting essentially of a compartment spun about a central axis to separate contained materials of different specific gravities or to separate colloidal particles suspended in a liquid.

cerebrospinal fluid Fluid within the subarachnoid space, the central canal of the spinal cord, and the four ventricles of the brain.

certification To attest as being true, as represented, or as meeting a standard; to have been tested,

usually by a third party, and awarded a certificate based on proven knowledge.

cerumen A waxy secretion in the ear canal; commonly called ear wax.

cervical Neck region containing seven cervical vertebrae.

chain of command A series of executive positions in order of authority.

channels Means of communication or expression; courses or directions of thought.

characteristics Distinguishing traits, qualities, or properties.

chief complaint The reason for the patient's seeking medical care.

chiropractic A medical discipline in which chiropractic physicians focus on the nervous system and painlessly, manually adjust the vertebral column to affect the nervous system, resulting in healthier patients.

cholesterol Substance produced by the liver and found in plant and animal fats that can produce fatty deposits or atherosclerotic plaques in the blood vessels.

chronic bronchitis Recurrent inflammation of the membranes lining the bronchial tubes.

chronological order Of, relating to, or arranged in or according to the order of time.

circumvent To manage to get around, especially by ingenuity or stratagem.

circumvention To manage to get around, especially by ingenuity or stratagem.

cited Quoted by way of example, authority, or proof or mentioned formally in commendation or praise.

Civilian Health and Medical Program of the Uniformed Services (CHAMPUS) A government-sponsored program wherein authorized dependents of military personnel receive medical care. This program is now referred to as TRICARE.

Civilian Health and Medical Program of the Veterans Administration (CHAMPVA) A health benefits program run by the Department of Veterans Affairs (VA) that helps eligible beneficiaries pay the cost of specific healthcare services/supplies.

clarity The quality or state of being clear.

clauses A group of words containing a subject and predicate and functioning as a member of a complex or compound sentence.

clean claim An insurance claim form that has been completed correctly (no errors or omissions) and can be processed and paid promptly if the claim meets the restrictions on covered services and items.

clearinghouse A centralized facility, sometimes called a *third-party administrator* (TPA), to whom insurance claims are transmitted. Clearinghouses separate, check, and redistribute claims electronically to various insurance carriers, and may offer additional services to the physician; networks of banks that exchange checks with each other.

clinical trials Research studies that test how well new medical treatments or other interventions work in the subjects, usually human beings.

clitoris Small, elongated erectile body situated above the urinary meatus at the superior point of the labia minora.

clubbing Abnormal enlargement of the distal phalanges (fingers and toes), associated with cyanotic heart disease or advanced chronic pulmonary disease.

coagulate Capable of being formed into clots.

"code also" When more than one code is necessary to fully identify a given condition, "code also" or "use additional code" is used.

"code if applicable" Notation meaning that the designated code may be principal if no casual condition is applicable or known.

Code of Federal Regulations (CFR) A coded delineation of the rules and regulations published in the Federal Register by the various departments and agencies of the federal government. The CFR is divided into 50 titles that represent broad subject areas, and then chapters that provide specific detail.

coding Converting verbal or written descriptions into numerical and alphanumerical designations.

cognitive Pertaining to the operation of the mind process by which we become aware of perceiving, thinking, and remembering.

cohesive The state of sticking together tightly; exhibiting or producing the cohesion.

coinsurance A policy provision frequently found in medical insurance whereby the policyholder and the insurance company share the cost of *covered* losses in a specified ratio (i.e., 80/20 means 80% is covered by the insurer and 20% by the insured).

coitus Sexual union between male and female, also known as intercourse.

collagen Protein that forms the inelastic fibers of tendons, ligaments, and fascia.

collect on delivery (COD) Method of payment used when an article or item is delivered and payment is expected before it is released.

collodion Preparation of cellulose nitrate that, when applied to the skin, dries to a strong, thin, protective, transparent film.

colloidal Pertaining to a gluelike substance.

colony forming units (CFU) Term used when reporting bacteriuria; one CFU represents one bacterium present in the urine sample.

colostrum Thin, yellow, milky fluid secreted by the mammary glands a few days before and after delivery.

coma An unconscious state from which the patient cannot be aroused.

comfort zone A place in the mind where an individual feels safe and confident.

commensurate Corresponding in size, amount, extent, or degree; equal in measure.

commercial insurance Plans (*sometimes called private insurance*) that reimburse the insured for expenses resulting from illness or injury according to a specific fee schedule as outlined in the insurance policy and on a fee-for-service basis.

comorbidities Preexisting conditions that will, because of their presence with a specific principal diagnosis, cause an increase in length of an inpatient hospital stay by at least 1 day in approximately 75% of cases.

competence The quality or state of being competent; having adequate or requisite capabilities.

competent Having adequate abilities or qualities; having the capacity to function or perform in a certain way.

complications Conditions that arise during a hospital stay that prolong the length of stay by at least 1 day in approximately 75% of cases.

component A constituent part; a part of a larger group.

compression The state of being pressed together.

computed tomography (CT) Computerized x-ray imaging modality providing axial and three-dimensional scans.

computer A machine that is designed to accept, store, process, and give out information.

concise Expressing much in brief form.

concurrently Occurring at the same time.

cones Structures found in the retina that make the perception of color possible.

congruence The verbal expression of the message matches the sender's nonverbal body language.

congruent Being in agreement, harmony, or correspondence; conforming to the circumstances or requirements of a situation.

connotation An implication; something suggested by a word or thing.

contaminated Soiled with pathogens or infectious material; nonsterile.

contamination A process by which something is made impure, unclean, or unfit for use by the introduction of unwholesome or undesirable elements; becoming unsterile by contact with any nonsterile material.

continuation pages The second and following pages of a letter.

continuing education units (CEUs) Credits for courses, classes, or seminars related to an individual's profession, designed to promote education and to keep the professional up-to-date on current procedures and trends in their field; often required for licensing.

continuity of care Care that continues smoothly from one provider to another, so that the patient receives the most benefit and no interruption in care.

contraindication Something, as a symptom or condition, that makes a particular treatment or procedure inadvisable.

contralateral Pertaining to the opposite side of the body.

contrast media Radiopaque substances used to enhance visualization of soft tissues in imaging studies.

contributory negligence Statutes in some states that may prevent a party from recovering damages if he or she contributed in any way to the injury or condition.

cookies Messages sent to a web browser from a web server that identify users and can prepare custom web pages for them, possibly displaying their name on return to the site.

coordination of benefits (COB) The mechanism used in group health insurance to designate the order in which multiple carriers are to pay benefits to prevent duplicate payments.

copayment A sum of money that is paid at the time of medical service; a form of coinsurance.

COPD Chronic obstructive pulmonary disease; a progressive and irreversible lung condition that results in diminished lung capacity.

copulation Sexual intercourse.

coronal plane Plane that divides the body into anterior and posterior parts.

corticosteroids Antiinflammatory hormones, natural or synthetic.

costal Pertaining to the ribs.

coulombs per kilogram (C/kg) International unit of radiation exposure.

counteroffer Return offer made by one who has rejected an offer or job.

creatinine Nitrogenous waste from muscle metabolism excreted in urine.

credentialing The act of extending professional or medical privileges to an individual; the process of verifying and evaluating that person's credentials.

credibility The quality or power of inspiring belief.

credit An entry on an account constituting an addition to a revenue, net worth, or liability account; the balance in a person's favor in an account.

crenate Forming notches or leaflike scalloped edges on an object.

crepitation Dry, crackling sound or sensation.

critical thinking The constant practice of considering all aspects of a situation when deciding what to believe or what to do.

cross-training Training in more than one area, so that a multitude of duties may be performed by one person, or so that substitutions of personnel may be made when necessary or in emergencies.

cryosurgery Technique of exposing tissue to extreme cold to produce a well-defined area of cell destruction.

cryptogenic Hidden origin.

cultivate To foster the growth of; to improve by labor, care, or study.

culture and sensitivity (C&S) A procedure performed in the microbiology laboratory in which a specimen is cultured on artificial media to detect bacterial or fungal growth, followed by appropriate screening for antibiotic sensitivity.

curettage Act of scraping a body cavity with a surgical instrument, such as a curette.

cursor A symbol appearing on the monitor that shows where the next character to be typed will appear.

curt Marked by rude or peremptory shortness.

cyanosis Blue color of the mucous membranes and body extremities caused by lack of oxygen.

cyberspace Describes the nonphysical space of the online world of computer networks in which communication takes place.

cyst A small capsule-like sac that encloses certain organisms in their dormant or larval stage.

cytology The study of cells using microscopic methods.

damages Loss or harm resulting from injury to person, property, or reputation; compensation in money imposed by law for losses or injuries.

database A collection of related files that serves as a foundation for retrieving information.

debit An entry on an account constituting an addition to an expense or asset account or a deduction from a revenue, a net worth, or a liability account.

debit cards A card that looks like a credit card and by which money may be withdrawn or the cost of purchases paid directly from the holder's bank account without the payment of interest.

debridement Removal of foreign material and dead, damaged tissue from a wound.

decedent A legal term for a deceased person.

decode To convert, as in a message, into intelligible form; to recognize and interpret.

decubitus ulcer A sore or ulcer over a bony prominence that is due to ischemia from prolonged pressure; a bedsore.

deductible A specific amount of money a patient must pay out-of-pocket before the insurance carrier begins paying. Usually this amount ranges from $100 to $500. This deductible amount is met on a yearly or per-incident basis.

default Failure to pay financial debts, such as a student loan.

defense mechanisms Psychological methods of dealing with stressful situations that are encountered in day-to-day living.

deferment Postponement, especially of a student loan.

defibrillator Machine used to deliver an electroshock to the heart through electrodes placed on the chest wall.

deficiencies Conditions caused by a below-normal intake of a particular substance.

demeanor Behavior toward others; outward manner.

demographic The statistical characteristics of human populations (as in age or income) used especially to identify markets.

dependents The spouse, children, and sometimes domestic partner or other individuals designated by the insured who are covered under a healthcare plan.

depleted To lessen markedly in quantity, content, power, or value.

detrimental Obviously harmful or damaging.

device driver The program or commands given to a device connected to a computer that enable the device to function. For instance, a printer may come equipped with a software program that must be loaded onto the computer first, so that the printer will work.

diabetes mellitus type 1 A disease in which the beta cells in the pancreas no longer produce insulin. Patients must rely on daily insulin administration to utilize glucose for energy and prevent complications.

diabetes mellitus type 2 A disease in which the body is unable to utilize glucose for energy as a result of either a lack of insulin production in the pancreas or resistance to insulin on the cellular level.

diagnosis Concise technical description of the cause, nature, or manifestations of a condition or problem. *Initial:* Physician's temporary impression, sometimes called a *working diagnosis*. *Differentiated diagnosis:* comparison of two or more diseases with similar signs and symptoms. *Final:* Conclusion physician reaches after evaluating all findings, including laboratory and other test results.

diaphoresis   The profuse excretion of sweat.

diaphysis   Midportion of a long bone containing the medullary cavity.

dictation   The act or manner of uttering words to be transcribed.

diction   The choice of words especially with regard to clearness, correctness, or effectiveness.

digestion   Process of converting food into chemical substances that can be used by the body.

digital signature   A signature used for electronic claims; it consists of lines of text or a text box and is attached through a software application.

digital subscriber line (DSL)   High-speed, sophisticated modulation scheme that operates over existing copper telephone wiring systems; often referred to as "last-mile technologies," because DSL is used for connections from a telephone switching station to a home or office, and not from between switching stations.

digital versatile disk or digital video disk (DVD)   An optical disk that holds approximately 28 times more information than a CD; a DVD is most commonly used to hold full-length movies. Compared with a CD, which holds approximately 600 megabytes, a DVD has the capacity to hold approximately 4.7 gigabytes.

dilatation   Opening or widening the circumference of a body orifice with a dilating instrument.

dilatation and curettage   The widening of the cervix and scraping of the endometrial wall of the uterus.

dilation   The opening of the cervix through the process of labor, measured as 0 to 10 cm dilated.

diluent   A liquid used to dilute a specimen or reagent.

dingy claim   A claim that is delayed because it cannot be processed, usually because the software used to transfer the claim or system changes make it incompatible with the receiving system.

diplopia   Double vision.

direct filing system   A filing system in which materials can be located without consulting an intermediary source of reference.

dirty claim   Claims that contain errors or omissions that cannot be processed or must be processed by hand because of OCR scanner rejection.

disability income insurance   Insurance that provides periodic payments to replace income when an insured person is unable to work as a result of illness, injury, or disease.

disbursements   Money (funds) paid out.

disbursements journal   A summary of accounts paid out.

discretion   The quality of being discrete; having or showing good judgment or conduct, especially in speech.

diseases   Pathological processes having a descriptive set of signs and symptoms.

disinfection   Destruction of pathogens by physical or chemical means.

disk   A removable device with a magnetic surface that is capable of storing computer programs, stored in a hard plastic square; also called diskettes, and early versions were called "floppy disks."

disk drives   Devices that load a program or data stored on a disk into the computer.

disorder   A disruption of normal system functions.

disparaging   Speak slightly about, with a negative or degrading tone.

disparities   Containing or made up of fundamentally different and often incongruous elements; markedly distinct in quality or character.

disposition   The tendency of something or someone to act in a certain manner under given circumstances.

disruption   An unexpected event that throws a plan into disorder; an interruption that prevents a system or process from continuing as usual or as expected.

dissect   To cut or separate tissue with a cutting instrument or scissors.

dissection   Separation into pieces and exposure of parts for scientific examination.

disseminate   To disperse throughout; to spread around.

diurnal rhythm   Patterns of activity or behavior that follow day-night cycles.

docket   A formal record of judicial proceedings; a list of legal causes to be tried.

domestic mail   Mail that is sent within the boundaries of the United States and its territories.

dosimeter   Badge for monitoring radiation exposure to personnel.

downcoding   A change in code done by the insurance company that receives a claim resulting in a lesser reimbursement. The change will usually be the code closest to the one submitted on the claim, because the code does not match in some way to the specifications of the insurance company.

drawee   Bank or facility on whom a check is drawn or written.

drawer   Person who writes a check.

due process   A fundamental constitutional guarantee that all legal proceedings will be fair; that one will be given notice of the proceedings and given an opportunity to be heard before the government acts to take away life, liberty, or property; a constitutional guarantee that a law will not be unreasonable or arbitrary.

duty   Obligatory tasks, conduct, service, or functions that arise from one's position, as in life or in a group.

dyspnea   Difficult or painful breathing.

e-banking   Electronic banking via computer modem or over the Internet.

ecchymosis   A hemorrhagic skin discoloration commonly called bruising; bluish-black skin discoloration produced by hemorrhagic areas.

ecommerce   An abbreviation for *electronic commerce*; used to describe the sale and purchase of goods and services over the Internet; doing business over the Internet.

ectopic   Originating outside of the normal tissue.

edema   Abnormal accumulation of fluid in the interstitial spaces of tissues; swelling between layers of tissue.

effacement   The thinning of the cervix during labor measured in percentages from 0 to 100 effaced.

effective date   The date on which an insurance policy or plan takes effect so that benefits are payable.

elastic pulse Pulse with regular alterations of weak and strong beats without changes in cycle.

elastin Essential part of elastic connective tissue that, when moist, is flexible and elastic.

electrodesiccation Destruction of cells and tissue by means of short high-frequency electrical sparks.

electronic claims Claims that are submitted to insurance processing facilities using a computerized medium, such as direct data entry, direct wire, dial-in telephone digital fax, or personal computer download/upload.

electronic data interchange The transfer of data back and forth between two or more entities using an electronic medium.

electronic signature A scanned signature or other such mark that is accepted as proof of approval and/or responsibility for the content of an electronic document.

email Communications transmitted via computer using a modem.

emancipated minor A person under legal age who is self-supporting and living apart from parents or guardian; a mature minor considered to possess a sufficient understanding of self-care and responsibility.

embezzlement Stealing from an employer; to appropriate goods, services, or funds for personal use without permission.

embolization Interventional technique using a catheter to block off a blood vessel to prevent hemorrhage.

embolus Foreign material blocking a blood vessel, frequently a blood clot that has broken away from some other part of the body.

emetic A substance that causes vomiting.

empathy Sensitivity to the individual needs and reactions of patients.

emphysema Pathological accumulation of air in the tissues or organs; in the lungs, the bronchioles become plugged with mucus and lose elasticity.

employer identification number (EIN) The number used by the Internal Revenue Service that identifies a business or individual functioning as a business entity for income tax reporting.

emulsification Dispersion of ingested fats into small globules by bile.

encode To convert from one system of communication to another; to convert a message into code.

encounter Any contact between a healthcare provider and a patient that results in treatment or evaluation of the patient's condition; not limited to in-person contact.

encroachments That which advances beyond the usual or proper limits.

encrypt To convert from one system of communication to another; encode.

endemic Disease or microorganism that is specific to a particular geographic area.

endocervical curettage The scraping of cells from the wall of the uterus.

endorser Person who signs his or her name on the back of a check for the purpose of transferring title to another person.

enteric-coated Drug formulation in which tablets are coated with a special compound that does not dissolve until the tablet is exposed to the fluids of the small intestine.

enunciate To utter articulate sounds; the act of being very distinct in speech.

enunciation Utterance of articulate, clear sounds.

environment The state of a computer, usually determined by the programs that are running as well as hardware and software characteristics.

enzymatic reaction Chemical reaction controlled by an enzyme.

enzyme Any of several complex proteins that are produced by cells and act as catalysts in specific biochemical reactions.

epiphysis End of a long bone.

equities The money value of a property or of an interest in a property in excess of claims or liens against it.

erroneous Containing or characterized by error or assumption.

erythropoietin Substance released from the kidney and liver that promotes red blood cell formation.

essential hypertension Elevated blood pressure of unknown cause that develops for no apparent reason; sometimes called primary hypertension.

established patients Patients who are returning to the office who have previously been seen by the physician.

etiology The cause of the disorder; a claim may be classified according to etiology.

eukaryote A single-celled or multicellular organism whose cells contain a distinct membrane-bound nucleus.

euthanasia The act or practice of killing or permitting the death of hopelessly sick or injured individuals in a relatively painless way for reasons of mercy.

exacerbation An increase in the seriousness of a disease marked by greater intensity in the signs and symptoms.

"excludes" Exclusion terms are always written in italics, and the word "excludes" is often enclosed in a box to draw particular attention to these instructions. Exclusion terms may apply to a chapter, a section, a category, or subcategory. The applicable code number usually follows the exclusion term.

exclusions Limitations on an insurance contract for which benefits are not payable.

expediency A means of achieving a particular end, as in a situation requiring haste or caution.

expert witness A person who provides testimony to a court as an expert in a certain field or subject to verify facts presented by one or both sides in a lawsuit, often compensated and used to refute or disprove the claims of one party.

external noise Sounds or factors outside the brain that interfere with the communication process.

externalization To attribute an event or occurrence to causes outside the self.

externship/internship A training program that is part of a course of study of an educational institution and is taken in the actual business setting in that field of study; these terms are often interchanged in reference to medical assisting.

extrinsic   External to a thing, its essential nature, or its original character.

exudates   Fluids with high concentration of protein and cellular debris that have escaped from the blood vessels and have been deposited in tissues or on tissue surfaces.

familial   Occurring in or affecting members of a family more than would be expected by chance.

fascia   Sheet or band of fibrous tissue located deep in the skin that covers muscles and body organs.

fastidious   Requiring specialized media or growth factors to grow.

fax   Abbreviation for *facsimile*; also, a document sent using a facsimile (fax) machine.

febrile   Pertaining to an elevated body temperature.

fecalith   A hard, impacted mass of feces in the colon.

fee for service   An established schedule of fees set for services performed by providers and paid by the patient.

fee profile   A compilation or average of physician fees over a given period of time.

fee schedule   A compilation of preestablished fee allowances for given services or procedures.

feedback   The transmission of evaluative or corrective information to the original or controlling source about an action, event, or process.

felony   A major crime, such as murder, rape, or burglary; punishable by a more stringent sentence than that given for a misdemeanor.

fermentation   An enzymatically controlled transformation of an organic compound.

fervent   Exhibiting or marked by great intensity of feeling.

fibrillation   Rapid, random, ineffective contractions of the heart.

fidelity   Faithfulness to something to which one is bound by pledge or duty.

filtrate   Fluid that remains after a liquid is passed through a membranous filter.

fine   A sum imposed as punishment for an offense; a forfeiture or penalty paid to an injured party or the government in a civil or criminal action.

fiscal agent   An organization under contract to the government as well as some private plans to act as financial representatives in handling insurance claims from providers of health care; also referred to as *fiscal intermediary*.

fiscal intermediary   An organization that contracts with the government to handle and mediate insurance claims from medical facilities, home health agencies, or providers of medical services or supplies.

fiscal year   An accounting period of 12 months.

fissures   Narrow slits or clefts in the abdominal wall.

fistula   Abnormal, tube-like passage between internal organs or from an internal organ to the body surface.

flagged   Marked in some way as to remind or remember that specific action needs to be taken.

flash   Animation technology often used on the opening page of a website to draw attention, excite, and impress the user.

flatus   Gas expelled through the anus.

fluoroscopy   Direct observation of the x-ray image in motion.

flush   Directly abutting or immediately adjacent, as set even with an edge of a type page or column; having no indention.

follicle-stimulating hormone (FSH)   A hormone secreted by the anterior pituitary; stimulates oogenesis and spermatogenesis.

font   A design for a set of type characters; a combination of typeface, spacing, pitch, and other qualities. Fonts are named; examples include Times Roman, Arial, and Garamond.

format   To magnetically create tracks on a disk where information will be stored, usually done by the manufacturer of the disk.

fovea centralis   A small pit in the center of the retina that is considered the center of clearest vision.

frontal projection   Radiographic view in which the coronal plane of the body or body part is parallel to the film plane; AP or PA.

gait   How a person walks; manner or style of walking.

gametes   Mature male or female germ cells usually possessing a haploid chromosome set and capable of initiating formation of a new diploid individual.

gangrene   Death of body tissue as a result of loss of nutritive supply and followed by bacteria invasion and putrefaction.

gantry   Doughnut-shaped portion of a scanner that surrounds the patient and functions, at least in part, to gather imaging data.

generic   Drugs that are not protected by trademark.

genome   The genetic material of an organism.

genuineness   Expressing sincerity and honest feeling.

germicides   Agents that destroy pathogenic organisms.

gigabyte   Approximately 1 billion bytes; abbreviated GB.

girth   A measure around a body or item.

gleaned   Gathered bit by bit (e.g., information or material); picked over in search of relevant material.

gluconeogenesis   The formation of glucose in the liver from proteins and fats.

glycogen   The sugar (starch) formed from glucose and stored mainly in the liver.

glycosuria   The abnormal presence of glucose in the urine.

goniometer   Instrument for measuring the degrees of motion in a joint.

government plan   An entitlement program or health-care plan that is sponsored and/or subsidized by the state or federal government, such as Medicaid and Medicare.

gradient   A change in response with distance from the stimulus.

grammar   The study of the classes of words, their inflections, and their functions and relations in the sentence; a study of what is to be preferred and what avoided in inflection and syntax.

Gray (Gy)   International unit of radiation dose.

grief   An unfortunate outcome; a deep distress caused by bereavement.

group policy   Insurance written under a policy that covers a number of people under a single master contract issued to their employer or to an association with which they are affiliated.

growth hormone (GH) Also called somatotropic hormone; stimulates tissue growth and restricts tissue glucose dependence when nutrients are not available.

guarantor The person who is responsible for paying a medical bill.

guardian ad litem Legal representative for a minor.

hard copy The readable paper copy or printout of information.

harmonious Marked by accord in sentiment or action; having the parts agreeably related.

health insurance Protection in return for periodic *premium* payments, which provides reimbursement of expenses resulting from illness or injury. Includes these forms of insurance: accident, disability income, medical expense, and accidental death and dismemberment. Also known as *accident and health insurance* or *disability income insurance*.

Health Insurance Portability and Accountability Act (HIPAA) The Kassebaum-Kennedy Act designed to improve portability and continuity of health insurance coverage; to combat waste, fraud, and abuse in health insurance and healthcare delivery; to promote the use of medical savings accounts; to improve access to long-term care services and coverage; to simplify the administration of health insurance; and for other purposes.

health maintenance organization (HMO) An organization that provides a wide range of comprehensive healthcare services for a specified group at a fixed periodic payment. HMOs can be sponsored by the government, medical schools, hospitals, employers, labor unions, consumer groups, insurance companies, and hospital-medical plans.

hematemesis Vomiting of bright red blood, indicating rapid upper gastrointestinal bleeding, associated with esophageal varices or peptic ulcer.

hematocrit The percentage by volume of packed red blood cells in a given sample of blood after centrifugation; volume percentage of erythrocytes in whole blood.

hematoma A sac filled with blood that may be the result of trauma.

hematuria Blood in the urine.

hemoconcentration A situation in which the concentration of blood cells is increased in proportion to the plasma.

hemoglobin Protein found in erythrocytes that transports molecular oxygen in the blood.

hemolysis The destruction or dissolution of red blood cells, with subsequent release of hemoglobin.

hemolyzed A term used to describe a blood sample in which the red blood cells have ruptured.

hepatomegaly Abnormal enlargement of the liver.

hereditary Pertaining to a characteristic, condition, or disease transmitted from parent to offspring on the DNA chain.

hermetically sealed Sealed so no air is allowed to enter.

holder Person presenting a check for payment.

holistic Related to or concerned with all of the systems of the body, rather than breaking it down into parts.

homeostasis Internal adaptation and change in response to environmental factors; maintaining constant internal environmental conditions compatible with life.

hormone A substance produced by one tissue and conveyed by the bloodstream to another to effect physiological activity, such as growth or metabolism.

HTML Acronym for HyperText Markup Language, which is the language used to create documents for use on the Internet.

HTTP Acronym for HyperText Transfer Protocol, which defines how messages are formatted and transmitted over the Internet. When a URL is entered into the computer, an HTTP command tells the web server to retrieve the requested web page.

hub A common connection point for devices in a network containing multiple ports, often used to connect segments of a LAN.

hydrocephaly Enlargement of the cranium caused by abnormal accumulation of cerebrospinal fluid within the cerebral system.

hydrogenated Combined with, treated with, or exposed to hydrogen.

hyperlipidemia Excess of fats or lipids in the blood plasma.

hyperplasia An increase in the number of cells.

hyperpnea Increase in the depth of breathing.

hypertension High blood pressure in which the systolic pressure is above 140 mm Hg or the diastolic pressure is above 90 mm Hg.

hyperventilation Abnormally prolonged and deep breathing usually associated with acute anxiety or emotional tension.

hypotension Blood pressure that is below normal (systolic pressure below 90 mm Hg and diastolic pressure below 50 mm Hg).

icon A picture, often on the desktop of a computer, that represents a program or an object. By clicking on the icon, the user is directed to the program.

idealism The practice of forming ideas or living under the influence of ideas.

idiopathic Without an apparent or known cause.

ileostomy Surgical formation of an opening of the ileum onto the surface of the abdomen through which fecal material is emptied.

immigrant A person who comes to a country to take up permanent residence.

immunotherapy Administering repeated injections of diluted extracts of the substance that causes an allergy; also called *desensitization*.

impenetrable Incapable of being penetrated or pierced; not capable of being damaged or harmed.

implied consent Presumed consent, such as when a patient offers an arm for a phlebotomy procedure.

in balance The total ending balances of patient ledgers equal total of accounts receivable control.

in vitro Refers to conditions outside of a living body; pertaining to a biological reaction that occurs in an artificial environment, such as in a test tube.

incentives   Something that incites or spurs to action; a reward or reason for performing a task.

"includes"   This term appearing under a subdivision, such as a category (three-digit code) or two-digit procedure code, indicates that the code and title include these terms. Other terms also classified to that particular code and title are listed in the Alphabetic Indexes.

incomplete claim   A claim that is missing information and is returned to the provider for correction and resubmission.

incontinence   Inability to control excretory functions.

indemnity plan   Traditional health insurance plan that pays for all or a share of the cost of covered services, regardless of which physician, hospital, or other licensed healthcare provider is used. Policyholders of indemnity plans and their dependents choose when and where to get healthcare services.

indicators   An important point or group of statistical values that, when evaluated, indicate the quality of care provided in a healthcare institution.

indicted   Charged with a crime by the finding or presentment of a jury with due process of law.

indigent   Totally lacking in something of need.

indirect filing system   A filing system in which an intermediary source of reference, such as a card file, must be consulted to locate specific files.

individual policy   An insurance policy designed specifically for the use of one person (and his or her dependents), not associated with the amenities of a group policy, namely higher premiums. Often called *personal insurance*.

induration   An abnormally hard, inflamed area.

infarction   Area of tissue that has died from lack of blood supply.

infection   Invasion of body tissues by microorganisms that then proliferate and damage tissues.

infertile   Not fertile or productive; not capable of reproducing.

inflammation   Tissue reaction to trauma or disease that includes redness, heat, swelling, and pain.

inflection   A change in pitch or loudness of the voice.

informed consent   A consent in which there is understanding of what treatment is to be undertaken and of the risks involved, why it should be done, and alternative methods of treatment available (including no treatment) and their attendant risks.

infraction   Breaking the law; a minor offense of the rules.

initiative   To cause or facilitate the beginning of; to initiate something into happening.

innate   Existing in, belonging to, or determined by factors present in an individual since birth.

input   Information entered into and used by the computer.

instigate   To goad or urge forward; to provoke.

insubordination   Disobedient to authority.

insured   An individual or organization who is covered by an insurance policy according to the policy terms, usually the individual or group who pays the premiums. Blue Cross/Blue Shield refers to this person or group as the subscriber.

intangibles   Incapable of being perceived, especially by touch; incapable of being precisely identified or realized by the mind.

integral   Essential; being an indispensable part of a whole.

interaction   A two-way communication; mutual or reciprocal action or influence.

intercom   A two-way communication system with a microphone and loudspeaker at each station for localized use.

intermittent   Coming and going at intervals; not continuous.

intermittent claudications   Recurring cramping in the calves caused by poor circulation of blood to the muscles of the lower leg.

intermittent pulse   Pulse in which beats are occasionally skipped.

internal noise   Factors inside the brain that interfere with the communication process.

International Classification of Diseases, Ninth Revision, Clinical Modification (ICD-9-CM)   System for classifying disease to facilitate collection of uniform and comparable health information, for statistical purposes and indexing medical records for data storage and retrieval.

International Classification of Diseases, Tenth Revision (ICD-10)   System containing the greatest number of changes in ICD's history. To allow more specific reporting of disease and newly recognized conditions, the ICD-10 contains approximately 5500 more codes than ICD-9.

international mail   Mail that is sent outside the boundaries of the United States and its territories.

interval   Space of time between events.

intolerable   Not tolerable or bearable.

intravenous urogram (IVU)   Radiographic examination of the urinary tract using intravenous injection of an iodine contrast medium.

intrinsic   Belonging to the essential nature or constitution of a thing; indwelling, inward; originating or due to causes within a body, organ, or part.

introspection   An inward, reflective examination of one's own thoughts and feelings.

invalid claim   A claim that is incorrect in some manner or does not present a logical picture of the patient's situation.

invariably   Consistent; not changing or capable of change.

invasive   Involving entry into the living body, as by incision or insertion of an instrument.

invoice   A paper describing a purchase and the amount due.

ipsilateral   Pertaining to the same side of the body.

irregular pulse   Pulse that varies in force and frequency.

ischemia   Decreased blood flow to a body part or organ, caused by constriction or plugging of the supplying artery.

ischemic   Characterized by temporary interruption in the blood supply to a tissue or organ.

jargon   The technical terminology or characteristic idiom of a particular group or special activity.

jaundice Yellowness of the skin and mucous membranes caused by deposition of bile pigment because of excess bilirubin in the blood; not a disease but a symptom of a number of diseases, especially liver disorders.

Java A commonly used object-oriented high-level programming language that is well suited for the Internet.

judicial Of or relating to a judgment, the function of judging, the administration of justice, or the judiciary.

jurisdiction A power constitutionally conferred on a judge or magistrate to decide cases according to law and to carry sentence into execution; jurisdiction is original when it is conferred on the court in the first instance, called original jurisdiction; or it is appellate, which is when an appeal is given from the judgment of another court.

jurisprudence The science or philosophy of law; a system or body of law or the course of court decisions.

keratin Very hard, tough protein found in hair, nails, and epidermal tissue.

keratinocytes Any one of the skin cells that synthesizes keratin.

kyphotic Relating to normal convex curvature of the thoracic spine region.

lacrimation The secretion or discharge of tears.

language barrier Any type of interference that inhibits the communication process that is related to languages spoken by the people attempting to communicate.

laryngoscopy Visual examination of the voice box area through an endoscope equipped with a light and mirrors for illumination.

latent image Invisible changes in exposed film that will become an image when the film is processed.

lateral projection Radiographic view in which the sagittal plane of the body or body part is parallel to the film.

law A binding custom or practice of a community; a rule of conduct or action prescribed or formally recognized as binding or enforceable by a controlling authority.

learning style The way that an individual perceives and processes information to learn new material.

leukoderma Lack of skin pigmentation, especially in patches.

liabilities Something that is owed; a debt.

liable Obligated according to law or equity; responsible for an act or circumstance.

libel A written defamatory statement or representation that conveys an unjustly unfavorable impression.

ligament A tough connective tissue band that holds joints together by attaching to the bones on either side of a joint.

ligation Process of tying off something to close it, usually a blood vessel during surgery, with a tie called a ligature.

limited radiography Limited-scope radiography practice, usually in an outpatient setting, that does not require the same credentials needed for professional radiologic technology; also called practical radiography.

lithotripsy A procedure for eliminating a stone by crushing or dissolving it in situ through the use of high intensity sound waves.

litigious Prone to engage in lawsuits.

loading dose Administering a double dose for the first dose of the medication; usually done with antibiotic therapy so that therapeutic blood levels are reached quickly.

lordotic Relating to normal concave curvature of the cervical and lumbar spine regions.

lower gastrointestinal (GI) series Fluoroscopic examination of the colon, usually employing rectal administration of barium sulfate as a contrast medium; also called a barium enema.

lumbar Lower back region containing five lumbar vertebrae.

lumen Open space, such as within a blood vessel, the intestine, the inside of a needle, or an examining instrument.

luteinizing hormone (LH) Hormone produced by the anterior pituitary gland; promotes ovulation.

luxation Dislocation of a bone from its normal anatomical location.

lymphadenopathy Any disorder of the lymph nodes or lymph vessels.

macromolecules The molecules needed for metabolism: carbohydrates, lipids, proteins, and nucleic acids.

magnetic resonance imaging (MRI) Imaging modality that uses a magnetic field and radiofrequency pulses to create computer images of both bones and soft tissues in multiple planes.

maker (of a check) Any individual, corporation, or legal party who signs a check or any type of negotiable instrument.

malaise Indefinite feeling of debility or lack of health, often indicative of or accompanying the onset of an illness.

malediction To speak evil of or curse.

malignant Cancerous.

managed care plans An umbrella term for all healthcare plans that provide healthcare in return for preset monthly payments and coordinated care through a defined network of primary care physicians and hospitals.

mandated Required by an authority or law.

mandatory Containing or constituting a command.

manifestation Something that is easily understood or recognized by the mind.

manipulation Moving or exercising a body part by an externally applied force.

Marfan syndrome An inherited condition characterized by elongation of the bones, joint hypermobility, abnormalities of the eyes, and development of aortic aneurysm.

marketing The process or technique of promoting, selling, and distributing a product or service.

matrix Something in which a thing originates, develops, takes shape, or is contained; a base on which to build.

m-banking Banking through the use of wireless devices, such as cellular phones and wireless Internet services.

media Term applied to agencies of mass communication, such as newspapers, magazines, and telecommunications.

mediastinum Space in the center of the chest under the sternum.

medical savings account A tax-deferred bank or savings account combined with a low-premium/high-deductible insurance policy, designed for individuals or families who choose to fund their own healthcare expenses and medical insurance.

medically indigent An individual who may be able to afford to pay for his or her normal daily living expenses but cannot afford adequate healthcare.

medically necessary Phrase indicating that the patient's symptoms and diagnosis justify or support specific medical services or procedures, as determined through a decision-making process used by third-party payors. Also known as medical necessity.

Medigap A term sometimes applied to private insurance products that supplement Medicare insurance.

medullary cavity Inner portion of diaphysis containing bone marrow.

megabyte Approximately 1 million bytes; abbreviated MB.

megahertz The measuring device for microprocessors, abbreviated MHz. A megahertz is 1 million cycles of electromagnetic currency alternation per second and is used as a unit of measure for the clock speed of computer microprocessors. The hertz is a unit of measure named after Heinrich Hertz, a German physicist.

meniscus The curved formation of liquids in a container.

mentor A trusted counselor or guide.

metabolite A substance produced by metabolism.

meticulous Marked by extreme or excessive care in the consideration or treatment of details.

microcephaly Small size of the head in relationship to the rest of the body.

microfilm A film bearing a photographic record on a reduced scale of printed or other graphic matter.

micromanage To manage with great or excessive control or attention to details.

microorganisms Living organisms of microscopic or submicroscopic size that can only be seen with a light microscope.

MIDI Acronym for Musical Instrument Digital Interface, a MIDI interface allows computers to record and manipulate sound.

miotic Any substance or medication that causes constriction of the pupil.

misdemeanor A minor crime, as opposed to a felony, punishable by fine or imprisonment in a city or county jail rather than in a penitentiary.

mnemonic A device, such as a sentence or rhyme, used as a memory aid (e.g., Roy G. Biv for remembering the colors of the spectrum: red-orange-yellow-green-blue-indigo-violet).

mock Simulated; intended for imitation or practice.

modem A device that allows information to be transmitted over telephone lines, at speeds measured in bits per second (bps); short for modulator-demodulator.

modifiers Code additions that explain circumstances that alter a service that has been provided and clarify exactly what was done to the patient.

molecule A group of like or different atoms held together by chemical forces.

monochromatic Having or consisting of one color or hue.

mononuclear white blood cell A leukocyte having an unsegmented nucleus; monocytes and lymphocytes in particular.

monotone A succession of syllables, words, or sentences in one unvaried key or pitch.

mons pubis Fat pad that covers the symphysis pubis.

morale The mental and emotional condition, such as enthusiasm, confidence, or loyalty, of an individual or group with regard to the function or tasks at hand.

morbidity The relative incidence of disease.

mortality The number of deaths in a given time or place.

motivation The process of inciting a person to some action or behavior.

multimedia The presentation of graphics, animation, video, sound, and text on a computer in an integrated way, or all at once. CD-ROMs are the most effective multimedia devices.

multiparous Pertaining to women who have had two or more pregnancies.

multitasking Performing multiple tasks at the same time.

municipal A court that sits in some cities and larger towns and that usually has civil and criminal jurisdiction over cases arising within the municipality.

murmur Abnormal sound heard when auscultating the heart that may or may not have a pathological origin.

myelography Fluoroscopic examination of the spinal canal with spinal injection of an iodine contrast medium.

myelomeningocele A herniation of a portion of the spinal cord and its meninges that protrudes through a congenital opening in the vertebral column.

myocardial Pertaining to the heart muscle.

myocardium The muscular lining of the heart.

myoglobinuria Abnormal presence of a hemoglobin-like chemical of muscle tissue in urine that is the result of muscle deterioration.

mysticism The experience of seeming to have direct communication with God or ultimate reality.

nanometer One billionth (10^{-9}) of a meter.

national provider identifier (NPI) A lifetime number consisting of 10 digits that Medicare will use to replace the provider identification number (PIN) and the unique physician identification number (UPIN).

naturopathy An alternative to conventional medicine in which holistic methods are used, as well as herbs and natural supplements, with the belief that the body will heal itself. Naturopathic physicians can currently be licensed in 12 states.

necrosis Pertaining to the death of cells or tissue.

negligence Failure to exercise the care that a prudent person usually exercises; implies inattention to one's duty or business; implies want of due or necessary diligence or care.

negotiable Legally transferable to another party.

networking Exchange of information or services among individuals, groups, or institutions; also, meeting and getting to know individuals in the same or similar career fields and sharing information about available opportunities.

neural tube defect Any of a group of congenital anomalies involving the brain and spinal column that are caused by failure of the neural tube to close during embryonic development.

nocturia Excessive urination during the night.

nodule Small lump, lesion, or swelling felt when palpating the skin.

nomogram A graph on which variables are plotted so that a particular value can be read on the appropriate line.

nonmaleficence Refraining from the act of harming or committing evil.

no-show A person who fails to keep an appointment without giving advance notice.

nosocomial Pertaining to or originating in the hospital, said of an infection not present or incubating before admittance to the hospital.

nosocomial infection Infection acquired during hospitalization or in a healthcare setting; often caused by *Escherichia coli*, hepatitis viruses, *Pseudomonas*, and *Staphylococcus* microorganisms.

"note" Notes are found in both the Alphabetic Index and the Tabular List as instructions or guides in classification assignments, defining category content or the use of subdivision codes.

NPO Nothing by mouth, from the Latin *nil per os*.

NSAIDs Nonsteroidal antiinflammatory drugs.

nuclear medicine Imaging modality that uses radioactive materials injected or ingested into the body to provide information about the function of organs and tissues.

numeric filing The filing of records, correspondence, or cards by number.

obesity An excessive accumulation of body fat (usually defined as more than 20% above the recommended body weight).

objective information Information that is gathered by watching or observation of a patient.

objectives Something toward which effort is directed; an aim, goal, or end of action.

oblique projection Radiographic view in which the body or part is rotated so that the projection is neither frontal nor lateral.

obliteration Act of making undecipherable or imperceptible by obscuring or wearing away.

obturator Metal rod with a smooth, rounded tip that is placed into hollow instruments to decrease injury to body tissues during insertion.

occlusion Complete blocking off of an opening.

"omit code" Term used primarily in Volume 3 of the ICD-9-CM when the procedure is the method of approach for an operation.

opaque Not translucent or transparent.

opinion A formal expression of judgment or advice by an expert; the formal expression of the legal reasons and principles on which a legal decision is based.

opportunistic infection Infections caused by a normally nonpathogenic organism in a host whose resistance has been decreased.

optic disc Region at the back of the eye at which the optic nerve meets the retina; considered the blind spot of the eye, because it contains only nerve fibers and no rods or cones and thus is insensitive to light.

optic nerve Second cranial nerve that carries impulses for the sense of sight.

optical character recognition (OCR) The electronic scanning of printed items as images and use of special software to recognize these images (or characters) as ASCII text.

ordinance An authoritative decree or direction; a law set forth by a governmental authority, specifically a municipal regulation.

organelle A differentiated structure within a cell, such as a mitochondrion, vacuole, or chloroplast, that performs a specific function.

orthopnea Difficulty breathing when in the supine position; individual must sit or stand to breathe comfortably.

orthostatic (postural) hypotension Temporary fall in blood pressure when a person rapidly changes from a recumbent position to a standing position.

osteopathy A medical discipline based primarily on the manual diagnosis and holistic treatment of impaired function resulting from loss of movement of all kinds of tissues.

osteoporosis Loss of bone density; lack of calcium intake is a major factor in its development.

other potentially infectious material (OPIM) Substances or material other than blood that has the potential to carry infectious pathogens, such as body fluid, urine, semen, and others.

otitis externa Inflammation or infection of the external auditory canal.

otosclerosis Formation of spongy bone in the labyrinth of the ear, often causing the auditory ossicles to become fixed and unable to vibrate when sound enters the ears.

ototoxic A substance or medication that damages the eighth cranial nerve or the organs of hearing and balance.

OUTfolder A folder used to provide space for the temporary filing of materials.

OUTguide A heavy guide that is used to replace a folder that has been temporarily moved from the filing space.

output Information that is processed by the computer and transmitted to a monitor, printer, or other device.

outreach The process of using marketing and education strategies to reach and involve diverse audiences through the use of key messages and effective programs.

over-the-counter drugs Medications sold without a prescription.

packing slip An itemized list of objects in a package.

palliative An agent that relieves or alleviates symptoms without curing the disease.

pandemic Affecting the majority of the people in a country or a number of countries.

paper claims Hard copies of insurance claims that have been completed and sent by surface mail.

papilledema Bulging of the optic disc and dilated retinal veins seen by ophthalmoscopic examination of the retina, a sign of increased intracranial pressure.

paraphrased A restatement of a text, passage, or work giving the meaning in another form.

paraphrasing To express an idea in different wording in an effort to enhance communication and clarify meaning.

parenteral Injection or introduction of substances into the body through any route other than the digestive tract such as subcutaneous, intravenous, or intramuscular administration.

paresthesia Abnormal sensation of burning, prickling, or stinging.

paroxysmal Pertaining to a sudden recurrent spasm of symptoms.

participating provider (PAR) A physician or other healthcare provider who enters into a contract with a specific insurance company or program, and by doing so, agrees to abide by certain rules and regulations set forth by that particular third-party payor.

parturition Act or process of giving birth to a child.

patency Open condition of a body cavity or canal.

pathogen An agent that causes disease, especially a living microorganism, such as a bacterium or fungus.

pathogenic Pertaining to disease-causing microorganisms.

pathophysiology Study of the biological and physical manifestations of disease as they are related to system abnormalities and physiologic disturbances.

payables The balance due to a creditor on an account.

payee Person named on a draft or check as the recipient of the amount shown.

payor Person who writes a check in favor of the payee.

peer review organizations A group of medical reviewers contracted by the Centers for Medicare and Medicaid Services (CMS) (formerly HCFA) to ensure quality control and medical necessity of services provided by a facility.

pegboard system Also called the *write-it-once system*; a method of tracking patient accounts that allows the figures to be proved accurate through mathematical formulas.

perceiving How an individual looks at information and sees it as real.

perception A quick, acute, and intuitive cognition; a capacity for comprehension; an awareness of the elements of the environment.

periosteum The thin, highly innervated, membranous covering of a bone.

peristalsis Wavelike movement by which the gastrointestinal tract moves food downward.

perjured testimony The voluntary violation of an oath or vow either by swearing to what is untrue or by omission to do what has been promised under oath; false testimony.

perks Extra advantages or benefits from working in a specific job that may or may not be commonplace in that particular profession; a shortened form of *perquisites*.

permeable Allows a substance to pass or soak through.

persona An individual's social facade or front that reflects the role in life the individual is playing; the personality that a person projects in public.

pertinent Having a clear, decisive relevance to the matter at hand.

petechiae Small, purplish hemorrhagic spots on the skin.

petty cash fund A fund maintained to pay small unpredictable cash expenditures.

phenylalanine Essential amino acid found in milk, eggs, and other foods.

philanthropist An individual who makes an active effort to promote human welfare.

philosopher A person who seeks wisdom or enlightenment; an expounder of a theory in a certain area of experience.

phlebotomy The invasive procedure used to obtain a blood specimen for testing, experimentation, or diagnosis of disease.

phonetic Constituting an alteration of ordinary spelling that better represents the spoken language, that employs only characters of the regular alphabet, and that is used in a context of conventional spelling.

phosphors Fluorescent crystals that give off light when exposed to x-rays.

photophobia Abnormal visual sensitivity to light.

physician office laboratories (POLs) Laboratories owned by a private physician or corporation, such as the lab inside a physician's office or a free-standing laboratory.

physiological noise Physiological interferences with the communication process.

pipet A cylindrical glass or plastic tube used to deliver fluids.

pitch The property of a sound, especially a musical tone, that is determined by the frequency of the waves producing it; the highness or lowness of sound.

plaque Abnormal accumulation of a fatty substance.

plasma The liquid portion of whole blood that contains active clotting agents.

policyholder A person who pays a premium to an insurance company and in whose name the policy is written in exchange for the insurance protection provided by a policy of insurance, usually applicable to an automobile policy.

polycythemia vera A condition marked by an abnormally large number of RBCs in the circulatory system.

polydipsia Excessive thirst.

polymorphonuclear white blood cell Leukocytes having a segmented nucleus. Also known as PMN (polymorphonuclear neutrophils) or segmented neutrophils.

polyphagia Increased appetite.

polyps Tumors on stems frequently found in the mucosal lining of the colon.

polyuria Excretion of an unusually large amount of urine.

portal hypertension An increased venous pressure in the portal circulation caused by cirrhosis or compression of the hepatic vascular system.

portfolio A set of pictures, drawings, documents, or photographs either bound in book form or loose in a folder.

posteroanterior (PA) Frontal projection in which the patient is prone or facing the x-ray film or image receptor.

posting Transferring or carrying from a book of original entry to a ledger; entering figures in an accounting system.

postmortem Done, collected, or occurring after death.

power of attorney A legal statement in which a person authorizes another person to act as his or her attorney or agent. The authority may be limited to the handling of specific procedures. The person authorized to act as the agent is known as the *attorney in fact.*

precedence To surpass in rank, dignity, or importance; to be, go, or come ahead or in front of.

precedents A person or thing that serves as a model; something done or said that may serve as an example or rule to authorize or justify a subsequent act of the same kind.

preexisting condition Physical condition of an insured person that existed before the issuance of the insurance policy.

premium The periodic (monthly, quarterly, or annual) payment of a specific sum of money to an insurance company for which the insurer, in return, agrees to provide certain benefits.

preponderance A superiority or excess in number or quantity; a majority.

preponderance of the evidence Evidence that is of greater weight or more convincing than the evidence offered in opposition to it; evidence that as a whole shows that the fact sought to be proven is more probable than not.

prerequisite Something that is necessary to an end or to carry out a function.

present illness The chief complaint, written in chronological sequence, with dates of onset.

preservatives Substances added to a specimen to prevent deterioration of cells or chemicals.

pressboard A strong, highly glazed composition board resembling vulcanized fiber; heavy card stock.

primary diagnosis The condition or chief complaint for which a patient is treated in an outpatient (physician's office or clinic) medical care setting.

principal A capital sum of money due as a debt or used as a fund for which interest is either charged or paid.

principal diagnosis A condition established after study that is chiefly responsible for the admission of a patient to the hospital. Used in coding inpatient hospital insurance claims.

processing How an individual internalizes new information and makes it his or her own.

procrastination Intentionally putting off doing something that should be done.

professional behaviors Those actions that identify the medical assistant as a member of a healthcare profession including dependability, respectful patient care, initiative, positive attitude, and teamwork.

professional courtesy Reduction or absence of fees to professional associates.

professionalism The conduct or qualities characterized by or conforming to the technical or ethical standards of a profession; exhibiting a courteous, conscientious, and generally businesslike manner in the workplace.

proficiency Competency as a result of training or practice.

profit sharing Offer of a part of the company's profits to employees or other designated individuals or groups.

progress notes Notes used in the patient chart to track the progress and condition of the patient.

prokaryote A unicellular organism having cells that lack a membrane-bound nucleus.

prolactin (PRL) Hormone secreted by the anterior pituitary gland; stimulates the development of the mammary gland.

proofread To read and mark corrections.

prosthesis Artificial replacement for a body part.

prosthetic The surgical or dental specialty concerned with the design, construction, and fitting of prostheses, which are artificial devices that replace missing parts of the body.

provider The company, individual, or group that provides medical services to a patient.

provider identification number (PIN) A number assigned to providers by carriers for use in submission of claims.

provisional diagnosis A temporary diagnosis made prior to receiving all test results.

proxemics The study of the nature, degree, and effect of the spatial separation individuals naturally maintain.

prudent Marked by wisdom or judiciousness; shrewd in the management of practical affairs.

psoriasis Usually chronic, recurrent skin disease marked by bright red patches covered with silvery scales.

psychosocial Pertaining to a combination of psychological and social factors.

public domain The realm embracing property rights that belong to the community at large, are unprotected by copyright or patent, and are subject to use or appropriation by anyone.

pulmonary consolidation Process of the lungs becoming solidified as they fill with exudates in pneumonia.

pulse deficit The radial pulse is less than the apical pulse; may indicate peripheral vascular abnormality.

pulse pressure Difference between the systolic and the diastolic blood pressures (less than 30 points or more than 50 points is considered normal).

pure culture A bacterial or fungal culture that contains a single organism.

putrefaction   Decomposition of animal matter that results in a foul smell.

pyemia   The presence of pus-forming organisms in the blood.

quackery   The pretense of curing disease.

quality assurance   Activities designed to increase the quality of a product or service through process or system changes that increase efficiency or effectiveness.

quality control   An aggregate of activities designed to ensure adequate quality, especially in manufactured products or in the service industries.

queries   Requests for information from a database.

rad   Conventional unit of radiation dose.

radiograph   An x-ray image.

radiographer   Person qualified to perform radiographic examinations.

radiography   Making diagnostic images using x-rays.

radiologist   Physician specialist in medical imaging or therapeutic applications of radiation.

radiolucent   Describing a substance that is easily penetrated by x-rays; these substances appear dark on radiographs.

radiopaque   Describing a substance that is not easily penetrated by x-rays; these substances appear light on radiographs.

rales   Abnormal or crackling breath sounds during inspiration.

ramifications   Consequence; outgrowth; something produced by a cause or necessarily following from a set of conditions.

rapport   Relationship of harmony and accord between the patient and the healthcare professional.

Raynaud's phenomenon   Intermittent attacks of ischemia of the extremities; results in cyanosis, numbness, tingling, and pain.

ream   A quantity of paper being 20 pounds or, variously, 480, 500, or 516 sheets.

reasonable doubt   Doubt based on reason and arising from evidence or lack of evidence; it is not doubt that is imagined or conjured up, but doubt that would cause reasonable persons to hesitate before acting.

receipts   Amounts paid on patient accounts.

receivables   Total monies received on accounts.

recipient   The receiver of some thing or item.

rectify   To correct by removing errors.

reduction   The return to correct anatomical position as in reduction of a fracture.

referral (reference) laboratory   A private or hospital-based laboratory that performs a wide variety of tests, many of them specialized; physicians often send specimens collected in the office to referral laboratories for testing.

reflection   The process of considering new information and internalizing it to create new ways of examining information.

refractile   Causing light to refract, thus creating a sharp boundary or image.

registered dietitian   Person with a minimum of a bachelor's degree in foods and nutrition who is concerned with the maintenance and promotion of health and the treatment of diseases through diet.

rejected claim   A claim returned to the provider for clarification of any question and that must be corrected prior to resubmission.

relapse   The recurrence of the symptoms of a disease after apparent recovery.

relevant   Having significant and demonstrable bearing on the matter at hand.

rem   Convention unit of radiation dose equivalent.

remission   The partial or complete disappearance of the clinical and subjective characteristics of a chronic or malignant disease.

remittent fever   Fever in which temperature fluctuates greatly but never falls to the normal level.

renal thresholds   Levels above which a substance cannot be reabsorbed by the renal tubules and is thus excreted in the urine.

reparations   The act of making amends, offering atonement, or giving satisfaction from a wrong or injury.

reprimands   Criticisms for a fault; a severe or formal reproof.

reproach   An expression of rebuke or disapproval; a cause or occasion of blame, discredit, or disgrace.

requisites   Something considered essential or necessary.

resolution   The ability of the eye to distinguish two objects that are very close together; the sharpness of an image.

resource-based relative value system (RBRVS)   A fee schedule designed to provide national uniform payment of Medicare benefits after being adjusted to reflect the differences in practice costs across geographic areas.

retention   To keep in possession or use; to keep in one's pay or service.

retention schedule   A method or plan for retaining or keeping medical records, and their movement from active, to inactive, to closed filing.

revenue   The total income produced by a given source.

rhinitis   Inflammation of the mucous membranes of the nose.

rhonchi   Abnormal rumbling sounds on expiration that indicate airway obstruction by thick secretions or spasms; continuous dry rattling in the throat or bronchial tube as a result of partial obstruction.

rider   A special provision or group of provisions that may be added to a policy to expand or limit the benefits otherwise payable. It may increase or decrease benefits, waive a condition or coverage, or in any other way amend the original contract.

robotics   Technology dealing with the design, construction, and operation of robots in automation.

rods   Structures located in the retina of the eye and forming the light-sensitive elements.

Roentgen (R)   Conventional unit of radiation exposure.

router   A device used to connect any number of LANs, which communicate with other routers and determine the best route between any two hosts.

sagittal plane   Plane that divides the body into right and left parts.

salutation An expression of greeting, goodwill, or courtesy by words or gestures.

sarcasm A sharp and often satirical response or ironic utterance designed to cut or give pain.

scanner Device that reads text or illustrations on a printed page and can translate the information on that page into a form that the computer can understand.

sclera White part of the eye that forms the orb.

scleroderma Autoimmune disorder that affects the blood vessels and connective tissue, causing fibrous degeneration of the major organs.

sclerotherapy Injection of sclerosing solutions in the treatment of hemorrhoids, varicose veins, or esophageal varices.

scoliosis Abnormal lateral curvature of the spine.

scored Tablet is manufactured with an indentation for division through the center.

screen Something that shields, protects, or hides; to select or eliminate through a screening process.

search engines Programs that search documents for keywords and return a list of documents containing those words.

seborrhea Excessive discharge of sebum from the sebaceous glands forming greasy scales or cheesy plugs on the body.

secondary hypertension Elevated blood pressure resulting from another condition.

"see" A direction given to the coder to look in another place. This term must always be followed and is found in the Alphabetic Index, Volumes 2 and 3.

"see also" A direction given to the coder to look elsewhere if the main term or subterm (or subterms) for that entry are not sufficient for coding the information. If a code number follows, "see also" is enclosed in parentheses. If there is no code number, "see also" is preceded by a dash.

"see category" A direction given to the coder to see a specific category (three-digit code). This must always be followed.

self-insured plan An insurance plan funded by an organization having a large enough employee base that they can afford to fund their own insurance program.

self-referral The act of a patient or insured individual who refers himself or herself to a specialist without requesting the referral to the primary provider, such as a woman seeking an annual gynecological examination. Managed care guidelines may require the patient to report the self-referral.

sensitivity The ability of a test to detect minute amounts of analyte.

sentinel event An unexpected occurrence involving death or serious physical or psychologic injury, or the risk thereof.

sequentially Of, relating to, or arranged in a sequence.

serial dilution A process in which a sample, such as serum, is diluted repeatedly for analysis. Most commonly, twofold or tenfold dilutions are prepared.

serous Thin, watery, serumlike drainage.

serum The liquid portion of whole blood that remains after the blood has clotted.

server A computer or device on a network that manages shared network resources.

service benefit plan Plan that provides its benefits in the form of certain surgical and medical services rendered, rather than cash. A service benefit plan is not restricted to a fee schedule.

sheath Covering surrounding the axon of the nerve cell that acts as an electrical insulator to speed the conduction of nerve impulses.

shelf filing A system that uses open shelves rather than cabinets for storing records.

shingling A method of filing whereby one report is laid on top of the older report, resembling the shingles of a roof.

Sievert (Sv) International unit of radiation dose equivalent.

sinoatrial (SA) node Pacemaker of the heart located in the right atrium.

sinus arrhythmia Irregular heartbeat originating in the sinoatrial node (pacemaker).

socioeconomic Relating to a combination of social and economic factors.

sociological Oriented or directed toward social needs and problems.

sonography Imaging modality that uses sound waves to produce images of soft tissues; also called diagnostic ultrasound.

sound card Device that allows a computer to output sound through speakers that are connected to the main circuitry board, or motherboard.

specific gravity Weight of urine compared with an equal volume of water.

specificity The ability of a particular antibody to combine with one antigen instead of another.

specimen A sample, as of tissue, blood, or urine, used for analysis and diagnosis.

spirometer Instrument that measures the volume of inhaled and exhaled air.

spores Thick-walled reproductive cells formed within bacteria and capable of withstanding unfavorable environmental conditions.

staff privileges Allowance of a healthcare professional to practice within a specific facility.

standards Established by authority, custom, or general consent as a model or example; something set up and established by authority as a rule for the measure of quantity, weight, extent, value, or quality.

stat A direction that an action is to be taken quickly (from the Latin word *statin*, meaning "at once"); an order found on a laboratory requisition indicating that the test must be done immediately.

statement A request for payment.

statement of income and expense A summary of all income and expenses for a given period.

stationers Sellers of stationery.

statute A law enacted by the legislative branch of a government.

stereotactic An x-ray procedure to guide the insertion of a needle into a specific area of the breast.

stereotype Something conforming to a fixed or general pattern; a standardized mental picture that is held in common by many and represents an oversimplified opinion, prejudiced attitude, or uncritical judgment.

sterilization   Complete destruction of all forms of microbial life.

stertorous   Strenuous respiratory effort that has a snoring sound.

stipulate   To specify as a condition or requirement of an agreement or offer; to make an agreement or covenant to do or forbear something.

stock option   Offer of stocks for purchase to a certain group of individuals or certain groups, such as employees of a for-profit hospital.

stressors   Stimulus that causes stress.

stridor   Shrill, harsh respiratory sound heard during inhalation in the presence of a laryngeal obstruction.

stroke   Sudden loss of consciousness or paralysis caused by extreme trauma or injury to an artery in the brain.

stylus   Metal probe that is inserted into or passed through a catheter, needle, or tube used for clearing purposes or to facilitate passage into a body orifice.

subjective information   Information that is gained by questioning the patient or taken from a form.

subluxation   Incomplete dislocation of a bone from its normal anatomical location.

subluxations   Slight misalignments of the vertebrae or a partial dislocation.

subordinate   Submissive to or controlled by authority; placed in or occupying a lower class, rank, or position.

subpoena   A writ or document commanding a person to appear in court under a penalty for failure to appear.

substance number   A number based on the weight of a ream of paper containing 500 sheets.

subtle   Difficult to understand or perceive; having or marked by keen insight and ability to penetrate deeply and thoroughly; ingenious; artful; delicate.

succinct   Marked by compact, precise expression without wasted words.

superbill   A form on which to list procedures and ICD-9-CM codes most frequently used in a specific practice. The encounter is marked off on this form at the time of patient checkout and utilized for billing purposes. This is usually called an encounter form.

superfluous   Exceeding what is sufficient or necessary.

suppurative   Characterized by formation and/or discharge of pus.

supravital   Of, relating to, or capable of staining living cells after their removal from a living or recently dead organism.

surrogate   A substitute; to put in place of another.

switch   In networks, a device that filters information between LAN segments and decreases overall network traffic and increases speed and bandwidth usage efficiency.

syncope   Fainting; a brief lapse in consciousness.

synopsis   Condensed statement or outline.

synovial fluid   Clear fluid found in joint cavities that facilitates smooth movements and nourishes joint structures.

systems software   The operating system and all utility programs that allow the computer to function and perform operations.

tachycardia   Rapid but regular heart rate exceeding 100 beats per minute.

tachypnea   Respirations that are rapid and shallow; hyperventilation.

tactful   Having a keen sense of what to do or say to maintain good relations with others or to avoid offense.

tangible   Capable of being appraised at an actual or approximate value; capable of being precisely identified or realized by the mind.

target market   A specific group of individuals to whom the marketing plan is focused.

targeted   Directed or used toward a target; directed toward a specific desire or position.

TCP/IP   Acronym for Transmission Control Protocol/ Internet Protocol; a suite of communications protocols used to connect users or hosts to the Internet.

tedious   Tiresome because of length or dullness.

telecommunication   The science and technology of communication by transmission of information from one location to another via telephone, television, telegraph, or satellite.

telemedicine   The use of telecommunications in the practice of medicine, in which great distances can exist between healthcare professionals, colleagues, patients, and students.

teleradiology   The use of telecommunications devices to enhance and improve the results of radiological procedures.

tendon   A tough band of connective tissue connecting muscle to bone.

teratogen   Any substance that interferes with normal prenatal development; substance that results in severe fetal deformities.

teratogenic   A substance that is known to cause birth defects.

testimony   A solemn declaration usually made orally by a witness under oath in response to interrogation by a lawyer or authorized public official.

thanatology   The description of the study of the phenomena of death and of psychological methods of coping with death.

third-party administrator   An organization that processes claims and performs other business-related functions for a health plan.

third-party payor   Someone other than the patient, spouse, or parent who is responsible for paying all or part of the patient's medical costs; an entity that makes a payment on an obligation or debt but is not a party of the contract that created the debt.

thixotropic gel   A material that appears to be a solid until subjected to a disturbance, such as centrifugation, upon which it becomes a liquid.

thoracic   The region of the back between the cervical and lumbar regions containing 12 thoracic vertebrae.

thready pulse   Pulse that is scarcely perceptible.

thrombus   Blood clot.

thyroid-stimulating hormone (TSH)   A hormone secreted by the anterior pituitary gland that stimulates the secretion of hormones produced by the thyroid gland.

tickler file   A chronological file used as a reminder that something must be taken care of on a certain date.

tinea   Any fungal skin disease that results in scaling, itching, and inflammation.

tissue culture   The technique or process of keeping tissue alive and growing in a culture medium.

toxemia   An abnormal condition of pregnancy characterized by hypertension, edema, and protein in the urine.

tracer   Radioactive substance administered to patient for nuclear medicine imaging procedure.

tracheostomy   Surgical opening through the neck into the trachea for breathing.

transaction   An exchange or transfer of goods, services, or funds.

transcription   To make a written copy of, either in longhand or by machine.

transducer   Part of the sonography machine that is in contact with the patient; the transducer sends high-frequency sound waves and receives the sound echoes that return from the patient's body.

transection   Cross-section: division by cutting across.

transient ischemic attack   Temporary neurological symptoms because of a gradual or partial occlusion of a cerebral blood vessel.

transillumination   Inspection of a cavity or organ by passing light through its walls.

transport medium   A medium used to keep an organism alive during transport to the laboratory.

transpose   To change the relative place or normal order of; to alter the sequence.

transverse plane   Plane that divides the body into superior and inferior parts.

trauma   Physical injury or wound caused by an external force or violence.

treatises   Systematic expositions or arguments in writing including a methodical discussion of the facts and principles involved and the conclusions reached.

triage   The sorting of and allocation of treatment to patients according to a system of priorities designed to maximize the number of survivors and treat the sickest patients first.

trial balance   A method of checking the accuracy of accounts.

TRICARE   See CHAMPUS.

triglycerides   Fatty acid and glycerol compounds that combine with a protein molecule to form high- and low-density lipoproteins.

truss   Elastic, canvas, or metallic device for retaining a reduced hernia within the abdominal cavity.

turgor   Resistance of the skin to being grasped between the fingers and released; refers to normal skin tension; is decreased in dehydration and increased with edema.

type and cross match   Tests performed to assess the compatibility of blood to be transfused.

unbundled codes   Separating the components of a procedure and reporting them separately.

unequal pulses   Pulse in which the beats vary in intensity.

Uniform Commercial Code (UCC)   A series of laws (regulations), adopted by most states, that regulate the fields of sales of goods; commercial paper, such as checks; secured transactions in personal property; and particular aspects of banking, letters of credit, warehouse receipts, bills of lading, and investment securities; a unified set of rules covering many business transactions; it has been adopted in all 50 states, the District of Columbia, and most U.S. territories.

unique identifiers   Codes used instead of names to protect the confidentiality of the patient in a method of anonymous HIV testing.

unique provider identification number (UPIN)   A number assigned by fiscal intermediaries to identify providers on claims for services.

unit dose   Method of preparing individual doses of medications by the pharmacy.

universal claim form   The form developed by the Health Care Financing Administration (HCFA) (now known as the Centers for Medicare and Medicaid Services [CMS]) and approved by the AMA for use in submitting all government-sponsored claims.

upcoding   A deliberate increase in a CPT code to receive higher reimbursements.

upper gastrointestinal (GI) series   Fluoroscopic examination of the esophagus, stomach, and duodenum using oral administration of barium sulfate as a contrast medium.

urea   The major nitrogenous end product of protein metabolism and the chief nitrogenous component of the urine.

urease   An enzyme that catalyzes the hydrolysis of urea to form ammonium carbonate.

uremia   Toxic renal condition characterized by an excess of urea, creatinine, and other nitrogenous end-products in the blood.

urgency   Sudden, compelling desire to urinate and the inability to control its release.

URL   Acronym for Uniform Resource Locator; specifies the global address of documents or information on the Internet. The URL provides the IP address and the domain name for the web page, such as *microsoft.com*.

urticaria   A skin eruption creating inflamed wheals; hives.

"use additional code"   This term appears only in volume 1 in those subdivisions in which the user should add further information by means of an additional code to give a more complete picture of the diagnosis. In some cases you will find "if desired" following the term. For the purpose of coding, the "if desired" phrase will not be used. When the term "use additional code...if desired" appears, you will disregard "if desired" and assign the appropriate additional code.

utilization   Related to the process of reviewing procedures and services for medical necessity.

utilization review   A review of individual cases by a committee to make sure that services are medically necessary and to study how providers use medical care resources.

Valsalva's maneuver   Occurs when one strains to defecate and urinate, uses the arms and upper trunk muscles to move up in bed, or strains during laughing, coughing, or vomiting; causes a trapping of blood in the great veins, preventing it from entering the chest and right atrium and may cause heart attack and death.

vasodilation   Increase in the diameter of a blood vessel.

vector   An animal, usually an insect or tick, that transmits the causative organisms of disease.

vehemently   Marked by forceful energy; intensely emotional.

ventricles   The two lower chambers of the heart.

veracity   A devotion to or conformity with the truth.

verdict   The finding or decision of a jury on a matter submitted to it in trial.

versatile   Embracing a variety of subjects, fields or skills; having a wide range of abilities.

vertigo   Dizziness; a sensation of faintness or an inability to maintain normal balance.

vested   Granted or endowed with a particular authority, right, or property; to have a special interest in.

viable   Capable of living, developing, or germinating under favorable conditions.

virtual reality   An artificial environment presented to a computer user that feels as if it were a real environment, often using special gloves, earphones, and goggles to enhance the experience.

virulent   Exceedingly pathogenic, noxious, or deadly.

viscosity   The quality of being thick and of lacking the capability of easy movement.

vocation   The work in which a person is regularly employed.

void   To urinate.

volatile   Easily aroused; tending to erupt in violence; an explosive substance's capacity to vaporize at a low temperature.

vulva   The external female genitalia, which begins at the mons pubis and terminates at the anus.

watermark   A marking in paper resulting from differences in thickness usually produced by the pressure of a projecting design in the mold or on a processing roll and visible when the paper is held up to the light.

wet mount   A slide preparation in which a drop of liquid specimen or the like is covered with a coverslip and observed with a microscope.

wheal   Localized area of edema or a raised lesion.

"with"   In the context of ICD-9-CM, the terms "with," "with mention of," and "associated with" in a title dictate that both parts of the title be present in the statement of the diagnosis order to assign the particular code.

workers' compensation   Insurance against liability imposed on certain employers to pay benefits and furnish care to employees who are injured and to pay benefits to dependents of employees killed in the course of or arising out of their employment.

Zip drive   A small, portable disk drive that is primarily used for backing up information and archiving computer files. A 100-megabyte Zip disk will hold the equivalent of about 70 floppy disks.

Index

Page references followed by "*f*" indicate figures and by "*t*" indicate tables.